Shnider and Levinson's

Anesthesia for Obstetrics

FIFTH EDITION

Shnider and Levinson's

Anesthesia for Obstetrics

FIFTH EDITION

Maya S. Suresh, MD

Professor and Chairman
Department of Anesthesiology
Baylor College of Medicine
Division Chief
Obstetrics and Gynecologic Anesthesiology
Ben Taub General Hospital
Houston, Texas

Scott Segal, MD, MHCM

Chair, Department of Anesthesiology
Tufts University School of Medicine
Anesthesiologist-in-Chief
Tufts Medical Center
Boston, Massachusetts

Roanne L. Preston, MD, FRCPC

Clinical Professor
Department of Anesthesiology
Pharmacology and Therapeutics
The University of British Columbia
Department Head
Department of Anesthesia
British Columbia Women's Hospital and Health Centre
Vancouver, British Columbia, Canada

Roshan Fernando, MB, BCh, FRCA

Consultant Anesthesiologist
University College London Hospitals NHS Trust
London, United Kingdom

C. LaToya Mason, MD

Assistant Professor
Department of Anesthesiology
Baylor College of Medicine
Attending Anesthesiologist
Department of Anesthesiology
Ben Taub General Hospital
Houston, Texas

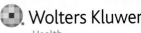 Wolters Kluwer | Lippincott Williams & Wilkins
Health

Philadelphia • Baltimore • New York • London
Buenos Aires • Hong Kong • Sydney • Tokyo

Acquisitions Editor: Brian Brown
Product Manager: Nicole Dernoski
Marketing Manager: Lisa Lawrence
Vendor Manager: Bridgett Dougherty
Designer: Stephen Druding
Compositor: Aptara, Inc.

Fifth Edition

351 West Camden Street   Two Commerce Square
Baltimore, MD 21201   2001 Market Street
                                Philadelphia, PA 19103 USA

Printed in China

9 8 7 6 5 4 3 2 1

Library of Congress Cataloging-in-Publication Data
Shnider and Levinson's anesthesia for obstetrics.—5th ed. / editor, Maya Suresh ; associate editors,
Roshan Fernando . . . [et al.].
     p. ; cm.
  Anesthesia for obstetrics
  Includes bibliographical references and index.
  ISBN 978-1-4511-1435-5 (hardback : alk. paper)
  I. Suresh, Maya. II. Shnider, Sol M., 1929- III. Title: Anesthesia for obstetrics.
  [DNLM: 1. Anesthesia, Obstetrical. WO 450]
  617.9′682—dc23

                                                    2012039413

To purchase additional copies of this book, call our customer service department at (800)
638-3030 or fax orders to (301) 223-2320. International customers should call (301) 223-2300.

Visit Lippincott Williams & Wilkins on the Internet: http://www.lww.com. Lippincott
Williams & Wilkins customer service representatives are available from 8:30 am to 6:00 pm, EST.

Katherine W. Arendt, MD
Assistant Professor
Department of Anesthesiology
Mayo Clinic College of Medicine
Consultant
Department of Anesthesiology
Mayo Clinic
Rochester, Minnesota

Valerie A. Arkoosh, MD, MPH
Professor of Clinical Anesthesiology
Professor of Clinical Obstetrics and Gynecology
Department of Anesthesiology and Critical Care
Perelman School of Medicine at the University of
    Pennsylvania
Attending Anesthesiologist
Anesthesiology and Critical Care Unit
Philadelphia, Pennsylvania

Sarah L. Armstrong, FRCA
Consultant Anaesthetist
Anaesthetic Department
Royal Surrey County Hospital
Guildford, United Kingdom

Emily J. Baird, MD, PhD
Assistant Professor
Department of Anesthesiology and Critical Care
University of Pennsylvania
Director of Obstetric Anesthesia
Department of Anesthesiology and Critical Care
Hospital of the University of Pennsylvania
Philadelphia, Pennsylvania

Mrinalini Balki, MD
Associate Professor
Department of Anesthesia and Pain Management
University of Toronto
Staff Anesthesiologist
Mount Sinai Hospital
Toronto, Canada

Venkata D. P. Bandi, MD
Associate Professor of Medicine
Department of Medicine
Pulmonary, Critical Care, and Sleep Medicine Section
Baylor College of Medicine
Associate Director, Medical ICU
Ben Taub General Hospital
Director, Intensive Care Unit
Texas Children's Hospital–Pavilion for Women
Houston, Texas

Curtis L. Baysinger, MD
Associate Professor
Department of Anesthesiology
Vanderbilt University School of Medicine
Chief, Obstetric Anesthesiology
Department of Anesthesiology
Vanderbilt University Medical Center
Nashville, Tennessee

Yaakov Beilin, MD
Professor and Vice Chair for Quality
Departments of Anesthesiology and Obstetrics and
    Gynecology
Mount Sinai School of Medicine
Co-Director of Obstetric Anesthesiology
Department of Anesthesiology
Mount Sinai Hospital
New York, New York

Brenda A. Bucklin, MD
Professor
Department of Anesthesiology
University of Colorado School of Medicine
Aurora, Colorado

William Camann, MD
Associate Professor
Department of Anesthesiology
Harvard Medical School
Director, Obstetric Anesthesia
Department of Anesthesiology
Brigham and Women's Hospital
Boston, Massachusetts

Christopher R. Cambic, MD
Assistant Professor
Department of Anesthesiology
Feinberg School of Medicine
Northwestern University
Staff Anesthesiologist
Department of Anesthesiology
Prentice Women's Hospital
Chicago, Illinois

David C. Campbell, MD, MSc, FRCPC
Professor and Chairman
Department of Anesthesiology, Perioperative Medicine and
    Pain Management
University of Saskatchewan
Chairman
Department of Anesthesiology
Saskatoon Health Region
Saskatoon, Saskatchewan, Canada

Thomas Chai, MD
Assistant Professor
Department of Pain Medicine
University of Texas MD. Anderson Cancer Center
Houston, Texas

Shobana Chandrasekhar, MD
Associate Professor
Department of Anesthesiology
Baylor College of Medicine
Houston, Texas

Katherine L. Cheesman, MBBS, FRCA, BSc
Consultant Anaesthetist
Department of Anaesthesia
Guy's & St. Thomas' NHS Trust
London, England

Edward T. Crosby, MD, FRCPC
Professor
Department of Anesthesiology
University of Ottawa
Staff Anesthesiologist
Department of Anesthesiology
The Ottawa Hospital
Ottawa, Ontario, Canada

Christina M. Davidson, MD
Assistant Professor
Department of Obstetrics and Gynecology
Division of Maternal Fetal Medicine
Baylor College of Medicine
Chief of Service
Department of Obstetrics and Gynecology
Ben Taub General Hospital
Houston, Texas

Oscar A. de Leon-Casasola, MD
Professor of Anesthesiology and Medicine
Department of Anesthesiology
University at Buffalo
Chief of Pain Medicine
Department of Anesthesiology
Roswell Park Cancer Institute
Buffalo, New York

Julio B. Delgado, MD
Staff Psychiatrist
Dual Diagnosis Attending Physician
Department of Psychiatry
Lake City VA Medical Center
Lake City, Florida

M. Joanne Douglas, MD, FRCPC
Clinical Professor
Department of Anesthesiology, Pharmacology and
    Therapeutics
University of British Columbia
Research Director
Department of Anesthesia
British Columbia's Women's Hospital and Health Centre
Vancouver, British Columbia, Canada

Roshan Fernando, MB, BCh, FRCA
Consultant Anesthesiologist
University College London Hospitals NHS Trust
London, United Kingdom

Pamela Flood, MD
Professor
Department of Anesthesia and Perioperative Care
Department of Obstetrics, Gynecology and Reproductive
    Science
University of California, San Francisco
Director of Obstetric Anesthesia
Department of Anesthesia and Perioperative Care
Moffitt Long Hospital
San Francisco General Hospital
San Francisco, California

Michael Frölich, MD, MS
Associate Professor
Department of Anesthesiology
Chair-Elect, Faculty Senate
The University of Alabama at Birmingham
Director, Fellowship Program for Obstetric Anesthesiology
    UAB Hospital
Birmingham, Alabama

Andrea J. Fuller, MD
Assistant Professor
Anesthesiology Department
University of Colorado School of Medicine
Aurora, Colorado

Rodolfo Gebhardt, MD
Associate Professor
Department of Pain Medicine
The University of Texas
Acute Pain Director
Department of Pain Medicine
MD. Anderson Cancer Center
Houston, Texas

Ravpreet Singh Gill, MD
Assistant Professor
Department of Anesthesiology
University of Tennessee Health Science Center
Anesthesiologist
Department of Anesthesiology
Regional Medical Center
Memphis, Tennessee

Laura Goetzl, MD, MPH
Associate Professor
Department of Obstetrics and Gynecology
Medical University of South Carolina
Charleston, South Carolina

Stephanie R. Goodman, MD
Associate Clinical Professor
Department of Anesthesiology
Columbia University
Associate Attending
Department of Anesthesiology
Columbia University Medical Center
New York, New York

Thomas A. Gough, MBChB, MRCP, FRCA
Specialist Registrar
Barts Health NHS Trust
The Royal London Hospital
London, United Kingdom

Stephen H. Halpern, MD, MSc, FRCPC

Professor
Departments of Anesthesia, Obstetrics, and Gynecology
University of Toronto
Division Head, Obstetrical Anesthesia
Department of Anesthesia
Sunnybrook Health Sciences Centre
Toronto, Canada

Joy L. Hawkins, MD

Professor
Associate Chair for Academic Affairs
Department of Anesthesiology
Denver School of Medicine, University of Colorado
Director of Obstetric Anesthesia
Department of Anesthesiology
University of Colorado Hospital
Aurora, Colorado

Paul Howell, BSc, MBChB, FRCA

Consultant Anaesthetist
St. Bartholomew's Hospital
London, United Kingdom

McCallum R. Hoyt, MD, MBA

Assistant Professor
Department of Anesthesiology, Perioperative and Pain
  Medicine
Harvard Medical School
Division Chief, Gynecologic and Ambulatory Anesthesia
Department of Anesthesiology, Perioperative & Pain
  Medicine
Brigham and Women's Hospital
Boston, Massachusetts

Bhavani Shankar Kodali, MD

Department of Anesthesiology
Brigham and Women's Hospital
Boston, Massachusetts

Ruth Landau, MD

Professor
Department of Anesthesiology and Pain Medicine
University of Washington
Chief, Director of Obstetric Anesthesia
Department of Anesthesiology and Pain Medicine
University of Washington Medical Center
Seattle, Washington

Ellen M. Lockhart, MD

Associate Professor
Department of Anesthesiology
Washington University
St. Louis, Missouri

Dennis T. Mangano, MD

Founder and Director
Ischemia Research and Education Foundation
Founder and Director
McSPI Research Group
San Mateo, California

Suzanne Wattenmaker Mankowitz, MD

Assistant Professor
Department of Anesthesiology
Columbia University
Faculty
Department of Anesthesiology
The New York–Presbyterian Hospital
New York, New York

David G. Mann, MD

Assistant Professor
Departments of Anesthesiology and Pediatrics
Baylor College of Medicine
Attending Anesthesiologist
Department of Anesthesiology
Texas Children's Hospital
Houston, Texas

C. LaToya Mason, MD

Assistant Professor
Department of Anesthesiology
Baylor College of Medicine
Attending Anesthesiologist
Department of Anesthesiology
Ben Taub General Hospital
Houston, Texas

Kenneth L. Mattox, MD

Distinguished Service Professor
Department of Surgery
Baylor College of Medicine
Chief of Staff, Chief of Surgery
Ben Taub General Hospital
Houston, Texas

Andrew D. Miller, MD

Instructor
Harvard Medical School
Staff Anesthesiologist
Department of Anesthesiology, Perioperative and Pain
  Medicine
Brigham and Women's Hospital
Boston, Massachusetts

Richard C. Month, MD

Assistant Professor of Clinical Anesthesiology
Department of Anesthesiology and Critical Care
Perelman School of Medicine
University of Pennsylvania
Attending Anesthesiologist
Department of Anesthesiology and Critical Care
University of Pennsylvania Health System
Philadelphia, Pennsylvania

Holly A. Muir, MD, FRPC

Assistant Professor
Department of Anesthesiology
Duke University
Vice Chair, Clinical Operations
Chief, Division of Women's Anesthesia
Department of Anesthesia
Duke University Hospital
Durham, North Carolina

Uma Munnur, MD
Associate Professor
Department of Anesthesiology
Baylor College of Medicine
Ben Taub Hospital
Houston, Texas

Olutoyin A. Olutoye, MD, MSc
Associate Professor
Department of Anesthesiology and Pediatrics
Baylor College of Medicine
Staff Anesthesiologist
Department of Anesthesiology and Pediatrics
Texas Children's Hospital
Houston, Texas

Geraldine O'Sullivan, MD, FRCA
Lead Clinician in Obstetric Anaesthesia
Department of Anaesthetics
Guy's and St Thomas' NHS Foundation Trust
King's College
London, United Kingdom

Alice L. Oswald, MD
Assistant Professor
Department of Anesthesiology
Baylor College of Medicine
Department of Obstetric and Gynecologic Anesthesiology
Ben Taub General Hospital
Houston, Texas

Medge D. Owen, MD
Professor
Department of Anesthesiology
Wake Forest School of Medicine
Director of Maternal and Infant Global Health Programs
Wake Forest School of Medicine
Winston-Salem, North Carolina

Michael Paech, DM, FANZCA
Winthrop Professor and Chair of Obstetric Anesthesia
School of Medicine and Pharmacology
The University of Western Australia
Senior Specialist Anaesthetist
Department of Anaesthesia and Pain Medicine
King Edward Memorial Hospital for Women
Perth, Western Australia

Quisqueya T. Palacios, MD
Associate Professor
Department of Anesthesiology
Assistant Professor
Department of Obstetrics and Gynecology
Baylor College of Medicine
Director of Patient Safety
Division of Obstetric and Gynecologic Anesthesiology
Baylor College of Medicine
Houston, Texas

Peter H. Pan, MD
Professor
Department of Anesthesiology
Wake Forest University School of Medicine
Wake Forest University Baptist Medical Center
Winston-Salem, North Carolina

Carlo Pancaro, MD
Assistant Professor
Department of Anesthesiology
Tufts University School of Medicine
Tufts Medical Center
Boston, Massachusetts

Moeen K. Panni, MD, PhD
Professor and Chair of Anesthesiology
Professor of Obstetrics and Gynecology
Chief of Perioperative Services
The University of Mississippi Medical Center
Jackson, Mississippi

Donald H. Penning, MD, MS, FRCP
Professor
Department of Anesthesiology
University of Colorado-Denver
Director of Anesthesia
Department of Anesthesiology
Denver Health
Denver, Colorado

Feyce M. Peralta, MD
Assistant Professor–Clinical
Department of Anesthesiology
The Ohio State University Wexner Medical Center
Columbus, Ohio

May C. M. Pian-Smith, MD, MS
Assistant Professor
Department of Anesthesia
Harvard Medical School
Obstetric Anesthesiologist
Department of Anesthesia, Critical Care and Pain Medicine
Massachusetts General Hospital
Boston, Massachusetts

Mihaela Podovei, MD
Instructor in Anesthesia
Harvard Medical School
Staff Anesthesiologist
Department of Anesthesiology, Perioperative and Pain Medicine
Brigham and Women's Hospital
Boston, Massachusetts

Stephen D. Pratt, MD
Assistant Professor
Department of Anesthesia
Harvard Medical School
Chief, Division of Quality and Safety
Department of Anesthesia, Critical Care, and Pain Medicine
Beth Israel Deaconess Medical Center
Boston, Massachusetts

Roanne L. Preston, MD, FRCPC
Clinical Professor
Department of Anesthesiology
Pharmacology and Therapeutics
The University of British Columbia
Department Head
Department of Anesthesia
British Columbia Women's Hospital and Health Centre
Vancouver, British Columbia, Canada

Jaya Ramanathan, MD

Professor
Department of Anesthesiology
The University of Tennessee Health Science Center
Director of Obstetric Anesthesia
Regional Medical Center at Memphis
Memphis, Tennessee

Sivam Ramanathan, MD (deceased)

Professor Emeritus
University of Pittsburgh
Director of OB Anesthesia Research
Associate Director OB Anesthesia Fellowship
Department of Anesthesiology
Cedars-Sinai Medical Center
Los Angeles, California

J. Sudharma Ranasinghe, MD, FFARCSI

Professor of Clinical Anesthesiology
Department of Anesthesiology
University of Miami Miller School of Medicine
Chief of Obstetric Anesthesia
Department of Anesthesiology
Jackson Memorial Medical Center
Miami, Florida

Sally Radelat Raty, MD, MHA

Associate Professor
Department of Anesthesiology
Baylor College of Medicine
Chief, Division of General and Trauma Anesthesia
Department of Anesthesiology
Ben Taub General Hospital
Houston, Texas

Elena Reitman-Ivashkov, MD

Assistant Professor
Anesthesiology Department
Columbia University
Staff
Anesthesiology Department
The Presbyterian Hospital
New York, New York

José M. Rivers, MD

Associate Professor
Department of Anesthesiology
Baylor College of Medicine
Faculty
Department of Anesthesia
Ben Taub Hospital
Houston, Texas

George R. Saade, MD

Professor
Department of Obstetrics and Gynecology
The University of Texas Medical Branch
Chief of Obstetrics and Maternal-Fetal Medicine
Department of Obstetrics and Gynecology
John Sealy Hospital
Galveston, Texas

Monica San Vicente, MD, FRCPC

Associate Professor
Department of Anesthesiology
Perioperative Medicine and Pain Management
University of Saskatchewan
Saskatoon, Saskatchewan, Canada

Barbara M. Scavone, MD

Professor
Department of Anesthesia and Critical Care
Department of Obstetrics and Gynecology
The University of Chicago
Chief
Division of Obstetric Anesthesia
University of Chicago Medical Center
Chicago, Illinois

Scott Segal, MD, MHCM

Chair, Department of Anesthesiology
Tufts University School of Medicine
Anesthesiologist-in-Chief
Tufts Medical Center
Boston, Massachusetts

Baha Sibai, MD

Professor
Department of Obstetrics and Gynecology
The University of Texas Medical School
Lyndon Baines Johnson General Hospital
Houston, Texas

Michelle Simon, MD

Assistant Professor
Department of Anesthesiology
Galveston, Texas

Julie A. Sparlin, MD

Clinical Instructor
Department of Anesthesiology
Creighton University School of Medicine
Associate Medical Director
Center for Comprehensive Pain Management
Valley Pain Consultants at St. Joseph's Hospital and Medical
    Center
Phoenix, Arizona

Margaret Srebrnjak, MD, FRCPC

Assistant Professor
Department of Anesthesia
University of Toronto
Toronto, Canada
Staff Anesthesiologist
Department of Anesthesia
The Credit Valley Hospital
Mississauga, Ontario, Canada

John T. Sullivan, MD, MBA

Residency Program Director
Department of Anesthesiology
Northwestern University Feinberg School of Medicine
Chicago, Illinois

William J. Sullivan, QC, LLB, MCL

Adjunct Professor
Faculty of Medicine
The University of British Columbia
Partner
Guild Yule, LLP Barristers and Solicitors
Vancouver, British Columbia, Canada

Maya S. Suresh, MD

Professor and Chairman
Department of Anesthesiology
Baylor College of Medicine
Division Chief
Obstetrics and Gynecologic Anesthesiology
Ben Taub General Hospital
Houston, Texas

Roulhac D. Toledano, MD, PhD

Assistant Clinical Professor
Department of Anesthesiology
SUNY–Downstate Medical Center
Director of Obstetric Anesthesia
Lutheran Medical Center
Brooklyn, New York

Daniel A. Tolpin, MD

Assistant Professor
Department of Anesthesia
Baylor College of Medicine
Attending Physician
Department of Cardiovascular Anesthesia
Texas Heart Institute
Houston, Texas

Ashley M. Tonidandel, MD

Assistant Professor
Department of Anesthesiology
Wake Forest University School of Medicine
Wake Forest University Baptist Medical Center
Winston-Salem, North Carolina

Connie Khanh Vu Lan Tran, MD

Associate Professor
Department of Anesthesiology
Baylor College of Medicine
Ben Taub General Hospital
Houston, Texas

Rakesh B. Vadhera, MD, FRCA, FFARCSI

Professor
Department of Anesthesiology
Galveston, Texas

Manuel C. Vallejo, MD, DMD

Professor
Department of Anesthesiology
University of Pittsburgh
Director, Obstetric Anesthesia
Department of Anesthesiology
Magee-Womens Hospital of UPMC
Pittsburgh, Pennsylvania

Ashutosh Wali, MD, FFARCSI

Associate Professor of Anesthesiology
Associate Professor of Obstetrics and Gynecology
Baylor College of Medicine
Director, Obstetric and Gynecologic Anesthesiology
Director, Advanced Airway Management
Ben Taub General Hospital
Houston, Texas

Jonathan H. Waters, MD

Professor
Departments of Anesthesiology and Bioengineering
University of Pittsburgh
Chief of Anesthesia Services
Department of Anesthesiology
Magee-Womens Hospital
Pittsburgh, Pennsylvania

Samantha J. Wilson, BSc, BMBCh, FRCA

Specialist Registrar
Department of Anaesthesia
University College Hospital
London, United Kingdom

David Wlody, MD

Medical Director and Vice President for Medical Affairs
Chief of Service, Department of Anesthesiology
State University of New York Downstate Medical Center
University Hospital of Brooklyn at Long Island College
    Hospital
Professor of Clinical Anesthesiology
Vice Chair for Clinical Affairs
Department of Anesthesiology
State University of New York Downstate Medical Center
Brooklyn, New York

Nikolaos Marios Zacharias, MD, FACOG

Assistant Professor
Department of Obstetrics and Gynecology, Maternal–Fetal
    Medicine Division
Baylor College of Medicine
Medical Director, Prenatal Ultrasound
Department of Obstetrics and Gynecology, Maternal–Fetal
    Medicine Division
Ben Taub General Hospital
Houston, Texas

Mark I. Zakowski, MD

Adjunct Associate Professor of Anesthesiology
Charles R. Drew University of Medicine and Science
Chief of Obstetric Anesthesia and Obstetric Anesthesiology
    Fellowship Director
Department of Anesthesiology
Cedars-Sinai Medical Center
Los Angeles, California

It has been ten years since the publication of the last edition of *Shnider and Levinson's Anesthesia for Obstetrics*. I am very pleased, as I am sure Dr. Shnider would be, that Dr. Suresh has undertaken the formidable task of updating and completely revising this textbook.

Reviewing the contents of the book's first edition, published in 1979, and each of the subsequent editions, provides an interesting review of the progress obstetric anesthesiologists have made in providing safe analgesia and anesthesia for women having babies. For example, when the book was first published, anesthesia was the third leading cause of maternal deaths, 45% of cesarean sections were performed under general anesthesia, less than 20% of women in the United States received epidural analgesia for labor, and epidural infusions and neuraxial opioids were not available.

Currently the majority of women having babies in the United States receive epidural anesthesia and many institutions report labor epidural rates between 80 and 90% of vaginal deliveries. The current practice of administering continuous epidural infusions with dilute concentrations of local anesthetics and low-dose opioids has made for much safer anesthesia with significantly greater patient satisfaction. General anesthesia for cesarean section is now a rarity, in many hospitals less than 5% of all cesarean sections, and typically is limited to patients with one of a few uncommon medical conditions or those requiring extremely emergent delivery. Despite increasing maternal age, with the inevitable increase in pre-existing maternal disease, the marked increase in maternal obesity, and the increase in cesarean section rates, anesthetic-related maternal mortality has fallen dramatically and is no longer one of the major culprits.

Anesthesia for Obstetrics was intended to be both a basic clinical guide and a reference source for students and practitioners. To accomplish this, great emphasis was placed on presenting in a lucid and concise fashion the various aspects of the pregnant women's modified response to anesthetic drugs, the fetal effects of both maternal physiologic alterations and placental transfer of these drugs, as well as understanding the unique perinatal and obstetric issues. In the fifth edition, Dr. Suresh has continued this approach and has produced an authoritative and comprehensive textbook of obstetric anesthesia. Those who practice and those who receive obstetric anesthesia should benefit greatly.

GERSHON LEVINSON, MD
SAN FRANCISCO, CALIFORNIA

Shnider and Levinson's Anesthesia for Obstetrics, Fifth Edition is the result of the contribution of several dedicated national and international experts in obstetric anesthesia, who have conceptualized the current evidence-based practice of modern obstetrical anesthesia in this textbook.

Dr. Sol M. Shnider, the first editor of this book, was born in Yorktown, Saskatchewan, Canada. Dr. Shnider received his medical degree from the University of Manitoba and underwent his residency training at the Columbia University in New York. He was the founding member of the Society for Obstetric Anesthesia and Perinatology and the recipient of numerous awards and honors. Indeed, he was one of the pioneers of modern obstetrical anesthesia. The first three editions were edited by Dr. Sol M. Shnider and Dr. Gershon Levinson. The fourth edition, published in 2002, was edited by the late Dr. Samuel C. Hughes, Dr. Gershon Levinson, and Dr. Mark Rosen. I am grateful to both Dr. Levinson and Dr. Mark Rosen for giving us approval to proceed with the publication of the fifth edition.

The fifth edition is unique due to the contributions of both national and international editors: Dr. Scott Segal (USA), Dr. Roanne Preston (Canada), Dr. Roshan Fernando (UK), and Dr. LaToya Mason (USA), who with their editing style have provided a global perspective to the practice of obstetric anesthesia. Since the first edition in 1979, this book has become the international standard in the field of obstetric anesthesia, with translations in Spanish, French, Portuguese, German, and Japanese; we hope to add other languages including Chinese translation and an electronic version. This textbook will continue, as in the past, to serve as a valuable guide and reference source for the present and next generation of anesthesia trainees, academic and private anesthesia practitioners, and other clinicians. The fifth edition is divided into eleven sections and comprises 50 chapters and 4 appendices. There are other textbooks on obstetric anesthesia that are complete and well written, whereas the focus and organization of the current *Sol M. Shnider Anesthesia for Obstetrics fifth edition* is in keeping with the vision of Dr. Sol M. Shnider; it reflects evidence-based, best practice approach and complete care of the obstetric patient. This book provides a comprehensive view of the role of the anesthesiologist as a physician responsible for sound judgment and for optimal and best outcomes for mother and baby, a view more in keeping with the approach to cutting-edge modern anesthesia practice.

Maternal mortality has emerged as one of the most challenging healthcare issues in the last decade; in addition, incidence of obesity has reached epidemic proportions in the USA and globally increasing the challenges confronted by the practitioner caring for obstetrical patients. Obstetric anesthesia practice has had an important albeit positive influence on maternal mortality. The contributing authors have made a conscious effort to address new technologies such as ultrasound-guided approach to regional anesthesia, new airway devices, and technologies in advanced airway management. Since the last edition, significant changes and advances have occurred; therefore, almost all the chapters have been rewritten. There are new chapters that address the challenges confronting the anesthesia practitioner in the United States and globally. These chapters include: "Global Perspective on Obstetric Anesthesia," "Near Misses and Mortality," "Utilization of Crisis Resource Management in Maternal and Neonatal Safety," "Jehovah's Witness: Ethical and Anesthetic-related Issue," "Anesthesia for Vaginal Birth after Cesarean Delivery," "Difficult and Failed Intubation: Strategies, Prevention and Management of Airway-related Catastrophes," and much more. The authors have also focused on postoperative pain management, "Postoperative Multimodal Acute Pain Management: Cesarean and Vaginal Delivery," and "Chronic Pain Issues in the Postpartum Period." Chapters on amniotic fluid embolism, thromboembolism, and hemorrhage have new information. The exciting field of in utero fetal surgery and EXIT procedure has been highlighted in this book. The authors and editors have attempted to present the information with key points at the end of every section in order to facilitate learning; it also makes it easy for the reader to understand, retain, and discuss the information cogently. The book also serves as a useful reference guide to the practicing anesthesiologists in academic centers, tertiary referral centers, and community hospitals.

At the outset, a major investment was made by the publisher of the textbook who recognized that the computer savvy as well as the millennial reader is accustomed to creative graphs and figures in color and therefore opted for enhanced visual aesthetics by having full color figures and graphical presentations throughout the book. We also hope that this book with the color illustrations will not only make it interesting for the reader, but it will also help the reader use the reference and illustrations to prepare lectures, slides, and other creative illustrative media.

We trust that this textbook will continue the tradition of high quality as in the previous editions. A comprehensive textbook of this depth and scope is not possible without the support and assistance of the family members, colleagues, friends, and support staff who have assisted the authors and editors in preparation of this textbook. I personally wish to thank all the authors and I am very grateful for their dedication and contribution to this illustrious textbook that bears the name of Sol M. Shnider, an Obstetric Anesthesiologist icon. I want to acknowledge our editors and express my utmost gratitude for their valuable time and dedication to the book; they have put in an enormous amount of time to enhance the quality of the contributions. I would like to acknowledge and thank Brian Brown for giving me the opportunity to be the lead senior editor. I also wish to acknowledge the masterful assistance of Tom Conville, Nicole Dernoski, and Ruchira Gupta for their skilled efficiency in organizing and managing the manuscripts, the illustrations, and obtaining permissions and trying to keep everyone on a tight timeline. Finally, I would like to express my sincere gratitude to my husband, my grandson, and my administrative secretary Annette Brieno for their continued support.

MAYA S. SURESH, MD

CONTENTS

CHAPTER

1

Physiologic Changes of Pregnancy

Brenda A. Bucklin • Andrea J. Fuller

Unique anatomic and physiologic modifications occur during pregnancy, labor, delivery, and the postpartum period. Every organ system undergoes changes—from the substantial increase in cardiac output observed throughout pregnancy and the peripartum period to the brain's increased sensitivity to anesthetic agents during pregnancy. The increased production of hormones from the ovaries and placenta and release of endorphins further impacts the physiologic changes. A thorough understanding of the anatomical and physiologic changes is a requirement for an anesthesia practitioner caring for women during this period in order to ensure safe and optimal outcomes for mother and baby.

■ CARDIOVASCULAR CHANGES OF PREGNANCY (TABLE 1-1)

The physiologic alterations of the cardiovascular system function to support fetal growth and metabolism, by significantly increasing uterine perfusion and also to prepare the parturient for blood loss at delivery.

Blood Volume

Both the intravascular and extravascular fluid volumes increase substantially during pregnancy. Much of the average 12.5 kg weight gain during pregnancy is attributed to the increase in the intravascular and extravascular fluid volumes. Significant increases in maternal blood volume occur, with plasma volume increasing 55% from 40 mL/kg to 70 mL/kg and red blood cell volume increasing approximately 17% from 25 mL/kg to 30 mL/kg (1,2) (Fig. 1-1). This increase in volume begins in the first few weeks of gestation, rises sharply in the second trimester, peaks early in the third trimester and decreases slightly by term (1). The rise in plasma volume is likely achieved by a decreased osmotic threshold for thirst and alterations in arginine vasopressin metabolism (3). A large portion of the increased blood volume perfuses the gravid uterus and 300 to 500 mL of blood may be forced back into the maternal circulation with contractions during labor (2,4). Blood volume returns to prepregnancy values at approximately 7 to 14 days postpartum (2).

Increased red blood cell production is stimulated by a rise in erythropoietin by the second month of gestation (5). The disproportionate increase in plasma volume to red blood cell

volume results in the "physiologic anemia of pregnancy" and a normal hemoglobin concentration of 11.6 gm/dL (6). Maternal anemia is present when the hemoglobin and hematocrit fall to less than 11 g/dL or 33% respectively, the most likely cause of which is iron deficiency.

The increase in blood volume during pregnancy prepares the parturient for normal blood loss at delivery. Blood loss is usually less than 500 mL for vaginal delivery and 1,000 mL for cesarean delivery. Hemodynamic changes due to blood loss are usually not observed until the blood loss is greater than 1,500 mL and transfusion is rarely required unless blood loss exceeds this amount. Blood volume decreases to 125% of prepregnancy levels in the first postpartum week and by the sixth to ninth postpartum week there is a more gradual decline in the blood volume to 110% of the prepregnancy level. The hemoglobin and hematocrit also decrease during the initial postpartum period and then gradually increase to prepregnancy levels by the sixth postpartum week.

Central Hemodynamics (Fig. 1-2)

Cardiac output begins to increase around 10 weeks' gestation (7). Serial assessment of maternal cardiac output by impedance cardiography and echocardiography demonstrates that changes in cardiac output start early in gestation with an increase of 35% to 40% by the end of first trimester. The cardiac output continues to increase during pregnancy until 34 weeks when it reaches 50% above prepregnant values and remains stable until term (8,9) (Fig. 1-3). During this time, the percentage of cardiac output devoted to uterine blood flow increases from 5% to 11% (8).

The increase in cardiac output is due to increases in heart rate and stroke volume. The initial increase in cardiac output is due to an increase in the heart rate which starts to occur as early as the fifth week of gestation. The heart rate rises steadily during pregnancy and is elevated approximately 10 to 20 bpm above baseline at term (Fig. 1-4). The hormonal changes and release of estrogens results in an early increase in stroke volume of approximately 20% as early as the fifth to eighth week of gestation. The stroke volume continues to increase by 25% to 30% from the first to third trimester of gestation.

During parturition, further demands are placed on the heart. Additional increases in cardiac output occur during labor and delivery as a result of elevated heart rate and stroke volume

TABLE 1-1 Changes in Cardiovascular System

Variable	Direction of Change	Average Change
Blood volume	↑	+35–40%
Plasma volume	↑	+50%
Red blood cell volume	↑	+20%
Cardiac output	↑	+40–50%
Stroke volume	↑	+30%
Heart rate	↑	+15–20%
Femoral venous pressure	↑	+15 mm Hg
Total peripheral resistance	↓	–15 mm Hg
Mean arterial blood pressure	↓	–15 mm Hg
Systolic blood pressure	↓	–0–15 mm Hg
Diastolic blood pressure	↓	–10–20 mm Hg
Central venous pressure	None	No change

Adapted from: Ueland K. Maternal cardiovascular dynamics. VII. Intrapartum blood volume changes. Am J Obstet Gynecol 1976;126:671–677; Pritchard J. Changes in blood volume during pregnancy and delivery. Anesthesiology 1965;26:393–399; Lindheimer M, Davison J. Osmoregulation, the secretion of arginine vasopressin and its metabolism during pregnancy. Eur J Endocrinol 1995;132:133–143; Hendricks C. Hemodynamics of a uterine contraction. Am J Obstet Gynecol 1958;76:968–982; Cotes P, Canning C, Lind T. Changes in serum immunoreactive erythropoietin during the menstrual cycle and normal pregnancy. Br J Obstet Gynaecol 1983;90:304–311; Clark S, Cotton D, Lee W. Central hemodynamic assessment of normal term pregnancy. Am J Obstet Gynecol 1989;161:1439–1442; Flo K, Wilsgaard T, Vartun A, et al. A longitudinal study of the relationship between maternal cardiac output measured by impedance cardiography and uterine artery blood flow in the second half of pregnancy. BJOG 2010;117:837–844; Mabie W, DiSessa T, Crocker L, et al. A longitudinal study of cardiac output in normal human pregnancy. Am J Obstet Gynecol 1994;174:1061–1064; Warner M, Fairhead A, Rawles J, et al. An investigation of the changes in aortic diameter and an evaluation of their effect on Doppler measurement of cardiac output in pregnancy. Int J Obstet Anesth 1996;5:73–78; Ueland K, Hansen J. Maternal cardiovascular dynamics. III. Labor and delivery under local and caudal analgesia. Am J Obstet Gynecol 1969;103:8–18; Ueland K, Hansen J. Maternal cardiovascular dynamics. II. Posture and uterine contractions. Am J Obstet Gynecol 1969;103:1–7; Seth R, Moss A, McNitt S, et al. Long QT syndrome and pregnancy. J Am Coll Cardiol 2007;49:1009–1018.

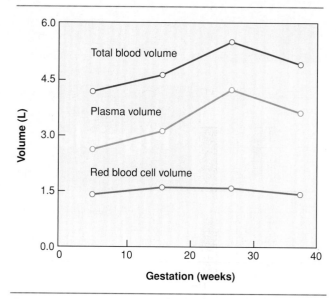

FIGURE 1-1 Changes in intravascular fluid volume (blood volume), plasma volume, and erythrocyte volume during progression of normal pregnancy. The disproportionate increase in plasma volume accounts for the relative anemia of pregnancy. Adapted from: Moir DD, Carty MJ. In: Moir DD, ed. *Obstetric Anesthesia and Analgesia*. Baltimore, MD: Williams & Wilkins; 1977.

(10,11). Cardiac output further increases 15% during the latent phase of labor, 30% during the active phase, and 45% during the expulsive stage of labor compared to prelabor values (11). Every uterine contraction results in an increase in cardiac output by an additional 10% to 25% (12). Immediately following cesarean delivery, cardiac index increases by 40% and systemic vascular resistance index (SVRI) decreases by 39%. However, the mean arterial pressure is maintained. These changes persist for approximately 10 minutes but may be present for up to 30 minutes after delivery, and return to baseline values by 2 to 5 days postpartum (13). Hemodynamic changes at delivery are

similar regardless of mode of delivery (13,14). While this substantial increase in cardiac work is well tolerated by most parturients, those with cardiac disease who are unable to increase cardiac output by meeting the large demands are often at highest risk for complications immediately postpartum.

Systemic vascular resistance decreases from approximately 1,530 dyn s/cm⁵ to 1,210 dyn s/cm⁵ during pregnancy by several mechanisms (7). The production of prostacyclin, a potent vasodilator, is increased during pregnancy (15). Progesterone also has a vasodilator effect on vascular smooth muscle. The low resistance placental circulation is in parallel with the systemic circulation. The sum of two resistances in parallel is less than either alone, which serves to decrease the afterload. The physiologic anemia of pregnancy results in a change in rheology resulting in decreased blood viscosity and improved blood flow, which also decreases afterload (16). Pulmonary vascular resistance (PVR) is also reduced by approximately 30% during pregnancy, presumably by similar mechanisms (7,17). This may have important implications in a patient with a shunt due to a congenital cardiac lesion as the balance between SVR and PVR may be disrupted during pregnancy.

The increase in cardiac output during gestation results in an overall increase in uteroplacental perfusion, renal perfusion, and lower y perfusion. Uterine blood flow increases gradually from 50 mL/min to 700 to 900 mL/min at term with over 90% of the blood flow going to the intervillous space. The remainder of the perfusion goes to the myometrium. At term, the skin blood flow increases by 3- to 4-fold thus resulting in an increase in the skin temperature.

Cardiac Evaluation

During gestation, the diaphragm is shifted upward by the gravid uterus. The result is a leftward shift in the position of the heart that can produce an enlarged appearance of the cardiac silhouette on chest radiograph (Fig. 1-5) as well as axis changes on the ECG. Echocardiographic studies reveal

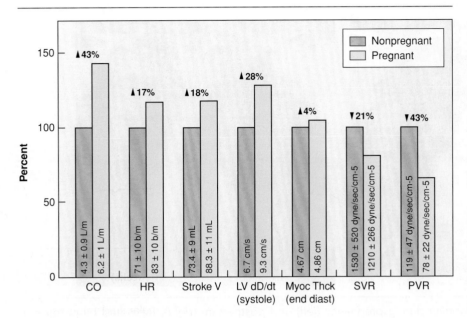

FIGURE 1-2 Hemodynamic changes of pregnancy from echocardiographic and pulmonary artery catheter monitoring in healthy women. CO, cardiac output; HR, heart rate; Stroke V, stroke volume; LV dD/dt (systole), left ventricle change (diameter/time); Myoc Thck (end diast), myocardial thickness; SVR, systemic vascular resistance; PVR, pulmonary vascular resistance. Data extracted from: Robson SC, Hunter S, Moore M, Dunlop W. Haemodynamic changes during the puerperium: A Doppler and M-mode echocardiographic study. *Br J Obstet Gynaecol* 1987;94:1028–1039; Clark SL, Cotton DB, Lee W, et al. Central hemodynamic assessment of normal term pregnancy. *Am J Obstet Gynecol* 1989;161:1439–1442.

left ventricular hypertrophy, demonstrated by increased end-diastolic chamber size and increased left ventricular wall thickness compared to nonpregnant women (18). The increase in cardiac mass is due to increased cardiac myocyte size rather than increased myocyte number (19). The left ventricular mass increases during gestation by 23% by the third trimester. Left ventricular end-diastolic volume also increases during gestation, with no change in the end-systolic volume thus resulting in a larger ejection fraction. When monitoring the hemodynamics, it should be noted that the central venous pressure, pulmonary artery diastolic pressure, and pulmonary capillary pressure are the same and comparable to the values in nonpregnant patients. Asymptomatic pericardial effusion has been reported in some parturients by echocardiographic studies (20).

Normal ECG findings in pregnancy include shortened PR and uncorrected QT interval, a shift in the QRS axis in any direction, a small right QRS axis deviation in the first trimester, a small leftward QRS axis deviation in the third

trimester, and transient S–T segment changes. Women with long QT syndrome experience fewer cardiac events during pregnancy but are at increased risk for cardiac events ranging from syncope to sudden death in the 9 months following delivery (21). The most common benign dysrhythmias in pregnancy are premature ectopic atrial and ventricular contractions and sinus tachycardia (22). These normal findings must be differentiated from those indicating heart disease which include: (a) Systolic murmur greater than grade III; (b) any diastolic murmur; (c) severe arrhythmias; and (d) unequivocal cardiac enlargement on radiographic examination (21,22). Regurgitation of the pulmonary and tricuspid valves is observed in 94% of normal pregnant women at term, while regurgitation of the mitral valve is present in

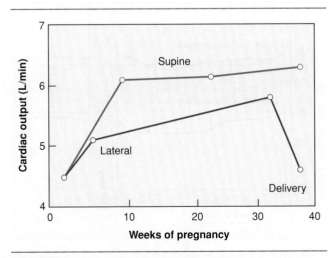

FIGURE 1-3 Changes in cardiac output during pregnancy. Adapted from: Lees MM, Taylor SH, Scott DB, et al. A Study of cardiac output at rest throughout pregnancy. *J Obstet Gynaecol Br Commonw* 1967;74:319.

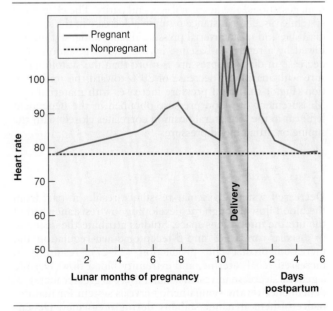

FIGURE 1-4 Changes in maternal heart rate during pregnancy. Adapted from: Burwell CS and Metcalfe JA: *Heart disease and Pregnancy: Physiology and Management.* Boston: Little, Brown and Co.; 1958.

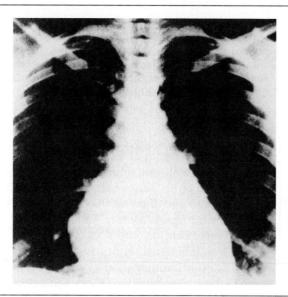
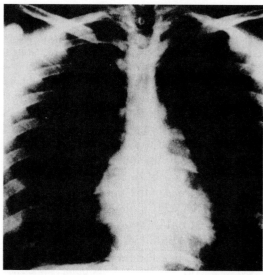

FIGURE 1-5 Chest radiograph of a woman during pregnancy (*left*) and postpartum (*right*). Reprinted by permission from: Burwell CS, McAnulty JH, Ueland K, eds. *Heart Disease in Pregnancy: Physiology and Management.* Boston: Little, Brown and Co;1986:60–63.

27% (23). Changes in heart sounds are not uncommon during pregnancy with an accentuation of the first heart sound and an exaggerated splitting of the mitral and tricuspid component. There are minimal changes in the second heart sound. In late pregnancy, a third heart sound may be heard as well (24). A murmur resulting from aortic regurgitation is not normally present in the pregnant patient (23), but grade I to II systolic heart murmurs caused by increased blood flow and tricuspid annulus dilation are commonly heard on auscultation of the heart (24).

Blood Pressure

The maternal blood pressure measurement is affected by position, gestational age, maternal age, and parity. The changes in systemic vascular resistance result in a decrease in the systolic, diastolic, and mean arterial pressure during midgestation followed by a return to baseline by the end of gestation. The decrease in diastolic pressure is more than the systolic pressure with maximum decrease of 20% toward the midgestation (Fig. 1-6). Blood pressure increases with maternal age. Measurement of blood pressure obtained in the dependent left arm in the left lateral position correlates closely with the supine or sitting blood pressure.

Sympathetic Nervous System

Decreased systemic vascular resistance results in part from the blood flow through the developing low resistance bed of the uterine intervillous space. Studies attribute the decrease in vascular tone to α- and β-receptor down-regulation and increased prostacyclin production (25–27), resulting in increased renal, uterine, and extremity blood flow. Despite a general decrease in vascular tone, there is greater maternal dependence on the sympathetic nervous system for maintenance of hemodynamic stability during pregnancy. Dependence increases progressively throughout pregnancy and peaks at term (28–30). The effects of decreased vascular tone are primarily observed on the venous capacitance system of the lower extremities. These effects counteract the untoward

effects of uterine compression of the inferior vena cava on venous return. Parasympathetic deactivation toward term is likely to contribute to increased heart rate and cardiac output at rest (31). Complex hormonal mediation results in depression of baroreflexes during pregnancy, making pregnant women even more susceptible to hypotension (32). In addition, some investigators suggest that an even greater decrease in vagal tone during pregnancy allows for relatively normal sympathetic function (33,34). This helps to explain why few women become severely bradycardic despite the high sympathectomy commonly seen at cesarean delivery. Although pharmacologic sympathectomy in term pregnant women can result in a marked decrease in blood pressure, there are minimal changes in blood pressure in nonpregnant women (28).

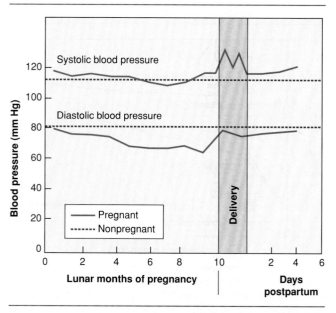

FIGURE 1-6 Changes in blood pressure during pregnancy.

Aortocaval Compression

Upon assuming the supine position, up to 15% of pregnant patients near term experience signs of shock, including hypotension, pallor, sweating, nausea, vomiting, and mental status changes. This constellation of symptoms is due to decreased venous return to the right ventricle and has been dubbed "supine-hypotension syndrome" (35). Imaging studies demonstrate complete or nearly complete occlusion of the inferior vena cava by the gravid uterus in the supine position (36,37). Partial compensation is accomplished by blood bypassing the obstructed inferior vena cava and returning to the heart via the paravertebral (epidural) veins emptying into the azygos system. However, the net result of occlusion of the inferior vena cava is decreased cardiac output and decreased organ perfusion in the supine position. Shifting from the supine to the lateral position partially relieves the obstruction of the vena cava (37) (Fig. 1-7). The collateral circulation is adequate enough to maintain right ventricular filling pressures in the lateral position.

Compression of the inferior vena cava is most common in late pregnancy before the fetal presenting part becomes fixed in the pelvis. The pooling of venous blood in the lower extremities results in a tendency toward phlebitis, venous varicosities, and lower extremity edema during pregnancy. Ankle edema, leg varicosities, and hemorrhoids indicate lower extremity venous engorgement. Blood flow to the uterus is proportional to perfusion pressure, i.e., uterine artery minus venous pressure. Compression of the inferior vena cava affects uteroplacental perfusion resulting in an overall decrease in perfusion. Increased uterine venous pressure further decreases uterine blood flow which can compromise fetal well-being. Even when maternal blood pressure is normal, uterine artery perfusion pressure decreases in the supine position because of increases in uterine venous pressure. While typically not associated with maternal symptoms, aortic compression results in increased maternal blood pressure measured in the upper extremity analogous to an aortic cross clamp. Partial occlusion of the aorta by the gravid uterus occurs in the supine position as well (38). At the same time, arterial hypotension is occurring in the lower extremities and uterine arteries. This results in decreased uterine blood flow to the fetus and fetal hypoxia (39). Therefore, even with normal upper extremity maternal blood pressure, uteroplacental perfusion may be decreased in the supine position. In fact, turning the term parturient from the supine to the left lateral position increases intervillous blood flow by 20% and increases fetal oxygen tension by 40% (40,41). Nonreassuring fetal heart rate patterns are more often observed in parturients in the supine position, particularly in the presence of neuraxial or general anesthesia (42).

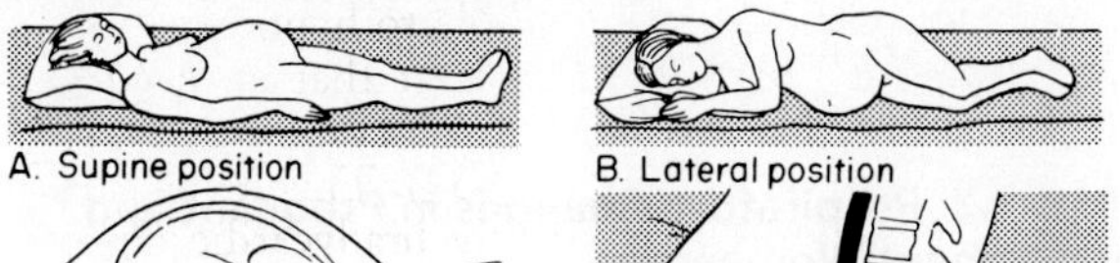

It is critical during anesthetic management to recognize the importance of aortocaval compression, the effects of which are observed as early as the 20th week of gestation. Drugs causing vasodilation, such as propofol and volatile anesthetics, or techniques resulting in sympathetic blockade, will further decrease venous return to the heart in the presence of vena cava obstruction. The presence of sympathetic blockade reduces or eliminates vasoconstriction in response to decreased venous return thus prevention of aortocaval compression is imperative. The vast majority of women avoid the supine position at night after 30 weeks (43). Therefore, it would do well to heed this natural instinct and avoid the supine position in a gravid patient. Maintaining the patient in lateral position with left uterine displacement (LUD) is essential to prevent aortocaval compression. This can be accomplished by manual displacement of the uterus, where the uterus is lifted and displaced to the left. Other alternatives include tilting the operating or delivery table 15 degrees or using sheets, a foam rubber wedge, or an inflatable bag to elevate the right buttock and back 10 to 15 cm. In the presence of conditions such as polyhydramnios or multiple gestations where the uterus is unusually large, more displacement (up to 30 degrees) may be required to relieve compression of the great vessels (44). Visual assessment of the position of the uterus is often invaluable—when the patient is in the supine position, the uterus should be visibly tilted away from the great vessels in the abdomen. Frequently, when maternal hypotension is present left uterine displacement is inadequate and repositioning the patient should be immediately considered. Occasionally, right uterine displacement or right lateral position may be at least as effective as left uterine displacement. Placement of the mother in LUD is imperative during cesarean delivery because neonates have less frequent and less severe depression of Apgar scores and are less likely to develop acidosis when LUD is employed (45). The Trendelenburg position without LUD is not an effective means to prevent or treat maternal hypotension and in fact, may worsen the maternal vital signs by shifting the uterus back further onto the vena cava and aorta. Maternal bearing down during the second stage of labor may also cause aortocaval compression and potentially decreased uterine perfusion (46). Any gravid patient near term with hypotension should be placed in LUD or the complete lateral position without delay as adequate venous return is essential to the success of any subsequent treatment. The anesthetic significance of the cardiovascular changes in pregnancy is summarized in Table 1-2.

FIGURE 1-7 Lateral and cross-sectional views of uterine aortocaval compression in the supine position and its resolution by lateral positioning of the pregnant woman. Reprinted by permission from: Bonica JJ, ed. *Obstetric Analgesia and Anesthesia*. Amsterdam: World Federation of Societies of Anaesthesiologists;1980.

TABLE 1-2 Cardiovascular Changes: Anesthetic Significance

A. Venodilation may increase the incidence of accidental epidural vein puncture.

B. Healthy parturients will tolerate up to 1,500 mL blood loss; transfusion rarely required (hemorrhage at delivery remains an important risk).

C. High hemoglobin levels (>14) indicate low-volume state caused by preeclampsia, hypertension, or inappropriate diuretics.

D. Cardiac output remains high in first few hours postpartum; women with cardiac or pulmonary disease remain at risk after delivery.

E. Epidural block reduces cardiac work during labor and may be beneficial in some cardiac disease states.

F. Maternal blood pressure of <90–95 mm Hg during regional block should be of concern because it may be associated with a proportional decrease in uterine blood flow.

G. ALWAYS AVOID AORTOCAVAL COMPRESSION: 70–80% of supine parturients with a T_4 sympathectomy develop significant hypotension.

■ RESPIRATORY CHANGES DURING PREGNANCY

Multiple significant anatomic and physiologic changes occur in the respiratory system during pregnancy which has a marked influence on the anesthetic management of these patients.

Upper Airway Changes and Implications for Airway Management

Upper airway changes begin early in the first trimester and increase progressively throughout the duration of the pregnancy (47). Capillary engorgement of the larynx, nasal, and oropharyngeal mucosa leads to increased mucosal friability and vascularity of the upper airway. Many patients appear to have symptoms of an upper respiratory tract infection as a result of respiratory tract swelling. Furthermore, many patients complain of shortness of breath due to nasal congestion (48). The hormonal influences of pregnancy and, in particular, the effects of estrogen result in an increase in airway connective tissue, increased blood volume, increased total body water, and an increase in interstitial fluid. These factors contribute to hypervascularity and edema of oropharynx, nasopharynx, and respiratory tract. The edematous changes in soft tissue of the airway may be markedly exacerbated by a mild upper respiratory infection, or fluid overload. Increased vascularity and consequent mucosal engorgement can be expected to be even greater in parturients with preeclampsia resulting in difficult endotracheal intubation especially in laboring women (49). All of these changes contribute to an increase in the Mallampati classification of the airway during pregnancy and labor resulting in a compromised airway (50). Manipulation of the airway should be approached with caution since all of these changes have important implications for airway management.

Although an 8 mm cuffed endotracheal tube many be suitable for a nonpregnant adult woman, pregnant women will typically require a smaller endotracheal tube, usually 6.0 to 6.5 mm because of increased vascularity and edema. Conse-

quently, mucosal injury during suctioning, airway placement, and laryngoscopy is more likely, and should such injury occur, there is an increased risk of excessive bleeding. Nasotracheal intubation and placement of nasogastric tubes should be avoided unless absolutely necessary, because of the potential for significant epistaxis.

Thoracic Changes during Pregnancy

The thorax also undergoes several important changes during pregnancy. Increases in both the anteroposterior and transverse diameters contribute to a 5 to 7 cm circumferential enlargement of the thoracic cage (47,51). Increased levels of relaxin causes structural changes in the ribcage resulting in relaxation of the ligamentous attachment of the ribs and an ~50% increase in the subcostal angle (52). Although the diaphragm is elevated by as much as 4 cm, diaphragmatic excursion is increased despite this change. These changes have important implications in the pregnant patient who sustains a penetrating thoracic injury resulting in a concurrent abdominal injury secondary to the elevated diaphragm.

Lung Volumes and Capacities (Table 1-3)

Lung volumes or capacities are not changed substantially during gestation. The total lung capacity is generally preserved or minimally decreased during pregnancy (53,54). Although changes in lung capacity are primarily due to a decrease in the functional residual capacity (15% to 20%) at term, tidal volume increases by nearly 45% during pregnancy. The majority of the increase occurs during the first trimester, and results in a increase in inspiratory reserve volume. In

TABLE 1-3 Respiratory Changes in Pregnant and Nonpregnant Women

Lung volumes	IRV	+5
	TV	+45
	ERV	−25
	RV	−15
Lung capacities	IC	+15
	FRC	−20
	VC	0
	TLC	−5
Ventilation	MV	+45
	AV	+45
	RR	0
	DS	+45
Respiratory mechanics	Pulmonary resistance	−50
	FEV_1	0
	FEV_1/FVC	0
	CC	0
	Flow volume loop	0

IRV, inspiratory reserve volume; TV, tidal volume; ERV, expiratory reserve volume; RV, residual volume; IC, inspiratory capacity; FRC, functional residual capacity; VC, vital capacity; TLC, total lung capacity; MV, minute ventilation; AV, alveolar ventilation; DS, dead space; FEV_1, forced expiratory volume in one second; FEV_1/FVC, ratio of forced expiratory volume in 1 second to forced vital capacity; CC, closing capacity. Reproduced from: Bucklin BA, Gambling DR, Wlody DJ. Practical Approach: Obstetric Anesthesia. Lippincott Williams and Wilkins; 2009.

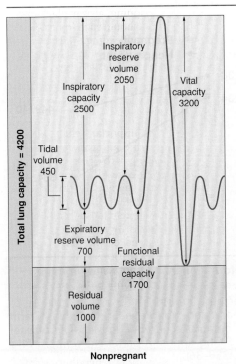
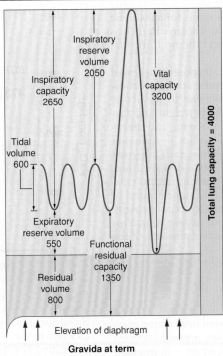

Nonpregnant   **Gravida at term**

FIGURE 1-8 Pulmonary volumes and capacities during pregnancy, labor, and postpartum period. Reprinted by permission from: Bonica JJ, ed. In: *Principles and Practice of Obstetric Analgesia and Anesthesia.* Philadelphia, PA: Davis; 1967:24.

addition, a decrease in residual volume helps to maintain the vital capacity. By the third trimester, the inspiratory capacity increases resulting from increases in both tidal volume and inspiratory reserve volumes (53,55). Consequently, expiratory reserve volume decreases (53,55).

Decreases in FRC result from elevation of the diaphragm and the enlarging uterus. These changes begin during the 20th week of pregnancy and are decreased 80% of prepregnancy by term (53,55,56). Functional residual capacity is reduced even further when parturients assume a supine position (Fig. 1-8). Vital capacity measurements in the upright position remain essentially unchanged; it also remains unchanged throughout pregnancy largely due to an increase in the inspiratory reserve volume. A measurable decrease in vital capacity occurs in obese parturients. The supine position markedly impairs the respiratory function in late pregnancy. Measurements of closing volume (lung volumes at which small airways begin to close in the dependent zones of the lungs) decrease by 30% to 50% in pregnant patients while they are in the supine position. Since the closing capacity will exceed the FRC, the parturient is at risk for hypoxemia and impaired organ perfusion in the supine position.

Ventilation and Arterial Blood Gasses (Table 1-4)

Minute ventilation is increased by 30% at the seventh week of pregnancy and approximately 50% at term (57–59). Hormonal changes (60) and greater CO_2 production (61) result in increased tidal volume with little change in respiratory rate and are responsible for the increased minute ventilation. Although the ratio of total dead space to tidal volume is unchanged during pregnancy, there is an increase in alveolar ventilation approximately 30% above baseline. Progesterone acts as a direct respiratory stimulant (62) and sensitizes central respiratory centers, increasing the ventilatory response to CO_2 and producing a leftward shift of the CO_2 curve (63). A recent study has shown that the hyperventilation of human pregnancy is the result of pregnancy-induced changes in wakefulness and central chemoreflex drives for breathing, acid–base balance, metabolic rate, and cerebral blood flow (64). Although CO_2 production at rest increases by about 300 mL/min during pregnancy (61), a normal pregnant $PaCO_2$ is 30 to 32 mm Hg, owing to the hyperventilation. Due to increased urinary excretion of bicarbonate (normal pregnant level 20 mm Hg), however, pH is partially corrected;

TABLE 1-4 Blood Gasses in Pregnancy

	Nonpregnant	Trimester		
		First	Second	Third
pH	7.40	7.41–7.44	7.41–7.44	7.41–7.44
pO₂ (mm Hg)	100	107	105	103
pCO₂ (mm Hg)	40	30–32	30–32	30–32
[HCO₃] (mEq/L)	24	21	20	20

Reproduced from: Bucklin BA, Gambling DR, Wlody DJ. Practical Approach: Obstetric Anesthesia. Lippincott Williams and Wilkins; 2009.

normal pH is 7.41 to 7.44 (65). These changes in the arterial blood gas analysis have important implications for anesthetic management. For example, if a pregnant woman's $PaCO_2$ is 40 mm Hg, this indicates hypercarbia and the need for further evaluation and treatment.

Oxygen uptake and consumption are markedly increased both at rest (about 20%) and during exercise at term as compared to nonpregnant patients. The increase in metabolic rate is out of proportion to changes in body weight and surface area. Per unit of weight, the fetus, placenta, and uterus together consume oxygen (and release carbon dioxide and heat) at a higher rate than the mother. Thus, each kilogram of maternal tissue consumes oxygen at a rate of 4 mL/min, whereas the fetoplacental unit and the growing uterus consume approximately 12 mL/min with the highest rates of fetal metabolism occurring during phases of rapid growth. Therefore, during pregnancy, the maternal oxygen consumption is the sum of the maternal metabolic rate plus that of the fetus, placenta, and uterus.

Pulmonary Function during Exercise in Pregnancy

Many women who are physically active want to continue exercise programs during pregnancy. However, pregnant women respond differently to exercise compared to nonpregnant women. Pregnancy increases exertional breathlessness. This results from an awareness of increased contractile respiratory muscle effort and mechanical adaptations of the respiratory system (66). The primary pulmonary changes associated with exercise during pregnancy include increased minute ventilation, tidal volume, oxygen consumption, CO_2 consumption and carbon monoxide diffusing capacity (DLCO) (67). Despite these changes, acid–base status remains unaltered.

Mechanisms of Hypoxemia in Pregnancy

Hyperventilation causes decreased alveolar CO_2 and greater alveolar ventilation, which, by the alveolar gas equation, leads to an increase in PaO_2 (normal 103 to 107 mm Hg) (68). However, due to the high metabolic demands of the enlarged uterus, the placenta, and the fetus, oxygen consumption increases throughout pregnancy (Table 1-5). By midgestation, pregnant women often demonstrate a PaO_2 of less than 100 mm Hg. In the supine position, FRC decreases further, and is exceeded by closing capacity. This leads to small airway closure, an increase in ventilation/perfusion (V/Q) mismatch, and decreased oxygen saturation (68). Decreased cardiac output in the supine position will cause decreased mixed venous saturation and therefore decreased arterial oxygen saturation. By changing the position from the supine to sitting or lateral decubitus, the alveolar-to-arterial oxygen gradient is usually

TABLE 1-5 Causes of Increased Oxygen Consumption during Pregnancy

Oxygen consumption ↑ by 40–60% during pregnancy as a result of:
1. Increased metabolic needs of:
   – Fetus
   – Uterus
   – Placenta
2. Increased respiratory work
3. Increased cardiac work

Reproduced from: Bucklin BA, Gambling DR, Wlody DJ. Practical Approach: Obstetric Anesthesia. Lippincott Williams and Wilkins; 2009.

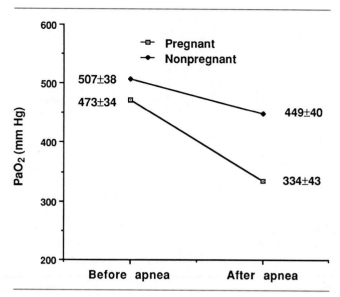

FIGURE 1-9 Decrease in arterial PO_2 after 1 minute of apnea in pregnant and nonpregnant patients. Graph developed from data in Archer GW Jr, Marx GF. Arterial oxygen tension during apnea in parturient women. *Br J Anaesth* 1974;46:358–360.

reduced and there is improvement in arterial oxygenation. At term, oxygen consumption increases 40% to 60% above prepregnancy levels (57).

Oxygen desaturation occurs much more rapidly during periods of apnea, e.g., during anesthetic induction or eclamptic seizures (Fig. 1-9). This effect is accentuated by changes in pulmonary volumes (q.v.). In a recent study, reduced apnea tolerance in pregnancy was demonstrated by simulating the physiologic changes of rapid sequence induction (69). The authors found **that after 99% denitrogenation, the time taken to decrease to SaO_2 <90% was 4 minutes in pregnant subjects and 7 minutes 25 seconds in nonpregnant subjects.** In addition, the time taken for SaO_2 to fall to 40% from 90% was 35 seconds in pregnant subjects and 45 seconds in nonpregnant subjects.

Sleep Disorders during Pregnancy

The physical and hormonal changes of pregnancy can profoundly change breathing patterns during sleep. While some of these changes may provide protection from sleep disorders, others may put women at risk. Sleep disturbances and snoring are common during pregnancy. A recent study evaluating sleep-disordered breathing and upper airway size in pregnancy confirmed increased snoring and showed narrower upper airways during the third trimester of pregnancy (70). Polysomnography in pregnant women reveals reduced slow-wave and REM phases of sleep, decreased total sleep time, and increased rates of awakening after the onset of sleep (71). Pregnancy-associated sleep disorder was first described by the American Academy of Sleep Medicine in 2000 (72). This disorder is defined as the occurrence of insomnia or excessive sleepiness that develops during pregnancy. Obstructive sleep apnea is another type of sleep disorder; however, the prevalence in pregnancy is unknown. Diagnosis during pregnancy may be difficult because sleep disturbance and daytime fatigue are common during pregnancy, especially near term. Obstructive sleep apnea should be suspected in women with BMI ≥35, neck circumference

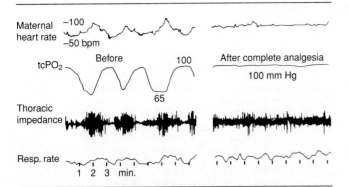

FIGURE 1-10 Maternal hyperventilation during painful uterine contractions results in hypoventilation between contractions with a corresponding decrease in transcutaneous oxygen pressure ($tcPO_2$) to 65 to 70 mm Hg. After effective epidural analgesia $tcPO_2$ is maintained at a stable 100 mm Hg. Reprinted by permission from: Huch R, Huch A, Lubbers DW, eds. In: *Transcutaneous PO_2*. New York, NY: Thieme-Stratton; 1981:139.

$\geq$16 in., frequent/loud snoring, periods of apnea during sleep, frequent arousals during sleep, or profound daytime somnolence. Prompt diagnosis by polysomnography and treatment with continuous positive airway pressure may be beneficial to reduce postoperative respiratory complications (73).

Respiratory Consequences of Uncontrolled Maternal Pain (Fig. 1-10)

When parturients are unmedicated and the pain is severe during labor, maternal minute ventilation can increase by as much as 70% to 140% during first stage of labor and by 120% to 200% in the second stage compared to the nonpregnant state (74,75). This results in marked maternal hypocarbia and alkalemia during painful contractions. The $PaCO_2$ can decrease to 10 to 15 mm Hg and this extreme degree of hypocarbia leads to maternal hypoventilation and a leftward shift of the oxyhemoglobin curve. This leftward shift causes oxygen to be more tightly bound to maternal hemoglobin thereby reducing oxygen availability to the fetus. At the same time oxygen consumption is increased (i.e., a doubling of ventilation by the parturient can increase oxygen consumption by as much as 50%) (75). As a result, significant hypoxemia can occur between contractions. Blood lactate also increases (76–78), indicating that maternal aerobic oxygen requirements exceed oxygen consumption during labor. Multiple studies have demonstrated that effective pain relief (e.g., epidural analgesia) can markedly diminish the maternal hyperventilation that occurs during painful contractions (76–79). This is an important consideration when the fetus is compromised and optimal oxygen delivery is paramount. The anesthetic implications of the respiratory changes in pregnancy are summarized in Table 1-6.

Hematologic Changes in Pregnancy

Oxygen transport is increased during pregnancy in an effort to deliver oxygen to the growing fetus. Although overall oxygen carrying capacity is decreased due to the lower hematocrit, other changes compensate for this. Maternal hyperventilation increases arterial oxygen tension to an average of

TABLE 1-6 Respiratory Changes: Anesthetic Significance

A. Airway management is more challenging:
  1. Weight gain and breast engorgement hinder laryngoscopy
  2. Swollen mucosa bleeds easily; avoid intranasal manipulation
  3. Use smaller endotracheal tube (6–7 mm)
B. Response to anesthetics:
  1. MAC decreased
  2. Decreased FRC results in faster induction with insoluble agents
  3. Increased VE speeds induction with soluble agents
  4. Overdose with loss of airway reflexes may occur more rapidly
C. Greater risk of hypoxemia:
  1. Decreased FRC causes less oxygen reserve during periods of apnea
  2. Increased oxygen consumption
  3. Rapid airway obstruction
D. Excessive mechanical hyperventilation ($P_{ET}CO_2$ <24) may reduce maternal cardiac output and uterine blood flow.
E. Maternal and fetal hypoxemia is associated with pain-induced hyper- and hypoventilation. Effective analgesia avoids these changes.

103 mm Hg. Blood flow to the uterus and other target organs increases due to increased cardiac output, vasodilation, and increased perfusion of the uterus and kidneys. Oxygen delivery to the fetus is facilitated by a shift in the maternal oxygen–hemoglobin dissociation curve to the right, with the maternal P50 shifting from 26 to 30 mm Hg (80). Fetal hemoglobin has a P50 of 18 mm Hg, which represents a higher oxygen affinity than maternal hemoglobin. This facilitates oxygen extraction from maternal hemoglobin and overall oxygen delivery to the fetus.

■ PLASMA PROTEINS

Plasma albumin begins to decrease in the first trimester and reaches a nadir of approximately 3.3 g/dL by term (81,82). The albumin-to-globulin ratio and total plasma protein concentration are both reduced in pregnancy (81). Plasma colloid oncotic pressure (COP) decreases approximately 14% during pregnancy, from 20.8 to 18 mm Hg. As a result, mild edema formation often occurs late in pregnancy (83).

Plasma COP to pulmonary capillary wedge pressure gradient declines approximately 28%, which indicates a tendency to develop pulmonary edema in the presence of changes in pulmonary capillary permeability or significantly increased cardiac preload (7). After delivery, high cardiac output and further decreases in COP may place women with severe preeclampsia and those who have recently been treated with β-agonist therapy at particular risk for postpartum pulmonary edema.

Coagulation System

Pregnancy is a compensated hypercoagulable state, with clotting factor substrates increasing with gestational age (84) (Table 1-7). Marked changes occur in nearly all aspects of hemostasis—the concentration of most clotting factors increase, levels of some anticoagulant proteins decrease,

TABLE 1-7 Changes in Coagulation Factors during Pregnancy

Unchanged	Decrease	Increase
Factor II (prothrombin)	Protein S	Fibrinogen
Factor V	Tissue plasminogen activator	Factors VII, VIII, IX, X, XII
Protein C	Factor XI (unchanged or decreased) Antithrombin III	Plasminogen Plasminogen activator inhibitor Thrombin activatable fibrinolysis inhibitor Prothrombin fragment 1 + 2 D-dimer Thrombin–antithrombin complex von Willebrand factor

and fibrinolytic activity is attenuated (85). Changes are most pronounced near term and immediately postpartum. While the teleologic value of the hypercoagulable state during pregnancy is to limit blood loss during parturition, in some women, the balance may be altered too much in favor of thrombosis and thrombotic disease occurs. In fact, the incidence of deep venous thrombosis is 5-fold higher during pregnancy and immediately postpartum (86). Levels of virtually all clotting factors increase during gestation, including factors VII, VIII, IX, X, and XII. The fibrinogen concentration increases by up to 50%, with a mean value in pregnancy of 450 mg/dL (nonpregnant mean 300 mg/dL) (84). Factor VIII and von Willebrand Factor (vWF) levels increase during pregnancy, causing a rise in the Factor VIII/vWF procoagulant complex (87). Prothrombin (factor II) and proaccelerin (factor V) are unchanged with pregnancy (88). The natural anticoagulant system is altered during pregnancy, with Protein S levels decreasing and an increase in activated protein C resistance. Protein C levels appear to be unchanged (89). Fibrinolysis is decreased during pregnancy, with levels of tissue plasminogen activator (t-PA) decreasing. In addition, there are increases in endothelial and placenta-derived plasminogen activators.

Most parturients have either a modest reduction (10%) or no change in platelet count (84). Increases in β-thromboglobulin and fibrinopeptide A during pregnancy reflect increased platelet activation (90). Increased platelet aggregation in response to epinephrine, arachidonic acid, collagen, and adenosine also occurs. Elevated mean platelet volume suggests increased platelet destruction during gestation, which is compensated for by increased platelet production (91,92). A small number of women have platelet counts of 90 to 100,000 cells/mm³ with no reduction in platelet function or activity. The diagnosis of "Gestational Thrombocytopenia" is a diagnosis of exclusion. It is generally considered to be benign and resolves spontaneously postpartum.

Immune System

Leukocyte levels increase beginning in the first trimester to as high as 6,000–16,000/mm³ (average 9,000–11,000) at term (84). This change is thought to be a result of increases in plasma-free cortisol and estrogen (93). The vast majority of the leukocyte increase is due to increases in polymorphonuclear cells, many of which are immature granulocytic cells such as myelocytes and metamyelocytes. Eosinophil, lymphocyte, and basophil levels fall during pregnancy while monocyte number remains unchanged. Further rises

in leukocyte levels are observed during labor and after delivery, with levels remaining above normal for 6 weeks or more postpartum. Leukocyte chemotaxis and adherence is impaired during pregnancy, which may account for the increased incidence of infection during gestation and reduced symptoms in some pregnant women with autoimmune disease (94,95). Serum levels of immunoglobulins A, G, and M do not change during pregnancy, while humoral antibody titers to viruses such as measles, herpes simplex, and influenza A are decreased (96).

The anesthetic significance of the hematologic changes in pregnancy is summarized in Table 1-8.

TABLE 1-8 Hematologic Changes: Anesthetic Significance

A. A disproportionate increase in plasma volume to red blood cell volume results in the "physiologic anemia of pregnancy."

B. In the absence of dietary iron supplementation, a hemoglobin concentration of 11.6 gm/dL is typical.

C. The increase in blood volume during pregnancy prepares the parturient for normal blood loss at delivery. Blood loss is usually less than 500 mL for vaginal delivery and 1,000 mL for cesarean delivery.

D. Hemodynamic changes due to blood loss are usually not observed until the blood loss exceeds 1,500 mL and transfusion is rarely required unless blood loss exceeds this amount.

E. Normal pregnancy is associated with profound alterations in the coagulation and fibrinolytic systems. Intrapartum blood loss is minimized but risk of thromboembolism is increased.

F. These changes are not detected by conventional tests (e.g., prothrombin time, activated partial thromboplastin time).

G. Most parturients have either a modest reduction (10%) or no change in platelet count. A routine platelet count in the NORMAL parturient is unnecessary prior to neuraxial anesthesia.

H. If thrombocytopenia is suspected (e.g., preeclampsia, gestational thrombocytopenia, idiopathic thrombocytopenic purpura), a platelet count should be obtained in addition to assessment for clinical signs of bleeding.

TABLE 1-9 Nervous System Changes: Anesthetic Significance

A. Anesthetic requirements as measured by minimal alveolar concentration (MAC), are decreased by as much as 30% from the nonpregnant state.

B. More rapid uptake of volatile anesthetics occurs due to decreased FRC and more rapid F_A/F_I rate of rise.

C. These changes are significant because inhaled concentrations of anesthetics that would be appropriate in a nonpregnant patient might have exaggerated effects in the pregnant patient.

D. A similar increased sensitivity to intravenous induction (e.g., propofol) and sedative (e.g., benzodiazepines) agents is also seen.

E. Neuraxial anesthetic requirements are decreased by approximately 40% at term. Both biochemical and mechanical changes are responsible for the decrease.

F. Increased neuronal sensitivity to local anesthetics results in decreased dose requirements for neuraxial anesthetics as early as the end of the first trimester suggesting a biochemical or hormonal mechanism.

G. Aortocaval compression results in epidural venous engorgement. This decreases the volume of the epidural space, and the volume of CSF per spinal segment.

H. For a given dose of epidural or intrathecal local anesthetic, there will be a greater degree of dermatomal spread.

■ THE NERVOUS SYSTEM

The anesthetic significance of the changes in the nervous system during pregnancy is summarized in Table 1-9.

General Anesthesia

Anesthetic requirements for the commonly used volatile anesthetic agents, as measured by minimal alveolar concentration (MAC), are decreased by as much as 30% from the nonpregnant state (97). Although proposed mechanisms for these changes include increased levels of plasma endorphins (98) and progesterone (10- to 20-fold during late pregnancy), progesterone is also known to have central nervous system depressant effects (99). Although the role of endorphins in pregnancy is not fully understood, maternal β-endorphin serum levels increase during gestation, labor, and delivery. These increases are proportional to the frequency of uterine contractions reflecting stress of labor but the effects of physiologic increases in β-endorphins on subjective responses to the pain of parturition or MAC are unclear.

Awareness of these changes in anesthetic requirements is significant because inhaled concentrations of anesthetics that would be appropriate in a nonpregnant patient might have exaggerated effects in the pregnant patient. For example, an inspired concentration of 50% N_2O used for supplementation of an inadequate neuraxial anesthesia during cesarean delivery might cause loss of consciousness and increase the risk of airway obstruction, vomiting, and aspiration. Although the mechanism for decreased MAC is uncertain, increased levels of progesterone during pregnancy cause sedation and even loss of consciousness in large doses (100). Anesthetic requirements for inhalation agents return to normal within 3 to 5 days following delivery (101). A similar increased sensitivity

to intravenous induction (e.g., thiopental) (102) and sedative (e.g., benzodiazepines) agents is also observed.

Neuraxial Anesthesia

Neuraxial anesthetic requirements are decreased by approximately 40% at term. Two mechanisms are thought to be responsible for these changes: First, pregnancy produces compression of the inferior vena cava resulting in distension of the epidural venous plexus by the enlarging uterus (103); second, the volume of epidural fat increases and contributes to a further reduction in subarachnoid cerebral spinal fluid (CSF) volume (104). These mechanical changes produce decreases in the volume of the epidural space, and also the volume of CSF per spinal segment. Thus, **a given dose of epidural or intrathecal local anesthetic will produce a greater degree of dermatomal spread.** Although the anatomic and mechanical changes in the vertebral column play an important role, biochemical changes are also responsible for alterations in neuraxial anesthetic requirements. The decreased dose requirements for neuraxial anesthesia occur as early as the end of the first trimester, long before significant epidural venous distension occurs. This suggests that a biochemical or hormonal mechanism may be at work. The concentration of local anesthetic required to block nerve conduction of in vitro vagus nerve obtained from male rabbits chronically exposed to progesterone is decreased (105). This effect is not observed in vagus nerve preparations acutely exposed to progesterone (106) suggesting that chronic exposure to progesterone causes alterations of receptor activity, modulation of sodium channels, or altered permeability within neuronal membranes leading to increased sensitivity to local anesthetics. Median nerve blockade with lidocaine is faster in pregnant (4 minutes) compared to nonpregnant women (11.5 minutes) (107). In addition, decreases in CSF specific gravity and acid–base changes also occur in the CSF. These factors may also influence the activity of local anesthetics in the subarachnoid space. Despite these changes, protein binding of CSF to local anesthetics does not appear to be altered in pregnancy. Local anesthetic requirements for spinal anesthesia return to normal 8 to 24 hours postpartum (108).

Pain Thresholds and Perception

Pain thresholds are increased during pregnancy, and even more so during labor, as a result of an increase in circulating β-endorphins and activated spinal cord κ-opioid receptors (109). Although one animal study determined that a progressive increase in pain tolerance was abolished by administration of an opioid antagonist (110), elevated concentrations of β-endorphins and enkephalins are found in the plasma and CSF of parturients (98). Thus, a pregnancy-induced activation of the endorphin system likely contributes to an increase in pain thresholds during pregnancy.

■ THE GASTROINTESTINAL SYSTEM

The anesthetic significance of the changes in the gastrointestinal system during pregnancy is summarized in Table 1-10.

Gastric Motility and Emptying

There have been long-standing concerns about delays in gastric motility and emptying throughout pregnancy, especially since pregnancy is associated with a shift in the position of the stomach caused by the gravid uterus (111). However, ultrasound studies demonstrate that gastric emptying remains normal throughout gestation, even in obese parturients (112). With the

TABLE 1-10 Gastrointestinal Changes: Anesthetic Significance

A. Despite long-standing concern, ultrasound studies demonstrate that gastric emptying remains normal throughout gestation, even in obese parturients.
B. With the onset of painful contractions, however, gastric emptying is slowed. Parenteral opioids have a similar effect.
C. Neuraxial analgesia during labor has no impact on gastric emptying unless fentanyl (or another opioid) is used to supplement the anesthetic.
D. The consumption of clear liquids appears to promote gastric emptying. Current ASA recommendations suggest that consumption of clear liquids by laboring patients without additional risk factors (e.g., morbid obesity, diabetes, difficult airway) is acceptable.
E. Ectopic gastrin (secreted by the placenta) has the potential to increase both the volume and acidity of gastric secretions. However, it has been shown by a number of studies that plasma gastrin levels are reduced or unchanged during pregnancy.
F. Progesterone and estrogen relax the smooth muscle of the lower esophageal sphincter (LES), decreasing the barrier pressure that normally prevents gastroesophageal reflux.
G. Elevation and rotation of the stomach by the enlarging uterus eliminates the "pinch valve" at the entry point of the esophagus through the diaphragm, further decreasing the barrier to reflux.
H. Changes in LES tone increase both the risk of regurgitation and aspiration of gastric contents, as well as the severity of the pulmonary injury that can be expected after aspiration.

onset of painful contractions, gastric emptying is slowed (113). Neuraxial analgesia during labor has no impact on gastric emptying unless fentanyl (or another opioid) is used to supplement the anesthetic (114). Epidural fentanyl in doses >100 mcg has been shown to have a significant effect on gastric emptying. In addition to parenteral opioids, a 25 mcg dose of intrathecal fentanyl will also impair gastric emptying (115). The consumption of clear liquids appears to promote gastric emptying, and current ASA recommendations suggest that consumption of clear liquids by laboring patients without additional risk factors (e.g., morbid obesity, diabetes, difficult airway) is acceptable (116). Gastric emptying returns to nonpregnant levels approximately 18 hours postpartum (117). Approximately 30% to 50% of pregnant women experience gastroesophageal reflux during pregnancy (118). Reflux can increase the risk for silent regurgitation, active vomiting, and aspiration during general anesthesia or if consciousness is impaired for any reason.

Gastric Secretions

Ectopic gastrin is secreted by the placenta beginning at 15 weeks' gestation (119). This has the potential to increase both the volume and acidity of gastric secretions. However, it has been shown by a number of studies that plasma gastrin levels are reduced or unchanged during pregnancy. The reduced gastric acid secretion, reaches its lowest levels at 20 to 30 weeks' gestation (120). Studies of gastric volume and pH in nonpregnant women undergoing elective surgery, and pregnant women at cesarean delivery, showed no difference between the two groups in terms of percentage of women with pH <2.5 (80%) and gastric volume >25 mL (50%) (121,122). The number of

women with both a low pH and high gastric volume was the same in both groups (40% to 50%). The same investigation of women at 15 weeks' gestation showed similar results (122).

Intragastric pressure is increased during the last weeks of pregnancy and reaches levels that exceed 40 cm H_2O, especially in the obese and parturients with, multiple gestation as well as polyhydramnios.

Lower Esophageal Sphincter Function

Progesterone and estrogen relax the smooth muscle of the lower esophageal sphincter (123), decreasing the barrier pressure that normally prevents gastroesophageal reflux. Elevation and rotation of the stomach by the enlarging uterus eliminates the "pinch valve" at the entry point of the esophagus through the diaphragm, further decreasing the barrier to reflux. In addition to these changes, pregnancy- and labor-related nausea, pain, fear, opioids, recent food ingestion, diabetes, and obesity and loss of airway reflexes increase both the risk of regurgitation and aspiration of gastric contents, as well as the severity of the pulmonary injury resulting from aspiration of gastric contents. Both opioids and anticholinergics are known to decrease gastroesophageal tone.

Hepatic Function

The anesthetic significance of the changes in hepatic function during pregnancy is summarized in Table 1-11.

TABLE 1-11 Hepatic Changes: Anesthetic Significance

A. Pregnancy induces reversible anatomic, physiologic, and functional changes in the liver as a result of an increase in serum estrogen and progesterone.
B. The amount of cardiac output distributed to the liver falls by 35% during pregnancy despite systemic increases in blood volume and cardiac output.
C. Pressure in the portal, and esophageal veins increases in the third trimester due to pressure of the gravid uterus on the intra-abdominal venous system.
D. These changes can be problematic if liver disease is present, since, for example spider naevi and palmar erythema are signs of liver disease, but may be seen in some pregnant women as a result of increased estrogen levels.
E. Telangiectasia and esophageal varices may appear in up to 60% of normal pregnancies, without evidence of liver dysfunction. Care should be used in placement of nasogastric tubes of esophageal temperature probes.
F. Serum transaminases can be increased to the upper limits of normal. Liver function tests are usually not affected by pregnancy except for the alkaline phosphatase (ALP). Due to increased production of fetal and placental ALP, maternal ALP can be increased up to 4 times normal which makes interpretation of these laboratory results difficult.
G. Average serum cholinesterase concentration is reduced by 24% before delivery perhaps due to the large volume of distribution. The apneic response to appropriate doses of succinylcholine is rarely prolonged.
H. Pseudocholinesterase activity appears to be normal in pregnancy.

Pregnancy induces reversible anatomic, physiologic, and functional changes in the liver as a result of an increase in serum estrogen and progesterone. Although the size of the liver does not normally increase during normal pregnancy and is usually not palpable, during late pregnancy the liver is displaced upward, posterior, and to the right. The amount of cardiac output distributed to the liver falls by 35% during pregnancy despite systemic increases in blood volume and cardiac output. Even though the proportion of blood flow to the liver decreases during pregnancy, pressure in the portal, and esophageal veins increases in the third trimester due to pressure of the gravid uterus on the intra-abdominal venous system. These changes can be problematic if liver disease is present, for example spider naevi and palmar erythema are signs of liver disease, but may be seen in some pregnant women as a result of increased estrogen levels. Telangiectasia and esophageal varices may appear in up to 60% of normal pregnancies (124), even though these patients have no evidence of liver dysfunction. However, these findings resolve postpartum. As a result of the large volume of distribution, the clearance of drugs dependent on hepatic blood flow is reduced.

During normal pregnancy, the serum transaminases can be slightly increased to the upper limits of normal (125) (Table 1-12). Liver function tests are usually not affected by pregnancy except for the alkaline phosphatase (ALP). Fetal and placental production of ALP increases; thus the maternal serum levels increase up to 4 times normal which makes interpretation of these laboratory results difficult. Serum albumin concentration decreases up to 60% from the increase in plasma volume, which leads to a 20% reduction in total serum protein by midpregnancy (126).

Although liver disease is present in approximately 3% of all pregnancies, biliary stasis and increased secretion of bile increase the risk of gallbladder disease during pregnancy.

Increased levels of progesterone also contribute to gallbladder hypomotility by inhibiting its contractility due to smooth muscle relaxation (127). Although the incidence of gallstones is 5% to 12% during pregnancy (128), bile acid composition returns rapidly to normal after delivery even in patients with preexisting gall stones. The incidence of cholecystectomy during pregnancy is between 1 in 1,600 and 1 in 10,000 (128).

Average serum cholinesterase concentration is reduced by 24% before delivery and by 33% at 3 days postpartum perhaps due to the large volume of distribution. Cholinesterase levels return to normal by 2 to 6 weeks postpartum. Despite the decreased levels, the apneic response to appropriate doses of succinylcholine is rarely prolonged. However, prolonged apnea after succinylcholine lasting more than 20 minutes has been reported in 2% to 6% of parturients who are genotypically normal but have low levels of serum pseudocholinesterase. Pseudocholinesterase is also required for the hydrolysis of 2-chloroprocaine which appears to be normal in pregnancy.

Physiologic Changes in the Kidney

The anesthetic significance of the changes in the renal system during pregnancy is summarized in Table 1-13.

Alterations in the kidney and upper urinary tract are among the earliest and most dramatic of the physiologic changes during pregnancy. Renal blood flow increases by approximately 50% to 80% above prepregnancy levels, rising sharply in the first trimester until 16 weeks. Peak renal blood flow occurs at approximately 26 weeks, and remains elevated until 34 weeks followed by a slight decline at term (129). These changes result in enlargement of the kidneys by up to 30% (129). Relaxin, which is a hormone produced in the corpus luteum and later in pregnancy by the placenta, mediates renal

TABLE 1-12 Liver Function Tests in Normal Pregnancy

Test	Pregnancy Effect	Trimester of Maximum Effect
Albumin	↓ 20–60%	2
α- and β-globulin	Slight ↑	3
γ-globulin	None to slight ↓	3
Fibrinogen	↓ 50%	2
Ceruloplasmin	↑	3
Transferring	↑	3
Bilirubin	None	—
ALP	2–4 × ↑	3
GGTP	↓	3
LDH	None or slight ↑	3
AST and ALT	None	—
5′ nucleotidase	None or slight ↑	2
bile acids		—
Triglycerides and cholesterol	2–3 × ↑	3

ALP, alkaline phosphatase; GGTP, γ-glutamyl-transpeptidase; LDH, lactate dehydrogenase; AST, aspartate aminotransferase; ALT, alanine aminotransferase.
Reproduced from: Bucklin BA, Gambling DR, Wlody DJ. Practical Approach: Obstetric Anesthesia. Lippincott Williams and Wilkins; 2009.

TABLE 1-13 Renal Changes: Anesthetic Significance

A. Alterations in the kidney and upper urinary tract are among the earliest and most dramatic of the physiologic changes during pregnancy. Renal blood flow increases by approximately 50–80% above prepregnancy levels. Kidneys enlarge by up to 30%.

B. Renal vasodilation results from increased levels of relaxin. Increases in progesterone are responsible for dilation of the ureters and renal pelvis.

C. The enlarged gravid uterus may obstruct the ureters leading to further dilation of the ureters. Approximately 80% of women have hydronephrosis by midpregnancy.

D. The result of these anatomic alterations is an increased risk of urinary stasis leading to infection and the potential for misinterpretation of diagnostic imaging studies.

E. Glomerular filtration rate and creatinine clearance are increased. Normal values for creatinine and BUN during pregnancy are 0.5 mg/dL and 9 mg/dL.

F. BUN and creatinine measurements that are normal or slightly elevated in nonpregnant individuals indicate poor renal function during pregnancy.

G. Increased GFR and tubular flow results in decreased proximal tubular reabsorption and a physiologic glucosuria. Glucosuria is normal.

H. Although proteinuria increases slightly and is due to the increased GFR, reduced proximal tubular reabsorption and perhaps alteration in the electrostatic charge of the glomerular filter, significant proteinuria is abnormal.

vasodilation during pregnancy (130). Hormonal changes, primarily increases in progesterone, are responsible for dilation of the ureters and renal pelvis by the end of the first trimester (129). Later in pregnancy, the enlarged gravid uterus may obstruct the ureters leading to further dilation of the ureters. Approximately 80% of women have hydronephrosis by mid-pregnancy (129,131). The net result of these anatomic alterations is an increased risk of urinary stasis leading to infection and the potential for misinterpretation of diagnostic imaging studies (131).

Changes in renal function also occur during pregnancy. The substantial increase in renal blood flow and reduced renal vascular resistance result in increased glomerular filtration rate (GFR) (130). The GFR increases from 100 to 150 mL/min (40% to 65% above the prepregnancy level) by the second trimester, which results in decreases in BUN and creatinine. Creatinine clearance is also increased from 120 mL/min to 150 to 200 mL/min (132). Because of these changes, BUN and creatinine measurements that are normal or slightly elevated in nonpregnant individuals indicate poor renal function during pregnancy. The normal values for creatinine and BUN during pregnancy are 0.5 mg/dL and 9 mg/dL, respectively (129).

The increased GFR decreased proximal reabsorption of protein, and possibly alterations in the electrostatic charge of the glomerular filter result in elevated protein excretion and proteinuria during pregnancy. During pregnancy the average 24-hour total protein excretion is 200 mg (upper limit 300 mg) and the average amount of albumin excreted is 12 mg (upper limit 20 mg) (133,134). Plasma levels of other substrates which require renal clearance and absorption are altered as well. Uric acid levels decrease during pregnancy by 25% to 35% due to increased renal clearance (135). Respiratory alterations during pregnancy result in increased minute ventilation and a respiratory alkalosis. The kidney responds by increasing urinary excretion of bicarbonate, leading to decreased serum bicarbonate and the potential for decreased buffering capacity in the blood.

Renal handling of glucose is altered during pregnancy. In nonpregnant individuals, glucose is filtered and almost completely reabsorbed in the proximal tubule by an active transport system, resulting in minimal urinary glucose excretion. During pregnancy, the increased GFR and tubular flow results in decreased proximal tubular reabsorption and a physiologic glucosuria (136). The amount of glucose excreted in the third trimester by normal women may be several times that of nonpregnant individuals. Therefore, screening of urine glucose levels to evaluate for impaired glucose tolerance during pregnancy is not routine.

■ CHANGES IN THE ENDOCRINE SYSTEM

The anesthetic significance of the changes in endocrine function during pregnancy is summarized in Table 1-14.

Thyroid Function

The thyroid gland enlarges up to 70% during pregnancy both from follicular hyperplasia and increased vascularity (137). Total T_3 and T_4 levels are increased by as much as 50% resulting from estrogen-induced increases in thyroid-binding globulin. This occurs during the first trimester and persists until term. Free T_3 and T_4 levels remain unchanged during pregnancy. Thyroid-stimulating hormone (TSH) levels decrease during the first trimester but return to nonpregnant levels and remain constant throughout the remainder of pregnancy. Subclinical hyperthyroidism occurs in approximately

TABLE 1-14 Endocrine Changes: Anesthetic Significance

A. Total T_3 AND T_4 levels increase due to estrogen-induced increases in thyroid binding globulin. Free T_3 AND T_4 remain unchanged during pregnancy.
B. TSH levels decrease during the first trimester and return to normal levels throughout the remainder of pregnancy.
C. Pregnancy is associated with reduced tissue sensitivity to insulin. Pregnant women will have higher blood glucose levels after a carbohydrate load.
D. The fetal placental unit has a higher glucose consumption which results in an altered response to fasting and exaggerated starvation ketosis.
E. Hyperplasia of the lactotrophic cells in the pituitary results in a state of hyperprolactinemia.
F. Active cortisol levels are increased 2.5 times above nonpregnant levels and result from increased production and decreased clearance of cortisol.

1.7% of all screened pregnant women. These women have suppressed TSH but normal T_4 levels. Subclinical hyperthyroidism is not associated with adverse pregnancy outcomes (138). Some studies have indicated that there are trimester-specific changes in some measures of thyroid function and if thyroid disease is suspected, an endocrinologist should be consulted (139,140).

Pancreatic Function and Glucose Metabolism

Although blood glucose concentrations remain near normal during pregnancy, pregnancy is associated with reduced tissue sensitivity to insulin. This diabetogenic effect is caused primarily by placental lactogen (141). This means that a pregnant woman will have higher blood glucose levels after a carbohydrate load than a nonpregnant woman, despite a hyperinsulinemic response in pregnancy. The fasting blood sugar during the third trimester is lower than in nonpregnant controls. This altered response to fasting during pregnancy is a result of higher glucose consumption by the fetoplacental unit. In addition to this relative hypoglycemic state and fasting hypoinsulinemia, pregnant women exhibit an exaggerated starvation ketosis. All of these changes resolve within 24 hours of delivery.

Pituitary Function

Normal pregnancy stimulates hyperplasia of the lactotrophic cells in the pituitary gland (142). Neuroendocrine control of prolactin secretion is markedly altered by pregnancy to allow a state of hyperprolactinemia. Placental lactogen and dopamine both play a role in this regard (143).

Adrenal Cortical Function

Plasma cortisol levels increase up to 100% above baseline during the first trimester and 200% at term. These changes are produced from increased concentrations of corticosteroid-binding globulin resulting from hormonally mediated increases in hepatic synthesis. Active cortisol levels are increased 2.5 times above nonpregnant levels. These increases result from increased production and decreased clearance of cortisol. Placental enzymes likely metabolize betamethasone resulting in lower systemic levels during pregnancy (144).

TABLE 1-15 Musculoskeletal Changes: Anesthetic Significance

A. The enlarging uterus and weight gain place significant stress on the musculoskeletal system due to shifts in the center of gravity of the body that results in strain on the spine and pelvic joints.

B. There is increased joint mobility during pregnancy secondary to the effects of the hormone relaxin.

C. Uterine growth results in significant lumbar lordosis, causing significant strain on the lower back and increasing the risk of falls. Labor and prolonged expulsive efforts also cause or exacerbate the back pain.

D. Low back pain is the most common musculoskeletal complaint during pregnancy and the puerperium.

E. Although there has been long-standing concern about a causal relationship between epidural anesthesia and development of long-term back pain, prospective studies have consistently demonstrated a noncausal relationship.

Pregnancy-associated Musculoskeletal Changes

The anesthetic significance of the changes in the musculoskeletal system during pregnancy is summarized in Table 1-15.

Changes in the musculoskeletal system during pregnancy have important implications; low back pain is the most common musculoskeletal complaint during pregnancy and the puerperium. The enlarging uterus and weight gain place significant stress on the musculoskeletal system due to shifts in the center of gravity of the body, resulting in strain on the spine and pelvic joints. Uterine growth results in significant lumbar lordosis, which can alter the patient's center of gravity over the legs, cause significant strain on the lower back and increase the risk of falls. In one longitudinal study, 98% of patients experienced back pain by 37 weeks' gestation (145). Labor and prolonged expulsive efforts also cause or exacerbate the back pain.

While the mechanism of the musculoskeletal changes during pregnancy is largely mechanical, the hormone relaxin also plays a role. Relaxin is produced by the corpus luteum in early pregnancy and later by the placenta and chorion. It is involved in the increased mobility of the sacroiliac, sacrococcygeal, and pubic joints, which occur in order for the fetus to pass during delivery (146). Relaxin causes the ligaments to stretch; however, the exact role of relaxin in many aspects of pregnancy-related changes is an area of active investigation. Although there has been long-standing concern about a causal relationship between epidural anesthesia and development of long-term back pain, prospective studies have consistently demonstrated a noncausal relationship.

■ ACKNOWLEDGMENT

The authors would like to acknowledge Theodore G. Cheek, M.D. and Brett B. Gutsche, M.D. for their contributions to this chapter.

KEY POINTS

■ Cardiac output increases throughout pregnancy and further increases are observed during labor and delivery.

■ After approximately 20 weeks' gestation, the supine position causes significantly decreased venous return with potentially detrimental decreases in cardiac output and uteroplacental perfusion.

■ Displacement of the uterus to the left relieves aortocaval compression and should be performed when parturients are supine. The supine position without uterine displacement should be avoided in all term parturients.

■ Uterine blood flow at term gestation is approximately 700 mL/min. Thus, uncontrolled uterine bleeding can rapidly lead to catastrophic hemorrhage.

■ Decreases in functional residual capacity and increases in oxygen consumption place the parturient at risk for significant hypoxia during periods of apnea.

■ Pain thresholds are increased during pregnancy. Consequently, parturients are more sensitive to both volatile and local anesthetics.

■ Airway changes such as increased edema and vascularity occur during pregnancy and labor may increase the risk of difficult airway management.

■ Glomerular filtration rate and renal blood flow increase early in gestation and are maintained throughout pregnancy. Under normal circumstances, blood creatinine decreases significantly. Therefore, a level which would be normal in nonpregnant individuals may represent impaired renal function.

■ Pregnancy increases the risk of gastroesophageal reflux. Under normal circumstances, gastric emptying is not changed in pregnancy but may be altered with obesity, recent food ingestion, and with the use of intravenous or neuraxial opioids to treat labor pain.

■ Pregnancy is a compensated hypercoagulable state in which most clotting factors are increased and the parturient is at high risk for thrombotic disease.

REFERENCES

1. Ueland K. Maternal cardiovascular dynamics. VII. Intrapartum blood volume changes. *Am J Obstet Gynecol* 1976;126:671–677.

2. Pritchard J. Changes in blood volume during pregnancy and delivery. *Anesthesiology* 1965;26:393–399.

3. Lindheimer M, Davison J. Osmoregulation, the secretion of arginine vasopressin and its metabolism during pregnancy. *Eur J Endocrinol* 1995;132:133–143.

4. Hendricks C. Hemodynamics of a uterine contraction. *Am J Obstet Gynecol* 1958;76:968–982.

5. Cotes P, Canning C, Lind T. Changes in serum immunoreactive erythropoietin during the menstrual cycle and normal pregnancy. *Br J Obstet Gynaecol* 1983;90:304–311.

6. Recommendations to prevent and control iron deficiency anemia in the United States. Centers for Disease Control and Prevention. *MMWR Recomm Rep* 1998;47:1–29.

7. Clark S, Cotton D, Lee W. Central hemodynamic assessment of normal term pregnancy. *Am J Obstet Gynecol* 1989;161:1439–1442.

8. Flo K, Wilsgaard T, Vartun A, et al. A longitudinal study of the relationship between maternal cardiac output measured by impedance cardiography and uterine artery blood flow in the second half of pregnancy. *BJOG* 2010;117:837–844.

9. Mabie W, DiSessa T, Crocker L, et al. A longitudinal study of cardiac output in normal human pregnancy. *Am J Obstet Gynecol* 1994;174:1061–1064.

10. Warner M, Fairhead A, Rawles J, et al. An investigation of the changes in aortic diameter and an evaluation of their effect on Doppler measurement of cardiac output in pregnancy. *Int J Obstet Anesth* 1996;5:73–78.

11. Ueland K, Hansen J. Maternal cardiovascular dynamics. III. Labor and delivery under local and caudal analgesia. *Am J Obstet Gynecol* 1969;103:8–18.

12. Ueland K, Hansen J. Maternal cardiovascular dynamics. II. Posture and uterine contractions. *Am J Obstet Gynecol* 1969;103:1–7.

13. Tihtonen K, Koobi T, Yli-Hankala A, et al. Maternal hemodynamics during cesarean delivery assessed by whole-body impedance cardiography. *Acta Obstet Gynecol Scand* 2005;84:355–361.

14. Niswonger J, Langmade C. Cardiovascular changes in vaginal deliveries and cesarean sections. *Am J Obstet Gynecol* 1970;107:337–344.

15. Ylikorala O, Jouppila P, Kirkinen P, et al. Prostacyclin production during pregnancy: comparison of production during normal pregnancy and pregnancy complicated by hypertension. *Am J Obstet Gynecol* 1982;142:817–822.

16. Scott DE. Anemia in pregnancy. *Obstet Gynecol Annu* 1972;1:219–244.

17. Poppas A, Shroff S, Korcarz C. Serial assessment of the cardiovascular system in normal pregnancy. Role of arterial compliance and pulsatile arterial load. *Circulation* 1997;95:2407–2415.

18. Robson S, Hunter S, Moore M, et al. Haemodynamic changes during the puerperium: A Doppler and M-mode echocardiographic study. *Br J Obstet Gynaecol* 1987;69:851–853.

19. Catalucci D, Latronico N, Ellingsen O, et al. Physiological myocardial hypertrophy: how and why? *Front Biosci* 2008;13:312–324.

20. Enein M, Zina A, Kassem M, et al. Echocardiography of the pericardium in pregnancy. *Obstet Gynecol* 1987;69:851–853.

21. Seth R, Moss A, McNitt S, et al. Long QT syndrome and pregnancy. *J Am Coll Cardiol* 2007;49:1009–1018.

22. Shotan A, Ostrzega E, Mehra A. Incidence of arrhythmias in normal pregnancy and relation to palpitations, dizziness, and syncope. *Am J Cardiol* 1997;79:1061–1064.

23. Campos O, Andrade J, Bocanegra J, et al. Physiologic multivalvular regurgitation during pregnancy: a longitudinal Doppler echocardiographic study. *Int J Cardiol* 1993;40:265–272.

24. Cutforth R, MacDonald C. Heart sounds and murmurs in pregnancy. *Am Heart J* 1966;71:741–747.

25. Goodman RP, Killam AP, Brash AR, et al. Prostacyclin production during pregnancy: comparison of production during normal pregnancy and pregnancy complicated by hypertension. *Am J Obstet Gynecol* 1982;142:817–822.

26. Ylikorkala O, Jouppila P, Kirkinen P, et al. Maternal prostacyclin, thromboxane, and placental blood flow. *Am J Obstet Gynecol* 1983;145:730–732.

27. Clark KE, Austin JE, Seeds AE. Effect of bisenoic prostaglandins and arachidonic acid on the uterine vasculature of pregnant sheep. *Am J Obstet Gynecol* 1982;142:261–268.

28. Assali NS, Prystowsky H. Studies on autonomic blockade. I. Comparison between the effects of tetraethylammonium chloride (TEAC) and high selective spinal anesthesia on blood pressure of normal and toxemic pregnancy. *J Clin Invest* 1950;29:1354–1366.

29. Tabsh K, Rudelstorfer R, Nuwayhid B, et al. Circulatory responses to hypovolemia in the pregnant and nonpregnant sheep after pharmacologic sympathectomy. *Am J Obstet Gynecol* 1986;154:411–419.

30. Goodlin RC. Venous reactivity and pregnancy abnormalities. *Acta Obstet Gynecol Scand* 1986;65:345–348.

31. Heiskanen N, Saarelainen H, Valtonen P, et al. Blood pressure and heart rate variability analysis of orthostatic challenge in normal human pregnancies. *Clin Physiol Funct Imaging* 2008;28:384–390.

32. Brooks VL, Dampney RA, Heesch CM. Pregnancy and the endocrine regulation of the baroreceptor reflex. *Am J Physiol Regul Integr Comp Physiol* 2010;299:R439–R451.

33. Ekholm EM, Piha SJ, Antila KJ, et al. Cardiovascular autonomic reflexes in mid-pregnancy. *Br J Obstet Gynaecol* 1993;100:177–182.

34. Kuo CD, Chen GY, Yang MJ, et al. The effect of position on autonomic nervous activity in late pregnancy. *Anaesthesia* 1997;52:1161–1165.

35. Howard B, Goodson J, Mengert W. Supine hypotension syndrome in late pregnancy. *Obstet Gynecol* 1953;1:371–377.

36. Marx G. Aortocaval compression: incidence and prevention. *Bull NY Acad Med* 1974;50:443–446.

37. Kerr M, Scott D, Samuel E. Studies of the inferior vena cava in late pregnancy. *Br Med J* 1964;1:532–533.

38. Bieniarz I, Crottogini J, Curachet E. Aortocaval compression by the uterus in late human pregnancy. *Am J Obstet Gynecol* 1968;100:203–217.

39. Drummond G, Scott S, Lees M, et al. Effects of posture on limb blood flow in late pregnancy. *Br Med J* 1974;2:587–588.

40. Kauppila A, Kokinen M, Puolakka J, et al. Decreased intervillous and unchanged myometrial blood flow in supine recumbency. *Obstet Gynecol* 1980;55:203–205.

41. Huch A, Huch R, Schneider H, et al. Continuous transcutaneous monitoring of fetal oxygen tension during labour. *Br J Obstet Gynaecol* 1977;84(suppl):1–39.

42. Preston R, Crosby E, Kotarba H, et al. Maternal positioning affects fetal heart rate changes after epidural analgesia for labour. *Can J Anaesth* 1993;40:1136–1141.

43. Mills G, Chaffe A. Sleeping position adopted by pregnant women of more than 30 weeks gestation. *Anaesthesia* 1994;49:249–250.

44. Kim Y, Chandra P, Marx G. Successful management of severe aortocaval compression in twin pregnancy. *Obstet Gynecol* 1975;46:362–364.

45. Crawford J. Anesthesia for section: further refinements of a technique. *Br J Obstet Gynecol* 1973;45:726–731.

46. Bassell G, Humayun S, Marx G. Maternal bearing down efforts–another fetal risk? *Obstet Gynecol* 1980;56:39–41.

47. Leontic EA. Respiratory disease in pregnancy. *Med Clin North Am* 1977;61:111–128.

48. Wise RA, Polito AJ, Krishnan V. Respiratory physiologic changes in pregnancy. *Immunol Allergy Clin North Am* 2006;26:1–12.

49. Heller PJ, Scheider EP, Marx GF. Pharyngolaryngeal edema as a presenting symptom in preeclampsia. *Obstet Gynecol* 1983;62:523–525.

50. Kodali BS, Chandrasekhar S, Bulich LN, et al. Airway changes during labor and delivery. *Anesthesiology* 2008;108:357–362.

51. Thomson KJ, Cohen ME. Studies on the circulation in pregnancy. II. Vital capacity observation in normal pregnant women. *Surg Gynaecol Obstet* 1938;66:591–603.

52. Goldsmith LT, Weiss G, Steinetz BG. Relaxin and its role in pregnancy. *Endocrinol Metab Clin North Am* 1995;24:171–186.

53. Alaily AB, Carrol KB. Pulmonary ventilation in pregnancy. *Br J Obstet Gynaecol* 1978;85:518–524.

54. Baldwin GR, Moorthi DS, Whelton JA, et al. New lung functions and pregnancy. *Am J Obstet Gynecol* 1977;127:235–239.

55. Gee JB, Packer BS, Millen JE, et al. Pulmonary mechanics during pregnancy. *J Clin Invest* 1967;46:945–952.

56. Russell IF, Chambers WA. Closing volume in normal pregnancy. *Br J Anaesth* 1981;53:1043–1047.

57. Prowse CM, Gaensler EA. Respiratory and acid-base changes during pregnancy. *Anesthesiology* 1965;26:381–392.

58. Pernoll ML, Metcalfe J, Kovach PA, et al. Ventilation during rest and exercise in pregnancy and postpartum. *Respir Physiol* 1975;25:295–310.

59. Clapp JF 3rd, Seaward BL, Sleamaker RH, et al. Maternal physiologic adaptations to early human pregnancy. *Am J Obstet Gynecol* 1988;159:1456–1460.

60. Machida H. Influence of progesterone on arterial blood and CSF acid-base balance in women. *J Appl Physiol* 1981;51:1433–1436.

61. Norregaard O, Schultz P, Ostergaard A, et al. Lung function and postural changes during pregnancy. *Respir Med* 1989;83:467–470.

62. Zwillich CW, Natalino MR, Sutton FD, et al. Effects of progesterone on chemosensitivity in normal men. *J Lab Clin Med* 1978;92:262–269.

63. Lyons HA, Antonio R. The sensitivity of the respiratory center in pregnancy and after the administration of progesterone. *Trans Assoc Am Physio* 1959;72:173–180.

64. Jensen D, Duffin J, Lam YM, et al. Physiological mechanisms of hyperventilation during human pregnancy. *Respir Physiol Neurobiol* 2008;161:76–86.

65. Lim VS, Katz AI, Lindheimer MD. Acid-base regulation in pregnancy. *Am J Physiol* 1976;231:1764–1769.

66. Jensen D, Webb KA, Davies GA, et al. Mechanical ventilatory constraints during incremental cycle exercise in human pregnancy: implications for respiratory sensation. *J Physiol* 2008;586:4735–4750.

67. Artal R, Wiswell R, Romem Y, et al. Pulmonary responses to exercise in pregnancy. *Am J Obstet Gynecol* 1986;154:378–383.

68. Templeton A, Kelman GR. Maternal blood-gases, PAo2–Pao2), hysiological shunt and VD/VT in normal pregnancy. *Br J Anaesth* 1976;48:1001–1004.

69. McClelland SH, Bogod DG, Hardman JG. Apnoea in pregnancy: an investigation using physiological modelling. *Anaesthesia* 2008;63:264–269.

70. Izci B, Vennelle M, Liston WA, et al. Sleep-disordered breathing and upper airway size in pregnancy and post-partum. *Eur Respir J* 2006;27:321–327.

71. Santiago JR, Nolledo MS, Kinzler W, et al. Sleep and sleep disorders in pregnancy. *Ann Intern Med* 2001;134:396–408.

72. American Academy of Sleep Medicine: International classification of sleep disorders. 2nd ed. Westchester, IL: American Academy of Sleep Medicine; 2005.

73. Gross JB, Bachenberg KL, Benumof JL, et al. Practice guidelines for the perioperative management of patients with obstructive sleep apnea: a report by the American Society of Anesthesiologists Task Force on Perioperative Management of patients with obstructive sleep apnea. *Anesthesiology* 2006;104:1081–1093.

74. Hagerdal M, Morgan CW, Sumner AE, et al. Minute ventilation and oxygen consumption during labor with epidural analgesia. *Anesthesiology* 1983;59:425–427.

75. Spatling L, Fallenstein F, Huch A, et al. The variability of cardiopulmonary adaptation to pregnancy at rest and during exercise. *Br J Obstet Gynaecol* 1992;99(Suppl 8):1–40.

76. Pearson JF, Davies P. The effect of continuous lumbar epidural analgesia on the acid-base status of maternal arterial blood during the first stage of labour. *J Obstet Gynaecol Br Commonw* 1973;80:218–224.

77. Jouppila R, Hollmen A. The effect of segmental epidural analgesia on maternal and foetal acid-base balance, lactate, serum potassium and creatine phosphokinase during labour. *Acta Anaesthesiol Scand* 1976;20:259–268.

78. Thalme B, Raabe N, Belfrage P. Lumbar epidural analgesia in labour. II. Effects on glucose, lactate, sodium, chloride, total protein, haematocrit and haemoglobin in maternal, fetal and neonatal blood. *Acta Obstet Gynecol Scand* 1974;53:113–119.

79. Pearson JF, Davies P. The effect on continuous lumbar epidural analgesia on maternal acid-base balance and arterial lactate concentration during the second stage of labour. *J Obstet Gynaecol Br Commonw* 1973;80:225–229.

80. Kambam J, Handte R, Brown W, et al. Effect of normal and preeclamptic pregnancies on the oxyhemoglobin dissociation curve. *Anesthesiology* 1986;65:426–427.

81. Coryell M, Beach E, Robinson A, et al. Metabolism of women during the reproductive cycle. XVII. Changes in electrophoretic patterns of plasma proteins throughout the cycle and following delivery. *J Clin Invest* 1950;29:1559–1567.

82. Mendenhall H. Serum protein concentrations in pregnancy. I. Concentrations in maternal serum. *Am J Obstet Gynecol* 1970;106:388–399.

83. Oian P, Maltau J, Noddeland H, et al. Oedema-preventing mechanisms in subcutaneous tissue of normal pregnant women. *Br J Obstet Gynaecol* 1985;92:1113–1119.

84. Abbassi-Ghanavati M, Greer L, Cunningham F. Pregnancy and laboratory studies: a reference table for clinicians. *Obstet Gynecol* 2009;114:1326–1331.

85. Franchini M. Haemostasis and pregnancy. *Thromb Haemost* 2006;95:401–413.

86. Toglia M, Weg J. Venous thromboembolism during pregnancy. *N Engl J Med* 1996;335:108–114.

87. Thorton C, Bonnar J. Factor VIII-related antigen and factor VIII coagulant activity in normal and preeclamptic pregnancy. *Br J Obstet Gynaecol* 1977;84(12):919–923.

88. Cadroy Y, Grandejean H, Pichon J, et al. Evaluation of six markers of haemostatic system in normal pregnancy and pregnancy complicated by hypertension or preeclampsia. *Br J Obstet Gynaecol* 1993;100:416–420.

89. Talbert L, Langdell R. Normal values of certain factors in the blood clotting mechanism in pregnancy. *Am J Obstet Gynecol* 1964;90:44–50.

90. Douglas J, Shah M, Lowe G, et al. Plasma fibrinopeptide A and b-thromboglobulin in preeclampsia and pregnancy hypertension. *Thromb Haemost* 1982;47:54–55.

91. Wallenburg HC, van Kessel PH. Platelet lifespan in normal pregnancy as determined by a nonradioisotopic technique. *Br J Obstet Gynaecol* 1978;85:33–36.

92. Fay R, Hughes A, Farron N. Platelets in pregnancy: hyperdestruction in pregnancy. *Obstet Gynecol* 1983;61:238–240.

93. Pitkin R, Witte D. Platelet and leukocyte counts in pregnancy. *JAMA* 1979;242:2696–2698.

94. Krause P, Ingardia C, Pontius L, et al. Host defense during pregnancy: neutrophil chemotaxis and adherence. *Am J Obstet Gynecol* 1987;157:743–751.

95. Taylor R. Immunobiology of human pregnancy. *Curr Probl Obstet Gynecol Fertil* 1998;21:743–751.

96. Baboonian C, Griffiths P. Is pregnancy immunosuppressive? Humoral immunity against viruses. *Br J Obstet Gynaecol* 1983;90:1168–1175.

97. Chan MT, Mainland P, Gin T. Minimum alveolar concentration of halothane and enflurane are decreased in early pregnancy. *Anesthesiology* 1996;85:782–786.

98. Abboud TK, Sarkis F, Hung TT, et al. Effects of epidural anesthesia during labor on maternal plasma beta-endorphin levels. *Anesthesiology* 1983;59:1–5.

99. Datta S, Hurley RJ, Naulty JS, et al. Plasma and cerebrospinal fluid progesterone concentrations in pregnant and nonpregnant women. *Anesth Analg* 1986;65:950–954.

100. Merryman W, Boiman R, Barnes L, et al. Progesterone anesthesia in human subjects. *J Clin Endocrinol Metab* 1954;14:1567–1569.

101. Chan MT, Gin T. Postpartum changes in the minimum alveolar concentration of isoflurane. *Anesthesiology* 1995;82:1360–1363.

102. Christensen JH, Andreasen F, Jansen JA. Pharmacokinetics of thiopental in caesarian section. *Acta Anaesthesiol Scand* 1981;25:174–179.

103. Kerr MG. The mechanical effects of the gravid uterus in late pregnancy. *J Obstet Gynaecol Br Commonw* 1965;72:513–529.

104. Igarashi T, Hirabayashi Y, Shimizu R, et al. The fiberscopic findings of the epidural space in pregnant women. *Anesthesiology* 2000;92:1631–1636.

105. Flanagan HL, Datta S, Lambert DH, et al. Effect of pregnancy on bupivacaine-induced conduction blockade in the isolated rabbit vagus nerve. *Anesth Analg* 1987;66:123–126.

106. Bader AM, Datta S, Moller RA, et al. Acute progesterone treatment has no effect on bupivacaine-induced conduction blockade in the isolated rabbit vagus nerve. *Anesth Analg* 1990;71:545–548.

107. Butterworth JFt, Walker FO, Lysak SZ. Pregnancy increases median nerve susceptibility to lidocaine. *Anesthesiology* 1990;72:962–965.

108. Abouleish EI. Postpartum tubal ligation requires more bupivacaine for spinal anesthesia than does cesarean section. *Anesth Analg* 1986;65:897–900.

109. Ohel I, Walfisch A, Shitenberg D, et al. A rise in pain threshold during labor: a prospective clinical trial. *Pain* 2007;132(Suppl 1):S104–S108.

110. Gintzler AR. Endorphin-mediated increases in pain threshold during pregnancy. *Science* 1980;210:193–195.

111. Vanner RG. Mechanisms of regurgitation and its prevention with cricoid pressure. *Int J Obstet Anesth* 1993;2:207–215.

112. Wong CA, McCarthy RJ, Fitzgerald PC, et al. Gastric emptying of water in obese pregnant women at term. *Anesth Analg* 2007;105:751–755.

113. Carp H, Jayaram A, Stoll M. Ultrasound examination of the stomach contents of parturients. *Anesth Analg* 1992;74:683–687.

114. Porter JS, Bonello E, Reynolds F. The influence of epidural administration of fentanyl infusion on gastric emptying in labour. *Anaesthesia* 1997;52:1151–1156.

115. Kelly MC, Carabine UA, Hill DA, et al. A comparison of the effect of intrathecal and extradural fentanyl on gastric emptying in laboring women. *Anesth Analg* 1997;85:834–838.

116. Practice guidelines for obstetric anesthesia: an updated report by the American Society of Anesthesiologists Task Force on Obstetric Anesthesia. *Anesthesiology* 2007;106:843–863.

117. Gin T, Cho AM, Lew JK, et al. Gastric emptying in the postpartum period. *Anaesth Intensive Care* 1991;19:521–524.

118. Richter JE. Review article: the management of heartburn in pregnancy. *Aliment Pharmacol Ther* 2005;22:749–757.

119. Attia RR, Ebeid AM, Fischer JE, et al. Maternal fetal and placental gastrin concentrations. *Anaesthesia* 1982;37:18–21.

120. Murray FA, Erskine JP, Fielding J. Gastric secretion in pregnancy. *J Obstet Gynaecol Br Emp* 1957;64:373–381.

121. Cohen SE, Jasson J, Talafre ML, et al. Does metoclopramide decrease the volume of gastric contents in patients undergoing cesarean section? *Anesthesiology* 1984;61:604–607.

122. Wyner J, Cohen SE. Gastric volume in early pregnancy: effect of metoclopramide. *Anesthesiology* 1982;57:209–212.

123. Shah S, Nathan L, Singh R, et al. E2 and not P4 increases NO release from NANC nerves of the gastrointestinal tract: implications in pregnancy. *Am J Physiol Regul Integr Comp Physiol* 2001;280:R1546–1554.

124. Angel Garcia AL. Effect of pregnancy on pre-existing liver disease physiological changes during pregnancy. *Ann Hepatol* 2006;5:184–186.

125. Romalis G, Claman AD. Serum enzymes in pregnancy. *Am J Obstet Gynecol* 1962;84:1104–1110.

126. Carter J. Liver function in normal pregnancy. *Aust N Z J Obstet Gynaecol* 1990;30:296–302.

127. Ryan JP, Pellecchia D. Effect of progesterone pretreatment on guinea pig gallbladder motility in vitro. *Gastroenterology* 1982;83:81–83.

128. Mendez-Sanchez N, Chavez-Tapia NC, Uribe M. Pregnancy and gallbladder disease. *Ann Hepatol* 2006;5:227–230.

129. Jeyabalan A, Lain K. Anatomic and functional changes of the upper urinary tract during pregnancy. *Urol Clin N Am* 2007;34:1–6.

130. Jeyabalan A, Conrad K. Renal function during normal pregnancy and preeclampsia. *Front Biosci* 2007;12:2425–2437.

131. Isfahani MR, Haghighat M. Measurable changes in hydronephrosis during pregnancy induced by positional changes: ultrasonic assessment and its diagnostic implication. *Urol J* 2005;2:97–101.

132. Sims E, Krantz K. Serial studies of renal function during pregnancy and the puerperium in normal women. *J Clin Invest* 1958;37:1764–1774.

133. Airoldi J, Weinstein L. Clinical significance of proteinuria in pregnancy. *Obstet Gynecol Surv* 2007;62:117–124.

134. Higby K, Suiter C, Phelps J, et al. Normal values of urinary albumin and total protein excretion during pregnancy. *Am J Obstet Gynecol* 1994;171:984–989.

135. Dunlop W, Davison J. The effect of normal pregnancy upon the renal handling of uric acid. *Br J Obstet Gynaecol* 1977;84:13–21.

136. Davison J, Hytten F. The effect of pregnancy on the renal handling of glucose. *Br J Obstet Gynaecol* 1975;82:374–381.

137. Abalovich M, Amino N, Barbour L, et al. Management of thyroid dysfunction during pregnancy and postpartum: An Endocrine Society Clinical Practice Guideline. *J Clin Endocrinol Metab* 2007;92:S1–S47.

138. Casey BM, Dashe JS, Wells CE, et al. Subclinical hyperthyroidism and pregnancy outcomes. *Obstet Gynecol* 2006;107:337–341.

139. Soldin OP, Tractenberg RE, Hollowell JG, et al. Trimester-specific changes in maternal thyroid hormone, thyrotropin, and thyroglobulin concentrations during gestation: trends and associations across trimesters in iodine sufficiency. *Thyroid* 2004;14:1084–1090.

140. Marwaha RK, Chopra S, Gopalakrishnan S, et al. Establishment of reference range for thyroid hormones in normal pregnant Indian women. *BJOG* 2008;115:602–606.

141. Fisher PM, Sutherland HW, Bewsher PD. The insulin response to glucose infusion in normal human pregnancy. *Diabetologia* 1980;19:15–20.

142. Scheithauer BW, Sano T, Kovacs KT, et al. The pituitary gland in pregnancy: a clinicopathologic and immunohistochemical study of 69 cases. *Mayo Clin Proc* 1990;65:461–474.

143. Grattan DR, Steyn FJ, Kokay IC, et al. Pregnancy-induced adaptation in the neuroendocrine control of prolactin secretion. *J Neuroendocrinol* 2008;20:497–507.

144. Pacheco LD, Ghulmiyyah LM, Snodgrass WR, et al. Pharmacokinetics of corticosteroids during pregnancy. *Am J Perinatol* 2007;24:79–82.

145. Quaresma C, Silva C, Secca M, et al. Back pain during pregnancy: a longitudinal study. 2010;35:346–351.

146. Becker L, Woodley S, Stringer M. The adult human pubic symphysis: a systematic review. *J Anat* 2010;217:475–487.

Uteroplacental Circulation and Respiratory Gas Exchange

Mark I. Zakowski • Sivam Ramanathan

The placenta is a union of maternal and fetal tissues for purposes of physiologic exchange of nutrients, respiration and metabolic waste. Since many stillbirths and depressed fetuses are the result of intrauterine asphyxia, the factors governing the adequacy of placental function, particularly respiratory gas exchange, assume great importance.

■ PLACENTAL ANATOMY AND CIRCULATION

The human placenta is a dynamic organ with vast changes from initial implantation in the uterine wall until birth. The human embryo initially implants into the uterus at the blastocyst stage. The human placenta grows initially in a low-oxygen environment, with PO_2 <20 mm Hg, following the historical development of species from the pre-oxygen atmosphere epoch. Prior to 10 weeks gestation, the uterine spiral arteries are blocked by extravillous trophoblasts, with an absence of blood flow on Doppler and in vivo oxygen tension <20 mm Hg (1). The placenta and burgeoning fetus are supplied by secretions from the endometrial glands, and perhaps should be described as deciduochorial during this time period (2). The low-oxygen milieu stimulates placental angiogenesis via hypoxia inducible factor-1α and its effect on vascular endothelial growth factor and placental growth factor protects against damage and congenital abnormalities during organogenesis by reactive oxygen species (ROS). ROS are highly reactive oxygen-based molecules with an unpaired valence shell electron that damage DNA, lipids, proteins, and enzymes. The endometrial endovascular trophoblastic plugs are normally lost at 10 to 12 weeks gestation with maternal blood flow occurring peripherally, and then centrally on the placenta. The remodeling results in high volume, low-resistance maternal blood flow within the intervillous space. Improper remodeling at this secondary invasion stage is a precursor of preeclampsia. Intervillous oxygen tension rises to 40 to 80 mm Hg, with higher oxygen tension in the central part of the placental lobule and lower at the periphery of the placenta (Fig. 2-1). The placenta adapts to changes in maternal blood flow and increased oxygen tension. The placenta increases the antioxidant enzymes catalase, glutathione peroxidase, and superoxide dismutase within the placenta to deal with the increase of ROS and oxidative stress of the increased blood flow and increased PO_2. Insufficient trophoblast invasion and lack of proper vascular remodeling in early pregnancy produces premature blood flow and increased

oxygenation in the intervillous space, which actually reduces maternal blood flow later in pregnancy (3).

The human placenta is classically described as a villous haemomonochorial type with only one layer of syncytiotrophoblast intervening between maternal and fetal circulation. The villi are projections of fetal tissue surrounded by chorion that are exposed to circulating maternal blood. The chorion is the outermost fetal tissue layer. At term, the human placenta weighs about 500 g and is disc shaped, with a diameter of approximately 20 cm and a thickness of 3 cm. The normal fetal-to-placental-weight ratio is approximately 6:1 at term. Before this, the placenta is relatively heavier and the ratio is less (e.g., 3:1 at 30 weeks of gestation).

Circulation of blood through the placenta is illustrated in Figure 2-2. The maternal blood is carried by the uterine arteries, which divide into spiral arteries in the basal plate. Blood is spurted from these arteries into the intervillous space. It traverses upward toward the chorionic plate, passing fetal villi where exchange takes place, and finally drains back to veins in the basal plate.

The fetal circulation within the placenta is quite different. Blood is carried into the placenta by two umbilical arteries that successively divide into smaller vessels within the fetal villi. Ultimately, capillaries traverse the tips of the fetal villi where exchange occurs with maternal blood within the intervillous space. The maternal–fetal blood flow pattern and vascular geometry consist more like a cross-current exchanger than the more efficient counter-current exchange mechanism. The blood is finally collected into a single umbilical vein in the umbilical cord, and this carries the oxygen, nutrient-rich and waste-poor blood to the fetus.

Fetal and maternal blood streams are separated by three microscopic tissue layers in the human placenta. The first layer is the fetal trophoblast, which consists of cytotrophoblast and syncytiotrophoblast. The syncytiotrophoblast is the metabolically active part of the placenta, where much of the endocrine function of the placenta occurs. The other tissue layers are fetal connective tissue, which serves to support the villi, and the endothelium of fetal capillaries (Fig. 2-3). As the placenta and fetus grow, the diffusion distance decreases as the rate of fetal capillary growth in the villi exceeds the trophoblast growth; thus placental oxygen diffusive conductance is matched to fetal weight (demand), which is also true for other species (4). At term, the ratio of cytotrophoblast to syncytiotrophoblast is significantly lower than earlier in pregnancy.

The quantitative relationship of fetal and maternal blood flow and relative concentrations of substances at any one point in the human placenta are quite complex. The relative rates of blood flow in various areas of the placenta are also quite variable, and there is a continually changing concentration of nutrients and waste materials in various areas of the placenta as exchange occurs (5).

Revised from the fourth edition, written by Julian T. Parer, Mark A. Rosen, and Gershon Levinson.

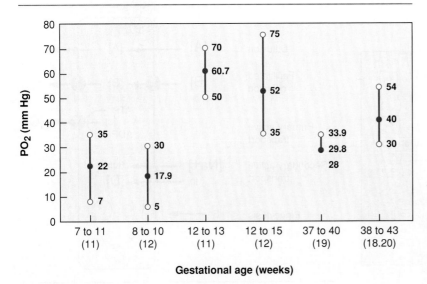

FIGURE 2-1 Intervillous partial pressure oxygen increases during pregnancy. Modified from: Tuuli MG, Longtine MS, Nelson DM. Oxygen and trophoblast biology—A source of controversy. *Placenta* 2011;32 (suppl 2):109–118.

■ MECHANISMS OF EXCHANGE

Substances are exchanged across the placental membrane by five mechanisms (Fig. 2-4): Diffusion (passive and facilitated), active transport, bulk flow, pinocytosis/phagocytosis, and barrier breaks (6). The placenta is a dynamic organ throughout pregnancy and these mechanisms of transfer vary at different stages of gestation. Placental stress states such as acidosis may cause placental cell damage, increasing placental permeability of substances (e.g., local anesthetics) (7).

Diffusion

Passive diffusion, a physicochemical process that requires no energy, occurs when substances pass from one area to another along a concentration gradient. The respiratory gases, oxygen and carbon dioxide, the fatty acids, and the smaller ions (e.g., Na^+ and Cl^-) are transported by this mechanism (6).

Facilitated diffusion describes the mechanism of passage of glucose and some other carbohydrates. With this mechanism, substances still pass down a concentration gradient, but the rate of passage is greater than can be explained by

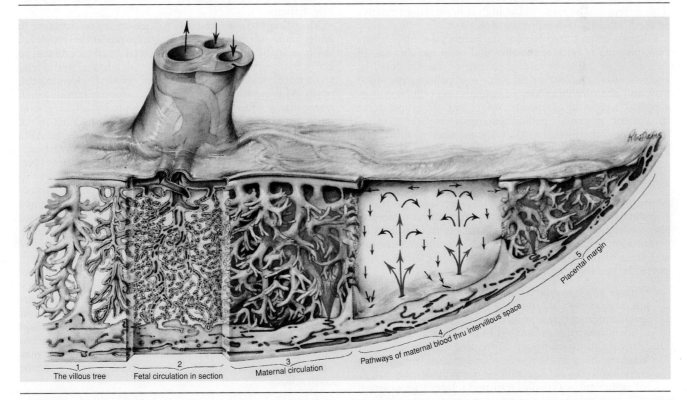

FIGURE 2-2 Composite drawing of the placenta showing its structure and circulation. *1*, villous tree; *2*, cross-section of the fetal circulation; *3* and *4*, hemodynamics of maternal circulation according to the concepts of Ramsey et al. From: Ramsey EM, and the Carnegie Institution of Washington. In: Greenhill JP. *Obstetrics*. 13th ed. Philadelphia, PA: WB Saunders Co; 1965.

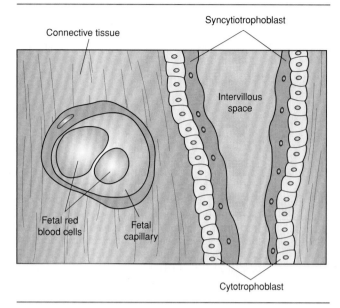

FIGURE 2-3 Drawing from an electron micrograph of cross-section through parts of two fetal villi, showing tissue layers that separate fetal and maternal blood in the human placenta. The cytotrophoblastic layer is much less distinct in the third trimester than is depicted here. Reprinted by courtesy of Berkeley Bio-Engineering, Inc., Berkeley, CA.

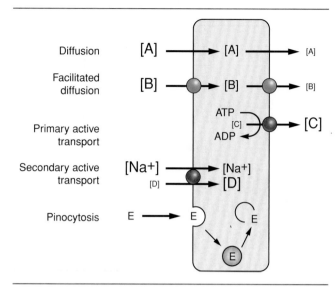

FIGURE 2-4 Modes of transport of molecules across the placenta.

the gradient alone. Possibly, carrier molecules are involved, and there may be need for energy expenditure. Facilitated diffusion does not use chemical energy in the form of ATP, but uses the gradient of another compound and a transporter. The system can be saturated at high concentrations relative to the Michaelis–Menten constant (Km).

Glucose crosses the placenta via facilitated-diffusion carriers inserted in both microvillus and basal membranes. In this mode of transport, the movement of glucose down its concentration gradient to the fetus is dependent on blood flow and plasma concentrations, and also on cellular energy supply. Changes in glucose transport and utilization occur in several placental pathophysiologies including intra-uterine growth restriction (IUGR), diabetes mellitus, and preeclampsia.

Active Transport

Active transport moves substances in a direction against the concentration gradient. Energy is required; carrier molecules are involved; and active transport is subject to inhibition by certain metabolites. The amino acids, water-soluble vitamins, and some of the larger ions (e.g., Ca^{++} and Fe^{++}) are transported by this mechanism.

    a. *Primary active transport*: Movement of a substance takes place against its concentration gradient (i.e., uphill) via a specific protein carrier, which uses the energy in the form of adenosine triphosphate (ATP) to drive transport.

    b. *Secondary active transport*: Movement of one transport substrate down its electrochemical gradient (e.g., sodium entry into cells) via a protein carrier provides the energy for movement of a coupled transport substrate via a carrier.

Amino acids are transported by a series of transporters with multiple substrate specificities. They can be divided into two types, those co-transported with sodium (secondary active transport) and those independent of sodium. Amino acids are

transported "uphill" against a concentration gradient from the maternal circulation into the fetal circulation.

Alterations in amino acid transport have been postulated in a number of placental pathophysiologies. Animal and human studies have shown clear deficits in certain classes of amino acids in IUGR. Studies on placental amino acid transporters from term and preterm human tissues have shown a greater than 5-fold increase in transport capacity between 10 and 40 weeks of gestation and decreases in amino acid transport capacity in both IUGR and macrosomic diabetes.

Most drugs that are transported are similar in structure to endogenous substrates. Active drug transporters are located in the maternal-brush border and the fetal-basal membrane; so active transporters exist in both maternal to fetal as well as fetal to maternal directions. Transporters include P-glycoprotein, of the ATP-binding cassette (ABC) transporter family, which transports a wide variety of drugs, typically uncharged or basic, between 200 and 1,800 Daltons and transports in the maternal to fetal direction. Other examples include the ABC transporter multidrug resistance protein family, breast cancer resistant protein, monoamine transporters, and novel Na^+ driven organic cation transporter 2.

The importance of efflux drug transporters in protection from fetotoxic effects of chemicals has been confirmed in transporter knockout animals (8) (Fig. 2-5). Transporter proteins are inducible by foreign compounds, natural compounds, and inflammatory diseases. Many cationic drugs like diphenhydramine, clonidine, and ranitidine compete with and inhibit choline uptake in a carrier-mediated fashion (9).

Smoking alters human placenta structure and transporters. Not all drugs transfer as predicted by simple models; buprenorphine, a highly lipophilic narcotic agonist–antagonist, has a low maternal to fetal transfer in vitro. Cocaine and amphetamines may compete with the norepinephrine transporter on placental surface. Elevated levels of maternal norepinephrine may cause uterine artery vasoconstriction and may induce uterine contractions.

Bulk Flow

This describes the passage of substances resulting from a hydrostatic or osmotic gradient. Water is transported by this

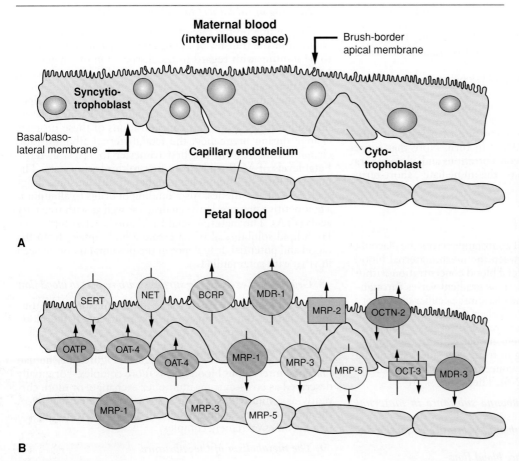

Maternal blood (intervillous space)

Brush-border apical membrane

Syncytio-trophoblast

Basal/baso-lateral membrane

Capillary endothelium

Cyto-trophoblast

Fetal blood

A

B

FIGURE 2-5 Various transporter proteins in the human placenta. **(A)** Placental Tissue layers **(B)** Transporter proteins and Locatioins in human placenta. BRCP, breast cancer resistance protein; MDR, multidrug resistance protein; MRP, multidrug resistance-associated protein; NET, noradrenalin transporter, OAT, organic anion transporter; OATP, organic anion-transporting polypeptide; OCTN, organic cation transporter; SER, serotonin transporter From: Vähäkangas K, Myllynen P. Transporters in human placenta. *Br J Pharmacology* 2009;158: 665–678.

mechanism and may also carry some solutes with it under the influence of this mechanism.

Water diffuses rapidly across the placenta in both directions. Fetal water acquisition (bulk flow) results from the maternal/fetal movement of water in response to an osmotic gradient. An osmotic gradient of less than 1 mOsm is sufficient to drive fetal water acquisition at term. The movement of water is dependent on the solute concentration and thus pumping of NaCl which requires ATP and may therefore be sensitive to conditions that produce reductions in cellular energy supply, such as hypoxia. Water permeabilities or the forces driving water movement may be altered in polyhydramnios, oligohydramnios, nonimmune fetal hydrops, or drinking excessive free water, as has been reported during labor. Transtrophoblastic channels which are usually 150 Angstroms wide, may become dilated when umbilical venous pressure rises and allow bulk pressure movement of water and proteins (e.g., albumin) (10).

Pinocytosis

Some large molecules such as the immune globulins are transported by being enclosed in small vesicles consisting of cell membranes. Phagocytosis and pinocytosis are thought to be relatively slow and not a primary determinant in transfer of drugs (11).

The cellular uptake of proteins (by endocytosis) involves binding of the protein to a specific receptor on the cell surface followed by the pinching off of a plasma membrane vesicle, which moves in the interior of the cell. Acidification of the endocytic vesicles releases the protein and the vesicle recycles to the cell surface. Efflux, or exocytosis, reverses this process. Sequestration of the specific protein into vesicles takes place followed by transfer of the vesicle to the cell surface, fusion with the plasma membrane, and release of the protein.

Iron circulates into an iron-binding protein, transferrin. Iron-bound transferrin binds specifically to transferrin receptors on the syncytiotrophoblast microvillus surface. These receptors are internalized in a plasma membrane (endocytic) vesicle and the iron is then released to the cell, while the iron-free transferrin, still bound to its receptor, is recycled back to the microvillus surface, along with the plasma membrane fragment.

Breaks

The delicate, filmy villi may at times break off within the intervillous space, and the contents may be extruded into the maternal circulation. It is also thought that maternal intravascular contents may be taken up by the fetal circulation at times. The most important result of this is seen when fetal Rh-positive red blood cells are deposited in the vascular system of an Rh-negative mother, resulting in alloimmunization and subsequent erythroblastosis fetalis. Fetal squamous cells have been reported in the maternal circulation without causing any maternal problems. When large amounts of fetal elements enter the maternal circulation, amniotic fluid embolism may occur.

■ DIFFUSION

When limitations of placental transfer occur in the human, they usually are first recognized as limitations of those substances that are exchanged by passive diffusion. For example, an acute decrease in placental function limits exchange of oxygen to and carbon dioxide between the fetus and the mother, resulting in fetal asphyxia. A more chronic decrease in placental function may limit the transfer of substances necessary for growth (e.g., carbohydrates), thus leading to IUGR. Hence, the process of diffusion is examined in some detail.

Fick's equation describes the physicochemical process of passive diffusion:

Rate of transfer (V_{diff}) = (concentration gradient × area × permeability)/membrane thickness

Each of the factors determining rate of passage of substances by diffusion is considered in turn. Note that some factors affect the steady state concentrations and while others have an effect predominantly on the immediate-, short-term transfer rates.

Concentration Gradient

The concentration gradient of a substance across the placenta is equal to the difference between the mean maternal blood concentration and the mean fetal blood concentration within each of the exchanging areas. This gradient varies throughout the placenta because of the placenta's peculiar circulatory anatomy. It probably varies from place to place and also from time to time in any particular area. However, by considering a simplified 2-compartment model with an exchanging membrane and blood flowing in from each side, each of the factors that would affect the concentration gradient can be conceptually discussed (Fig. 2-6). These factors are

1. *Concentration of free, unbound substance in maternal arterial blood*
2. *Concentration of free, unbound substance in fetal arterial blood*
3. *Maternal intervillous space blood flow*
4. *Fetal–placental blood flow*

Note that pathologic conditions such as elevated umbilical venous pressure has been associated with reduced drug transfer.

5. *Diffusing capacity of the placenta for the substance*
6. *Ratio of maternal to fetal blood flow in exchanging areas*

This is analogous to ventilation-to-perfusion ratios as applied to the lung. Inequalities in the ratio give rise to decreased efficiency of transfer. Exchange of substances is optimal if the flows are evenly matched. The blood flow will affect the transfer of some substances. A freely diffusible substance is considered flow limited; the transfer is limited by the blood flow (e.g., carbon dioxide). A slowly transferred substance is not affected by changes in blood flow; the transfer is diffusion limited.

7. *Binding of substances to molecules and dissociation rates*

Depending on the rate of dissociation, this reaction time could limit the transfer of a substance. This does not appear to be limiting with regard to the dissociation of oxygen and hemoglobin. The ultimate ratio in fetal versus maternal circulation can be greatly influenced by the protein binding of the substance. Generally, albumin binds acidic, lipophilic drugs while α_1-acid glycoprotein (AGP) binds basic, lipophilic drugs. Note that concentrations of these proteins change during pregnancy; the fetal:maternal albumin ratio changes from 30% in the first trimester to 120% at term. Fetal levels of AGP triple from first to third trimesters. The maternal form of albumin has a higher affinity for some drugs such as local anesthetics. Also, binding of drugs to albumin is a competitive process, between drugs as well as with free fatty acids (FFA). The maternal:fetal FFA ratio is 3:1 at term (11). High lipid solubility also can create a high uptake from the blood and potential drug depot in the placental tissue, as seen in vitro with sufentanil (12).

8. *Geometry of exchanging surfaces with respect to blood flow*

If the blood flows are traveling in the same direction during exchange, the system is called concurrent. If the blood flows are traveling in opposite directions, the system is called counter-current. This latter system is the most efficient from the exchange point of view. As seen in Figure 2-2, human placental intervillous blood flow is more complex—originally described as cross-current multiplier exchange, or more currently as a multivillus stream system (5). The evaluation of the mean concentration gradient of any nutrient in this system becomes extremely complex.

9. *The metabolism of the substance*

If a substance is consumed within the placenta, its rate of passage across the placenta will not be reflected by the concentration gradient. For example, oxygen is consumed in considerable quantities by the trophoblast and the rate of passage appears to be relatively inefficient when based on oxygen tension gradients alone. Although the human placenta contains enzymes related to drug oxidation, reduction, hydrolysis and conjugation, they are primarily geared to steroid metabolism; the fetal liver is more active in drug breakdown.

Area of the Placenta

The villous surface area of the human term placenta increases from 3.4 m^2 at 28 weeks (11) to over 11 m^2 at term (13). In comparison, the lung has an alveolar surface area of 70 m^2. The area of actual exchange, the vasculosyncytial membrane – that is, the area where fetal capillaries approach closely

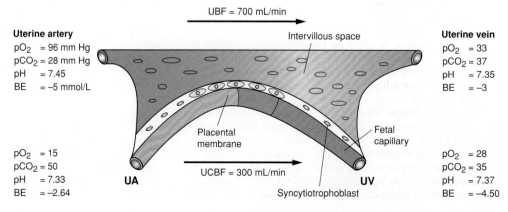

FIGURE 2-6 Uteroplacental gas exchange. Data for healthy women, breathing room air at time of cesarean section. Crosscurrent Multiplier Geometry, Flow, and Values. UA, umbilical artery; UV, umbilical vein; UCBF, umbilical cord blood flow.

UBF = 700 mL/min

Uterine artery
pO$_2$ = 96 mm Hg
pCO$_2$ = 28 mm Hg
pH = 7.45
BE = −5 mmol/L

Intervillous space

Uterine vein
pO$_2$ = 33
pCO$_2$ = 37
pH = 7.35
BE = −3

Placental membrane

Fetal capillary

pO$_2$ = 15
pCO$_2$ = 50
pH = 7.33
BE = −2.64

UA

UCBF = 300 mL/min

UV

Syncytiotrophoblast

pO$_2$ = 28
pCO$_2$ = 35
pH = 7.37
BE = −4.50

enough to the surface to exchange materials with maternal blood—is 1.8 m^2.

Placental area is decreased in a number of clinical situations. An acute decrease occurs with abruptio placentae. A minor separation of the placenta may not always lead to intrauterine fetal demise as a result of asphyxia. The ability of the fetus to survive depends on the placental reserve that existed before the onset of abruption. Some placentas, particularly those in cases of maternal hypertension or those that have infarcted fibrotic areas, have a reduced area available for exchange and, hence, lowered reserve. Thus, the placenta of a mother with long-term hypertension is likely to be smaller than expected, resulting in IUGR. The placental infarctions are thought to be caused by maternal arteriolar deficiencies leading to necrosis and fibrosis of certain villi and even entire cotyledons. Analogous to hypoxic pulmonary vasoconstriction in areas of lung V/Q mismatch, villous fibrosis may improve exchange by fibrosis of nonperfused areas. In addition, in certain cases of intrauterine infection or congenital defects, the placentas are decreased in size and area. Large placentas are found in erythroblastosis fetalis and in some diabetics. In the former case, most of the increased placental mass is thought to be hydropic in origin and, hence, is unlikely to improve the exchange characteristics of the placenta. In the latter case, it is not certain whether the increased area improves the transfer of nutrients to the fetus.

Permeability of the Placental Membrane

The permeability of a membrane to a substance depends on characteristics of both the membrane and the substance that is being exchanged. The units for permeability can be found by a transposition of Fick's diffusion equation. There are three major determinants of permeability:

1. *Molecular size.* The term placental barrier is a relative misnomer because many substances pass through the placenta to reach the fetus. A molecular weight of 1,000 is a rough dividing line between those substances that cross the placenta by diffusion and those that are relatively impermeable by diffusion. Below a molecular weight of 1,000, the rate of passage of the molecule is related to its weight unless other properties (see below) prevent or hasten rate of passage. A common clinical example is found in cases in which it is necessary to use anticoagulants in a pregnant woman. If one uses heparin, with a molecular weight above 6,000, one does not concomitantly heparinize the fetus. However, warfarin (Coumadin), with a molecular weight of 330, will readily pass through the placenta and raise the fetal INR leading to intrapartum bleeding. Also, warfarin is a well-known teratogen in the first trimester.
2. *Lipid solubility.* A lipid-soluble substance traverses the lipid bilayers of cell membranes, including those in the placenta more rapidly than a substance that has limited lipid solubility. Most local anesthetic are weak bases with a pK$_a$ greater than 7.4. Thus, local anesthetics generally cross into nerves and the placenta in the more lipophilic, unionized form, but then equilibrate with the ionized form in the fetus. Fetal acidosis can increase transfer due to ion trapping of local anesthetics. High lipid solubility also can create a high uptake and potential drug deposition in placental tissue, as seen with sufentanil (12).
3. *Electrical charge.* This deters the passage of a substance across the placenta. For example, succinylcholine, commonly used for rapid sequence intubation, is highly ionized and is poorly diffusible across the placenta despite its molecular weight of 361. Thiopental, with a molecular weight of 264, is lipid soluble, relatively unionized, and moves very rapidly into the fetal circulation.

Substances are classified into those in which the rate of passage is either "permeability limited" or "flow limited" (14). A substance that has poor permeability is limited in its rate of passage across the placenta by permeability and not by rates of blood flow. Hence, increasing the rate of blood flow will not improve its rate of passage by much. The majority of biologic molecules are limited in their rate of passage across the placenta by resistance of diffusion. However, substances that are highly permeable are limited by the rate of blood flow. Oxygen and carbon dioxide are examples of this. Decreasing the rate of blood flow decreases the rate of exchange considerably.

Diffusion Distance

The average distance for diffusion across the placenta (13) has been measured as approximately 3.5 μm. This contrasts with the much smaller distance from alveolus to pulmonary capillary in the lung (0.5 μm). The diffusion distance decreases as the placenta matures, from 50–100 μm to less than 5 μm, meeting the increasing metabolic demands of the fetus. The distance is increased in several conditions, such as erythroblastosis fetalis and congenital syphilis. This increased distance probably is due to villous edema and presumably decreases the organ's efficiency for exchange. Fibrous or calcified deposits in the placental vasculature, such as the ones found in diabetes mellitus or preeclampsia, presumably increase diffusion distance. Diabetic placentas have fibrin thrombi, villous edema, hyperplasia, and thickening of basement membranes (15). Insulin stimulates fetal aerobic glucose metabolism and thus oxygen demand. However, diabetic pregnancies have reduced oxygen delivery to the fetus due to higher oxygen affinity of glycosylated hemoglobin, thickening of placenta basement membrane, and reduced blood flow. Reduced oxygen stimulates angiogenesis and hypercapillarization of fetal vessels within the placenta lobules. Women with gestational diabetes mellitus (GDM) have 20% to 50% chance of developing type 2 diabetes 5 to 10 years after pregnancy and their offspring have greater incidence of diabetes and obesity (16). Even in well-controlled gestational diabetes, fetuses were significantly more hypoxic, with increased glucose and lactate at birth compared to nondiabetic controls (17).

▪ UTERINE BLOOD FLOW

Since uterine blood flow is one of the prime determinants of passage of a number of critical substances across the placenta, its characteristics, the factors affecting it, and the effects of anesthesia on uterine blood flow are discussed in the latter portion of this chapter.

Uterine blood flow rises progressively throughout pregnancy from 50 mL/min at 10 weeks to approximately 700 mL/min at term (Fig. 2-7). This represents about 10% of the maternal cardiac output. Approximately 70% to 90% of the uterine blood flow passes through the intervillous space, and the remainder largely supplies the myometrium. About 150 mL blood is in the intervillous space at term.

The uterine vascular bed is thought to be almost maximally dilated under normal conditions, with little capacity to dilate further (18). It is not autoregulated, so flow is proportional to the mean perfusion pressure. However, it is capable of marked vasoconstriction by α-adrenergic action. The uterine blood flow is determined by the following relationship:

Uterine blood flow
  = (uterine arterial pressure − uterine venous pressure)/
    uterine vascular resistance

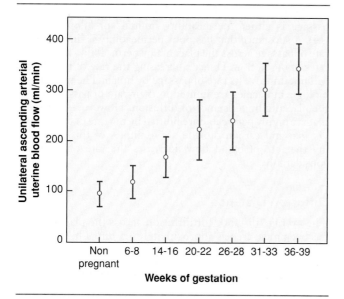

FIGURE 2-7 Changes in uterine blood flow during pregnancy. Assuming equal flow in both uterine arteries, total uterine blood flow as measured by a transvaginal duplex Doppler ultrasound would be about 700 mL/min. Reprinted with permission from: Thaler I, Manor D, Itskovitz J, et al. Changes in uterine blood flow during human pregnancy. *Am J Obstet Gynecol* 1990;162:121–125.

Many factors affect uterine blood flow. A number of causes of decreased uterine blood flow are shown in Table 2-1.

Uterine contractions decrease uterine blood flow as a result of increased uterine venous pressure brought about by increased intramural pressure of the uterus. There may also be a decrease in uterine arterial pressure with contractions. Uterine hypertonus or tachysystole (too frequent contractions) causes a decreased uterine blood flow through the same mechanism.

In sheep, if uterine arterial perfusion pressure is altered without changing the resistance of the uterine vascular bed, there is a direct relationship between uterine blood flow and the pressure (18). Hence, hypotension through any of the mechanisms noted in Table 2-1 will cause a decrease in blood flow.

In the case of maternal arterial hypertension, both chronic and acute, there is a concomitant increased vascular resistance by the uterine vascular bed, decreasing uterine blood flow. Either endogenous or exogenous vasoconstriction results in decreased blood flow because of increased uterine vascular resistance.

There are a few useful means of increasing uterine blood flow when it is known to be suboptimal. The most important clinical considerations are the avoidance or correction of factors responsible for an acute decrease in blood flow (e.g., excessive uterine activity or maternal hypotension). Uterine blood flow can generally be increased by decreasing uterine tone (if increased), by increasing maternal BP (if low), decreasing uterine vascular resistance (if increased), and by using hemodynamic alterations which increase cardiac output (see Table 2-2).

Some of the β-mimetic agents that are used as uterine relaxants for preterm labor may increase uterine blood flow, but this effect, if it occurs, is small and may only be a result of decreased uterine tonus. There are a number of experimen-

TABLE 2-1 Factors Causing Decreased Uterine Blood Flow

Uterine contractions
Hypertonus
  Abruptio placentae
  Tetanic contraction
  Tachysystole (overstimulation with or without oxytocin)
  α-adrenergic agonists including epinephrine IV, norepinephrine

Hypotension
  Sympathetic block
  Hypovolemia
  Supine hypotensive syndrome
  Low cardiac output
    Contractility decreased (e.g., cardiomyopathy of pregnancy)
    Preload decreased (e.g., bleeding, regional anesthesia)
    Afterload increased (e.g., phenylephrine in large amounts, preeclampsia)
    Heart rate decreased (e.g., maternal bradycardia after spinal)

Hypertension
  Essential
  Preeclamptic
  Medication–induced
  Cocaine

Vasoconstriction, endogenous
  Sympathetic discharge
  Adrenal medullary activity

Vasoconstrictors, exogenous
  Most sympathomimetics (α-adrenergic effects)
  Consider: Decreased blood pressure, increased vascular resistance, decreased cardiac output
  Exception is ephedrine (primarily β-adrenergic effect)

tal means of increasing uterine blood flow, sometimes transiently, but these have no real clinical use. Examples of such treatments include estrogens, acetylcholine, nitroglycerin, cyanide, ischemia, and mild hypoxia, the latter either acute or chronic (19). Antihypertensives such as hydralazine can improve uterine blood flow. Similarly, epidural anesthesia during labor will increase uterine blood flow.

Clinically, it has been known for many years that maternal bed rest may improve the outcome in suspected fetal growth restriction. There is some evidence that bed rest does improve fetal growth, as evidenced by increasing estriol excretion (20).

■ UMBILICAL BLOOD FLOW

The umbilical blood flow in the undisturbed fetus at term is about 120 mL/kg/min or 360 mL/min by noninvasive ultrasound techniques (21). Lower values are obtained immediately after birth, but are probably affected by cord manipulation during the birth process. Ultrasound can be used to calculate the peak systolic-to-diastolic (S/D) ratio, which is a reflection of vascular resistance distal to the point of measurement.

TABLE 2-2 Maximization of Uterine Blood Flow

Uterine tone—relax if contracted or tachysystole
  Remove uterotonics—oxytocin, prostaglandin
    cervical ripening
  β-adrenergic agonist (terbutaline 0.25 mg IV/SQ)
  Nitroglycerin (nitric oxide donor, dose 100–400 mcg
    IV/SL)

Hypertension (presumed increased SVR/uterine
  vascular resistance)
  Decrease afterload/SVR—hydralazine 5 mg IV,
    alpha-methyldopa 250 mg IV
  Decrease circulating catecholamines—pain relief,
    anxiety
  HTN with possible increased stroke volume
    Hypervolemia—consider diuresis
    Hyperdynamic—consider beta blockade with
      labetalol
  HTN with increased HR
  β-blockers generally not used during pregnancy/
    delivery—labetalol OK

Hypotension
  Hypovolemia—give fluids, crystalloid or colloid,
    blood as indicated
  Supine hypotensive syndrome—left uterine dis-
    placement, full lateral position
  Inferior vena cava compression—laparoscopic insuf-
    flation >16 mm Hg
  Sympathetic tone decreased (regional anesthesia)—
    fluids, vasopressors (ephedrine, phenylephrine)

Low cardiac output
  Raise HR if low—ephedrine, glycopyrrolate
  Raise SV if low—fluids, increased contractility –
    catecholamine (ephedrine)
  Reduce afterload (SVR) if elevated

Oxygenation
  Supplemental oxygen
  V/Q mismatch—pulmonary embolism, morbid
    obesity supine position
  Pulmonary edema
  Pulmonary disease, e.g., pneumonia

The umbilical blood flow in human is considerably less than that of sheep, where it is approximately 200 mL/kg/min (22). The differences may be explained by the somewhat higher metabolic rate of sheep (body temperature 39°C) and differences in hemoglobin concentrations (sheep, 10 g/dL vs. human, 15 g/dL). It is important to recognize this species difference because the bulk of our information regarding fetal circulatory physiology comes from the chronically instrumented sheep fetus. In sheep, the umbilical blood flow is approximately 45% of the combined ventricular output (22), and about 20% of this blood flow is "shunted," that is, it does not exchange with maternal blood (5).

Umbilical blood flow is unaffected by acute moderate hypoxia but is decreased by severe hypoxia (23). Only the most proximal segment of the umbilical cord is innervated; however, the smooth muscle cells are responsive to paracrine effects and umbilical blood flow decreases with the administration of catecholamines. It is also decreased by acute cord occlusion. There are no known means of increasing umbilical flow in patients in whom it is thought to be decreased chronically. However, certain fetal heart rate patterns (i.e., variable decelerations) have been ascribed to transient umbilical cord compression in the fetus during

labor. Manipulation of maternal position either to the lateral or Trendelenburg position can sometimes abolish these patterns, the implication being that cord compression has been relieved.

Blood Flow Studies in the Human Fetus

Blood Velocity Wave Forms

Real-time directed Doppler ultrasound has been used to investigate human fetal, placental, and uterine blood flows (24). Doppler ultrasound allows for measurement of velocity waveforms of red blood cells traveling in vessels. The velocity data can be used to make inferences about blood flow, vascular resistance, and myocardial contractility. Blood flow velocity waveforms have a characteristic appearance that varies from vessel to vessel. The observed waveform shape is affected by the pumping ability of the heart, the heart rate, the elasticity of the vessel wall, the outflow impedance, and the blood viscosity. Waveforms in arteries supplying low-resistance vascular beds have a characteristically high forward velocity during diastole, whereas absent or reverse diastolic flow is seen in arteries supplying high-resistance vascular beds. These observations prompted the definition of indices of flow that could be related to the vascular resistance of a downstream vascular bed. The most commonly used indices are:

$$\text{Pulsatility index, PI} = (V_{max} - V_{min})/V_{mean}$$
$$\text{Resistive index, RI} = (V_{max} - V_{min})/V_{max}$$
$$\text{Pourcelot ratio, PR} = (V_{max} - V_{min})/V_{max}$$
$$\text{AB (S/D) ratio, AB} = V_{max}/V_{min}$$

where

V_{max} = Point of maximal blood flow velocity/cardiac cycle
V_{min} = Point of minimal blood flow velocity/cardiac cycle
V_{mean} = Mean blood flow velocity/cardiac cycle

Blood Flow

Doppler ultrasound permits the estimation of blood flows in the human fetus. Blood flow is calculated using the formula:

$$Q = (V \times A) \cos \theta$$

where V = Mean velocity as averaged over many cardiac cycles (cm/s)

A = Estimated cross-sectional area of the vessel (cm^2)

θ = Angle between the Doppler beam and the direction of flow of the blood

This calculation is complicated by the variation in the velocity of blood cells across a vascular lumen. Cells flow faster in the center of the vessel and slower near the vessel wall. The overall flow in a vessel is the sum of the different flows across the lumen. For this reason, satisfactory volume flow measurements can best be made on large vessels (4 to 10 mm in diameter) with appropriate Doppler angles (30 to 60 degrees). The two-dimensional echo Doppler provides a means of estimating fetal cardiac output by quantifying blood flow volume at the atrioventricular valve orifices. The estimated cardiac output of the human fetus (553 mL^{-1} kg^{-1} min^{-1}) is higher than that of the sheep (450 mL^{-1} kg^{-1} min^{-1}). In addition, the right and left ventricular outputs are more similar in the human, as compared with the sheep. The ratio of right-to-left ventricular outputs decreases with advancing gestation, from 1.3 at 15 weeks to 1.1 at 40 weeks. In normal pregnancy, high forward velocity levels in the umbilical artery are maintained throughout diastole. A lowered diastolic flow, as seen in severe IUGR, may reflect raised placental resistance (25). Marx et al. used Doppler ultrasound waveform analysis to demonstrate a significant reduction in umbilical artery vascular resistance (S/D ratio) with epidural analgesia in healthy laboring women, a beneficial effect (26). Youngstrom et al. (27) investigated the effect of more extensive epidural anesthesia (and maternal sympathetic blockade) on umbilical artery flow velocity waveforms in healthy, nonlaboring women undergoing elective cesarean section. They found no statistically significant change in umbilical artery resistance (S/D ratio), probably due to the lack of pain and associated release of catecholamines. Recent studies have suggested that changes in PI/RI/ uterine artery notching at 24 weeks' gestation may be predictive of preeclampsia development later in pregnancy (28).

■ OXYGEN TRANSFER TO THE FETUS

Most stillbirths and cases of fetal depression are likely the result of inadequate exchange of the respiratory gases. Oxygen has the lowest storage-to-utilization ratio of any nutrient in the fetus. From animal data, it can be calculated that a term fetus has approximately 42 mL of oxygen with a normal oxygen consumption of approximately 21 mL/min (23). In theory, the fetus has a 2-minute supply of oxygen. However, fetuses do not consume the total quantity of oxygen in their body within 2 minutes, nor do they die after this time. In fact, irreversible brain damage does not start to occur until about 10 minutes have elapsed (29). This is because the fetus has a number of important compensatory mechanisms that enable it to survive on a lesser quantity of oxygen for longer periods. Clinical situations in which there is total cessation of oxygen delivery are rare. These include sudden total abruption of the placenta or complete umbilical cord compression, generally after prolapse of the cord.

Animal experiments show that the compensations that occur in the hypoxic fetus are (a) redistribution of blood flow to vital organs, including heart, brain, and placenta; (b) decreased total oxygen consumption (e.g., with moderate hypoxia, the fetal oxygen consumption drops to 50% of the normal level); and (c) dependence of certain vascular beds on anaerobic metabolism. These compensatory mechanisms appear to be initiated with mild hypoxia and result in the maintenance of oxygen supply to vital organs during times of oxygen limitation (23).

The factors that determine oxygen transfer from mother to fetus are listed in Table 2-3. Since the transfer of oxygen to the fetus depends on rates of blood flow and not limitations to diffusion, the respective blood flow on each side of the placenta assumes major importance for maintenance of fetal oxygenation. Animal studies suggest that in the normal placenta there is a "safety factor" of approximately 50% of the total uterine blood flow. That is, the uterine blood flow will drop to half its normal value before severe fetal acidosis becomes evident (30) and oxygen uptake declines (31). This applies only to the normal situation with normal placental reserve and is unlikely to be the case in pathologic situations, such as in the infant of a hypertensive mother. In such situations, the placental function may be adequate for oxygenation but not for fetal growth, and a growth-restricted infant may result from such a pregnancy. Furthermore, with superimposition of uterine contractions on such a fetus, there may be transient inadequacy of uterine blood flow during the uterine contractions; this may be recognized by responses of the fetal heart rate (i.e., late decelerations).

During labor, uterine contractions reduce uterine blood flow and can lead to episodes of hypoxia–reperfusion stress; increased levels of lipid peroxidation were noted compared

TABLE 2-3 Factors Affecting Oxygen Transfer from Mother to Fetus

Intervillous blood flow
Fetal–placental blood flow
Oxygen tension in maternal arterial blood
Oxygen tension in fetal arterial blood
Oxygen affinity of maternal blood
Oxygen affinity of fetal blood
Hemoglobin concentration or oxygen capacity of maternal blood
Hemoglobin concentration or oxygen capacity of fetal blood
Maternal and fetal blood pH and P_{CO_2} (Bohr effect)
Placental diffusing capacity
Placental vascular geometry
Ratio of maternal to fetal blood flow in exchanging areas
Shunting around exchange sites
Placental oxygen consumption

to elective cesarean section (2). The increased activity of xanthine oxidase, a marker of hypoxia–reperfusion, and decreased vitamin C levels, which typically scavenge ROS, help compensate. Preeclamptic placentas also show these changes (2). Indeed, the oxidative stress that occurs in preeclampsia leads to release of proinflammatory cytokines and angiogenic factors that affect the maternal endothelial cells. Normal placental tissue exposed to hypoxia showed similar metabolites as preeclamptic placental tissue, supporting the role of hypoxia and oxidative stress, as well as possible future diagnostic testing (32).

Additional important determinants of fetal oxygenation include oxygen tension in maternal arterial and fetal arterial blood. In general, maternal arterial oxygen tension depends on adequate ventilation and pulmonary integrity. Disruptions of this function are relatively rare in obstetrics, although they can occur with pulmonary diseases such as asthma, with congestive heart failure, or in mothers with congenital cardiac defects. The oxygen affinity and oxygen capacity of maternal and fetal blood are also important determinants of fetal oxygen transfer. At a given oxygen tension, the quantity of oxygen carried by blood depends on the oxygen capacity, which depends on the hemoglobin concentration and oxygen affinity. The oxygen affinity of fetal hemoglobin (p50 at 18 mm Hg) is greater than that of maternal hemoglobin (p50 at 27 mm Hg) (Fig. 2-8). That is, the oxygen dissociation curve of the fetus is to the left of that of the mother. In addition, the hemoglobin concentration of fetal blood is approximately 15 g/100 mL in the term fetus, whereas that of the mother is approximately 12 g/100 mL. Both of these factors, an increased oxygen affinity and higher oxygen capacity, confer advantages to the fetus for oxygen uptake across the placenta (Fig. 2-9). During acidosis and increased tissue oxygen demand, fetal hemoglobin was more efficient in delivering oxygen to tissues (33).

Both the Bohr and Haldane effects enhance the exchange of oxygen and carbon dioxide across the placenta (Fig. 2-10). The Bohr effect describes the shift of the hemoglobin dissociation curve to the right by hydrogen ions, which reduces the affinity of hemoglobin for oxygen. The Haldane effect

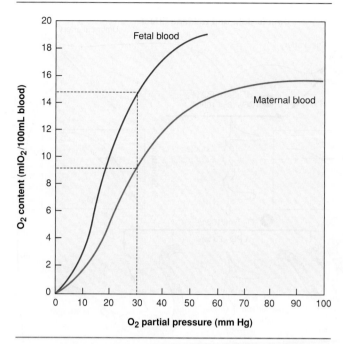

FIGURE 2-8 Oxygen dissociation curves of maternal and fetal blood. *Vertical broken line* illustrates the higher oxygen affinity of fetal blood—fetal blood is more highly saturated with oxygen than is maternal blood at the same oxygen partial pressure. Reprinted with permission from: Parer JT, ed. Uteroplacental physiology and exchange. In: *Handbook of Fetal Heart Rate Monitoring*. Philadelphia, PA: WB Saunders; 1997:40.

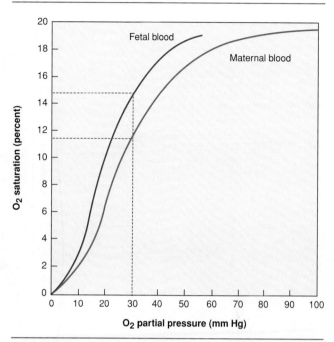

FIGURE 2-9 Oxygen dissociation curves relating oxygen content of blood to oxygen partial pressure in maternal and fetal blood. This relationship illustrates the even greater oxygen content of fetal blood when the greater hemoglobin content of fetal blood is taken into account. Reprinted with permission from: Parer JT. Uteroplacental physiology and exchange. In: *Handbook of Fetal Heart Rate Monitoring*. Philadelphia, PA: WB Saunders; 1997:41.

describes the increased ability of deoxygenated blood to carry more carbon dioxide. The carbon dioxide from the fetal side diffuses into the maternal blood, causing an increase in maternal intervillous hydrogen ion, which reduces the affinity of maternal hemoglobin for oxygen, increasing oxygen transfer to the fetus. At the same time, the relative decrease in carbon dioxide on the fetal side causes the fetal blood to become slightly more alkaline, increasing the fetal hemoglobin uptake of oxygen. Since the Bohr effect occurs on both sides of oxygen delivery/uptake, it has been called the double Bohr effect. Likewise, the double Haldane effect describes maternal and fetal changes in carbon dioxide and oxygen uptake. The fetal hemoglobin becomes oxygenated and releases carbon dioxide, which has increased binding to the maternal hemoglobin that has just deoxygenated. The double Bohr effect occurs functionally by the slight opening and closing of the hemoglobin chain allowing or blocking entry of oxygen to the iron-heme–binding site. Carbon dioxide binding to the sentinel histidine on the hemoglobin chain can block access of oxygen to the heme-binding site (see Fig. 2-10).

Since most measurements have been made in the human fetus during or after labor, the values of oxygen saturation, oxygen tension, and pH are generally decreased compared with those of the mother. In fact, investigations on chronically instrumented animals have shown that the oxygen saturation and content of fetal blood and acid–base status is very close to that of maternal blood; only the Po_2 is lower. Note that the quantity of oxygen delivered or taken up by each 100 mL of circulating blood in the placenta is approximately equal in the mother and fetus. A number of additional miscellaneous factors determine the rate of oxygen transfer across

the placenta; they are listed in Table 2-3 as the last six determinants. They appear to be relatively minor compared with the major factors already outlined.

CARBON DIOXIDE AND ACID–BASE BALANCE

Carbon dioxide crosses the placenta even more readily than does oxygen; the diffusion coefficient is 20 times greater than oxygen. In general, the determinants for oxygen transfer also apply to carbon dioxide transfer across the placenta. It is limited by rate of blood flow and not by resistance to diffusion. The carbon dioxide tension in fetal blood in the undisturbed state is close to 40 mm Hg (5). It is well known that the maternal arterial carbon dioxide tension is approximately 34 mm Hg, and the mother is in a state of compensated respiratory alkalosis (lowered serum bicarbonate by the kidneys). The pH of fetal blood under undisturbed conditions is probably close to 7.4, and the bicarbonate concentration is close to that of maternal blood.

Bicarbonate and the fixed acids cross the placenta much more slowly than does carbon dioxide; that is, equilibration takes a matter of hours rather than seconds. There is a situation analogous to "respiratory acidosis" that occurs in the fetus when blood flow, either uterine or umbilical, is acutely compromised. In such cases, carbon dioxide tension acutely increases causing a drop in pH, but the metabolic acid–base status remains unchanged. This occurs during severe or profound fetal decelerations (called variable decelerations) in association with certain uterine contractions, especially during the second stage of labor. These acid–base changes are generally rapidly resolved with cessation of the contraction and

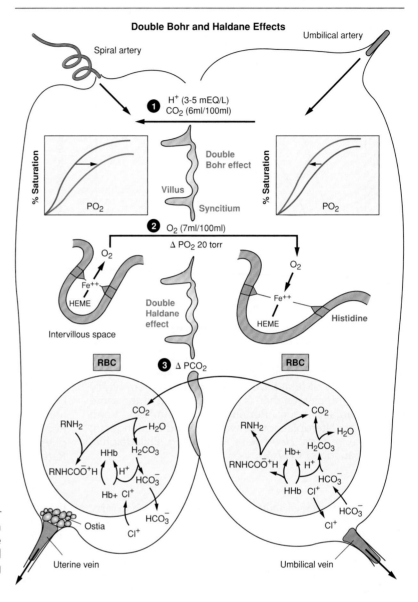

Double Bohr and Haldane Effects

FIGURE 2-10 Bohr and Haldane effect on oxygen and carbon dioxide exchange. Note that carbon dioxide can bind to the amino acid histidine on the hemoglobin chain, restricting access to binding by oxygen.

the bradycardia. However, as noted earlier, if there is a significant oxygen lack that is unrelieved, the fetus will decrease its oxygen consumption, redistribute blood flow, and depend partly on anaerobic metabolism to supply its energy needs, albeit with decreased efficiency. Under these conditions, lactate (an end product of anaerobic metabolism) is produced, resulting in metabolic acidosis. The acidosis may also be aggravated by combined respiratory acidosis because of retained carbon dioxide. Unlike carbon dioxide, lactate is lost slowly from the fetus.

Lactate is transported by specific, pH-dependent carriers, while protons pass to the maternal circulation via channels, lipid diffusion, co-transport, and specific proton-pumping ATPases.

■ CLINICAL IMPLICATIONS

Fetal compromise results from an alteration of normal placental exchange mechanisms. With a knowledge of the components involved in exchange of nutrients and waste materials across the placenta, potential problems can be recognized and corrections made.

The most important components of placental exchange are the rates of blood flow on each side of the placenta and

the area available for exchange. Uterine blood flow will decline in the presence of factors causing decreased perfusion pressure or increased uterine vascular resistance. Common clinical occurrences are hypotension, hypertension, endogenous or exogenous vasoconstriction, and severe psychological stress. The uterine vascular bed is not autoregulated and normally has little capacity to dilate further. However, hypertensive states (e.g., preeclampsia) and high catecholamine levels (e.g., stress, pain) can cause increased uterine vascular resistance. During labor, it is most likely that the rate of uterine blood flow is a common limiting factor in cases of fetal compromise because of the intermittent decline in uterine blood flow with each uterine contraction. In addition, transient or persistent umbilical cord compression may cause fetal asphyxia.

■ OBSTETRIC ANESTHESIA AND UTERINE BLOOD FLOW

Obstetric anesthesia and analgesia may directly affect uterine blood flow or may alter the response of the uteroplacental circulation to noxious stimuli and to various pharmacologic agents (Table 2-4). Uterine blood flow varies directly with the perfusion pressure (i.e., uterine arterial minus

TABLE 2-4 Drug Effects on Uterine/Placental Blood Flow[a]

Drug	Model and Technique	Dosage/Blood Level	Effect	Reference
Induction Agents				
Thiopental	Microsphere—ewe	Standard	40% initial decrease UBF	26
Thiopental	Xenon—human	Standard	Marked decrease placental BF	27
Propofol	Microsphere—ewe	≤450 mg/kg/min	No change UBF from baseline	26
Diazepam	Sheep gravid	0.5 mg/kg	No change utero/placental flow	28
Ketamine	Sheep gravid	0.7 mg/kg	UBF constant	34
Ketamine	Sheep gravid	≤5 mg/kg	Dose-related decrease UBF, increase uterine tone	35
Ketamine	Human recommendations	0.25–1 mg/kg	No adverse effect	37–40
Inhalation Drugs				
Halothane	Sheep gravid	Up to 1.5%	No effect or slight increase UBF	51
Halothane	Monkey and sheep	>2 MAC	Dose-related decrease UBF	51, 53
Isoflurane	Sheep gravid	1%	25% increase UBF	51
Desflurane	No UBF studies			
Sevoflurane	No UBF studies			
Local Anesthetics				
Lidocaine	Uterine artery (human)	400 μg/mL	Vasoconstriction (supraclinical dose)	54
Lidocaine	Sheep gravid	2–4 μg/mL blood level	No change UBF	60
2 CP	Guinea pigs	2 mg/kg	No change UBF	61
Bupivacaine	Human/ultrasound	≈140 mg epidural	No change UBF	63
Ropivacaine	Human/ultrasound	≈140 mg epidural	No change UBF	63
Cocaine	Sheep gravid	0.5–2.8 mg/kg	Dose-related decrease UBF	66
Epidural Block				
Uncomplicated by hypotension			No change UBF	69, 77–80
Catecholamines				
Epinephrine 1:200K	Human/xenon	10 mL w 2CP epidural	No change intervillous BF	87
Epinephrine	Sheep gravid	20 μg IV	Decrease UBF 40% for 60 s	82
Epinephrine	Guinea pig	0.2–1 μg/kg	Dose-related decrease UBF	83
Isoproterenol	Pregnant ewe	4, 16, 80 μg IV	Dose-related transient decrease UBF	182
Stress	Monkey/flow probe	Severe stress	Marked reduction UBF	91
	Human	Very anxious	Higher catechols and abnormal FHT	93
Vasopressors				
Ephedrine	Monkey/flow probe	10–15 mg IV	Restores UBF better than other pressors	99
Ephedrine	Gravid sheep	5–10 mg IV	Restores UBF after SAB	98
Ephedrine	Xenon–human	25 mg IV	No decrease IVBF	74
Phenylephrine	Human clinical outcome	20–100 μg IV	Restored maternal BP and possibly UBF	101, 183, 184
Dopamine	Sheep gravid	Doses to correct BP	Decrease UBF	105, 106
Ritodrine	Sheep gravid	Therapeutic doses	Decrease UBF	83, 110
Terbutaline	Sheep gravid	Therapeutic doses	Decrease UBF	111

(continued)

TABLE 2-4 Drug Effects on Uterine/Placental Blood Flow[a] (Continued)

Drug	Model and Technique	Dosage/Blood Level	Effect	Reference
Antihypertensives				
Hydralazine	Hypertensive sheep	Dose to normalize BP	Increase UBF while decreasing BP	112
Hydralazine	Human hypertension/xenon	125 µg/min	Increase umbilical BF, no change IVBF	115
Nitroglycerin	Hypertensive sheep	Infusion	Increase UBF while decreasing BP	116
Nitroprusside	Hypertensive sheep	Infusion	Decrease UBF, restrict to induction use	113, 185
Labetalol	Human/PEC/xenon/US	1 mg/kg	No change in IVBF or fetal BF	127
Calcium Channel Blockers				
Verapamil	Pregnant ewe	0.2 mg/kg	25% decrease UBF 2 min	130
Nicardipine	Pregnant rabbit	Low and high dose	Dose-related decrease UBF	131
Nifedipine	Pregnant ewe	5–10 µg/kg 90 min	UBF decrease transient, fetal hypoxia	186
Magnesium sulfate	Pregnant ewe	4 g load, 2–4 g/h	Initial decrease UBF, then normalization	143
Epidural Opioids				
MS, Fentanyl, Sufentanil	Pregnant ewe	Clinical doses	No effect UBF	146–148
Clonidine	Pregnant ewe	300 µg epidural	No significant change UBF	187
Clonidine	Pregnant ewe	300 µg IV	Significant decrease UBF, fetal hypoxia	187
Dantrolene	Pregnant ewe	1.2–2.4 mg/kg	No change UBF	166
Respiratory Gases				
Hypocapnia	Pregnant ewe	Mechanical hyperventilation	Decrease UBF 25%	171
Hypercapnia	Pregnant ewe	Arterial P_{CO_2} >60 mm Hg	Decrease UBF	169

[a]Table prepared by Dr. T. Cheek.

uterine venous pressure) and inversely with uterine vascular resistance. Obstetric anesthesia may affect uterine blood flow by (a) changing the perfusion pressure, that is, altering the uterine arterial or venous pressure; or (b) changing uterine vascular resistance either directly through changes in vascular tone or indirectly by altering uterine contractions or uterine muscle tone; or (c) changing the maternal cardiac output.

Direct measurement of human uterine blood flow is not easy because of the relative inaccessibility of the human uteroplacental circulation. Clinically, changes in uterine blood flow are presumed from assessment of fetal and neonatal acid–base and heart rate status. Both the intervillous and myometrial components of human uterine blood flow were measured based on the clearance of xenon-133 given intravenously (34,35).

Currently, the most common technique for assessing uteroplacental circulation is Doppler ultrasound. Actual measurements of blood flow require precise measurement of the cross-sectional areas of the vessel. An additional problem in converting velocity measurements to actual flows is the difficulty in precisely measuring the angle between the ultrasound beam and the vessel. Describing the relationship between the Doppler waveform during systole and diastole – that is, the S/D ratio – allows one to study *relative* changes without actually measuring absolute flow.

Doppler arterial waveforms in most vessels show high systolic velocity and little or no diastolic velocity. During pregnancy, maternal uteroplacental vessels show continuous forward diastolic flow. Any decrease, absence, or reversal of end-diastolic flow velocity is considered abnormal. The use of a true mean velocity measurement that is more accurate has improved the quality of this technique (36).

The vast majority of information on the effects of anesthesia on uteroplacental circulation has been derived mainly from animal experiments. The development of chronic maternal–fetal animal preparations has allowed precise measurement of changes in uterine and placental blood flow and of the effect of these changes on fetal cardiovascular and acid–base status (Fig. 2-11) using various techniques (37). The following section reviews the effects of commonly used anesthetic agents, techniques, and adjuvants, and of anesthetic complications on uterine blood flow.

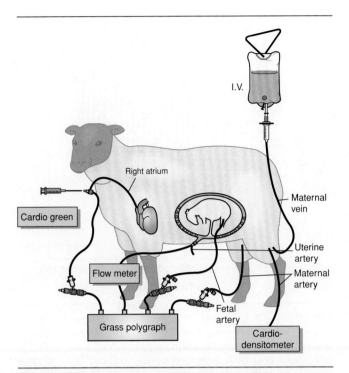

FIGURE 2-11 Diagram of sheep experimental preparation with chronically implanted maternal and fetal intravascular catheters and an electromagnetic flow probe around a branch of uterine artery. Reprinted with permission from: Ralston DH, Shnider SM, DeLorimier AA. Effects of equipotent ephedrine, metaraminol, mephentermine and methoxamine on uterine blood flow in the pregnant ewe. *Anesthesiology* 1974;40:354–370.

■ INTRAVENOUS INDUCTION AGENTS

Barbiturates

Ultrashort-acting barbiturates may be used for induction of anesthesia and are usually followed by endotracheal intubation and nitrous oxide maintenance. Palahniuk and Cumming (38) studied this sequence and reported that uterine blood flow decreased by 20% after induction of anesthesia without a significant decrease in maternal arterial blood pressure. Fetal oxygen saturation and pH also decreased. They postulated that the increase in uterine vascular resistance was due to maternal catecholamine release during light anesthesia.

Shnider et al. (39) reported that, in sheep, intravenous induction of anesthesia with thiopental and succinylcholine followed by direct laryngoscopy and endotracheal intubation resulted in an increase in arterial plasma norepinephrine of 89% from control. Blood pressure rose by 65%, uterine vascular resistance rose by 42%, and uterine blood flow fell by 24%. These acute cardiovascular changes quickly diminished with the termination of airway manipulation. Alon et al. (40), also studying pregnant sheep, reported that uterine blood flow decreased by about 40% during thiopental induction and endotracheal intubation, then rapidly increased significantly to a point approximately 28% ± 27% above baseline values during anesthetic maintenance with isoflurane. Jouppila et al. (41), using the radioactive xenon technique, corroborated these findings in humans. During the induction of general anesthesia for cesarean section, they found a marked decrease in placental blood flow with a mean reduction of 35%.

Propofol

In contrast to thiopental, uterine blood flow demonstrated no change during induction of anesthesia with propofol (2 mg/kg) despite a significant increase in mean arterial blood pressure. Unlike the uterine blood flow response during maintenance of anesthesia with isoflurane, maintenance of anesthesia with infusions of propofol at either 150, 300, or 450 μg^{-1} kg^{-1} min^{-1} (40) did not change uterine blood flow from preinduction baseline values, and it remained stable throughout anesthesia.

Diazepam

In pregnant sheep, diazepam in doses as high as 0.5 mg/kg did not alter maternal or fetal cardiovascular function or uteroplacental blood flow (42). However, larger doses produced an 8% to 12% decrease in arterial pressure with an equivalent decrease in uterine blood flow. Fetal oxygenation was not affected. Cosmi (43) also observed that the bolus injection of diazepam to the ewe in doses of 0.18 mg/kg had no deleterious effects on maternal or fetal blood pressure or acid–base status.

Ketamine

Ketamine usually increases arterial blood pressure. Greiss and Van Wilkes (44) and Ralston et al. (45) demonstrated that drugs that increase maternal arterial blood pressure as a result of vasoconstriction may lead to a decrease in uterine blood flow with consequent fetal hypoxia and acidosis. Levinson et al. (46) administered 5 mg/kg of ketamine to a group of pregnant ewes near term. They found a 15% increase in mean maternal blood pressure and a 10% increase in uterine blood flow. Eng et al. (47) reported similar results in monkeys. Craft et al. (48) administered 0.7 mg/kg ketamine to pregnant sheep and noted similar results. Maternal effects consisted of a slight increase in blood pressure and cardiac output (up to 16%) and a moderate increase in uterine resting tone, whereas uterine blood flow remained relatively constant.

Cosmi (49) evaluated the effects of ketamine in pregnant sheep not in labor and during labor. In the ewes not in labor (condition resembling that of elective cesarean section), the drug was administered intravenously in doses of 1.8 to 2.2 mg/kg. Anesthesia was maintained with nitrous oxide and oxygen, and ventilation was controlled. Under these conditions, ketamine produced increases in mean maternal blood pressure and heart rate and in uterine blood flow without significant changes in fetal cardiovascular and acid–base status. However, when ketamine in doses of 0.9 to 5 mg/kg was given to the ewes in labor, Cosmi observed a marked increase of maternal ventilation, as well as increases in uterine tone and frequency and intensity of uterine contractions, and a slight decrease of uterine blood flow. These changes were dose related and were accompanied by fetal tachycardia and acidosis. Similarly, Galloon (50) reported a dose-related increase in uterine muscle tone after ketamine administration in patients undergoing therapeutic abortion during the second trimester.

Therefore, there appears to be some variability in the maternal circulatory response to ketamine related in part to the presence or absence of labor, the dosage, and the stage of gestation. It would appear, however, that ketamine in the usual clinical doses (0.25 to 1 mg/kg) does not adversely affect uterine blood flow. Several studies report normal neonatal clinical and acid–base conditions after the administration of ketamine in doses up to 1 mg/kg for vaginal and abdominal delivery (49). Doses of 2 mg/kg or above may increase uterine muscle tone.

Etomidate

Etomidate administration did not depress cardiovascular function in the pregnant ewe or fetus and during an infusion of etomidate, raised maternal HR and blood pressure (51). Etomidate crossed the placenta rapidly, with similar rates of metabolism and redistribution in ewe and fetus (52). Although etomidate has been reported to produce adrenal suppression, especially in patients with sepsis (53), its use in parturients with chorioamnionitis has not been associated with problems.

Dexmedetomidine

Dexmedetomidine, a selective α_2-agonist, is more lipophilic and had a greater placental uptake and lower fetal transport into the circulation than the α_1-agonist clonidine (54).

■ HALOGENATED INHALATION AGENTS

The effect of inhalation analgesia–anesthesia on the uteroplacental circulation and on the fetus is still a controversial matter. Some authors (55), report fetal asphyxia, whereas others (46) indicate that well-conducted inhalation anesthesia produces no effects on the fetus or the uteroplacental circulation.

Halogenated agents have a unique and specific place in obstetric anesthesia because of their potent uterine relaxant properties. Hence, they are the agent of choice when uterine relaxation is required—for example, for version and extraction, breech delivery, retained placenta, tetanic contractions, and surgical manipulations (56). Attempts to improve fetal oxygenation by increasing maternal inspired oxygen concentration (57) stimulated interest in the use of halothane with lower concentrations of nitrous oxide for cesarean section. In addition, its use has also been recommended to improve fetal oxygenation in case of fetal distress caused by uterine tetany.

Several investigators have studied the effect of halothane on uterine blood flow. Palahniuk and Shnider (58) found that in the pregnant ewe during light and moderately deep anesthesia (1 and 1.5 minimum alveolar concentration [MAC]), maternal blood pressure was slightly depressed (less than 20% from control), but uterine vasodilation occurred and uteroplacental blood flow was maintained. Neither fetal hypoxemia nor metabolic acidosis occurred. Deep levels of anesthesia (2 MAC) produced greater reductions in maternal blood pressure and cardiac output. Despite uterine vasodilation, uterine blood flow decreased and the fetuses became hypoxic and acidotic. Similar results have been reported by Carenza and Cosmi (59) in pregnant sheep and by Eng et al. (60) in pregnant monkeys. Furthermore, Cosmi and Marx (55) reported that in humans, light-to-moderate planes of halothane anesthesia (i.e., 0.5 to 1 vol/100 mL) did not alter either maternal cardiovascular function or fetal acid–base status. In contrast, deep planes (i.e., 1.5 vol/100 mL or greater) produced maternal hypotension and fetal acidosis.

Shnider et al. (39) studied the effects in pregnant ewes of halothane 0.5% inspired combined with 50% nitrous oxide and oxygen. They reported a 22% increase in uterine blood flow during the 1-hour administration period. Thus, it seems that low concentrations of halothane do not adversely affect uteroplacental circulation and, in fact, produce uterine vasodilation. Increasing concentrations produce progressive decreases in the uterine blood flow due to maternal hypotension.

Studies by Palahniuk and Shnider (58) indicate that isoflurane is essentially indistinguishable from halothane in its effects on maternal and fetal cardiovascular and acid–base

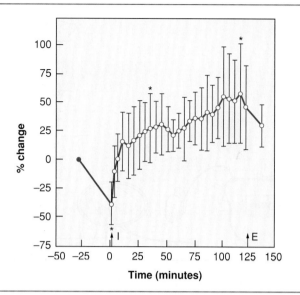

FIGURE 2-12 Changes in uterine blood flow following induction with 5 mg/kg thiopental, 1.5 mg/kg succinylcholine, endotracheal intubation, and maintenance with 1% isoflurane and 50% (inspired concentration) N_2O in oxygen. *I*, intubation; *E*, extubation; *asterisk*, statistically significant differences from control values (p<05). Reprinted with permission from: Alon E, Ball RH, Gillie MH, et al. Effects of propofol and thiopental on maternal and cardiovascular and acid–base variables in the pregnant ewe. *Anesthesiology* 1993;78:562–576.

status. Light planes of anesthesia do not decrease uterine blood flow, but deep planes do. Similarly, Alon et al. (40) reported that, in pregnant ewes, light anesthesia produced by inhalation of isoflurane 1% combined with 50% nitrous oxide and oxygen produced a 25% increase in uterine blood flow (Fig. 2-12).

Available data suggest equipotent doses of enflurane, desflurane, and sevoflurane act similarly to halothane and isoflurane with respect to their effects on uterine tone, uterine vasculature, and perfusion. All inhalation agents have dose-dependent effects on uterine tone. In human pregnant myometrium, relaxation was equivalent for sevoflurane, desflurane, halothane with ED50 about 1.5 MAC and required more for isoflurane, with an ED50 2.3 MAC (61). In clinical situations when uterine tone is increased (e.g., uterine hyperstimulation, tetanic contraction), halogenated agents will decrease uterine tone, and if maternal blood pressure is maintained, result in improved uteroplacental perfusion. In humans, 1.5 MAC desflurane produced adequate uterine relaxation with propofol and remifentanil supplementation for fetal surgery, while 2.5 MAC produced left ventricular dysfunction and fetal bradycardia (62). This fetal effect was confirmed in sheep, where 1.5 to 2 MAC of sevoflurane and isoflurane decreased uterine blood flow, and significantly decreased fetal blood pressure and heart rate. Sevoflurane produced fetoplacental vasodilation in vitro, mediated in part by lipoxygenase-generated eicosanoids and not mediated by nitric oxide (63). In summary, the potent inhalational agents should be kept at <1.5 MAC during pregnancy.

■ LOCAL ANESTHETICS

Gibbs and Noel (64) demonstrated a vasoconstricting effect of both lidocaine and mepivacaine using an in vitro preparation

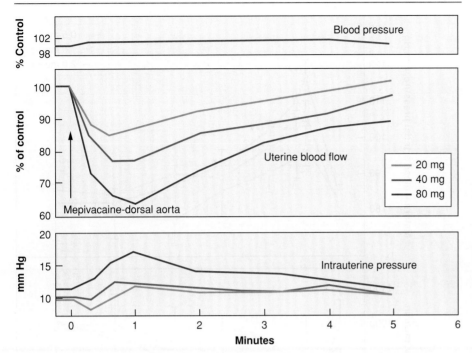

FIGURE 2-13 Effects of increasing intra-aortic doses of mepivacaine on uterine blood flow and intra-uterine pressure in pregnant ewes near term. Note the progressive decrease in uterine blood flow with similar inverse changes in intra-uterine pressure. Reprinted with permission from: Greiss FC Jr, Still JG, Anderson SG. Effects of local anesthetic agents on the uterine vasculatures and myometrium. *Am J Obstet Gynecol* 1976;124: 889–899.

of human uterine artery segments obtained from cesarean hysterectomy specimens. The concentrations of local anesthetics ranged from 400 to 1000 µg/mL, concentrations well above levels achieved during clinical use. Uterine vasoconstriction was not seen with lower concentrations or in uterine arteries taken from nonpregnant hysterectomy specimens, indicating that the response was dose related and occurred only during pregnancy. Pretreatment of the strips with phenoxybenzamine (an α-adrenergic blocker) did not abolish the vasoconstrictive response.

Greiss et al. (65), injecting 20, 40, and 80 mg boluses of either lidocaine or mepivacaine into the dorsal aorta of eight anesthetized pregnant ewes, found a dose-related, transient (2 to 3 minutes) decrease in uterine blood flow and a simultaneous increase in intrauterine pressure (Fig. 2-13). Uterine arterial blood levels were not measured. These investigators also infused lidocaine, mepivacaine, bupivacaine, and procaine directly into the uterine artery of nonpregnant ewes. The following uterine arterial concentrations reduced mean uterine blood flow by 40%: Bupivacaine 5 µg/mL, mepivacaine 40 µg/mL, procaine 40 µg/mL, and lidocaine 200 µg/mL. Such enormously high concentrations could not occur during epidural anesthesia in the absence of an intravenous injection.

Subsequent studies in the pregnant ewe by Fishburne et al. (66) produced similar findings of uterine vasoconstriction occurring only at very high blood levels, which might be found in the uterine vasculature during paracervical blocks (close proximity of the injected drugs to the uterine arteries) or during systemic toxic reactions. Morishima et al. (67) found that during lidocaine-induced maternal convulsions in the pregnant ewe, uterine blood flow was reduced by 55% to 71% of control values. The lack of uterine vasoconstriction with low blood levels of lidocaine was demonstrated by Biehl et al. (68). These investigators infused the local anesthetic intravenously to produce blood levels (2 to 4 µg/mL) in the pregnant ewe comparable to those usually found in the human parturient undergoing epidural anesthesia during the first and second stages of labor. They found that a 2-hour exposure to these

low concentrations of lidocaine did not significantly decrease uterine blood flow or increase intra-amniotic pressure.

Similarly, lidocaine in a dose of 0.4 mg/kg or 2-chloroprocaine in doses up to 2 mg/kg administered intravenously to guinea pigs did not significantly decrease uterine blood flow velocity (69).

In a clinical study of women undergoing cesarean section with epidural anesthesia, Alahuhta et al. demonstrated that 115 to 140 mg of 0.5% ropivacaine epidurally had no effect on uterine blood flow (70).

Cocaine is a potent local anesthetic with unique vasoconstrictive properties. Studies on the effect of intravenous cocaine on uterine blood flow have shown that cocaine at doses between 0.5 and 2.8 mg/kg produced a dose-related reduction in uterine blood flow (Fig. 2-14) (71). Cocaine may significantly decrease uterine blood flow and thus should be avoided or administered cautiously and sparingly to human parturients. In addition, cocaine may cause hypertensive crises, placental abruption, and altered response to medications.

■ REGIONAL ANESTHESIA

The most frequent complication of spinal, lumbar epidural, and caudal anesthesia is systemic hypotension. The decrease in mean arterial blood pressure reduces uterine blood flow proportionately (72). However, epidural anesthesia uncomplicated by arterial hypotension is associated with no alterations in uterine blood flow (73).

Jouppila et al. (35), extensively studied the effect of regional anesthesia for labor or cesarean section on uteroplacental perfusion. Studies in healthy women not in labor undergoing cesarean section indicated that neither epidural (74) nor spinal (35) anesthesia uncomplicated by hypotension is associated with changes in intervillous blood flow. However, women with preeclampsia showed an improvement in intervillous blood flow following initiation of regional anesthesia.

Healthy women in labor showed a 35% increase in intervillous blood flow following the epidural administration of 10 mL of either 0.25% bupivacaine or 2% chloroprocaine

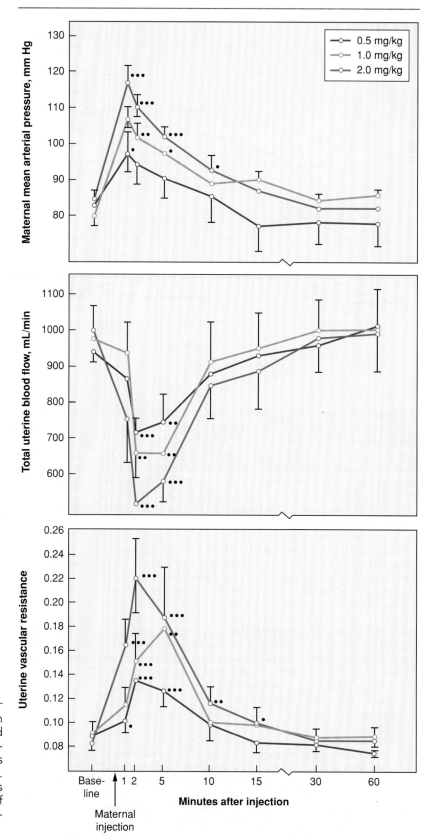

FIGURE 2-14 Responses of maternal mean arterial pressure (*top*), total uterine blood flow (*middle*), and uterine vascular resistance (*bottom*) to maternal administrations of cocaine. Single asterisks indicate *p* <001. Reprinted with permission from: Woods JR Jr, Plessinger MA, Clark KE. Effect of cocaine on uterine blood flow and fetal oxygenation. *JAMA* 1987;257:957–961.

(Fig. 2-15) (75). In patients with pregnancy-induced hypertension, the epidural injection of 10 mL 0.25% bupivacaine resulted in a much more significant improvement in intervillous blood flow; the increase amounted to 77% (76). The investigators (75,77) using smaller volumes of drug (e.g., 4 mL 0.5% bupivacaine with or without epinephrine 1:200,000), found no improvement in placental blood flow. The authors postulated that the more widespread sympathectomy obtained with larger volumes, together with the relief of pain and anxiety, tends to

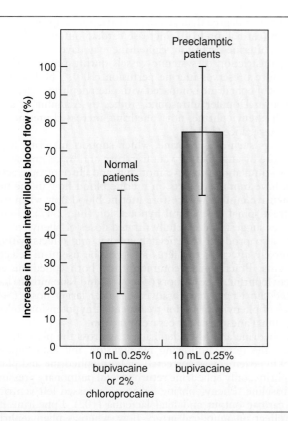

FIGURE 2-15 Percentage increase in mean intervillous blood flow values (±SE) after epidural anesthesia for labor in normal and preeclamptic patients. Redrawn with permission from: Hollmén A, Jouppila R, Jouppila P, et al. Effect of extradural analgesia using bupivacaine and 2-chloroprocaine on intervillous blood flow during normal labour. *Br J Anaesth* 1982;54:837–842; Jouppila P, Jouppila R, Hollmén A, et al. Lumbar epidural analgesia to improve intervillous blood flow during labor in severe preeclampsia. *Obstet Gynecol* 1982;59:158–161.

restore uterine blood flow to its normal nonstressed basal condition.

Studies using Doppler ultrasound to measure uteroplacental arterial flow velocity waveforms have confirmed, with rare exception (78), the lack of deleterious effects of epidural anesthesia on uterine blood flow (79). These studies involved women receiving epidural blocks to T3 to T5 dermatome levels for elective cesarean sections. These women were prehydrated with 1 to 2 L balanced salt solution, positioned with left uterine tilt, and received either lidocaine 2% or bupivacaine 0.5%, both with and without epinephrine 1:200,000.

■ CATECHOLAMINES AND STRESS

Adrenergic stimulation produced by either exogenous or endogenous catecholamines can constrict uterine vessels and reduce uterine blood flow. Exogenous catecholamines (primarily epinephrine) are administered with local anesthetics to produce vasoconstriction at the site of injection. Endogenous catecholamines (both epinephrine and norepinephrine) are released during anxiety and pain. Vasopressors (e.g., ephedrine, phenylephrine) are frequently used to prevent or treat spinal or epidural hypotension. Stress, pain, and even smoking can increase levels of circulating catecholamines.

Epinephrine

Epinephrine has significant effects on both α- and β-adrenergic receptors. High epinephrine blood levels achieved by accidental intravascular injection of epinephrine-containing local anesthetics produce α-adrenergic effects, including hypertension, increased total peripheral resistance, uterine vasoconstriction, increased uterine activity, and decreased uterine blood flow. In ewes given 0.10 to 1 μg^{-1} kg^{-1} min^{-1} epinephrine, maternal pressure rose 65% above control and uterine blood flow fell by 55% to 75% (80). Injection of epinephrine 20 μg in pregnant ewes decreased uterine blood flow by 40% for about 60 seconds (81).

Low blood levels of epinephrine, such as occurring from systemic absorption during caudal or epidural block, have been shown to produce a generalized β-adrenergic response that becomes maximal 15 minutes after epidural injection (82). A number of studies of the β-adrenergic effects of epinephrine on the uterine vessels have produced conflicting results.

Rosenfeld et al. (83) infused 50 to 100 μg epinephrine intravenously over a 5-minute period into pregnant ewes and produced a generalized β-adrenergic effect with tachycardia and increased cardiac output and blood flow to skeletal muscles. However, although blood pressure did not change, uterine blood flow decreased almost 50%. These investigators postulated that the uterine artery in the pregnant ewe may be more sensitive to the α-adrenergic effects of epinephrine, while vasculature of skeletal muscle, adipose tissue, and other visceral organs may be more sensitive to the β-adrenergic effects.

Albright et al. (84) did not corroborate these latter findings in humans. These investigators reported that 10 mL epidural chloroprocaine with 1:200,000 epinephrine did not alter *human* intervillous blood flow during epidural anesthesia for labor despite a reduction in mean blood pressure of 11 mm Hg. Levinson et al. (85) compared 2% lidocaine alone to 2% lidocaine with 1:200,000 epinephrine administered for epidural anesthesia for cesarean section. They found no adverse effects of epinephrine on the mother or neonate as ascertained by the incidence of hypotension, low Apgar scores, or abnormal fetal acid–base status. Ramanathan et al. (86) found that plasma epinephrine levels increased 400% following epidural bupivacaine with epinephrine in women undergoing elective cesarean, while plasma norepinephrine increased 80% in both epinephrine and non—epinephrine-containing groups. Cascio et al. (87) found both intrathecal fentanyl as well as epidural lidocaine for pain relief during labor reduced maternal plasma epinephrine levels 52%, while norepinephrine levels rose 25% to 30% over 30 minutes. Rapid pain relief has been associated with uterine hyperstimulation and short-term fetal bradycardia, possibly due to the decreased epinephrine (less uterine relaxing β-adrenergic effect) and/or increased norepinephrine (more uterine contracting α-adrenergic stimulation).

In summary, there may be transient fluctuations in uterine blood flow after epidural anesthesia with epinephrine-containing solutions. However, these have little effect on the healthy fetus.

Stress

Myers (88) reported that maternal stress and anxiety in the pregnant rhesus monkey produced fetal asphyxia, likely due to uterine vasoconstriction as a consequence of maternal catecholamine release. Shnider et al. (89) found that stress sufficient to produce maternal hypertension resulted in a precipitous fall in uterine blood flow and an increase in plasma norepinephrine in pregnant ewes. Similarly, Martin and Gingerich (90) found a marked reduction in uterine blood flow in response to severe stress in the pregnant rhesus monkey.

Lederman et al. (91) reported that both primiparous and multiparous parturients who were very anxious during labor had increased circulating epinephrine blood levels and a higher incidence of abnormal fetal heart rate patterns compared with those who were less anxious. Again, we presume that these findings are due to uterine hypoperfusion. Stress increased systolic and diastolic blood pressure in African-American women, and an increased diastolic pressure was associated with lower birthweight (92). Stress has also been shown to increase preterm births by 50% to 100% (93).

Vasopressors

Vasopressors with predominant α-adrenergic activity reduce uterine blood flow and may adversely affect the fetus (94). Methoxamine, phenylephrine, angiotensin, or norepinephrine treatment of spinal hypotension in animals diminishes uterine blood flow and leads to fetal asphyxia (94,95). Ephedrine, mephentermine, and metaraminol restore uterine blood flow toward normal (Fig. 2-16) (96,97).

Studies of treatment of spinal or epidural hypotension using either low-dose phenylephrine (20 to 100 μg), or ephedrine (10 to 15 mg) in elective cesarean sections have not confirmed the animal data (98,99). Using an impedance cardiograph to measure stroke volume, ejection fraction, and end-diastolic volume, Ramanathan and Grant (98) showed that both ephedrine and phenylephrine produce venoconstriction to a greater degree than arterial constriction, improve venous return (cardiac preload), increase cardiac output, and likely restore uterine perfusion. Ephedrine may have a more selective constriction of systemic vessels during pregnancy, and therefore preserves uterine perfusion (100). The beneficial effects of ephedrine compared with phenylephrine have been shown in Doppler ultrasound studies by Alahuhta et al. in which phenylephrine, not ephedrine, increased uterine vascular resistance (101).

Drugs such as ephedrine, which support maternal blood pressure by augmenting venous return and by central adrenergic stimulation (positive inotropic and chronotropic activity), have minimal effects on uterine blood flow in the normotensive mother and restore uterine blood flow when used to treat spinal or epidural hypotension (Fig. 2-17). Human studies suggest that carefully titrated doses of phenylephrine may also produce beneficial hemodynamic effects without adversely affecting the fetus and may be useful in selected patients. Practitioners commonly use both ephedrine and phenylephrine. The authors (Zakowski and Ramanthan) have noted short-term fetal bradycardia after larger doses (>600 mcg) of phenylephrine for treatment of hypotension following spinal anesthesia for cesarean section.

Ephedrine and phenylephrine may cross the placenta and affect the fetus. Following hypotension and fetal hypoxia, fetal hypoxemia was corrected by both ephedrine and phenylephrine, only ephedrine returned fetal pulmonary pressures to baseline. Phenylephrine led to a decreased left ventricular cardiac output and fetal lactemia (102). Ephedrine had no effect on umbilical artery flow, whereas phenylephrine

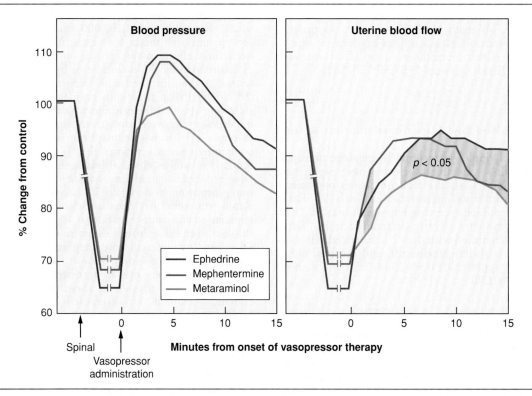

FIGURE 2-16 Average response patterns to ephedrine and slow infusions of mephentermine and metaraminol after hypotension induced by spinal anesthesia. After 4 minutes, uterine blood flow was significantly higher with ephedrine and mephentermine than with metaraminol therapy. Reprinted with permission from: James FM 3rd, Greiss FC Jr, Kemp RA. An evaluation of vasopressor therapy for maternal hypotension during spinal anesthesia. *Anesthesiology* 1970;33:25–34.

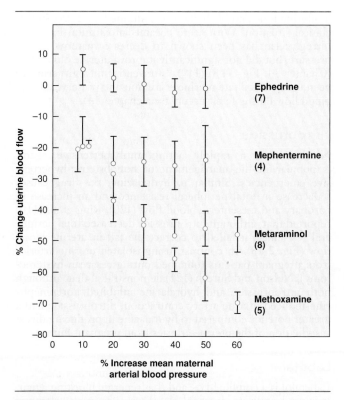

FIGURE 2-17 Mean changes in uterine blood flow at equal elevations of mean arterial blood pressure after vasopressor administration. Reprinted with permission from: Ralston DH, Shnider SM, DeLorimier AA. Effects of equipotent ephedrine, metaraminol, mephentermine and methoxamine on uterine blood flow in the pregnant ewe. *Anesthesiology* 1974;40:354–370.

decreased umbilical artery flow after prolonged administration (103). However, recent studies in humans have suggested that ephedrine crosses the placenta, increasing fetal oxygen consumption via β-adrenergic agonist effects; phenylephrine was associated with a higher umbilical artery pH at birth and lower lactate levels (104).

Dopamine, a catecholamine that stimulates dopaminergic and α- and β-adrenergic receptors, has predominantly different adrenergic receptor effects at different dosages. In normotensive sheep, Callender et al. (105) reported that doses that increase maternal blood pressure and cardiac output decrease uterine blood flow. Rolbin et al. (106) reported that dopamine, when used to treat spinal hypotension, corrected maternal blood pressure but resulted in a further decrease in uterine blood flow. This was due to a significant increase in uterine vascular resistance despite minimal changes in total peripheral resistance. Conflicting results were reported by Cabalum et al. (107), who found that dopamine infusion in doses similar to those used by Rolbin restored uterine blood flow with the correction of hypotension. A vasoconstrictive effect on uterine blood vessels has been reported with β-adrenergic drugs such as isoxsuprine, ritodrine, and terbutaline (108). The effects of dopamine on the uterine vessels likely represent an increased sensitivity of these vessels to dopamine's α-adrenergic stimulation.

■ ANTIHYPERTENSIVE AGENTS

Hypertensive disorders of pregnancy frequently require therapy. Ideally, drugs used to treat maternal hypertension

should reduce blood pressure and uterine vascular resistance so that uterine blood flow is either unchanged or increased. Blood pressure is commonly used as a surrogate for uterine blood flow, which is difficult to measure. However, cardiac output can also be used as a surrogate marker for uterine blood flow; thus any cardiovascular manipulations should maintain or increase cardiac output. Recall that blood pressure equals cardiac output times systemic vascular resistance, and cardiac output equals heart rate times stroke volume. High-dose phenylephrine following hypotension may decrease cardiac output while increasing blood pressure by increased vascular resistance and reduced heart rate. Cardiac output may be a better indicator for uterine artery perfusion. The authors (Zakowski, Ramanathan) have observed fetal bradycardia following return of maternal blood pressure after larger doses of phenylephrine (>600 mcg total) administration for hypotension during spinal anesthesia for cesarean delivery.

Hydralazine

Hydralazine, a slow-acting antihypertensive drug, is used widely in the treatment of gestational hypertension. The effects of hydralazine on uterine blood flow in the hypertensive pregnant ewe have been studied by Brinkman and Assali (109). These investigators induced severe hypertension and reduction in uterine blood flow by placing a modified Goldblatt clamp around one renal artery and removing the contralateral kidney. Hydralazine, in this preparation, reduced blood pressure while increasing uterine blood flow. Similarly, in a study by Ring et al. (110) on phenylephrine-induced hypertension, hydralazine slowly lowered the blood pressure while significantly increasing uterine blood flow, although uterine blood flow did not return to normal (Fig. 2-18). During cocaine-induced hypertension in the pregnant ewe, hydralazine did not restore uterine blood flow as maternal blood pressure returned to normal (Fig. 2-19) (111). In humans, the effects of intravenously infused hydralazine (incremental doses up to 125 μg/min during 60 minutes) were studied by Jouppila et al. (112) in 10 women with acute or superimposed severe preeclampsia. The intervillous and umbilical vein blood flows were measured before and during hydralazine infusion with the xenon-133 method and with a combination of real-time and Doppler ultrasound equipment, respectively. Maternal blood pressure decreased and pulse rate increased during the infusion. Hydralazine did not change the intervillous blood flow but increased the blood flow in the umbilical vein. The results indicated that hydralazine affected the placental and fetal circulations differently.

Alpha-methyldopa

Alpha-methyldopa, the classic antihypertensive agent used during pregnancy, is still used today for chronic hypertension during pregnancy and pregnancy-induced hypertension. The drug is metabolized to alpha-methylnorepinephrine, an agonist of the presynaptic CNS α_2-adrenergic receptors, which inhibits sympathetic nervous system outflow and lowers blood pressure. The other mechanism of action is due to inhibition of the enzyme that converts L-DOPA into dopamine, the precursor for norepinephrine and epinephrine. Alpha-methyldopa showed no significant effect on human umbilical arterial rings in vitro (113). Pulsatility index in the umbilical artery, a measure of placental vascular resistance was significantly decreased by alpha-methyldopa in mild preeclamptic and chronic hypertensive women (114). In women with pregnancies with hypertensive disorders,

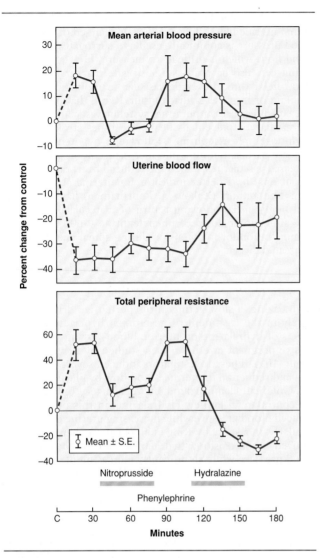

FIGURE 2-18 Percentage change from control of maternal mean arterial blood pressure, uterine blood flow, and total peripheral resistance during phenylephrine-induced hypertension and correction of hypertension with nitroprusside and hydralazine. Hydralazine, but not nitroprusside, resulted in a significant increase in uterine blood flow ($p < 05$). Reprinted with permission from: Ring G, Krames E, Shnider SM, et al. Comparison of nitroprusside and hydralazine in hypertensive pregnant ewes. *Obstet Gynecol* 1977;50:598–602.

alpha-methyldopa did not significantly change uterine artery PI and thus resistance to blood flow (115). In another study, in preeclamptic women, alpha-methyldopa decreased uterine artery resistance but did not affect the umbilical and fetal middle cerebral artery resistance (116).

Nitroglycerin

Craft et al. (117) found that a nitroglycerin infusion administered to pregnant ewes during phenylephrine-induced hypertension resulted in a reduction in blood pressure associated with improved uterine blood flow. Sublingual nitroglycerin has been used to relax the uterus in patients with uterine hyperstimulation and fetal heart rate decelerations (118). Intravenous nitroglycerin may also prove useful when managing fetal bradycardia reported in conjunction with intrathecal opioids. Nitroglycerin appears to bring about a decrease

in uterine tone and likely increases uterine blood flow in this clinical situation. With acute cocaine intoxication in sheep, nitroglycerin has been shown to decrease maternal blood pressure, but did not significantly improve uterine blood flow (Chapter 34, Fig. 34.8) (119). Intravenous nitroglycerin has been used to facilitate uterine relaxation and preserve uterine blood flow during fetal surgery (see Chapter 14).

Nitroprusside

Nitroprusside, a rapidly acting antihypertensive agent, is popular in the management of nonobstetric-hypertensive emergencies. Similar to hydralazine, the drug causes a decrease in total peripheral resistance and an increase in coronary and mesenteric blood flow (120). Ring et al. (110) reported that, although nitroprusside decreased total peripheral resistance, it failed to correct the fall in uterine blood flow (Fig. 2-18). In contrast, using isolated uterine arteries from pregnant patients (obtained during cesarean-hysterectomy), Nelson and Suresh (121) demonstrated that, although both nitroprusside and hydralazine inhibited norepinephrine-induced uterine artery contraction, nitroprusside had a greater potency compared to hydralazine in producing direct vasodilation of the uterine arteries from pregnant humans.

Labetalol

Labetalol is a combined α- and β-adrenergic blocking agent. It is used orally to decrease blood pressure in preeclamptic women (122). It is also used intravenously to rapidly decrease blood pressure in severely preeclamptic women and to attenuate the hemodynamic response to tracheal intubation (123). Intravenously administered, labetalol does not alter uterine blood flow in preeclamptic women at rest (124), nor does it alter placental perfusion in pregnant hypertensive rats (125). In the near-term pregnant ewe, intravenous-bolus administration of labetalol ameliorated the effects of increased circulating norepinephrine on maternal arterial pressure and uterine blood flow and produced less adrenergic blockade in the fetus than in the mother (126).

■ CALCIUM CHANNEL BLOCKING DRUGS

Calcium channel blocking drugs are potentially useful in obstetrics. They produce arteriolar vasodilation and may be effective agents in the management of preeclampsia. They slow atrioventricular conduction and may have a role in maternal and fetal supraventricular tachyarrhythmias. In addition, they inhibit uterine contractility and thus may be useful in the treatment of preterm labor.

Murad et al. (127) studied the hemodynamic effects of verapamil in the awake pregnant ewe. Verapamil (0.2 mg/kg) administered intravenously over 3 minutes resulted in a variety of maternal cardiovascular changes: a transient (2 to 5 minutes) decrease in systolic, diastolic, and mean blood pressures; and increase in central venous, mean pulmonary artery, and pulmonary capillary wedge pressures. These results are consistent with the negative inotropic and peripheral vasodilating effects of verapamil. Cardiac output, systemic peripheral vascular resistance, and pulmonary vascular resistance were unaffected. Uterine blood flow decreased by 25% at 2 minutes, then remained slightly below control levels for 30 minutes after drug injection. Thus, the effects of verapamil on uterine blood flow suggest that the drug should be used with caution in cases of uteroplacental insufficiency.

Studies of nicardipine in animals (128) have shown that these drugs decrease uteroplacental blood flow. On the other hand, studies in humans using Doppler ultrasound have shown that

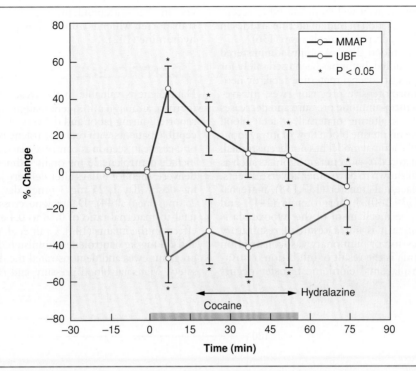

FIGURE 2-19 Effect of hydralazine therapy on cocaine-induced maternal hypertension. Percentage change in maternal mean arterial pressure (*MMAP*) and uterine blood flow (*UBF*) during cocaine administration and hydralazine therapy (n = 10). The arrow represents the time of hydralazine treatment. Both drugs were discontinued at 55 minutes. Values are expressed as ± SD. Changes are compared to baseline values with significance noted (*asterisk = p* <05). Reprinted with permission from: Vertommen JD, Hughes SC, Rosen MA, et al. Hydralazine does not restore uterine blood flow during cocaine-induced hypertension in the pregnant ewe. *Anesthesiology* 1992;76:580–587.

short-term oral administration does not significantly alter uteroplacental circulation (129). Nifedipine has been increasingly used for management of preterm labor (130).

■ MAGNESIUM SULFATE

Since its first use in obstetrics reported in 1925, magnesium sulfate has been used parenterally as an adjunct in the management of certain hypertensive diseases of pregnancy, especially preeclampsia and eclampsia. Its effects on the central and peripheral nervous systems and on neuromuscular transmission are discussed in Chapters 16 and 17. Its action on the maternal and fetal cardiovascular systems and uteroplacental circulation has been investigated in pregnant normotensive and hypertensive ewes (131).

Magnesium sulfate was administered to the mother in amounts sufficient to produce a constant serum concentration of 5 to 12 mEq/L in a study by Dandavino et al. (131) and 5 to 7 mEq/L in a study by Krames et al. (132). Dandavino et al. found that magnesium sulfate produced a fall in the systemic arterial blood pressure in both hypertensive and normotensive animals. However, this effect was transient, lasting less than 10 minutes. The uteroplacental blood flow increased by about 10%. Administration of high doses of magnesium sulfate (a 4 g bolus injection followed by a 2 to 4 g/h infusion) produced an initial and transitory decrease of maternal arterial pressure that was greater in the hypertensive than in the normotensive animals. However, 5 to 10 minutes after the start of the infusion, the mean arterial pressure in both groups had returned to control values. The uteroplacental blood flow increased by an average of 13.5% in the normotensive and 7.7% in the hypertensive animals. Krames

et al. found that magnesium sulfate produced a decrease in mean arterial blood pressure of 7% with a 7% rise in uterine vascular conductance, thereby resulting in no change in uterine blood flow.

The results of these studies suggest that magnesium sulfate has only a mild and transient effect on maternal arterial pressure and uterine blood flow.

■ INTRASPINAL OPIOIDS

Epidural opioids are widely used for the treatment of labor pain. Studying pregnant ewes near term, Rosen et al. (133) administered 20 mg morphine into the epidural space. These investigators found no significant changes in uterine blood flow nor, indeed, in any maternal or fetal cardiovascular or acid–base variable during a 2-hour study period. Craft et al. (134) confirmed these findings. They found no significant deleterious effects on uterine blood flow or maternal or fetal hemodynamic or acid–base parameters following administration to the awake pregnant ewe of 50, 75, or 100 μg fentanyl (135) or 10 or 20 μg sufentanil (Craft JB Jr, unpublished data). However, intrathecal opioids may cause acute hypotension in 10% to 15% of parturients and this could decrease uterine blood flow if untreated (see Chapter 9). Hypotension is typically not seen in non-catecholamine elevated states (e.g., pain).

■ CLONIDINE

Clonidine is used orally as an antihypertensive agent, intravenously to rapidly control hypertensive emergencies, and epidurally to produce analgesia by an opiate-independent mechanism. It acts primarily by stimulation of α_2-adrenergic receptors, although in high concentrations it will stimulate other receptor subtypes. It causes constriction of human uterine arteries in vitro by a mixed α_1- and α_2-adrenergic mechanism (136).

The effects on uterine blood flow of orally administered clonidine have not been studied, but it has been used safely for many years without apparent adverse maternal, fetal, or neonatal effects (137). In normotensive pregnant ewes, intravenous clonidine increases intra-amniotic pressure and decreases uterine blood flow without altering maternal or fetal blood pressure (138). The effect on uterine blood flow of intravenous clonidine in a hypertensive animal model has not been studied.

Intravenously administered α_2-adrenergic agonists such as clonidine have also been shown to have other adverse effects. These include rapid placental transfer (137,138), maternal and fetal hypoxemia (139,140), hyperglycemia (141), and decreased heart rate. The mechanism of the hypoxemia is not well understood since it is not a result of respiratory or cardiovascular depression or pulmonary vasoconstriction (140). The hyperglycemia is the result of inhibition of insulin release (141). Transplacental clonidine transfer occurs

via an Na^+-independent, but H^+-dependent transporter transporter, which is inhibited by cationic drugs like diphenhydramine (142).

■ DANTROLENE

Dantrolene is valuable in the treatment of malignant hyperthermia, although infrequent malignant hyperthermia has been reported during labor and delivery (143). Pretreatment of susceptible patients with oral dantrolene before induction of labor or a cesarean section is controversial. Recommended regimens include dantrolene 25 mg orally 4 times a day for 5 days before delivery, then for 3 days after delivery in progressively decreasing doses (day 1, 25 mg 3 times; day 2, 25 mg twice; day 3, 25 mg once) (144). Dantrolene crosses the placenta with a fetal-to-maternal ratio of 0.18 to 0.4 and no apparent adverse effects in the infants (144). Craft et al. (145) studied 1.2 mg/kg and 2.4 mg/kg dantrolene administered intravenously to awake pregnant ewes and demonstrated the drug's maternal and fetal safety. Maternal blood pressure and cardiac output increased

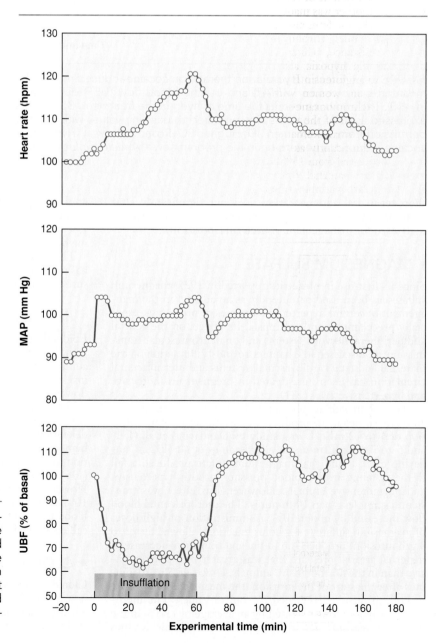

FIGURE 2-20 The effect of abdominal carbon dioxide insufflation on ewe hemodynamics, including uterine blood flow. From: Uemura K, McClaine RJ, de la Fuente SG, et al. Maternal insufflation during the second trimester equivalent produces hypercapnia, acidosis, and prolonged hypoxia in fetal sheep. *Anesthesiology* 2004;101:1332–1338.

slightly, but no significant changes were observed in maternal heart rate, central venous pressure, or uterine blood flow. Fetal heart rate decreased by 25% at 3 minutes but returned to normal at 10 minutes. No clinically significant changes in maternal or fetal acid–base status were noted.

■ RESPIRATORY GASES

Contrary to earlier beliefs, *moderate* hypoxia, hypercapnia, and hypocapnia do not affect uteroplacental blood flow (146). On the other hand, marked changes in respiratory gases decrease placental perfusion. Dilts et al. (147) measured uterine blood flow in pregnant sheep during severe maternal hypoxia induced by ventilating the lungs with 6% or 12% oxygen gas mixtures. When the lungs were ventilated with a gas mixture containing 6% oxygen, there was an increase in cardiac output and a decrease in maternal systemic vascular resistance. Uteroplacental vascular resistance increased, and uterine blood flow decreased markedly. Milder hypoxia induced with 12% oxygen produced changes that were qualitatively smaller. These investigators attributed these hemodynamic changes to the enhanced output of catecholamines induced by hypoxia. When the mother was made hypoxic by reducing arterial Po_2 to 40 mm Hg, the fetus also became hypoxic.

In a rat model, chronic hypoxia increased fetoplacental vascular resistance, which was unresponsive to nitroprusside. Chronic hypoxia also increased the vasoconstrictor response to angiotensin II and acute hypoxic episodes (148). Placentas from women with IUGR showed an increased response to thromboxane-induced contractions with hypoxia and involvement of the voltage-dependent potassium channel (149). In vitro, human placental fetal arterial pressure increased significantly as the perfused placental tissue had oxygen decreased from 15% to 0% (150).

Effects of maternal *hypercapnia* on the uteroplacental circulation are variable ranging from an increase (151), decrease (152), or no change. Walker et al. (153), using chronic unanesthetized sheep preparations, found that by increasing the arterial Pco_2 to 60 mm Hg, uterine blood flow increased. Mean arterial pressure rose, while uterine vascular resistance was unchanged. However, at $Paco_2$ levels above 60 mm Hg, uterine vascular resistance increased progressively and uterine blood flow fell despite further increases in mean arterial pressure. In second trimester sheep, pneumoperitoneum with CO_2 produced a decrease in uterine blood flow by 30%, increased maternal $Paco_2$, decreased maternal pH and also produced fetal decreases in heart rate, MAP, oxygen saturation, and pH with an increased $Paco_2$ (154) (see Fig. 2-20).

Maternal *hypocapnia* is a frequent phenomenon in pregnant women. It may occur spontaneously as a result of painful uterine contractions, anxiety, and apprehension during labor, or improperly performed Lamaze breathing technique. Controlled ventilation during anesthesia may also accidentally produce severe maternal alkalemia. Controversy still exists regarding its effects on the fetus and the uteroplacental circulation. Some investigators have reported that marked hyperventilation ($Paco_2$ of 17 mm Hg or less) causes uteroplacental vasoconstriction, decreases uteroplacental blood flow, and induces fetal hypoxia, acidosis, and neonatal depression (155). Others have denied that maternal hyperventilation, even of marked degree, is harmful to the fetus. These investigators found minimal changes in the acid–base status of the fetus and no significant effect on uteroplacental blood flow (30,156). Levinson et al. (150) studied changes in uterine blood flow and fetal oxygenation in unanesthetized pregnant ewes during mechanical hyperventilation. In order to evaluate separately the effects of maternal hypocapnia and positive-pressure ventilation, carbon dioxide was added to the inspired air during mechanical hyperventilation to produce normocapnia and hypercapnia. Uterine blood flow decreased by approximately 25% during all hyperventilation periods (Fig. 2-21). Since the

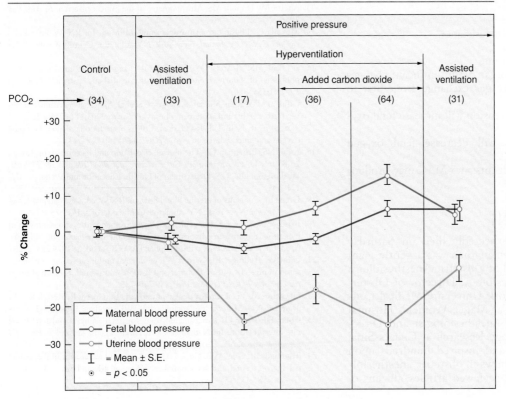

FIGURE 2-21 Changes from control values in mean maternal and fetal arterial blood pressure and uterine blood flow during five periods of positive-pressure ventilation. Mean maternal $Paco_2$ during each period is indicated at the *top* of the figure. Reprinted with permission from: Levinson G, Shnider SM, DeLorimier AA, et al. Effects of maternal hyperventilation on uterine blood flow and fetal oxygenation and acid–base status. *Anesthesiology* 1974;40:340–347.

reduction in uterine blood flow was unrelated to changes in maternal $Paco_2$ (range: 17 to 64 mm Hg) or pH (range: 7.74 to 7.24), the decrease probably was caused by the mechanical effect of positive-pressure ventilation.

Metabolic alkalosis may also be detrimental to the fetus as a result of decreased uteroplacental blood flow and displacement of the maternal oxygen–hemoglobin dissociation curve to the left, resulting in increased affinity of maternal hemoglobin for oxygen and decreased release at the placenta (157,158). In the pregnant ewe, Cosmi (43) found that maternal metabolic alkalosis induced by intravenous infusion of trishydroxymethylaminomethane caused maternal bradycardia and hypotension, decreased uterine blood flow, and induced fetal hypoxia and acidosis. Ralston et al. (157) produced maternal alkalemia with the infusion of sodium bicarbonate in normal pregnant ewes and found a 16% reduction in uterine blood flow with a concomitant decrease in fetal oxygenation and pH. In contrast, in Cosmi's study (43), the infusion of small doses of sodium bicarbonate (e.g., 100 mEq over 12 minutes) to the acidotic ewe did not alter uterine blood flow.

SUMMARY

Intravenous induction agents, inhalation and local anesthetics, endogenous and exogenous catecholamines and vasopressors, antihypertensive agents and magnesium sulfate, respiratory gases, and metabolic alkalosis can all alter uterine blood flow. Their net effect on uterine blood flow ultimately depends on how these agents alter uterine perfusion pressure relative to uterine vascular resistance. The effects of anesthetic drugs are summarized in Table 2-4.

KEY POINTS

- Placental circulation is not autoregulated.
- Factors which would reduce uteroplacental blood flow include:
  - Decreased blood pressure
  - Increased systemic vascular resistance
  - Decreased cardiac output
  - Supine hypotensive syndrome
- The placenta is a dynamic organ, with significant changes in structure and respiratory gas exchange from first to third trimesters.
- Increased maternal oxygen tension will increase fetal oxygen stores.
- Maternal hyperventilation will decrease fetal oxygen uptake.
- Use of potent inhalational agents >1.5 MAC may produce fetal cardiac depression.

ACKNOWLEDGMENT

Dr. Sivam Ramanathan unexpectedly died on Saturday night, May 26, 2012. Dr. Ramanathan was a gentle giant of a man, beloved in the field of Obstetric Anesthesiology. He was Professor of Anesthesiology, Director of Obstetric Anesthesiology at New York University Medical Center, Chief of Anesthesiology at Magee Women's Hospital in Pittsburg, and Attending Anesthesiologist and Director of Obstetric Anesthesiology Research at Cedars-Sinai Medical Center. He taught and inspired hundreds upon hundreds of residents and fellows in obstetric anesthesiology, authored over 120 peer-reviewed articles, dozens of

textbook chapters, as well as solely authored the textbook, Obstetric Anesthesia in 1988. Dr. Ramanathan won several teaching awards, including the National Society for Obstetric Anesthesia and Perinatology Teacher of the Year, and the prestigious Nils Lofgren Award for Outstanding Service to Obstetric Anesthesia.

Dr. Ramanathan loved to travel, enjoyed wines, and was lovingly devoted to and proud of his wife Sita and their daughter Radha and son Kumar. Sivam will always be remembered for his great sense of humor, phenomenal knowledge, willingness to help, and his ability to mentor and inspire others.

REFERENCES

1. Tuuli MG, Longtine MS, Nelson DM. Review: Oxygen and trophoblast biology—A source of controversy. *Placenta* 2011;32(suppl 2):109–118.
2. Burton GJ. Oxygen, the Janus gas; its effects on human placental development and function. *J Anat* 2009;215:27–35.
3. Pringle KG, Kind KL, Sferruzzi-Perri AN, et al. Beyond oxygen: complex regulation and activity of hypoxia inducible factors in pregnancy. *Hum Reprod Update* 2010;16:415–431.
4. Mayhew TM. Allometric studies on growth and development of the human placenta: growth of tissue compartments and diffusive conductances in relation to placental volume and fetal mass. *J Anat* 2006;208:785–794.
5. Metcalfe J, Bartels H, Moll W. Gas exchange in the pregnant uterus. *Physiol Rev* 1967;47:782–838.
6. Longo L. Placental transfer mechanisms: An overview. *Obstet Gynecol Annu* 1972;1:103–138.
7. Ueki R, Tatara T, Kariya N, et al. Comparison of placental transfer of local anesthetics in perfusates with different pH values in a human cotyledon model. *J Anesth* 2009;23:526–529.
8. Vahakangas K, Myllynen P. Drug transporters in the human blood-placental barrier. *Br J Pharmacol* 2009;158:665–678.
9. Muller J, Born I, Neubert RH, et al. Apical uptake of choline and cationic drugs in epithelial cell lines derived from human placenta. *Placenta* 2005;26:183–189.
10. Schneider H. In vitro perfusion of human placental tissue/International workshop on in vitro perfusion of human placental tissue. *Gynecology and Obstetrics:* Karger Basel, 1985.
11. Syme MR, Paxton JW, Keelan JA. Drug transfer and metabolism by the human placenta. *Clin Pharmacokinet* 2004;43:487–514.
12. Krishna BR, Zakowski MI, Grant GJ. Sufentanil transfer in the human placenta during in vitro perfusion. *Can J Anaesth* 1997;44:996–1001.
13. Aherne W, Dunnill MS. Morphometry of the human placenta. *Br Med Bull* 1966;22:5–8.
14. Meschia G. Physiology of transplacental diffusion. In: RN W, ed. *Obstetrics and Gynecology Annual.* New York, NY: Appleton-Century-Crofts; 1976: 21–38.
15. al-Okail MS, al-Attas OS. Histological changes in placental syncytiotrophoblasts of poorly controlled gestational diabetic patients. *Endocr J* 1994;41:355–360.
16. Gillman MW, Rifas-Shiman S, Berkey CS, et al. Maternal gestational diabetes, birth weight, and adolescent obesity. *Pediatrics* 2003;111:e221–e226.
17. Taricco E, Radaelli T, Rossi G, et al. Effects of gestational diabetes on fetal oxygen and glucose levels in vivo. *BJOG* 2009;116:1729–1735.
18. Assali NS, Brinkman CI. The uterine circulation and its control. In: Longo L, Bartels H, eds. *Respiratory Gas Exchange and Blood Flow in the Placenta.* Washington, DC: U.S. Department of Health, Education and Welfare; 1972: 121–141.
19. Greiss FJ. Concepts of uterine blood flow. In: RN W, ed. *Obstetrics and Gynecology Annual.* New York, NY: Appleton-Century-Crofts; 1973:55–83.
20. Beischer N, Drew J, JM K, et al. The effect of rest and intravenous infusion of hypertonic dextrose on subnormal estriol excretion in pregnancy. In: Milunsky A, ed. *Clinics in Perinatology.* Philadelphia, PA: WB Saunders; 1974:253–272.
21. Gill RW, Trudinger BJ, Garrett WJ, et al. Fetal umbilical venous flow measured in utero by pulsed Doppler and B-mode ultrasound. I. Normal pregnancies. *Am J Obstet Gynecol* 1981;139:720–725.
22. Heymann M. Fetal cardiovascular physiology. In: Creasy R, Resnik R, eds. *Maternal-Fetal Medicine.* Philadelphia, PA: WB Saunders; 1984:259–273.
23. Court DJ, Parer JT. Experimental studies in fetal asphyxia and fetal heart rate interpretation. In: Nathanielsz PW, Parer JT, eds. *Research in Perinatal Medicine.* Ithaca, NY: Perinatology Press; 1985:114–164.
24. Trudinger BJ, Giles WB, Cook CM. Flow velocity waveforms in the maternal uteroplacental and fetal umbilical placental circulations. *Am J Obstet Gynecol* 1985;152:155–163.

25. Fleischer A, Schulman H, Farmakides G, et al. Umbilical artery velocity waveforms and intrauterine growth retardation. *Am J Obstet Gynecol.* 1985;151: 502–505.

26. Marx GF, Patel S, Berman JA, et al. Umbilical blood flow velocity waveforms in different maternal positions and with epidural analgesia. *Obstet Gynecol* 1986;68:61–64.

27. Youngstrom P VJ, Kanaan C, Wilson B. Umbilical artery flow velocity waveforms before and during epidural anesthesia for cesarean section. *Anesthesiology* 1988;69:A704.

28. Espinoza J, Kusanovic JP, Bahado-Singh R, et al. Should bilateral uterine artery notching be used in the risk assessment for preeclampsia, small-for-gestational-age, and gestational hypertension? *J Ultrasound Med* 2010:29: 1103–1115.

29. Myers RE. Two patterns of perinatal brain damage and their conditions of occurrence. *Am J Obstet Gynecol* 1972;112:246–276.

30. Parer JT, Behrman RE. The influence of uterine blood flow on the acid-base status of the rhesus monkey. *Am J Obstet Gynecol* 1970;107:1241–1249.

31. Wilkening R, Meschia G. Fetal oxygen uptake, oxygenation and acid-base balance as a function of uterine blood flow. *Am J Physiol* 1983;24: H749–H755.

32. Haezell AE, Brown M, Worton SA, et al. Review: The effects of oxygen on normal and pre-eclamptic placental tissue – insights from metabolomics. *Placenta* 2010;32(suppl 2):S119–S124.

33. Kwasiborski PJ, Kowalczyk P, Zielinski J, et al. [Role of hemoglobin affinity to oxygen in adaptation to hypoxemia]. *Pol Merkur Lekarski* 2010;28:260–264.

34. Rekonen A, Luotola H, Pitkanen M, et al. Measurement of intervillous and myometrial blood flow by an intravenous 133Xe method. *Br J Obstet Gynaecol* 1976;83:723–728.

35. Jouppila P, Jouppila R, Barinoff T, et al. Placental blood flow during caesarean section performed under subarachnoid blockade. *Br J Anaesth* 1984;56:1379–1383.

36. Palmer S, Zamudio S, Coffin C, et al. Quantitative estimation of human artery blood flow redistribution in pregnancy. *Obstet Gynecol* 1992;80:1000–1006.

37. McParland P, Pearce JM. Doppler blood flow in pregnancy. *Placenta* 1988;9:427–450.

38. Palahniuk RJ, Cumming M. Foetal deterioration following thiopentone-nitrous oxide anaesthesia in the pregnant ewe. *Can Anaesth Soc J* 1977;24: 361–370.

39. Shnider SM, Wright RG, Levinson G, et al. Plasma norepinephrine and uterine blood flow changes during endotracheal intubation and general anesthesia in the pregnant ewe. Abstracts of Scientific Papers: American Society of Anesthesiologists 1978;115.

40. Alon E, Ball RH, Gillie MH, et al. Effects of propofol and thiopental on maternal and fetal cardiovascular and acid-base variables in the pregnant ewe. *Anesthesiology* 1993;78:562–576.

41. Jouppila P, Kuikka J, Jouppila R, et al. Effect of induction of general anesthesia for cesarean section on intervillous blood flow. *Acta Obstet Gynecol Scand* 1979;58:249–253.

42. Mofid M, Brinkman CR 3rd, Assali NS. Effects of diazepam on uteroplacental and fetal hemodynamics and metabolism. *Obstet Gynecol* 1973;41:364–368.

43. Cosmi EV. Fetal homeostasis. In: Scarpelli E, Auld P, eds. *Pulmonary Physiology of the Fetus, Newborn and Child.* Philadelphia, PA: Lea & Febiger; 1975:61.

44. Greiss FC Jr., Van W. Effects of Sympathomimetic drugs and angiotensin on the uterine vascular bed. *Obstet Gynecol* 1964;23:925–930.

45. Ralston DH, Shnider SM, DeLorimier AA. Effects of equipotent ephedrine, metaraminol, mephentermine, and methoxamine on uterine blood flow in the pregnant ewe. *Anesthesiology* 1974;40:354–370.

46. Levinson G, Shnider SM, Gildea JE, et al. Maternal and foetal cardiovascular and acid-base changes during ketamine anaesthesia in pregnant ewes. *Br J Anaesth* 1973;45:1111–1115.

47. Eng M, Berges PU, Bonica JJ. The effects of ketamine on uterine blood flow in the monkey. Abstracts of Scientific Papers: Society for Gynecological Investigation 1973;48.

48. Craft JB Jr., Coaldrake LA, Yonekura ML, et al. Ketamine, catecholamines, and uterine tone in pregnant ewes. *Am J Obstet Gynecol* 1983;146:429–434.

49. Cosmi E. Effetti della ketamina sulla madre e sul feto. Studio sperimentale e clinico. *Minerva Anestesiol* 1977;49:19.

50. Galloon S. Ketamine for obstetric delivery. *Anesthesiology* 1976;44:522–524.

51. Fresno L, Andaluz A, Moll X, et al. The effects on maternal and fetal cardiovascular and acid-base variables after the administration of etomidate in the pregnant ewe. *Vet J* 2008;177:94–103.

52. Fresno L, Andaluz A, Moll X, et al. Placental transfer of etomidate in pregnant ewes after an intravenous bolus dose and continuous infusion. *Vet J* 2008;175:395–402.

53. Edwin SB, Walker PL. Controversies surrounding the use of etomidate for rapid sequence intubation in patients with suspected sepsis. *Ann Pharmacother* 2010;44:1307–1313.

54. Ala-Kokko TI, Pienimaki P, Lampela E, et al. Transfer of clonidine and dexmedetomidine across the isolated perfused human placenta. *Acta Anaesthesiol Scand* 1997;41:313–319.

55. Cosmi EV, Marx GF. The effect of anesthesia on the acid-base status of the fetus. *Anesthesiology* 1969;30:238–242.

56. Allard E, Guimond C.. Líhalothane en obstetrique. *Can Anaesth Soc J* 1964;11:83–87.

57. Marx GF, Mateo CV. Effects of different oxygen concentrations during general anaesthesia for elective caesarean section. *Can Anaesth Soc J* 1971;18:587–593.

58. Palahniuk RJ, Shnider SM. Maternal and fetal cardiovascular and acid-base changes during halothane and isoflurane anesthesia in the pregnant ewe. *Anesthesiology* 1974;41:462–472.

59. Carenza I, Cosmi EV. Analgo-anetesia in travaglio e nel parto: Valutazione des metosi e del farmaci. 58th Congress of the Italian Society of Obstetrics and Gynecology 1977;286.

60. Eng M, Bonica JJ, Akamatsu TJ, et al. Maternal and fetal responses to halothane in pregnant monkeys. *Acta Anaesthesiol Scand* 1975;19:154–158.

61. Yoo KY, Lee JC, Yoon MH, et al. The effects of volatile anesthetics on spontaneous contractility of isolated human pregnant uterine muscle: a comparison among sevoflurane, desflurane, isoflurane, and halothane. *Anesth Analg* 2006;103:443–447, table of contents.

62. Boat A, Mahmoud M, Michelfelder EC, et al. Supplementing desflurane with intravenous anesthesia reduces fetal cardiac dysfunction during open fetal surgery. *Paediatr Anaesth* 2010;20:748–756.

63. Farragher R, Maharaj CH, Higgins BD, et al. Sevoflurane and the feto-placental vasculature: The role of nitric oxide and vasoactive eicosanoids. *Anesth Analg* 2008;107:171–177.

64. Gibbs CP, Noel SC. Human uterine artery responses to lidocaine. *Am J Obstet Gynecol* 1976;126:313–315.

65. Greiss FC Jr., Still JG, Anderson SG. Effects of local anesthetic agents on the uterine vasculatures and myometrium. *Am J Obstet Gynecol* 1976;124: 889–899.

66. Fishburne J, Hopkinson R, Greiss F Jr. Responses of gravid uterine vasculature to arterial levels of local anesthetic agents. *Abstracts of Scientific Papers. Society for Obstetric Anesthesia and Perinatology;* 1977:37.

67. Morishima HO, Gutsche B, Keenaghan J, et al. The effect of lidocaine-induced maternal convulsions on the fetal lamb. *Abstracts of Scientific Papers.* New Orleans, LA: *American Society of Anesthesiologists;* 1977:293.

68. Biehl D, Shnider SM, Levinson G, et al. The direct effects of circulating lidocaine on uterine blood flow and foetal well-being in the pregnant ewe. *Can Anaesth Soc J* 1977;24:445–451.

69. Chestnut DH, Weiner CP, Martin JG, et al. Effect of intravenous epinephrine on uterine artery blood flow velocity in the pregnant guinea pig. *Anesthesiology* 1986;65:633–636.

70. Alahuhta S, Rasanen J, Jouppila P, et al. The effects of epidural ropivacaine and bupivacaine for cesarean section on uteroplacental and fetal circulation. *Anesthesiology* 1995;83:23–32.

71. Woods JR Jr., Plessinger MA, Clark KE. Effect of cocaine on uterine blood flow and fetal oxygenation. *JAMA* 1987;257:957–961.

72. Greiss FC, Crandell DL. Therapy for hypotension induced by spinal anesthesia during pregnancy: observations on gravid ewes. *JAMA* 1965;191:793–796.

73. Wallis KL, Shnider SM, Hicks JS, et al. Epidural anesthesia in the normotensive pregnant ewe: Effects on uterine blood flow and fetal acid-base status. *Anesthesiology* 1976;44:481–487.

74. Jouppila R, Jouppila P, Kuikka J, et al. Placental blood flow during caesarean section under lumbar extradural analgesia. *Br J Anaesth* 1978;50:275–279.

75. Hollmen AI, Jouppila R, Jouppila P, et al. Effect of extradural analgesia using bupivacaine and 2-chloroprocaine on intervillous blood flow during normal labour. *Br J Anaesth* 1982;54:837–842.

76. Jouppila P, Jouppila R, Hollmen A, et al. Lumbar epidural analgesia to improve intervillous blood flow during labor in severe preeclampsia. *Obstet Gynecol* 1982;59:158–161.

77. Jouppila R, Jouppila P, Hollmen A, et al. Effect of segmental extradural analgesia on placental blood flow during normal labour. *Br J Anaesth* 1978;50:563–567.

78. Baumann H, Alon E, Atanassoff P, et al. Effect of epidural anesthesia for cesarean delivery on maternal femoral arterial and venous, uteroplacental, and umbilical blood flow velocities and waveforms. *Obstet Gynecol* 1990;75:194–198.

79. Giles WB, Lah FX, Trudinger BJ. The effect of epidural anaesthesia for caesarean section on maternal uterine and fetal umbilical artery blood flow velocity waveforms. *Br J Obstet Gynaecol* 1987;94:55–59.

80. Barton MD, Killam AP, Meschia G. Response of ovine uterine blood flow to epinephrine and norepinephrine. *Proc Soc Exp Biol Med* 1974;145:996–1003.

81. Hood DD, Dewan DM, James FM 3rd. Maternal and fetal effects of epinephrine in gravid ewes. *Anesthesiology* 1986;64:610–613.

82. Bonica JJ, Berges PU, Morikawa K, et al. Circulatory effects of peridural block effects of epinephrine. *Anesthesiology* 1972;34:514–522.

83. Rosenfeld CR, Barton MD, Meschia G. Effects of epinephrine on distribution of blood flow in the pregnant ewe. *Am J Obstet Gynecol* 1976;124:156–163.

84. Albright GA, Jouppila R, Hollmen AI, et al. Epinephrine does not alter human intervillous blood flow during epidural anesthesia. *Anesthesiology* 1981;54:131–135.

85. Levinson G, Shnider SM, Krames E, et al. Epidural anesthesia for cesarean section: Effects of epinephrine in the local anesthetic solution. *Abstracts of Scientific Papers.* Chicago, IL: American Society of Anesthesiologists; 1975:285.

86. Ramanathan S, Desai NS, Zakowski M. Systemic vascular uptake of epinephrine from the lumbar epidural space in parturients. *Reg Anesth* 1995;20:199–205.

87. Cascio M, Pygon B, Bernett C, et al. Labour analgesia with intrathecal fentanyl decreases maternal stress. *Can J Anaesth* 1997;44:605–609.

88. Myers RE. Maternal psychological stress and fetal asphyxia: a study in the monkey. *Am J Obstet Gynecol* 1975;122:47–59.

89. Shnider SM, Wright RG, Levinson G, et al. Uterine blood flow and plasma norepinephrine changes during maternal stress in the pregnant ewe. *Anesthesiology* 1979;50:524–527.

90. Martin CB Jr., Gingerich B. Uteroplacental physiology. *JOGN Nurs* 1976;5:16s–25s.

91. Lederman RP, Lederman E, Work B Jr., et al. Anxiety and epinephrine in multiparous women in labor: relationship to duration of labor and fetal heart rate pattern. *Am J Obstet Gynecol* 1985;153:870–877.

92. Hilmert CJ, Schetter CD, Dominguez TP, et al. Stress and blood pressure during pregnancy: racial differences and associations with birthweight. *Psychosom Med* 2008;70:57–64.

93. Hobel C, Culhane J. Role of psychosocial and nutritional stress on poor pregnancy outcome. *J Nutr* 2003;133:1709S–1717S.

94. Eng M, Berges PU, Ueland K, et al. The effects of methoxamine and ephedrine in normotensive pregnant primates. *Anesthesiology* 1971;35:354–360.

95. Shnider SM, DeLorimier AA, Asling JH, et al. Vasopressors in obstetrics. II. Fetal hazards of methoxamine administration during obstetric spinal anesthesia. *Am J Obstet Gynecol* 1970;106:680–686.

96. Eng M, Berges PU, Parer JT, et al. Spinal anesthesia and ephedrine in pregnant monkeys. *Am J Obstet Gynecol* 1973;115:1095–1099.

97. Shnider SM, de Lorimier AA, Steffenson JL. Vasopressors in obstetrics. 3. Fetal effects of metaraminol infusion during obstetric spinal hypotension. *Am J Obstet Gynecol* 1970;108:1017–1022.

98. Ramanathan S, Grant GJ. Vasopressor therapy for hypotension due to epidural anesthesia for cesarean section. *Acta Anaesthesiol Scand* 1988;32:559–565.

99. Moran DH PM, Bader AM, Datta S. Phenylephrine in treating maternal hypotension secondary to spinal anesthesia. *Anesthesiology* 1989;71:A857.

100. Tong C, Eisenach JC. The vascular mechanism of ephedrine's beneficial effect on uterine perfusion during pregnancy. *Anesthesiology* 1992;76:792–798.

101. Alahuhta S, Rasanen J, Jouppila P, et al. Ephedrine and phenylephrine for avoiding maternal hypotension due to spinal anaesthesia for caesarean section. Effects on uteroplacental and fetal haemodynamics. *Int J Obstet Anesth* 1992;1:129–134.

102. Erkinaro T, Makikallio K, Acharya G, et al. Divergent effects of ephedrine and phenylephrine on cardiovascular hemodynamics of near-term fetal sheep exposed to hypoxemia and maternal hypotension. *Acta Anaesthesiol Scand* 2007;51:922–928.

103. Erkinaro T, Makikallio K, Kavasmaa T, et al. Effects of ephedrine and phenylephrine on uterine and placental circulations and fetal outcome following fetal hypoxaemia and epidural-induced hypotension in a sheep model. *Br J Anaesth* 2004;93:825–832.

104. Ngan Kee WD, Khaw KS, Tan PE, et al. Placental transfer and fetal metabolic effects of phenylephrine and ephedrine during spinal anesthesia for cesarean delivery. *Anesthesiology* 2009;111:506–512.

105. Callender K, Levinson G, Shnider SM, et al. Dopamine administration in the normotensive pregnant ewe. *Obstet Gynecol* 1978;51:586–589.

106. Rolbin SH, Levinson G, Shnider SM, et al. Dopamine treatment of spinal hypotension decreases uterine blood flow in the pregnant ewe. *Anesthesiology* 1979;51:37–40.

107. Cabalum T, Zugaib M, Lieb S, et al. Effect of dopamine on hypotension induced by spinal anesthesia. *Am J Obstet Gynecol* 1979;133:630–634.

108. Chestnut DH, Weiner CP, Wang JP, et al. The effect of ephedrine upon uterine artery blood flow velocity in the pregnant guinea pig subjected to terbutaline infusion and acute hemorrhage. *Anesthesiology* 1987;66:508–512.

109. Brinkman CI, Assali N. Uteroplacental hemodynamic response to antihypertensive drugs in hypertensive pregnant sheep. In: Lindheimer M, Katz A, Zuspan F, eds. *Hypertension in Pregnancy.* New York, NY: John Wiley; 1976:363–375.

110. Ring G, Krames E, Shnider SM, et al. Comparison of nitroprusside and hydralazine in hypertensive pregnant ewes. *Obstet Gynecol* 1977;50:598–602.

111. Vertommen JD, Hughes SC, Rosen MA, et al. Hydralazine does not restore uterine blood flow during cocaine-induced hypertension in the pregnant ewe. *Anesthesiology* 1992;76:580–587.

112. Jouppila P, Kirkinen P, Koivula A, et al. Effects of dihydralazine infusion on the fetoplacental blood flow and maternal prostanoids. *Obstet Gynecol* 1985;65:115–118.

113. Houlihan DD, Dennedy MC, Ravikumar N, et al. Anti-hypertensive therapy and the feto-placental circulation: effects on umbilical artery resistance. *J Perinat Med* 2004;32:315–319.

114. Rey E. Effects of methyldopa on umbilical and placental artery blood flow velocity waveforms. *Obstet Gynecol* 1992;80:783–787.

115. Khalil A, Harrington K, Muttukrishna S, et al. Effect of antihypertensive therapy with alpha-methyldopa on uterine artery Doppler in pregnancies with hypertensive disorders. *Ultrasound Obstet Gynecol* 2010;35:688–694.

116. Gunenc O, Cicek N, Gorkemli H, et al. The effect of methyldopa treatment on uterine, umbilical and fetal middle cerebral artery blood flows in preeclamptic patients. *Arch Gynecol Obstet* 2002;266:141–144.

117. Craft JB Jr., Co EG, Yonekura ML, et al. Nitroglycerin therapy for phenylephrine-induced hypertension in pregnant ewes. *Anesth Analg* 1980;59:494–499.

118. Bell E. Nitroglycerin and uterine relaxation. *Anesthesiology* 1996;85:683.

119. Kessin CHS, Rosen MA, Johnson JL, et al. Nitroglycerin improves decreased uterine blood flow in the pregnant ewe with cocaine-induced hypertension. *Anesthesiology* 1995;83:A937.

120. Styles M, Coleman AJ, Leary WP. Some hemodynamic effects of sodium nitroprusside. *Anesthesiology* 1973;38:173–176.

121. Nelson SH, Suresh MS. Comparison of nitroprusside and hydralazine in isolated uterine arteries from pregnant and nonpregnant patients. *Anesthesiology* 1988;68:541–547.

122. Pickles CJ, Symonds EM, Broughton Pipkin F. The fetal outcome in a randomized double-blind controlled trial of labetalol versus placebo in pregnancy-induced hypertension. *Br J Obstet Gynaecol* 1989;96:38–43.

123. Ramanathan J, Sibai BM, Mabie WC, et al. The use of labetalol for attenuation of the hypertensive response of endotracheal intubation in preeclampsia. *Am J Obstet Gynecol* 1988;159:650–654.

124. Jouppila P, Kirkinen P, Koivula A, et al. Labetalol does not alter the placental and fetal blood flow or maternal prostanoids in pre-eclampsia. *Br J Obstet Gynaecol* 1986;93:543–547.

125. Ahokas RA, Mabie WC, Sibai BM, et al. Labetalol does not decrease placental perfusion in the hypertensive term-pregnant rat. *Am J Obstet Gynecol* 1989;160:480–484.

126. Eisenach JC, Mandell G, Dewan DM. Maternal and fetal effects of labetalol in pregnant ewes. *Anesthesiology* 1991;74:292–297.

127. Murad SH, Tabsh KM, Shilyanski G, et al. Effects of verapamil on uterine blood flow and maternal cardiovascular function in the awake pregnant ewe. *Anesth Analg* 1985;64:7–10.

128. Lirette MHR, Katz M. Cardiovascular and uterine blood flow changes during nicardipine HCl tocolysis in the rabbit. *Obstet Gynecol* 1987;69:79–82.

129. Mari G, Kirshon B, Moise KJ Jr., et al. Doppler assessment of the fetal and uteroplacental circulation during nifedipine therapy for preterm labor. *Am J Obstet Gynecol* 1989;161:1514–1518.

130. Papatsonis DN, Kok JH, van Geijn HP, et al. Neonatal effects of nifedipine and ritodrine for preterm labor. *Obstet Gynecol* 2000;95:477–481.

131. Dandavino A, Woods JR Jr., Murayama K, et al. Circulatory effects of magnesium sulfate in normotensive and renal hypertensive pregnant sheep. *Am J Obstet Gynecol* 1977;127:769–774.

132. Krames E, Ring G, Wallis KL, et al. The effect of magnesium sulfate on uterine blood flow and fetal well-being in the pregnant ewe. *Abstracts of Scientific Papers.* Chicago, IL: American Society of Anesthesiologists; 1975:287.

133. Rosen MA HS, Curtis JD, Norton M, et al. Effects of epidural morphine on uterine blood flow and acid-base status in the pregnant ewe. *Anesthesiology* 1982;57:A383.

134. Craft JB Jr., Bolan JC, Coaldrake LA, et al. The maternal and fetal cardiovascular effects of epidural morphine in the sheep model. *Am J Obstet Gynecol* 1982;142:835–839.

135. Craft JB Jr., Robichaux AG, Kim HS, et al. The maternal and fetal cardiovascular effects of epidural fentanyl in the sheep model. *Am J Obstet Gynecol* 1984;148:1098–1104.

136. Ribeiro CA, Macedo TA. Pharmacological characterization of the postsynaptic alpha-adrenoceptors in human uterine artery. *J Pharm Pharmacol* 1986;38:600–605.

137. Huisjes HJ, Hadders-Algra M, Touwen BC. Is clonidine a behavioural teratogen in the human? *Early Hum Dev* 1986;14:43–48.

138. Eisenach JC, Castro MI, Dewan DM, et al. Intravenous clonidine hydrochloride toxicity in pregnant ewes. *Am J Obstet Gynecol* 1989;160:471–476.

139. Jansen CA, Lowe KC, Nathanielsz PW. The effects of xylazine on uterine activity, fetal and maternal oxygenation, cardiovascular function, and fetal breathing. *Am J Obstet Gynecol* 1984;148:386–390.

140. Eisenach JC. Intravenous clonidine produces hypoxemia by a peripheral alpha-2 adrenergic mechanism. *J Pharmacol Exp Ther* 1988;244:247–252.

141. Metz SA, Halter JB, Robertson RP. Induction of defective insulin secretion and impaired glucose tolerance by clonidine. Selective stimulation of metabolic alpha-adrenergic pathways. *Diabetes* 1978;27:554–562.

142. Muller J, Neubert R, Brandsch M. Transport of clonidine at cultured epithelial cells (JEG-3) of the human placenta. *Pharm Res* 2004;21:692–694.

143. Douglas MJ, McMorland GH. The anaesthetic management of the malignant hyperthermia susceptible parturient. *Can Anaesth Soc J* 1986;33:371–378.

144. Shime J, Gare D, Andrews J, et al. Dantrolene in pregnancy: lack of adverse effects on the fetus and newborn infant. *Am J Obstet Gynecol* 1988;159:831–834.

145. Craft JB Jr., Goldberg NH, Lim M, et al. Cardiovascular effects and placental passage of dantrolene in the maternal-fetal sheep model. *Anesthesiology* 1988;68:68–72.

146. Makowski EL, Hertz RH, Meschia G. Effects of acute maternal hypoxia and hyperoxia on the blood flow to the pregnant uterus. *Am J Obstet Gynecol* 1973;115:624–631.

147. Dilts PV Jr., Brinkman CR 3rd, Kirschbaum TH, et al. Uterine and systemic hemodynamic interrelationships and their response to hypoxia. *Am J Obstet Gynecol* 1969;103:138–157.

148. Jakoubek V, Bibova J, Herget J, et al. Chronic hypoxia increases fetoplacental vascular resistance and vasoconstrictor reactivity in the rat. *Am J Physiol Heart Circ Physiol* 2008;294:H1638–H1644.

149. Wareing M, Greenwood SL, Fyfe GK, et al. Reactivity of human placental chorionic plate vessels from pregnancies complicated by intrauterine growth restriction (IUGR). *Biol Reprod* 2006;75:518–523.

150. Ramasubramanian R, Johnson RF, Downing JW, et al. Hypoxemic fetoplacental vasoconstriction: a graduated response to reduced oxygen conditions in the human placenta. *Anesth Analg* 2006;103:439–442, table of contents.

151. Assali NS HL, Sehgal N. Hemodynamic changes in fetal lambs in utero in response to asphyxia, hypoxia and hypercapnia. *Circ Res* 1962;11:423–430.

152. Levinson G, Shnider SM, DeLorimier AA, et al. Effects of maternal hyperventilation on uterine blood flow and fetal oxygenation and acid-base status. *Anesthesiology* 1974;40:340–347.

153. Walker AM, Oakes GK, Ehrenkranz R, et al. Effects of hypercapnia on uterine and umbilical circulations in conscious pregnant sheep. *J Appl Physiol* 1976;41:727–733.

154. Uemura K, McClaine RJ, de la Fuente SG, et al. Maternal insufflation during the second trimester equivalent produces hypercapnia, acidosis, and prolonged hypoxia in fetal sheep. *Anesthesiology* 2004;101:1332–1338.

155. Morishima HO, Daniel S, Adamsons KJ, et al. Effects of positive pressure ventilation of the mother upon the acid-base state of the fetus. *Am J Obstet Gynecol* 1965;93:269–273.

156. Lumley J, Renou P, Newman W, et al. Hyperventilation in obstetrics. *Am J Obstet Gynecol* 1969;103:847–855.

157. Ralston DH, Shnider SM, DeLorimier AA. Uterine blood flow and fetal acid-base changes after bicarbonate administration to the pregnant ewe. *Anesthesiology* 1974;40:348–353.

158. Buss D, Bisgard E, Rawlings C, et al. Uteroplacental blood flow during alkalosis in the sheep. *Am J Physiol* 1975;228:1497–1500.

Placental Transfer of Drugs and Perinatal Pharmacology

David C. Campbell • Monica San Vicente

■ INTRODUCTION

Walter Channing, Professor of Obstetrics and Dean of the School of Medicine at Harvard, described one of the first reports of the effects of anesthesia on the neonate in 1847. Based upon his inability to smell ether at the cut ends of the umbilical cord, Dr. Channing suggested that anesthesia had negligible effects on the fetus (1). Sir John Snow, one of the founders of anesthesia, eventually brought this opinion into question. Sir Snow detected ether on exhalation of infants whose mothers had been exposed to ether. It was not until the 1850s that experimental evidence was generated to prove that drugs are able to cross the placenta (1). This quest for knowledge has continued to this day.

The placenta provides a vital link between the mother and the fetus. It plays the fundamental role of transferring nutrients and oxygen from the mother to the developing fetus. It also allows waste products and carbon dioxide to be removed from the fetus and returned to the mother. In addition, it plays a role in the synthesis of hormones that are important in maintaining a successful pregnancy.

The placenta was at one time considered to provide an impenetrable barrier of protection to the fetus against drugs administered to the mother. However, it has been shown that the majority of drugs given to the mother during pregnancy will enter the fetal circulation to some degree. Studies have used many different models in an effort to better understand the function and mechanism of nutrient and drug transport across the placenta. The mammalian organ exhibits the greatest variation in placental structure among species. Mammalian placentas may be classified based upon the number of layers between the maternal and fetal circulations: (i) Hemochorial, (ii) endotheliochorial, and (iii) epitheliochorial (2). The placentas of guinea pigs and rabbits are frequently selected for studies due to the similarity of their hemochorial placenta to the human placenta (3). The sheep placenta has also been used in multiple studies. Although fewer parallels exist between the epitheliochorial sheep placenta and the hemochorial human placenta, the sheep placenta has been utilized because it allows for the performance of intricate surgery and the collection of large samples for chemical analysis (3). The effects in the human placenta must be extrapolated from these studies. For both ethical and technical reasons, in vivo studies on human placental drug transfer are limited to drug administration near the time of delivery and collection of maternal venous samples and fetal umbilical samples at delivery (4). Comparison of the drug concentration in the fetus to the drug concentration in maternal plasma at a given time provides an idea of the amount of drug administered to the mother that may eventually reach the fetus. The need for a more accurate model of human placental drug transfer has led to the development of models using perfused human placentas including the ex vivo dually perfused placental cotyledon model (5).

■ MECHANISMS OF DRUG TRANSFER

Drugs cross the placenta by one of the four possible mechanisms: (1) Simple diffusion, (2) facilitated diffusion, (3) active transport, and (4) pinocytosis.

Simple Diffusion

Most drugs cross the placenta by simple diffusion (6). Simple diffusion occurs without the use of energy. The following parameters have been shown to influence the extent of placental transfer: The physicochemical characteristics of the drug, the concentration gradient between maternal and fetal blood, the surface area and thickness of the placental membrane, placental blood flow, the pH of the maternal and fetal blood, and the degree of protein binding (7).

The physicochemical characteristics of a drug include molecular weight, lipid solubility, and degree of ionization. Size does not frequently limit the rate of placental drug transfer because most drugs have a molecular weight <500 daltons (Da). Incomplete placental transfer is observed in drugs with a molecular weight >500 Da and drugs with a molecular weight >1,000 Da cross very poorly. In general, lipophilic drugs readily diffuse across biologic membranes while polar drugs diffuse more slowly across membranes (6). Polar molecules have been shown to cross the placenta at a rate that is inversely dependent on their molecular size (8).

Simple diffusion occurs down a concentration gradient. The concentration gradient is influenced by maternal factors such as the drug administration rate, the volume of drug distribution, and the rate of drug clearance (6). Maintenance of placental blood flow is integral in establishing a concentration gradient across the placenta. However, one study demonstrated that the umbilical circulation is more important in facilitating drug transfer than maternal circulation (9).

The pH of the fetal plasma also influences the rate of drug transfer across the placenta. The fetal plasma is typically ~0.1 of a pH unit lower than the maternal plasma pH (6). In the maternal plasma, weakly acidic drugs are more ionized. It is the unionized component of a drug that equilibrates across the placenta. This results in a tendency of the fetal/maternal (F/M) plasma drug concentration ratio of the acidic drug to be less than 1. In contrast, weakly basic drugs are more ionized in fetal plasma and tend to have an F/M ratio greater than 1 (6). Hence, it follows that a distressed fetus that progressively becomes more acidotic will tend to accumulate basic drugs. This phenomenon is referred to as "ion-trapping" (10).

Protein binding plays a role in determining the amount of free drug that is available to cross the placenta, because it is the free fraction of drug that eventually crosses the placenta. Drugs may be bound to either albumin or alpha-1-acid glycoprotein (AAG). One of the characteristic physiologic changes of pregnancy includes the reduction in plasma albumin levels. Krauer et al. observed the gradual rise in fetal plasma protein concentrations that occurs with increasing gestational age. In their study, the mean F/M ratio of albumin was found to be 0.38 at 12 to 15 weeks' gestation, 0.66 at 16 to 25 weeks, 0.97 at 26 to 35 weeks, and 1.2 at >35 weeks' gestation (11). These values demonstrate that fetal albumin concentrations progressively increase during fetal development to the point of being higher than maternal values by the time term gestation is reached. Regarding AAG levels, maternal serum AAG concentrations were quite variable while fetal AAG concentrations showed a constant rate of increase without ever attaining maternal values. The average term F/M ratio of AAG was found to be 0.37 (11). For drugs that are highly bound to plasma proteins, the changes of protein concentrations in the maternal and fetal plasma may result in variable drug binding and variable free drug concentrations in the maternal and fetal blood at different gestational ages.

Facilitated Diffusion

Facilitated diffusion is a form of passive transport that is dependent on transmembrane proteins. These proteins assist the transport of polar molecules and charged ions that are unable to passively cross a biologic membrane. The carrier proteins do not require energy but do require a concentration gradient. They are also saturable and may be inhibited by structural analogs of carrier molecule substrates (12). Drugs that are structurally related to an endogenous substance are assumed to use this form of diffusion (7). This transport mechanism allows the concentration to equilibrate in both maternal and fetal circulations.

Active Transport

Active transport has characteristics similar to facilitated diffusion in that it is carrier mediated. In addition, its carriers are saturable and can be inhibited by structural analogs. However, active transport requires cellular energy and the transport of substances occurs across an electrochemical or concentration gradient (12).

Pinocytosis

Pinocytosis and phagocytosis are processes that involve solutes being invaginated into the cell membrane and then transferred across the membrane to the opposite side (7). Pinocytosis and phagocytosis are thought to be too slow to have any significant impact on fetal drug concentrations (13).

■ DRUG TRANSFER

The F/M ratio provides a quantitative measurement that helps delineate the degree of fetal exposure to drugs administered to the mother during pregnancy. The following section profiles some of the pharmacologic agents used by obstetric anesthesia providers. Specifically, F/M ratios are presented in conjunction with other pertinent pharmacodynamic and pharmacokinetic information to aid in one's better understanding of transplacental drug transfer (Table 3-1).

■ INDUCTION AGENTS

Thiopental—The rapid transfer of thiopental across the placenta is attributed to the drug's high lipid solubility. Despite this characteristic, the newborn of the mother who has received thiopental is often vigorous and cries spontaneously following its use in cesarean deliveries. This inconsistency has been attributed to the extensive uptake of thiopental into the fetal liver with decreased plasma levels reaching the fetal brain (14). The highly lipid soluble nature of this drug has been demonstrated in studies with an F/M ratio of approximately 1 (15) while other studies have found an F/M ratio of 0.43 (16). The wide range of values is likely due to the short dose delivery time and rapid redistribution in the maternal circulation. Thiopental is also highly bound to albumin—a factor that influences the pharmacokinetics of the drug (6).

Ketamine—Ketamine is a weak base that readily crosses the placenta. Less than half of the drug is bound to plasma proteins. An F/M ratio of 1.26 was observed following intravenous bolus dosing for cesarean delivery (17). It has also been demonstrated that the umbilical cord gasses were similar when small doses of ketamine were used for vaginal delivery compared to spinal anesthesia for vaginal delivery (18). In their study, Houlton et al. observed similarly comparable blood gasses although thiopentone showed better fetal oxygenation when compared to ketamine for induction of anesthesia for cesarean delivery (19).

Propofol—A broad range of F/M ratios following bolus doses of propofol given for cesarean delivery has been noted in many studies varying as much as 0.74 to 1.13 depending on the albumin concentration in the fetal perfusate (20–22). Another study found that increasing uterine blood flow rates resulted in increased maternal venous concentrations. This finding was attributed to decreased extraction of propofol from the maternal circulation possibly due to either shortened contact time with placental tissues or to saturation of placental binding sites with propofol (21). In contrast, increased propofol placental transfer was noted during increased umbilical blood flow rates—likely due to increased clearance of propofol (21). It could then be presumed that the amount of propofol received by a fit fetus with adequate umbilical blood flow rates would be higher than the amount received by a distressed fetus with poor umbilical blood flow. Another proposed reason for the wide variation of F/M ratios observed following a bolus dose of propofol is the wide spectrum of time taken to deliver the fetus following administration of an induction dose (22).

Etomidate—In a study that compared etomidate to thiopentone for induction of anesthesia for cesarean delivery, similarities were observed in Apgar scores as well as in F/M ratios (etomidate F/M ratio ~0.5 and thiopentone F/M ratio 0.6). Despite these similarities, the clinical status of the newborns in the etomidate group was deemed superior by the investigators (23–25).

■ INHALATIONAL AGENTS

Inhalational agents are usually administered to the mother under steady-state conditions during general anesthesia while bolus dosing is utilized in administration of induction agents; hence, the F/M ratios of inhalational agents tend to have less erratic values (6). These agents have been shown to readily cross the placenta and have equal solubility in fetal and maternal blood; therefore, longer maternal exposure to an inhalational agent corresponds to a higher fetal exposure to the agent (26).

Halothane—Dwyer et al. studied the uptake of halothane by mother and infant during cesarean delivery. With an induction-to-delivery time averaging 10.8 minutes, an F/M ratio for halothane of 0.71 was reported after exposure to 0.5% halothane (27). There was a correlation of the duration of exposure to halothane and the measured F/M ratio (28). However, it appears that the volatile anesthetic received by the newborn

TABLE 3-1 Reported Fetal/Maternal Drug Ratios

Drug	F/M Ratio	Reference(s)
INDUCTION AGENTS		
Thiopental	0.43–1.1	14–16, 23
Propofol	0.74–1.13	20–22
Ketamine	1.26	17–19
Etomidate	0.5	23–25
NEUROMUSCULAR BLOCKING AGENTS		
Succinylcholine	undetected[a]	63–65
Rocuronium	0.16	72, 73
Atracurium	0.12	66, 67
Pancuronium	0.19	69–71
Vecuronium	0.056–0.11	68, 69
INHALATION AGENTS		
Desflurane	NR	
Sevoflurane	NR	
Nitrous oxide	0.785–0.812	34–36
Isoflurane	0.71	27
Halothane	0.71–0.87	27, 28
Enflurane	0.6	30
OPIOIDS		
Fentanyl	0.37	38
Sufentanil	0.4	37
Remifentanil	0.88	50
Alfentanil	0.28–0.31	51–53
Meperidine	0.35–1.5	45, 46
Morphine	0.61	48
Nalbuphine	0.69–0.75	54, 55
LOCAL ANESTHETICS		
Lidocaine	0.76–0.9	125, 126, 130, 133
Bupivacaine	0.3–0.56	6, 125, 130–133
Ropivacaine	0.25	133
Mepivacaine	0.53	133, 138
Chloroprocaine	NR	
ANTICHOLINERGIC AGENTS		
Atropine	1.0	78, 80
Glycopyrrolate	0.13	78, 80
Scopolamine	1.0	81
ANTICHOLINESTERASE AGENTS		
Neostigmine	NR	
Edrophonium	NR	
VASOPRESSOR AGENTS		
Ephedrine	0.71	74
Phenylephrine	0.17	77
BENZODIAZEPINES		
Diazepam	2.0	56, 57
Midazolam	0.15–0.28	15, 59
Lorazepam	1.0	61
ANTIHYPERTENSIVE AGENTS		
Propranolol	1.0[a]	109, 110
Sotalol	1.1	105
Phenoxybenzamine	1.6	118
Labetalol	0.38	103
Hydralazine	0.72	115
Metoprolol	1.0	111
Atenolol	0.94	113
Esmolol	0.2	106
Methyldopa	1.17	116
Clonidine	1.04	79
Dexmedetomidine	0.88	79
Nitroglycerine	0.18	119
Nitroprusside	1.0	121

0.26[a] after single dose

TABLE 3-1 Reported Fetal/Maternal Drug Ratios (*continued*)

Drug	F/M Ratio	Reference(s)
ANTIEMETICS		
Ondansetron	0.41	95
Metoclopramide	NR	
Gravol	NR	
Dexamethasone	NR	
ORAL HYPOGLYCEMICS		
Glyburide	<0.3	87–92
Metformin	0.3	93

NR, not reported

[a]undetected in umbilical vein if maternal dose of succinylcholine <300 mg.

is quickly eliminated since the blood–gas partition coefficient has been found to be less in the newborn versus adult subjects. Consequently, as soon as respiration has been established, the elimination of the volatile anesthetic is rapid (29).

Isoflurane—Isoflurane 0.8% rapidly crosses the placenta resulting in an F/M ratio of 0.71 (27). As isoflurane is less soluble in blood than halothane, the elimination should be even faster.

Enflurane—It was found that enflurane has an F/M ratio of approximately 0.6 (30).

Sevoflurane—In a study by Okutomi et al., sevoflurane and isoflurane were given to gravid sheep to determine the hemodynamic effects of these volatile agents as well as their effect on the blood gasses. Although the blood gasses showed little change from exposure to the volatile anesthetics, the agents produced decreases in maternal and fetal arterial pressure (31). In another study in which sevoflurane was compared to other inhalational anesthetics (including halothane, enflurane, and isoflurane), there were no differences in any of the following: Blood pressure, heart rate, Apgar score, blood loss, uterine contractility, maternal arterial blood gas, umbilical venous gas, anesthetic recovery time, and intraoperative awareness (32). This study deemed sevoflurane to be as safe as the other volatile anesthetic agents used for cesarean delivery.

Desflurane—In a comparison of desflurane and sevoflurane, neonatal Apgar scores and the neurologic and adaptive capacity score (NACS) were similar between the two agents. Parturients receiving desflurane did have a statistically significant greater mean heart rate than the sevoflurane group although the heart rate remained within normal limits. This did not correlate to any clinical significance for the mother or fetus (33).

Nitrous oxide—The reported F/M ratio of nitrous oxide was 0.812 for cesarean delivery and 0.785 for vaginal birth (34–36). This study showed no correlation between the F/M ratio and the duration of exposure to nitrous oxide after the first 2 minutes. A previous study (26) reported an increased incidence of newborn respiratory depression when the fetus was exposed to nitrous oxide for longer than 15 to 17 minutes during cesarean delivery. Although the possibility of newborn sedation due to nitrous oxide is considered, there is a concern that nitrous oxide in the setting of low oxygen tension may lead to diffusion hypoxia in the newborn with resulting respiratory insufficiency.

■ OPIOIDS

Sufentanil—The F/M ratio for sufentanil was initially reported to be 0.81 (37) although a subsequent investigation reported the F/M ratio to be 0.4 (38). The maternal to fetal transfer was increased during times of fetal acidosis although the sufentanil accumulated in placental tissue reducing the total amount of

drug that reached the fetus (38). In addition, sufentanil was highly affected by maternal protein binding (38).

Fentanyl—Fentanyl is highly lipid soluble and bound to plasma proteins (39). It reaches peak concentrations in maternal plasma within 10 to 15 minutes of epidural injection (40). Fentanyl has an F/M ratio that was originally reported as ranging from 0.6 to 0.7 (41,42) to as high as 1.12 (43). However, a subsequent study (37) suggested an F/M ratio of 0.37 that is more reflective of clinical observations of little to no effect on neonates. A comparison between bupivacaine alone versus bupivacaine combined with 80 mcg of fentanyl for epidural analgesia showed no statistical difference in Apgar scores between the two groups (44). An additional investigation reported that epidural doses of 2 mcg/mL of fentanyl produced plasma concentrations well below that required for systemic effects to be manifested in the newborn. This finding provides further evidence that epidural administration of fentanyl has little effect on the newborn (43).

Meperidine—Meperidine has an F/M ratio of 0.61 following administration of 100 mg intramuscularly (45). A second study reported a large range of F/M ratios (0.35 to 1.5) dependent upon the dose delivery time interval (46). While maternal peak plasma concentration of the drug occurs approximately 30 to 60 minutes post administration, fetal peak plasma concentration occurs between 1 and 5 hours following the maternal dose (46). These findings are consistent with the observations of Apgar scores less than 8 when the newborn was delivered between 1 and 6 hours after the maternal intramuscular injection of 1.5 mg/kg dose (47).

Morphine—The F/M ratio for morphine was found to be approximately 0.61 following 10 or 15 mg of maternally administered intramuscular morphine in fetuses that were between 28 and 35 weeks' gestation requiring diagnostic or therapeutic blood sampling (48). The blood samples were taken between 30 and 71 minutes following the maternal morphine injection. The morphine-exposed fetuses had absent or decreased fetal breathing movements and non-reactive non-stress tests (48). The impact of 1,000 mcg of intrathecal morphine resulted in very low umbilical levels of morphine. No adverse effects were observed in the fetus (49).

Remifentanil—According to Kan et al., the mean remifentanil F/M ratio is 0.88; this finding indicates that a significant degree of placental transfer occurs (50). This study also demonstrated an umbilical artery to umbilical vein ratio of 0.29 suggesting rapid metabolism and redistribution of remifentanil in the fetus. Apgar scores and adaptive capacity scores indicated alert neonates who showed minimal clinical effects of the maternal drug administration despite the clinical presence of maternal sedation (50).

Alfentanil—Following an intravenous dose of alfentanil (30 mcg/kg) in patients scheduled for elective cesarean delivery, the investigators reported an F/M ratio of 0.31 (51). This ratio decreased to 0.28 in patients who received epidural analgesia for labor that consisted of a 30 mcg/kg loading dose followed by a 30 mcg/kg/h maintenance infusion of alfentanil (52). Following the administration of intravenous alfentanil (10 mcg/kg) for cesarean delivery performed under general anesthesia, no detectable adverse effects on the newborns were identified (53).

Nalbuphine—Nalbuphine is a mixed agonist–antagonist opioid. Examining the effects of intramuscular nalbuphine (0.29 mg/kg) and intravenous nalbuphine (0.1 mg/kg), the F/M ratios were found to be 0.69 and 0.75 respectively (54). The investigators found that all newborns had Apgar scores of 10 at 5 minutes even though the half-life of nalbuphine was longer in the newborn than in the mother. In addition, loss of fetal heart rate tracing variability occurred in 54% of the subjects but did not appear to be related to the drug dose or blood concentration of the drug (54,55).

■ BENZODIAZEPINES

Diazepam—The F/M ratio of diazepam has been reported to be as high as 2 (56). This suggests that diazepam readily crosses the placenta and accumulates in the fetus. It appears in the cord blood within 30 to 60 seconds after maternal injection; equilibrium across the placenta occurs within 5 to 10 minutes (57). However, a maternal intravenous dose of diazepam (5 mg) did not result in impairment in the Apgar scores according to a study by Ridd et al. (58).

Midazolam—The F/M ratio of midazolam and its metabolite, 1-hydroxymethylmidazolam, has been reported to range from 0.15 to 0.28 (15,59). The distribution and elimination half-lives for midazolam and its metabolite were the same (59). Use of midazolam has not been associated with newborn sedation (60).

Lorazepam—The F/M ratio for lorazepam has been reported to be 1.0 (61). The elimination half-life of lorazepam is slow in the newborn. A term infant has been found to excrete detectable amounts of the drug for up to 8 days post exposure (62).

■ NEUROMUSCULAR BLOCKING AGENTS

Succinylcholine—Although it was once believed that succinylcholine did not cross the placenta, studies have now demonstrated that transfer across the placenta occurs quite rapidly. Peak fetal concentrations have been detected at intervals occurring 5 and 10 minutes following maternal intravenous administration (63,64). In a study conducted by Drabkova et al., a fetal plasma concentration of 0.6 mcg/mL was observed in macaca mulatta monkeys. While this plasma concentration is likely high enough to affect a fetal EMG, it would be unlikely to result in neonatal respiratory depression (65).

Atracurium—In a study of 15 women who received intravenous atracurium, 7 of the patients had drug levels below the limit of detection while the other 8 patients reflected an F/M ratio averaging approximately 0.12 (66,67). None of the newborns showed signs of adverse effects from the maternally administered atracurium (66).

Vecuronium—Vecuronium has a profile similar to other nondepolarizing muscle relaxants in that very little of it passes across the placenta. The F/M ratio of vecuronium is reported to range from 0.056 (68) to 0.11 (69). Consequently, the newborns of mothers who received vecuronium had normal Apgar scores and normal NACS (69). It was determined that the degree of placental transfer decreases as the time interval from maternal injection to delivery of the newborn decreases (68).

Pancuronium—Pancuronium has an F/M ratio of 0.19. No effect has been observed on newborn Apgar scores or NACS (69,70,71).

Rocuronium—Rocuronium has an F/M ratio of 0.16 (72). In a study by Abouleish et al., all Apgar scores at 5 minutes were normal following a 0.6 mg/kg dose of rocuronium (72). It has been reported that intubation was easily performed in 50% of patients receiving ketamine–rocuronium for induction versus only 25% of patients receiving a thiopental–rocuronium combination. Apgar scores were the same between the two groups (73).

■ VASOACTIVE DRUGS

Ephedrine—The F/M ratio has been found to be 0.71 (74) with the placental transfer resulting in increased fetal heart rate and beat-to-beat variability (75). Ephedrine has been widely used in obstetric anesthesia to treat hypotension specifically related to neuraxial anesthesia. It has been reported that the administration of significant amounts of ephedrine may lead to decrease in both fetal pH and umbilical arterial oxygen content (76). These fetal metabolic effects are postulated to be a direct effect of ephedrine. The observation of increased concentrations of lactate, glucose, epinephrine, and norepinephrine in the fetuses born to mothers who have been treated with ephedrine compared to those treated with phenylephrine offers further evidence of the direct effects of ephedrine (77).

Phenylephrine—Phenylephrine does not readily cross the placenta. It has an F/M ratio of 0.17 (77). Traditionally, ephedrine has been the drug of choice for the treatment of maternal hypotension caused by neuraxial anesthesia or analgesia. Recently, however, this practice has been re-evaluated and has resulted in the introduction of phenylephrine as a routine drug for treatment of maternal hypotension. Although fetuses exposed to ephedrine show increased levels of products of metabolism in comparison to phenylephrine, the umbilical arterial pCO_2 and umbilical venous pO_2 have been found to be greater in the ephedrine group. Consequently, it has been suggested that phenylephrine causes greater vasoconstriction in the uteroplacental circulation than ephedrine. The clinical relevance of these metabolic differences remains unclear as no difference in Apgar scores has been observed (77).

■ ANTICHOLINERGIC AGENTS

Atropine—In a study of pregnant ewe that received intravenous atropine (0.05 mg/kg), an F/M ratio of 1.0 was observed (78). Although atropine rapidly crosses the placenta (79), no effects on the fetal arterial pressure, heart rate, or beat-to-beat variability were observed despite a 25% increase in maternal heart rate (78).

Glycopyrrolate—Following administration of intravenous glycopyrrolate (0.025 mg/kg) to a pregnant ewe, an F/M ratio of 0.13 was reported, indicating that glycopyrrolate does not cross the placenta to any significant degree (78,80).

Scopolamine—Similar to atropine, scopolamine readily crosses the placenta. This is reflected by its F/M ratio of 1.0 following intramuscular administration (81).

■ ANTICHOLINESTERASE AGENTS

Neostigmine—Neostigmine is an ionized, quaternary ammonium compound that undergoes minimal placental transfer (80). Despite this, a case report by Clark et al. suggested that a 5 mg maternal dose of neostigmine given as a part of general anesthesia for elbow surgery resulted in a prolonged (~1 hour) decrease in fetal heart rate from 130 beats/min to 90 to 110 beats/min (80). General anesthesia was again required for re-operation of the patient's elbow just days later. In that anesthetic encounter, the anesthesiologist opted to use 5 mg neostigmine with 0.4 mg atropine. There were no effects on the fetal heart rate. Hence, it was concluded that atropine, which readily crosses the placenta, prevented the drop in fetal heart rate caused by neostigmine. In contrast, there have been case reports of parturients with myasthenia gravis being treated with neostigmine throughout their pregnancy without any adverse fetal effects (82).

Edrophonium—Edrophonium is an ionized, quaternary ammonium compound that undergoes minimal placental transfer (80). Edrophonium has been associated with preterm labor (83).

■ ANTICOAGULANTS

Warfarin—Although warfarin is a weak acid that readily crosses the placenta, no known F/M ratio for warfarin has been reported. Warfarin has been associated with spontaneous abortion as well as teratogenic defects of the brain, face, and eyes, especially when the fetus is exposed during the first trimester. Warfarin has also been identified as a causative agent in chondrodysplasia punctata (6).

Heparin—Heparin has a large molecular weight of 20,000 to 40,000 Da, making it too large to cross the placenta in any significant amount (6). Therefore, it is routine practice to have patients requiring anticoagulation during pregnancy to either discontinue the use of warfarin in favor of heparin or start with the use of heparin if the patient does not require anticoagulation prior to the pregnancy.

Tinzaparin—Tinzaparin is a low molecular weight heparin formed by the enzymatic degradation of porcine unfractionated heparin. In a study of direct fetal blood sampling under ultrasound, tinzaparin did not cross the placenta by 3 hours following maternal injection (84). Given this observation, serious doubt is raised with regard to case reports suggesting that it is an agent of teratogenicity that causes aplasia cutis congenita in neonates born to mothers who have a history of postpartum pulmonary embolism and are treated with prophylactic Tinzaparin (4,500 IU daily) starting at 10 weeks' gestation (85).

Enoxaparin—In a study of patients receiving enoxaparin for venous thromboembolism, there were no significant amounts of enoxaparin detected in fetal venous and arterial samples. This finding indicates the absence of placental transfer (86).

■ ANTIHYPERGLYCEMIC AGENTS

Insulin—Glucose is able to cross the placenta by facilitated diffusion. Therefore, insulin-dependent diabetic parturients need to maintain tight plasma glucose control during pregnancy. Insulin is a polypeptide with a molecular weight of 6,000 Da that cannot cross the placenta (6). In parturients who have poorly controlled diabetes, large amounts of glucose readily cross the placenta into the fetus thereby stimulating the fetal production of endogenous insulin. This can lead to fetal macrosomia as well as neonatal hyperinsulinemia that predisposes the newborn to hypoglycemia in the first days of life (6).

Glyburide—Despite previous assertions that oral hypoglycemics should be considered contraindicated in pregnancy, there was no difference in the incidence of macrosomia, neonatal hypoglycemia, or cesarean delivery in parturients who received glyburide compared to those who received insulin (87). Clinically, glyburide produced adequate plasma glucose control with significantly less hypoglycemia than insulin (87). Glyburide was initially thought to cross the placenta; recent investigations have demonstrated glyburide placental transfer with an F/M ratio of less than 0.3 (88). The placental transfer of glyburide is limited by several factors: High protein binding

(89), placental microsomal metabolism (90), rapid clearance rate (91), and placental efflux receptors including the breast cancer resistant protein (BRCP) (92).

Metformin—Like glyburide, metformin also crosses the placenta with a 0.3 F/M ratio having been reported (93). The use of metformin for the treatment of gestational diabetes was not associated with increased adverse neonatal effects when compared to insulin (94). However, the clinical benefit of metformin has been questioned due to the finding that 46.3% of the patients receiving metformin required supplemental insulin for inadequate glucose control. This requirement essentially eliminates any benefit of taking an oral hypoglycemic agent to avoid daily insulin injections (94).

■ ANTIEMETIC AGENTS

Ondansetron—The F/M ratio of ondansetron is reportedly 0.41 during the first trimester of pregnancy (95). A review of 176 women exposed to ondansetron during pregnancy concluded that there was no difference in the occurrence of major neonatal malformations in the ondansetron group compared to control subjects (96).

Metoclopramide—The prokinetic agent, metoclopramide, has been used for nausea and vomiting in pregnancy. A prospective multicenter trial found that metoclopramide use in the first trimester of pregnancy is not associated with an increased risk of malformations, spontaneous abortions, or decreased birth weights (97).

Dimenhydrinate—Dimenhydrinate, a chemical salt of diphenhydramine and 8-chlorotheophylline, is used to prevent nausea and motion sickness. A case control study found no increased incidence of teratogenicity in mothers who had been exposed to dimenhydrinate during pregnancy (98).

Dexamethasone—Dexamethasone is a synthetic glucocorticoid. In a meta-analysis of four studies, the use of glucocorticoids was associated with a three- to four-fold increased incidence of cleft lip (with or without cleft palate) when used before 10 weeks' gestation (99).

■ ANTIHYPERTENSIVE AGENTS

Hypertension in pregnancy can have detrimental effects on both the mother and fetus. Multiple drugs have been used to treat hypertension in pregnancy. Houlihan et al. investigated the effects of many commonly used antihypertensive agents on umbilical artery resistance; this study was performed in order to address concerns that lowering blood pressure could compromise feto-placental circulation, fetal growth, and fetal development (100). It was observed that nifedipine, magnesium sulfate, hydralazine, and labetalol all had direct vasodilatory effects on the umbilical artery. Alpha-methyldopa had minimal non-significant vasodilatory effects. As alpha-methyldopa has the least effects on uteroplacental hemodynamics, the authors concluded that it could be an ideal option for the treatment of hypertension in the parturient population.

Beta-blockers can cross the placenta and may lead to increased levels of insulin and a decrease in glucagon (101). Both of these physiologic responses can lead to hypoglycemia in the newborn. However, maternal exposure to beta-blockers has not been associated with an increased risk of congenital anomalies (102).

Labetalol—Labetalol, a mixed alpha/beta-adrenergic antagonist, has an F/M ratio of 0.38. It has been associated with mild neonatal bradycardia determined to be clinically insignificant (103). In one study, patients were exposed to 600 to 1,200 mg of labetalol per day and fetal heart rates remained within normal limits (104). There were no cases of fetal bradycardia following exposure to labetalol. In a separate investigation comparing labetalol to atenolol, neonatal weights were significantly higher in the group treated with labetalol. Apgar scores higher than 8 (at 5 minutes) were observed with both drugs (104). This suggests that labetalol is more effective than atenolol in reducing the fetal growth restriction that can occur in maternal hypertensive disorders.

Sotalol—Sotalol, a hydrophilic non-selective beta-adrenergic blocker, has a reported F/M ratio of 1.1 (105). Interestingly, due to its high F/M ratio, sotalol has been used for the specific purpose of treating fetal tachycardia (105). Importantly, sotalol has not been associated with fetal growth restriction.

Esmolol—Esmolol is a selective beta-1-adrenergic blocking agent that has a very short duration of action due to its rapid elimination by red blood cell esterases; it has a reported F/M ratio of 0.2 (106). Esmolol has not been routinely used in the pregnant population. This practice is formally endorsed in an isolated case report of emergency cesarean delivery performed for fetal bradycardia following a maternal dose of 0.5 mg/kg esmolol in an attempt to treat maternal supraventricular tachycardia (SVT) (107). The author was unable to determine if the fetal bradycardia was secondary to reduced placental blood flow or to an inability of the fetus to compensate to decreased placental perfusion. Despite esmolol's small degree of placental transfer, the hemodynamic effects appear to be similar in both the mother and fetus (101).

Propranolol—Propranolol is a non-selective beta-blocker that is highly lipid soluble (101). Its reported F/M ratios range from 0.26 after single dose administration (108) to 1.0 or greater following long-term maternal administration (109). Profound newborn hypoglycemia and respiratory depression have been reported following a daily propranolol dose of 160 mg during pregnancy (109).

Metoprolol—Metoprolol is a cardioselective beta-1-blocker that has low lipid solubility and 12% protein binding (101); it has been reported to have an F/M ratio of 1.0 (110). Similar concentrations have been observed in the maternal plasma and in the umbilical cord. There have been no observed adverse effects on fetal heart rate, glucose homeostasis, or growth (111). Teratogenicity has also not been reported (101).

Atenolol—Atenolol is a hydrophilic cardioselective beta-blocker with a reported F/M ratio of 0.94 (112). Although studies have not found evidence of an association with hypoglycemia, respiratory distress, or an altered fetal response to a stress (101), there have been reports of women treated with atenolol in early pregnancy delivering low birth weight neonates (113).

Hydralazine—Hydralazine reportedly crosses the placenta by simple diffusion resulting in an F/M ratio of 0.72 (114). Magee and Bawdon observed the following in their study of the placental transfer and vasoactive properties of hydralazine: An accumulation of hydralazine in fetal tissue that reached a maximum concentration that was 40% of the maternal concentration (114) as well as a statistically significant drop in fetal blood pressure following the maternal administration of hydralazine.

Methyldopa—The alpha-2-adrenergic agonist, methyldopa, has a reported F/M ratio of 1.17 (115).

Clonidine—The alpha-2-adrenergic agonist, clonidine, has a reported F/M ratio of 1.04 (79). There have been no significant adverse effects on the fetus or newborn due to the use of clonidine (79).

Dexmedetomidine—Dexmedetomidine is a potent alpha-2-selective agonist reported to have an F/M ratio of 0.88 (79). When administered as an adjunct for labor analgesia, dexmedetomidine was reportedly devoid of maternal hypotension or bradycardia. There were also no observed adverse effects on the fetus (116).

Phenoxybenzamine—According to a case report of a parturient diagnosed with pheochromocytoma and treated with phenoxybenzamine, phenoxybenzamine has an F/M ratio of 1.6 (117). In this report, the authors endorsed close monitoring of the newborn for transient hypotension in the first few days of life.

Nitroglycerin—The reported F/M ratio for nitroglycerin is 0.18 (118). In a report by DeRosayro et al., the use of nitroglycerin was found to reduce uterine blood flow in pregnant ewes as a consequence of a decrease in maternal blood pressure (119). There were no documented adverse effects on the fetus. There was, however, a statistically significant decrease in the fetal PaO_2 when compared to the control group.

Nitroprusside—The reported F/M ratio in the ewe model has been reported as 1.0 as nitroprusside rapidly crosses the placenta (120). Nitroprusside has been associated with transient fetal bradycardia (121). There has been no association with congenital defects. The primary concern with the use of nitroprusside resides primarily in the potential for fetal cyanide accumulation. This concern, however, has been refuted since excessive accumulation has not been identified in the fetal liver (122). Although sodium thiosulfate has not been observed to cross the placenta, it may be useful in treating fetal cyanide toxicity as it decreases maternal cyanide levels (123).

■ LOCAL ANESTHETICS

Lidocaine—The F/M ratio for lidocaine was reported to be 0.9 in a perfused human cotyledon after 2 hours (124). In an earlier model, variation in the degree of placental transfer of lidocaine was demonstrated such that the F/M ratio increased from 0.76 to 1.1 with fetal acidosis (125). Despite the accumulation of lidocaine in the acidotic fetus, lidocaine did not alter fetal heart rate, blood pressure, arterial pH, and blood gas responses to asphyxia (126). There is very little back-transfer of lidocaine from the fetal circulation back to the maternal circulation; therefore, following inadvertent intravascular injection of lidocaine, there is no need to delay the delivery of the fetus in hopes that lidocaine will transfer out of the fetal circulation back to the mother (127).

Bupivacaine—The F/M ratio for lidocaine was reported to be 0.56 in a perfused human cotyledon after 2 hours (124). This was slightly higher than the previously reported F/M ratio of 0.3 (6). A dually perfused human placenta model suggested that the mode of placental transfer of bupivacaine is primarily by passive diffusion (128). Fetal bupivacaine plasma concentrations tend to rise with increasing maternal doses. However, when bupivacaine is given via a continuous epidural infusion, the maternal plasma concentrations remain relatively stable resulting in F/M ratios that show little variation with time (129). The F/M ratio is highly influenced by the transplacental AAG gradient given that bupivacaine is highly protein bound (6). Placental transfer is increased in the presence of fetal acidosis (9); however, the addition of epinephrine to bupivacaine does not alter the placental transfer (130).

The placenta has been shown to accumulate bupivacaine at concentrations five times higher than the perfusate concentration. This finding was demonstrated to be independent of protein binding and direction of drug transfer (128). Interestingly, significant back-transfer of bupivacaine from the fetal circulation to the maternal circulation has been observed (125). Therefore, there may be a theoretical advantage to delaying delivery following an inadvertent accidental intravascular injection of bupivacaine immediately prior to delivery, assuming adequate fetal and maternal circulations, in an effort to facilitate back-transfer to the maternal circulation (127).

Ropivacaine—The F/M ratio of ropivacaine has been reported to be 0.25. This value was primarily dependent upon the concentration of unionized ropivacaine in the maternal circulation (131). A similar placental transfer of ropivacaine and bupivacaine throughout a spectrum of maternal and fetal pH changes was also observed (131). This has led to the suggestion that ropivacaine might be a better choice due to evidence of less cardiotoxicity (132). In contrast, another investigation observed no significant association between maternal free fraction of ropivacaine, umbilical venous concentrations, or on placental transfer of ropivacaine (133). The investigators concluded that factors other than maternal free fraction of ropivacaine must dictate the placental transfer rate.

Chloroprocaine—Due to the rapid hydrolysis of chloroprocaine in maternal blood, minimal placental transfer occurs (134). Furthermore, placental transfer of chloroprocaine has not been observed to be influenced by fetal acidosis (135). A comparison of bupivacaine, chloroprocaine, and etidocaine found no significant differences in neuro-behavioral performances, Apgar scores, or acid–base status between bupivacaine and chloroprocaine (134). Chloroprocaine had the advantage of having a faster onset of action and a shorter administration-to-onset interval than bupivacaine (134).

Mepivacaine—The F/M ratio of mepivacaine has been reported to be 0.53. Investigations that compared the placental transfers of mepivacaine, lidocaine, bupivacaine, and ropivacaine found that the F/M ratio of mepivacaine was higher than the other local anesthetics regardless of the perfusate pH (131). Previously, an F/M ratio of 0.56 was reported when mepivacaine was utilized for spinal anesthesia in elective cesarean deliveries (136).

KEY POINTS

- Careful review of existing literature suggests that the majority of drugs are transferred across the placenta to some degree; however, the extent of their placental transfer varies considerably.
- Much of what is known regarding the degree of placental transfer of drugs has been obtained via extrapolation of data from animal studies to humans. Data has been inferred from single measurements of drug concentrations in maternal and newborn blood samples taken at the time of delivery. More recently, data has been inferred from human placental models.
- Drugs cross the placenta by one of four possible mechanisms: (1) Simple diffusion, (2) facilitated diffusion, (3) active transport, and (4) pinocytosis.
- Parameters that have been shown to influence the extent of placental transfer include the following: Molecular weight; lipid solubility; degree of ionization; degree of protein binding; the concentration gradient between maternal and fetal blood (F/M ratio); the surface area and thickness of the placental membrane, placental blood flow; and the pH of the maternal and fetal blood.
- The F/M ratio provides a comparison of drug concentration in maternal and fetal plasma; hence, it gives an idea of exposure of the fetus to maternally administered drugs.
- A thorough understanding of placental transfer improves the efficacy and safety of drug administration in pregnancy.

REFERENCES

1. Caton D. Obstetric anesthesia and concepts of placental transport: a historical review of the nineteenth century. *Anesthesiology* 1977;46:132–137.
2. Faber JJ, Thornburg KL. Structural features of placental exchange. In: Faber JJ, Thornburg KL, eds. *Placental physiology: Structure and function of fetomaternal exchange.* New York, NY: Raven Press. Inc; 1983:1–32.
3. Omarini D, Pistotti V, Bonati M. Placental perfusion: An overview of the literature. *JPM* 1992;25(2):61–66.
4. Reynolds F, Knott C. Pharmacokinetics in pregnancy and placental drug transfer. *Oxf Rev Reprod Biol* 1989;11:389–449.
5. Ala-Kokko TI, Myllynen P, Vahakangas K. Ex vivo perfusion of the human placental cotyledon: implications for anesthetic pharmacology. *IJOA* 2000; 9(26):26–38.
6. Reynolds F. Placental transfer of drugs. *Curr Anaesth Crit Care* 1991;2:108–116.
7. Ven der Aa EM, Peereboom-Stegeman J, Noordhoek J, et al. Mechanisms of drug transfer across the human placenta. *Pharm World Sci* 1998;20(4):139–148.
8. Illsley NP, Hall S, Penfold P, et al. Diffusional permeability of the human placenta. *Contrib Gynec Obstet* 1985;13:92–97.
9. Gaylard DG, Carson RJ, Reynolds F. The effect of umbilical perfusate pH and controlled maternal hypotension on placental drug transfer in the rabbit. *Anesth Analg* 1990;71:42–48.
10. Johnson R, Herman N, Hohnson HV, et al. Effects of fetal pH on local anesthetic transfer across the human placenta. *Anesthesiology* 1996;85:608–615.
11. Krauer B, Dayer P, Anner R. Changes in serum albumin and alpha-1-acid glycoprotein concentrations during pregnancy: an analysis of fetal-maternal pairs. *Br J Obs Gynecol* 1984;91:875–881.
12. Unadkat JD, Dahlin A, Vijay S. Placental drug transporters. *Curr Drug Metab* 2004;5(1):125–131.
13. Syme M, Paxton J, Keelan J. Drug transfer and metabolism by the human placenta. *Clin Pharmacokinet* 2004;43(8):487–514.
14. Finster M, Perel JM, Papper EM. Uptake of thiopental by fetal tissue and the placenta. *Fed Proc* 1968;27:706.
15. Bach V, Carl P, Ravlo O, et al. A randomized comparison between midazolam and thiopental for elective cesarean section anesthesia: III placental transfer and elimination in neonates. *Anesth Analg* 1989;68:238–242.
16. Gaspari F, Marraro G, Penna GF, et al. Elimination kinetics of thiopentone in mothers and their newborn infants. *Eur J Clin Pharmacol* 1985;28:321–325.
17. Ellingson A, Haram K, Sagen N, et al. Transplacental passage of ketamine after intravenous administration. *Acta Anaesth Scand* 1977;21:41–44.
18. Maduska AL, Hajghassemali M. Arterial blood gases in mother and infants during ketamine anesthesia for vaginal delivery. *Anesth Analg* 1978;57:121–123.
19. Houlton PC, Downing JW, Buley RJ, et al. Anaestheic induction of caesarean section with thiopentone, methohexitone and ketamine. *S Afr Med J* 1978;54(20):818–820.
20. He Y, Tsujimoto S, Tanimoto M, et al. Effects of protein binding on the placental transfer of propofol in the human dually-perfused cotyledon. *Br J Anaesth* 2000;85:281–286.
21. He Y, Seno H, Tsujimoto S, et al. The effects of uterine and umbilical blood flows on the transfer of propofol across the human placenta during in vitro perfusion. *Anesth Analg* 2001;93:151–156.
22. Sanchez-Alcaraz A, Quintana MB, Laguarda M et al. Placental transfer and neonatal effects of propofol in caesarean section. *J Clin Pharm Ther* 1998; 23:19–23.
23. Downing JW, Buley RJR, Brock-Utne JG, et al. Etomidate for induction of anaesthesia at caesarean section: Comparison with thiopentone. *Br J Anaesth* 1979;51:135.
24. Gregory MA, Davidson DG. Plasma etomidate levels in mother and fetus. *Anaesthesia* 1991;46:716–718.
25. Fresno L, Andaluz A, Moll X, et al. Placental transfer of etomidate in pregnant ewes after an intravenous bolus dose and continuous infusion. *Vet J* 2008;175:395–402.
26. Stenger VG, Blechner JN, Prystowsky H. A study of prolongation of obstetric anesthesia. *Am J Obstet Gynecol* 1969;103:901–907.
27. Dwyer R, Fee JPH, Moore J. Uptake of halothane and isoflurane by mother and baby during caesarean section. *Br J Anaesth* 1995;74:379–383.
28. Kangas L, Erkkola R, Kanto J, et al. Halothane anaesthesia in caesarean section. *Acta Anaesthesiol Scan* 1976;20:189–194.
29. Gibbs CP, Munson ES, Tham MK. Anesthetic solubility coefficients for maternal and fetal blood. *Anesthesiology* 1975;43:100–103.
30. Dick W, Knoche E, Traub E. Clinical investigations concerning the use of Ethrane for cesarean section. *J Perinat Med* 1979;7:125–133.
31. Okutomi T, Whittington R, Stein D, et al. Comparison of the effects of sevoflurane and isoflurane anesthesia on the maternal–fetal unit in sheep. *J Anesth* 2009;23:392–398.
32. Keiichi K, Shigihara A, Tase C, et al. Comparison of sevoflurane and other volatile anesthetics for cesarean section. *J Anesth* 1995;9:363–365.
33. Karaman S, Akercan F, Aldemir O, et al. The maternal and neonatal effects of the volatile anaesthetic agents desflurane and sevoflurane in caesarean section: a prospective, randomized clinical study. *J Int Med Res* 2006;34:183–192.
34. Marx GF, Joshi CW, Orkin LR. Placental transmission of nitrous oxide. *Anesthesiology* 1970;32:429–432.
35. Polvi HJ, Pirhonen JP, Erkkola RU. Nitrous oxide inhalation: Effects on maternal and fetal circulations at term. *Obstet Gynecol* 1996;87:1045–1048.

36. Mankowitz E, Brock-Utne JG, Downing JW. Nitrous oxide elimination by the newborn. *Anaesthesia* 1981;36:1014–1016.

37. Loftus JR, Hill H, Cohen SE. Placental transfer and neonatal effects of epidural sufentanil and fentanyl administered with bupivacaine during labor. *Anesthesiology* 1995;83:300–308.

38. Johnson RF, Herman N, Arney T, et al. The placental transfer of sufentanil: effects of fetal pH, protein binding, and sufentanil concentration. *Anesth Analg* 1997;84:1262–1268.

39. Bower S. Plasma protein binding of fentanyl. *J Pharm Pharmacol* 1981;33:507–514.

40. Desprats R, Dumas JC, Giroux M, et al. Maternal and umbilical cord concentrations of fentanyl after epidural analgesia for cesarean section. *Eur J Obstet Gynecol Reprod Biol* 1991;42:89–94.

41. Rayburn W, Rathke A, Leuschen P, et al. Fentanyl citrate analgesia during labor. *Am J Obstet Gynecol* 1989;161:202–206.

42. Bang U, Helbo-Hansen HS, Lindholm P, et al. Placental transfer and neonatal effects of epidural fentanyl–bupivacaine for caesarean section (abstract). *Anesthesiology* 1991;75:AA847.

43. Fernando R, Bonello E, Gill P, et al. Neonatal welfare and placental transfer of fentanyl and bupivacaine during ambulatory combined spinal epidural analgesia for labour. *Anaesthesia* 1997;52:517–524.

44. Justins D, Francis DM, Houlton PG, et al. A controlled trial of extradural fentanyl in labour. *Br J Anaesth* 1982;54:409–414.

45. Wilson CM, McClean E, Moore J, et al. A double-blind comparison of intramuscular pethidine and nalbuphine in labour. *Anaesthesia* 1986;41(12):1207–1213.

46. Tomson G, Garle R, Thalme B, et al. Maternal kinetics and transplacental passage of pethidine during labour. *Br J Clin Pharmac* 1982;13:653–659.

47. Bundsen P, Peterson LE, Selstam U. Pain relief during labour. An evaluation of conventional methods. *Acta Obstet Gynecol Scand* 1982;61(4):289–297.

48. Kopecky E, Ryan ML, Barrett J, et al. Fetal response to maternally administered morphine. *Am J Obstet Gynecol* 2000;183:424–430.

49. Hee P, Sorensen S, Bock J, et al. Intrathecal administration of morphine for the relief of pains in labour and estimation of maternal and fetal plasma concentration of morphine (abstract). *Eur J Ostet Gynecol Reprod Biol* 1987;25:195–201.

50. Kan R, Hughes S, Rosen M, et al. Intravenous remifentanil: placental transfer, maternal and neonatal effects. *Anesthesiology* 1998;88:467–474.

51. Gepts E, Heytens L, Camu F. Pharmacokinetics and placental transfer of intravenous and epidural alfentanil in parturient women. *Anesth Analg* 1986;65:1155–1160.

52. Zakowski MI, Ham AA, Grant GJ. Transfer and uptake of alfentanil in the human placenta during in vitro perfusion. *Anesth Analg* 1994;79:1089–1093.

53. Cartwright DP, Dann WL, Hutchinson A. Placental transfer of alfentanil at caesarean section. *Eur J Anaesthesiol* 1989;6:103–109.

54. Nicolle E, Devillier P, Delanoy B, et al. Therapeutic monitoring of nalbuphine: transplacental transfer and estimated pharmacokinetics in the neonate. *Eur J Clin Pharmacol* 1996;49:485–489.

55. Wilson SJ, Errick JK, Balkon J. Pharmacokinetics of nalbuphine during parturition. *Am J Obstet Gynecol* 1986;155:340–345.

56. Erkkola R, Kangas L, Pekkarinen A. The transfer of diazepam across the placenta during labour. *Acta Obstet Gynecol Scand* 1973;52:167–170.

57. Bakke OM, Haram K. Time-course of transplacental passage of diazepam: influence of injection-delivery interval on neonatal drug concentration. *Clin Pharm* 1982;7:353–362.

58. Ridd M, Brown K, Nation R, et al. The disposition and placental transfer of diazepam in cesarean section. *Clin Pharmacol* 1989;45:506–512.

59. Vree TB, Reekers-Kettling JJ, Fragen RJ, et al. Placental transfer of midazolam and its metabolite 1-hydroxymethylmidazolam in the pregnant ewe. *Anesth Analg* 1984;63:31–34.

60. Crawford ME, Carl P, Bach V, et al. A randomized comparison between midazolam and thiopental for elective cesarean section anesthesia. I. Mothers. *Anesth Analg* 1989;68:229–233.

61. McBride RJ, Dundee JW, Moore J, et al. A study of the plasma concentrations of lorazepam in mother and neonate. *Br J Anaesth* 1979;51:971–978.

62. Whitelaw AGL, Cummings AJ, McFadyen IR. Effect of maternal lorazepam on the neonate. *Br Med J* 1981;282:1106–1108.

63. Moya F, Kvisselgaard N. The placental transmission of succinylcholine. *Anesthesiology* 1961;22:1–6.

64. Kvisselgaard N, Moya F. Investigation of placental thresholds to succinylcholine. *Anesthesiology* 1961;22:7–10.

65. Drabkova C, Van Der Kleijn E. Placental transfer of C14 labelled succinylcholine in near term macaca mulatta monkeys. *Br J Anesth* 1973;45:1087–1096.

66. Flynn P, Frank M, Hughes R. Use of atracurium in cesarean section. *Br J Anaesth* 1984;56:599.

67. Shearer ES, Fahy LT, O'Sullivan EP, et al. Transplacental distribution of atracurium, laudanosine and monoquaternary alcohol during elective caesarean section. *Br J Anaesth* 1991;66:551–556.

68. Iwama H, Kaneko T, Tobishima S, et al. Time dependency of the ratio of umbilical vein/maternal artery concentrations of vecuronium in caesarean section. *Acta Anaesthesiol Scand* 1999;43:9–12.

69. Dailey P, Fisher D, Shnider S, et al. Pharmacokinetics, placental transfer, and neonatal effects of vecuronium and pancuronium administered during cesarean section. *Anesthesiology* 1984;60:569–574.

70. Duvaldestin P, Demetriou M, Henzel D, et al. The placental transfer of pancuronium and its pharmacokinetics during caesarean section. *Acta Anaesthesiol Scand* 1978;22:327–333.

71. Abouleish E, Wingard LB Jr, de la Vega S, et al. Pancuronium in caesarean section and its placental transfer. *Br J Anaesth* 1980;52:531–536.

72. Abouleish E, Abboud T, Lechevalier T, et al. Rocuronium for caesarean section. *Br J Anaesth* 1994;73:336–341.

73. Baraka AS, Sayyid SS, Assaf BA. Thiopental-rocuronium versus ketamine-rocuronium for rapid-sequence intubation in parturients undergoing cesarean section. *Anesth Analg* 1997;84:1104–1107.

74. Hughes S, Ward M, Levinson G, et al. Placental transfer of ephedrine does not affect neonatal outcome. *Anesthesiology* 1985;63:217–219.

75. Wright RG, Shnider SM, Levinson G, et al. The effect of maternal administration of ephedrine on fetal heart rate and variability. *Am J Obstet Gynecol* 1981;57:734–738.

76. Ngan Kee WD, Lee A, Khaw KS, et al. A randomized double-blinded comparison of phenylephrine and ephedrine infusion combinations to maintain blood pressure during spinal anesthesia for cesarean delivery: the effects on fetal acid–base status and hemodynamic control. *Anesth Analg* 2008;107:1295–1302.

77. Ngan Kee WD, Khaw KS, Tan PE, et al. Placental transfer and fetal metabolic effects of phenylephrine and ephedrine during spinal anesthesia for cesarean delivery. *Anesthesiology* 2009;111:506–512.

78. Murad S, Conklin K, Tabsh K, et al. Atropine and glycopyrrolate. Hemodynamic effects and placental transfer in the pregnant ewe. *Anesth Analg* 1981;60:710–714.

79. Ala-Kokko TI, Pienimaki P, Lampela E, et al. Transfer of clonidine and dexmedetomidine across the isolated perfused human placenta. *Acta Anaesthesiol Scand* 1997;41:313–319.

80. Clark RB, Brown MA, Lattin DL. Neostigmine, atropine, and glycopyrrolate: does neostigmine cross the placenta? *Anesthesiology* 1996;84:450–452.

81. Kanto J, Kentala E, Kaila T, et al. Pharmacokinetics of scopolamine during caesarean section: Relationship between serum concentration and effect. *Acta Anaesthesiol Scand* 1989;33:482–486.

82. Lefvert AK, Osterman PO. Newborn infants to myasthenic mothers: a clinical study and an investigation of acetylcholine receptor antibodies in 17 children. *Neurology* 1983;33:133–138.

83. McNall PG, Jafarnia MR. Management of myasthenia gravis in the obstetric patient. *Am J Obstet Gynecol* 1965;92:182–185.

84. Forestier F, Daffos F, Capella-Pavlovsky M. Low molecular weight heparin (PK 10169) does not cross the placenta during the second trimester of pregnancy: study by direct fetal blood sampling under ultrasound. *Thromb Res* 1984;34:557–560.

85. Sharif S, Hay C, Clayton-Smith J. Aplasia cutis congenital and low molecular weight heparin. *BJOG* 2005;112:256–258.

86. Lagrange F, Vergnes C, Brun J, et al. Absence of placental transfer of pentasaccharide (fondaparinux, Arixtra) in the dually perfused human cotyledon in vitro. *Thromb Haemost* 2002;87:831–835.

87. Langer O, Conway DL, Berkus MD, et al. A comparison of glyburide and insulin in women with gestational diabetes mellitus. *N Engl J Med* 2000;343:1134–1138.

88. Kraemer J, Klein J, Lubetsky A, et al. Perfusion studies of glyburide transfer across the human placenta: Implications for fetal safety. *Am J Obstet Gynecol* 2006;195:270–274.

89. Nanovskaya TN, Nekhayeva I, Hankins GDV, et al. Effect of human serum albumin on transplacental transfer of glyburide. *Biochem Pharmacol* 2006;72:632–639.

90. Jain S, Zharikova OL, Ravindran S, et al. Glyburide metabolism by placentas of healthy and gestational diabetics. *Am J Perinatology* 2008;25(3):169–174.

91. Gedeon C, Behravan J, Koren G, et al. Transport of glyburide by placental ABC transporters: Implication in fetal drug exposure. *Placenta* 2006;27:1096–1102.

92. Pollex EK, Feig DS, Koren G. Oral hypoglycemic therapy: understanding the mechanisms of transplacental transfer. *J Matern Fetal Neonatal Med* 2010;23(3):224–228.

93. Nanovskaya TN, Nekhayeva IA, Patrikeeva SL, et al. Transfer of metformin across the dually perfused human placental lobule. *Am J Obstet Gynecol* 2006;195:1081–1085.

94. Rowan JA, Hague W, Gao W, et al. Metformin versus insulin for the treatment of gestational diabetes. *NEJM* 2008;358:2003–2015.

95. Siu S, Chan M, Lau T. Placental transfer of ondansetron during early human pregnancy. *Clin Pharmacokinet* 2006;45:419–423.

96. Einarson A, Maltepe C, Navioz Y, et al. The safety of ondansetron for nausea and vomiting of pregnancy: a prospective comparative study. *BJOG* 2004;111:940–943.

97. Berkovitch M, Mazzota P, Greenberg R, et al. Metoclopramide for nausea and vomiting of pregnancy: a prospective multicenter international study (abstract). *Amer J Perinatol* 2002;19:311–316.

98. Czeizel AE, Vargha P. A case-control study of congenital abnormality and dimenhydrinate usage during pregnancy. *Arch Gynecol Obstet* 2005;271:113–118.

99. Park-Wyllie L, Mazzotta P, Pastuszak A, et al. Birth defects after maternal exposure to corticosteroids: prospective cohort study and meta-analysis of epidemiological studies. *Teratology* 2000;62:385–392.

100. Houlihan D, Dennedy M, Ravikumar N, et al. Anti-hypertensive therapy and the feto-placental circulation: effects on umbilical artery resistance. *J Perinat Med* 2004;32:315–319.

101. Bricelj V. Use of adrenergic beta-blockers in pregnancy. *Heart Views* 1999;1(4):130–132.

102. Davis R, Eastman D, McPhillips H, et al. Risks of congenital malformations and perinatal events among infants exposed to calcium channel and beta-blockers during pregnancy. *Pharmacoepidemiol Drug Saf* 2010 [Epub ahead of print].

103. Macpherson M, Broughton-Pipkin F, Rutter N. The effect of maternal labetalol on the newborn infant. *Br J Obstet Gynaecol* 1986;93:539–542.

104. Lardoux H, Gerard J, Blazquez G, et al. Hypertension in pregnancy: evaluation of two beta blockers atenolol and labetalol. *Eur Heart J* 1983;4:35–40.

105. Oudijk M, Ruskamp J, Ververs T, et al. Treatment of fetal tachycardia with sotalol: transplacental pharmacokinetics and pharmacodynamics. *J Am Coll Cardiol* 2003;42(4):765–770.

106. Östman PL, Chestnut DH, Robillard JE, et al. Transplacental passage and hemodynamic effects of esmolol in gravid ewe. *Anesthesiology* 1988;69:738–741.

107. Ducey J, Knape K. Maternal esmolol administration resulting in fetal distress and cesarean section in a term pregnancy. *Anesthesiology* 1992;77:829–832.

108. Erkkola R, Lammintausta R, Liukko P, et al. Transfer of propranolol and sotalol across the human placenta, their effect on maternal and fetal plasma renin activity. *Acta Obstet Gynecol Scand* 1982;61:31–34.

109. Cottrill C, McAllister R, Gettes L, et al. Propranolol therapy during pregnancy, labor, and delivery: Evidence for transplacental drug transfer and impaired neonatal drug disposition. *J Pediatr* 1977;91:812–814.

110. Lindeberg S, Sandström B, Lundborg P, et al. Disposition of the adrenergic blocker metoprolol in the late-pregnant woman, the amniotic fluid, the cord blood and the neonate. *Acta Obstet Gynaecol* 1984;118:61–64.

111. Cox J, Gardner M. Treatment of cardiac arrhythmias during pregnancy. *Prog Cardiovasc Dis* 1993;137–178.

112. Melander A, Niklasson B. Ingemarsson I, et al. Transplacental passage of atenolol in man. *Eur J Clin Pharmacol* 1978;14:93–94.

113. Gregory YH, Beevers M, Churchill D, et al. Effect of atenolol on birth weight. *Am J Cardiol* 1997;79:1436–1438.

114. Magee K, Bawdon R. Ex vivo human placental transfer and the vasoactive properties of hydralazine. *Am J Obstet Gynecol* 2000;182:167–169.

115. Jones HMR, Cummings AJ, Setchell KD, et al. A study of the disposition of alpha-methyldopa in newborn infants following its administration to the mother for treatment of hypertension during pregnancy. *Br J Clin Pharmacol* 1979;8:433–440.

116. Palanisamy A, Klickovich RJ, Ramsay M, et al. Intravenous dexmedetomidine as an adjunct for labor analgesia and cesarean delivery anesthesia in a parturient with a tethered spinal cord. *IJOA* 2009;18:258–261.

117. Santeiro ML, Stromquist C, Wyble L. Phenoxybenzamine placental transfer during the third trimester. *Ann Pharmacother* 1996;30:1249–1251.

118. Bootstaylor BS, Roman C, Parer JT, et al. Fetal and maternal hemodynamic and metabolic effects of maternal nitroglycerin infusion in sheep. *Am J Obstet Gynecol* 1997;176:644–650.

119. De Rosayro M, Nahrwold ML, Hill AB, et al. Plasma levels and cardiovascular effects of nitroglycerin in pregnant sheep. *Can J Anesth* 1980;27:560–564.

120. Naulty J, Cefalo RC, Lewis PE. Fetal toxicity of nitroprusside in the pregnant ewe. *Am J Obstet Gynecol* 1981;139(6):708–711.

121. Donchin Y, Amirav B, Sahar A, et al. Sodium nitroprusside for aneurysm surgery in pregnancy. *Br J Anaesth* 1978;50:849–851.

122. Shoemaker CT, Meyers M. Sodium nitroprusside for control of severe hypertensive disease of pregnancy: a case report and discussion of potential toxicity. *Am J Obstet Gynecol* 1984;149:1713.

123. Graeme KA, Curry SC, Bikin DS, et al. The lack of transplacental movement of the cyanide antidote thiosulfate in gravid ewes. *Aneth Analg* 1999;89(6):1448–1452.

124. Ala-Kokko TI, Pienimaki P, Herva R, et al. Transfer of lidocaine and bupivacaine across the isolated perfused human placenta. *Pharmacol Toxicol* 1995;77(2):142–148.

125. Biehl D, Shnider S, Levinson G, et al. Placental transfer of lidocaine: effects of fetal acidosis. *Anesthesiology* 1978;48:409–412.

126. Morishima H, Santos A, Pedersen H, et al. Effect of lidocaine on the asphyxial responses in the mature fetal lamb. *Anesthesiology* 1987;66:502–507.

127. Kennedy R, Bell J, Miller R, et al. Uptake and distribution of lidocaine in fetal lambs. *Anesthesiology* 1990;72:483–489.

128. Johnson R, Herman N, Arney T, et al. Bupivacaine transfer across the human term placenta. *Anesthesiology* 1995;82:459–468.

129. Reynolds F, Laishley R, Morgan B, et al. The effect of time and adrenaline on the transplacental distribution of bupivacaine. *Br J Anaesth* 1989;62:509–514.

130. Laishley R, Carson R, Reynolds F. Effect of adrenaline on placental transfer of bupivacaine in the perfused in situ rabbit placenta. *Br J Anaesth* 1989;63:439–443.

131. Ueki R, Tatara T, Kariya N, et al. Comparison of placental transfer of local anesthetics in perfusates with different pH values in a human cotyledon model. *J Anesth* 2009;23:526–529.

132. Reiz S, Haggmark G, Johansson G, et al. Cardiotoxicity of ropivacaine—a new amide local anaesthetic agent. *Acta Anaesthesiol Scand* 1989;33:93–98.

133. Porter JM, Kelleher N, Flynn R, et al. Epidural ropivacaine hydrochloride during labour: protein binding, placental transfer and neonatal outcome. *Anaesthesia* 2001;56:418–423.

134. Datta S, Corke B, Alper M, et al. Epidrual anesthesia for cesarean section: a comparison of bupivacaine, chloroprocaine and etidocaine. *Anesthesiology* 1980;52:48–51.

135. Philipson EH, Kuhnert BR, Syracuse CD. Fetal acidosis, 2-chloroprocaine, and epidural anesthesia for cesarean section. *Am J Obstet Gynecol* 1985;151:322–324.

136. Bremerich DH, Schlosser RL, L'Allemand N, et al. Mepivacaine for spinal anesthesia in parturients undergoing elective cesarean and neonatal plasma concentrations and neonatal outcome. *Zentralbl Gynakol* 2003;125:518–521.

ASSESSMENT OF THE FETUS

CHAPTER

4

Antenatal Fetal Assessment, Therapy, and Outcomes

Christina M. Davidson

The mean duration of pregnancy calculated from the first day of the last normal menstrual period is very close to 280 days or 40 weeks. Pregnancy is then divided into three trimesters of equal duration. The first trimester extends through completion of 14 weeks, the second through 28 weeks, and the third includes the 29th to 42nd weeks of pregnancy. Since precise knowledge of fetal age is imperative for ideal obstetrical management, the clinically appropriate unit is weeks of gestation completed. Clinicians designate gestational age using completed weeks and days, for example 32^{+2} weeks for 32 completed weeks and 2 days (1).

■ FIRST TRIMESTER FETAL ASSESSMENT

Ultrasonography

Indications for first trimester ultrasound are listed in Table 4-1. When used for gestational age assessment, first trimester crown–rump measurement is the most accurate means for ultrasound dating of pregnancy (2). Ultrasonography may be considered to confirm menstrual dates if there is a gestational age agreement within 1 week by crown–rump measurements (2) (Fig. 4-1). Maximum embryo length at 6 to 10 weeks of gestation and crown–rump length, which represents the maximum length of the fetus from the top of the head to the rump region, are the most accurate at determining gestational age (3).

If a multiple gestation is detected, the first trimester is the optimal period to determine chorionicity (number of placentas) and amnionicity (number of amniotic sacs). Accurate determination of this is critical for the determination of fetal surveillance and timing of delivery in a twin gestation.

Prenatal Diagnosis of Fetal Aneuploidy

Screening

Historically, maternal age of 35 years or older at the time of delivery was used to identify women at highest risk of having a child with Down syndrome, and these women were offered genetic counseling and invasive testing (chorionic villus sampling [CVS] or amniocentesis) (4). Many additional screening tests for Down syndrome have since become available, including serum biochemical tests in both the first and second trimesters and ultrasound assessment of "nuchal translucency." Current recommendations are that all women should be offered aneuploidy screening before 20 weeks of gestation, regardless of maternal age, and that all women, regardless of age, should have the option of invasive testing (4).

In the first trimester, a combination of nuchal translucency (NT) measurement, serum markers (pregnancy-associated plasma protein A [PAPP-A] and free beta-human chorionic gonadotropin [free beta-HCG]), and maternal age is a very effective screening test for Down syndrome (4). The NT is a fluid-filled space in the posterior fetal nuchal area (Fig. 4-2). The excess skin of individuals with Down syndrome can be visualized by ultrasonography as increased NT in the first 3 months of intrauterine life (5) (Fig. 4-3), and the optimal gestational age for measurement is 11 to 14 weeks of gestation.

Women with an increased risk of aneuploidy with first trimester screening should be offered genetic counseling and diagnostic testing by CVS or a second trimester amniocentesis (5).

Diagnostic Techniques: Chorionic Villus Sampling

CVS involves sampling of placental villi through transcervical or transabdominal access to the placenta, thus allowing for cytogenetic analysis of fetal cells. It is generally performed at 10 to 13 weeks of gestation. The primary advantage of CVS is that a diagnosis of fetal aneuploidy can be made in the first trimester, thus allowing for earlier and safer termination of pregnancy if desired.

■ SECOND TRIMESTER FETAL ASSESSMENT

Ultrasonography

There are many indications for second and third trimester ultrasound (Table 4-2). When used for assessment of gestational age, ultrasound may be considered confirmatory of menstrual dates if there is a gestational age agreement within 10 days by an average of multiple fetal biometric measurements obtained in the second trimester (up to 20 weeks of gestation) (6). Determination of gestational age by ultrasonographic biometry alone in the first half of pregnancy has been shown to be a more accurate predictor of the delivery date than using menstrual data alone or in combination with ultrasonography (7–9). The biparietal diameter (BPD), head circumference, abdominal circumference, and femoral diaphysis length are the parameters used to estimate gestational age and fetal weight to (Figs. 4-4 to 4-6).

In the absence of specific indications, ultrasound examination between 18 and 20 weeks of gestation allows for a reasonable survey of fetal anatomy and an accurate estimation of gestational age. At this gestational age, anatomically complex organs, such as the fetal heart and brain, can be imaged with

TABLE 4-1 Indications for First Trimester Ultrasonography

- To confirm the presence of an intrauterine pregnancy
- To evaluate a suspected ectopic pregnancy
- To evaluate vaginal bleeding
- To estimate gestational age
- To diagnosis or evaluate multiple gestations
- To confirm cardiac activity
- As adjunct to chorionic villus sampling, embryo transfer, or localization and removal of an intrauterine device
- To assess for certain fetal anomalies, such as anencephaly, in patients at high risk
- To evaluate maternal pelvic or adnexal masses or uterine abnormalities
- To screen for fetal aneuploidy
- To evaluate suspected hydatidiform mole

Adapted from American College of Radiology. ACR practice guideline for the performance of obstetrical ultrasound. Available at: http://www.acr.org/SecondaryMainMenuCategories/quality_safety/guidelines/us/us_obstetrical.aspx. Last accessed October 31, 2011.

sufficient clarity to allow detection of many major malformations at a time when termination of pregnancy may still be an option (2). The essential elements of a standard fetal anatomic survey are listed in Table 4-3.

Prenatal Diagnosis of Fetal Aneuploidy

Screening

Multiple maternal serum markers are used to differentiate pregnancies affected by trisomy 18 and 21 (Down syndrome) that differ from those utilized with first trimester serum screening. Specifically, maternal serum alpha-fetoprotein (AFP), HCG, unconjugated estriol, and inhibin A are useful only in the second trimester. This "quad test" can detect 70% of Down syndrome fetuses (4). The inclusion of the maternal serum AFP aids in the identification of fetuses at increased risk for a neural tube defect (NTD), as amniotic fluid and

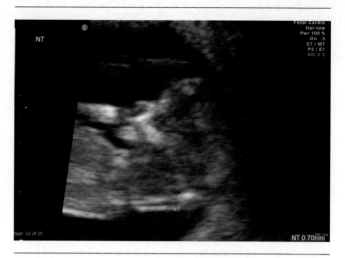

FIGURE 4-2 Normal nuchal translucency (NT) on ultrasound image. NT shows the measurement between cross marks.

maternal serum AFP levels are elevated in 89% to 100% of pregnancies complicated by fetal NTDs (10).

Diagnostic Techniques: Amniocentesis

Genetic amniocentesis is usually offered between 15 and 20 weeks of gestation. In the United States, it is the procedure most commonly used to diagnose fetal aneuploidy and other genetic disorders (11). A needle is inserted through the woman's abdominal wall and into the amniotic sac around the fetus, under ultrasound guidance, and a sample of amniotic fluid is collected. The cells in the amniotic fluid have been shed from the surface of the fetus and membranes. Once these cells have been cultured, fetal karyotyping can be performed (12).

■ FETAL THERAPY

Antenatal Corticosteroids for Fetal Maturity

Preterm birth is defined as delivery prior to 37 weeks of gestation. In the United States, it affects 12% of all births and is the leading cause of neonatal mortality and cerebral palsy. Despite advances in medicine, preterm births have increased by one-third over the last 25 years. The rate was 9.5% in 1981, 10.6% in 1990, 12.7% in 2005, and 12.8% in 2006 (13).

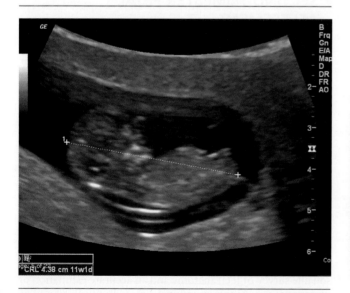

FIGURE 4-1 Crown–rump length (CRL) measurement on ultrasound image. Measured distance shown between cross marks.

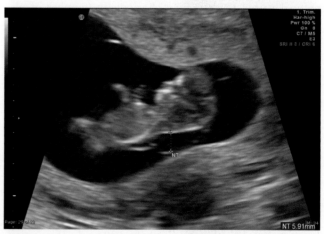

FIGURE 4-3 Increased nuchal translucency (NT) on ultrasound image. NT shows the measurement between cross marks.

TABLE 4-2 Indications for Second and Third Trimester Ultrasonography

- Estimation of gestational age
- Evaluation of fetal growth
- Evaluation of vaginal bleeding
- Evaluation of cervical insufficiency
- Evaluation of abdominal and pelvic pain
- Determination of fetal presentation
- Evaluation of suspected multiple gestation
- Adjunct to amniocentesis or other procedure
- Significant discrepancy between uterine size and clinical dates
- Evaluation of pelvic mass
- Examination of suspected hydatidiform mole
- Adjunct to cervical cerclage placement
- Evaluation of suspected ectopic pregnancy
- Evaluation of suspected fetal death
- Evaluation of suspected uterine abnormality
- Evaluation for fetal well-being
- Evaluation of suspected amniotic fluid abnormalities
- Evaluation of suspected placental abruption
- Adjunct to external cephalic version
- Evaluation for premature rupture of membranes or premature labor
- Evaluation for abnormal biochemical markers
- Follow-up evaluation of a fetal anomaly
- Follow-up evaluation of placental location for suspected placenta previa
- Evaluation for those with a history of previous congenital anomaly
- Evaluation of fetal condition in late registrants for prenatal care
- To assess findings that may increase the risk of aneuploidy
- To screen for fetal anomalies

Adapted from American College of Radiology. ACR practice guideline for the performance of obstetrical ultrasound. Available at: http://www.acr.org/SecondaryMainMenuCategories/quality_safety/guidelines/us/us_obstetrical.aspx. Last accessed October 31, 2011.

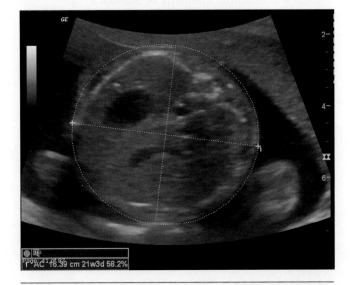

FIGURE 4-5 Abdominal circumference (AC) measurement on ultrasound image.

This increase has been attributed to the increased number of late preterm births (between 34 and 36 weeks of gestation) and the increased number of multi-fetal gestations secondary to fertility therapies (13–16).

Since 1970s, antenatal corticosteroid administration has been one of the most effective and cost-efficient prenatal interventions for preventing perinatal morbidity and mortality related to preterm birth (17). Antenatal corticosteroid therapy leads to improvement in neonatal lung function by enhancing maturational changes in lung architecture and by inducing type II alveolar cells that increase surfactant production (18). Antenatal corticosteroid therapy reduces the incidence of respiratory distress syndrome (RDS), intraventricular hemorrhage, necrotizing enterocolitis, sepsis, and neonatal mortality by approximately 50% (17). Maximum benefit is seen if delivery occurs more than 24 hours and less than 7 days after initiation of therapy. These effects are not limited by infant gender or race (19), however efficacy in multi-fetal gestations is less clear. A course

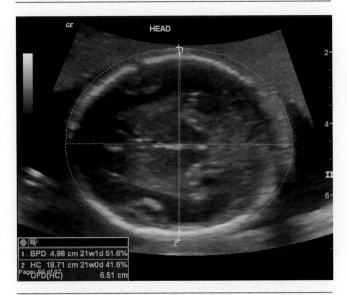

FIGURE 4-4 Head circumference (HC) and biparietal diameter (BPD) measurements on ultrasound image.

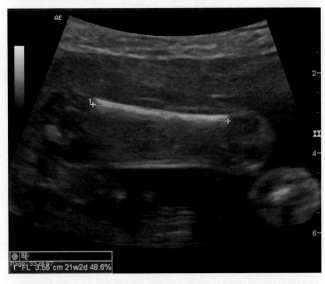

FIGURE 4-6 Femur length (FL) measurement on ultrasound image. Measured distance shown between cross marks.

TABLE 4-3 Essential Elements of Standard Examination of Fetal Anatomy

- Head, face, and neck
  - Cerebellum
  - Choroid plexus
  - Cistern magna
  - Lateral cerebral ventricles
  - Midline falx
  - Cavum septi pellucidum
  - Upper lip
- Chest–heart
  - 4-chamber view
  - Attempted visualization of the left and right outflow tracts
- Abdomen
  - Stomach (presence, size, and situs)
  - Kidneys
  - Bladder
  - Umbilical cord insertion site into the fetal abdomen
  - Umbilical cord vessel number
- Spine
  - Cervical
  - Thoracic
  - Lumbar
  - Sacral
- Extremities
  - Presence or absence of legs and arms
- Sex
  - Medically indicated in low-risk pregnancies only for the evaluation of multiple gestations

Adapted from American College of Radiology. ACR practice guideline for the performance of obstetrical ultrasound. Available at: http://www.acr.org/SecondaryMainMenuCategories/quality_safety/guidelines/us/us_obstetrical.aspx. Last accessed October 31, 2011.

of antenatal corticosteroids consists of 12 mg betamethasone intramuscularly every 24 hours for two doses or 6 mg dexamethasone intramuscularly every 12 hours for four doses (20,21). The American College of Obstetricians and Gynecologists (ACOG) recommends a single course of corticosteroids be given to all pregnant women between 24 and 34 weeks of gestation who are at risk of preterm delivery within 7 days. A single course of antenatal corticosteroids should be administered to women with preterm premature rupture of membranes (PPROM) before 32 weeks of gestation. The efficacy of antenatal corticosteroid use at 32 to 33 weeks of gestation for PPROM is unclear based on available evidence, but treatment may be beneficial, particularly if pulmonary immaturity is documented (20).

The lower limit of estimated gestational age for corticosteroid administration is approximately 24 weeks since there is a presumed inability of type II alveolar cells to respond at earlier gestational ages (22). Earlier administration might be justifiable only if aggressive perinatal interventions are planned for deliveries at 23 to 24 weeks of gestation. In a retrospective cohort study of neonates born at 23 weeks of gestation between 1998 and 2007, the authors concluded that neonates whose mothers completed a full course of antenatal corticosteroids had an associated 82% reduction in odds of death. Since RDS was uniform throughout their study population and 50% of the neonates exposed to steroids and survived to discharge experienced necrotizing enterocolitis or intraventricular hemorrhage or both, it was postulated that the survival benefit at this early gestational age may primarily be related to the beneficial effects of antenatal corticosteroids in tissues outside of the lung (18,23).

Magnesium Sulfate for Neuroprotection of the Fetus

Approximately one-third of the cases of cerebral palsy are associated with early preterm birth. Observational studies in the 1990s found that children born preterm who were exposed prenatally to magnesium sulfate for obstetric indications such as seizure prophylaxis (in preeclampsia) or tocolysis (in threatened preterm birth) had decreased rates of cerebral palsy as compared with children born preterm to women not exposed to magnesium sulfate (24–26). Magnesium sulfate is thought to induce its neuroprotective effects by reducing vascular instability, preventing hypoxic damage and mitigating cytokine or excitatory amino acid damage, all of which threaten the vulnerable preterm brain. Subsequently, several large randomized prospective clinical trials were performed to evaluate the utility of magnesium sulfate for fetal and neonatal neuroprotection (27–31).

In the most recent multicenter, placebo-controlled, randomized trial by Rouse et al. that was conducted at 20 participating NICHHD and Maternal Fetal Medicine Unit sites across the United States, 2,241 women at imminent risk for preterm birth between 24 and 32 weeks of gestation were randomly assigned to receive either IV magnesium sulfate or placebo (31). The risks for preterm birth included PPROM (87%), advanced preterm labor (10%), or indicated preterm delivery (3%). Although the composite study endpoint of neonatal death or cerebral palsy at 2 years of age was not found to be different between the magnesium and placebo treatment groups, a significant reduction in moderate or severe cerebral palsy among children whose mothers received magnesium sulfate (1.9% vs. 3.5%; relative risk, 0.55; 95% CI, 0.32 to 0.95) was noted. In contrast to previous trials, retreatment with magnesium sulfate was permitted in this study.

The Cochrane review (32) on the use of magnesium sulfate for neuroprotection of the fetus in women at risk for preterm birth included five randomized, placebo-controlled trials involving 6,145 babies and concluded that "the neuroprotective role for antenatal magnesium sulfate therapy given to women at risk of preterm birth for the preterm fetus is now established." There was a reduction in cerebral palsy for all the five studies (5,357 infants) that recruited women at less than 34 weeks gestation (RR 0.69, 95% CI 0.54 to 0.88). The number of women needed-to-be- treated to benefit one baby by avoiding cerebral palsy was 63. In addition, secondary analyses of some of the studies demonstrated an improvement in gross motor function (33).

Since the available evidence suggests that magnesium sulfate given before anticipated early preterm birth (up to 34 weeks of gestation) reduces the risk of cerebral palsy in surviving infants (34), ACOG recommends that physicians electing to use magnesium sulfate for fetal neuroprotection should develop specific guidelines regarding inclusion criteria, treatment regimens, management of concurrent tocolysis, and monitoring requirements in accordance with one of the larger trials (29–31).

■ THIRD TRIMESTER FETAL ASSESSMENT

Sonographic Evaluation of Fetal Growth and Amniotic Fluid Volume

Indications for third trimester ultrasound are listed in Table 4-2. A common use of third trimester ultrasound is assessment of fetal growth and amniotic fluid volume (AFV). Fetal growth is assessed indirectly throughout gestation with use of fundal height measurements during the prenatal care visits. Between 20 and 34 weeks of gestation, the height of the uterine fundus measured in centimeters correlates closely with gestational

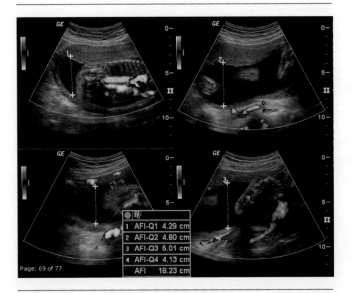

FIGURE 4-7 Amniotic fluid index (AFI). Four ultrasound images showing measurements of maximum vertical pockets of amniotic fluid in each of the four quadrants of the uterus with sum of the measurements equaling the AFI, as shown in the box.

age in weeks (35–37). Human fetal growth is characterized by sequential patterns of tissue and organ growth, differentiation and maturation. Development is determined by maternal provision of substrate, placental transfer of these substrates, and fetal growth potential governed by the genome (38). The fetus grows at a rate of approximately 5 g/day at 15 weeks of gestation, 15 to 20 g/day at 24 weeks of gestation, and 30 to 35 g/day at 34 weeks of gestation, however there is considerable biological variation in the velocity of fetal growth (39).

Amniotic fluid creates a physical space for the fetal skeleton to shape normally, promotes normal fetal lung development, and helps to avert compression of the umbilical cord (40). Normally, AFV reaches 1 L by 36 weeks of gestation and decreases thereafter to less than 200 mL at 42 weeks of gestation (41). Diminished fluid is termed oligohydramnios and excessive fluid is termed polyhydramnios. AFV is estimated using ultrasonography by either measurement of the single deepest vertical pocket of fluid, which is free of fetal extremities and umbilical cord, or measurement of the amniotic fluid index (AFI) (Fig. 4-7), which is the sum of the maximum vertical pockets in each of the four quadrants of the uterus (42–44). One widely used definition of oligohydramnios is no measurable vertical pocket of amniotic fluid greater than 2 cm (45) and another is an AFI of 5 cm or less (46). Polyhydramnios is defined as an AFI of 24 cm or more or a maximum vertical pocket of 8 cm or more (47).

Between 18 and 30 weeks, the uterine fundal height in centimeters coincides within 2 weeks of gestational age. Thus, if the measurement is more than 2 to 3 cm from the expected height, inappropriate fetal growth and/or abnormal AFV should be suspected (38). When discrepancies exist between fundal height and gestational age, an ultrasound is performed to investigate the cause; a lower than expected fundal height may represent fetal growth restriction (FGR) and/or oligohydramnios whereas a greater than expected fundal height may represent fetal macrosomia and/or polyhydramnios.

Fetal Growth Restriction
FGR is most commonly defined as an estimated fetal weight of less than the 10th percentile. This definition will include normal fetuses at the lower end of the growth spectrum as well as those with specific clinical conditions in which the fetus fails to achieve its inherent growth potential as a consequence of either pathologic extrinsic influences (such as maternal smoking) or intrinsic genetic defects (such as fetal aneuploidy) (48). Suboptimal fetal growth, which may or may not result in FGR, is evident by a reduction in growth percentiles as compared between estimated fetal weight estimates determined on ultrasound examinations performed at least 2 weeks apart.

Fetal Macrosomia
Excessive fetal growth is termed fetal macrosomia, however there is no uniform diagnosis of this condition. ACOG defines fetal macrosomia as growth beyond a specific weight of 4,500 g (49). The prenatal diagnosis of fetal macrosomia is very imprecise, however, as ultrasound's accuracy in predicting macrosomia has been found unreliable (50–52) and the superiority of ultrasound-derived estimates of fetal weight over clinical estimates has not been established (53–55). In fact, parous women are able to predict the weight of their newborns as well as clinicians who use ultrasound measurements or abdominal palpation (Leopold's maneuvers) (56).

Antenatal Surveillance in High-risk Pregnancies
The rate of stillbirth is 6.2/1,000 live births and fetal deaths in the United States, accounting for more than 55% of perinatal mortality (57). Fetal hypoxia and acidosis represent the final common pathways to fetal injury and death in many high-risk pregnancies (58). The goal of antenatal fetal surveillance (AFS) is to prevent fetal death and avoid unnecessary interventions. It relies on the premise that the fetus whose oxygenation in utero is challenged will respond with a series of detectable physiologic adaptive or decompensatory signs as hypoxemia or frank metabolic academia develop (59). It is generally used to assess the risk of fetal death in pregnancies at increased risk for antepartum fetal demise. This may be due to preexisting maternal conditions that pose a risk for uteroplacental insufficiency or from complications that develop during gestation. Table 4-4 lists factors that should prompt scheduled fetal surveillance.

Several AFS techniques, or tests, are used. The test selected, gestational age upon initiation of testing, and frequency of testing may vary by hospital and by institution. The most frequently used tests include non-stress test (NST), biophysical profile (BPP), modified BPP, contraction stress test (CST), and umbilical artery Doppler velocimetry. AFS is typically performed once or twice weekly, beginning at 32 to 34 weeks of gestation until delivery. A normal test result is considered reassuring (Table 4-5).

Non-stress Test
The NST is a recording of the fetal heart rate (FHR) with simultaneous documentation of uterine activity. Interpretation of the NST is on the basis of the premise that the heart rate of the fetus that is not acidotic or neurologically depressed will temporarily accelerate with fetal movement (60). FHR acceleration is defined as a visually apparent abrupt increase (onset to peak in less than 30 seconds) with a peak of 15 beats/min or more above the FHR baseline and a duration of 15 seconds or more from onset to return in a fetus of 32 weeks of gestation or more (61). NST results are categorized as being either reactive (normal) or nonreactive. Reactivity is said to occur if at least two accelerations are observed in a 20-minute period (Fig. 4-8). If reactivity has not occurred during the first 20 minutes, FHR and contraction monitoring may be continued for an additional 20 minutes. A nonreactive NST is one that lacks sufficient FHR accelerations over a 40-minute period (61).

TABLE 4-4 Indications for Antenatal Fetal Surveillance

Maternal Conditions	Pregnancy-induced Conditions
Antiphospholipid syndrome	Preeclampsia
Poorly controlled thyroid disease	Gestational hypertension
Hemoglobinopathies	Gestational diabetes mellitus requiring pharmacotherapy (A2)
Cyanotic heart disease	Amniotic fluid abnormalities
Systemic lupus erythematosus	Fetal growth restriction
Chronic renal disease	Alloimmunization
Pre-gestational diabetes mellitus (type I and type II)	Monochorionic/diamnionic twin gestation
Chronic hypertension	Dichorionic/diamnionic twin gestation with growth abnormality of one or both fetuses Decreased fetal movement Prior stillbirth Postterm pregnancy Fetal anomalies at increased risk for stillbirth Cholestasis of pregnancy Unexplained abnormal maternal serum screen analysis results

Biophysical Profile

The BPP consists of an NST combined with four observations made by real-time ultrasonography. These four components involve an assessment of fetal movements, fetal breathing, fetal tone, and AFV. The presence of a normal biophysical activity is indirect evidence that a given portion of the central nervous system that controls the activity is intact and functioning and therefore non-hypoxemic. The absence of a given fetal biophysical activity, however, is much more difficult to interpret, since it may reflect either pathologic depression or normal periodicity (62). The biophysical activities that become active first in fetal development are the last to disappear when asphyxia arrests all biophysical activities. The fetal tone center is the earliest to function in utero, at 7.5 to 8.5 weeks of gestation. The fetal movement center starts functioning at approximately 9 weeks of gestation. Diaphragmatic contraction and regular fetal breathing do not occur until 20 to 21 weeks of gestation. The FHR reactivity center, which starts operating by the end of the second trimester or

TABLE 4-5 False-negative Rate of Antepartum Fetal Surveillance[a]

- NST: 1.9/1,000
- BPP: 0.8/1,000
- Modified BPP: 0.8/1,000
- CST: 0.3/1,000

[a]*Defined* as incidence of stillbirth occurring within 1 week of normal test. NST, non-stress test; BPP, biophysical profile; CST, contraction stress test. Compiled from: Freeman RK, Anderson G, Dorchester W. A prospective multi-institutional study of antepartum fetal heart rate monitoring. I. Risk of perinatal mortality and morbidity according to antepartum fetal heart rate test results. *Am J Obstet Gynecol* 1982;143:771–777. Manning FA, Morrison I, Harman CR, et al. Fetal assessment based on fetal biophysical profile scoring: experience in 19,221 referred high-risk pregnancies. II. An analysis of false-negative fetal deaths. *Am J Obstet Gynecol* 1987;157:880–884. Miller DA, Rabello YA, Paul RH. The modified biophysical profile: antepartum testing in the 1990s. *Am J Obstet Gynecol* 1996;174:812–817.

early third trimester, is the most sensitive to hypoxia, whereas the fetal tone is the last to disappear during asphyxia (62). In the antepartum fetal evaluation, the presence or absence of the acute markers of the fetal condition (NST, fetal breathing movements, fetal movements, and fetal tone) will determine the level of fetal compromise at the time of testing. The fetus with suboptimal oxygenation will usually present with nonreactive non-stress testing and absence of fetal breathing at the initial stages of hypoxia. If hypoxia becomes worse, the fetal body movements and fetal tone will be abolished (gradual hypoxia concept). AFV, unlike the other biophysical variables, is not acutely influenced by alterations in fetal central nervous system function (62). Rather, it is a chronic marker of the fetal condition with oligohydramnios resulting from fetal oliguria secondary to hypoxia-induced redistribution of fetal blood flow (63).

Each of the five components of the BPP is assigned a score of either 2 (normal or present) or 0 (abnormal, absent, or insufficient) (Table 4-6). A composite score of 8 (with normal amniotic fluid) or 10 is normal, indicating no fetal indication exists for intervention. A score of 6 is considered equivocal, posing a possible risk of fetal asphyxia, and generally prompts delivery in the term fetus. In a preterm fetus, a repeat BPP may be considered in 24 hours (64). A score of 4 or less is abnormal, suggesting probable fetal asphyxia, and generally warrants delivery.

Modified BPP

The modified BPP combines the NST as a short-term indicator of fetal acid–base status with an assessment of AFV, which, as discussed previously, is an indicator of long-term placental function (65). An AFI greater than 5 cm represents an adequate volume of amniotic fluid (46). Thus, the modified BPP is considered normal if the NST is reactive and the AFI is more than 5, and abnormal if either the NST is nonreactive or the AFI is 5 or less (60).

Contraction Stress Test

The CST is based on the response of the FHR to uterine contractions, in contrast to the NST. It relies on the premise that fetal oxygenation will be transiently worsened by

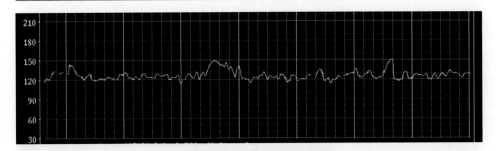

FIGURE 4-8 Reactive non-stress test (NST) tracing.

uterine contractions. In the suboptimally oxygenated fetus, the resultant intermittent worsening in oxygenation will, in turn, lead to the FHR pattern of late decelerations (60). Contractions may be induced with either oxytocin or nipple stimulation until three contractions of 40 seconds' duration each or longer are present in a 10-minute period. If this occurs spontaneously, no uterine stimulation is necessary. The CST is then interpreted according to the presence or absence of late FHR decelerations (Table 4-7). Relative contraindications to the CST generally include conditions associated with an increased risk of preterm labor and delivery, uterine rupture, or uterine bleeding, such as preterm labor or certain patients at high risk of preterm labor, PPROM, history of extensive uterine surgery or classical cesarean delivery, or known placenta previa (66).

Umbilical Artery Doppler Velocimetry

The umbilical arteries arise from the common iliac arteries and represent the dominant outflow of the distal aortic circulation. They are a reflection of the downstream resistance of the placental circulation. Normal umbilical artery (UA) resistance falls progressively throughout pregnancy (67), so increased resistance in the UA represents placental injury. As UA resistance rises, diastolic velocities fall, and ultimately these are absent (absent end-diastolic velocities) (68). As resistance rises even further, an elastic component is added, which will induce reversed end-diastolic flow, as the insufficient, rigid placental circulation recoils after being distended by pulse pressure (69).

UA Doppler flow velocimetry assessments are considered most useful for monitoring early onset FGR (less than 32 to 34 weeks of gestation) due to uteroplacental insufficiency

(70) based on the observation that flow velocity waveforms in the UA of normally growing fetuses differ from those of growth-restricted fetuses. Normally growing fetuses are characterized by high-velocity diastolic flow (Fig. 4-9). In contrast, when FGR exists as a result of uteroplacental insufficiency, UA diastolic flow is diminished, absent (Fig. 4-10), or reversed (Fig. 4-11) in severe cases (71).

Abnormal flow velocity waveforms have been correlated with fetal hypoxia and acidosis, as well as with perinatal morbidity and mortality (7273). Absent end-diastolic velocity may progress to reversed end-diastolic flow. Since reversed end-diastolic flow is considered a terminal condition, preparations for delivery are often made once abnormal UA Doppler flow is detected. The best test for determining the optimal timing of delivery for a preterm fetus with growth restriction is not yet known, however abnormal UA flow generally prompts admission to the hospital for administration of antenatal corticosteroids and daily BPP and FHR monitoring. The fetus with reversal of flow in the UA is often delivered after administration of corticosteroids, however in the fetus with only absent end-diastolic flow, delivery may be delayed up to 34 weeks of gestation if the BPPs and NSTs remain reassuring (74).

Assessment of Fetal Lung Maturity and Timing of Elective Delivery

To prevent iatrogenic prematurity, fetal pulmonary maturity should be confirmed before elective delivery at less than 39 weeks of gestation unless fetal maturity can be inferred from any of the following criteria: (1) ultrasound measurement at less than 20 weeks of gestation supports gestational

TABLE 4-6 **Biophysical Profile Components**

Component	Score 2	Score 0
NST	≥2 accelerations of ≥15 BPM for ≥15 s w/in 20–40 min	0 or 1 acceleration w/in 20–40 min
Fetal breathing	≥1 episode of rhythmic breathing lasting ≥30 s w/in 30 min	<30 s of breathing w/in 30 min
Fetal movement	≥3 discrete body or limb movements w/in 30 min	<3 discrete movements
Fetal tone	≥episode of extremity extension and subsequent return to flexion	0 extension/flexion events
Amniotic fluid volume	A pocket of amniotic fluid that measures at least 2 cm in two planes perpendicular to each other (2 × 2 cm pocket)	Largest single vertical pocket ≤2 cm

NST, non-stress test; BPM, breaths/minute.
Adapted from: Manning FA, Platt LD, Sipos L. Antepartum fetal evaluation: Development of a fetal biophysical profile. *Am J Obstet Gynecol* 1980;136:787–795.

TABLE 4-7 CST Interpretation

- Negative: no late or significant variable decelerations
- Positive: late decelerations following ≥50% of contractions (even if contraction frequency is <3 in 10 min)
- Equivocal suspicious: intermittent late decelerations or significant variable decelerations
- Equivocal hyperstimulatory: FHR decelerations that occur in the presence of contractions more frequent than every 2 min or lasting longer than 90 s
- Unsatisfactory: <3 contractions in 10 min or an uninterpretable tracing

age of 39 weeks or greater; (2) fetal heart tones have been documented as present for 30 weeks by Doppler ultrasonography; (3) it has been 36 weeks since a serum or urine HCG pregnancy test was found to be positive by a reliable laboratory test. If any of these criteria confirms a gestational age of 39 weeks or more, it is appropriate to schedule delivery at that time (6).

If fetal lung maturity testing is required, amniocentesis may be performed for amniotic fluid analysis of either the concentration of particular components of pulmonary surfactant (biochemical tests) or the surface-active effects of these phospholipids (biophysical tests) (6). A commonly used fetal lung maturity test is fluorescence polarization (TDx-FLM II), however other tests are available as well. A TDx-FLM II value of 55 mg/g or greater has a 96% to 100% positive predictive value of pulmonary maturity (6). In a study that sought to determine the weekly increment in TDx-FLM ratio during the third trimester, the mean value was 14.4 ± 9.9 mg/g (median 12.7 mg/g), and was not impacted by maternal race, diabetic status or fetal gender (75). Studies that have investigated the association between elective cesarean deliveries and neonatal respiratory morbidity have demonstrated an increased risk with decreasing gestational age. If elective cesarean delivery is performed after 39 weeks of gestation, respiratory morbidity

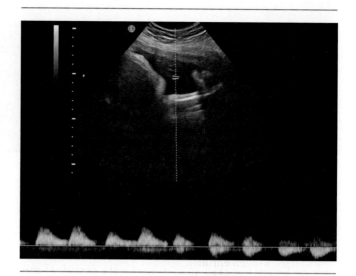

FIGURE 4-10 Absent end-diastolic flow in umbilical artery. Flow tracing shows end-diastolic flow at zero baseline.

is lower than if performed between 37 and 39 weeks of gestation (76–80). In one study, the incidence of respiratory morbidity decreased from 8.4% at 37 weeks to 1.8% after 39 weeks (77). There is also evidence that the risk of respiratory morbidity is reduced with labor before cesarean delivery (81–83). A reduction in the incidence of respiratory morbidity from 30% of neonates delivered before labor compared with 11.2% delivered after the onset of labor has been demonstrated (81). Therefore, awaiting the onset of spontaneous labor to determine the timing of repeat cesarean delivery in women at term is an effective way of preventing iatrogenic neonatal RDS (83).

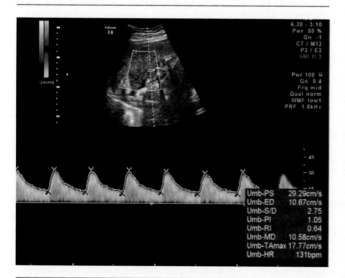

FIGURE 4-9 Normal umbilical artery Doppler flow. Ultrasound image shows direction of scan with direction of blood flow indicated by red and blue colors. Flow tracing shows normal systolic peaks (PS) and diastolic troughs (ED) of flow through the umbilical artery.

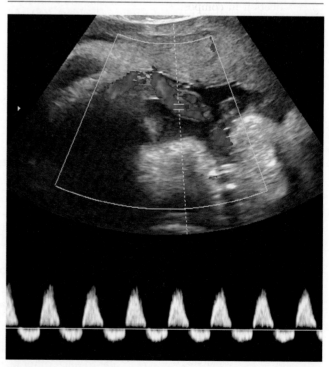

FIGURE 4-11 Reversed end-diastolic flow. Flow tracing shows diastolic flow as negative which represents reversal of flow in the umbilical artery during diastole.

■ FETAL THERAPY

Antenatal Corticosteroids for Fetal Maturity

Although antenatal corticosteroids for fetal maturity are recommended for all pregnant women between 24 and 34 weeks of gestation who are at risk for preterm delivery within 7 days (20), approximately 50% of patients given an initial course of antenatal corticosteroids remain undelivered 7 to 10 days later (84). Since some of these women remain at high risk for preterm birth and obstetricians are inaccurate at predicting who will deliver preterm and when, investigators looked at the administration of repeat courses of corticosteroids. Clinical trials investigating repeat doses of antenatal corticosteroids have shown an association with higher rates of cerebral palsy (85) and a decrease in birth weight, birth length, and head circumference, especially after four courses of steroids (86). Because of insufficient scientific evidence, repeat corticosteroid courses should not be used routinely but should be reserved for women enrolled in clinical trials (20).

Since routine weekly administration of antenatal corticosteroids may have deleterious effects on the neonate, another strategy that has been investigated is administration of a "rescue" course of steroids. In this approach, an initial course of steroids is administered when preterm birth is first anticipated. If the patient does not deliver over the next 7 to 14 days and preterm delivery is again imminent, a repeat steroid course is given. Recently, a small randomized placebo-controlled trial evaluated the impact of a single "rescue course" of steroids in 247 pregnancies with intact membranes (87). Participants had initiated the first steroid course at least 14 days before enrollment and at a gestational age less than 30 weeks and were once again considered at risk for preterm delivery within a week from enrollment. In spite of that entry criterion, the mean interval between randomization and delivery was about 25 days. Delivery occurred at less than 34 weeks of gestation in 56% of women receiving rescue corticosteroids and 55% of those receiving placebo. A significant reduction in composite neonatal morbidity, including decreased RDS, ventilator support, and surfactant use, was observed in the retreated group, without perinatal survival benefit or any long-term data.

In addition to use of antenatal corticosteroids for women at risk for preterm birth up to 34 weeks of gestation, there may be a role for their administration between 34 and 37 weeks of gestation as well. The same investigators that looked at the mean weekly increment in TDx-FLM II have recently estimated the effect of antenatal glucocorticoid administration on fetal lung maturity in pregnancies with known fetal lung immaturity (by amniocentesis) between 34th and 37th weeks of gestation (88). Administration of steroids to women with a TDx-FLM II of less than 45 mg/g between 34 and 37 weeks of gestation resulted in a mean increase in 1 week of 28.37 mg/g as opposed to 9.76 mg/g with no treatment ($p <$ 0.002). Therefore, a single course of antenatal corticosteroids may be considered between 34 and 37 weeks of gestation in women with proven pulmonary immaturity and obstetrical indication for prompt delivery.

Since prelabor cesarean delivery, especially those performed at term but prior to 39 weeks of gestation, has been associated with increased respiratory morbidity in the newborn, the antenatal steroids for term cesarean sections (ASTECS) randomized trial was conducted to evaluate whether giving the recommended two doses of betamethasone before delivery reduces the incidence of respiratory distress in babies delivered by elective cesarean at term (89). Corticosteroids significantly decreased the rate of admission to the special care nursery for respiratory distress (RR, 0.46; 95% CI, 0.23 to 0.93), however RDS in this study was unconventionally defined as transient tachypnea of the newborn (respiratory rate >60) with grunting, recession, or nasal flaring. Although suggestive, the number needed to treat to prevent one case of RDS or even one NICU admission would exceed 100 at term (90).

Magnesium Sulfate for Neuroprotection of the Fetus

As previously stated, since the available evidence suggests that magnesium sulfate given before anticipated early preterm birth (up to 34 weeks of gestation) reduces the risk of cerebral palsy in surviving infants (34), ACOG recommends that physicians electing to use magnesium sulfate for fetal neuroprotection should develop specific guidelines regarding inclusion criteria, treatment regimens, concurrent tocolysis, and monitoring in accordance with one of the larger trials (29–31).

KEY POINTS

- When used for gestational age assessment, first trimester crown–rump measurement is the most accurate means for ultrasound dating of pregnancy.
- Current recommendations are that all women should be offered aneuploidy screening before 20 weeks of gestation, regardless of maternal age, and that all women, regardless of age, should have the option of invasive testing.
- In the absence of specific indications, ultrasound examination between 18 and 20 weeks of gestation allows for a reasonable survey of fetal anatomy and an accurate estimation of gestational age.
- Antenatal corticosteroid therapy reduces the incidence of RDS, intraventricular hemorrhage, necrotizing enterocolitis, sepsis, and neonatal mortality by approximately 50%. ACOG recommends a single course of corticosteroids be given to all pregnant women between 24 and 34 weeks of gestation who are at risk of preterm delivery within 7 days. A single rescue course of antenatal corticosteroids may be considered if the antecedent treatment was given more than 2 weeks prior, the gestational age is less than 32^{+6} weeks, and the women are judged by the clinician to be likely to give birth within the next week.
- The Cochrane review on the use of magnesium sulfate for neuroprotection of the fetus in women at risk for preterm birth concluded that "the neuroprotective role for antenatal magnesium sulfate therapy given to women at risk of preterm birth for the preterm fetus is now established."
- The goal of AFS is to prevent fetal death and avoid unnecessary interventions. It relies on the premise that the fetus whose oxygenation in utero is challenged will respond with a series of detectable physiologic adaptive or decompensatory signs as hypoxemia or frank metabolic academia develop.
- To prevent iatrogenic prematurity, fetal pulmonary maturity should be confirmed before elective delivery at less than 39 weeks of gestation.

REFERENCES

1. Hauth JC, Rouse DJ, Spong CY. Prenatal Care. In: Cunningham GF, Leveno KJ, Bloom SL, et al., eds. *Williams Obstetrics.* 23rd ed. New York, NY: McGraw-Hill; 2010:189–214.
2. American College of Obstetricians and Gynecologists. ACOG Practice Bulletin No. 101: Ultrasonography in pregnancy. *Obstet Gynecol* 2009;113(2 Pt 1):451–461.
3. Wisser J, Dirschedl P, Krone S. Estimation of gestational age by transvaginal sonographic measurement of greatest embryonic length in dated human embryos. *Ultrasound Obstet Gynecol* 1994;4:457–462.

4. ACOG Committee on Practice Bulletins. ACOG Practice Bulletin No. 77: Screening for fetal chromosomal abnormalities. *Obstet Gynecol* 2007;109(1):217–227.
5. Nicolaides KH, Azar G, Byrne D, et al. Fetal nuchal translucency: ultrasound screening for chromosomal defects in first trimester of pregnancy. *BMJ* 1992;5:15–19.
6. American College of Obstetricians and Gynecologists. ACOG Practice Bulletin No. 97: Fetal lung maturity. *Obstet Gynecol* 2008;112(3):717–726.
7. Mongelli M, Wilcox M, Gardosi J. Estimating the date of confinement: ultrasonographic biometry versus certain menstrual dates. *Am J Obstet Gynecol* 1996;174:278–281.
8. Savitz DA, Terry JW, Dole N, et al. Comparison of pregnancy dating by last menstrual period, ultrasound scanning, and their combination. *Am J Obstet Gynecol* 2002;187:1660–1666.
9. Mul T, Mongelli M, Gardosi J. A comparative analysis of second-trimester ultrasound dating formulae in pregnancies conceived with artificial reproductive techniques. *Ultrasound Obstet Gynecol* 1996;8:397–402.
10. Milunsky A. Maternal serum screening for neural tube and other defects. In: *Genetic Disorders and the Fetus: Diagnosis, Prevention, and Treatment.* 4th ed. Baltimore, MD: Johns Hopkins University Press; 1998:635–701.
11. Hauth JC, Rouse DJ, Spong CY. Prenatal diagnosis and fetal therapy. In: Cunningham GF, Leveno KJ, Bloom SL, et al., eds. *Williams Obstetrics.* 23rd ed. New York, NY: McGraw-Hill; 2010:287–311.
12. Gianluigi P. Prenatal diagnostic techniques. In: Nyberg DA, McGahan JP, Pretorius DH, et al., eds. *Diagnostic Imaging of Fetal Anomalies.* Philadelphia, PA: Lippincott Williams and Wilkins; 2003:943–968.
13. Hamilton BE, Martin JA, Sutton PD, et al. Births: Final data for 2005. *Natl Vital Stat Rep* 2007;56(6):4.
14. Martin JA, Hamilton BE, Sutton PD, et al. Births. Final data for 2004. *Natl Vital Stat Rep* 2006;55(1):80–81.
15. Wright VC, Schieve LA, Reynolds MA, et al. Assisted reproductive technology surveillance, United States, 2000. *MMWR Morb Mortal Wkly Rep* 2000;52(SS 9):1–16.
16. March of Dimes Peristats 2008. Rates of preterm birth in multifetal pregnancies 1990–2004. Available at http://www.marchofdimes.com/peristats/ Last accessed October 14, 2011.
17. Liggins GC, Howie RN. A controlled trial of antepartum glucocorticoid treatment for prevention of the respiratory distress syndrome in premature infants. *Pediatrics* 1972;50:515–525.
18. Ballard PL, Ballard RA. Scientific basis and therapeutic regimens for use of antenatal glucocorticoids. *Am J Obstet Gynecol* 1995;173:254–262.
19. Crowley PA. Antenatal corticosteroid therapy: a meta-analysis of the randomized trials, 1972–1994. *Am J Obstet Gynecol* 1995;173:322.
20. ACOG Committee on Obstetric Practice. ACOG Committee Opinion No. 475: Antenatal corticosteroid therapy for fetal maturation.. *Obstet Gynecol* 2011;117(2 Pt 1):422–424.
21. Report of the Consensus Development Conference on the Effect of Corticosteroids for Fetal Maturation on Perinatal Outcomes. National Institute of Child Health and Human Development. November 1994. NIH Publication No. 95-3784.
22. Jobe A. The respiratory system: Part 1. Lung development. In: Fanaroff A, Martin R, eds. *Neonatal-Perinatal Medicine: Diseases of the Fetus and Infant.* 7th ed. St. Louis, MO: Mosby; 2002:973–991.
23. Hayes EJ, Paul DA, Stahl GE, et al. Effect of antenatal corticosteroids on survival for neonates born at 23 weeks of gestation. *Obstet Gynecol* 2008;111:921–926.
24. Nelson KB, Grether JK. Can magnesium sulfate reduce the risk of cerebral palsy in very low birthweight infants? *Pediatrics* 1995;95:263–269.
25. Schendel DE, Berg CJ, Yeargin-Allsopp M, et al. Prenatal magnesium sulfate exposure and the risk for cerebral palsy or mental retardation among very low-birth-weight children aged 3 to 5 years. *JAMA* 1996;276:1805–1810.
26. Paneth N, Jetton J, Pinto-Martin J, et al. Magnesium sulfate in labor and risk of neonatal brain lesions and cerebral palsy in low birth weight infants. The Neonatal Brain Hemorrhage Study Analysis Group. *Pediatrics* 1997;99:E1.
27. Mittendorf R, Covert R, Boman J, et al. Is tocolytic magnesium sulphate associated with increased total paediatric mortality? *Lancet* 1997;350:1517–1518.
28. Mittendorf R, Dambrosia J, Pryde PG, et al. Association between the use of antenatal magnesium sulfate in preterm labor and adverse health outcomes in infants. *Am J Obstet Gynecol* 2002;186:1111–1118.
29. Crowther CA, Hiller JE, Doyle LW, et al. Effect of magnesium sulfate given for neuroprotection before preterm birth: a randomized controlled trial. Australasian Collaborative Trial of Magnesium Sulphate (ACTOMgSO4) Collaborative Group. *JAMA* 2003;290:2669–2676.
30. Marret S, Marpeau L, Zupan-Simunek V, et al. Magnesium sulphate given before very-preterm birth to protect infant brain: the randomised controlled PREMAG trial group. *BJOG* 2007;114:310–318.
31. Rouse DJ, Hirtz DG, Thom E, et al. A randomized, controlled trial of magnesium sulfate for the prevention of cerebral palsy. Eunice Kennedy Shriver NICHD Maternal-Fetal Medicine Units Network. *N Engl J Med* 2008;359:895–905.
32. Doyle LW, Crowther CA, Middleton P, et al. Magnesium sulphate for women at risk of preterm birth for neuroprotection of the fetus. *Cochrane Database Syst Rev* 2009;21(1):CD004661.
33. Marret S, Marpeau L, Follet-Bouhamed C, et al. Effect of magnesium sulphate on mortality and neurologic morbidity of the very-preterm newborn (of less than 33 weeks) with two-year neurological outcome: results of the prospective PREMAG trial. [French]. *Gynecol Obstet Fertil* 2008;36:278–288.
34. Conde-Agudelo A, Romero R. Antenatal magnesium sulfate for the prevention of cerebral palsy in preterm infants less than 34 weeks' gestation: a systematic review and metaanalysis. *Am J Obstet Gynecol* 2009;200(6):595–609.
35. Calvert JP, Crean EE, Newcombe RG, et al. Antenatal screening by measurement of symphysis-fundus height. *BMJ* 1982;285:846.
36. Jimenez J, Tyson JE, Reisch JS. Clinical measures of gestational age in normal pregnancies. *Obstet Gynecol* 1983;61:438.
37. Quaranta P, Currell R, Redman CWG, et al. Prediction of small-for-dates infants by measurement of symphysial-fundal height. *Br J Obstet Gynaecol* 1981;88:115.
38. Hauth JC, Rouse DJ, Spong CY. Fetal Growth Disorders. In: Cunningham GF, Leveno KJ, Bloom SL, et al., eds. *Williams Obstetrics.* 23rd ed. New York, NY: McGraw-Hill; 2010:842–858.
39. Williams RL, Creasy RK, Cunningham GC, et al. Fetal growth and perinatal viability in California. *Obstet Gynecol* 1982;59:624.
40. Hauth JC, Rouse DJ, Spong CY. Disorders of Amnionic Fluid Volume. In: Cunningham GF, Leveno KJ, Bloom SL, et al., eds. *Williams Obstetrics.* 23rd ed. New York, NY: McGraw-Hill; 2010:490–499.
41. Queenan JT. Polyhydramnios and oligohydramnios. *Contemp Obstet Gynecol* 1991;36:60.
42. Manning FA, Platt LD, Sipos L. Antepartum fetal evaluation: development of a fetal biophysical profile score. *Am J Obstet Gynecol* 1980;136:787–795.
43. Phelan JP, Ahn MO, Smith CV, et al. Amniotic fluid index measurements during pregnancy. *J Reprod Med* 1987;32:601–604.
44. Phelan JP, Smith CV, Broussard P, et al. Amniotic fluid volume assessment with the four-quadrant technique at 36–42 weeks' gestation. *J Reprod Med* 1987;32:540–542.
45. Chamberlain PF, Manning FA, Morrison I, et al. Ultrasound evaluation of amniotic fluid volume. I. The relationship of marginal and decreased amniotic fluid volumes to perinatal outcome. *Am J Obstet Gynecol* 1984;150:245–249.
46. Rutherford SE, Phelan JP, Smith CV, et al. The four-quadrant assessment of amniotic fluid volume: an adjunct to antepartum fetal heart rate testing. *Obstet Gynecol* 1987;70:353–356.
47. Gianluigi P. Abnormalities of Amniotic Fluid. In: Nyberg DA, McGahan JP, Pretorius DH, et al., eds. *Diagnostic Imaging of Fetal Anomalies.* Philadelphia, PA: Lippincott Williams and Wilkins; 2003:59–84.
48. American College of Obstetricians and Gynecologists. Intrauterine growth restriction. Clinical management guidelines for obstetricians-gynecologists. *Int J Gynaecol Obstet* 2001;72(1):85–96.
49. ACOG Practice Bulletin No. 22. Fetal Macrosomia. *Obstet Gynecol* 2000;96(5). (reaffirmed 2010)
50. Deter RL, Hadlock FP. Use of ultrasound in the detection of macrosomia: a review. *J Clin Ultrasound* 1985;13:519–524.
51. Rossavik IK, Joslin GL. Macrosomatia and ultrasonography: what is the problem? *South Med J* 1993;86:1129–1132.
52. Sandmire HF. Whither ultrasonic prediction of fetal macrosomia? *Obstet Gynecol* 1993;82:860–862.
53. Chauhan SP, Cowan BD, Magann EF, et al. Intrapartum detection of a macrosomic fetus: clinical versus 8 sonographic models. *Aust N Z J Obstet Gynaecol* 1995;35(3):266–270.
54. Johnstone FD, Prescott RJ, Steel JM, et al. Clinical and ultrasound prediction of macrosomia in diabetic pregnancy. *Br J Obstet Gynaecol* 1996;103:747–754.
55. Chauhan SP, Hendrix NW, Magann EF, et al. Limitations of clinical and sonographic estimates of birth weight: experience with 1034 parturients. *Obstet Gynecol* 1998;91:72–77.
56. Chauhan SP, Sullivan CA, Lutton TD, et al. Parous patients' estimate of birth weight in postterm pregnancy. *J Perinatol* 1995;15:192–194.
57. Mac Dorman MF, Munson ML, Kirmeyer S. Fetal and perinatal mortality, United States, 2004. *Natl Vital Stat Rep* 2007;56:1–19.
58. Vintzileos A, Campbell W, Rodis H, et al. The relationship between fetal biophysical assessment, umbilical artery velocimetry, and fetal acidosis. *Obstet Gynecol* 1991;77:622–626.
59. Signore C, Freeman R, Spong C. Antenatal Testing-A Reevaluation. *Obstet Gynecol* 2009;113:687–701.
60. ACOG Practice Bulletin No. 9. Antepartum Fetal Surveillance. *Obstet Gynecol* 1999;94(4). (reaffirmed 2009)
61. American College of Obstetricians and Gynecologists. ACOG Practice Bulletin No. 106: Intrapartum fetal heart rate monitoring: nomenclature, interpretation, and general management principles. *Obstet Gynecol* 2009;114(1):192–202.

62. Vintzileos A, Campbell W, Nochimson D, et al. The use and misuse of the fetal biophysical profile. *Am J Obstet Gynecol* 1987;156:527–533.

63. Groome LJ, Owen J, Neely CL. Oligohydramnios: antepartum fetal urine production and intrapartum fetal distress. *Am J Obstet Gynecol* 1991;165:1077.

64. Manning FA, Harman CR, Morrison I, et al. Fetal assessment based on fetal biophysical profile scoring. IV. An analysis of perinatal morbidity and mortality. *Am J Obstet Gynecol* 1990;162:703–709.

65. Clark SL, Sabey P, Jolley K. Nonstress testing with acoustic stimulation and amniotic fluid volume assessment: 5973 tests without unexpected fetal death. *Am J Obstet Gynecol* 1989;160:694–697.

66. Free RK. The use of the oxytocin challenge test for antepartum clinical evaluation of uteroplacental respiratory function. *Am J Obstet Gynecol* 1975;121:481–489.

67. Stuart B, Drumm J, Fitzgerald DE, et al. Fetal blood velocity waveforms in normal pregnancy. *BJOG* 1980;87:780.

68. Trudinger BJ, Stevens D, Connelly A, et al. Umbilical artery flow velocity waveforms and placental resistance: the effects of embolization of the umbilical circulation. *Am J Obstet Gynecol* 1987;157:1443.

69. Arabin B, Siebert M, Jimenez R, et al. Obstetrical characteristics of a loss of end diastolic velocities in the fetal aorta and/or umbilical artery using Doppler ultrasound. *Gynecol Obstet Invest* 1988;25:173.

70. Kontopoulos EV, Vintzileos AM. Condition-specific antepartum fetal testing. *Am J Obstet Gynecol* 2004;191:1546–1551.

71. Gudmundsson S, Marsal K. Umbilical and uteroplacental blood flow velocity waveforms in pregnancies with fetal growth retardation. *Eur J Obstet Gynecol Reprod Biol* 1988;27:187–196.

72. Karsdorp VH, van Vugt JM, van Geijn HP, et al. Clinical significance of absent or reversed end diastolic velocity waveforms in umbilical artery. *Lancet* 1997;344:1664–1668.

73. Nicolaides KH, Bilardo CM, Soothill PW, et al. Absence of end diastolic frequencies in umbilical artery: a sign of fetal hypoxia and acidosis. *BMJ* 1988;297:1026–1027.

74. Mari G, Hanif F. Intrauterine growth restriction: how to manage and when to deliver. *Clin Obstet Gynecol* 2007;50:497–509.

75. Bildirici I, Moga CN, Gronowski AM, et al. The mean weekly increment of amniotic fluid TDx-FLM II ratio is constant during the latter part of pregnancy. *Am J Obstet Gynecol* 2005;193:1685–1690.

76. Hansen AK, Wisborg K, Uldbjerg N, et al. Risk of respiratory morbidity in term infants delivered by elective caesarean section: cohort study. *BMJ* 2008;336(7635):85–87.

77. Van den Berg A, Van Elburg RM, Van Geijn HP, et al. Neonatal respiratory morbidity following elective caesarean section in term infants; a 5-year retrospective study and review of the literature. *Eur J Obstet Gynecol Reprod Biol* 2001;98(1):9–13.

78. Zanardo V, Simbi AK, Franzoi M, et al. Neonatal respiratory morbidity risk and mode of delivery at term: influence of timing of elective caesarean delivery. *Acta Paediatr* 2004;93:643–647.

79. Zanardo V, Simbi AK, Vedovato S, et al. The influence of timing of elective cesarean section on neonatal resuscitation risk. *Pediatr Crit Care Med* 2004;5(6):566–570.

80. Yee W, Amin H, Wood S. Elective cesarean delivery, neonatal intensive care unit admission, and neonatal respiratory distress. *Obstet Gynecol* 2008;111:823–828.

81. Cohen M, Carson BS. Respiratory morbidity benefit of awaiting onset of labor after elective cesarean section. *Obstet Gynecol* 1985;65(6):818–824.

82. Gerten KA, Coonrod DV, Bay RC, et al. Cesarean delivery and respiratory distress syndrome: Does labor make a difference? *Am J Obstet Gynecol* 2005;193:1061–1064.

83. Bowers SK, MacDonald HM, Shapiro ED. Prevention of iatrogenic neonatal respiratory distress syndrome: elective repeat cesarean section and spontaneous labor. *Am J Obstet Gynecol* 1982;143:186–189.

84. Modi N, Lewis H, Al-Naqeeb N, et al. The effects of repeated antenatal glucocorticoid therapy on the developing brain. *Pediatr Res* 2001;50:581–585.

85. Wapner RJ, Sorokin Y, Mele L, et al. Long-term outcomes after repeat doses of antenatal corticosteroids. *N Engl J Med* 2007;357:1190–1198.

86. Murphy KE, Hannah ME, Willan AR, et al. Multiple courses of antenatal corticosteroids for preterm birth (MACS): a randomised controlled trial. *Lancet* 2008;372:2143–2151.

87. Garite TJ, Kurtzman J, Maurel K, et al. Impact of a "rescue course" of antenatal corticosteroids: a multicenter randomized placebo-controlled trial. *Am J Obstet Gynecol* 2009;200:248.e1–248.e9.

88. Shanks A, Gross G, Shim T, et al. Administration of steroids after 34 weeks of gestation enhances fetal lung maturity profiles. *Am J Obstet Gynecol* 2010;203:47.e1–47.e5.

89. Stutchfield P, Whitaker R, Russell I. Antenatal betamethasone and incidence of neonatal respiratory distress after elective caesarean section: pragmatic randomised trial. *BMJ* 2005;331(7518):662.

90. Sinclair JC. Meta-analysis of randomized controlled trials of antenatal corticosteroid for the prevention of respiratory distress syndrome: discussion. *Am J Obstet Gynecol* 1995;173:335–344.

Intrapartum Fetal Monitoring: Old and New Concepts

Michelle Simon • Rakesh B. Vadhera • George R. Saade

■ BACKGROUND

The original goal among obstetric practice and basis for intrapartum fetal monitoring was the prevention of cerebral palsy (CP), hypoxic ischemic encephalopathy (HIE), neonatal encephalopathy, and perinatal death. Any of these morbidities and mortality of a term or near-term infant not only produces a wide array of long-term sequelae and disabilities, they are also a prominent cause of medicolegal claims against the health care system both in economic terms and in the length of time it takes to resolve them (1). Over five decades since its introduction, electronic fetal monitoring (EFM) became synonymous with intrapartum fetal monitoring and fetal heart rate (FHR) interpretation became the most common tool available for fetal surveillance. Although it is very sensitive for detecting a nonhypoxic fetus, it has repeatedly been shown to have a very poor predictive value for accurately identifying a hypoxic fetus or one that will develop CP (2). This may be partly related to a lack of standardized protocol for interpretation of FHR and high interobserver and intraobserver variability interpreting FHR tracings even in the presence of guidelines. Recent data indicate that compared to other peripartum causes, the incidence of CP secondary to intrapartum hypoxia is very low (2–4). There are very few tools available to predict a fetus at risk as insult may occur prior to the onset of labor, labor itself may not be tolerated, or the fetus is in an unhealthy environment that requires prompt delivery. Recently published new guidelines on standardizing the approach to the interpretation of FHR tracings and additional complementary tests to predict a fetus at risk for intrapartum hypoxia are the basis of current monitoring strategies and research discussed below.

■ GOALS OF INTRAPARTUM MONITORING

The ideal goals of intrapartum fetal monitoring are to 1. assure fetal well-being and improve perinatal outcome; specifically by decreasing incidence of stillbirth and neonatal seizures and preventing injury to the fetal central nervous system and long-term neurologic impairments such as CP; 2. serve as a screening test to detect episodes, trends, and severity of hypoxia and metabolic acidemia, their effect on cardiac rhythm, variability, and depression which may also result in neurologic damage or fetal death; 3. identify and differentiate the fetus that is not affected by labor from the one that is negatively affected by labor but has enough reserve to tolerate it, and the fetus that lacks the reserve to compensate the insult of labor and can be harmed by it; 4. allow for timely interventions, such as prompt delivery, to avoid any morbidity and mortality in infants; and 5. minimize unnecessary obstetric interventions such as operative vaginal and cesarean deliveries. In conclusion, the ideal monitor should aim to reduce CP rates and fetal or neonatal deaths without increasing maternal morbidity and interventions. To this date, EFM has not been able to fulfill these objectives (5).

Intrapartum continuous EFM was introduced into obstetric practice in the 1960s for complicated pregnancies with the idea that it would prevent perinatal asphyxia and mortality (6). By 1978, almost 66% of all women in the United States were being monitored with EFM during labor, whether their pregnancy was complicated or not (7); and by 2002 over 85% of women in the United States underwent EFM during labor (8).

Although monitoring FHR is widely used and accepted, it has very poor interobserver and intraobserver reliability, uncertain efficacy, and a high false-positive rate (2).

■ DEFINITIONS AND INCIDENCE OF FETAL HYPOXIC ENCEPHALOPATHY AND CEREBRAL PALSY

According to ACOG's task force on neonatal encephalopathy and cerebral palsy, *neonatal encephalopathy* is defined in term and near-term infants as "a constellation of findings to include a combination of abnormal consciousness, tone and reflexes, feeding, respiration, or seizures and can result from a myriad of conditions" (9–11). It is a clinical syndrome of disturbed neurologic function of the term and near-term infant in the early neonatal period, manifested by respiratory difficulties, depression of tone and reflexes, obtundation, and frequent seizures (10,12). The etiology is varied and can include multiple genetic and metabolic conditions that present with similar clinical signs (3). It is only called HIE if there is evidence that intrapartum asphyxia is the cause of the encephalopathy which resulted in neurologic depression or seizures. In order to define an acute intrapartum event sufficient to cause CP and intrapartum asphyxia, ACOG and the American Academy of Pediatrics Task Force on Neonatal Encephalopathy and Cerebral Palsy defined several criteria that must be met (Table 5-1) (13). While these criteria are still current as of writing of this chapter, revised criteria are expected and may be published by the time this textbook is published or shortly thereafter. It is important to note that over 75% of cases of neonatal encephalopathy have no clinical signs of intrapartum hypoxia (11).

Cerebral palsy (CP) is a static neurologic condition resulting from brain injury that mostly occurs before cerebral development is complete. It can occur during the prenatal, perinatal, or postnatal periods, during the time the brain is developing (14). It is described as an aberrant control of movement or posture that is nonprogressive and permanent, appearing in early life secondary to a defect or lesion in the immature brain (15). The onset occurs no later

TABLE 5-1 Acute Intrapartum Events Most Likely to Cause CP

Must fulfill all four essential criteria:
1. Exclude trauma, coagulation disorders, infectious conditions, or genetic disorders.
2. Fetal metabolic acidosis (pH < 7 and base deficit >12 mmol/L in umbilical arterial blood)
3. Spastic quadriplegic or diskinetic CP in infants born at ≥34 weeks
4. Moderate to severe neonatal encephalopathy

Additional evidence to suggest an intrapartum insult:
1. Apgar scores ≤3 beyond 5 minutes
2. Evidence of multisystem insult within three days of birth
3. A hypoxic sentinel peripartum event
4. A sudden and sustained fetal bradycardia or the absence of FHR variability in the presence of category II or III tracing, following a sentinel event.
5. Acute nonfocal cerebral abnormality on radiologic studies.

Adapted from: American College of Obstetricians and Gynecologists, *Neonatal encephalopathy and cerebral palsy: defining the pathogenesis and pathophysiology.* 1st ed. Washington, DC: ACOG; 2003.

than 1 year of age and the definite diagnosis is preferably reserved until the age of 4 and 5 (16). It affects 2/1,000 liveborn children and its incidence has remained constant over the past 30 years.

In 1861–1862 William J. Little, an orthopedic surgeon, proposed the hypothesis that cerebral palsy was primarily caused by prematurity, birth trauma, and asphyxia neonatorum (3,17). This hypothesis was accepted as soon as it was proposed, without any significant scientific evidence to confirm it, and it was not challenged for many years. Although many people continue to believe this original hypothesis about the etiology of CP, there is substantial evidence that 70% to 80% of cerebral palsy cases in term and preterm infants arise during pregnancy due to antenatal factors long before the onset of labor (15,18–22). Birth complications including asphyxia account for only about 8% to 28% of the cases of CP (3,12,15,23). Only 24% of all term children with CP had a history of neonatal encephalopathy, which means 76% had a normal intrapartum and newborn course. Among the children that survived moderate to severe neonatal encephalopathy at term, the overall rate of those who developed CP was 13%, and the rate was higher in the group that presented with neonatal seizures (18,24). It is now believed that as few as 4% of moderate and severe neonatal encephalopathy cases which are attributable to hypoxia incurred solely during the intrapartum period, explaining the estimated low overall incidence of neonatal encephalopathy due to intrapartum hypoxia (1.6 per 10,000 births) (25).

FACTORS CONTROLLING FETAL HEART RATE

FHR analysis and its variability are the primary means by which the fetus is evaluated for adequacy of oxygenation. Variability of FHR results from the interaction of the sympathetic and parasympathetic autonomic nervous sys-

tem. The fetal brain is known to modulate the heart rate through a series of interactions between the sympathetic and parasympathetic systems; as a result, if the fetal brain is hypoxic, FHR changes would reflect the insult. FHR variability is believed to represent an intact neurologic pathway that includes the fetal cerebral cortex, midbrain, vagus nerve, and cardiac conduction system. It has prognostic importance clinically, and valuable empiric interpretations can be made according to its presence or absence. A fetus with unexplained minimal or absent FHR variability and no periodic changes can fall into one of several categories: (a) quiet sleep state; (b) idiopathic reduced FHR variability with no obvious explanation but without evidence of asphyxia or central nervous system compromise; (c) centrally acting drugs given to the mother, for example, opioids; (d) congenital neurologic abnormality due to either a developmental CNS defect or an in utero infection or asphyxic event (26); (e) abnormal cardiac conduction system, for example, complete heart block; or (f) deep asphyxia with inability of the heart to manifest periodic changes (27). Severely growth restricted fetuses can also have minimal FHR variability without any demonstrable asphyxia. It is important to consider that a fetus with an abnormal cardiac conduction system, anencephaly, or other congenital neurologic deficit may present with minimal or absent variability. In the case of congenital neurologic impairment, this FHR pattern may actually represent asphyxia that occurred during the antepartum period (11).

Sympathetic outflow in the fetus is thought to be relatively tonic. The vagus nerve, hence the vagal tone, is responsible for FHR variability, and blocking it with atropine results in disappearance of this variability (28). Modulation in vagal tone occurs in response to changes in blood pressure detected by baroreceptors in the aortic arch and to changes detected in chemoreceptors on the carotid bodies detecting oxygen and carbon dioxide fluctuations. The sympathetic influence is tonic and helps improve pumping activity in the heart during intermittent stressful situations by increasing the FHR. As with the vagal tone, the sympathetic tone influence increases during fetal hypoxia.

The term asphyxia is defined experimentally as impaired respiratory gas exchange accompanied by the development of metabolic acidosis. In the clinical setting, it is a continuum of oxygen deficit. One side of this spectrum includes transient or intermittent hypoxemia, which if repeated, continued, or prolonged may progressively lead to hypercarbia, metabolic acidemia, and acidosis especially in a fetus with already reduced reserve (29–32). During periods of asphyxia, fetal response can vary from physiologic compensatory mechanisms to asphyxia damage.

Alpha adrenergic activity alters the distribution of blood flow to specific organs during hypoxia causing vasoconstriction to certain vascular beds such as the intestines, liver, and lung, hence improving perfusion to vital organs such as the brain, heart, adrenals, and placenta (33,34). It is known that hypoxia in the fetus causes bradycardia with hypertension (35). Umbilical blood flow is unaffected by acute moderate hypoxia but is decreased by severe hypoxia. Umbilical blood flow is also affected by the administration of catecholamines and acute cord occlusion.

Brief reduction of intervillous blood flow during uterine contractions and temporary cord occlusion causing transient hypoxemia is common during labor. During these periods there is hyperemia-induced redistribution of blood flow favoring the heart, brain, and adrenal glands (33,36). These transient events decrease the arterial and venous oxygen concentration gradient across the myocardial and cerebral circulation but increase the respective blood flow, thus maintaining constant oxygen consumption in the heart and brain (33,37–39). This compensation is achieved by reducing blood flow to other vascular beds thereby inducing anaerobic metabolism.

During repetitive hypoxic events, the fetus develops metabolic acidosis from accumulation of lactic acid which is often an end result of vasoconstriction and anaerobic oxidation in certain vascular beds. Increase in carbon dioxide tension superimposes a respiratory component to this acidosis (40). These compensating mechanisms allow the fetus to survive moderately long periods of limited oxygen supply (up to 30 minutes) without affecting vital organs like the brain and heart (38,39).

When asphyxia becomes severe and fetal acidemia ensues, the protective mechanisms become overwhelmed, and vasoconstriction becomes severe and extensive. At this point, oxygen delivery and consumption by all organs is decreased, even in the organs previously favored. Fetal bradycardia mostly accompanied by hypotension is marked at this point, and in a short period of time death can occur. It is thought that hypoxic organ damage occurs during this period of physiologic decompensation (41).

During labor, there are four major mechanisms by which a fetus can have decreased oxygen delivery: (a) inadequate uterine blood flow (UBF) to the intervillous space, (b) interruption of umbilical blood flow, (c) decrease in maternal oxygen tension, and (d) fetal pathology.

UBF is one of the major determinants of oxygen exchange across the placenta. Reducing UBF beyond a certain level will result in inadequate fetal oxygen uptake. This reduction may occur acutely, for example, in cases of abruptio placenta or hypotension following spinal anesthesia; chronically, as in cases of pregnancy-induced hypertension; or intermittently, during maternal hypotension secondary to supine positioning.

Once oxygen has been transported from the maternal to the fetal side of the placenta, the adequacy of *umbilical blood flow* will determine its availability to the fetus. When umbilical cord occlusion occurs, it results in fetal hypertension, which initiates a vagal response with subsequent bradycardia. If the occlusion is intermittent in an otherwise healthy fetus, the FHR will intermittently decrease as evidence of a variable deceleration.

A decrease in *maternal oxygen tension* is a rare cause of fetal asphyxia during the intrapartum period. It can be caused during maternal apnea, pulmonary edema, amniotic fluid embolism, venous air embolism, or severe asthma. Another rare cause of asphyxia or hypoxemia is abnormal *fetal pathology* with either increased metabolic rate (e.g., pyrexia) or with decreased oxygen carrying capacity (e.g., anemia from Rh sensitization). These fetuses and the preterm fetus can be less tolerant of the decreased oxygen delivery during uterine contractions in labor and may develop metabolic acidosis sooner.

■ ELECTRONIC FETAL MONITORING

Since the 1970s EFM became widely available and its use disseminated rapidly. Interpretations of FHR tracings were empirical and with time the tracings that were considered abnormal were the ones where a depressed baby was delivered. Believing that intrapartum asphyxia was the main cause of CP, proponents of EFM hoped that by using this monitor fetuses at risk of asphyxia would be recognized easily and delivered promptly, therefore reducing the rate of CP. Studies have shown that the use of EFM has neither decreased the rate of CP nor proven to be a precise tool for predicting

either fetal metabolic acidosis or HIE (42,43). In fact, relevant clinical trials argue that EFM as it exists today, does not decrease neonatal morbidity or mortality related to intrapartum acidosis or hypoxia, but rather increases the risks to mothers and babies of having additional surgical or instrumental deliveries (44).

Even though EFM has not been able to prove substantial benefits to both mother and fetus, it is still the commonest obstetric procedure performed in the United States, used in about 85% of all births in 2002 (45).

The most commonly used monitors for fetal well-being during labor consist of three complementary techniques:

1. *external (indirect)* ultrasound (Doppler) monitoring of the FHR and uterine contractions, that can be obtained either continuously or intermittently;
2. *internal (direct)* fetal electrocardiogram (ECG) and uterine contraction monitoring, that is invasive, continuous and is obtained by passage of electrodes and an intrauterine pressure catheter (IUPC) through the cervical os;
3. *fetal scalp blood sampling* through the cervical os to determine fetal blood pH.

In addition to these techniques, during labor the use of the ultrasound to verify FHR and fetal movements can be used and some mothers and care givers still use intermittent auscultation of the FHR with a Doppler monitor or fetoscope during labor to assess the fetus. Other complementary techniques used to assess the fetus include the use of ultrasound for a biophysical profile (BPP) and newer techniques such as fetal ECG monitoring using fetal ST segment analysis and fetal oximetry monitoring. Some of these techniques require validation and are currently undergoing clinical trials to confirm their utility.

The use of FHR monitoring is not without risks. The increase in operative deliveries and cesarean deliveries is not negligible and imposes risks for the mother and the fetus (46,47). There are also infectious complications associated with invasive fetal monitoring that include endometritis, chorioamnionitis, and direct fetal infections. The use of an IUPC has been associated with uterine perforation, placental laceration, abruption, placental vessel perforation, cord entanglement, and possible amniotic fluid embolism (48,49). Monitoring has also been blamed for affecting women's and partners' experience of labor, changing the interaction with healthcare practitioners, and has been considered by some patients intrusive and dehumanizing during a natural event of labor and delivery.

The EFM device has two components: one for the FHR and one for uterine contractions. The FHR can be recorded directly or indirectly. The indirect method can be used throughout pregnancy and has no contraindications. This indirect method utilizes ultrasound waves (approximately 2.5 MHz) originating from a transducer, that reflect from the moving structures of the heart and return to the transducer and are interpreted as electrical signals (Fig. 5-1). The direct method utilizes an ECG electrode placed subcutaneously on the fetus that detects the electrical impulses originating in the fetal heart, the R wave of the fetal ECG complex is detected and amplified and the interval between two complexes is used to calculate the FHR. This direct method requires the cervix to be at least 1 cm dilated, rupture of the fetal membranes, and the insertion of a probe into the fetal scalp, which carries a small risk of infection, and should only be used when the benefit of it outweighs the risk.

Uterine contractions can also be detected and measured directly or indirectly. In the indirect method a tocodynamometer (pressure transducer) is applied tightly to the

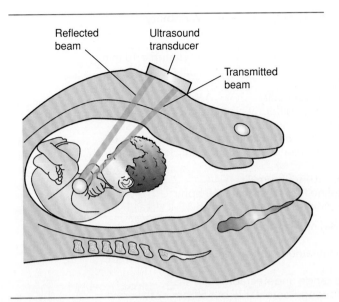

FIGURE 5-1 The Doppler ultrasound device for detecting cardiac activity.

mother's abdominal wall and recognizes the tightening of the maternal abdomen during contractions. These signals are converted and plotted into the uterine activity graph. This indirect method is noninvasive and can be performed throughout pregnancy but its information is limited to determining contraction frequency, but not strength, and is further limited in morbidly obese women. The direct method is obtained using a thin, flexible IUPC placed transcervically in the intra-amniotic cavity. Pressure is transmitted through a pressure transducer and the measurements plotted on a graph that allows reading of both the frequency and strength of contractions. This method requires ruptured membranes and is an invasive method that should only be used when benefits outweigh the risks.

■ FETAL HEART RATE PATTERNS: NOMENCLATURE, INTERPRETATION, AND GUIDELINES

When assessing FHR patterns, basic guidelines dictated by ACOG and the National Institute of Child Health and Human Development have been updated (2,50). The assessment of uterine contractions and FHR and its baseline, variability, presence of accelerations and decelerations, and the changes of these over time are necessary for the interpretation of intrapartum FHR monitoring. The data of FHR and uterine contractions are plotted on paper that is moving at a rate of 3 cm/min; the vertical scale of this paper is standardized to a scale of 30 beats/min/cm. The characteristics of the plotted information are used to analyze and interpret FHR patterns and draw conclusions about the status of the fetus at a given point in time.

Terminology is very important when assessing FHR patterns. The term *"nonreassuring fetal heart status"* has been adopted by ACOG instead of the term "fetal distress" which is an inaccurate term that implies much more than it is able to predict. Clinical signs of a nonreassuring FHR poorly predict a compromised fetus, and the use of "fetal distress" may encourage wrong assumptions or inappropriate management (11).

Uterine contractions are quantified as the number of contractions present in a 10-minute window, averaged over a 30-minute period. In clinical practice, not only is frequency important, but also duration, intensity, and relaxation time between contractions. *Normal* uterine activity is defined as five contractions or less in 10 minutes, averaged over 30 minutes. *Tachysystole* is defined as more than five contractions in 10 minutes averaged over 30 minutes. Adequate uterine contractions in labor have an intensity of 50 to 70 mm Hg at their peak or may be expressed as 250 to 300 Montevideo units (contractions/10 min multiplied by peak pressure over baseline, measured by an IUPC).

The *normal baseline FHR* is between 110 and 160 beats per minute (bpm), with *bradycardia* defined as any FHR below 110 bpm and *tachycardia* as FHR above 160 bpm (2). The baseline is established during a 10-minute segment, for a minimum of 2 minutes. *Baseline variability* is defined as fluctuations in the baseline FHR that are irregular in amplitude and frequency and are determined in a 10-minute window, excluding acceleration and decelerations. Accelerations and decelerations are noted as well as other patterns. Variability is the most sensitive marker for fetal well-being and is currently assessed visually, as a whole, quantitated as the amplitude of peak to trough in bpm, and classified as *absent, minimal, moderate (normal)*, or *marked* (50) (Table 5-2).

Acceleration is a visually apparent abrupt increase in FHR, from onset to peak in <30 seconds. The peak must be at least 15 bpm above baseline and it must last at least 15 seconds from its onset to the return to baseline. A prolonged acceleration lasts longer than 2 minutes but less than 10 minutes. If acceleration lasts longer than 10 minutes it is called a change in baseline.

Decelerations can be classified as *late, early,* or *variable* based on their characteristic timing relative to uterine contractions (Table 5-3). *Early decelerations* mirror a simultaneous uterine contraction, with the FHR nadir occurring within 30 seconds and simultaneously with the peak of the contraction. They are felt to be related to reflexes initiated by fetal head compression and are treated as benign. *Variable decelerations* can be accompanied by several different patterns that require further investigation to assess their clinical relevance (e.g., slow return of FHR after the end of the contraction, biphasic decelerations, or tachycardia after the deceleration often called overshoot or shoulder). *Prolonged decelerations* are present when the FHR decreases from baseline more than 15 bpm longer than 2 minutes, but less than 10 minutes. Deceleration lasting longer than 10 minutes is deemed a baseline change.

Late decelerations are considered to be caused by a decrease in UBF during the contraction that pushes which exceeds the capacity of the fetus to extract oxygen. The relatively deoxygenated blood transported from the placenta to the fetus during the contraction causes fetal hyperemia, which results in chemoreceptor-mediated vagal discharge causing a transient deceleration. They are thought to start late relative to the peak of the uterine contraction because the progressive decrease in oxygen tension must reach a certain threshold to induce increased vagal activity. In extreme cases direct myocardial hypoxic depression can produce late decelerations (28,51).

A *sinusoidal FHR pattern* is defined as having a visually apparent smooth sine wave-like undulating pattern in FHR with a frequency of 3 to 5 per minute that persists for over 20 minutes. It is considered an ominous pattern and immediate action is required to deliver a fetus with this pattern.

Principles of management of FHR monitoring should consider that it correlates with fetal acid–base status at the time of observation, but it does not predict CP, and the clinician

TABLE 5-2 Electronic Fetal Monitoring Definitions of Baseline and Variability

Pattern	Definition

Baseline	• The mean FHR rounded to increments of 5 bpm during a 10 min segment, excluding:
	  • Periodic or episodic changes
	  • Periods of marked FHR variability
	  • Segments of baseline that differ by more than 25 bpm
	• The baseline must be for a minimum of 2 min in any 10 min segment, or the baseline for that time period is indeterminate. In this case, one may refer to the prior 10 min window for determination of baseline.
	• Normal FHR baseline: 110–160 bpm
	• Tachycardia: FHR baseline is greater than 160 bpm
	• Bradycardia: FHR baseline is less than 110 bpm

Baseline variability	• Fluctuations in the baseline FHR that are irregular in amplitude and frequency
	• Variability is visually quantitated as the amplitude of peak-to-trough in bpm
	  • Absent—amplitude range undetectable
	  • Minimal—amplitude range detectable but 5 bpm or fewer
	  • Moderate (normal)—amplitude range 6–25 bpm
	  • Marked—amplitude range greater than 25 bpm

FHR, fetal heart rate.
Reprinted with permission from: Macones GA, Hankins GD, Spong CY, et al. The 2008 National Institute of Child Health and Human Development workshop report on electronic fetal monitoring: update on definitions, interpretation, and research guidelines. *Obstet Gynecol* 2008;112:661–666.

should always consider its evolution over time and correlation with the entire clinical scenario.

FHR tracings during intrapartum fetal monitoring have recently been organized into a three-tier classification system and depending on this classification different actions are recommended to try to minimize fetal risk. They group the tracings as *category I, category II,* and *category III* tracings. The three categories can be summarized as classifying the tracings as normal (*category I*), abnormal (*category III*), or in a "middle category" (*category II*) that is considered equivocal, indeterminate, suspicious, atypical, and intermediate (Table 5-4).

A *category I FHR tracing* is considered *normal* and includes tracings with normal baseline FHR, moderate variability, absent variable or late decelerations, and with or without early decelerations and accelerations (Fig. 5-2). These category

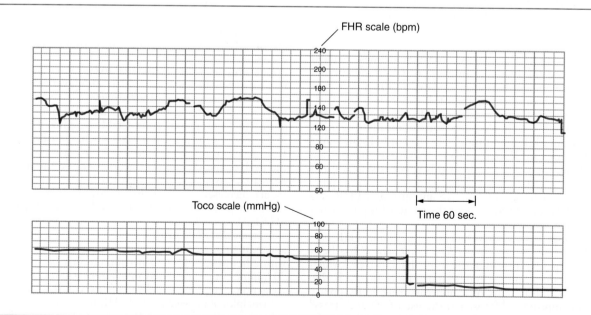

FIGURE 5.2 Example of a Category I tracing with moderate variability, normal baseline, and accelerations. Note the scales used on the standardized paper for recording FHR and the lack of contractions on the tocodynamometer scale.

TABLE 5-3 Electronic Fetal Monitoring Definitions for Acceleration and Different Decelerations

Pattern	Definition
Acceleration	• A visually apparent abrupt increase (onset to peak in less than 30 s) in the FHR • At 32 wks of gestation and beyond, acceleration has a peak of 15 bpm or more above baseline, with a duration of 15 s or more but less than 2 min from onset to return • Before 32 wks of gestation, acceleration has a peak of 10 bpm or more above baseline, with a duration of 10 s or more but less than 2 min from onset to return • Prolonged acceleration lasts 2 min or more but less than 10 min in duration • If acceleration lasts 10 min or longer, it is a baseline change
Early deceleration	• Visually apparent usually symmetrical gradual decrease and return of the FHR associated with a uterine contraction • A gradual FHR decrease is defined as from the onset to the FHR nadir of 30 s or more • The decrease in FHR is calculated from the onset to the nadir of the deceleration • The nadir of the deceleration occurs at the same time as the peak of the contraction • In most cases the onset, nadir, and recovery of the deceleration are coincident with the beginning, peak, and ending of the contraction, respectively
Late deceleration	• Visually apparent usually symmetrical gradual decrease and return of the FHR associated with a uterine contraction • A gradual FHR decrease is defined as from the onset to the FHR nadir of 30 s or more • The decrease in FHR is calculated from the onset to the nadir of the deceleration • The deceleration is delayed in timing, with the nadir of the deceleration occurring after the peak of the contraction • In most cases, the onset, nadir, and recovery of the deceleration occur after the beginning, peak, and ending of the contraction, respectively
Variable deceleration	• Visually apparent abrupt decrease in FHR • An abrupt FHR decrease is defined as from the onset of the deceleration to the beginning of the FHR nadir of less than 30 s • The decrease in FHR is calculated from the onset to the nadir of the deceleration • The decrease in FHR is 15 bpm or greater, lasting 15 s or greater, and less than 2 min in duration • When variable decelerations are associated with uterine contractions, their onset, depth, and duration commonly vary with successive uterine contractions
Prolonged deceleration	• Visually apparent decrease in the FHR below the baseline • Decrease in FHR from the baseline that is 15 bpm or more, lasting 2 min or more but less than 10 min in duration • If a deceleration lasts 10 min or longer, it is a baseline change
Sinusoidal pattern	• Visually apparent, smooth, sine wave-like undulating pattern in FHR baseline with a cycle frequency of 3–5 per min which persists for 20 min or more

FHR, fetal heart rate.
Reprinted with permission from: Macones GA, Hankins GD, Spong CY, et al. The 2008 National Institute of Child Health and Human Development workshop report on electronic fetal monitoring: update on definitions, interpretation, and research guidelines. *Obstet Gynecol* 2008;112:661–666.

I tracings may be monitored in a regular manner and do not require any specific action.

A *category III FHR tracing* is considered *abnormal* and is associated with fetal acid–base abnormalities at the time of observation. Depending on the clinical scenario, efforts to expeditiously resolve this pattern are needed, such as providing maternal oxygen, changing maternal position, discontinuation of labor stimulation, treatment of maternal hypotension, and treatment of tachysystole. If these efforts do not resolve the category III FHR tracing, the fetus should be delivered (2). FHR tracings in this category are usually extreme cases, for example, repetitive late decelerations with absent variability (Fig. 5-3).

A *category II FHR tracing* is considered *indeterminate* and is not predictive of fetal acid–base abnormality; it may be also considered equivocal, indeterminate, suspicious, or atypical. Such tracings require constant re-evaluation and surveillance, taking into consideration the clinical circumstances of the patient and the fetus (2). Most nonreassuring FHR tracings will be in this category, and given the high false-positive rate and other limitations of EFM, it is recommended to use more

tests to reassess the fetal status and to continue with nonsurgical interventions. A backup test available is fetal scalp pH and lactate measurement, but according to the ACOG survey of US hospitals, it is currently used in less than 3% of labor and delivery units. Fetal oximetry or computerized ST analysis are possible backup tests for the future; both of the latter are currently undergoing clinical trials to evaluate their efficacy for this purpose.

ACOG recommends that during the first stage of labor in uncomplicated pregnancies, the FHR tracing should be reviewed every 30 minutes and during the second stage of labor every 15 minutes. When monitoring complicated pregnancies, the frequency of evaluation of the tracings should be every 15 minutes during the first stage and every 5 minutes during the second stage (2).

■ EFFICACY AND OUTCOMES

Since its introduction in the 1960s, EFM has been shown to increase cesarean delivery (CS) rates but has not shown benefits in neonatal outcome. Some have argued that it can

TABLE 5-4 Three-tiered Fetal Heart Rate Interpretation and Classification System

Category I

Category I FHR tracings include all of the following
- Baseline rate: 110–160 bpm
- Baseline FHR variability: Moderate
- Late or variable decelerations: Absent
- Early decelerations: Present or absent
- Accelerations: Present or absent

Category II

Category II FHR tracings includes all FHR tracings not categorized as Category I or Category III. Category II tracings may represent an appreciable fraction of those encountered in clinical care. Examples of Category II FHR tracings include any of the following

Baseline rate
- Bradycardia not accompanied by absent baseline variability
- Tachycardia

Baseline FHR variability
- Minimal baseline variability
- Absent baseline variability with no recurrent decelerations
- Marked baseline variability

Accelerations
- Absence of induced accelerations after fetal stimulation

Periodic or episodic decelerations
- Recurrent variable decelerations accompanied by minimal or moderate baseline variability
- Prolonged deceleration more than 2 min but less than 10 min
- Recurrent late decelerations with moderate baseline variability
- Variable decelerations with other characteristics such as slow return to baseline, overshoots, or "shoulders"

Category III

Category III FHR tracings include either
- Absent baseline FHR variability and any of the following
  - Recurrent late decelerations
  - Recurrent variable decelerations
  - Bradycardia
- Sinusoidal pattern

FHR, fetal heart rate.
Reprinted with permission from: Macones GA, Hankins GD, Spong CY, et al. The 2008 National Institute of Child Health and Human Development workshop report on electronic fetal monitoring: update on definitions, interpretation, and research guidelines. *Obstet Gynecol* 2008;112:661–666.

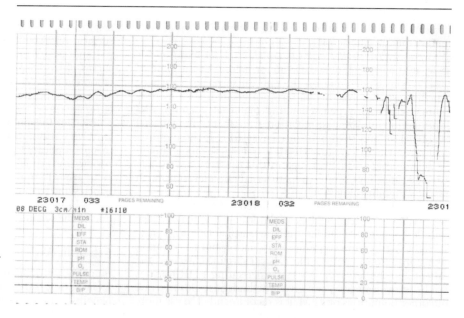

FIGURE 5-3 Category III tracing with absent variability, normal baseline, and recurrent variable decelerations.

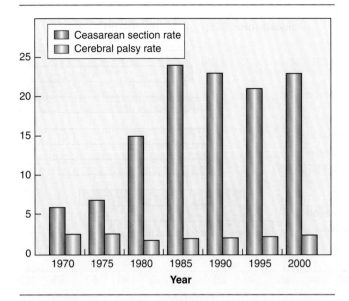

FIGURE 5-4 Increase in cesarean section trends and constant cerebral palsy rates in the past three decades. Reprinted with permission from: Clark SL, Hankins GD. Temporal and demographic trends in cerebral palsy—fact and fiction. *Am J Obstet Gynecol* 2003;188:628–633.

cause harm to mothers due to the increased CS rates and instrumental vaginal deliveries (US preventive task force grade D) (2). Since the end of the 1970s, several clinical trials have shown that EFM has no effect on perinatal morbidity or mortality and its benefits have been sharply questioned (7). The incidence of CP has remained constant throughout the past four decades at 2 to 2.5 cases per 1,000 live-born children despite the use of these monitoring techniques and a fivefold increase in the cesarean delivery rate (Fig. 5-4) (15,52–56). The increasing survival rates of premature infants have also not had a significant change in CP rates in developed countries.

There are no high quality randomized controlled trials comparing the benefits of EFM to any other form of monitoring during labor (2). Recent meta-analyses have compared the benefits of EFM with intermittent auscultation, with fetal scalp lactate sampling and in some cases to no monitoring. The outcomes have been disappointing, and in general show no improvement in outcomes with the use of traditional

EFM, in terms of decreasing neonatal deaths, adverse neurologic outcomes including CP, or decrease in unnecessary maternal obstetric interventions.

In a meta-analysis, Grivell et al. compared traditional EFM with no fetal monitoring, including four studies from publications in 1980s and 1990s, and found there was no difference in perinatal mortality (EFM 2.3% vs. no EFM 1.1%, risk ratio [RR] 2.05, 95% confidence interval [CI] 0.95 to 4.42, four studies, $n = 1,627$) or potentially preventable deaths (RR 2.46, 95% CI, 0.96 to 6.30, four studies, $n = 1,627$). They also found no significant difference in cesarean delivery rates (19.7% vs. 18.5%, RR 1.06, 95% CI, 0.88 to 1.28, three trials, $n = 1,279$). They also compared traditional EFM with computerized analysis of EFM, and they did show promising results with the use of computerized EFM in the reduction of perinatal mortality (0.9% vs. 4.2%, RR 0.20, 95% CI, 0.04 to 0.88, two studies, 469 women). However, the included studies and meta-analysis were underpowered to detect a significant difference in potentially preventable deaths (RR 0.23, 95% CI, 0.04 to 1.29) (57).

Another meta-analysis compared intermittent auscultation (IA) with continuous EFM (44). It included twelve trials enrolling over 37,000 women and showed that continuous EFM did decrease neonatal seizures (RR 0.50, 95% CI 0.31 to 0.80, $n = 32,386$, nine trials). However, continuous EFM did not affect the incidence of CP (RR 1.74, 95% CI 0.97 to 3.11, $n = 13,252$, two trials) or perinatal death rate (RR 0.85, 95% CI 0.59 to 1.23, $n = 33,513$, 11 trials). It did show a significant increase in the rate of cesarean deliveries (RR 1.66, 95% CI 1.30 to 2.13, $n = 18,761$, 10 trials) and instrumental vaginal birth (RR 1.16, 95% CI 1.01 to 1.32, $n = 18,151$, nine trials) (44,57).

Access to fetal scalp blood sampling did not appear to influence the difference in neonatal outcomes, including seizures, low Apgar scores at 5 minutes, admission to neonatal intensive care units, neonatal encephalopathy, umbilical cord blood pH, base deficit, or metabolic acidemia in a meta-analysis of two randomized trials involving over 3,000 deliveries (58).

It has long been known that during EFM most abnormal FHR tracings do not result in acidosis (Fig. 5-5) (59). It is also known that the poor sensitivity and specificity of these FHR patterns in identifying or predicting CP would be unacceptable for any screening or diagnostic test. Moreover, the positive predictive value of an abnormal tracing is extremely low, with a false-positive rate of 99.8% (Table 5-5) (42). EFM also has very high intra- and inter-observer variability and ability to predict acidosis in labor, both for identification of basic FHR features like decelerations, variability, and classification of tracings (Table 5-6) (60,61).

TABLE 5-5 Multiple Late Decelerations and/or Decreased Variability in Prediction of Cerebral Palsy in Singleton Children with Birth Weights ≥2,500 g, According to Risk Group: Sensitivity and Specificity of FHR Tracings in Predicting Cerebral Palsy

Risk Group	% of Population	Prevalence of Cerebral Palsy (Per 10,000)	Sensitivity (%)	Specificity (%)	Positive Predictive Value (%)
Low	69	3.6	13.8	91.3	0.05
High	31	13.8	34.7	89.1	0.25
Total	100	6.8	26.9	90.7	0.14

Reprinted from: Nelson KB, Dambrosia JM, Ting TY, et al. Uncertain value of electronic fetal monitoring in predicting cerebral palsy. *N Eng J Med* 1996;334:613–618.

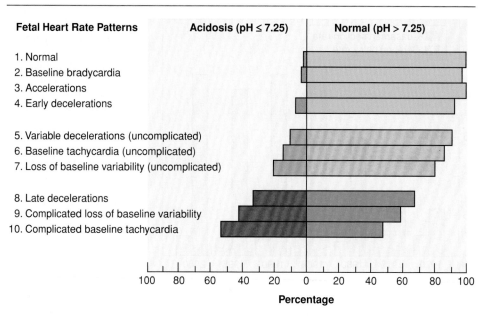

FIGURE 5-5 Significance of changes in FHR tracings and their relationship to fetal acidosis after birth. Reprinted with permission from: Beard RW, Filshie GM, Knight CA, et al. The significance of the changes in the continuous fetal heart rate in the first stage of labour. *J Obstet Gynaecol Br Commonw* 1971;78:865–881.

■ FUTURE MONITORING STRATEGIES

Fetal ECG Monitoring

Fetal cardiac muscle can function under conditions of aerobic or anaerobic metabolism. Aerobic glucose metabolism normally efficiently provides energy for cardiac muscle activity and its growth produces carbon dioxide and water as waste products. When excess glucose is available, it is stored in the cell as glycogen. During hypoxia, the fetus is capable of supporting the energy requirements of the cardiac muscle cells with anaerobic metabolism, using blood glucose and the stored glycogen to produce the energy required for its basal activities. During anaerobic metabolism lactic acid and ions such as potassium are released locally as the waste products. The amount of energy produced during anaerobic metabolism from glucose is only

TABLE 5-6 Inter-observer Variability of Intrapartum FHR Tracings

Agreement	Kappa Coefficient	Early Labor[a]	Before Delivery[b]
Poor	0.00–0.19	Baseline Accelerations Bradycardia Beat-to-beat variability, decreased Beat-to-beat variability, absent Recurrent prolonged decelerations Variable deceleration with slow return —	Baseline Accelerations Bradycardia Beat-to-beat variability, decreased — Recurrent prolonged decelerations Variable decelerations with slow return Recurrent late decelerations
Fair	0.20–0.29	Recurrent late decelerations Recurrent severe variable decelerations	Beat-to-beat variability, absent
Moderate	0.30–0.43	—	Recurrent severe variable decelerations
Good	0.44–0.59	Tachycardia	Tachycardia
Substantial	0.60–0.80	—	—
Almost perfect	0.81–1.00	—	—

[a]FHR tracing of 1 hour duration, before the onset of periodic decelerations.
[b]FHR tracing of 1 hour before birth.
Reprinted with Permission from: Chauhan SP, Klauser CK, Woodring TC, et al. Intrapartum nonreassuring fetal heart rate tracing and prediction of adverse outcomes: inter-observer variability. *Am J Obstet Gynecol* 2008;199:623.e1–623.e5.

Myocardial Metabolic Paths

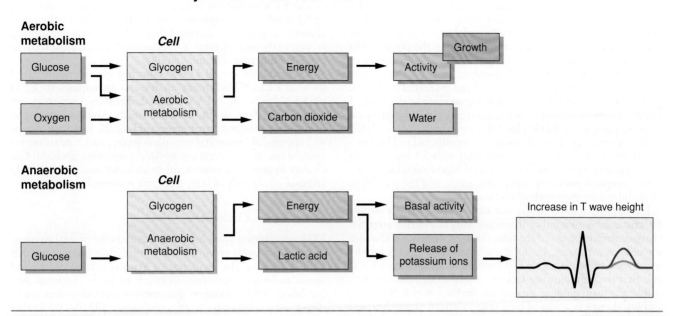

FIGURE 5-6 Myocardial metabolic pathways and changes in T wave. Reprinted with permission from: Fetal Monitoring and ST Analysis. Neoventa Medical AB. © Neoventa Medical 2012.

5% of the energy produced compared to aerobic metabolism.

The concept of fetal ECG monitoring and ST–T wave analysis is based on adult cardiac stress testing analogizing from treadmill exercise to the stress of labor. During labor, when the fetus is under stress and oxygen supply is not enough to sustain cardiac aerobic metabolism, the change to anaerobic metabolism and the release of potassium ions during anaerobic metabolism causes a change in the T wave and the ST interval of the fetal ECG during this time

(Fig. 5-6) (62). The analysis of these changes (Fig. 5-7) provides continuous information about the ability of the fetal heart muscle to respond to the changing requirements during the stress of labor. An elevation of the ST segment and T wave, quantified by the ratio between the T wave and QRS amplitude (T/QRS) (Fig. 5-7), identifies fetal heart muscle responding to hypoxia by a surge of stress hormones, like catecholamines, which lead to utilization of glycogen. ST segment depression can indicate a situation where the heart is not fully able to compensate (63).

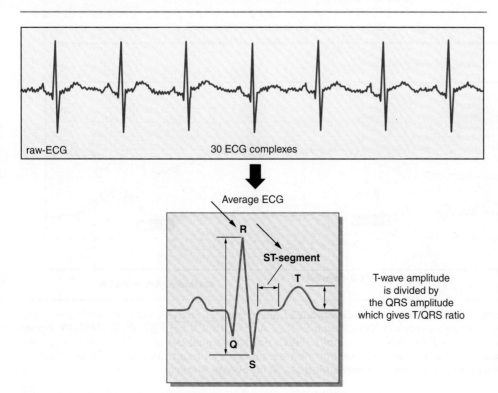

FIGURE 5-7 Fetal EKG information and calculation of the T/QRS ratio by ST analysis monitor. Reprinted with permission from: Fetal Monitoring and ST Analysis. Neoventa Medical. © Neoventa Medical 2012.

The analysis of the fetal ECG during labor has been a work in progress since the 1970s. Since 1975, studies in animals, such as guinea pigs, lamb, and cat fetuses, have shown the relationship between fetal hypoxia and changes in FHR and ECG (64–66). This type of monitor during labor is intended to be used as an adjunct to FHR monitoring to aid the physician in decision making and in identifying the fetus at increased risk.

The ST waveform signal monitor (STAN; Neoventa, Gothenburg, Sweden) has been used and evaluated in clinical trials in Europe and currently is being studied in the United States. A systematic review of the first three clinical trials from Europe comparing FHR plus ST monitoring with isolated FHR monitoring showed promising results (62). The concomitant use of both FHR monitoring with ST monitoring was shown to reduce the rates of fetal blood sampling, neonatal encephalopathy, operative deliveries, and the incidence of umbilical artery metabolic acidosis (67).

It is important to recognize that some fetuses may not display ST changes because either the monitoring has started after ST changes already began or the fetus does not display ST changes for unknown reasons. Under these circumstances it is important to remember that fetal ECG analysis is an adjunct to EFM and that tracings showing lack of variability or reactivity will still be the main guide in identifying the fetus at risk (68).

This change is assessed by a computerized algorithm and results in an ST event alarm. The clinician can then use these ST events to aide in the differentiation of the category II strips and make clinical decisions based on this additional information (Fig. 5-8).

The ST wave analysis for the fetal ECG monitor is intended to be used as a complement to EFM, to aide in the decision-making process during labor. ST segment monitoring is currently undergoing a randomized controlled trial to assess its functionality and viability.

This trial will enroll 11,000 laboring women randomized to fetal ECG ST segment analysis as an adjunct to EFM or EFM with the STAN masked. Primary outcomes are intrapartum fetal death, neonatal death, Apgar scores <3 at 5 minutes, seizures, cord artery pH <7.05 and base deficit >12 mmols/dL, neonatal encephalopathy, and intubation for ventilation at delivery; secondary outcomes include CS, change in practice patterns, other neonatal outcomes (NICU admissions, length of stay, etc.), and maternal outcomes.

Fetal Pulse Oximetry

FHR monitoring is an indirect measurement of fetal oxygenation. Pulse oximetry in pediatric and adult populations has helped decrease the incidence of hypoxic-related deaths and seems to be an alternative approach to assess the fetus during labor. A fetal monitor that continuously measures either direct fetal oxygenation or continuous pH or preferably both together may better identify fetuses that are oxygen deprived or have an altered pH status. Current fetal pulse

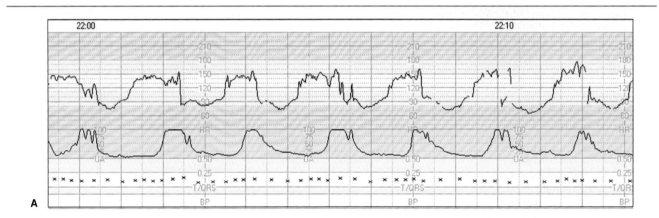

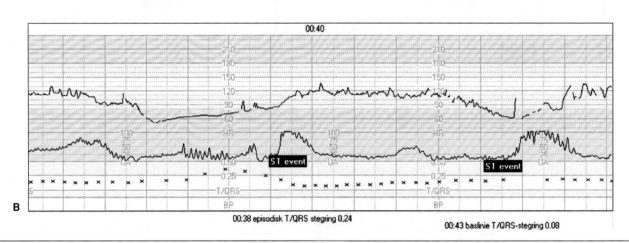

FIGURE 5-8 Examples of category II STAN tracings with and without ST alerts from ST analysis monitor: Decisions made and outcome of newborn. (**A**) Second stage recoding NVD, Apgar 9–10; CA pH 7.18; CV pH 7.27. (**B**) CS NRFHR, Apgar 8–9; CA pH 7.14, Bdef 8.7 mmol/LCV pH 7.34, Bdef 6.3 mmol/L. NVD, normal vaginal delivery; CA, cord gas arterial result; CV, cord gas venous result; CS NRFHR, cesarean section nonreassuring fetal heart rate; Bdef, Base deficit on blood gas. Tracings reprinted with permission from: Neoventa Medical. © Neoventa Medical 2012.

oximetry yields a continuous assessment of the fetal oxygen saturation. The difficulties to access the fetus, and obtain an appropriate surface to monitor oximetry levels, and the difference in fetal physiology with smaller pulse wave, lower fetal saturation, and low signal amplitude have complicated the development of such a monitor (69). Another important difference in the development of fetal oximetry has been the lack of available tissue on which to use a conventional transmission oximetry monitor. A probe has been developed that utilizes reflectance oximetry, in which light is emitted and reflected from the underlying tissue to a photosensor in the same probe.

To monitor fetal pulse oximetry, a probe similar to an IUPC is placed transvaginally between the uterine wall and the face of the fetus. It has two low voltage, light-emitting diodes as light sources and one photodetector. One of the diodes emits a red light at 735 nm and the other infrared light at 890 nm. The photosensor measures the reflected or nonabsorbed light using a process similar to conventional pulse oximetry. The ratio between the amount of each wavelength absorbed is related to oxy- and deoxyhemoglobin, and fetal saturation is determined from this ratio.

Several studies have linked fetal oximetry levels lower than 30% to acidemia, especially when maintained for two or more minutes (70–74). These studies were conducted in fetal lambs and humans, comparing saturation results with umbilical artery pH.

Garite et al. studied fetal oximetry as an adjuvant in nonreassuring FHR tracings (75). They allowed labor to continue if oximetry was above 30%. They found a reduction in CS for fetal intolerance of labor, but an increase in CS for fetal dystocia; overall there was no difference in the rate of CS or outcomes. Similar results were obtained by Bloom et al. (76). A systematic review of fetal pulse oximetry as an adjuvant during EFM showed no decrease in the overall rate of CS or differences in fetal or maternal outcomes when combining both techniques (77).

Technical issues, including capillary stasis in the fetal scalp during labor, as well as the risks involved with an invasive device to reach the fetus, has limited their usefulness to date. Currently ACOG does not endorse fetal oximetry.

The ideal fetal monitor is yet to be developed. It should be able to distinguish between an acute insult and a chronic one, combinations of acute and chronic insults, and reliably detect fetal hypoxia. It should decrease fetal morbidity and mortality and decrease obstetric maternal interventions. Traditional FHR monitoring fails far short of this ideal, and promising technologies including fetal ECG analysis and pulse oximetry have not yet advanced our ability sufficiently to enter clinical practice.

KEY POINTS

- The original goal for fetal monitoring was the prevention of cerebral palsy (CP), hypoxic ischemic encephalopathy, neonatal encephalopathy and perinatal death.
- The ideal goals for fetal monitoring are: assure fetal wellbeing and improve perinatal outcome, serve as a screening test to detect hypoxia and acidemia, identify fetal reserve for labor, allow for timely interventions to avoid morbidity and mortality in infants and minimize unnecessary obstetric interventions.
- Over 5 decades, electronic fetal monitoring (EFM) became synonymous with intrapartum fetal monitoring and fetal heart rate interpretation and became the most common tool available for fetal surveillance.
- EFM has been shown to have very poor predictive value for identifying the hypoxic fetus and predicting fetus that will develop CP—this may be due to the lack of standardization.

- Neonatal encephalopathy is only called hypoxic ischemic encephalopathy (HIE) if there is evidence that intrapartum asphyxia is the cause of the encephalopathy that which resulted in neurologic depression or seizures. Over 75% of neonatal encephalopathy cases have no clinical signs of intrapartum hypoxia.
- Neonatal encephalopathy is present only in 24% of term children with CP.
- Fetal heart rate (FHR) variability is believed to represent an intact neurologic pathway that includes fetal cerebral cortex, midbrain, vagus nerve, and cardiac conduction system—if the fetal brain is hypoxic FHR changes would be noted.
- Most common monitors to assess intrapartum fetal wellbeing are ultrasound monitoring, fetal heart rate monitors (external or internal), uterine contraction monitors (external or internal) and fetal scalp blood sampling.
- Normal FHR is between 110–160 beats per minute. Plotted information is analyzed and interpreted to determine fetal status. Baseline variability is the most sensitive marker for fetal well being.
- FHR correlates with fetal acid-base status at the time of observation, but it does not predict CP and should be evaluated over time and clinical scenario.
- Current classification of FHR patterns have a three-tier system organizing them as category I (normal), category II (middle or intermediate) or category III (abnormal) tracings. Specific management recommendations are suggested for each category.
- Future monitoring strategies currently undergoing validation and reviews include fetal ECG monitoring and fetal pulse oximetry monitoring.

REFERENCES

1. Hankins GD. The long journey: defining the true pathogenesis and pathophysiology of neonatal encephalopathy and cerebral palsy. *Obstet Gynecol Surv* 2003;58:435–437.
2. ACOG Practice Bulletin No. 106: Intrapartum fetal heart rate monitoring: nomenclature, interpretation, and general management principles. *Obstet Gynecol* 2009;114:192–202.
3. Hankins GD, Speer M. Defining the pathogenesis and pathophysiology of neonatal encephalopathy and cerebral palsy. *Obstet Gynecol* 2003;102:628–636.
4. Morgan MA, Hankins GD, Zinberg S, et al. Neonatal encephalopathy and cerebral palsy revisited: the current state of knowledge and the impact of american college of obstetricians and gynecologists task force report. *J Perinatol* 2005;25(8):519–525.
5. Bernardes J, Ayres-de-Campos D. The persistent challenge of foetal heart rate monitoring. *Curr Opin Obstet Gynecol* 2010;22:104–109.
6. Hon EH. The electronic evaluation of the fetal heart rate; preliminary report. *Am J Obstet Gynecol* 1958;75:1215–1230.
7. Banta HD, Thacker SB. Policies toward medical technology: the case of electronic fetal monitoring. *Am J Public Health* 1979;69:931–935.
8. Martin JA, Hamilton BE, Sutton PD, et al. Births: final data for 2002. *Natl Vital Stat Rep* 2003;52:1–113.
9. Leviton A, Nelson KB. Problems with definitions and classifications of newborn encephalopathy. *Pediatr Neurol* 1992;8:85–90.
10. Nelson KB, Leviton A. How much of neonatal encephalopathy is due to birth asphyxia? *Am J Dis Child* 1991;145:1325–1331.
11. MacLennan A. A template for defining a causal relation between acute intrapartum events and cerebral palsy: international consensus statement. *BMJ* 1999;319:1054–1059.
12. Kumar S, Paterson-Brown S. Obstetric aspects of hypoxic ischemic encephalopathy. *Early Hum Dev* 2010;86:339–344.
13. American College of Obstetricians and Gynecologists' Task Force on Neonatal Encephalopathy and Cerebral Palsy, American College of Obstetricians and Gynecologists, American Academy of Pediatrics. *Neonatal Encephalopathy and Cerebral Palsy: Defining the Pathogenesis and Pathophysiology.* Washington: American College of Obstetricians and Gynecologists;2003.
14. Krigger KW. Cerebral palsy: an overview. *Am Fam Physician* 2006;73:91–100.
15. Clark SM, Ghulmiyyah LM, Hankins GD. Antenatal antecedents and the impact of obstetric care in the etiology of cerebral palsy. *Clin Obstet Gynecol* 2008;51:775–786.

16. Hagberg B, Hagberg G, Beckung E, et al. Changing panorama of cerebral palsy in Sweden. VIII. Prevalence and origin in the birth year period 1991-94. *Acta Paediatr* 2001;90:271–277.
17. Little WJ. On the influence of abnormal parturition, difficult labours, premature birth, and asphyxia neonatorum, on the mental and physical condition of the child, especially in relation to deformities. *Clin Orthop Relat Res* 1966;46:7–22.
18. Keogh JM, Badawi N. The origins of cerebral palsy. *Curr Opin Neurol* 2006;19(2):129–134.
19. Nelson KB, Chang T. Is cerebral palsy preventable? *Curr Opin Neurol* 2008;21:129–135.
20. Blair E, Stanley FJ. Intrapartum asphyxia: a rare cause of cerebral palsy. *J Pediatr* 1988;112:515–519.
21. Blair E, Stanley F, Hockey A. Intrapartum asphyxia and cerebral palsy. *J Pediatr* 1992;121:170–171.
22. Blair E, Stanley F. When can cerebral palsy be prevented? The generation of causal hypotheses by multivariate analysis of a case-control study. *Paediatr Perinat Epidemiol* 1993;7:272–301.
23. Rennie JM, Hagmann CF, Robertson NJ. Outcome after intrapartum hypoxic ischaemia at term. *Semin Fetal Neonatal Med* 2007;12(5):398–407.
24. Dixon G, Badawi N, Kurinczuk JJ, et al. Early developmental outcomes after newborn encephalopathy. *Pediatrics* 2002;109:26–33.
25. Miller R, Depp R. Minimizing perinatal neurologic injury at term: is cesarean section the answer? *Clin Perinatol* 2008;35:549–559, xi.
26. Phelan JP, Ahn MO. Perinatal observations in forty-eight neurologically impaired term infants. *Am J Obstet Gynecol* 1994;171(2):424–431.
27. Schifrin BS, Hamilton-Rubinstein T, Shields JR. Fetal heart rate patterns and the timing of fetal injury. *J Perinatol* 1994;14:174–181.
28. Martin CB Jr., de Haan J, van der Wildt B, et al. Mechanisms of late decelerations in the fetal heart rate. A study with autonomic blocking agents in fetal lambs. *Eur J Obstet Gynecol Reprod Biol* 1979;9:361–373.
29. Bax M. Birth asphyxia. *Dev Med Child Neurol* 1992;34:283–284.
30. Bax M, Nelson KB. Birth asphyxia: a statement. World Federation of Neurology Group. *Dev Med Child Neurol* 1993;35:1022–1024.
31. Low JA. Intrapartum fetal asphyxia: definition, diagnosis, and classification. *Am J Obstet Gynecol* 1997;176:957–959.
32. Low JA. Determining the contribution of asphyxia to brain damage in the neonate. *J Obstet Gynaecol Res* 2004;30:276–286.
33. Cohn HE, Sacks EJ, Heymann MA, et al. Cardiovascular responses to hypoxemia and acidemia in fetal lambs. *Am J Obstet Gynecol* 1974;120:817–824.
34. Thakor AS, Giussani DA. Effects of acute acidemia on the fetal cardiovascular defense to acute hypoxemia. *Am J Physiol Regul Integr Comp Physiol* 2009;296(1):R90–R99.
35. Hanson MA. The importance of baro- and chemoreflexes in the control of the fetal cardiovascular system. *J Dev Physiol* 1988;10:491–511.
36. Jensen A, Garnier Y, Berger R. Dynamics of fetal circulatory responses to hypoxia and asphyxia. *Eur J Obstet Gynecol Reprod Biol* 1999:155–172.
37. Jensen A, Berger R. Fetal circulatory responses to oxygen lack. *J Dev Physiol* 1991;16:181–207.
38. Fisher DJ, Heymann MA, Rudolph AM. Fetal myocardial oxygen and carbohydrate consumption during acutely induced hypoxemia. *Am J Physiol* 1982;242:H657–H661.
39. Jones M Jr., Sheldon RE, Peeters LL, et al. Fetal cerebral oxygen consumption at different levels of oxygenation. *J Appl Physiol* 1977;43:1080–1084.
40. Mann LI. Effects in sheep of hypoxia on levels of lactate, pyruvate, and glucose in blood of mothers and fetus. *Pediatr Res* 1970;4:46–54.
41. Yaffe H, Parer JT, Block BS, et al. Cardiorespiratory responses to graded reductions of uterine blood flow in the sheep fetus. *J Dev Physiol* 1987;9:325–336.
42. Nelson KB, Dambrosia JM, Ting TY, et al. Uncertain value of electronic fetal monitoring in predicting cerebral palsy. *N Engl J Med* 1996;334:613–618.
43. Freeman RK. Problems with intrapartum fetal heart rate monitoring interpretation and patient management. *Obstet Gynecol* 2002;100:813–826.
44. Alfirevic Z, Devane D, Gyte GM. Continuous cardiotocography (CTG) as a form of electronic fetal monitoring (EFM) for fetal assessment during labour. *Cochrane Database Syst Rev* 2006;3:CD006066.
45. American College of Obstetricians and Gynecologists. ACOG Practice Bulletin. Clinical Management Guidelines for Obstetrician-Gynecologists, Number 106, July 2009 (Replaces Practice Bulletin Number 70, December 2005). Intrapartum fetal heart rate monitoring: nomenclature, interpretation, and general management principles. *Obstet Gynecol* 2009;114(1):192–202.
46. Thacker SB, Stroup DF, Peterson HB. Efficacy and safety of intrapartum electronic fetal monitoring: an update. *Obstet Gynecol* 1995;86:613–620.
47. Thacker SB, Stroup D, Chang M. Continuous electronic heart rate monitoring for fetal assessment during labor. *Cochrane Database Syst Rev* 2001: CD000063.
48. Harbison L, Bell L. Anaphylactoid syndrome after intrauterine pressure catheter placement. *Obstet Gynecol* 2010;115:407–408.
49. Matsuo K, Lynch MA, Kopelman JN, et al. Anaphylactoid syndrome of pregnancy immediately after intrauterine pressure catheter placement. *Am J Obstet Gynecol* 2008;198:e8–e9.
50. Macones GA, Hankins GD, Spong CY, et al. The 2008 National Institute of Child Health and Human Development workshop report on electronic fetal monitoring: update on definitions, interpretation, and research guidelines. *J Obstet Gynecol Neonatal Nurs* 2008;37:510–515.
51. Harris JL, Krueger TR, Parer JT. Mechanisms of late decelerations of the fetal heart rate during hypoxia. *Am J Obstet Gynecol* 1982;144(5):491–496.
52. Clark SL, Hankins GD. Temporal and demographic trends in cerebral palsy—fact and fiction. *Am J Obstet Gynecol* 2003;188:628–633.
53. Ozturk A, Demirci F, Yavuz T, et al. Antenatal and delivery risk factors and prevalence of cerebral palsy in Duzce (Turkey). *Brain Dev* 2007:39–42.
54. Jacobsson B, Hagberg G. Antenatal risk factors for cerebral palsy. *Best Pract Res Clin Obstet Gynaecol* 2004;18(3):425–436.
55. Graham E, Ruis K, Hartman A, et al. A systematic review of the role of intrapartum hypoxia-ischemia in the causation of neonatal encephalopathy. *Am J Obstet Gynecol* 2008;199:587–595.
56. Clark SL. Elective induction: an analysis of economic and health consequences. *Am J Obstet Gynecol* 2003;188:1664–1665; author reply 1665.
57. Grivell RM, Alfirevic Z, Gyte GM, et al. Antenatal cardiotocography for fetal assessment. *Cochrane Database Syst Rev* 2010;(1):CD007863.
58. East CE, Leader LR, Sheehan P, et al. Intrapartum fetal scalp lactate sampling for fetal assessment in the presence of a non-reassuring fetal heart rate trace. *Cochrane Database Syst Rev* 2010;(3):CD006174.
59. Beard RW, Filshie GM, Knight CA, et al. The significance of the changes in the continuous fetal heart rate in the first stage of labour. *J Obstet Gynaecol Br Commonw* 1971;78:865–881.
60. Chauhan SP, Klauser CK, Woodring TC, et al. Intrapartum nonreassuring fetal heart rate tracing and prediction of adverse outcomes: interobserver variability. *Am J Obstet Gynecol* 2008;199:623.e1–623.e5.
61. Ayres-de-Campos D, Bernardes J, Costa-Pereira A, et al. Inconsistencies in classification by experts of cardiotocograms and subsequent clinical decision. *Br J Obstet Gynaecol* 1999;106:1307–1310.
62. Fetal Monitoring and ST Analysis: Neoventa Medical AB, 2010.
63. Rosen KG, Amer-Wahlin I, Luzietti R, et al. Fetal ECG waveform analysis. *Best Pract Res Clin Obstet Gynaecol* 2004;18:485–514.
64. Rosen KG, Kjellmer I. Changes in the fetal heart rate and ECG during hypoxia. *Acta Physiol Scand* 1975;93:59–66.
65. Rosen KG, Hokegard KH, Kjellmer I. A study of the relationship between the electrocardiogram and hemodynamics in the fetal lamb during asphyxia. *Acta Physiol Scand* 1976;98:275–284.
66. Rosen KG, Dagbjartsson A, Henriksson BA, et al. The relationship between circulating catecholamines and ST waveform in the fetal lamb electrocardiogram during hypoxia. *Am J Obstet Gynecol* 1984;149(2):190–195.
67. Neilson JP. Fetal electrocardiogram (ECG) for fetal monitoring during labour. *Cochrane Database Syst Rev* 2006;3:CD000116.
68. Rosen KG. Fetal electrocardiogram waveform analysis in labour. *Curr Opin Obstet Gynecol* 2005;17:147–150.
69. Seeds JW, Cefalo RC, Proctor HJ, et al. The relationship of intracranial infrared light absorbance to fetal oxygenation. I: Methodology. *Am J Obstet Gynecol* 1984;149:679–684.
70. Dildy GA, van den Berg PP, Katz M, et al. Intrapartum fetal pulse oximetry: fetal oxygen saturation trends during labor and relation to delivery outcome. *Am J Obstet Gynecol* 1994;171:679–684.
71. Dildy GA, Thorp JA, Yeast JD, et al. The relationship between oxygen saturation and pH in umbilical blood: implications for intrapartum fetal oxygen saturation monitoring. *Am J Obstet Gynecol* 1996;175:682–687.
72. Bloom SL, Swindle RG, McIntire DD, et al. Fetal pulse oximetry: duration of desaturation and intrapartum outcome. *Obstet Gynecol* 1999;93:1036–1040.
73. Nijland R, Jongsma HW, Crevels J, et al. Transmission pulse oximetry in the fetal lamb: is there a universal calibration? *Pediatr Res* 1996;39:464–469.
74. Kühnert M, Seelbach-Göebel B, Butterwegge M. Predictive agreement between the fetal arterial oxygen saturation and fetal scalp pH: results of the German multicenter study. *Am J Obstet Gynecol* 1998;178:330–335.
75. Garite TJ, Dildy GA, McNamara H, et al. A multicenter controlled trial of fetal pulse oximetry in the intrapartum management of nonreassuring fetal heart rate patterns. *Am J Obstet Gynecol* 2000;183:1049–1058.
76. Bloom SL, Spong CY, Thom E, et al. Fetal pulse oximetry and cesarean delivery. *N Engl J Med* 2006;355(21):2195–2202.
77. East CE, Chan FY, Colditz PB, et al. Fetal pulse oximetry for fetal assessment in labour. *Cochrane Database Syst Rev* 2007:CD004075.

CHAPTER

6

Alternative (Non-pharmacologic) Methods of Labor Analgesia

Katherine W. Arendt • William Camann

■ INTRODUCTION

Not every woman in labor needs or wants pharmacologic pain relief or regional analgesic techniques. For centuries, a variety of non-pharmacologic techniques have been used to assist women during labor. Many of these methods are available and becoming increasingly utilized in labor units today. Familiarity and respect for these philosophies and techniques can assist obstetric anesthesiologists in providing satisfying and respectful birth experiences for all women who deliver under their care.

The patient who desires non-pharmacologic labor pain relief often presents unique and difficult challenges for the obstetric anesthesiologist, because these patients' goals often seem irrational compared to what we usually do in our customary practice of providing effective and total pain relief. Moreover, many patients who have successfully achieved a non-medicated, but extraordinarily painful, birth are very satisfied. This is an observation which is also difficult for many anesthesiologists to understand. On the other hand, some patients enter labor with unrealistic expectations; consequently, when pharmacologic analgesia is requested and received, satisfaction may not be ideal even if the pain relief was excellent (1). The psychological and social dynamics of the non-pharmacologic childbirth population are complex and often shaped by previous experiences and/or a variety of information. This information is oftentimes inaccurate as it may be obtained from various non-authoritative sources such as the internet, books, television, magazines, friends, childbirth education classes, and others.

The use of regional analgesia is rarely precluded by the use of other non-pharmacologic techniques. Regional analgesic techniques are quite compatible and complimentary to many of the other pain relief methods utilized in labor. Furthermore, obstetric anesthesiologists play an important role in the childbirth process for this population. When and if urgent delivery or resuscitation is required for mother and/or baby, it is the job of obstetric anesthesiologists to ensure safety for both patients.

■ COMPLEMENTARY AND ALTERNATIVE MEDICINE

The National Institutes of Health (NIH) National Center for Complementary and Alternative Medicine (NCCAM) has specific definitions surrounding complementary and alternative medicine (CAM) (2). *Conventional medicine* (also called Western or allopathic medicine) is medicine as practiced by providers with M.D. and D.O. degrees and by allied health professionals, such as physical therapists, psychologists, and registered nurses. *Complementary medicine* refers to the use of CAM in conjunction with conventional medicine. *Alternative medicine* refers to the use of CAM instead of conventional medicine. *Integrative medicine* refers to a practice that combines both conventional and CAM treatments for which there is evidence of safety and effectiveness. The NCCAM states that "the boundaries between CAM and conventional medicine are not absolute, and specific CAM practices may, over time, become widely accepted."

In this chapter, we work to apply the scientific rigor of conventional medicine to the basic principles of CAM for labor analgesia or labor satisfaction. Through our evaluation of the clinical investigations that have been performed to assess the safety and efficacy of various CAM philosophies and techniques, we will discuss the evidence (or lack thereof) supporting these practices in the labor setting.

Complementary and Alternative Medicine in Obstetrics

Moxibustion and Acupuncture for Breech Presentation: An example of the challenge of evaluating CAM techniques by scientific standards.

There are examples of CAM techniques widely used in obstetrics throughout the world that illustrate the challenges of evaluating CAM with the rigor of evidence-based medicine (EBM). The use of moxibustion techniques for the treatment of breech presentation provides a nice example of such challenges because the outcome is objective, unlike analgesic outcomes in which the outcome can be quite subjective.

Generally speaking, moxibustion (moxa) refers to the traditional Chinese medicine (TCM) technique of igniting slow-burning substances on or near certain acupuncture points for the purpose of stimulating or maintaining a particular desired health outcome. Specifically, moxibustion involving the burning of herbal preparations of mugwort (*Artemisia vulgaris*) to acupoint bladder (BL) 67 (Zhi Yin, located at the outside corner of the fifth toenail) has been used since ancient times to promote cephalic version of fetuses in the breech position. In 1998, Cardini and Weixin reported in the Journal of the American Medical Association (JAMA) that among Chinese primigravidas with breech presentation at 33 weeks' gestation, moxibustion increased fetal activity during treatment and resulted in cephalic presentation after the 7- to 14-day treatment period as well as the cephalic presentation at delivery in comparison to observation alone (3).

Since this study, Cardini et al. attempted to evaluate the efficacy of moxibustion on a non-Chinese population by performing a similar study at six Italian hospitals. They found difficulties in evaluating this CAM in its nontraditional setting (4). Because of a "high number of treatment interruptions," only 46% of the planned sample was able to be recruited and no difference was found between the groups. Further, it was noted that 27 out of 65 women in the moxa group complained of unpleasant side effects with 14 interrupting treatment as a result. Interestingly, the authors go on to conclude that "the significance of this study is to underline several problems concerning the ability to transfer the investigated treatment from the original ethnic, social and cultural context . . . and to draw some deductions on methodology of clinical research in traditional medicine." The inability to blind patients, a placebo effect, or even positive thinking and "buy in" from subjects in evaluating CAM techniques in obstetrics must be noted as randomized controlled trials (RCTs) are evaluated in the context of CAM techniques.

Since the 1998 JAMA article, others have found moxibustion, acupuncture, electroacupuncture, or laser stimulation at BL 67 to be more effective in correcting breech presentation than observation (5,6) or knee to chest positioning (7) in women willing to be randomized in a moxibustion study. However, a 2005 Cochrane review attempted to evaluate cephalic version by moxibustion (only) for breech presentation. The authors used stricter inclusion criteria, did not include the Chinese sources of studies, and looked only at moxibustion stimulation of BL 67. The authors determined that because of differences in interventions and small sample size it was not appropriate to perform a meta-analysis to determine the efficacy of moxibustion for cephalic version (8). It is important to note that this therapy appears to be safe. Fetal cardiotocography of 12 women receiving moxibustion therapy demonstrated no non-reassuring interpretations (9).

Overall, it appears that stimulation at BL 67 is safe and possibly effective in cephalic version of breech presentation. However, it seems to be more accepted by the Chinese than Western culture (3,4). If prior to the technique, the parturient, partner, and provider are accepting of this CAM, the therapy generally is well tolerated (10). Studies evaluating the analgesic efficacy of CAM techniques for labor pain are plagued by similar difficulties, cultural and regional differences in acceptance of various analgesic techniques, selection bias within studies (women willing to be in the studies may be more likely to "buy in" to alternative therapies), and differences in techniques in the performance of alternative therapies.

Complementary and Alternative Medicine in Labor: Defining Outcomes

When discussing efficacy of CAM techniques or birth philosophies for decreasing pain during labor, the subjective nature of the outcome must be considered. While anesthesiologists may provide neuraxial techniques to decrease pain with a potential goal of a *pain-free* birth, proponents of CAM techniques or alternative birth philosophies may work with a parturient toward the goal of giving a woman the tools and strength to mitigate and *cope* with the pain. The role of this type of caregiver may not be to decrease pain, but instead to *decrease suffering*. Since *suffering* is defined individually by each parturient, the pain of childbirth to some women may not be something to eliminate or avoid. Therefore, outcomes of CAM techniques may include decreasing suffering and increasing satisfaction, which may or may not involve the mitigation of physical pain.

Women may have a variety of reasons for choosing (or avoiding) certain interventions or types of birthing experiences. Spiritually, emotionally, physically, or culturally, a non-

medicated birth experience holds significant value for many parturients (11). There may be the desire for a woman to birth her child in the same way that her own mother birthed her. There may be the desire to set the particular goal of a non-medicated childbirth and then to have the satisfaction of achieving the goal. There may be the belief that a woman may feel more bonded to her child if she does not mask the pain of the labor. Whatever the reason, we do know that women who have the goal of a non-medicated childbirth and are successful in achieving it are more satisfied than those who do not achieve their goal and use epidural analgesia—even though they report significantly lower pain scores (1). Thus, the elimination of pain is not synonymous with childbirth satisfaction for some women. To add further complexity, the elimination of pain may not be synonymous with one's satisfaction with pain relief.

A woman's *birth philosophy* reflects her individual beliefs and values surrounding childbirth and labor pain. When assessing CAM techniques, it is important that we look at the outcome that a particular study evaluated carefully. Pain relief or elimination, maternal satisfaction with analgesic options, and maternal satisfaction with the childbirth experience are all separate outcomes and should be evaluated accordingly. Proponents of CAM techniques and philosophies believe the latter outcome to be the most important.

Complementary and Alternative Medicine in Labor: General Efficacy

It is difficult to scientifically prove if CAM techniques are efficacious in reducing pain in labor. It is even more difficult to prove if one technique is more effective than another. A 2002 literature review by Simkin evaluated five non-pharmacologic methods of labor analgesia: Continuous labor support, baths, touch and massage, maternal movement and positioning, and intradermal water blocks for back pain relief. It was concluded that all five of these techniques were safe although further studies are required to clarify their efficacy (12). A 2004 systematic review of 12 trials utilizing acupuncture, biofeedback, hypnosis, intracutaneous sterile water injections, massage, and respiratory autogenic training concluded that there is insufficient evidence for the efficacy of any of these techniques (with the exception of sterile water injections) in decreasing labor pain (13). In a Cochrane review, Smith and colleagues found acupuncture and hypnosis to be beneficial for the management of pain during labor, but they conceded that the number of women studied has been small (14). Other complementary therapies evaluated in this review included audio-analgesia, acupressure, aromatherapy, hypnosis, massage, and relaxation. The authors concluded that these therapies have not been subjected to proper scientific study to draw conclusions at this time. A 2006 review concluded the following regarding the utility of alternative methods in decreasing labor pain and/or reducing the need for conventional analgesic methods: Efficacy for acupressure and sterile water blocks, possible efficacy for acupuncture and hydrotherapy, and no efficacy established at this time for other CAM therapies (15).

Hypnosis, acupressure, acupuncture, hydrotherapy, and sterile water injections are thought by some to have scientific evidence to support their analgesic efficacy. Of note, reduction of labor pain has been conclusively established with neuraxial anesthesia (16). However, in a 2005 Cochrane review of epidural versus non-epidural or no analgesia in labor, *maternal satisfaction with pain relief* could not be established (RR 1.18, 95% CI 0.92 to 1.50, 5 trials, 1,940 women). These findings appear to be consistent with what proponents of CAM techniques and philosophies emphasize, that is, pain relief is not the same as satisfaction. Therefore, CAM techniques and philosophies may have a role in improving parturients' satisfaction with their pain relief as well as their overall birth experience.

Complementary and Alternative Medicine in Labor: Benefits

As anesthesiologists, it is important to be open to various CAM techniques and birth philosophies that hold value to individual parturients. Such techniques do not threaten our practice and, in fact, can be used in conjunction with neuraxial or systemic analgesia to achieve greater maternal satisfaction. Such techniques can be used prior to the onset of neuraxial analgesia—especially when the anesthesiologist is delayed. They can also be used when neuraxial techniques are contraindicated, during the time interval between epidural placement and analgesic onset, or in the rare situation that neuraxial anesthesia fails.

Negative attitudes toward CAM techniques or birth philosophies may threaten our patients' satisfaction with their childbirth experience. A systematic review of 137 reports of factors that influenced women's evaluations of their child birth experiences (including RCTs and systematic reviews of intrapartum interventions) found that personal expectations, the amount of support from caregivers, the quality of the caregiver–patient relationship, and the patient's involvement in decision making were so important that they surpassed the influences of demographic differences, childbirth preparation, their degree of experienced pain, medical interventions, their physical birth environment, and continuity of care (17). Therefore, for some patients, respecting and supporting an individual parturient's decisions regarding her pain relief, keeping the parturient involved and in control of her analgesic decisions, and creating a positive caregiver–patient relationship may be more important for the anesthesiologist than eliminating pain with neuraxial analgesia.

■ BIRTH PHILOSOPHIES

Lamaze® Philosophy

Lamaze® is the most recognized childbirth philosophy in the United States. It was developed in the 1960s by Dr. Fernand Lamaze, a French obstetrician, as a technique of "psychoprophylaxis" in which breathing and relaxation techniques were employed by parturients in order to experience "childbirth without pain." Since this time, Lamaze has developed from breathing and relaxation techniques into an entire philosophy of pregnancy, childbirth, and parenting (see Tables 6-1–6-4). The main tenet of this philosophy is that birth is "normal, natural, and healthy" and provides "a

TABLE 6-1 The Lamaze® Philosophy Approach to Birth (18)

- Birth is normal, natural, and healthy.
- The experience of birth profoundly affects women and their families.
- Women's inner wisdom guides them through birth.
- Women's confidence and ability to give birth is either enhanced or diminished by the care provider and place of birth.
- Women have a right to give birth free from routine medical intervention.
- Birth can safely take place in homes, birth centers, and hospitals.
- Childbirth education empowers women to make informed choices in health care, to assume responsibility for their health, and to trust their inner wisdom.

TABLE 6-2 The Lamaze® Philosophy Health Birth Practices (18)

- Let labor begin on its own.
- Walk, move around, and change positions throughout labor.
- Bring a loved one, friend, or doula for continuous support.
- Avoid interventions that are not medically necessary.
- Avoid giving birth on your back, and follow your body's urges to push.
- Keep mother and baby together—it is best for mother, baby, and breastfeeding.

foundation and direction for women as they prepare to give birth and become mothers" (18). Lamaze educators no longer teach that the Lamaze techniques result in a pain-free birth experience. Lamaze educators are certified by Lamaze International and accredited by the National Organization of Competency Assurance (NOCA).

When Lamaze techniques were first introduced throughout the United States in the 1960s and 1970s, a woman's birth experience was quite different from a typical birth experience in a United States hospital now. Introduction of the Lamaze philosophy created a movement of parturients who actively prepared themselves for childbirth, of fathers who participated in the preparation process, and of caregivers who empowered birthing women with information and choices. Such philosophies are now recommended and largely practiced by the obstetric medical community in the United States today. One of the early studies evaluating Lamaze assessed obstetric outcomes in 500 consecutive Lamaze-prepared patients and compared them to 500 controls with no childbirth preparation. The Lamaze-prepared patients had one-fourth the number of cesarean deliveries and one-fifth the amount of fetal distress (P < 0.005), one-third the incidence of postpartum infection (P < 0.005), and fewer perineal lacerations with those that occurred not as serious as those in the control patients (P < 0.005). The control patients had three times as many cases of preeclampsia (P < 0.005) and twice as many cases of prematurity (P < 0.05) (19). Although selection bias may exist in this study, it did indicate that childbirth preparation for women was likely not harmful and perhaps helpful.

TABLE 6-3 The Lamaze® Approach to Pregnancy (18)

- Pregnancy is a normal, natural life event.
- Women's bodies are perfectly designed to nourish and nurture their babies through pregnancy.
- The months of pregnancy are necessary for babies to develop and grow, for women's bodies to prepare for birth, and for women to become mothers.
- Pregnancy provides an opportunity for mothers and fathers to begin forming lifelong bonds with their babies.
- A good support system, a healthy lifestyle, and the ability to cope with the stresses of life promote a healthy pregnancy, a healthy birth, and a healthy baby.
- The healthcare system and care provider can increase or decrease a woman's confidence in the normality of pregnancy and in her ability to have a healthy baby.
- Lamaze education empowers women to gain confidence in their bodies, trust their inner wisdom, and make informed decisions about pregnancy, birth, breastfeeding, and parenting.

TABLE 6-4 The Lamaze® Approach to Parenting (18)

- Good parenting is vital to the physical, emotional, and spiritual health of our children, ourselves, and our society.
- Parenting is a joyful, important, challenging, and deeply satisfying work that is worthy of everyone's best efforts.
- Parenting begins before birth. The intimate connection between children and their parents must be respected and protected from the moment of birth throughout life.
- Mothers and fathers play unique, irreplaceable roles in their children's lives.
- Babies and children thrive in close, consistent interaction with their parents.
- Parenting is a learned art; our most important teachers are our own parents, our family, and our children.
- Good parenting requires the support of family, friends, and community.
- Knowledge and support enhance parents' confidence and ability to make informed decisions that meet the needs of their children and themselves.

A 1984 study found only a slight decrease in average pain score that was not statistically significant between women prepared with Lamaze versus a control group (20). However, a 1985 study measuring levels of plasma beta endorphin levels (which have been found to be reduced in effective analgesic techniques such as epidural or intrathecal analgesia) found that in 26 patients who had Lamaze preparation compared to 28 patients who had no Lamaze classes, the Lamaze group had significantly lower plasma beta-endorphin immunoreactivity (37.2 vs. 68.5 pg/mL; p < 0.02) as well as shorter first stages of labor (8.28 hours vs. 9.86 hours; p < 0.02) (21). Lamaze childbirth preparation is well accepted by women. According to a 1990 publication by Mackey, 95% of Lamaze-prepared women who were interviewed stated that being informed through Lamaze education decreased their fear, increased their relaxation, reduced tension, and increased their chances of managing their labor well (22). Furthermore, the philosophy itself does not necessarily recommend against pharmacologic pain relief for women but instead empowers women to make their own choices throughout their birth experience. Many of the Lamaze techniques work well in conjunction with intravenous or neuraxial analgesia.

The Bradley Method®

Dr. Robert Bradley, an obstetrician and natural childbirth proponent, published his book *Husband-Coached Childbirth* in 1965 (23). In the most recent version of this book he states, "New research brings new impetus and new justification for bringing babies into the world in an ideal state: babies who are breast-fed immediately and unhandicapped by the ill effects of drugs. It is a basic human right to be so born. What better endowment could we give a child?" (24).

This quote encompasses the birth philosophy that has become known as the Bradley method. Bradley method instructors are certified by the American Academy of Husband-Coached Childbirth (AAHCC). The method teaches the husband or partner to coach the laboring woman in her breathing and to keep the labor environment free of distractions. The philosophy emphasizes education, preparation, the participation of a supportive, loving coach, and the importance of keeping women healthy and low-risk to avoid complications which could lead to medical intervention. The goal of the Bradley method is achieving a "natural childbirth"—a birth without surgery, medication, or medical intervention. Therefore, the Bradley method *does not* support the use of intravenous or neuraxial analgesia for laboring parturients.

The Bradley method students are taught techniques of deep abdominal breathing and concentrated awareness to work through the pain. The Bradley method works to give couples an understanding of the labor and delivery process prior to childbirth. However, it has also been thought by some to foster a sense of suspicion of health care providers because of its emphasis on "consumerism" which they define as patients/parents taking responsibility for their safety and the safety of the baby. No RCTs have been done evaluating the Bradley method.

Other Birth Philosophies

Other less well-known birth philosophies also exist. Grantly Dick-Read introduced a philosophy of "natural childbirth" in 1933 in which the pain of childbirth was thought to be a pathologic response by women because they were fearful and tense (25). Through teaching the facts of childbirth and instructing them in relaxation techniques, Dick-Read believed that the pain of childbirth could be diminished.

Frederic Leboyer published a book in 1974 entitled *Birth Without Violence* which established his philosophy inspired by Indian yoga in which an environment of tranquility is established (26). The mother, father, and professionals are all to remain quiet and calm. The mother is to keep her attention focused on the baby throughout the process to increase her pain threshold. The room is to have little noise and light and the baby is to be given a warm bath upon birth. Although neither Dick-Read's nor Leboyer's philosophies have been well studied, some of their general principles are incorporated into modern natural childbirth teachings.

■ COMPLEMENTARY AND ALTERNATIVE MEDICINE ANALGESIC TECHNIQUES

Water Immersion and Birth

The use of birthing pools, tubs, or whirlpools during labor is becoming more popular in many hospitals and birthing centers in the United States. (Fig. 6-1). Immersion in warm water appears to provide comfort to many women in labor.

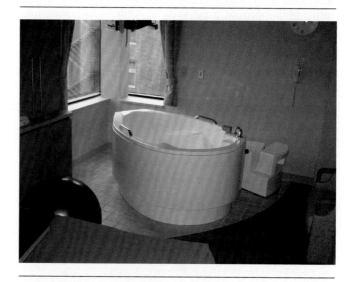

FIGURE 6-1 A typical labor tub.

The mechanism of the analgesia is unknown—possibly the buoyancy as well as the warmth and soothing atmosphere are helpful. In addition, the warmth and flotation may influence nociceptive input with resultant analgesic effects.

Restrictions as to which patients can use hydrotherapy during labor vary from hospital to hospital. For most hospitals, contraindications to hydrotherapy in labor may include premature labor, multiple gestation, patients undergoing a trial of labor after cesarean (TOLAC), induced labor, active genital herpes or other infections, ruptured membranes and/or the presence of meconium-stained amniotic fluid, or vaginal bleeding. Some institutions allow a parturient to only labor but not birth in the tub; others allow both labor and birth. Most hospitals also have guidelines for water temperature and length of immersion. A study by Geissbuehler et al. does not support such guidelines and reports no significant thermal risks to mother or baby when mothers choose their own temperature and duration of immersion (27). New monitors allow continuous fetal heart rate monitoring even while the parturient is submerged in water. In general, anesthesiologists agree that a laboring patient with an epidural is not allowed to use a tub or shower.

A 1983 observational study suggested that women who labor in water have faster labors, less perineal tears, and less requirement for other analgesics (28). Other studies have also suggested decreased rates of tears, episiotomies, blood loss (29), or obstetrical intervention such as augmentation, amniotomy, episiotomy, or operative delivery (30). A randomized trial involving 108 parturients in Brazil supported the analgesic benefits of laboring in water (31). Studies have also found less frequent use of conventional analgesic medications or techniques (such as neuraxial or intravenous analgesia) during hydrotherapy (30,32,33). It is interesting to note that hydrotherapy may offer greater benefit during early labor and lesser benefit at the time of birth (30). Some studies suggest that labor pain with hydrotherapy seems to escalate more slowly; however, the pain experienced in the end of the birthing process is similar to that experienced by women undergoing conventional birth (31,34). A Cochrane review including 11 trials (*n* = 3,146) found that there was significant reduction in the epidural, spinal, or paracervical analgesia rate amongst women randomized to water immersion compared to controls (odds ratio 0.82, 95% confidence interval 0.70 to 0.98). There were no differences in rates of assisted vaginal deliveries, cesarean deliveries, perineal trauma, or maternal infection (35).

Because of the nature of water immersion, it is impossible to blind the parturient and caregiver to the intervention. Therefore, with the subjective nature of pain, the analgesic effects are difficult to assess. However, some studies do show greater satisfaction (30) and greater relaxation during labor with hydrotherapy when compared to conventional labor (30,34). Further, a single study indicated that after utilizing hydrotherapy once, most women prefer it for subsequent deliveries (34).

There are concerns about complications caused by bathing in water during labor and birth. A hospital in New Zealand reported four cases of neonates born in water who purportedly aspirated at birth, experienced moderate to severe respiratory distress, and displayed subsequent pulmonary edema on chest radiograph with "features typical of fresh-water near-drowning in children" (36). Infectious risks, however, have been the most widely reported complications of water births. *Pseudomonas aeruginosa* and *Klebsiella pneumoniae* have been documented in the water in birthing tubs (37), in filling hoses (38), and in heating systems (39). Anecdotal case reports exist describing such occurrences of infection in both neonates and parturients (40,41). One case report describes

an 11-hour-old neonate who developed signs and symptoms of septicemia.

P. aeruginosa grew from swab samples taken from the neonate's ear and umbilicus. The specimen matched the serotype of *P. aeruginosa* grown from specimens taken from the birthing tub, filling hose, taps, exit hose, and disposable lining of the tub into which the baby was born (42). The neonate was treated with antibiotics and recovered.

In spite of these case reports, multiple studies have been performed which do not reveal worse neonatal outcomes (including incidence of infection) in neonates whose mothers labored in water (33,34,43). None of these studies involved a power analysis. Only some of the mothers *birthed* (versus just labored) in water; in total, they comprise only 988 women utilizing hydrotherapy. A surveillance study of all pediatricians and postal survey of all National Health Service maternity units in the United Kingdom found that among 4,032 deliveries, no neonatal deaths were attributable to delivery in water. Two admissions to special care nursery for water aspiration were reported (44). When compared to regional data, the relative risk for perinatal mortality associated with delivery in water was 0.9 (99% confidence interval 0.2 to 3.6). For low-risk, spontaneous, normal vaginal deliveries at term, the authors concluded that perinatal mortality was not higher among babies delivered in water than those who delivered conventionally. A Cochrane review also supports the safety of hydrotherapy concluding that there are no differences in Apgar scores, neonatal unit admissions, or infection rates amongst women who use hydrotherapy during labor and/or birth (35).

In summary, hydrotherapy is generally safe; however, it must be used by experienced caregivers with awareness of the neonatal risks in order to avoid aspiration or neonatal infection. Proper sanitation of the facilities cannot be overemphasized. Many women find the practice relaxing and satisfying. Although the data is not yet strong enough to claim that it provides significant analgesic effects, fewer neuraxial or intravenous analgesic techniques are utilized by women who labor and/or birth in water.

Hypnosis

First described in 1960 (45), there has been a recent surge in the popularity of patients utilizing hypnosis-based techniques for labor analgesia. Various consumer-oriented programs are available such as "hypnobirthing" or "hypnobabies." Patients utilizing this modality typically have taken a course of varying length during pregnancy to prepare for the labor experience. Sometimes a hypnosis instructor will accompany the patient during labor, and other times the patient and her partner will rely on her learned techniques. Hypnotic-based techniques use a variety of focusing techniques, guided imagery, and relaxation audio tapes to achieve a state of focused concentration in which a parturient is relatively unaware but not entirely blind to her surroundings. Many of these techniques involve using words which appear "softer" than our typical terminology to help relax the mind of the parturient. Some examples include uterine "surge" instead of contraction; "pressure/sensation/tightening" rather than pain; membrane "release" rather than rupture; "breathing down" rather than pushing; "birthing companion" rather than coach; and "blossoming" rather than dilation. Hypnosis is a useful technique for the motivated patient. It is well received and popular among its advocates, and it has been described as a successful form of analgesia when a neuraxial technique was contraindicated (46). The use of hypnotic techniques is also entirely compatible with the concomitant use of regional analgesic techniques.

Hypnosis has become scientifically accepted as a form of pain control (47). Hypnosis modulates pain via suppression of neural activity in the anterior cingulate gyrus as demonstrated by positron emission tomography (48). In evaluation of labor pain, a 2004 systematic review of the evidence suggests that hypnosis may be associated with a reduced need for pharmacologic labor analgesia (relative risk = 0.51; 95% CI 0.28, 0.95), although the authors emphasize that an adequately powered randomized trial has yet to be performed (49). This systematic review also suggested a lower incidence of oxytocin labor augmentation and an increased incidence of spontaneous vaginal delivery amongst women using hypnosis (50). Similar findings were demonstrated in a pilot study evaluating self-hypnosis in which birth outcomes of self–hypnosis-prepared women were compared with routinely managed parturients (51). This small study found that of the women taught antenatal self-hypnosis, nulliparous parturients used fewer epidurals: 36% (18/50) vs. 53% (765/1,436), relative risk = 0.68 (95% CI 0.47, 0.98) and required less oxytocin augmentation: 18% (9/50) vs. 36% (523/1,436), relative risk = 0.48 (95% CI 0.27, 0.90).

Acupuncture

Acupuncture is a branch of TCM wherein a type of energy ("Qi," or chi) flows through the body over channels known as meridians. Many medical conditions are considered to be due to disorders, disruptions, imbalances, or obstructions of this energy flow. According to TCM, insertion of fine needles along appropriate meridians will restore the harmony of the Qi and can be used to treat a variety of disorders and promote health. It is well recognized, even by practitioners of TCM, that these meridians and energy flows have no known anatomic, neurologic, pharmacologic, or physiologic correlates in traditional Western medical thinking.

Several trials have suggested efficacy of acupuncture and acupressure for a variety of uses during pregnancy and birth. Acupuncture has been shown to provide relief from hyperemesis during the first trimester (52). It may increase rates of pregnancy and live birth when used among women undergoing in vitro fertilization (53). Acupuncture and moxibustion (burning of *A. vulgaris* near acupoint BL67 on the outer corner of the little toe) therapy have been shown in a randomized trial to be useful for turning a breech baby to the vertex position (1). It has also been suggested that acupuncture can assist in labor induction (54). There has been recent interest in the use of acupoint P6 (on the inner wrist) for treatment of nausea encountered during pregnancy, delivery, and anesthetic administration. The results are mixed although somewhat suggestive of a possible effect (55). See Figure 6-2 which shows a partial list of selected acupoints that have been used for various obstetrical and anesthetic indications.

RCTs of acupuncture during labor have shown a modest—if any—decrease in maternal pain scores, decreased need for other pharmacologic analgesics, and an increase in maternal relaxation (56). A 2010 systematic review and meta-analysis of acupuncture for pain relief in labor including ten RCTs ($n = 2,038$) found that acupuncture was not superior to minimal acupuncture (placing needles in areas that are not acupoints) at 1 hour (pooled mean difference −8.02; 95% CI −21.88, 5.84; $I^2 = 94\%$) and at 2 hours (pooled mean difference −10.15; 95% CI −23.18, 2.87; $I^2 = 92\%$). VAS pain scores were found to be reduced by 4% and 6% during electroacupuncture treatment versus placebo at 15 minutes (pooled mean difference −4.09; 95% CI −8.05, −0.12) and 30 minutes (pooled mean difference −5.94; 95% CI −9.83, −2.06). When compared to no intervention, acupuncture reduced pain by 11% at 30 minutes (pooled mean difference −10.56; 95% CI

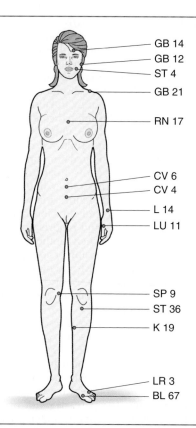

FIGURE 6-2 Selected acupoint sites relevant to obstetrics and anesthesia (artwork courtesy of Marlena Bocian).

Wonggu GB12, Yangbai GB14 & Taichang LR3; headache, including PDPH.

Dicang ST4; Bell's Palsy.

Jianjing GB21 & Shanzhang RN17; breastfeeding and labor induction.

Guanyuan CV 4; contraception.

Qihai CV 6; infertility.

Neiguan P6; nausea.

Hegu L14 & Zhiyin BL 67; labor pain and hypertension.

Shaoshang LU11; laryngospasm.

Yinlingquan SP 9; sore throat.

Zusanli ST36; Edema.

Zhubin K19; anxiety.

Zhi yin BL 67; breech and labor induction.

−16.08, −5.03) (57). Less meperidine (pooled risk ratio 0.20; 95% CI 0.12, 0.33) and other analgesic methods (0.75; 95% CI 0.66, 0.85) were required for the acupuncture group.

Most of the studies included in this meta-analysis are weakened by lack of blinding. Blinding is difficult to employ in acupuncture studies. There are placebo or sham acupuncture intervention devices in which the procedure is mimicked without a needle being inserted into the skin (58). There is a study evaluating acupuncture analgesia efficacy using such a device (59). This study showed that patients who actually receive acupuncture are less likely to request meperidine (14.14% vs. 35.29%; p < 0.001) or epidural analgesia (10.38% vs. 10.47%; p < 0.01); furthermore, the patients report decreased pain on visual analog scale (p < 0.05) versus patients undergoing sham acupuncture.

Another method to achieve blinding in acupuncture studies is to use "minimal acupuncture" or to insert needles in places that are not regarded as acupoints. A single study evaluating labor analgesic benefits utilized this methodology and found that visual analog scale pain scores were lower in the real acupuncture group after 2 hours, but the visual analog scale scores *averaged* over the first 2 hours were not significantly different (60). This study also evaluated length of labor and augmentation requirements and showed that the acupuncture group had a shorter duration of the active phase of labor and required less oxytocin for labor augmentation. This finding has (61) and has not (62) been demonstrated in other randomized control trials evaluating length of labor and augmentation.

Acupuncture is generally a safe technique. Very few complications have been reported (63,64). None have been described when it has been used specifically in labor. The use of acupuncture for labor analgesia is largely dependent on a motivated patient and the availability of trained, licensed acupuncturists. The exact mechanism of action is unclear, but the neuroendocrine system is likely involved. A recent randomized controlled trial allocated 36 laboring parturients to either an electroacupuncture group or a control group (65). Those who received electroacupuncture demonstrated lower pain intensity (p = 0.018), greater relaxation (p = 0.031), and greater concentrations of beta-endorphin (p = 0.037) and 5-hydroxytryptamine (p = 0.030) in peripheral blood samples than the control group (65). Interestingly, needling of certain acupoints that are thought to cause an increase in uterine blood flow or fetal activity (e.g., BL 67) is relatively contraindicated during early pregnancy due to the possibility of inducing miscarriage or preterm labor. Needling may be indicated later in gestation for very specific circumstances such as labor induction at term or turning of a breech baby.

Labor Support

Continuous one-on-one intrapartum support of women during labor has been shown to shorten labor, improve rates of spontaneous vaginal birth, reduce rates of intrapartum analgesia, and increase women's satisfaction with their childbirth experience (66). A labor support person may provide emotional support (continuous presence and reassurance), physical support (comfort measures such as a glass of water or a back rub), information, advice, and/or advocacy. The better outcomes for parturients with continuous support are theorized to involve anxiety. Anxiety is known to lead to endogenous catecholamine release which lessens uterine contractility and decreases placental blood flow. The theory is that women who are well-supported experience less anxiety which leads to more efficient uterine contractions and improved placental blood flow. Studies have evaluated the efficacy of untrained lay women, trained lay women (doulas), female relatives, and nurses in the role of a labor support person (67). No particular type of labor support provider has been shown to be consistently more effective than another.

The studies evaluating labor support are difficult to control and difficult to evaluate because of cultural and regional differences. For example, an early study on labor support was performed in Guatemala where family members and friends were not normally allowed to be with women during labor. The labor area was crowded, and nurse staffing was minimal (68). This study showed that parturients with intrapartum support had markedly fewer cesarean delivery rates, less meconium staining, shorter length of labors, and better bonding with their babies. However, in this study, the overall environment was exceptionally stressful and the control parturients were alone; therefore, the effect of a labor support person may have been exaggerated. A different study showed that young, nulliparous, disadvantaged women in a crowded obstetric unit in the United States have improved outcomes

when attended to by a doula (69). Another study in which low-income pregnant women were randomized to choose a female friend to receive lay doula training and support them during their labor illustrated that the supported women had a shorter labor (70). Contrarily, one study involving women who were privately insured did not show the benefits demonstrated by studies involving lower socioeconomic groups (71).

A doula is a woman experienced and professionally trained in labor support. Doulas are usually of lay background but often have worked as labor nurses, childbirth educators, or in other obstetric areas. They provide the parturient with praise, reassurance, comfort measures, and companionship. The word "doula" is derived from the Greek word for "woman servant." Doulas are to be distinguished from labor nurses; they perform no clinical tasks nor do they assist with traditional nursing functions. Doulas are also to be distinguished from midwives or obstetricians as they perform no medical tasks nor do they assist in the actual physical act of the birth. Labor nurses are frequently required to render care to several patients simultaneously. Similarly, midwives and obstetricians are generally not in constant attendance with the laboring woman. Despite love, devotion, childbirth education classes, and best intentions, even the parturient's partner may be of only limited (but certainly not unimportant) help during the actual laboring process. In fact, one study illustrated that women consistently find doulas helpful even when the parturient is accompanied by her partner (72). Another randomized trial of hospital-based doulas found that over half the women rated the doula as being more useful than their husband during labor (71).

A low-cost alternative to a professional doula could be a female relative or a friend. One study evaluated such women who attended a 2-hour class with the patient about providing non-medical, continuous support to a laboring woman (73). Overall, the women randomized to be supported by such minimally trained "doulas" (versus standard care) were more likely to report positive perceptions of themselves, their infants, and satisfaction with their care at the hospital. These women were also more likely to be breastfeeding at 6 weeks' postpartum.

Many doulas are strongly committed to non-pharmacologic methods of pain control, and many patients who seek doula support are equally committed to attempting a medication-free labor. Nonetheless, an increasing recognition of the importance of emotional support during labor, combined with the ever increasing popularity and safety of modern regional analgesic techniques for labor, has resulted in some women requesting doula support even with the intention of receiving regional analgesia in labor. While some doulas will limit their client base to those women who only desire to labor without medications, it is not the role of the doula to make this decision for the woman. Excerpts from the *Doulas of North America* Code of Ethics and Standards of Practice include: "Doulas do not offer second opinions or give medical advice. Doulas do not make decisions for their clients; they do not project their own values and goals onto the laboring woman. The doula's goal is to help the woman have a safe and satisfying childbirth *as the woman defines it.* (Italics added) Many women choose or need pharmacologic pain relief. It is not the role of the doula to discourage the mother from her choices. The comfort and reassurance offered by the doula are beneficial regardless of the use of pain medication" (18).

Some patients may hire a doula if they are planning epidural analgesia for their labor. Relief of pain does not obviate all emotional distress and anxiety during labor. Concerns about welfare of the neonate, length of labor, fear of return of pain, fear and anticipation of the approaching second stage of labor, fear of alterations in body image, and loss of dignity during childbirth—among many others—are all valid sources of anxiety, even in the presence of a well-functioning epidural analgesic. Support and reassurance, as professionally provided by a doula, can be invaluable to some women in these circumstances. Nonetheless, doulas can, on occasion, interfere with delivery room routines, and their role needs to be clearly defined in order to facilitate cordial interactions on the labor unit. Some doulas may be very militant about their role and advocacy for their patients. The exact nature of the role of the doula in hospital births is still a matter of much discussion.

Sterile Water Papules

A little known technique often advocated by midwives and doulas is the cutaneous injection of sterile water papules also known as "intradermal water blocks." Several observational as well as randomized trials have confirmed that these injections can provide analgesia specifically for severe back pain or "back labor" often associated with a posterior presenting fetus. The technique for the injections is to place four small (0.1 mL) papules of sterile water in a square pattern several centimeters above the sacrum using a 1 mL syringe and 25 gauge needle (Fig. 6-3). The analgesia is transient, usually lasting 45 minutes to 2 hours. The mechanism may involve some sort of distraction technique similar to transcutaneous electrical nerve stimulation (TENS) or the gate control theory (74). It may involve a mechanism similar to acupuncture in which needling increases levels of beta-endorphins or it may involve a combination of these theories. Interestingly, a controlled trial of 128 parturients randomized to analgesia by either acupuncture or sterile water papules during labor found that sterile water injections provided greater pain relief (p < 0.001), a greater degree of relaxation (p < 0.001), and was favored by the parturients (p < 0.001) (75).

The RCTs evaluating this technique have demonstrated decreased low back pain by visual analog scale after 10 minutes (74,76,77), 45 minutes (74,77), 60 minutes (76,78), 90 minutes (74), and 120 minutes (78). There were no differences demonstrated in intravenous opioid (74,76,78) or epidural use (74,76) in comparison to control groups not receiving sterile water papules. Interestingly, when sterile water is compared to saline papules, both solutions demonstrate effective analgesia but sterile water is more effective (79). Of further interest, a 2009 systematic review and meta-analysis evaluated the effect of sterile water papules on cesarean delivery rate (80). It included eight RCTs (n = 828) and found the cesarean delivery rate to be 4.6% in the sterile water injection group and 9.9% in the control group (RR 0.51, 95% CI 0.30, 0.87). The authors recommend further studies that are tightly controlled and more robust.

Transcutaneous Electrical Nerve Stimulation

Transcutaneous electrical nerve stimulation (TENS) units emit low-voltage electrical impulses which, when applied to the lower back of laboring women, are believed to provide pain relief (Fig. 6-4). This method of non-pharmacologic pain relief for labor has been used since the 1970s. Some estimate that in the United Kingdom the device may be used in up to 25% of deliveries (81,82). One of the mechanisms by which TENS is believed to relieve pain includes the "gate control theory." According to this theory, electrical impulses stimulate large afferent nerve fibers traveling toward the central nervous system and thereby inhibit other painful stimuli from traveling in that path. It has also been postulated that TENS may increase endorphin release in the brain (83). In doing so, it may provide distraction from the pain, increase a woman's sense of control, and decrease anxiety thereby reducing pain in labor (84).

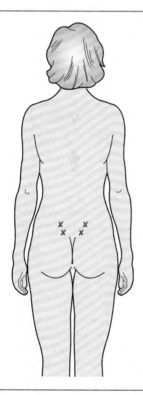

FIGURE 6-3 Sterile water papule placement (artwork courtesy of Marlena Bocian).

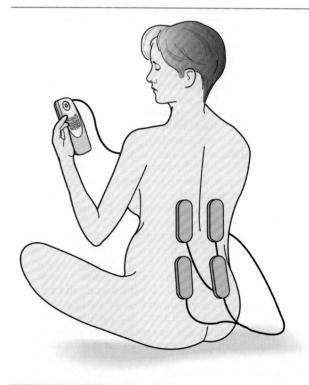

FIGURE 6-4 Transcutaneous electrical nerve stimulation electrode placement when used for labor analgesia (artwork courtesy of Marlena Bocian).

RCTs have not demonstrated significant analgesic benefits from TENS. A meta-analysis and systematic review which included 19 studies ($n = 1,671$) found little difference in pain ratings between women who labored with TENS and control subjects (85). TENS also provided no additional benefit when used as an adjunct to epidural analgesia. This study did find, however, that when TENS was performed at acupuncture points, women were less likely to report severe pain (risk ratio 0.41, 95% CI 0.32, 0.55). TENS has not been found to have any impact on the outcomes of labor such as length of labor, interventions in labor, or well-being of the mother and/or baby.

Position Changes, Touch, Massage, Music, and Aromatherapy

A variety of soothing touch and massage techniques may be utilized by the parturient seeking non-pharmacologic pain relief during childbirth. The literature regarding effects of position changes is conflicting. There is much anecdotal evidence that upright posture, ambulation, or activities such as sitting on a birthing ball are beneficial. The nature of the conflict is that it is not clear if these activities are truly analgesic, or if women who are having easier, less painful labors are more likely to avail themselves of these options. A systematic review and meta-analysis reviewing if women encouraged to assume upright positions versus recumbent positions in the first stage of labor had an effect on labor outcomes included 21 studies totaling 3,706 women (86). Women who were randomized to upright positions had labors that were about 1 hour shorter (Mean difference −0.99, 95% CI −0.61, 0.39) and were less likely to have epidural analgesia (RR 0.83, 95% CI 0.72, 0.96). Otherwise, there were no differences in mode of delivery, length of second stage, or well-being of the mother or baby between the groups. Of note, there were no differences in any outcomes (including labor length) for women with epidurals who were randomized to upright versus supine positions.

Aromatherapy, or application of scented fragrances and essential oils, is popular among some patients. Certain essences (such as lavender, rose, peppermint, eucalyptus, and others) can be massaged into the temples or other areas to create a calm and soothing environment. Music, massage, and other relaxation techniques are likewise common for women during childbirth. Although little analgesia may actually ensue, the effect on stress relief may be significant. These techniques all present little or no risk to the mother and baby. Furthermore, a motivated patient and a capable provider can use these measures to enhance the birth experience, and all are entirely compatible with regional analgesia.

■ CONCLUSION

Virtually all of the non-pharmacologic techniques are entirely compatible with a patient who also wishes to receive epidural analgesia during labor. Educated, well-informed patients accompanied by supportive, open-minded caregivers are the best modalities to ensure a safe and comfortable birth. Obstetric anesthesiologists should be conversant with the wide range of popular non-pharmacologic modalities used during pregnancy and labor. They should understand that pain mitigation may not be the goal of all parturients and instead respect the broader goal of maternal satisfaction. Besides maternal and fetal safety, little is more important than empowering mothers and couples as they begin their important roles as parents (84,87).

KEY POINTS

- Virtually all non-pharmacologic labor analgesic techniques are entirely compatible with a patient who also wishes to receive epidural analgesia during labor.
- Outcomes of CAM techniques during labor may include decreasing suffering and increasing satisfaction, which may or may not involve the mitigation of physical pain.
- A woman's *birth philosophy* reflects her individual beliefs and values surrounding childbirth and labor pain.
- Lamaze® is the most recognized birth philosophy in the United States and teaches that birth is "normal, natural, and healthy." Lamaze does not recommend against pharmacologic pain relief. In fact, many of the Lamaze techniques work well in conjunction with intravenous or neuraxial analgesia.
- The Bradley method, also known as husband-coached childbirth, is a birth philosophy that emphasizes education, preparation, the participation of a supportive coach, and the importance of keeping women healthy. The goal of the Bradley method is achieving a "natural childbirth"— a birth without surgery, medication, or medical intervention. Therefore, the Bradley method *does not* support the use of intravenous or neuraxial analgesia for laboring parturients.
- Hydrotherapy must be used by experienced caregivers with awareness of the neonatal risks in order to avoid neonatal aspiration or infection. Many parturients find the practice satisfying with studies indicating analgesic benefits that may decrease intravenous or neuraxial analgesic requirements.
- Some studies have shown that continuous one-on-one intrapartum support of women during labor can shorten labor, improve rates of spontaneous vaginal birth, reduce rates of intrapartum analgesia, and increase women's satisfaction with their childbirth experience.
- Studies indicate that sterile water papules can provide analgesia for severe back pain or "back labor" often associated with a posterior presenting fetus.
- Hypnosis, acupressure, acupuncture, hydrotherapy, and sterile water injections are thought by some to have scientific evidence to support their analgesic efficacy.
- Familiarity and respect for non-pharmacologic methods of labor analgesia can assist obstetric anesthesiologists in providing satisfying and respectful birth experiences for women who deliver under their care.

■ ACKNOWLEDGMENTS

For all their patience in continuously teaching me their art of providing non-pharmacologic modes of childbirth pain relief, I would like to thank the excellent Mayo Clinic Family Birth Center midwifery staff including Susan M. Skinner, C.N.M.; Lisa M. Bowman, C.N.M.; DeAnna L. Griebenow, C.N.M.; Patricia J. Hinck, C.N.M.; Laurel A. McKeever, C.N.M.; Mary M. Murry, C.N.M.; and Candi L. Nelson, C.N.M.

REFERENCES

1. Kannan S, Jamison RN, Datta S. Maternal satisfaction and pain control in women electing natural childbirth. *Reg Anesth Pain Med* 2001;26:468–472.
2. What Is Complementary and Alternative Medicine? National Institutes of Health, U.S. Department of Health and Human Services, National Center for Complementary and Alternative Medicine, Bethesda, Maryland 2010. http://nccam.nih.gov/health/whatiscam/#definingcam. Accessed 11/29/11.
3. Cardini F, Weixin H. Moxibustion for correction of breech presentation: a randomized controlled trial. *JAMA* 1998;280:1580–1584.

4. Cardini F, Lombardo P, Regalia AL, et al. A randomised controlled trial of moxibustion for breech presentation. *Br J Obstet Gynaecol* 2005;112:743–747.

5. Neri I, Airola G, Contu G, et al. Acupuncture plus moxibustion to resolve breech presentation: a randomized controlled study. *J Matern Fetal Neona* 2004;15:247–252.

6. van den Berg I, Bosch JL, Jacobs B, et al. Effectiveness of acupuncture-type interventions versus expectant management to correct breech presentation: a systematic review. *Complement Ther Med* 2008;16:92–100.

7. Li X, Hu J, Wang X, et al. Moxibustion and other acupuncture point stimulation methods to treat breech presentation: a systematic review of clinical trials. *Chin Med* 2009;4:4.

8. Coyle ME, Smith CA, Peat B. Cephalic version by moxibustion for breech presentation. *Cochrane Database Syst Rev* 2005:CD003928.

9. Guittier MJ, Klein TJ, Dong H, et al. Side-effects of moxibustion for cephalic version of breech presentation. *J Altern Complement Med* 2008;14:1231–1233.

10. Mitchell M, Allen K. An exploratory study of women's experiences and key stakeholders views of moxibustion for cephalic version in breech presentation. *Complement Ther Clin Pract* 2008;14:264–272.

11. Roberts L, Gulliver B, Fisher J, et al. The coping with labor algorithm: an alternate pain assessment tool for the laboring woman. *J Midwifery Womens Health* 2010;55:107–116.

12. Simkin PP, O'Hara M. Nonpharmacologic relief of pain during labor: systematic reviews of five methods. *Am J Obstet Gynecol* 2002;186:S131–S159.

13. Huntley AL, Coon JT, Ernst E. Complementary and alternative medicine for labor pain: a systematic review. *Am J Obstet Gynecol* 2004;191:36–44.

14. Smith CA, Collins CT, Cyna AM, et al. Complementary and alternative therapies for pain management in labour. *Cochrane Database Syst Rev* 2006: CD003521.

15. Tournaire M, Theau-Yonneau A. Complementary and alternative approaches to pain relief during labor. *Evid Based Complement Alternat Med* 2007;4:409–417.

16. Anim-Somuah M, Smyth R, Howell C. Epidural versus non-epidural or no analgesia in labour. *Cochrane Database Syst Rev* 2005:CD000331.

17. Hodnett ED. Pain and women's satisfaction with the experience of childbirth: a systematic review. *Am J Obstet Gynecol* 2002;186:S160–S172.

18. Lamaze International Position Paper: Lamaze for the 21st Century. Originally published by the Lamaze International Education Council Governing Body in 2001. Reviewed and updated 2007. http://www.lamaze.org. Accessed 11/29/2011.

19. Hughey MJ, McElin TW, Young T. Maternal and fetal outcome of Lamaze-prepared patients. *Obstet Gynecol* 1978;51:643–647.

20. Melzack R. The myth of painless childbirth (the John J. Bonica lecture). *Pain* 1984;19:321–337.

21. Delke I, Minkoff H, Grunebaum A. Effect of Lamaze childbirth preparation on maternal plasma beta-endorphin immunoreactivity in active labor. *Am J Perinatol* 1985;2:317–319.

22. Mackey MC. Women's preparation for the childbirth experience. *Matern Child Nurs J* 1990;19:143–173.

23. Bradley RA. *Husband-Coached Childbirth.* New York, NY: Harper & Row; 1965.

24. Bradley RA. *Husband-Coached Childbirth: The Bradley Method of Natural Childbirth.* New York, NY: Bandam Dell; 2008.

25. Dick-Read G. *Natural Childbirth.* London: William Heinemann; 1933.

26. Leboyer F. *Birth without Violence.* New York, NY: Random House; 1975.

27. Geissbuehler V, Eberhard J, Lebrecht A. Waterbirth: water temperature and bathing time—mother knows best. *J Perinat Med* 2002;30:371–378.

28. Odent M. Birth under water. *Lancet* 1983;2:1476–1477.

29. Geissbuhler V, Eberhard J. Waterbirths: a comparative study. A prospective study on more than 2,000 waterbirths. *Fetal Diagn Ther* 2000;15:291–300.

30. Cluett ER, Pickering RM, Getliffe K, et al. Randomised controlled trial of labouring in water compared with standard of augmentation for management of dystocia in first stage of labour. *BMJ* 2004;328:314.

31. da Silva FM, de Oliveira SM, Nobre MR. A randomised controlled trial evaluating the effect of immersion bath on labour pain. *Midwifery* 2009;25:286–294.

32. Mackey MM. Use of water in labor and birth. *Clin Obstet Gynecol* 2001;44:733–749.

33. Rush J, Burlock S, Lambert K, et al. The effects of whirlpools baths in labor: a randomized, controlled trial. *Birth* 1996;23:136–143.

34. Cammu H, Clasen K, Van Wettere L, et al. 'To bathe or not to bathe' during the first stage of labor. *Acta Obstet Gynecol Scand* 1994;73:468–472.

35. Cluett ER, Burns E. Immersion in water in labour and birth. *Cochrane Database Syst Rev* 2009:CD000111.

36. Nguyen S, Kuschel C, Teele R, et al. Water birth—a near-drowning experience. *Pediatrics* 2002;110:411–413.

37. George R. Bacteria in birthing tubs (letter). *Nurs Times* 1990;86:14.

38. Robb EJ, Spiby H, Stewart P, et al. Hygiene in birthing pools. *Nurs Times* 1991;87:14.

39. Loomes SA FR. Breeding ground for bacteria (letter). *Nurs Times* 1990;86:14–15.

40. Franzin L, Scolfaro C, Cabodi D, et al. Legionella pneumophila pneumonia in a newborn after water birth: a new mode of transmission. *Clin Infect Dis* 2001;33:e103–e104.

41. Nagai T, Sobajima H, Iwasa M, et al. Neonatal sudden death due to Legionella pneumonia associated with water birth in a domestic spa bath. *J Clin Microbiol* 2003;41:2227–2229.

42. Rawal J, Shah A, Stirk F, et al. Water birth and infection in babies. *BMJ* 1994;309:511.

43. Schorn MN, McAllister JL, Blanco JD. Water immersion and the effect on labor. *J Nurse Midwifery* 1993;38:336–342.

44. Gilbert RE, Tookey PA. Perinatal mortality and morbidity among babies delivered in water: surveillance study and postal survey. *BMJ* 1999;319:483–487.

45. August RV. Obstetric hypnoanesthesia. *Am J Obstet Gynecol* 1960;79:1131–1138.

46. Cyna AM. Hypno-analgesia for a labouring parturient with contra-indications to central neuraxial block. *Anaesthesia* 2003;58:101–102.

47. Nash MR. The truth and the hype of hypnosis. *Sci Am* 2001;285:46–49, 52–45.

48. Rainville P, Duncan GH, Price DD, et al. Pain affect encoded in human anterior cingulate but not somatosensory cortex. *Science* 1997;277:968–971.

49. Cyna AM, Andrew MI, McAuliffe GL. Antenatal hypnosis for labour analgesia. *Int J Obstet Anesth* 2005;14:365–366.

50. Cyna AM, McAuliffe GL, Andrew MI. Hypnosis for pain relief in labour and childbirth: a systematic review. *Br J Anaesth* 2004;93:505–511.

51. Cyna AM, Andrew MI, McAuliffe GL. Antenatal self-hypnosis for labour and childbirth: a pilot study. *Anaesth Intensive Care* 2006;34:464–469.

52. Carlsson CP, Axemo P, Bodin A, et al. Manual acupuncture reduces hyperemesis gravidarum: a placebo-controlled, randomized, single-blind, crossover study. *J Pain Symptom Manage* 2000;20:273–279.

53. Manheimer E, Zhang G, Udoff L, et al. Effects of acupuncture on rates of pregnancy and live birth among women undergoing in vitro fertilisation: systematic review and meta-analysis. *BMJ* 2008;336:545–549.

54. Smith CA, Crowther CA. Acupuncture for induction of labour. *Cochrane Database Syst Rev* 2004:CD002962.

55. Allen TK, Habib AS. P6 stimulation for the prevention of nausea and vomiting associated with cesarean delivery under neuraxial anesthesia: a systematic review of randomized controlled trials. *Anesth Analg* 2008;107:1308–1312.

56. Lee H, Ernst E. Acupuncture for labor pain management: A systematic review. *Am J Obstet Gynecol* 2004;191:1573–1579.

57. Cho SH, Lee H, Ernst E. Acupuncture for pain relief in labour: a systematic review and meta-analysis. *Br J Obstet Gynaecol* 2010;117:907–920.

58. Vickers AJ. Placebo controls in randomized trials of acupuncture. *Eval Health Prof* 2002;25:421–435.

59. Skilnand E, Fossen D, Heiberg E. Acupuncture in the management of pain in labor. *Acta Obstet Gynecol Scand* 2002;81:943–948.

60. Hantoushzadeh S, Alhusseini N, Lebaschi AH. The effects of acupuncture during labour on nulliparous women: a randomised controlled trial. *Aust N Z J Obstet Gynaecol* 2007;47:26–30.

61. Gaudernack LC, Forbord S, Hole E. Acupuncture administered after spontaneous rupture of membranes at term significantly reduces the length of birth and use of oxytocin. A randomized controlled trial. *Acta Obstet Gynecol Scand* 2006;85:1348–1353.

62. Borup L, Wurlitzer W, Hedegaard M, et al. Acupuncture as pain relief during delivery: a randomized controlled trial. *Birth* 2009;36:5–12.

63. Ernst G, Strzyz H, Hagmeister H. Incidence of adverse effects during acupuncture therapy—a multicentre survey. *Complement Ther Med* 2003;11:93–97.

64. Norheim AJ. Adverse effects of acupuncture: a study of the literature for the years 1981–1994. *J Altern Complement Med* 1996;2:291–297.

65. Qu F, Zhou J. Electro-acupuncture in relieving labor pain. *Evid Based Complement Alternat Med* 2007;4:125–130.

66. Hodnett ED, Gates S, Hofmeyr GJ, et al. Continuous support for women during childbirth. *Cochrane Database Syst Rev* 2011:CD003766.

67. Rosen P. Supporting women in labor: analysis of different types of caregivers. *J Midwifery Womens Health* 2004;49:24–31.

68. Sosa R, Kennell J, Klaus M, et al. The effect of a supportive companion on perinatal problems, length of labor, and mother–infant interaction. *N Engl J Med* 1980;303:597–600.

69. Kennell J, Klaus M, McGrath S, et al. Continuous emotional support during labor in a US hospital. A randomized controlled trial. *JAMA* 1991;265:2197–2201.

70. Campbell DA, Lake MF, Falk M, et al. A randomized control trial of continuous support in labor by a lay doula. *J Obstet Gynecol Neonatal Nurs* 2006;35:456–464.

71. Gordon NP, Walton D, McAdam E, et al. Effects of providing hospital-based doulas in health maintenance organization hospitals. *Obstet Gynecol* 1999;93:422–426.
72. McGrath SK, Kennell JH. A randomized controlled trial of continuous labor support for middle-class couples: effect on cesarean delivery rates. *Birth* 2008;35:92–97.
73. Campbell D, Scott KD, Klaus MH, et al. Female relatives or friends trained as labor doulas: outcomes at 6 to 8 weeks postpartum. *Birth* 2007;34:220–227.
74. Ader L, Hansson B, Wallin G. Parturition pain treated by intracutaneous injections of sterile water. *Pain* 1990;41:133–138.
75. Martensson L, Stener-Victorin E, Wallin G. Acupuncture versus subcutaneous injections of sterile water as treatment for labour pain. *Acta Obstet Gynecol Scand* 2008;87:171–177.
76. Labrecque M, Nouwen A, Bergeron M, et al. A randomized controlled trial of nonpharmacologic approaches for relief of low back pain during labor. *J Fam Pract* 1999;48:259–263.
77. Martensson L, Wallin G. Labour pain treated with cutaneous injections of sterile water: a randomised controlled trial. *Br J Obstet Gynaecol* 1999;106:633–637.
78. Trolle B, Moller M, Kronborg H, et al. The effect of sterile water blocks on low back labor pain. *Am J Obstet Gynecol* 1991;164:1277–1281.
79. Kushtagi P, Bhanu BT. Effectiveness of subcutaneous injection of sterile water to the lower back for pain relief in labor. *Acta Obstet Gynecol Scand* 2009;88:231–233.
80. Hutton EK, Kasperink M, Rutten M, et al. Sterile water injection for labour pain: a systematic review and meta-analysis of randomised controlled trials. *Br J Obstet Gynaecol* 2009;116:1158–1166.
81. Augustinsson LE, Bohlin P, Bundsen P, et al. Pain relief during delivery by transcutaneous electrical nerve stimulation. *Pain* 1977;4:59–65.
82. McMunn V BC, Neilson J, Jones A, et al. A national survey of the use of TENS in labour. *Br J Midwifery* 2009;17:492–495.
83. Lechner W, Jarosch E, Solder E, et al. [Beta-endorphins during childbirth under transcutaneous electric nerve stimulation]. *Zentralbl Gynakol* 1991;113:439–442.
84. Simkin P, Bolding A. Update on nonpharmacologic approaches to relieve labor pain and prevent suffering. *J Midwifery Womens Health* 2004;49:489–504.
85. Dowswell T, Bedwell C, Lavender T, et al. Transcutaneous electrical nerve stimulation (TENS) for pain relief in labour. *Cochrane Database Syst Rev* 2009:CD007214.
86. Lawrence A, Lewis L, Hofmeyr GJ, et al. Maternal positions and mobility during first stage labour. *Cochrane Database Syst Rev* 2009:CD003934.
87. Ewies AA, Olah KS. The sharp end of medical practice: the use of acupuncture in obstetrics and gynaecology. *Br J Obstet Gynaecol* 2002;109:1–4.

Systemic and Inhalational Agents for Labor Analgesia

Samantha J. Wilson • Roshan Fernando

■ INTRODUCTION

The use of drugs to provide pain relief during labor dates back to 1847, when James Young Simpson anesthetized a parturient with a deformed pelvis using diethyl ether. Both the use of heavy sedation during labor and general anesthesia during uncomplicated vaginal delivery have since then been abandoned due to an increasing awareness of neonatal effects and the wish for women to be actively involved in childbirth. However, given that less than 10% of laboring women in the United States underwent childbirth without analgesia in 2001 (Table 7-1), analgesia plays an important role in labor.

Central neuraxial analgesia in the form of an epidural is currently the gold standard, providing effective maternal pain relief with few adverse effects on the mother and infant and have replaced systemic analgesics as the preferred techniques for many patients, with epidural uptake rates of up to 61% in major maternity centers in the United States (1).

However, although rates of epidural analgesia have been shown to be increasing with increasing availability of epidurals across all types of facilities worldwide, systemic analgesia use in labor remains a common practice. In the United Kingdom (UK), the NHS Maternity Statistics of 2005–2006 (2) show that only a third of parturients received regional techniques during their labor and delivery.

Several reasons exist for this continued use of systemic analgesia during labor. Firstly, epidural analgesia is not without well-documented risks. Unrecognized incorrect placement can be associated with serious consequences. Reports exist of intravascular, intrathecal, and subdural placements with incidences of 1 in 5,000, 1 in 2,900, and 1 in 4,200, respectively (3).

Regional analgesia may also be medically contraindicated, for example, if there is a coagulopathy or technical difficulty (e.g., following surgery to the lumbar spine). It may also be declined by some women on the basis of personal preference. Finally, although regional analgesia is becoming more and more accessible across all sorts of medical facilities, women will naturally continue to labor in places where epidurals may not be available.

■ COMMONLY USED LABOR ANALGESICS

Systemic Agents: Opioids

Opioids are the most commonly used systemic medications for labor analgesia, and although they do not typically provide complete analgesia, they do allow the parturient to better tolerate labor pain. In addition, they are easily accessible worldwide, and easy to administer in most facilities as their use does not usually need any specialized equipment or personnel. Factors acting against their popularity include the frequency of side effects experienced by the parturient (e.g., nausea, vomiting, delayed gastric emptying, dysphoria, drowsiness, hypoventilation) combined with the concerning potential for adverse effects on the neonate.

Despite the longstanding tradition of the use of systemic opioids for labor analgesia, there has been a paucity of evidence to promote the use of one opioid over another and it appears to be the case that often the selection of an opioid has been based on institutional tradition and/or personal preference rather than having a scientific basis. The efficacy of systemic opioid analgesia and the incidence of side effects appear to be largely dose dependent rather than drug dependent.

The risks of neonatal respiratory depression and neurobehavioral changes exist with the use of all opioids due to several factors. Firstly, opioids easily cross the placenta by diffusion due to their lipid solubility and low molecular weight, and secondly, the metabolism and elimination of opioids are prolonged in neonates compared to adults. Thirdly, the blood–brain barrier is also less well developed and due to this there can be additional direct effects of opioids on the respiratory center of the neonate. The likelihood of neonatal respiratory depression at delivery is dependent on the dose and timing of opioid administration. In utero effects on the fetus can also be seen in the form of decreased beat-to-beat variability of the fetal heart rate (FHR). This change does not, however, usually reflect a worsening of fetal oxygenation or acid–base status.

The neonatal effects of maternal opioid administration can also be much more subtle than obvious neonatal depression at birth. For example, there may be slight changes in neonatal neurobehavior for several days, although the long-term clinical significance of these changes is unclear. Reynolds et al. (4) performed a meta-analysis of studies comparing epidural analgesia with systemic opioid analgesia using meperidine, butorphanol, or fentanyl. The authors concluded that lumbar epidural analgesia was associated with improved neonatal acid–base status. In addition, a multicenter randomized controlled trial by Halpern et al. (5) compared patient-controlled epidural analgesia to intravenous patient-controlled opioid analgesia and demonstrated a higher need for active neonatal resuscitation in the opioid group (52% vs. 31%).

Routes and Techniques of Administration

Opioids may be administered as intermittent bolus doses to the parturient, or as patient-controlled analgesia. The suitability of various types of opioids to these differing administration techniques will be discussed below and can be seen to be both dependent on, and affect the pharmacokinetic and dynamic properties of the drugs involved.

Intermittent Bolus Technique

Opioids may be administered intermittently by subcutaneous (SC), intramuscular (IM) or intravenous (IV) administration,

TABLE 7-1 **Type of Labor Analgesia Used by Parturients Stratified by Births Per Annum**

Labor Analgesia	Stratum 1 (>1,500 births per annum)			Stratum 2 (500–1,500 births per annum)			Stratum 3 (100–500 births per annum)		
	1981	1992	2001	1981	1992	2001	1981	1992	2001
None	27	11	6	33	14	10	45	33	12
Parenteral	52	48	34	53	60	42	37	48	37
Epidural	22	51	61	13	33	42	9	17	35

Modified from: Bucklin BA, Hawkins JL, Anderson JR, et al. Obstetric Anesthesia Workforce Survey. *Anesthesiology* 2005;103:645–653.

and the route and timing of this administration influence both maternal uptake and placental transfer. SC and IM injections have the advantage of relative safety and simplicity but can be painful and are associated with a variable absorption depending on the site of the injection. The injection itself is inevitably followed by a delay in the onset of analgesia. Therefore, delivery via SC or IM injection results in analgesia of variable onset, quality, and duration. The IV route of administration offers several advantages. Firstly, there is less variability in the peak plasma concentration of the drug; secondly, there is a faster onset of analgesia; and thirdly, the ability to titrate dose to effect tends to be much more achievable.

Patient-Controlled Intravenous Analgesic Technique
Patient-controlled intravenous analgesia (PCIA) is widely and effectively used in the management of postoperative pain and has also been applied to the management of labor analgesia, with a recent survey of UK practice showing that 49% obstetric units offer PCIA for labor analgesia (6). Advantages of the PCIA technique over that of intermittent boluses have been shown to be plentiful with smaller, more frequent dosing resulting in a more stable plasma drug concentration and having a more consistent analgesic effect (7). Other advantages include superior pain relief with lower doses of drug, less risk of maternal respiratory depression, less placental transfer of drug, less need for antiemetic agents, and higher patient satisfaction (7).

PCIA can offer an attractive alternative for labor analgesia in hospitals when epidural anesthesia is unavailable or when contraindicated or unsuccessful. The mother can theoretically adjust the analgesic dose to her individual needs and achieve a greater perceived control over the situation. PCIA use has resulted in higher patient satisfaction scores than other methods of opioid administration. However, studies have not concurrently demonstrated either a reduced use of drug or improved analgesia with PCIA as compared with intravenous administration of an opioid by the obstetric nurse (8).

PCIA use for labor does have some limitations, as even frequent administration of small doses of opioid proves to not always be effective for the fluctuating intensity of labor pains, especially in the late first or second stage of labor (7). Many of the studies in this area have used variable, non-comparable methods to assess the risks to the neonate making the true risks to the fetus and neonate difficult to assess. In addition, variable doses and dosing intervals have also been used, including both the use of a background infusion with an added PCIA bolus as well as PCIA bolus alone, which can make comparison across different studies using a variety of opioids difficult. The most appropriate drug, drug dose, and dosing schedules have not necessarily yet been thoroughly defined with a wide variety being used (Table 7-2).

Individual Agents
Meperidine
Meperidine (pethidine, Demerol™) is the most widely used opioid for labor analgesia worldwide, with 84% of UK units prescribing meperidine for labor analgesia (9), usually at a dose of 100 mg IM 4 hourly for 2 doses. Onset of analgesia is 30 to 45 minutes with a 2- to 3-hour duration. Its popularity and widespread use are perpetuated by familiarity, ease of administration, low cost and until recently perhaps, a lack of extensive evidence that alternative opioids showed any significant superiority.

The use of meperidine has been investigated by Tsui et al. (10), who conducted the first double-blind, randomized, placebo-controlled study of IM meperidine for labor analgesia. The study was terminated prematurely when interim analysis revealed significantly greater reduction in visual analog scale

TABLE 7-2 **Different Patient-Controlled Intravenous Labor Analgesia Regimens**

Drug	Patient-Controlled IV Dose	Lockout Period (min)
Meperidine	10–15 mg	8–20
Nalbuphine	1–3 mg	6–10
Morphine	1–2 mg	3–6
Diamorphine	1 mg	6
Alfentanil	250 μg	3–5
Fentanyl	10–25 μg	5–12
Remifentanil (bolus only)	0.4–0.5 μg/kg	2–3
Remifentanil (background infusion with bolus)	0.05 μg/kg/min with bolus 0.25 μg/kg	2–3

Modified from collated data: Saravanakumar K, Garstang JS, Hasan K. Intravenous patient-controlled analgesia for labor: a survey of UK practice. *Int J Obstet Anesth* 2007;16:221–225 and Douma MR, Verwey RA, Kam-Endtz CE, et al. Obstetric analgesia: a comparison of patient-controlled meperidine, remifentanil and fentanyl in labour. *Br J Anaesth* 2010;104(2):209–215.

TABLE 7-3 Fetal and Neonatal Effects of Meperidine

Fetal Effects	Reduced	Muscular Activity
Aortic blood flow		
Oxygen saturation		
Short-term heart rate variability		
Neonatal Effects	Depressed	Apgar Scores
Respiration		
Neurobehavioral scores		
Muscle tone and suckling		
A detrimental effect on breast feeding		

From: Reynolds F. Labour analgesia and the baby: good news is no news. *Intl J Obstet Anesth* 2011;20:38–50.

(VAS) pain scores with 100 mg IM meperidine versus saline control. The analgesic effect was found to be modest, however, with a median change in VAS pain score of 11 mm (95% CI 2 to 26 mm) at 30 minutes.

Maternal, fetal, and neonatal side effects are ongoing concerns with meperidine use. Maternal nausea, vomiting, and sedation all occur frequently. Fetal and neonatal effects relate to the pharmacokinetic properties of meperidine and are shown in Table 7-3, as well as being discussed below. It is a synthetic opioid which readily crosses the placenta by passive diffusion, equilibrating between materno-fetal compartments in 6 minutes (11). Decreased FHR variability occurs 25 to 40 minutes after administration and resolves within an hour (12). Maternal half-life is 2.5 to 3 hours but neonatal half-life is prolonged at 18 to 23 hours (13). It is metabolized in the liver to produce normeperidine, a pharmacologically active metabolite which is a potent respiratory depressant. This crosses the placenta and is also produced by the neonate's own metabolism of meperidine.

Normeperidine has a half-life of 60 hours in the neonate (14). Neonatal complications relate to the total dose and dose-delivery time. Maximal fetal uptake of meperidine occurs 2 to 3 hours after maternal IM administration and studies have shown that infants born within this time have increased risk of respiratory depression (15,16). Normeperidine accumulates after multiple doses or after prolonged dose–delivery interval (17) and may be associated with altered neonatal neurobehavior including reduced duration of wakefulness, reduced attentiveness, and impaired breast feeding (18–20).

The efficacy of meperidine use in labor with variable administration techniques was investigated by Isenor and Penny-McGillivray (21), who compared intermittent bolus IM meperidine (50 to 100 mg 2 hourly) and PCIA meperidine with background infusion 60 mg/h and bolus 25 mg up to a maximum of 200 mg. They found that pain scores were significantly lower in the PCIA group and that there was no difference in maternal side effects, FHR or neonatal Apgars in this small group. However, when meperidine PCIA is compared with shorter acting opioids, it has been shown to have disadvantages. Volikas et al. (22) compared 10 mg meperidine with 5-minute lockout to 0.5 μg/kg remifentanil with a 2-minute lockout. The study was terminated after 17 subjects due to concern about poor neonatal Apgar scores in the meperidine group (median score 5.5 at 1 minute, and 7.5 at 5 minutes). Blair et al. (23) also compared meperidine PCIA (15 mg,

10-minute lockout) to remifentanil PCIA (40 μg, 2-minute lockout). VAS pain scores were similar in both groups but neurologic and adaptive capacity scores were significantly lower in the meperidine group. These studies show a clear advantage to the use of shorter acting opioids, such as remifentanil, in the PCIA technique as compared to meperidine.

Morphine
Historically, morphine had been administered in combination with scopolamine to provide "twilight sleep" during labor and delivery, with good analgesia being obtained at the expense of excessive maternal sedation and neonatal depression. Morphine is also used in the present day in some North American hospitals as a single agent in early labor, at doses of 5 to 10 mg IM or 2 to 5 mg IV with a time of onset at 20 to 40 minutes or 3 to 5 minutes, respectively, and a duration of 3 to 4 hours (24).

Morphine is metabolized by conjugation to its major inactive and active metabolites. Morphine-3-glucuronide is the major inactive metabolite and is excreted in the urine with 66% clearance in 6 hours if renal function is normal (24,25). Morphine-6-glucuronide is the active metabolite, which is produced in smaller amounts (1:4). This has significant analgesic properties but also a respiratory depressant effect (26,27). Morphine rapidly crosses the placenta with a fetal to maternal blood concentration ratio of 0.96 at 5 minutes (28). The elimination half-life is increased in neonates (at 6.5 +/− 2.8 hours) as compared to adults (at 2.0 +/− 1.8 hours) (28,29). FHR variability decreases as with other opioids.

Oloffson et al. (30) assessed the analgesic efficacy of IV morphine during labor (0.05 mg/kg every third contraction to a maximum of 0.2 mg/kg) and found clinically insignificant reductions in pain intensity. The group's further work (31) compared IV morphine (up to 0.15 mg/kg) to IV meperidine (up to 1.5 mg/kg) and found high pain scores were maintained in both groups despite high levels of sedation. Way et al. (32) showed that IM morphine given to newborns caused greater respiratory depression than an equipotent dose of meperidine when response to CO_2 was measured, and attributed it to an increased permeability of the neonatal brain to morphine.

The concern regarding using morphine PCIA in labor is the accumulation of the active metabolite, morphine-6-glucuronide, a respiratory depressant, which may increase the incidence of neonatal adverse events. There are no studies to compare modes of administration of morphine in labor. Morphine PCIA is not routinely used in labor when there is a viable fetus.

Diamorphine
Diamorphine (3,6-diacetylmorphine, heroin) is a synthetic derivative of morphine used as a labor analgesic and has been reported to provide rapid, effective analgesia with euphoria and reduced nausea and vomiting. Although it is not available legally anywhere other than the UK, it is used in 34% UK obstetric units, and in some areas of the country, it is used more frequently than meperidine (9). Diamorphine is rapidly metabolized to 6 monoacetylmorphine via hydrolytic ester cleavage (33). The greater lipid solubility as compared to morphine accounts for its rapid onset. A significant proportion of analgesic activity is due to the metabolite 6-monoacetylmorphine, which crosses the placenta and is associated with respiratory depression. Further breakdown to morphine occurs and this is metabolized by conjugation as already described (34). Typically, a dose of 5 to 7.5 mg IM diamorphine is used, with the administration of higher doses being linked to neonatal respiratory depression (35).

Rawal et al. (35) investigated the effects of a single dose of diamorphine on free morphine concentrations in the umbilical cord at delivery. Following diamorphine 7.5 mg IM, they found evidence of rapid fetal exposure to morphine and a significant correlation between dose–delivery interval and umbilical cord morphine levels. There was a trend toward lower 1-minute Apgar scores, the need for resuscitation, and higher morphine concentrations in those infants born after a short dose–delivery interval.

In 1999, Fairlie et al. (36) compared IM meperidine (150 mg) to IM diamorphine (7.5 mg) and found significantly more of the meperidine group reported no or poor pain relief at 60 minutes. The trial was small, but suggested that diamorphine conferred some benefits over meperidine with regard to maternal side effects, notably vomiting, and neonatal condition as assessed by Apgar scores at 1 minute. High numbers in both groups required analgesia in addition to meperidine though, suggesting poor efficacy of analgesia achieved by both meperidine and diamorphine.

Diamorphine PCIA has been found to be associated with higher pain scores and lower satisfaction scores when compared to intermittent IM bolus in labor (37). As is the case for morphine, diamorphine PCIA is also not frequently used for labor.

Fentanyl

Fentanyl is a highly lipid soluble, highly protein bound synthetic opioid with an analgesic potency 100 times that of morphine and 800 times that of meperidine. Its rapid onset (peak effect 3 to 4 minutes), short duration of action and lack of active metabolites make it attractive for labor analgesia. However, large doses of fentanyl may accumulate, and the context sensitive half-time (the time for plasma concentration to decrease by 50% after stopping an infusion which had achieved steady-state plasma concentration) of fentanyl increases with the length of infusion.

Fentanyl readily crosses the placenta but the average umbilical to maternal concentration ratio remains low at 0.31. Eisele et al. (38) found that 1 μg/kg fentanyl provided good analgesia without significant hemodynamic effect and with no adverse effect on Apgar scores, acid–base status or neurobehavioral scores at 2 and 24 hours. Rayburn et al. (39) administered 50 to 100 μg fentanyl IV as often as hourly at maternal request during labor. All patients experienced transient analgesia and sedation. Reduced FHR variability occurred but there was no difference, when compared with a group of infants unexposed to analgesia, with regard to Apgar scores, respiratory depression, or neurologic and adaptive capacity scores at 2 to 4 hours or 24 hours. Rayburn et al. (40) also compared fentanyl (50 to 100 μg IV hourly) and an equi-analgesic dose of meperidine (25 to 50 mg IV 2 to 3 hourly). The authors found less sedation, vomiting, and significantly less naloxone use for neonatal respiratory depression with fentanyl but no difference in neurologic and adaptive capacity scores. Unfortunately, both groups had similarly high pain scores, suggesting poor efficacy of both analgesics.

The pharmacokinetic profile of fentanyl with rapid onset, high potency, short duration, and absence of active metabolites makes it particularly suitable for PCIA mode of delivery and because of this is one of the most common opioids for labor PCIA. In the UK it was found to be used in 26% of the units which offer PCIA for labor (6).

Rayburn et al. (40) compared PCIA fentanyl (10 μg, 12-minute lockout) to intermittent IV fentanyl (50 to 100 μg hourly) and found equivalent analgesia and sedation between the groups. Unfortunately, however, both groups had incomplete analgesia in late labor. Neonatal Apgar scores, naloxone requirement, and neuroadaptive tests were comparable. Morley-Forster and Weberpals (41) found a 44% incidence of moderate neonatal depression (1-minute Apgar <6) in a retrospective review of 32 neonates after maternal fentanyl

PCIA. They found a significant difference in total dose of fentanyl in the mothers of neonates who required naloxone (mean $770 \pm$ SD 233 μg vs. 298 ± 287 μg).

Alfentanil

Alfentanil is a fentanyl derivative with reduced potency (10 times less than fentanyl). Alfentanil is less lipophilic and more protein bound, so has a low volume of distribution, which results in a rapid onset (within 1 minute), short duration of action, and rapid clearance (elimination half-life is only 90 minutes). It has a shorter context sensitive half-life than fentanyl. It has, however, been associated with greater depression of neonatal scores than meperidine (42). Morley-Forster et al. (43) compared PCIA alfentanil (200 μg bolus, 5-minute lockout and 200 μg/h basal infusion) to PCIA fentanyl (20 μg bolus, 5-minute lockout and 20 μg/h basal rate). PCIA alfentanil failed to provide adequate analgesia late in labor as compared to fentanyl. There were no significant differences in maternal side effects or neonatal outcome. They concluded that alfentanil was less effective as PCIA than fentanyl.

Remifentanil

Remifentanil is a novel ultra-short acting mu-receptor agonist with a rapid onset of action (brain–blood equilibration occurs in 1.2 to 1.4 minutes) and is rapidly metabolized by plasma and tissue esterases to an inactive metabolite (44). It has a constant context sensitive half-life of 3.5 minutes, which is independent of the duration of infusion. The effective analgesia half-life is longer at 6 minutes allowing effective analgesia for several consecutive painful uterine contractions (45).

Plasma concentrations in pregnancy are about half that of the non-pregnant state. This may be due to the increased volume of distribution, with higher blood volume and reduced protein binding, and greater clearance due to increased cardiac output and renal perfusion with higher esterase activity. Remifentanil crosses the placenta rapidly; the umbilical vein to maternal blood ratio is 0.85. However, umbilical artery to vein concentration ratio is low, at 0.29, demonstrating that the drug is rapidly redistributed and metabolized by the fetus (46). Remifentanil was introduced into obstetric analgesia at the end of the 1990s and has many advantages as an opioid PCIA for this purpose. In 2007, 33% of UK obstetric units that offered labor PCIA were using remifentanil (47) and this is likely to increase as clinical confidence with the technique grows.

Analgesic Efficacy

Remifentanil has been assessed in comparison to many other analgesics and a growing body of evidence exists to suggest its efficacy (Table 7-4). Thurlow et al. (48) compared remifentanil (20 μg IV bolus, 3-minute lockout) to the most commonly used opioid analgesic, meperidine 100 mg IM. Significantly, lower pain scores were found in the remifentanil group with a median pain score of 48 versus 72 ($P = 0.004$). Maternal side effects included mild sedation and more episodes of desaturation to less than 94% but there was reduced nausea and vomiting. No significant difference in neonatal Apgar scores was found. In addition, Volmanen et al. (49) performed a double-blind crossover trial (subjects used both analgesics in random order) comparing remifentanil 0.4 μg/kg and 1-minute lockout with 50% nitrous oxide. They showed a significant reduction in pain scores with remifentanil, yet no difference in maternal side effects other than sedation.

Blair et al. (23), on evaluating the efficacy of remifentanil versus meperidine PCIA, found that VAS pain scores were similar but that patient satisfaction was higher with remifentanil. In 2005, Evron et al. (50) performed a double-blind, randomized controlled trial comparing the analgesic effects of remifentanil PCIA with an IV infusion of meperidine in

TABLE 7-4 Summary of Studies on Remifentanil for Labor Analgesia

	Remifentanil PCIA Bolus Dose[a]	N	Comparator Group	Lockout Interval (min)	Nitrous Oxide Used	Median or Reduction in Pain Scores	Conversion to Neuraxial Analgesia
Blair (57)	0.25–0.5 µg/kg	21	None	2	No	Median 50 mm	4 of 21
Thurlow (48)	0.2 µg/kg	18	IM meperidine	2	Yes	Median 48 mm	7 of 18
Volmanen (49)	0.4 µg/kg	20	Nitrous oxide	1		Reduction of 15 mm	Not reported
Blair (23)	40 µg	20	PCIA meperidine	2	Yes	Median 64 mm	2 of 20
Volmanen (54)	0.2–0.8 µg/kg	17	None	1	No	Reduction of 42 mm	Not reported
Evron (50)	0.27–0.93 µg/kg	43	meperidine infusion	3	No	Median 35 mm	4 of 43
Volikas (54)	0.5 µg/kg	50	None	2	No	Mean 46 mm	5 of 50
Balki (56)	0.25–1.0 µg/kg variable bolus + fixed IV infusion	20	0.025–0.1 µg/kg/min variable infusion + fixed IV bolus	2	No	Reduction of 56 mm vs. 41 mm (variable bolus vs. variable infusion)	1 of 20
Volmanen (58)	0.3–0.7 µg/kg	24	Epidural	1	No	Median 73 mm	Not reported
Douma (51)	40 µg	52	PCIA meperidine, PCIA fentanyl	2	No	Mean 46 mm at 1 h Mean 57 mm at 2 h Mean 72 mm at 3 h	7 or 52

All pain scores reported in millimeter (0–100 mm scale) for comparison between studies.
[a]When indicated, most bolus doses were administered over 1 min.
PCIA, patient-controlled intravenous analgesia; IM, intramuscular.

early labor. More effective analgesia was achieved with remifentanil PCIA with lower VAS pain scores (36 vs. 59 mm) and higher patient satisfaction scores (3.9 vs. 1.9 using a 4 point scale, 1 = poor and 4 = excellent analgesia). In addition, the need to convert to epidural analgesia because of inadequate pain relief was less with remifentanil (11% vs. 39%).

The evidence for increased analgesic efficacy of remifentanil over and above other opioids is unclear. Douma et al. (51) compared the efficacy of remifentanil PCIA with that of meperidine and fentanyl at equipotent doses and found that although the remifentanil PCIA was associated with the greatest decrease in VAS pain scores, this difference was only significant at 1 hour. Marwah et al. (52) recently published a retrospective 5-year review of PCIA remifentanil versus PCIA fentanyl for labor analgesia at their institution. Ninety-eight women were included and overall results showed that both remifentanil and fentanyl provided moderate analgesia with no difference in VAS pain scores. Remifentanil was associated with more transient maternal desaturation than fentanyl (13% vs. 2%, respectively; odds ratio, 7.32; 95% confidence interval [CI], 0.85 to 63.3), and fentanyl was associated with an increased rate of neonatal resuscitation (59% vs. 25%, respectively; odds ratio, 4.33; 95% CI, 1.75 to 10.76).

Optimal Dosing Regimens
Timing of Bolus Dose. Efficacy of remifentanil is dependent on both the dose and the way in which it is given. Notably, the timing of each remifentanil PCIA dose is thought to be of paramount importance with an IV bolus dose delivered at the beginning of a contraction (which lasts 70 seconds on average) being likely to provide analgesia for the following contraction (48). Accordingly, much work has been done to

attempt to optimize timing for PCIA bolus doses, although most recently, Volmanen et al. were unable to increase the analgesic effect or reduce side effects by optimizing the timing of the remifentanil bolus within the uterine contraction cycle (53). They were unable to prove the hypothesis that a remifentanil bolus dose administered between contractions may confer optimal analgesic benefits due to peak concentrations being achieved at the peak of the following contraction.

Bolus Dose Size. Volikas et al. (54) found that a PCIA dose of 0.5 mg/kg with a 2-minute lockout was effective in 86% subjects and that this dose was associated with acceptable levels of maternal side effects and minimal neonatal side effects. Volmanen et al. (55) found a median effective remifentanil dose to be 0.4 mg/kg with wide individual variation of 0.2 to 0.8 mg/kg. This was associated with a median VAS pain score of 3–5/10 but desaturation below 94% occurred in 10 of 17 subjects. As is illustrated in Table 7-4, reported remifentanil bolus dose sizes vary with the majority using a weight-dependent bolus size. However, some choose a fixed bolus dose regardless of patient weight (23,51).

Bolus Dose Titration. Volmanen commented on the comparative improvement in pain scores when remifentanil bolus dose was titrated to patient request rather than being fixed (55). Allowing titration of the bolus dose to account for inter-individual variability in response to pain, as well as the escalation in pain intensity through the course of labor, seems to be beneficial. Volmanen achieved median pain intensity difference of −4.2 with a titrated dose of remifentanil as opposed to −1.5 with a fixed dose of 0.4 µg/kg. Similarly,

Evron et al. (50) also used a regimen to titrate analgesia against response, which involved an initial bolus of 20 μg, regardless of patient weight, with a 3-minute lockout, followed by an increase in the bolus dose of 5 μg every 15 minutes on patient request until adequate analgesia was achieved.

Rate of Administration of Bolus Dose. As well as the timing, the rate of administration of a bolus dose in remifentanil PCIA delivery also appears to be an important aspect in achieving adequate pain relief in labor. Blair et al. (23) delivered the remifentanil bolus dose in "stat" mode through the PCIA device over 18 seconds, whereas other investigators administered a bolus over 1 minute (49,56).

Background Infusion. It is not entirely clear as to whether or not a background infusion confers any analgesic advantage as is seen by conflicting evidence from various studies. Balki et al. (57) aimed to establish the ideal infusion regimen of remifentanil by comparing a group that received a fixed bolus with a titratable background infusion to a group who received a fixed background infusion with a titratable bolus dose. The starting point was a 0.025 μg/kg/min background infusion with a 0.25 μg/kg bolus dose and 2-minute lockout. Either the background infusion rate or the bolus dose was increased in a stepwise fashion on patient request to a maximum of 0.1 μg/kg/min or 1 μg/kg bolus. Mean pain and satisfaction scores were similar in both groups as was the cumulative remifentanil dose. There was only a 5% crossover to epidural analgesia. Neonatal side effects were similar with only one infant having a 1-minute Apgar below 9. However, maternal side effects were significantly higher in the escalating bolus group with 100% drowsiness as compared to 30% in the escalating background infusion group. This group also desaturated below 95% and required oxygen supplementation more frequently (60% vs. 40%). The authors therefore advocated the use of an increasing background infusion within the range 0.025 to 0.1 μg/kg/min with a constant bolus of 0.25 μg/kg and a 2-minute lockout. In contrast, Blair et al. (56) reported that a background infusion of remifentanil did not improve analgesia but caused more maternal side effects.

Maternal Adverse Effects
Usually, opioid doses are limited by the side effects and this often results in administration of ineffective doses. Remifentanil's fast onset and offset allows easy titration. Rapid elimination in parturients and newborns also reduces concern regarding adverse events. Volikas et al. (54) investigated the maternal and neonatal effects of a remifentanil PCIA (0.5 μg/kg bolus, 2-minute lockout) in 50 women. Drowsiness was the most common problem with 44% being drowsy, though alert to voice. There was no change in nausea incidence and no evidence of cardiovascular instability apart from a decrease in heart rate of greater than 15% in five women who required no intervention. No muscle rigidity or hypoventilation occurred and the lowest saturations recorded were 93%.

FHR changes, as monitored by cardiotocography (CTG), occurred in ten women 20 minutes after starting the PCIA but none required intervention. Median 1- and 5-minute Apgar scores were 9, umbilical cord gasses and neurologic examination were all within normal limits.

In addition, Blair et al. (23) found a similar incidence of maternal desaturation, defined as oxygen saturation levels below 95%, when remifentanil PCIA was compared to meperidine PCIA, and Evron et al. (50) showed a significantly lower maternal oxygen saturation with IV meperidine compared with remifentanil (94.2% vs. 97.5%).

When reviewing the literature on remifentanil PCIA analgesia for labor, it is clear that the need for oxygen supplementation due to maternal desaturation may be more common than with the use of alternative methods of labor analgesia. This potential for respiratory depression does mandate close respiratory monitoring in order to be used safely and effectively.

Neonatal Adverse Effects
Neonatal side effects are shown to be similarly encouraging, with fewer non-reassuring FHR patterns and better neurobehavioral scores with remifentanil PCIAs compared to meperidine PCIA (23). In addition, in the study by Evron et al. (50), the baseline FHR remained reactive in 90% in the remifentanil group versus 38% in the meperidine group.

PCIA Remifentanil versus Epidural Analgesia
The encouraging results with remifentanil PCIA led Volmanen et al. (58) to hypothesize that it may provide comparable analgesia to epidural. They compared a titrated remifentanil bolus with mean effective bolus 0.5 μg/kg (with individual variation of 0.3 to 0.7 μg/kg) and 1-minute lockout to lumbar epidural using 20 mL low dose mixture (0.625 mg/mL levobupivacaine and 2 μg/mL fentanyl) in a randomized, double-blind study. Twenty-six percent of the remifentanil group and 52% of the epidural group reached acceptable pain scores. Some of the remifentanil group were reluctant to escalate the dose further to achieve lower pain levels, as they were concerned about over-sedation. Fifty-four percent of the remifentanil group required supplementary oxygen and this was associated with doses greater than 0.5 μg/kg. There was no difference in fetal or neonatal outcome. They therefore concluded that epidural analgesia remains superior, even to the "optimal" PCIA opioid.

Safety Precautions
Practically, remifentanil PCIA is now the most commonly used opioid PCIA for live births in the UK and Northern Ireland (47). It remains unlicensed for this use and requires local guidelines for safe practice. Ulster Community and Hospitals Trust, Northern Ireland has good safety guidelines (Table 7-5). Midwives have a period of supervised practice with remifentanil PCIA until they are assessed as competent. Women must not have received other opioids in the previous 4 hours

**TABLE 7-5 Ulster Community and Hospitals Trust—Remifentanil for Labor Analgesia.
Guideline for Remifentanil PCA = 40 μg Bolus with a 2-min Lockout**

Continuous Observations	30-min Observations	Indications for Contacting the Anesthetist
Oxygen saturations 1:1 supervision	Sedation score Respiratory rate Pain score	Sedation score <3 (not rousable to voice) Respiratory rate <8/min Oxygen saturations <90% despite oxygen

and are fully informed of potential side effects including the need for oxygen supplementation. A dedicated IV cannula is used solely for the PCIA. Continuous oxygen saturation monitoring is established and sedation scores recorded every 30 minutes with clear triggers for contacting anesthetic assistance. One to one supervision is essential.

In summary, although the analgesic efficacy of remifentanil has been demonstrated, it is not complete, or equivalent to neuraxial blockade, and many women continue to use 50% nitrous oxide in oxygen (Entonox) in addition to remifentanil PCIA. A recently published meta-analysis of 12 randomized controlled trials comparing remifentanil versus any other method of labor analgesia confirmed the superiority of remifentanil to meperidine and the superiority of epidural analgesia to remifentanil (59). The optimal method of delivery may require dose titration against individual patient response as well as dose escalation as labor progresses. Studies to date infer a good safety profile for parturients and neonates but remifentanil requires careful monitoring and continuous supervision by a midwife or labor nurse because of the potential for maternal adverse events. Further developments may include synchronization of the remifentanil PCIA bolus dose to the tocodynamometer recording to enable the maximum analgesic effect of the drug coinciding with the peak of uterine contraction.

Inhalational Agents

In the United States, the use of inhalational analgesia for labor is uncommon. This is not the case in Canada and the UK, however, with Entonox available in 100% of obstetric units in the UK and administered by midwives (60). Although many of the inhalational anesthetic agents used in surgery have been tried for pain relief in childbirth, only nitrous oxide continues to remain in regular use. There has been recent interest in sevoflurane as a labor analgesic, which will be discussed in more detail later in the chapter.

Nitrous Oxide

Intermittent inhalation of nitrous oxide can provide analgesia for labor although it does not completely eliminate the pain of uterine contractions. In recent years, the efficacy of Entonox for labor analgesia has been questioned, with several studies on intrapartum analgesia noting that 30% to 40% of mothers reported little or no benefit from Entonox (60). Others argue that, when properly timed, inhalation of 50% nitrous oxide provides significant pain relief in as many as half of parturients (61). To achieve substantial pain relief with nitrous oxide, maternal cooperation is required. There must be an analgesic concentration of nitrous oxide in the blood (and thus the brain) at the peak of the contraction. The patient is encouraged to breathe Entonox from the very beginning of the contraction and to continue until the end of the contraction. Nitrous oxide does not interfere with uterine activity (62).

Suitable equipment must be available to provide safe and satisfactory inhalation analgesia with nitrous oxide. An apparatus that limits the concentration of nitrous oxide (e.g., a nitrous oxide/oxygen blender or a premixed 1:1 cylinder) is required, and it must be checked periodically to prevent the unintentional administration of a high concentration of nitrous oxide and a resultant hypoxic concentration of gas. Inhalation may occur through a mask or a mouthpiece with a one-way valve to limit pollution of the labor suite with unscavenged gasses. Environmental pollution from the unscavenged nitrous oxide may be significant (63) and may lead its ultimate disappearance as a labor analgesic. It is unclear whether occupational exposure to subanesthetic concentrations of nitrous oxide results in significant health risks for health care workers (64).

Some physicians have expressed concern about the possibility of diffusion hypoxia after the administration of a nitrous oxide/oxygen mixture, which may lead to hypoxemia during labor. The overall evidence for this is however limited. In fact, Carstoniu et al. (65) compared parturients breathing 50% nitrous oxide in oxygen with a similar group of women breathing compressed air. Maternal oxygen saturation measurements between contractions were slightly higher in the nitrous oxide/oxygen group than in the group breathing compressed air. Of note, there was no difference between the two groups in mean pain scores. By contrast, other physicians have observed episodes of maternal hypoxemia with the use of nitrous oxide analgesia during labor (66).

Some studies have indicated that maternal hypoxemia may not be entirely due to diffusional hypoxia associated with nitrous oxide use, with the suggestion that the combined use of nitrous oxide and opioids increases the risk of maternal hypoxemia during labor (67,68). Also of interest is a study looking at rates of maternal desaturation in parturients receiving different modes of analgesia showing that desaturation was most commonly seen in the second stage of labor when parturients were receiving no analgesia for labor at all, as compared with parturients receiving either a combination of IM meperidine and Entonox, epidural bupivacaine/fentanyl mixtures, or plain epidural bupivacaine (69).

It may therefore be possible to conclude that although there has been some evidence to show that maternal desaturation may occur with the use of nitrous oxide, similar desaturation rates have also been seen with alternative labor analgesics as well as during normal labor without the use of any analgesics.

Another theoretical risk for the fetus with the use of nitrous oxide is the associated inhibition of the enzyme methionine synthase seen in prolonged administration (70). However, as the use of nitrous oxide in labor analgesia is generally intermittent in nature and not associated with prolonged high exposure levels or accumulation over time, this is likely to be no more than a theoretical risk, with the neonate eliminating most of the gas within minutes of birth. Used in this way, nitrous oxide does not depress neonatal respiration or affect neonatal neurobehavior (71).

On balance, the use of nitrous oxide in oxygen for labor analgesia has a good safety profile and continues to be widely used.

■ LESS COMMONLY USED LABOR ANALGESICS

Systemic Agents

Opioid Agonist–Antagonists and Others
Nalbuphine

Nalbuphine (Nubain) is a mixed agonist/antagonist opioid analgesic. Romagnoli et al. demonstrated that nalbuphine and morphine are of similar potency but that nalbuphine had an added safety feature, with nalbuphine showing a ceiling effect for respiratory depression beyond that induced for morphine. Nalbuphine doses in excess of 30 mg/70 kg failed to increase respiratory depression beyond that induced by morphine 20 mg/70 kg (72). This additional safety aspect of nalbuphine was however not of great clinical importance as the doses used in labor were typically 10 to 20 mg every 4 to 6 hours. The onset of analgesia occurs within 2 to 3 minutes of IV administration and within 15 minutes of IM or SC administration. The duration of analgesia ranges from 3 to 6 hours (73). Concerns that nalbuphine may have an antanalgesic effect led to nalbuphine being discontinued in the UK in 2003.

Wilson et al. (74) performed a randomized, double-blind comparison of 20 mg IM nalbuphine and 100 mg IM meperidine for labor analgesia. Although analgesia was comparable between the groups, nalbuphine was associated with less nausea and vomiting and more maternal sedation than meperidine. Neonatal neurobehavioral scores at 2 to 4 hours were lower in the nalbuphine group but there was no difference at 24 hours. The mean umbilical vein to maternal blood concentration ration was higher for nalbuphine (0.78 ± 0.03) than meperidine (0.61 ± 0.02).

Giannina et al. (75) compared effects of nalbuphine and meperidine on intrapartum FHR recordings. Nalbuphine significantly reduced the number of accelerations and variability. Meperidine had little significant effect. Case reports of a variety of non-reassuring FHR changes have been reported after maternal administration of nalbuphine.

Patient satisfaction was increased by using nalbuphine PCA (1 mg bolus, 6- to 10-minute lockout) as compared to intermittent IV bolus (10 to 20 mg 4 to 6 hourly) (76). Analgesia and Apgar scores were similar between groups and no neonates required naloxone. Moreover, when compared to meperidine PCIA (15 mg bolus, 10-minute lockout), Frank et al. (77) found that nalbuphine (3 mg bolus, 10-minute lockout) provided better analgesia. Maternal sedation scores were similar and there was no difference in neonatal outcome as assessed by Apgar scores, time to sustained respiration or neurobehavioral assessment at 6 to 10 hours post-delivery.

Butorphanol
Butorphanol is an opioid with agonist–antagonist properties. It is five times as potent as morphine and 40 times as potent as meperidine (78). The typical dose during labor is 1 to 2 mg IV or IM. Butorphanol is 95% metabolized in the liver to inactive metabolites. Excretion is primarily renal. Butorphanol and morphine result in similar respiratory depression at equi-analgesic doses. Butorphanol 2 mg produces respiratory depression similar to that which occurs with morphine 10 mg or meperidine 70 mg. However, butorphanol 4 mg results in less respiratory depression than morphine 20 mg or meperidine 140 mg (78).

Butorphanol has been described as a good labor analgesic due to its short half-life and inactive metabolites, combined with good analgesic effects. Maduska and Hajghassemali (79) compared butorphanol (1 to 2 mg) with meperidine (40 to 80 mg) and found that they resulted in similar efficacy of labor analgesia. They noted rapid placental transfer of butorphanol with a mean umbilical vein to maternal blood concentration ratio of 0.84 at 30 to 210 minutes post-IM injection (similar to that of meperidine). No differences in FHR changes, Apgar scores, time to sustained respiration or cord gas measurements were found.

In addition, Quilligan et al. (80) performed a double-blind comparison of intravenous butorphanol (1 or 2 mg) and meperidine (40 or 80 mg) during labor. They noted better analgesia at 30 minutes and 1 hour after the administration of butorphanol. There was no difference in Apgar scores between the two groups of infants.

Nelson and Eisenach (81) investigated the possible synergistic effect of combining butorphanol with meperidine as opposed to each drug alone as an IV bolus. All three groups showed similar reduction in pain intensity (25% to 35%) and there was no difference in maternal side effects or Apgar scores. They concluded that there was no improvement in therapeutic benefit from combining the two drugs.

Meptazinol
Meptazinol (Meptid) is a partial opioid agonist specific to mu-1 receptors with mixed agonist/antagonist activity. It has a short onset of action, with effect in 15 minutes after IM administration, with a similar duration of action to meperidine. It is used at a dose of 100 mg IM. Its partial agonist activity is thought to confer less sedation, respiratory depression and risk of dependence (82). Meptazinol is metabolized by glucuronidation in the liver, a process which is less immature in neonates than the metabolic pathway for meperidine. Neonatal half-life is 3.4 hours compared to the adult half-life of 2.2 hours (83). Rapid elimination should in theory be associated with benefit to neonatal outcome following use of meptazinol as a labor analgesic.

Nicholas and Robson (84) compared 100 mg IM meptazinol with 100 mg IM meperidine in a large randomized, blinded study. They demonstrated significantly better pain relief at 45 and 60 minutes with meptazinol with a trend toward fewer side effects (28% compared to 35% in the meperidine group). There was no significant difference in neonatal outcomes but the use of meptazinol was associated with an increased incidence of 1-minute Apgar score being greater than 7.

Morrison et al. (85) failed to find much benefit of meptazinol over meperidine in a large study involving 1,100 patients, with similar pain scores being recorded at 60 minutes post-IM dose. Drowsiness was significantly less than meperidine but the incidence of vomiting was higher. FHR changes were similar and neonatal outcomes in the form of need for resuscitation, Apgar scores and suckling ability were comparable across the two groups. Overall use of naloxone was similar between groups, but if dose–delivery interval exceeded 180 minutes, significantly more neonates in the meperidine group required naloxone.

de Boer et al. (86) compared neonatal gas and acid–base status in neonates following maternal administration of IM meptazinol or meperidine in labor (both at 1.5 mg/kg). Heel prick gasses at 10 minutes showed significantly lower pH and higher CO_2 in the meperidine group although this had resolved by 60 minutes. These findings suggest that meptazinol has less depressant effect on neonatal respiration.

Overall, meptazinol may confer some benefits to neonatal outcome as compared to meperidine but it is not as widely available or as widely used. Cost of meptazinol is considerably more than meperidine.

Pentazocine
Pentazocine (Talwin) has both agonist and weak antagonist properties. Pentazocine 30 to 60 mg is equipotent to morphine 10 mg. Peak analgesia occurs within 10 minutes after IV administration, and plasma levels peak at 15 to 60 minutes after IM administration (87). A ceiling effect for respiratory depression occurs at doses of 40 to 60 mg. Clinical studies have demonstrated that a single injection of meperidine 100 mg or pentazocine 40 to 45 mg produces similar degrees of neonatal respiratory depression. However, repeated maternal doses of pentazocine do not increase neonatal respiratory depression proportionally, whereas the respiratory depression with repeated doses of meperidine is cumulative (88). Psychomimetic effects may occur with standard doses, but they occur more frequently after larger doses. The potential for psychomimetic side effects has limited the popularity of pentazocine in obstetrics.

Tramadol
Tramadol (Tramal, Zydol) is an atypical weak opioid. It has low mu-receptor affinity with 10% the potency of morphine as well as also exerting GABAergic, noradrenergic and serotonergic effects. It causes no clinically significant respiratory depression at normal doses. The analgesic effect of 100 mg IM tramadol occurs within 10 minutes and has a duration of 2 hours. Tramadol is metabolized by the liver to an active

metabolite, M1, which has a longer elimination half-life at 9 hours than that of tramadol (89).

Claahsen van der Grinten et al. (90) demonstrated high placental permeability for tramadol with a maternal to umbilical vein ratio of 0.97. The neonates possessed complete hepatic capacity for metabolism of tramadol into its active metabolite M1. The elimination profile of M1 suggests a terminal half-life of 85 hours which is due to its requirement for renal elimination, an immature process in neonates. Neonatal outcome, assessed by Apgar and the Neurologic and Adaptive Capacity Score, was within normal limits and showed no correlation to tramadol or M1 concentrations.

Keskin et al. (91) compared IM tramadol 100 mg to IM meperidine 100 mg for labor analgesia. The 30- and 60-minute pain scores were significantly lower in the meperidine group and tramadol was associated with higher nausea levels. There was no significant difference in neonatal outcomes but more of the tramadol group required oxygen for respiratory distress and hypoxemia. The authors concluded that meperidine provided superior analgesia to tramadol as well as being associated with a better side-effect profile.

Opioid Antagonists

Naloxone (Narcan) is the opioid antagonist of choice to reverse the neonatal effects of maternal opioid administration. There is no neonatal benefit to the maternal administration of naloxone during labor or just before delivery and this practice has been shown to antagonize maternal analgesia during labor or at delivery without causing a decrease in opioid-related maternal side effects (92). In addition, it provides at best, uncertain and/or incomplete reversal of the depressive effects on the neonate. When maternal administration of an opioid is anticipated to result in neonatal respiratory depression, it is best to administer naloxone directly to the newborn. Naloxone reverses opioid depression of newborn minute ventilation and increases the slope of the CO_2-response curve in infants affected by the maternal administration of an opioid (93). It may precipitate a withdrawal reaction in the newborn of the opioid-dependent mother. The recommended dose of naloxone is 0.1 mg/kg or a 1 mg/mL or 0.4 mg/mL solution and it should be given IV or intratracheally, if possible. It may also be given IM or SC; however, absorption of the agent may be delayed and unpredictable in the infant who is stressed and vasoconstricted (93).

Analgesic Adjuncts and Sedatives

Historically, many drugs (e.g., barbiturates, hydroxyzine, scopolamine) have been used as adjuncts to parenteral opioid analgesia. Most of these cause sedation and neonatal depression and are now used infrequently as adequate analgesia is now possible using labor epidurals or PCIA opioid techniques.

Barbiturates are sedative and have no analgesic effect. They are lipid soluble, rapidly cross the placenta and are measurable in fetal blood. There is a risk of neonatal depression, especially if combined with systemic analgesics (94).

Phenothiazines may be used in combination with opioids to cause sedation and reduce nausea and vomiting. They rapidly cross the placenta and reduce FHR variability but there is no evidence of neonatal respiratory depression. Neurobehavioral outcomes are poorly studied. Phenothiazines such as chlorpromazine may cause unacceptable hypotension from alpha-adrenergic blockade. Promethazine (Phenergan) can be used at a dose of 25 to 50 mg IV/IM and is found to produce sedation which can be profound, and a mild respiratory stimulation which may counteract opioid respiratory depression. Promethazine appears in fetal blood 1 to 2 minutes after maternal IV administration and equilibrates within 15 minutes (95). Propiomazine (Largon) is a mild respiratory

depressant which may further depress maternal ventilation after opioids. It has a shorter onset and duration than promethazine. Only two studies suggest that phenothiazines may potentiate the effect of meperidine (96,97).

Metoclopramide is a dopamine D2 receptor antagonist and a mixed 5-HT3 receptor antagonist/5-HT4 receptor agonist which is non-sedative and used to reduce nausea and vomiting and increase gastric emptying (98). Vella et al. (99) observed that administration of metoclopramide reduced requirements for nitrous oxide during labor, as well as also showing that women who received both meperidine and metoclopramide had slightly better pain scores than women who received meperidine alone.

Benzodiazepines have been used for sedation in obstetric patients but are associated with significant side effects. Diazepam (Valium) rapidly crosses the placenta and accumulates in the fetus at concentrations which may exceed maternal. It has a long elimination half-life (24 to 48 hours) and has a slightly less potent active metabolite with an elimination half-life of 51 to 120 hours (100). Administration of diazepam during labor has been associated with neonatal hypotonicity, respiratory depression, and impairment of neonatal thermoregulation and stress responses; these may be dose-related effects (101). Lorazepam (Ativan) has a shorter half-life at 12 hours and is metabolized to produce an inactive glucuronide. McAuley et al. (102) gave lorazepam 2 mg or placebo prior to meperidine 100 mg IM as needed for analgesia. Analgesia was better in the lorazepam group but there was an increase in respiratory depression, although this was not statistically significant. Neonatal neurobehavioral scores were similar across the 2 groups. Maternal amnesia was common with lorazepam, with 14/20 patients given lorazepam having difficulty in recall of events of labor compared with 4/20 in the unpremedicated group. Midazolam (Versed) has a rapid onset and short duration of action with inactive metabolites. It has been shown to cross the placenta and, at high doses used for induction of general anesthesia, it causes neonatal hypotonia (103). Due to maternal and neonatal side effects seen with benzodiazepine administration in labor along with the lack of need for sedation in laboring parturient, these are not widely used agents.

Ketamine is a phencyclidine derivative. Small doses administered intravenously or intramuscularly provide a dissociative state of analgesia with or without amnesia and larger doses (1 mg/kg) are used to induce general anesthesia. Ketamine is best avoided in the preeclamptic patient, as it causes sympathetic nervous system stimulation and may exacerbate hypertension. However, it is the induction agent of choice for patients with hypovolemia or asthma. Although small doses of ketamine have not been shown to result in neonatal depression, high doses have been associated with low Apgar scores and abnormal neonatal muscle tone (104).

Intravenous ketamine has a rapid onset of action (30 seconds) and a short duration of action (3 to 5 minutes). It may provide effective analgesia for labor by administration of a 0.1 mg/kg bolus dose on initiation of labor pain followed by an infusion of 0.2 mg/kg/h, with the infusion rate being adjusted up or down in 1 to 2 mL/h increments to provide ongoing analgesia. Such doses have not been associated with hallucinations or unpleasant dreams (105).

Inhalational Agents

The potential use of volatile halogenated anesthetic agents in labor has been studied, both as sole agents as well as adjuncts to nitrous oxide. Most, but not all, of this research has focused on sevoflurane, most probably due to its non-irritant quality on inhalation and its common use in inhalational induction of anesthesia. All volatile halogenated agents cause dose-related relaxation of uterine smooth muscle. A recent study identified the minimum alveolar concentration (MAC) for each agent at which 50% inhibition of contractile function of uterine muscle occurred in vitro: Isoflurane at 2.35 MAC, sevoflurane at 1.7 MAC, desflurane at 1.4 MAC and halothane at 1.66 MAC (106). The administration of greater concentrations may decrease the smooth muscle response to the administration of oxytocin.

An important consideration with the use of inhalational anesthetic agents for labor analgesia is prevention of exposure of those in the labor room to the agent. An accurate delivery system to avoid overdose, demand valve, and scavenging system are necessary.

Enflurane

Abboud et al. (107) compared 0.25% to 1.25% enflurane in oxygen to 30% to 60% nitrous oxide during the second stage of labor. Approximately 89% of the enflurane group and 76% of the nitrous oxide group rated their analgesia as satisfactory and amnesia rates were similar at 7% to 10%. There were no differences in blood loss, Apgar scores, or cord gas results.

Isoflurane

After studies by McLeod (108), Arora (109) and Wee (110) suggested better pain relief scores with levels of drowsiness that did not confer a clinical problem and Ross et al. (111) performed a study of 221 parturients comparing 0.25% isoflurane in Entonox versus Entonox alone. A demand valve from pre-mixed cylinders was used. Previous studies had used draw-over vaporizers in circuit with Entonox. No mother became unduly sedated and there was no increased need for neonatal resuscitation except in infants where maternal opioids had also been administered. Blood loss was no higher than expected (mean 200 mL). The rate of intolerance to the odor was 8% and 14% eventually requested epidural analgesia. The same authors have assessed the clinical safety of the cylinder system to verify clinically acceptable performance (112).

Desflurane

Desflurane is associated with rapid onset and recovery due to its low solubility. Abboud et al. (113) found similar analgesia scores when comparing 1% to 4% desflurane in oxygen with 30% to 60% nitrous oxide with amnesia rates up to 23%. Neonatal outcomes were similar between groups.

Sevoflurane

Sevoflurane is the volatile agent most commonly used for gas induction of anesthesia. It has short onset and offset of action but is less irritating and has a less unpleasant odor than other volatiles. Toscano's pilot study in 2003 (114) included 50 parturients breathing intermittent 2% to 3% sevoflurane in oxygen/air mix via a small anesthesia system. They aimed for an expired end-tidal concentration of 1% to 1.5% at the peak of uterine contraction. Mean VAS pain score before sevoflurane was 8.7 ± 1, post-sevoflurane 3.3 ± 1.5 ($p < 0.05$). No desaturations or loss of consciousness occurred and blood loss was unremarkable. FHR was unchanged and mean neonatal Apgar scores were 9 at 1 minute (range: 5 to 9) and 10 at 5 minutes (range: 8 to 10).

Yeo et al. (115) compared 0.8% sevoflurane with Entonox in 32 parturients using crossover comparisons. Two patients could not tolerate the odor of sevoflurane and five requested epidurals during the Entonox phase. Median pain relief scores were significantly higher for sevoflurane at 67 (interquartile range [IQR]: 55 to 74) than Entonox at 51 (IQR 41 to 70) on 100 mm scales. In addition, nausea and vomiting were more common in the Entonox group (relative risk 2.7 [95% CI 1.3 to 5.7]; $P = 0.004$). Although there was significantly more sedation with sevoflurane than with Entonox (median score 74 mm [IQR 66.5 to 81 [range: 32.5 to 100]]) vs. 51 mm (IQR 41 to 69.5 [range: 13 to 100]), respectively; $P < 0.001$), 29 out of 32 patients preferred sevoflurane to Entonox and found its sedative effects helpful. There were no other adverse events: No desaturations, apnea, or change in end-tidal CO_2. They concluded that sevoflurane can provide useful analgesia for labor.

The routine use of inhalational analgesia may be limited for several reasons including the need for specialized equipment, concern regarding pollution, the potential for maternal amnesia and the loss of protective airway reflexes. Although sedation occurs during intermittent use of volatile anesthetic agents, none profound enough to jeopardize airway reflexes has been reported. Further research into intermittent volatile inhalation for providing labor analgesia may demonstrate good maternal safety profiles and allow development of this technique for cases where regional anesthesia is contraindicated.

As this chapter has illustrated, many agents have been used to provide labor analgesia with varying success. Meperidine has long been used worldwide but due to its poor analgesic properties and safety profile is being eliminated from common practice. From the evidence and experience to date, the remifentanil PCIA, when used in conjunction with appropriate monitoring and safety measures, currently appears to be establishing itself as the current best alternative available to epidural analgesia. Sevoflurane is also a potentially promising agent in the treatment of labor analgesia and its use maybe seen to increase in the near future, given initial promising results in terms of effect and safety profile.

KEY POINTS

- Systemic analgesics are still commonly used.
- All opioid analgesic drugs rapidly cross the placenta and cause transient reduced FHR variability.
- Meperidine is most commonly used as an intermittent bolus. Its active metabolite is associated with neonatal respiratory depression and neurobehavioral differences.
- Remifentanil PCIA use in labor is associated with high maternal satisfaction scores. It provides good, although incomplete, analgesia and has minimal effect on neonatal outcome. Its use requires intensive monitoring due to maternal sedation and the potential for serious complications.
- Inhalation analgesia is less common in the United States than other countries. Nitrous oxide may provide some analgesia and can be used to supplement other techniques.
- Intermittent inhalation of volatile anesthetic agents is rarely used but has provided good analgesia with minimal side effects in studies to date.

REFERENCES

1. Bucklin BA, Hawkins JL, Anderson JR, et al. Obstetric Anesthesia Workforce Survey. *Anesthesiology* 2005;103:645–653.
2. Maternity. The Information Centre. www.ic.nhs.uk/pubs/maternity, last accessed 23/7/11.
3. Jenkins JG. Some immediate serious complications of obstetric epidural analgesia and anaesthesia: a prospective study of 145550 epidurals. *Int J Obstet Anesth* 2005;14:47–42.
4. Reynolds F, Sharma SK, Seed PT. Analgesia in labour and fetal acid–base balance: A meta-analysis comparing epidural with systemic opioid analgesia. *BJOG* 2002;109:1344–1353.

5. Halpern SH, Muir H, Breen TW, et al. A multicenter randomized controlled trial comparing patient-controlled epidural with intravenous analgesia for pain relief in labor. *Anesth Analg* 2004;99:1532–1538.

6. Saravanakumar K, Garstang JS, Hasan K. Intravenous patient-controlled analgesia for labour: a survey of UK practice. *Int J Obstet Anesth* 2007;16:221–225.

7. McIntosh DG, Rayburn WF. Patient-controlled analgesia in obstetrics and gynecology. *Obstet Gynecol* 1991;78:1129–1135.

8. Rayburn WF, Smith CV, Leuschen MP, et al. Comparison of patient-controlled and nurse administered analgesia using intravenous fentanyl during labor. *Anesth Rev* 1991;18:31–36.

9. Tuckey JP, Prout RE, Wee MYK. Prescribing intramuscular opioids for labour analgesia in consultant-led maternity units: a survey of UK practice. *Int J Obstet Anesth* 2008;17:3–8.

10. Tsui MHY, Ngan Kee WD, Ng FF, et al. A double blinded randomised placebo-controlled study of intramuscular pethidine for pain relief in the first stage of labour. *BJOG* 2004;111:648–655.

11. Shnider SM, Way EL, Lord MJ. Rate of appearance and disappearance of meperidine in fetal blood after administration of narcotic to the mother. *Anesthesiology* 1966;27:227–228.

12. Kariniemi V, Pirkko A. Effects of intramuscular pethidine on fetal heart rate variability. *Br J Obstet Gynaecol* 1981;88:718–720.

13. Kuhnert BR, Kuhnert PM, Tu AL, et al. Meperidine and normeperidine levels following meperidine administration during labor. I. Mother. *Am J Obstet Gynecol* 1979;133:904–913.

14. Caldwell J, Wakile LA, Notarianni LJ, et al. Maternal and neonatal disposition of pethidine in childbirth: A study using quantitative gas chromatography–mass spectrometry. *Life Sci* 1978;22:589–596.

15. Shnider SM, Moya F. Effect of meperidine on the newborn infant. *Am J Obstet Gynecol* 1964;89:1008–1015.

16. Kuhnert BJ, Kuhnert PM, Philipson EH, et al. Disposition of meperidine and normeperidine following multiple doses during labor. II. Fetus and neonate. *Am J Obstet Gynecol* 1985;151:410–415.

17. Belfrage P, Boréus LO, Hartvig P, et al. Neonatal depression after obstetrical analgesia with pethidine: The role of the injection-delivery time interval and of the plasma concentrations of pethidine and norpethidine. *Acta Obstet Gynecol Scand* 1981;60:43–49.

18. Hodgkinson R, Bhatt M, Wang CN. Double-blinded comparison of neurobehavior of neonates following the administration of different doses of meperidine to the mother. *Can Anaesth Soc J* 1978;25:405–411.

19. Belsey EM, Rosenblatt DB, Lieberman BA, et al. The influence of maternal analgesia in neonatal behaviour. I. Pethidine. *Br J Obstet Gynaecol* 1981;88:398–406.

20. Kuhnert BR, Linn PL, Kennard MJ, et al. Effects of low doses of meperidine on neonatal behavior. *Anesth Analg* 1985;63:301–308.

21. Isenor L, Penny-McGillivray T. Intravenous meperidine infusion for obstetric analgesia. *J Obstet Gynecol Neonatal Nurs* 1993;22:349–356.

22. Volikas I, Male D. A comparison of pethidine and remifentail patient-controlled analgesia in labour. *Int J Obstet Anesth* 2001;10:86–90.

23. Blair JM, Dobson GT, Hill DA, et al. Patient controlled analgesia for labour: a comparison of remifentanil with pethidine. *Anaesthesia* 2005;60:22–27.

24. Stoelting RK. Opioid agonists and antagonists. In: Stoelting RK, ed. *Pharmacology and Physiology in Anesthetic Practice.* 4th ed. Philadelphia, PA: J.B. Lippincott; 2006:92–105.

25. Brunk FS, Delle M. Morphine metabolism in man. *Clin Pharmacol Ther* 1974;16:51.

26. Osborne R, Thompson P, Joel S, et al. The analgesic activity of morphine-6-glucuronide. *Br J Clin Pharm* 1992;34:130–138.

27. Peat SJ, Hanna MH, Woodham M, et al. Morphine-6-glucuronide: effects on ventilation in normal volunteers. *Pain* 1991;45:101–104.

28. Gerdin E, Rane A, Lindberg B. Transplacental transfer of morphine in man. *J Perinat Med* 1990;18:305.

29. Kart T, Christrup LL, Rasmussen M. Recommended use of morphine in neonates, infants and children based on a literature review: Part 1—Pharmacokinetics. *Paediatr Anaesth* 1997;7:5–11.

30. Olofsson C, Ekblom A, Ekman-Ordeberg G, et al. Analgesic efficacy of intravenous morphine in labour pain: A reappraisal. *Int J Obstet Anesth* 1996;5:176–180.

31. Olofsson C, Ekblom A, Ekman-Ordeberg G, et al. Lack of analgesic effect of systemically administered morphine or pethidine on labour pain. *Br J Obstet Gynaecol* 1996;103:968–972.

32. Way WL, Costley EC, Way EL. Respiratory sensitivity of the newborn infant to meperidine and morphine. *Clin Pharm Ther* 1965;6:454–461.

33. Boerner U. The metabolism of morphine and heroin in man. *Drug Metabol Rev* 1975;4:39–73.

34. Barrett DA, Barker DP, Rutter N, et al. Morphine, morphine-6-glucuronide and morphine-3-glucuronide pharmacokinetics in newborn infants receiving diamorphine infusions. *Br J Clin Pharm* 1996;41:531–537.

35. Rawal N, Tomlinson AJ, Gibson GJ, et al. Umbilical cord plasma concentrations of free morphine following single-dose diamorphine analgesia and their relationship to dose-delivery time interval, Apgar scores and neonatal respiration. *Eur J Obstet Gynecol Reprod Biol* 2007;133:30–33.

36. Fairlie FM, Marshall L, Walker JJ, et al. Intramuscular opioids for maternal pain relief in labour: a randomised controlled trial comparing pethidine to diamorphine. *Br J Obstet Gynaecol* 1999;106:1181–1187.

37. McInnes RJ, Hillan E, Clark D, et al. Diamorphine for pain relief in labour: a randomised controlled trial comparing intramuscular injection and patient-controlled analgesia. *BJOG* 2004;111:1081–1089.

38. Eisele JH, Wright R, Rogge P. Newborn and maternal fentanyl levels at cesarean section. *Anesth Analg* 1982;61:179–180.

39. Rayburn W, Rathke A, Leuschen P, et al. Fentanyl citrate analgesia during labor. *Am J Obstet Gynecol* 1989;161:202–206.

40. Rayburn WF, Smith CV, Parriott JE, et al. Randomized comparison of meperidine and fentanyl during labor. *Obstet Gynecol* 1989;74:604–606.

41. Morley-Forster PK, Weberpals J. Neonatal effects of patient-controlled analgesia using fentanyl in labor. *Int J Obstet Anesth* 1998;7:103–107.

42. Gepts E, Heytens L, Camu F. Pharmacokinetics and placental transfer of intravenous and epidural alfentanil in parturient women. *Anesth Analg* 1986;65:1155–1160.

43. Morley-Forster PK, Reid DW, Vandeberghe H. A comparison of patient-controlled analgesia fentanyl and alfentanil for labor analgesia. *Can J Anesth* 2000;47:113–119.

44. Egan TD, Minto CF, Hermann DJ, et al. Remifentanil versus alfentanil. *Anesthesiology* 1996;84:821–833.

45. Glass SA, Hardman D, Kamiyama Y, et al. Preliminary pharmacokinetics and pharmacodynamics of an ultra-short-acting opioid: remifentanil. *Anesth Analg* 1993;77:1031–1040.

46. Kan RE, Hughes SC, Rosen MA, et al. Intravenous remifentanil: Placental transfer, maternal and neonatal effects. *Anesthesiology* 1998;88:1467–1474.

47. Hill D. The use of remifentanil in obstetrics. *Anesthesiol Clin* 2008;26:169–182.

48. Thurlow JA, Laxton CH, Dick A, et al. Remifentanil by patient-controlled analgesia compared with intramuscular meperidine for pain relief in labour. *Br J Anaesth* 2002;88:374–378.

49. Volmanen P, Akural E, Raudaskoski T, et al. Comparison of remifentanil and nitrous oxide in labour analgesia. *Acta Anaesthesiol Scand* 2005;49:453–458.

50. Evron S, Glezerman M, Sadan O, et al. Remifentanil: a novel systemic analgesic for labor pain. *Anesth Analg* 2005;100:233–238.

51. Douma MR, Verwey RA, Kam-Endtz CE, et al. Obstetric analgesia: a comparison of patient-controlled meperidine, remifentanil, and fentanyl in labour. *Br J Anaesth* 2010;104:209–215.

52. Marwah R, Hassan S, Carvalho JC, et al. Remifentanil versus fentanyl for intravenous patient-controlled labour analgesia: an observational study. *Can J Anesth* 2012;59(3):246–254.

53. Volmanen PVE, Akural EI, Raudaskoski T, et al. Timing of intravenous patient-controlled remifentanil bolus during early labour. *Acta Anaesthesiol Scand* 2011;55:486–494.

54. Volikas I, Butwick A, Wilinson C, et al. Maternal and neonatal side-effects of remifentanil patient-controlled analgesia in labour. *Br J Anaesth* 2005;95:504–509.

55. Volmanen P, Akural EI, Raudaskoski T, et al. Remifentanil in obstetric analgesia: A dose finding study. *Anesth Analg* 2002;94:913–917.

56. Blair JM, Hill DA, Fee JP. Patient-controlled analgesia for labor using remifentanil: a feasability study. *Br J Anaesth* 2001;87:415–420.

57. Balki M, Kasodekar S, Dhumne S, et al. Remifentanil patient-controlled analgesia for labour: optimising drug delivery regimens. *Can J Anesth* 2007;54:626–633.

58. Volmanen P, Sarvela J, Akural EI, et al. Intravenous remifentanil vs. epidural levobupivacaine with fentanyl for pain relief in early labour: a randomised, controlled, double-blinded study. *Acta Anaesthesiol Scand* 2008;52(2):249–255.

59. Schnabel A, Hahn N, Broscheit A, et al. Remifentanil for labour analgesia: a meta-analysis of randomised controlled trials. *Eur J Anaesthesiol* 2012;29(4):177–185.

60. Yentis SM. The use of Entonox® for labour pain should be abandoned. *Int J Obstet Anesth* 2001:10;25–28.

61. Rosen M. Recent advances in pain relief in childbirth: Inhalation and systemic analgesia. *Br J Anaesth* 1971;43:837–848.

62. Marx GF, Katsnelson T. The introduction of nitrous oxide into obstetrics. *Obstet Gynecol* 1992;80:715–718.

63. Mills GH, Singh D, Longan M, et al. Nitrous oxide exposure on the labour ward. *Int J Obstet Anesth* 1996;5:160–164.

64. Bernow J, Bjordal J, Wiklund KE. Pollution of delivery ward air by nitrous oxide: Effects of various modes of room ventilation, excess and close scavenging. *Acta Anaesthesiol Scand* 1984;28:119–123.

65. Carstoniu J, Levytam S, Norman P, et al. Nitrous oxide in labour: Safety and efficacy assessed by a double-blind placebo controlled study. *Anesthesiology* 1994;80:30–35.

66. Lucas DN, Siemaszko O, Yentis SM. Maternal hypoxemia associated with the use of Entonox in labour. *Int J Obstet Anesth* 2000;9:270–272.

67. Deckart R, Fembacher PM, Schneider KTM, et al. Maternal arterial oxygen saturation during labor and delivery: Pain dependent alteration and effects on the newborn. *Obstet Gynecol* 1987;70:21–25.

68. Irestadi L. Current status for nitrous oxide for obstetric pain relief. *Acta Anesthesiol Scand* 1994;38:771–772.

69. Griffin RP, Reynolds F. Maternal hypoxaemia during labour and delivery: the influence of analgesia and effect on neonatal outcome. *Anaesthesia* 1995;50:151–156.

70. Reynolds F. Labour analgesia and the baby: good news is no news. *Int J Obstet Anesth* 2011;20:38–50.

71. Stefani SJ, Hughes SC, Shnider SM, et al. Neonatal neurobehavioral effects of inhalation analgesia for vaginal delivery. *Anesthesiology* 1982;56:351–355.

72. Romagnoli A, Keats AS. Ceiling effect for respiratory depression by nalbuphine. *Clin Pharmacol Ther* 1980;27:478–485.

73. Gunion MW, Marchionne AM, Anderson CTM. Use of the mixed agonist–antagonist nalbuphine in opioid based analgesia. *Acute Pain* 2004;6:29–39.

74. Wilson CM, McClean E, Moore J, et al. A double-blind comparison of intramuscular pethidine and nalbuphine in labour. *Anaesthesia* 1986;41:207–213.

75. Giannina G, Guzman ER, Yu-Ling L, et al. Comparison of the effects of meperidine and nalbuphine on intrapartum fetal heart rate tracings. *Obstet Gynecol* 1995;86:441–445.

76. Podlas J, Breland BD. Patient-controlled analgesia with nalbuphine during labor. *Obstet Gynecol* 1987;70:202–204.

77. Frank M, McAteer EJ, Cattermole R, et al. Nalbuphine for obstetric analgesia: A comparison of nalbuphine with pethidine for pain relief in labour when administered by patient-controlled analgesia. *Anaesthesia* 1987;42:697–703.

78. Kallos T, Caruso FS. Respiratory effects of butorphanol and pethidine. *Anaesthesia* 1979;34:633–637.

79. Maduska AL, Hajghassemali M. A double-blind comparison of butorphanol and meperidine in labour: Maternal pain relief and effects on the newborn. *Can Anaesth Soc J* 1978;25:398–404.

80. Quilligan EJ, Keegan KA, Donahue MJ. Double-blind comparison of intravenously injected butorphanol and meperidine in parturients. *Int J Gynaecol Obstet* 1980;18:363–367.

81. Nelson KE, Eisenach JC. Intravenous butorphanol, meperidine and their combination relieve pain and distress in women in labor. *Anesthesiology* 2005;102:1008–1013.

82. Holmes B, Ward A. Meptazinol. A review of its pharmacodynamic and pharmacokinetic properties and therapeutic efficacy. *Drugs* 1985;30:285–312.

83. Franklin RA, Frost T, Robson PJ, et al. Preliminary studies on the disposition of meptazinol in the neonate. *Br J Clin Pharmacol* 1981;12:88–90.

84. Nicholas AD, Robson PJ. Double-blind comparison of meptazinol and pethidine in labour. *Br J Obstet Gynaecol* 1987;94:256–261.

85. Morrison CE, Dutton D, Howie H, et al. Pethidine compared with meptazinol during labour. *Anaesthesia* 1987;42:7–14.

86. de Boer FC, Shortland D, Simpson RL, et al. A comparison of the effects of maternal administration of meptazinol and pethidine on neonatal acid–base status. *Br J Obstet Gynaecol* 1987;94:256–261.

87. Jaffe JH, Martin WR. Opioids with mixed actions: Partial agonists. In: Gilman AG, Rall TW, Nies AS, Taylor P, eds. *The Pharmacological Basis of Therapeutics*. 8th ed. New York, NY: Pergamon Press; 1990:512–514.

88. Refstad SO, Lindbaek E. Ventilatory depression of the newborn of women receiving pethidine or pentazocine. *Br J Anaesth* 1980;52:265–271.

89. Lee CR, McTavish D, Sorkin EM. Tramadol. A preliminary review of its pharmacodynamic and pharmacokinetic and therapeutic potential in acute and chronic pain states. *Drugs* 1993;46:313–340.

90. Claahsen-van der Grinten HL, Verbruggen I, van den Berg PP, et al. Different pharmacokinetics of tramadol in mothers treated for labour pain and in their neonates. *Eur J Clin Pharmacol* 2005;61:523–529.

91. Keskin HL, Aktepe Keskin E, Avsar AF, et al. Pethidine versus tramadol for pain relief during labour. *Int J Gynecol Obstet* 2003;82:11–16.

92. Girvan CB, Moore J, Dundee JW. Pethidine compared with pethidine–naloxone administered during labor. *Br J Anaesth* 1976;48:563–569.

93. Gerhardt T, Bancalari E, Cohen H, et al. Use of naloxone to reverse narcotic respiratory depression in the newborn infant. *J Pediatr* 1977;90:1009–1012.

94. Althaus J, Wax J. Analgesia and anesthesia in labor. *Obstet Gynecol Clin North Am* 2005;32:231–244.

95. Clark RB, Seifen AB. Systemic medication during labor and delivery. *Obstet Gynecol* 1983;12:165–197.

96. Powe CE, Kien IM, Fromhagen C, et al. Propiomazine hydrochloride in obstetrical analgesia. *JAMA* 1962;181:290–294.

97. Ullery JC, Bair JR. Maternal–fetal effects of propiomazine–meperidine analgesia. *Am J Obstet Gynecol* 1962;84:1051–1056.

98. Rang HP, Dale MM, Ritter JM, et al. The gastrointestinal tract. In: Rang HP, Dale MM, Ritter JM, Flower RJ, Henderson J, eds. *Rang & Dale's Pharmacology*. 7th ed. [e-book]. Oxford: Churchill Livingstone; 2012:29.

99. Vella L, Francis D, Houlton P, et al. Comparison of the antiemetics metoclopramide and promethazine in labour. *Br Med J (Clin Res Ed)* 1985;290:1173–1175.

100. Mandelli M, Tognoni G, Garatini S. Clinical pharmacokinetics of diazepam. *Clin Pharmacokinet* 1978;3:72–91.

101. McElhatton PR. The effects of benzodiazepine use during pregnancy and lactation. *Reprod Toxicol* 1994;8:461–475.

102. McAuley DM, O'Neill MP, Moore J, et al. Lorazepam premedication for labour. *Br J Obstet Gynaecol* 1982;89:149–154.

103. Ravlo O, Carl P, Crawford ME, et al. A randomized comparison between midazolam and thiopental for elective caesarean section anaesthesia. *Anesth Analg* 1989;68:234–237.

104. Akamatsu TJ, Bonica JJ, Rehmet R, et al. Experiences with the use of ketamine for parturition. I. Primary anesthesia for vaginal delivery. *Anesth Analg* 1974;53:284–287.

105. Joselyn AS, Cherian VT, Joel S. Ketamine for labour analgesia. *Intl J Obstet Anesth* 2010:19;122–123.

106. Yoo KY, Lee JC, Yoon MH, et al. The effects of volatile anesthetics on spontaneous contraction of isolated human pregnant uterine muscle: A comparison among Sevoflurane, Desflurane, Isoflurane and Halothane. *Anesth Analg* 2006;103:443–447.

107. Abboud TK, Shnider SM, Wright RG, et al. Enflurane analgesia in obstetrics. *Anesth Analg* 1981;60:133–137.

108. McLeod DD, Ramayya GP, Turnstall ME. Self-administered isoflurane in labour. *Anaesthesia* 1985;40:424–426.

109. Arora S, Turnstall M, Ross J. Self-administered mixture of Entonox and isoflurane in labour. *Int J Obstet Anesth* 1992;1:199–202.

110. Wee MYK, Hasan MA, Thomas TA. Isoflurane in labor. *Anaesthesia* 1993;48:369–372.

111. Ross JA, Tunstall ME, Campbell DM, et al. The use of 0.25% isoflurane premixed in 50% nitrous oxide and oxygen for pain relief in labour. *Anaesthesia* 1999;54:1166–1172.

112. Ross JA, Tunstall ME. Simulated use of premixed 0.25% isoflurane in 50% nitrous oxide and 50% oxygen. *Br J Anaesth* 2002;89:820–824.

113. Abboud TK, Swart F, Zhu J, et al. Desflurane analgesia for vaginal delivery. *Acta Anaethesiol Scand* 1995;39:259–261.

114. Toscano A, Pancaro C, Giovannoni S, et al. Sevoflurane analgesia in obstetrics: a pilot study. *Int J Obstet Anesth* 2003;12:79–82.

115. Yeo ST, Holdcroft A, Yentis S, et al. Analgesia with sevoflurane during labour: ii. Sevoflurane compared with Entonox for labour analgesia. *Br J Anaesth* 2007;98:110–115.

Local Anesthetics in Obstetrics: Evidence-based Applications, Controversies, Toxicity, and Current Therapies

Barbara M. Scavone

■ INTRODUCTION

A wide variety of local anesthetic drugs are employed in obstetric anesthesia practice. These agents are administered during intrathecal and epidural anesthesia, during peripheral nerve blockade procedures such as pudendal nerve block, and subcutaneously. Safe use of these medications necessitates knowledge of their chemical properties, pharmacodynamics, and pharmacokinetics. The clinician must also become familiar with the diagnosis and treatment of various adverse reactions, the most serious of which is local anesthetic systemic toxicity. Understanding these pharmacologic principles will allow for a rational approach to the use of these therapeutic agents.

■ LOCAL ANESTHETIC CHEMICAL STRUCTURE AND MECHANISM OF ACTION

The commonly used local anesthetics possess a similar chemical structure consisting of a lipid soluble aromatic ring, a hydrocarbon chain, and a terminal amine group, with various R chains throughout (Fig. 8-1). Amino-ester local anesthetics contain an amide bond between the aromatic ring and the hydrocarbon chain. Commonly used amino-ester anesthetics include procaine, chloroprocaine, tetracaine, and cocaine. (Cocaine is not commonly administered to parturients due to teratogenicity.) Amino-amide local anesthetics have an amide group linking the aromatic ring and the hydrocarbon chain. Lidocaine, bupivacaine, levobupivacaine, ropivacaine, and mepivacaine are examples of amino-amides.

Local anesthetics reversibly block neural conduction when administered near central or peripheral nerves; they do so by reversibly binding a specific receptor site on voltage-gated Na^+ channels, preventing influx of Na^+ into the cell, and thus preventing generation of an action potential (Fig. 8-2) (1–3). The clinical properties of the individual local anesthetics are determined by interplay of many factors including the drug's charge, pKa, lipid solubility, and protein binding (Table 8-1). First, the local anesthetic must gain entry into the cell; only the uncharged form of the molecule can enter the cell in significant amounts (4,5). Clinically used local anesthetics are weak bases; the molecule accepts a proton at its terminal amine group to become charged. The pKa is the pH at which a molecule exists equally in the charged and the uncharged forms. Since local anesthetics have pKa's greater than physiologic pH, the human body is a relatively acidic environment, favoring formation of the protonated charged moiety. The further away from physiologic pH the pKa of the drug, the greater the proportion that is ionized,

unable to cross the cell membrane. Therefore, the pKa of a local anesthetic partially determines its speed of action, such that those with a lower pKa (closer to physiologic pH, less charged) tend to have a faster onset. (An exception to this general rule concerns chloroprocaine, which has a short onset latency despite its high pKa.)

Lipid solubility augments the passing of the molecule into and through the cell membrane, and thus, in part determines the local anesthetic's potency (6).

Once inside the neuron, the charged form of the local anesthetic binds the voltage-gated Na^+ channel at a specific receptor site on its inner surface (4,5). Binding interferes with conformational changes in the Na^+ channel necessary for opening, and thus prevents the translocation of Na^+ ions into the cell; an action potential is not generated when threshold depolarization is reached. The local anesthetic demonstrates a higher likelihood of binding to the channel when it is in its open/activated or closed/inactivated state (the states associated with depolarization), rather than its resting state (1). This contributes to the phenomenon known as "phasic block" or "use-dependent" or "frequency-dependent" blockade: The tendency for nerves that fire action potentials frequently to be more sensitive to the effects of local anesthetics than those that do not fire as often.

Eventually the local anesthetic dissociates from the binding site, leaves the cell and is metabolized. Smaller molecules leave the site quickly; very large ones, slowly. Intermediate-sized local anesthetics enter the cell relatively rapidly, and leave at rates dependent on the drug's shape, structural flexibility and lipophilicity. Moderate lipophilicity (e.g., lidocaine) augments drug departure, and extreme lipophilicity (e.g., bupivacaine) tends to favor continued binding (7). In addition, agents that are soluble into perineural lipids and/or tightly bound to perineural proteins demonstrate slower rates of absorption into the intravascular compartment and thus, both lipid solubility and protein binding influence duration (8,9).

■ DIFFERENTIAL BLOCKADE

Differential blockade refers to the tendency of nerves among different classes to exhibit varying degrees of susceptibility to local anesthetic blockade. It is a result of axon myelination, diameter, and function (Table 8-2). Myelination causes a neuron to be more sensitive to local anesthetics. In unmyelinated fibers, action potential generation causes the area adjacent to reach threshold potential, and thus, the action potential is propagated. A large length of nerve axon must be blocked in order to prevent propagation in this manner. In contrast, in myelinated nerves, one

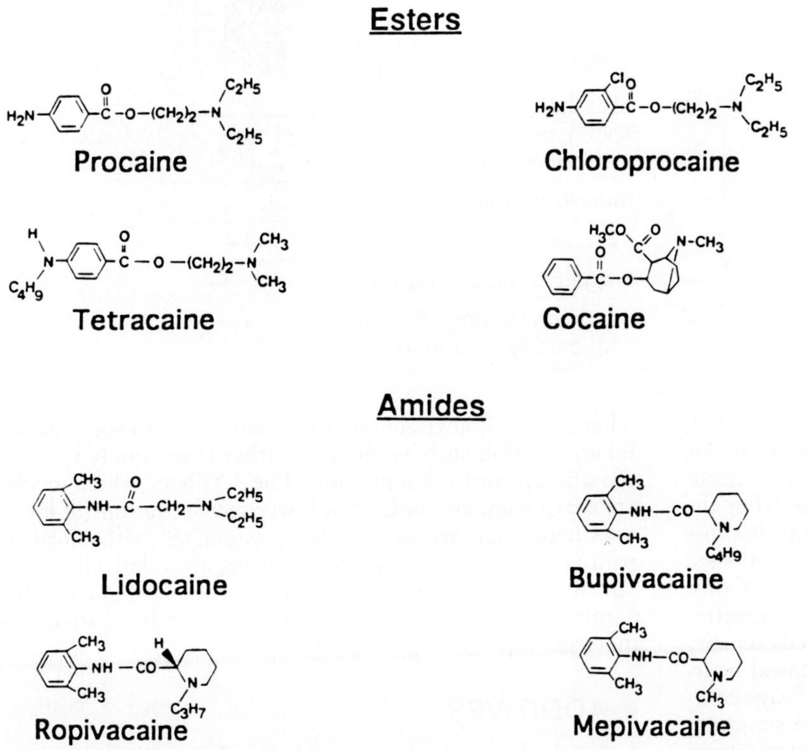

Esters

Procaine

Chloroprocaine

Tetracaine

Cocaine

Amides

Lidocaine

Bupivacaine

Ropivacaine

Mepivacaine

FIGURE 8-1 Local anesthetic chemical structure: Note the aromatic ring, hydrocarbon chain and terminal amine groups. Amino-ester local anesthetics contain an ester bond between the aromatic ring and the hydrocarbon chain. Amino-amide local anesthetics contain an amide bond between the aromatic ring and the hydrocarbon chain.

need block only three successive nodes of Ranvier to block action potential propagation (generally a shorter length of the neuron) (10).

Large diameter axons demonstrate resistance to blockade as compared to axons of small diameter. This may be a function of the diameter itself, but may also represent the fact that the nodes of Ranvier are placed at intervals farther apart in large diameter nerves, and therefore a greater axonal length must be exposed to anesthetic before three successive nodes are blocked (10–12).

It is possible that rates of differential blockade that seem to correlate with axon diameter and myelination status actually vary according to functional class of the nerve, and are due to anatomic and physiologic differences that exist among nerves of varying functions. This might include variations in the density and gating behavior of particular ion channels, the density of ion pumps, or characteristics of the myelination (13).

Anatomic features such as the location of a nerve within a trunk may determine some blockade features. Also, the principle of phasic block dictates that rapidly firing nerves are more sensitive to conduction blockade than nerves that fire less frequently. Preganglionic sympathetic nerve fibers have a high rate of tonic firing and are easily blocked; sensory neurons fire more frequently than motor neurons, and are more affected by local anesthetics.

Several important implications follow from the concept of differential blockade. During spinal and epidural anesthesia,

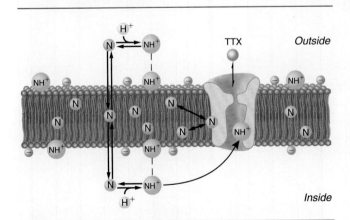

FIGURE 8-2 The local anesthetic exists in equilibrium between its charged and uncharged moieties. The neutral molecule crosses the epineurium; intracellularly, the ionized molecule binds a specific receptor protein on the sodium channel. Adapted from: Strichartz GR: Neural physiology and local anesthetics, Neural blockade in Clinical Anesthesia and Management of Pain. Edited by Cousins MJ Bridenbaugh PO, Philadelphia, PA: Lippincott-Raven 1998, p 35.

TABLE 8-1 Chemical Properties of Local Anesthetics

Local Anesthetic	pKa	Relative Lipid Solubility	Relative Protein Binding
Procaine[a]	8.9	—	—
Chloroprocaine[a]	8.7	—	—
Tetracaine[a]	8.5	++	++
Lidocaine[b]	7.8	++	++
Bupivacaine[b]	8.1	++++	+++
Ropivacaine[b]	8.1	+++	+++
Mepivacaine[b]	7.6	++	++

[a]Amino-ester anesthetics.
[b]Amino-amide anesthetics.

TABLE 8-2 Neuronal Properties that Determine Local Anesthetic Sensitivity

Fiber Classification	Myelination	Relative Diameter	Function	Relative Sensitivity
Aα	+	Largest	Motor, proprioception	+
Aβ	+	↓	Touch, pressure, proprioception	++
Aγ	+	↓	Muscle spindle	++
Aδ	+	↓	Pain, touch, pressure	+++
B	+	↓	Preganglionic sympathetic	++++
C	—	Smallest	Pain, temperature, postganglionic sympathetic	+++

a site of maximal concentration of local anesthetic exists, termed the epicenter, which is dependent on injection site, patient position, drug baracity, etc. Anesthetic concentration then decreases as a function of distance from the epicenter. Zones of differential blockade develop, because the sympathetic nerves (most sensitive) may be affected along the entire concentration gradient, but the motor nerves (least sensitive), only at sites of greatest concentration density. Sympathetic blockade usually exceeds sensory blockade by several dermatome levels during central neuraxial anesthesia, even if sympathectomy is not always complete (Fig. 8-3) (14–16). Decreased temperature sensation occurs at a higher dermatome level than decreased sensation of sharp pain, which exceeds light touch (Fig. 8-4) (17,18).

Therefore it is advisable to assess sensitivity to some painful stimulation such as pinprick rather than simply to cold sensation prior to skin incision. The Aδ fibers, which mediate sharp pain, are blocked at lower concentrations of local anesthetic than are the C fibers, associated with burning pain (13). Lastly, since motor neurons are relatively resistant to blockade, dilute solutions of local anesthetic can be administered to provide labor pain relief without affecting maternal expulsive efforts (19).

■ ADDITIVES

Labor analgesia is often provided with intrathecal and/or epidural opioids added to the local anesthetic. The inclusion

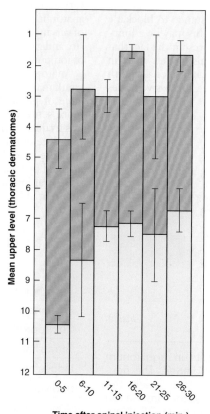

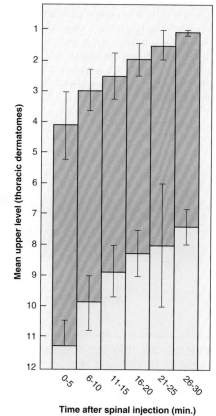

FIGURE 8-3 Mean sympathetic and sensory blockade levels over time after intrathecal administration of lidocaine (*left*) and tetracaine (*right*). Reprinted with permission from: Chamberlain DP, Chamberlain BD. Changes in the skin temperature of the trunk and their relationship to sympathetic blockade during spinal anesthesia. *Anesthesiology* 1986;65:139–143.

Legend:
- Sympathetic level
- Sensory level
- ⊥ S.E.

LIDOCAINE — Time after spinal injection (min.)

TETRACAINE — Time after spinal injection (min.)

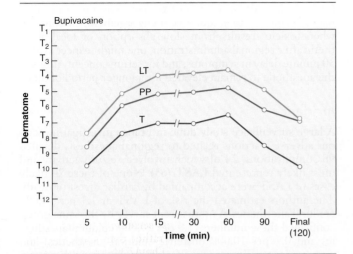

FIGURE 8-4 Blockade levels of light touch (*LT*), pin prick (*PP*), and temperature (*T*) over time after intrathecal administration of bupivacaine. Reprinted with permission from: Brull SJ, Greene NM. Time-courses of zones of differential sensory blockade during spinal anesthesia with hyperbaric tetracaine or bupivacaine. *Anesth Analg* 1989;69:342–347.

of opioids in labor analgesia solutions allows for the use of lower local anesthetic concentrations, thus decreasing motor weakness and the incidence of instrumental vaginal delivery (20,21). Fentanyl added to spinal anesthesia for cesarean delivery increases intraoperative comfort, decreases need for intraoperative analgesic supplementation, and helps prevent intraoperative nausea (22–24).

As explained above, local anesthetics are weak bases with pKa's higher than 7.4, and so tend towards ionization at physiologic pH. Many commercial local anesthetic preparations are formulated as hydrochloride salts for stability, and are therefore acidic, favoring ionization. The addition of bicarbonate to the local anesthetic solution adjusts pH of the local environment closer to pKa, thus favoring non-ionization and hastening speed of onset of sensory blockade which can be advantageous in emergent situations.

Addition of epinephrine to spinal anesthetics increases density and duration of block, and slows block regression time (25–27). When epinephrine is added to epidurally administered drugs, onset is faster, analgesia is more dense, and duration is longer (28,29). Explanations for this are twofold: Epinephrine's α-2-agonism directly enhances neuraxial anesthesia (30). In addition, epinephrine is vasoconstrictive and decreases clearance from nonneural tissues, thus amplifying blockade and prolonging duration of blockade (30). Inclusion of epinephrine in epidural lidocaine or bupivacaine solutions reduces peak plasma concentrations of the agents (31). Addition of epinephrine to labor analgesia solutions may intensify motor block (32). Phenylephrine is no longer used as a vasoconstrictor additive due to its association with transient neurologic symptoms (TNS) (33).

Use of the α_2-agonist clonidine with local anesthetics enhances intrathecal and epidural labor analgesia; however, it increases maternal hypotension and sedation (34–36). Addition of neostigmine to labor analgesia regimens is associated with high rates of nausea and vomiting and its routine use is not recommended (37,38). The benefits of additives must be weighed against increased costs and a theoretical potential for error when multiple medications are administered.

■ EFFECT OF PREGNANCY

It has been observed that women in the second and third trimesters of pregnancy experience higher cephalad blockade in response to intrathecal hyperbaric local anesthetics than nonpregnant women and it has been suggested that the same effect is also seen after epidural administration of local anesthetics (39,40). The effects of pregnancy on local anesthetic action are twofold: (1) Anatomical changes in the central neuraxiom favor cephalad spread of injected local anesthetics. (2) In addition, neuronal susceptibility to local anesthetic blockade increases.

Magnetic resonance imaging reveals that epidural vein engorgement which occurs during pregnancy due to vena cava compression by the gravid uterus causes posterior displacement of the vertebral canal, resulting in a decrease in cerebrospinal fluid volume (41,42). Administration of standard local anesthetic doses into this smaller intrathecal volume results in a greater dermatomal spread and a higher block. Vein engorgement also impedes leakage of injected epidural solutions through the foramina, thus promoting longitudinal spread of epidural administered medications (43).

In addition to these anatomical factors, the nerves per se appear to have heightened sensitivity to local anesthetic action during pregnancy. Parturients demonstrate intensified blockade of the median nerve at the wrist compared to nonpregnant women who receive the same dose of lidocaine (44). In vitro studies reveal that nerves from pregnant animals are more quickly and easily blocked by local anesthetics than those from nonpregnant animals (45,46). This effect is not due to differences in local anesthetic neuronal uptake and is presumed to be a pharmacodynamic effect, possibly mediated by progesterone (47,48). The acid–base changes that occur in cerebrospinal fluid during the pregnancy probably exert little effect (49). Protein binding of local anesthetics in CSF is not altered in pregnancy.

■ PHARMACOKINETICS

Understanding the pharmacokinetics of local anesthetics requires knowledge of the principle of absorption as well as the commonly discussed pharmacokinetic variables governing elimination (8,50). Since local anesthetics are placed regionally, absorption from the site of injection must be taken into account when discussing drug elimination. The maximal serum concentration after administration (C_{max}) and the time at which C_{max} occurs (t_{max}) characterize absorption. Absorption is dependent on local blood flow which varies by site of injection in the following order (greatest blood flow/highest absorption to least blood flow/lowest absorption): Intercostal > caudal > epidural > peripheral nerve block > subcutaneous injection. The addition of vasoconstrictors decreases C_{max} and may prolong t_{max} and one may expect that this effect is most pronounced in highly vascular tissues such as the epidural space (31). Absorption is also dependent upon local tissue binding: As stated above, drugs that are soluble into perineural lipids and/or tightly bound to perineural proteins demonstrate slower rates of absorption (lower C_{max} and longer t_{max}) (8,9). Systemic uptake from the epidural space is biphasic: A rapid uptake phase is followed by a longer, slower phase, the latter phase being relatively more prolonged for highly lipid soluble drugs such as bupivacaine than the less lipid soluble lidocaine (51). Continued absorption into the intravascular compartment offsets elimination as compared to that which occurs during intravenous administration of the drug (51). If rate of absorption from site of injection is slower than $t_{1/2}$ (as is for clinically relevant local anesthetics and injection sites) then it is more useful to discuss mean body residence time (how long the medication stays in the body) than serum $t_{1/2}$.

Serum elimination $t_{1/2}$ varies directly with volume of distribution (V_d) and indirectly with clearance. V_d is related to the relative amounts of plasma and blood cell binding versus tissue binding, and is relatively low for the highly protein bound bupivacaine. Clearance differs for amino-ester versus amino-amide local anesthetics. The esters are quickly hydrolyzed by pseudocholinesterase and other plasma esterases. Despite the decrease in pseudocholinesterase during pregnancy the serum half-life of 2-chloroprocaine in vitro is 11 seconds. The half-life of 2-chloroprocaine injection after epidural administration is longer and ranges from 1.5 to 6.4 minutes because of continued absorption from the site of administration (52,53).

In contrast, the amide local anesthetics are metabolized in the liver over several hours. Lidocaine, with a particularly high hepatic extraction ratio, demonstrates a clearance predominantly determined by hepatic blood flow and the elimination half-life of lidocaine following epidural administration during pregnancy is 114 minutes (54). However, the majority of amino-amides possess intermediate hepatic extraction ratios, and thus clearance depends on both hepatic blood flow and enzymatic activity (50).

Serum levels of bupivacaine and ropivacaine increase over time during prolonged epidural infusion (55,56). This may be partially offset by increases in protein binding that occur in the postoperative period, so that free drug concentrations remain stable (57,58).

Pregnancy decreases both V_d and clearance, such that $t_{1/2}$ remains unchanged (59). Thus, inadvertent intravascular administration of a large dose of local anesthetic to a parturient might result in a higher initial serum concentration but unchanged $t_{1/2}$.

■ PLACENTAL TRANSFER AND EFFECTS ON BLOOD FLOW AND THE FETUS

Local anesthetics rapidly cross the placenta and can be found in fetal serum (60). In the case of fetal acidemia, maternally administered and absorbed local anesthetic could become ionized and "trapped" in the fetal circulation. It seems prudent to avoid lidocaine in the setting of fetal academia, as it has more potential for placental passage. Bupivacaine is found in only very low concentrations in the umbilical vein, even after several hours of epidural administration (61). Since chloroprocaine is cleared from the circulation so rapidly, its potential for accumulation in the fetus is virtually nonexistent (52,53).

Animal studies demonstrate no effect of local anesthetics on uterine artery blood flow at clinically relevant doses (60). Clinical studies confirm that epidural administration of either bupivacaine or ropivacaine does not cause changes in either uterine artery or umbilical artery Doppler blood flow (62). In contrast, toxic doses of local anesthetics, as might occur during inadvertent intravascular injection may increase uterine tone, thereby decreasing uterine blood flow.

With the exception of cocaine, local anesthetics are not considered teratogenic in man at clinically relevant doses.

■ LOCAL ANESTHETIC SYSTEMIC TOXICITY

Local anesthetic systemic toxicity (LAST) remains a feared complication of regional anesthesia. When local anesthetic drugs are accidentally injected or otherwise absorbed into the intravascular space in toxic amounts, the result can be devastating due to effects on the central nervous and cardiovascular systems. Unintentional venous injection may be associated with a rapid onset of seizure activity and may be more likely during administration of epidural anesthesia in pregnancy secondary to epidural vein engorgement. In contrast, when toxicity results from slow absorption of local anesthetic after regional administration, one might expect a 20 to 30 minute delay in symptoms, and for serum concentrations of the anesthetic to remain elevated for a longer period of time.

Incidence

A large surveillance study done in France investigating serious adverse reactions related to regional anesthesia detailed 98 complications, 24 of which involved seizure activity and most likely represented LAST (63). None of these 24 likely cases of LAST were accompanied by cardiac arrest or death. The authors estimated the risk of LAST at 1.3 per 10,000 epidural anesthetics. A more recent survey by the same group confirmed these numbers (1.8 per 10,000 epidural anesthetics and 0.7 per 10,000 obstetric epidural anesthetics) and once again, toxicity was manifested by seizures without cardiac arrest (64). A recent examination of anesthesia-related maternal mortality in the United States revealed a risk of 3.8 deaths per million regional anesthetics administered for cesarean delivery, including 0.7 per million which were due to a "drug reaction"—presumably LAST (65). The incidence of LAST is declining in both the general and obstetric populations (65–67). The most recent obstetric anesthesia closed claims analysis included no cases of malpractice payment on behalf of an anesthesiologist due to LAST (68). Authors attribute this decline to the withdrawal of 0.75% bupivacaine from the market for obstetric use, an increased awareness of LAST, increased use of safety measures such as test dosing and slow incremental injection, and new treatment options with lipid emulsion solutions (65).

Clinical Presentation

Symptoms of LAST are due to blockade of voltage-gated Na^+ channels in the central nervous system (CNS) and cardiovascular system. Symptoms are dose dependent (Table 8-3). CNS effects reflect local anesthetic action on the brain: At low serum concentrations, local anesthetics inhibit the inhibitory neurons in the CNS, and thus a period of excitation ensues. The patient may experience tongue numbness and a vague lightheadedness or dizziness, followed by agitation and muscular twitching, and eventual generalized tonic–clonic seizure activity. At higher serum levels, generalized CNS inhibition occurs, which is manifested by coma and depression of brainstem cardiorespiratory centers, and may result in death.

TABLE 8-3 Dose-dependent Symptoms of Lidocaine Toxicity

Plasma Concentration ($\mu g/mL$)	Effect
1–5	Analgesia
5–10	Lightheadedness Tinnitus Numbness of tongue
10–15	Seizures Unconsciousness
15–25	Coma Respiratory arrest
>25	Cardiovascular depression

Reprinted with permission from: Barash Clinical Anesthesia, I (2009 6th edition).

Local anesthetics bear both direct and indirect effects on the cardiovascular system: Direct effects include myocardial depression; indirect effects are mediated through the CNS and are biphasic such that during the CNS excitatory phase sympathetic activation occurs and during the CNS depressant phase, vasomotor depression appears (69–72). The end result is that at subconvulsant doses of local anesthetics, one sees a small decrease in cardiac contractility, cardiac output, and systemic blood pressure. At convulsant levels, increases in heart rate, contractility, cardiac output, systemic vascular resistance, and blood pressure occur. Supraconvulsant concentrations are followed by decreases in contractility, cardiac output, and systemic blood pressure. In addition, bradycardias and wide complex arrhythmias develop.

A review of published case reports over the past 30 years reveals that the clinical presentation of LAST can be quite variable (73). Patients suffering LAST were more likely to be at the extremes of age and have co-morbidities, particularly cardiac, pulmonary, neurologic, and/or metabolic disease. Forty-one percent of published cases involved some type of "atypical presentation": 25% had a delay of >5 minutes in symptoms, fewer than 20% had a prodrome (e.g., perioral numbness, dizziness, etc.) prior to seizure onset, cardiovascular symptoms occurred simultaneously with CNS symptoms in some cases, and without evidence of CNS toxicity at all in 11% of patients. The authors of this report recommend adopting a low threshold for the diagnosis of LAST, and furthermore, point out that LAST symptoms and signs can recur minutes to hours after initial resolution, underscoring the need for a period of prolonged observation (73).

Relative Toxicities

CNS toxicity varies directly with drug potency, meaning that different local anesthetics given in equipotent doses have equal propensity to cause seizures. An exception involves the L-isomer of bupivacaine, which is less potent regarding seizure generation than the equipotent racemic mixture of the drug (74). In contrast, tendency to cause cardiovascular toxicity varies among different agents. When animals are given intravenous doses of lidocaine, bupivacaine, and ropivacaine, lidocaine has a greater safety margin. The ratio of fatal doses is 9:1:2, respectively, although the ratio of therapeutic doses is closer to 4:1:1.7, respectively (75). Mechanism of death differs among the medications used. Lidocaine treated animals suffer respiratory arrest and progressive hypotension and cardiac pump failure without evidence of arrhythmias. Bupivacaine and ropivacaine animals experience more arrhythmias, including ventricular tachycardia/fibrillatory arrest (75,76). Highly lipophilic drugs such as bupivacaine and ropivacaine bind to the receptor during or shortly after systole, when it is in its open/activated or closed/inactivated state, and then do not dissociate during diastole, accumulating inside the cell with each subsequent depolarization (termed "fast-in slow-out" binding); lidocaine both binds and dissociates quickly (termed "fast-in fast-out" binding), leaving little potential for accumulation inside the myocyte (77). This phenomenon takes place when heart rate lies between 60 and 150, the normal clinical range (77). (L-bupivacaine is less arrhythmogenic than racemic bupivacaine but unfortunately is no longer available in the United States.)

While it is well established that lidocaine is less toxic than the long-acting lipophilic local anesthetics, it remains controversial as to whether ropivacaine carries less cardiac toxicity than racemic bupivacaine. Ropivacaine is less often associated with ventricular dysrhythmia than bupivacaine (76,78,79). However, many toxicity studies have not accounted for potency differences, and ropivacaine appears to be less potent than

bupivacaine. Using an up-down sequential allocation technique, Polley et al. measured the median effective concentration of a 20 mL volume of local anesthetic that provides epidural labor analgesia (median local anesthetic concentration, or MLAC, an approximation of ED_{50}) and determined the ropivacaine:bupivacaine potency ratio to be 0.6 (80). These findings were confirmed by another group of investigators and similar data exist regarding intrathecal labor analgesia (81,82). However, D'Angelo has questioned the validity of using MLAC data to determine potency ratios, arguing that since ED_{50} is not the clinically significant dosage, full dose response curves must be mapped to determine comparative ED_{95}'s (83). One group of investigators determined the full dose response curves of intrathecal bupivacaine and ropivacaine added to sufentanil for labor analgesia and concluded that the ropivacaine:bupivacaine potency ratio was 0.69 at the ED_{95} (84). Conversely, another group determined that the ED_{90}'s of bupivacaine and ropivacaine for epidural labor analgesia were similar (85).

Despite the literature's lack of agreement regarding potency, evidence exists to suggest that ropivacaine is less toxic than bupivacaine, even accounting for possible differences in potency. In dogs, administration of twice the seizure dose of bupivacaine versus ropivacaine was more likely to cause arrhythmias; bupivacaine animals were also less likely to be resuscitated in response to advanced cardiac life support, although the small number (6 dogs per group) precluded statistical significance (70,76). Similarly, when dogs received infusions of bupivacaine or ropivacaine to the point of cardiovascular collapse and were then treated with advanced cardiac life support which included open-chest massage, dogs in the bupivacaine group were more likely to develop ventricular fibrillation ($P < 0.05$); the apparent differences in mortality were not statistically different, possibly because of the small number of study subjects (86). Finally, utilizing a rat model, investigators infused bupivacaine 3 mg/kg/min versus ropivacaine 3 mg/kg/min versus ropivacaine 4.5 mg/kg/min (thus accounting for possible potency differences) and measured time to certain toxic events. The times required to produce bradycardia, dysrhythmias, hypotension and cardiac arrest were more for both ropivacaine groups (Fig. 8-5) (87).

Effect of Pregnancy

Several studies have examined the effect of pregnancy on vulnerability to toxicity. One investigation in pregnant ewes that demonstrated an increase in susceptibility was hampered by a small number of subjects and lack of blinding of investigators (88). Santos et al. performed a series of experiments in an ovine model which consistently demonstrated lack of effect of pregnancy on cardiac toxicity, although some possible augmentation of seizure susceptibility (89–91). The effect of pregnancy on susceptibility to LAST is minimal, if present at all.

Prevention of LAST

The American Society of Regional Anesthesia and Pain Medicine Practice Advisory on Local Anesthetic Systemic Toxicity stresses "the primacy of prevention" regarding LAST (92). Aspiration of epidural catheters prior to injection is recommended, although the reader is cautioned that the false negative rate is 0.6% to 2.3% (93). Aspiration of a multiport catheter decreases the incidence of false negatives and is associated with fewer false positives than performing a standard lidocaine and epinephrine test dose in parturients (94). Although slow incremental injection is not studied well, it follows from basic pharmacokinetic principles and authors advocate it because diagnosis of LAST in its early stages

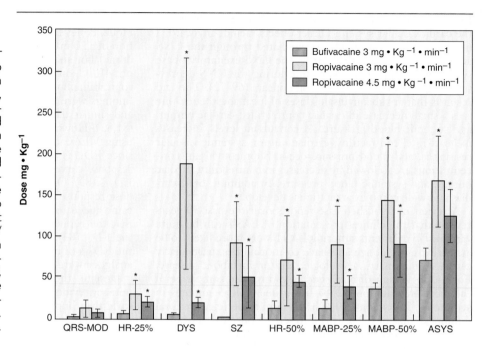

FIGURE 8-5 Doses required to produce the first QRS modification (*QRS-MOD*), dysrhythmia (*DYS*), seizure (*SZ*), 25% and 50% reduction in heart rate (*HR-25%* and *HR-50%*), 25% and 50% reduction in mean arterial blood pressure (*MABP-25%* and *MABP-50%*), and final systole (*ASYS*) in the bupivacaine group (3mg/kg/min), in the equivalent dose ropivacaine group (3 mg/kg/min), and the equipotent dose ropivacaine group (4.5 mg/kg/min). *, $P < 0.05$ compared with bupivacaine. Reprinted with permission from: Dony P, Dewinde V, Vanderick B, et al. The comparative toxicity of ropivacaine and bupivacaine at equipotent doses in rats. *Anesth Analg* 2000;91:1489–1492.

limits the total dose given and slow administration of any given dose limits peak serum concentration (93).

The practitioner is advised to incorporate an intravascular marker (i.e., a test dose) into clinical practice. Several such tests of intravascular placement have been proposed but there exists a lack of conclusive supporting data in the literature. Mulroy suggests basing test dosing regimens on two or more randomized controlled trials at two or more institutions. Using that standard, he concludes that intravascular epinephrine at a dose of 15 mcg will increase heart rate by 10 beats per minute and systolic blood pressure by 15 mm Hg, with 80% sensitivity and positive predictive value (93). Epinephrine may be less sensitive and specific in laboring patients due to baseline heart rate variability, although its use is still advocated (95,96). Concurrent use of general anesthesia, sedation, or β-blockade further limits the sensitivity and specificity of epinephrine as an intravascular marker (93).

Small doses of local anesthetics included in the test dose solution produce subjective symptoms of low level toxicity (lightheadedness, perioral numbness, etc.). Authors recommend doses of 100 mg lidocaine, 100 mg chloroprocaine, or 25 mg bupivacaine to reliably assess intravascular injection (93). Administration of local anesthetics at these doses into the intrathecal space would result in dangerously high blocks, and so, a divided test dose should be performed: Initially, one administers a small dose of local anesthetic to rule out intrathecal placement of the catheter, and then administers the higher dose to rule out intravascular location.

The air test dose has been described in parturients. The Doppler ultrasound probe is temporarily moved from the patient's abdomen to her precordium and 1 mL air is injected through the epidural catheter. Intravascular injection produces a characteristic change in the quality of the maternal heart sounds termed a "mill wheel murmur" (97,98). Fentanyl 100 mcg can also be administered as a test dose. If inadvertently administered intravenously, it will produce subjective symptoms of dizziness or drowsiness within 3 minutes (99).

Total dose administered at one time should be limited to reduce serious toxicity sequelae (Table 8-4). The reader is cautioned that safe dose is affected by the site of injection—epidural administration being associated with intermediate

levels of absorption as noted above—addition of vasoconstrictors, and patient-related factors such as extremes of age, and co-existing disease (9). Renal dysfunction represents a hyperdynamic state and so is associated with increased absorption; in addition, decreased clearance of metabolites may occur and so caution is warranted especially during continuous infusion (9). Decreased clearance may also occur in the settings of severe hepatic disease and heart failure (9).

Treatment of LAST

Weinberg emphasizes the "primacy of airway management" in the treatment of local anesthetic toxicity (100). In vitro data indicate that hypoxemia and acidosis enhance bupivacaine-associated myocardial depression and bradyarrhythmogenic effects (101). Likewise, in animals, severe hypoxia augments both CNS and cardiovascular toxicity from bupivacaine; it also increases the likelihood that bupivacaine will induce arrhythmias before seizures (102). (It is noted that severe hypocapnia may prolong the arrhythmogenic period and so maintaining normocapnia is recommended [103]). *Therefore, it is of paramount importance to control seizure activity, so as to gain airway control and ensure oxygenation and ventilation, as well as ameliorate the metabolic acidosis that may accompany generalized tonic–clonic seizures.* Small doses of benzodiazepines suffice for this purpose; small doses of propofol also

TABLE 8-4 Recommended Maximum Doses of Local Anesthetics in a Healthy 70 kg Adult

Local Anesthetic	Plain	With Epinephrine
Procaine	1000	N/A
Chloroprocaine	800	N/A
Lidocaine	300	500
Bupivacaine	175	225
Ropivacaine	200	N/A
Mepivacaine	400	500

treat seizures, but have more untoward cardiovascular effects than benzodiazepines. Succinylcholine aids the anesthesiologist in airway management.

The clinician must provide circulatory support in order to maintain an adequate coronary perfusion pressure to prevent/treat myocardial hypoxia/acidosis and remove bupivacaine from the myocytes (100). Guidelines for basic and advanced cardiac life support should be followed (92). Ventricular arrhythmias may respond to treatment with amiodarone rather than local anesthetics (104). The wash out of bupivacaine from the heart may require prolonged resuscitation efforts. Indeed, institution of cardiopulmonary bypass may be used to provide circulatory support during several hours of resuscitation (105). Cardiopulmonary bypass has been referred to as "the patient's last hope" (100).

The effective use of lipid emulsion in the treatment of LAST has recently been reviewed (106). In 1998, Weinberg et al. first reported a potential role for lipid therapy during LAST (107). Employing a rat model, the investigators utilized saline placebo or varying doses of lipid for prophylaxis of bupivacaine toxicity; asystole and/or death occurred at higher doses of bupivacaine in lipid treated animals, in a dose-dependent fashion. In the same study treatment with lipid decreased bupivacaine-induced mortality compared to saline placebo. Similarly, when dogs were resuscitated with lipid versus saline, survival was 6 out of 6 versus 0 out of 6, respectively (*P* < 0.01) (108).

The first report of the clinical administration of lipid emulsion involved a patient who received an interscalene block with 20 mL 0.5% bupivacaine and 20 mL 1.5% mepivacaine. Generalized tonic–clonic seizures, arrhythmias and arrest occurred. Resuscitation efforts were unsuccessful for approximately 20 minutes, until lipid was given, at which time the practitioners successfully defibrillated the patient within less than 1 minute (109). Another report describes a patient who received 10 mL 0.5% bupivacaine for cesarean delivery and quickly developed signs of CNS toxicity including seizure activity, which resolved within 30 seconds of lipid administration (110). This account is interesting not only because it is the first report of lipid use in a parturient, but also because it demonstrates an increased proclivity to provide lipid therapy early in the course of LAST. Although one can draw only limited conclusions from uncontrolled case report communications of this sort, numerous publications concerning the apparently successful use of lipid infusion exist, and seem to indicate a role for this therapy to combat the signs and symptoms of LAST and possibly to decrease mortality (111–113).

The mechanism of action of lipid therapy is debated. It may be that the lipid acts as a "sink," drawing the highly fat soluble local anesthetics out of the myocytes and into the lipid substrate in the blood. During lipid treatment, clinical improvement does parallel a decrease in myocardial bupivacaine concentrations and a partitioning of bupivacaine into the lipid compartment (107,114,115). This effect is dose dependent (115). An alternate or additional mechanism may lie in the fact that bupivacaine inhibits acylcarnitine translocase in the cell. This decreases the transfer of fatty acids into cardiac mitochondria, resulting in a loss of substrate and energy production at the cellular level. Lipid may provide an alternate energy source (116). A third possibility is that lipids increase intracellular calcium concentrations, and improve cardiac contractility (117).

It remains unclear how lipid therapy fits into current resuscitation algorithms (106). In a series of experiments using a rat model, Weinberg and DiGregorio et al. compared lipid to epinephrine, vasopressin, and combination epinephrine/vasopressin treatment and demonstrated better hemodynamic

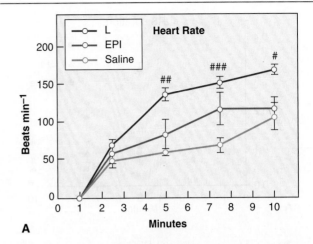

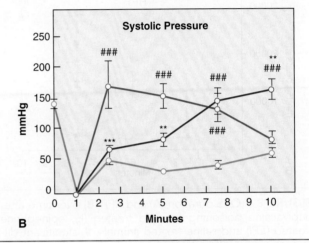

FIGURE 8-6 Heart rate (**A**) and systolic blood pressure (**B**) over time after bupivacaine poisoning for lipid treated (L), epinephrine treated (*EPI*) and saline treated animals. #, significant difference versus saline treated animals; *, significant difference versus epinephrine treated animals. Reprinted with permission from: Weinberg GL, Di Gregorio G, Ripper R, et al. Resuscitation with lipid versus epinephrine in a rat model of bupivacaine overdose. *Anesthesiology* 2008;108:907–913.

recovery (as measured by rate–pressure product [RPP]), superior metabolic recovery (as demonstrated by higher arterial and mixed venous oxygen tensions), and faster recovery of QRS duration in the lipid treated animals (Figs. 8-6 and 8-7) (118,119). Epinephrine alone resulted in better early recovery, but it was not sustained, and animals developed persistent arrhythmias, lactic acidosis, and pulmonary edema (118). Vasopressin therapy was also associated with higher lung water content (119). In contrast to this, Mayr et al., using a porcine model, showed superior results for combination epinephrine/vasopressin therapy compared to lipid: 5 of 5 pigs treated with epinephrine and vasopressin had spontaneous return of circulation (defined as systolic blood pressure ≥80 mm Hg for ≥5 minutes), versus 0 of 5 pigs given lipids (120).

Differences in experimental protocol help to explain these contradictory results. Mayr used a smaller lipid dose than others. In addition, the porcine model included a period of asphyxia prior to arrest and resuscitation. Lipid therapy is useful only for toxin-associated arrest, and, in fact, impedes recovery after asphyxia-induced arrest (121). Species differences most likely exist between dogs (used for Weinberg's initial lipid experiments), rats (utilized in the investigations

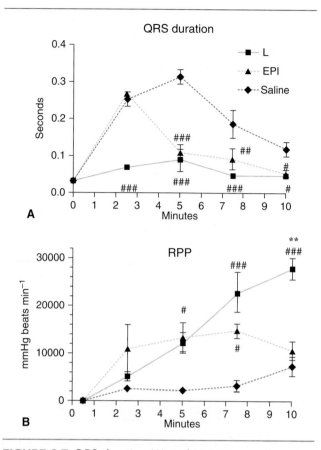

A

B

FIGURE 8-7 QRS duration (**A**) and RPP (**B**) over time after bupivacaine poisoning for lipid treated (L), epinephrine treated (*EPI*) and saline treated animals; #, significant difference versus saline treated animals. *, significant difference versus epinephrine treated animals. Reprinted with permission: Weinberg GL, Di Gregorio G, Ripper R, et al. Resuscitation with lipid versus epinephrine in a rat model of bupivacaine overdose. *Anesthesiology* 2008;108:907–913.

demonstrating lipid's superiority) and pigs (employed when outcomes with lipid treatment were inferior). Dogs have more collateral circulation and are more easily resuscitated than other animals. Also, resuscitation in the dog model included open-chest massage, which provides for more adequate chest compressions, and better coronary perfusion pressure, a primary determinant of outcome.

It has been suggested that when human patients undergo traditional basic and advanced cardiac life support in the clinical setting (i.e., with closed-chest compressions), vasopressors are essential to increase coronary perfusion pressure during resuscitation (122). The clinical implications seem to be that one should avoid asphyxia, and use lipid therapy early in the course of the event, prior to when cardiac arrest takes place. If arrest occurs, it is recommended that one include vasopressors in resuscitation algorithms so as to maintain adequate coronary perfusion pressure, but limit administration to the minimal effective dose (123). When rats were resuscitated with lipid and escalating doses of epinephrine, the animals had a more rapid return of spontaneous circulation when the regimen included epinephrine; however, above a certain threshold dose (epinephrine 10 mcg/kg), they had poorer later outcomes, associated with lactic acidosis and evidence of pulmonary edema (124). One study that demonstrated no benefit to lipid after bupivacaine-induced cardiac arrest called for high-dose epinephrine, and so some attribute

lack of lipid efficacy in that study to the high doses of epinephrine used (124,125).

The LD$_{50}$ of lipid is orders of magnitude higher than recommended doses (126). Occasional metabolic disturbances that occur such as elevated triglycerides and/or amylase appear transient (127). Events such as volume overload and fat embolism are theoretical risks but do not appear troublesome during short-term use of currently available preparations (128). Allergic reactions may occur (128). A recent report describes a patient with LAST who had an initial positive response to lipid infusion, but the reappearance of cardiac symptoms 40 minutes later, indicating that prolonged monitoring and treatment are called for (127).

Recommendations call for an initial bolus dose of 20% lipid emulsion of 1.5 mL/kg, followed by a maintenance infusion at 0.25 mL/kg/min. The bolus dose may be repeated once or twice for continued cardiovascular instability and the infusion rate may be increased to 0.50 mL/kg/min. Administration should continue for a minimum of 10 minutes after cardiovascular stability has been achieved. The reader is referred to Figure 8-8 for a summary of the current American Society of Regional Anesthesia and Pain Medicine practice advisory on treatment of LAST. A copy of this is available for download at http://links.lww.com/AAP/A17 or http://links.lww.com/AAP/A18. It can be printed, laminated, and posted in the labor and delivery suite. A registry collecting data on the clinical use of lipid therapy can be found at http://www.lipidrescue.org. Reporting to this confidential registry is encouraged, as controlled trials in humans will be limited.

OTHER ADVERSE REACTIONS

All local anesthetics are neurotoxic if applied directly to nerves in high enough concentrations for a long enough period of time (129,130). Lidocaine may possess more intrinsic neurotoxic potential than other local anesthetics (131). Several case reports describe cauda equina syndrome after continuous spinal anesthesia with lidocaine (132,133). Common to these reports is repeated administration of lidocaine through the small diameter–high resistance catheter with minimal dermatomal blockade, presumed evidence of maldistribution in the cerebrospinal fluid, and pooling of high concentrations of lidocaine at the cauda equina. It seems prudent to avoid unusually high dosing of lidocaine in the intrathecal space. Small-gauge intrathecal catheters are no longer available for use in the United States as a result of these reports.

In spite of these concerns, prospective surveys reveal that nerve damage occurs rarely, albeit more frequently after spinal than epidural anesthetics, and more frequently after lidocaine than other local anesthetics (63,64). Permanent neurologic deficits after regional anesthesia are more likely due to needle trauma or other factors, and not due to neurotoxicity. The clinician is advised to monitor patients carefully for symptoms of paresthesia and to avoid injecting local anesthetic solutions when paresthesias are reported.

TNS may occur after spinal anesthesia with local anesthetics. Patients complain of burning pain in the buttocks radiating to the lower extremities; symptoms are sometimes severe, and begin after resolution of the anesthetic and usually resolve within 72 hours (134). Outpatient status and lithotomy position during surgery represent risk factors for development of TNS (134). Authors of a systematic review concluded that the syndrome is over four times more likely to occur after lidocaine compared to other local anesthetic agents (135). TNS is seen in almost 12% of patients who experience lidocaine spinal anesthesia and its incidence is not affected by lidocaine dose, osmolarity, nor concentration

---

The Pharmacologic Treatment of Local Anesthetic Systemic Toxicity (LAST) is Different from Other Cardiac Arrest Scenarios

❑ **Get Help**
❑ **Initial Focus**
  ❑ **Airway management:** ventilate with 100% oxygen
  ❑ **Seizure suppression:** benzodiazepines are preferred; **AVOID propofol** in patients having signs of cardiovascular instability
  ❑ **Alert** the nearest facility having **cardiopulmonary bypass** capability
❑ **Management of Cardiac Arrhythmias**
  ❑ **Basic and Advanced Cardiac Life Support (ACLS)** will require adjustment of medications and perhaps prolonged effort
  ❑ **AVOID vasopressin, calcium channel blockers, beta blockers, or local anesthetic**
  ❑ **REDUCE individual epinephrine doses to <1 mcg/kg**
❑ **Lipid Emulsion (20%) Therapy** (values in parenthesis are for 70 kg patient)
  ❑ **Bolus 1.5 mL/kg** (lean body mass) intravenously over 1 minute (~100 mL)
  ❑ **Continuous infusion 0.25 mL/kg/min** (~18 mL/min; adjust by roller clamp)
  ❑ Repeat bolus once or twice for persistent cardiovascular collapse
  ❑ Double the infusion rate to 0.5 mL/kg/min if blood pressure remains low
  ❑ **Continue infusion** for at least 10 minutes after attaining circulatory stability
  ❑ Recommended upper limit: Approximately 10 mL/kg lipid emulsion over the first 30 minutes
❑ **Post LAST events at** www.lipidrescue.org and report use of lipid to www.lipidregistry.org

---

BE PREPARED

- We strongly advise that those using local anesthetics (LA) in doses sufficient to produce local anesthetic systemic toxicity (LAST) establish a plan for managing this complication. Making *Local Anesthetic Toxicity Kit* and posting instructions for its use are encouraged

RISK REDUCTION (*BE SENSIBLE*)

- Use the least dose of LA necessary to achieve the desired extent and duration of block.
- Local anesthetic blood levels are influenced by site of injection and dose. Factors that can increase the likelihood of LAST include: advanced age, heart failure, ischemic heart disease, conduction abnormalities, metabolic (e.g., mitochondrial) disease, liver disease, low plasma protein concentration, metabolic or respiratory acidosis, medications that inhibit sodium channels. Patients with severe cardiac dysfunction, particularly very low ejection fraction, are more sensitive to LAST and also more prone to 'stacked' injections (with resulting elevated LA tissue concentrations) due to slowed circulation time.
- Consider using a pharmacologic marker and/or test dose, e.g. epinephrine 5 mcg/mL of LA. Know the expected response, onset, duration, and limitations of "test dose" in identifying intravascular injection.
- Aspirate the syringe prior to *each* injection while observing for blood.
- Inject incrementally, while observing for signs and querying for symptoms of toxicity between each injection.

DETECTION (*BE VIGILANT*)

- Use standard American Society of Anesthesiologists (ASA) monitors.
- Monitor the patient during and after completing injection as clinical toxicity can be delayed up to 30 minutes.
- Communicate frequently with the patient to query for symptoms of toxicity.
- Consider LAST in any patient with altered mental status, neurological symptoms or cardiovascular instability after a regional anesthetic.

- Central nervous system signs (may be subtle or absent)
  o *Excitation* (agitation, confusion, muscle twitching, seizure)
  o *Depression* (drowsiness, obtundation, coma *or* apnea)
  o *Non-specific* (metallic taste, circumoral numbness, diplopia, tinnitus, dizziness)
- Cardiovascular signs (often the only manifestation of severe LAST)
  o *Initially may be hyperdynamic* (hypertension, tachycardia, ventricular arrhythmias), then
  o *Progressive hypotension*
  o *Conduction block, bradycardia or asystole*
  o *Ventricular arrhythmia* (ventricular tachycardia, Torsades de Pointes, ventricular fibrillation)
- Sedative hypnotic drugs reduce seizure risk but even light sedation may abolish the patient's ability to recognize or report symptoms of rising LA concentrations.

TREATMENT

- Timing of lipid infusion in LAST is controversial. The most conservative approach, waiting until after ACLS has proven unsuccessful, is unreasonable because early treatment can prevent cardiovascular collapse. Infusing lipid at the earliest sign of LAST can result in unnecessary treatment since only a fraction of patients will progress to severe toxicity. The most reasonable approach is to implement lipid therapy on the basis of clinical severity and rate of progression of LAST.
- There is laboratory evidence that epinephrine can impair resuscitation from LAST and reduce the efficacy of lipid rescue. Therefore it is recommended to avoid high doses of epinephrine and use smaller doses, e.g., < 1mcg/kg, for treating hypotension.
- Propofol *should not be used* when there are signs of cardiovascular instability. Propofol is a cardiovascular depressant with lipid content too low to provide benefit. Its use is discouraged when there is a risk of progression to cardiovascular collapse.
- Prolonged monitoring (>12 hours) is recommended after any signs of systemic LA toxicity, since cardiovascular depression due to local anesthetics can persist or recur after treatment.

FIGURE 8-8 ASRA Practice Advisory on LAST. Reprinted with permission from: The American Society of Regional Anesthesia and Pain Management Practice Advisory on Treatment of Local Anesthetic Systemic Toxicity. Copyright 2012 The American Society of Regional Anesthesia and Pain Management. Copies which can be laminated and posted in the practice area are available for download at http://links.lww.com/AAP/A17 or http://links.lww.com/AAP/A18

(134,136–139). The etiology of TNS remains to be elucidated but does not appear to be related to neurologic dysfunction or toxicity (140). The incidence of TNS among parturients is low. Wong and Slavenas interviewed 303 patients who underwent spinal anesthesia with lidocaine, bupivacaine or tetracaine for obstetric procedures and did not discover any cases of TNS (141).

Allergic reactions to local anesthetics do occur, but only rarely. Most reported allergic reactions are not immune-mediated reactions at all, but instead represent other responses such as epinephrine absorption, LAST, etc. Among 177 patients who reported adverse reactions to local anesthetics, allergy testing (skin rick, intracutaneous and subcutaneous challenges, and radioimmunoassay to detect IgE) identified only 3 who had positive responses, none of which were IgE mediated (142). Allergies are more common after amino-ester administration because metabolism of ester compounds yields para-aminobenzoic acid (PABA) a known allergen; cross-reactivity between different ester local anesthetics is expected (143). Allergic responses to the paraben or sulfite preservatives present in some formulations may also occur (143). Obstetric patients who present with a local anesthetic "allergy" should be sent for consultation with clinicians who specialize in the diagnosis and treatment of allergic conditions. Standardized provocative testing, performed by specialists in this area, may avoid unnecessarily depriving patients of the benefits of neuraxial analgesia/anesthesia, although results of such tests are sometimes equivocal.

If an allergic reaction is suspected the causative agent should be discontinued immediately. A patent airway should be ensured, and ventilation with 100% oxygen should ensue. Intravenous volume expansion will aid support of the circulation. Intravenous epinephrine may be titrated to effect, using initial doses of 5 to 10 mcg for mild symptoms and 50 to 100 mcg for more severe anaphylactic/anaphylactoid reactions. Epinephrine is useful due to its α-1-mediated vasoconstriction, β-1-mediated increases in myocardial contractility, β-2-mediated bronchodilation, and β-2-mediated inhibition of mast cell and basophil degranulation. Secondary treatment options to be considered include histamine blockers and inhaled β-2 agonists and/or anticholinergic agents for bronchospasm. Corticosteroids may prevent delayed symptoms which sometimes occur; either hydrocortisone 0.5 to 1 g or methylprednisolone 1 to 2 g may be administered intravenously.

■ LOCAL ANESTHETICS COMMONLY USED IN OBSTETRIC ANESTHESIA (TABLE 8-5)

Hyperbaric or isobaric bupivacaine is often administered into the intrathecal space for surgical procedures, such as cesarean delivery. It is not commonly used for epidural anesthesia for surgical procedures because of concerns regarding systemic toxicity when concentrations of ≥0.75% are administered into the epidural space of pregnant women. Bupivacaine is often given for neuraxial labor analgesia. The goal during labor analgesia is to provide adequate maternal analgesia and satisfaction along with minimal motor blockade, as advised in the American Society of Anesthesiologists' Obstetric Anesthesia Practice Guidelines (21). Therefore the practitioner may employ low concentrations of bupivacaine (e.g., 0.0625% to 125%) for both initiation and maintenance of epidural labor analgesia; the addition of opioids to the local anesthetic solution allows for a lower concentration of bupivacaine to be administered, for maximal preservation of motor strength (19). During combined spinal–epidural labor analgesia, the addition of bupivacaine (1 to 2.5 mg) to intrathecal opioid improves analgesia and decreases opioid-associated itching (144,145).

Ropivacaine is used in much the same manner as bupivacaine in obstetrics. Some authors find it preferable to the latter due to its purported greater sensory–motor differential blockade and its lesser potential for systemic toxicity (146). However, others find no advantage to ropivacaine over bupivacaine, citing a lack of convincing data regarding differences in motor blockade at equipotent doses, and a minimal potential for toxicity when bupivacaine is administered in very low concentrations, as is in obstetrics (147). These authors also point out that even if ropivacaine does preserve motor strength to a greater degree than bupivacaine, it carries no outcome advantages regarding maternal analgesia or satisfaction, ability to ambulate, or rates of instrumental vaginal delivery (147). Ropivacaine is more costly than bupivacaine.

Lidocaine (usually hyperbaric) is another option for intrathecal administration for surgical procedures, particularly those of short duration such as postpartum tubal ligation and curettage of retained products of conception. In addition, it is often used when one wishes to extend epidural labor analgesia for cesarean delivery. Concentrations of 2% are common in this setting; alkalization of the local anesthetic provides a faster onset time, and epinephrine (typically 5 mcg/mL)

TABLE 8-5 Commonly used Local Anesthetics and Doses for Obstetric Anesthesia

Local Anesthetic	Cesarean Delivery		Labor and Delivery Analgesia			
	Intrathecal	Epidural	Intrathecal Initiation	Epidural Initiation	Epidural Maintenance Infusion	Instrumental Vaginal Delivery
Bupivacaine	9–12 mg[a]	N/A	1–2.5 mg[a]	10–20 mL 0.0625–0.125%[a]	0.0625–0.1%[a]	N/A
Ropivacaine	18–25 mg[a]	N/A	1–2.5 mg[a]	10–15 mL 0.1%[a]	0.1%[a]	N/A
Lidocaine	75 mg	20 mL 2%[b]	N/A	N/A	N/A	10 mL 1–2%
Chloroprocaine	N/A	20 mL 3%[c]	N/A	N/A	N/A	10 mL 2–3%

[a]Opioid commonly added.
[b]Epinephrine and bicarbonate commonly added.
[c]Bicarbonate commonly added.

intensifies block and extends duration. Concentrations of 1% to 2% may be employed to increase density of epidural blockade for instrumental vaginal delivery.

With its short onset latency and minimal accumulation in the fetus, chloroprocaine, with or without added bicarbonate, is used when one wishes to very quickly extend epidural anesthesia for an urgent or emergent cesarean delivery. When 25 mL of 3% chloroprocaine with bicarbonate is administered to a patient who has previously been receiving an epidural infusion for labor analgesia, surgical conditions are routinely achieved within less than 5 minutes (148). Chloroprocaine possesses a slightly faster onset time than lidocaine (148). In addition, it may take more time to prepare lidocaine due to the need for inclusion of additives bicarbonate and epinephrine. An additional theoretical advantage of chloroprocaine over lidocaine exists in the setting of nonreassuring fetal well-being, which may signify fetal acidemia: Due to its rapid metabolism, chloroprocaine does not accumulate, even in an acidotic fetus, whereas lidocaine, which crosses the placenta readily, has the potential to accumulate and become ion-trapped in this clinical setting (149,150). Chloroprocaine provides an alternative to lidocaine when one wishes to intensify blockade for instrumental vaginal delivery.

Chloroprocaine has been associated with adhesive arachnoiditis when large doses meant for the epidural space are accidentally injected intrathecally, as might occur during intrathecal migration of an epidural catheter. The complication is thought to be due to the presence of the preservative sodium metabisulfite at an acidic pH, although not all authors agree regarding this mechanism (151,152). A formulation with the preservative disodium ethylenediaminetetraacetic acid (EDTA) results in back pain that is poorly localized, aching or burning, and can be severe, especially if large volumes are used (153). Back pain may be due to EDTA chelation of calcium and resultant tetanic muscle contractions. It seems reasonable to avoid the use of preservatives and to minimize the volume of chloroprocaine administered. The short duration of chloroprocaine necessitates redosing of the epidural catheter after 30 to 40 minutes during surgical procedures; to minimize the amount administered, one might choose to switch to lidocaine at the time of redose.

KEY POINTS

- The molecular properties of local anesthetics determine their clinical actions and utility.
  - The pKa governs speed of onset.
  - Lipid solubility determines potency and duration.
  - Protein binding further impacts duration.
  - Various additives modify onset time, density, and duration of blockade.
- The concept of differential blockade:
  - Implies that sympathetic exceeds sensory blockade level;
  - Allows the anesthesiologist to provide labor analgesia with minimal motor blockade through the use of dilute concentrations of local anesthetics mixed with opioids.
- Pregnancy enhances local anesthetic sensitivity due to anatomic and pharmacodynamic effects.
- Safe use of local anesthetics requires knowledge of the adverse reactions that may accompany administration, especially LAST syndrome.
  - LAST presentation can vary, so the clinician must have a low threshold for its diagnosis.
  - Lidocaine is less cardiotoxic than the lipophilic anesthetics such as bupivacaine and ropivacaine; ropivacaine is most likely less cardiotoxic than bupivacaine.

- Prevention of LAST through catheter aspiration, slow incremental injection and the use of an intravascular test dose is of paramount importance.
- Treatment of LAST centers on airway management, hemodynamic support and early administration of lipid emulsion.
- It is advisable to post algorithms for LAST treatment which include dosing regimens for lipid administration in the clinical area where regional anesthesia takes place.
- Bupivacaine, ropivacaine, lidocaine and chloroprocaine are all commonly administered to obstetric patients.

■ ACKNOWLEDGMENT

The author wishes to thank Sandra Nunnally for her assistance in the preparation of this chapter.

REFERENCES

1. Butterworth JF, Strichartz GR. Molecular mechanisms of local anesthesia: a review. *Anesthesiology* 1990;72:711–734.
2. Catterall WA. From ionic currents to molecular mechanisms: the structure and function of voltage-gated sodium channels. *Neuron* 2000;26:13–25.
3. Jackson T, McLure HA. Pharmacology of local anesthetics. *Ophthalmol Clin N Am* 2006;19:155–161.
4. Narahashi T, Frazier DT, Yamada M. The site of action and active form of local anesthetics. I. Theory and pH experiments with tertiary compounds. *J Pharmacol Exp Ther* 1970;171:32–44.
5. Frazier DT, Narahashi T, Yamada M. The site of action and active form of local anesthetics. II. Experiments with quaternary compounds. *J Pharmacol Exp Ther* 1970;171:45–51.
6. Strichartz GR, Sanchez V, Arthur GR, et al. Fundamental properties of local anesthetics. II. Measured octanol: buffer partition coefficients and pKa values of clinically used drugs. *Anesth Analg* 1990;71:158–170.
7. Courtney KR. Size-dependent kinetics associated with drug block of sodium current. *Biophys J* 1984;45:42–44.
8. Tucker GT. Pharmacokinetics of local anaesthetics. *Br J Anaesth* 1986;58:717–731.
9. Rosenberg PH, Veering BT, Urmey WF. Maximum recommended doses of local anesthetics: a multifactorial concept. *Reg Anesth Pain Med* 2004;29:564–575.
10. Franz DN, Perry RS. Mechanisms for differential block among single myelinated and non-myelinated axons by procaine. *J Physiol* 1974;236:193–210.
11. Fink BR, Cairns AM. Differential slowing and block of conduction by lidocaine in individual afferent myelinated and unmyelinated axons. *Anesthesiology* 1984;60:111–120.
12. Fink BR. Mechanisms of differential axial blockade in epidural and subarachnoid anesthesia. *Anesthesiology* 1989;70:851–858.
13. Huang JH, Thalhammer JG, Raymond SA, et al. Susceptibility to lidocaine of impulses in different somatosensory afferent fibers of rat sciatic nerve. *J Pharmacol Exp Ther* 1997;292:802–811.
14. Chamberlain DP, Chamberlain BD. Changes in the skin temperature of the trunk and their relationship to sympathetic blockade during spinal anesthesia. *Anesthesiology* 1986;65:139–143.
15. Malmqvist LA, Bengtsson M, Bjornsson G, et al. Sympathetic activity and haemodynamic variables during spinal analgesia in man. *Acta Anaesthesiol Scand* 1987;31:467–473.
16. Cook PR, Malmqvist LA, Bengtsson M, et al. Vagal and sympathetic activity during spinal analgesia. *Acta Anaesthesiol Scand* 1990;34:271–275.
17. Brull SJ, Greene NM. Time-courses of zones of differential sensory blockade during spinal anesthesia with hyperbaric tetracaine or bupivacaine. *Anesth Analg* 1989;69:342–347.
18. Brull SJ, Greene NM. Zones of differential sensory block during extradural anaesthesia. *Br J Anaesth* 1991;66:651–655.
19. Chestnut DH, Laszewski LJ, Pollack KL, et al. Continuous epidural infusion of 0.0625% bupivacaine-0.0002% fentanyl during the second stage of labor. *Anesthesiology* 1990;72:613–618.
20. Comparative Obstetric Mobile Epidural Trial (COMET) Study Group UK. Effect of low-dose mobile versus traditional epidural techniques on mode of delivery: a randomised controlled trial. *Lancet* 2001;358:19–23.
21. American Society of Anesthesiologists Task Force on Obstetric Anesthesia. Practice guidelines for obstetric anesthesia: an updated report by the American Society of Anesthesiologists Task Force on Obstetric Anesthesia. *Anesthesiology* 2007;106:843–863.
22. Hunt CO, Naulty JS, Bader AM, et al. Perioperative analgesia with subarachnoid fentanyl-bupivacaine for cesarean delivery. *Anesthesiology* 1989;71:535–540.

23. Shende D, Cooper GM, Bowden MI. The influence of intrathecal fentanyl on the characteristics of subarachnoid block for caesarean section. *Anaesthesia* 1998;53:702–710.

24. Manullang TR, Viscomi CM, Pace NL. Intrathecal fentanyl is superior to intravenous ondansetron for the prevention of perioperative nausea during cesarean delivery with spinal anesthesia. *Anesth Analg* 2000;90:1162–1166.

25. Racle JP, Benkhadra A, Poy JY, et al. Prolongation of isobaric bupivacaine spinal anesthesia with epinephrine and clonidine for hip surgery in the elderly. *Anesth Analg* 1987;66:442–446.

26. Racle JP, Benkhadra A, Poy JY, et al. Effect of increasing amounts of epinephrine during isobaric bupivacaine spinal anesthesia in elderly patients. *Anesth Analg* 1987;66:882–886.

27. Chiu AA, Liu S, Carpenter RL, et al. The effects of epinephrine on lidocaine spinal anesthesia: a cross-over study. *Anesth Analg* 1995;80:735–739.

28. Eisenach JC. Grice SC, Dewan DM. Epinephrine enhances analgesia produced by epidural bupivacaine during labor. *Anesth Analg* 1987;66:447–451.

29. Polly LS, Columb MO, Naughton NN, et al. Effect of epidural epinephrine on the minimum local analgesic concentration of epidural bupivacaine in labor. *Anesthesiology* 2002;96:1123–1128.

30. Neal JM. Effects of epinephrine in local anesthetics on the central and peripheral nervous systems: Neurotoxicity and neural blood flow. *Reg Anesth Pain Med* 2003;28:124–134.

31. Burm AG, van Kleff JW, Gladines MP, et al. Epidural Anesthesia with lidocaine and bupivacaine: effects of epinephrine on the plasma concentration profiles. *Anesth Analg* 1986;65:1281–1284.

32. Campbell DC, Banner R, Crone LA, et al. Addition of epinephrine to intrathecal bupivacaine and sufentanil for ambulatory labor analgesia. *Anesthesiology* 1997;86:525–531.

33. Sakura S, Sumi M, Sakaguchi Y, et al. The addition of phenylephrine contributes to the development of transient neurologic symptoms after spinal anesthesia with 0.5% tetracaine. *Anesthesiology* 1997;87:771–778.

34. Mercier FJ, Dounas M, Bouaziz H, et al. The effect of adding a minidose of clonidine to intrathecal sufentanil for labor analgesia. *Anesthesiology* 1998;89:594–601.

35. Tremlett MR, Kelly PJ, Parkins J, et al. Low-dose clonidine infusion during labor. *Br J Anaesth* 1999;83:257–261.

36. Sia AT. Optimal dose of intrathecal clonidine added to sufentanil plus bupivacaine for labour analgesia. *Can J Anaesth* 2000;47:875–880.

37. Owen MD, Ozsarac O, Sahin S, et al. Low-dose clonidine and neostigmine prolong the duration of intrathecal bupivacaine-fentanyl for labor analgesia. *Anesthesiology* 2000;92:361–366.

38. Nelson KE, D'Angelo R, Foss ML, et al. Intrathecal neostigmine and sufentanil for early labor analgesia. *Anesthesiology* 1999;91:1293–1298.

39. Hirabayashi Y, Shimizu R, Saitoh K, et al. Spread of subarachnoid hyperbaric amethocaine in pregnant women. *Br J Anaesth* 1995;74:384–386.

40. Greene NM. Distribution of local anesthetic solutions within the subarachnoid space. *Anesth Analg* 1985;64:715–730.

41. Hirabayashi Y, Shimizu R, Fukuda H, et al. Soft tissue anatomy within the vertebral canal in pregnant women. *Br J Anaesth* 1996;77:153–156.

42. Takiguchi T, Yamaguchi S, Tezuka M, et al. Compression of the subarachnoid space by the engorged epidural venous plexus in pregnant women. *Anesthesiology* 2006;105:848–851.

43. Higuchi H, Takagi S, Onuki E, et al. Distribution of epidural saline upon injection and the epidural volume effect in pregnant women. *Anesthesiology* 2011;114:1155–1161.

44. Butterworth JF, Walker FO, Lysak SZ. Pregnancy increases median nerve susceptibility to lidocaine. *Anesthesiology* 1990;72:962–965.

45. Datta S, Lambert DH, Gregus J, et al. Differential sensitivities of mammalian nerve fibers during pregnancy. *Anesth Analg* 1983;62:1070–1072.

46. Flanagan HL, Datta S, Lambert DH, et al. Effect of pregnancy on bupivacaine-induced conduction blockade in the isolated rabbit vagus nerve. *Anesth Analg* 1987;66:123–126.

47. Popitz-Bergez FA, Leason S, Thalhammer JG, et al. Intraneural lidocaine uptake compared with analgesic differences between pregnant and nonpregnant rats. *Reg Anesth* 1997;22:363–371.

48. Datta S, Hurley RJ, Naulty JS, et al. Plasma and cerebrospinal fluid progesterone concentrations in pregnant and nonpregnant women. *Anesth Analg* 1986;65:950–954.

49. Hirabayashi Y, Shimizu R, Saitoh K, et al. Acid-base state of cerebrospinal fluid during pregnancy and its effect on spread of spinal anesthesia. *Br J Anaesth* 1996;77:352–355.

50. Thomas JM, Schug SA. Recent advances in the pharmacokinetics of local anaesthetics: Long-acting amide enantiomers and continuous infusions. *Clin Pharmacokinet* 1999;36:67–83.

51. Burm AG, Vermeulen NP, van Kleff JW, et al. Pharmacokinetics of lignocaine and bupivacaine in surgical patients following epidural administration. Simultaneous investigation of absorption and disposition kinetics using stable isotopes. *Clin Pharmacokinet* 1987;13:191–203.

52. Kuhnert BR, Kuhnert PM, Prochaska AL, et al. Plasma levels of 2-chloroprocaine in obstetric patients and their neonates after epidural anesthesia. *Anesthesiology* 1980;53:21–25.

53. Kuhnert BR, Kuhnert PM, Philipson EH, et al. The half-life of 2-chloroprocaine. *Anesth Analg* 1986;65:273–278.

54. Downing JW, Johnson HV, Fonzalez HF, et al. The pharmacokinetics of epidural lidocaine and bupivacaine during cesarean section. *Anesth Analg* 1997;84:527–532.

55. Richter O, Klein K, Abel J, et al. The kinetics of bupivacaine (Carbostesin) plasma concentrations during epidural anesthesia following intraoperative bolus injection and subsequent continuous infusion. *Int J Clin Pharmacol Ther Toxicol* 1984;22:611–617.

56. Emanuelsson BM, Zaric D, Nydahl PA, et al. Pharmacokinetics of ropivacaine and bupivacaine during 21 hours of continuous epidural infusion in healthy male volunteers. *Anesth Analg* 1995;81:1163–1168.

57. Erichsen CJ, Sjovall J, Kehlet H, et al. Pharmacokinetics and analgesic effect of ropivacaine during continuous epidural infusion for postoperative pain relief. *Anesthesiology* 1996;84:834–842.

58. Burm AG, Stienstra R, Brouwer RP, et al. Epidural infusion of ropivacaine for postoperative analgesia after major orthopedic surgery: pharmacokinetic evaluation. *Anesthesiology* 2000;93:395–403.

59. Santos AC, Arthur GR, Lehning EJ, et al. Comparative pharmacokinetics of ropivacaine and bupivacaine in nonpregnant and pregnant ewes. *Anesth Analg* 1997;85:87–93.

60. Santos AC, Karpel B, Noble G. The placental transfer and fetal effects of levobupivacaine, racemic bupivacaine, and ropivacaine. *Anesthesiology* 1999;90:1698–1703.

61. Bader AM, Fragnetto R, Terui K, et al. Maternal and neonatal fentanyl and bupivacaine concentrations after epidural infusion during labor. *Anesth Analg* 1995;81:829–832.

62. Alahuta S, Rasanen J, Jouppila P, et al. The effects of epidural ropivacaine and bupivacaine for cesarean section on uteroplacental and fetal circulation. *Anesthesiology* 1995;83:23–32.

63. Auroy Y, Narchi P, Messiah A, et al. Serious complications related to regional anesthesia: Results of a prospective survey in France. *Anesthesiology* 1997;87:479–486.

64. Auroy Y, Benhamou D, Bargues L, et al. Major complications of regional anesthesia in France: The SOS regional anesthesia hotline service. *Anesthesiology* 2002;97:1274–1280.

65. Hawkins JL, Chang J, Palmer SK, et al. Anesthesia-related maternal mortality in the United States: 1979–2002. *Obstet Gynecol* 2011;117:69–74.

66. Hawkins JL, Koonin LM, Palmer SK, et al. Anesthesia-related deaths during obstetric delivery in the United States, 1979–1990. *Anesthesiology* 1997;86:277–284.

67. Faccenda KA, Finucane BT. Complications of regional anaesthesia: Incidence and prevention. *Drug Saf* 2001;24:413–442.

68. Davies JM, Posner KL, Lee LA, et al. Liability associated with obstetric anesthesia: a closed claims analysis. *Anesthesiology* 2009;110:131–139.

69. Rutten AJ, Nancarrow C, Mather LE, et al. Hemodynamic and central nervous system effects of intravenous bolus doses of lidocaine, bupivacaine, and ropivacaine in sheep. *Anesth Analg* 1989;69:291–299.

70. Feldman HS, Arthur GR, Pitkanen M, et al. Treatment of acute systemic toxicity after the rapid intravenous injection of ropivacaine and bupivacaine in the conscious dog. *Anesth Analg* 1991;73:373–384.

71. Huang YF, Upton RN, Rutten AJ, et al. I.V. bolus administration of subconvulsive doses of lignocaine to conscious sheep: effects on circulatory function. *Br J Anaesth* 1992;69:368–374.

72. Chang DH, Ladd LA, Copeland S, et al. Direct cardiac effects of intracoronary bupivacaine, levobupivacaine and ropivacaine in the sheep. *Br J Pharmacol* 2001;132:649–658.

73. Di Gregorio G, Neal JM, Rosenquist RW, et al. Clinical presentation of local anesthetic systemic toxicity: a review of published cases, 1979 to 2009. *Reg Anesth Pain Med* 2010;35:181–187.

74. Mather LE, Copeland SE, Ladd LA. Acute toxicity of local anesthetics: underlying pharmacokinetic and pharmacodynamics concepts. *Reg Anesth Pain Med* 2005;30:553–566.

75. Nancarrow C, Rutten AJ, Runciman WB, et al. Myocardial and cerebral drug concentrations and the mechanisms of death after fatal intravenous doses of lidocaine, bupivacaine, and ropivacaine in sheep. *Anesth Analg* 1989;69:276–283.

76. Feldman HS, Arthur GR, Covino BG. Comparative systemic toxicity of convulsant and supraconvulsant doses of intravenous ropivacaine, bupivacaine and lidocaine in the conscious dog. *Anesth Analg* 1989;69:794–801.

77. Clarkson CW, Hondeghem LM. Mechanism for bupivacaine depression of cardiac conduction: fast block of sodium channels during the action potential with slow recovery from block during diastole. *Anesthesiology* 1985;62:396–405.

78. Knudsen K, Beckman Suurkula M, Blomberg S, et al. Central nervous and cardiovascular effects of i.v. infusions of ropivacaine, bupivacaine and placebo in volunteers. *Br J Anaesth* 1997;78:507–514.

79. Morrison SG, Dominguez JJ, Frascarolo P, et al. A comparison of the electro-cardiographic cardiotoxic effects of racemic bupivacaine, levobupivacaine, and ropivacaine in anesthetized swine. *Anesth Analg* 2000;90:1308–1314.

80. Polley LS, Columb MO, Naughton NN, et al. Relative analgesic potencies of ropivacaine and bupivacaine for epidural analgesia in labor: Implications for therapeutic indexes. *Anesthesiology* 1999;90:944–950.

81. Capogna G, Celleno D, Fusco P, et al. Relative potencies of bupivacaine and ropivacaine for analgesia in labour. *Br Jr Anaesth* 1999;82:371–373.

82. Camorcia M, Capogna G, Columb MO. Minimum local analgesic doses of ropivacaine, levobupivacaine, and bupivacaine for intrathecal labor analgesia. *Anesthesiology* 2005;102:646–650.

83. D'Angelo R, James RL. Is ropivacaine less potent than bupivacaine? *Anesthesiology* 1999;90:941–943.

84. Van de Velde M, Dreelinck R, Dubois J, et al. Determination of the full dose-response relation of intrathecal bupivacaine, levobupivacaine, and ropivacaine, combined with sufentanil, for labor analgesia. *Anesthesiology* 2007;106:149–156.

85. Kee WD, Ng FF, Khaw KS, et al. Determination and comparison of graded dose-response curves for epidural bupivacaine and ropivacaine for analgesia in laboring nulliparous women. *Anesthesiology* 2010;113:445–453.

86. Groban L, Deal DD, Vernon JC, et al. Cardiac resuscitation after incremental overdosage with lidocaine, bupivacaine, levobupivacaine, and ropivacaine in anesthetized dogs. *Anesth Analg* 2001;92:37–43.

87. Dony P, Dewinde V, Vanderick B, et al. The comparative toxicity of ropivacaine and bupivacaine at equipotent doses in rats. *Anesth Analg* 2000;91:1489–1492.

88. Morishima HO, Pedersen H, Finster M, et al. Bupivacaine toxicity in pregnant and nonpregnant ewes. *Anesthesiology* 1985;63:134–139.

89. Santos AC, Arthur GR, Pedersen H, et al. Systemic toxicity of ropivacaine during ovine pregnancy. *Anesthesiology* 1991;75:137–141.

90. Santos AC, Arthur GR, Wlody D, et al. Comparative systemic toxicity of ropivacaine and bupivacaine in nonpregnant and pregnant ewes. *Anesthesiology* 1995;82:734–740.

91. Santos AC, DeArmas PI. Systemic toxicity of levobupivacaine, bupivacaine and ropivacaine during continuous intravenous infusion to nonpregnant and pregnant ewes. *Anesthesiology* 2001;95:1256–1264.

92. Neal JM, Bernards CM, Butterworth JF, et al. ASRA Practice Advisory on local anesthetic systemic toxicity. *Reg Anesth Pain Med* 2010;35:152–161.

93. Mulroy MF, Hejtmanek MR. Prevention of local anesthetic systemic toxicity. *Reg Anesth Pain Med* 2010;35:177–180.

94. Norris MC, Ferrenbach D, Dalman H, et al. Does epinephrine improve diagnostic accuracy of aspiration during labor epidural analgesia? *Anesth Analg* 1999;88:1073–1076.

95. Leighton BL, Norris MC, Sosis M, et al. Limitations of epinephrine as a marker of intravascular injection in laboring women. *Anesthesiology* 1987;66:688–691.

96. Birnbach DJ, Chestnut DH. The epidural test does in obstetric patients: has it outlived its usefulness? *Anesth Analg* 1999;88:971–972.

97. Leighton BL, Gross JB. Air: an effective indicator of intravenously located epidural catheters. *Anesthesiology* 1989;71:848–851.

98. Leighton BL, Norris MC, DeSimone CA, et al. The air test as a clinically useful indicator of intravenously placed epidural catheters. *Anesthesiology* 1990;73:610–613.

99. Yoshii WY, Miller M, Rottman RL, et al. Fentanyl for epidural intravascular test dose in obstetrics. *Reg Anesth* 1993;18:296–299.

100. Weinberg GL. Treatment of local anesthetic systemic toxicity (LAST). *Reg Anesth Pain Med* 2010;35:188–193.

101. Sage DJ, Feldman HS, Arthur GR, et al. Influence of lidocaine and bupivacaine on isolated guinea pig atria in the presence of acidosis and hypoxia. *Anesth Analg* 1984;63:1–7.

102. Heavner JE, Dryden CF, Sanghani V, et al. Severe hypoxia enhances central nervous system and cardiovascular toxicity of bupivacaine in lightly anesthetized pigs. *Anesthesiology* 1992;77:142–147.

103. Mochizuki T, Sato S. Hypocapnia prolongs bradycardia induced by bupivacaine or levobupivacaine in isolated rat hearts. *Can J Anesth* 2008;55:836–846.

104. Haasio J, Pitkanen MT, Kytta J, et al. Treatment of bupivacaine-induced cardiac arrhythmias in hypoxic and hypercarbic pigs with amiodarone or bretylium. *Reg Anesth* 1990;15:174–179.

105. Long WB, Rosenblum S, Grady IP. Successful resuscitation of bupivacaine-induced cardiac arrest using cardiopulmonary bypass. *Anesth Analg* 1989;69:403–406.

106. Toledo P. The role of lipid emulsion during advanced cardiac life support for local anesthetic toxicity. *Int J Obstet Anesth* 2011;20:60–63.

107. Weinberg GL, VadeBoncouer T, Ramaraju GA, et al. Pretreatment of resuscitation with a lipid infusion shifts the dose-response to bupivacaine-induced asystole in rats. *Anesthesiology* 1998;88:1071–1075.

108. Weinberg G, Ripper R, Feinstein DL, et al. Lipid emulsion infusion rescues dogs from bupivacaine-induced cardiac toxicity. *Reg Anesth Pain Med* 2003;28:198–202.

109. Rosenblatt MA, Abel M, Fischer GW, et al. Successful use of 20% lipid emulsion to resuscitate a patient after a presumed bupivacaine-related cardiac arrest. *Anesthesiology* 2006;105:217–218.

110. Spence AG. Lipid reversal of central nervous system symptoms of bupivacaine toxicity. *Anesthesiology* 2007;107:516–517.

111. Litz RJ, Popp M, Stehr SN, et al. Successful resuscitation of a patient with ropivacaine-induced asystole after axillary plexus block using lipid infusion. *Anaesthesia* 2006;61:800–801.

112. Litz RJ, Roessel T, Heller AR, et al. Reversal of central nervous system and cardiac toxicity after local anesthetic intoxication by lipid emulsion injection. *Anesth Analg* 2008;106:1575–1577.

113. Warren JA, Thoma RB, Georgescu A, et al. Intravenous lipid infusion in the successful resuscitation of local anesthetic-induced cardiovascular collapse after supraclavicular brachial plexus block. *Anesth Analg* 2008;106:1578–1580.

114. Weinberg GL, Ripper R, Murphy P, et al. Lipid infusion accelerates removal of bupivacaine and recovery from bupivacaine toxicity in the isolated rat heart. *Reg Anesth Pain Med* 2006;31:296–303.

115. Chen Y, Xia Y, Liu L, et al. Lipid emulsion reverses bupivacaine-induced asystole in isolated rat hearts. *Anesthesiology* 2010;113:1320–1325.

116. Drasner K. Local anesthetic systemic toxicity. *Reg Anesth Pain Med* 2010;35:162–166.

117. Huang JM, Xian H, Bacaner M. Long-chain fatty acids activate calcium channels in ventricular myocytes. *Proc Natl Acad Sci USA* 1992;89:6452–6456.

118. Weinberg GL, Di Gregorio G, Ripper R, et al. Resuscitation with lipid versus epinephrine in a rat model of bupivacaine overdose. *Anesthesiology* 2008;108:907–913.

119. Di Gregorio G, Schwartz D, Ripper R, et al. Lipid emulsion in superior to vasopressin in a rodent model of resuscitation from toxin-induced cardiac arrest. *Crit Care Med* 2009;37:993–999.

120. Mayr VD, Mitterschiffthaler L, Neurauter A, et al. A comparison of the combination of epinephrine and vasopressin with lipid emulsion in a porcine model of asphyxial cardiac arrest after intravenous injection of bupivacaine. *Anesth Analg* 2008;106:1566–1571.

121. Harvey M, Cave G, Kazemi A. Intralipid infusion diminishes return of spontaneous circulation after hypoxic cardiac arrest in rabbits. *Anesth Analg* 2009;108:1163–1168.

122. Harvey M, Cave G, Prince G, et al. Epinephrine injection in lipid-based resuscitation from bupivacaine-induced cardiac arrest: Transient circulatory return in rabbits. *Anesth Analg* 2010;111:791–796.

123. Harvey M. Bupivacaine-induced cardiac arrest: fat is good—is epinephrine really bad? *Anesthesiology* 2009;111:467–469.

124. Hiller DB, Di Gregio G, Ripper R, et al. Epinephrine impairs lipid resuscitation from bupivacaine overdose. *Anesthesiology* 2009;111:498–505.

125. Hicks SD, Salcido DD, Logue ES, et al. Lipid emulsion combined with epinephrine and vasopressin does not improve survival in a swine model of bupivacaine-induced cardiac arrest. *Anesthesiology* 2009;111:138–146.

126. Hiller DB, Di Gregorio G, Kelly K, et al. Safety of high volume lipid emulsion infusion: a first approximation of LD_{50} in rats. *Reg Anesth Pain Med* 2010;35:140–144.

127. Marwick PC, Levine AI, Coetzee AR. Recurrence of cardiotoxicity after lipid rescue from bupivacaine-induced cardiac arrest. *Anesth Analg* 2009;108:1344–1346.

128. Brull SJ. Lipid emulsion for the treatment of local anesthetic toxicity: patient safety implications. *Anesth Analg* 2008;106:1337–1339.

129. Lambert LA, Lambert DH, Strichartz GR. Irreversible conduction block in isolated nerve by high concentrations of local anesthetics. *Anesthesiology* 1994;80:1082–1093.

130. Kanai Y, Katsuki H, Takasaki M. Lidocaine disrupts axonal membrane of rate sciatic nerve in vitro. *Anesth Analg* 2000;91:944–948.

131. Johnson ME. Potential neurotoxicity of spinal anesthesia with lidocaine. *Mayo Clin Proc* 2000;75:921–932.

132. Schell RM, Brauer FS, Cole DJ, et al. Persistent sacral nerve root deficits after continuous spinal anaesthesia. *Can J Anaesth* 1991;38:908–911.

133. Rigler ML, Drasner K, Krejcie TC, et al. Cauda equina syndrome after continuous spinal anesthesia. *Anesth Analg* 1991;72:275–281.

134. Freedman JM, Li D, Drasner K, et al. Transient neurologic symptoms after spinal anesthesia: an epidemiologic study of 1,863 patients. *Anesthesiology* 1998;89:633–641.

135. Zaric D, Christiansen C, Pace NL, et al. Transient neurologic symptoms after spinal anesthesia with lidocaine versus other local anesthetics: a systematic review of randomized, controlled trials. *Anesth Analg* 2005;100:1811–1816.

136. Hampl KF, Schneider MC, Thorin D, et al. Hyperosmolarity does not contribute to transient radicular irritation after spinal anesthesia with hyperbaric 5% lidocaine. *Reg Anesth* 1995;20:363–368.

137. Hampl KF, Schneider MC, Pargger H, et al. A similar incidence of transient neurologic symptoms after spinal anesthesia with 2% and 5% lidocaine. *Anesth Analg* 1996;83:1051–1054.

138. Pollock JE, Liu SS, Neal JM, et al. Dilution of spinal lidocaine does not alter the incidence of transient neurologic symptoms. *Anesthesiology* 1999;90:445–450.

139. Tong D, Wong J, Chung F, et al. Prospective study on incidence and functional impact of transient neurologic symptoms associated with 1% versus 5% hyperbaric lidocaine in short urologic procedures. *Anesthesiology* 2003;98:485–494.

140. Pollock JE, Burkhead D, Neal JM, et al. Spinal nerve function in five volunteers experiencing transient neurologic symptoms after lidocaine subarachnoid anesthesia. *Anesth Analg* 2000;90:658–665.

141. Wong CA, Slavenas P. The incidence of transient radicular irritation after spinal anesthesia in obstetric patients. *Reg Anesth Pain Med* 1999;24:55–58.

142. Gall H, Kaufmann R, Kalveram CM. Adverse reactions to local anesthetics: analysis of 197 cases. *J Allergy Clin Immunol* 1996;97:933–937.

143. Finucane BT. Allergies to local anesthetics—the real truth. *Can J Anesth* 2003; 50:869–874.

144. Asokumar C, Newman LM, McCarthy RJ, et al. Intrathecal bupivacaine reduces pruritus and prolongs duration of fentanyl analgesia during labor: a prospective randomized controlled trial. *Anesth Analg* 1998;87:1309–1315.

145. Shah MK, Sia ST, Chong JL. The effect of the addition of ropivacaine or bupivacaine upon pruritus induced by intrathecal fentanyl in labour. *Anaesthesia* 2000;55:1008–1013.

146. Stienstra R. Clinical application of ropivacaine in obstetrics. *Curr Top Med Chem* 2001;1:215–218.

147. Beilin Y, Halpern S. Ropivacaine versus bupivacaine for epidural labor analgesia. *Anesth Analg* 2010;111:482–487.

148. Gaiser RR, Cheek TG, Adams HK, et al. Epidural lidocaine for cesarean delivery of the distressed fetus. *Int J Obstet Anesth* 1998;7:27–31.

149. Philipson EH, Kuhnert BR, Syracuse CD. Fetal acidosis, 2-chloroprocaine, and epidural anesthesia for cesarean section. *Am J Obstet Gynecol* 1985; 151:322–324.

150. Morishima HO, Santos AC, Pedersen H, et al. Effect of lidocaine on the asphyxial responses in the mature fetal lamb. *Anesthesiology* 1987;66:502–507.

151. Gissen AJ, Datta S, Lambert D. The chloroprocaine controversy II. Is chloroprocaine neurotoxic? *Reg Anesth* 1984;9:135–145.

152. Taniguchi M, Bollen AW, Drasner K. Sodium bisulfite: scapegoat for chloroprocaine neurotoxicity? *Anesthesiology* 2004;100:85–91.

153. Stevens RA, Urmey WF, Urquhart BL, et al. Back pain after epidural anesthesia with chloroprocaine. *Anesthesiology* 1993;78:492–497.

Regional Analgesia/Anesthesia Techniques in Obstetrics

Manuel C. Vallejo

Regional anesthetic techniques are commonly used and are very effective for intrapartum analgesia. These techniques provide analgesia while allowing the parturient to remain awake and participate in her labor and delivery experience. Properly conducted, these techniques provide superior analgesia to alternative methods and are very safe (Table 9-1). In contrast to parenteral or general inhalation anesthesia techniques, regional anesthesia decreases the likelihood of fetal drug depression and maternal aspiration pneumonitis, and more reliably reduces the cycle of maternal hyperventilation associated with painful uterine contractions and hypoventilation between contractions (1,2). Labor analgesia decreases maternal catecholamines and improves uteroplacental perfusion, which can be particularly beneficial for the parturient with pregnancy-induced hypertension. Effective analgesia blunts the hemodynamic effects associated with painful uterine contractions, which may be detrimental to patients with certain medical conditions such as cardiac valvular disease (see Chapter 26) or intracranial vascular disease (see Chapter 29). Furthermore, epidural analgesia can provide assistance with complicated delivery, such as vaginal breech, preterm, or twin delivery (see Chapter 15).

The most common forms of regional anesthesia are lumbar epidural, spinal, combined spinal–epidural (CSE), pudendal, and local perineal infiltration (Fig. 9-1). Other techniques for providing analgesia include caudal, paracervical, lumbar sympathetic, and paravertebral somatic nerve blocks (Table 9-2). Each regional technique can be used to block most of the nerves carrying pain impulses during the first or second stage of labor, or both.

PAIN PATHWAYS

The pain of labor arises primarily from nociceptors in the uterine and perineal structures.

Visceral afferent nerve fibers transmitting pain sensation during the first stage of labor result primarily from uterine contractions and cervical dilation, and travel with sympathetic fibers to enter the neuraxis at the tenth, eleventh, and twelfth thoracic and first lumbar spinal segments (Figs. 9-1 and 9-2). These afferent fibers synapse in the dorsal horn and make connections with other ascending and descending fibers, particularly in lamina V (Figs. 9-2 and 9-3). In late first and second stages of labor, pain impulses increasingly originate from pain-sensitive areas in the perineum (pelvic floor distention, vagina) and travel via somatic nerve fibers of the pudendal nerve to enter the neuraxis at the second, third, and fourth sacral segments. The afferent sensory component of pain can be largely relieved by blockade of the neural pathways at several anatomic sites (Figs. 9-1 and 9-4).

PREPARATION FOR REGIONAL BLOCKADE

Guidelines for safe patient care in regional anesthesia in obstetrics have been put forth by the ASA and are contained in Appendix A. Before initiating a regional block, preparation must be made for potential complications, which could include total spinal anesthesia, systemic toxicity from local anesthetics accidentally injected intravenously, and hemodynamic or airway sequelae. Regional anesthesia must be initiated and maintained only in an area where resuscitation equipment and drugs are immediately available. Equipment, facilities, and support personnel available in the labor and delivery operating suite should be similar to those available in the main operating suite (3). Necessary equipment includes a positive-pressure breathing apparatus for ventilating with 100% oxygen, appropriate suction device, airway equipment (including oral and nasal airways, laryngoscopes, endotracheal tubes, and stylets), and drugs for managing the airway and supporting the circulation to manage procedurally related complications of regional anesthesia. Alternative devices for securing the airway such as the laryngeal mask airway (LMA) should be readily available. In addition, each labor room should be equipped with an oxygen supply and suction, and a bed that rapidly can be placed in the Trendelenburg (head-down) position. An equipment list that should be readily available for maternal resuscitation is listed in Table 9-3.

TECHNIQUES OF REGIONAL ANESTHESIA

Lumbar Epidural Anesthesia (Table 9-4 and Figs. 9-4–9-6)

Lumbar epidural analgesic techniques for labor are characterized by numerous variations of drug regimens, including those with and without local anesthetics, opioids, and/or epinephrine, and some that include other, more novel agents such as clonidine. Advocates and rationale for various regimens depend on many factors, including patient expectations, staffing and availability of anesthesiologists, and institutional expectations. Below are recommended techniques commonly used for the provision of lumbar epidural anesthesia.

Once labor has been well established, and the obstetrician or midwife has consulted the patient, and the patient has requested epidural analgesia for pain relief, has been evaluated, and consent obtained, a continuous epidural infusion (CEI), patient controlled epidural analgesia (PCEA), or CSE may be administered. Epidural analgesia is appropriate at any time of labor when the parturient experiences painful uterine contractions, providing there are no medical or obstetric

TABLE 9-1 Regional Anesthesia Advantages

Provides superior pain relief during first and second stages of labor
Facilitates patient cooperation during labor and delivery
Decreases maternal hyperventilation and improves fetal acid–base status
Decreases maternal plasma catecholamines
Optimizes uteroplacental circulation, oxygenation, and function
Allows for an awake mother who can interact immediately with her baby
Decreases risk of airway loss, apnea, and aspiration associated with general anesthesia
Provides anesthesia for episiotomy or instrumental vaginal delivery
Allows extension of anesthesia for cesarean delivery
Avoids opioid-induced maternal and neonatal respiratory depression

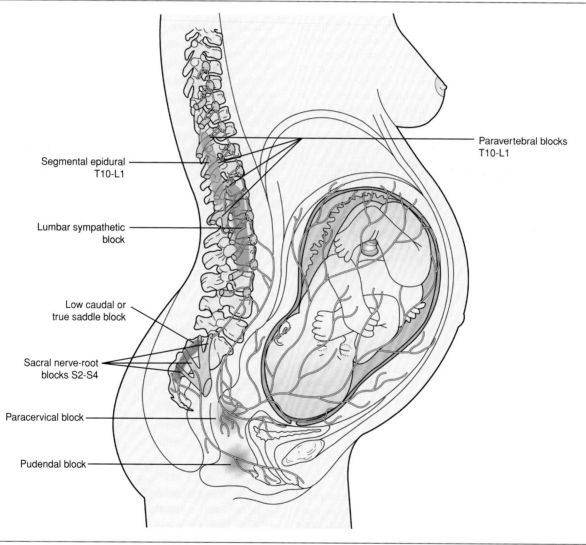

FIGURE 9-1 Specific blocks and pathways of labor pain. Labor pain has a visceral component and a somatic component. Uterine contractions may result in myometrial ischemia, causing the release of potassium, bradykinin, histamine, and serotonin. In addition, stretching and distention of the lower segments of the uterus and the cervix stimulate mechanoreceptors. These noxious impulses follow sensory-nerve fibers that accompany sympathetic nerve endings, traveling through the paracervical region and the pelvic and hypogastric plexus to enter the lumbar sympathetic chain. Through the white rami communicantes of the T10, T11, T12, and L1 spinal nerves, they enter the dorsal horn of the spinal cord. These pathways could be mapped successfully by a demonstration that blockade at different levels along this path (sacral nerve-root blocks S2 through S4, pudendal block, paracervical block, low caudal or true saddle block, lumbar sympathetic block, segmental epidural blocks T10 through L1, and paravertebral blocks T10 through L1) can alleviate the visceral component of labor pain. Reprinted with permission from: Eltzschig HK, Lieberman ES, Camann WR. Regional anesthesia and analgesia for labor and delivery. *N Engl J Med* 2003;348(4):320.

TABLE 9-2 Labor Analgesia Techniques

Continuous Epidural Infusion (CEI)
Patient Controlled Epidural Analgesia (PCEA)
Combined Spinal–Epidural (CSE)
Intravenous/Patient Controlled Analgesia (PCA) Narcotics
Nitrous-oxide inhalation (Nitronox®, Entonox®)
Other Inhalation Agents (sevoflurane)
Trancutaneous Electrical Nerve Stimulation (TENS)
Acupuncture
Lamaze
Birthing Ball
Hypnosis
Doula (Coach)

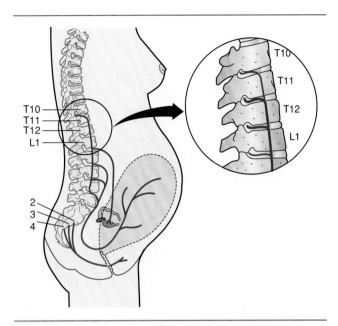

FIGURE 9-2 Parturition pain pathways. Afferent pain impulses from the cervix and uterus are carried by nerves that accompany sympathetic fibers and enter the neuraxis at T10, T11, T12, and L1 spinal levels. Pain pathways from the perineum travel to S2, S3, and S4 via the pudendal nerve. Reprinted with permission from: Bonica JJ. The nature of pain of parturition. *Clin Obstet Gynaecol* 1975;2:511.

contraindications. In the past, epidural analgesia had been withheld until a parturient was in the active phase of labor (4 to 6 cm dilated), or was experiencing strong uterine contractions lasting 1 minute or longer at regular intervals of 3 minutes. This has been the source of considerable controversy, but there is no evidence that administering an epidural analgesic in early labor is harmful (4). Both the ASA and the American College of Obstetricians and Gynecologists (ACOG) endorse practice guidelines which advocate that neuraxial analgesia should not be withheld on the basis of achieving an arbitrary cervical dilation, and neuraxial analgesia should be offered on an individual basis and on patient request (3).

After placement of a needle or catheter in the epidural space, either a specific test dose or testing regimen (see later) must be used to help rule out accidental subarachnoid or intravenous (IV) placement (Table 9-4). Analgesia is then established by injecting a local anesthetic and/or opioid (Table 9-4). The mother is tilted to her side to prevent

aortocaval compression. If unilateral analgesia occurs, the patient is turned to the opposite side and more local anesthetic (5 to 10 mL) is injected. When continuous infusion techniques are used, sufficient perineal anesthesia is usually achieved by the time of delivery and a perineal dose of local anesthetic is usually not required for spontaneous vaginal delivery. When intermittent injections are used during labor, segmental analgesia is provided during labor with repeated injections until perineal anesthesia is required. When

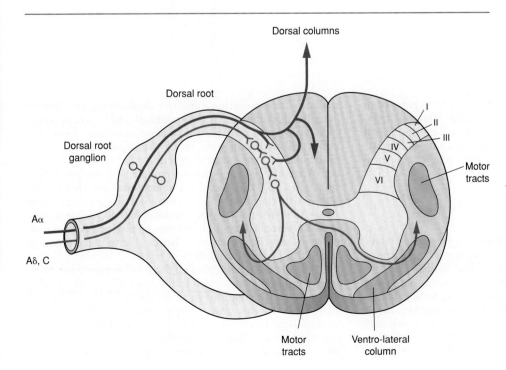

FIGURE 9-3 Schematic cross section of the spinal cord. A-delta and C fibers make multiple synaptic connections in the dorsal horn. Cell bodies in lamina V send axons to the ipsilateral and contralateral ventral column to make up the spinothalamic system. Reprinted with permission from: Bonica JJ. The nature of pain of parturition. *Clin Obstet Gynaecol* 1975;2:500.

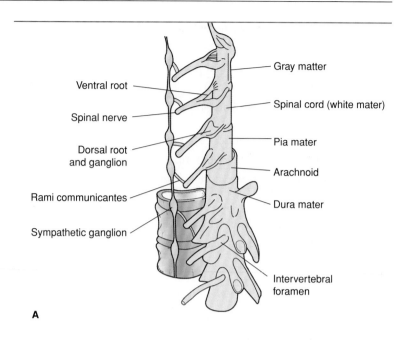

A

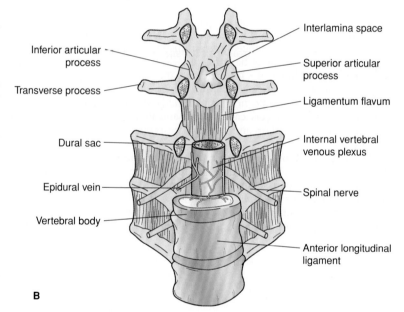

B

FIGURE 9-4 A: The spinal cord and its related structures. Reprinted with permission from: Bridenbaugh PO, Greene NM, Brull SJ. Spinal (subarachnoid) neural blockade. In: Cousins MJ, Bridenbaugh PO, eds. *Neural Blockade in Clinical Anesthesia and Management of Pain.* Philadelphia, PA: Lippincott–Raven Publishers; 1998:203–241. **B:** An anterior view demonstrates the relationship between the epidural space, dura, arachnoid, and pia membranes. Note the large number of veins that are in continuity with the veins draining the vertebral body. Reprinted with permission from: Macintosh RR. Lumbar puncture and spinal analgesia. Edinburgh: E & S Livingstone, 1957. Reprinted in Cousins MJ, Veering BT. Epidural neural blockade. In: Cousins MJ, Bridenbaugh PO, eds. *Neural Blockade in Clinical Anesthesia and Management of Pain.* Philadelphia, PA: Lippincott–Raven Publishers; 1998:243–321.

there is perineal distention by the fetal presenting part, 10 to 15 mL of drug can be administered; either lidocaine 1.0% to 2.0% or 2-chloroprocaine 2% or 3% will produce rapid onset of profound analgesia and muscle relaxation. Bupivacaine 0.125% or 0.25% can also be used to augment perineal analgesia.

Continuous Infusion Lumbar Epidural Anesthesia (Tables 9-4 and 9-5)

The use of a CEI of epidural local anesthetics provides greater quality of analgesia compared with parenteral (i.e., intravenous or intramuscular) opioids (1,3). The addition of opioids to epidural local anesthetics has been shown to improve analgesia with reduced motor block and maternal side effects (e.g., hypotension) compared with higher concentrations of local anesthetics without opioids (3). The lowest concentration of local anesthetic infusion (i.e., ≤0.125% bupivacaine) with or without an opioid that provides adequate maternal

analgesia and satisfaction should be administered to minimize potential side effects such as motor block and hypotension (3).

A CEI allows a stable therapeutic anesthetic level, and avoids fluctuations in pain relief often found with conventional intermittent epidural injections during labor. A number of studies have suggested significant advantages to this approach (5,6). Because of the dilute local anesthetic solutions used, the amount of motor block is minimal. This allows the parturient greater mobility in bed. Pelvic muscle tone is maintained, possibly decreasing the incidence of malposition, and the parturient is better able to make expulsive efforts during the second stage of labor.

Compared to intermittent epidural bolus injections, there are fewer hypotensive episodes during CEIs (5–8), possibly due to fewer fluctuations in sympathetic block. CEI offers advantages to the busy anesthesiologist in that without intermittent injections, there is no need for the time-consuming repeat test doses or the necessary close monitoring of the patient after a reinjection. This does not mean,

TABLE 9-3 Suggested Resources for Airway Management during Initial Provision of Neuraxial Anesthesia

Positive-pressure breathing apparatus
Pulse oximeter
Laryngoscope and various sized assorted curved and straight blades
Endotracheal tubes (adult—6.0, 6.5, 7.0, 7.5) with stylets
Qualitative carbon dioxide detector
Oral and nasal airways
Laryngeal mask airways
Video laryngoscope (e.g., Glidoscope®, C-Mac®)
Supplies for venous access and fluid resuscitation
Oxygen supply, suction, and bed capable of rapid Trendelenburg position
Equipment and drugs for CPR (including a defribrillator)

however, that the anesthesiologist can ignore the patient following establishment of the block (Table 9-6). To safely achieve optimum analgesia and patient satisfaction, the anesthesiologist should examine and interview the patient at regular intervals. At those times, he or she can make necessary adjustments in the infusion rate or concentration of local anesthetic, and detect any signs of intravascular or subarachnoid migration of the catheter. Between visits, trained labor and delivery nurses must closely monitor the patient.

A variety of infusion devices may be used for delivery of continuous epidural analgesia. However, it is important that the device used has a number of safety features. The flow rate should be accurate, adjustable, and locked so that the flow rate cannot be changed by accident. The solution reservoir and tubing should be clearly and prominently labeled, and precautions must be taken to eliminate the possibility of unintentional injection of other drugs by mistake.

Potential complications of this technique are intravascular or subarachnoid migration of the catheter during the infusion, or the development of progressively higher levels of anesthesia with resulting hypotension and respiratory difficulties. It is unlikely that serious complications would occur with the

TABLE 9-4 Lumbar Epidural Anesthesia for Labor and Vaginal Delivery: Suggested Technique

1. Evaluate patient and obtain consent.
2. Verify that the patient has been examined by an individual qualified in obstetrics; the maternal and fetal status and progress of labor have been evaluated, and a physician is readily available to manage any obstetric complications that arise.
3. Check resuscitation equipment and oxygen-delivery system.
4. Assure adequate venous access (18 gauge plastic indwelling catheter is usually sufficient) and proper functioning. Administration of a fixed volume of intravenous fluid is not required before epidural catheter placement.
5. Apply blood pressure cuff and check baseline maternal pressure.
6. Position patient: sitting position (useful in very obese patients) or lateral position. Have labor and delivery nurse available to reassure patient, to help with positioning and monitoring, and to prevent patient movement during placement of the block.
7. Palpate lumbar spinous processes and choose widest vertebral interspace below L3.
8. Wash back with an appropriate antiseptic solution and drape the lumbar area.
9. Confirm area of insertion by palpating insertion point and give local anesthesia.
10. Place an epidural needle (17 gauge to 18 gauge) in the epidural space in the usual manner.
    a. Midline approach is most popular but lateral or paramedian approach can also be used.
    b. Use loss-of-resistance technique with saline- (or air-)filled syringe.
11. Administer 3–5 mL preservative-free saline or dilute local anesthetic to facilitate passage of the catheter.
12. Insert epidural catheter and remove needle. Catheter should be threaded 3–5 mL into the epidural space (threading further may increase incidence of one-sided or single dermatome blocks; threading less makes dislodgement from epidural space more common).
13. Aspirate for blood or cerebrospinal fluid.
14. Administer a test dose (see text for discussion). Use of a 3 mL test dose of local anesthetic containing epinephrine 1:200,000 (5 μg mL^{-1}) is most common. Observe for heart rate increase within 60 s or evidence of spinal blockade within 3–5 min. If test dose is negative, administer additional drug in divided doses as required to obtain desired pain relief.
15. Maintain patient in lateral tilted (nonsupine) position throughout labor to prevent aortocaval compression.
16. Monitor blood pressure every 1–2 min for the first 10 min after injection of local anesthetic, then every 10–30 min until the block wars off. In some patients, more frequent assessments may be indicated.
17. During the first 20 min after the initial dose, the patient must be monitored and not left unattended. Hypotension or other sequelae may also occur after a top-up dose, and the patient should be appropriately monitored.
18. If hypotension occurs (decrease in systolic blood pressure greater than 20–30% of baseline or below 100 mm Hg), ensure LUD, infuse intravenous fluids rapidly, and, if necessary, administer ephedrine 5–15 mg IV or phenylephrine 40–160 μ IV. If hypotension persists, administer additional vasopressor and oxygen.
19. Monitor fetal heart rate and uterine contractions continuously by electronic means before and after instituting an epidural block.
20. Aspirate catheter for blood or cerebrospinal fluid before each top-up dose. Consider a test dose. Bolus doses should be fractionated.
21. After delivery, remove catheter and ensure the tip of the catheter is removed intact.

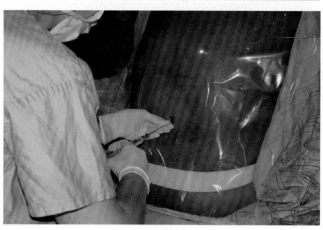

FIGURE 9-5 Loss-of-resistance technique for identifying the epidural space. Needle is placed in the interspinous ligament, and resistance to pressure on plunger of syringe is determined. Needle is stabilized with left hand, while thumb of right hand apples intermittent pressure to the plunger. Needle is slowly advanced with both hands to prevent too rapid progression and inadvertent dural puncture. Following each incremental advance, intermittent pressure is applied to the plunger until loss-of-resistance is felt.

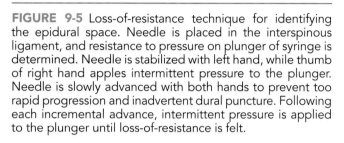

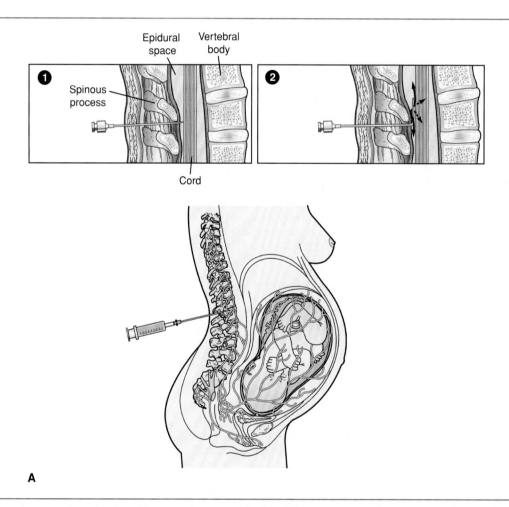

FIGURE 9-6 Technique of Epidural analgesia and CSE. Epidural analgesia (Panel A) is achieved by placement of a catheter into the lumbar epidural space (1). After the desired intervertebral space (e.g., between L3 and L4) has been identified and infiltrated with local anesthetic, a hollow epidural needle is placed in the intervertebral ligaments. These ligaments are characterized by a high degree of resistance to penetration. A syringe connected to the epidural needle allows the anesthesiologist to confirm the resistance of these ligaments. In contrast, the epidural space has a low degree of resistance. When the anesthesiologist slowly advances the needle while feeling for resistance, he or she recognizes the epidural space by a sudden loss of resistance as the epidural needle enters the epidural space (2). Next, an epidural catheter is advanced into the space. Solutions of a local anesthetic, opioids, or a combination of the two can now be administered through the catheter. (*continued*)

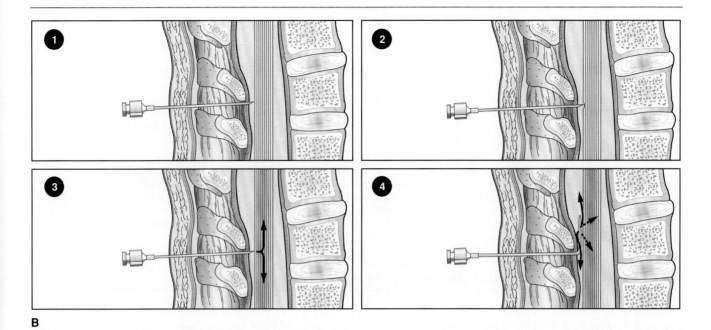

B

FIGURE 9-6 (*Continued*) For CSE (Panel B), the lumbar epidural space is also identified with an epidural needle (1). Next, a very thin spinal needle is introduced through the epidural needle into the subarachnoid space (2). Correct placement can be confirmed by free flow of cerebrospinal fluid. A single bolus of local anesthetic, opioid, or a combination of the two is injected through this needle into the subarachnoid space (3). Subsequently, the needle is removed, and a catheter is advanced into the epidural space through the epidural needle (4). When the single-shot spinal analgesic wears off, the epidural catheter can be used for the continuation of pain relief. Reprinted with permission from: Eltzschig HK, Lieberman ES, Camann WR. Regional anesthesia and analgesia for labor and delivery. *N Engl J Med* 2003;348(4):323.

technique as outlined above. Significant systemic toxicity is usually avoided if the catheter migrates into a blood vessel because of the very low infusion rate and low concentration of local anesthetic. The principal "side effect" would be loss of pain relief. For example, bupivacaine 0.125% infused at 10 mL/h would only inject 12.5 mg of drug per hour—an amount that would not cause systemic toxicity, but which would not produce any analgesic effect.

Should the epidural catheter accidently be sited intrathecally, the onset of motor block would be slow and easily diagnosed. For example, bupivacaine 0.125% infused at 10 mL/h over a 30-minute period would deliver 6.25 mg bupivacaine into the subarachnoid space, an amount that would prevent the patient from raising her legs, thereby alerting the staff to an intrathecal injection. Even with higher infusion rates of dilute solutions, the unexpectedly and generally slowly ascending sensory level would be easily recognized. Despite the inherent safety of continuous infusion for obstetric anesthesia, mishaps can still occur. Experienced, trained, vigilant medical and nursing staff must be immediately and readily available to manage possible complications of epidural analgesia.

TABLE 9-5 CEI and PCEA Drug Regimens for Lumbar Epidural Anesthesia for Labor and Vaginal Delivery

1. Epidural catheter is positioned and placement verified as described in Table 9-4.
2. Following (usually) a test dose with lidocaine 1.5% + epinephrine 1:200,000, initial bolus options include:
   a. Bupivacaine 0.06–0.125% (10–15 mL) ± fentanyl 50–100 μg (or sufentanil 5–10 μg)
   b. Ropivacaine 0.1–0.2% (10–15 mL) ± fentanyl 50–100 μg (or sufentanil 5–10 μg)
3. Subsequent analgesia options include:
   a. Intermittent boluses—repeat as above, as necessary, to maintain maternal comfort
   b. Continuous infusions—10–15 mL/h
      i. Bupivacaine 0.0625–0.125% + fentanyl 1–2 μg mL^{-1} (or sufentanil 0.1–0.3, 1–2 μg mL^{-1})
   c. PCEA
      i.   Initial bolus as in 2a or 2b above
      ii. Basal infusion of 5–10 mL/h bupivacaine as in 3b (continuous infusion) above
      iii. Demand bolus dose of 5–10 mL bupivacaine as in 3b (continuous infusion) above
      iv. Lockout interval of 5–15 min
      v.   Total 1 h lockout of 20–25 mL or 4 h lockout of 80–100 mL
4. If perineal anesthesia is required, administer 10–15 mL local anesthetic, lidocaine 1.0–2.0% or chloroprocaine 2–3% or bupivacaine 0.25%

Note: Equipotent doses of local anesthetics, including bupivacaine, chloroprocaine, lidocaine, levobupivacaine, and ropivacaine, can be used interchangeably.
PCEA, patient controlled epidural analgesia.

TABLE 9-6 Labor Epidural Analgesia Monitoring

1. Place epidural catheter in usual manner.
2. Use appropriate test dose regimen to rule out accidental intravascular or subarachnoid injection.
3. Start infusion at appropriate time (depending on agent used for initial block).
4. Check sensory level and adequacy of anesthesia regularly. Adjust infusion rate based on dermatomal level. Increase concentration of local anesthetic or add opioid if block is not adequate.
5. Maintain patient in lateral tilted position throughout labor to prevent aortocaval compression. Patient should turn from side to side approximately every 1 h to avoid an asymmetric block.
6. Monitor blood pressure every 1–2 min for the first 10 min after initial injection of local anesthetic, then every 10–30 min during the infusion and until the block wears off.
7. Ability of the patient to lift legs should be checked regularly to monitor motor block.
8. Careful nursing supervision is mandatory.
9. Diminishing analgesia may indicate intravascular migration. A repeat test dose should be administered before any bolus injections.
10. Development of dense motor block may indicate subarachnoid migration. Catheter location should be verified by aspiration, careful sensory motor examination, and, if necessary, cautious administration of a test dose.

Patient Controlled Epidural Analgesia (PCEA) (Table 9-5)

Gambling in 1988 was the first to describe PCEA (9). PCEA can be provided as demand dose only or in combination with a continuous background infusion. Compared to CEI, advantages of PCEA include less local anesthetic consumption (3,9–11), decreased anesthesia personnel work-load with fewer anesthetic interventions, equivalent or improved analgesia (3,9), increased patient satisfaction (3,9), greater patient participation, control, and autonomy over pain relief (9), and less motor blockade (3). PCEA may be used with or without a background infusion (3); however, a fixed continuous background infusion may allow for a more stable therapeutic analgesic level with improved analgesia and less need for intervention (i.e., "top-ups") by the anesthesia provider (3,12).

Solutions used for PCEA are the same as those used for CEI analgesia. The anesthesia provider can manipulate the infusion solution (local anesthesia/opioid concentration), patient controlled bolus volume, lockout interval, background infusion rate, and maximum allowable dose per hour. It should be noted that the ideal PCEA parameters (i.e., bolus dose, lockout interval, background infusion rate) have not been determined. Recommended PCEA drug regimens and infusion parameters are presented in Table 9-5.

In a meta-analysis of nine randomized controlled trials comparing PCEA without a background infusion versus CEI, van der Vyer et al. (11) found there were fewer anesthetic interventions, less local anesthetic requirement, and less motor block, equivalent maternal satisfaction, and no differences in maternal or neonatal outcome.

In summary, PCEA offers many advantages over CEI and provides a highly effective and flexible approach for the maintenance of labor analgesia (3).

Programmed Intermittent Epidural Bolus (PIEB)

Programmed intermittent epidural bolus (PIEB) dosing compared with CEI used with or without PCEA has been studied. It seems that when larger epidural volumes are administered under high pressure, distribution of anesthetic solutions in the epidural space is more uniform. In a study on cadavers, Hogan noticed that epidural spread is much more uniform when larger volumes are given with corresponding higher injectate pressures, while low-pressure continuous infusions

are associated with uneven distribution in the epidural space (13). Similarly, in comparing CEI to an intermittent hourly bolus dose of the same solution, Fettes et al. (14) found that regular intermittent epidural administration is associated with reduced need for epidural rescue medication, less epidural drug use, and equivalent pain relief when compared with CEI. Fettes concluded that intermittent boluses result in more uniform spread, giving more reliable analgesia than CEI (14).

In a clinical study, Wong et al. (15) compared automated PIEB every 30 minutes beginning 45 minutes after the intrathecal injection in multiparous patients with CEI (12 mL/h infusion) in laboring parturients, and found that PIEB combined with PCEA provided similar analgesia, but with a smaller bupivacaine dose, fewer manual rescue boluses, and better patient satisfaction compared with CEI. Likewise, Sia et al. (16) found that PIEB delivered as an automated bolus every hour combined with PCEA reduced analgesic consumption and the need for parturients' self-bolus of analgesics compared with CEI. In both studies, the total dose of local anesthetic was smaller in the automated bolus groups than in the continuous infusion groups. In another PIEB study by Wong et al. (17), they compared PIEB alone (without the combination of PCEA) and found that extending the PIEB interval and volume from 15 to 60 minutes, and 2.5 to 10 mL decreased bupivacaine consumption without decreasing patient comfort or satisfaction.

In summary PIEB can result in less local anesthetic consumption, less breakthrough pain, and improved patient satisfaction compared with CEI or PCEA with a continuous basal infusion. However, the greatest impediment to implementation of PIEB analgesia is the lack of commercial pumps designed to deliver timed boluses or time boluses with PCEA. Further studies are needed to determine the optimal combination of bolus volume, time interval, and drug concentrations for use with this technique.

Spinal Anesthesia

Spinal anesthesia, also referred to as a saddle block, is often administered when a patient is in advanced labor. It can provide immediate analgesia when there is not enough time for placement of an epidural catheter. For a true saddle block, a small dose of hyperbaric local anesthetic (e.g., bupivacaine 4 to 5 mg, lidocaine 15 to 20 mg, or tetracaine 3 mg, with or without fentanyl 10 to 25 μg, or sufentanil 2.5 to 5 μg) is injected into the subarachnoid space with the patient in the sitting position, to accomplish sacral-only anesthesia.

More commonly, however, a wider dermatomal anesthetic distribution (T10 to S5) is desired and can be accomplished with slightly larger doses of bupivacaine (7.5 mg), lidocaine (30 mg), or tetracaine (4 mg) with or without an opioid (fentanyl 10 to 25 μg, or sufentanil 2.5 to 5 μg). Small-bore, pencil-point spinal needles will decrease the incidence of postdural puncture headache (PDPH) (18–20).

The degree to which spinal anesthesia can be confined to sacral, or even to low thoracic dermatomes is limited and not directly related to the dose of subarachnoid local anesthetic (21). Hyperbaric solutions tend to ascend to mid- or upper thoracic dermatomes regardless of dose. One-shot spinal anesthesia is therefore rarely used in modern practice.

Intermittent and Continuous Spinal Anesthesia (Table 9-7)

Passing a catheter into the subarachnoid space has several potential advantages: (1) Provision of rapid analgesia or anesthesia, (2) allows flexibility in medication dosing of small amounts of local anesthetic or opioid, *perhaps* limiting the degree of sympathectomy and hypotension, which can be particularly useful for high-risk patients in whom an unplanned high block may produce serious cardiovascular or respiratory problems, (3) the morbidly obese parturient in whom placement of an epidural is technically difficult or impossible (22), and (4) placing an epidural catheter into the subarachnoid space following an accidental dural puncture during a planned epidural ("wet tap"). When this situation occurs, the anesthesiologist may choose to insert the epidural catheter into the subarachnoid space proceed with intermittent or continuous spinal anesthesia. After delivery, the intrathecal catheter can be left in place for 24 hours before removal, which has been shown in some but not all studies to decrease the incidence of PDPH (19).

Disadvantages of the technique include the increased risk for infection (meningitis, arachnoiditis) and nerve trauma, which have not proven to be a significant problem in clinical practice. Concern regarding the use of a large-bore needle commonly used for continuous techniques producing an unacceptably high incidence of PDPH also has not been consistently supported by clinical studies in nonpregnant patients (23–25). However, many obstetric anesthesiologists find the rate of PDPH when unintentional dural puncture occurs and is managed with an intrathecal (epidural) catheter to be too high to allow for routine elective use.

Spinal microcatheters that pass through a standard 25 or 26 gauge spinal needle have been investigated in the past, and are not currently marketed in the United States. In 1992, the US Food and Drug Administration removed intrathecal microcatheters (27 to 32 gauge) from clinical use after reports of neurologic injury in nonobstetric patients (26–30). Larger gauge spinal catheters have been investigated (31). Alonso studied continuous spinal anesthesia using an over-the-needle 22 or 2 -gauge spinal catheter and found an unacceptably high block failure rate and PDPH rate (31).

More recently, in a prospective, randomized, multicenter trial, Arkoosh et al. (32) examined the safety and efficacy of a 28 gauge intrathecal catheter for labor analgesia using bupivacaine and sufentanil compared to conventional epidural analgesia and found that the intrathecal technique was associated with increased technical difficulties (more difficult to remove) and catheter failures compared with traditional epidural analgesia. Importantly, there were zero cases of adverse neurologic sequelae. Nonetheless, spinal microcatheters have not found a market in the United States after the earlier failures. Novel devices for continuous spinal anesthesia have been explored, including the Wiley spinal device (an over-the-needle system utilizing a small-bore pencil-point needle for the dural puncture) and may be promising alternatives (33).

Combined Spinal–epidural Analgesia (Table 9-8 and Figs. 9-6 and 9-7)

CSE analgesia in labor has become a popular technique in many obstetric centers. The CSE technique combines the benefits of spinal anesthesia including rapid onset of analgesia and confirmation of correct needle placement (CSF flow) with the benefits of epidural anesthesia (34–36). After the spinal anesthesia wears off, the epidural catheter can be dosed in the usual fashion and used for labor analgesia or anesthesia. The CSE technique can also be used to provide anesthesia for cesarean delivery and other surgical procedures (37).

CSE kits can be purchased individually from several manufacturers. The CSE technique can also be performed by placing a standard epidural needle in the usual manner at L3–L4 or L4–L5, and then placing a long spinal needle (24 gauge or smaller and 124 mm or longer) through the epidural needle to enter the subarachnoid space. For labor analgesia, an opioid such as fentanyl (10 to 25 μg) or sufentanil (2.5 to 10 μg) may be injected alone or in combination with a local anesthetic such as plain bupivacaine (1 to 2.5 mg) to provide pain relief for approximately 90 minutes (range: 20 to 245 minutes) (34–36).

TABLE 9-7 Continuous Spinal Anesthesia

1. Lumbar puncture is performed in the usual manner. Any approach to the subarachnoid space may be used. A standard epidural needle is placed.
2. The bevel of the epidural needle can be positioned laterally (i.e., parallel to the long axis of the spinal cord) until the dura is pierced, then directed cephalad.
3. The catheter is passed only 2–3 cm beyond the tip of the needle. This distance is sufficient to prevent accidental dislodgement but short enough to prevent curling or passage of the catheter into a dural sleeve. If the catheter cannot be threaded into the subarachnoid space, the needle and the catheter should be withdrawn together and the procedure repeated. A catheter should never be withdrawn through a needle because a portion of it may be sheared off. The use of spinal microcatheters is not currently recommended.
4. After the catheter has been inserted, the needle is slowly withdrawn over the catheter, taking care not to simultaneously remove the catheter.
5. Aspiration of cerebrospinal fluid indicates proper placement of the catheter.
6. A local anesthetic solution or opioid may be used. Drugs are usually administered in a volume of at least 1.0–1.5 mL.
7. Suggested drugs are hyperbaric lidocaine (15–30 mg), bupivacaine (2.5–7.5 mg), sufentanil (2.5–5–10 μg), fentanyl (10–25 μg), or morphine (25–100 μg).

TABLE 9-8 CSE Analgesia for Vaginal Delivery: Suggested Technique

1. Check resuscitation equipment and anesthesia machine prior to block.
2. Assure intravenous access and administer a fluid bolus before starting block.
3. Apply blood pressure cuff and check baseline blood pressure.
4. Position patient. The sitting position is most common. Lateral decubitus with reverse Trendelenburg may be used, especially if there is a preterm infant or a multigravida in whom fetal descent may be very rapid.
5. Prepare and drape lumbar area.
6. Palpate lumbar spinous process and choose widest interspace below L3.
7. Place epidural needle as described in Table 9.4 using loss of resistance technique. Next, insert long 124 mm (5 in.) small-gauge (22–27), noncutting, pencil-point needle through epidural needle into the intrathecal space.
8. Inject opioid (fentanyl 15–25 μg or sufentanil 5–10 μg) with or without plain bupivacaine 1.5–2.5 mg between uterine contractions.
9. Monitor blood pressure every 1–2 min for the first 10 min after injection of local anesthetic, then every 5–10 min.
10. If hypotension occurs (decrease in systolic blood pressure greater than 20–30% of baseline or below 100 mm Hg), ensure LUD, infuse intravenous fluids rapidly, and place patient in 10–20-degree Trendelenburg position. If blood pressure is not restored promptly, administer ephedrine 5–15 mm Hg or phenylephrine 40–160 μg intravenously. If hypotension persists, administer additional vasopressor and oxygen.

In many institutions, intrathecal fentanyl alone is a common choice for CSE. In one study, the median effective dose was 14 μg (95% confidence interval, 13 to 15 μg), and there was no benefit shown in increasing the dose beyond 25 μg (35). In another study, the mean duration of intrathecal sufentanil (10 μg) for labor analgesia was 102 $\pm$ 49.8 minutes (36), though lower doses (5 μg) may be sufficient. After the intrathecal dose is administered, an epidural catheter is then placed for further administration of local anesthetic for labor analgesia or instrumental surgical delivery as needed. For labor, an epidural infusion initiated with a bolus of bupivacaine 0.0625% to 0.125% with 0.0002% fentanyl (2 μg/mL) or an equivalent dose of ropivacaine or levobupivacaine. Alternatively, a continuous infusion or PCEA may be initiated without a bolus

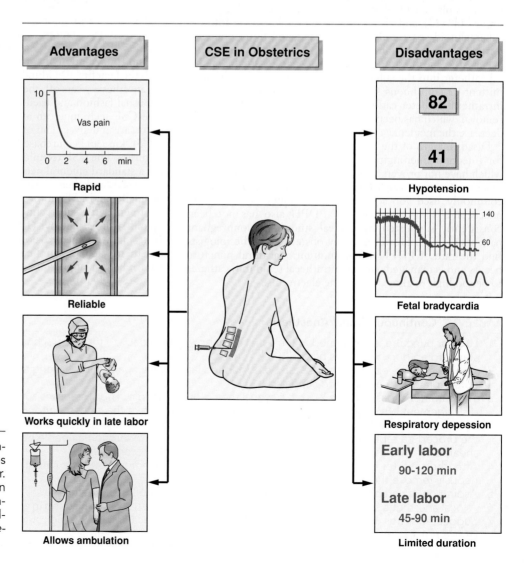

FIGURE 9-7 The advantages and disadvantages of CSE analgesia for labor. Reprinted with permission from: Eisenach JC. Combined spinal-epidural analgesia in obstetrics. *Anesthesiology* 1999;91:299–302.

immediately following the intrathecal injection and insertion of the epidural catheter. The transition from intrathecal to epidural analgesia is typically nearly seamless.

When the CSE technique is used for labor, it has the benefit of allowing maternal ambulation if desired, and is often referred to as the walking epidural. While walking itself with CSE (38), or without neuraxial analgesia (39), may not offer any real advantages with respect to labor duration, augmentation with oxytocin, delivery outcome, maternal, or fetal complications, walking using the CSE technique can be safely done and may be appealing to some parturients (40,41). However, specific criteria to allow walking must be developed and followed if accidents are to be avoided (42). Even if ambulation is not encouraged, establishing analgesia promptly with minimal initial motor blockade is not only satisfying to the patient, but to the obstetricians and nurses as well.

In comparing labor analgesia using epidural anesthesia or CSE in nulliparous and parous women, no significant differences were observed in duration of labor, mode of delivery, local anesthetic consumed, or maternal or fetal complications (42–44).

Side Effects of CSE (Fig. 9-7)

The side effects of the CSE technique are similar to those encountered with epidural or intrathecal opioids combined with those of spinal anesthesia. They include pruritus, nausea, vomiting, hypotension, respiratory depression, PDPH, urinary retention, and fetal heart rate (FHR) abnormalities (Table 9-9) (45). The most common side effect of the CSE is pruritus, which has been reported to occur in 80% of patients

receiving intrathecal sufentanil (45,46); however, few of these patients require treatment. Hypotension occurs in 5% to 10% of patients who receive intrathecal fentanyl or sufentanil (47,48). The incidence of hypotension is similar to that seen with routine labor epidural analgesia and is treated in the same manner. Nausea and vomiting (2% to 3%), respiratory depression (very rare), and PDPH (1% or less) are not common and can be managed fairly easily (Table 9-9).

However, FHR abnormalities with the CSE technique are more common (47,49,50). Three nonrandomized studies have reported that the risk of fetal bradycardia is similar after intrathecal sufentanil or epidural bupivacaine (51–53). Meta-analysis of multiple randomized trials comparing intrathecal and epidural analgesia found a modest increase in FHR abnormalities (odds ratio 1.8 [95% confidence interval 1.0 to 3.1], number-needed-to-harm 28) but not in adverse fetal outcomes or emergency cesarean delivery (54). FHR abnormalities occur commonly during labor and have been reported to occur with IV meperidine, paracervical blocks, epidural local anesthetics, and intrathecal opioids (55). It has also been suggested that women in severe pain, or with induced labor may be at a greater risk for FHR changes (53), and that a selection bias may be created by administering CSE to these women (55). Management of FHR changes can include treatment of maternal hypotension, maternal position change (left uterine displacement [LUD]), supplemental oxygen administration, IV fluid bolus, and treatment of uterine hyperstimulation. Uterine hyperstimulation has been postulated as a possible mechanism for fetal bradycardia associated with the CSE technique (see Chapter 9) (50,55). Terbutaline (1.25 to 2.5 mg IV or subcutaneously) or nitroglycerin (50 to 200 μg IV or 400 to 800 g [two puffs]

TABLE 9-9 Side Effects of Intrathecal Opioids-CSE

Problems	Treatments	Comments
Pruritus	• Naloxone 40–100 μg IV • Nalbuphine 5–10 mg IV • Diphenhydramine 25 mg IV • Propofol 10 mg IV • Droperidol 0.0625 mg IV • Ondansetron 8 mg IV	10–25% may need some therapy, but few (<5%) have sever pruritus; more problematic with intrathecal morphine; treat early if patient is concerned
Hypotension	• IV fluids, maternal Positioning (LUD), and vasopressors (ephedrine, phenylephrine), as usual	Occurs in 5–10% of laboring women with intrathecal opioids; probably catecholamine mediated but cause unproven
Respiratory depression	• O$_2$ as needed (ventilation rarely necessary) • Naloxone 40–100 μg or more as indicated when previously opioids administered	Rarely clinically significant but has occurred with sufentanil 10 μg (lower dose [5 μg] may decrease incidence); depression immediately or at 0.5–5 h; more common
Nausea and vomiting	• Naloxone 40–100 μg, IV • Metoclopramide 5–10 mg, IV • Droperidol 0.0625 mg, IV • Other agents—ondansetron, Dolasetron, propofol (also see Pruritus above)	Often hard to differentiate from obstetric causes; use lowest effective dose of opioid
PDPH	• Postpartum management as needed; epidural blood patch highly effective	Headache uncommon (<1%); incidence similar to that with the use of routine epidural technique
Urinary retention	• Catheterization • Naloxone 400–800 μg may be required for treatment	Catheterization (single time) often provides resolution
FHR	• Maintain maternal BP, saturation, LUD • Fluids and ephedrine • Nitroglycerin (50–200 μg IV or 400–800 μg [1–2 puffs] sublingual)	Incidence unclear; mechanism not defined—sudden catecholamine changes and/or increased uterine tone implicated

LUD, left uterine displacement; PDPH, postdural puncture headache; FHR, fetal heart rate; BP, blood pressure; IV, intravenous.

TABLE 9-10 **Caudal Block for Labor and Vaginal Delivery**

1. Prepare as for epidural block (Table 9.4).
2. Position patient: Lateral is most commonly used, but prone position with bolster under hips is also popular. Have nurse available to reassure patient, to help with positioning, and to prevent movement during placement of the block.
3. Prepare and drape the caudal area.
4. Using the coccyx as a landmark for the midline, palpate the sacral hiatus and the sacrococcygeal ligament.
5. Place a 16 to 18 gauge epidural needle in the caudal canal in the usual manner.
    a. After positioning the needle, remove drapes and perform rectal examination to exclude the possibility of inadvertent puncture of the rectum, cervix, and fetal presenting part, and subsequent anesthetic intoxication of the fetus.
    b. Change glove, replace drape, and pass catheter through needle.
6. Aspirate for blood or cerebrospinal fluid.
7. Administer local anesthetic as for epidural anesthetic. For a T10 level, a total volume of 15–20 mL local anesthetic is often necessary.

sublingual) can be useful for treatment of uterine hyperstimulation. An alternative hypothesis is transient uterine vascular constriction following changes in maternal catecholamines (56). FHR abnormalities usually respond to this management and in a large retrospective review the incidence of emergency cesarean sections was no different in women receiving CSE for labor analgesia compared with either no regional technique or systemic medication (1.3% vs. 1.4%) (57). As noted earlier, the rate of emergency cesarean delivery also did not differ in a meta-analysis of RCTs comparing CSE to conventional epidural analgesia (54).

Caudal Anesthesia (Table 9-10 and Figs. 9-8–9-11)

A caudal block may be administered after labor is established. Caudal blocks are performed with patients positioned either on their side (Fig. 9-8) or prone with a bolster place under the thighs. Using the coccyx as a landmark for the midline, the sacral cornu and sacrococcygeal ligament are palpated (Figs. 9-9 and 9-10). When a caudal block is performed late in labor, or when the fetal head is in the perineum, a maternal rectal examination can be performed to exclude the possibility of accidental puncture of the fetal presenting part and subsequent anesthetic intoxication of the fetus (Fig. 9-11) (58). After aspiration, a test dose of local anesthetic is given through the needle and/or catheter, because it is possible to puncture the dural sac that ends at the second vertebra or a dural sleeve of a sacral nerve root, and thus produce spinal anesthesia. This area is a highly vascular space as well, and inadvertent IV injection is possible. In a review of obstetric epidural analgesia, signs of central nervous system toxicity occurred more frequently with the caudal approach (1 in 600) than with the lumbar route (1 in 3,500) (59). The volume of

local anesthetic necessary to provide a T10 block usually varies between 15 and 20 mL, with subsequent doses of 15 mL to maintain analgesia. Placing the patient in a head-down position, it may be necessary to achieve a T10 block with smaller volumes of drug. Very large volumes would be needed for a cesarean delivery, and thus the caudal block technique is an imprudent choice except for labor analgesia.

Insertion of two catheters (double-catheter technique), a lumbar epidural catheter for labor and a caudal catheter for vaginal delivery, was popular many years ago. It permitted one to achieve a segmental block (T10–L1) early in labor and then, at the time of delivery, by not injecting the lumbar epidural catheter but instead activating the caudal catheter, the mother would feel contractions, have maximal ability to push, and still have profound perineal analgesia. This technique is now rarely used because similar analgesia can be achieved with other techniques.

Lumbar epidural is preferable to caudal anesthesia for the following reasons: (1) Segmental T10 to T12 levels can be achieved in early labor when sacral anesthesia is not required, (2) less drug is needed during labor, (3) pelvic muscles retain their tone, and rotation of the fetal head is more easily accomplished, and (4) even though there is an increased risk of dural puncture, often a lumbar epidural is technically easier for the anesthesiologist to administer and less painful for the patient during the placement of the needle than a caudal anesthetic. Caudal anesthesia administered just before delivery was formerly recommended over lumbar epidural anesthesia in that the onset of perineal anesthesia and muscle relaxation is more rapid. However, use of the CSE technique in this setting allows for the rapid onset of analgesia with epidural catheter placement for potential surgical intervention. Thus, caudal anesthesia is rarely used today for analgesia during labor unless a lumbar epidural is contraindicated or technically difficult.

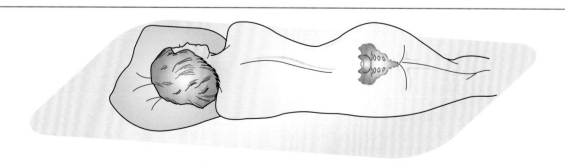

FIGURE 9-8 Lateral position for caudal block. Note forward tilt of upper hip. For the right-handed physician, the patient should lie on her left side.

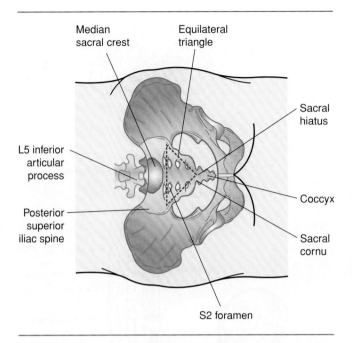

FIGURE 9-9 Sacrum, showing bony landmarks for identifying sacral cornua and sacral hiatus. Sacral hiatus is usually located 2.5 in. above the tip of coccyx or at the apex of an equilateral triangle formed by posterior-superior iliac spine and sacrococcygeal ligament.

Paracervical Block Anesthesia

Paracervical block is a relatively simple method used by obstetricians to provide analgesia during labor. Local anesthesia is injected submucosally into the fornix of the vagina lateral to the cervix. Frankenhauser's ganglion, containing all the visceral

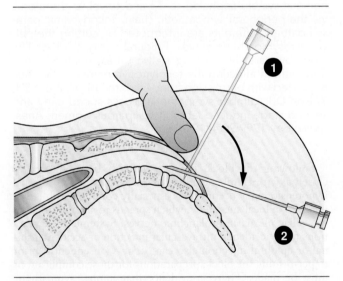

FIGURE 9-10 Technique of caudal anesthesia. Thumb is placed between sacral cornua at apex of sacral hiatus. Needle is inserted through sacrococcygeal ligament at an angle of approximately 45 degrees (needle position 1). Once the ligament is penetrated, the needle is repositioned as shown and advanced 1 to 2 cm into the caudal canal (needle position 2). The position of the caudal canal can be verified by rapidly injecting a 2 to 3 mL bolus of saline and not palpating an impulse under the fingertips.

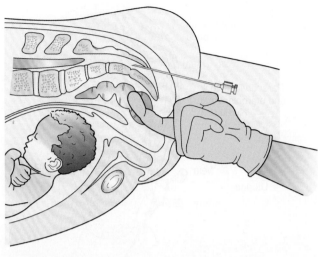

FIGURE 9-11 Prior to injection of medication or placement of catheter, a rectal examination is performed to rule out inadvertent misplacement of needle with rectal or fetal puncture.

sensory nerve fibers from the uterus, cervix, and upper vagina, is anesthetized. The somatic sensory fibers from the perineum are not blocked; thus, the technique is only effective during the first stage of labor. The major disadvantage of paracervical block anesthesia is the relatively high frequency of fetal bradycardia following the block. This bradycardia is associated with decreased fetal oxygenation fetal acidosis, and an increased likelihood of neonatal depression. Bradycardia usually develops within 2 to 10 minutes and lasts from 3 to 30 minutes. The etiology of bradycardia is still unclear, but evidence suggests that it is primarily related to decreased uterine blood flow from uterine vasoconstriction induced by the local anesthetic applied in close proximity to the artery (Fig. 9-12) (60,61).

Fetal bradycardia may be exacerbated by high fetal blood levels of local anesthetics (62). Fetal drug levels in infants with bradycardia are occasionally higher than simultaneously drawn maternal level, suggesting that local anesthetics may reach the fetus by a more direct route than maternal system absorption. Some investigators have postulated that high concentrations of local anesthetics reach the fetus by diffusion across the uterine arteries.

Although the precise cause of fetal bradycardia may be controversial, the significance is not. Paracervical block bradycardia indicates decreased fetal oxygenation. Incased neonatal morbidity and, mortality occur when bradycardia follows paracervical block. Because of the potential fetal and neonatal hazards, this technique should not be used when there is known uteroplacental insufficiency or preexisting concern for fetal well-being (e.g., an abnormal FHR tracing). There may be exceptions if other anesthetic techniques are contraindicated or pose a greater hazard to the mother or fetus.

When the technique is used, the drug dosage must be kept to a minimum. Safe use of this technique requires that injections be superficial (i.e., just below the mucosa), aspiration is performed before injection, and FHR is monitored closely after the injection. The block is performed with the patient in the lithotomy position. A needle is placed through the vaginal mucosa just later to the cervix at the 3 o'clock position. After aspiration for blood, 5 to 10 mL, low concentration local anesthetic is injected. If there is no fetal bradycardia, the block is repeated on the other side, just lateral to the cervix

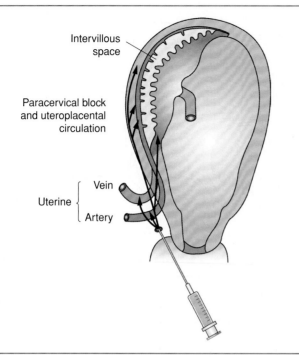

FIGURE 9-12 Diagram of paracervical area in relation to uteroplacental circulation. Reprinted with permission from: Asling JH, Shnider SM, Margolis AJ, et al. Paracervical block anesthesia in obstetrics. II. Etiology of fetal bradycardia following paracervical block anesthesia. *Am J Obstet Gynecol* 1970;107:626–634.

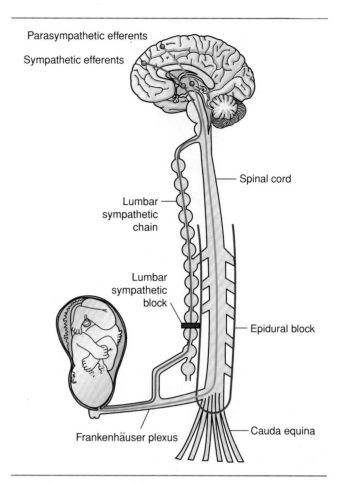

FIGURE 9-13 Proposed pathway of tocolytic sympathetic and tocodynamic parasympathetic efferents. Nerve transaction experiments in pregnant and postpartum dogs suggest that tocolytic sympathetic efferents exit the central nervous system cephalad to T3 and travel to the uterus via the peripheral sympathetic chain. Tocodynamic parasympathetic efferents are interrupted by cutting the pelvic parasympathetic nerves. Epidural analgesia may slow labor by partially blocking pelvic parasympathetic outflow without affecting the tocolytic sympathetic efferents. Reprinted with permission from: Leighton BL, Halpern SH, Wilson DB. Lumbar sympathetic blocks speed early and second stage induced labor in nulliparous women. *Anesthesiology* 1999;90(4):1044.

at the 9 o'clock position with the same volume of drug. FHR and maternal blood pressure are monitored closely during the next 10 minutes. This technique will reduce the incidence of fetal bradycardia; however, the occurrence of postblockade fetal bradycardia cannot be entirely eliminated (63). The duration of pain relief will vary from 40 minutes with 1.5% chloroprocaine to 90 minutes with 1% mepivacaine. In the United States, bupivacaine is considered contraindicated for paracervical block anesthesia in obstetrics due to maternal systemic absorption. The block may be repeated at intervals depending on the duration of action of the local anesthetic. If the cervix has reached 8 cm of dilation, the block should be used with caution to avoid injection into the fetal scalp.

Lumbar Sympathetic Block (Fig. 9-13)

Bilateral lumbar sympathetic block interrupts the pain impulses from the uterus, cervix, and upper third of the vagina without motor blockade, and may be used to provide analgesia during the first stage of labor (Fig. 9-13). For relief of perineal pain during the second stage, a pudendal nerve block or subarachnoid block must be added.

The lumbar sympathetic block is performed at the level of the second lumbar vertebra. Using a 22 gauge, 10 cm needle, the transverse process is located; the needle is then redirected and advanced an additional 5 cm so that the tip is at the anterolateral surface of the vertebral column just anterior to the medial attachment of the psoas muscle (64). The needle is aspirated in two planes to detect blood or CSF, and then following a test dose a total of 10 mL of local anesthetic is injected in fractionated amounts. This volume will allow the anesthetic to spread along the length of the sympathetic chain. The procedure must be performed on both sides. Bupivacaine 0.5% will provide 2 to 3 hours of anesthesia.

Following the block, the patient must be monitored as closely as with a lumbar epidural or caudal anesthetic. Maternal hypotension may occur and is especially common with larger volumes of local anesthetic, which spreads to and anesthetizes the celiac plexus and splanchnic nerves. Systemic toxic reactions from accidental intravascular injection or accidental spinal or epidural injection also can occur. Consequently, prior to performing the block, preparations for those complications must be made. There is evidence that lumbar sympathetic block accelerates the first stage of labor (65), and it should be used cautiously in the presence of rapidly progressive labor, to avoid tumultuous contractions. A single randomized trial showed that lumbar sympathetic blocks were associated with an increased speed of labor compared with epidural blocks in nulliparous women whose labor was induced (66).

Compared to continuous lumbar epidural analgesia, PCEA and CSE, lumbar sympathetic block is technically more difficult to perform, involves more painful needle placement, and does not provide second-stage analgesia. Consequently, it is seldom performed in obstetrics. Furthermore, few anesthesiologists have proficiency in performing this block and the goals of analgesia with minimal motor blockade can be achieved by epidural techniques. However, it may be useful for a parturient with a history of back surgery in which successful epidural analgesia has failed or is precluded.

Pudendal Block and Local Perineal Infiltration Anesthesia

These blocks are usually administered by the obstetrician during the second stage of labor or just before delivery to alleviate the pain form distention of the lower vagina, vulva, and perineum. They are useful for spontaneous vaginal delivery and outlet forceps and vacuum deliveries, but may not provide sufficient anesthesia for midpelvic instrumental delivery, or procedures such as repair of a cervical or upper-vaginal laceration or manual removal of a retained placenta. Pudendal nerve block also causes motor blockade to the perineal muscles and the external anal sphincter. Pudendal block is most commonly performed transvaginally. With the patient in the lithotomy position, the physician palpates the ischial spine, places a needle guide (Iowa trumpet) under the spine, and introduces a 20 gauge needle through the guide until the point rests on the vaginal mucosa. The needle is advanced approximately 1 cm, piercing the sacrospinous ligament; after aspirating for blood, 10 mL of local anesthetic (lidocaine or mepivacaine 1% or chloroprocaine 2%) is injected. The technique is then repeated on the opposite side. Unfortunately, efficacy of pudendal block even in experienced hands is limited for labor pain and is inferior to neuraxial analgesia (67).

■ PREVENTION AND MANAGEMENT OF COMPLICATIONS

Contraindication to Epidural, Caudal, and Spinal Anesthesia

There are relatively few absolute contraindications to major conduction anesthesia. These include: (1) Patient refusal, (2) infection at the site of needle insertion, (3) sepsis, (4) hypovolemic shock, and (5) significant coagulopathy.

Overt sepsis is usually considered a contraindication to instrumentation of the spinal or epidural spaces for analgesia because of the possibility of hematogenous spread of infection to the CNS. The same concern applies to localized infection at the planned insertion site. However, there is little direct human data to support or refute these concerns. Most epidemiologic evidence suggests that meningitis following spinal anesthesia is more likely traced to lapses in sterile technique, as opposed to spread from the perispinal vasculature (68). Some guidance is found from animal experiments. In a study in rats, Carp and Bailey (69) found that dural puncture in rats made bacteremic from an abdominal abscess resulted in meningitis in 12/40 animals. None of 40 septic animals without dural puncture, and none of 30 uninfected animals that underwent dural puncture, developed meningitis. Importantly, a dose of antibiotic given just prior to dural puncture in bacteremic rats completely prevented the development of meningitis. Based largely on this study, it is generally felt that laboring women who are suspected to be infected can safely undergo regional anesthesia, provided appropriate antibiotics have previously been administered.

Coagulopathies most commonly affecting parturients include thrombocytopenia and use of heparins. A specific platelet count that is predictive of a higher incidence of

regional anesthetic complications has not been determined (3,70). The anesthesiologist's decision to order or require a platelet count should be individualized and based on a patient's history, physical examination, and clinical signs (3). Conversely, the platelet count at which most anesthesiologists will administer conduction anesthesia has gradually declined in recent decades and many are comfortable doing so if the count exceeds 80×10^9/L (71,72).

The decision to administer an epidural or spinal anesthetic to a patient receiving low-molecular-weight heparin (LMWH) must be made on an individual basis. The recommendations of a consensus conference of the American Society of Regional Anesthesia (73,74) include the following: In patients receiving LMWH, needle placement should not occur for at least 10 to 12 hours after low dose LMWH (e.g., enoxaparin 0.5 mg/kg daily). Patients receiving higher doses of LMWH (e.g., enoxaparin 1 mg kg^{-1} twice daily) require longer delays (24 hours). If possible, epidural catheters should be removed prior to the initiation of LMWH thromboprophylaxis. If not, catheter removal should be delayed until 10 to 12 hours after a dose of LMWH. Subsequent dosing should not occur for at least 2 hours after catheter removal. Modern advanced coagulation monitors, such as thromboelastography (TEG), can be used to assess and manage coagulation defects as well as aid in determining if a parturient can undergo neuraxial anesthesia (75).

Preexisting neurologic disease of the spinal cord or peripheral nerves is a relative contraindication, but at times regional anesthesia may be in the best interest of the mother and neonate. Each case should be evaluated individually.

Inadequate or Failed Blocks

Epidural techniques for labor analgesia are extremely effective in skilled hands. However, a failure rate as high as 2% to 5% may occur with incomplete pain relief in 10% to 15% of patients (76,77). Failed or inadequate blocks typically result from failure to identify the epidural space or from malposition of the catheter. The higher failure rates may be related to inexperience of the practitioner (particularly those in training) or rapid progression of labor. In some instances, for example, there is no time to repeat the placement of a failed epidural catheter.

When there is a question concerning the correct placement of an epidural catheter in labor, the clinician might inject 5 to 10 mL of a more concentrated local anesthetic (1.5% lidocaine; 2% to 3% 2-chloroprocaine) in divided doses to verify correct placement. If this does not promptly provide significant analgesia, the epidural catheter should be replaced without prolonged attempts to verify placement.

A unilateral epidural block in labor is not uncommon and can occur despite the use of a good technique. In a prospective analysis ($n = 10,995$), Paech et al. noted that 1.3% of epidural catheters placed for labor or cesarean section needed to be replaced for unilateral or asymmetric blocks (59). While this problem has previously been attributed to obstruction in the epidural space (dorsomedian connective tissue) (78), anatomical causes are less likely than patient position (prolonged time on one side) or excessive catheter length in the epidural space. Withdrawal of the catheter by 1 to 2 cm and injection with a larger volume of dilute local anesthetic usually resolves the problem. In prospective studies, the ideal length for a multiorifice catheter insertion in the epidural space has been determined to be 2 to 6 cm (79,80).

In the obese parturient, epidural block is typically initiated with the patient in the sitting position. The catheter should not be fixed with tape until the patient has returned to her side or lateral position since the magnitude of catheter movement with position change can be more than 4 cm in the obese parturient (81). The patient in labor often experiences a great deal of movement compared to a patient undergoing a cesarean delivery, for example, and catheters can become dislodged despite careful placement. Therefore, catheters may need to be replaced on occasion particularly during prolonged labor or in the obese parturient. In a review of anesthesia outcome in the morbidly obese parturient, it was noted that 94% of these patients ultimately obtained successful epidural anesthesia despite the technical difficulties. However, the epidural catheters needed to be replaced once in 46% of the patients and two or more times in 21% of the patients (22).

When surgery is contemplated in a parturient with a "questionable" epidural catheter, a spinal anesthetic may be preferable to continued use of the epidural catheter. However, high spinal anesthesia has been reported when spinal anesthesia follows a failed ("spotty") epidural anesthetic, and caution is indicated (82–84).

When an epidural anesthetic is used for a cesarean delivery and anesthesia is found to be incomplete after the incision is made, several choices are possible to remedy the situation. Often, simply waiting for the epidural block to take effect will be successful, particularly if bupivacaine or ropivacaine has been used. Other choices include administration of additional local anesthetic to reinforce the block (5 to 10 mL), administration of small IV doses of an analgesic (50 to 100 μg fentanyl), or IV ketamine (0.25 mg kg^{-1}). One or two doses of ketamine may provide adequate analgesia until the onset of a "slow" but otherwise successful epidural. Alternatively, the surgical team might infiltrate locally in the surgical field with a local anesthetic if it appears there is a missed segment. Finally, low-dose inhalation analgesia with nitrous oxide may be helpful. The risk of aspiration must be kept in mind with use of supplemental IV and/or inhalation agent. Regardless of the approach, adequate anesthesia must be provided, and the use of general anesthesia may be necessary in some cases, particularly if the surgery is urgent or an incision has been made and the patient is in pain.

Test Dose Regimens

An epidural needle or catheter may be unintentionally placed in either the subarachnoid space or a blood vessel. A variety of regimens have been suggested for testing an epidural to allow the anesthesiologist to recognize this misplacement before a subarachnoid or intravascular injection of an inappropriately large amount of drug. These tests include aspiration, incremental injection of dilute local anesthetics, injection of local anesthetics with epinephrine, injection of air, or injection of fentanyl. Ideal characteristics of a test dose include: (1) The test regimen should be safe, (2) it should employ readily available drugs or equipment, and (3) it should have high sensitivity and specificity, that is, few false-positive or false-negative findings. Fulfilling these ideal criteria is difficult, and controversy exists regarding which regimen to use.

Aspiration of the needle or catheter is the simplest way to detect intravascular or subarachnoid placement and should be universally employed. However, there are numerous case reports of unintentional intravascular or subarachnoid injections occurring after negative aspiration (85–88). Aspiration does not appear to be reliable with single end-hole epidural catheters (89), but some claim aspiration always detects IV placement of multiple-orifice epidural catheters (90,91).

Norris et al. (92) studied 1,029 laboring women, using multiple-orifice epidural catheters with incremental injections of dilute solutions of local anesthetic agent and opioids, and aspiration as the sole test of intravascular placement and concluded that no additional test dose was necessary. The

catheters were also tested with 2 mL plain local anesthetic to identify possible subarachnoid placement. In a subsequent study (93), these investigators found only one intravascular catheter detected by epinephrine that was not found by aspiration, and 7/10 others which represented false-positives (the catheters subsequently provided bilateral analgesia). Nonetheless, an accompanying editorial review recommended that **careful aspiration followed by an appropriate test dose would increase the likelihood that an intravascular catheter will be detected** (94).

Thus, currently, the most commonly used test dose is local anesthetic, typically lidocaine, with 15 to 25 μg epinephrine, that is, 3 to 5 mL of a 1:200,000 solution. Since the function of a test dose is to allow recognition of either an accidental dural or intravascular puncture, a local anesthetic test dose should contain an amount of drug sufficient to rapidly produce a low spinal block if injected into the subarachnoid space and also should provide a reliable indication of an accidental intravascular injection.

Lidocaine appears to be the preferred local anesthetic for use in an epidural test dose. When 3 mL of 1.5% hyperbaric lidocaine is injected into the subarachnoid space at the L2–3 or L3–4 lumbar level, sensory anesthesia at the S2 dermatome level occurs within 2 minutes (87). Lidocaine 2% with epinephrine at a dose of 60 mg (3 mL) reliably induced motor block when injected spinally (95). Bupivacaine and ropivacaine do not appear as reliable in producing similar effects (96,97).

Epinephrine is the most commonly used drug for identifying intravascular misplacement of an epidural catheter. The landmark study of the use of 15 μg epinephrine with local anesthetic showed that this dose injected intravascularly rapidly produced a transient increase in heart rate of 20 to 30 beats per minute (bpm) and usually a slight increase in blood pressure (98). Although initially demonstrated in nonobstetric patients, similar changes occur in the parturient when an epidural vein is accidentally cannulated and epinephrine injected (Fig. 9-14) (99,100). However, in the parturient, the heart rate response to an IV injection of epinephrine 15 μg has an acceleratory phase of 1.2 bpm/s (i.e., the rate of increase in maternal heart rate (MHR) is faster than 1.2 bpm for each second), which is different from the 0.69 bpm acceleration induced by labor pain (100). **In the obstetric patient, the epinephrine test dose should be injected during uterine diastole, preferably soon after a uterine contraction.**

Criticisms of using epinephrine as a test dose to determine accidental intravascular injection in the parturient include a high incidence of false-positive (101) and false-negative results (100–102), and possible adverse effects on uterine blood flow and fetal well-being (101,103), particularly in preeclampsia (104).

There are several proposed alternatives to epinephrine. Subconvulsant doses of local anesthetics, such as 100 mg lidocaine, or 2-chloroprocaine, rely on the subjective responses of the mother, which may be unreliable in the anxious parturient. Furthermore, if injected subarachnoid, this dose may produce an unacceptably high block. Other catecholamines that may produce a greater increase in MHR without adverse effects on uterine blood flow, such as isoproterenol (5 μg) (105,106), involve the preparation of impractical dilution of available drugs. Injection of air (1 mL) and the use of the FHR Doppler monitor over the heart have also been suggested (107) but have not achieved widespread popularity. The Doppler test has a low false-positive rate and a high positive predictive value in practiced hands, but it requires a subjective interpretation of Doppler sound changes, requires additional personnel to position and hold the Doppler transducer, cannot be easily performed with the patient on her side, and precludes continuous monitoring of the fetus during injection unless a

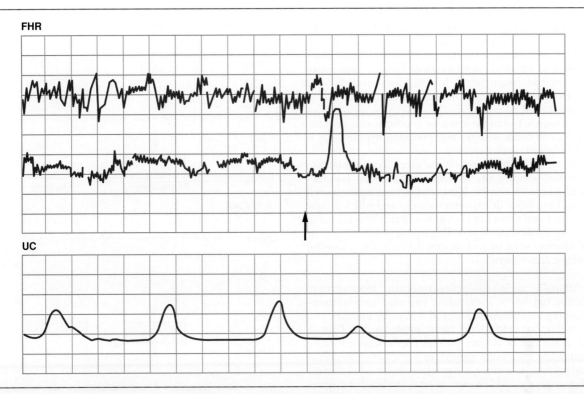

FIGURE 9-14 A peak increase in maternal heart rate lasting 40 seconds in a laboring woman during intravenous injection of 12.5 mg bupivacaine plus 12.5 μg epinephrine in 10 mL physiologic saline, recorded with the use of a direct electrocardiogram mode of fetal monitoring with dual heart rate capacity. Arrow shows start of injection. Thirty second is represented between each pair of vertical lines. Reprinted with permission from: Van Zundert AA, Vaes LE, De Wolf AM. ECG monitoring of mother and fetus during epidural anesthesia. *Anesthesiology* 1987;66(4):584–585.

second external FHR monitor is available. Intrathecal injection of a small amount of air is safe, as is intravenous injection.

Hypotension

Hypotension is the most common side effect of major conduction anesthesia for vaginal delivery (108). Mild to moderate reductions in maternal blood pressure that do not adversely affect the mother may have adverse effects on uterine blood flow and fetal well-being. When delivery occurs shortly after induction of conduction anesthesia, as during cesarean delivery, these effects may be clinically important. The prevention and treatment of hypotension during regional anesthesia for cesarean delivery is discussed in detail in Chapter 12.

Despite an increased blood volume of 40% above prepregnancy levels, the parturient at term is particularly susceptible to hypotension during major conduction anesthesia (109). Partial or complete inferior vena cava and aortic occlusion from compression by the gravid uterus is present in the majority of parturients lying in the supine position (110,111). Vena caval obstruction not only impedes venous return to the heart, thereby causing hypotension, but also increases uterine venous pressure, further decreasing uterine blood flow. In most parturients, an increase in resting sympathetic tone compensates for the effects of caval compression and blood pressure is maintained. However, when sympathetic tone is abolished acutely, as with spinal or epidural anesthesia, marked deceases in blood pressure may result. It is believed by many that hypotension occurs less frequently and may be less severe with epidural than with spinal anesthesia. This is likely due, in large part, to the gradual onset of epidural anesthesia, allowing time for compensatory mechanisms to

modify the cardiovascular effects produced. The addition of sodium bicarbonate to local anesthetics to increase the speed of onset of epidural blockade is common (112), and with faster onset, there may be a greater incidence of hypotension (113). **In general, the higher level of sympathetic blockade, the greater the incidence and severity of hypotension.** Diminished intravascular volume—frequently found with preeclampsia, antepartum bleeding, or dehydration—may further promote maternal hypotension.

Most healthy parturients tolerate systolic blood pressures of 80 to 90 mm Hg without ill effects. The fetus, however, is highly sensitive to decreased maternal arterial blood pressure. In contrast to other vital organs, with acute decreases in maternal blood pressure, there is no autoregulation of blood flow to the uterus. With spinal- or epidural-induced hypotension, uterine blood flow decease linearly with blood pressure (114,115).

The fetal consequences of the reduced uterine blood flow depend on the degree and duration of the fall and the preexisting status of the uteroplacental circulation. When uterine blood flow is inadequate, fetal asphyxia will develop (116–118). The precise degree and duration of hypotension necessary to cause fetal distress seems to be variable. Conduction anesthesia producing a maternal systolic blood pressure of less than 70 mm Hg consistently produced sustained fetal bradycardia (119). When maternal systolic blood pressure was between 70 and 80 mm Hg for 4 minutes or longer, some fetuses developed sustained bradycardia. With maternal systolic blood pressure less than 100 mm Hg for 5 minutes, abnormal FHR patterns developed (120,121). A systolic pressure of less than 100 mm Hg for 10 to 15 minutes may lead to fetal acidosis and bradycardia (122). **In all these studies, FHR returned to normal with correction of hypotension.**

In a classic study published in 1969, Marx et al. (123) found better fetal biochemical and neonatal clinical conditions when spinal hypotension was prevented rather than treated. However, direct application of these results to today's practice should be made with caution because preventive measures for and treatment of hypotension have changed significantly since that time. Other investigators (124–126) have demonstrated no significant differences in Apgar scores or blood gasses between neonates of mothers who become hypotensive and those who do not, provided hypotension is detected early and treated quickly.

Several preventive measures can be taken to minimize the incidence and severity of hypotension following conduction anesthesia in obstetrics. Most studies investigating such maneuvers have been in cesarean delivery and often in spinal anesthesia, and there has been considerably less attention paid to labor epidural analgesia. Regarding routine spinal or epidural blocks for labor and vaginal delivery, the following measures are recommended:

1. Traditionally anesthesiologists routinely intravenously administered 500 to 1,000 mL of balanced, nondextrose-containing solution administered within 30 minutes of a low epidural or saddle block (dermatome level of T10). A modest amount of volume preload does not appear to be harmful and may make significant decreases in maternal blood pressure less likely, less precipitous, or easier to treat with vasopressors. However, several studies have questioned the value of volume preloading with crystalloid in preventing hypotension, even with spinal anesthesia for cesarean section (127,128). Nonetheless, the ASA task force on Obstetric Anesthesia states that intravenous fluid preloading for spinal anesthesia reduces the frequency of maternal hypotension when compared with no fluid preloading (3). But, the task force also states that initiation of spinal anesthesia should not be delayed to administer a fixed volume of intravenous fluid (3). To effectively prevent hypotension associated with a sympathetic block, IV volume administration must produce a large enough increase in blood volume to result in a significant increase in cardiac output (129). Sufficient amounts of IV crystalloid administered rapidly produce an increase in cardiac filling pressures; however, the intravascular half-life is short and this increase is quickly reversed after the onset of sympathetic blockade (130,131). A fluid bolus during labor may produce a transient decrease in the frequency of uterine contractions (132,133). This transient decrease (about 20 minutes) was found to occur with rapid administration of 1,000 mL crystalloid, but not with 500 mL. In both of these studies, hydration of 500 or 1,000 mL did not further decrease the low incidence of hypotension.

   Although dextrose-containing solutions may be useful in reducing maternal ketosis (134), they are undesirable in the large volumes required for acute IV loading prior to regional anesthesia. Adverse effects include maternal hyperglycemia (often associated with an osmotic dieresis), fetal hyperglycemia, and subsequent neonatal hyperinsulinemia and hypoglycemia (135–137). There is evidence indicating that hyperglycemia increases the fetal brain's susceptibility to anoxic injury, and is further a cause for avoiding hyperglycemia during labor and delivery (138).

2. Vasopressor prophylaxis is not recommended for epidural analgesia for labor. The incidence of hypotension is not great, and when it does occur, it is usually mild and easily treated. Furthermore, placental transfer of ephedrine is efficient (Fig. 9-15) and may increase FHR and variability, making interpretation of the FHR tracing during labor more difficult (139).

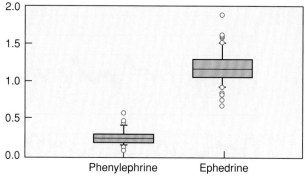

A. UV/MA

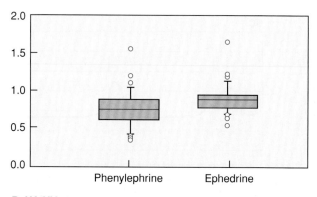

B. UA/UV

FIGURE 9-15 Plasma concentration ratios for phenylephrine and ephedrine. Data are shown for (**A**) umbilical venous to maternal arterial (UV/MA) and (**B**) umbilical arterial to umbilical venous (UA/UV) ratios. *Box plots* display the 25th, 50th, and 75th percentiles as *horizontal lines* on a bar, *whiskers* above and below the box indicate the 90th and 10th percentiles, and data beyond the 10th and 90th percentiles are displayed as individual points. Data were significantly different between groups (*P* < 0.001) for both concentration ratios. Reprinted with permission from: Ngan Kee WD, Khaw KS, Tan PE, et al. Placental transfer and fetal metabolic effects of phenylephrine and ephedrine during spinal anesthesia for cesarean delivery. *Anesthesiology* 2009;111(3):506–512.

3. Continuous LUD should be applied to minimize aortocaval compression. Laboring patients should remain in the lateral or semilateral position.
4. Frequent monitoring of arterial blood pressure is mandatory after institution of epidural or spinal analgesia for labor. This will allow early recognition and prompt therapy of hypotension.

Therapy for epidural or spinal hypotension includes more LUD, or a change in position, rapid IV fluid infusion, the Trendelenburg position to increase venous return, IV phenylephrine or ephedrine, and oxygen administration. For additional discussion of pressor choices, see Chapter 12.

Vasopressor-induced Hypertension

The interaction of vasoactive drugs and ergot derivatives may lead to severe maternal hypertension and possible cerebrovascular accidents (140). Particularly dangerous is the combination of a purely α-adrenergic agent, such as methoxamine, and the ergot derivatives ergonovine and methylergonovine. Ergot derivatives, when used alone, also may be associated with postpartum hypertension (141). However, these drugs may be life-saving in the face of maternal hemorrhage (see Chapter 23). Prophylactic vasopressors or ergot derivatives should be used with caution in parturients with hypertension. If acute postpartum hypertension occurs, treatment might include (a) labetalol 10 to 20 mg intravenously, repeated or escalated (40 to 80 mg/dose, up to 300 mg total) every 5 minutes up to 1 mg kg^{-1}, (b) hydralazine 10 to 20 mg intravenously, which can be repeated every 15 minutes, or (c) in extreme cases nitroprusside infusion, nitroglycerin infusion or sublingual spray 0.4 to 0.8 mg, or other agents such as phentolamine.

Local Anesthetic Convulsions

Central nervous system toxicity occurs when a critical brain tissue concentration of local anesthetic is exceeded. These excessive brain tissue concentrations are almost invariably associated with high blood levels that result from accidental intravascular injection, accumulation of local anesthetic during repeated injections over a prolonged period of time, or rapid systemic absorption of local anesthetic from a highly vascular area. The rate of administration, the total dose of drug, and the physical status of the patient affect tolerance to local anesthetics (142). Accidental intravascular injection may occur with any regional anesthetic technique, including paracervical and pudendal blocks (143). Therefore, when a needle or catheter is placed, a test regimen should be used (described earlier) to include aspiration of the catheter to determine whether a blood vessel has been entered before drug injection (93). When local anesthetics are injected, particularly large volumes of concentrated local anesthetics (e.g., for cesarean delivery), they should be administered in divided (fractionated) doses at no more that 3 to 5 mL at a time, while observing for signs of systemic toxicity and the onset of spinal anesthesia.

The elimination half-life of amide local anesthetics is 2 to 3 hours. Therefore, systemic accumulation of amide local anesthetics to near-toxic levels may occur with large doses repeated at frequent intervals. During properly conducted regional anesthesia, toxic concentrations of local anesthetic resulting from absorption are rarely seen (59,141,142). The current use of more dilute local anesthetics for labor analgesia further reduces this risk.

The reported incidence of convulsions during obstetric regional anesthesia varies widely from 0% to 0.5% (59,144–147). In more recent reports, convulsions due to local anesthetic toxicity have become increasingly rare, with an incidence of 1:5,000 to 9,000 (148,149). In most clinical circumstances of convulsions associated with obstetric regional anesthesia, prompt recognition and treatment usually result in full recovery of the mother and fetus. While the number of claims involving convulsions in the United States has decreased since 1984 (150), this remains a significant potential complication. The toxicity of local anesthetics, including the cardiotoxicity of bupivacaine, is discussed in Chapter 8. A summary of the signs and symptoms of local anesthetic toxic reactions is shown in Table 9-11.

Treatment Involves

Early recognition of the reaction. By constant observation of the patient, her vital signs, and her ability to communicate,

TABLE 9-11 Signs and Symptoms of Local Anesthetic-induced Systemic Toxicity

Central nervous system
  Cerebral cortex
    Stimulation—restlessness, nervousness, incoherent speech, metallic taste, dizziness, blurred vision, tremors, and convulsions
    Depression—unconsciousness
  Medulla
    Stimulation—increased blood pressure, heart and respiratory rate, nausea, and vomiting
    Depression—hypotension, apnea, and asystole
Cardiovascular
  Heart—bradycardia, ventricular tachycardia and fibrillation, decreased contractility
  Blood vessels—vasodilatation and hypotension
Uterus
  Uterine vasoconstriction and uterine hypertonus resulting in fetal distress

it is possible to become aware of an impending toxic reaction and to take steps to prevent it from becoming serious.

Prevention of progression of the reaction. Small doses of propofol given intravenously may prevent convulsions. The depressant effect of the propofol may intensify the cardiovascular and respiratory depression that results from the local anesthetic, but small doses of diazepam (5 mg), or midazolam (1 to 2 mg), repeated as needed, are probably safe. At the same time, oxygen should be given by a facemask so that the patient is well oxygenated should a convulsion occur. Successful use of lipid emulsion therapy for the treatment of local anesthesia toxicity has also been reported and can result in a successful outcome (151).

Maintenance of oxygenation despite convulsions and/ or vomiting. Convulsions are not lethal, but the anoxia and acidosis that they produce may be. The airway should be cleared of foreign material and the patient ventilated with 100% oxygen with a positive-pressure breathing apparatus. Ventilating the unparalyzed and convulsing patient may be difficult and it may be necessary to paralyze the patient with succinylcholine (80 to 100 mg). Tracheal intubation with a cuffed endotracheal tube to facilitate ventilation and/or protect the airway from aspiration may also be necessary.

Support of circulation. Elevation of the legs, displacement of the uterus off the vena cava and aorta, and rapid administration of IV fluids and vasopressors (e.g., ephedrine, phenylephrine, epinephrine) may be needed to support the depressed circulation.

Treatment of cardiac arrest. Cardiac arrest should be treated using standard advanced cardiac life-support (ACLS) protocols. Appropriate equipment and medication should be immediately available in the labor and delivery unit (Table 9-3) (3). LUD should be maintained if possible. Delivery of the fetus, by relieving vena caval obstruction, may facilitate cardiopulmonary resuscitation (CPR) (152,153). The American Heart Association has stated: "Several authors now recommend that the decision to perform a peripartum cesarean section should be made rapidly with delivery effected within 4 to 5 minutes of arrest" (154). While an emergency cesarean delivery has the best chance of improving the outcome for the other and newborn, this decision must be considered carefully to include (a) the differential diagnosis of cardiac arrest, (b) the age of the fetus, and (c) the availability of equipment and supplies.

Consideration of the fetus. As soon as possible after the convulsion, the condition of the fetus should be assessed to decide the subsequent course of delivery. Prompt maternal resuscitation will usually restore uterine blood flow and fetal oxygenation, allow fetal excretion of local anesthetic to the mother via the placenta, and obviate the need for emergent cesarean delivery (155).

High Block and Total Spinal

Total spinal anesthesia or profoundly high block may occur from an excessive spread of local anesthetic administered intrathecally, extradurally, or subdurally (in the potential space between dura mater and arachnoid mater). Dural perforation by an epidural catheter may occur when the catheter is initially inserted or during the course of a previously uneventful, continuous epidural anesthetic by migration of the catheter (148,156). The incidence has been estimated at 1:1,400 to 1:4,500 (59,148). A total or high spinal may lead to profound hypotension, dyspnea, inability to speak, and ultimately a loss of consciousness. The subdural space has been referred to as the "third space to go astray" and also can lead to a high block (Fig. 9-16) (157). Acute, life-threatening respiratory depression has been reported after an opioid was injected through an epidural catheter placed, and initially used successfully as part of a CSE for cesarean delivery (158). The catheter appeared to have migrated subdurally in the postoperative period. While placement of an epidural catheter during the CSE technique seems extremely safe, accidental intrathecal insertion of an epidural catheter is possible, as well as migration of a catheter, and thus the catheter must always be aspirated and tested to rule out this rare but real possibility (159).

Subdural injection of a local anesthetic leads to an unexpectedly high but inconsistent ("patchy") block (157,160). A subdural block has a variable spread that ultimately is quite extensive for the volume of local anesthetic injected. It is often a patchy block, has a delayed onset, and has a relatively mild motor component (161). The subdural space is the potential space between the dura mater and the arachnoid mater and extends intracranially, so that the cranial nerves

may be involved (Fig. 9-16). A retrospective review in non-obstetric patients suggested that the incidence of subdural injection may be as high as 0.82% (162).

Although infrequent, the possibility of total spinal anesthesia or other high block necessitates the immediate presence of personnel who can promptly diagnose and treat this complication, with immediate availability of necessary equipment. Treatment consists of establishing an airway, ventilation with oxygen, and provision of cardiovascular support. Tracheal intubation should be performed as soon as possible to protect the airway from aspiration. A total spinal block will not necessarily produce relaxation of the jaw muscles and succinylcholine may be required for intubation. The Trendelenburg position and LUD should be used to increase venous return to the heart, fluids and vasopressors administered to maintain maternal hemodynamic stability and provide adequate uteroplacental perfusion to the fetus (154).

Dense or Prolonged Epidural Block

The goal of epidural analgesia for labor is to achieve pain relief; motor blockade is usually not needed or desired. Thus, increasingly dilute epidural solutions, as well as the CSE technique, have become increasingly popular (see Chapter 9) (6,163). However, more concentrated local anesthetics (bupivacaine 0.125% to 0.25%, or lidocaine 1.0% to 2.0%) are sometimes required for the treatment of incomplete analgesia or top-up doses. After long continuous infusions or repeated bolus dosing, significant motor block can develop and may be bothersome to the patient and the nursing staff (164). This may also make voluntary maternal expulsive efforts more difficult during the second stage of labor and lead to prolonged epidural blocks in the postpartum period, particularly if epinephrine is added to the anesthetic solution. A dense block during the course of labor epidural analgesia can be easily managed by decreasing the epidural infusion rate or decreasing the concentration of the local anesthetic. If a dense block is bothersome, discontinuing the infusion for 30 minutes may be helpful, followed by restarting the infusion with a more dilute local anesthetic solution, and/or a lower infusion rate, or eliminating the background infusion in a PCEA regimen. An unexpectedly prolonged block is most often related to the prolonged administration of a concentrated local anesthetic with epinephrine. This occurred more often with etidocaine, which is no longer commonly used (165,166).

In the differential diagnosis of a prolonged block, neurologic complications of both labor and delivery itself, as well as regional analgesia, must also be considered (see Chapter 26) (167). While an epidural hematoma is often considered in this situation, it is extremely unlikely without a coagulation abnormality or the administration of an anticoagulant. The reported incidence of epidural hematomas is 0.2 to 3.7 per 100,000 epidural blocks for obstetric patients (167). A block that does not progress or slowly regresses would suggest diagnoses other than an epidural hematoma. A dense, one-sided block would also make this diagnosis unlikely. However, consultation with a neurologist is appropriate if the more routine cause of a prolonged block does not explain the clinical findings. The increasing use of dilute local anesthetic solutions for labor should decrease the incidence of this problem.

Cardiac Arrest

Severe bradycardia progressing to cardiac asystole has been reported in young healthy patients not premedicated with atropine (168,169). In 1997, a large French study reported a cardiac arrest rate of 6.4 ± 1.2 per 10,000 patients receiving spinal anesthesia (170). In 2005, a Mayo Clinic retrospective

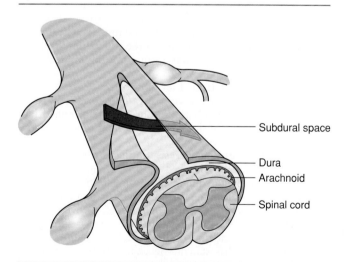

FIGURE 9-16 The subdural space exists as a potential space encircling the arachnoid membrane and contained within the dura. Reprinted with permission from: Lubenow T, Keh-Wong E, Kristof K, et al. Inadvertent subdural injection: a complication of an epidural block. *Anesth Analg* 1988;67(2):179.

Subdural space

Dura
Arachnoid

Spinal cord

study reported a rate of 2.9 per 10,000 patients receiving spinal anesthesia (171). Decreases in heart rate to less than 60 bpm should be promptly treated by increasing venous return and, if necessary, by promptly administering atropine and/or ephedrine. Some cases of brady-asystolic arrest following onset of regional anesthesia do not appear to be vagally mediated (172). If conventional doses of atropine or ephedrine are not effective, IV epinephrine should be administered (173).

In cases of **cardiac arrest** associated with high spinal anesthesia, poor neurologic outcome has been reported with routine (basic) CPR (169). Of 14 healthy patients who suffered cardiac arrest during spinal anesthesia in the ASA closed claims analysis, Caplan et al. found bradycardia was the first sign in seven (50%). While all patients were resuscitated after cardiac arrest, six suffered neurologic injury and died in the hospital. Of the eight survivors, only one recovered to perform routine daily self-care. It is believed that high sympathetic blockade allows increased peripheral blood flow during CPR and inhibits the usual preferential perfusion of the brain. In the cases cited by Caplan, epinephrine was not administered for an average of 8 minutes after the onset of asystole. Epinephrine should be given "early" in the management of sudden bradycardia (Fig. 9-17). It is speculated that early administration of epinephrine may improve cerebral perfusion during CPR and decrease the high incidence of neurologic damage that occurs in these circumstances. It is recommended that a full resuscitation dose of epinephrine be given immediately upon recognition of cardiac arrest during a spinal or epidural anesthetic (169,173).

Underlying, undiagnosed medical problems also must be considered in these circumstances. In a case report of cardiac arrest that occurred during spinal anesthesia for cesarean delivery, a cardiomyopathy was ultimately diagnosed (174). Prompt endotracheal intubation, delivery of the infant, CPR including epinephrine (1 mg IV) and atropine, as well as an epinephrine infusion and intensive care management, led to a good recovery of the mother and newborn in this case. Thus, concomitant medical problems also must be considered, as well as a differential diagnosis that includes anaphylactic shock, eclampsia, amniotic fluid, air or thromboembolism, and extreme aortocaval compression.

Backache

Local tenderness at the site of epidural or spinal placement and transient backache are relatively common, particularly if placement of the block was difficult. This usually clears within several days to 3 weeks and may be related to superficial irritation of the skin or periosteal irritation or injury. However, postpartum backache that persists several months or longer has been reported (175,176). Although these reports received a great deal of attention, postpartum backache is common, with or without regional anesthesia. Postpartum backache may be related to hormonal changes, softening of maternal ligaments, and mechanical changes (e.g., exaggerated lumbar lordosis and maternal weight gain). In studies by MacArthur et al., data were obtained from a mailed questionnaire to 11,701 women who had delivered 1 to 9 years earlier. They found back pain was more common in those who delivered vaginally using epidural analgesia than in those who delivered vaginally without epidural analgesia (18.9% vs. 10.5%). However, this study has been questioned for a number of reasons, including the accuracy and possible recall and response bias in mailed questionnaires (177). Prospective studies of postpartum backache have not supported the data obtained from retrospective surveys. In a prospective study of 1,042 parturients, Breen et al. found the incidence of back pain 1 to 2 months after delivery was 44% in women who received epidural anesthesia and 45% in those who did not (178). These results were supported by Russell et al. who found that about 33% of women reported backache that lasted for at least 3 months postpartum, whether they received epidural analgesia or not (179). The principal risk factor for backache within the first 3 months postpartum appears to be antenatal backache (178,179). Weight gain during the pregnancy also may be a factor (178). Although postpartum back pain is common, it does not appear related to the use of regional analgesia or a particular epidural technique (178,179).

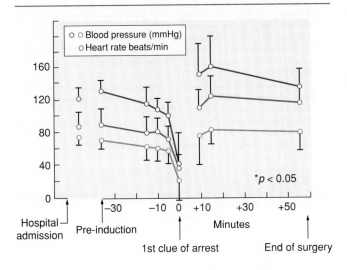

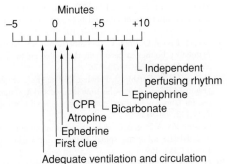

FIGURE 9-17 Composite display of vital signs (*upper graph*) and key events (*lower graph*) in 14 cases of cardiac arrest during spinal anesthesia. Events are shown in relation to the first clue of impending cardiac arrest (located at 0 minutes on the time scale). The values for systolic blood pressure (closed circles) are mean ± SD. *P < 0.05 versus hospital admission values. Reprinted with permission from: Caplan RA, Ward RJ, Posner K, et al. Unexpected cardiac arrest during spinal anesthesia: a closed claims analysis of predisposing factors. *Anesthesiology* 1988;68:5–11.

Urinary Retention

Urinary retention during labor is not uncommon but appears to be more likely with regional analgesia. However, in a study of women receiving dilute epidural local anesthetic solution with opioids demonstrated that women were able to void in most cases (6). In an older study, it was noted that 14.2% of women had bladder dysfunction after a normal vaginal delivery compared with 37.5% of women who had an instrumental vaginal delivery. None of these women had regional anesthesia (180). More recent examination of this problem found a much lower overall incidence. Among women who self-selected epidural analgesia, the incidence was 2.7%

compared with 0.1% in women without regional anesthesia (181). Although it has been demonstrated that epidural opioids likely cause urinary retention by their direct sacral spinal action and effect on the detrusor muscle (182), urinary retention is less likely in routine practice with dilute local anesthetic and opioid infusions for labor.

Clearly in a nonrandomized design, the two groups may not have had comparable baseline risk of postpartum urinary retention. Urinary retention during labor and postpartum is no doubt affected by numerous obstetric factors, including perineal trauma, edema, lengthy labor, prolonged second stage, instrumental delivery, and pain. Patients in labor and postpartum should be observed for possible bladder distention and urinary bladder catheterization performed as indicated.

Although epidural analgesia for labor is most often highly effective, its use requires skill and practice, acceptance of the occasional failed block, and the knowledge and skill to implement alternative approaches when necessary.

Note: The current ASA Guidelines for Regional Anesthesia in Obstetrics are included in Appendices A through C.

KEY POINTS

- Regional anesthetic techniques are very effective for intrapartum analgesia.
- Labor analgesia decreases maternal catecholamines and improves uteroplacental perfusion.
- Equipment, facilities, and support personnel available in the labor and delivery operating suite should be similar to those available in the main operating suite.
- Aspiration of the needle or catheter is the simplest, but not always most reliable, way to detect intravascular or subarachnoid placement. Careful aspiration followed by an appropriate test dose increases the likelihood that an intravascular catheter will be detected.
- The epinephrine test dose should be injected during uterine diastole. A sudden and fast acceleration in MHR of at least 10 bpm occurring within 1 minute of injection indicates an IV injection.
- Intermittent bolus or CEIs , CSE, and PCEA are popular options for labor analgesia. PCEA and CSE may offer advantages over traditional continuous infusions, which are in turn superior to intermittent boluses. Continuous spinal and lumbar sympathetic block techniques are technically more challenging and associated with more frequent side effects.
- Hypotension is the most common side effect of major conduction anesthesia for vaginal delivery. Vasopressor prophylaxis is not recommended for epidural analgesia for labor.
- Therapy for epidural or spinal hypotension includes more LUD, or a change in position, rapid IV fluid infusion, the Trendelenburg position to increase venous return, IV phenylephrine or ephedrine, and oxygen administration.
- Intravenous ephedrine and phenylephrine are both acceptable drugs for treating hypotension during neuraxial anesthesia. In the absence of maternal bradycardia, phenylephrine may be preferable because of improved fetal acid–base status in uncomplicated pregnancies.
- When local anesthetics are injected, particularly large volumes of concentrated local anesthetics (e.g., for cesarean delivery), they should be administered in divided (fractionated) doses at no more than 3 to 5 mL at a time, while observing for signs of systemic toxicity and the onset of spinal anesthesia.
- Epidural analgesia for labor fails in up to 5% of blocks and may be incomplete in 10% or more. A subdural block is often patchy, has a delayed onset, and has a relatively mild motor block. It may be considerably more common than previously recognized.
- In a maternal arrest situation, unmodified ACLS and LUD are essential; the decision to perform an emergency peripartum cesarean delivery should be made rapidly with delivery within 4 to 5 minutes of the arrest.

REFERENCES

1. Eltzschig HK, Lieberman ES, Camann WR. Regional anesthesia and analgesia for labor and delivery. *N Engl J Med* 2003;348:319–332.
2. Halpern SH, Muir H, Breen TW, et al. A multicenter randomized controlled trial comparing patient-controlled epidural with intravenous analgesia for pain relief in labor. *Anesth Analg* 2004;99:1532–1538.
3. American Society of Anesthesiologists Task Force on Obstetric Anesthesia. Practice guidelines for obstetric anesthesia: an updated report by the American Society of Anesthesiologists Task Force on Obstetric Anesthesia. *Anesthesiology* 2007;106:843–863.
4. Wong CA, McCarthy RJ, Sullivan JT, et al. Early compared with late neuraxial analgesia in nulliparous labor induction: a randomized controlled trial. *Obstet Gynecol* 2009;113:1066–1074.
5. Morison DH, Smedstad KG. Continuous infusion epidurals for obstetric analgesia. *Can Anaesth Soc J* 1985;32:101–104.
6. Cohen SE, Yeh JY, Riley ET, et al. Walking with labor epidural analgesia: the impact of bupivacaine concentration and a lidocaine-epinephrine test dose. *Anesthesiology* 2000; 92:387–392.
7. Rosenblatt R, Wright R, Denson D, et al. Continuous epidural infusions for obstetric analgesia. *Reg Anesth* 1983;8:10–15.
8. Chestnut DH, Owen CL, Bates JN, et al. Continuous infusion epidural analgesia during labor: a randomized, double-blind comparison of 0.0625% bupivacaine/0.0002% fentanyl versus 0.125% bupivacaine. *Anesthesiology* 1988; 68:754–759.
9. Gambling DR, Yu P, Cole C, et al. A comparative study of patient controlled epidural analgesia (PCEA) and continuous infusion epidural analgesia (CIEA) during labour. *Can J Anaesth* 1988;35:249–254.
10. Vallejo MC, Ramesh V, Phelps AL, et al. Epidural labor analgesia: continuous infusion versus patient-controlled epidural analgesia with background infusion versus without a background infusion. *J Pain* 2007;8:970–975.
11. van der Vyver M, Halpern S, Joseph G. Patient-controlled epidural analgesia versus continuous infusion for labour analgesia: a meta-analysis. *Br J Anaesth* 2002;89:459–465.
12. Halpern S. Recent advances in patient-controlled epidural analgesia for labour. *Curr Opin Anaesthesiol* 2005;18:247–251.
13. Hogan Q. Distribution of solution in the epidural space: examination by cryomicrotome section. *Reg Anesth Pain Med* 2002;27:150–156.
14. Fettes PD, Moore CS, Whiteside JB, et al. Intermittent vs continuous administration of epidural ropivacaine with fentanyl for analgesia during labour. *Br J Anaesth* 2006;97:359–364.
15. Wong CA, Ratliff JT, Sullivan JT, et al. A randomized comparison of programmed intermittent epidural bolus with continuous epidural infusion for labor analgesia. *Anesth Analg* 2006;102:904–909.
16. Sia AT, Lim Y, Ocampo C. A comparison of a basal infusion with automated mandatory boluses in parturient-controlled epidural analgesia during labor. *Anesth Analg* 2007;104:673–678.
17. Wong CA, McCarthy RJ, Hewlett B. The effect of manipulation of the programmed intermittent bolus time interval and injection volume on total drug use for labor epidural analgesia: a randomized controlled trial. *Anesth Analg* 2011;112:904–911.
18. Greene BA. A 26 gauge lumbar puncture needle: its value in the prophylaxis of headache following spinal analgesia for vaginal delivery. *Anesthesiology* 1950;11:464–469.
19. Halpern S, Preston R. Postdural puncture headache and spinal needle design. Metaanalyses. *Anesthesiology* 1994;81:1376–1383.
20. Vallejo MC, Mandell GL, Sabo DP, et al. Postdural puncture headache: a randomized comparison of five spinal needles in obstetric patients. *Anesth Analg* 2000;91:916–920.
21. Stienstra R, Greene NM. Factors affecting the subarachnoid spread of local anesthetic solutions. *Reg Anesth* 1991;16:1–6.
22. Hood DD, Dewan DM. Anesthetic and obstetric outcome in morbidly obese parturients. *Anesthesiology* 1993;79:1210–1218.
23. Peterson DO, Borup JL, Chestnut JS. Continuous spinal anesthesia: Case review and discussion. *Reg Anesth* 1983;8:109–113.
24. Kallos T, Smith TC. Continuous spinal anesthesia with hypobaric tetracaine for hip surgery in lateral decubitus. *Anesth Analg* 1972;51:766–771.

25. Denny N, Masters R, Pearson D, et al. Postdural puncture headache after continuous spinal anesthesia. *Anesth Analg* 1987;66:791–794.
26. Rigler ML, Drasner K. Distribution of catheter-injected local anesthetic in a model of the subarachnoid space. *Anesthesiology* 1991;75:684–692.
27. Rigler ML, Drasner K, Krejcie TC, et al. Cauda equina syndrome after continuous spinal anesthesia. *Anesth Analg* 1991;72:275–281.
28. Ross BK, Coda B, Heath CH. Local anesthetic distribution in a spinal model: a possible mechanism of neurologic injury after continuous spinal anesthesia. *Reg Anesth* 1992;17:69–77.
29. Lambert LA, Lambert DH, Strichartz GR. Irreversible conduction block in isolated nerve by high concentrations of local anesthetics. *Anesthesiology* 1994;80:1082–1093.
30. Schneider M, Ettlin T, Kaufmann M, et al. Transient neurologic toxicity after hyperbaric subarachnoid anesthesia with 5% lidocaine. *Anesth Analg* 1993;76:1154–1157.
31. Alonso E, Gilsanz F, Gredilla E, et al. Observational study of continuous spinal anesthesia with the catheter-over-needle technique for cesarean delivery. *Int J Obstet Anesth* 2009;18:137–141.
32. Arkoosh VA, Palmer CM, Yun EM, et al. A randomized, double-masked, multicenter comparison of the safety of continuous intrathecal labor analgesia using a 28-gauge catheter versus continuous epidural labor analgesia. *Anesthesiology* 2008;108:286–298.
33. Tao W, Nguyen AP, Ogunnaike BO, et al. Use of a 23-gauge continuous spinal catheter for labor analgesia: a case series. *Int J Obstet Anesth* 2011;20:351–354.
34. Collis RE, Baxandall ML, Srikantharajah ID, et al. Combined spinal epidural (CSE) analgesia: technique, management, and outcome of 300 mothers. *Int J Obstet Anesth* 1994;3:75–81.
35. Palmer CM, Cork RC, Hays R, et al. The dose-response relation of intrathecal fentanyl for labor analgesia. *Anesthesiology* 1998;88:355–361.
36. Norris MC, Grieco WM, Borkowski M, et al. Complications of labor analgesia: epidural versus combined spinal epidural techniques. *Anesth Analg* 1994;79:529–537.
37. Rawal N, Van Zundert A, Holmström B, et al. Combined spinal-epidural technique. *Reg Anesth* 1997;22:406–423.
38. Nageotte MP, Larson D, Rumney PJ, et al. Epidural analgesia compared with combined spinal-epidural analgesia during labor in nulliparous women. *N Engl J Med* 1997;337:1715–1719.
39. Bloom SL, McIntire DD, Kelly MA, et al. Lack of effect of walking on labor and delivery. *N Engl J Med* 1998;339:76–79.
40. Parry MG, Fernando R, Bawa GP, et al. Dorsal column function after epidural and spinal blockade: implications for the safety of walking following low-dose regional analgesia for labour. *Anaesthesia* 1998;53:382–403.
41. Pickering AE, Parry MG, Ousta B, et al. Effect of combined spinal-epidural ambulatory labor analgesia on balance. *Anesthesiology* 1999;91:436–441.
42. Douglas MJ. Walking epidural analgesia in labour. *Can J Anaesth* 1998;45:607–611.
43. Aneiros F, Vazquez M, Valiño C, et al. Does epidural versus combined spinal-epidural analgesia prolong labor and increase the risk of instrumental and cesarean delivery in nulliparous women? *J Clin Anesth* 2009;21:94–97.
44. Simmons SW, Cyna AM, Dennis AT, et al. Combined spinal-epidural versus epidural analgesia in labour. *Cochrane Database Syst Rev* 2007;3:CD003401.
45. Eisenach JC. Combined spinal-epidural analgesia in obstetrics. *Anesthesiology* 1999;91:299–302.
46. Campbell DC, Camann WR, Datta S. The addition of bupivacaine to intrathecal sufentanil for labor analgesia. *Anesth Analg* 1995;81:305–309.
47. Cohen SE, Cherry CM, Holbrook RH Jr, et al. Intrathecal sufentanil for labor analgesia—sensory changes, side effects, and fetal heart rate changes. *Anesth Analg* 1993;77:1155–1160.
48. Riley ET, Ratner EF, Cohen SE. Intrathecal sufentanil for labor analgesia: do sensory changes predict better analgesia and greater hypotension? *Anesth Analg* 1997;84:346–351.
49. Honet JE, Arkoosh VA, Norris MC, et al. Comparison among intrathecal fentanyl, meperidine, and sufentanil for labor analgesia. *Anesth Analg* 1992;75:734–739.
50. Clarke VT, Smiley RM, Finster M. Uterine hyperactivity after intrathecal injection of fentanyl for analgesia during labor: a cause of fetal bradycardia? *Anesthesiology* 1994;81:1083.
51. Nielsen PE, Erickson JR, Abouleish EI, et al. Fetal heart rate changes after intrathecal sufentanil or epidural bupivacaine for labor analgesia: incidence and clinical significance. *Anesth Analg* 1996;83:742–746.
52. Palmer CM, Maciulla JE, Cork RC, et al. The incidence of fetal heart rate changes after intrathecal fentanyl labor analgesia. *Anesth Analg* 1999;88:577–581.
53. Eberle RL, Norris MC, Eberle AM, et al. The effect of maternal position on fetal heart rate during epidural or intrathecal labor analgesia. *Am J Obstet Gynecol* 1998;179:150–155.
54. Mardirosoff C, Dumont L, Boulvain M, et al. Fetal bradycardia due to intrathecal opioids for labour analgesia: a systematic review. *BJOG* 2002;109:274–281.
55. Norris MC. Intrathecal opioids and fetal bradycardia: Is there a link? *Int J Obstet Anesth* 2000;9:264–269.
56. Segal S, Wang SY. The effect of maternal catecholamines on the caliber of gravid uterine microvessels. *Anesth Analg* 2008;106:888–892.
57. Albright GA, Forster RM. The safety and efficacy of combined spinal and epidural analgesia/anesthesia (6,002 blocks) in a community hospital. *Reg Anesth Pain Med* 1999;24:117–125.
58. Sinclair JC, Fox HA, Lentz JF, et al. Intoxication of the fetus by a local anesthetic. A newly recognized complication of maternal caudal anesthesia. *N Engl J Med* 1965;273:1173–1177.
59. Paech MJ, Godkin R, Webster S. Complications of obstetric epidural analgesia and anaesthesia: a prospective analysis of 10,995 cases. *Int J Obstet Anesth* 1998;7:5–11.
60. Asling JH, Shnider SM, Margolis AJ, et al. Paracervical block anesthesia in obstetrics. II. Etiology of fetal bradycardia following paracervical block anesthesia. *Am J Obstet Gynecol* 1970;107:626–634.
61. Manninen T, Aantaa R, Salonen M, et al. A comparison of the hemodynamic effects of paracervical block and epidural anesthesia for labor analgesia. *Acta Anaesthesiol Scand* 2000;44:441–445.
62. Ralston DH, Shnider SM. The fetal and neonatal effects of regional anesthesia in obstetrics. *Anesthesiology* 1978;48:34–64.
63. Ranta P, Jouppila P, Spalding M, et al. Paracervical block—a viable alternative for labor pain relief? *Acta Obstet Gynecol Scand* 1995;74:122–126.
64. Bonica J. *Principles and Practice of Obstetric Analgesia and Anesthesia*. Philadelphia, PA: Davis; 1967:520–526.
65. Hunter CA. Uterine motility studies during labor. Observations on bilateral sympathetic nerve block in the normal and abnormal first stage of labor. *Am J Obstet Gynecol* 1963;85:681–686.
66. Leighton BL, Halpern SH, Wilson DB. Lumbar sympathetic blocks speed early and second stage induced labor in nulliparous women. *Anesthesiology* 1999;90:1039–1046.
67. Pace MC, Aurilio C, Bulletti C, et al. Subarachnoid analgesia in advanced labor: a comparison of subarachnoid analgesia and pudendal block in advanced labor: analgesic quality and obstetric outcome. *Ann N Y Acad Sci* 2004;1034:356–363.
68. Kilpatrick ME, Girgis NL. Meningitis—a complication of spinal anesthesia. *Anesth Analg* 1983;62:513–515.
69. Carp H, Bailey S. The association between meningitis and dural puncture in bacteremic rats. *Anesthesiology* 1992;76:739–742.
70. Douglas MJ. Platelets, the parturient and regional anesthesia. *Int J Obstet Anesth* 2001;10:113–120.
71. Wee L, Sinha P, Lewis M. Central nerve block and coagulation: a survey of obstetric anaesthetists. *Int J Obstet Anesth* 2002;11:170–175.
72. van Veen JJ, Nokes TJ, Makris M. The risk of spinal haematoma following neuraxial anaesthesia or lumbar puncture in thrombocytopenic individuals. *Br J Haematol* 2010;148:15–25.
73. Horlocker TT, Wedel DJ, Rowlingson JC, et al. Regional anesthesia in the patient receiving antithrombotic or thrombolytic therapy: American Society of Regional Anesthesia and Pain Medicine Evidence-Based Guidelines (Third Edition). *Reg Anesth Pain Med* 2010;35:64–101.
74. Horlocker TT, Heit JA. Low molecular weight heparin: biochemistry, pharmacology, perioperative prophylaxis regimens, and guidelines for regional anesthetic management. *Anesth Analg* 1997;85:874–885.
75. Sharma SK, Philip J, Whitten CW, et al. Assessment of changes in coagulation in parturients with preeclampsia using thromboelastography. *Anesthesiology* 1999;90:385–390.
76. Eappen S, Blinn A, Segal S. Incidence of epidural catheter replacement in parturients: a retrospective chart review. *Int J Obstet Anesth* 1998;7:220–225.
77. Morrison LM, Buchan AS. Comparison of complications associated with single-holed and multi-holed extradural catheters. *Br J Anaesth* 1990;64:183–185.
78. Narang VP, Linter SP. Failure of extradural blockade in obstetrics. A new hypothesis. *Br J Anaesth* 1988;60:402–404.
79. Beilin Y, Bernstein HH, Zucker-Pinchoff B. The optimal distance that a multiorifice epidural catheter should be threaded into the epidural space. *Anesth Analg* 1995;81:301–304.
80. D'Angelo R, Berkebile BL, Gerancher JC. Prospective examination of epidural catheter insertion. *Anesthesiology* 1996;84:88–93.
81. Hamilton CL, Riley ET, Cohen SE. Changes in the position of epidural catheters associated with patient movement. *Anesthesiology* 1997;86:778–784.
82. Mets B, Broccoli E, Brown AR. Is spinal anesthesia after failed epidural anesthesia contraindicated for cesarean section? *Anesth Analg* 1993;77:629–631.
83. Goldstein MM, Dewan DM. Spinal anesthesia after failed epidural anesthesia. *Anesth Analg* 1994;79:1206–1207.
84. Kick O, Böhrer H. Unexpectedly high spinal anaesthesia following failed extradural anaesthesia for caesarean section. *Anaesthesia* 1993;48:271.
85. Carr MF, Hehre FW. Complications of continuous lumbar peridural anesthesia. I. Inadvertent lumbar puncture. *Anesth Analg* 1962;41:349–353.

86. Kenepp NB, Gutsche BB. Inadvertent intravascular injections during lumbar epidural anesthesia. *Anesthesiology* 1981;54:172–173.

87. Abraham RA, Harris AP, Maxwell LG, et al. The efficacy of 1.5% lidocaine with 7.5% dextrose and epinephrine as an epidural test dose for obstetrics. *Anesthesiology* 1986;64:116–119.

88. Vallejo MC, Beaman ST, Ramanathan S. Blurred vision as the only symptom of a positive epidural test dose. *Anesth Analg* 2006;102:973–974.

89. Leighton BL, Norris MC, DeSimone CA, et al. The air test as a clinically useful indicator of intravenously placed epidural catheters. *Anesthesiology* 1990;73:610–613.

90. Michael S, Richmond MN, Birks RJ. A comparison between open-end (single hole) and closed-end (three lateral holes) epidural catheters. Complications and quality of sensory blockade. *Anaesthesia* 1989;44:578–580.

91. Reynolds F. Epidural catheter migration during labour. *Anaesthesia* 1988;43:69.

92. Norris MC, Fogel ST, Dalman H, et al. Labor epidural analgesia without an intravascular "test dose." *Anesthesiology* 1998;88:1495–1501.

93. Norris MC, Ferrenbach D, Dalman H, et al. Does epinephrine improve the diagnostic accuracy of aspiration during labor epidural analgesia? *Anesth Analg* 1999;88:1073–1076.

94. Birnbach DJ, Chestnut DH. The epidural test dose in obstetric patients: has it outlived its usefulness? *Anesth Analg* 1999;88:971–972.

95. Poblete B, Van Gessel EF, Gaggero G, et al. Efficacy of three test doses to detect epidural catheter misplacement. *Can J Anaesth* 1999;46:34–39.

96. Prince GD, Shetty GR, Miles M. Safety and efficacy of a low volume extradural test dose of bupivacaine in labour. *Br J Anaesth* 1989;62:503–508.

97. Morton CPJ, McClure JH. Ropivacaine test dose in extradural anaesthesia. *Br J Anaesth* 1997;79:813.

98. Moore DC, Batra MS. The components of an effective test dose prior to epidural block. *Anesthesiology* 1981;55:693–696.

99. Colonna-Romano P, Lingaraju N, Godfrey SD, et al. Epidural test dose and intravascular injection in obstetrics: sensitivity, specificity, and lowest effective dose. *Anesth Analg* 1992;75:372–376.

100. Colonna-Romano P, Salvage R, Lingaraju N, et al. Epinephrine-induced tachycardia is different from contraction-associated tachycardia in laboring patients. *Anesth Analg* 1996;82:294–296.

101. Cartwright PD, McCarroll SM, Antzaka C. Maternal heart rate changes with a plain epidural test dose. *Anesthesiology* 1986;65:226–228.

102. Leighton BL, Norris MC, Sosis M, et al. Limitations of epinephrine as a marker of intravascular injection in laboring women. *Anesthesiology* 1987;66:688–691.

103. Hood DD, Dewan DM, James FM 3rd. Maternal and fetal effects of epinephrine in gravid ewes. *Anesthesiology* 1986;64:610–613.

104. Schobel HP, Fischer T, Heuszer K, et al. Preeclampsia—a state of sympathetic overactivity. *N Engl J Med* 1996;335:1480–1485.

105. Cleaveland CR, Rangno RE, Shand DG. A standardized isoproterenol sensitivity test. The effects of sinus arrhythmia, atropine, and propranolol. *Arch Intern Med* 1972;130:47–52.

106. Leighton BL, DeSimone CA, Norris MC, et al. Isoproterenol is an effective marker of intravenous injection in laboring women. *Anesthesiology* 1989;71:206–209.

107. Leighton BL, Topkis WG, Gross JB, et al. Multiport epidural catheters: does the air test work? *Anesthesiology* 2000;92:1617–1620.

108. Shnider S. Experience with regional anesthesia for vaginal delivery. In: Shnider S, Moya F, eds. *The Anesthesiologist, Mother and Newborn.* Baltimore, MD: Williams and Wilkins; 1974:38.

109. Bromage PR. Physiology and pharmacology of epidural analgesia. *Anesthesiology* 1967;28:592–622.

110. Eckstein KL, Marx GF. Aortocaval compression and uterine displacement. *Anesthesiology* 1974;40:92–96.

111. Kerr MG, Scott DB, Samuel E. Studies of the inferior vena cava in late pregnancy. *Br Med J* 1964;1:532–533.

112. DiFazio CA, Carron H, Grosslight KR, et al. Comparison of pH-adjusted lidocaine solutions for epidural anesthesia. *Anesth Analg* 1986;65:760–764.

113. Parnass SM, Curran MJ, Becker GL. Incidence of hypotension associated with epidural anesthesia using alkalinized and nonalkalinized lidocaine for cesarean section. *Anesth Analg* 1987;66:1148–1150.

114. Greiss FC, Crandell DL. Therapy for hypotension induced by spinal anesthesia during pregnancy: observations on gravid ewes. *JAMA* 1965;191:793–796.

115. Greiss FC. Pressure-flow relationship in the gravid uterine vascular bed. *Am J Obstet Gynecol* 1966;96:41–47.

116. Adams FH, Assali N, Cushman M, et al. Interrelationships of maternal and fetal circulations. I. Flow-pressure responses to vasoactive drugs in sheep. *Pediatrics* 1961;27:627–635.

117. Lucas W, Kirschbaum T, Assali NS. Spinal shock and fetal oxygenation. *Am J Obstet Gynecol* 1965;93:583–587.

118. Myers RE. Two patterns of perinatal brain damage and their conditions of occurrence. *Am J Obstet Gynecol* 1972;112:246–276.

119. Ebner H, Barcohana J, Bartoshuk AK. Influence of postspinal hypotension on the fetal electrocardiogram. *Am J Obstet Gynecol* 1960;80:569–572.

120. Hon EH, Reid BL, Hehre FW. The electronic evaluation of fetal heart rate. II. Changes with maternal hypotension. *Am J Obstet Gynecol* 1960;79:209–215.

121. Bonica J, Hon E. Fetal distress. In: Bonica J, ed. *Principles and Practice of Obstetric Analgesia and Anesthesia.* Philadelphia, PA: Davis; 1964:1252.

122. Zilianti M, Salazar JR, Aller J, et al. Fetal heart rate and pH of fetal capillary blood during epidural analgesia in labor. *Obstet Gynecol* 1970;36:881–886.

123. Marx GF, Cosmi EV, Wollman SB. Biochemical status and clinical condition of mother and infant at cesarean section. *Anesth Analg* 1969;48:986–994.

124. Brizgys RV, Dailey PA, Shnider SM, et al. The incidence and neonatal effects of maternal hypotension during epidural anesthesia for cesarean section. *Anesthesiology* 1987;67:782–786.

125. Datta S, Alper MH, Ostheimer GW, et al. Method of ephedrine administration and nausea and hypotension during spinal anesthesia for cesarean section. *Anesthesiology* 1982;56:68–70.

126. Norris MC. Hypotension during spinal anesthesia for cesarean section: does it affect neonatal outcome? *Reg Anesth* 1987;12:191–194.

127. Jackson R, Reid JA, Thorburn J. Volume preloading is not essential to prevent spinal-induced hypotension at caesarean section. *Br J Anaesth* 1995;75:262–265.

128. Rout CC, Rocke DA, Levin J, et al. A reevaluation of the role of crystalloid preload in the prevention of hypotension associated with spinal anesthesia for elective cesarean section. *Anesthesiology* 1993;79:262–269.

129. Ueyama H, He YL, Tanigami H, et al. Effects of crystalloid and colloid preload on blood volume in the parturient undergoing spinal anesthesia for elective cesarean section. *Anesthesiology* 1999;91:1571–1576.

130. Rout CC, Akoojee SS, Rocke DA, et al. Rapid administration of crystalloid preload does not decrease the incidence of hypotension after spinal anaesthesia for elective caesarean section. *Br J Anaesth* 1992;68:394–397.

131. Karinen J, Räsänen J, Alahuhta S, et al. Effect of crystalloid and colloid preloading on uteroplacental and maternal haemodynamic state during spinal anaesthesia for caesarean section. *Br J Anaesth* 1995;75:531–535.

132. Cheek TG, Samuels P, Miller F, et al. Normal saline i.v. fluid load decreases uterine activity in active labour. *Br J Anaesth* 1996;77:632–635.

133. Zamora JE, Rosaeg OP, Lindsay MP, et al. Haemodynamic consequences and uterine contractions following 0.5 or 1.0 litre crystalloid infusion before obstetric epidural analgesia. *Can J Anaesth* 1996;43:347–352.

134. Evans SE, Crawford JS, Stevens ID, et al. Fluid therapy for induced labour under epidural analgesia: biochemical consequences for mother and infant. *Br J Obstet Gynaecol* 1986;93:329–333.

135. Kenepp NB, Kumar S, Shelley WC, et al. Fetal and neonatal hazards of maternal hydration with 5% dextrose before caesarean section. *Lancet* 1982;1:1150–1152.

136. Mendiola J, Grylack LJ, Scanlon JW. Effects of intrapartum maternal glucose infusion on the normal fetus and newborn. *Anesth Analg* 1982;61:32–35.

137. Morton KE, Jackson MC, Gillmer MD. A comparison of the effects of four intravenous solutions for the treatment of ketonuria during labour. *Br J Obstet Gynaecol* 1985;92:473–479.

138. Lanier WL, Stangland KJ, Scheithauer BW, et al. The effects of dextrose infusion and head position on neurologic outcome after complete cerebral ischemia in primates: examination of a model. *Anesthesiology* 1987;66:39–48.

139. Wright RG, Shnider SM, Levinson G, et al. The effect of maternal administration of ephedrine on fetal heart rate and variability. *Obstet Gynecol* 1981;57:734–738.

140. Casady GN, Moore DC, Bridenbaugh LD. Postpartum hypertension after use of vasoconstrictor and oxytocic drugs. Etiology, incidence, complications, and treatment. *J Am Med Assoc* 1960;172:1011–1015.

141. Poppers PJ. Evaluation of local anaesthetic agents for regional anaesthesia in obstetrics. *Br J Anaesth* 1975;47:322–327.

142. Moore DC, Bridenbaugh LD, Thompson GE, et al. Factors determining dosages of amide-type local anesthetic drugs. *Anesthesiology* 1977;47:263–268.

143. Grimes DA, Cates W Jr. Deaths from paracervical anesthesia used for first-trimester abortion, 1972–1975. *N Engl J Med* 1976;295:1397–1399.

144. Adamson DH. Continuous epidural anaesthesia in the community hospital. *Can Anaesth Soc J* 1973;20:687–692.

145. Crawford JS. The second thousand epidural blocks in an obstetric hospital practice. *Br J Anaesth* 1972;44:1277–1287.

146. Kandel PF, Spoerel WE, Kinch RA. Continuous epidural analgesia for labour and delivery: review of 1000 cases. *Can Med Assoc J* 1966;95:947–953.

147. Bush RC. Caudal analgesia for vaginal delivery. II. Analysis of complications. *Anesthesiology* 1959;20:186–191.

148. Crawford JS. Some maternal complications of epidural analgesia for labour. *Anaesthesia* 1985;40:1219–1225.

149. Brown DL, Ransom DM, Hall JA, et al. Regional anesthesia and local anesthetic-induced systemic toxicity: seizure frequency and accompanying cardiovascular changes. *Anesth Analg* 1995;81:321–328.

150. Chadwick HS. An analysis of obstetric anesthesia cases from the American society of anesthesiologists closed claims project database. *Int J Obstet Anesth* 1996;5:258–263.

151. Espinet AJ, Emmerton MT. The successful use of intralipid for treatment of local anesthetic-induced central nervous system toxicity: Some considerations for administration of intralipid in an emergency. *Clin J Pain* 2009;25:808–809.

152. Marx GF. Cardiopulmonary resuscitation of late-pregnant women. *Anesthesiology* 1982;56:156.

153. Finegold H, Darwich A, Romeo R, et al. Successful resuscitation after maternal cardiac arrest by immediate cesarean section in the labor room. *Anesthesiology* 2002;96:1278.

154. Vanden Hoek TL, Morrison LJ, Shuster M, et al. Part 12: cardiac arrest in special situations: 2010 American Heart Association guidelines for cardiopulmonary resuscitation and emergency cardiovascular care. *Circulation* 2010;122: S829–S861.

155. Morishima HO, Adamsons K. Placental clearance of mepivacaine following administration to the guinea pig fetus. *Anesthesiology* 1967;28:343–348.

156. Philip JH, Brown WU. Total spinal anesthesia late in the course of obstetric bupivacaine epidural block. *Anesthesiology* 1976;44:340–341.

157. Reynolds F, Speedy HM. The subdural space: the third place to go astray. *Anaesthesia* 1990;45:120–123.

158. Ferguson S, Brighouse D, Valentine S. An unusual complication following combined spinal-epidural anaesthesia for caesarean section. *Int J Obstet Anesth* 1997;6:190–193.

159. Robbins PM, Fernando R, Lim GH. Accidental intrathecal insertion of an extradural catheter during combined spinal-extradural anaesthesia for caesarean section. *Br J Anaesth* 1995;75:355–357.

160. Morgan B. Unexpectedly extensive conduction blocks in obstetric epidural analgesia. *Anaesthesia* 1990;45:148–152.

161. Collier C. Total spinal or massive subdural block? *Anaesth Intensive Care* 1982; 10:92–93.

162. Lubenow T, Keh-Wong E, Kristof K, et al. Inadvertent subdural injection: a complication of an epidural block. *Anesth Analg* 1988;67:175–179.

163. Vallejo MC, Firestone LL, Mandell GL, et al. Effect of epidural analgesia with ambulation on labor duration. *Anesthesiology* 2001;95:857–861.

164. Russell R. Assessment of motor blockade during epidural analgesia in labour. *Int J Obstet Anesth* 1992;1:230–234.

165. Bromage PR, Datta S, Dunford LA. Etidocaine: an evaluation in epidural analgesia for obstetrics. *Can Anaesth Soc J* 1974;21:535–545.

166. Bromage PR. An evaluation of bupivacaine in epidural analgesia for obstetrics. *Can Anaesth Soc J* 1969;16:46–56.

167. Loo CC, Dahlgren G, Irestedt L. Neurological complications in obstetric regional anaesthesia. *Int J Obstet Anesth* 2000;9:99–124.

168. Wetstone DL, Wong KC. Sinus bradycardia and asystole during spinal anesthesia. *Anesthesiology* 1974;41:87–88.

169. Caplan RA, Ward RJ, Posner K, et al. Unexpected cardiac arrest during spinal anesthesia: a closed claims analysis of predisposing factors. *Anesthesiology* 1988;68:5–11.

170. Auroy Y, Narchi P, Messiah A, et al. Serious complications related to regional anesthesia: results of a prospective survey in France. *Anesthesiology* 1997; 87:479–486.

171. Kopp SL, Horlocker TT, Warner ME, et al. Cardiac arrest during neuraxial anesthesia: frequency and predisposing factors associated with survival. *Anesth Analg* 2005;100:855–865.

172. Arendt KW, Segal S. Present and emerging strategies for reducing anesthesia-related maternal morbidity and mortality. *Curr Opin Anaesthesiol* 2009;22:330–335.

173. Scull TJ, Carli F. Cardiac arrest after caesarean section under subarachnoid block. *Br J Anaesth* 1996;77:274–276.

174. Hawthorne L, Lyons G. Cardiac arrest complicating spinal anaesthesia for caesarean section. *Int J Obstet Anesth* 1997;6:126–129.

175. MacArthur C, Lewis M, Knox EG, et al. Epidural anaesthesia and long term backache after childbirth. *BMJ* 1990;301:9–12.

176. MacArthur C, Lewis M, Knox EG. Investigation of long term problems after obstetric epidural anaesthesia. *BMJ* 1992;304:1279–1282.

177. Svensson HO, Andersson GB, Hagstad A, et al. The relationship of low-back pain to pregnancy and gynecologic factors. *Spine* 1990;15:371–375.

178. Breen TW, Ransil BJ, Groves PA, et al. Factors associated with back pain after childbirth. *Anesthesiology* 1994;81:29–34.

179. Russell R, Dundas R, Reynolds F. Long term backache after childbirth: prospective search for causative factors. *BMJ* 1996;312:1384–1388.

180. Grove LH. Backache, headache and bladder dysfunction after delivery. *Br J Anaesth* 1973;45:1147–1149.

181. Olofsson CI, Ekblom AO, Ekman-Ordeberg GE, et al. Post-partum urinary retention: a comparison between two methods of epidural analgesia. *Eur J Obstet Gynecol Reprod Biol* 1996;71:31–34.

182. Rawal N, Möllefors K, Axelsson K, et al. An experimental study of urodynamic effects of epidural morphine and of naloxone reversal. *Anesth Analg* 1983;62:641–647.

Anesthesia for Vaginal Birth After Cesarean Delivery

C. LaToya Mason • Nikolaos Marios Zacharias

■ INTRODUCTION

Vaginal birth after cesarean (VBAC) is the term used to describe vaginal delivery by a woman who has had a previous cesarean delivery. This topic is largely an issue directly related to obstetrical management. However, its discussion is merited in this context because anesthesia providers are routinely called upon to play a role in the care of women undergoing a trial of labor after cesarean delivery (TOLAC). Historically, the question of how to best approach subsequent delivery of this patient population has been the subject of much debate. In 1916, Edward Cragin pronounced the dictum "once a cesarean, always a cesarean" (1). In 1997, Bruce Flamm modified this phrase to "once a cesarean, always a controversy" (2). Undoubtedly, this topic continues to be controversial and complex. The NIH Consensus Development Conference convened in 2010 with the objective of providing health care providers, expecting couples, and the general public with a responsible assessment of currently available data on TOLAC/VBAC (3).

In the past decade, impactful statements have been published by the American College of Obstetricians and Gynecologists (ACOG)—renamed in 2010 the American Congress of Obstetricians and Gynecologists—as well as the professional obstetrical societies of other countries, affecting the choices of obstetricians and expecting couples (4,5). Reasonable recommendations regarding capacity for emergency abdominal delivery in hospitals offering TOLAC and avoidance of prostaglandins and oxytocin for labor induction/augmentation in women with prior cesarean delivery (CD) have led to even further distancing of practicing US obstetricians from TOLAC. The most recent ACOG practice bulletin on this topic (August 2010) was meant to invigorate the practice of TOLAC in the United States, but it essentially re-interprets prior evidence aiming to curtail the US cesarean delivery rate, without new convincing data (6). This document is unlikely to have any significant impact on the established trends (too little, too late). A factor that cannot be underestimated is the evolution of modern US society and its values; focus on maternal autonomy, convenience, quality of life (e.g., avoiding intrapartum asphyxia with neurologic sequelae, and maternal pelvic floor defects with incontinence) and perinatal risk-aversion, in the midst of an obesity epidemic, delayed childbearing and declining fertility have all helped frame a particular context for prenatal informed consent that may well be the main underlying cause of the observed CD trends in this country.

The determination of which women are appropriate candidates to attempt a trial of labor after prior cesarean delivery is a delicate decision that takes into consideration numerous factors. Although it is the obstetrician who is primarily responsible for helping the gravida make this decision, it is of utmost importance that anesthesia providers understand the implications of such decisions as well as how the complex confluence of factors—medical and non-medical—interplay in the provision of care for these women. In order to ensure optimal patient outcomes, it is essential that anesthesia providers have a thorough understanding of the clinical benefits and risks associated with VBAC. This chapter will provide an evidence-based discussion of the aforementioned topics as well as provide management recommendations for the anesthesia provider who is charged with the arduous task of caring for the woman planning VBAC.

■ BACKGROUND INFORMATION

Relevant Terminology

Anesthesia providers may have varying degrees of familiarity with certain terms relevant to this topic that are often used in conflicting and confusing ways by obstetricians, family practitioners, nurse midwives, investigators, and expecting couples. The following definitions and acronyms are offered to promote clarity and to provide consistency throughout this discussion (3,6):

- Trial of labor after previous cesarean delivery (TOLAC): A planned attempt to labor by a woman who has had a previous cesarean delivery (CD).
- VBAC delivery: Vaginal delivery after TOLAC; that is, a successful TOLAC.
- Unsuccessful or failed TOLAC: Cesarean delivery after TOLAC.
- Prelabor repeat cesarean delivery (PRCD): Also referred to as elective repeat cesarean delivery; this term describes planned repeat CD without TOLAC attempt at 39 weeks.

Rates and Practice Patterns

The past four decades have seen a remarkable swing of the pendulum regarding overall CD rates and VBAC in the United States, and worldwide. Cesarean delivery represents the most commonly performed surgical procedure in the United States. According to data from the National Center for Health Statistics, nearly one-third (32%) of all births in 2007 were cesarean deliveries (7) (Fig. 10-1). This rate represents an all-time high. The United States CD rate was approximately 5% in 1970 and has been rising since with ever-increasing prospects. The VBAC rate has played an important role in this trend: When recommendations favoring TOLAC were published by ACOG in 1988 and 1994, the number of women delivering by VBAC with a prior CD rose from 5% in 1985 to almost 29% in 1996, and the total CD rate declined to 20%. Since then, reports of increasing uterine rupture and TOLAC complications in an

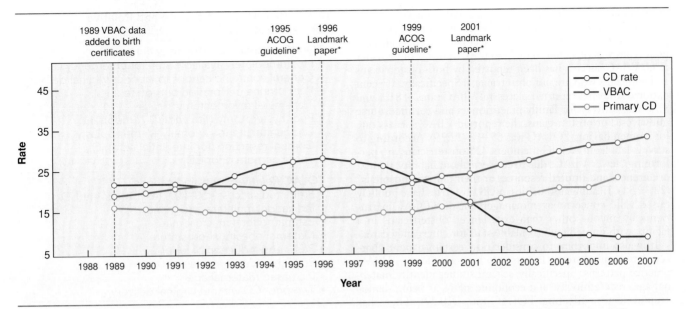

FIGURE 10-1 Rates of VBAC, total cesarean deliveries (CD rates), and primary cesarean deliveries (Primary CD).

adverse medicolegal climate and large epidemiologic studies documenting the maternal–fetal safety of PRCD dissuaded many obstetricians and expecting couples from attempting TOLAC. US data from 2006 show that only 8% of women with prior CD delivered by VBAC. It appears that modern obstetrics has returned via a convoluted path to Dr. Cragin's century-old dictum (8,9).

Several factors contribute to the increased rate of cesarean delivery. Roughly one-third of nulliparous women undergo operative delivery (10). In addition, an estimated 40% of cesarean deliveries performed are planned repeat procedures. PRCD performed due to a previous scar is the most commonly cited reason for cesarean delivery (11). The coinciding decrease in the number of TOLAC attempts also significantly contributes to the overall increase in the rate of cesarean delivery (3). Other contributing factors include changes in practice environment such as the introduction of electronic fetal monitoring, the extinction of vaginal breech deliveries, and the declining use of operative vaginal deliveries (12–14). There is an ever-growing body of evidence providing clinical reasons to substantiate the increased performance of CD. Nonetheless, the short- and long-term benefits and risks presented to both mother and infant have been the subject of intense debate for several decades (15). Similarly, the mode of delivery for subsequent pregnancy among women who have undergone a previous CD has divided the scientific community for years.

VBAC is not a novel concept. There are reports of successful VBAC dating back to the 1950s in Europe—the United Kingdom in particular. Publications addressing the appropriateness of VBACs have ranged from isolated case reports to large clinical trials. VBAC has been widely practiced in UK since the standardization of the low transverse (Kerr) hysterotomy as the incision of choice (16). However, it was not until the time period spanning from 1981 to 1996 that US obstetric providers really embraced this practice. During that time, VBAC grew in popularity in the United States primarily due to concerns regarding the growing cesarean delivery rate. In 1982, the first statement published after the National Institutes of Health Consensus Conference endorsed VBAC as being an "acceptable option" to repeat cesarean delivery for many women. It was then stated that measures should be taken to ensure careful selection of patients, proper facilities, and immediate availability of appropriate staff including in-house obstetrician and anesthesia provider (17). At its peak in 1996, VBAC rates were reported to be more than 28% in the United States. These rates were short-lived though as concerns quickly grew about the potentially serious complications of TOLAC (18). Quite notably, there was marked concern regarding adverse outcomes associated with failed TOLAC including but not limited to uterine rupture, hysterectomy, transfusion, maternal, and perinatal mortality. The current VBAC rate in the United States is reported to be approximately 8.5% (19). Concerns about patient safety and physician liability have thus led to more restrictive policies and the coinciding decline in VBAC use in the United States.

Factors Influencing TOLAC/VBAC Practice Patterns

TOLAC rates are highly variable; they range from 28% to 70% with an overall US rate of 58% (20). The Royal College of Obstetricians and Gynaecologists (RCOG) reports a successful VBAC rate of 72% to 76% after one cesarean delivery (5). A Canadian study reported similar results, citing a VBAC success rate of 76.6% (21). Globally speaking, TOLAC results in VBAC 60% to 80% of the time although physicians in Europe, Asia, and Africa are more inclined than those in the United States and Canada to attempt TOLAC (22). There are several factors—medical and non-medical—that can be used as predictors of VBAC success and hence influence VBAC practice patterns. Practice patterns may vary according to geographic region, hospital setting, provider preference, and patient characteristics. VBAC has an inverse relationship to CD rates; high VBAC rate is invariably associated with lower CD rates (23). Geographically speaking, recent data trends suggest that Southern states have the lowest VBAC rates and Western states have the highest VBAC rates (23–25). In terms of hospital setting, TOLAC is more likely to be attempted in hospitals with higher delivery volumes, academic tertiary care centers, and teaching hospitals with residency programs. As a result, lower rates of cesarean delivery are observed in such facilities (26,27). A study by DeFranco et al. further demonstrates greater VBAC attempts at university and community hospitals with obstetrics training programs than in community hospitals without training programs (61% vs. 50.4%). The success rate across all hospital types was reported to be 75% (28). In terms of provider type, VBAC success has been reported by both obstetricians and clinicians who are not obstetricians. Specifically, a recent national study has reported successful VBAC rates of 81% and 87% respectively for family practitioners and certified nurse midwives. For obstetricians, the reported VBAC success rate for women having TOLAC was 65.4% (22,29). According to survey data from ACOG members, US obstetricians are performing "fewer VBACs due to concern about liability, patient preference, and limited resources at their delivery hospitals" (22,30,31). Leading authorities in US obstetrics have publicly raised valid concerns over management of TOLAC parturients by anyone other than experienced obstetricians in a facility with immediately available staff for emergency care.

It is also important to consider how certain patient characteristics and obstetric factors may have an effect on VBAC practice patterns. Specifically, several studies identify maternal age, race/ethnicity, and economic status as being demographic factors affecting TOLAC rates (20,29). There has been a decrease in VBAC use across all age groups (18,19). Similarly, the VBAC rate has declined for all racial and ethnic groups (19,23,25). It is interesting to note, however, that non-white women are more likely to attempt TOLAC but less likely to be successful at VBAC (32). In terms of obstetric factors, women with a prior vaginal delivery had greater than twice the chance of a TOLAC (odds ratio: 1.51 to 6.67) (23,33–35). Eleven cohort studies consistently reported that a prior history of vaginal delivery increases the chance of VBAC (35–45). Furthermore, women with a history of prior VBAC were three to seven times more likely to have a VBAC for their current delivery compared with women with no prior vaginal deliveries (38,40–44,46,47). As alluded to earlier, non-clinical factors are influential and relate to the likelihood of TOLAC. NIH data suggest variance in VBAC rates by insurance status; privately insured women have lower VBAC rates and higher cesarean delivery rates than their Medicaid counterparts (26). Contrarily, analyses of datasets from the Nationwide Inpatient Sample (NIS) for years 2000, 2003, and 2005 found no difference in VBAC process measures by insurance type. It has been postulated that the low use of VBAC is independent of insurance type but rather it is dependent upon hospital resources (23,34). The interaction of the many factors—medical and non-medical—that influence TOLAC utilization and VBAC practice patterns are quite complex and constitute an important component in decision-making and quality of patient care. Certainly, a better understanding of these factors and the significance of their impact on TOLAC/VBAC is warranted (20).

■ DETERMINING PATIENT ELIGIBILITY FOR TOLAC

Absolute and Relative Contraindications

There are several (absolute or relative) contraindications to TOLAC: Unavailability of staff for emergency abdominal delivery (home birth, understaffed small hospital), general contraindications to labor or vaginal delivery (e.g., placenta or vasa previa, obstructed birth canal [e.g., fibroids], active herpetic infection in the birth canal, severe maternal cardiovascular pathology, intrapartum malpresentation [singleton or multifetal], Ehlers–Danlos syndrome type IV), prior uterine perforation or open fetal surgery, prior hysterotomy with any vertical component (documented or suspected by history), transmural myomectomy, cornual resection (for interstitial

TABLE 10-1 TOLAC Absolute and Relative Contraindications

TOLAC Absolute Contraindications
- No immediately available staff for emergency care
- General contraindications to labor or vaginal delivery
- Prior uterine perforation or rupture
- Transmural myomectomy
- Prior hysterotomy with vertical component
- Congenital uterine anomaly +/−metroplasty
- Cornual resection (for interstitial ectopic)
- Three or more prior CD

TOLAC Relative Contraindications
- Predicted success <50–60% (e.g., recurrent CD indication, multifetal pregnancy)
- Estimated fetal macrosomia
- Maternal obesity, short stature
- Post-term induction of labor
- Prior shoulder dystocia
- Increased maternal age
- Two prior CD without vaginal delivery

ectopic), prior uterine rupture or hysterotomy scar dehiscence, congenital uterine anomaly with or without metroplasty, three or more previous CD, two previous CD without vaginal delivery, prior shoulder dystocia, fetal macrosomia (estimated fetal weight >4 kg), maternal obesity, short stature, and post-term induction of labor (or combinations thereof—in order of decreasing criterion firmness) (48,49) (Table 10-1).

The risk of symptomatic uterine rupture during TOLAC varies considerably by prior hysterotomy type: It is 0.2% to 1.5% with Kerr (low transverse), 1% to 7% with Krönig (low vertical) and 4% to 9% with classical/T/J-shaped incisions (Fig. 10-2). As most expecting couples and obstetricians in the United States consider a risk of catastrophic uterine rupture greater than 1% to be excessive, in practical terms only women with prior known or estimated Kerr hysterotomy are considered TOLAC candidates. Limited literature has addressed the issue of mode of delivery among women with two prior Kerr hysterotomies and prior vaginal delivery; it suggests that these women have similar chance of successful VBAC and moderately increased major morbidity when compared to women with one prior CD. Thus, ACOG now states that women with two previous Kerr hysterotomies may be considered TOLAC candidates (6).

Most other women with a prior CD via documented or estimated Kerr hysterotomy carrying a singleton pregnancy may be TOLAC candidates and should expect at least a 2/3 to 3/4 chance of successful VBAC, especially if they have had a prior vaginal delivery (VBAC chance may be as high as 4/5 in such cases). They should be counseled accordingly in a non-directive fashion during prenatal care, as recommended by a 2010 NIH panel. Expecting couples should realize that both PRCD and TOLAC carry maternal–fetal benefits and risks and the two options should be compared on the basis of data analyzed by prospective intention-to-deliver (not actual delivery mode, which is only known post hoc).

Benefits from intended TOLAC in comparison to intended PRCD include avoidance of major abdominal surgery with prolonged physical recovery, and return to lower-risk status for all future pregnancies. It may, thus, be more appealing to younger women considering larger families, by offering lower likelihood of: Surgical morbidity (bowel, bladder, or ureter injury), future abnormal placental implantation (previa, accreta/increta/percreta), secondary infertility, and perhaps future fetal loss (50,51).

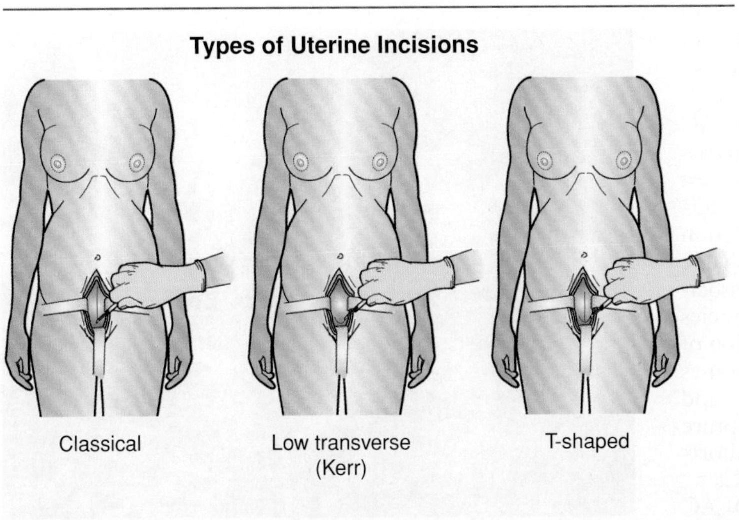

Types of Uterine Incisions

Classical

Low transverse
(Kerr)

T-shaped

FIGURE 10-2 Types of uterine incisions.

Benefits from intended PRCD in comparison to intended TOLAC include increased control over delivery timing (convenience) and significantly lower risks for: Symptomatic uterine rupture and its sequelae (0% vs. 0.9%), endometritis (1.8% vs. 2.9%), hypoxic ischemic encephalopathy (0% vs. 0.78%), and perinatal mortality (0.01% vs. 0.13%). It may, thus, be more appealing to most couples eager to minimize perinatal risks—especially older couples considering smaller families (1 to 2 children, with or without in vitro fertilization assistance)—and to women who have never entered active labor and are concerned about preserving their pelvic floor function.

Benefits aside, the prenatal counseling should identify and incorporate risk factors for TOLAC failure requiring urgent CD, because that is by far the most common morbid outcome in such attempts. Analysis of the literature confirms that several factors influence VBAC chance; spontaneous labor and prior vaginal birth increase the likelihood of successful VBAC. Conversely, recurring indication for CD (labor dystocia, cephalopelvic disproportion), short stature, maternal obesity, increasing age, fetal macrosomia, post-term pregnancy (>40 weeks), and labor induction/augmentation all decrease the likelihood of successful VBAC. A clinically useful online calculator for eligible couple counseling (one prior Kerr hysterotomy, currently with singleton, cephalic fetus) is derived from data of the US Maternal–Fetal Medicine Units Network (MFMU) and is available at: http://www.bsc.gwu.edu/mfmu/vagbirth.html. When the predicted likelihood of VBAC is <60%, there is evidence that morbidity is greater with planned TOLAC than PRCD; as an example, induction of labor in women with a prior CD, no prior vaginal delivery, and an unfavorable cervix has a 45% chance of successful VBAC and should be discouraged (52). On the other hand, it is appropriate to revisit the mode of delivery topic when women planning for PRCD present in advanced spontaneous labor (term or preterm), as they have fewer benefits from CD (no longer prelabor) and greater likelihood of successful VBAC (even if the antepartum prognostic score was unfavorable).

■ CONCERNS FOR PATIENT WELL-BEING

Short-term Maternal Outcomes

TOLAC is a reasonable and safe choice for the majority of eligible women. High-grade evidence evaluated during the NIH Consensus Development Conference of 2010 purports that women who attempt TOLAC are at decreased risk of maternal mortality compared to those who proceed directly with PRCD. Maternal mortality is estimated to be 3.8/100,000 live births for women undergoing TOLAC

compared with 13.4/100,000 live births for elective repeat cesarean delivery (3,20). The majority (60% to 80%) of women who attempt TOLAC will achieve VBAC. Women who successfully achieve VBAC may also experience the following distinct benefits when compared to those who proceed directly with planned PRCD: Lower rates of hysterectomies, lower rates of thromboembolic events, lower rates of blood transfusion, and shorter durations of hospital stay (11). Despite these known benefits, the rate of TOLAC attempts remains low. This is largely attributed to the potential occurrence of short- and long-term adverse outcomes women may be predisposed to if their attempts at TOLAC fail.

Presently, there is no existing model to accurately and absolutely predict which candidates will successfully achieve VBAC. A minority of women attempting TOLAC will require emergent repeat cesarean delivery that may be associated with serious adverse outcomes. Anesthesia providers, obstetric providers, and women contemplating TOLAC should be cognizant of these potential yet serious risks. Uterine rupture, hysterectomy, thromboembolic disease, operative injury, and maternal death are amongst the most severe outcomes reported in the literature (11,35,53–57). Figure 10-3 demonstrates left broad ligament hematoma caused by uterine rupture that resulted in intrauterine fetal demise. Less severe outcomes that have been cited include postpartum hemorrhage requiring blood transfusion, infectious

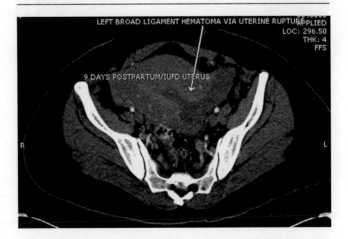

FIGURE 10-3 This CT image demonstrates left broad ligament hematoma caused by uterine rupture that resulted in intrauterine fetal demise.

morbidity (i.e., endometritis, wound infections, puerperal fever), and prolonged hospitalization (53–56,58,59). Symptomatic uterine rupture occurs almost exclusively in the setting of unsuccessful TOLAC. The rate of hysterectomy is similar for successful VBAC (0.1%), unsuccessful TOLAC (0.5%), and PRCD (0.3%). The frequency of blood transfusion and the risk for endometritis appears to be greatest among women with an unsuccessful TOLAC. Both maternal death and thromboembolic disease are rarely reported in the literature and their frequency is not easily distinguishable between these groups. However, intended PRCD is associated with one excess maternal death per 10,000 pregnancies when compared to intended TOLAC. With the exception of uterine rupture, data is scarce regarding maternal outcomes associated with successful VBAC, unsuccessful TOLAC, and PRCD. Hence, this discussion will focus upon uterine rupture as it is considered by many to be the most devastating short-term complication associated with attempting a TOLAC.

The less frequent but most feared outcome of TOLAC is symptomatic uterine rupture with its potentially lethal maternal–fetal sequelae. Symptomatic uterine rupture is practically never observed in PRCD. It is challenging to ascertain the exact rate of uterine rupture, because studies often combine symptomatic uterine ruptures with asymptomatic uterine scar dehiscences in their reporting. The 2010 NIH Development Consensus offers the following estimates for uterine rupture rate. The incidence of uterine rupture is 0.3% (325/100,000) in women undergoing TOLAC when all gestational ages are considered. This rate increases to 0.77% (778/100,000) in term women who attempt TOLAC. Uterine rupture risk is 0.026% (26/100,000) in women who undergo PRCD (3,20). Symptomatic rupture of the unscarred gravid uterus is a rare event, estimated to occur in 1 per 5 to 10,000 pregnancies. That rate is greater by two orders of magnitude in women with one prior CD attempting TOLAC. Risk factors for symptomatic uterine rupture in women with a prior CD include some of the same risk factors as for failed TOLAC: Vaginal nulliparity, multiple prior CD, labor induction or augmentation, post-term pregnancy, and thinning of the uterovesical septum on prenatal sonography (less than 2.3 mm) (Fig. 10-4) (60).

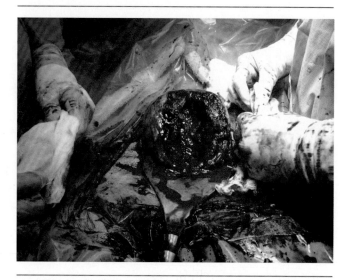

FIGURE 10-5 Uterine rupture.

It is paramount to distinguish between symptomatic uterine rupture and uterine scar dehiscence. Symptomatic uterine rupture and its intraoperative repair are photographed in Figure 10-5 and Figure 10-6. By definition, symptomatic uterine rupture describes a complete disruption of the entire thickness of the uterine wall (decidua, myometrium, and serosa), typically leading to (overt or covert) hemorrhage and occasionally to at least partial extrusion of the fetoplacental unit with resultant fetal heart rate abnormalities. A major impediment to interpreting literature on this topic is that different authors use the terms complete/incomplete uterine rupture, uterine scar dehiscence, and symptomatic uterine rupture interchangeably. In uterine scar dehiscence, the serosa is intact and maternal–fetal consequences are minimal—a stark contrast to symptomatic uterine rupture. Most of the TOLAC-associated cases in the literature represent symptomatic uterine ruptures (dehiscence would have remained undiagnosed without laparotomy in a successful VBAC) whereas the PRCD cases represent incidentally documented uterine scar dehiscence during repeat laparotomy (symptomatic uterine ruptures are not delivered via prelabor planned CD but are surgical emergencies). This has been shown in several studies, where TOLAC was

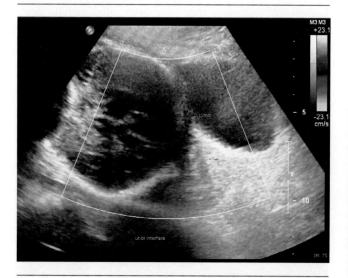

FIGURE 10-4 Thinning of the myometrium (<2.3 mm) at the site of six prior Kerr hysterotomies in a woman found to have uterine scar dehiscence at the time of her seventh repeat cesarean delivery.

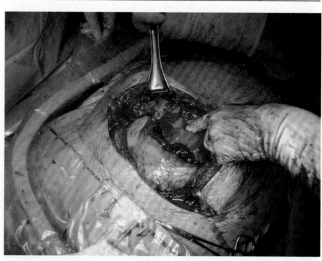

FIGURE 10-6 Uterine rupture repair.

associated with 3 to 4 additional symptomatic uterine ruptures per 1,000 cases in excess of PRCD—whereas the rate of asymptomatic uterine scar dehiscence was comparable between the two intended modes of delivery. In fact, women should expect practically no symptomatic uterine rupture and no hypoxic ischemic encephalopathy of their offspring if they deliver by PRCD; this is clearly the safest option for the index baby. PRCD is not, however, the safest option for the mother (1 excess death per 10,000 pregnancies, compared to planned TOLAC) and may jeopardize potential future pregnancies (placenta previa/accreta with resulting bladder injury and transfusion, secondary infertility, future fetal wastage—all increase exponentially with the number of CD) (61–63).

True uterine rupture may result in deleterious maternal–fetal consequences unless emergent care is promptly initiated. The close relationship that uterine rupture shares with maternal and perinatal morbidity and mortality makes it an area of great interest among healthcare providers, hospitals, policymakers, and expecting couples. Recognizing this, there is growing concern regarding what, if any, management factors may reduce its occurrence and/or severity (3). The rates of uterine rupture vary significantly and are dependent upon a variety of clinical risk factors. The type and location of the prior uterine incision is probably the most important factor to consider (Fig. 10-2). Previous vertical (classical and J/T-shaped) incisions significantly increase this risk (4% to 9%) (33). Prior low vertical incision (Krönig) carries a 1% to 7% risk of symptomatic uterine rupture. In addition to uterine scar type, the following characteristics of the obstetrical history have all been reported to affect the rate and risk of uterine rupture: Number of previous cesarean deliveries, previous vaginal delivery, interdelivery interval, and gestational age at delivery (61,64). Clearly, there are several identifiable factors associated with uterine rupture that may prove useful in counseling women and helping them to make informed decisions regarding their individual risks. There is unfortunately no perfect prospective risk calculator at this time despite attempts to develop an accurate model to estimate individual specific risk for uterine rupture during TOLAC (65).

Long-term Maternal Outcomes

The discussion of adverse outcomes associated with TOLAC attempts is not complete without the mention of potential long-term maternal outcomes. The majority of existing scientific literature focuses upon those adverse outcomes frequently observed in the short-term setting. It is equally important, however, to acknowledge associated long-term maternal complications when weighing the risk-to-benefit ratio for women considering TOLAC/VBAC. Women who undergo cesarean delivery and repeat cesarean delivery for that matter may experience a variety of chronic problems. These women are at increased risk for development of chronic pelvic pain, surgical adhesions, gastrointestinal symptoms, secondary infertility, and increased fetal wastage with future pregnancies; these morbidities occur in increasing frequency with the number of prior CDs (50,51). Quite noteworthy to mention is the fact that women undergoing multiple repeat CD—whether emergent or planned—are at markedly increased risk for placenta previa and accreta/increta/percreta accreta with the resultant life-threatening hemorrhage and morbidity risks (66). This condition and its anesthetic management are addressed in "*Chapter 21: Antepartum Hemorrhage and Blood Conservation Therapy; Postpartum Hemorrhage, Massive Transfusion Protocols, and Novel Therapeutic Interventions*". Even if placenta accreta is not present, the MFMU Network cohort study reports an association between increasing numbers of cesarean deliveries with increasing occurrences of

the following complications: Hysterectomy, placenta previa, cystotomy, operative injury, ileus, blood transfusion of four or more units, postoperative ventilation requirements, and prolonged duration of hospital stay (67,68). On the other hand, TOLAC +/– VBAC increase the likelihood of maternal pelvic floor dysfunction, urinary/fecal incontinence and pelvic organ prolapse several years later, thus undermining the quality of life for those affected. All in all, possible long-term complications must be considered as well as short-term complications when the decision is being made of whether or not TOLAC is the optimal choice for a particular expecting couple. Knowing what factors to take into account when evaluating the risk of adverse outcomes is important to providers and expectant mothers who want to make safe and wise management choices for childbirth.

■ OBSTETRIC MANAGEMENT APPROACH

Intrapartum Monitoring/ACOG Recommendations

Parturients attempting TOLAC are at high-risk for life-threatening maternal–fetal complications and should be managed accordingly. A multidisciplinary approach should be utilized in the management of such parturients (Fig. 10-7); that is, they should be cared for in facilities with immediately available staff (obstetrician, perinatal anesthesiologist, neonatologist, blood bank, and operating room) to provide emergency care (4,67). Continuous external fetal monitoring and tocodynamometry with real-time interpretation by an experienced obstetrician, epidural anesthesia, and a low threshold for repeat CD are the cornerstones of successful TOLAC management.

Symptomatic uterine rupture typically occurs intrapartum, although it can rarely happen in the antepartum period or first manifest postpartum (Fig. 10-3). Intrapartum presentation is usually heralded by fetal heart rate abnormalities (in up to 87% of cases: Bradycardia, decelerations or tachycardia) but may also manifest with maternal abdominal pain, tachycardia, hypotension/shock, cessation of uterine contractions, loss of station of the presenting fetus, uterine scar tenderness, and change in uterine shape. Diagnosis relies on maternal–fetal heart rate findings and not solely on maternal pain. Confirmation of the diagnosis occurs in the operating room during emergent laparotomy, and treatment is initiated at that time; continuous obstetrical vigilance and timely operative action are essential to optimize the perinatal outcome. After abdominal delivery of the fetus, the decision of uterine rupture repair versus

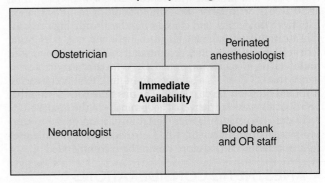

Multidisciplinary Management

Obstetrician	Perinated anesthesiologist
	Immediate Availability	
Neonatologist	Blood bank and OR staff

FIGURE 10-7 A multidisciplinary approach should be utilized in the management of parturients attempting TOLAC.

hysterectomy rests with the operating obstetrician and depends on maternal hemodynamic and coagulation parameters.

Intrauterine pressure catheter is not generally required for TOLAC management (unless oxytocin is being infused—controversial, but good practice point to allow careful titration to effect); fetal scalp electrode may be advisable if external fetal monitoring is unreliable, as with any other parturient (e.g., in obesity). Epidural anesthesia is highly recommended in women undergoing TOLAC because it is a safe comfort that takes the fear of painful contractions out of the equation of mode of delivery counseling and provides rapid access to surgical anesthesia—should that become necessary.

Prostaglandin use is contraindicated in women with prior hysterotomy undergoing third trimester TOLAC, as it has been associated with increased risk for symptomatic uterine rupture and its potentially lethal sequelae (4). ACOG states that misoprostol should not be used for third trimester cervical ripening or labor induction in women with a viable fetus and a prior CD or major uterine surgery. Of note, misoprostol may still be safely used for evacuation of the midtrimester gravid uterus (e.g., for lethal fetal anomalies) and for delivery of fetal demise in the third trimester with symptomatic uterine rupture rate <1%.

If labor induction is required in women with a prior CD and a viable fetus, the mode of delivery counseling should be revisited and informed consent should be obtained to reflect the decreased likelihood of successful VBAC (especially with unfavorable cervical examination) and increased risk of perinatal complications. Amniotic membrane stripping in GBS negative women around 38 weeks may be a good practice point to stimulate labor at term, but is not an evidence-based approach in women with prior CD, and may not always be practical as several medical indications for labor induction cannot be reliably predicted. Mechanical cervical ripening (Foley catheter) followed by amniotomy and continuous close monitoring is probably the safest approach for women desiring TOLAC after appropriate counseling in such situations, reserving oxytocin infusion for a select subgroup of women with prior vaginal delivery and favorable cervical examination. The oxytocin infusion rate and its duration should both be kept at a minimum on the basis of adequate contraction frequency and strength by intrauterine pressure catheter data—at the discretion of experienced obstetricians. No evidence-based recommendations currently exist regarding oxytocin use in the setting of TOLAC (for either induction or augmentation of labor). Therefore, careful maternal–fetal and labor monitoring along with sound clinical judgment and a low threshold for repeat CD are advisable (4).

In the absence of reliable data on external cephalic version (ECV) in women with prior CD, most obstetricians shy away from ECV and proceed with repeat CD for malpresentation at 39 weeks or in labor. By extrapolation of malpresentation data from singletons, and considering the already high risk for CD in multifetal pregnancies (to benefit the non-presenting fetus[es]), most authorities recommend PRCD in women with multifetal pregnancies and prior CD. As there is no reliable evidence that TOLAC is a safe option in multifetal pregnancies, it should probably be discouraged at this time considering that >80% of all twins are delivered abdominally in the modern US.

There is no evidence that digital inspection of the hysterotomy scar after successful VBAC provides any clinically useful information. It therefore cannot be recommended.

■ ANESTHETIC CONSIDERATIONS

Role of the Anesthesia Provider

Anesthesia providers play an integral role on the multidisciplinary teams that provide care for women attempting TOLAC. This role may solely mean the provision of epidural analgesia during labor for women who successfully achieve VBAC. In past decades, there has been concern regarding the utility of labor analgesia via epidural in this clinical setting. This concern stemmed primarily from the hypothesis that its use in labor interferes with the detection and treatment of uterine rupture. Obstetric clinicians rely heavily upon identification of the classically described signs and symptoms of uterine rupture that include fetal heart rate abnormalities, vaginal bleeding, maternal pain, and maternal hemodynamic instability (6,69–72). Specifically, there was great concern regarding whether the maternal pain caused by uterine rupture is blunted and not easily detected in the setting of epidural use. Evidence now exists to prove that this is not the case. Epidural dosing patterns may actually serve as a marker for impending or evolving uterine rupture. In 2010, Cahill et al. sought to estimate the association between epidural dosing patterns and the risk of uterine rupture in women who attempt VBAC in a nested case-control study within a multicenter retrospective cohort study of more than 25,000 women. This study observed increased requirements for epidural dosing immediately before uterine rupture relative to the women who did not experience uterine rupture. Women who experienced uterine rupture received more epidural doses on average than those who did not (4.1 vs. 3.5 doses, respectively; P = 0.04). These findings argue against the belief that women who undergo TOLAC with epidural anesthesia cannot perceive the pain that accompanies uterine rupture (72). These findings may be of significant use to those involved in the intrapartum management of women attempting TOLAC.

Good and consistent evidence support the recommendation that epidural analgesia for labor is appropriate for use in women attempting TOLAC (69). Epidural analgesia is not a causal risk factor for an unsuccessful TOLAC (6,68,73,74). While its use does not appear to enhance success rates, its use is certainly not contraindicated. Epidural analgesia should be used in TOLAC attempts. ACOG endorses the use of epidural analgesia during TOLAC upon maternal request. ACOG also acknowledges that the ability of epidurals to provide adequate pain relief during labor may encourage more women to opt for TOLAC. Most importantly, epidural analgesia should not be expected to mask the signs and symptoms of uterine rupture (55,61,64). In actuality, the perinatal care team should be cognizant of increased epidural dosing requirements in women attempting TOLAC as this may represent a surrogate marker for impending/evolving uterine rupture.

For those whose TOLAC attempts are unsuccessful due to failure to progress or other non-emergent obstetric indications, the anesthesia provider's role may translate to the provision of surgical anesthesia for uncomplicated repeat cesarean delivery. If the maternal–fetal status is reassuring, the anesthetic technique may be handled in the same manner as any other non-emergent repeat cesarean delivery. If an epidural catheter is in place and has been functioning well, it may be dosed appropriately to achieve surgical anesthesia.

In other cases where attempts at TOLAC go awry and dire obstetric emergencies are at hand, the role of the anesthesia provider may be extended further to include the provision of surgical anesthesia for emergent cesarean delivery. The choice of anesthetic technique should be made on a case-by-case basis (Fig. 10-8). Depending upon the clinical situation, a regional technique may be reasonable or induction of general endotracheal anesthesia may be mandated. In many cases, it may also become necessary for anesthesia providers to aid in the management of serious complications that may occur. Anesthesia providers are also responsible for managing fluid and electrolyte resuscitation,

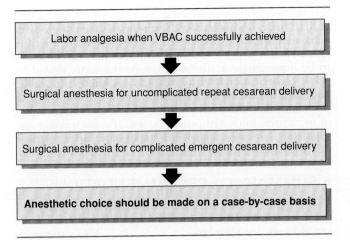

FIGURE 10-8 Role of the anesthesia provider.

administering blood products, and providing overall supportive care as indicated.

In a woman opting for TOLAC, the exact course of labor cannot be reliably be predicted on an individual basis. Therefore, anesthesia providers should make every effort to be thoroughly prepared to ensure optimal peripartum outcomes. It is recommended that a complete pre-anesthetic evaluation be performed including assessment of the maternal airway. Informed consent should also be obtained from all women undergoing TOLAC. In addition, large-bore intravenous access should be established early. Cross-matched blood products should be readily available at all times, preferably with an institutional massive transfusion protocol in place. The execution

TABLE 10-2 Highlights from "Optimal Goals for Anesthesia Care in Obstetrics"

ASA and ACOG Joint Statement
- Immediate availability of appropriate facilities and personnel, including obstetric anesthesia, nursing personnel, and a physician capable of monitoring labor and performing cesarean delivery, including an emergency cesarean delivery in cases of vaginal birth after cesarean (VBAC) delivery.
- Availability of anesthesia and surgical personnel to permit the start of a cesarean delivery within 30 min of the decision to perform the procedure.

of such measures is strongly encouraged given the potential for rapid and catastrophic blood loss should symptomatic uterine rupture or other peripartum emergencies occur.

ASA and ACOG Joint Recommendations

In 2008, a joint statement was issued by ASA and ACOG—"Optimal Goals for Anesthesia Care in Obstetrics" (75). This statement addresses issues of concern to both specialties and presents goals that all hospitals providing obstetric services should strive to achieve. The portions of this joint statement that directly pertain to the provision of TOLAC/VBAC services appear in Table 10-2.

Availability of Anesthesia Personnel

As stated previously, both ASA and ACOG advocate the "immediate availability" of appropriate personnel and equipment to facilitate an emergency cesarean delivery should the

TABLE 10-3 Summary of Recommendations for Delivery After Cesarean Delivery

Recommendation	Evidence Grade
TOLAC may be a reasonable option for many women with one prior Kerr CD and should be offered to appropriately selected candidates.	Level A
Improved access to care, patient education, and a reversal of the adverse medicolegal climate are needed in order to improve VBAC rates in the United States.	Level C
The determination of which women are appropriate candidates to attempt TOLAC is a complex, delicate decision best left to the expecting couple and their obstetrician.	Level C
Symptomatic uterine rupture is one of the most devastating short-term complications associated with TOLAC and occurs exclusively in unsuccessful TOLAC.	Level B
Women with documented or estimated previous vertical uterine scar should not be offered TOLAC, as these incisions are most frequently associated with symptomatic uterine rupture.	Level B
Epidural analgesia is safe and should be offered to all parturients attempting TOLAC.	Level A
A pattern of increasing epidural dosing requirements in women attempting TOLAC may represent a warning for impending/evolving uterine rupture.	Level B
Both ASA and ACOG endorse immediate availability of appropriate facilities and personnel, including perinatal anesthesia, nursing personnel, and an experienced obstetrician capable of monitoring TOLAC and performing emergency cesarean delivery.	Level C
A multidisciplinary approach is necessary in order to ensure the most optimal perinatal outcomes in women attempting TOLAC.	Level C

need arise. What exactly is meant by this concept of "immediate availability" and is it possible to achieve in all hospitals offering TOLAC? Certainly, these and other important questions can be raised when one examines this issue in depth. Inherently, the question that must be asked is whether or not there are sufficient anesthesia personnel to accommodate this requirement. Birnbach and colleagues recently addressed three areas of interest to anesthesia providers: "The current ability of anesthesiologists in the United States to provide immediate availability for TOLAC/VBAC at all delivery locations; the workforce estimates for anesthesiology staffing in the future; and the barriers to the immediate availability of anesthesiologists in all hospitals that provide obstetrical care (76)." The availability of anesthesiologists is affected by many factors. It has tremendous regional variation. There is not only an increased demand for obstetric anesthesia providers. There is also an overall increased demand for the service that anesthesia providers render in general due to growing numbers of procedures being scheduled in operating rooms, endoscopy and interventional radiology suites, and other remote settings. Compounding the anesthesiologist availability and staffing issues even more are increasing patterns of job sharing, part-time employment, individual workload reduction, early retirement, and flexibility in scheduling.

The Joint Commission endorses team training and simulation exercises on the labor and delivery suite to improve patient safety. Until data can be generated to clearly delineate

this complex issue and according to the review by Birnbach et al., "there do not currently appear to be enough extra personnel to radically shift staffing patterns throughout the United States to provide anesthesia personnel at all hospitals to be immediately available." Perhaps the focus should be upon "consolidation of obstetrical services wherever possible, improved patient education, development of protocols and guidelines that allow stratification of risk and optimization of workforce, improved processes, use of team training and simulation for labor and delivery staff, and further patient safety research" (76).

■ SUMMARY OF RECOMMENDATIONS

Based upon review of the best existing evidence, management recommendations pertinent to delivery after cesarean delivery are presented in Table 10-3. These summary statements should be strongly considered when one is faced with the task of providing anesthetic care for the parturient planning TOLAC/VBAC. Recommendation statements are graded according to the following categories: *Level A, Level B,* or *Level C. Level A* recommendations are based on good and consistent scientific evidence. *Level B* recommendations are based on limited or inconsistent evidence. *Level C* recommendations are based on consensus and expert opinion.

Table 10-4 provides a summary of the TOLAC recommendations for several professional societies including American

TABLE 10-4 TOLAC Recommendations of Professional Societies

Society	VBAC Counseling	Facilities and Personnel	Other Recommendations
ACOG	VBAC should be offered to most women with one previous CD with low transverse incision; consider those with two previous low transverse CD.	Safest where staff can provide immediate emergency CD, but patients should be allowed to accept increased risk when such resources are not available.	Twins, macrosomia, postdatism, low vertical incision, and unknown type of uterine incision should not preclude.
RCOG	Women with one prior low segment CD should be able to discuss option of VBAC; final decision between woman and her obstetrician.	Should be conducted in suitably staffed and equipped delivery suite with continuous intrapartum care and monitoring and available resources for immediate CD and advanced neonatal resuscitation.	Caution with twins and macrosomia (uncertainty due to underpowered studies).
SOGC	VBAC should be offered to women with one previous CD with low transverse incision.	In hospital where a timely CD is available; an approximate timeframe of 30 min should be considered adequate for urgent laparotomy.	Not addressed.
AAFP	VBAC should be offered to women with one previous CD with low transverse incision.	Should not be restricted only to those facilities with available surgical teams present throughout labor because there is no evidence that these additional resources result in improved outcome.	Not addressed.
AHRQ	VBAC is a reasonable choice for the majority of women with prior cesarean delivery.	Not addressed.	Not addressed.

VBAC, vaginal birth after cesarean delivery; CD, cesarean delivery; ACOG, American Congress (formerly College) of Obstetricians and Gynecologists; RCOG, Royal College of Obstetricians and Gynaecologists, UK; SOGC, Society of Obstetricians and Gynecologists of Canada; AAFP, American Academy of Family Physicians; AHRQ, US Health and Human Services Agency for Healthcare Research and Quality.
Modified from: Scott JR. Vaginal birth after cesarean delivery: a common-sense approach. *Obstet Gynecol* 2011;118:342. Copyright 2011 Lippincott Williams & Wilkins.

Congress (formerly College) of Obstetricians and Gynecologists (ACOG), RCOG, Society of Obstetricians and Gynecologists of Canada (SOGC), American Academy of Family Physicians (AAFP), and US Department of Health and Human Services Agency for Healthcare Research and Quality (AHRQ).

KEY POINTS

- TOLAC may be a reasonable option for many women with one prior Kerr CD and should be offered to appropriately selected candidates.
- Improved access to care, patient education, and a reversal of the adverse medicolegal climate are needed in order to improve VBAC rates in the United States and worldwide.
- The determination of which women are appropriate candidates to attempt TOLAC is a complex, delicate decision best left to the expecting couple and their obstetrician.
- Symptomatic uterine rupture is one of the most devastating short-term complications associated with TOLAC and occurs exclusively in unsuccessful TOLAC.
- Women with documented or estimated previous vertical uterine scar should not be offered TOLAC, as these incisions are most frequently associated with symptomatic uterine rupture.
- Epidural analgesia is safe and should be offered to all parturients attempting TOLAC.
- A pattern of increasing epidural dosing requirements in women attempting TOLAC may represent a warning for impending/evolving uterine rupture.
- Both ASA and ACOG endorse immediate availability of appropriate facilities and personnel, including perinatal anesthesia, nursing personnel, and an experienced obstetrician capable of monitoring TOLAC and performing emergency cesarean delivery.
- A multidisciplinary approach is necessary in order to ensure the most optimal perinatal outcomes in women attempting TOLAC.

REFERENCES

1. Cragin EB. Conservatism in obstetrics. *N Y Med J* 1916;104:1–3.
2. Flamm BL. Once a cesarean, always a controversy. *Obstet Gynecol* 1997;90(2):312–315.
3. National institutes of health consensus development conference statement: Vaginal birth after cesarean: New insights march 8–10, 2010. *Semin Perinatol* 2010;34(4):293–307.
4. Scott JR. Vaginal birth after cesarean delivery: A common-sense approach. *Obstet Gynecol* 2011;118(2 Pt 1):342–350.
5. Royal College of Obstetricians and Gynaecologists. Birth after previous cesarean birth. Green-top guideline number 45. *Royal College of Obstetricians and Gynaecologists* 2007;(45):1.
6. American College of Obstetricians and Gynecologists. ACOG practice bulletin no. 115: Vaginal birth after previous cesarean delivery. *Obstet Gynecol* 2010;116(2 Pt 1):450–463.
7. Menacker F, Hamilton BE. Recent trends in cesarean delivery in the United States. *NCHS Data Brief* 2010;(35):1–8.
8. Centers for Disease Control and Prevention (CDC). Rates of cesarean delivery—United States, 1991. *MMWR Morb Mortal Wkly Rep* 1993;42(15):285–289.
9. Hamilton BE, Martin JA, Ventura SJ. Births: Preliminary data for 2007. *Nat'l Vital Stat Rep* 2009;57(12):1–23.
10. Zhang J, Troendle J, Reddy UM, et al. Contemporary cesarean delivery practice in the United States. *Am J Obstet Gynecol* 2010;203(4):326.e1–326.e10.
11. Lydon-Rochelle MT, Cahill AG, Spong CY. Birth after previous cesarean delivery: Short-term maternal outcomes. *Semin Perinatol* 2010;34(4):249–257.
12. Clark SL, Hankins GD. Temporal and demographic trends in cerebral palsy—fact and fiction. *Am J Obstet Gynecol* 2003;188(3):628–633.
13. Lee HC, El-Sayed YY, Gould JB. Population trends in cesarean delivery for breech presentation in the United States, 1997–2003. *Am J Obstet Gynecol* 2008;199(1):59.e1–59.e8.
14. Goetzinger KR, Macones GA. Operative vaginal delivery: Current trends in obstetrics. *Womens Health (Lond Engl)* 2008;4(3):281–290.
15. Department of Health and Human Services. Cesarean childbirth: Report of a Consensus development conference sponsored by the national institute of child health and human development in conjunction with the national center for health care technology. September 22–24, 1980. *NIH Publication* 1981;82–2067.
16. Case BD, Corcoran R, Jeffcoate N, et al. Caesarean section and its place in modern obstetric practice. *J Obstet Gynaecol Br Commonw* 1971;78(3):203–214.
17. American College of Obstetricians and Gynecologists. Guidelines for vaginal delivery after a cesarean childbirth. 1982.
18. Cohen B, Atkins M. Brief history of vaginal birth after cesarean section. *Clin Obstet Gynecol* 2001;44(3):604–608.
19. Martin JA, Hamilton BE, Sutton PD. Births: Final data for 2006. *Nat'l Vital Stat Rep* 2009;57.
20. Guise JM, Eden K, Emeis C, et al. Vaginal birth after cesarean: New insights. *Evid Rep Technol Assess (Full Rep)* 2010;(191):1–397.
21. Martel MJ, MacKinnon CJ, Clinical Practice Obstetrics Committee, Society of Obstetricians and Gynaecologists of Canada. Guidelines for vaginal birth after previous caesarean birth. *J Obstet Gynaecol Can* 2005;27(2):164–188.
22. Russillo B, Sewitch MJ, Cardinal L, et al. Comparing rates of trial of labour attempts, VBAC success, and fetal and maternal complications among family physicians and obstetricians. *J Obstet Gynaecol Can* 2008;30(2):123–128.
23. Gregory KD, Fridman M, Korst L. Trends and patterns of vaginal birth after cesarean availability in the united states. *Semin Perinatol* 2010;34(4):237–243.
24. Taffel SM. State variation in VBAC delivery: 1994, vol 77. *Stat Bull Metrop Insurance Co* 1996:28–36.
25. Martin JA, Hamilton BE, Sutton PD, et al. Births: Final data for 2004. *Nat'l Vital Stat Rep* 2006;55(1):1–101.
26. National Institutes of Health. National institutes of health, consensus development conference on cesarean childbirth. 1981.
27. Stafford RS, Sullivan SD, Gardner LB. Trends in cesarean section use in California, 1983 to 1990. *Am J Obstet Gynecol* 1993;168(4):1297–1302.
28. DeFranco EA, Rampersad R, Atkins KL, et al. Do vaginal birth after cesarean outcomes differ based on hospital setting? *Am J Obstet Gynecol* 2007;197(4):400.e1–400.e6.
29. MacDorman MF, Menacker F, Declercq E. Cesarean birth in the united states: Epidemiology, trends, and outcomes. *Clin Perinatol* 2008;35(2):293,307, v.
30. Lieberman E, Ernst EK, Rooks JP, et al. Results of the national study of vaginal birth after cesarean in birth centers. *Obstet Gynecol* 2004;104(5 Pt 1):933–942.
31. Coleman VH, Erickson K, Schulkin J, et al. Vaginal birth after cesarean delivery: Practice patterns of obstetrician-gynecologists. *J Reprod Med* 2005;50(4):261–266.
32. Bais JM, van der Borden DM, Pel M, et al. Vaginal birth after caesarean section in a population with a low overall caesarean section rate. *Eur J Obstet Gynecol Reprod Biol* 2001;96(2):158–162.
33. Naef RW 3rd, Ray MA, Chauhan SP, et al. Trial of labor after cesarean delivery with a lower-segment, vertical uterine incision: Is it safe? *Am J Obstet Gynecol* 1995;172(6):1666,73; discussion 1673–1674.
34. Misra A. Impact of the HealthChoice program on cesarean section and vaginal birth after C-section deliveries: A retrospective analysis. *Matern Child Health J* 2008;12(2):266–274.
35. Blanchette H, Blanchette M, McCabe J, et al. Is vaginal birth after cesarean safe? Experience at a community hospital. *Am J Obstet Gynecol* 2001;184(7):1478,84; discussion 1484–1487.
36. Ravasia DJ, Wood SL, Pollard JK. Uterine rupture during induced trial of labor among women with previous cesarean delivery. *Am J Obstet Gynecol* 2000;183(5):1176–1179.
37. Quinones JN, Stamilio DM, Pare E, et al. The effect of prematurity on vaginal birth after cesarean delivery: Success and maternal morbidity. *Obstet Gynecol* 2005;105(3):519–524.
38. Weinstein D, Benshushan A, Tanos V, et al. Predictive score for vaginal birth after cesarean section. *Am J Obstet Gynecol* 1996;174(1 Pt 1):192–198.
39. Buhimschi CS, Buhimschi IA, Patel S, et al. Rupture of the uterine scar during term labour: Contractility or biochemistry? *BJOG* 2005;112(1):38–42.
40. Leung AS, Leung EK, Paul RH. Uterine rupture after previous cesarean delivery: Maternal and fetal consequences. *Am J Obstet Gynecol* 1993;169(4):945–950.
41. Gyamfi C, Juhasz G, Gyamfi P, et al. Increased success of trial of labor after previous vaginal birth after cesarean. *Obstet Gynecol* 2004;104(4):715–719.
42. Harper LM, Cahill AG, Stamilio DM, et al. Effect of gestational age at the prior cesarean delivery on maternal morbidity in subsequent VBAC attempt. *Am J Obstet Gynecol* 2009;200(3):276.e1–276.e6.
43. Hendler I, Bujold E. Effect of prior vaginal delivery or prior vaginal birth after cesarean delivery on obstetric outcomes in women undergoing trial of labor. *Obstet Gynecol* 2004;104(2):273–277.
44. Huang WH, Nakashima DK, Rumney PJ. Interdelivery interval and the success of vaginal birth after cesarean delivery. *Obstet Gynecol* 2004;99(10):41–44.

45. Kabir AA, Pridjian G, Steinmann WC, et al. Racial differences in cesareans: An analysis of U.S. 2001 national inpatient sample data. *Obstet Gynecol* 2005;105(4):710–718.

46. Selo-Ojeme D, Abulhassan N, Mandal R, et al. Preferred and actual delivery mode after a cesarean in London, UK. *Int J Gynaecol Obstet* 2008;102(2):156–159.

47. Learman LA, Evertson LR, Shiboski S. Predictors of repeat cesarean delivery after trial of labor: Do any exist? *J Am Coll Surg* 1996;182(3):257–262.

48. Smith GC, Pell JP, Cameron AD, et al. Risk of perinatal death associated with labor after previous cesarean delivery in uncomplicated term pregnancies. *JAMA* 2002;287(20):2684–2690.

49. Smith GC, Pell JP, Pasupathy D, et al. Factors predisposing to perinatal death related to uterine rupture during attempted vaginal birth after caesarean section: Retrospective cohort study. *BMJ* 2004;329(7462):375.

50. Smith GC, Wood A. Previous caesarean and the risk of antepartum stillbirth. *BJOG* 2008;115(11):1458; author reply 1458–1459.

51. Smith GC, Wood AM, Pell JP, et al. First cesarean birth and subsequent fertility. *Fertil Steril* 2006;85(1):90–95.

52. Grobman WA, Gilbert S, Landon MB, et al. Outcomes of induction of labor after one prior cesarean. *Obstet Gynecol* 2007;109(2 Pt 1):262–269.

53. El-Sayed YY, Watkins MM, Fix M, et al. Perinatal outcomes after successful and failed trials of labor after cesarean delivery. *Am J Obstet Gynecol* 2007;196(6):583.e1– 583.e5; discussion 583.e5.

54. Gregory KD, Korst LM, Fridman M, et al. Vaginal birth after cesarean: Clinical risk factors associated with adverse outcome. *Am J Obstet Gynecol* 2008;198(4):452.e1– 452.e10; discussion 452.e10–452.e12.

55. Landon MB, Hauth JC, Leveno KJ, et al. Maternal and perinatal outcomes associated with a trial of labor after prior cesarean delivery. *N Engl J Med* 2004;351(25):2581–2589.

56. Macones GA, Peipert J, Nelson DB, et al. Maternal complications with vaginal birth after cesarean delivery: A multicenter study. *Am J Obstet Gynecol* 2005;193(5):1656–1662.

57. Lydon-Rochelle M, Holt VL, Easterling TR, et al. Risk of uterine rupture during labor among women with a prior cesarean delivery. *N Engl J Med* 2001;345(1):3–8.

58. Wen SW, Rusen ID, Walker M, et al. Comparison of maternal mortality and morbidity between trial of labor and elective cesarean section among women with previous cesarean delivery. *Am J Obstet Gynecol* 2004;191(4):1263–1269.

59. Quiroz LH, Chang H, Blomquist JL, et al. Scheduled cesarean delivery: Maternal and neonatal risks in primiparous women in a community hospital setting. *Am J Perinatol* 2009;26(4):271–277.

60. Bujold E, Jastrow N, Simoneau J, et al. Prediction of complete uterine rupture by sonographic evaluation of the lower uterine segment. *Am J Obstet Gynecol* 2009;201(3):320.e1–320.e6.

61. Landon MB. Vaginal birth after cesarean delivery. *Clin Perinatol* 2008; 35(3):491–504, ix–x.

62. Guise JM, McDonagh MS, Osterweil P, et al. Systematic review of the incidence and consequences of uterine rupture in women with previous caesarean section. *BMJ* 2004;329(7456):19–25.

63. Greene MF. Vaginal delivery after cesarean section—is the risk acceptable? *N Engl J Med* 2001;345(1):54–55.

64. Landon MB. Predicting uterine rupture in women undergoing trial of labor after prior cesarean delivery. *Semin Perinatol* 2010;34(4):267–271.

65. Smith GC, White IR, Pell JP, et al. Predicting cesarean section and uterine rupture among women attempting vaginal birth after prior cesarean section. *PLoS Med* 2005;2(9):e252.

66. Delivery after previous cesarean: Long-term maternal outcomes. *Semin Perinatol* 2010;34(4):258–266.

67. Silver RM, Landon MB, Rouse DJ, et al. Maternal morbidity associated with multiple repeat cesarean deliveries. *Obstet Gynecol* 2006;107(6):1226–1232.

68. Landon MB, Leindecker S, Spong CY, et al. The MFMU cesarean registry: Factors affecting the success of trial of labor after previous cesarean delivery. *Am J Obstet Gynecol* 2005;193(3 Pt 2):1016–1023.

69. Kuehn BM. Obstetrics group relaxes guideline for trial of labor after cesarean delivery. *JAMA* 2010;304(9):951–952.

70. Kieser KE, Baskett TF. A 10-year population-based study of uterine rupture. *Obstet Gynecol* 2002;100(4):749–753.

71. Ridgeway JJ, Weyrich DL, Benedetti TJ. Fetal heart rate changes associated with uterine rupture. *Obstet Gynecol* 2004;103(3):506–512.

72. Cahill AG, Odibo AO, Allsworth JE, et al. Frequent epidural dosing as a marker for impending uterine rupture in patients who attempt vaginal birth after cesarean delivery. *Am J Obstet Gynecol* 2010;202(4):355.e1–355.e5.

73. Flamm BL, Lim OW, Jones C, et al. Vaginal birth after cesarean section: Results of a multicenter study. *Am J Obstet Gynecol* 1988;158(5):1079–1084.

74. Stovall TG, Shaver DC, Solomon SK, et al. Trial of labor in previous cesarean section patients, excluding classical cesarean sections. *Obstet Gynecol* 1987; 70(5):713–717.

75. American Society of Anesthesiologists. Optimal goals for anesthesia care in obstetrics. *Obstetrical Anesthesia Committee* 2008.

76. Birnbach DJ, Bucklin BA, Dexter F. Impact of anesthesiologists on the incidence of vaginal birth after cesarean in the United States: Role of anesthesia availability, productivity, guidelines, and patient safety. *Semin Perinatol* 2010;34(5):318–324.

Effects of Anesthesia on Uterine Activity, Progress in Labor and Outcomes

Elena Reitman-Ivashkov • Pamela Flood • Mrinalini Balki

Medications that are used for anesthesia and analgesia during pregnancy and labor may have variable effects on uterine contractility. This chapter will review the mechanisms known to be involved in uterine contractility, and to delineate the effects of anesthesia on labor and uterine contractility during cesarean section.

■ MECHANISMS OF PARTURITION

The uterus is composed of smooth muscles, which normally contract throughout gestation with variable frequencies and intensity. Prior to the onset of labor, changes occur in the uterine cervix including ingrowth of afferent C fibers and activation of biochemical signaling pathways that lead to the breakdown of collagen, changing the structural integrity of the cervix. During labor, or parturition, the contractions increase in frequency and intensity to cause thinning and dilation of the cervix allowing passage of the fetus from the uterus through the birth canal (1).

Labor is classically divided into three stages. The *first stage* can be considered the cervical stage during which cervical effacement and dilation occur. The *second stage* is the pelvic stage when the fetus descends through the pelvis. The *third stage* is the placental stage during which the placenta is expelled. Some authorities identify a *fourth stage* of labor, corresponding to the first postpartum hour, during which uterine contraction leads to volume expansion and postpartum hemorrhage is most likely to occur (2).

■ MECHANISMS OF LABOR PAIN

Pain during the *first stage of labor* is predominantly visceral in nature, arising from afferents in the uterine corpus and cervix during contractions (3). The uterus and cervix are supplied by afferents accompanying sympathetic nerves in the uterine and cervical plexuses; the inferior, middle, and superior hypogastric plexuses; and the aortic plexus. Small unmyelinated "C" fibers (4) transmit nociception through lumbar and lower thoracic sympathetic chains to the posterior nerve roots of the 10th, 11th, and 12th thoracic and also the 1st lumbar nerves to synapse in the dorsal horn (3). As the labor progresses, severe pain is referred to dermatomes supplied by T10 and L1. The severity of pain is related to the duration and intensity of contraction (5) but there is enormous variability among women (6,7).

Pain during the *second stage of labor*, is due to somatic factors added to the visceral pain of the first stage. Pressure on the parietal peritoneum, traction on uterine ligaments, urethra, bladder, rectum, lumbosacral plexus, fascia, and muscles of the pelvic floor may increase the intensity of pain. In the second stage, the direct pressure exerted by the fetal presenting part against the lumbosacral plexus may cause neuropathic pain. Stretching of the vagina and perineum results in activation of the pudendal nerve (S2 to S4) via fine, myelinated, rapidly transmitting "A delta" fibers (4). From these areas, the nociceptive impulses pass to dorsal horn cells up the spinothalamic tract to the brain where they are finally interpreted as pain.

There is some suggestion from animal models that labor pain possibly affects uterine contractility. In rodents, if the hypogastric nerve is severed, the amplitude of uterine contractility is increased, potentially increasing the rate of labor (8). It is unknown whether this feedback system is relevant in human labor.

■ NORMAL LABOR PROGRESS

A critical task for the obstetrical management is to determine whether labor is progressing normally and, if not, to determine the significance of the delay and what the response should be. Emmanuel Friedman's model for labor progress and its modifications has classically been used by obstetricians to predict labor progress. His approach was straightforward: He graphed cervical dilation on the y-axis and elapsed time on the x-axis for thousands of labors (9). The original Friedman model was sigmoidal consisting of a latent phase of labor before 4 cm dilation, an active phase followed by a deceleration stage just before full cervical dilation at 10 cm. The presence of the deceleration stage has been debated, and the active and latent phases of labor have commonly been simplified as linear. Friedman's most important contribution is his separation of the latent phase from the active phase of the first stage of labor. Many hours of regular, painful uterine contractions may take place with significant cervical effacement but little change in cervical dilation. The Friedman model was modified by Philpott as an alert line at dilation less than 1 cm/h, which represented the lowest 10 percentile rate for nulliparous patients. This has been developed into the WHO partograph, designed to predict obstructed labor in low resource environments (10).

The Friedman model has been useful for the study of labor progress in different populations. However, for the individual woman, the transition from the latent to the active phase of the first stage of labor, does not occur abruptly at an arbitrary cervical dilation but rather occurs as a change in slope of the cervical dilation curve (7,11,12). Recently, two new approaches have been applied to labor progress modeling. Zhang and colleagues have used repeated measures regression with a multi-order polynomial function (11). Flood, Reitman, and colleagues have used a bi-exponential model of labor progress to detect factors that significantly influence labor progress (7,12). Each of these methodologies has strengths and limitations that are beyond the scope of this chapter.

There is enormous variability in the length of the latent phase of labor. A prolonged latent phase alone is not associated with fetal compromise or cephalopelvic disproportion. However, primary dysfunctional labor and arrest of dilation during the active phase may indicate cephalopelvic disproportion (9,13,14). Friedman's original work suggested that an arrest of dilation during the active phase was associated with the need for cesarean delivery nearly half of the time. Later studies suggest a lower percentage, but it is clear that women who experience active-phase arrest of dilation are more likely to require abdominal delivery than women with normal labor progress during the active phase. However, obstetrical convention may contribute to these numbers. Recent work by Zhang and colleagues in a large contemporary cohort suggests that the active phase of labor may not begin until 6 cm dilation in many patients and slow progress before 6 cm dilation may not be an indication of abnormal labor progress (15). Clearly, individualization of expectations for normal labor progress would contribute to more efficient use of resources and may decrease the rate of unnecessary operative deliveries.

■ VOLATILE ANESTHETICS

In modern obstetric anesthesia, regional techniques are favored because of advantages for both the mother and the newborn baby. However, conditions such as coagulopathy, serious infection, hypovolemia, and neurologic anomaly may shift the balance of risk toward general anesthesia for safe delivery.

All volatile anesthetics, including sevoflurane, desflurane, isoflurane, halothane, and ethanol, inhibit spontaneous contractility of gravid human uterine muscle in a dose-dependent manner. Uterine relaxation or atony results in increased blood loss after delivery. Therefore, large concentrations of volatile anesthetics that may cause profound uterine relaxation are best avoided during cesarean delivery (16,17). However, this well-known side effect of volatile anesthetics may be paradoxically used to achieve uterine relaxation to facilitate complicated deliveries in some instances (18,19).

Historically, parenteral ethanol was introduced by Fuchs (20) during the mid-60s as a tocolytic agent for preterm labor and, despite the alternatives available, was still in clinical use up until 1981 (21). It was reported that for ethanol to be effective, blood levels between 1.2 and 1.8 g/L were needed. However, higher blood levels may cause maternal anesthesia and respiratory depression with risk of aspiration pneumonitis. Hypotension and incontinence, although uncommon, can also occur. Most women on ethanol experienced nausea and required the routine use of an anti-emetic drug.

Sevoflurane and desflurane have gained widespread acceptance in obstetric anesthesia. Their inhibitory effects on myometrial contractility have been documented in rat (22,23), and human preparations (24,25). The degree of inhibition induced by sevoflurane and desflurane is comparable to that of halothane, whereas that induced by isoflurane is less. This might be explained by differences in their mechanism of action. The inhibitory effects of isoflurane may be related, at least in part, to its ability to modulate K_{ATP} channels, whereas effects of other volatile anesthetics may involve other pathways including transmembrane Ca^{2+} flux (26). The inhibitory effect of volatile anesthetics occurs in a concentration-dependent manner. The uterine contractility abolished by these volatile agents is seen only at lower concentration of anesthetics (below 1 minimum alveolar concentration [MAC]) (26) and the contractility can be restored by the administration of oxytocin.

Desflurane and sevoflurane are promising agents for use in cesarean section, because they have low blood–gas partition coefficients, allowing rapid uptake and elimination. Both agents appear to have a similar relaxant effect on the uterus to those of older agents at equivalent MACs, although their rapid clearance at the end of the operation may minimize the duration of uterine relaxation. The declining use of general anesthesia for cesarean section means that few data are available on these agents. Gambling et al. compared 1% sevoflurane with 0.5% isoflurane for elective cesarean section (27). They found no difference in cardiovascular parameters, blood loss, uterine tone, perioperative complications, emergence time, or neonatal outcome. Abboud et al. compared desflurane (3% and 6%) with enflurane 0.6% for cesarean section anesthesia (28) and found no difference in uterine contractility. The use of desflurane for cesarean sections is relatively new and knowledge about its maternal and neonatal effects is being accumulated. Karaman et al. (29) compared maternal and neonatal outcomes in women undergoing elective cesarean section with desflurane, sevoflurane, or epidural anesthesia, and found no differences among the three groups.

Volatile halogenated agents provide distinct advantages, because they can be easily titrated and reduce the risk of intraoperative awareness. However, there is little evidence to guide the specific choice of modern agent (isoflurane, sevoflurane, or desflurane) routine for cesarean delivery. In patients undergoing cesarean delivery, uterine contractility typically can be maintained with a small concentration of a volatile agent (and concurrent infusion of oxytocin), but in the presence of obstetric hemorrhage due to uterine atony, it is prudent to minimize the concentration of the volatile halogenated agent or convert to an intravenous anesthetic technique.

A modification of cesarean delivery to allow various interventions during birth is called ex utero intrapartum therapy (EXIT procedure) (30). This sequence is most often employed to allow for a fetal procedure while gas exchange continues in the placenta (placental bypass). The EXIT procedure enables the prevention of postnatal asphyxia in the setting of lesions such as cystic hygroma, lymphangioma, cervical teratoma, and congenital syndromes in which securing an airway after birth can be problematic. The procedure is also used as a bridge to extracorporeal membrane oxygenation (ECMO) for a fetus with cardiopulmonary disease that is at risk for postnatal cardiac failure and resulting hypoxia. The EXIT procedure has become a widely practiced fetal intervention for a growing list of indications. The myometrial relaxant properties of volatile anesthetics are used to advantage in the EXIT procedure and similarly to facilitate fetal surgery. The EXIT procedure is conducted under general anesthesia; however, unlike normal cesarean delivery, sufficient time must be allowed after induction of anesthesia—before surgery commences—to achieve the high steady-state end-tidal concentration of the volatile halogenated agent needed to ensure uterine relaxation and to allow time for fetal anesthesia. After adequate uterine relaxation has been achieved, a uterine incision is made with the stapling device, and the fetal head and shoulders are delivered in preparation for tracheal intubation. Once the umbilical cord is clamped and the fetus delivered, the maternal anesthetic technique is changed to reduce uterine relaxation rapidly in order to avoid postpartum hemorrhage. The inspired concentration of the volatile halogenated agent is reduced or eliminated and nitrous oxide 70%, opioids, and/or a propofol infusion can be instituted (2).

Both low concentration of volatile anesthetics and nitrous oxide have been used for labor analgesia. Abboud et al. (31) compared administration of 0.25% to 1.25% enflurane in oxygen with administration of 30% to 60% nitrous oxide during the second stage of labor. Approximately 89% of the enflurane group and 76% of the nitrous oxide group rated their analgesia as satisfactory. The rates of amnesia were similar (7% and 10%). There were no differences in blood loss, Apgar scores, or umbilical cord blood–gas measurements. Unlike the volatile anesthetics, nitrous oxide appears to have no effect on uterine contractility (32).

■ INTRAVENOUS ANESTHETICS

In addition to cesarean section, non-obstetrical surgical procedures may be required during pregnancy. Intravenous anesthetics may be used to complement volatile anesthetics or alone as total intravenous anesthesia (TIVA) techniques. The effects of these agents on uterine contractions and placental blood flow are very important to anticipate. The unexpected relaxation or contraction of myometrium can be harmful to fetus and continuing pregnancy.

The effect of general anesthesia on surgical blood loss was compared in patients anesthetized with isoflurane or propofol TIVA regimens for voluntary termination of pregnancy in the first trimester in a double-blind clinical trial (33). The mean blood loss was significantly lower in the propofol TIVA group, 148 (123 to 177) mL compared to the isoflurane group, 244 (198 to 301) mL. This difference remained significant even after controlling age, body weight, and uterus size. However, propofol has been found to decrease uterine muscle contractility in a dose-dependent manner in in vitro studies (34,35). Although propofol has not been approved by the FDA for use in pregnancy, because of the lack of availability of thiopental in the United States, it is now commonly used in clinical practice in pregnant patients and several published clinical studies attest to the safety of propofol for induction of cesarean sections (36–38). Propofol is rapidly distributed across the placenta, with an umbilical venous concentration/maternal venous concentration ratio of 0.65 (37).

Midazolam is a short-acting, water-soluble benzodiazepine that has few adverse hemodynamic effects and provides hypnosis and amnesia. It is used commonly in small doses (1 to 2 mg) to provide anxiolysis as an adjunct to regional anesthesia for cesarean section. While midazolam clearly crosses the placenta, at these doses, there is no evidence for a negative effect on fetal well-being (39). Although most commonly used as a premedicant prior to anesthesia, midazolam can be used in higher doses as an induction agent for cesarean delivery. The effect of midazolam on human uterine contractility has not been directly studied, but it has been shown to reduce the contractility of rat uterine muscle in in vitro preparations (40).

Ketamine is useful as an analgesic and/or sedative supplement to general or regional anesthesia for obstetric surgery. It causes limited cardiovascular and respiratory depression in the mother and may reduce opioid side effects in the newborn (41,42). Ketamine's analgesic effects are likely related to antagonism of the N-methyl-D-aspartate (NMDA) receptor. Animal studies suggest that the use of ketamine is not associated with a reduction in uterine blood flow (43–45). Ketamine is associated with dose-dependent increases in uterine tone in vitro, but a single induction dose does not increase uterine tone at term gestation (46). Ketamine is suitable for induction of general anesthesia for cesarean section and has compared favorably with thiopental in terms of maternal hemodynamics, wakefulness, and neonatal outcome (47–49). It rapidly crosses the placenta but neonatal depression is not observed with doses less than 1 mg/kg (41,50). However, the emergence delirium and hallucinations experienced with ketamine, particularly in the unpremedicated patient, limit the routine use of ketamine as an induction agent for cesarean delivery (51). If ketamine is used, a benzodiazepine should be administered to decrease the incidence of these psychomimetic effects (52).

Although many different systemic opioids have been used for labor analgesia, little scientific evidence suggests that one drug is intrinsically better than another for this purpose; most often the selection of an opioid is based on institutional tradition and/or pharmacokinetics. Ex vivo studies on isolated human pregnant uterine muscle strips demonstrate that opioids such as fentanyl, meperidine, remifentanil, and alfentanil may directly inhibit uterine contractility, though at concentrations higher than those used for analgesia (40,53,54). At analgesic concentrations, they do not have a significant effect on spontaneous contractions of gravid human uterine muscle. Interestingly, morphine and sufentanil had no effect on uterine contractility even at much higher than clinically relevant levels (53). Prospective comparison of the effects of neuraxial analgesia and parenteral opioid analgesia on cesarean delivery rates showed that there was no difference in the rate of cesarean delivery for dystocia (55,56). A meta-analysis of trials that randomized patients to receiving neuraxial analgesia or parenteral opioids suggested that patients receiving neuraxial analgesia had slightly longer labor, but, also higher satisfaction and better neonatal outcome. A low umbilical artery pH (<7.15 or 7.20) was recorded more commonly among neonates born after parenteral opioids than after epidural analgesia (57).

■ NEURAXIAL BLOCKADE FOR CESAREAN DELIVERIES

Neuraxial anesthesia and analgesia has become increasingly popular for obstetrics. The foremost reason is evidence that it is safer than general anesthesia for most pregnant women. The most common anesthesia-related contribution to maternal mortality is inability to secure a difficult airway, the incidence of which has been increasing in pregnancy (58,59). Maternal mortality significantly decreased during the period between 1991 and 2002 compared to 1979 and 1990, potentially partially as a result of increased use of neuraxial anesthesia for cesarean deliveries (60,61).

Due to the smaller amount of drug required for spinal anesthesia and the resulting reduction in systemic exposure, there is little direct effect of spinal anesthetic medication on the uterus/fetus or neonate (62). Hypotension and increased uterine tone that can be side effects of neuraxial anesthesia can potentially adversely affect placental blood flow. Since uterine blood flow is not autoregulated, uteroplacental perfusion is directly dependent on maternal perfusion pressure. Untreated reduction in maternal blood pressure may not be very well tolerated by the fetus. A meta-analysis of studies comparing spinal and epidural anesthesia for cesarean delivery revealed that the severity of hypotension is greater with spinal anesthesia (63). Another review that compared different modes of anesthesia found that spinal anesthesia compared to both general and epidural anesthesia was associated with lower umbilical pH and higher base deficit (64). There is no evidence, however, that this statistical difference in fetal acid–base status results in clinically different neonatal outcome. It should also be noted that none of the reviews mentioned considered treatment of sympathectomy with modern methods that include administration of phenylephrine infusion.

When a spinal dose was first added to epidural analgesia for labor, as part of a combined spinal–epidural technique, an increase in the incidence of transient fetal heart rate abnormalities was observed. In some settings these were clearly related to maternal hypotension but in many cases maternal blood pressure was largely unchanged while the rate of uterine contractility was noted to increase, including case reports of uterine hyperactivity (65). This hypothesis has been recently supported by the results of a randomized clinical trial in patients who had intrauterine pressure catheters (66). The uterus expresses β2-adrenergic receptors that are activated by endogenous epinephrine to result in tonic uterine relaxation. Systemic epinephrine concentrations are rapidly reduced after neuraxial anesthesia. When that tonic break on uterine tone is released in the setting of neuraxial anesthesia, the baseline contractile activity increases. Treatment with intramuscular ephedrine (25 mg) prior to combined spinal–epidural analgesia has been shown to reduce the incidence of late and variable fetal decelerations independent of maternal blood pressure (67). A direct relationship to uterine tone cannot be inferred however as the patients who were studied did not have intrauterine pressure catheters in place.

■ NEURAXIAL ANALGESIA FOR LABOR

Administered with modern protocols, neuraxial labor analgesia does not increase maternal or perinatal morbidity and mortality and is not associated with an increased risk of cesarean delivery (68,69).

First Stage of Labor

As discussed previously, pain during the first stage of labor is visceral and diffuse in localization. In order to block the enhanced afferent response that occurs during cervical ripening and labor, analgesia covering the T10 to L1 dermatomes is necessary.

The effect of neuraxial labor analgesia on the duration of the first stage of labor has been addressed as a secondary outcome variable in many prospective randomized controlled trials. A meta-analysis (70) of nine studies found no difference in the duration of the first stage of labor between women who were randomly assigned to receive epidural analgesia and those assigned to receive systemic opioid analgesia. There was significant heterogeneity in the outcome because of the mixed parity of the patient populations and differences among studies in the definition of the duration of the first stage of labor. In contrast, the individual meta-analysis of the Parkland Hospital data showed a significant but small prolongation of the first stage of labor (approximately 0.5 hour) in nulliparous women who were randomly assigned to receive epidural analgesia (71). Wong et al. (55) and Ohel et al. (72) assessed duration of labor as a secondary outcome in their randomized controlled trials of the initiation of neuraxial analgesia during early labor. Both groups of investigators determined that the duration of the first stage of labor was significantly *shorter* in women randomly assigned to receive early labor neuraxial analgesia than in those assigned to receive systemic opioid analgesia. Multiple factors may influence the duration of the first stage of labor. Clinicians have noted enhanced uterine activity in some patients for approximately 30 minutes after the initiation of neuraxial analgesia, whereas uterine activity appears to be reduced in other patients. Cheek et al. (73) noted that uterine activity decreased after the intravenous infusion of 1 L of crystalloid solution, but not after infusion of 0.5 L or maintenance fluid alone. There was no decrease in uterine activity after the administration of epidural anesthesia without a fluid load. Zamora et al. (74) made similar observations.

In a prospective study, Rahm et al. (75) observed that treatment with epidural bupivacaine with sufentanil was associated with lower plasma oxytocin levels at 60 minutes after initiation of analgesia than in healthy controls who did not receive epidural analgesia. Behrens et al. (76) noted that epidural analgesia during the first stage of labor significantly reduced the release of prostaglandin $F_{2\alpha}$ and impeded the normal

progressive increase in uterine activity. In contrast, Nielsen et al. (77) measured upper and lower uterine segment intrauterine pressures for 50 minutes before and after the administration of epidural bupivacaine analgesia in 11 nulliparous women during spontaneous labor. The investigators observed no significant difference in the number of contractions before and after epidural analgesia. There was greater intrauterine pressure in the upper uterine segment than in the lower segment (consistent with fundal dominance) both before and after initiation of epidural analgesia. Furthermore, in this study, fundal dominance was more pronounced after epidural analgesia than in the pre-analgesia period.

The epidural administration of a local anesthetic with epinephrine is followed by systemic absorption of both drugs. Some physicians have expressed concern that the epinephrine may exert a systemic β-adrenergic activity effect that could slow labor. Early studies, in which large doses of epinephrine were used, suggested that the caudal epidural administration of a local anesthetic with epinephrine prolonged the first stage of labor and increased the number of patients who required oxytocin augmentation of labor (78). However, more modern studies have suggested that the addition of epinephrine 1.25 to 5 μg/mL (1:800,000 to 1:200,000) to the local anesthetic solution does not affect the progress of labor or method of delivery (79–82).

Fetal bradycardia after intrathecal opioid injection has been associated with increased resting uterine tone (83). A suggested mechanism is the acute decrease in circulating maternal catecholamine concentrations that occurs after establishment of analgesia. Since epinephrine has tocolytic effects via β2-adrenergic activation, a sudden decrease in circulating concentrations may result in an increase in uterine tone, decreased uteroplacental perfusion, and fetal bradycardia. Usually uterine hypertonus resolves within 4 to 8 minutes with treatment and an emergency cesarean delivery is not necessary.

In summary, neuraxial analgesia appears to have a variable effect on the duration of labor. It may shorten labor in some women and lengthen it in others. However, analgesia-related mild prolongation of the first stage of labor, if it occurs, has not been shown to have adverse maternal or neonatal effects and is probably of minimal clinical significance (2).

Second Stage of Labor

Contraction of the uterus and distension of the lower uterine segments are predominately responsible for nociceptive stimulation during the second stage of labor. The fascia and subcutaneous tissues of the lower birth canal begin to stretch and may tear as the perineum distends, and pressure is applied to the perineal skeletal muscles. The pain is sharply localized to the perineum. In order to provide analgesia during the second stage of labor, the cephalad extent of blockade should extend to T10, and caudal extent must include pudendal nerve, which is derived from the anterior primary division of S2 to S4 (83).

Traditional epidural analgesia is associated with a longer second stage of labor.

The ACOG has defined a prolonged second stage in nulliparous women as lasting more than 3 hours with neuraxial analgesia and more than 2 hours without neuraxial analgesia; for parous women, it is more than 2 hours in those with neuraxial analgesia and more than 1 hour in those without neuraxial analgesia (84). Meta-analyses of randomized controlled trials comparing neuraxial with systemic opioid analgesia support this clinical observation (69,70). However, the average increase in duration of the second stage is relatively short, approximately 15 minutes longer in women randomly assigned to receive neuraxial analgesia than in women assigned to receive systemic opioid analgesia.

A recent study compared the intermittent bolus technique with PCEA (85). The latter provided better pain relief during the first and second stages of labor; however, the rate of cesarean delivery was higher in the PCEA group (although the rate of vacuum deliveries was lower). Continuous epidural infusion of bupivacaine 0.125 % at 10 to 14 mL/h was associated with prolonged labor due to motor blockade (86). Also, some studies have shown that parturients with background infusion may require outlet forceps for delivery more often than parturients receiving intermittent boluses; midforceps and cesarean delivery rates are similar in both groups (87).

■ UTEROTONIC AGENTS

Uterotonic drugs are used to induce or augment labor. More importantly, they are instrumental in preventing and treating postpartum hemorrhage due to uterine atony. These drugs can be associated with some harmful maternal side effects, and therefore need judicious administration. Understanding the uterine actions of these drugs and their systemic effects is essential for the anesthesiologist to optimize drug therapy and prevent maternal morbidity.

Oxytocin

Oxytocin is a neurohypophysial hormone, naturally synthesized during pregnancy, which plays a central role in the contraction of uterine smooth muscles during labor. Oxytocin mediates its action by binding with oxytocin receptors (OTRs) on the uterine surface. The oxytocin–OTR complex induces uterine contractility through the activation of phospholipase C, and the release of inositol 1,4,5-triphosphate, 1,2-diacylglycerol, and intracellular calcium (88). Pharmacokinetic studies of oxytocin suggest a half-life of 5 to 15 minutes (89,90) time to steady-state plasma concentration of 40 minutes (89,91) and a steady-state uterine response of around 30 minutes (92).

Oxytocin is commonly employed to induce or augment the process of labor with the objective of achieving a normal vaginal delivery; it is also used as the first-line drug to restore uterine contractility and minimize blood loss following delivery. Despite its widespread use, there are no standardized protocols for the use of oxytocin during labor and delivery, leading to inconsistent practices in its administration (93). A meta-analysis of 11 randomized clinical trials on the use of oxytocin for labor induction demonstrated that low-dose oxytocin protocols, in which doses were not increased more frequently than every 30 minutes, resulted in fewer episodes of uterine hyperstimulation, a higher rate of spontaneous vaginal delivery, less postpartum maternal infection, and less postpartum hemorrhage, compared with more aggressive or high-dose regimens (94). These studies, however, involved a wide range of oxytocin protocols. On the other hand, a recent systematic review on oxytocin for labor augmentation, which included 10 studies differentiating high- versus low-dose regimens based on the initial starting dose (above or below 4 mU/min) and the rate of dose increments, suggested that high-dose oxytocin protocol was associated with a moderate decrease in the risk of cesarean delivery and a decrease in the labor duration, although with a high rate of uterine hyperstimulation (95). Compared with normal uterine activity, uterine hyperstimulation has been shown to be associated with significant fetal desaturation and significantly more non-reassuring fetal heart rate patterns (96,97). In addition, oxytocin administration in the form of boluses is associated with significant adverse maternal hemodynamic effects, such as hypotension, tachycardia, and signs of myocardial ischemia, that are dose-related (98–100). In the Confidential Enquiries into Maternal Deaths

in the United Kingdom, 1997 to 1999, two deaths were reported from cardiovascular instability following an intravenous bolus of 10 IU oxytocin (101). Other adverse effects from the use of high dose of oxytocin include decreased free water clearance, peripheral flushing, nausea and emesis (93). Therefore, an approach based on patient safety favors the use of a low-dose oxytocin infusion that can be used without compromising the clinical efficacy of the drug.

Oxytocin exhibits a dose-related effect on uterine activity; however, when administered in non-laboring women undergoing cesarean delivery, a "ceiling effect" is witnessed at a dose of 5 IU, beyond which no further improvement in uterine contractility or blood loss is observed (102). A small loading dose of oxytocin (ED 90 = 0.35 IU) has been determined to be sufficient in producing adequate uterine contractions during elective cesarean deliveries in non-laboring women (103). Laboring women who have received oxytocin for augmentation of their labor, however, require a 9 times higher loading dose (ED 90 = 2.99 IU), and despite this higher dose, they have greater blood loss after delivery (104). Similar to the meta-analysis mentioned above, a recent study has demonstrated a higher incidence of severe postpartum hemorrhage secondary to uterine atony when oxytocin is used for labor augmentation in higher doses and for longer durations (105). These clinical findings can be explained by the molecular mechanism of OTR desensitization and signal attenuation that occur with exposure of the OTRs to oxytocin during labor in a time- and concentration-dependent manner (106–109).

■ OXYTOCIN DESENSITIZATION PHENOMENON

OTRs belong to the family of G-protein–coupled receptors (GPCRs), and like other GPCRs, undergo rapid molecular desensitization due to homologous stimulation (110). Upon binding with the OTR, the receptor rapidly internalizes and uncouples from its G protein, thereby limiting further oxytocin signaling. The oxytocin-induced desensitization of the OTRs in human culture reduces the ability of cells to respond to subsequent administration of oxytocin (107) and is characterized by the reduction in the concentration of myometrial oxytocin-binding sites and OTR mRNA (108). In vitro studies in pregnant rat model myometrial strips further demonstrated this desensitization phenomenon, in the form of inhibition of the oxytocin-induced myometrial contractions after pretreatment with oxytocin (109). Similarly, continued high-dose oxytocin exposure in the postpartum period may also lead to acute receptor desensitization and render the myometrium less responsive to additional oxytocin (109). In view of the fact that repeated doses of oxytocin may become increasingly ineffective, second-line uterotonic agents should be considered early in the event of postpartum bleeding. As the oxytocin-induced desensitization phenomenon is homologous, the uterotonic effects of ergonovine and prostaglandin $F_{2\alpha}$ that act through other receptors do not appear to be affected by this phenomenon in rat myometrial strips (111,112). Interestingly, despite the effect of desensitization, the contractions induced by oxytocin in oxytocin-exposed rat myometrium are still superior compared to other uterotonic drugs (111,112).

Carbetocin

Carbetocin is a long-acting synthetic analogue of oxytocin that produces uterine contractions by binding with the OTR on the myometrium (113,114). In vivo studies have shown its potency to be 1/10th that of oxytocin (115), while in vitro studies in rat models show that its myometrial contractile activity is only 1/30th that of oxytocin, albeit with a prolonged nature of effect (114). The low uterotonic activity of carbetocin could be due to a reduced ability of the ligand–receptor complex to induce intrinsic activity in the myometrial cells (114). Its increased half-life in plasma and at the OTR (4 to 10 times that of oxytocin) and reduced degradation by enzymes due to its structural modification seem to contribute to its prolonged uterotonic activity (113–115).

The clinical studies done with carbetocin over the last decade, on the contrary, have shown either a higher or equivalent efficacy in the prevention of postpartum hemorrhage compared to oxytocin (116–120). The side effects of carbetocin appear to be similar to that of oxytocin. The dose–response profile of this drug and the issue of receptor desensitization after oxytocin exposure during labor are as yet unstudied, and further work on the efficacy of carbetocin is necessary.

Ergot Alkaloids

Ergonovine maleate causes tonic contractions of both the upper and lower uterine segments and has a long duration of action. It acts via calcium channel or α-receptor in the inner myometrial layer, and is also a partial agonist at α-adrenergic, 5HT-1, and dopamine receptors (121). It increases the myometrial contractility in a dose-dependent manner (111,122) but higher doses may be associated with more side effects. Clinical studies comparing ergonovine with oxytocin have shown little differences in the mean blood loss and the incidence of postpartum hemorrhage (123). Currently ergonovine remains the second-line agent in the management of postpartum hemorrhage, if uterine atony persists after oxytocin administration during delivery. The use of ergonovine is relatively contraindicated in patients with preeclampsia or hypertension due to its potential to cause an exaggerated hypertensive response leading to cerebral hemorrhage (124). A low titrated dose of this drug is advisable under such circumstances and it should be administered only after checking the blood pressure (124).

Prostaglandins

Prostaglandins (PGs) have been established as effective uterotonic agents in term labor induction trials and pregnancy termination, as well as in the treatment of postpartum hemorrhage due to uterine atony. PGs exert their effect via G-protein–coupled prostanoid receptors, several subtypes of which are known (125). $PGF_{2\alpha}$ produces uterine contraction via FP receptor linked to the mobilization of calcium from intracellular stores (126), and also by augmenting OTR expression (127). It produces dose-dependent increase in the uterine contractions in in vitro pregnant rat myometrium. The myometrial contractions produced by $PGF_{2\alpha}$ are superior compared to other types of PGs but not compared to similar concentrations of oxytocin (112). Carboprost tromethamine, a methylated analogue of $PGF_{2\alpha}$, has been shown to be a more potent uterotonic agent with longer duration of action than the parent compound (128). It is indicated for the treatment of postpartum hemorrhage due to uterine atony that has not responded to conventional methods of management. It may be associated with bronchospasm, ventilation–perfusion mismatch, and hypoxemia, and hence caution should be exercised in patients with respiratory disorders (129,130).

Misoprostol, a prostaglandin E1 analogue, is a uterotonic agent that selectively binds with EP_2 or EP_3 prostanoid receptors (131). It is useful for induction of labor or abortion, cervical priming, and also for the prevention of postpartum hemorrhage. In in vitro pregnant rat myometrial samples, it produces weak contractions compared to $PGF_{2\alpha}$ and oxytocin (112). It shows promising results in reducing blood loss

after delivery when compared to placebo; however, it is not preferable to conventional injectable uterotonics as part of the management of the third stage of labor, especially for low-risk women (132). As the side effects are dose-related, more research directed toward establishing the lowest effective dose for routine use is advocated.

Drugs used in Hypertensive Disorders of Pregnancy

The antihypertensive drugs used in the treatment of hypertensive disorders of pregnancy, including magnesium sulfate, nifedipine, nitroglycerine, and labetalol, have mainly relaxant effects on uterine tone. Some of them are also used for tocolysis.

Magnesium sulfate remains the drug of choice for prevention and treatment of seizures in patients with severe preeclampsia. Clinically, it has also been used as a tocolytic agent, although it has been strongly argued as ineffective in that context (133). It has been recently established that antenatal magnesium sulfate therapy given to women at risk of preterm birth has a neuroprotective role for the preterm fetus (134). In vitro, magnesium sulfate has been shown to decrease the frequency followed by the amplitude of spontaneous myometrial contractions in the pregnant non-laboring human uterus. The reduction is dose-dependent and time progressive, with complete arrest of spontaneous contractions at high concentrations. Oxytocin-induced myometrial contractions are also reduced in response to magnesium sulfate, although the effect is not as pronounced and requires doses of magnesium much higher than those used in clinical practice (135). Further studies are warranted to clarify the discrepancy between in vitro and in vivo studies.

Calcium channel blockers such as nifedipine have been shown to cause more frequent successful prolongation of pregnancy in cases of preterm labor compared to magnesium with few neonatal problems (136).

Nitroglycerin, used in the treatment of severe hypertension of pregnancy, also has a uterine relaxant effect. It is commonly employed for the removal of retained placenta, assisting difficult fetal extraction during delivery, facilitation of external cephalic version, twin manipulation, correction of fetal heart rate abnormalities from uterine hypertonus, and correction of uterine inversion. Its uterine relaxing effect is mainly due to its active compound nitric oxide (137). Nitroglycerine is a potent human uterine relaxant in vitro, but its tocolytic effect can easily be reversed by uterotonic agents (138). Despite its wide use in clinical practice, its superiority over currently used tocolytic agents is questioned (139).

The contractile effects of labetalol on in vitro term human myometrium samples have been studied, and any tocolytic effect of labetalol is only observed at concentrations higher than used clinically for hypertension. The mild uterine relaxant effect of labetalol is likely the result of a direct myometrial depression (140). However, clinically, labetalol does not seem to have any effect on the duration of pregnancy or the process of labor.

KEY POINTS

- Labor is a dynamic process characterized by structural and functional changes in the uterus. Various methods have been proposed to predict the progress of labor.
- All volatile anesthetics including sevoflurane, desflurane, isoflurane, halothane, and ethanol produce dose-dependent inhibition of uterine contractility; their actions

can be reversed by oxytocin only at lower concentrations (below 1 MAC).

■ Propofol decreases uterine contractility in a dose-dependent manner. The increase in uterine tone by ket-amine is not clinically significant, when it is administered as a single dose for induction of anesthesia.

■ At analgesic concentrations, systemic opioids such as fen-tanyl, meperidine, remifentanil, and alfentanil do not have a significant effect on spontaneous uterine contractions. They may directly inhibit uterine contractility at concentrations higher than those used for analgesia; however, even at higher doses morphine and sufentanil have no effect on the uterus.

■ Combined spinal–epidural anesthesia may increase uter-ine tone with sympathectomy due to a decrease in plasma epinephrine levels, thereby increasing the baseline uterine activity.

■ Low-dose neuraxial labor analgesia administered in current practice is not associated with maternal or perinatal morbid-ity or mortality, nor an increased risk of cesarean delivery.

■ Neuraxial analgesia appears to have a variable effect on the duration of labor, with a shortening of labor in some and a lengthening in others. The first stage of labor is not affected by epidural anesthesia, and even if it is slightly prolonged, it does not have adverse maternal or neonatal effects.

■ Epidural analgesia may be associated with a longer second stage of labor, but the average increase in duration of the second stage is relatively short. Continuous epidural infu-sion of bupivacaine 0.125% at 10 to 14 mL/h increases the chance of prolonged labor and instrumental delivery due to motor blockade.

■ All uterotonic drugs produce uterine contractions and sys-temic effects that are dose-dependent. Large doses of oxy-tocin when administered for induction or augmentation of labor may lead to poor uterine tone postpartum, possibly as a result of the desensitization phenomenon.

■ Antihypertensive agents such as magnesium sulfate, nife-dipine, nitroglycerine, and labetalol, used in the treatment of hypertensive diseases of pregnancy, have a relaxant effect of variable magnitudes on uterine muscle. This may poten-tially result in reduced uterine contractility; however, the clinical significance of this property is not well recognized.

REFERENCES

1. Smith R. Parturition. *N Engl J Med* 2007;356:271–283.
2. Chestnut D, Polley LS, Tsen L, Wong C. *Chestnut's Obstetric Anesthesia: Principles and Practice*. Mosby Elsevier; Philadelphia, 2009.
3. Bonica JJ. Peripheral mechanisms and pathways of parturition pain. *Br J Anaesth* 1979;51:3S–9S.
4. Rowlands S, Permezel M. Physiology of pain in labour. *Baillieres Clin Obstet Gynaecol* 1998;12:347–362.
5. Gibb DM, Arulkumaran S, Lun KC, et al. Characteristics of uterine activity in nulliparous labour. *Br J Obstet Gynaecol* 1984;91(3):220–227.
6. Conell-Price J, Evans JB, Hong D, et al. The development and validation of a dynamic model to account for the progress of labor in the assessment of pain. *Anesth Analg* 2008;106:1509–1515.
7. Debiec J, Conell-Price J, Evansmith J, et al. Mathematical modeling of the pain and progress of the first stage of nulliparous labor. *Anesthesiology* 2009; 111:1093–1110 .
8. Dmitrieva N, Johnson OL, Berkley KJ. Bladder inflammation and hypogastric neurectomy influence uterine motility in the rat. *Neurosci Lett* 2001;313:49–52.
9. Friedman E. *Labor: Clinical Evaluation and Management*. Appleton-Century-Crofts; New York, 1978.
10. Mathai M. The partograph for the prevention of obstructed labor. *Clin Obstet Gynecol* 2009;52:256–269.
11. Zhang J, Troendle JF, Yancey MK. Reassessing the labor curve in nulliparous women. *Am J Obstet Gynecol* 2002;187:824–828.
12. Reitman E, Conell-Price J, Evansmith J, et al. Beta-2-adrenergic receptor genotype and other variables that contribute to labor pain and progress. *Anesthesiology* 2011;114:927–939.
13. Bottoms SF, Sokol RJ, Rosen MG. Short arrest of cervical dilatation: A risk for maternal/fetal/infant morbidity. *Am J Obstet Gynecol* 1981;140:108–116.
14. Bottoms SF, Hirsch VJ, Sokol RJ. Medical management of arrest disorders of labor: A current overview. *Am J Obstet Gynecol* 1987;156:935–939.
15. Zhang J, Landy HJ, Ware Branch D, et al. Contemporary patterns of spontane-ous labor with normal neonatal outcomes. *Obstet Gynecol* 2010;116:1281–1287.
16. Gilstrap LC 3rd, Hauth JC, Hankins GD, et al. Effect of type of anesthesia on blood loss at cesarean section. *Obstet Gynecol* 1987;69:328–332.
17. Stallabrass P. Halothane and blood loss at delivery. *Acta Anaesthesiol Scand Suppl* 1965;25:376.
18. Rolbin SH, Hew EM, Bernstein A. Uterine relaxation can be life saving. *Can J Anaesth* 1991;38:939–940.
19. Gaiser RR, Cheek TG, Kurth CD. Anesthetic management of cesarean deliv-ery complicated by ex utero intrapartum treatment of the fetus. *Anesth Analg* 1997;84:1150–1153.
20. Fuchs F, Fuchs AR, Poblete VF Jr, et al. Effect of alcohol on threatened pre-mature labor. *Am J Obstet Gynecol* 1967;99:627–637.
21. Fuchs AR, Fuchs F. Ethanol for prevention of preterm birth. *Semin Perinatol* 1981;5:236–251.
22. Dogru K, Dalgic H, Yildiz K, et al. The direct depressant effects of desflurane and sevoflurane on spontaneous contractions of isolated gravid rat myome-trium. *Int J Obstet Anesth* 2003;12:74–78.
23. Dogru K, Yildiz K, Dalgic H, et al. Inhibitory effects of desflurane and sevo-flurane on contractions of isolated gravid rat myometrium under oxytocin stimulation. *Acta Anaesthesiol Scand* 2003;47:472–474.
24. Turner RJ, Lambros M, Holmes C, et al. The effects of sevoflurane on iso-lated gravid human myometrium. *Anaesth Intensive Care* 2002;30:591–596.
25. Turner RJ, Lambros M, Kenway L, et al. The in-vitro effects of sevoflurane and desflurane on the contractility of pregnant human uterine muscle. *Int J Obstet Anesth* 2002;11:246–251.
26. Yoo KY, Lee JC, Yoon MH, et al. The effects of volatile anesthetics on spon-taneous contractility of isolated human pregnant uterine muscle: A compari-son among sevoflurane, desflurane, isoflurane, and halothane. *Anesth Analg* 2006;103:443–447.
27. Gambling DR, Sharma SK, White PF, et al. Use of sevoflurane during elec-tive cesarean birth: a comparison with isoflurane and spinal anesthesia. *Anesth Analg* 1995;81:90–95.
28. Abboud TK, Zhu J, Richardson M, et al. Desflurane: a new volatile anesthetic for cesarean section. Maternal and neonatal effects. *Acta Anaesthesiol Scand* 1995; 39:723–726.
29. Karaman S, Akercan F, Aldemir O, et al. The maternal and neonatal effects of the volatile anaesthetic agents desflurane and sevoflurane in caesarean section: A prospective, randomized clinical study. *J Int Med Res* 2006;34:183–192.
30. Mychaliska GB, Bealer JF, Graf JL, et al. Operating on placental support: The ex utero intrapartum treatment procedure. *J Pediatr Surg* 1997;32:227–231.
31. Abboud TK, Shnider SM, Wright RG, et al. Enflurane Analgesia in Obstet-rics. *Anesth Analg* 1981;60:133–137.
32. Munson ES. Maier WR, Caton D. Effects of halothane, cyclopropane and nitrous oxide on isolated human uterine muscle. *J Obstet Gynecol Br Com-monw* 1969;76:27–33.
33. Kumarasinghe N, Harpin R, Stewart AW. Blood loss during suction termina-tion of pregnancy with two different anaesthetic techniques. *Anaesth Intensive Care* 1997;25:48–50.
34. Luo D, Wang QY, Huang W, et al. [The effect of propofol on isolated human pregnant uterine muscles]. *Sichuan Da Xue Xue Bao Yi Xue Ban* 2004;35:668–670.
35. Thind AS, Turner RJ. In vitro effects of propofol on gravid human myome-trium. *Anaesth Intensive Care* 2008;36:802–806.
36. Valtonen M, Kanto J, Rosenberg P. Comparison of propofol and thiopen-tone for induction of anaesthesia for elective caesarean section. *Anaesthesia* 1989;44:758–762.
37. Kanto J, Rosenberg P. Propofol in cesarean section. A pharmacokinetic and pharmacodynamic study. *Methods Find Exp Clin Pharmacol* 1990;12:707–711.
38. Gregory MA, Gin T, Yau G, et al. Propofol infusion anaesthesia for caesarean section. *Can J Anaesth* 1990;37:514–520.
39. Frolich MA, Burchfield DJ, Euliano TY, et al. A single dose of fentanyl and midazolam prior to Cesarean section have no adverse neonatal effects. *Can J Anaesth* 2006;53:79–85.
40. Nacitarhan C, Sadan G, Kayacan N, et al. The effects of opioids, local anes-thetics and adjuvants on isolated pregnant rat uterine muscles. *Methods Find Exp Clin Pharmacol* 2007;29:273–276.
41. Little B, Chang T, Chucot L, et al. Study of ketamine as an obstetric anes-thetic agent. *Am J Obstet Gynecol* 1972;113:247–260.
42. Hodgkinson R, Marx GF. Ketamine for delivery. *Anesthesiology* 1976;45:694–695.
43. Strümper D, Gogarten W, Durieux ME, et al. The effects of S+-ketamine and racemic ketamine on uterine blood flow in chronically instrumented pregnant sheep. *Anesth Analg* 2004;98:497–502, table of contents

44. Craft JB Jr., Coaldrake LA, Yonekura ML, et al. Ketamine, catecholamines, and uterine tone in pregnant ewes. *Am J Obstet Gynecol* 1983;146:429–434.

45. Levinson G, Shnider SM, Gildea JE, et al. Maternal and foetal cardiovascular and acid-base changes during ketamine anaesthesia in pregnant ewes. *Br J Anaesth* 1973;45:1111–1115.

46. Oats JN, Vasey DP, Waldron BA. Effects of ketamine on the pregnant uterus. *Br J Anaesth* 1979;51:1163–1166.

47. Wanna O, Werawatganon T, Piriyakitphaiboon S, et al. A comparison of propofol and ketamine as induction agents for cesarean section. *J Med Assoc Thai* 2004;87:774–779.

48. Schultetus RR, Hill CR, Dharamraj CM, et al. Wakefulness during cesarean section after anesthetic induction with ketamine, thiopental, or ketamine and thiopental combined. *Anesth Analg* 1986;65:723–728.

49. Baraka A, Louis F, Noueihid R, et al. Awareness following different techniques of general anaesthesia for caesarean section. *Br J Anaesth* 1989;62:645–648.

50. Janeczko GF, El-Etr AA, Younes S. Low-dose ketamine anesthesia for obstetrical delivery. *Anesth Analg* 1974;53:828–831.

51. Bovill JG, Coppel DL, Dundee JW, et al. Current status of ketamine anaesthesia. *Lancet* 1971;1:1285–1288.

52. Dich-Nielsen J, Holasek J. Ketamine as induction agent for caesarean section. *Acta Anaesthesiol Scand* 1982;26:139–142.

53. Yoo KY, Lee J, Kim HS, et al. The effects of opioids on isolated human pregnant uterine muscles. *Anesth Analg* 2001;92:1006–1009.

54. Kayacan N, Ertugrul F, Arici G, et al. In vitro effects of opioids on pregnant uterine muscle. *Adv Ther* 2007;24:368–375.

55. Wong CA, Scavone BM, Peaceman AM, et al. The risk of cesarean delivery with neuraxial analgesia given early versus late in labor. *N Engl J Med* 2005;352:655–665.

56. Wang F, Shen X, Guo X, et al. Epidural analgesia in the latent phase of labor and the risk of cesarean delivery: a five-year randomized controlled trial. *Anesthesiology* 2009;111:871–880.

57. Halpern SH, Leighton BL, Ohlsson A, et al. Effect of epidural vs parenteral opioid analgesia on the progress of labor. *JAMA* 1998;280:2105–2110.

58. Pilkington S, Carli F, Dakin MJ, et al. Increase in Mallampati score during pregnancy. *Br J Anaesth* 1995;74:638–642.

59. Boutonnet M, Faitot V, Katz A, et al. Mallampati class changes during pregnancy, labour, and after delivery: Can these be predicted? *Br J Anaesth* 2010;104:67–70.

60. Hawkins JL, Koonin LM, Palmer SK, et al. Anesthesia-related deaths during obstetric delivery in the United States, 1979–1990. *Anesthesiology* 1997;86:277–284.

61. Hawkins JL, Chang J, Palmer SK, et al. Anesthesia-related maternal mortality in the United States: 1979–2002. *Obstet Gynecol* 2011;117:69–74.

62. Gupta RC. *Toxicology of the Placenta.* John Wiley & Sons, Ltd; Chichester, UK, 2009.

63. Ng K, Parsons J, Cyna AM, et al. Spinal versus epidural anaesthesia for caesarean section. *Cochrane Database Sys Rev* 2004;(2):CD003765.

64. Reynolds F, Seed PT. Anaesthesia for caesarean section and neonatal acid-base status: A meta-analysis. *Anaesthesia* 2005;60:636–653.

65. Friedlander JD, Fox HE, Cain CF, et al. Fetal bradycardia and uterine hyperactivity following subarachnoid administration of fentanyl during labor. *Reg Anesth* 1997;22(4):378–381.

66. Abrao KC, Francisco RP, Miyadahira S, et al. Elevation of uterine basal tone and fetal heart rate abnormalities after labor analgesia: A randomized controlled trial. *Obstet Gynecol* 2009;113(1):41–47.

67. Cleary-Goldman J, Negron M, Scott J, et al. Prophylactic ephedrine and combined spinal epidural: maternal blood pressure and fetal heart rate patterns. *Obstet Gynecol* 2005;106(3):466–472.

68. Halpern SH, Leighton BL. Epidural analgesia and risk of caesarean section. *Lancet* 1999;353:1801–1802.

69. Zhang J, Yancey MK, Klebanoff MA, et al. Does epidural analgesia prolong labor and increase risk of cesarean delivery? A natural experiment. *Am J Obstet Gynecol* 2001;185:128–134.

70. Leighton BL, Halpern SH. Epidural analgesia and the progress of labor. In Halpern SH, Douglas MJ (editors). *Evidence-based obstetric anesthesia.* Blackwell Publishing Ltd; Oxford, UK, 2007.

71. Sharma SK, McIntire DD, Wiley J, et al. Labor analgesia and cesarean delivery: An individual patient meta-analysis of nulliparous women. *Anesthesiology* 2004;100:142–148.

72. Ohel G, Gonen R, Vaida S, et al. Early versus late initiation of epidural analgesia in labor: Does it increase the risk of cesarean section? A randomized trial. *Am J Obstet Gynecol* 2006;194:600–605.

73. Cheek TG, Samuels P, Miller F, et al. Normal saline i.v. fluid load decreases uterine activity in active labour. *Br J Anaesth* 1996;77:632–635.

74. Zamora JE, Rosaeg OP, Lindsay MP, et al. Haemodynamic consequences and uterine contractions following 0.5 or 1.0 litre crystalloid infusion before obstetric epidural analgesia. *Can J Anaesth* 1996;43:347–352.

75. Rahm VA, Hallgren A, Högberg H, et al. Plasma oxytocin levels in women during labor with or without epidural analgesia: A prospective study. *Acta Obstet Gynecol Scand* 2002;81:1033–1039.

76. Behrens O, Goeschen K, Luck HJ, et al. Effects of lumbar epidural analgesia on prostaglandin F2 alpha release and oxytocin secretion during labor. *Prostaglandins* 1993;45:285–296.

77. Nielsen PE, Abouleish E, Meyer BA, et al. Effect of epidural analgesia on fundal dominance during spontaneous active-phase nulliparous labor. *Anesthesiology* 1996;84:540–544.

78. Gunther RE, Bauman J. Obstetrical caudal anesthesia: I. A randomized study comparing 1% mepivacaine with 1% lidocaine plus epinephrine. *Anesthesiology* 1969;31:5–19.

79. Eisenach JC, Grice SC, Dewan DM. Epinephrine enhances analgesia produced by epidural bupivacaine during labor. *Anesth Analg* 1987;66:447–451.

80. Grice SC, Eisenach JC, Dewan DM. Labor analgesia with epidural bupivacaine plus fentanyl: enhancement with epinephrine and inhibition with 2-chloroprocaine. *Anesthesiology* 1990;72:623–628.

81. Abboud TK, Sheik-ol-Eslam A, Yanagi T, et al. Safety and efficacy of epinephrine added to bupivacaine for lumbar epidural analgesia in obstetrics. *Anesth Analg* 1985;64:585–591.

82. Abboud TK, David S, Nagappala S, et al. Maternal, fetal, and neonatal effects of lidocaine with and without epinephrine for epidural anesthesia in obstetrics. *Anesth Analg* 1984;63:973–979.

83. Van de Velde M, Teunkens A, Hanssens M, et al. Intrathecal sufentanil and fetal heart rate abnormalities: A double-blind, double placebo-controlled trial comparing two forms of combined spinal epidural analgesia with epidural analgesia in labor. *Anesth Analg* 2004;98:1153–1159.

84. Birnbach D, Hernandez M. Neuraxial analgesia for labor. In Wong C (editor). *Spinal and epidural anesthesia.* The McGraw-Hill Companies; New York, 2007.

85. Halonen P, Sarvela J, Saisto T, et al. Patient-controlled epidural technique improves analgesia for labor but increases cesarean delivery rate compared with the intermittent bolus technique. *Acta Anaesthesiol Scand* 2004;48:732–737.

86. Bogod DG, Rosen M, Rees GA. Extradural infusion of 0.125% bupivacaine at 10 ml h-1 to women during labour. *Br J Anaesth* 1987;59:325–330.

87. Smedstad KG, Morison DH. A comparative study of continuous and intermittent epidural analgesia for labour and delivery. *Can J Anaesth* 1988;35:234–241.

88. Gimpl G, Fahrenholz F. The oxytocin receptor system: structure, function, and regulation. *Physiol Rev* 2001;81:629–683.

89. Dawood MY, Ylikorkala O, Trivedi D, et al. Oxytocin levels and disappearance rate and plasma follicle-stimulating hormone and luteinizing hormone after oxytocin infusion in men. *J Clin Endocrinol Metab* 1980;50:397–400.

90. Leake RD, Weitzman RE, Fisher DA. Pharmacokinetics of oxytocin in the human subject. *Obstet Gynecol* 1980;56:701–704.

91. Seitchik J, Amico J, Robinson AG, et al. Oxytocin augmentation of dysfunctional labor. IV. Oxytocin pharmacokinetics. *Am J Obstet Gynecol* 1984;150:225–228.

92. Seitchik J, Castillo M. Oxytocin augmentation of dysfunctional labor. II. Uterine activity data. *Am J Obstet Gynecol* 1983;145:526–529.

93. Tsen L, Balki M. Oxytocin protocols during cesarean delivery: Time to acknowledge the risk/benefit ratio? *Int J Obstet Anesth* 2010;19:243–245.

94. Crane JMG, Young DC. Metanalysis of low dose versus high dose oxytocin for labour induction. *J Obstet Gynaecol Can* 1998;20:1215–1523.

95. Wei SQ, Luo ZC, Qi HP, et al. High-dose vs low-dose oxytocin for labor augmentation: a systematic review. *Am J Obstet Gynecol* 2010;203:296–304.

96. Simpson KR, James DC. Effects of oxytocin-induced uterine hyperstimulation during labor on fetal oxygen status and fetal heart rate patterns. *Am J Obstet Gynecol* 2008;199:34.e1–34.e5.

97. Johnson N, van Oudgaarden E, Montague I, et al. The effect of oxytocin-induced hyperstimulation on fetal oxygen. *Br J Obstet Gynaecol* 1994;101:805–807.

98. Thomas JS, Koh SH, Cooper GM. Haemodynamic effects of oxytocin given as i.v. bolus or infusion on women undergoing caesarean section. *Br J Anaesth* 2007;98:116–119.

99. Svanstrom MC, Biber B, Hanes M, et al. Signs of myocardial ischaemia after injection of oxytocin: a randomized double-blind comparison of oxytocin and methylergometrine during caesarean section. *Br J Anaesth* 2008;100:683–689.

100. Pinder AJ, Dresner M, Calow C, et al. Haemodynamic changes caused by oxytocin during caesarean section under spinal anaesthesia. *Int J Obstet Anesth* 2002;11:156–159.

101. Thomas TA, Cooper GM. Anaesthesia. In: Lewis G, ed. *Why Mothers Die 1997–1999. The Confidential Enquiry Into Maternal Deaths in the United Kingdom.* London: RCOG Press; 2001:135–137.

102. Sarna MC, Soni AK, Gomez M, et al. Intravenous oxytocin in patients undergoing elective cesarean section. *Anesth Analg* 1997;84:753–756.

103. Carvalho JC, Balki M, Kingdom J, et al. Oxytocin requirements at elective cesarean delivery: a dose-finding study. *Obstet Gynecol* 2004;104:1005–1010.

104. Balki M, Ronayne M, Davies S, et al. Minimum oxytocin dose requirement after cesarean delivery for labor arrest. *Obstet Gynecol* 2006;107:45–50.

105. Grotegut CA, Paglia MJ, Johnson LNC, et al. Oxytocin exposure during labor among women with postpartum hemorrhage secondary to uterine atony. *Am J Obstet Gynecol* 2011;204(1):56.e1–56.e6.

106. Phaneuf S, Asboth G, Carrasco MP, et al. Desensitization of oxytocin receptors in human myometrium. *Hum Reprod Update* 1998;4:625–633.

107. Robinson C, Schumann R, Zhang P, et al. Oxytocin-induced desensitization of the oxytocin receptor. *Am J Obstet Gynecol* 2003;188:497–502.

108. Phaneuf S, Rodríguez Liñares B, TambyRaja RL, et al. Loss of myometrial oxytocin receptors during oxytocin-induced and oxytocin-augmented labour. *J Reprod Fertil* 2000;120:91–97.

109. Magalhaes JK, Carvalho JC, Parkes RK, et al. Oxytocin pretreatment decreases oxytocin-induced myometrial contractions in pregnant rats in a concentration-dependent but not time-dependent manner. *Reprod Sci* 2009;16:501–508.

110. Zingg HH, Laporte SA. The oxytocin receptor. *Trends Endocrinol Metab* 2003;14:222–227.

111. Balki M, Cristian AL, Kingdom J, et al. Oxytocin pretreatment of pregnant rat myometrium reduces the efficacy of oxytocin but not of ergonovine maleate or prostaglandin F2 alpha. *Reprod Sci* 2010;17:269–277.

112. Balki M, Kanwal N, Erik-Soussi M, et al. Contractile efficacy of various prostaglandins in pregnant rat myometrium pretreated with oxytocin. *Reprod Sci* 2012. [Epub ahead of print]

113. Engstrom T, Barth T, Melin P, et al. Oxytocin receptor binding and uterotonic activity of carbetocin and its metabolites following enzymatic degradation. *Eur J Pharmacol* 1998;355:201–210.

114. Atke A, Vilhardt H. Uterotonic activity and myometrial receptor affinity of 1-deamino-1-carba-2-tyrosine (O-methyl)-oxytocin. *Acta endocrinol (Copenh)* 1987;115:155–160.

115. Hunter DJS, Schulz P, Wassenaar W. Effect of carbetocin, a long-acting oxytocin analog the postpartum uterus. *Clin Pharmacol Ther* 1992;52:60–67.

116. Peters NC, Duvekot JJ. Carbetocin for the prevention of postpartum hemorrhage—A systematic review. *Obstet Gynecol Surv* 2009;64:129–135.

117. Dansereau J, Joshi AK, Helewa ME, et al. Double-blind comparison of carbetocin versus oxytocin in prevention of uterine atony after cesarean section. *Am J Obstet Gynecol* 1999;180:670–676.

118. Borruto F, Treisser A, Comparetto C. Utilization of carbetocin for prevention of postpartum hemorrhage after cesarean section: a randomized clinical trial. *Arch Gynecol Obstet* 2009;280:707–712.

119. Boucher M, Horbay GL, Griffin P, et al. Double-blind, randomized comparison of the effect of carbetocin and oxytocin on intraoperative blood loss and uterine tone of patients undergoing cesarean section. *J Perinatol* 1998;18:202–207.

120. Attilakos G, Psaroudakis D, Ash J, et al. Carbetocin versus oxytocin for the prevention of postpartum haemorrhage following caesarean section: the results of a double-blind randomised trial. *BJOG* 2010;117:929–936.

121. De Groot AN, van Dongen PW, Vree TB, et al. Ergot alkaloids. Current status and review of clinical pharmacology and therapeutic use compared with other oxytocics in obstetrics and gynaecology. *Drugs* 1998;56:523–535.

122. Myerscough PR, Schild HO. Quantitative assays of oxytocic drugs on the human postpartum uterus. *Br J Pharmacol Chemother* 1958;13:207–212.

123. Sloan N, Durocher J, Aldrich T, et al. What measured blood loss tells us about postpartum bleeding: a systematic review. *BJOG* 2010;117:788–800.

124. Lewis G, ed. *The confidential enquiry into maternal and child health (CEMACH). Saving Mothers' Lives: Reviewing maternal deaths to make motherhood safer—2003–2005.* The Seventh Report of the Confidential Enquiries into Maternal Deaths in the United Kingdom. London: CEMACH; 2007.

125. Wright DH, Abran D, Bhattacharya M, et al. Prostanoid receptors: Ontogeny and implications in vascular physiology. *Am J Physiol Regul Integr Comp Physiol* 2001;281:R1343–R1360.

126. Narumiya S, Sugimoto Y, Ushikubi F. Prostanoid receptors: structures, properties, and functions. *Physiol Rev* 1999;79:1193–1226.

127. Mirando MA, Prince BC, Tysseling KA, et al. Proposed role for oxytocin in regulation of endometrial prostaglandin $F_2\alpha$ secretion during luteolysis in swine. *Adv Exp Med Biol* 1995;395:421–433.

128. Bygdeman M. Pharmacokinetics of prostaglandins. *Best Pract Res Clin Obstet Gynaecol* 2003;17:707–716.

129. Harber CR, Levy DM, Chidambaram S, et al. Lifethreatening bronchospasm after intramuscular carboprost for postpartum haemorrhage. *BJOG* 2007;114:366–368.

130. Andersen LH, Secher NJ. Pattern of total and regional lung function in subjects with bronchoconstriction induced by 15-me PGF2 alpha. *Thorax* 1976;31:685–692.

131. Senior J, Marshall K, Sangha R, et al. In vitro characterization of prostanoid receptors on human myometrium at term pregnancy. *Br J Pharmacol* 1993;108:501–506.

132. Mousa HA, Alfirevic Z. Treatment for primary postpartum haemorrhage. *Cochrane Database Syst Rev* 2007;(1):CD003249.

133. Han S, Crowther CA, Moore V. Magnesium maintenance therapy for preventing preterm birth after threatened preterm labour. *Cochrane Database Syst Rev* 2010;7(7):CD000940.

134. Doyle LW, Crowther CA, Middleton P, et al. Magnesium sulphate for women at risk of preterm birth for neuroprotection of the fetus. *Cochrane Database Syst Rev* 2009;21(1):CD004661.

135. Tica VI, Tica AA, Carlig V, et al. Magnesium ion inhibits spontaneous and induced contractions of isolated uterine muscle. *Gynecol Endocrinol* 2007;23:368–372.

136. King JF, Flenady VJ, Papatsonis DN, et al. Calcium channel blockers for inhibiting preterm labour. *Cochrane Database Syst Rev* 2003;(1):CD002255.

137. Cameron IT, Cambell S. Nitric oxide in the endometrium. *Humn Repro Update* 1998; 4:565–569.

138. Lau LC, Adaikan PG, Arulkumaran S, et al. Oxytocics reverse the tocolytic effect of glyceryl trinitrate on the human uterus. *BJOG* 2001;108:164–168.

139. Morgan PJ, Kung R, Tarshis J. Nitroglycerin as a uterine relaxant: a systematic review. *J Obstet Gynaecol Can* 2002;24:403–409.

140. Thulesius O, Lunell NO, Ibrahim M, et al. The effect of labetalol on contractility of human myometrial preparations. *Acta Obstet Gynecol Scand* 1987;66:237–240.

CHAPTER

12

Anesthesia for Cesarean Delivery

McCallum R. Hoyt

Cesarean deliveries have become one of the most commonly performed surgical procedures. This is largely due to the fact that its incidence has exploded over the past few decades, especially in developed countries (1). The choice of anesthetic most appropriate for a cesarean depends on many factors, not the least of which are the urgency of the situation, maternal medical conditions, and any contraindications for a particular technique. Obstetric anesthesia practice has adapted as a better understanding of maternofetal conditions, risks and benefits have developed. As a result, neuraxial techniques are the anesthetic of choice for cesarean delivery most often, especially in the non-emergent situation (2). Practice has shifted so much that residents may never perform a general anesthetic for a cesarean delivery (3,4), which makes it all the more important that they have an understanding of the reasons for, performance of, and risks and benefits of a general anesthesic for cesarean while in training. Other concepts that are impacting anesthesic practice are new information on oxytocin administration as well as studies on maternal oxygenation during surgery and perceived benefits to the fetus.

■ INCIDENCE AND ETIOLOGY OF CESAREAN DELIVERY

The incidence of cesarean delivery has increased significantly over the past several decades. What has led to the explosive increase in cesarean deliveries in most developed countries appears to be a combination of many factors, and current international data suggest that strong regional influences may affect both cesarean delivery rates and maternal mortality numbers. In a report published in 2007, the international cumulative rate was cited as 15%, with the United States and many other industrialized countries reporting much higher rates (1). Unfortunately, this same international data suggest that there exists a worrisome relationship between maternal mortality and higher cesarean delivery rates. The data show that there comes a point where maternal and fetal mortality rates no longer improve with higher cesarean delivery rates but rather worsen. Whether the current high rates can be lowered is speculative despite evidence that higher cesarean delivery rates do not positively correlate with improved outcomes (5).

Cesarean Delivery Rates

An international survey on cesarean delivery rates showed dramatic variability among regions as well as between developed and less developed countries (1). The survey collected data on maternal, fetal and neonatal mortality, incidence as a percentage of births and the presence of a trained health professional, which represented a measure of obstetric care afforded to the population. Data were collected for 126 countries and the authors estimated that they were able to capture 89% of all live births for 2002. Those countries were organized into regional and subregional categories using United Nations criteria, and the cesarean delivery rates were reported within those categories (Table 12-1). Taken together, the surveys indicated an overall international incidence of 15%. However, there was significant variance between and within regional categories and level of development among countries.

In developed regions such as Western Europe, North America, Australia, and New Zealand, cesarean rates averaged well over the worldwide figure of 15%. Taking developed countries as a whole, the mean rate was reported as 21.1%. In the United States, primary and repeat rates have increased steadily from 5.5% in 1970 to 32% in 2007 (6,7). Zhang et al. (8) reported an overall cesarean rate of 30.5% in the United States between 2002 and 2008. But cesarean deliveries varied significantly among the various hospitals surveyed with rates ranging from 20% to 44%. In other regions such as Canada, rates increased from 17.8% to 19.1% from 1994 to 1997 (9), and in England and Wales, the rate increased from 16% to 19% to 21.5% in 1995, 1999, and 2000, respectively (10).

In less developed regions, the mean cesarean delivery rate hovered about 15%, again with marked variation among regions and subregions. In the least developed regions, as defined by 49 countries located mostly in Africa, the average cesarean delivery rate was 2% (1). Here, an association of low cesarean delivery rates and high maternal mortality rates was supported, with some exceptions.

Alarmed at the rapid rise in cesarean delivery rates, in 1985 the World Health Organization made the recommendation that information about cesarean delivery rates at obstetric institutions should be made available to the public (11). The assumption was that by informing mothers of the potential negative effects of cesarean deliveries and then publishing institutional data, those rates would fall. The WHO report noted that countries with rates less than 10% had some of the lowest perinatal mortality rates in the world, stating "there is no justification for any region to have a rate higher than 10–15%." Despite this very public attempt to reduce cesarean delivery rates, the trend has shown a distinctive increase.

TABLE 12-1 Cesarean Delivery Rates by Region and Subregion and Coverage of the Estimates

Region/Subregion[a]	Births by Cesarean Section %	Range, Minimum to Maximum %	Coverage of Estimates[b] %
Africa	3.5	0.4–15.4	83
Eastern Africa	2.3	0.6–7.4	93
Middle Africa	1.8	0.4–6.0	26
Northern Africa	7.6	3.5–11.4	84
Southern Africa	14.5	6.9–15.4	93
Western Africa	1.9	0.6–6.0	95
Asia	15.9	1.0–40.5	89 (65)[c]
Eastern Asia	40.5	27.4–40.5	90 (0.31)[c]
South-central Asia	5.8	1.0–10.8	93
South-eastern Asia	6.8	1.0–17.4	83
Western Asia	11.7	1.5–23.3	75
Europe	19.0	6.2–36.0	99
Eastern Europe	15.2	6.2–24.7	100
Northern Europe	20.1	14.9–23.3	100
Southern Europe	24.0	8.0–36.0	97
Western Europe	20.2	13.5–24.3	100
Latin America and the Caribbean	29.2	1.7–39.1	92
Caribbean	18.1	1.7–31.3	78
Central America	31.0	7.9–39.1	98
South America	29.3	12.9–36.7	90
Northern America	24.3	22.5–24.4	100
Oceania	14.9	4.7–21.9	92
Australia/New Zealand	21.6	20.4–21.9	100
Melanesia	4.9	4.7–7.1	87
Micronesia	N/A	N/A	0
Polynesia	N/A	N/A	0
World total	15.0	0.4–40.5	89 (74)[c]
More developed regions	21.1	6.2–36.0	90
Less developed countries	14.3	0.4–40.5	89 (72)[c]
Least developed countries	2.0	0.4–6.0	74

[a]Countries categorized according to the UN classification. Countries with a population of less than 140,000 in 2,000 are not included.
[b]Refers to the proportion of live births for which nationally representative data were available.
[c]Figures in brackets represent coverage excluding data from China.
N/A, data not available.
Reprinted from: Betrán AP, Merialdi M, Lauer JA, et al. Rates of caesarean section: Analysis of global, regional and national estimates. *Paediatric and Perinatal Epidem* 2007;21(2):98–113.

Cesarean Delivery Indications

The reasons for the rising cesarean rates in developed countries appear to be complex and numerous but do not vary greatly among most industrialized countries suggesting a commonality of influences. Joseph et al. (9) reviewed the indications for all primary cesarean deliveries in Nova Scotia, Canada between 1988 and 2000. They found that changes in maternal characteristics, maternal comorbidities, and obstetric practice were responsible for the rise in primary cesarean delivery rates (Table 12-2). The maternal characteristics identified were increasing age, lower parity, higher prepregnancy weight and greater weight gain during pregnancy. Of reasons cited for a primary cesarean delivery, the most significant increases were for dystocia and breech presentation. Concurrent maternal comorbidities contributing to greater maternal risk were also implicated in driving the rate upward. These findings were supported by others noting that more women were choosing to follow a career path

TABLE 12-2 Identified Risks Associated with a Cesarean Delivery

Maternal Characteristics	Changes in Obstetric Practice
Advanced age	Reduced forceps use
Comorbidities	Breech delivery by cesarean
Prepregnancy obesity	Non-indicated elective inductions
Excessive Antepartum Weight Gain	Increased Use of Technology
Litigation	Routine electronic fetal monitoring
Maternal Requests	Medical Society Guidelines

and delay marriage and family. Thus, the average age of nulliparity has risen over the past two decades and public health analyses confirm that women of advanced maternal age are more likely to have a cesarean delivery (12). Menacker et al. concurred with all of the aforementioned reasons and added concerns over litigation and more conservative recommendations from medical associations as contributing to the rising rate from 1991 to 2007 in the United States. Cesarean delivery rates in 2007 were at the highest ever recorded in the United States at 32%, and represented a 53% increase from rates 16 years previously (13). In some states, rates increased by over 70%.

Obstetric practice has changed over time with more technology available to assist in labor management, and a better awareness by obstetric providers of maternal safety and outcomes. Breech presentations are rarely performed vaginally for a variety of reasons including poor maternal and neonatal outcomes, fear of litigation, and obstetric society publications suggesting a better outcome with cesarean delivery (14,15). The decreased use of forceps as well as the greater use of fetal monitoring in obstetric practice leading to variable interpretations of abnormal fetal traces have led to more cesarean deliveries (6,9,13). In the United States in 2004, fully one in three nulliparous women were delivered by cesarean delivery (8). In this report by Zhang et al., a statistically significant contributing factor was the elective induction of labor especially without a clear obstetric or medical indication.

When the 1985 WHO recommendations were published, along with promulgating a 10% to 15% cesarean delivery rate, the concept of always requiring a cesarean following the first was debunked (11). As a means to achieve a lower surgical delivery rate, the concept of a vaginal birth after cesarean (VBAC) was endorsed. There followed a brief drop in the overall rate during the early 1990s as women were counseled to attempt a VBAC. However, VBAC rates began to drop off in 1996 and cesarean rates rose for reasons of perceived maternal safety. Macones et al. (16) performed a retrospective observational study of more than 25,000 women who had previously had cesarean delivery. They reported that the incidence of uterine rupture for a low transverse incision was 9.8/1,000, and that if a woman had a previous successful VBAC, the incidence of uterine rupture was further lowered. Regardless, VBAC rates fell and in an editorial response 3 years later to an article on the diminishing rate of VBAC delivery in the United States, Macones (17) suggested that the factor driving the decision making among obstetricians and their patients was an overly emphasized concern about uterine rupture. He pointed out that the current evidence-based rates placed the risk of uterine rupture at 0.5% to 1%, and the neonatal risk of hypoxic ischemic encephalopathy at 12/15,000. Macones also stressed the longer-term risks of placenta previa or placenta accreta with increasing numbers of cesarean deliveries. Despite the data, more current numbers show that VBAC rates remain low. Women with a previous cesarean delivery undergo a trial of labor in 28.8% of possible cases when estimates are that two-thirds of women with uterine scars are eligible (8). Among those who attempt a VBAC, only 57.1% of them have a successful vaginal birth. Thus, 83.6% of women in 2004, who had a previous cesarean delivery, were delivered by repeat cesarean delivery.

An oft-quoted explanation for the rise in cesarean deliveries is the corresponding rise in litigation for poor maternal or neonatal outcomes (9,18,19). Litigation pressures are positively correlated with rising cesarean delivery rates in industrialized countries including the United States and negatively correlated with VBAC delivery (18). Murthy et al. reported that an indirect measure of the effect of litigation on medical practice is to measure the professional liability premiums.

They analyzed the rate of rise of medical professional liability premiums in Illinois between 1998 and 2003 against the primary cesarean delivery over that same time period and reported a positive correlation between rising primary cesarean rates and rising premiums both in nulliparous and multiparous women (19).

Another relatively recent yet concerning trend has been the occurrence of maternal request for an elective cesarean delivery, thereby avoiding a vaginal attempt. Habiba et al. (20) surveyed obstetricians from eight European countries and inquired how they would respond to a woman's request for elective cesarean delivery without any obstetric or medical indication. Countries whose obstetricians were likely to agree to such a request were Germany and the United Kingdom. Those countries where obstetricians were least likely to consent to the same were Spain and France. These authors suggested that cultural differences and fear of litigation were important factors in determining whether the providers in a particular country would be willing to perform an elective cesarean without indication. Some suggest that the mother's perception of the optimal delivery method for her baby influences her decision of the mode of delivery. With this in mind, a Lancet editorial written in response to the growing national debate over maternal request in the United Kingdom suggested that a mother who is well informed about the indications and consequences of cesarean delivery would be less inclined to want cesarean delivery when it was not indicated, and if well informed would be more amenable to undergoing a trial of labor after cesarean delivery (TOLAC). However, a survey quoted in that editorial reported that when the female obstetricians in 31 hospitals in the United Kingdom were asked what mode of delivery they would prefer if they were pregnant, 31% answered they would choose an elective cesarean delivery despite a lack of indication. This suggested that even the well-informed mother may make requests based on personal preference despite the evidence of no benefit but substantially more risk of morbidity and mortality (21).

Maternal Risks and Complications

Whether elective or not, cesarean deliveries expose the mother to an assortment of potential short- and long-term risks. Kainu et al. demonstrated in a cohort study of 600 patients that persistent pain 1 year after delivery was more common in those who had a cesarean delivery compared to a vaginal birth (22). Although rare, bladder and ureteral injuries are greater with cesarean than vaginal delivery and there is a significantly increased risk of postpartum endometritis in patients who have undergone surgery over a vaginal delivery (23). Women are less likely to have symptoms of urinary incontinence or pelvic floor dysfunction after elective cesarean delivery provided no labor has occurred as compared to women who have labored. This statistic is quoted at times as the reason for maternal request. Yet it has been shown that if a woman has a cesarean delivery for obstructed labor, she risks a similar incidence of urinary incontinence as those who had a vaginal delivery (24). As the presence of a uterine scar increases the risk of abnormal implantation of the placenta, the increased risk of a placenta previa and/or accreta is significant for future pregnancies (17).

Overall maternal mortality has decreased significantly over the last century but not necessarily because of the rise in cesarean delivery. Deneaux et al. (25) performed a case-control analysis of the incidence of postpartum maternal death in French women who had a cesarean delivery and compared the rate of death following a vaginal delivery. They reported that the risk of postpartum death was 3.6 times higher following a cesarean compared to a vaginal delivery. Anesthetic causes were implicated in four cases of maternal death during a cesarean delivery of which general anesthesia was implicated in three cases and spinal anesthesia in only one. Studies in other countries also report an increased risk to a mother's health with cesarean delivery over vaginal. The 2001 Confidential Enquiry into Maternal Deaths, a triennial report from the Royal College of Obstetricians and Gynaecologists on adverse maternal outcomes in Great Britain, calculated that an elective cesarean delivery is associated with a 2.84 times greater incidence of maternal death than a vaginal delivery.

Regardless of the mode of delivery, the maternal mortality rate in the United States in 2007 was 12.7/100,000 live births (26). Clark et al. (27) specifically investigated the causes of maternal death in the United States between 2000 and 2006 that were related to cesarean delivery. They reported that the maternal mortality rate from all causes was 0.2/100,000 vaginal deliveries and 2.2/100,000 cesarean deliveries. Upon examination of the causes of deaths, they reported that a significant number were due to thromboembolic complications. They further calculated that if these thromboembolic events had been prevented, the incidence of maternal death due to cesarean delivery would fall to 0.9/100,000 cesarean deliveries. This would make the maternal mortality rate between cesarean and vaginal deliveries comparable. Even with such preventative measures, Clark et al. noted that whether the delivery mode is vaginal or surgical, most maternal deaths are not preventable.

Fetal Complications

There is no evidence that a cesarean delivery leads to a better neonatal outcome over a vaginal delivery. The epidemiologic study of Villar et al. (5) that involved 97,095 births within eight Latin American countries suggested that as the cesarean delivery rate rose from 10% to 20%, there was an increase in the number of admissions to the neonatal intensive care units (ICU) for 7 days or longer. There may be an optimum cesarean delivery rate at which overall maternal and fetal morbidity and mortality are minimized but this has not yet been defined. Several reports indicate that a cesarean delivery rate greater than 15% may be associated with increased maternal and fetal morbidity and mortality (1,7,11).

Other studies have examined whether cesarean delivery has a negative association on the long-term outcome of neonates. Leung et al. (28) questioned whether cesarean delivery impacted pediatric morbidity by looking at outpatient care or hospital admission (15). This epidemiologic study involved 5,449 term singleton infants from a Chinese post-industrialized community. Once all potential confounders were accounted for, the authors found no association between cesarean delivery and the frequency of outpatient visits or hospital admissions during the first 18 months of the child's life. They concluded that the mode of delivery did not have an effect on the morbidity or mortality of an infant's life during the first 18 months.

Ways to Reduce the Cesarean Delivery Rate

The incidence of cesarean delivery is increasing worldwide particularly in developed countries. The reasons for this increase are complex as discussed. It has been suggested that the best way to slow the increasing cesarean delivery rate is to target low risk mothers with term, singleton, and vertex presentations. Evidence suggests that permitting only indicated inductions or allowing spontaneous labor would improve vaginal delivery numbers. Also, not acceding to maternal requests for non-indicated surgical deliveries would be a significant influence. Another group of parturients to target

are those with a previous cesarean delivery who qualify for a TOLAC (13). Under the correct conditions, maternal risks are minimal and a TOLAC can be performed safely with a reasonable expectation of success. This would prevent these patients from being relegated to cesarean delivery for future deliveries with its associated risks.

■ PREPARATION FOR CESAREAN DELIVERY

Many patients undergoing a cesarean delivery will have a relatively benign medical history and will require a no more than a routine approach as described below (Table 12-3). Considering just the healthy patient population, the necessary bedside procedures are performance of a routine history and physical examination, discussion of the risks, benefits and alternatives to the proposed anesthetic plan, and obtaining the informed consent. Before taking the patient to the operating area, final checks should include a review of any ordered laboratory tests, assurance that the patient has a large-bore intravenous catheter that is reliable and secure, a check that aspiration concerns are addressed, and information on what antibiotic will be given and when. For those with a more complex history, greater preparation is necessary but the same basic steps are followed.

Patient Evaluation and Consent

Because the unexpected can occur quickly in obstetrics, it is always best to have a baseline assessment before any procedure. Thus a complete preanesthetic evaluation should include not only a thorough history but a physical examination that evaluates the airway, lungs, and heart, at the very least. Examination of other areas should be directed by the patient's history and anesthetic plan. For a complete discussion of the airway examination and approaches to the difficult airway, please see Chapter 23.

Informed consent is a discussion with the patient that consists of five components: A presentation of the proposed

TABLE 12-3 Preparation for Cesarean Delivery

Complete History	
Physical examination	Airway
	Heart
	Lungs
	As indicated by history and anesthetic plan
Informed consent	Presentation of the anesthetic plan
	Discussion of benefits
	Discussion of risks
	Presentation of alternatives
	Question and answer
Check on ordered labs and blood bank sample	
Provide aspiration prophylaxis	H_2 Antagonist 30 minutes before
	Non-particulate antacid immediately before
Antibiotic	Confirm choice
	Administer completely immediately before incision

anesthetic, a discussion of the risks and benefits, a presentation of the alternatives to the plan, and the opportunity for the patient to have all her questions asked and answered to her satisfaction. The question has been raised whether the obstetric patient can make an informed decision while experiencing labor pain or coping with an urgent or emergency situation requiring a rapid response. Opinion at this time is that there is no evidence that she cannot. Thus, unless the situation presents an immediate threat to the life of the mother or fetus, every parturient should go through the informed consent process prior to any anesthetic.

Preoperative Laboratory Tests and Blood Products

There is no evidence that any particular laboratory test such as a platelet count or hematocrit is necessary for a healthy parturient undergoing a routine cesarean delivery. The selection of laboratory studies should be determined by the maternal history or clinical situation. Although it has been common practice in the past to routinely request a platelet count prior to the initiation of a neuraxial anesthetic, best evidence shows that doing so is unwarranted in a patient with a benign history and examination (29). Equally unnecessary is to have a full type and crossmatch completed prior to a routine surgical delivery. However, having a completed type and screen or blood sample in the blood bank is considered reasonable.

If the patient's history warrants a platelet count prior to a neuraxial block, the next issue to consider is what the lower limit to the count is placement contraindicated because of concerns of a hematoma. The "100,000-rule" that was adhered to for so long has no scientific basis, and it is now felt by most anesthesiologists that 80×10^9/L ("80,000") is safe. However, there is no objective or outcome-based evidence for that belief either, and unfortunately there are no established bedside tests that can be used to evaluate platelet function. The bleeding time of old is no longer considered valid but neither the platelet function analyzer (PFA) nor the thromboelastogram (TEG) has been validated by adequate study designs and sample sizes either. Studies to evaluate the usefulness of these two methods have been based on small population sizes. Thus, more work is necessary before any recommendations on these devices can be made (30).

Both the US and British Hematological Societies have suggested a lower count that is tolerable in situations of idiopathic thrombocytopenic purpura. The British Committee for Standards in Haematology published guidelines stating that platelet counts of 50×10^9/L are safe for a vaginal delivery and 80×10^9/L for cesarean delivery and neuraxial anesthesia (31). The American College for Hematology guidelines state 50×10^9/L as safe, and make no distinction between vaginal delivery, cesarean delivery, and neuraxial anesthesia (32). There remains a lack of adequate data behind these recommendations, but increasing numbers of anesthesia providers are comfortable performing a neuraxial block in the presence of a count below 100×10^9/L in a patient without a bleeding history (30), and some recommend as low as 50×10^9/L in parturients with non-preeclamptic thrombocytopenia (33,34).

Intravenous Access and Fluid Loads

Intravenous access must be adequate to allow for effective resuscitation in the event of hemorrhage. Large-bore intravenous catheters (16 or 18 gauge) allow for rapid fluid resuscitation and blood administration if the need arises. Preloading with fluid prior to the initiation of neuraxial anesthesia is not obligatory and should not preclude the initiation of the block. Dyer et al. (35) demonstrated that rapid co-loading

with 20 mL/kg crystalloid at the time of neuraxial placement was as effective as preloading. Although significant hypotension following a spinal anesthetic is a common complication, not all parturients have this complication to a significant extent, and it is difficult to predict who will. Regardless, this complication is readily corrected with fluids and vasopressors, of which ephedrine, phenylephrine, or a combination of both are preferred in the United States (29).

Monitors and Equipment

The ASA Practice Guidelines for Obstetric Anesthesia state that equipment, monitors, facilities, and support personnel should be similar to those available in the main operating room facility (29). Patients undergoing a cesarean delivery or any operative procedure should be monitored as defined by ASA standards and fetal monitors and neonatal resuscitative equipment should be in or adjacent to all operative sites. Equipment necessary for maternal resuscitation should also meet facility standards, and items such as an air warmer, fluid warmer, rapid infuser, and resuscitative equipment should be in the operating room or nearby and ready for use. Given the greater potential difficulties of the obstetric airway, a "Difficult Airway Cart" should be fully stocked, routinely checked, and immediately available to the operating area.

Aspiration Prophylaxis

The risk of aspiration, techniques of prophylaxis, and consideration of NPO policies are discussed extensively in Chapter 24. In this section, the specific practices for prophylaxis relating to cesarean delivery are considered. Modern obstetric anesthesia practice and guidelines have changed with a better understanding of gastrointestinal physiology in the pregnant patient (29). Current recommendations allow for the consumption of modest amounts of clear liquids until 2 hours before an uncomplicated elective cesarean delivery in non-laboring patients. Obviously, those with known gastric dysfunction or risk factors for aspiration will require more prolonged fasting or treatment as "full stomach" (at risk for aspiration). As for the ingestion of solid foods, current recommendations are that patients should fast for 6 to 8 hours depending on the fat content of the meal consumed prior to an elective uncomplicated cesarean delivery. Because any laboring patient may need an urgent or emergent cesarean, and because it has been shown that eating even light solid food during labor increases gastric volume and amount of vomitus (36), it is common practice in many centers to discourage solid intake during labor. When it may not be possible to wait the recommended 6 to 8 hours in a non-elective cesarean situation, it may be prudent to allow as much time to elapse as is safe, and agents to neutralize gastric acid and perhaps to promote gastric emptying should be utilized.

Early studies supported the effectiveness of non-particulate antacids such as sodium citrate to increase gastric pH but did so at the cost of increasing gastric volume. However, effectiveness is related to timing of administration. Dewan et al. (37) evaluated the optimal timing and efficacy of sodium citrate in increasing gastric pH prior to cesarean delivery. They randomized 32 patients receiving general anesthesia to receive 30 mL 0.3 M sodium citrate either less than 60 minutes before surgery, greater than 60 minutes before surgery, or immediately after delivery of the baby. Their results demonstrated that sodium citrate must be administered within 60 minutes of the start of surgery in order to be effective in raising pH, although gastric volumes were similar in all groups. As H_2 receptor antagonists became available, studies determined that they are effective in increasing gastric pH and do not add to gastric volumes. Rout et al. (38) studied whether it was best to use both or only one agent. They evaluated the efficacy of ranitidine and sodium citrate compared to citrate alone. Patients scheduled to undergo a non-elective cesarean delivery with general anesthesia received ranitidine or placebo at the time of the decision to operate followed by sodium citrate as they entered the operating room. The authors found that if 30 minutes had elapsed from the administration of ranitidine to induction of anesthesia, patients were at significantly less risk for aspiration, though defined by liberal criteria (pH >3.5, volume >25 mL), and only pre-extubation and not post-intubation. Lin et al. (39) compared the efficacy of H_2 receptor antagonists and proton pump inhibitors in neutralizing gastric acidity in patients undergoing an elective cesarean delivery under spinal anesthesia. They randomized 160 patients to receive orally either a placebo, famotidine 40 mg, ranitidine 300 mg, or omeprazole 40 mg at least 3 hours before surgery. They determined that omeprazole was not effective at neutralizing gastric acid and that it resulted in the largest gastric volumes. However, the H_2 antagonists, famotidine and ranitidine, were equally effective.

A recent Cochrane review evaluated current evidence of the effectiveness of prophylactic agents against acid aspiration (40). The authors reported that although the available studies were of poor quality, current evidence supports the combination of H_2 receptor antagonists and antacids as being more effective than either one alone or no prophylaxis. Proton pump inhibitors were not very effective, and the prokinetic drug, metoclopramide, did not seem useful either. Moreover, de Souza et al. (41) have argued against cricoid pressure in preventing aspiration in elective cesarean delivery. Taken together, best evidence suggests that administering some agent for aspiration prophylaxis is likely warranted, particularly in laboring patients, and that multimodal therapy is better than a single agent in raising surrogate measures of aspiration risk such as gastric pH. The best support is for the use of an H_2 antagonist 30 minutes before and a non-particulate antacid closer to the procedure. The lack of evidence for differences in outcome, however, suggests that other regimens should be considered acceptable.

Antibiotic Administration

Postpartum infection is 5 to 20 times more frequent in patients who have had cesarean delivery than in those who have had a vaginal delivery (42). Which antibiotic is the best choice and when to give it are important issues to determine before proceeding with cesarean delivery. Currently, the antibiotic of choice in the United States is a cephalosporin. How-ever, a recent Cochrane review reported that cephalosporins are equivalent to penicillins in preventing immediate post-cesarean infections (43). This was supported by evidence from 25 randomized controlled trials but the quality of the trials was reported as weak. They also noted that there were no data to support an antibiotic class that was best to prevent neonatal or late maternal infections.

Until recently, all antibiotics for a cesarean delivery were given after the cord was clamped to avoid exposing the neonate to antibiotics and thus potentially cloud signs of impending sepsis. Current national standards in the United States promote pre-incisional timing of antibiotic as an important practice to prevent postoperative infections. Tita et al. (44) reviewed the current literature examining antibiotic prophylaxis during cesarean delivery. They performed a meta-analysis of various randomized controlled trials and other meta-analyses and found that whether a narrow spectrum antibiotic such as cefazolin was given prior to surgical incision or an extended-spectrum antibiotic such as azithromycin or metronidazole was given after clamping of the umbilical cord, both approaches appeared equally effective in preventing postoperative infection by 50%. This was in contrast to the traditional practice of administering a narrower spectrum antibiotic such as cefazolin after clamping of the umbilical cord. However, they reported no evidence on the risk of infection in the neonate or infection due to resistant bacteria. Numerous other randomized trials have confirmed the advantage of pre-incision administration (45) and ACOG now recommends this timing (46). As it is less expensive to administer a cephalosporin, current recommendations are to give cefazolin 2 g before the incision. If the patient is cephalosporin-allergic, clindamycin together with gentamicin is the preferred choice regardless of any other antibiotic given earlier for another infection source.

■ NEURAXIAL TECHNIQUES FOR CESAREAN DELIVERY

Neuraxial techniques in obstetric anesthetic practice have dominated over the past several decades both on the labor floor and in the operating areas. Once the default choice for all cesarean deliveries, general anesthesia represented less than 5% of anesthetics for elective cesarean delivery in the United States in 2001 (Fig. 12-1) (2). Spinal anesthesia became the dominant choice in 2001, and although the choice of epidural anesthesia increased from 1981 to 1992, its use declined as spinal anesthesia became more popular. Not all local anesthetics are suitable for neuraxial use and only a few have been investigated for use

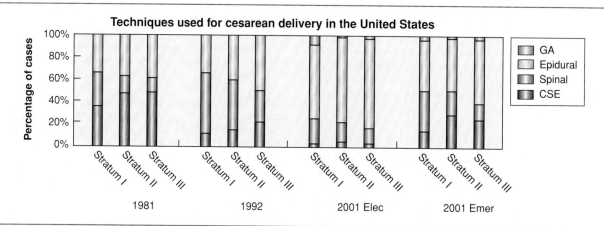

FIGURE 12-1 Rates of techniques used for cesarean delivery.

in obstetric practice. Characteristics to consider when choosing a local anesthetic include not only the onset and length of action but also the fetal exposure. In addition, which agent is a "best choice" may depend on the situation and availability within an institution. Neuraxial opioids are popularly added to local anesthetics because they have been shown to improve and prolong surgical anesthesia (47,48), and provide postoperative analgesia (49–51). Fentanyl and sufentanil are the best-studied, short-acting opioids and are most commonly used for their intraoperative effects. Morphine has little intraoperative effect but is the opioid of choice for postoperative pain management. Adjuvant agents are routinely combined with local anesthetic agents, but not all agents improve all local anesthetics, so choices and combinations vary.

This chapter will provide an overview of techniques and medications. It will focus more on issues with neuraxial techniques that are unique to the cesarean delivery situation. For a more in-depth discussion on neuraxial techniques and their contraindications, local anesthetics and postoperative pain management, see Chapters 8 and 9.

Techniques

Spinal Anesthesia

Spinal anesthesia provides a rapid onset of dense anesthesia and has an obvious endpoint of visual cerebrospinal fluid (CSF) return. It is performed as a "single-shot" technique, meaning the needle is introduced, the intrathecal space is identified by CSF return, medication is injected, and the needle is removed. Although quickly performed with a fast onset, its disadvantage is that there is no way to extend its action beyond that dictated by the pharmacologic choices made at injection. The technique is usually performed at the L3 to L4 interspace or lower to reduce the risk of damage to the spinal cord, which typically ends at L1 to L2. However, there is a small subset of the population whose cord ends one space lower. Moreover, there is evidence of substantial inaccuracy of identification of various interspaces (52), so the lowest acceptable space should generally be utilized.

The resurgence in popularity of spinal anesthesia is partly due to the technologic advances in spinal needles that reduce the incidence of post-dural-puncture headache to less than 1%. It has become the preferred anesthetic in many institutions because of the superior quality of surgical anesthesia, shorter onset time, less patient discomfort and fewer complications over epidurals (53). Spinal anesthesia is also associated with the least absorption of local anesthetic into the maternal circulation and thus least fetal exposure. It should be noted that all agents injected into the intrathecal space should be preservative free to minimize the chance of neurotoxicity.

Epidural Anesthesia

It is common practice to utilize an indwelling epidural catheter placed for labor analgesia when converting to surgical anesthesia for cesarean delivery. Epidural anesthesia for elective cesarean delivery has declined in use as spinal anesthesia is technically easier and provides a faster and more complete block. However, it can be the best choice if a slow onset and avoidance of hypotension is important to the anesthetic plan. Its best advantage over an intrathecal technique is that it can be maintained when a surgical procedure is prolonged.

To be effective for patient comfort for a cesarean, the level needs to be extended from the labor analgesic level (approximately T10) to T4. Motor block with an epidural is generally not as dense as that achieved with a spinal injection but typically adequate enough for surgical exposure. However, patients should be informed that they may be aware of surgical manipulation ("pulls and tugs") during the procedure.

Combined Spinal–Epidural Anesthesia

The combined spinal–epidural (CSE) technique has the benefits of a rapid onset with the spinal portion and option of maintenance of anesthesia through the epidural component. It is a useful technique if the anticipated surgery may be longer than the anesthetic a spinal medication can provide. The technique may be performed at two separate interspaces, one for the intrathecal injection and usually a lower space for the epidural catheter placement. Since CSE-compatible and CSE-specific needle designs are readily available, most practitioners use the needle-through-needle technique at a single interspace.

Despite the simple concept, studies show that combining these two neuraxial techniques may change the characteristics of the anesthetic. Ithnin et al. (54) conducted a study in which 30 patients received hyperbaric bupivacaine intrathecally either as part of a single-shot spinal (SSS) or a CSE in which the epidural space was located but the catheter was not placed. The maximum sensory block achieved for the SSS averaged a T3 level, but the CSE technique averaged a C6 level. Time to establish a maximum sensory block was longer with the CSE technique, but regression of the sensory block was similar as the incidences of nausea, vomiting, and hypotension. The authors postulated that with the SSS technique, the negative pressure within the epidural space was preserved. This would not be the case with the CSE approach. Lim et al. (55) postulated that laboring patients would have different epidural pressures from non-laboring parturients. The authors randomized 40 laboring patients without labor analgesia scheduled for cesarean delivery to receive either SSS or CSE. Both groups of patients received hyperbaric bupivacaine intrathecally and with the CSE group, the epidural space was located and a catheter inserted but not used to administer medications. The authors found no difference in the maximum sensory blocks between the two groups. They concluded that the theory of a pressure differential in the epidural space influencing the sensory spread of spinal anesthetics may be valid, but that in laboring patients this differential is lost and thus no dose adjustment is necessary.

Epidural Volume Extension

Epidural volume extension (EVE) is the concept that the injection of a volume of any fluid into the epidural space immediately after an intrathecal injection will influence the characteristics of the spinal. Lew et al. (56) recruited patients scheduled for an elective cesarean delivery to receive either an SSS technique or a CSE. All patients received the same intrathecal dose but the CSE group received 6 mL of saline through the epidural catheter 5 minutes later. Those with the CSE had a faster recovery from their motor block but the motor block itself was less dense. There were no differences in peak sensory level, analgesia for the procedure, time for sensory regression, or the time to first analgesic request. Tyagi et al. (57) compared three neuraxial techniques: SSS, CSE without epidural use, and CSE with EVE. All patients were undergoing elective cesarean delivery and had the same intrathecal dose. Those in the CSE with EVE group were the only ones to have an epidural catheter placed and received 5 mL of normal saline through the catheter over 15 seconds as soon as it was placed. Those in the SSS group had a more rapid onset to maximal sensory and motor blocks. Other studied parameters such as the extent and duration of sensory and motor blocks and the incidence of adverse effects were similar across all groups. The clinical utility of the technique was questioned by Kucukguclu et al. (58), who randomized patients undergoing elective cesarean delivery to spinal bupivacaine, either hyper- or isobaric, and EVE or no epidural saline. They found no difference in the sensory or motor blocks from EVE with either spinal solution.

Sequential CSE

Sequential CSE is a variant on the traditional approach where the intrathecal injection is intentionally low so that the block height will have to be extended with injection through the epidural catheter. Its reported advantage is that it produces a more hemodynamically stable induction period. It has been successfully used in patients with significant cardiac disease where stability is crucial (59).

Drugs and Doses

Local Anesthetics

The local anesthetics that can be used for intrathecal injection are not necessarily the same that can be used for epidural injection. Any medication that will be injected into the spinal space should be preservative free to avoid neurotoxicity or adhesive arachnoiditis. Many epidural preparations contain preservatives to prolong shelf life. The concentration of a local anesthetic is not always the same between techniques as well. The classic example is bupivacaine where the 0.75% preparation is routinely used for intrathecal injection but not for epidural injection. Use of 0.75% bupivacaine for epidural use was disapproved by the FDA after documented maternal cardiac arrests were caused by unintentional intravenous injection of this very cardiotoxic medication. Doses are also very different as epidural administration requires much larger medication amounts because of anatomy, pharmacokinetics, and pharmacodynamics.

The most commonly used local anesthetics for intrathecal injection for cesarean purposes are noted in Table 12-4. Ropivacaine is not approved for intrathecal use in the United States but can be used for epidural administration, and has been used off-label for spinal anesthesia. Lidocaine and mepivacaine have also been used successfully but their shorter duration of action requires confidence that the surgical procedure will be brief. Lidocaine has recently fallen out of favor in many institutions because of concerns that it causes a transient neurologic syndrome at an unacceptably high rate, although others have argued that pregnancy is relatively protective (60). Of all the agents, bupivacaine is most widely used and studies support the choice of bupivacaine because it consistently produces adequate spinal anesthesia of longer duration and better motor block than either ropivacaine or levobupivacaine (61).

Local anesthetics used for epidural anesthesia for cesarean delivery are noted in Table 12-5. These agents vary in their speed of onset and their duration of action, and when epidural administration is the only technique; speed of onset usually defines the preferred local anesthetic. Chloroprocaine provides a faster onset time compared to lidocaine but the onset (as well as depth of the block) of the latter can be improved with the addition of bicarbonate (62). However, due to the rapid metabolism and short duration of action of

TABLE 12-5 Agents for Epidural Dosing

	Concentration	Dose[b]
Bupivacaine	0.25%–0.5%	50–100 mg
Levobupivacaine	0.5%	75–150 mg
Ropivacaine	0.5%–0.75%	100–150 mg
Chloroprocaine	2%–3%	600–800 mg
Lidocaine	1.5%–2%	300–400 mg
Mepivacaine	1%–2%	300–400 mg
Fentanyl	N/A	50–100 mcg
Sufentanil	N/A	5 mcg
Morphine	N/A	3–5 mg

[a]Doses presume no previous labor epidural anesthetic or an intrathecal injection given.
[b]Upper amount reported is the maximum dose.
N/A, data not available.

chloroprocaine, repeated dosing may be necessary during the cesarean delivery. Also, chloroprocaine administration is associated with decreased responsiveness to amide local anesthetics and opioids, which can have a negative impact on intraoperative neuraxial opioid effectiveness and potentially postoperatively as well (see Chapter 8). Mepivacaine is similar to lidocaine in its characteristics and epidural mepivacaine has been compared to 2-chloroprocaine (63). There was no significant difference in onset or duration of anesthesia, hypotension, Apgar, or neurobehavioral scores. However, there was a significantly shorter induction to delivery interval in the patients who received chloroprocaine.

Bupivacaine and levobupivacaine are significantly slower in onset than lidocaine but have a longer duration of action. However, racemic bupivacaine also has greater potential for cardiotoxicity than other agents and the risk of inadvertent intravascular injection resulting in cardiotoxicity may dissuade some from choosing these agents. The anesthetic characteristics of bupivacaine and levobupivacaine are similar (64). Ropivacaine is a relatively newer local anesthetic, similar in onset and duration to bupivacaine and levobupivacaine, and reportedly less cardiotoxic than the other agents. Ropivacaine has been compared to bupivacaine for cesarean delivery and was not found to be superior to bupivacaine with respect to block quality, hypotension, nausea, or neonatal condition (65).

Neuraxial Opioids

Fentanyl and sufentanil are fast-onset, shorter-acting opioids that have been shown to be a useful addition to local anesthetics for their intraoperative effects. Studies show that they can decrease local anesthetic needs (66,67), improve intraoperative anesthesia, and prolong duration of action (47,48,68,69). The optimal intrathecal dose of either opioid is hard to define as studies have shown more patient discomfort with lower doses but a greater incidence of side effects with higher doses (47,68). Thus, there is a range of suggested doses as noted in Tables 12-4 and 12-5. Neither of these opioids impact postoperative pain relief because of their short action, so morphine is commonly administered in addition to either of the other two. Morphine has little impact on intraoperative anesthesia because it has such a prolonged onset but it provides significant postoperative analgesia (49) and is the agent of choice. At doses of 100 to 200 mcg, it can provide about 18 hours of effective pain relief (50,51).

Neuraxial opioids have well-known side effects of which most are more annoying than life-threatening. These side

TABLE 12-4 Agents for Intrathecal Dosing

	Concentration	Dose
Bupivacaine	0.5%–0.75%	7.5–15 mg
Levobupivacaine	0.5%	7.5–15 mg
Lidocaine	2%–5%	75 mg
Fentanyl	N/A	10–20 mcg
Sufentanil	N/A	1.25–2.5 mcg
Morphine	N/A	100–200 mcg

N/A, data not available.

effects are pruritus, nausea, vomiting, delayed gastric empty-ing, urinary retention, sedation, and respiratory depression. All three opioids can produce significant pruritus. Nausea and vomiting are less common, although very distressing when present and urinary retention is clinically irrelevant as cesarean delivery patients typically have urinary catheters in place for the first 24 hours. Although sedation by short-acting opioids is a concern, under the typical monitoring conditions during cesarean delivery, such effects can be easily detected and treated. The concern and focus of many studies has always been on the potentially life-threatening, delayed respiratory depressive effects of morphine. For a more com-plete discussion, see Chapter 13. However, within the doses of 100 to 200 mcg that are recommended, depression is exceedingly rare (47,49,50).

Other Added Agents

Adjuvant agents are those added to local anesthetics to influ-ence their characteristics, most typically to speed onset or prolong action. The most commonly added agents other than opioids are epinephrine and sodium bicarbonate. Epi-nephrine is frequently added to intrathecal injections to make the block denser and to prolong its duration. This is accom-plished in two ways: A set amount of epinephrine is drawn into the syringe (5 to 15 mcg) or an "epi wash" is performed where an ampule of epinephrine is drawn into a syringe and then removed. This action is thought to coat the insides of the syringe with epinephrine. The syringe is then filled with the chosen local anesthetic. This provides an indetermi-nate amount of epinephrine which is thought to be enough to extend the local anesthetic's duration. Epinephrine is also used as a means of determining if an epidural injection is intravascular. It is added to a local anesthetic as a 1:200,000 dilution, which delivers 15 mcg with a 3 mL injection. This is enough to raise the heart rate if the 3mL test injection is intravascular, although the pain of labor may not make this a reliable test (see Chapter 9). A similar concentration given in a spinal injection can reportedly increase the density of the block and significantly increase its duration of action. Another reason to add epinephrine is to reduce absorption of the local anesthetic. However, one study showed that adding epineph-rine in varying concentrations of 1:200,000 to 1:400,000 to an epidural dose decreased the amount of lidocaine required for the cesarean but did not reduce maternal plasma levels when compared against injections without the epinephrine (70).

Sodium bicarbonate is added to local anesthetics for epidural injection to speed the onset of action. It is not added to intra-thecal injections. Adding 8.4% bicarbonate raises the pH of the local anesthetic closer to physiologic pH and thus increases the speed of action (see Chapter 8). Adding it to bupivacaine is problematic as the bupivacaine rapidly precipitates with small doses of bicarbonate, which negatively impacts the quality of the block. However, bicarbonate added to lidocaine reduces the onset time from about 10 minutes to 5 minutes (71). Alka-linization of chloroprocaine can also accelerate its onset time (72), but as it already has a fast onset, the addition of bicar-bonate may not hasten onset in a clinically significant manner. Bicarbonate also likely potentiates local anesthetic action via mechanisms distinct from its alkalinizing effect (73).

■ NON-ELECTIVE CESAREAN DELIVERY MANAGEMENT

Urgent and Emergent Cesarean Delivery

When a non-elective cesarean delivery is indicated, surgical anesthesia must be obtained in a manner that expedites the safe delivery of the fetus without compromising the mother.

The American College of Obstetricians and Gynecologists (ACOG) and the American Society of Anesthesiologists (ASA) issued a joint statement that the time from the request for an urgent cesarean delivery to incision should be no lon-ger than 30 minutes. There is significant controversy, how-ever, regarding both the feasibility of this standard (74–76) and the neonatal effects of this guideline, and several stud-ies have failed to find good correlation between decision to delivery interval of less than 30 minutes and neonatal condi-tion (77,78). Communication between the patient's provid-ers is crucial as not all non-elective cesareans are the same. Needing a cesarean for an arrested first stage does not follow as tight of a time restriction as a prolapsed cord, but it should not be unnecessarily delayed either. Neither the patient nor the fetus should be placed at any unnecessary risk as prepara-tions are made for the surgery. If a functioning labor epidural is in place, bicarbonate is often added to a rapidly acting local anesthetic to further shorten the time of onset. Depending on which local anesthetic is chosen, a short-acting opioid may be added to improve the quality of the block.

A spinal anesthetic can be attempted in an emergent situ-ation but the patient should be hemodynamically stable and the spinal must be placed expeditiously or the plan changed to a general anesthetic. Retrospective (77,79) and simula-tion (80) studies suggest that general anesthesia is marginally faster at achieving surgical anesthesia than spinal anesthesia.

Epidural Anesthesia in the Setting of a Compromised Fetal Status

A non-reassuring fetal heart rate pattern may imply compro-mised uteroplacental perfusion and fetal acidosis (see Chap-ter 5). Use of a rapidly acting local anesthetic is required for expeditious conversion of a labor epidural to a surgical anes-thetic. With the understanding that local anesthetics cross the placenta, the question becomes which is the best choice without further compromising the fetus. Chloroprocaine has traditionally been the local anesthetic of choice because it will not accumulate in an acidotic fetus as lidocaine might, but it may also compromise the effectiveness of opioids (Chapter 8). Gaiser et al. (81) studied the effects of epidural administra-tion of 3% chloroprocaine compared to 1.5% lidocaine with bicarbonate and 1:200,000 epinephrine in cesarean delivery of the distressed fetus. They reported similar Apgar scores and umbilical cord pH between the two groups indicating a lack of fetal compromise. The same group evaluated the effects of alkalinized 3% chloroprocaine and 1.5% lidocaine with epi-nephrine on neonatal outcome. A surgical level was achieved in 3.1 and 4.4 minutes with chloroprocaine and lidocaine respectively, and again there were no differences in neonatal Apgar score or umbilical cord pH between the two groups (82). These results suggest that lidocaine with bicarbonate is clini-cally as rapid and effective as chloroprocaine in situations of cesarean delivery for non-reassuring fetal heart rate patterns.

■ NEURAXIAL ANESTHESIA FOR HIGH RISK PATIENTS

Traditionally certain patients have been thought not to be candidates for regional anesthesia. In recent years, however, these previous contraindications have been questioned, and many such patients can be safely managed with epidural or spinal anesthesia. This population would include those with severe preeclampsia or medical conditions such as multiple sclerosis or cardiac disease.

Hood et al. (83) reported on a series of patients diagnosed with severe preeclampsia who received neuraxial anesthesia for cesarean delivery. Approximately one quarter had an epidural anesthetic and the remainder received a spinal. Although epidural use in this population was already considered appropriate, spinal anesthesia was avoided because of concerns that the sympathectomy would create a dangerous hemodynamic situation. These authors found that the blood pressure changes were similar with both anesthetics as were the Apgar scores demonstrating that either form of neuraxial anesthetic could be used safely in patients with severe preeclampsia provided there is normal platelet function present to initiate the block. Similarly, Wallace et al. (84) randomly assigned 80 women with severe preeclampsia to receive epidural, spinal, or general anesthesia for cesarean delivery. They found equivalent maternal and fetal outcomes in all three groups. For a more extensive discussion of anesthetic considerations in preeclampsia, see Chapter 27.

Bader et al. (85) published a retrospective review where they reported the outcomes of parturients with multiple sclerosis who received either an epidural or general anesthetic for cesarean delivery. They reported no difference in the relapse rate among parturients for either anesthetic. Drake et al. (86) sent a questionnaire to anesthesiologists in the United Kingdom to gauge their willingness to perform neuraxial anesthesia on patients with multiple sclerosis. Most reported being comfortable but their experience with such cases was limited. For a more extensive discussion of the anesthetic implications of multiple sclerosis and other neurologic conditions, see Chapters 31 and 32.

The number of women presenting to an obstetrician with a cardiac condition has exploded. Given the older ages of women starting a family, some may have a preexisting state such as hypertension, coronary, or valvular disease. Many more are now presenting with a history of a congenital condition for which they have had corrective or palliative surgery. Most such patients are now managed successfully with regional anesthesia, though perhaps with greater use of invasive hemodynamic monitoring (87). For a more extensive discussion of the anesthetic implications of cardiac disease, see Chapter 29.

■ SIDE EFFECTS, COMPLICATIONS, AND MANAGEMENT

Side effects, complications, and management will be discussed here as they pertain to neuraxial techniques for cesarean delivery. More detailed discussion can be found in Chapters 8 and 9.

Hypotension is the most common side effect of spinal anesthesia because of the profound sympathectomy produced. It can be seen with extension of a labor epidural for a cesarean delivery but typically is not as dramatic as a partial sympathectomy is already in place. This hypotension can be clinically significant and produce maternal side effects such as nausea and vomiting. If not treated, it can lead to fetal acidosis because of diminished uteroplacental flow. Studies attempting to identify patients who might be most at risk for severe hypotension have not succeeded in making that determination (87,88).

Prophylaxis and treatment of hypotension is a combination of proper patient positioning, fluids and vasopressor support. All patients of 20 weeks or more gestation should have a left lateral tilt because aortocaval compression can occur this early in the pregnancy leading to compromised uteroplacental flow. Fluid administration has classically been considered the first line treatment for prevention and treatment of hypotension. Crystalloid preloads with 500 to 1,000 mL are traditional. Numerous studies, however, have disputed the usefulness of this common technique. Rout et al. (89) first questioned fluid loading and found only minimal benefit

of 20 mL/kg crystalloid preloading compared to no preload, and no differences in neonatal outcome. Meta-analysis of 75 trials of over 4,600 women (90) found slightly decreased incidence of hypotension with crystalloid preloading (RR 0.78, 95% CI 0.60 to 1.0). Colloid solutions were somewhat more effective. No effects of various doses, timing regimens, or rates of administration were found. It is likely that some women may benefit from fluid loading more than others, for example, those with volume deficits or those with particularly high resting sympathetic tone or greater decreases after initiating spinal anesthesia. A more recent variation in technique is co-loading, the administration of fluid immediately coincident with the onset of spinal anesthesia, and early studies suggested superiority to preloading (35). Meta-analysis of five randomized trials enrolling over 500 subjects, however, found no benefit (91).

For years, ephedrine was believed to be the only appropriate vasopressor for use with maternal hypotension. This practice was based on sheep studies showing that of the available vasopressors, only ephedrine improved maternal hypotension without diminishing uteroplacental blood flow. However, animal studies do not always translate well to humans and the use of ephedrine was noted to result in maternal tachycardia and rebound hypertension. Newer studies have called into question which is the better vasopressor agent when treating maternal hypotension. Lee et al. (92) performed a meta-analysis of randomized controlled trials comparing the efficacy and safety of ephedrine and phenylephrine both as prophylactic and management medications for hypotension following spinal anesthesia for cesarean delivery. They found that ephedrine was similar to phenylephrine for the purposes of prophylaxis and treatment of hypotension. They also noted that maternal bradycardia was more common with phenylephrine and that the umbilical arterial pH was 0.03 lower in the patients who received ephedrine. However, neither agent was associated with a true fetal acidosis nor was there any difference in Apgar scores. Ngan Kee et al. (93) analyzed the effect of varying infusion rates of crystalloid fluids in patients with spinal anesthesia in which a background infusion of a phenylephrine at 100 mcg/min was in place and titrated to maintain systolic blood pressure near normal values until the uterus was incised. Patients were randomized to receive a rapid infusion of crystalloid up to 2 L until uterine incision or a baseline maintenance infusion. Patients, who received the rapid infusion of crystalloid required less phenylephrine, had higher systolic blood pressures and normal heart rates. Lee et al. (94) in another study examined the efficacy of prophylactic ephedrine in preventing hypotension during cesarean delivery under spinal anesthesia. They evaluated five studies and concluded that prophylactic ephedrine was ineffective in preventing hypotension.

The Cochrane database review (90) evaluated the available randomized studies that examined prophylactic interventions to prevent hypotension after spinal anesthesia for cesarean delivery. In addition to the results noted above on fluid administration, ephedrine was more effective than no vasopressor or crystalloid alone, as was phenylephrine, and mechanical devices such as lower limb compressors were better than no intervention but not to a large degree. Ephedrine and phenylephrine were equivocal in their efficacy at preventing hypotension. Most notably, no intervention was able to prevent the hypotension experienced during spinal anesthesia for cesarean delivery. Two other more recent reviews concluded that phenylephrine, particularly when given as a prophylactic infusion, was the preferred technique for prevention of hypotension (95,96). For additional discussion of prevention and treatment of hypotension, see Chapter 9.

Conversion of a Neuraxial Block to General Anesthetic for Cesarean Delivery

On occasion, a neuraxial anesthetic either is not extended or proves inadequate for surgery. This might be apparent before the case starts or during the course of the operation. Halpern et al. (97) studied the proportion of unsuccessful labor epidural analgesia conversions to surgical anesthetics for nonelective cesarean delivery in an academic hospital. The overall rate of conversion to general anesthesia was 4.1%. The most common reasons for conversion were insufficient anesthesia intraoperatively (71%), insufficient time to administer the local anesthetics through the epidural catheter (14%), and maternal request (10%). One-third of patients with insufficient epidural anesthesia had a repeat neuraxial procedure for the surgery. Of these 66% received a single-shot spinal, 22% received a CSE, and 12% received a repeat epidural. The authors noted an association between the number of top-ups during labor and failure of the epidural to convert for surgery.

The UK Royal College of Anesthetists published guidelines recommending a less than 3% conversion rate to general anesthesia but some institutions find this an unrealistic number, noting the conversion rate varies considerably between reports. Rafi et al. (98) performed a retrospective audit of conversion rates to general anesthesia at an academic institution. They reported that for elective cesarean deliveries, there were almost no conversions to general anesthesia. However, for urgent-emergent cesarean deliveries, conversion was 5.4%. These occurred primarily in category 1 cesarean deliveries in which there is an urgent threat to the life of the mother or the fetus. This was the only category that did not demonstrate a reduction in conversion rates over the 4 years of the audit despite the 3% guideline. Another retrospective study of neuraxial anesthesia failure accounted for 16% of cesarean delivery cases requiring general anesthesia. These failures accounted for 4% of all neuraxial techniques performed. These failures were also the highest in an emergency situation where surgical anesthesia was attempted through conversion of the labor epidural (99). Similarly, Campbell and Tran (100) found 12.4% of labor epidurals failed to convert to surgical anesthesia, but >80% of the remainder were rescued by manipulation of the catheter and only 1.2% to 5.6% required conversion to general anesthesia, depending on the experience of the practitioner.

High Spinal Following Epidural Analgesia

Conversion of a failed epidural to a spinal can also be hazardous. There have been many case reports of a high spinal level following such a conversion. The question is how large an intrathecal dose should be given in the face of a partial epidural block. Furst et al. (101) performed a retrospective audit of the incidence of high spinal anesthesia following conversion of an inadequate epidural to a spinal anesthetic. They analyzed almost 1,400 deliveries over a 2-year period. Of those epidurals that failed, 84% received a single-shot spinal at the institution's usual dose and the remainder received general anesthesia. There was an 11% incidence of high spinal anesthesia following a single-shot spinal. Another report (102) found no occurrences of high spinal among patients who received a single-shot spinal following an unsuccessful attempt at extending a labor epidural. However, the authors' usual practice was to replace an epidural with a single-shot spinal whenever a cesarean delivery was called for and time allowed, rather than attempting to extend the epidural. Thus, they evaluated the placement of a spinal anesthetic in the absence of a large bolus of local anesthetic in the epidural space (102).

Inadequate labor analgesia conversion to surgical anesthesia has a varying incidence between institutions and practitioners. Whether failure to convert results in a high spinal or an inadequate block, conversion to a general anesthetic is more likely to occur during an emergency. A full complement of equipment and agents should always be ready to allow for the provision of a general anesthetic in a safe and expeditious manner.

■ GENERAL ANESTHESIA FOR CESAREAN DELIVERY

General anesthesia was the primary technique used for cesarean delivery until the literature showed epidural anesthesia for labor could be rapidly extended for surgery, neuraxial opioids could provide excellent postoperative relief and were safe (50,51), and the reduction in maternal risk by avoiding airway mishap was demonstrated in closed claims analyses (103). Nevertheless, there are times when general anesthesia may be the only indicated choice, for example, when neuraxial anesthesia is contraindicated or fails; on maternal request; or when an emergency requires such rapid responses that induction of a neuraxial technique would prolong the time to delivery. Thus, it is important to understand how various anesthetic agents might impact the mother or neonate and what the risks may be. Airway management will not be covered here but is discussed in Chapter 23.

Sedative/Hypnotics

The ideal induction agent should provide a rapid and smooth intravenous induction, maintain hemodynamic stability, and have minimal adverse effects on uterine tone or the fetus. Such an agent does not yet exist. Studies have focused on delineating and comparing the positive and negative attributes of available medications. Those that are currently used for induction are thiopental, propofol, ketamine, and etomidate. Midazolam has been used as an induction agent in the past.

Until recently, thiopental was the traditional intravenous agent used for induction. It was preferred because it worked quickly, provided hemodynamic stability, and although it definitely crossed the placenta, it did not produce neonatal depression at the normal induction doses of 4 mg/kg. Compared to ketamine, its use resulted in better Apgar scores and acid–base profiles in the neonate (104). Compared to etomidate, which produced more stable maternal hemodynamics, it crossed the placenta to suppress cortisol production in the neonate (105). Recently, thiopental has become increasingly scarce as production in the United States has been halted, and at present there are no signs that production will resume in the near future, which may cause thiopental to become of historical interest only.

Ketamine is a popular choice for induction when there is asthma present or cardiovascular instability due to hypovolemia. It has vasopressor effects that can support blood pressure in a hemorrhaging patient but it should not be used in patients with a hypertensive disorder. Despite its pressor effects, it has not been shown to decrease uterine blood flow in animal models (106). However, ketamine given early in pregnancy has been shown to increase uterine tone. This effect disappears in late pregnancy (107). Ketamine crosses the placenta but at induction doses of 1 mg/kg does not produce neonatal depression. However, it is known to cause unpleasant dreams in the mothers (108).

Propofol has become the most commonly used induction agent when maternal conditions do not require a less cardiodepressive medication. Even in those situations, it may be used in lower doses and combined with another medication such as an opioid. Propofol has a similar profile to thiopental and appears to be a suitable replacement should thiopental disappear all together. Placental transfer appears to be similar to thiopental at normal induction doses of 2 to 3 mg/kg, and as with thiopental, the minimal effect seen on the neonate is presumed due to rapid redistribution in the mother and metabolism of the drug by the fetal liver.

Opioids

Concerns about the use of opioids during general anesthesia revolve around the potential effects these drugs might have on the fetus as they cross the placenta. Opioid use in the general population is commonly employed during induction to obtund the neuroendocrine stress response and stabilize hemodynamics. Short-acting opioids may allow for titration to maternal hemodynamic responses with shorter-lived effects in the neonate. Fentanyl unquestionably crosses the placenta but how quickly this occurs and whether it precludes its use for a cesarean delivery is not as clear. Eisele et al. (109) measured fentanyl plasma levels in the umbilical vein and non-intravenous maternal vein at delivery after administering 1 mcg/kg fentanyl upon induction of general anesthesia or under neuraxial anesthesia for elective cesarean deliveries. All deliveries occurred within 10 minutes of administration, and umbilical vein concentrations never achieved analgesic levels despite the high lipophilicity of fentanyl. Apgar and neurobehavioral scores were normal. The results suggested that the high protein binding properties of fentanyl reduced the amount of drug crossing the placenta, possibly limiting fetal exposure if given shortly before delivery.

Remifentanil is an ultra-short–acting opioid that has gained wide popularity in non-obstetric anesthesia. Because it can be titrated to a patient's hemodynamic needs and stress responses, it appears to be a desirable choice for induction of general anesthesia in the parturient with the assumption that its rapid action would have minimal effect on the fetus. Draisci et al. (110) studied 42 parturients undergoing a general anesthetic who were randomized to receive either fentanyl or remifentanil. Patients receiving fentanyl were not given the drug until after delivery of the neonate but those receiving remifentanil received a bolus for induction followed by an infusion until peritoneal incision. The infusion was restarted after delivery of the neonate. Maternal stress responses to surgery were greater in patients who received fentanyl after delivery. However, of those mothers who received remifentanil, three neonates required intubation for apnea for a very short period and overall Apgar scores were lower than in the fentanyl group. Orme et al. (111) considered whether remifentanil might be the opioid of choice in critical situations where maternal hemodynamics take a priority over fetal concerns. They presented a series of four patients with critical aortic stenosis who required cesarean delivery under general anesthesia. Remifentanil was used for induction and an infusion was maintained. They reported that this anesthetic regimen provided the hemodynamic stability they sought while having little neonatal effect. These two studies would suggest that remifentanil is an acceptable opioid choice should maternal hemodynamic stability take precedence, but there must be neonatal resuscitative equipment and personnel readily available for temporary neonatal support.

Neuromuscular Blocking Drugs

Because of concerns of aspiration in obstetric patients, intubating conditions for general anesthesia have generally been achieved with a rapidly acting agent to speed the time from induction to intubation (see Chapter 24). Those conditions are most often achieved with succinylcholine. Although plasma cholinesterase levels are decreased in pregnancy, the duration of action of a single injection of succinylcholine does not demonstrate clinically significant prolongation.

Non-depolarizing neuromuscular blocking drugs are often used for maintenance relaxation after intubation. They have been compared against each other for length of duration and placental transfer. Vecuronium was compared to pancuronium, and vecuronium had the more favorable profile (112). It had a relatively short duration of action with a half-life of 36 minutes and very little drug transfer across the placenta. Rocuronium is another non-depolarizing agent touted to provide intubating conditions as rapidly as succinylcholine. Magorian et al. (113) compared the effects of rocuronium, vecuronium, and suxamethonium for time to and adequacy of intubating conditions in 50 patients. They found that rocuronium at doses of 0.9 mg/kg and 1.2 mg/kg provided intubating conditions similar to suxamethonium. However, the duration of rocuronium was longer, particularly at 1.2 mg/kg. This would suggest that rocuronium is a suitable alternative to succinylcholine when the latter drug is contraindicated. However, one must be confident of being able to secure the airway in view of its prolonged action.

Volatile Anesthetics
Minimal Alveolar Concentration

The minimum alveolar concentration (MAC) of volatile anesthetics in parturients appears to be reduced. The reasons may be multifactorial. Early animal studies demonstrated reduced MAC requirements but did not elucidate why. Datta et al. examined the question of whether rising progesterone levels might be involved, noting that progesterone levels increase in pregnancy (113). They simulated this increase by administering progesterone to ovariectomized rabbits and compared the MAC requirements to non-ovariectomized and ovariectomized rabbits without progesterone injections. They found an association between increased progesterone levels and decreased halothane requirements, and suggested that there might be an inverse linear association between progesterone levels and MAC requirements. In humans, Gin et al. (114) compared MAC requirements for isoflurane of women in early pregnancy undergoing termination to similar but nonpregnant women. All patients underwent an inhalational induction and maintenance with isoflurane. They determined that the MAC of isoflurane was decreased by 28% at 8 to 12 weeks gestation but in their discussion suggested there was not a linear association as proposed by Datta. They suggested that, based on the results of studies published at the time, there may possibly be a threshold value of progesterone associated with decreased MAC requirements. These same authors showed a reduction of 27% and 30% in the MAC of parturients for halothane and enflurane, respectively (115). Thus it appears that maternal anesthetic requirements in early pregnancy are reduced for multiple volatile agents.

MAC appears to return to normal relatively quickly after delivery. Gin et al. evaluated the MAC requirements for isoflurane in parturients having a postpartum tubal ligation (116). They found that MAC remained reduced until 24 to 36 hours postpartum and then increased to normal levels by 72 hours.

Effects on Uterine Tone

Volatile anesthetics negatively impact uterine muscle contraction. Munson demonstrated that with human myometrial fibers exposed to as little as 0.5 MAC of enflurane, isoflurane, or halothane, contractions were reduced from baseline and further reduced in a dose-dependent manner (117). Early studies also showed that this effect could not be reversed with oxytocin, posing an increased risk for postpartum hemorrhage. Dogru et al. (118) studied the effects of the newer volatiles, desflurane and sevoflurane on oxytocin-stimulated myometrial contractions in a rat model. At 2 MAC of desflurane and sevoflurane, the duration, amplitude, and frequency of uterine contractions were nearly abolished despite the presence of oxytocin. This study was replicated using isolated human myometrial fibers stimulated by oxytocin and exposed to varying concentrations of desflurane and sevoflurane. Upon exposure to 0.5, 1, and 2 MAC of desflurane and sevoflurane, the frequency and amplitude of contractions decreased. However, desflurane inhibited the oxytocin-induced contractions less than sevoflurane at 1 MAC (119). Thus, it appears that despite the reduced MAC requirements of the parturient, exposure to volatile anesthetic levels as low as 0.5 MAC can negatively impact uterine contractions even in the presence of oxytocin.

Awareness and the Obstetric Population

General anesthesia for cesarean delivery is thought to be associated with a higher incidence of intraoperative awareness than seen in the general surgical population. There are many reasons proposed for this including a high maternal cardiac output that rapidly redistributes intravenous induction agents and delays end-organ effects, and administration of lower MAC multiples to minimize uterine relaxation, or concerns of effects on the fetus by anesthetic agents. The manner of induction of a general anesthetic in the obstetric population is designed to avoid fetal effect. It is common to wait until the patient is prepped and draped before inducing, using a typical rapid sequence technique. During the prep and drape, the patient is preoxygenated and then anesthesia is induced when the surgical team is completely prepared to begin. The skin incision usually follows immediately after intubation, about a minute after the induction medications are given. King et al. (120) studied how this induction style might contribute to awareness. They designed a complex study whereby patients newly induced could respond via a tourniquet-isolated forearm by flexing fingers in response to taped instructions by earphones every minute up to 10 minutes after induction. They interviewed patients afterward for signs of recall. During the procedure, 96% indicated awareness at skin incision, 76% 1 minute later, 20% 2 minutes later and 6.7% 3 minutes later. There were no indications of awareness after 3 minutes, and upon the postoperative interview, no patient *recalled* being aware. Unfortunately, this study was not sufficiently powered to determine the incidence of awareness or recall in clinical situations. Paech et al. (121) reported a multicenter, prospective, observational study of awareness in patients undergoing general anesthesia for both elective and urgent cesarean delivery. Inductions were with thiopental or propofol, sometimes supplemented with opioid or midazolam, and the maintenance volatile anesthetic was sevoflurane. A bispectral index (BIS) monitor was used in 32% of the cases. There were two cases positively identified of awareness for an incidence of 0.26% and three more cases deemed possible for awareness.

BIS has been suggested for monitoring the level of consciousness. Readings less than 60 are thought to reduce the potential for awareness during general anesthesia, though outcome studies have produced conflicting results (122). Although there is some literature on the use of BIS in the obstetric population, the purpose of the studies has been to determine that current practice is not associated with high BIS values (123) or to compare MAC levels against BIS numbers (124). Much more needs to be done to determine the usefulness of the BIS monitor in obstetric practice.

General Anesthesia and Maternal Mortality

Maternal mortality is covered in more depth elsewhere (see Chapter 46) but it should be noted that general anesthesia for cesarean delivery is associated with greater mortality compared to neuraxial anesthesia. This was first suggested by the triennial reports from the United Kingdom, the Confidential Enquiries into Maternal Deaths. These serial reports showed a significant decline in anesthesia-related deaths, which were primarily due to airway mishaps, as more neuraxial and less general anesthesia were provided.

More recently, Hawkins et al. (125) published a follow-up observational study to their 1997 article of deaths due to obstetric anesthesia in the United States. The more recent study compared the periods 1979 to 1990 to 1991 to 2002. They noted that although the overall rate of anesthesia-related deaths decreased by 59%, 86% of those deaths occurred during cesarean delivery. Deaths under general anesthesia have decreased during the 1991 to 2002 time frame and still occur primarily during induction or with airway management. Deaths under neuraxial anesthesia for cesarean delivery have also increased, unfortunately. The authors suggested that some of these deaths were due to unrecognized intrathecal catheters or the inability to treat emergencies because of a lack of readily available equipment.

■ MATERNAL OXYGEN ADMINISTRATION AND FETAL OUTCOMES

It has been traditional in many institutions to administer oxygen to the mother during a cesarean delivery even though the literature has never established that this is a safe practice or improves outcomes. Some of the earliest literature suggested that high concentrations delivered to the mother while under general anesthesia either did not increase fetal PO_2 or reached a plateau (126,127). Yet other studies with women receiving oxygen and with an epidural anesthetic showed an improved fetal acid–base balance (128,129). The discrepancy in findings was attributed to technique. Newer studies have re-examined this issue and now suggest that high oxygen concentrations administered to the parturient during cesarean delivery may have deleterious effects on the fetus.

It has long been established that high FiO_2 administration to the preterm neonate results in a number of serious medical conditions. The pediatric literature has now established that high FiO_2 concentrations delivered for resuscitation to a term neonate can also be deleterious, and the 6th edition of the Neonatal Resuscitation Program (NRP) now teaches that resuscitations should be started on room air or a low FiO_2 (130). But is there harm to the fetus if the mother is given supplemental oxygen just prior to delivery?

Khaw and colleagues (131) have performed the bulk of the work examining this question. In one of the earliest studies, they compared the effects of room air against supplemental oxygen given to the mother on maternal and fetal oxygenation and free radical formation. All mothers underwent an elective cesarean delivery by neuraxial technique and those randomized to supplemental oxygen received an FiO_2 of 60% by face mask. Although fetal oxygen levels were modestly elevated in the supplemental oxygen group, free radical activity was increased in both the mothers and fetuses. Cogliano et al. (132) also examined whether supplemental oxygen was of benefit to fetuses under an elective cesarean situation. They randomized mothers to receive 40% oxygen by face mask, room air (by face mask), or 2 L/min oxygen by nasal cannula. They measured the umbilical arterial and venous pH, and oxygen concentrations. They found that supplemental oxygen did not alter pH values or umbilical arterial or improve fetal oxygenation. Backe et al. (133) evaluated the effect of supplemental maternal oxygen on neonatal outcome. They randomized 60 women undergoing elective cesarean delivery to receive either 21% to 25% or 40% to 60% oxygen by face mask during cesarean delivery. They measured the neonatal neurologic adaptive capacity scores between the two groups and found no significant difference. Khaw et al. (134) also studied whether maternal supplemental oxygen improved fetal oxygenation in cases of prolonged uterine incision to delivery times under conditions of an elective cesarean. They defined a prolonged time as any time over 180 seconds. They determined that even under these conditions fetal oxygenation was not increased.

The obvious next question is whether the use of supplemental maternal oxygen is of benefit under conditions of an emergency cesarean delivery. The group from Hong Kong, once again, published a study looking at just this question (135). Under conditions of an emergency cesarean that did not require a general anesthetic, Khaw et al. randomized patients to receive 60% supplemental oxygen by face mask or room air. They measured length of oxygen administration to delivery, umbilical arterial and venous blood gases and oxygen content, and by-products of free radical activity. They also noted whether fetal compromise was present. They found that those fetuses whose mothers received supplemental oxygen had higher UA and UV PO_2 values and O_2 content. pH values were similar between the groups and there were no measurable signs of free radical activity. However, they attributed that finding to the shorter time from incision to delivery that occurs in an emergency situation compared to an elective procedure. These findings held whether or not fetal compromise was present, and no neonate required extensive resuscitation such as chest compressions or intubation. Apgar scores were similar between the groups. Thus they concluded that under emergency conditions where a neuraxial technique can be used, supplemental oxygen delivery to the mother may benefit the fetus, whether or not fetal compromise is present.

Thus, supplemental maternal oxygenation may increase fetal oxygenation but may be associated with concomitant harmful effects on the fetus if administered beyond an undetermined amount of time. Under elective conditions there does not appear to be a benefit to the fetus, but under emergency conditions there is some improvement in fetal oxygen content but no other measured impact. In addition, there is little evidence of neonatal benefits in the early postpartum period.

■ OXYTOCIN ADMINISTRATION

Oxytocin is a nonapeptide that is similar in structure to vasopressin and secreted from the posterior pituitary. It is the first polypeptide hormone ever synthesized and is best known for its actions in vivo in women of uterine smooth muscle contraction and lactation. Oxytocin receptors are most numerous in the uterus and increase exponentially during pregnancy, peaking at term (136). However, these receptors are present elsewhere, and best described is the heart where activation of oxytocin receptors leads to the release of atrial natriuretic peptide (ANP) and brain natriuretic peptide (BNP). These natriuretic peptides have actions similar to each other and cause natriuresis, diuresis, and vasodilation. The result can be hypovolemia and hypotension. Paradoxically, because the oxytocin structure is similar to vasopressin, oxytocin administration in higher concentrations can activate those vasopressin receptors resulting in an antidiuretic and presser effect. This can explain the diverse side effects ascribed to oxytocin infusions and boluses (137) (Table 12-6).

TABLE 12-6 Oxytocin Protocol for Cesarean Delivery: "Rule of Threes"

3 IU oxytocin intravenous loading dose[a] (administered no faster than 15s[12]).
3 min assessment intervals. If inadequate uterine tone, give 3 IU oxytocin intravenous rescue dose.
3 total doses of oxytocin (initial load + 2 rescue doses).
3 IU oxytocin intravenous maintenance dose (3 IU/L at 100 mL/h).
3 pharmacologic options (e.g., ergonovine, carboprost, and misoprostol) if inadequate uterine tone persists.

[a]An initial dose of 3 IU oxytocin is sufficient for effective uterine contractions for both non-laboring[12,21] and laboring[23] women. Preferably, this dose should be administered in the form of a rapid infusion, rather than a bolus. Maintenance oxytocin infusion can be administered for up to 8 h following delivery.
Reprinted with permission from: Tsen LT, Balki M. Oxytocin protocols during cesarean delivery: time to acknowledge the risk/benefit ratio? *Int J Obstet Anesth* 2010;19(3):243–245.

Recent attention on the significant side effects of oxytocin and outcomes has prompted a review of the drug and how it is administered. Clark et al. (138) pointed out that charges of oxytocin misuse are currently cited in over 50% of obstetric lawsuits and that the drug has been placed on the Institute for Safe Medication Practices (ISMP) list of 12 drugs that "bear a heightened risk of harm."

During a cesarean procedure, oxytocin is almost universally administered at the time of delivery to encourage uterine contraction and reduce the risk of hemorrhage. However, how it is administered and how much is given varies considerably worldwide. Some countries such as the United Kingdom suggest a bolus dose of 5 units of oxytocin administered by slow intravenous injection, yet bolus doses as high as 10 units have been described. In the United States, it is common to start an infusion of 40 to 60 units/L of oxytocin at an undefined rate that may or may not include small boluses of 2 to 5 units as well (136).

What is the therapeutic dose of oxytocin for cesarean delivery? Two studies have defined the effective dose for a 90% response (ED90) in women undergoing an elective cesarean delivery or those undergoing cesarean after a period of labor (136,139). Carvalho et al. (139) performed a randomized, single-blinded study with 40 women undergoing an elective cesarean delivery who never experienced labor. Oxytocin was administered by bolus injection following a dose–response protocol. They determined that the ED90 of oxytocin was 0.35 units, which is considerably less than the dose commonly administered in clinical practice. Balki et al. (136) conducted a similarly designed study to define the ED90 of women who required a cesarean delivery for labor arrest despite oxytocin augmentation. They determined that in this defined clinical situation, the ED90 of oxytocin was 2.99 units. They opined that the difference in oxytocin requirements compared with Carvalho's study was due to desensitization of the oxytocin receptors following exposure to an oxytocin infusion. Of interest is that the dose defined as the ED90 is still far less than doses administered in most cesarean deliveries. This suggests that a lack of response to 3 units should not prompt administration of more oxytocin but rather use of a second line drug (see Chapter 33).

Best evidence strongly suggests that oxytocin must be administered judiciously to minimize the adverse effects of the medication while achieving the benefits (Table 12-7). Consideration should be given early to other uterotonic agents

TABLE 12-7 Adverse Effects of Oxytocin

Hypotension	Nausea/vomiting
Chest pain	Arrhythmias
EKG changes	Elevated pulmonary pressures
Flushing	Headache
Shortness of breath	Pulmonary edema
Myocardial ischemia	Maternal death

if uterine tone remains poor. In an editorial, Tsen and Balki suggested an algorithm for rational oxytocin use in a cesarean delivery (140). In it, they propose the "Rule of Threes" as a more evidence-based way to administer oxytocin (see Table 12-5). Also, evidence supports the use of infusions over boluses to avoid the potential side effects as much as possible.

KEY POINTS

- There has been an explosive increase in cesarean deliveries in most developed countries that appears due to a combination of factors and strong regional influences. In developed countries, trends driving the cesarean delivery rate appear to be changes in obstetric practice, fear of litigation, changing maternal demographics, and maternal request.
- The assumption that a higher surgery rate equates with improved maternal and neonatal outcomes is not true. Rates above the recommended 15% are associated with worsening outcomes for both the mother and the neonate.
- Although none of the methods for aspiration prophylaxis have been proven to be effective, there is reasonable evidence that precautions should be taken. The best recommendation currently is to use both an H_2 blocker and non-particulate antacid. Other protocols may be reasonable, given the lack of outcome data.
- Neuraxial techniques are the anesthetic choice for cesarean delivery for most patients, especially for those having elective surgery. They are associated with lower risks of mortality and complications for the mother, and less exposure to lipid-soluble medications for the fetus. The spinal technique is currently more commonly used than an epidural technique in an elective situation and opioids are typically added to improve the quality of the block and possibly the duration. Morphine is the opioid of choice for postoperative pain management.
- All agents used for induction of general anesthesia cross the placenta, and as little as 0.5 MAC of a volatile agent can relax uterine muscle causing atony unresponsive to oxytocin. Induction is performed in a manner to limit fetal exposure. As a result, maternal awareness is a concern but recall probably does not occur as frequently.
- Under elective conditions, giving the mother supplemental oxygen does not appear to benefit the fetus. But under emergency conditions there is improvement in fetal oxygen content but no other measured impact.
- Oxytocin is on the ISMP list of drugs that "bear a heightened risk of harm." Best evidence supports infusion and not bolusing of oxytocin and no more than 3 units infused for a cesarean delivery to avoid potentially serious side effects. If there is little response, then a second line uterotonic should be administered.

REFERENCES

1. Betrán AP, Merialdi M, Lauer JA, et al. Rates of caesarean section: Analysis of global, regional and national estimates. *Paediatr Perinat Epidemiol.* 2007;21:98–113.
2. Bucklin BA, Hawkins JL, Anderson JR, et al. Obstetric anesthesia workforce survey: Twenty year update. *Anesthesiology* 2005;103(3):645–653.
3. Johnson RV, Lyons GR, Wilson RC, et al. Training in obstetric anesthesia: A vanishing act? *Anaesthesia* 2000;55(2):179–183.
4. Searle RD, Lyons G. Vanishing experience in training for obstetric general anaesthesia: An observational study. *Int J Obstet Anesth* 2008;17(3):233–237.
5. Villar J, Valladares W, Wojdyla D, et al. Caesarean delivery rates and pregnancy outcomes: the 2005 WHO global survey on maternal and perinatal health in Latin America. *Lancet* 2006;367(9525):1819–1829.
6. Placek PJ, Taffel S. Trends in cesarean section rates for the United States, 1970–1978. *Public Health Rep* 1980;95(6):540–548.
7. Menacker F. Trends in cesarean rates for first births and repeat cesarean births for low-risk women: United States, 1990–2003. *Natl Vital Stat Rep* 2005; 54(4):1–8.
8. Zhang J, Troendle J, Reddy UM, et al. Contemporary cesarean delivery practice in the United States. *Am J Obstet Gynecol* 2010;203(4):326.e1–326.e10.
9. Joseph KS, Young DC, Dodds L, et al. Changes in maternal characteristics and obstetric practice and recent increases in primary cesarean delivery. *Obstet Gynecol* 2003;102(4):791–800.
10. Dobson R. Caesarean section rate in England and Wales hits 21%. *BMJ* 2001;323(7319):951.
11. The World Health Association. Appropriate technology for birth. *Lancet* 1985;2(8452):436–437.
12. Declerq E, Menacker F, MacDorman M. Maternal risk profiles and the primary cesarean rate in the United States, 1991–2002. *Am J Public Health* 2006;96(5):867–872.
13. Menacker F, Hamilton BE. Recent trends in cesarean delivery in the United States. *NCHS Data Brief* 2010;35:1–8.
14. Kotaska A, Menticoglou S, Gagnon R, et al. SOCG clinical practice guideline: Vaginal delivery of breech presentation: No. 226, June 2009. *Int J Gynaecol Obstet* 2009;107(2):169–176.
15. ACOG Committee on Obstetric Practice. ACOG Committee Opinion No. 340. Mode of term singleton breech delivery. *Obstet Gynecol* 2006;108(1):235–237.
16. Macones GA, Peipert J, Nelson DB, et al. Maternal complications with vaginal birth after cesarean delivery: A multicenter study. *Am J Obstet Gynecol* 2005; 193(5):1656–1662.
17. Macones GA. Clinical outcomes in VBAC attempts: What to say to patients? *Am J Obstet Gynecol* 2008;199(1):1–2.
18. Yang YT, Mello MM, Subramanian SV, et al. Relationship between malpractice litigation pressure and rates of cesarean section and vaginal birth after cesarean section. *Med Care* 2009;47(2):234–242.
19. Murthy K, Grobman WA, Lee TA, et al. Association between rising professional liability insurance premiums and primary cesarean delivery rates. *Obstet Gynecol* 2007;110(6):1264–1269.
20. Habiba M, Kaminski M, Da Fre M, et al. Caesarean section on request: A comparison of obstetricians' attitudes in eight European Countries. *BJOG* 2006; 113(6):647–656.
21. Anonymous editorial. What is the right number of caesarean sections? *Lancet* 1997;349(9055):815.
22. Kainu JP, Sarvela J, Tiippana E, et al. Persistent pain after caesarean section and vaginal birth: A cohort study. *Int J Obstet Anesth* 2010;19(1):4–9.
23. Chaim W, Bashiri A, Bar-David J, et al. Prevalence and clinical significance of postpartum endometritis and wound infection. *Infect Dis Obstet Gynecol* 2000; 8(2):77–82.
24. Groutz A, Rimon E, Peled S, et al. Cesarean section: Does it really prevent the development of postpartum stress urinary incontinence? A prospective study of 363 women one year after their first delivery. *Neurourol Urodyn* 2004;23(1):2–6.
25. Deneux-Thomas C, Carmona E, Bouvier-Colle MH, et al. Postpartum maternal mortality and cesarean delivery. *Obstet Gynecol* 2006;108(3):541–548.
26. Arias E, Rostron BL, Tejada-Vera B. United States life tables, 2005. *Natl Vital Stat Rep* 2010;58(10):1–132.
27. Clark SL, Belfort MA, Dildy GA, et al. Maternal death in the 21st century: Causes, prevention, and relationship to cesarean delivery. *Am J Obstet Gynecol* 2008;199(1):36.e1–e5.
28. Leung GM, Ho LM, Tin K, et al. Health care consequences of cesarean birth during the first 18 months of life. *Epidemiology* 2007;18(4):479–484.
29. American Society of Anesthesiologists Task Force on Obstetric Anesthesia. Practice guidelines for obstetric anesthesia: An updated report by the American Society of Anesthesiologists Task Force on Obstetric Anesthesia. *Anesthesiology* 2007;106(4):843–863.
30. Douglas MJ. The use of neuraxial anesthesia in parturients with thrombocytopenia: What is an adequate platelet count? In: Halpern SH, Douglas MJ, eds. *Evidence-Based Obstetric Anesthesia.* Oxford: Blackwell Publishing Ltd; 2005:165–177.

31. Provan D, Stasi R, Newland A, et al. International consensus report on the investigation and management of primary idiopathic thrombocytopenic purpura. *Blood* 2010;115(2):168–186.

32. George JN, Woolf SH, Raskob GE, et al. Idiopathic thrombocytopenic purpura: A practice guideline developed by explicit methods for the American Society of Hematology. *Blood* 1996;88(1):3–40.

33. Beilin Y, Zahn J, Comerford M. Safe epidural analgesia in thirty parturients with platelet counts between 69,000 and 98,000 mm^{-3}. *Anesth Analg* 1997;85(2):385–388.

34. Tanaka M, Balki M, McLeod A, et al. Regional anesthesia and non-preeclamptic thrombocytopenia: Time to re-think the safe platelet count. *Rev Bras Anestesiol* 2009;59(2):142–153.

35. Dyer RA, Farina Z, Joubert IA, et al. Crystalloid preload versus rapid crystalloid administration after induction of spinal anaesthesia (coload) for elective caesarean section. *Anaesth Intensive Care* 2004;32(3):351–357.

36. Scrutton MJ, Metcalfe GA, Lowy C, et al. Eating in labour. A randomised controlled trial assessing the risks and benefits. *Anaesthesia* 1999;54(4):329–334.

37. Dewan DM, Floyd HM, Thistlewood JM, et al. Sodium citrate pretreatment in elective cesarean section patients. *Anesth Analg* 1985;64(1):34–37.

38. Rout CC, Rocke DA, Gouws E. Intravenous ranitidine reduces the risk of acid aspiration of gastric contents at emergency cesarean section. *Anesth Analg* 1993;76(1):156–161.

39. Lin CJ, Huang CL, Hsu HW, et al. Prophylaxis against acid aspiration in regional anesthesia for elective cesarean section: A comparison between oral single-dose ranitidine, famotidine, and omeprazole assessed with fiberoptic gastric aspiration. *Acta Anaesthesiol Sin* 1996;34(4):179–184.

40. Paranjothy S, Griffiths JD, Broughton HK, et al. Interventions at caesarean section for reducing the risk of aspiration pneumonitis. *Cochrane Database Syst Rev* 2010;CD004943.

41. de Souza DG, Doar LH, Mehta SH, et al. Aspiration prophylaxis and rapid sequence induction for elective cesarean delivery: Time to reassess an old dogma? *Anesth Analg* 2010;110(5):1503–1505.

42. Gibbs RS. Clinical risk factors for puerperal infection. *Obstet Gynecol* 1980;55(5):178S–184S.

43. Alfirevic Z, Gyte GM, Dou L. Different classes of antibiotics given to women routinely for preventing infection at caesarean section. *Cochrane Database Syst Rev* 2010;CD008726.

44. Tita ATN, Rouse DJ, Blackwell S, et al. Emerging concepts in antibiotic prophylaxis for cesarean delivery: A systematic review. *Obstet Gynecol* 2009;113(3):675–682.

45. Costantine MM, Rahman M, Ghulmiyah L, et al. Timing of perioperative antibiotics for cesarean delivery: a metaanalysis. *Am J Obstet Gynecol* 2008;199(3):301.e1–e6.

46. Committee opinion no. 465: antimicrobial prophylaxis for cesarean delivery: timing of administration. *Obstet Gynecol* 2010;116(3):791–792.

47. Hunt CO, Naulty JS, Bader AM, et al. Perioperative analgesia with subarachnoid fentanyl-bupivacaine for cesarean delivery. *Anesthesiology* 1989;71(4):535–450.

48. Shende D, Cooper GM, Bowden MI. The influence of intrathecal fentanyl on the characteristics of subarachnoid block for caesarean section. *Anaesthesia* 1998;53(7):706–710.

49. Dahl JB, Jeppesen IS, Jørgensen H, et al. Intraoperative and postoperative analgesic efficacy and adverse effects of intrathecal opioids in patients undergoing cesarean section with spinal anesthesia: A qualitative and quantitative systematic review of randomized controlled trials. *Anesthesiology* 1999;91(6):1919–1927.

50. Palmer CM, Emerson S, Volgoropolous D, et al. Dose-response relationship of intrathecal morphine for post-cesarean analgesia. *Anesthesiology* 1999;90(2):437–444.

51. Abboud TK, Dror A, Mosaad P, et al. Mini-dose intrathecal morphine for the relief of post-cesarean section pain: Safety, efficacy, and ventilatory responses to carbon dioxide. *Anesth Analg* 1988;67(2):137–143.

52. Broadbent CR, Maxwell WB, Ferrie R, et al. Ability of anaesthetists to identify a marked lumbar interspace. *Anaesthesia* 2000;55(11):1122–1126.

53. Riley ET, Cohen SE, Macario A, et al. Spinal versus epidural anesthesia for cesarean section: A comparison of time efficiency, costs, charges, and complications. *Anesth Analg* 1995;80(4):709–712.

54. Ithnin F, Lim Y, Sia AT, et al. Combined spinal epidural causes higher level of block than equivalent single-shot spinal anesthesia in elective cesarean patients. *Anesth Analg* 2006;102(2):577–580.

55. Lim Y, Teoh W, Sia AT. Combined spinal epidural does not cause a higher sensory block than single shot spinal technique for cesarean delivery in laboring women. *Anesth Analg* 2006;103(6):1540–1542.

56. Lew E, Yeo SW, Thomas E. Combined spinal-epidural anesthesia using epidural volume extension leads to faster motor recovery after elective cesarean delivery: A prospective, randomized, double-blind study. *Anesth Analg* 2004;98(3):810–814.

57. Tyagi A, Girotra G, Kumar A, et al. Single-shot spinal anaesthesia, combined spinal-epidural and epidural volume extension for elective cesarean section: A randomized comparison. *Int J Obstet Anesth* 2009;18(3):231–236.

58. Kucukguclu S, Unlugenc H, Gunenc F, et al. The influence of epidural volume extension on spinal block with hyperbaric or plain bupivacaine for caesarean delivery. *Eur J Anaesthesiol* 2008;25(4):307–313.

59. Hamlyn EL, Douglass CA, Plaat F, et al. Low-dose sequential combined spinal-epidural: An anaesthetic technique for caesarean section in patients with significant cardiac disease. *Int J Obstet Anesth* 2005;14(4):355–361.

60. Aouad MT, Siddik SS, Jalbout MI, et al. Does pregnancy protect against intrathecal lidocaine-induced transient neurologic symptoms? *Anesth Analg* 2001;92(2):401–404.

61. Gautier P, De Kock M, Huberty L, et al. Comparison of the effects of intrathecal ropivacaine, levobupivacaine, and bupivacaine for caesarean section. *Br J Anaesth* 2003;91(5):684–689.

62. Curatolo M, Petersen-Felix S, Arendt-Nielsen L, et al. Adding sodium bicarbonate to lidocaine enhances the depth of epidural blockade. *Anesth Analg* 1998;86(2):341–347.

63. Abboud TK, Moore MJ, Jacobs J, et al. Epidural mepivacaine for cesarean section: Maternal and neonatal effects. *Reg Anesth Pain Med* 1987;12(2):76–79.

64. Bader AM, Tsen LC, Camann WR, et al. Clinical effects and maternal and fetal plasma concentrations of 0.5% epidural levobupivacaine versus bupivacaine for cesarean delivery. *Anesthesiology* 1999;90(6):1596–1601.

65. Crosby E, Sandler A, Finucane B, et al. Comparison of epidural anaesthesia with ropivacaine 0.5% and bupivacaine 0.5% for caesarean section. *Can J Anaesth* 1998;45(11):1066–1071.

66. Parpaglioni R, Baldassini B, Barbati G, et al. Adding sufentanil to levobupivacaine or ropivacaine intrathecal anaesthesia effects the minimum local anaesthetic dose required. *Acta Anaesthesiol Scand* 2009;53(9):1214–1220.

67. Chen X, Qian X, Fu F, et al. Intrathecal sufentanil decreases the median effective dose (ED 50) of intrathecal hyperbaric bupivacaine for caesarean delivery. *Acta Anaesthesiol Scand* 2010;54(3):284–290.

68. Demiraran Y, Ozdemir I, Kocaman B, et al. Intrathecal sufentanil (1.5 mcg) added to hyperbaric bupivacaine (0.5%) for elective caesarean section provides adequate analgesia without need for pruritus therapy. *J Anesth* 2006;20(4):274–278.

69. Dahlgren G, Hultstrand C, Jakobsson J, et al. Intrathecal sufentanil, fentanyl, or placebo added to bupivacaine for cesarean section. *Anesth Analg* 1997;85(6):1288–1293.

70. Brose WG, Cohen SE. Epidural lidocaine for cesarean section: Effect of varying epinephrine concentration. *Anesthesiology* 1988;69(6):936–940.

71. Lam DT, Ngan Kee WD, Khaw KS. Extension of epidural blockade in labour for emergency caesarean section using 2% lidocaine with epinephrine and fentanyl, with or without alkalinisation. *Anaesthesia* 2001;56(8):790–794.

72. Ackerman WE, Denson DD, Juneja MM, et al. Alkalinization of chloroprocaine for epidural anesthesia: Effects of pCO2 at constant pH. *Reg Anesth* 1990;15(2):89–93.

73. Wong K, Strichartz GR, Raymond SA. On the mechanisms of potentiation of local anesthetics by bicarbonate buffer: Drug structure-activity studies on isolated peripheral nerve. *Anesth Analg* 1993;76(1):131–143.

74. Lurie S, Sulema V, Kohen-Sacher B, et al. The decision to delivery interval in emergency and non-urgent cesarean sections. *Eur J Obstet Gynecol Reprod Biol* 2004;113(2):182–185.

75. Huissoud C, Dupont C, Canoui-Poitrine F, et al. Decision-to-delivery interval for emergency caesareans in the Aurore perinatal network. *Eur J Obstet Gynecol Reprod Biol* 2010;149(2):159–164.

76. Chauleur C, Collet F, Furtos C, et al. Identification of factors influencing the decision-to-delivery interval in emergency caesarean sections. *Gynecol Obstet Invest* 2009;68(4):248–254.

77. Holcroft CJ, Graham EM, Aina-Mumuney A, et al. Cord gas analysis, decision-to-delivery interval, and the 30-minute rule for emergency cesareans. *J Perinatol* 2005;25(4):229–235.

78. Bloom SL, Leveno KJ, Spong CY, et al; National Institute of Child Health and Human Development Maternal-Fetal Medicine Units Network. Decision-to-incision times and maternal and infant outcomes. *Obstet Gynecol* 2006;108(1):6–11.

79. Harte C, McCaul C, Hayes N. Decision to delivery interval in emergency caesarean section: a prospective observational study. *Int J Obstet Anesth* 2011;20:S40.

80. Douglas J, Kathirgamanathan A, Tyler J, et al. How fast are we? General versus spinal anesthesia for emergency cesarean section. Society for Obstetric Anesthesia and Perinatology Annual Meeting 2010;A34.

81. Gaiser RR, Cheek TG, Gutsche BB. Epidural lidocaine versus 2-chloroprocaine for fetal distress requiring urgent cesarean section. *Int J Obstet Anesth* 1994;3(4):208–210.

82. Gaiser RR, Cheek TG, Adams HK, et al. Epidural lidocaine for cesarean delivery of the distressed fetus. *Int J Obstet Anesth* 1998;7(1):27–31.

83. Hood DD, Curry R. Spinal versus epidural for cesarean section in severely preeclamptic patients: A retrospective survey. *Anesthesiology* 1999;90(5):1276–1282.

84. Wallace DH, Leveno KJ, Cunningham FG, et al. Randomized comparison of general and regional anesthesia for cesarean delivery in pregnancies complicated by severe preeclampsia. *Obstet Gynecol* 1995;86(2):193–199.

85. Bader AM, Hunt CO, Datta S, et al. Anesthesia for the obstetric patient with multiple sclerosis. *J Clin Anesth* 1988;1(1):21–24.

86. Drake E, Drake M, Bird J, et al. Obstetric regional blocks for women with multiple sclerosis: A survey of UK experience. *Int J Obstet Anesth* 2006;15(2):115–123.

87. Kinsella SM, Norris MC. Advance prediction of hypotension at cesarean delivery under spinal anesthesia. *Int J Obstet Anesth* 1996;5(1):3–7.

88. Dahlgren G, Granath F, Wessel H, et al. Prediction of hypotension during spinal anesthesia for cesarean section and its relation to the effect of crystalloid or colloid preload. *Int J Obstet Anesth* 2007;16(2):128–134.

89. Rout CC, Rocke DA, Levin J, et al. A reevaluation of the role of crystalloid preload in the prevention of hypotension associated with spinal anesthesia for elective cesarean section. *Anesthesiology* 1993;79(2):262–269.

90. Cyna AM, Andrew M, Emmett RS, et al. Techniques for preventing hypotension during spinal anaesthesia for caesarean section. *Cochrane Database Syst Rev* 2006;CD002251.

91. Banerjee A, Stocche RM, Angle P, et al. Preload or coload for spinal anesthesia for elective cesarean delivery: a meta-analysis. *Can J Anaesth* 2010;57(1):24–31.

92. Lee A, Ngan Kee WD, Gin T. A quantitative, systematic review of randomized controlled trials of ephedrine versus phenylephrine for the management of hypotension during spinal anesthesia for cesarean delivery. *Anesth Analg* 2002;94(4):920–926.

93. Ngan Kee WD, Khaw KS, Ng FF. Prevention of hypotension during spinal anesthesia for cesarean delivery: An effective technique using combination phenylephrine infusion and crystalloid cohydration. *Anesthesiology* 2005; 103(4):744–750.

94. Lee A, Ngan Kee WD, Gin T. A Dose-response meta-analysis of prophylactic intravenous ephedrine for the prevention of hypotension during spinal anesthesia for elective cesarean delivery. *Anesth Analg* 2004;98(2):483–490.

95. Ngan Kee WD. Prevention of maternal hypotension after regional anaesthesia for caesarean section. *Curr Opin Anaesthesiol* 2010;23(3):304–309.

96. Habib AS. A review of the impact of phenylephrine administration on maternal hemodynamics and maternal and neonatal outcomes in women undergoing cesarean delivery under spinal anesthesia. *Anesth Analg* 2012;114(2):377–390.

97. Halpern SH, Soliman A, Yee J, et al. Conversion of epidural labour analgesia to anaesthesia for caesarean section: A prospective study of the incidence and determinants of failure. *Br J Anaesth* 2009;102(2):240–243.

98. Rafi M, Arfeen Z, Misra U. Conversion of regional to general anaesthesia at caesarean section: Increasing the use of regional anaesthesia through continuous prospective audit. *Int J Obstet Anesth* 2010;19(2):179–182.

99. Kan RK, Lew E, Yeo SW, et al. General anesthesia for cesarean section in a Singapore maternity hospital: A retrospective survey. *Int J Obstet Anesth* 2004; 13(4):221–226.

100. Campbell DC, Tran T. Conversion of epidural labour analgesia to epidural anesthesia for intrapartum cesarean delivery. *Can J Anaesth* 2009;56(1):19–26.

101. Furst SR, Reisner LS. Risk of high spinal anesthesia following failed epidural block for cesarean delivery. *J Clin Anesth* 1995;7(1):71–74.

102. Visser WA, Dijkstra A, Albayrak M, et al. Spinal anesthesia for intrapartum cesarean delivery following epidural labor analgesia: A retrospective cohort study. *Can J Anaesth* 2009;56(8):577–583.

103. Hawkins JL, Koonin LM, Palmer SK, et al. Anesthesia-related deaths during obstetric delivery in the United States, 1979–1990. *Anesthesiology* 1997;86 (2):277–284.

104. Downing JW, Mahomedy MC, Jeal DE, et al. Anaesthesia for caesarean section with ketamine. *Anaesthesia* 1976;31(7):883–892.

105. Crozier TA, Flamm C, Speer CP, et al. Effects of etomidate on the adrenocortical and metabolic adaptation of the neonate. *Br J Anaesth* 1993;70(1):47–53.

106. Craft JB, Coaldrake LA, Yonekura ML, et al. Ketamine, catecholamines, and uterine tone in pregnant ewes. *Am J Obstet Gynecol* 1983;146(4):429–434.

107. Oats JN, Vasey DP, Waldron BA. Effects of ketamine on the pregnant uterus. *Br J Anaesth* 1979;51(12):1163–1166.

108. Dich-Nielsen J, Holasek J. Ketamine as induction agent for caesarean section. *Acta Anaesthesiol Scand* 1982;26(2):139–142.

109. Eisele J, Wright R, Rogge P. Newborn and maternal fentanyl levels at cesarean section. *Anesth Analg* 1982;61:179–180.

110. Draisci G, Valente A, Suppa E, et al. Remifentanil for cesarean section under general anesthesia: Effects on maternal stress hormone secretion and neonatal well-being: A randomized trial. *Int J Obstet Anesth* 2008;17(2):130–136.

111. Orme RM, Grange CS, Ainsworth QP, et al. General anaesthesia using remifentanil for caesarean section in parturients with critical aortic stenosis: A series of four cases. *Int J Obstet Anesth* 2004;13(3):183–187.

112. Dailey PA, Fisher DM, Shnider SM, et al. Pharmacokinetics, placental transfer, and neonatal effects of vecuronium and pancuronium administered during cesarean section. *Anesthesiology* 1984;60(6):569–574.

113. Datta S, Migliozzi RP, Flanagan HL, et al. Chronically administered progesterone decreases halothane requirements in rabbits. *Anesth Analg* 1989;68(1): 46–50.

114. Gin T, Chan MT. Decreased minimum alveolar concentration of isoflurane in pregnant humans. *Anesthesiology* 1994;81(4):829–832.

115. Chan MT, Mainland P, Gin T. Minimum alveolar concentration of halothane and enflurane are decreased in early pregnancy. *Anesthesiology* 1996;85(4): 782–786.

116. Chan MT, Gin T. Postpartum changes in the minimum alveolar concentration of isoflurane. *Anesthesiology* 1995;82(6):1360–1363.

117. Munson ES, Embro WJ. Enflurane, isoflurane, and halothane and isolated human uterine muscle. *Anesthesiology* 1977;46(1):11–14.

118. Dogru K, Yildiz K, Dalgiç H, et al. Inhibitory effects of desflurane and sevoflurane on contractions of isolated gravid rat myometrium under oxytocin stimulation. *Acta Anaesthesiol Scand* 2003;47(4):472–474.

119. Yildiz K, Dogru K, Dalgic H, et al. Inhibitory effects of desflurane and sevoflurane on oxytocin-induced contractions of isolated pregnant human myometrium. *Acta Anaesthesiol Scand* 2005;49(9):1355–1359.

120. King H, Ashley S, Brathwaite D, et al. Adequacy of general anesthesia for cesarean section. *Anesth Analg* 1993;77(1):84–88.

121. Paech M, Scott K, Clavisi O, et al. A prospective study of awareness and recall associated with general anaesthesia for caesarean section. *Int J Obstet Anesth* 2008;17(4):298–303.

122. Monk TG, Weldon BC. Does depth of anesthesia monitoring improve postoperative outcomes? *Curr Opin Anaesthesiol* 2011;24(6):665–669.

123. Yeo SN, Lo WK. Bispectral index in assessment of adequacy of general anaesthesia for lower segment caesarean section. *Anaesth Intensive Care* 2002; 30(1):36–40.

124. Ittichaikulthol W, Sriswasdi S, Prachanpanich N, et al. Bispectral index in assessment of 3% and 4.5% desflurane in 50% N2O for caesarean section. *J Med Assoc Thai* 2007;90(8):1546–1550.

125. Hawkins JL, Chang J, Palmer SK, et al. Anesthesia-related maternal mortality in the United States: 1979–2002. *Obstet Gynecol* 2011;117(1):69–74.

126. Marx GF, Mateo CV. Effects of different oxygen concentrations during general anaesthesia for elective caesarean section. *Can Anaesth Soc J* 1971;18(6): 587–593.

127. Rorke MJ, Davey DA, Du Toit HJ. Foetal oxygenation during caesarean section. *Anaesthesia* 1968;23(4):585–596.

128. Fox GS, Houle GL. Acid–base studies in elective caesarean sections during epidural and general anaesthesia. *Can Anaesth Soc J* 1971;18(1):60–71.

129. Ramanathan S, Gandhi S, Arismendy J, et al. Oxygen transfer from mother to fetus during cesarean section under epidural anesthesia. *Anesth Analg* 1982; 61(7):576–581.

130. 2005 International Consensus Conference on cardiopulmonary resuscitation and emergency cardiovascular care science with treatment recommendations. Neonatal resuscitation. *Circulation* 2005;112(suppl 12):III-91–III-99. http://ovidsp.tx.ovid.com.ezp-prod1.hul.harvard.edu/sp-3.6.0b/ovidweb.cgi?&S=PNOFFPBAIADDGJHNNCPKMGFBDIEJAA00&Complete+Reference=S.sh.18.19.23.27%7c7%7c1

131. Khaw KS, Wang CC, Ngan Kee WD, et al. Effects of high inspired oxygen fraction during elective caesarean section under spinal anaesthesia on maternal and fetal oxygenation and lipid peroxidation. *Br J Anaesth* 2002;88(1):18–23.

132. Cogliano MS, Graham AC, Clark VA. Supplementary oxygen administration for elective caesarean section under spinal anaesthesia. *Anaesthesia* 2002; 57(1):66–69.

133. Backe SK, Kocarev M, Wilson RC, et al. Effect of maternal facial oxygen on neonatal behavioural scores during elective caesarean section with spinal anaesthesia. *Eur J Anaesthesiol* 2007;24(1):66–70.

134. Khaw KS, Ngan Kee WD, Lee A, et al. Supplementary oxygen for elective caesarean section under spinal anaesthesia: Useful in prolonged uterine incision-to-delivery interval? *Br J Anaesth* 2004;92(4):518–522.

135. Khaw KS, Wang CC, Ngan Kee WD, et al. Supplementary oxygen for emergency caesarean section under regional anaesthesia. *Br J Anaesth* 2009;102(1):90–96.

136. Balki M, Ronayne M, Davies S, et al. Minimum oxytocin dose requirement after cesarean delivery for labor arrest. *Obstet Gynecol* 2006;107(1):45–50.

137. Dyer RA, van Dyk D, Dresner A. The use of uterotonic drugs during caesarean section. *Int J Obstet Anesth* 2010;19(3):313–319.

138. Clark SL, Simpson KR, Knox E, et al. Oxytocin: New perspectives on an old drug. *Am J Obstet Gynecol* 2009;200(1):35.e1–e6.

139. Carvalho JCA, Balki M, Kingdom J, et al. Oxytocin requirements at elective cesarean delivery: A dose-finding study. *Obstet Gynecol* 2004;104(5):1005–1010.

140. Tsen LT, Balki M. Oxytocin protocols during cesarean delivery: Time to acknowledge the risk/benefit ratio? *Int J Obstet Anesth* 2010;19(3):243–245.

Postoperative Multimodal Acute Pain Management: Cesarean and Vaginal Delivery

Rodolfo Gebhardt • Sarah L. Armstrong • Oscar A. de Leon-Casasola • Thomas Chai • Julie A. Sparlin • José M. Rivers • Roshan Fernando

▪ INTRODUCTION

Over the last two decades the number of cesarean deliveries performed around the world has increased dramatically and acute postoperative pain is a predominant feature for the majority of these patients. Acute pain can be defined as an unpleasant sensory and emotional experience associated with actual or potential tissue damage. Failure to treat acute postoperative pain can have adverse physical and psychological consequences for the patient. Results from a US national survey suggests that a patient has a 50% to 71% chance of experiencing moderate to severe pain after surgery (1). Furthermore, inadequate treatment of acute pain can progress to a persistent, chronic pain state (2). High-quality postoperative analgesia after cesarean delivery is important because the new mother must recover from major intra-abdominal surgery while also caring for her newborn. Many analgesic treatment options are available but tailoring the method to the individual patient can be problematic due to the difficulty of predicting the severity of the postoperative pain and the individual's response to the regimen. A variety of factors influence the analgesic regimen such as the patient's preferences and expectations, surgical difficulty and duration, and experience of the practitioner. Some of these predictors may be quantifiable at the bedside and amenable to modulation (3). Several studies demonstrate that patient education increases the efficacy of analgesic techniques after cesarean delivery (4,5).

▪ PAIN PATHWAYS

In a healthy individual, pain is a complex sensory experience associated with actual or potential tissue damage. Noxious inputs stimulate the unspecialized, peripheral nociceptors. Both nerve types C and A delta, transmit signals to the dorsal horn. Unmyelinated, small C fibers, conduct electrical impulses induced by thermal, pressure, and chemical stimuli generally at a rate <1 m/s. Myelinated, medium A delta fibers transmit a faster impulse (5 to 30 m/s) when activated by the same stimuli (6). At the molecular level, pain stimulates the release of many mediators from keratinocytes and blood vessels in the dermis, including prostaglandins, substance P, and calcitonin gene–related peptide (CGRP). These neurotransmitters bind to receptors on the nociceptive fibers, cause depolarization and the subsequent transmission of signals to the central nervous system (CNS) as well as the release of neurotransmitters from the nerve itself into the periphery. This phenomenon, called axon reflex, causes vasodilation and inflammation and results in a positive feedback loop that begins to recruit silent nociceptors and pain fibers in close proximity to the initially activated nerve (6).

Pain fibers synapse with their secondary fibers at the superficial laminae (Rexed's I and II) of the dorsal horn where neuropeptides such as tachykinins (substance P and neurokinin A) and glutamate are released at the presynaptic level. The tachykinins bind to the postsynaptic neurokinin receptors NK_1 and NK_2 leading via GTP protein activation, to depolarization and changes in second messengers (Fig. 13-1).

Depolarization of the first-order neuron induces the opening of voltage-gated calcium channels at the body of this cell, allowing the influx of calcium. Calcium binds to vesicles containing neurotransmitters and stimulates their release. The neurotransmitters bind to their corresponding receptors on the postsynaptic or secondary neurons and induce an excitatory event there. Second-order neurons cross the spinal cord and carry their impulses via the spinothalamic tract to the thalamus on the contralateral side. Opioid receptors and their ligands are present on the superficial dorsal horn, particularly on Rexed's lamina II, also known as the substantia gelatinosa. Since their identification, opioid receptors have had a variety of names. The current nomenclature (approved by the International Union of Pharmacology) for identification of the opioid receptors is as follows:

MOP (mu opioid peptide receptor)
KOP (kappa opioid peptide receptor)
DOP (delta opioid peptide receptor) and
NOP (nociceptin/orphanin FQ peptide receptor)

A number of different subtypes of each receptor exist; two MOP, three KOP, and two DOP. The sigmoid receptor is no longer classified as it fails to meet all the criteria for an opioid receptor.

Opioids have both presynaptic (indirect) and postsynaptic (direct) facilitatory and inhibitory actions on synaptic transmission in many regions of the nervous system via G-protein coupled receptors. These effector systems can be divided into two categories: Short-term effectors involving potassium and calcium channels, and longer-term effects involving second messengers such as cyclic adenosine monophosphate (cAMP). All opioid receptors can inhibit the voltage-gated calcium channel opening while MOP and DOP receptors activate inwardly rectifying potassium channels. MOP receptor activation can also directly increase calcium entry and therefore intracellular concentration in neurons (7). Potassium channel activation leads to hyperpolarization of neuronal membranes, decreased synaptic transmission, and inhibition of conduction of pain signals while neurotransmitter mobilization and release is modulated by intracellular calcium concentrations (6). Spinal opioids exert their analgesic effects by reducing neurotransmitter release at the presynaptic level, and by hyperpolarizing the membrane of dorsal horn neurons at the postsynaptic level (8).

Synaptic Transmission

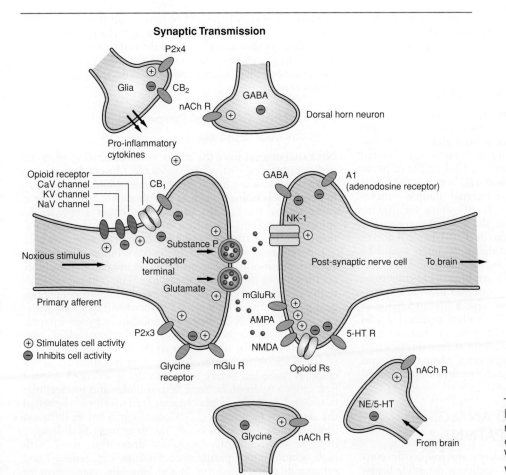

FIGURE 13-1 Synaptic transmission. Copyright© 2010 Board of Regents of the University of Wisconsin System, reprinted with permission.

Opioid receptor activation can inhibit the release of CGRP, glutamate, and substance P from nerves, thereby preventing the feed-forward mechanism of pain that typically results in sensitization at the site of injury (9). These injury-induced neuromodifications which may include microglial cell activation can be perceived as allodynia (pain due to a stimulus which does not normally provoke pain) or hyperalgesia (an increased response to a normally painful stimulus). Moreover, peripheral sensitization drives the repeated release of molecular mediators at the dorsal horn, causing secondary hyperalgesia (Fig. 13-2).

Descending pathways from the somatosensory cortex also modulate the perception of pain. The activation of cells within the periaqueductal gray (PAG) and rostral ventromedial medulla (RVM) stimulate descending fibers to release serotonin and norepinephrine at the level of the spinal cord (10). This event modulates spinal nociceptive conduction (10). Opioids exerting their effect at the supraspinal level promote descending pain modulation by increasing the release of aminobutyric acid, or GABA, an inhibitory neurotransmitter in the brain (11). In this mechanism, called *opioid disinhibition*, opioids release GABA from the PAG, RVM, and other

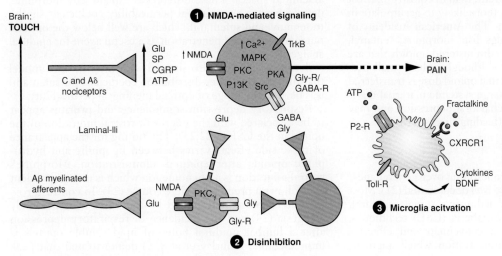

FIGURE 13-2 Cellular and molecular mechanisms of pain. Reprinted with permission from: Basbaum AI, Bautista DM, Scherrer G, et al. Cellular and molecular mechanisms of pain. *Cell* 2009;139(2): 267–284.

centers, activating the descending inhibitory pathways and increasing the concentrations of serotonin and norepinephrine at the presynaptic level thereby modulating pain signals at the spinal cord.

Pain Pathways after Cesarean Delivery

Postcesarean pain has both somatic and visceral components. Somatic pain arises from nociceptors within the abdominal wound and has both cutaneous and deep components, which are transmitted within the anterior divisions of the spinal segmental nerves, usually T10–L1. These nerve fibers run laterally in the abdominal wall between the layers of the transversus abdominis and internal oblique muscles (12). Visceral uterine nociceptive stimuli return via afferent nerve fibers that ascend through the inferior hypogastric plexus and enter the spinal cord via the T10-L1 spinal nerves (13,14). An ideal postcesarean analgesic regimen would be one that is cost-effective, simple to implement, and has minimal impact on staff workload. It would provide consistent and high-quality pain relief while catering to wide interpatient variabilities, and would also have a low incidence of side effects and complications. This ideal regimen would not interfere with the maternal care of the newborn or with breastfeeding, and there would be minimal drug transfer into the breast milk and consequently minimal adverse effects on the newborn. Achieving these goals requires a multimodal approach (15,16).

■ BREASTFEEDING AND ANALGESIA FOR THE OBSTETRIC PATIENT

Mothers who breastfeed their infants are frequently concerned about neonatal exposure to analgesic drugs via breast milk. There has been much debate in the literature about the effect of neuraxial analgesia on the initiation of breastfeeding. Breastfeeding ability is multifactorial and it has been suggested therefore that the role played by neuraxial blockade in influencing this is small. However, there is a paucity of randomized controlled trials (RCTs) investigating this relationship (17).

There is little objective information on the effect of systemic opioids administered to the mother on her breastfeeding newborn. Drug excretion into human milk may occur when a drug binds to the milk proteins or adheres to the milk fat globules. Several factors, including the timing of breastfeeding relative to drug administration, and breast milk contents, influence drug excretion into the human milk. Lipid soluble drugs are more likely to accumulate in mature milk, which has a higher fat content, than in colostrum. Most opioids are weak bases and are more likely to accumulate in mature milk than in colostrum. The American Academy of Pediatrics Committee on Drugs lists morphine, fentanyl, and butorphanol as maternally administered opioids that are compatible with breastfeeding. Although only a small percentage (1% to 3%) of the maternal opioid dose is transferred to the neonate in breast milk, large systemic maternal doses may result in neonatal neurobehavioral depression and may potentially interfere with breastfeeding success (18–20).

Neuraxial Techniques

The safety benefits of regional anesthesia over general anesthesia in the pregnant patient are well documented (21). Most cesarean deliveries are performed using spinal, epidural, or combined spinal–epidural anesthesia (CSE) techniques. These methods also provide a convenient and effective route for neuraxial opioid administration which augment

intraoperative anesthesia and optimize postoperative analgesia. Potency, onset, duration of action, and side effects vary depending on the opioid used and the route of its administration. Pruritus, nausea, and vomiting are the most common side effects of these agents and cause a decrease in maternal satisfaction.

Physical and Chemical Properties of Neuraxial Opioids

Neuraxial opioids have the advantage of producing analgesia without motor or sympathetic blockade. Onset of analgesia is more rapid with the highly lipid soluble opioids. Conversely, lipid insoluble opioids, such as morphine, are retained in the cerebrospinal fluid (CSF), providing a longer supply to the spinal cord and consequently a slower onset, but longer duration of analgesia after the administration of a single dose (22).

Lipophilicity, as assessed by octanol/buffer distribution coefficient, does correlate with the meningeal permeability coefficient but in a nonlinear fashion. The optimal octanol/buffer distribution coefficient that results in maximal meningeal permeability is between 129 (alfentanil) and 560 (bupivacaine) (22). This biphasic relationship between lipophilicity and a drug's meningeal permeability coefficient, may be explained by the dual nature of the arachnoid membrane which is the main barrier. After a drug is deposited in the epidural space but before it reaches the spinal cord, it must first cross a hydrophilic zone (extracellular and intracellular fluids) and then a hydrophobic zone (cell membrane lipids) of the arachnoid membrane (22). Consequently before diffusion through these two areas occur, the drug must first dissolve in those environments. Lipophilic drugs (i.e., those with high octanol/buffer partition coefficients, e.g., fentanyl and sufentanil) readily dissolve in the lipophilic component of arachnoid mater and can cross the region easily. Conversely, they penetrate the hydrophilic zone with difficulty creating the rate-limiting factor in their diffusion through the arachnoid membrane. Drugs with intermediate lipophilicity move more readily between the lipid and the aqueous zones, and their meningeal permeability coefficients are correspondingly greater (e.g., alfentanil, hydromorphone, meperidine) (22). These physical and chemical properties of the opioids will also determine vascular permeability. Opioids with high octanol/buffer distribution coefficients, such as fentanyl and sufentanil move more easily to the intravascular compartment than to the subarachnoid compartment. In this way spinal cord concentrations of an opioid following epidural administration are the result of the net difference between the rate of uptake and distribution to the vascular and subarachnoid spaces. These differences explain why morphine, despite having a meningeal permeability coefficient similar to fentanyl and sufentanil, which are well below the optimal range of meningeal penetration, is a useful agent for epidural analgesia.

Bernards and Hill also showed with their in vitro model that the octanol/buffer distribution coefficient for sufentanil was beyond the range of optimal meningeal permeability.

Respiratory depression somnolence and pruritus appear to be associated with the degree of rostral migration of the opioid in the CSF (8,22,23). The timing for the appearance of these side effects varies between lipophilic and hydrophilic opioids after epidural administration. Morphine's rostral migration is a phenomenon which is dose dependent and follows a predictable time course (23). In contrast, rostral migration as determined by the onset of upper body analgesia (24) and the incidence of respiratory depression after a lumbar epidural bolus of lipid soluble opioids is unpredictable. Gourlay et al. (25) demonstrated that peak

TABLE 13-1 Octanol/buffer Coefficients, Meningeal Permeability Coefficients, and Minimum Effective Analgesic Concentrations (MEAC) for Opioids

Opioids	Octanol/buffer Distribution Coefficient	Meningeal Permeability Coefficient[a]	MEAC[b] (ng/mL)
Morphine	1[67]	0.6[9]	30.00[8]
Meperidine	525[68]	NA	455.00[9]
Hydromorphone	525[67]	NA	4.00
Fentanyl	955[67]	0.9[9]	0.60[66]
Sufentanil	1737[67]	0.75[9]	0.04[31]
Alfentanil	129[67]	2.3[9]	41.00[52]
Bupivacaine	560[9]	1.6[9]	Nap

[a]cm/min × 10^{-3}.
[b]MEAC represents a range of plasma levels and not a specific value. MEAC plasma levels may vary up to fivefold between different individuals with time and activity in a patient. The values depicted in this table are the values more frequently utilized.
NA, data not available.
Nap, not applicable.

cervical CSF concentrations of fentanyl occurred as early as 10 minutes after lumbar epidural administration and averaged 10% of the peak lumbar CSF concentrations. However, in two of the six patients, peak cervical CSF concentrations were twice the level found in the rest of the patients. In another study, sufentanil concentrations were measured after 72 hours of a continuous infusion of 14 µg/h via a low thoracic epidural catheter (26). Sufentanil concentrations in plasma and the cisterna magna CSF were 56% and 82% respectively the concentrations measured in the lumbar CSF. Lipophilic opioids also exhibit rostral migration, but in a less predictable manner than morphine. This difference suggests that the same level of care used for monitoring respiratory depression after epidural administration of morphine should also be utilized when lipophilic opioids are administered for postoperative epidural analgesia. The American Society of Anesthesiologists Task Force has published specific guidelines for the prevention, detection, and management of respiratory depression associated with neuraxial opioid administration (27).

The octanol/buffer partition coefficients and meningeal permeability coefficients for several opioids are presented in Table 13-1.

◾ NEURAXIAL ANALGESIA FOR CESAREAN DELIVERY

More than 90% of cesarean deliveries in the United States are performed under regional anesthesia. Similarly, data from the United Kingdom shows that regional anesthesia is used for 94.9% of elective and 86.7% of emergent cesarean deliveries (28).

The first report of intraspinal opioid administration in humans occurred in 1979. Since then, neuraxial administration of opioids has become a popular technique for postoperative analgesia. It has been reported that more than 90% of obstetric anesthesiologists administer subarachnoid or epidural opioids to parturients undergoing cesarean deliveries under spinal, epidural or CSE (5,29,30). Administration of subarachnoid or epidural opioids offer several advantages to parturients recovering from cesarean delivery. These include excellent postoperative analgesia with a decrease in total dose of opioid required, a low level of sedation, minimal accumulation of the drug in breast milk, facilitation of early ambulation, and early return of bowel function.

◾ INTRATHECAL OPIOIDS

Opioids, especially preservative-free morphine, are central to many intrathecal-based analgesic regimens. They appear to act principally on MOP receptors in the substantia gelatinosa of the dorsal horn by suppressing the release of excitatory neuropeptides from C fibers (31). Lipid solubility of the individual drug determines the degree of uptake from the CSF by the dorsal horn. Lipid soluble drugs like fentanyl or sufentanil enjoy greater direct diffusion into neural tissue as well as greater delivery to the dorsal horn by spinal segmental arteries. Highly soluble fentanyl, for instance, has a relatively rapid uptake into the lipid-rich dorsal horn and consequently has a swift onset of action but a short duration. Studies that measure 24-hour opioid consumption confirm its limitations for adequate postoperative analgesia (32). The short analgesic duration of action of fentanyl contrasts with the long duration from morphine, which is less lipid soluble and so takes longer to penetrate neural tissues. A significant drawback, however, is the longer time that morphine resides within the CSF, allowing it to spread rostrally and from which complications such as respiratory depression arise (33).

Intrathecal Morphine

Morphine was the first opioid approved by the United States Food and Drug Administration (US FDA) for intraspinal administration. Morphine is highly ionized and hydrophilic and does not penetrate lipid-rich tissues as rapidly as fentanyl. Morphine remains within the CSF for a prolonged period of time, spreading rostrally and reaching the trigeminal nerve distribution as early as 3 hours after intrathecal injection in healthy volunteers (24). Morphine requires 45 to 60 minutes to achieve a peak effect, and the duration of analgesia is 14 to 36 hours. This duration may be dose dependent. A variety of intrathecal morphine doses have been investigated. No clear dose–response relationship has been demonstrated using doses greater than 100 µg. Palmer et al. studied patients receiving intrathecal doses from 25 to 500 µg and found a ceiling effect with doses greater than 75 µg, as measured by patient-controlled intravenous morphine use (34). Higher doses conferred no additional analgesic benefit but caused a dose-dependent increase in side effects, particularly pruritus. Palmer et al. also noted that despite high doses of intrathecal morphine, most parturients continued to administer additional opioid analgesia at a low but constant rate, possibly explaining the interaction between spinal and supraspinal sites of action.

Yang et al. administered 100 or 250 μg of morphine as a component of spinal anesthesia to 60 women undergoing elective cesarean delivery. Women also received 20 μg of spinal fentanyl and perioperative and postoperative nonsteroidal anti-inflammatory drugs (NSAIDs) routinely. There was no significant difference between the small- and large-dose morphine groups in pain relief, as measured by visual analog pain scores (35). Adverse effects of intrathecal morphine have been reported widely and include pruritus, nausea and vomiting, urinary retention, and early or delayed respiratory depression. The most common side effect, pruritus, increased in severity as morphine doses increased. If a morphine dose of 100 μg is used, it is estimated that 43% of women will experience pruritus, and 12% will experience nausea and vomiting (33). Neuraxial morphine administration has also been linked to reactivation of oral herpes simplex. In a study of women with a past history of oral herpes simplex, reactivation occurred in 38% receiving intrathecal morphine compared with 16% of those receiving intravenous morphine (36).

Respiratory depression is an uncommon but potentially serious side effect, though the incidence in the obstetric population is difficult to determine. Abouleish et al. studied 856 parturients who received 200 μg of intrathecal morphine during cesarean delivery and found respiratory depression, as defined by SpO_2 <85% or respiratory rate of less than 10 breaths per minute, in eight patients (0.93%), all of whom were obese (37). The physiologic changes of pregnancy, specifically the higher respiratory rate associated with elevated progesterone levels, may provide a greater margin of safety in comparison to other patient populations. It should be noted however that smaller dosages of intrathecal morphine (75 μg) therapy may result in a reduced duration of analgesia and may therefore require an increased need for supplemental analgesics. Also, due to the variability in patient response to intrathecal morphine, some patients may additionally experience inadequate postoperative analgesia and/or opioid-related side effects.

Intrathecal Fentanyl

Fentanyl is arguably one of the most commonly administered intrathecal opioids worldwide. Its relative high lipid solubility results in a greater restriction of segmental activity and rapid onset of action when compared to morphine. Although intrathecal fentanyl offers a relatively short duration of analgesia, it is shown to improve intraoperative analgesia, especially during uterine exteriorization, and provides the patient with a better postoperative transition to other pain medications during recovery from spinal anesthesia. Shende et al. performed a randomized study where 40 healthy patients scheduled for elective cesarean delivery were randomly allocated to receive either saline or 15 μg of fentanyl added to 2.5 mL of hyperbaric bupivacaine intrathecally. They found that the fentanyl group had significantly improved intraoperative analgesia and a longer block regression time. (38). Chu et al. looked at 75 women undergoing elective cesarean delivery and randomized them to receive intrathecally bupivacaine 5 mg alone, or bupivacaine with 7.5, 10, 12.5 or 15 μg of fentanyl. They found that with increasing doses of fentanyl, surgical analgesia was improved and postoperative analgesia lasted longer. They concluded that a ceiling effect was reached at a dose of 12.5 μg. (39). Intrathecal fentanyl also may offer a longer-term analgesic benefit when administered alongside a local anesthetic at the time of cesarean

delivery (40). In contrast to morphine, intrathecal fentanyl does not appear to predispose the patient to nausea and vomiting following cesarean delivery. Fentanyl has been shown to cause pruritus in a dose-related manner, though less severely than morphine (32). The risk of delayed respiratory depression is relatively small with intrathecal fentanyl given its segmental effect and lack of rostral spread. A recent large-scale meta-analysis resulted in no reported cases of respiratory depression associated with intrathecal fentanyl at cesarean delivery (33). If respiratory depression does occur however, it usually tends to manifest within the first 30 minutes.

Intrathecal Sufentanil

Sufentanil is a thienyl derivative of fentanyl but has higher potency due to greater lipid solubility. The octanol:water partition coefficient of sufentanil is 1,778 and is 91% protein bound. Fentanyl has an octanol:water partition coefficient 813 with protein binding 84%, illustrating the differences in pharmacokinetics. Intrathecal sufentanil offers some theoretical advantages over fentanyl including faster onset, reduced rostral spread, and a lower level of placental transfer. Several studies have been performed comparing fentanyl and sufentanil for analgesia for caesarean delivery and have found them to be equivalent but those women in the sufentanil groups experienced more pruritus (41–43). The optimal dose of sufentanil in the subarachnoid space is less than 5 μg with side effects (particularly pruritus) occurring in a dose-dependent manner (44).

Alternative Intrathecal Opioids

Other less-commonly used intrathecal opioids include meperidine, diamorphine, buprenorphine, and, nalbuphine. Meperidine is the only member of the opioid family with local anesthetic-like effects and it has a tendency to sometimes result in motor block. Meperidine has historically been used as a sole spinal drug for cesarean delivery (45).

Diamorphine (3,6-diacetylmorphine) also known as morphine diacetate is a semisynthetic opioid produced by acetylation of morphine. The administration of neuraxial diamorphine for the treatment of pain relief after cesarean section is a common practice in the United Kingdom (46). In contrast, in the United States diamorphine is unavailable for clinical use. Diamorphine has many of the ideal physicochemical properties to provide good pain relief after surgery with the potential to decrease side effects. The intermediate lipid solubility of diamorphine (oil/water partition coefficient 280), increases permeability to both hydrophobic and hydrophilic tissue compartments when compared either with morphine or fentanyl. Diamorphine undergoes metabolism within spinal cord tissue, generating active compounds (6-acetylmorphine and morphine) which increases the analgesic effects, these metabolites are less lipid soluble than the parent drug, that limit their back diffusion into the CSF. Other important physicochemical characteristics of diamorphine are lower PKa (PKa 7.8), low protein binding (40%), and a high unionized fraction (27%) that increases the bioavailability for opioid receptors within the spinal cord and increases clearance from CSF decreasing the potential for serious side effects, such as respiratory depression (47). There is a wealth of data on the use and safety of diamorphine for cesarean delivery in the literature. Cowan et al. looked at 74 parturients for elective cesarean delivery who were randomized to receive either 20 μg fentanyl or 300 μg diamorphine intrathecally using hyperbaric bupivacaine (48). The authors looked at supplemental intraoperative analgesia requirements and found no difference between the groups. When they looked at postoperative analgesia requirements they found that the diamorphine group had reduced visual analog scale (VAS) scores 12 hours postoperatively but fentanyl reduced VAS only 1 hour postoperatively. They found no difference in pruritus postoperatively between the opioid groups.

There have been three well-reported, dose-finding studies looking at intrathecal diamorphine doses for cesarean delivery (49–51). Skilton et al. and Kelly et al. looked at doses up to 0.375 mg and found improved analgesia (as determined by the amount of rescue analgesia required) as the dose increased without a ceiling effect. (49,50). Stacey et al. randomly allocated 40 women undergoing elective caesarean delivery to receive either 0.5 mg or 1 mg of intrathecal diamorphine intrathecally. They found the time to rescue analgesia and 24-hour morphine consumption was significantly lower in the 1 mg group (45% using no opioids postoperatively at all) and that pain scores in this group tended to be lower. Minor side effects were found to be present in both groups but incidence did not differ between groups (51).

■ EPIDURAL OPIOIDS

Morphine

Palmer et al. performed a dose–response study looking at 0 to 5 mg epidural morphine on postcesarean pain and found a ceiling effect in terms of analgesia. They found no difference in cumulative systemic morphine use above 3.75 mg used epidurally. 3 mg of morphine epidurally appeared equivalent to 100 μg intrathecally and was found to provide analgesia for 12 to 24 hours (52). There are several studies in the literature comparing epidural and intrathecal morphine for postcesarean analgesia. Sarvela et al. performed a double-blinded, RCT comparing 3 mg epidural morphine with either 100 μg or 200 μg intrathecal morphine and found no significant differences in pain scores. However, rescue analgesia was requested more frequently in the 100 μg group suggesting this dose was less effective for postcesarean analgesia and perhaps unsurprisingly this group were shown to have less pruritus (53).

Due to its prolonged analgesic effects epidural morphine can be administered as an intermittent bolus or as a continuous infusion. It appears that some clinical advantages in using continuous epidural morphine infusions over intermittent bolus for epidural analgesia exist. Studies in the non-obstetric population evaluating morphine's cephalad migration after a lumbar epidural bolus suggest that respiratory depression may occur as a result of significant amount of the drug reaching the respiratory center in the brain stem after the administration of a bolus dose in the lumbar epidural area (22,23). In fact, large-scale studies suggest that respiratory depression requiring treatment may be higher with intermittent bolus than with continuous infusions (54,55). When mean doses between 7 to 13 mg/d were utilized in the intermittent bolus group and mean doses of 6 to 14 mg/d were used in the continuous infusion group, the incidence of respiratory depression was different. In the bolus study group, the incidence of respiratory depression was 1:500 (54). In contrast, in the continuous infusion group, the incidence was 1:1,500 (55). Based on these data, in the non-obstetric population the maximum risk of respiratory depression within the 95% confidence intervals are 1:100 versus 1:5,000 respectively. Moreover, the concurrent use of parenteral opioids for breakthrough pain, a practice which has been discouraged when intermittent dosing of epidural morphine is used (23), may be administered without an increased risk of delayed respiratory depression even on the surgical wards (54).

Interestingly, the quality of analgesia appears to be more complete when utilizing continuous infusions compared with an intermittent bolus. A study evaluating the quality of analgesia produced by epidural morphine administered either as bolus doses or via continuous infusion demonstrated that patients who received continuous infusion of epidural morphine experienced a higher quality of analgesia than those who received intermittent bolus injections (56). Based on apparent greater clinical efficacy and a lower incidence of respiratory depression it would appear that patients would derive a greater benefit from receiving epidural morphine via a continuous infusion. A recent systematic review of ten studies comparing analgesia efficacy and/or adverse effects of a single epidural morphine administration versus systemic opioids after elective cesarean delivery proved that a single bolus of epidural morphine provides better analgesia than parenteral opioids but with an effect limited to the first postoperative day after cesarean delivery and with an increase in side effects (57). Based on this study and others, the general practice is to use 3 mg of preservative-free morphine in the epidural space.

Hydromorphone

The quality of analgesia experienced after hydromorphone administration appears to be similar to that produced by morphine (58). Based on unpublished clinical observations, a ratio of 5:1 between morphine and hydromorphone has been utilized when administering the drug in a bolus form, and a ratio of 3:1 has been recommended for continuous infusions (58). Hydromorphone appears to have a faster onset and shorter duration of action than morphine with a lower incidence of pruritus.

Fentanyl

Fentanyl, which has a high octanol/buffer coefficient, appears to undergo preferential vascular absorption than meningeal penetration after epidural administration. In fact, the value of utilizing fentanyl for epidural analgesia is controversial. Several studies have demonstrated that the quality of analgesia, the incidence of side effects, daily fentanyl utilization, and plasma levels after 24 hours of infusion are similar between patients receiving either epidural or intravenous therapy after cesarean delivery (59–62).

Sevarino et al. performed a double-blinded, randomized study on 40 ASA I/II women undergoing elective cesarean delivery under lidocaine epidural anesthesia who received after delivery either saline or 100 μg fentanyl through the epidural catheter (63). All patients were provided with an intravenous meperidine patient-controlled analgesia (PCA) postoperatively and it was noted that no differences in PCA use were recorded between the groups. The authors concluded that a single bolus of fentanyl does not provide an advantage for postoperative pain relief in this patient population.

Ginosar et al. examined the hypothesis that in the presence of epidural bupivacaine, continuous infusions of epidural fentanyl elicit analgesia by a spinal mechanism (64). They performed a prospective, randomized, double-blinded study in which women in active labor received epidural bupivacaine until pain free. The women were then randomized to receive either IV or epidural fentanyl infusions. It was found that an equivalent dose of fentanyl was more than three times as potent when administered epidurally than by the intravenous route, suggesting a predominantly spinal mechanism of opioid action.

Sufentanil

Just like fentanyl, sufentanil produces analgesia via both spinal and supraspinal effects (65–67). Studies comparing postoperative analgesia with IV or epidural sufentanil have shown that both the quality of analgesia, and plasma levels are similar after either route of administration. However, the incidence of respiratory depression (judged by high CO_2 levels in 6/26 vs. 1/24 patients) (68) and sedation (in 4/15 vs. 0/15 patients) (66) appears to be greater in the IV group.

Grass et al. performed a randomized, double-blinded study comparing epidural fentanyl versus sufentanil analgesia after cesarean delivery. Eighty women undergoing elective cesarean delivery with epidural 2% lidocaine with epinephrine received either fentanyl (25, 50, 100, or 200 μg) or sufentanil (5, 10, 20, or 30 μg) when they experienced pain. Visual analogue and sedation scores were used to assess response. A dose–response relationship was demonstrated for both opioids with fentanyl 100 and 200 μg and sufentanil 20 and 30 μg all achieving VAS scores of <10 mm with no difference in the time to 50% reduction of VAS. They suggested that the 50% and 95% effective doses for each opioids to achieve a VAS score of <10 mm were 33 μg and 92 μg fentanyl respectively and 6.7 and 17.5 μg of sufentanil respectively. They found no differences in the onset, duration, and effectiveness of analgesia where equianalgesia doses were administered postoperatively (69).

■ LOCAL ANESTHETIC/OPIOID COMBINATIONS

Clinically, the objectives of coadministering epidural opioids with subanesthetic concentrations of local anesthetics are important for three reasons: (1) Reduction in the dose of both drugs is achieved, (2) maintenance or enhancement of the degree of pain relief is realized, and (3) reduction in the incidence of adverse effects produced by both opioids and/or local anesthetics is experienced. Chestnut and collaborators have demonstrated that these three goals could be achieved when fentanyl, 2 μg/mL was added to 0.0625% bupivacaine (70). They reported that the quality of analgesia was comparable while the degree of motor blockade was less with bupivacaine/fentanyl than when 0.125% bupivacaine was administered alone. Since the concentrations of fentanyl and bupivacaine used in this study are below the doses needed to achieve analgesia when either of these two agents are used alone, their results suggest potentiation between the two drugs. However, this study was performed in a laboring population making their conclusions not applicable to the surgical population due to the high levels of progesterone seen in these patients.

By administering lower doses of epidural opioids, the incidence of side effects may be lower than that experienced with the intravenous route. However, properly conducted dose-ranging studies in humans to determine the ideal equimolar ratios between opioids and local anesthetics have not been performed. It is important to note that the equimolar ratio at which the opioid and the local anesthetic are administered is important. Tejwani et al. found that the enhancement of spinal morphine antinociception produced by bupivacaine is dose dependent (71). Although increasing the binding of morphine to kappa opioid receptors is its most prominent effect, the binding of opioid ligands to all spinal receptors is inhibited at high doses of bupivacaine. It may be important to consider this limitation when coadministering epidural local anesthetics and opioids.

■ SINGLE-DOSE EXTENDED-RELEASE EPIDURAL MORPHINE

The goal of current postoperative pain research and development is to find a medication that can work locally to give long-lasting pain relief at the site of surgical focus with as little negative impact as possible. Single-dose, extended-release epidural morphine (EREM) (DepoDur, Endo Pharmaceuticals, Chadds Ford, PA) is a recently developed drug that delivers conventional morphine sulfate using DepoFoam (SkypePharma, San Diego, CA) technology. DepoFoam is a revolutionary drug delivery system containing multivesicular lipid particles comprised of nonconcentric aqueous chambers that fully encapsulate the active drug. These naturally occurring lipids are broken down by erosion and reorganization, resulting in a locally contained morphine depository for up to 48 hours after a single administration (72).

Clinical studies within the obstetric population show EREM's postoperative analgesia consistently extending into the second day with no significant side effects. This is of notable benefit as a single dose of neuraxial morphine would lose its efficacy in this time frame and peak postcesarean delivery pain levels are not typically reached until 24 to 48 hours following surgery (73). When an EREM dosage of 10 mg was compared to that of a standard 4 mg dose of epidural morphine, the supplemental opioid dose usage during 24 to 48 hours postoperatively was significantly decreased by 60% in patients receiving EREM. In addition, no significant differences in the occurrence of nausea, pruritus, sedation, respiratory depression or hypoxic events were observed between these two groups. In September 2009, the FDA approved safety labeling revisions for morphine sulfate extended-release liposome injection (DepoDur) to emphasize the need for individualized dosing adjustments, as well as the need for monitoring capabilities, resuscitative equipment, and opioid antagonist availability. When EREM is given correctly in the epidural space, monitoring should be continued for up to 48 hours. While the prolonged analgesic effect during the first 48 hours is quite attractive, this advantage must be weighed against the potential disadvantages associated with EREM administration including the instability of Lipofoam in the presence of local anesthetics, the need for prolonged monitoring of patients following its administration, and the cost of the formulation (74).

Clinical trials have demonstrated the efficacy of EREM for postoperative pain relief following hip arthroplasty (75) and elective cesarean delivery (76). Recent pharmacokinetic data obtained by Gambling et al. have described the effective use of EREM following injection of an epidural anesthetic (77). They designed a controlled, dose-ranging study of 144 patients administered EREM for analgesia following lower abdominal surgery. The authors observed that the best balance of maximum analgesia with the lowest occurrence of side effects was achieved by administration of 15 mg of EREM and as such recommended that a multimodal pain management approach—such as the addition of a NSAID to the regimen—could further reduce the dose required to provide effective analgesia and concomitantly the occurrence of adverse side effects.

Benefits of Neuraxial Techniques

Using random sampling to evaluate mortality and major morbidity outcomes in high-risk patients undergoing non-obstetric surgeries, the Multicentre Australian Study of Epidural Anaesthesia and Analgesia in Major Surgery (MASTER) trial is the largest prospective study to date comparing epidural and PCA for postoperative analgesia (78). Of the seven predefined major morbidity complications assessed in this study, respiratory failure was the only outcome with a lower incidence in the epidural infusion group than in the PCA group. An extensive retrospective cohort study performed over a 15-year period assessed 30-day mortality in over 250,000 intermediate- and high-risk patients having non-cardiac surgery and treated with either epidural infusion or systemic analgesics for postoperative pain management. While the researchers described a significant reduction in mortality in the epidural group, the small sample size limited its applicability and specific morbidity complications were not detailed. However, the proportion of patients requiring mechanical ventilation postoperatively was similar between the two groups (79).

Neuraxial analgesic techniques appear more likely to reduce perioperative morbidity in high-risk obstetric patients than systemic analgesic techniques. The benefits include a lower rate of perioperative cardiovascular complications, a lowered incidence of pulmonary infections and pulmonary embolism, a faster return of gastrointestinal function, fewer coagulation disturbances, and reduction in inflammatory and stress responses to surgery (80). Other indirect benefits include the mother's ability to ambulate and interact with her infant after cesarean delivery by negating the need for a general anesthetic (17).

Patient-controlled Analgesia (PCA)

Different opioids can be delivered utilizing a PCA pump, including fentanyl, morphine, and hydromorphone. It is usually used for those patients who did not receive any neuraxial opioids such as in cesarean delivery under general anesthesia and in whom potent analgesia via the intravenous route is required.

Cooper et al. performed a randomized, double-blinded controlled trail to compare epidural fentanyl and patient-controlled IV morphine after cesarean delivery in 84 patients (81). All patients received an epidural and IV PCA device. PCA use was found to be less in the epidural fentanyl group and there was also less nausea and drowsiness in this group. There was no difference in pruritus between the groups.

A study by Howell et al. compared PCA fentanyl with PCA morphine for postcesarean delivery analgesia (82). Both analgesic solutions provided effective analgesia for a mean of 37 hours postoperatively with high levels of patient satisfaction with no differences in VAS pain scores between groups. However, more patients in the fentanyl group required supplementary boluses or alterations to the PCA settings and one patient in this group had to be removed from the study due to inadequate analgesia. The authors concluded that morphine PCA should be used in preference to fentanyl PCA for routine use after cesarean delivery.

PCA, which permits the patient to self-administer small doses of opioid analgesic intravenously at frequent intervals, often provides effective and sustained analgesia after major surgery. PCA is associated with all the usual opioid-related side effects, including potentially lethal respiratory depression, so we recommend close monitoring including continuous pulse oximetry and frequent nursing assessments.

Multimodal Analgesia

The concept of multimodal analgesia was first proposed in the mid-1990s and is now well established in clinical practice. It is based on the recognition that acute postoperative pain is rarely purely nociceptive pain. More likely, there are components of neuropathic, visceral, and inflammatory pain, as well as muscle spasms. Thus, appropriate management requires a balanced approach using multiple agents that act in different ways and at different sites (Figs. 13-3 and 13-4). By using multiple agents, it is possible to reduce the doses of any single drug, improve analgesia by the additive or synergistic effects, and reduce the dose effects that occur when using a single drug. For example, nonsteroidal anti-inflammatory medications combined with intravenous patient-controlled

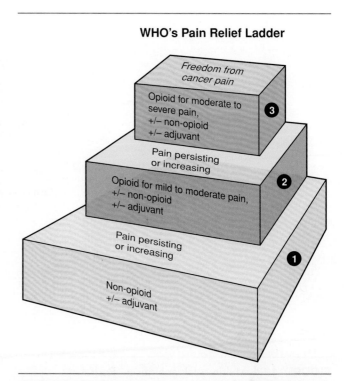

FIGURE 13-3 World Health Organization (WHO) analgesic ladder. Copyright© 2012 WHO. Reprinted with permission.

morphine administration may decrease nausea and sedation in patients when compared with those using patient-controlled morphine alone (83). Different classes of analgesics with different routes of administration (i.e., intravenous vs. epidural methods) are used to produce fewer side effects such as sedation, nausea, vomiting, pruritus, and constipation, and also improve pain relief. Multimodal analgesia also produces opioid sparing and helps to speed recovery, reduce hospital stay, and decrease length of convalescence. A multimodal approach is therefore critical for effective pain management. The development of newer agents for postoperative pain control provides for more effective combinations in multimodal analgesia (84) which emphasize the differences between routes of administration of opioid and non-opioid analgesics, neuraxial techniques, neuraxial adjuncts, wound infiltration, and nerve blocks.

Opioids and epidurals have been described before. Other types of regional anesthetics used for obstetric or gynecologic surgery include rectus abdominis sheath block and transversus abdominis plane (TAP) block. These can be performed at the bedside either blind or now, more frequently, with the aid of ultrasound to direct the needle to the correct location and see the local anesthetic spread. Both of these blocks help reduce the perceived pain originating from the abdominal wall after surgery.

■ TRANSVERSUS ABDOMINIS PLANE BLOCK

The TAP block is performed by introducing local anesthetics into the plane between the fascia of the transversus abdominis muscle and the internal oblique muscle. It is possible to block the sensory nerves of the anterior abdominal wall before they leave this plane and pierce the musculature to innervate the anterior abdominal wall (Fig. 13-5). Using an ultrasound to localize this fascial plane, you can guide and direct the advancement of

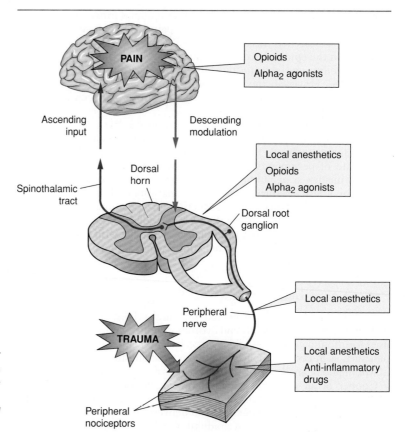

FIGURE 13-4 Multimodal analgesia. Redrawn with permission from: Kehlet H, Dahl JB. The value of "multimodal" or "balanced analgesia" in postoperative pain treatment. *Anesth Analg* 1993;77(5):1049.

a needle to the desired location and then watch the spread of the injectate along the correct fascial plane. Duration of action is dependent on the type of local anesthetic used and if prolonged analgesia is needed a catheter for continuous infusion can also be placed using ultrasound imaging.

There are a number of studies in the literature looking at TAP blocks for analgesia after cesarean delivery. McDonnell et al. randomized 50 women to receive either bilateral TAP blocks with 0.75% ropivacaine or saline placebo (85). They found that the median time to the first morphine request was extended from 90 to 220 minutes in the TAP group. The TAP group were also found to have lower morphine requirements in the first 48 hours postoperatively and a corresponding reduction in sedation and nausea. However, not all studies

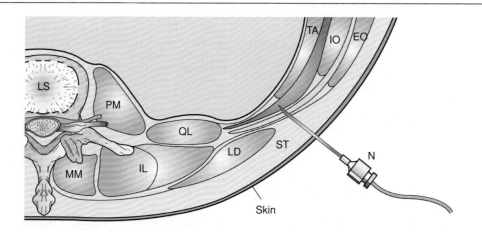

FIGURE 13-5 Transversus abdominis plane block. The floor of the triangle is composed, from superficial to deep, of the fascial extensions of external oblique, internal oblique, and transversus abdominis, respectively, and the peritoneum. The needle is inserted through the triangle, using the loss-of-resistance technique. The needle is shown in the transversus abdominis plane, and the fascial layers have separated as a result of the injection of local anesthetic. *LS,* lumbar spine; *LD,* latissimus dorsi; *PM,* psoas major; *QL,* quadratus lumborum; *MM,* multifidus muscle; *IL,* longissimus iliocostalis; *TA,* transversus abdominis; *IO,* internal oblique; *EO,* external oblique; *ST,* subcutaneous tissue. Reprinted with permission from: Carney, J, McDonnell JG, Ochana A, et al. The transversus abdominis plane block provides effective postoperative analgesia in patients undergoing total abdominal hysterectomy. *Anesth Analg* 2008;107(6):2056–2060.

have confirmed this finding. Belavy et al. performed a similar study which showed a decrease in postoperative intravenous opioid use between groups (86) but no difference in pain scores whereas Costello et al. found no difference between groups in either opioid use or pain scores with the additional TAP block (87). McMorrow et al. compared the TAP block to intrathecal morphine for analgesia postcesarean delivery (88). They randomized 80 patients to one of the four groups to receive (in addition to spinal anesthesia) either spinal morphine 100 μg or saline and a postoperative bilateral TAP block with either 2 mg/kg bupivacaine or saline. Pain on movement and early morphine consumption were lowest in the groups receiving spinal morphine and were not improved by TAP block. From these studies it would seem reasonable to conclude that TAP blocks should not be used in preference to neuraxial opioids for postcesarean analgesia and should probably be reserved for a parturient undergoing general anesthesia.

■ WOUND INFILTRATION

There has been recent interest in wound infiltration using both local anesthetic and NSAIDs. Results after general abdominal surgery are mixed probably due to differences in the site of catheter placement, the drugs used, and the outcome with continuous versus bolus techniques. A Cochrane review in 2009 looked at 20 studies involving local anesthetic wound infiltration during cesarean deliveries and found that:

1. Local anesthetic infiltration and abdominal nerve blocks as adjuncts to regional and general anesthesia are of benefit by reducing opioid consumption;
2. NSAIDS as an adjuvant in the local anesthetic mixture may confer additional pain relief (89).

Lavand'homme et al. found that diclofenac alone via a wound infusion catheter decreases 48-hour morphine requirements compared with ropivacaine infusion or intravenous diclofenac, suggesting that diclofenac may have peripheral analgesic properties in addition to its systemic effects (90). Further studies are required to assess local anesthetic infusions and NSAIDs on outcomes beyond analgesic efficacy such as wound healing and the formation of adhesions.

Oral Opioids and Adjuvant Analgesics

Once patients are tolerating an oral diet, analgesics are given via the oral route as a convenient "step-down" after primary management with neuraxial or intravenous opioids as part of a multimodal regimen.

Common regimens used include the following:

Hydrocodone (dihydrocodeine) + acetaminophen (paracetamol)
Oxycodone + acetaminophen
Hydromorphone
Oxycodone
Oral morphine

There are a number of studies looking at these regimens in the literature. Davis et al. performed an RCT comparing intravenous patient-controlled morphine with oral oxycodone–acetaminophen after cesarean delivery (91). They assessed pain at 6 and 24 hours after delivery and found that the oral group experienced less pain at both time intervals. They also found that this group had less nausea and drowsiness at 6 hours but slightly more nausea at 24 hours. Another study by Jakobi et al. assessed patient satisfaction with oral analgesia following cesarean delivery and found that it provided

satisfactory pain relief, was easily administered and was substantially less expensive compared to intravenous methods of analgesia (92).

Acetaminophen (Paracetamol)

Alhashemi et al. compared the effects of IV acetaminophen with those of oral ibuprofen with respect to pain control and morphine requirements in patients receiving PCA morphine after cesarean delivery (93). They measured both VAS scores and patient satisfaction. VAS scores were found to decrease similarly in both groups over time however there were no differences between groups at any time. Patient satisfaction was high in both groups. They concluded that IV acetaminophen was a reasonable adjunct to IV PCA morphine. There have been surprisingly few trials looking at acetaminophen alone after cesarean delivery. Munishankar et al. compared oral acetaminophen, diclofenac, or the combination for pain relief after cesarean in a double-blinded, RCT of acetaminophen (94). Patients given the combination of diclofenac and acetaminophen required 38% less morphine than patients given acetaminophen alone. Morphine use in patients given diclofenac alone was not significantly different from morphine use in the other two groups. Nauta et al. performed a systematic review of randomized trials comparing a combination of codeine–acetaminophen versus NSAIDs in the treatment of postoperative abdominal pain (95). They found that none of the studies showed the codeine–acetaminophen to be superior to NSAIDs in controlling post-laparotomy pain and that fewer adverse effects were reported in the NSAID group. There are currently no similar studies that have been performed in obstetric patients.

Non-steroidal Anti-inflammatory Drugs
Diclofenac Sodium

This is an NSAID commonly used to treat pain, inflammatory disorders, dysmenorrhea, endometriosis, and mild to moderate postoperative or post-traumatic pain. As with similar NSAIDs, it predisposes to gastrointestinal bleeding but is amongst the better tolerated NSAIDs. It has anti-inflammatory, antipyretic, and analgesic action due to the inhibition of prostaglandin synthesis by inhibition of cyclooxygenase. There is some evidence that diclofenac inhibits lipoxygenase pathways, thus reducing leukotriene formation and may also inhibit phospholipase A_2. These actions may explain the high potency of diclofenac—it is the most potent NSAID on a broad basis (96). Approximately half of the diclofenac dose is metabolized during first pass hepatic metabolism. 60% is excreted renally, with 1% unchanged in the urine. Diclofenac has been classified as FDA category B in the first two trimesters but pregnancy risk category D if used in the third trimester or near delivery.

Diclofenac has been shown previously to confer significant pain relief when used in combination with acetaminophen. Mitra et al. compared this combination with a diclofenac–tramadol combination when considering pain relief after cesarean section in a randomized, double-blinded parallel-group controlled trial involving 204 parturients (97). They found both combinations to provide satisfactory postoperative pain relief after cesarean section. The diclofenac–tramadol combination was overall more efficacious but associated with a higher incidence of postoperative nausea.

Celecoxib

Celecoxib is an NSAID indicated for osteoarthritis and primary dysmenorrhea, among other pain conditions. Celecoxib, as with all NSAIDs, has analgesic, antipyretic, and anti-inflammatory properties. Celecoxib works by selectively inhibiting the cyclooxygenase-2 (COX-2) enzyme, which is involved in prostaglandin synthesis as part of the inflammatory response pathway. COX-2-specific inhibition both reduces the risk of gastrointestinal adverse events and lacks effect on platelet aggregation, in comparison to nonselective cyclooxygenase inhibitors (that block both the COX-1 and COX-2 enzymes), such as naproxen or ibuprofen. Celecoxib is supplied as 50 mg, 100 mg, 200 mg, and 400 mg capsules. It is metabolized hepatically and thus dosage adjustments must be made in those with impairment in hepatic function. It should be used with great caution in those with renal insufficiency, as NSAIDs may decrease renal perfusion. It is a Pregnancy Category C drug prior to 30 weeks gestation and Pregnancy Category D drug starting at 30 weeks gestation. Therefore in late gestation, celecoxib should be avoided as it may cause premature closure of the ductus arteriosus. Celecoxib should not be used in those with sulfa allergy. Celecoxib carries an FDA black box warning for possible increased risk of serious cardiovascular and gastrointestinal adverse events.

Celecoxib has been used in the perioperative period as an adjuvant analgesic since it has the advantage over nonselective NSAIDs of not inhibiting platelet aggregation, although there is questionable effect on bone healing.

A Cochrane review evaluated the efficacy of a single dose of oral celecoxib for postoperative pain (98). Eight trials were included. A 200 mg dose of celecoxib was as effective as 600/650 mg of aspirin and 1,000 mg of acetaminophen for relieving postoperative pain. A dose of 400 mg of celecoxib was as effective as 400 mg of ibuprofen. Adverse event rates were similar with celecoxib and placebo. The conclusion of the study was that a single dose of celecoxib was effective for postoperative pain relief. A 400 mg dose was recommended for acute pain.

Ketorolac

Ketorolac is an NSAID indicated for short-term use (5 days or less due to gastric ulceration, bleeding, and perforation risk) in managing moderate-to-severe acute pain. It is thought to inhibit prostaglandin synthetase, thereby exerting analgesic, anti-pyretic, and anti-inflammatory effects. Routes of administration are oral, IV, or IM. When given intravenously, usual adult dosing is 15 to 30 mg IV every 6 hours, with a maximum of 120 mg in 24 hours. Side effects and adverse effects are similar to other NSAIDs. It is a Pregnancy Category C drug and is not recommended during breastfeeding.

Ketorolac has been evaluated as a perioperative analgesic, as it appears to have greater potency (similar to opioids) than other NSAIDs and an opioid-sparing effect. El-Tahan et al. studied the effect of preoperative ketorolac for cesarean delivery, randomly assigning 90 patients to receive either IV ketorolac bolus at 15 mg prior to induction followed by infusion at 7.5 mg/h, or saline placebo (99). The results showed, in part, that 15.6% of patients in the ketorolac group requested postoperative tramadol for analgesia, compared with 31.1% in the control group. The conclusion was that prophylactic ketorolac improved analgesia after cesarean delivery. A randomized, controlled trial by Lowder et al. compared ketorolac with placebo after cesarean section in 44 patients (100). The ketorolac group was found to have significantly reduced morphine IV PCA requirements at 24 hours compared to the control group. It was concluded that ketorolac reduced opioid usage and reduced postoperative pain. Another study was performed by Tzeng and Mok to determine the analgesic effect from a combination of ketorolac and low-dose epidural morphine after cesarean delivery (101). Ninety patients were enrolled in the study and randomized to three groups to receive

postoperatively either (A) Epidural morphine 2 mg and IV placebo, (B) epidural morphine 2 mg and IM ketorolac 30 mg, or (C) epidural saline placebo and IM ketorolac 30 mg. Group B had significant superior pain relief compared to the other two groups. The addition of ketorolac was thought to enhance the analgesic effect of low-dose epidural morphine.

■ SELECT ADJUVANT ANALGESICS

Ketamine

Ketamine is a non-barbiturate anesthetic indicated for procedures that do not require skeletal muscle relaxation. It can be used for anesthesia induction prior to administration of general anesthesia, or less frequently as a general anesthetic. It is metabolized by the liver and excreted renally. Its exact mechanism of action is unknown; however, it acts on limbic and cortical receptors to produce "dissociative" anesthesia, characterized by analgesia, amnesia, and catalepsy. Side effects include psychotomimetic effects such as hallucinations, vivid dreams, and emergence confusion, among others, usually in doses greater than 2 mg/kg. Ketamine is a Pregnancy Category B drug; however, since its safe use in pregnancy has not been established, such use cannot be recommended in the obstetric setting. Ketamine is known to work, in part, through its interaction with the N-methyl-D-aspartate (NMDA) receptor, specifically as an antagonist. The NMDA receptor is an excitatory amino acid receptor involved in the processing of pain, leading to sensitization of the CNS to painful stimuli. Drugs that work against this receptor, therefore, have been shown to decrease central sensitization and consequently decrease the experience of pain. Ketamine can be administered in subanesthetic dosages (less than 1 mg/kg intravenously) for use specifically as a co-analgesic in the perioperative setting. A recent Cochrane systematic review of 37 trials (102) of perioperative IV ketamine for acute postoperative pain concluded that ketamine was effective in reducing morphine requirements during the first 24 hours post-surgery. Ketamine also appeared to reduce postoperative nausea and vomiting. The route of administration in these studies was mostly intravenous, and the timing of administration varied, to include preincision, intraoperative, and postoperative administration.

One study, by Kwok et al. evaluated ketamine use as a preemptive analgesic, the idea being that preoperative administration of ketamine would prevent central sensitization and thereby reduce postoperative pain (103). The study recruited 135 patients who were to undergo gynecologic laparoscopic surgery. The patients were randomly assigned to one of the three groups. The first group received preincision IV ketamine (0.15 mg/kg); the second group received postoperative IV ketamine at the same dose; the third group, placebo. The results of this study demonstrated a reduction in early postoperative pain as assessed by VAS and a reduction in opioid consumption in the preincision group, suggesting that ketamine did indeed provide a preemptive analgesic effect.

Another study performed by Zakine, et al. evaluated the postoperative opioid-sparing effect of ketamine administration in those undergoing major abdominal surgery (104). Patients in this study were prospectively randomized in a double-blinded fashion to one of the three groups—the first group ("PERI" group) receiving both intraoperative and 48-hour duration postoperative ketamine intravenous infusion (0.5 mg/kg IV bolus, followed by 2 μg/kg/min infusion); the second group ("INTRA" group) receiving only intraoperative ketamine IV infusion; and the third group ("CTRL" group) receiving placebo. Postoperative morphine consumption data was then collected, showing significantly lower morphine use in the "PERI" group compared to the control group. The study also showed significantly lower VAS scores and a lower incidence of nausea in both ketamine groups ("PERI" and "INTRA") compared to the placebo group. No differences in sedation or psychotomimetic effects were demonstrated between the three groups.

Magnesium

Magnesium (Mg^{++}) is a cofactor for enzymatic reactions and therefore is important for neurochemical transmission and muscular excitability.

It is available as magnesium sulfate injection that can be administered by the intravenous route as an electrolyte replenisher or anticonvulsant to treat a number of conditions, including hypomagnesemia, preeclampsia/eclampsia, and torsade de pointes, among others. Magnesium sulfate injection is a Pregnancy Category A drug. Magnesium crosses the placenta and is found in breast milk.

Magnesium may be useful as an analgesic adjuvant in the perioperative period. Its antinociceptive mechanism is explained in part by inhibition of calcium's entry into the cell by blocking the NMDA receptor. The NMDA receptor is an excitatory amino acid receptor involved in the processing of pain, leading to sensitization of the CNS to painful stimuli. Drugs that work against this receptor, therefore, have been shown to decrease central sensitization and consequently decrease the experience of pain. Magnesium is an antagonist of the NMDA receptor and therefore has been studied to determine its effectiveness as an adjuvant in perioperative analgesia, with inconsistent, but many promising findings thus far. Results from a study by Ghrab et al. suggest that magnesium sulfate added to intrathecal morphine improves postoperative analgesia (105). The authors recruited 105 patients postcesarean section surgery receiving intrathecal analgesia and randomly allocated them into one of the three groups—Group morphine received intrathecal bupivacaine 10 mg at 0.5% with morphine 0.1 mg and fentanyl 10 μg; Group magnesium received bupivacaine 10 mg at 0.5% with 100 mg of magnesium sulfate at 10% and fentanyl 10 μg; and Group morphine + magnesium receiving bupivacaine, morphine, magnesium, and fentanyl at the aforementioned doses. Pain scores were statistically lower in Group morphine + magnesium compared to the other two groups.

A prospective double-blinded, randomized study by Yousef and Amr included 90 patients to evaluate the analgesic effect of adding 500 mg of magnesium sulfate to CSE in elective cesarean section surgery (106). Their study showed a significant reduction of postoperative analgesic requirement in the group that received magnesium.

Gabapentin

Gabapentin is clinically indicated for epilepsy and postherpetic neuralgia. It has been prescribed for a number of other pain states, particularly for neuropathic-type pain.

The mechanism by which it exerts analgesia is unknown; however, animal model studies have demonstrated prevention of allodynia and hyperalgesia. Gabapentin also has been shown to prevent pain-related responses in several neuropathic pain states and after peripheral inflammation.

Structurally, it is related to the neurotransmitter GABA, but it does not act on GABA receptors. It does, however, bind to voltage-activated calcium channels, acting as a membrane stabilizer. Gabapentin is supplied as capsules of 100 mg, 300 mg, and 400 mg; tablets of 600 mg and 800 mg; and oral solution containing 250 mg per 5 mL.

Gabapentin is not appreciably metabolized and is eliminated through renal excretion as unchanged drug. Dosing adjustments must be made in patients with renal insufficiency.

It is considered a Pregnancy Category C drug and is secreted in human milk; thus, the risk–benefit ratio must be considered carefully for use during pregnancy or lactation.

Adverse reactions include dizziness, somnolence, and peripheral edema, usually seen with rapid titration or higher doses. To avoid withdrawal symptoms, weaning is recommended when discontinuing the medication.

In addition to its US FDA-approved clinical indications for use, gabapentin has also been studied as a multimodal agent in the perioperative period. One such study was by Turan et al. in which the analgesic effects of gabapentin after total abdominal hysterectomy were investigated (107). Fifty patients were enrolled in this randomized, placebo-controlled, double-blinded study. One group received oral gabapentin 1,200 mg prior to surgery; the other, placebo. Postoperatively, all patients received IV tramadol through a PCA device. Postoperative VAS scores during sitting and supine were found to be statistically significantly lower in the gabapentin group compared to the placebo group. Sedation scores were similar between groups at all times. 24-hour postoperative tramadol consumption was significantly less in the gabapentin group as well. The conclusion of the study was that preoperative oral gabapentin appeared to enhance the analgesic effect of tramadol, resulting in a decrease in its use.

A randomized, double-blinded, placebo-controlled study by Moore et al. was conducted to evaluate efficacy of adding gabapentin to a multimodal pain medication regimen for postcesarean delivery patients. (108). Forty-six patients were randomized to receive 600 mg of gabapentin or a lactose placebo pill 1 hour prior to surgery. The primary outcome measure was VAS pain score at 24 hours. It was concluded that preoperative gabapentin in the setting of a multimodal analgesic regimen results in a significant reduction in postcesarean delivery pain. In addition, maternal satisfaction ratings were higher than placebo, and there were no adverse effects on the neonate.

Another study by Sen et al. compared gabapentin with ketamine for perioperative supplemental analgesia following elective hysterectomy (109). Sixty patients were randomly assigned to one of the three groups—the control group receiving pre-surgery oral placebo capsule and IV saline bolus/infusion; the ketamine group receiving pre-surgery oral placebo capsule and pre-incision IV bolus of ketamine at 0.3 mg/kg, followed by 0.05 mg/kg/h infusion until the end of surgery; and the gabapentin group receiving 1,200 mg of oral gabapentin plus bolus/infusion of saline. Postoperative assessments included verbal rating scale(VRS) scores for pain and morphine consumption, among other outcome measures. Postoperative VRS pain scores were significantly lower in the gabapentin group (at 24 hours) compared to both the ketamine group (up to 16 hours) and the placebo group. Total morphine consumption (at 24 hours postop) in the treatment groups (gabapentin group and ketamine group) were significantly reduced compared to the placebo group. The conclusion was that both gabapentin and ketamine were similar in both early postop pain control and postop opioid consumption.

Gilron et al. performed a placebo-controlled, randomized clinical trial to study the effects of perioperative administration of gabapentin, rofecoxib (a non-steroidal anti-inflammatory medication), and their combination on pain evoked with movement in patients after abdominal hysterectomy surgery (110). 110 patients were enrolled to receive, starting 1 hour preoperatively, either placebo, gabapentin (1,800 mg/d), rofecoxib (50 mg/d), or the combination (gabapentin 1,800 mg/d plus rofecoxib 50 mg/d). The medications were continued for 72 hours. Outcome measures were recorded for 24 hours and included pain at rest and movement-evoked pain (sitting), among others. Morphine consumption was recorded for 48 hours. The results showed that the combination group and rofecoxib group significantly reduced movement-induced pain and morphine consumption. The conclusion drawn was that a gabapentin–rofecoxib combination was superior to either as a single agent for post-hysterectomy pain elicited by sitting and provided more consistent analgesia (Note: In September 2004 rofecoxib was voluntarily removed from the market due to concerns about increased risk of cardiovascular events with long-term, high-dose use). A systematic review of randomized clinical trials and meta-analysis by Kong and Irwin was performed to evaluate gabapentin (and pregabalin, a gabapentinoid drug) for acute postoperative pain (111). There were a total of 663 patients from seven original randomized trials. 333 subjects received oral gabapentin, while 330 received placebo. Outcome measures were obtained for postoperative opioid consumption, pain score at rest, and pain score during activity. Those who received gabapentin had significantly reduced postoperative opioid requirement in the first 24 hours post-surgery in 6 out of the 7 trials. Mean pain scores at rest were reduced significantly within 6 hours post-surgery in 3 out of 7 studies. Mean pain scores during activity were significantly reduced in 2 out of 4 studies. A meta-analysis of 719 patients from 8 original RCTs evaluated gabapentin in acute postoperative pain management. Pooled analysis showed no significant differences in adverse effects from analgesia or gabapentin. Meta-analysis of the analgesic effect of perioperative gabapentin was performed on data from 12 RCTs. 449 subjects received oral gabapentin and 447 received placebo. There was a significantly higher incidence of sedation with gabapentin, decrease in postoperative pain scores, and opioid consumption. A pooled analysis of 1,151 patients (614 patients receiving gabapentin) from 16 studies showed that a single preoperative dose of gabapentin (1,200 mg or less), but not multiple perioperative doses of gabapentin, significantly decreased pain intensity at 6 hours and 24 hours postop. 24-hour postop cumulative opioid consumption was significantly decreased, however, in all groups (those who received 1,200 mg of gabapentin, those who received <1,200 mg of gabapentin, and those who received multiple doses of gabapentin).

Tramadol

Tramadol is a synthetic, centrally acting analgesic, acting as a weak serotonin and norepinephrine reuptake inhibitor as well as a weak MOP opioid receptor agonist. It is indicated for moderate to severe pain. It is supplied as 50 mg tablets (immediate release) and 100 mg, 200 mg, and 300 mg tablets (extended release). Side effects may include nausea/vomiting, dizziness, constipation, among others. There is an increased risk of seizure in those with a history of epilepsy. It should be avoided in those with anaphylactoid reactions to codeine and used with caution in those on medications that affect serotonin (risk of serotonin syndrome). Dosage adjustments should be made in those with renal or hepatic impairment and in those with advanced age. In severe impairment, it should be avoided. It is labeled as a Pregnancy Category C drug and should not be used during breastfeeding.

A randomized clinical trial by Olle Fortuny et al. compared tramadol to ketorolac for postoperative pain after abdominal hysterectomy (112). Seventy-six women were enrolled for this study and two treatment groups were formed: The tramadol (TRA) group received 100 mg of tramadol orally, while the ketorolac (KET) group received 30 mg of ketorolac intravenously every 6 hours. During the first 12 hours after surgery, the 100 mg dose of tramadol was shown to be more effective for pain relief compared to the 30 mg ketorolac every 6 hours. There was, however, increased incidence of postoperative vomiting in the TRA group.

APPENDIX

United States Food and Drug Administration Categories of Drugs Taken During Pregnancy and Lactation

FDA Classification of Drugs Taken in Pregnancy

Category	
A	Adequate and well-controlled human studies have failed to demonstrate a risk to the fetus in the first trimester of pregnancy (and there is no evidence of risk in later trimesters).
B	Animal reproduction studies have failed to demonstrate a risk to the fetus and there are no adequate and well-controlled studies in pregnant women OR animal studies have shown an adverse effect, but adequate and well-controlled studies in pregnant women have failed to demonstrate a risk to the fetus in any trimester.
C	Animal reproduction studies have shown an adverse effect on the fetus and there are no adequate and well-controlled studies in humans, but potential benefits may warrant use of the drug in pregnant women despite potential risks.
D	There is positive evidence of human fetal risk based on adverse reaction data from investigational or marketing experience or studies in humans, but potential benefits may warrant use of the drug in pregnant women despite potential risks.
X	Studies in animals or humans have demonstrated fetal abnormalities and/or there is positive evidence of human fetal risk based on adverse reaction data from investigational or marketing experience, and the risks involved in use of the drug in pregnant women clearly outweigh potential benefits.
N	FDA has not classified this drug.

NB: This classification system is currently under review by the FDA.

FDA Classification of Drugs Taken During Lactation

Category	
S	Safe
NS	Not safe
U	Unknown

■ MORPHINE

Pregnancy Category C
Lactation Category S
Fetal Considerations

There are no adequate reports or well-controlled studies in human fetuses. Morphine rapidly crosses the human placenta achieving an F:M ratio approximating unity. Alterations in fetal biophysical profile parameters should be expected. Placental retention of morphine may prolong fetal exposure explaining in part its prolonged effect on fetal behavior relative to the maternal concentration. Infants born to opioid-abusing mothers are more often SGA, have decreased ventilatory response to CO_2 and increased risk of neonatal abstinence syndrome with sleep–wake abnormalities, feeding difficulties, weight loss, and seizures. Animal studies suggest that prolong in utero exposure causes long-term alterations in adult brain behavior. Short-term exposure in animal studies are generally reassuring, revealing no evidence of teratogenicity.

Breastfeeding Safety

Morphine is excreted in human breast milk. The amount taken by the neonate depends on the maternal plasma concentration, quantity of milk ingested, and the extent of first-pass metabolism. Intrathecal morphine is not associated with clinically relevant maternal plasma and milk morphine concentrations. The milk concentration after routine doses of morphine PCA is small, supporting the safety of breastfeeding.

■ FENTANYL

Pregnancy Category C
Lactation Category S
Fetal Considerations

There are no adequate reports or well-controlled studies in human fetuses. Fentanyl readily crosses the human placenta achieving an F:M ratio of 1. Alterations in fetal biophysical profile parameters should be expected. Animal studies are generally reassuring, revealing no evidence of teratogenicity or IUGR.

Breastfeeding Safety

There are no adequate reports or well-controlled studies in nursing women. Fentanyl enters human breast milk, but is not likely to pose a risk to the neonate of an alert, breastfeeding woman.

■ CLONIDINE

Pregnancy Category C
Lactation Category NS?
Fetal Considerations

There are no adequate reports or well-controlled studies in human fetuses. Clonidine readily crosses the placenta achieving an F:M ratio of 1. Amniotic fluid concentrations are four times higher than in serum. Neonates of women receiving clonidine during labor may experience mild hypotension. Animal studies are reassuring revealing no evidence of teratogenicity or IUGR.

Breastfeeding Safety

Clonidine is concentrated in human breast milk reaching an M:P ratio of 2.

■ KETAMINE

Pregnancy Category D
Lactation Category U
Fetal Considerations

There are no adequate reports or well-controlled studies in human fetuses. Animal studies suggest ketamine may alter postnatal behavior.

Breastfeeding Safety

There are no adequate reports or well-controlled studies in nursing women. It is unknown whether ketamine enters human breast milk.

■ NSAIDs

Pregnancy Category C
Lactation Category U?
Fetal Considerations

There are no adequate reports or well-controlled studies in human fetuses. It is unknown whether NSAIDs cross the placenta. They can produce fetal oliguria and ductal constriction in a dose and are gestational age dependent. Animal studies are reassuring revealing no evidence of teratogenicity or IUGR.

Breastfeeding Safety

Small quantities of NSAID enters human breast milk. It seems unlikely the breastfeeding neonate would ingest a clinically relevant amount.

■ GABAPENTIN AND PREGABALIN

Pregnancy Category C
Lactation Category S?
Fetal Considerations

There are no adequate reports or well-controlled studies in human fetuses. It is unknown whether gabapentin/pregabalin crosses the human placenta. Animal studies reveal and increased prevalence of minor malformations including skeletal abnormalities and hydronephrosis.

Breastfeeding Safety

Excreted into human breast milk, though the content likely to be subclinical. It seems unlikely the breastfeeding neonate would ingest a clinically relevant amount.

KEY POINTS

- Failure to treat acute postoperative pain can have adverse physical and psychological consequences for the patient and the potential to progress to a persistent, chronic pain state.
- Neuraxial opioids provide excellent postoperative analgesia with a decrease in total dose of parenteral opioid, low level of sedation, early ambulation, early return of bowel function with better maternal–infant bonding and minimal accumulation of the drug in breast milk.
- Neuraxial opioids may have side effects and complications including pruritus, nausea and vomiting, urinary retention, somnolence, respiratory depression, and reactivation of oral herpes simplex.
- Oral analgesia has an important role in the step-down management of post-delivery pain after primary management with neuraxial opioids.
- Adjuvant analgesics may have an additional role to play in postoperative pain relief after cesarean delivery.
- Magnesium sulfate injection is a Pregnancy Category A drug. Patients receiving magnesium have shown significantly lower postoperative pain scores, cumulative analgesic use, and shivering incidents, compared to a placebo group.
- Tramadol is a synthetic, centrally acting analgesic, acting as a weak serotonin and norepinephrine reuptake inhibitor, as well as a weak mu opioid receptor agonist. It is indicated for moderate to severe pain. Tramadol is a Pregnancy Category C drug and should not be used during breastfeeding.

REFERENCES

1. Apfelbaum JL, Chen C, Mehta SS, et al. Postoperative pain experience: Results from a national survey suggest postoperative pain continues to be undermanaged. *Anesth Analg* 2003;97(2):534–540, table of contents.
2. Macrae WA. Chronic post-surgical pain: 10 years on. *Br J Anaesth* 2008; 101(1):77–86.
3. Pan PH, Coghill R, Houle TT, et al. Multifactorial preoperative predictors for postcesarean section pain and analgesic requirement. *Anesthesiology* 2006; 104(3):417–425.
4. Kuczkowski KM. Postoperative pain control in the parturient: New challenges in the new millennium. *J Matern Fetal Neonatal Med* 2011;24(2):301–304.
5. Leung AY. Postoperative pain management in obstetric anesthesia—new challenges and solutions. *J Clin Anesth* 2004;16(1):57–65.
6. Merskey HBN, ed. *IASP task force on taxonomy, classification of chronic pain.* 2nd ed. Seattle, WA: IASP Press; 1994.
7. Wandless AL, Smart D, Lambert DG. Fentanyl increases intracellular Ca2+ concentrations in SH-SY5Y cells. *Br J Anaesth* 1996;76(3):461–463.
8. Gourlay GK, Cherry DA, Cousins MJ. Cephalad migration of morphine in CSF following lumbar epidural administration in patients with cancer pain. *Pain* 1985;23(4): 317–326.
9. Julius D, Basbaum AI. Molecular mechanisms of nociception. *Nature* 2001; 413(6852):203–210.
10. Woolf CJ. Pain: Moving from symptom control toward mechanism-specific pharmacologic management. *Ann Intern Med* 2004;140(6): 441–451.
11. Devor M. Neurobiology of normal and pathophysiological pain. In: Aronoff GM, ed. *Evaluation and Treatment of Chronic Pain.* Baltimore, MD: Williams and Wilkins; 1998:11–27.
12. Moore KA, Kohno T, Karchewski LA, et al. Partial peripheral nerve injury promotes a selective loss of GABAergic inhibition in the superficial dorsal horn of the spinal cord. *J Neurosci* 2002;22(15):6724–6731.
13. McDonnell NJ, Keating ML, Muchatuta NA, et al. Analgesia after caesarean delivery. *Anaesth Intensive Care* 2009;37(4):539–551.
14. Tingaker BK, Irestedt L. Changes in uterine innervation in pregnancy and during labour. *Curr Opin Anaesthesiol* 2010;23(3):300–303.
15. Lavand'homme P. Postcesarean analgesia: Effective strategies and association with chronic pain. *Curr Opin Anaesthesiol* 2006;19(3):244–248.
16. Pan PH. Post cesarean delivery pain management: Multimodal approach. *Int J Obstet Anesth* 2006;15(3):185–188.
17. Reynolds F. Labour analgesia and the baby: Good news is no news. *Int J Obstet Anesth* 2011;20(1):38–50.
18. Hirose M, Hara Y, Hosokawa T, et al. The effect of postoperative analgesia with continuous epidural bupivacaine after cesarean section on the amount of breast feeding and infant weight gain. *Anesth Analg* 1996;82(6):1166–1169.
19. Spigset O. Anaesthetic agents and excretion in breast milk. *Acta Anaesthesiol Scand* 1994;38(2):94–103.
20. Hale TW. Anesthetic medications in breastfeeding mothers. *J Hum Lact* 1999;15(3):185–194.
21. Hawkins JL, Koonin LM, Palmer SK, et al. Anesthesia-related deaths during obstetric delivery in the United States, 1979–1990. *Anesthesiology* 1997; 86(2):277–284.
22. Bernards CM, Hill HF. Physical and chemical properties of drug molecules governing their diffusion through the spinal meninges. *Anesthesiology* 1992;77(4):750–756.
23. Thomas DA, Williams GM, Iwata K, et al. The medullary dorsal horn. A site of action of morphine in producing facial scratching in monkeys. *Anesthesiology* 1993;79(3):548–554.
24. Bromage PR, Camporesi EM, Durant PA, et al. Rostral spread of epidural morphine. *Anesthesiology* 1982;56(6):431–436.
25. Gourlay GK, et al. Pharmacokinetics of fentanyl in lumbar and cervical CSF following lumbar epidural and intravenous administration. *Pain* 1989; 38(3):253–259.
26. de Leon-Casasola OA, Lema MJ. Epidural sufentanil for acute pain control in a patient with extreme opioid dependency. *Anesthesiology* 1992;76(5):853–856.
27. Horlocker TT, Burton AW, Connis RT, et al. Practice guidelines for the prevention, detection, and management of respiratory depression associated with neuraxial opioid administration. *Anesthesiology* 2009;110(2):218–130.
28. Jenkins JG, Khan MM. Anaesthesia for Caesarean section: A survey in a UK region from 1992 to 2002. *Anaesthesia* 2003;58(11):1114–1118.
29. Kuczkowski KM. Postoperative pain control in the parturient: New challenges (and their solutions). *J Clin Anesth* 2004;16(1):1–3.
30. Draisci G, Frassanito L, Pinto R, et al. Safety and effectiveness of coadministration of intrathecal sufentanil and morphine in hyperbaric bupivacaine-based spinal anesthesia for cesarean section. *J Opioid Manag* 2009;5(4):197–202.
31. Cousins MJ, Mather LE. Intrathecal and epidural administration of opioids. *Anesthesiology* 1984;61(3):276–310.
32. Belzarena SD. Clinical effects of intrathecally administered fentanyl in patients undergoing cesarean section. *Anesth Analg* 1992;74(5):653–657.
33. Dahl JB, Jeppesen IS, Jørgensen H, et al. Intraoperative and postoperative analgesic efficacy and adverse effects of intrathecal opioids in patients undergoing cesarean section with spinal anesthesia: A qualitative and quantitative systematic review of randomized controlled trials. *Anesthesiology* 1999; 91(6):1919–1927.
34. Palmer CM, Emerson S, Volgoropolous D, et al. Dose-response relationship of intrathecal morphine for postcesarean analgesia. *Anesthesiology* 1999; 90(2):437–444.
35. Yang T, Breen TW, Archer D, et al. Comparison of 0.25 mg and 0.1 mg intrathecal morphine for analgesia after Cesarean section. *Can J Anaesth* 1999; 46(9):856–860.
36. Davies PW, Vallejo MC, Shannon KT, et al. Oral herpes simplex reactivation after intrathecal morphine: A prospective randomized trial in an obstetric population. *Anesth Analg* 2005;100(5):1472–1476, table of contents.
37. Abouleish E., Rawal N, Rashad MN. The addition of 0.2 mg subarachnoid morphine to hyperbaric bupivacaine for cesarean delivery: A prospective study of 856 cases. *Reg Anesth* 1991;16(3):137–140.
38. Shende D, Cooper GM, Bowden MI. The influence of intrathecal fentanyl on the characteristics of subarachnoid block for caesarean section. *Anaesthesia* 1998;53(7):706–710.
39. Chu CC, Shu SS, Lin SM, et al. The effect of intrathecal bupivacaine with combined fentanyl in cesarean section. *Acta Anaesthesiol Sin* 1995;33(3):149–154.
40. Siddik-Sayyid SM, Aouad MT, Jalbout MI, et al. Intrathecal versus intravenous fentanyl for supplementation of subarachnoid block during cesarean delivery. *Anesth Analg* 2002;95(1):209–213, table of contents.
41. Lee, JH, Chung KH, Lee JY, et al. Comparison of fentanyl and sufentanil added to 0.5% hyperbaric bupivacaine for spinal anesthesia in patients undergoing cesarean section. *Korean J Anesthesiol* 2011;60(2):103–108.
42. Ngiam SK, Chong JL. The addition of intrathecal sufentanil and fentanyl to bupivacaine for caesarean section. *Singapore Med J* 1998;39(7):290–294.
43. Dahlgren G, Hultstrand C, Jakobsson J, et al. Intrathecal sufentanil, fentanyl, or placebo added to bupivacaine for cesarean section. *Anesth Analg* 1997; 85(6):1288–1293.
44. Demiraran Y, Ozdemir I, Kocaman B, et al. Intrathecal sufentanil (1.5 microg) added to hyperbaric bupivacaine (0.5%) for elective cesarean section provides adequate analgesia without need for pruritus therapy. *J Anesth* 2006;20(4):274–278.
45. Kafle SK. Intrathecal meperidine for elective caesarean section: A comparison with lidocaine. *Can J Anaesth* 1993;40(8):718–721.

46. Giovannelli M, Bedforth N, Aitkenhead A. Survey of intrathecal opioid usage in the UK. *Eur J Anaesthesiol* 2008;25(2):118–122.

47. Hallworth SP, Fernando R, Bell R, et al. Comparison of intrathecal and epidural diamorphine for elective caesarean section using a combined spinal-epidural technique. *Br J Anaesth* 1999;82(2):228–232.

48. Cowan CM, Kendall JB, Barclay PM, et al. Comparison of intrathecal fentanyl and diamorphine in addition to bupivacaine for caesarean section under spinal anaesthesia. *Br J Anaesth* 2002;89(3):452–458.

49. Skilton RW, Kinsella SM, Smith A, et al. Dose response study of subarachnoid diamorphine for analgesia after elective caesarean section. *Int J Obstet Anesth* 1999;8(4):231–235.

50. Kelly MC, Carabine UA, Mirakhur RK. Intrathecal diamorphine for analgesia after caesarean section. A dose finding study and assessment of side-effects. *Anaesthesia* 1998;53(3):231–237.

51. Stacey R, Jones R, Kar G, et al. High-dose intrathecal diamorphine for analgesia after Caesarean section. *Anaesthesia* 2001;56(1):54–60.

52. Palmer CM, Nogami WM, Van Maren G, et al. Postcesarean epidural morphine: A dose-response study. *Anesth Analg* 2000;90(4):887–891.

53. Sarvela J, Halonen P, Soikkeli A, et al. A double-blinded, randomized comparison of intrathecal and epidural morphine for elective cesarean delivery. *Anesth Analg* 2002;95(2):436–440, table of contents.

54. Ready LB, Loper KA, Nessly M, et al. Postoperative epidural morphine is safe on surgical wards. *Anesthesiology* 1991;75(3):452–456.

55. de Leon-Casasola OA, Parker B, Lema MJ, et al. Postoperative epidural bupivacaine-morphine therapy. Experience with 4,227 surgical cancer patients. *Anesthesiology* 1994;81(2):368–375.

56. Rauck RL, Raj PP, Knarr DC, et al. Comparison of the efficacy of epidural morphine given by intermittent injection or continuous infusion for the management of postoperative pain. *Reg Anesth* 1994;19(5):316–324.

57. Bonnet MP, Mignon A, Mazoit JX, et al. Analgesic efficacy and adverse effects of epidural morphine compared to parenteral opioids after elective caesarean section: A systematic review. *Eur J Pain* 2010;14(9):894 e1–e9.

58. Chaplan SR, Duncan SR, Brodsky JB, et al. Morphine and hydromorphone epidural analgesia. A prospective, randomized comparison. *Anesthesiology* 1992; 77(6):1090–1094.

59. Glass PS, Estok P, Ginsberg B, et al. Use of patient-controlled analgesia to compare the efficacy of epidural to intravenous fentanyl administration. *Anesth Analg* 1992;74(3):345–351.

60. Sandler AN, Stringer D, Panos L, et al. A randomized, double-blind comparison of lumbar epidural and intravenous fentanyl infusions for postthoracotomy pain relief. Analgesic, pharmacokinetic, and respiratory effects. *Anesthesiology* 1992;77(4):626–634.

61. Loper KA, Ready LB, Downey M, et al. Epidural and intravenous fentanyl infusions are clinically equivalent after knee surgery. *Anesth Analg* 1990;70(1):72–75.

62. Ellis DJ, Millar WL, Reisner LS. A randomized double-blind comparison of epidural versus intravenous fentanyl infusion for analgesia after cesarean section. *Anesthesiology* 1990;72(6):981–986.

63. Sevarino FB, McFarlane C, Sinatra RS. Epidural fentanyl does not influence intravenous PCA requirements in the post-caesarean patient. *Can J Anaesth* 1991;38(4 pt 1):450–453.

64. Ginosar Y, Columb MO, Cohen SE, et al. The site of action of epidural fentanyl infusions in the presence of local anesthetics: A minimum local analgesic concentration infusion study in nulliparous labor. *Anesth Analg* 2003;97(5):1439–1445.

65. Geller, E., Chrubasik J, Graf R, et al. A randomized double-blind comparison of epidural sufentanil versus intravenous sufentanil or epidural fentanyl analgesia after major abdominal surgery. *Anesth Analg* 1993;76(6):1243–1250.

66. Miguel R, Barlow I, Morrell M, et al. A prospective, randomized, double-blind comparison of epidural and intravenous sufentanil infusions. *Anesthesiology* 1994;81(2):346–352; discussion 25A-26A.

67. Swenson JD, Hullander RM, Bready RJ, et al. A comparison of patient controlled epidural analgesia with sufentanil by the lumbar versus thoracic route after thoracotomy. *Anesth Analg* 1994;78(2):215–218.

68. Grant RP, Dolman JF, Harper JA, et al. Patient-controlled lumbar epidural fentanyl compared with patient-controlled intravenous fentanyl for post-thoracotomy pain. *Can J Anaesth* 1992;39(3):214–219.

69. Grass JA, Sakima NT, Schmidt R, et al. A randomized, double-blind, dose-response comparison of epidural fentanyl versus sufentanil analgesia after cesarean section. *Anesth Analg* 1997;85(2):365–371.

70. Chestnut DH, Owen CL, Bates JN, et al. Continuous infusion epidural analgesia during labor: A randomized, double-blind comparison of 0.0625% bupivacaine/0.0002% fentanyl versus 0.125% bupivacaine. *Anesthesiology* 1988; 68(5):754–759.

71. Tejwani GA, Rattan AK, McDonald JS. Role of spinal opioid receptors in the antinociceptive interactions between intrathecal morphine and bupivacaine. *Anesth Analg* 1992;74(5):726–734.

72. Sumida S, Lesley MR, Hanna MN, et al. Meta-analysis of the effect of extended-release epidural morphine versus intravenous patient-controlled analgesia on respiratory depression. *J Opioid Manag* 2009;5(5):301–305.

73. Carvalho B, Roland LM, Chu LF, et al. Single-dose, extended-release epidural morphine (DepoDur) compared to conventional epidural morphine for post-cesarean pain. *Anesth Analg* 2007;105(1):176–183.

74. Atkinson Ralls L, Drover DR, Clavijo CF, et al. Prior epidural lidocaine alters the pharmacokinetics and drug effects of extended-release epidural morphine (DepoDur®) after cesarean delivery. *Anesth Analg* 2011;113(2):251–258.

75. Hartrick CT, Hartrick KA. Extended-release epidural morphine (DepoDur): Review and safety analysis. *Expert Rev Neurother* 2008;8(11):1641–1648.

76. Carvalho B, Riley E, Cohen SE, et al. Single-dose, sustained-release epidural morphine in the management of postoperative pain after elective cesarean delivery: Results of a multicenter randomized controlled study. *Anesth Analg* 2005;100(4):1150–1158.

77. Gambling DR, Hughes TL, Manvelian GZ. Extended-release epidural morphine (DepoDur) following epidural bupivacaine in patients undergoing lower abdominal surgery: A randomized controlled pharmacokinetic study. *Reg Anesth Pain Med* 2009;34(4):316–325.

78. Rigg JR, Jamrozik K, Myles PS, et al. Epidural anaesthesia and analgesia and outcome of major surgery: A randomised trial. *Lancet* 2002;359(9314):1276–1282.

79. Wijeysundera DN, Beattie WS, Austin PC, et al. Epidural anaesthesia and survival after intermediate-to-high risk non-cardiac surgery: A population-based cohort study. *Lancet* 2008;372(9638):562–569.

80. Guay J. The benefits of adding epidural analgesia to general anesthesia: A metaanalysis. *J Anesth* 2006;20(4):335–340.

81. Cooper DW, Saleh U, Taylor M, et al. Patient-controlled analgesia: Epidural fentanyl and i.v. morphine compared after caesarean section. *Br J Anaesth* 1999;82(3):366–370.

82. Howell PR, Gambling DR, Pavy T, et al. Patient-controlled analgesia following caesarean section under general anaesthesia: A comparison of fentanyl with morphine. *Can J Anaesth* 1995;42(1):41–45.

83. Elia N, Lysakowski C, Tramer MR. Does multimodal analgesia with acetaminophen, nonsteroidal antiinflammatory drugs, or selective cyclooxygenase-2 inhibitors and patient-controlled analgesia morphine offer advantages over morphine alone? Meta-analyses of randomized trials. *Anesthesiology* 2005;103(6):1296–1304.

84. Vadivelu N, Mitra S, Narayan D. Recent advances in postoperative pain management. *Yale J Biol Med* 2010;83(1):11–25.

85. McDonnell JG, Curley G, Carney J, et al. The analgesic efficacy of transversus abdominis plane block after cesarean delivery: A randomized controlled trial. *Anesth Analg* 2008;106(1):186–191, table of contents.

86. Belavy D, Cowlishaw PJ, Howes M, et al. Ultrasound-guided transversus abdominis plane block for analgesia after Caesarean delivery. *Br J Anaesth* 2009;103(5):726–730.

87. Costello JF, Moore AR, Wieczorek PM, et al. The transversus abdominis plane block, when used as part of a multimodal regimen inclusive of intrathecal morphine, does not improve analgesia after cesarean delivery. *Reg Anesth Pain Med* 2009;34(6):586–589.

88. McMorrow RC, Ni Mhuircheartaigh RJ, Ahmed KA, et al. Comparison of transversus abdominis plane block vs spinal morphine for pain relief after Caesarean section. *Br J Anaesth* 2011;106(5):706–712.

89. Bamigboye AA, Hofmeyr GJ. Local anaesthetic wound infiltration and abdominal nerves block during caesarean section for postoperative pain relief. *Cochrane Database Syst Rev* 2009;(3):CD006954.

90. Lavand'homme PM, Roelants F, Waterloos H, et al. Postoperative analgesic effects of continuous wound infiltration with diclofenac after elective cesarean delivery. *Anesthesiology* 2007;106(6):1220–1225.

91. Davis KM, Esposito MA, Meyer BA. Oral analgesia compared with intravenous patient-controlled analgesia for pain after cesarean delivery: A randomized controlled trial. *Am J Obstet Gynecol* 2006;194(4):967–971.

92. Jakobi P, Weiner Z, Solt I, et al. Oral analgesia in the treatment of post-cesarean pain. *Eur J Obstet Gynecol Reprod Biol* 2000;93(1):61–64.

93. Alhashemi JA, Alotaibi QA, Mashaat MS, et al. Intravenous acetaminophen vs oral ibuprofen in combination with morphine PCIA after Cesarean delivery. *Can J Anaesth* 2006;53(12):1200–1206.

94. Munishankar B, Fettes P, Moore C, et al. A double-blind randomised controlled trial of paracetamol, diclofenac or the combination for pain relief after caesarean section. *Int J Obstet Anesth* 2008;17(1):9–14.

95. Nauta M, Landsmeer ML, Koren G. Codeine-acetaminophen versus nonsteroidal anti-inflammatory drugs in the treatment of post-abdominal surgery pain: A systematic review of randomized trials. *Am J Surg* 2009;198(2):256–261.

96. Scholer DW, Ku EC, Boettcher I, et al. Pharmacology of diclofenac sodium. *Am J Med* 1986;80(4B):34–38.

97. Mitra S, Khandelwal P, Sehgal A. Diclofenac-tramadol vs. diclofenac-acetaminophen combinations for pain relief after caesarean section. *Acta Anaesthesiol Scand* 2012;56(6):706–711.

98. Derry S, Barden J, McQuay HJ, et al. Single dose oral celecoxib for acute postoperative pain in adults. *Cochrane Database Syst Rev*, 2008;(4):CD004233.

99. El-Tahan MR, Warda OM, Yasseen AM, et al. A randomized study of the effects of preoperative ketorolac on general anaesthesia for caesarean section. *Int J Obstet Anesth* 2007;16(3):214–220.

100. Lowder JL, Shackelford DP, Holbert D, et al. A randomized, controlled trial to compare ketorolac tromethamine versus placebo after cesarean section to reduce pain and narcotic usage. *Am J Obstet Gynecol* 2003;189(6):1559–1562; discussion 1562.

101. Tzeng JI, Mok MS. Combination of intramuscular Ketorolac and low dose epidural morphine for the relief of post-caesarean pain. *Ann Acad Med Singapore* 1994;23(6 suppl):10–13.

102. Bell RF, Dahl JB, Moore RA, et al. Perioperative ketamine for acute postoperative pain. *Cochrane Database Syst Rev* 2006;(1):CD004603.

103. Kwok RF, Lim J, Chan MT, et al. Preoperative ketamine improves postoperative analgesia after gynecologic laparoscopic surgery. *Anesth Analg* 2004;98(4):1044–1049, table of contents.

104. Zakine J, Samarcq D, Lorne E, et al. Postoperative ketamine administration decreases morphine consumption in major abdominal surgery: A prospective, randomized, double-blind, controlled study. *Anesth Analg* 2008;106(6):1856–1861.

105. Ghrab BE, Maatoug M, Kallel N, et al. (Does combination of intrathecal magnesium sulfate and morphine improve postcaesarean section analgesia?). *Ann Fr Anesth Reanim* 2009;28(5):454–459.

106. Yousef AA, Amr YM. The effect of adding magnesium sulphate to epidural bupivacaine and fentanyl in elective caesarean section using combined spinal-epidural anaesthesia: A prospective double blind randomised study. *Int J Obstet Anesth* 2010;19(4):401–404.

107. Turan, A., Karamanlioğlu B, Memiş D, et al. The analgesic effects of gabapentin after total abdominal hysterectomy. *Anesth Analg* 2004;98(5):1370–1373, table of contents.

108. Moore A, Costello J, Wieczorek P, et al. Gabapentin improves postcesarean delivery pain management: A randomized, placebo-controlled trial. *Anesth Analg* 2011;112(1):167–173.

109. Sen H, Sizlan A, Yanarates O, et al. A comparison of gabapentin and ketamine in acute and chronic pain after hysterectomy. *Anesth Analg* 2009;109(5):1645–1650.

110. Gilron I, Orr E, Tu D, et al. A placebo-controlled randomized clinical trial of perioperative administration of gabapentin, rofecoxib and their combination for spontaneous and movement-evoked pain after abdominal hysterectomy. *Pain* 2005;113(1–2):191–200.

111. Kong, VK, Irwin MG. Gabapentin: A multimodal perioperative drug? *Br J Anaesth* 2007;99(6):775–786.

112. Ollé Fortuny GOJL, Oferil Riera F, Sánchez Pallarés M, et al. Ketorolac versus tramadol: Comparative study of analgesic efficacy in the postoperative pain in abdominal hysterectomy. *Rev Esp Anestesiol Reanim* 2000;47(4):162–167.

14

Chronic Pain Issues After Cesarean Delivery

Ruth Landau

■ INTRODUCTION

In 1994, the International Association for the Study of Pain (IASP) defined pain as *"an unpleasant sensory and emotional experience associated with actual or potential tissue damage or described in terms of such damage."*

Acute pain is defined as pain of short duration that is primarily caused by peripheral tissue injury. Chronic pain is empirically defined as pain lasting for an extended period of 3 months, or alternatively as *persisting beyond the expected healing time*. Substantial progress has occurred in the last decades in the understanding of the neurobiologic basis of clinical painful conditions. The distinctions between *pain* (a sensory and unpleasant experience) and *noxious stimulus* (an actually or potentially tissue-damaging event) were underlined in the IASP Basic Pain Terminology published by the IASP Task Force on Taxonomy (Table 14-1) (1).

"Real Women, Real Pain" was a campaign launched in 2007 by IASP to empower women and raise awareness of pain issues affecting women worldwide. That year (2007 to 2008) was declared the "Global Year Against Pain in Women." Obstetric pain was reported as *"pain related to childbirth that may present (a) during pregnancy, (b) during labor when more than 95% of women report pain, (c) occasionally during cesarean delivery if there is poor quality of nerve block or prolonged surgery, and (d) after delivery when more than 70% of mothers report acute or chronic pain."*

With over 4 million deliveries annually in the United States alone with a cesarean delivery rate above 30% (2), labor and delivery is likely to have a huge impact on the occurrence of acute pain and possibly chronic pain issues in the postpartum. Recent awareness that chronic pain may occur after childbirth has prompted clinicians and researchers to investigate this topic. Clearly, obstetric anesthesiologists have a unique opportunity to make a real difference in women's experience of labor and delivery. With a constant increase in cesarean delivery rate and evidence that severe acute post-operative pain may result in chronic pain after surgery, obstetric anesthesia has to embrace its new role to provide optimal post-cesarean analgesia not only to improve short-term outcomes but also to prevent severe acute pain from becoming chronic and incapacitating in a constantly growing number of women.

In this chapter, a review of the vast body of knowledge accumulated in recent decades on chronic post-surgical pain, and more specifically the emerging concern that cesarean delivery may well be resulting in chronic pain in some women, as well as ways to predict and prevent this potentially devastating outcome are presented.

In order to treat something, we first must learn to recognize it.

—*Sir William Osler*

■ CHRONIC PAIN AFTER SURGERY

The concept that tissue trauma from surgery could result in chronic pain was described approximately four decades ago. The first reports related to long-term phantom pain after limb amputations (3) and were followed shortly by publications on phantom breast pain after mastectomy (4), chronic pain post-thoracotomy (5,6), post-cholecystectomy (7), and post-inguinal hernia repair (8). It became apparent in the mid-1990s that one in five patients referred to a chronic pain clinic implicated surgery as a cause of their chronic pain (9). Soon after, chronic post-surgical pain was recognized as an entity in its own (10–12). The incidence of chronic pain after surgery has been shown to depend on the surgical procedure and ranges between 4% and 50% (Table 14-2) (10).

The need for adequate pain control post-surgery was well established and "acute pain services" have thrived since the early 90s with the objective to reduce surgical stress, promote an early return to normal function, and improve overall post-surgical outcomes (13). The premise that acute post-operative pain may result in "wind-up" and pain hypersensitivity prompted anesthesiologists to offer preemptive analgesia and promote multi-modal strategies to enhance post-surgical analgesia (14,15). While there is overwhelming evidence that acute post-operative pain is associated with persistent pain and a high rate of chronic post-surgical pain, whether this describes a causal link or that individuals are simply more susceptible to develop both acute and chronic pain after surgery is still under investigation to this day. Management of acute post-operative pain in itself remains an ongoing challenge as it appears to be undermanaged (16). It has been proposed that applying procedure-specific analgesic recommendations may improve short and even long-term outcomes (17,18).

Definition of Chronic Post-surgical Pain

Several criteria (listed below) are required to meet the definition of chronic post-surgical pain so that preexisting pain that persists beyond the post-surgical recovery time is not misclassified as chronic post-surgical pain (19).

- The pain developed after a surgical procedure
- The pain has been lasting for at least 2 to 3 months
- Other causes for the pain have been excluded (e.g., ongoing cancer pain, chronic infection)
- The pain is not continuing from a preexisting painful condition (aggravation of pain attributed to the surgery is difficult to distinguish in this situation)

TABLE 14-1 IASP Basic Pain Terminology Published by the IASP Task Force on Taxonomy (1)

Pain	An unpleasant sensory and emotional experience associated with actual or potential tissue damage, or described in terms of such damage.
Allodynia*	Pain due to a stimulus that does not normally provoke pain.
Analgesia	Absence of pain in response to stimulation which would normally be painful.
Anesthesia dolorosa	Pain in an area or region which is anesthetic.
Causalgia	A syndrome of sustained burning pain, allodynia, and hyperpathia after a traumatic nerve lesion, often combined with vasomotor and sudomotor dysfunction and later trophic changes.
Central pain	Pain initiated or caused by a primary lesion or dysfunction in the central nervous system.
Dysesthesia	An unpleasant abnormal sensation, whether spontaneous or evoked.
Hyperalgesia*	Increased pain from a stimulus that normally provokes pain.
Hyperesthesia	Increased sensitivity to stimulation, excluding the special senses.
Hyperpathia	A painful syndrome characterized by an abnormally painful reaction to a stimulus, especially a repetitive stimulus, as well as an increased threshold.
Hypoalgesia	Diminished pain in response to a normally painful stimulus.

The implications of some of the above definitions may be summarized for convenience as follows:

Allodynia	Lowered threshold	Stimulus and response mode differ
Hyperalgesia	Increased response	Stimulus and response mode are the same
Hyperpathia	Raised threshold: Increased response	Stimulus and response mode may be the same or different
Hypoalgesia	Raised threshold: Lowered response	Stimulus and response mode are the same

Hypoesthesia	Decreased sensitivity to stimulation, excluding the special senses.
Neuralgia	Pain in the distribution of a nerve or nerves.
Neuritis	Inflammation of a nerve or nerves.
Neuropathic pain*	Pain caused by a lesion or disease of the somatosensory nervous system.
Central neuropathic pain*	Pain caused by a lesion or disease of the central somatosensory nervous system.
Peripheral neuropathic pain*	Pain caused by a lesion or disease of the peripheral somatosensory nervous system.
Neuropathy	A disturbance of function or pathologic change in a nerve: In one nerve, mononeuropathy; in several nerves, mononeuropathy multiplex; if diffuse and bilateral, polyneuropathy.
Nociception*	The neural process of encoding noxious stimuli.
Nociceptive neuron*	A central or peripheral neuron of the somatosensory nervous system that is capable of encoding noxious stimuli.
Nociceptive pain*	Pain that arises from actual or threatened damage to non-neural tissue and is due to the activation of nociceptors.
Nociceptive stimulus*	An actually or potentially tissue-damaging event transduced and encoded by nociceptors.
Nociceptor*	A high-threshold sensory receptor of the peripheral somatosensory nervous system that is capable of transducing and encoding noxious stimuli.
Noxious stimulus*	A stimulus that is damaging or threatens damage to normal tissues.
Pain threshold*	The minimum intensity of a stimulus that is perceived as painful.
Pain tolerance level*	The maximum intensity of a pain-producing stimulus that a subject is willing to accept in a given situation.
Paresthesia	An abnormal sensation, whether spontaneous or evoked.
Sensitization*	Increased responsiveness of nociceptive neurons to their normal input, and/or recruitment of a response to normally subthreshold inputs.
Central sensitization*	Increased responsiveness of nociceptive neurons in the central nervous system to their normal or subthreshold afferent input.
Peripheral sensitization*	Increased responsiveness and reduced threshold of nociceptive neurons in the periphery to the stimulation of their receptive fields.

Note: An asterisk (*) indicates that the term is either newly introduced or the definition or accompanying note has been revised since the 1994 publication.
Reprinted with permission from: "Part III: Pain Terms, A Current List with Definitions and Notes on Usage" (pp. 209–214) Classification of Chronic Pain, Second Edition, IASP Task Force on Taxonomy, edited by H. Merskey and N. Bogduk, IASP Press, Seattle, © 1994.

TABLE 14-2 Incidence of Chronic Pain After Surgery (10)

	Estimated Incidence of Chronic Pain	Estimated Disabling Chronic Pain (Pain Score above 5, on a Scale from 0–10)	US Surgical Volumes (1,000)
Amputation (phantom pain)	30–50%	5–10%	159 (lower limb only)
Breast surgery (lumpectomy and mastectomy)	20–30%	5–10%	479
Thoracotomy	30–40%	10%	N/A
Inguinal hernia repair	10%	2–4%	609
Coronary artery bypass surgery	30–50%	5–10%	598
C-section	10%	4%	1,400[a]

[a]Estimated volume in 2007.
Reprinted from: Kehlet H, Jensen TS, Woolf CJ. Persistent postsurgical pain: Risk factors and prevention. *Lancet* 2006;367:1618–1625, with permission from Elsevier.

Mechanisms Involved with the Development of Chronic Pain

Chronic post-surgical pain is similar to other chronic pain syndromes in that it is clearly multifactorial and complex. As emphasized above, it is considered as "abnormal" pain that persists beyond the expected time of healing. The current paradigm of chronic post-surgical pain emphasizes a transitional period during which acute pain evolves into chronic pain, or that individuals whose pain persists long term have inherent and/or induced deficiencies in endogenous pain inhibition that allow central sensitization to occur unopposed after injury.

Nociceptive pain refers to acute pain perception evoked by short-lasting noxious stimuli in intact tissue, in the absence of peripheral or central sensitization. Acute pain usually arises in response to activation of peripheral nociceptors, also called primary afferents. This "normal" or expected unpleasant sensation signals the presence, location, intensity and duration of a noxious stimulus and fades when the stimulus is removed. Nociception is a protective process that helps prevent injury by generating both a reflex withdrawal from the stimulus and a sensation so unpleasant that it results in complex behavioral strategies to avoid further contact with such stimuli. Sensitization of the nociceptive system is an additional phenomenon that occurs after repeated or particularly intense noxious stimuli, so that the threshold for its activation falls and responses to subsequent inputs are amplified. In the absence of ongoing tissue injury, this state of heightened sensitivity returns over time to the normal baseline.

With surgical trauma, besides the obvious nociceptive pain, inflammation and nerve injury also occur (Fig. 14-1). Ongoing inflammation and nerve damage are two factors that have been associated with hyperalgesia, central sensitization, and persistent pain.

Inflammatory pain refers to pain following tissue injury but with no neural injury. It results from the release of inflammatory mediators in response to tissue injury and inflammation. Peripheral sensitization occurs as sensitizing inflammatory mediators reduce the threshold of nociceptors that innervate the inflamed tissue. This hypersensitivity reduces the intensity of the peripheral stimulus needed to activate nociceptors at the site of inflammation and is called primary hyperalgesia. Peripheral sensitization is due to the reduction in threshold and enhanced responsiveness of nociceptors that occurs when the peripheral terminals of high-threshold primary sensory neurons are exposed to inflammatory mediators

and damaged tissue. It is elicited by activation of nociceptors that play a major role in altered heat hypersensitivity and is restricted to the site of tissue injury. Central sensitization is an increase in the excitability of neurons within the central nervous system, so that normal inputs begin to produce abnormal responses. It results from changes in the properties of neurons in the central nervous system. The pain is no longer coupled to the presence, intensity, or duration of nociceptive stimuli. Instead, central sensitization represents an abnormal state of responsiveness or increased gain of the nociceptive system. Clinical manifestations of inflammatory pain often include spontaneous pain in the inflamed area, tactile allodynia, heat hyperalgesia, and throbbing pain. These exaggerated responses to normal sensory inputs usually outlast the tissue injury for hours and days but are usually reversible and normal sensitivity is eventually restored.

Neuropathic pain refers to pain after neural injury (peripheral or central). It is distinct from nociceptive and inflammatory pain conditions by the fact that the injury itself is neuronal. Neuropathic pain conditions are usually associated with abnormal neuronal activity at the site of injury as well as with central sensitization. A key feature of neuropathic pain is the combination of sensory loss with paradoxical hypersensitivity. Clinical features of neuropathic pain include hypoesthesia, dysesthesia, allodynia (often to cold), hyperalgesia, hyperpathia (bursts), and burning pain. The current paradigm is that not all patients with nerve damage will experience neuropathic pain. In some patients, the type of nerve injury may explain both the increase in acute pain and chronic pain, but the extent of pain will be mediated by other factors, including genetic, psychological, and physiologic factors that heighten pain sensitivity and impair pain modulation. It has been proposed that individuals whose pain persists long term have inherent and/or induced deficiencies in endogenous pain inhibition that allow central sensitization to occur unopposed very soon after the surgical injury. If that is the case, that would explain why examining pathways that inhibit pain, such as descending inhibitory pathways, could help predict patients with a higher risk for developing chronic post-surgical pain (20).

While it is a known phenomenon that stress induces analgesia, the opposite can also occur under particular condition, that is, non-painful stress can actually induce hyperalgesia. In a series of studies, Rivat et al. demonstrated in a rat model of pain that long-lasting hyperalgesia following inflammation or a surgical incision is enhanced by a single opioid dose (opioid-induced hyperalgesia); animals with inflammatory

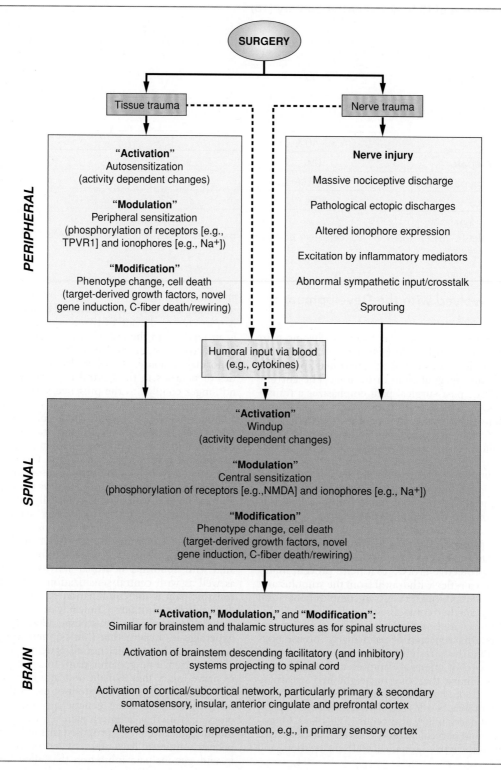

FIGURE 14-1 Mechanisms of nociception-induced hyperalgesia (102).

pain experienced enhanced hyperalgesia in response to the same injury when this was repeated 1 week later (21). This exaggerated response was blocked by the administration of N-methyl-D-aspartate (NMDA) receptor antagonists (such as ketamine) indicating that opioid-induced hyperalgesia after inflammatory and surgical pain in rats treated with fentanyl is mediated by NMDA-dependent pro-nociceptive systems (21–24). Finally, rats exposed to inflammatory pain and/or opioid treatment in a repetitive manner (several

weeks apart) as a model to explore opioid-induced hyperalgesia under non-naïve conditions (equivalent to "prior life events") were shown to have persistent sensitization that was enhanced after each repeated 1exposure to painful stimulation in opioid-exposed rats. That phenomenon was preventable by a single dose of NMDA antagonist such as ketamine (Fig. 14-2) (25).

The potential clinical relevance of these animal experiments is that repetitive exposure to post-operative pain

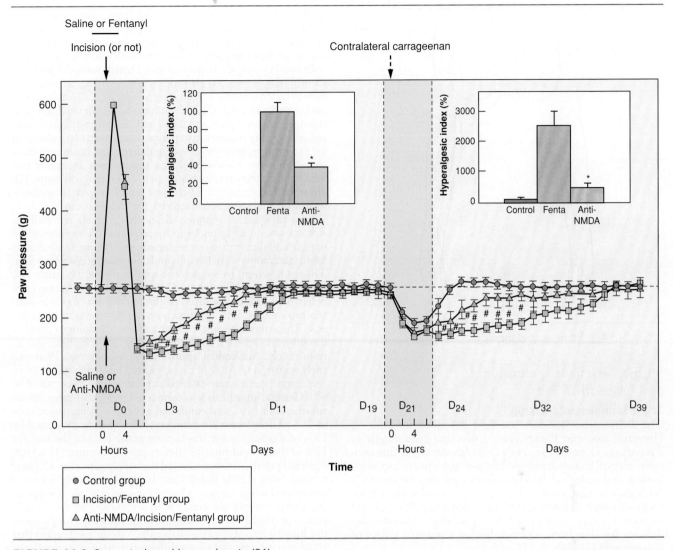

FIGURE 14-2 Stress-induced hyperalgesia (21).

treated with opioids may well result in central sensitization and wound hyperalgesia with a growing number of surgical procedures. One could therefore speculate that chronic post-operative pain may actually occur in patients after a second painful "hit" rather than in opioid-naïve unsensitized patients. If these concepts are confirmed in humans, then repeat cesarean deliveries could be the ultimate model to replicate the conditions examined by Rivat *et al* in their rat model. This would set the basis for a theory whereby women may develop chronic pain only after their second cesarean delivery if hypersensitization and/or opioid-induced hyperalgesia occurred at the time of the first cesarean delivery.

Chronic Pelvic Pain

Chronic pelvic pain is a common entity defined as *non-menstrual pain in the lower abdomen present for at least 6 months* (26,27). Gynecologic factors that have been associated with this disabling condition in women include endometriosis, intrapelvic adhesions, and chronic pelvic inflammatory disease. Diagnostic interventions often include a laparoscopy to identify anatomical anomalies, even though it is well known that pelvic anatomical anomalies do not necessarily cause pain. In particular, not all adhesions result in chronic pelvic pain. Neurologic factors have also been associated with chronic pelvic pain syndromes such as

pudendal neuropathy and neuropathy secondary to the Pfannenstiel incision.

Almeida et al. were the first to report that a history of cesarean delivery may predispose to development of chronic pelvic pain (28). In a retrospective cohort study of Brazilian women scheduled to undergo a laparoscopy, findings in women with pelvic pain ($n = 116$) were compared to those of healthy women with no history of pain scheduled for a surgical tubal ligation ($N = 83$). A significantly higher proportion of women with a history of cesarean delivery was found in the group with chronic pain (67%) compared with the women in the control group (39%) (OR 3.7, 95% CI 1.7–7.7; $p = 0.0006$). Other predictors for chronic pelvic pain identified during the laparoscopy were the presence of endometriosis and sequelae of pelvic inflammatory disease. The presence of adhesions did not seem to be related with complaints of chronic pelvic pain.

Factors thought to be involved in the remodeling process that may cause pelvic adhesions include ischemia and an imbalance of proteolytic enzyme cells in the extracellular matrix (29). While pelvic surgery is associated with a very high occurrence of pelvic adhesions, it has been suggested that pregnancy may confer some protection from the risk of developing pelvic adhesions when compared to other gynecologic procedures, due to the increase in plasminogen activator activity that occurs in pregnancy (29).

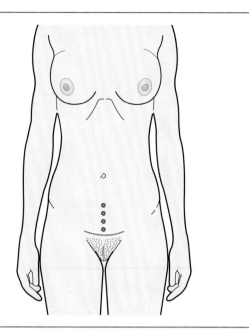

FIGURE 14-3 Pfannenstiel incision.

Surgical Factors: Gynecologic and Obstetrical Procedures

The Pfannenstiel Incision

The Pfannenstiel incision was first described in 1900 by Hermann Johannes Pfannenstiel, a German gynecologist in a report on 51 cases (Fig. 14-3) (30). Advantages of this then novel surgical approach included the low incidence of incisional hernias and esthetical benefits (also called the "bikini-cut"). Nonetheless, chronic pain has been associated with entrapment of lower abdominal wall nerves and the Pfannenstiel incision as a surgical approach for gynecologic and cesarean delivery has now been acknowledged as a possible source of chronic pain (31–34).

In a series of studies, Brandsborg et al. reported that 5% to 32% of women suffer chronic pain after hysterectomy. Eleven studies were identified in a review of the literature evaluating studies that included the following keywords: Pain, chronic pain, pelvic pain, neuropathic pain, visceral pain, neuroplasticity, post-surgical, post-operative, gynecology, hysterectomy, Pfannenstiel, Joel-Cohen, vertical incision, nerve entrapment, incisional hernia, and incisional endometriosis (33). Pain as a preoperative symptom was present in 60% to 100% of women, and the pain prevalence 1 to 2 years after hysterectomy was 5% to 32%. Newly developed pain was reported in 1% to 15%, and exacerbated pain was found in 3% to 5% of women with preoperative pelvic pain. Factors reported to be associated with chronic pain included preoperative depression, preoperative pelvic pain, two or more pregnancies, previous cesarean delivery, and poor socio-economical status. The surgical approach (abdominal vs. vaginal or laparoscopy), incision type (vertical vs. Pfannenstiel), or anesthesia type (general vs. spinal) were not consistently associated with an increased risk for chronic post-hysterectomy pain. The authors suggest a list of parameters to enable comparisons between future studies and optimal assessment of chronic post-hysterectomy pain that include preoperative factors (indication for hysterectomy, previous pelvic disease/surgery, pain characteristics, analgesic consumption, psychological profiling and quantitative sensory testing, socio-demographics, genetics); intra- and early post-operative parameters (anesthesia, surgical procedure and complications, histopathology, acute post-operative pain and analgesic consumption); and post-operative parameters at more than 3 months post-hysterectomy (pain characteristics and analgesic consumption, post-operative complications including infection and reoperation, psychological profiling and quantitative sensory testing, and socio-demographics).

Brandsborg et al. as part of the Danish national audit to identify risk factors for chronic pain after hysterectomy contacted 1,299 women 1 year after surgery (32). Analysis was performed on a total of 1,135 women (87%) out of which 32% reported chronic pain and 23% had pain that affected daily activities. Only preoperative pelvic pain, pain as an indication for the surgery, previous cesarean delivery, and pain problems elsewhere were associated with a significantly increased risk for chronic post-hysterectomy pain. The surgical approach did not affect incidence of chronic pain but spinal anesthesia was associated with a reduced risk for chronic pain.

In a prospective manner, Brandsborg et al. enrolled 90 women scheduled to undergo hysterectomy. The women did not have endometriosis or malignancy. The main indications for hysterectomy were fibroids and abnormal uterine bleeding. The study sought to assess more specifically perioperative risk factors for the development of chronic pain (31). Preoperative pelvic pain (mostly localized to the middle of the pelvic area) was reported by 51% of women and 32% were taking analgesics. The attending gynecologist and anesthesiologist decided the surgical approach for hysterectomy and anesthesia mode, respectively. Abdominal approach (Joel-Cohen or Pfannenstiel) occurred in 63% of cases, vaginal approach occurred in 28%, and laparoscopic-assisted vaginal approach occurred in 9%. General anesthesia was conducted in 39% of cases, spinal anesthesia in 14%, and combined general–epidural anesthesia in 47%. Three weeks after surgery, pelvic pain was reported by 53% of women, and it was located at the level of the scar for 12% of them. Four months after surgery, 15 women (17%) still reported pelvic pain that affected their daily activities, and four women (4%) clearly stated that the pain was newly acquired and related to the surgery. Due to the small sample size, spinal anesthesia was not associated with a reduced risk for chronic pain as previously described by the same authors. This prospective longitudinal study is probably the only detailed report that avoided recall bias and allows differentiation of exacerbation of preexisting pelvic pain from new onset persistent post-surgical pain. The fact that only a relatively small proportion of women actually attributed their pelvic pain to the surgery itself sheds new insights into the incidence of chronic post-hysterectomy pain and associated risk factors. Preexisting pain and poor self-perceived control of pain along with acute post-operative pain were associated with persistent pain 4 months after hysterectomy rather than the surgical procedure itself. While nerve entrapment can occur with a Pfannenstiel incision, scar pain is unlikely to be a major contributor for persistent pain. This is consistent with the premise that abnormal pain modulation due to physiologic and psychosocial factors are involved in the development of chronic pain after hysterectomy as has been described for other surgical procedures as well.

In a survey to evaluate the prevalence and identify risk factors for post-Pfannenstiel pain syndromes, Loos et al. contacted 866 women who had a Pfannenstiel incision for either a hysterectomy (7%) or cesarean delivery (93%) in the previous 2 years (34). The Pfannenstiel incision was described to follow a standardized procedure that involved a 12 to 15 cm transverse incision approximately 2 to 3 cm cranial to the symphysis pubis with diathermal incision of subcutaneous fat and rectus sheath. If needed, the incision was extended laterally by cutting the fibrous sheath containing the aponeuroses of the external, internal oblique, and transverse abdominal muscles. The anterior fascia and linea alba was separated from underlying rectus and pyramidalis muscles over the entire distance between symphysis and umbilicus. Abdominal rectus muscles were then separated in the

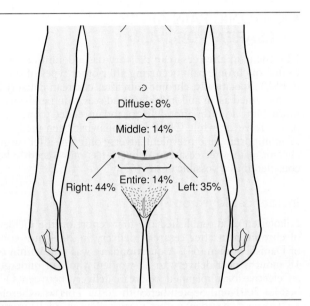

FIGURE 14-4 Location of persistent pain after a Pfannenstiel incision (34).

midline, followed by division of the preperitoneal fat tissue and the opening of the peritoneum. No retractors were used. Once the abdominal procedure was completed, absorbable running sutures were used to approximate facial and muscle layers. The skin was closed intradermally. The questionnaire used to quantify and qualify pain was one used in several studies (see Appendix). It also included a schematic drawing on which women were instructed to mark the exact location of pain (Fig. 14-4). More than 90% of women described pain at the level of the incision, and in 70% the pain was at the lateral ends. Both neuropathic descriptors ("prickling" or "stabbing") as well as non-neuropathic descriptors ("nagging" or "pulling") were used in equal frequency to qualify the pain. Out of 690 responders (80%), 223 women (33%) stated that the incision site was still painful within the preceding month (median time from surgery was 26 months) with 9% reporting moderate to severe pain. Women with moderate or severe pain ($n = 61$) were invited for a follow-up at the institution's outpatient clinic, and 32 women were extensively evaluated. Neuropathic pain caused by an entrapment of the iliohypogastric or ilioinguinal nerve was present in 17 women (53%). Nine women accepted a diagnostic nerve block that led to a significant pain reduction in six of them. The initial pain reduction persisted for at least 12 months in two of these six women. The remaining eight women refused injection. A diagnostic classification of chronic post-Pfannenstiel pain in these 32 women was presented. This finding suggests neuropathic pain in 53% of women, non-neuropathic non-gynecologic pain in 37% of women (diffuse scar pain in seven cases, musculotendinous pain in two cases, abdominal wall atrophy with bulging in one case, keloid in one case, fat necrosis in one case), and non-neuropathic gynecologic pain in 9% of women (endometriosis in one case, secondary vaginismus in one case, dysmenorrhea in one case). The incidence of nerve entrapment in women with moderate to severe pain was relatively high (17/32 women) but represented only a low occurrence within the entire cohort (less than 3%). Overall, numbness at the incision site, recurrent Pfannenstiel incisions, and emergency cesarean delivery were significant predictors for chronic post-Pfannenstiel pain. While length of incision did not as such predict chronic pain, a substantial proportion of women reported pain in the lateral portions of the scar. The innervating nerves of the suprapubic area and lower abdomi-

nal portions can be damaged or trapped when the incision is extended beyond lateral edges of the rectus sheath, and nerve entrapment was found to be common in women with moderate to severe pain.

Loos et al. also reported that neurectomy of the ilioinguinal and/or iliohypogastric nerve(s) provides good to excellent results in a series of 27 women (post-cesarean delivery in 19 of these cases) suffering from Pfannenstiel-induced neuralgic pain (35).

The Joel-Cohen Incision

The Joel-Cohen incision is a transverse skin incision that is placed about 3 cm below the line joining the anterior superior iliac spines, making it higher than the traditional Pfannenstiel incision. It has been proposed as a surgical approach to reduce surgical time and bleeding. However, its impact on infectious complications is still debated (36–40).

In a longitudinal prospective randomized clinical trial to compare the Joel-Cohen approach versus the Pfannenstiel approach for a primary cesarean delivery (mostly under general anesthesia), Nabhan et al. enrolled 600 Egyptian women. Sixty-two women in each group were further evaluated when a repeat cesarean delivery was scheduled (41). At the preoperative evaluation for the repeat cesarean delivery, four women in each group (7%) reported long-term pain. Patchy numb sensations were present in two women in the Joel-Cohen group and three women in the Pfannenstiel group. Intra-operative outcomes were significantly more complicated in the Pfannenstiel group, with a higher percentage of severe adhesions (bladder adherent to uterus) resulting in a longer surgical time and increased blood loss.

Options in surgical technique other than the abdominal skin incision type include blunt versus sharp abdominal entry, exteriorization of the uterus versus abdominal in situ repair, single- versus double-layer closure of the uterine incision, closure versus non-closure of the pelvic peritoneum, and liberal versus restricted use of a sub-rectus sheath drain. Studies assessing these surgical alternatives have evaluated primarily serious intra-operative and post-operative complications including organ damage, organ failure, significant sepsis, thromboembolism, high-care unit admission, blood loss, blood transfusion, and death (42–46). Evaluation of maternal satisfaction, pain outcomes, and analgesic use in the immediate postpartum are often scarce in these studies.

Peritoneal Closure

The benefits of closure versus non-closure of the visceral and/or parietal peritoneum to reduce pelvic adhesions have been evaluated in several studies and remain controversial (29,42,47). It has been suggested that more severe adhesions that require adhesiolysis prior to uterine incision occur more frequently when the peritoneum has been closed in a prior cesarean delivery (48). The impact of closure versus non-closure of the parietal peritoneum closure on severe acute post-operative pain (49,50) and chronic post-cesarean pain (51) has been evaluated.

Shahin et al. tested the hypothesis that non-closure of the parietal peritoneum would reduce the incidence of persistent post-cesarean pain (51). In a randomized clinical trial, Egyptian women were randomized to parietal peritoneum closure or non-closure during elective primary cesarean delivery under spinal anesthesia with hyperbaric bupivacaine (no opioid). In the closure group ($n = 161$), acute abdominal pain was present in 40% of women, with 29% of women reporting pain at 15 days postpartum and 25% reporting pain at 8 months postpartum. In the non-closure group ($n = 16$), only 18% reported severe acute pain, 12% at 15 days and 10% at 8 months. There was higher morphine consumption for management of acute post-operative pain in women in the closure group. At 8 months, 14% of women in the closure group were taking analgesics compared to 4% in the non-closure group. When specifically assessing pain at the level of the incision, there was no difference at 8 months between the two groups; scar pain was present in 7% of women in the closure group and 2% of women in the non-closure group. Irrespective of surgical technique (and with no uterine exteriorization), this large prospective trial demonstrates that 18% of women report chronic abdominal pain at 8 months despite conventional multi-modal post-operative analgesia (NSAIDs, acetaminophen, and morphine for breakthrough pain). Better pain outcomes following peritoneal non-closure have been attributed to the rich nerve supply and poor blood supply of the peritoneum. Stretching, traction, suturing, and reapproximation of the peritoneum may cause ischemia which could explain high reports of visceral and epigastric pain.

Uterine Exteriorization

Uterine exteriorization is a common practice in North America and is thought to provide better exposure of the angles that may result in an easier and faster uterine closure, overall shorter surgical time, decreased blood loss, and decreased post-operative infection rate. It is important to note, however, that these purported advantages remain debated (52–56). Uterine exteriorization is also associated with increased intra-operative discomfort and pain (55,57,58), increased intra-operative nausea and vomiting (59), hemodynamic changes (59), and potentially fatal air embolism (60).

Nafisi et al. evaluated in a randomized clinical trial the effect of uterine exteriorization on acute post-operative pain in Iranian women who were scheduled for a cesarean delivery under general anesthesia (58). Visceral peritoneal closure was performed in all cases, and parietal peritoneal closure was performed in some cases (although which case and the proportion between the two groups were not specified). Ratings of visceral pain during the first two nights post-delivery and the number of women requiring supplemental opioids for breakthrough pain were significantly higher in women with uterine exteriorization ($n = 102$) versus women with in situ closure ($n = 104$). There was no difference in ratings of incisional pain between the two groups. Explanations for increased post-delivery pain with uterine exteriorization include peritoneal stretching. When added to that caused by parietal peritoneal closure, this factor may be consequential in this study.

Single-layer versus Double-layer Uterine Closure

Few studies have assessed this surgical parameter with pain outcomes after cesarean delivery. It has been suggested in one study that single-layer closure may marginally reduce the occurrence of severe post-operative pain on the first day post-delivery (61). On the other hand, this surgical technique may increase the risk for uterine rupture in subsequent pregnancies (62).

In summary, no study to date has been strictly designed to evaluate acute post-operative pain as a primary outcome combining all the various surgical options under optimal anesthesia. Nonetheless, surgical factors and the mechanisms whereby they appear to increase the likelihood for visceral pain, severe post-operative pain, and increased post-operative analgesic requirements include:

- Larger surgical incisions (increases risk for lateral nerve entrapment and neuromas)
- Uterine exteriorization (peritoneal stretching)
- Parietal peritoneal closure (peritoneal stretching)
- Repeated surgical procedure (hypersensitization)

■ CHRONIC PAIN AFTER CESAREAN DELIVERY

Chronic pain after cesarean delivery has a definition similar to that of chronic pain occurring after other types of surgery (CPSP). Specifically, chronic pain after cesarean delivery has been defined as an abdominal wound scar pain persisting for more than 3 months after delivery and unrelated to menstrual pain. However, while CPSP has somewhat been recognized as an important and prevalent adverse outcome after surgery, chronic pain after cesarean delivery has only recently been considered as a possible entity (63).

Incidence: Myth or Reality?

Nikolajsen et al. published the first report on the incidence of chronic pain after cesarean delivery in 2004 in a cohort of Danish women (64). A questionnaire was sent within 6 to 18 months post-delivery to all women who had undergone an elective or unplanned cesarean delivery between October 1st 2001 and September 30th 2002. This was therefore a retrospective survey with a mean follow-up of 10 months. Two hundred and forty-four women were contacted, and the response rate was 90% ($n = 220$). Pain resolved in most women within 3 months. However, 19% of women reported that post-operative abdominal scar pain had lasted for more than 3 months, and at the time of the interview, pain was still present in 12% of women. Information about anesthetic technique and post-cesarean analgesia strategies (in particular, the administration of intrathecal morphine) was not provided. Several factors (i.e., previous abdominal surgery including cesarean delivery, presence of an indwelling epidural catheter for labor analgesia, indication for cesarean delivery [scheduled/unplanned], incision type, post-operative wound infection, maternal weight and height, and time of interview) were similar in women with and without chronic pain. Identified risk factors for persistent pain included general anesthesia, pain issues elsewhere, and recall of severe acute post-operative pain. This survey was important not only as the first study reporting on the incidence of chronic pain; it also provided a questionnaire (see Appendix) that has been utilized since then by other investigators in subsequent studies.

Eisenach et al. undertook a prospective longitudinal cohort study to describe the incidence of acute pain and chronic pain after delivery and possibly identify risk factors for the development of chronic pain (65). They enrolled 1,228 women who had delivered vaginally ($n = 837$), with or without neuraxial labor analgesia, as well as women who had undergone cesarean delivery ($n = 391$), either scheduled or unplanned (with or without a trial of labor). Unlike the previous report by Nikolajsen et al., women were questioned within 36 hours after delivery to assess for the presence of acute pain and to record preexisting pain, pain treatment before or during pregnancy, and degree of somatization using a 10-point scale (66). Delivery data including analgesic and anesthetic requirements were noted. At 8 weeks after delivery, the presence of persistent pain and its characteristics as well as features of postpartum depression based on the Edinburgh Postnatal Depression scale (67,68) were evaluated via phone interview. The major findings of this large prospective trial were that 20% of women after a cesarean delivery and 8% of women after a vaginal delivery reported severe acute pain in the immediate postpartum period that was associated with persistent pain and postpartum depression that had a significant impact on women's ability to perform daily activities in the postpartum period. These observations stress the need for both better acute pain management at the time of delivery and studies that may help identify women at risk as well as validate interventions that may reduce persistent pain and depression.

Sia et al. examined the incidence of chronic pain after cesarean delivery as an extension of their studies on acute post-cesarean analgesia, ethnicity, and genetic polymorphisms (69,70). In one study on the association between μ-opioid receptor genotype (OPRM1) and the clinical efficacy of intravenous morphine in 1,066 Asian women undergoing a cesarean delivery under spinal anesthesia with intrathecal morphine, 857 (80%) agreed to answer a survey that was based on Nikolajsen's questionnaire (71). The median follow-up between the delivery and the phone interview was 14 months (12 to 20 months). The number of women reporting pain for more than 3 months but not present at the time of the survey was 28 (3%) and an additional 51 women (6%) reported pain still present at the time of the survey, resulting in a chronic pain rate of 9%. There was no association of chronic pain with the presence of other abdominal surgery or previous cesarean delivery, maternal age, gestational age, maternal weight or height, wound infection, duration of surgery, pain at 24 hours, or total morphine consumption post-cesarean. However, pain recall in the immediate post-operative period, pain present elsewhere (back pain and migraines most commonly), and non-private insurance were independent risk factors for the development of chronic pain. Since there was a higher recall of post-operative pain without a recorded difference in 24 hours post-cesarean pain scores or morphine consumption in women with chronic pain, this strongly suggested over reporting and recall bias; indeed some women were surveyed up to 20 months post-delivery. However, as noted by the authors, this could be a true effect as pain scores were not recorded beyond the first 24 hours post-cesarean and subsequent analgesia may have been ineffective.

In a second study by the same authors focusing on Chinese Han women, 631 women were enrolled for a genetic association study on polymorphisms of the ATP-binding cassette sub-family B member-1 (ABCB1) gene and acute and chronic pain after intrathecal morphine for cesarean delivery (72). Five hundred and three women (80%) agreed to take the Nikolajsen questionnaire. At 6 months post-delivery, 33% of women recalled wound pain at 1 month, 25% up to 3 months post-delivery, and 4% (20 women) between 3 and 6 months. Pain was still present at the time of the survey in 4% (18 women), with 1.2% (6 women) requiring analgesia for moderate to severe pain, and 0.6% (3 women) reporting daily pain. The incidence of chronic pain was 8%, which was essentially similar to the previous report by the same authors if one takes into account recall bias. The relatively low incidence of chronic pain in both reports in Asian women could be due to differences in ethnicity, genetics, and the surgical technique (no exteriorization of uterus and non-closure of peritoneum).

In a cohort of Finnish women, 600 consecutive mothers were surveyed within 12 months of their delivery to determine whether the incidence of persistent pain was more common after cesarean delivery than after vaginal birth (73). A sample size of 184 women per group would enable investigators to detect an increase in persistent pain from 5% after vaginal birth to 15% after cesarean delivery at a 0.05 significance level with 90% power. The response rate was 76% ($n = 229$) in the cesarean delivery group and 70% ($n = 209$) in the vaginal delivery group. Scheduled (37%) and unplanned cesarean deliveries (63%) were done under spinal anesthesia that contained morphine (120 to 160 μg), epidural anesthesia, or general anesthesia (14% of women). Labor epidural analgesia was provided to 66% of women with a vaginal delivery. Postpartum pain lasted significantly longer after cesarean delivery than after vaginal delivery; pain resolved by

2 months in 70% of women after cesarean delivery and 83% of women delivering vaginally. The major finding was that chronic pain was more frequent after cesarean delivery; pain at 12 months was reported by 18% of women after cesarean versus 10% after vaginal delivery ($p = 0.011$; odds ratio 2.1, 95% confidence interval 1.2 to 3.7). A trial of labor prior to cesarean delivery did not affect the incidence of chronic pain. Labor epidural analgesia did not affect the incidence of chronic pain in women delivering vaginally. While the intensity of the pain was rated overall as being mild in both groups, it affected daily life in 14% of women with a cesarean delivery and 15% of women delivering vaginally. Constant or daily pain at 12 months was present in 4% of women after cesarean delivery and in 1% of women with a vaginal delivery. Women with chronic pain at 12 months had a higher recall of pain in the first postpartum day regardless of mode of delivery and other risk factors included a history of chronic disease and previous pain (i.e., back pain).

Overall, most of these studies have relied on recall of pain at the time of delivery to quantify the incidence of acute and chronic post-cesarean pain. The incidence of chronic pain ranges between 3% and 18% according to the studies (Table 14-3).

Risk Factors

Based mostly on retrospective surveys and some prospective studies, risk factors for chronic pain postpartum include personal characteristics, preoperative factors, intra-operative factors, and post-operative factors (Table 14-4).

Oxytocin: Its Potential Role in Protecting Women During Childbirth

Oxytocin is a nonapeptide hormone best known for its role in parturition and lactation, social behaviors (memory, recognition, affiliation, sexual behavior, aggression), non-social behaviors (learning, stress, anxiety, depression, feeding, and human behaviors (love, bonding, and trust) (74). Oxytocin is primarily synthesized in the paraventricular nucleus and the supraoptic nucleus of the hypothalamus. The paraventricular nucleus projects nerve fibers excreting oxytocin to various areas of the central nervous system including the spinal cord (75). In the spinal cord, nociceptive afferent messages originating from C and Aδ primary afferents are inhibited by a pathway that begins with oxytocin being released from the paraventricular nucleus and exciting a subpopulation of glutamatergic interneurons in the most superficial layer of the dorsal horn, which subsequently distribute their excitation to all GABAergic neurons. In numerous animal models, oxytocin has long been shown to possess antinociceptive effects with some renewed interest (75–81).

Despite robust evidence from animal studies that oxytocin exhibits antihyperalgesic properties, and suggestions that given centrally (intrathecally) it could be advantageous perioperatively, human studies are very scarce and anecdotal. Intraventricular administration of oxytocin has been shown to relieve cancer pain in one terminally ill patient (82) and intrathecal oxytocin appears to reduce low back pain (83). Local administration of oxytocin in the colon increases the pain threshold to colonic distention in patients with irritable bowel syndrome (84). Prolonged treatment with nasal inhalation of oxytocin has a beneficial effect on abdominal pain, discomfort, and mood in women with refractory constipation (85). Plasma oxytocin levels were assessed in several clinical pain syndromes. In a cohort of women suffering from fibromyalgia, it appears that oxytocin has a pain-processing role and

TABLE 14-3 Incidence of Chronic Pain After Cesarean Delivery

References	Study Design	Acute Pain	Chronic Pain >3 mos		Associated Factors
Observational Study—Chronic Pain as Primary Outcome					
(3)	Retrospective (6–17 mos) Danish CS N = 222	At 1 mo: 55% 1–3 mos: 26.4%	3–6 mos: 18.6% >6 mos: 12.3%		General anesthesia Pain elsewhere Severe pain post-CS
(4)	Prospective CS N = 391 VD N = 837 Multicentric (USA)	At 24 h, VAS >7/10: 17% CS and 8% VD At 8 wks: 9.2% CS and 10% VD			Severe pain at delivery Postpartum depression
(5)	Retrospective (12–20 mos) Mixed Asian CS N = 857	N/A	3–12 mos: 3.2% >12 mos: 6% (Total: 9.2%)		Severe pain post-CS Pain elsewhere Non-private insurance
(6)	"Prospective" recall (6 mos) Chinese CS N = 503	At 1 mo: 33% At 3 mos: 25%	3–6 mos: 4% At 6 mos: 3.6% (Total: 7.6%)		ABCB1 genetics
(7)	Retrospective (12 mos) Finnish CS N = 229 VD N = 209	Within 3 wks 37% CS 51% VD 3 wks–2 mos 33% CS 32% VD	2–5 mos 9% CS 9% VD At 1 yr 18% CS 10% VD		Severe pain post-delivery Previous pain Chronic disease CS >VD
(8)	Prospective (12 mos) China CS N = 301 VD N = 301	N/A	6 &12 mos Waist/back pain: 20% CS vs. 17% VD Abdominal pain CS 4% vs. VD 2%		Abdominal pain CS vs. VD RR 3.6 (95% CI 1.2–11.0)
RCT—Persistent/Chronic Pain as Secondary Outcome					**Outcome**
(9)	Parietal peritoneal closure vs. nonclosure Egypt, N = 340 Spinal anesthesia (no IT morphine)	At 2 wks Closure: 29% pain Nonclosure: 12% pain	8 mos (18%)		Parietal peritoneal closure increased chronic pain
			Closure: Pain 26% (treated 14%) Epigastric 8% (treated 5%)	Nonclosure: Pain 10% (treated 4%) Epigastric 3% (treated 2%)	
(10)	IT clonidine (no IT morphine) Belgium, N = 96	IT Clo 150 µg Clo 75-Suf 2 µg No Clo	At 3 mos 3% 22% 17%	At 6 mos 3% 12% 7%	IT clonidine reduced 48 h hyperalgesia
(11)	IW diclofenac 48 h (no IT morphine) Belgium, N = 92		At 6 mos IW ROP: 10% IW DIC: 3% IV DIC: 23%		IW diclofenac more effective than IV diclofenac As effective as IW ROP with IV DIC
(12)	IW ropivacaine 48 h above vs. below fascia France, N = 50	At 1 mo Above: 2 patients Below: 1 patient	At 6 mos Above: 1 patient Below: 1 patient		Improved analgesia when catheter is below the fascia
(13)	TAP block (ropivacaine) vs. placebo Canada, N = 100	At 6 wks: Pain in 8.3% (only 1 patient needed pain medication)			No added benefit of TAP when IT morphine is given
(14)	PO gabapentin vs. placebo Canada, N = 44	GABA reduced pain scores in the first 48 h (no morphine-sparing)	At 3 mos GABA: 2/16 (12%) Placebo: 4/20 (20%)		GABA improves analgesia in the first 48 h
(15)	IV MgSO₄ 24h Australia, N = 120	At 6 wks Persistent pain: 16% "Wind-up" pain: 12% Hyperalgesia: 8% (MgSO₄ 9%, placebo 5%)			No benefit of MgSO₄ on acute or persistent pain

IW, intrawound; CS, C-section; Clo, clonidine; MgSO₄, magnesium sulfate IT, intrathecal; VD, vaginal delivery; ROP, ropivacaine; GABA, gabapentin TAP, transversus abdominis plane; DIC, diclofenac.

TABLE 14-4 Risk Factors Associated with Acute/Chronic Pain After Cesarean Delivery

Preoperative	Specific Parameter	References
Psychosocial factors	Somatization score	(4)
	Pain Catastrophizing Scale (PCS)	(16,17)
Preceding pain/ other pain	Back pain	(3,5,7)
	Migraines	(5)
	Menstrual pain	(4)
	Scar hyperalgesia from previous cesarean delivery	(18)
Chronic disease		(7)
Genetic susceptibility	ABCB1	(6)
Intra-operative		
Type of anesthesia	General anesthesia	(3)
Surgical factors	Emergency cesarean delivery	(19)
	Repeat incision >2	(19)
	Length of Pfannenstiel incision	(19)
	Uterine exteriorization	(20,21)
	Closure of peritoneum	(9,22,23)
Post-operative		
Acute pain		(3–5,7,24)
Depression		(4)

may explain some of the symptoms associated with fibromyalgia such as pain, stress, and depression (86). Plasma oxytocin levels were shown to be decreased in children with recurrent abdominal pain versus a control of healthy children (87).

To provide a potential mechanistic explanation for the relatively low incidence of chronic pain after childbirth and in particular, after cesarean delivery compared with that after other types of surgical procedures (10), it has been proposed that endogenous secretion of oxytocin during labor and delivery may confer specific protection. Preliminary work in rats by Eisenach et al. to examine the potential protective effect of oxytocin during childbirth suggests that it could well modulate post-surgical pain but is unlikely to have an effect on labor pain (88,89). In addition, spinal oxytocin levels in 12 women undergoing a postpartum tubal ligation under spinal anesthesia were not different from that of 12 healthy women undergoing non-obstetric surgery under spinal anesthesia (90), and could therefore not explain the relatively low incidence of chronic pain found in a cohort of 978 women followed up to 1 year postpartum. Chronic pain was present in only 2% (18 women) of this cohort at 6 months, declining to 0.3% (3 women) at 12 months (90). More work is needed to understand and substantiate the antihyperalgesic effects of endogenous oxytocin at the time of labor and delivery and examine the potential use of intrathecal oxytocin to reduce chronic post-surgical pain.

Prevention of Chronic Pain After Cesarean Delivery

Substantial evidence has been generated over the last decade suggesting that severe acute pain after delivery and specifically after cesarean delivery may not be a myth and requires effective management to prevent potential devastating long-term outcomes (91); these include persistent debilitating pain that can last beyond the expected period of healing, as well as postpartum depression (65).

Numerous targets to provide optimal multi-modal post-operative analgesia have been suggested (Fig. 14-5). However, even with gold-standard multi-modal regimens

(spinal or epidural morphine in conjunction with acetaminophen and NSAIDs), the proportion of women who suffer severe acute pain post-cesarean is still remarkably high (65) and women's fear of post-cesarean pain is ranked as being their most important concern (92). Despite numerous studies to improve immediate post-operative analgesia, targeted strategies to prevent hyperalgesia and chronic pain are scarce.

Carvalho et al. conducted two studies looking at the effects of an extended-release epidural morphine (EREM) formulation for post-cesarean analgesia (93,94). In their second randomized clinical trial, they compared EREM (10 mg) with epidural morphine (4 mg) in a setting reflecting current obstetric anesthesia practice in a multi-modal fashion (94). The authors found a significant morphine-sparing effect between 24 and 48 hours after delivery, with superior functional activity in the EREM group. The incidence of side effects and respiratory depression were similar in both groups. Despite the initial excitement generated by liposomal drug delivery, EREM might not be the panacea for post-cesarean analgesia and requires more research to define its benefits. It has not been defined yet whether EREM justifies routinely placing combined-spinal epidurals to allow its delivery in the epidural space rather than performing single shot spinals for elective cesarean deliveries. Lastly, some concern about inadvertent administration of EREM in the subarachnoid space remains to be resolved.

■ ANALGESIC OPTIONS TO PREVENT CHRONIC PAIN AFTER CESAREAN DELIVERY

Intrathecal Clonidine

Several studies have added clonidine to the intrathecal anesthetic solution for cesarean deliveries with various goals and outcomes (Table 14-5) (95–98). Intrathecal clonidine has a potent α2-adrenergic receptor-mediated antinociceptive effect in descending pathways to the dorsal horn of the spinal cord. It is effective for both somatic and visceral pain (99). Intrathecal clonidine added to local anesthetics for surgery prolongs the

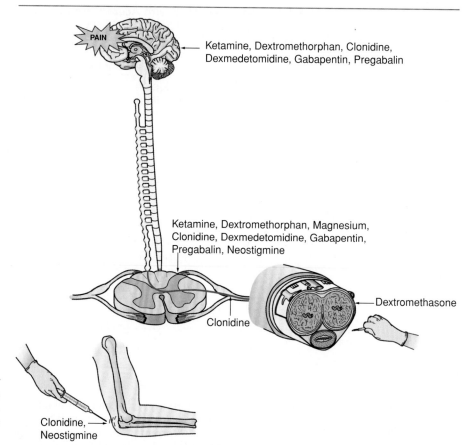

FIGURE 14-5 Numerous targets to enhance opioids or local anesthetics to reduce post-operative pain have been suggested.

surgical block time (sensory regression to L2 and duration of motor block) and the time to first analgesic request (100).

Benhamou et al., in a randomized clinical trial to assess intra-operative pain, compared the effects of hyperbaric bupivacaine administered alone, with fentanyl 15 µg, and/or clonidine 75 µg (95). Dermatomal spread was significantly increased by the addition of clonidine, and no woman receiving the clonidine–fentanyl solution reported any pain during the cesarean delivery. Duration of the surgical block was significantly prolonged and time to first analgesic request was substantially

longer in the clonidine–fentanyl group. Intra-operative nausea and vomiting was lower in women who received clonidine (with or without fentanyl). Sedation was more frequent in the clonidine–fentanyl group. Hypotension and ephedrine use were not different between groups. The solution with the best anesthetic profile was clearly the bupivacaine with fentanyl–clonidine combination. Acute pain scores and persistent pain were not evaluated in this early study.

Paech et al. evaluated various anesthetic solutions combining bupivacaine, fentanyl, morphine, and clonidine (97).

TABLE 14-5 Effect of Intrathecal Clonidine on Post-Cesarean Analgesia

References	Study Design	IT Clonidine	Primary Outcome	Findings
(25)	N = 78 RCT BUP 10 mg ±Fent 15 µg no morphine	± 75 µg	Intra-operative pain	Fent–Clo best combination Delayed first rescue Sedation
(26)	N = 240 RCT BUP 10 mg Fent 15 µg Mo 100 µg	60–150 µg	Morphine iv PCA → 48 h	Morphine 100 µg–Clo 60 µg best combination Sedation Vomiting
(27)	N = 106 BUP 10 mg No fentanyl No morphine	± 75 µg	Time to first request Morphine iv PCA dose	↑ Surgical time Delayed first rescue No morphine-sparing
(10)	N = 96 RCT BUP 10 mg Suf 2 µg No morphine	± 75–150 µg	Time to first request Morphine iv PCA dose Pain → 48 h Pain at 6 mos	↑ Surgical time Delayed first rescue Antihyperalgesic Pain at 6 mos 12%

BUP, bupivacaine; Fent, fentanyl; Suf, sufentanil; Mo, morphine; Clo, clonidine.

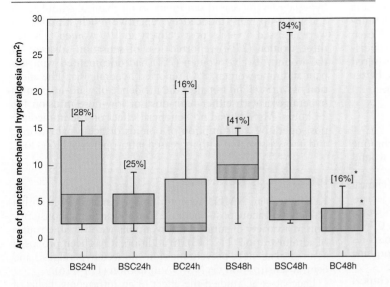

FIGURE 14-6 Antihyperalgesic effect of spinal clonidine (96).

Morphine consumption with intravenous patient-controlled analgesia (PCA) in the first 48 hours was compared. The combination of 100 μg morphine and 60 μg clonidine increased the duration of post-cesarean analgesia, reduced pain scores up to 12 hours post-operative, and decreased intravenous morphine consumption. Intra-operative sedation was found in women receiving clonidine. There was no difference in pain score between groups beyond 12 hours and up to 36 hours post-cesarean. Persistent pain was not evaluated.

van Tuijl et al., in a placebo-controlled randomized clinical trial, compared intrathecal bupivacaine alone to intrathecal bupivacaine with 75 μg clonidine (98). Total post-operative intravenous morphine consumption was similar in both groups and so were pain scores in the first 24 hours; however, the time to first analgesic request was substantially longer. The authors concluded that adding 75 μg clonidine to hyperbaric bupivacaine prolongs spinal analgesia and motor block after cesarean delivery without any major side effects but does not have effects that last beyond the first 2 hours. Persistent pain was not evaluated.

Lavand'homme et al., in a placebo-controlled randomized clinical trial, compared intrathecal bupivacaine alone to a low-dose of clonidine (75 μg) with sufentanil (2 μg) or a high-dose of clonidine (150 μg) (96). For the first time, the primary outcome was to evaluate the extent of peri-incisional punctate mechanical hyperalgesia, using a von Frey filament to map the scar (101) as a marker of central sensitization (hyperexcitation) that may predict persistent pain. The major finding of this study was that clonidine (150 μg) decreased the incidence and the extent of wound hyperalgesia at 48 hours (Fig. 14-6). First request for additional analgesia was substantially delayed in the group receiving clonidine–sufentanil. Ephedrine use was similar between groups, although the incidence of hypotension (between 30 and 45 minutes after spinal injection) was higher in the group receiving 150 μg clonidine. One month after delivery, 30% of all women reported mild pain, mostly at the level of the scar (although one-third of those reported visceral pain). There was no difference between groups in the incidence of pain, although there was a slight trend with less pain in the group of women allocated to receive the higher dose of clonidine. At 3 months, 17% of women in the placebo group, 22% of women receiving low-dose clonidine, and only 3% receiving high-dose clonidine reported mild pain, and only one of them was still taking analgesics. At 6 months, 7% of women in the placebo group, 12% of women receiving low-dose clonidine, and only 3% receiving high-dose clonidine reported mild pain, and one of them was still taking

analgesics. The addition of clonidine did not seem to reduce the risk for chronic pain, although this study was certainly underpowered for this specific outcome. The finding that the incidence and extent of post-operative mechanical hyperalgesia could be reduced by the addition of a high-dose of clonidine is of interest, especially since wound hyperalgesia associated with central sensitization may induce permanent modifications and promote the development of persistent pain (102).

Intrawound Diclofenac

Other novel strategies to optimize analgesia after cesarean delivery tested the short- and long-term benefits of intrawound infusion of NSAIDs with or without local anesthetics (103). Lavand'homme et al. tested the hypothesis that diclofenac has peripheral analgesic properties in addition to systemic effects that could reduce local expression of mediators that sensitize nociceptors (104). In their clinical trial, women scheduled for a cesarean delivery under spinal anesthesia were randomized to one of three groups: Intrawound infusion of diclofenac with an elastomeric pump connected to a multi-hole 20 G catheter (Pain Buster®; I-Flow Corporation, Lake Forest, Ca.) inserted superficial to the fascia, intrawound infusion of ropivacaine with intravenous diclofenac, or intrawound saline infusion with intravenous diclofenac. Continuous intrawound infusion of diclofenac resulted in greater opioid-sparing and better post-operative analgesia than the same dose administered as an intermittent intravenous bolus, and it produced similar analgesia to that of ropivacaine infusion with intravenous diclofenac. There was no benefit of either solution beyond 24 hours, and no long-term benefit was demonstrated. Although this study was clearly underpowered to test any difference in long-term outcomes, the incidence of persistent pain at 6 months post-cesarean was not statistically different between groups, but chronic pain was present in 14% of women.

Mignon et al. tested the effect of solutions containing local anesthetics and NSAIDs in a randomized clinical trial including 50 women undergoing elective cesarean deliveries and provided a follow-up at 6 months after delivery (105). The specific modality of leaving an indwelling catheter for 48 hours with a solution containing both a local anesthetic (ropivacaine) and an NSAID (ketoprofen) while comparing the efficacy of this cocktail in two different planes is novel. The authors report that below-the-fascia infusion through a 20 G multi-hole catheter (PAINfusor 7.5 cm) of 450 mg of ropivacaine and 20 mg ketoprofen provide better analgesia than above-the-fascia infusion of the same solution over 48 hours, with lower pain scores at rest up to 36 hours post-cesarean and lower rescue doses of morphine for breakthrough pain up to 48 hours after surgery. The authors report no difference in morphine-related side effects or long-term benefits; one woman in each group of 25 women reported post-operative residual pain or discomfort at 6 months. The question that remains to be answered is whether below-the-fascia wound instillation provides better pain relief than other local anesthetic injection techniques.

Transversus Abdominis Plane (TAP) Block

The TAP block is another recently investigated technique that is simple to manage and probably less costly than wound instillations with promising results (106–109).

McDonnell et al., in a placebo-controlled randomized clinical trial in 50 Irish women scheduled for cesarean delivery under spinal anesthesia (bupivacaine and fentanyl), evaluated pain scores and duration of TAP blocks (1.5 mg/kg of ropivacaine 0.75% per side) using the loss-of-resistance technique (109). Pain scores were higher in the placebo group up to 48 hours, and morphine consumption was higher up to 36 hours post-TAP block.

Belavy et al., in a placebo-controlled randomized clinical trial in 50 Australian women scheduled for cesarean delivery under spinal anesthesia (bupivacaine and fentanyl), evaluated the post-operative morphine-sparing effect of ultrasound (US)-guided TAP blocks (20 mL ropivacaine 0.5% per side) (106). The morphine consumption over the first 24 hours was significantly higher in women allocated to the placebo group and so was the anti-emetic use.

Kanazi et al. compared the analgesic effect of a US-guided TAP block (20 mL per side of bupivacaine 0.375% with epinephrine 5 μg/mL) to spinal morphine (0.2 mg) in a randomized clinical trial in 57 Lebanese women scheduled for elective cesarean delivery under spinal anesthesia (bupivacaine and fentanyl) (108). Spinal morphine provided longer post-operative analgesia, improved early visceral pain scores, and reduced analgesic consumption for breakthrough pain in the initial 12 hours but at the expense of nausea, vomiting, and pruritus.

Costello et al. evaluated the benefits of adding an US-guided TAP block (ropivacaine 0.375% 20 mL per side) in a placebo-controlled randomized clinical trial in 87 North American women undergoing an elective cesarean delivery under spinal anesthesia (bupivacaine, fentanyl, and morphine 0.1 mg) (107). Pain scores with movement and at rest as well as analgesic consumption were similar in both groups over 48 hours. Residual abdominal pain at 6 weeks was 8.4%.

Questions still remaining unanswered include the optimal solution (which adjuvant to add to the local anesthetic), the ideal duration of the infiltration, and the possible benefit of leaving an indwelling TAP catheter for reinjection. These techniques may be found to reduce the extent and incidence of wound hyperalgesia and could reduce the incidence of persistent pain.

IV Magnesium Sulfate

The magnesium ion is able to modulate NMDA receptor activation and acts as a non-competitive NMDA antagonist. In an animal model of tissue injury and central sensitization, systemic administration of magnesium with morphine increased opioid analgesic effect (110).

Paech et al. conducted a placebo-controlled randomized clinical trial to test the hypothesis that IV magnesium sulfate (MgSO4) may reduce post-operative opioid consumption, acute post-operative pain, and wound hyperalgesia (111). Saline versus a low-dose (1 g/h) infusion of MgSO4 started 1 hour preoperatively and continued up to 24 hours post-delivery was compared to a high-dose (2 g/h) infusion. Using a von Frey filament to map the scar (101), punctate mechanical

hyperalgesia (increased sensitivity to mechanical stimulation) and wind-up pain (induced by repetitive touch stimulation) were assessed 6 weeks post-delivery in 104 women. Thirty-three women (27%) reported loss of sensation adjacent to the wound. Twelve women (7%) had documented wind-up pain and nine women (8%) reported hyperalgesia. The addition of MgSO4 did not alter the incidence of wind-up pain or hyperalgesia with either high-dose or low-dose infusion for 24 hours. MgSO4 had no beneficial effect on the immediate post-operative consumption of opioids or acute pain scores, and it was associated with increased intra-operative blood loss.

Intravenous Ketamine

Ketamine is an NMDA receptor antagonist associated with a reduction in acute post-operative pain and analgesic consumption in a variety of surgical interventions with variable routes of administration (112,113). In addition, it has been proposed as an ideal agent to prevent incision-induced hyperalgesia and central sensitization via NMDA inhibition (114–116).

Bauchat et al. studied the effect of an intravenous bolus of 10 mg ketamine immediately post-delivery as part of a multi-modal strategy in 174 women undergoing elective cesarean delivery under spinal anesthesia (bupivacaine 12 mg, fentanyl 15 μg, and morphine 150 μg) in a placebo-controlled randomized clinical trial (117). The aim of the study was to evaluate post-operative breakthrough pain in the first 24 hours post-cesarean and the need for rescue medication. There was no difference in the immediate outcome parameters (breakthrough pain, time to first analgesic request, analgesic rescue doses, nausea and vomiting); however, more women allocated to receive ketamine were either restless or drowsy and 35% of them reported feeling lightheaded, dizzy, or seeing double. There were no reports of disturbing dreams in the 72 hours that followed ketamine dosing. Despite not having any measurable analgesic benefits in the first 24 hours, women receiving ketamine had lower pain scores 2 weeks post-cesarean. The use of systemic multi-modal analgesia in addition to spinal morphine may have masked the potential benefits of ketamine and the post-delivery timing may have precluded any preemptive effects. Nonetheless, the beneficial effects reported at 2 weeks suggest that it may be useful in a subset of women that may be at risk for chronic pain. Further studies with a different dosing regimen may reveal more tangible effects, particularly long term.

Oral Gabapentin and Pregabalin

Gabapentin and pregabalin have been shown to reduce post-surgical allodynia and hyperalgesia, and clinical studies have demonstrated an opioid-sparing effect (118). The mechanisms involved in the analgesic efficacy of these (and other) anticonvulsant agents include sodium and calcium channel antagonism and decreased glutamate transmission. The efficacy of gabapentin as part of a multi-modal regimen to reduce chronic post-surgical pain after breast surgery (119) and abdominal hysterectomy (120–122) has recently been shown. One randomized clinical trial in women undergoing hysterectomy compared the analgesic efficacy of gabapentin to that of ketamine and found that gabapentin reduced more effectively pain scores 6 months post-surgery than ketamine (123). Pregabalin has also been proposed as an effective drug to decrease the incidence of chronic pain when neuropathic-type acute pain is anticipated post-surgery (124).

Moore et al. evaluated the analgesic effect of gabapentin in a placebo-controlled randomized clinical trial in women undergoing elective cesarean delivery under spinal anesthesia (bupivacaine 12 mg, fentanyl 10 μg, and morphine 100 μg) with multi-modal analgesia (oral acetaminophen, diclofenac, and systemic opioids for breakthrough pain). The primary outcome was maternal pain on movement at 24 hours. They found that a single dose of 600 mg oral gabapentin given 1 hour prior to cesarean delivery improved pain scores and patient satisfaction in the first 48 hours. Persistence of pain at 3 months was assessed in a subset of women that agreed to be contacted. In the gabapentin group, two women (12%) had persistent pain and three (19%) reported abnormal wound sensation. In the placebo group, four women (20%) had persistent pain and nine (45%) reported abnormal wound sensation. The study was underpowered to detect differences in long-term outcomes.

Prediction of Chronic Pain After Cesarean Delivery

The current body of evidence emphasizes that the percentage of patients who develop chronic pain post-surgery varies greatly and depends upon the type of surgery as well as numerous biologic, psychological, and social/environmental factors (10,125). Clinical interventions to reduce the incidence and severity of chronic post-surgical pain have not been consistently effective. Likely explanations are that the tested drugs were truly ineffective (ineffective drug, inadequate dose, wrong timing) or that the effect was too modest because with a low incidence of chronic pain, any study trying to "make a difference" is likely to be underpowered and fail to demonstrate an effect. Therefore, since not all women require preemptive/preventive interventional therapies, preoperative testing that may identify patients vulnerable to pain may be highly beneficial. In other words, if women at risk for pain-induced sensitization and deficient pain inhibition were identified prior to delivery, then a more robust effect and tangible benefit could be achieved with targeted analgesic interventions in these "susceptible" women.

Quantitative Sensory Testing

Quantitative sensory testing (QSTs) encompass a series of different tests that can measure an individual's response to various painful stimuli with different modalities (thermal, mechanical, electrical, and chemical) (126). The more traditional tests have mainly focused on measuring the "static" response to evoked pain: Threshold, tolerance, and suprathreshold. More advanced tests explore more complex "dynamic" components of pain processing: Peripheral and central sensitization, wind-up pain, temporal summation (TS), and descending noxious inhibiting control (DNIC). Recent recommendations on the taxonomy and practice of these tests emphasized the need for more standardized and uniform tests to allow comparisons between clinical trials, and the DNIC paradigm has been renamed "conditioned pain modulation" (127).

Numerous recent studies have utilized QST to predict acute post-operative pain and chronic pain. Several pain modalities have been used as well as varying populations undergoing different surgical procedures. In a qualitative systematic review, Abrishami et al. identified 13 studies that examined preoperative pain sensitivity to predict acute postoperative pain and analgesic consumption and two studies that evaluated persistent/chronic post-surgical pain (128). An important finding was that the response to suprathreshold heat pain reliably predicted post-operative pain outcomes, whereas no significant correlation was consistently found between heat pain threshold and post-operative pain. It was suggested that suprathreshold painful stimulation, which is at a level between pain threshold and tolerance, may more closely mimic the pain experience caused by surgical trauma.

Yarnitsky et al. published a landmark study in 2008 that described for the first time the use of the DNIC paradigm to predict chronic post-surgical pain (129). Patients with deficient pain inhibition as demonstrated by a "bad" DNIC test preoperatively were at risk for chronic pain post-thoracotomy. Lundblad et al. also found an association between preoperative testing (using an electrical stimulus to evaluate pain threshold) and chronic pain after total knee replacement (130). Lower thresholds indicated a higher risk for chronic post-surgical pain.

Pregnancy-induced analgesia has been suggested as a "coping mechanism" that allows women to tolerate/survive the intense pain endured during labor and delivery. Pregnancy-induced analgesia may have interesting implications for the understanding of pain modulation at the time of labor and delivery; in particular, it may offer insight as to why some women are able to tolerate this intense pain while others are not. The proposed mechanism for this phenomenon is based on animal studies that have demonstrated activation of the opioid system at the spinal level in response to the pregnant state (131). However, human studies looking into pregnancy-induced analgesia have reported inconsistent findings. Some authors found that women in late pregnancy or during labor have decreased sensitivity to evoked pain (132–135) while others have found no such effect (136,137) or even reported an increase in sensitivity to noxious stimuli during pregnancy (138,139). Fear of labor was also suggested to affect evoked pain tolerance during pregnancy as well as in the postpartum period (140) and adds a new dimension to this already complex concept of testing women's response to evoked pain to predict pain outcomes during labor and delivery.

To date, four studies have evaluated models that involved preoperative pain tests to predict pain severity and analgesic consumption after cesarean delivery. Granot et al. tested preoperative thermal pain thresholds in 58 Israeli women scheduled for a cesarean delivery (141). Suprathreshold pain was associated with increased pain at 24 hours, and a stimulus of 48°C predicted best the level of post-operative pain both at rest and with movement.

Pan et al. evaluated a model in a North American cohort of 34 healthy women that includes preoperative parameters and thermal threshold to predict post-cesarean pain and analgesic consumption (142). Six predictive factors were identified: (1) Pain and unpleasantness of a heat stimuli of 49°C applied on the arm and the back, (2) preoperative blood pressure, (3) preexisting pain and unpleasantness during pregnancy, (4) expectation of post-cesarean pain and amount of analgesics needed, (5) thermal pain threshold on the arm and in the back, and (6) intraoperative factors (duration of surgery and upper sensory dermatomal level at the time of incision). Resting post-cesarean pain was best predicted by two factors (pain and unpleasantness of the thermal stimuli and patient expectation). The authors concluded that a combination of preoperative physical and psychosocial tests results in a model that could predict post-operative pain and analgesic needs.

Nielsen et al. evaluated pain threshold with an electrical stimuli in 39 healthy Danish women and found that the pain threshold before caesarean delivery predicts the intensity of post-operative pain at rest and with movement (143).

Strulov et al. found in 47 Israeli women that pain on the first day post-cesarean was predicted by the intensity of pain during a 1-minute tonic (continuous) heat stimulus of 46°C, while pain on the second day post-cesarean was best predicted by preoperative pain catastrophizing. The pain catastrophizing scale (PCS) is a questionnaire that evaluates 13 items that include rumination (ruminative thoughts, worry, and an inability to inhibit pain-related thoughts), magnification (of the unpleasantness of painful situations and expectation of negative outcomes), and helplessness (reflecting the inability to cope with painful situations) (144). Preoperative pain catastrophizing predicts acute post-operative pain (145) and pain catastrophizing during labor has been shown to be associated with postpartum depression and social functioning (146).

Lavand'homme et al. reported preliminary data suggesting that the presence of abnormal temporal summation preoperatively is associated with increased post-cesarean pain with movement and uterine cramping at 24 hours, an increased incidence of wound (peri-incisional) hyperalgesia, and an increased risk for persistent pain 2 months postpartum (147). In addition, in women with preoperative temporal summation, intravenous ketamine had a beneficial effect on uterine cramping and pain with movement.

Landau et al. are testing clinical predictors along with genetic factors in an ongoing multicentric international prospective observational study to predict acute post-cesarean pain, wound hyperalgesia, and chronic pain up to 10-year postpartum (148). Preliminary data suggests that preoperative testing of DNIC and mechanical temporal summation (mTS) allows identification of women with an increased risk for severe acute pain and wound hyperalgesia (149). In addition, a substantial proportion of women undergoing a repeat cesarean delivery appear to have abnormal scar mapping *prior* to the repeat procedure. Furthermore, preoperative hyperalgesia was associated with abnormal preoperative mTS, higher post-operative pain scores, and post-operative wound hyperalgesia (Fig. 14-7) (150). The combination of several QST that all substantiate central sensitization (hyperexcitation) suggests abnormal pain modulation in these women. Preoperative wound mapping may allow prediction of women at higher risk for severe acute and possibly persistent pain that would justify anti-hyperalgesic drugs such as neuraxial clonidine and/or intravenous ketamine in addition to the provision of standard multi-modal analgesia.

Genetic Factors

Over the last decade, a myriad of genetic variants have been suggested to play a key role in pain perception, coping strategies, response to opioids, and chronic pain. Human (151) and animal (152–156) databases describing pain genes to help researchers conduct phenotype–genotype pain association

studies are available. In particular, the μ-opioid receptor gene (*OPRM1*) (69,70,157–170), the catechol-*O*-methyltransferase gene (*COMT*) (171–179), the guanosine triphosphate cyclohydrolase 1 gene (*GCH1*) (180–187), the β2-adrenergic receptor gene (*ADRB2*) (188,189), the *ABCB1* (190,191), the melanocortin-1 receptor gene (*MCR1*) responsible for the redhead phenotype (192–196), and sodium channel gene (SCN9A) (197–205) have been evaluated in the context of pain perception and analgesia. In addition, the first genome wide association study (GWAS) of acute post-surgical pain in humans has recently been reported (206) as well as the novel discovery of a gene that is involved in the development of chronic pain after nerve injury, the CACNG2 gene (207).

Sia et al. evaluated the potential association of several common variants of the ABCB1 gene with acute post-cesarean pain, analgesic consumption, and chronic pain in a Chinese cohort of 631 women followed up to 6 months after cesarean delivery (72). None of the single nucleotide polymorphisms (SNPs) of the ABCB1 gene influenced post-operative morphine consumption, pain scores, or side effects in the first 24 hours after cesarean delivery. However, there was a trend toward a higher risk of persistent pain after surgery in women homozygous for the T allele of C3435T polymorphism (18% of women in this cohort), although this failed to reach statistical significance. The overall incidence of chronic pain in this study was 8%.

While there is no doubt that inherited differences impact upon the experience of pain and that genetic variants influence pain sensitivity, pain modulation, response to analgesics, and the risk for chronic pain, no human study has established a strong association that allows selected genes to be integrated in a clinical and genetic predictive model. An ongoing study is currently evaluating preoperative testing of DNIC and mTS, with scar mapping for women with repeat cesarean deliveries along with questionnaires, to assess pain catastrophizing and anxiety levels (148). Genetic analysis involves sequencing of polymorphisms of the *OPRM1* gene, the *COMT* gene, the

Scar mapping technique
Stimulation with 180g von Frey filament starts from outside the scar and moved in ≈0.5 inch increments toward the scar every inch until a painful, sore, or sharp sensation is reported. The distance to the incision is measured. If no change in sensation occurs, stimulation is stopped 0.3 inch from the incision.

The Hyperalgesia Index (HI) is calculated as:
Σ **distances to scar from point of hyperalgesia/length of incision**

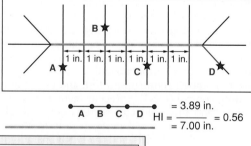

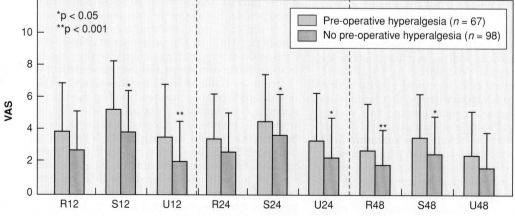

Pain at rest (R), sitting (S) and uterine cramping (U) at 12, 24 and 48 hours post-CS

FIGURE 14-7 Preoperative scar mapping in repeat cesarean delivery (150). Hyperalgesia was associated with increase pain scores at 12, 24, and 48 hours.

oxytocin receptor gene (*OXTR*) and potentially genome wide sequencing. These parameters will be included in a model to predict acute post-operative pain, analgesic consumption, wound hyperalgesia, and chronic pain up to 1-year postpartum. The ultimate goal of this project is to provide a robust predictive tool to identify susceptible women that could most benefit from targeted post-cesarean anti-hyperalgesic therapies (tailored individualized preemptive analgesia).

■ FUTURE DIRECTIONS

There is still much debate about the underlying mechanisms, the nature, and even the definition of persistent post-surgical pain; therefore, better designed clinical trials are needed to confirm the incidence of chronic pain and identify preventative measures that are truly effective and safe (208–211).

APPENDIX

Questionnaire Translated into English from Nikolajsen et al. (64)

1. Did you have an epidural catheter to treat labor pain?   ☐ Yes   ☐ No   ☐ Do not know

2. What type of C-section did you have?   ☐ Emergency   ☐ Planned   ☐ Do not know

3. Did you have general anesthesia or spinal anesthesia for the C-section?
   ☐ General   ☐ Spinal   ☐ Do not know

4. Did you experience much pain in the immediate post-operative period?
   ☐ Yes   ☐ No   ☐ Do not know

5. Did you experience infection in the wound?
   ☐ Yes   ☐ No   ☐ Do not know

6. Have you had a Caesarean section previously?
   ☐ Yes   ☐ No

7. Have you ever had any other abdominal operations?
   ☐ Yes   ☐ No If yes, please specify.

8. What is your present weight and height?   Weight: _____   Height: _____

9. What was the duration of post-operative abdominal wound pain?
   ☐ Less than 1 month   ☐ 1 to 3 months   ☐ More than 3 months   ☐ Pain is still present

   If you still have pain located to the scar, please proceed with questions 10 to 18.
   If you have no more pain, only answer the last two questions 17 and 18

10. How often is the pain present?
    ☐ Constantly   ☐ Daily   ☐ With days interval   ☐ With weeks interval

11. What is the intensity of pain?
    At rest: ☐ Not present   ☐ Mild   ☐ Moderate   ☐ Severe
    During physical activity: ☐ Not present   ☐ Mild   ☐ Moderate   ☐ Severe

12. Please state whether pain is a problem when carrying out the following activities:
    Rising from a low chair?   ☐ Yes   ☐ No
    Sitting down >30 min?   ☐ Yes   ☐ No
    Standing up >30 min?   ☐ Yes   ☐ No
    Walking on stairs?   ☐ Yes   ☐ No
    Carrying heavy bags or the baby?   ☐ Yes   ☐ No
    Driving?   ☐ Yes   ☐ No   ☐ Do not drive
    Doing sports?   ☐ Yes   ☐ No   ☐ Do not do sports
    Working?   ☐ Yes   ☐ No   ☐ Do not work

13. Does the pain disturb your sleep?   ☐ Yes   ☐ No

14. Does the pain have impact on your mood?   ☐ Yes   ☐ No

15. Have you taken any medication because of pain in the operated area within the last 3 months?
    ☐ Yes   ☐ No If yes, please specify.

16. Have you seen a doctor because of pain in the operated area within the last 3 months?
    ☐ Yes   ☐ No

17. Do you have pain problems elsewhere, e.g., back pain, migraine?   ☐ Yes   ☐ No If yes, please specify.

18. How often is the pain present?
    ☐ Constantly   ☐ Daily   ☐ With days interval   ☐ With weeks interval

KEY POINTS

- Evaluating pain that persists beyond the expected time of recovery after childbirth has proven to be complex and challenging, and the definition of what constitutes chronic pain in this specific context of healthy young women still remains to be defined.
- The recovery expectations of women after childbirth are very different from that of women undergoing breast surgery for cancer; therefore, any study assessing post-surgical pain outcomes should take this into account.
- Women's perceptions of pain may be different if their cesarean delivery was urgent and unplanned rather than elective and scheduled; hence, they are more likely to be unprepared and unwilling to suffer any discomfort that will deter from the joys of motherhood.
- Pregnancy-induced analgesia and possibly oxytocin may confer protection against persistent pain. Therefore, standard tools and criteria to define persistent incapacitating pain and failed prevention to reduce chronic pain may need to be adapted to this unique population and post-surgical context.
- With an increased trend for repeat cesarean delivery, cesarean deliveries may constitute a unique surgical model that allows the testing of women's residual hypersensitization from the previous surgery and identification of women at risk for subsequent chronic pain. Therefore, further research to identify valid models to predict chronic pain are needed to allow targeted interventions to women who are most likely to need more tailored anti-hyperalgesic therapies.

REFERENCES

1. Loeser JD, Treede RD. The Kyoto protocol of IASP Basic Pain Terminology. *Pain* 2008;137:473–477.
2. Zhang J, Troendle J, Reddy UM, et al. Contemporary cesarean delivery practice in the United States. *Am J Obstet Gynecol* 2010;203:326 e1–326 e10.
3. Sherman RA, Sherman CJ, Parker L. Chronic phantom and stump pain among American veterans: results of a survey. *Pain* 1984;18:83–95.
4. Kroner K, Krebs B, Skov J, et al. Immediate and long-term phantom breast syndrome after mastectomy: incidence, clinical characteristics and relationship to pre-mastectomy breast pain. *Pain* 1989;36:327–334.
5. Katz J, Jackson M, Kavanagh BP, et al. Acute pain after thoracic surgery predicts long-term post-thoracotomy pain. *Clin J Pain* 1996;12:50–55.
6. Keller SM, Carp NZ, Levy MN, et al. Chronic post thoracotomy pain. *J Cardiovasc Surg (Torino)* 1994;35:161–164.
7. Bates T, Ebbs SR, Harrison M, et al. Influence of cholecystectomy on symptoms. *Br J Surg* 1991;78:964–967.
8. Callesen T, Bech K, Kehlet H. Prospective study of chronic pain after groin hernia repair. *Br J Surg* 1999;86:1528–1531.
9. Crombie IK, Davies HT, Macrae WA. Cut and thrust: antecedent surgery and trauma among patients attending a chronic pain clinic. *Pain* 1998;76:167–171.
10. Kehlet H, Jensen TS, Woolf CJ. Persistent postsurgical pain: risk factors and prevention. *Lancet* 2006;367:1618–1625.
11. Macrae WA. Chronic pain after surgery. *Br J Anaesth* 2001;87:88–98.
12. Perkins FM, Kehlet H. Chronic pain as an outcome of surgery. A review of predictive factors. *Anesthesiology* 2000;93:1123–1133.
13. Kehlet H. Postoperative pain relief—what is the issue? *Br J Anaesth* 1994;72:375–378.
14. Dahl JB, Kehlet H. The value of pre-emptive analgesia in the treatment of postoperative pain. *Br J Anaesth* 1993;70:434–439.
15. Kehlet H, Dahl JB. The value of "multimodal" or "balanced analgesia" in postoperative pain treatment. *Anesth Analg* 1993;77:1048–1056.
16. Apfelbaum JL, Chen C, Mehta SS, et al. Postoperative pain experience: results from a national survey suggest postoperative pain continues to be undermanaged. *Anesth Analg* 2003;97:534–540.
17. Kehlet H. Procedure-specific postoperative pain management. *Anesthesiol Clin North America* 2005;23:203–210.
18. Kehlet H, Wilkinson RC, Fischer HB, et al. PROSPECT: evidence-based, procedure-specific postoperative pain management. *Best Pract Res Clin Anaesthesiol* 2007;21:149–159.
19. Macrae WA, Davies HT. Chronic postsurgical pain. In: Crombie IK, Linton S, Croft P, Von Korff M, LeResche L, eds. *Epidemiology of Pain*. Seattle: International Association for the Study of Pain; 1999:125–142.
20. Granot M. Can we predict persistent postoperative pain by testing preoperative experimental pain? *Curr Opin Anaesthesiol* 2009;22:425–430.
21. Rivat C, Laulin JP, Corcuff JB, et al. Fentanyl enhancement of carrageenan-induced long-lasting hyperalgesia in rats: prevention by the N-methyl-D-aspartate receptor antagonist ketamine. *Anesthesiology* 2002;96:381–391.
22. Celerier E, Rivat C, Jun Y, et al. Long-lasting hyperalgesia induced by fentanyl in rats: preventive effect of ketamine. *Anesthesiology* 2000;92:465–472.
23. Laulin JP, Maurette P, Corcuff JB, et al. The role of ketamine in preventing fentanyl-induced hyperalgesia and subsequent acute morphine tolerance. *Anesth Analg* 2002;94:1263–1269.
24. Richebe P, Rivat C, Laulin JP, et al. Ketamine improves the management of exaggerated postoperative pain observed in perioperative fentanyl-treated rats. *Anesthesiology* 2005;102:421–428.
25. Rivat C, Laboureyras E, Laulin JP, et al. Non-nociceptive environmental stress induces hyperalgesia, not analgesia, in pain and opioid-experienced rats. *Neuropsychopharmacology* 2007;32:2217–2228.
26. Scott M Fishman, Jane C Ballantyne, James P Rathmell, eds. *Bonica's Management of Pain*. 4th ed. Philadelphia, PA: Wolters Kluwer/Lippincott, Williams and Wilkins; 2010.
27. de Leon J, Dinsmore L, Wedlund P. Adverse drug reactions to oxycodone and hydrocodone in CYP2D6 ultrarapid metabolizers. *J Clin Psychopharmacol* 2003;23:420–421.
28. Almeida EC, Nogueira AA, Candido dos Reis FJ, et al. Cesarean section as a cause of chronic pelvic pain. *Int J Gynaecol Obstet* 2002;79:101–104.
29. Alpay Z, Saed GM, Diamond MP. Postoperative adhesions: from formation to prevention. *Semin Reprod Med* 2008;26:313–321.
30. Pfannenstiel HJ. On the advantages of the symphyseal transverse fascial incision for gynecological caliotomies as well as the contribution to the surgical indications. *Samml Klin Vortr* 1900;268.
31. Brandsborg B, Dueholm M, Nikolajsen L, et al. A prospective study of risk factors for pain persisting 4 months after hysterectomy. *Clin J Pain* 2009;25:263–268.
32. Brandsborg B, Nikolajsen L, Hansen CT, et al. Risk factors for chronic pain after hysterectomy: a nationwide questionnaire and database study. *Anesthesiology* 2007;106:1003–1012.
33. Brandsborg B, Nikolajsen L, Kehlet H, et al. Chronic pain after hysterectomy. *Acta Anaesthesiol Scand* 2008;52:327–331.
34. Loos MJ, Scheltinga MR, Mulders LG, et al. The Pfannenstiel incision as a source of chronic pain. *Obstet Gynecol* 2008;111:839–846.
35. Loos MJ, Scheltinga MR, Roumen RM. Surgical management of inguinal neuralgia after a low transverse Pfannenstiel incision. *Ann Surg* 2008;248:880–885.
36. Dumas AM, Girard R, Ayzac L, et al. Maternal infection rates after cesarean delivery by Pfannenstiel or Joel-Cohen incision: a multicenter surveillance study. *Eur J Obstet Gynecol Reprod Biol* 2009;147:139–143.
37. Franchi M, Ghezzi F, Balestreri D, et al. A randomized clinical trial of two surgical techniques for cesarean section. *Am J Perinatol* 1998;15:589–594.
38. Franchi M, Ghezzi F, Raio L, et al. Joel-Cohen or Pfannenstiel incision at cesarean delivery: does it make a difference? *Acta Obstet Gynecol Scand* 2002;81:1040–1046.
39. Malvasi A, Tinelli A, Serio G, et al. Comparison between the use of the Joel-Cohen incision and its modification during Stark's cesarean section. *J Matern Fetal Neonatal Med* 2007;20:757–761.
40. Stark M, Finkel AR. Comparison between the Joel-Cohen and Pfannenstiel incisions in cesarean section. *Eur J Obstet Gynecol Reprod Biol* 1994;53:121–122.
41. Nabhan AF. Long-term outcomes of two different surgical techniques for cesarean. *Int J Gynaecol Obstet* 2008;100:69–75.
42. Caesarean section surgical techniques: a randomised factorial trial (CAESAR). *BJOG* 2010;117:1366–1376.
43. The CORONIS Trial. International study of caesarean section surgical techniques: a randomised fractional, factorial trial. *BMC Pregnancy Childbirth* 2007;7:24.
44. Dodd JM, Anderson ER, Gates S. Surgical techniques for uterine incision and uterine closure at the time of caesarean section. *Cochrane Database Syst Rev* 2008:CD004732.
45. Hofmeyr JG, Novikova N, Mathai M, et al. Techniques for cesarean section. *Am J Obstet Gynecol* 2009;201:431–444.
46. Mathai M, Hofmeyr GJ. Abdominal surgical incisions for caesarean section. *Cochrane Database Syst Rev* 2007:CD004453.
47. Cheong YC, Premkumar G, Metwally M, et al. To close or not to close? A systematic review and a meta-analysis of peritoneal non-closure and adhesion formation after caesarean section. *Eur J Obstet Gynecol Reprod Biol* 2009; 147:3–8.
48. Komoto Y, Shimoya K, Shimizu T, et al. Prospective study of non-closure or closure of the peritoneum at cesarean delivery in 124 women: Impact of

prior peritoneal closure at primary cesarean on the interval time between first cesarean section and the next pregnancy and significant adhesion at second cesarean. *J Obstet Gynaecol Res* 2006;32:396–402.

49. Rafique Z, Shibli KU, Russell IF, et al. A randomised controlled trial of the closure or non-closure of peritoneum at caesarean section: effect on postoperative pain. *BJOG* 2002;109:694–698.

50. Malvasi A, Tinelli A, Guido M, et al. Should the visceral peritoneum at the bladder flap closed at cesarean sections? A post-partum sonographic and clinical assessment. *J Matern Fetal Neonatal Med* 2010;23:662–669.

51. Shahin AY, Osman AM. Parietal peritoneal closure and persistent postcesarean pain. *Int J Gynaecol Obstet* 2009;104:135–139.

52. Wilkinson C, Enkin MW. Uterine exteriorization versus intraperitoneal repair at caesarean section. *Cochrane Database Syst Rev* 2000:CD000085.

53. Magann EF, Washburne JF, Harris RL, et al. Infectious morbidity, operative blood loss, and length of the operative procedure after cesarean delivery by method of placental removal and site of uterine repair. *J Am Coll Surg* 1995;181:517–520.

54. Baksu A, Kalan A, Ozkan A, et al. The effect of placental removal method and site of uterine repair on postcesarean endometritis and operative blood loss. *Acta Obstet Gynecol Scand* 2005;84:266–269.

55. Edi-Osagie EC, Hopkins RE, Ogbo V, et al. Uterine exteriorisation at caesarean section: influence on maternal morbidity. *Br J Obstet Gynaecol* 1998; 105:1070–1078.

56. Magann EF, Dodson MK, Allbert JR, et al. Blood loss at time of cesarean section by method of placental removal and exteriorization versus in situ repair of the uterine incision. *Surg Gynecol Obstet* 1993;177:389–392.

57. Coutinho IC, Ramos de Amorim MM, Katz L, et al. Uterine exteriorization compared with in situ repair at cesarean delivery: a randomized controlled trial. *Obstet Gynecol* 2008;111:639–647.

58. Nafisi S. Influence of uterine exteriorization versus in situ repair on post-cesarean maternal pain: a randomized trial. *Int J Obstet Anesth* 2007;16:135–138.

59. Siddiqui M, Goldszmidt E, Fallah S, et al. Complications of exteriorized compared with in situ uterine repair at cesarean delivery under spinal anesthesia: a randomized controlled trial. *Obstet Gynecol* 2007;110:570–575.

60. Stock RJ, Skelton H. Fatal pulmonary embolism occurring two hours after exteriorization of the uterus for repair following cesarean section. *Mil Med* 1985;150:549–551.

61. Ferrari AG, Frigerio LG, Candotti G, et al. Can Joel-Cohen incision and single layer reconstruction reduce cesarean section morbidity? *Int J Gynaecol Obstet* 2001;72:135–143.

62. Bujold E, Goyet M, Marcoux S, et al. The role of uterine closure in the risk of uterine rupture. *Obstet Gynecol* 2010;116:43–50.

63. Lavand'homme P. Chronic pain after vaginal and cesarean delivery: a reality questioning our daily practice of obstetric anesthesia. *Int J Obstet Anesth* 2010;19:1–2.

64. Nikolajsen L, Sorensen HC, Jensen TS, et al. Chronic pain following caesarean section. *Acta Anaesthesiol Scand* 2004;48:111–116.

65. Eisenach JC, Pan PH, Smiley R, et al. Severity of acute pain after childbirth, but not type of delivery, predicts persistent pain and postpartum depression. *Pain* 2008;140:87–94.

66. Barsky AJ, Wyshak G, Klerman GL. The somatosensory amplification scale and its relationship to hypochondriasis. *J Psychiatr Res* 1990;24:323–334.

67. Roy A, Gang P, Cole K, et al. Use of Edinburgh Postnatal Depression Scale in a North American population. *Prog Neuropsychopharmacol Biol Psychiatry* 1993;17:501–504.

68. Vincenti GE. Edinburgh Post-natal Depression Scale. *Br J Psychiatry* 1987; 151:865.

69. Sia AT, Lim Y, Lim EC, et al. A118G single nucleotide polymorphism of human mu-opioid receptor gene influences pain perception and patient-controlled intravenous morphine consumption after intrathecal morphine for postcesarean analgesia. *Anesthesiology* 2008;109:520–526.

70. Tan EC, Lim EC, Teo YY, et al. Ethnicity and OPRM variant independently predict pain perception and patient-controlled analgesia usage for post-operative pain. *Mol Pain* 2009;5:32.

71. Sng BL, Sia AT, Quek K, et al. Incidence and risk factors for chronic pain after caesarean section under spinal anaesthesia. *Anaesth Intensive Care* 2009;37:748–752.

72. Sia AT, Sng BL, Lim EC, et al. The influence of ATP-binding cassette subfamily B member-1 (ABCB1) genetic polymorphisms on acute and chronic pain after intrathecal morphine for caesarean section: a prospective cohort study. *Int J Obstet Anesth* 2010;19:254–260.

73. Kainu JP, Sarvela J, Tiippana E, et al. Persistent pain after caesarean section and vaginal birth: a cohort study. *Int J Obstet Anesth* 2010;19:4–9.

74. Dworkin RH, Turk DC, Revicki DA, et al. Development and initial validation of an expanded and revised version of the Short-form McGill Pain Questionnaire (SF-MPQ-2). *Pain* 2009;144:35–42.

75. Breton JD, Veinante P, Uhl-Bronner S, et al. Oxytocin-induced antinociception in the spinal cord is mediated by a subpopulation of glutamatergic neurons in lamina I–II which amplify GABAergic inhibition. *Mol Pain* 2008;4:19.

76. DeLaTorre S, Rojas-Piloni G, Martinez-Lorenzana G, et al. Paraventricular oxytocinergic hypothalamic prevention or interruption of long-term potentiation in dorsal horn nociceptive neurons: electrophysiological and behavioral evidence. *Pain* 2009;144:320–328.

77. Gu XL, Yu LC. Involvement of opioid receptors in oxytocin-induced antinociception in the nucleus accumbens of rats. *J Pain* 2007;8:85–90.

78. Han Y, Yu LC. Involvement of oxytocin and its receptor in nociceptive modulation in the central nucleus of amygdala of rats. *Neurosci Lett* 2009;454:101–104.

79. Lundeberg T, Uvnas-Moberg K, Agren G, et al. Anti-nociceptive effects of oxytocin in rats and mice. *Neurosci Lett* 1994;170:153–157.

80. Millan MJ, Schmauss C, Millan MH, et al. Vasopressin and oxytocin in the rat spinal cord: analysis of their role in the control of nociception. *Brain Res* 1984;309:384–388.

81. Schorscher-Petcu A, Sotocinal S, Ciura S, et al. Oxytocin-induced analgesia and scratching are mediated by the vasopressin-1A receptor in the mouse. *J Neurosci* 2010;30:8274–8284.

82. Madrazo I, Franco-Bourland RE, Leon-Meza VM, et al. Intraventricular somatostatin-14, arginine vasopressin, and oxytocin: analgesic effect in a patient with intractable cancer pain. *Appl Neurophysiol* 1987;50:427–431.

83. Yang J. Intrathecal administration of oxytocin induces analgesia in low back pain involving the endogenous opiate peptide system. *Spine (Phila Pa 1976)* 1994;19:867–871.

84. Louvel D, Delvaux M, Felez A, et al. Oxytocin increases thresholds of colonic visceral perception in patients with irritable bowel syndrome. *Gut* 1996;39:741–747.

85. Ohlsson B, Truedsson M, Bengtsson M, et al. Effects of long-term treatment with oxytocin in chronic constipation; a double blind, placebo-controlled pilot trial. *Neurogastroenterol Motil* 2005;17:697–704.

86. Anderberg UM, Uvnas-Moberg K. Plasma oxytocin levels in female fibromyalgia syndrome patients. *Z Rheumatol* 2000;59:373–379.

87. Alfven G. Plasma oxytocin in children with recurrent abdominal pain. *J Pediatr Gastroenterol Nutr* 2004;38:513–517.

88. Eisenach JC, Hobo S, Boada MD. Oxytocin reduces excitability of sensory afferents. *SOAP* abstract A-70 2010.

89. Eisenach JC, Liu B, Tong C. Central oxytocin reduces hypersensitivity from injury, but not labor pain. *SOAP* abstract A-125 2010.

90. Taylor NL, Eisenach JC, Pan P. Incidence of chronic pain after delivery and postpartum spinal oxytocin level—are they related? *SOAP* abstract A-11 2010.

91. Lavand'homme P. Postcesarean analgesia: effective strategies and association with chronic pain. *Curr Opin Anaesthesiol* 2006;19:244–248.

92. Carvalho B, Cohen SE, Lipman SS, et al. Patient preferences for anesthesia outcomes associated with cesarean delivery. *Anesth Analg* 2005;101:1182–1187.

93. Carvalho B, Riley E, Cohen SE, et al. Single-dose, sustained-release epidural morphine in the management of postoperative pain after elective cesarean delivery: results of a multicenter randomized controlled study. *Anesth Analg* 2005;100:1150–1158.

94. Carvalho B, Roland LM, Chu LF, et al. Single-dose, extended-release epidural morphine (DepoDur) compared to conventional epidural morphine for post-cesarean pain. *Anesth Analg* 2007;105:176–183.

95. Benhamou D, Thorin D, Brichant JF, et al. Intrathecal clonidine and fentanyl with hyperbaric bupivacaine improves analgesia during cesarean section. *Anesth Analg* 1998;87:609–613.

96. Lavand'homme PM, Roelants F, Waterloos H, et al. An evaluation of the postoperative antihyperalgesic and analgesic effects of intrathecal clonidine administered during elective cesarean delivery. *Anesth Analg* 2008;107:948–955.

97. Paech MJ, Pavy TJ, Orlikowski CE, et al. Postcesarean analgesia with spinal morphine, clonidine, or their combination. *Anesth Analg* 2004;98:1460–1466.

98. van Tuijl I, van Klei WA, van der Werff DB, et al. The effect of addition of intrathecal clonidine to hyperbaric bupivacaine on postoperative pain and morphine requirements after caesarean section: a randomized controlled trial. *Br J Anaesth* 2006;97:365–370.

99. Eisenach JC, De Kock M, Klimscha W. alpha(2)-adrenergic agonists for regional anesthesia. A clinical review of clonidine (1984–1995). *Anesthesiology* 1996;85:655–674.

100. Elia N, Culebras X, Mazza C, et al. Clonidine as an adjuvant to intrathecal local anesthetics for surgery: systematic review of randomized trials. *Reg Anesth Pain Med* 2008;33:159–167.

101. Stubhaug A, Breivik H, Eide PK, et al. Mapping of punctuate hyperalgesia around a surgical incision demonstrates that ketamine is a powerful suppressor of central sensitization to pain following surgery. *Acta Anaesthesiol Scand* 1997;41:1124–1132.

102. Wilder-Smith OH, Arendt-Nielsen L. Postoperative hyperalgesia: its clinical importance and relevance. *Anesthesiology* 2006;104:601–607.

103. Bamigboye AA, Hofmeyr GJ. Local anaesthetic wound infiltration and abdominal nerves block during caesarean section for postoperative pain relief. *Cochrane Database Syst Rev* 2009:CD006954.

104. Lavand'homme PM, Roelants F, Waterloos H, et al. Postoperative analgesic effects of continuous wound infiltration with diclofenac after elective cesarean delivery. *Anesthesiology* 2007;106:1220–1225.

105. Rackelboom T, Le Strat S, Silvera S, et al. Improving continuous wound infusion effectiveness for postoperative analgesia after cesarean delivery: a randomized controlled trial. *Obstet Gynecol* 2010;116:893–900.

106. Belavy D, Cowlishaw PJ, Howes M, et al. Ultrasound-guided transversus abdominis plane block for analgesia after caesarean delivery. *Br J Anaesth* 2009;103:726–730.

107. Costello JF, Moore AR, Wieczorek PM, et al. The transversus abdominis plane block, when used as part of a multimodal regimen inclusive of intrathecal morphine, does not improve analgesia after cesarean delivery. *Reg Anesth Pain Med* 2009;34:586–589.

108. Kanazi GE, Aouad MT, Abdallah FW, et al. The analgesic efficacy of subarachnoid morphine in comparison with ultrasound-guided transversus abdominis plane block after cesarean delivery: a randomized controlled trial. *Anesth Analg* 2010;111:475–481.

109. McDonnell JG, Curley G, Carney J, et al. The analgesic efficacy of transversus abdominis plane block after cesarean delivery: a randomized controlled trial. *Anesth Analg* 2008;106:186–191.

110. Begon S, Pickering G, Eschalier A, et al. Magnesium increases morphine analgesic effect in different experimental models of pain. *Anesthesiology* 2002;96:627–632.

111. Paech MJ, Magann EF, Doherty DA, et al. Does magnesium sulfate reduce the short- and long-term requirements for pain relief after caesarean delivery? A double-blind placebo-controlled trial. *Am J Obstet Gynecol* 2006;194:1596–1602; discussion 602–603.

112. Elia N, Tramer MR. Ketamine and postoperative pain—a quantitative systematic review of randomised trials. *Pain* 2005;113:61–70.

113. Bell RF, Dahl JB, Moore RA, et al. Perioperative ketamine for acute postoperative pain. *Cochrane Database Syst Rev* 2006:CD004603.

114. Brennan TJ, Kehlet H. Preventive analgesia to reduce wound hyperalgesia and persistent postsurgical pain: not an easy path. *Anesthesiology* 2005;103:681–683.

115. De Kock MF, Lavand'homme PM. The clinical role of NMDA receptor antagonists for the treatment of postoperative pain. *Best Pract Res Clin Anaesthesiol* 2007;21:85–98.

116. Lavand'homme P, De Kock M, Waterloos H. Intraoperative epidural analgesia combined with ketamine provides effective preventive analgesia in patients undergoing major digestive surgery. *Anesthesiology* 2005;103:813–820.

117. Bauchat JR, Higgins N, Wojciechowski KG, et al. Low-dose ketamine with multimodal postcesarean delivery analgesia: a randomized controlled trial. *Int J Obstet Anesth* 2011;20:3–9.

118. Dauri M, Faria S, Gatti A, et al. Gabapentin and pregabalin for the acute post-operative pain management. A systematic-narrative review of the recent clinical evidences. *Curr Drug Targets* 2009;10:716–733.

119. Fassoulaki A, Triga A, Melemeni A, et al. Multimodal analgesia with gabapentin and local anesthetics prevents acute and chronic pain after breast surgery for cancer. *Anesth Analg* 2005;101:1427–1432.

120. Fassoulaki A, Melemeni A, Stamatakis E, et al. A combination of gabapentin and local anaesthetics attenuates acute and late pain after abdominal hysterectomy. *Eur J Anaesthesiol* 2007;24:521–528.

121. Fassoulaki A, Stamatakis E, Petropoulos G, et al. Gabapentin attenuates late but not acute pain after abdominal hysterectomy. *Eur J Anaesthesiol* 2006;23:136–141.

122. Gilron I, Orr E, Tu D, et al. A placebo-controlled randomized clinical trial of perioperative administration of gabapentin, rofecoxib and their combination for spontaneous and movement-evoked pain after abdominal hysterectomy. *Pain* 2005;113:191–200.

123. Sen H, Sizlan A, Yanarates O, et al. A comparison of gabapentin and ketamine in acute and chronic pain after hysterectomy. *Anesth Analg* 2009;109:1645–1650.

124. Durkin B, Page C, Glass P. Pregabalin for the treatment of postsurgical pain. *Expert Opin Pharmacother* 2010;11:2751–2758.

125. Katz J, Seltzer Z. Transition from acute to chronic postsurgical pain: risk factors and protective factors. *Expert Rev Neurother* 2009;9:723–744.

126. Arendt-Nielsen L, Yarnitsky D. Experimental and clinical applications of quantitative sensory testing applied to skin, muscles and viscera. *J Pain* 2009;10:556–572.

127. Yarnitsky D, Arendt-Nielsen L, Bouhassira D, et al. Recommendations on terminology and practice of psychophysical DNIC testing. *Eur J Pain* 2010;14:339.

128. Abrishami A, Chan J, Chung F, et al. Preoperative pain sensitivity and its correlation with postoperative pain and analgesic consumption: a qualitative systematic review. *Anesthesiology* 2011;114:445–457.

129. Yarnitsky D, Crispel Y, Eisenberg E, et al. Prediction of chronic post-operative pain: pre-operative DNIC testing identifies patients at risk. *Pain* 2008;138:22–28.

130. Lundblad H, Kreicbergs A, Jansson KA. Prediction of persistent pain after total knee replacement for osteoarthritis. *J Bone Joint Surg Br* 2008;90:166–171.

131. Sander HW, Gintzler AR. Spinal cord mediation of the opioid analgesia of pregnancy. *Brain Res* 1987;408:389–393.

132. Cogan R, Spinnato JA. Pain and discomfort thresholds in late pregnancy. *Pain* 1986;27:63–68.

133. Whipple B, Josimovich JB, Komisaruk BR. Sensory thresholds during the antepartum, intrapartum and postpartum periods. *Int J Nurs Stud* 1990;27:213–221.

134. Carvalho B, Angst MS, Fuller AJ, et al. Experimental heat pain for detecting pregnancy-induced analgesia in humans. *Anesth Analg* 2006;103:1283–1287.

135. Ohel I, Walfisch A, Shitenberg D, et al. A rise in pain threshold during labor: a prospective clinical trial. *Pain* 2007;132(Suppl 1):S104–S108.

136. Dunbar AH, Price DD, Newton RA. An assessment of pain responses to thermal stimuli during stages of pregnancy. *Pain* 1988;35:265–269.

137. Shapira SC, Magora F, Chrubasik S, et al. Assessment of pain threshold and pain tolerance in women in labour and in the early post-partum period by pressure algometry. *Eur J Anaesthesiol* 1995;12:495–499.

138. Goolkasian P, Rimer BA. Pain reactions in pregnant women. *Pain* 1984;20:87–95.

139. Sengupta P, Nielsen M. The effect of labour and epidural analgesia on pain threshold. *Anaesthesia* 1984;39:982–986.

140. Saisto T, Kaaja R, Ylikorkala O, et al. Reduced pain tolerance during and after pregnancy in women suffering from fear of labor. *Pain* 2001;93:123–127.

141. Granot M, Lowenstein L, Yarnitsky D, et al. Postcesarean section pain prediction by preoperative experimental pain assessment. *Anesthesiology* 2003;98:1422–1426.

142. Pan PH, Coghill R, Houle TT, et al. Multifactorial preoperative predictors for postcesarean section pain and analgesic requirement. *Anesthesiology* 2006;104:417–425.

143. Nielsen PR, Norgaard L, Rasmussen LS, et al. Prediction of post-operative pain by an electrical pain stimulus. *Acta Anaesthesiol Scand* 2007;51:582–586.

144. Sullivan MJ, Thorn B, Haythornthwaite JA, et al. Theoretical perspectives on the relation between catastrophizing and pain. *Clin J Pain* 2001;17:52–64.

145. Pavlin DJ, Sullivan MJ, Freund PR, et al. Catastrophizing: a risk factor for postsurgical pain. *Clin J Pain* 2005;21:83–90.

146. Ferber SG, Granot M, Zimmer EZ. Catastrophizing labor pain compromises later maternity adjustments. *Am J Obstet Gynecol* 2005;192:826–831.

147. Lavand'homme P, Roelants F. Effect of a low dose of ketamine on postoperative pain after elective cesarean delivery according to the presence of a preoperative temporal summation. *SOAP* abstract A-258 2009.

148. Landau R, Kraft JC, Flint LY, et al. An experimental paradigm for the prediction of Post-Operative Pain (PPOP). *J Vis Exp* 2010.

149. Landau R, Cardoso M, Lavand'homme P, et al. Prediction of acute postcesarean pain: preliminary data from a multicenter project on the prediction of post-operative pain (PPOP). *SOAP* abstract 2010.

150. Ortner CM, Granot M, Richebe P, et al. Preoperative scar hyperalgesia is associated with post-operative pain in women undergoing a repeat Caesarean delivery. *Eur J Pain* 2012;June 13 (epub ahead of print).

151. Foulkes T, Wood JN. Pain genes. *PLoS Genet* 2008;4:e1000086.

152. Lacroix-Fralish ML, Ledoux JB, Mogil JS. The Pain Genes Database: An interactive web browser of pain-related transgenic knockout studies. *Pain* 2007;131:3e1–3e4.

153. Lacroix-Fralish ML, Mogil JS. Progress in genetic studies of pain and analgesia. *Annu Rev Pharmacol Toxicol* 2009;49:97–121.

154. Lariviere WR, Mogil JS. The genetics of pain and analgesia in laboratory animals. *Methods Mol Biol* 2010;617:261–278.

155. Mogil JS. Animal models of pain: progress and challenges. *Nat Rev Neurosci* 2009;10:283–294.

156. Mogil JS, Davis KD, Derbyshire SW. The necessity of animal models in pain research. *Pain* 2010;151:12–17.

157. Chou WY, Wang CH, Liu PH, et al. Human opioid receptor A118G polymorphism affects intravenous patient-controlled analgesia morphine consumption after total abdominal hysterectomy. *Anesthesiology* 2006;105:334–337.

158. Chou WY, Yang LC, Lu HF, et al. Association of mu-opioid receptor gene polymorphism (A118G) with variations in morphine consumption for analgesia after total knee arthroplasty. *Acta Anaesthesiol Scand* 2006;50:787–792.

159. Fillingim RB, Kaplan L, Staud R, et al. The A118G single nucleotide polymorphism of the mu-opioid receptor gene (OPRM1) is associated with pressure pain sensitivity in humans. *J Pain* 2005;6:159–167.

160. Lotsch J, Zimmermann M, Darimont J, et al. Does the A118G polymorphism at the mu-opioid receptor gene protect against morphine-6-glucuronide toxicity? *Anesthesiology* 2002;97:814–819.

161. Oertel BG, Schmidt R, Schneider A, et al. The mu-opioid receptor gene polymorphism 118A>G depletes alfentanil-induced analgesia and protects against respiratory depression in homozygous carriers. *Pharmacogenet Genomics* 2006;16:625–636.

162. Walter C, Lotsch J. Meta-analysis of the relevance of the OPRM1 118A>G genetic variant for pain treatment. *Pain* 2009;146:270–275.

163. Beyer A, Koch T, Schroder H, et al. Effect of the A118G polymorphism on binding affinity, potency and agonist-mediated endocytosis, desensitization,

and resensitization of the human mu-opioid receptor. *J Neurochem* 2004; 89:553–560.

164. Bond C, LaForge KS, Tian M, et al. Single-nucleotide polymorphism in the human mu opioid receptor gene alters beta-endorphin binding and activity: possible implications for opiate addiction. *Proc Natl Acad Sci U S A* 1998;95:9608–9613.

165. Chong RY, Oswald L, Yang X, et al. The mu-opioid receptor polymorphism A118G predicts cortisol responses to naloxone and stress. *Neuropsychopharmacology* 2006;31:204–211.

166. Janicki PK, Schuler G, Francis D, et al. A genetic association study of the functional A118G polymorphism of the human mu-opioid receptor gene in patients with acute and chronic pain. *Anesth Analg* 2006;103:1011–1017.

167. Wand GS, McCaul M, Yang X, et al. The mu-opioid receptor gene polymorphism (A118G) alters HPA axis activation induced by opioid receptor blockade. *Neuropsychopharmacology* 2002;26:106–114.

168. Landau R, Kern C, Columb MO, et al. Genetic variability of the mu-opioid receptor influences intrathecal fentanyl analgesia requirements in laboring women. *Pain* 2008;139:5–14.

169. Mague SD, Blendy JA. OPRM1 SNP (A118G): involvement in disease development, treatment response, and animal models. *Drug Alcohol Depend* 2010;108:172–182.

170. Wong CA, McCarthy RJ, Blouin J, et al. Observational study of the effect of mu-opioid receptor genetic polymorphism on intrathecal opioid labor analgesia and post-cesarean delivery analgesia. *Int J Obstet Anesth* 2010;19:246–253.

171. Andersen S, Skorpen F. Variation in the COMT gene: implications for pain perception and pain treatment. *Pharmacogenomics* 2009;10:669–684.

172. Dai F, Belfer I, Schwartz CE, et al. Association of catechol-O-methyltransferase genetic variants with outcome in patients undergoing surgical treatment for lumbar degenerative disc disease. *Spine J* 2010;10:949–957.

173. Diatchenko L, Nackley AG, Slade GD, et al. Catechol-O-methyltransferase gene polymorphisms are associated with multiple pain-evoking stimuli. *Pain* 2006;125:216–224.

174. Jensen KB, Lonsdorf TB, Schalling M, et al. Increased sensitivity to thermal pain following a single opiate dose is influenced by the COMT val(158)met polymorphism. *PLoS One* 2009;4:e6016.

175. Lee PJ, Delaney P, Keogh J, et al. Catecholamine-O-methyltransferase polymorphisms are associated with postoperative pain intensity. *Clin J Pain* 2011;27:93–101.

176. Rakvag TT, Klepstad P, Baar C, et al. The Val158Met polymorphism of the human catechol-O-methyltransferase (COMT) gene may influence morphine requirements in cancer pain patients. *Pain* 2005;116:73–78.

177. Reyes-Gibby CC, Shete S, Rakvag T, et al. Exploring joint effects of genes and the clinical efficacy of morphine for cancer pain: OPRM1 and COMT gene. *Pain* 2007;130:25–30.

178. Zubieta JK, Heitzeg MM, Smith YR, et al. COMT val158met genotype affects mu-opioid neurotransmitter responses to a pain stressor. *Science* 2003; 299:1240–1243.

179. Kolesnikov Y, Gabovits B, Levin A, et al. Combined catechol-O-methyltransferase and {micro}-opioid receptor gene polymorphisms affect morphine postoperative analgesia and central side effects. *Anesth Analg* 2011;112:448–453.

180. Doehring A, Antoniades C, Channon KM, et al. Clinical genetics of functionally mild non-coding GTP cyclohydrolase 1 (GCH1) polymorphisms modulating pain and cardiovascular risk. *Mutat Res* 2008;659:195–201.

181. Campbell CM, Edwards RR, Carmona C, et al. Polymorphisms in the GTP cyclohydrolase gene (GCH1) are associated with ratings of capsaicin pain. *Pain* 2009;141:114–118.

182. Kim DH, Dai F, Belfer I, et al. Polymorphic variation of the guanosine triphosphate cyclohydrolase 1 gene predicts outcome in patients undergoing surgical treatment for lumbar degenerative disc disease. *Spine (Phila Pa 1976)* 2010;35:1909–1914.

183. Lotsch J, Klepstad P, Doehring A, et al. A GTP cyclohydrolase 1 genetic variant delays cancer pain. *Pain* 2010;148:103–106.

184. Smith HS. The role of genomic oxidative–reductive balance as predictor of complex regional pain syndrome development: a novel theory. *Pain Physician* 2010;13:79–90.

185. Tegeder I, Adolph J, Schmidt H, et al. Reduced hyperalgesia in homozygous carriers of a GTP cyclohydrolase 1 haplotype. *Eur J Pain* 2008;12:1069–1077.

186. Tegeder I, Costigan M, Griffin RS, et al. GTP cyclohydrolase and tetrahydrobiopterin regulate pain sensitivity and persistence. *Nat Med* 2006;12:1269–1277.

187. Dabo F, Gronbladh A, Nyberg F, et al. Different SNP combinations in the GCH1 gene and use of labor analgesia. *Mol Pain* 2010;6:41.

188. Diatchenko L, Anderson AD, Slade GD, et al. Three major haplotypes of the beta2 adrenergic receptor define psychological profile, blood pressure, and the risk for development of a common musculoskeletal pain disorder. *Am J Med Genet B Neuropsychiatr Genet* 2006;141:449–462.

189. Hocking LJ, Smith BH, Jones GT, et al. Genetic variation in the beta2-adrenergic receptor but not catecholamine-O-methyltransferase predisposes to chronic pain: results from the 1958 British Birth Cohort Study. *Pain* 2010;149:143–151.

190. Campa D, Gioia A, Tomei A, et al. Association of ABCB1/MDR1 and OPRM1 gene polymorphisms with morphine pain relief. *Clin Pharmacol Ther* 2008;83:559–566.

191. Zwisler ST, Enggaard TP, Noehr-Jensen L, et al. The antinociceptive effect and adverse drug reactions of oxycodone in human experimental pain in relation to genetic variations in the OPRM1 and ABCB1 genes. *Fundam Clin Pharmacol* 2010;24:517–524.

192. Delaney A, Keighren M, Fleetwood-Walker SM, et al. Involvement of the melanocortin-1 receptor in acute pain and pain of inflammatory but not neuropathic origin. *PLoS One* 2010;5:e12498.

193. Mogil JS, Ritchie J, Smith SB, et al. Melanocortin-1 receptor gene variants affect pain and mu-opioid analgesia in mice and humans. *J Med Genet* 2005;42:583–587.

194. Carroll L, Voisey J, van Daal A. Gene polymorphisms and their effects in the melanocortin system. *Peptides* 2005;26:1871–1885.

195. Beltramo M, Campanella M, Tarozzo G, et al. Gene expression profiling of melanocortin system in neuropathic rats supports a role in nociception. *Brain Res Mol Brain Res* 2003;118:111–118.

196. Mogil JS, Wilson SG, Chesler EJ, et al. The melanocortin-1 receptor gene mediates female-specific mechanisms of analgesia in mice and humans. *Proc Natl Acad Sci U S A* 2003;100:4867–4872.

197. Reimann F, Cox JJ, Belfer I, et al. Pain perception is altered by a nucleotide polymorphism in SCN9A. *Proc Natl Acad Sci U S A* 2010;107:5148–5153.

198. Estacion M, Harty TP, Choi JS, et al. A sodium channel gene SCN9A polymorphism that increases nociceptor excitability. *Ann Neurol* 2009;66:862–866.

199. Nilsen KB, Nicholas AK, Woods CG, et al. Two novel SCN9A mutations causing insensitivity to pain. *Pain* 2009;143:155–158.

200. Oertel B, Lotsch J. Genetic mutations that prevent pain: implications for future pain medication. *Pharmacogenomics* 2008;9:179–194.

201. Waxman SG. Nav1.7, its mutations, and the syndromes that they cause. *Neurology* 2007;69:505–507.

202. Ahmad S, Dahllund L, Eriksson AB, et al. A stop codon mutation in SCN9A causes lack of pain sensation. *Hum Mol Genet* 2007;16:2114–2121.

203. Goldberg YP, MacFarlane J, MacDonald ML, et al. Loss-of-function mutations in the Nav1.7 gene underlie congenital indifference to pain in multiple human populations. *Clin Genet* 2007;71:311–319.

204. Cox JJ, Reimann F, Nicholas AK, et al. An SCN9A channelopathy causes congenital inability to experience pain. *Nature* 2006;444:894–898.

205. Rush AM, Dib-Hajj SD, Liu S, et al. A single sodium channel mutation produces hyper- or hypoexcitability in different types of neurons. *Proc Natl Acad Sci U S A* 2006;103:8245–8250.

206. Kim H, Ramsay E, Lee H, et al. Genome-wide association study of acute post-surgical pain in humans. *Pharmacogenomics* 2009;10:171–179.

207. Nissenbaum J, Devor M, Seltzer Z, et al. Susceptibility to chronic pain following nerve injury is genetically affected by CACNG2. *Genome Res* 2010;20:1180–1190.

208. Dworkin RH, McDermott MP, Raja SN. Preventing chronic postsurgical pain: how much of a difference makes a difference? *Anesthesiology* 2010; 112:516–518.

209. Kehlet H, Rathmell JP. Persistent postsurgical pain: the path forward through better design of clinical studies. *Anesthesiology* 2010;112:514–515.

210. Scholz J, Yaksh TL. Preclinical research on persistent postsurgical pain: what we don't know, but should start studying. *Anesthesiology* 2010;112:511–513.

211. Wicksell RK, Olsson GL. Predicting and preventing chronic postsurgical pain and disability. *Anesthesiology* 2010;113:1260–1261.

Anesthesia for Nondelivery Obstetric Procedures

Christopher R. Cambic • Feyce M. Peralta

Anesthesia providers occasionally provide care for women undergoing obstetric-related procedures not directly connected to labor and delivery. These procedures include cerclage for cervical insufficiency, external cephalic version (ECV) for nonvertex presentation, postpartum tubal sterilization, and assisted reproductive technologies, which is covered in Chapter 48. Despite each procedure presenting a unique set of anesthetic issues, the impact of pregnancy-induced physiologic changes on maternal and fetal well-being still remains a priority in the management of these patients.

■ CERCLAGE

Cervical insufficiency is the inability to sustain a pregnancy to term due to dysfunction of the uterine cervix. It is characterized by painless dilation and/or shortening of the cervix during the second trimester of pregnancy, resulting in preterm delivery and recurring pregnancy loss. The incidence of cervical insufficiency is difficult to determine due to poorly defined clinical criteria for the diagnosis. Instead, the frequency of cervical cerclage is used as a surrogate to estimate the incidence of cervical insufficiency. Martin et al. reported that the rate of cervical cerclage is of 4.4/1,000 live births in the United States (1). Risk factors for the development of cervical insufficiency include familial inheritance (e.g., connective tissue disorders such as Ehlers–Danlos and Marfan syndromes), African-American race, intrauterine infections, hormonal abnormalities, congenital uterine abnormalities (e.g., in utero maternal exposure to diethylstilbestrol), and diagnostic or therapeutic surgical interventions (2–6). Structural damage to the uterine cervix from biopsies, cauterization, conization, and mechanical dilation and curettage are also associated with cervical insufficiency.

Diagnosis of cervical insufficiency is one of exclusion, based on medical history and clinical assessment. History of previous pregnancy losses during the second trimester, cervical shortening, painless cervical dilation, and the presence of known risk factors should point toward this diagnosis. The patient may report vaginal pressure, caused by the protruding membranes, urinary frequency, and increased mucoid vaginal discharge. If left untreated, eventual rupture of fetal membrane may occur, which will likely proceed to the delivery of a premature and/or nonviable neonate (7).

Ultrasound can aid in assessing cervical length, as the risk of spontaneous preterm labor/delivery is higher with shorter sonographic cervical length in the mid-second trimester (8). Since only a small fraction of all patients who will have a spontaneous preterm birth have a shortened cervix in the mid-second trimester, surveillance of the cervical length by ultrasound should only be considered in patients at high risk for cervical insufficiency (7,9).

Although controversial, management of cervical insufficiency is centered on cerclage placement. Current evidence suggests that the subgroups of patients that may benefit from cerclage placement are those with clinical presentation of acute cervical insufficiency, or those with a previous history of cervical insufficiency and progressive shortening of the cervix as demonstrated by ultrasound (7,10,11). Other therapies that have been used in combination with cervical cerclage for the management of cervical insufficiency include administration of progesterone, tocolytic drugs, and perioperative antibiotics (12–14). In a study published by the National Institute of Child Health and Human Development Maternal-Fetal Medicine Units Network, the authors concluded that, when compared to placebo, weekly injections of progesterone resulted in a substantial reduction in the rate of recurrent preterm delivery in the at-risk patient (14). Information regarding other adjunct therapies is less well defined.

Cerclage placement can be considered elective, urgent, or an emergency (15). Elective cerclage is typically performed between 13 and 16 weeks of gestation in asymptomatic patients with a history of cervical insufficiency or multiple risk factors. Urgent cerclage is performed after ultrasonographic findings of decreasing cervical length (<25 mm) in asymptomatic patients between 20 and 24 weeks of gestation. Emergency cerclage is performed for symptomatic patients with advanced cervical dilation (>2 cm), with or without bulging of the fetal membranes, in the absence of labor. Emergency cerclage is controversial since it carries a higher procedural risk of fetal membrane rupture. The timing for cervical cerclages in relation to neonatal outcome is also debated, as it has not been adequately studied in large, randomized trials.

The optimal surgical technique for cerclage placement is unclear. In general, two approaches are used: transvaginal or transabdominal. The McDonald and the modified Shirodkar are the most common techniques for cerclage placement. Both of these surgical techniques are done by a transvaginal approach and have similar fetal outcomes (16). The McDonald cerclage is less invasive with a purse-string suture placed at the cervicovaginal junction, without bladder mobilization (Fig. 15-1). The Shirodkar cerclage differs from the McDonald in that the suture is placed following bladder mobilization, to allow for a higher insertion level (15,17). In addition, removal of a McDonald cerclage can usually be accomplished without the need for pain medication, whereas a Shirodkar cerclage is more invasive, and removal typically requires analgesia and possibly anesthesia. Transabdominal cerclage, which requires a laparotomy or laparoscopy, serves as an alternative for patients in whom placement of a transvaginal cerclage is exceedingly challenging (e.g., previous cervical surgery) or those who have had a failed transvaginal approach. A systematic review

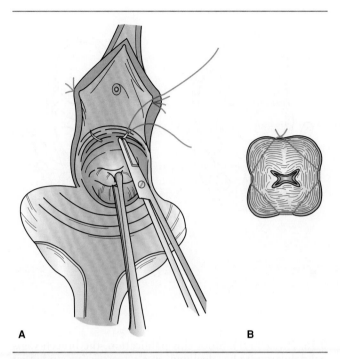

FIGURE 15-1 McDonald cerclage procedure. **A:** Suture is placed in four areas around the junction of the vaginal mucosa and cervix. **B:** Cross-sectional view of the cervix with cerclage in place. Reproduced with permission from: Rock J, Jones HW III. *TeLinde's Operative Gynecology.* 10th ed. Philadelphia, PA: Lippincott Williams & Wilkins; 2008.

comparing pregnancy outcomes after a transabdominal versus a transvaginal cerclage in patients with a failed transvaginal cerclage during a previous pregnancy concluded that the risk of perinatal death and delivery before 24 weeks was lower for women who received a transabdominal cerclage (6.0% vs. 12.5%, respectively) (18). However, transabdominal cerclage was also associated with a higher incidence of serious operative complications compared to the transvaginal approach (3.4% vs. 0%; 95% CI 0.01% to 6.8%). Cesarean delivery is typically the mode of delivery for patients with a transabdominal cerclage.

The most frequent procedural risks associated with cervical cerclages include iatrogenic rupture of membranes, chorioamnionitis, hemorrhage, cervical stenosis, and cervical laceration. Cervical cerclages also increase the number of obstetrical interventions (e.g., administration of tocolytics, cesarean delivery, etc.) and the need for repeat cerclage in the future (19). Moreover, a meta-analysis of eight studies demonstrated that women who underwent cervical cerclage placement had a slightly higher rate of cesarean delivery compared to women who received other forms of treatment for cervical incompetency (relative risk [RR] 1.19; 95% CI 1.01 to 1.40) (20). Cervical cerclage should not be performed in the setting of maternal hemodynamic instability, rupture of fetal membranes, intra-amniotic or vaginal infection, abnormal placentation, active maternal or fetal bleeding, uterine contractions or preterm labor, intrauterine fetal demise, major fetal abnormality incompatible with life, and gestational age >28 weeks (19).

The anesthetic management for cerclage placement will depend on the technical approach and timing of the procedure. Transvaginal cerclages are typically performed with spinal, epidural, or general anesthesia, while the transabdominal is more frequently done under general anesthesia. The procedure is usually performed in the outpatient setting,

requires 30 to 45 minutes for completion, and a T10 to L1 and S2 to S4 sensory blockade is desired to provide coverage of the cervix, vagina, and perineum. Among the different neuraxial techniques, spinal anesthesia is the preferred choice as it provides a faster and denser block compared to epidural anesthesia. A hyperbaric solution of lidocaine 30 to 70 mg, hyperbaric bupivacaine 5.25 to 12 mg, or mepivacaine 45 to 60 mg are reasonable options for spinal anesthesia. Lee et al. observed that the spread of analgesic effects of spinally administered hyperbaric bupivacaine was enhanced in women in the second trimester compared to the nonpregnant state (21). Lipophilic opioids (e.g., fentanyl 10 to 20 μg) are often used to reduce local anesthetic requirements and duration (22,23).

Although lidocaine may be a better option for cervical cerclage placement in terms of its duration, increased concern for transient neurologic syndrome (TNS) after intrathecal administration has dissuaded many providers from using hyperbaric lidocaine for cerclage placement. Indeed, the incidence of TNS in nonpregnant patients is higher with lidocaine than bupivacaine, and this risk of TNS is not decreased by decreasing the concentration (24,25). Although not completely exempt from the risk of TNS, parturients may be at decreased risk compared to nonpregnant patients. In a prospective study, Wong and Slavenas reported a 0% incidence (95% CI 0% to 4.5%) of TNS in 67 parturients who received hyperbaric 5% lidocaine for cerclage placement (26). Although no cases of TNS were detected, the 95% confidence interval is still less than the 10% to 37% incidence reported in the nonobstetric population (25). In another study, Aouad et al. randomized patients undergoing cesarean delivery to spinal anesthesia with hyperbaric 5% lidocaine or hyperbaric 0.75% bupivacaine, reporting a 0% incidence of TNS (95% CI 0% to 3%) (27). Finally, Philip et al. randomized patients to receive intrathecal hyperbaric 5% lidocaine versus hyperbaric 0.75% bupivacaine for postpartum tubal ligation (28). The authors reported no difference in the incidence of TNS with lidocaine versus bupivacaine (3% vs. 7%) in this patient population. Overall, the evidence suggests that the use of hyperbaric lidocaine intrathecally in pregnant women is likely safe in terms of TNS risk and that this risk is likely less than that in the nonpregnant population, and comparable to the intrathecal administration of other local anesthetics.

Low-dose epidural anesthesia can also be used to provide surgical anesthesia for cervical cerclages (29). Lidocaine 2% with epinephrine 5 μg/mL, 10 to 15 mL, typically provides adequate sensory coverage; fentanyl 50 to 100 μg can be added through the epidural catheter to increase the density of the neuraxial block. Finally, paracervical block is another option for a McDonald cerclage, but it has fallen out of favor due to the potential for fetal bradycardia after local anesthesia injection, with a reported incidence of 2% to 10% (30–32). Regardless of the anesthetic technique, postoperative analgesic requirements are none to minimal after transvaginal placement of a cervical cerclage.

General anesthesia is more likely to be used for emergency cerclage as the use of volatile anesthetics provides uterine relaxation, potentially reducing cervical protrusion of fetal membranes. In addition, this anesthetic technique does not require a sitting or lateral position for administration, positions which may not be possible if protruding fetal membranes are present. Mask anesthesia or a laryngeal mask airway (LMA) is an acceptable option for healthy, fasted patients before 18 to 20 weeks of gestation. However, women of 18 to 20 weeks of gestation and later are at increased risk of aspiration, and therefore should undergo endotracheal intubation. If intubation is performed, beware that coughing

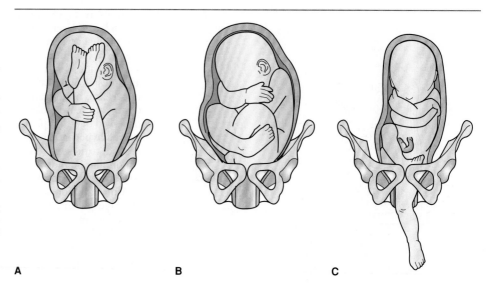

FIGURE 15-2 Types of breech presentations. **A: Frank Breech**—the lower extremities of the fetus are flexed at the hips and extended at the knees. **B: Complete Breech**—both the hips and knees of the fetus are flexed. **C: Incomplete Breech**—one or both of the lower extremities of the fetus are extended at the hips. Reproduced with permission from: Evans, AT. *Manual of Obstetrics.* 7th ed. Philadelphia, PA: Lippincott Williams & Wilkins; 2007.

and vomiting increase intra-abdominal and intrauterine pressures, precipitating or worsening protrusion of the fetal membranes, or even promoting membrane rupture. Steps should be taken to ensure these perianesthesia events are avoided.

■ EXTERNAL CEPHALIC VERSION

The incidence of breech presentation for term, singleton pregnancies is estimated to be between 3% and 4% (33). Breech fetal presentation occurs when the fetal head is in the fundus of the uterus with the buttocks, legs, or feet presenting. There are three main types of breech presentations: frank, complete, and incomplete (Fig. 15-2). A frank breech occurs when the fetus's lower extremities are flexed at the hips and extended at the knees so that the feet are against the face and the buttocks only are the presenting part. A complete breech occurs when the fetus's hips and knees are flexed but the feet do not extend below the buttocks. An incomplete breech (also known as footling breech) occurs when one or both fetal lower extremities are extended and one or both feet present in the vagina.

Although the causes of breech presentation are unclear, there are both fetal and maternal factors that increase this likelihood (Table 15-1). A relative increase in the uterine volume (e.g., prematurity, low birth weight) prevents the accommodation of the fetus to the shape of the uterine cavity leading to malpresentation. Multiparity, multiple gestation, and polyhydramnios are also associated with breech presentation due to increased uterine relaxation. Finally, limited uterine space (e.g., pelvic tumors, uterine anomalies, abnormal placentation, oligohydramnios) and fetal muscular disorders (e.g., muscular dystrophy) can result in fetal malpresentation. In all of these situations, cephalic rotation of the fetus may not occur prior to delivery (34–36).

Multiple delivery options exist for fetuses in breech presentation, including cesarean delivery, trial of labor with vaginal delivery, or ECV, each with its respective benefits and risks. The Term Breech Trial (TBT) randomized more than 2,000 women with a singleton fetus in breech presentation to cesarean or vaginal delivery (37), and demonstrated better neonatal outcomes after a cesarean delivery than after vaginal delivery for breech-presenting fetuses, (1.6% vs. 5%, respectively); (RR 0.33; 95% CI 0.19 to

0.56; $P < 0.0001$). Since this publication, the breech vaginal delivery rate has declined. In a retrospective study that assessed the vaginal delivery rate of breech term pregnancies in the 8 years before and after the TBT, the authors observed that the rate of vaginal delivery in nulliparous and multiparous women decreased from 15.3% to 7.2% in the former group, and from approximately 32.6% to 14.8% in the latter group (38).

Since cesarean and vaginal breech deliveries increase maternal and perinatal morbidity and mortality compared to vaginal vertex deliveries. The American College of Obstetricians and Gynecologists (ACOG) recommends the use of ECV to rotate the fetus to a vertex presentation at term (37,39–41). ECV is an obstetrical procedure performed for the purpose of changing a nonvertex (typically breech) fetal presentation to vertex by external rotation through the maternal abdominal wall. According to a systematic review of randomized controlled trials, the overall success rate of ECV is 60%, with results ranging from 35% to 85% depending if tocolytics are used (42,43). If successful, ECV not only reduces the need for cesarean delivery, but also results in improved maternal and perinatal outcomes (44,45).

TABLE 15-1 Predisposing Factors for Breech Presentation

Fetal	Maternal
Prematurity	Uterine relaxation (e.g., high parity, multiple fetuses, polyhydramnios)
Fetal neurologic impairments (e.g., muscular dystrophy)	Abnormal placentation
Fetal congenital anomalies (e.g., hydrocephalus, anencephaly)	Contracted maternal pelvis
Short umbilical cord	Mullerian duct anomalies
Oligohydramnios	Uterine anomalies Pelvic tumors Previous breech delivery

Timing of ECV

Several studies have addressed the issue of appropriate timing for ECV procedures. A Cochrane systematic review demonstrated that ECV performed early in the third trimester (i.e., between 32 and 34 weeks of gestation) did not reduce the number of breech fetuses at term, nor did it reduce the number of cesarean deliveries (15). However, the authors were unable to make any definitive recommendations regarding the use of ECV at 34 to 36 weeks of gestation versus 37 weeks or later.

Two randomized controlled trials, the ECV1 and early ECV2 trials, investigated this issue. The ECV1 trial randomized 232 patients with singleton breech fetus to undergo ECV between 34 and 36 weeks of gestation (early group) or between 37 and 38 weeks of gestation (delayed group) (46). Although the authors demonstrated that malpresentation at delivery was lower in the early group than in the delayed group (56.9% vs. 66.4%, respectively), the results were not statistically significant, likely due to the study being underpowered. As such, the authors performed the early ECV2 trial, in which more than 1,500 women with a singleton breech fetus were randomized to undergo ECV between 34 and 36 weeks of gestation or at or after 37 weeks (47). The authors demonstrated that fewer fetuses were in a noncephalic presentation at birth in the early ECV group (41%) versus (49%) in the late ECV group (RR 0.84; 95% CI 0.75 to 0.94; $P = 0.002$). Despite this difference, there was no difference in the rate of cesarean delivery between groups. Similarly, there were no differences in the rate of preterm birth or risk of maternal or neonatal morbidity between groups. The authors concluded that even though ECV at an early gestation increases the likelihood of cephalic presentation at birth, it does not result in decreased cesarean delivery rates. Currently, ACOG recommendations state that ECV should be offered to eligible patients at term, defined as after completion of 36 weeks of gestation, due to concerns regarding fetal size, spontaneous versions, spontaneous reversions, and well-being of the preterm fetus (39).

Safety

Despite the fact that ECV reduces the rate of noncephalic presentation at term, as well as maternal and neonatal morbidity associated with cesarean and vaginal breech deliveries, there is resistance by both physicians and women to attempt this procedure. Studies have reported that the number of women suitable for ECV who were not offered an attempted procedure ranges from 4% to 33% (46,48). Even when offered, rates of maternal refusal of ECV range from 18% to 76% (49,50). In addition, ECV may not always be beneficial to the mother and/or fetus. ECV is contraindicated whenever the procedure may pose significant harm to the fetus, if the likelihood of success after an attempt is very low, or when the indication for cesarean delivery is not limited to breech presentation (Table 15-2).

Concerns about the safety of ECV are one issue that may dissuade obstetric providers and mothers. However, available evidence suggests that the overall rate of severe complications is relatively low. In a meta-analysis by Collaris et al. of 44 studies involving more than 7,000 women, the most frequently reported complication was transient fetal heart rate changes, occurring in 5.7% of ECV attempts (51). Persistent fetal heart rate changes, vaginal bleeding, and placental abruption occurred much less frequently (0.37%, 0.47%, and 0.12%, respectively). Similarly, the rate of emergent cesarean delivery and perinatal mortality were also low at 0.43% and 0.16%, respectively. However, there was also a 3% risk of

TABLE 15-2 Absolute and Relative Contraindication to External Cephalic Version

Absolute Contraindications	Multiple gestation Severe fetal or uterine anomalies Ruptured fetal membranes Intrauterine growth restriction Nonreassuring fetal status Isoimmunization Placenta previa Placental abruption
Relative Contraindications	Early labor Oligohydramnios Small for gestational age fetus Presence of uterine scar Maternal obesity

spontaneous reversion to breech presentation after successful ECV at or beyond 36 weeks of gestation. Similar findings were also reported in a systematic review of 84 studies of 12,955 ECV-related complications for singleton breech pregnancies after 36 weeks of gestation. In this meta-analysis, the authors found a pooled complication rate of 6.1% (95% CI 4.7 to 7.8), with a risk of serious complications (e.g., placental abruption, fetal death) occurring in 1/417 ECV attempts, and emergent cesarean delivery occurring in 1/286 (52). Overall, the risk of complications from ECV was found to be no different between successful and failed attempts (OR 1.24; 95% CI 0.93 to 1.7) (Fig. 15-3).

Predictors of ECV Success

The overall success rate of ECV can be predicted by the presence of several clinical and ultrasound factors. Known clinical factors associated with successful ECV include multiparity, low body mass index, a relaxed uterus, and a nonengaged fetal head (53). Interestingly, fundal height and gestational age have no impact on the outcome of ECV (54). Posterior placental location, complete breech presentation, and increased amniotic fluid index are ultrasound parameter predictors of successful ECV (55).

Cluver et al. performed a meta-analysis of 25 studies involving more than 2,500 women, comparing several interventions used to increase the success of ECV (42). The interventions included the use of tocolytic drugs, regional anesthesia, vibroacoustic stimulation, amnioinfusion, and systemic opioids. Of these interventions the authors concluded that only tocolytics improved the success rate of ECV. In addition, the use of regional anesthesia with tocolytics was superior in increasing the ECV success rate than use of tocolytics alone. There was insufficient data to make recommendations on the use of vibroacoustic stimulation, amnioinfusion, and systemic opioids for ECV. Recently, Kok et al. developed a predictive model to calculate the chance of successful ECV. Although this model still requires external validation, it appears to discriminate between women with a poor chance of successful ECV (less than 20%) and women with a good chance of success (more than 60%) in breech pregnancies after 36 weeks of gestation age (56).

Tocolysis

Various tocolytic agents have been used to provide uterine relaxation during ECV. When compared to control groups neither ritodrine, salbutamol, nor nitroglycerin have been found to increase the success rate of ECV after their administration

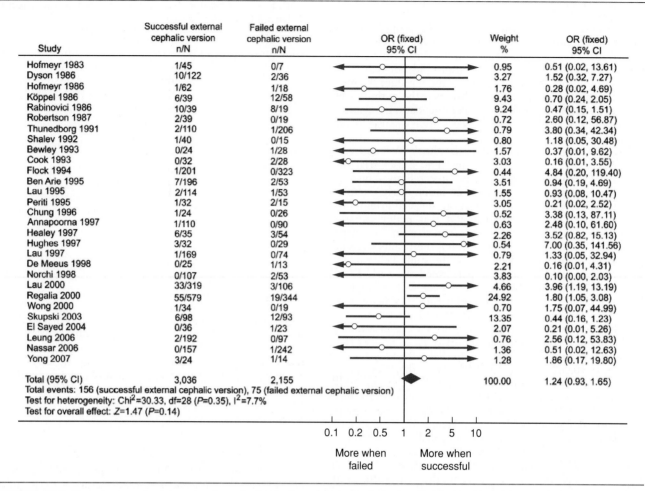

FIGURE 15-3 Forest plot of odds ratios from individual studies reporting on all complications related to ECV in relation to the ECV outcome. OR, odds ratio; CI, confidence interval. Reproduced with permission from: Grootscholten K, Kok M, Oei SG, et al. External cephalic version-related risks: a meta-analysis. *Obstet Gynecol* 2008;112:1143–1151.

(57–59). In a prospective study by Fernandez et al., terbutaline was found to increase the success rate of ECV when compared to placebo (52% vs. 27%, respectively; RR of 1.9; 95% CI 1.3 to 6.5, P = 0.01) (60). In a systematic review, Wilcox et al. observed that patients that received nifedipine compared to terbutaline, had lower rates of successful ECV (pooled risk ratio = 0.67; 95% CI 0.48 to 0.93, P = 0.016) (61). Based on the available evidence, terbutaline is the tocolytic recommended for ECV procedures.

Analgesic Options

Several studies have investigated the impact of intravenous analgesia, neuraxial *analgesia*, and neuraxial *anesthesia* on ECV success rates. Yoshida et al. assessed the ECV success rate as they changed their practice, from the time when they performed ECV without neuraxial anesthesia to when it was offered (62). The authors reported that not only did the overall ECV success rate increase from 56% to 79% after regional anesthesia was offered, but also the cesarean delivery rate in the term breech population decreased from 50% to 33%. Similarly, in a systematic review of six randomized controlled trials, Goetzinger et al. concluded that regional anesthesia was associated with a higher ECV success rate compared with intravenous or no analgesia (59.7% compared with 37.6%) (Fig. 15-4) (63).

Neuraxial Techniques

Compared to no or intravenous analgesia, neuraxial techniques provide several benefits for patients undergoing ECV. First, they allow for relaxation of the maternal abdominal wall, prevention of involuntary abdominal tensing, and improvement of maternal tolerance to the procedure, potentially increasing the success rate of ECV. In addition, maternal pain scores are significantly lower in patients that received neuraxial blockade compared to control groups in several randomized controlled studies (64–66). Sullivan et al. demonstrated that patient satisfaction scores were significantly higher in patients who received a combined spinal–epidural technique versus those who received intravenous (IV) fentanyl (10 vs. 7, P < 0.005) (66). Maternal discomfort in control groups can also lead to ECV discontinuation in some cases (65,67). The ability to rapidly extend epidural analgesia to a surgical level of anesthesia for emergent cesarean delivery is particularly beneficial, as it circumvents the need for general anesthesia and its inherent risks. Finally, in patients who undergo a trial of labor after ECV, the presence of a functioning epidural catheter allows for the provision of labor analgesia without the need for a second anesthetic technique.

Several studies have attempted to elucidate the impact of neuraxial anesthesia on ECV success rates. However, the heterogeneity of these studies has led to conflicting results not

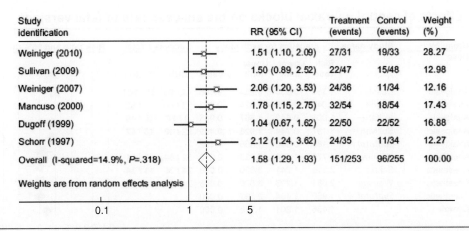

Study identification	RR (95% CI)	Treatment (events)	Control (events)	Weight (%)
Weiniger (2010)	1.51 (1.10, 2.09)	27/31	19/33	28.27
Sullivan (2009)	1.50 (0.89, 2.52)	22/47	15/48	12.98
Weiniger (2007)	2.06 (1.20, 3.53)	24/36	11/34	12.16
Mancuso (2000)	1.78 (1.15, 2.75)	32/54	18/54	17.43
Dugoff (1999)	1.04 (0.67, 1.62)	22/50	22/52	16.88
Schorr (1997)	2.12 (1.24, 3.62)	24/35	11/34	12.27
Overall (I-squared=14.9%, P=.318)	1.58 (1.29, 1.93)	151/253	96/255	100.00

Weights are from random effects analysis

FIGURE 15-4 Meta-analysis of the outcome of successful ECV comparing neuraxial anesthesia with intravenous or no anesthesia. The pooled risk ratio (RR) is 1.58 (95% confidence interval [CI] 1.29–1.93), I^2 = 14.9%. Reproduced with permission from: Goetzinger KR, Harper LM, Tuuli MG, et al. Effect of regional anesthesia on the success rate of external cephalic version: a systematic review and meta-analysis. *Obstet Gynecol* 2011;118:1137–1144.

only on the impact of analgesic and anesthetic techniques on ECV success rates, but also on its impact on maternal and fetal safety. Factors where studies differ include parity, timing of ECV in relation to gestational age, type and route of administration of tocolytics, local anesthetics used, and dose variations of neuraxially administered medications.

Low-dose Neuraxial Techniques

Low-dose intrathecal bupivacaine (i.e., 2.5 mg) with opioid have been shown not to improve the success of ECV. Dugoff et al. compared the success rate of ECV in patients who randomized to spinal anesthesia (0.5% bupivacaine 2.5 mg and sufentanil 10 μg) or no analgesia, and demonstrated no difference in overall ECV success rate between groups (44% spinal vs. 42% no spinal, $P = 0.86$) (67). Similarly, Sullivan et al. randomized patients to CSE technique (0.5% bupivacaine 2.5 mg and fentanyl 15 μg) versus intravenous fentanyl 50 μg before the procedure (66). The authors reported an ECV success rate of 47% with CSE compared to 31% in the intravenous group, although this result was not statistically significant.

Intermediate-dose Neuraxial Techniques

Weiniger et al. investigated the effect of a higher dose of intrathecal bupivacaine (7.5 mg) on ECV success rates in two separate studies that controlled for parity. The first study randomized term, nulliparous women to spinal dosage of bupivacaine 7.5 mg or no analgesia (65). The success rate of ECV was 67% in the spinal group compared to 34% in the control group, ($P = 0.004$). The follow-up study also randomized term, multiparous patients to spinal analgesia (bupivacaine 7.5 mg) or no analgesia, resulting in similar success rates of 87% in the spinal group compared to 57% in the control group, ($P = 0.009$) (64).

High-dose Neuraxial Techniques

Schorr et al. randomized term parturients scheduled for ECV to receive an epidural or no epidural anesthesia (68). Lidocaine 2% with 1:200,000 epinephrine was administered through the epidural catheter with the goal of achieving a T6 level. The success rate was higher for the epidural group,

with 69% compared with 32% in the control group ($P = 0.01$). Mancuso et al. performed a similar study with epidural anesthesia, obtaining comparable results (69).

A systematic review and meta-analysis of randomized trials by Goetzinger et al. suggest that neuraxial blockade is associated with an increased success rate of ECV (60% compared with 38%; RR 1.58; 95% CI [1.29 to 1.93]) but the risk of cesarean delivery was not significantly different for parturients that received neuraxial blockade compared to those that received intravenous or no analgesia (48% compared with 59%; RR 0.8; 95% CI 0.55 to 1.17) (63). Similar results were reported in a 2012 Cochrane Collaboration regarding interventions that improved the success rate of ECV. The authors concluded that regional analgesia, in addition to tocolytics, increased the success rate of ECV. Cephalic presentation in labor or cesarean delivery rate, however, was not different (42).

Results regarding the ideal neuraxial technique to improve the success rate of ECV are inconclusive. In Goetzinger's study the association between regional anesthesia and higher ECV success rate prevailed when the data was further divided into spinal and epidural groups, with epidural technique associated with a higher chance of ECV success (RR 1.91, 95% CI 1.29 to 1.93) than a spinal or CSE technique (RR 1.46, 95% CI 1.14 to 1.87), although this difference may be explained by the higher doses of local anesthetic used in the epidural groups (63). Lavoie and Guay performed a meta-analysis that compared randomized controlled trials on ECV success rates after neuraxial blockade with analgesic versus anesthetic doses, and concluded that the success rate for ECV is only increased by a neuraxial blockade in anesthetic doses (Fig. 15-5) (70).

There are several limitations to many of these studies. Neuraxial blockade is poorly defined, as the terms analgesia and anesthesia are used arbitrarily. Different tocolytics have been used at different doses and routes of administration. While β-mimetics increase the success rate of ECV, information regarding the effectiveness of other tocolytics (e.g., calcium channel blockers and nitric acid donor) is limited (42). Multiparity increases the success rate of ECV and by not controlling for parity the success rate may not achieve the same positive effect.

Although most of the current studies seem to indicate that anesthetic doses can improve the success rate of ECV, the authors' opinion is that the risk-to-benefit ratio to both

Effects of central neuraxial blocks on the success rate of fetal versions

Group by Dose	Study name	Statistics for each study				Success / Total		Risk ratio and 95% CI
		Risk ratio	Lower limit	Upper limit	p-Value	CNB	Control	
Analgesic	Delisle	1.363	0.936	1.984	0.106	41 / 99	31 / 102	
Analgesic	Dugoff	1.040	0.666	1.624	0.863	22 / 50	22 / 52	
Analgesic	Hollard	1.006	0.542	1.867	0.985	9 / 17	10 / 19	
Analgesic	Sullivan	1.197	0.744	1.926	0.459	22 / 48	18 / 47	
Analgesic	Subtotal	1.182	0.940	1.485	0.152			
Anesthetic	Mancuso	1.778	1.148	2.753	0.010	32 / 54	18 / 54	
Anesthetic	Schorr	2.119	1.241	3.620	0.006	24 / 35	11 / 34	
Anesthetic	Weiniger	2.061	1.203	3.529	0.008	24 / 36	11 / 34	
Anesthetic	Subtotal	1.950	1.464	2.597	0.000			
Overall		1.436	1.201	1.716	0.000			

0.1 0.2 0.5 1 2 5 10

Favours control favours CNB

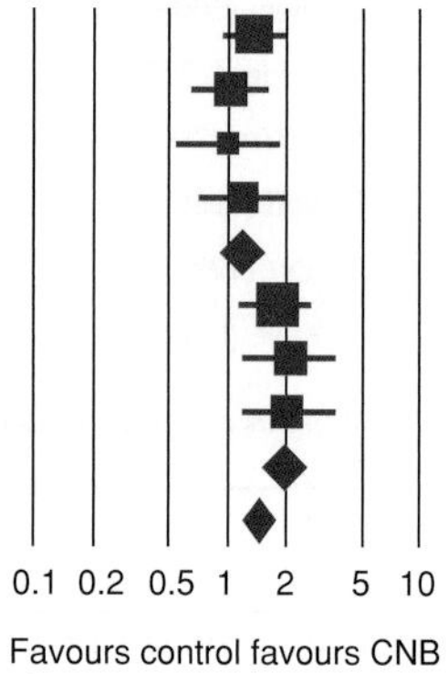

Mixed effects models

FIGURE 15-5 Meta-analysis investigating the effect of neuraxial anesthetic technique on the success rate of ECV. $I^2 = 30.25\%$ for the overall analysis and 0% for each subgroup. The two subgroups are significantly different from each other ($P = 0.007$). Reproduced with permission from: Lavoie A, Guay J. Anesthetic dose neuraxial blockade increases the success rate of external fetal version: a meta-analysis. *Can J Anaesth* 2010;57:408–414.

the mother and the fetus as well as the costs engaged after the administration of an anesthetic dose should all be considered before final recommendations are made.

Overall, the available evidence is inconclusive to recommend a specific neuraxial technique or dosage of local anesthetic which increases the success of ECV. Well-designed randomized controlled trials that specifically address the effect of neuraxial techniques on ECV outcomes and control for confounding factors are needed before any firm recommendations can be made. Nevertheless, the majority of studies suggest a strong association between higher neuraxial doses of local anesthetic and improved ECV success rates. Moreover, a CSE technique seems to be a better alternative to a spinal or epidural technique, in that it offers the benefit of a spinal anesthetic (e.g., rapid onset, dense and reliable block, lower doses of local anesthetic needed) with the versatility of an epidural catheter (e.g., ability to quickly augment block to surgical level of anesthesia, ability to be used for labor analgesia).

■ COST-EFFECTIVENESS

Tan et al. studied the cost-effectiveness, from society's perspective, of ECV compared to schedule cesarean delivery for term breech presentation. Cost-effectiveness, defined by a certain quality-adjusted life year, was less for ECV compared to scheduled cesarean deliveries for breech presentation. However, this only held true if the probability of successful ECV was >32% (71). Moreover, Bolaji and colleague demonstrated that even if the use of a neuraxial technique would increase the number of successful ECV by 15%, this would result in more than $33,000 in savings due to the decreased rates of cesarean delivery and its complications (72).

■ LOGISTICS

ECV should be attempted in the operating room or in the labor and delivery unit with an operating room available in case an emergent cesarean delivery becomes necessary.

However, considering the cost of utilizing an operating room, it may be cost effective to perform this procedure in the labor and delivery unit. In addition, both mother and fetus should be monitored throughout the procedure. Blood pressure and pulse oximetry should be used for the mother, while fetal monitoring should be performed before and after each ECV attempt. Moreover, left uterine displacement should be ensured whenever the patient is supine, and providers should have the ability to rapidly treat hypotension if it develops. Finally, ECV should be performed at times that do not detract from the care of the rest of the patients in the labor and delivery unit (Table 15-3).

TABLE 15-3 General Recommendations for External Cephalic Version

- Fetal presentation should be reassessed before preparing the patient for ECV.
- Verify nil per os (NPO) status of the patient.
- Discuss with the obstetrician the delivery plan for each scenario, if the ECV is successful or not.
- Consider placing an epidural catheter if the plan is to deliver the fetus after the ECV, regardless of success of the procedure, to provide either labor analgesia for induction of labor, or anesthesia for a cesarean delivery.
- Perform ECV in the labor and delivery room, preoperative holding area or postoperative unit, after confirming that there is an operating room available for emergent cesarean delivery.
- Plan for routine noninvasive monitoring of the mother, especially when neuraxial blockade is performed.
- Maintain left uterine displacement throughout the procedure.
- Fetal heart rate monitoring before and after each ECV attempt is recommended.

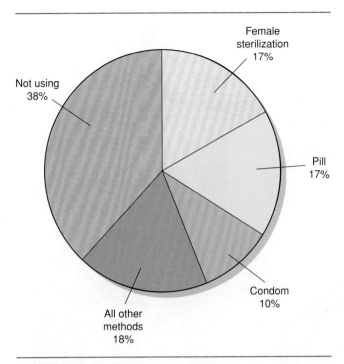

FIGURE 15-6 Percent distribution of women aged 15 to 44 years, by current contraceptive status: United States, 2006 to 2008. Data from The National Survey of Family Growth. From: Mosher WD, Jones J. Use of contraception in the United States: 1982–2008. *Vital Health Stat 23* 2010;29:1–44.

■ POSTPARTUM TUBAL STERILIZATION

Tubal sterilization is a highly effective form of female birth control, with a failure rate of <1%. Due to its reliability and permanence, this form of contraception was utilized by 16.7% of women in the United States between 2006 and 2008, second only to oral contraception in frequency of use among women (Fig. 15-6) (73). It is also one of the most commonly performed operations in the United States with 643,000 patients undergoing this procedure in 2006, approximately 340,000 of which are performed postpartum (74). Since more than 50% of tubal sterilizations are performed during the early postpartum period, anesthesiologists providing obstetric care to women are frequently called upon to provide care for this procedure.

Surgical Considerations

Performing tubal sterilizations during the postpartum period offers several advantages. First, the fallopian tubes are right below the abdominal wall at the level of the umbilicus, allowing for easy access. Second, abdominal wall laxity allows for manipulation of the incision to be located above each uterine cornu. Third, the patient is already an inpatient, forgoing the additional inconvenience and cost of a second hospital visit. Moreover, many women tend to have epidural labor analgesia, which can usually be augmented to a surgical level of anesthesia, eliminating the need for a second anesthetic. There is also a lower failure rate (7.5 pregnancies/1,000 sterilizations) with tubal ligations performed during the postpartum period compared to interval procedures, i.e., tubal ligations performed more than 6 to 8 weeks of postpartum (75). Finally, women who do not receive a requested postpartum tubal ligation are more likely to become pregnant again

within 1 year after delivery than women who did not request one, resulting in increased economic and social burdens on both the patient and the community (76).

However, there are some disadvantages to performing tubal sterilization during the immediate postpartum period. First, there may not be enough time to allow for proper newborn assessment after vaginal or cesarean delivery. If there is any adverse neonatal outcome, a mother may wish to have additional children, which would be more challenging if permanent tubal sterilization is performed immediately postpartum. Similarly, a national, multicenter cohort study in the United States demonstrated that women who underwent tubal sterilization during cesarean delivery or immediately after vaginal delivery had a higher probability of regretting her decision 3 to 7 years later, than if she would have had the procedure performed at a later time (77). This risk of regret increases if the patient is 30 years old or younger, or reports substantial conflict with her husband prior to the procedure (78). Finally, immediate postpartum sterilization may not be safe in women with obstetric complications or comorbid medical conditions. Women may be at increased risk for uterine atony and postpartum hemorrhage immediately after delivery, rendering a patient hemodynamically unstable. In addition, since there is a significant increase in afterload, cardiac output, and venous return immediately postpartum, women with cardiac disease may have deterioration in their hemodynamic status, making it unsafe to proceed with this procedure.

Several surgical techniques are utilized for tubal sterilization, each with their respective benefits and drawbacks (Fig. 15-7). Of these techniques, the Parkland and Pomeroy methods are the most commonly employed for postpartum tubal ligations (79). Typically, a mini-laparotomy approach is used during the postpartum procedure, although laparoscopy may also be considered. Although the risk of major morbidity (e.g., bowel perforation, vascular injury) is similar between two methods, minor morbidity and operative times have been shown to be less with the laparoscopic approach (80). Failure rates of the different techniques depend on patient age at the time of sterilization, as well as the method of tubal occlusion (75). However, compared to other forms of female contraception, the failure rate from tubal ligation, regardless of surgical technique, is significantly lower.

Anesthetic Considerations

Despite external demands to perform postpartum tubal ligations relatively soon after delivery (e.g., obstetrician availability, hospital costs, avoidance of prolonged hospital stay, presence of functioning anesthetic technique with labor epidural analgesia), they are considered to be an elective procedure. As such, these procedures should only be performed if the patient is medically stable, meets appropriate fasting guidelines, and can be performed without compromising other aspects of patient care on the labor and delivery unit. In 2007, the American Society of Anesthesiologists (ASA) Task Force on Obstetric Anesthesia published an updated report on systemic recommendations for the anesthetic management of obstetric patients, including five guidelines for postpartum tubal ligation (81):

1. For postpartum tubal ligation, the patient should have no oral intake of solid foods within 6 to 8 hours of the surgery, depending on the type of food ingested (e.g., fat content).
2. Aspiration prophylaxis should be considered.
3. Both the timing of the procedure and the decision to use a particular anesthetic technique (i.e., neuraxial vs. general) should be individualized based on anesthetic risk factors, obstetric risk factors (e.g., blood loss), and patient preferences.

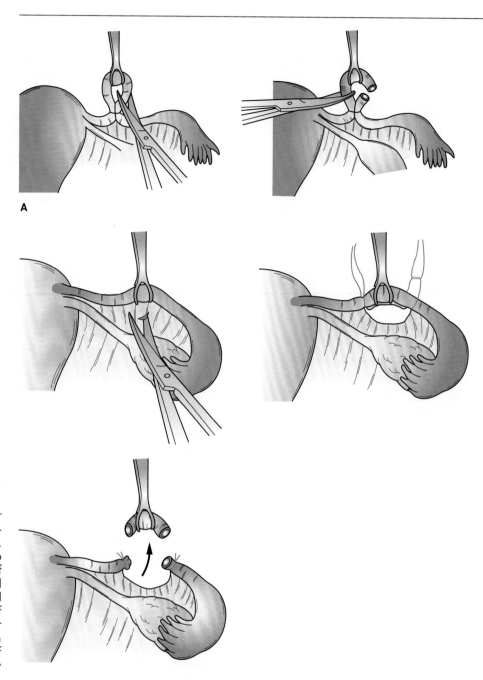

FIGURE 15-7 Common techniques for tubal sterilization. **A: Pomeroy Procedure**—a loop is created in the mid-segment of the tube, which is then ligated and resected. **B: Parkland Procedure**—after separation of the tube from an avascular site on the mesosalpinx, a 2 cm segment of the mid portion of the tube is ligated proximately and distally and then excised. (*continued*)

4. Neuraxial techniques are preferred to general anesthesia for most postpartum tubal ligations. The anesthesia provider should be aware that gastric emptying will be delayed in patients who have received opioids during labor and that an epidural catheter may be more likely to fail with longer postdelivery time.

5. If a postpartum tubal ligation is to be performed before the patient is discharged from the hospital, the procedure should not be attempted at a time when it might compromise other aspects of patient care on the labor and delivery unit.

In addition, the Task Force recommends a basic preoperative evaluation on any obstetric patient before providing anesthesia care, including: (1) Maternal health and anesthetic history; (2) relevant obstetric history; (3) baseline blood pressure measurement, as well as airway, heart, lung, and back examinations. Even if the patient has had a prior preoperative evaluation for labor analgesia, her medical history, focused physical examination, and intra- and postpartum courses (including blood loss from delivery) should be reviewed before proceeding as these may have changed in the interim.

Physiologic Changes of the Puerperium

Pregnancy is associated with significant physiologic changes in virtually all organ systems. The onset of labor and subsequent delivery further alter these changes, which persist into the postpartum period. Anesthesia providers caring for women need to be aware of these changes and their impact on anesthetic management.

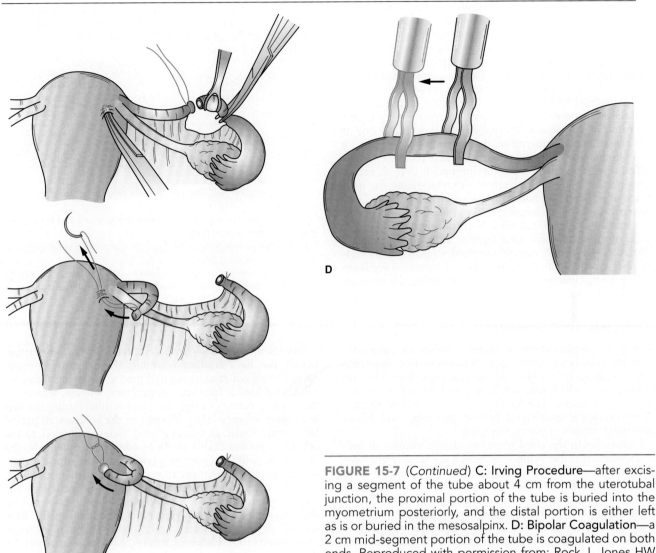

C

D

FIGURE 15-7 (*Continued*) **C: Irving Procedure**—after excising a segment of the tube about 4 cm from the uterotubal junction, the proximal portion of the tube is buried into the myometrium posteriorly, and the distal portion is either left as is or buried in the mesosalpinx. **D: Bipolar Coagulation**—a 2 cm mid-segment portion of the tube is coagulated on both ends. Reproduced with permission from: Rock J, Jones HW III. *TeLinde's Operative Gynecology*. 10th ed. Philadelphia, PA: Lippincott Williams & Wilkins; 2008.

Cardiovascular Changes

Women who present for surgery in the immediate postpartum period demonstrate pregnancy-induced changes in cardiovascular physiology. At term, parturients have a 50% increase in their cardiac output compared to the nonpregnant state; this change is due to a relative increase in both stroke volume and heart rate (82). With the onset of labor, cardiac output increases by another 10% during the early first stage, and continues to increase by 25% in the late first stage to 40% in the second stage, compared to prelabor values (83–85). These alterations occur due to increased sympathetic drive, increased venous return, and uterine autotransfusion during contractions. Immediately after delivery, cardiac output increases by as much as 75% of prelabor values, due to relief of vena caval compression, increase in central blood volume due to a contracted uterus, and decreased lower extremity venous pressure (85,86). Although cardiac output returns to prelabor values approximately 24 hours after delivery, pre-pregnancy values do not occur until 12 to 24 weeks postpartum (83,87). Heart rate does not approach prepregnancy values until 2 weeks postpartum, although it does significantly decrease soon after delivery due to decreased sympathetic drive and increased venous return (84,87).

Respiratory Changes

Pregnancy is associated with a 45% increase in minute ventilation, primarily due to an increase in tidal volumes, and resulting in a partially compensated respiratory alkalosis (88). Compared to prepregnancy levels, this increase in minute ventilation can increase by up to 200% during labor, especially in unmedicated labor (89). Oxygen consumption also increases during pregnancy as the metabolic demands of the mother and fetus grow, increasing by as much as 75% during labor. This increase in oxygen consumption is due to increased metabolic demands from increased uterine activity, hyperventilation secondary to pain, and expulsive efforts during the second stage of labor. Finally, functional residual capacity (FRC) progressively decreases during pregnancy due to diaphragmatic elevation from the enlarging uterus. At term, this change in FRC decreases by 80% of prepregnancy values, and reduces even further when a parturient is placed in the supine position (88). Following delivery, minute ventilation and oxygen consumption remain elevated until 6 to 8 weeks postpartum (90). FRC increases after delivery as the impact of the enlarged uterus on the diaphragm is lessened, but it does not return to prepregnancy values until 1 to 2 weeks postpartum. This delay in FRC improvement, along with the persistent increase in oxygen consumption, continues to place the postpartum patient at increased risk of rapid oxygen desaturation during periods of apnea.

Pregnancy is also associated with changes in maternal airway anatomy. Vascular engorgement of the airway results in oropharyngeal, laryngeal, and tracheal edema, resulting in potential difficulties with intubation and mask ventilation, as well as mucosal friability (91,92). During the course of labor and delivery, studies have demonstrated that airway edema can result in a change in Mallampati classification by one or two classes (93). Furthermore, these changes can persist up to 48 hours after delivery, potentially increasing the risk of difficult mask ventilation and/or intubation (94). A recent retrospective study by McKeen et al. investigating the incidence of difficult and failed intubations in more than 2,600 obstetric patients undergoing general anesthesia, reported two cases of failed intubation, both occurring in patients undergoing postpartum tubal ligation after vaginal delivery (95). Although these cases did not result in maternal mortality, they do highlight the importance of increased vigilance during airway management for women during the postpartum period.

Gastrointestinal Changes

Maternal aspiration of gastric contents has been a major concern for anesthesiologists since Mendelson first described this complication in 1946 (96). Several physiologic changes of pregnancy, which may not be resolved immediately upon delivery, are responsible for this increased risk, and include decreased lower esophageal barrier pressures, and labor-induced decreases in gastric emptying.

Parturients in the third trimester often complain of gastroesophageal reflux symptoms, which are usually attributable to decreased lower esophageal barrier pressure from upward displacement of the stomach and increased progesterone (97). Although lower esophageal barrier tone reaches its nadir around 36 weeks of gestation and does not reach prepregnancy levels until 1 to 4 weeks postpartum, progesterone levels quickly decline after delivery of the placenta, reaching luteal phase levels 24-hours postpartum, suggesting a limited contribution of progesterone to decreased lower barrier pressures postpartum (98). Vanner and Goodman reported that 17 out of 25 parturients had gastroesophageal reflux at term, based on lower esophageal pH measurements, but only five continued to have evidence of reflux on postpartum day 2 (99). However, since the authors failed to define the "normal" incidence of reflux before or 6 to 8 weeks after pregnancy, the incidence of gastroesophageal reflux in the postpartum period remains uncertain, and women in the postpartum period should be considered to be at increased risk.

Several studies have demonstrated that gastric emptying during pregnancy remains unchanged (100,101). However, due to the increased sympathetic drive that occurs with the onset of labor, gastric emptying decreases (102,103). In addition, the administration of opioids for labor analgesia, either systemically or intrathecally, contributes to decreased gastric motility, which may not be reversed with metoclopramide administration (104–106). Interestingly, studies investigating the effect of epidurally administered opioids on gastric emptying are conflicting. Porter et al. showed that epidural infusion of low-dose bupivacaine and fentanyl 2.5 μg/mL without a preceding epidural fentanyl bolus did not slow gastric emptying during labor (107). However, other studies have demonstrated delayed gastric emptying in laboring women receiving epidurally administered fentanyl or diamorphine (108,109).

TABLE 15-4 Gastric Emptying Times of 500 mL of Water in Female Volunteers, Women in the Third Trimester of Pregnancy, and Women in the Immediate Postpartum Period

	Nonpregnant (n = 15)	Third Trimester (n = 30)	Postpartum (n = 23)
$T_{0.7}$ (min)	5.2 ± 0.6	4.4 ± 0.5	8.8 ± 1.6[a]
$T_{0.5}$ (min)	8.3 ± 0.9	7.2 ± 0.6	13.0 ± 1.9[a]
$T_{0.3}$ (min)	11.1 ± 1.3	9.8 ± 0.8	15.8 ± 2.3[b]

Values are mean ± SEM.
[a]$P < 0.05$ between subjects immediately postpartum and the other two groups.
[b]$P < 0.05$ between subjects immediately postpartum and the women in the third trimester of pregnancy.
$T_{0.7}$, 70% gastric emptying time; $T_{0.5}$, 50% gastric emptying time; $T_{0.3}$, 30% gastric emptying time.
Modified with permission from: O'Sullivan GM, Sutton AJ, Thompson SA, et al. Noninvasive measurement of gastric emptying in obstetric patients. *Anesth Analg* 1987;66:505–511.

Studies investigating gastric emptying in the postpartum period also have conflicting results. Using gastric impedance, O'Sullivan et al. compared gastric emptying times for solids and liquids between nonpregnant women, women in the third trimester of pregnancy, and women during the first hour after delivery (110). Women in the postpartum period had longer mean gastric emptying times compared to the other two groups (Table 15-4). In addition, women who did not receive intramuscular meperidine intrapartum had gastric emptying rates similar to nonpregnant patients; women who did receive intrapartum opioids had decreased gastric emptying rates (Table 15-5). Whitehead et al. observed no difference in gastric emptying rates in women in the first, second, or third trimester, and women 18 hours or more postpartum (100). However, women 2 hours postpartum did demonstrate increased gastric emptying times. Moreover, 4 of the 17 women in this group received meperidine and promethazine during labor, suggesting that the intrapartum administration of opioids delays gastric emptying within 2 hours of delivery.

Despite delayed gastric emptying, laboring women often do not have increased gastric volume. Several studies have investigated the relationship between increased intrapartum and postpartum gastric volumes. Lam et al. demonstrated no

TABLE 15-5 Gastric Emptying Times in the Postpartum Subjects who did and did not Receive Opiate Analgesia

	No Analgesia or Epidural Analgesia (n = 15)	Intravenous Analgesia (n = 8)	P Value
$T_{0.7}$ (min)	6.6 ± 1.4	13.1 ± 3.0	<0.05
$T_{0.5}$ (min)	10.3 ± 1.4	18.2 ± 4.0	<0.05
$T_{0.3}$ (min)	12.9 ± 1.5	21.8 ± 5.6	<0.05

Values are mean ± SEM.
$T_{0.7}$, 70% gastric emptying time; $T_{0.5}$, 50% gastric emptying time; $T_{0.3}$, 30% gastric emptying time.
Modified with permission from: O'Sullivan GM, Sutton AJ, Thompson SA, et al. Noninvasive measurement of gastric emptying in obstetric patients. *Anesth Analg* 1987;66:505–511.

difference in gastric volumes in women administered 150 mL of water 2 to 3 hours before tubal ligation 1 to 5 days postpartum, and women who were postpartum or nonpregnant women who fasted after midnight (111). Similarly, James et al. compared gastric volume and pH in women 1 to 8 hours, 9 to 23 hours, and 24 to 45 hours postpartum to nonpregnant women undergoing elective surgery (112). The authors found no difference between the four groups in the percentage of women with gastric volume >25 mL or gastric pH <2.5, suggesting no difference in risk or severity of aspiration pneumonitis between postpartum women and those undergoing elective surgery.

The type of substance ingested likely affects gastric volumes and rate of gastric emptying. Clear liquids are unlikely to increase the risk of postpartum aspiration. Kubli et al. found that postpartum gastric volumes were no different in parturients who consumed water in labor compared to those who consumed an isotonic sports drink (113). However, there is evidence that gastric transit times for liquids and solids are different, with liquids leaving the stomach faster (114). This observation was demonstrated in laboring women by Scrutton et al. who randomized women presenting in early labor to receive either a light diet or only water during labor (115). The authors found that those who received a light diet had more gastric distension on ultrasound and were more likely to vomit, compared to those who only received water (Table 15-6). Similarly, Jayaram et al. found that 19 out of 20 postpartum women, compared to 4 of 21 nonpregnant women, had solid food particles in the stomach 4 hours after a standardized meal (116). Of note, mean time of last narcotic administration in the postpartum group was 14.7 ± 6.9 hours. However, a 2009 study by O'Sullivan et al. randomized more than 2,000 laboring women to a light diet or water, and found no difference in the incidence of vomiting (35% vs. 34%, RR 1.05; 95% CI 0.94 to 1.17), although the study was likely underpowered to detect a difference as this was not the primary outcome (117).

Overall, the data on gastric function during the postpartum period suggests that:

1. Despite an unknown incidence during the postpartum period, women undergoing postpartum tubal ligation should be considered to be at increased risk of gastroesophageal reflux.
2. Gastric emptying is likely delayed during the immediate postpartum period if intrapartum opioids were administered. There is little data on gastric emptying during the first 8 hours postpartum.

3. Gastric emptying of solid foods is delayed during the postpartum period in all patients, regardless of intrapartum opioid administration. Gastric emptying of liquids is likely delayed, unless intrapartum opioids were given.

Based on these findings, it is reasonable to assume that no defined time period will decrease or increase a postpartum patient's risk of gastric aspiration. Nevertheless, it seems prudent to still administer aspiration prophylaxis (e.g., H_2-receptor antagonist, metoclopramide, and/or nonparticulate antacid) before proceeding, as the benefit of this intervention greatly outweighs the risk. Patients with conditions known to increase the risk of aspiration (e.g., diabetes mellitus, obesity) should receive prophylaxis with all three medications. Finally, adherence to a nil per os (NPO) status of 6 to 8 hours for solids for all women undergoing postpartum tubal ligation, and 2 hours for liquids in women who received intrapartum opioids, will likely decrease the risk of gastric aspiration in this patient population.

Anesthetic Management

Local, neuraxial, and general anesthesia have all been successfully utilized for postpartum tubal sterilization. The decision of which anesthetic technique to use depends on several factors, including patient and provider preference, time interval between delivery and tubal sterilization, obstetric and anesthetic risk factors, and presence of a functioning epidural catheter.

Anesthetic Risk for Postpartum Tubal Sterilization

The true anesthetic risk of performing tubal sterilization immediately postpartum (i.e., within 8 hours after delivery) is unknown. In 1983, Peterson et al. reported 29 deaths out of 3 million tubal sterilizations (both postpartum and interval procedures) in the United States between 1977 and 1981 (118). Eleven deaths were attributable to complications from general anesthesia, with six deaths due to hypoventilation and the remaining due to cardiorespiratory arrest of unknown etiology. Although five of the eleven deaths occurred during this postpartum period and all six of the hypoventilation deaths occurred in nonintubated patients, none were due to aspiration. Higher rates of intra- and postoperative complications (although no deaths) have also been reported in patients undergoing interval tubal ligation procedures undergoing general anesthesia, compared to local or neuraxial anesthetic techniques (119,120).

Since these initial reports, significant advances in airway management techniques, improvements in intraoperative monitoring of oxygenation and ventilation, as well as the increase utilization of neuraxial techniques, have resulted in decreased rates of anesthesia-related maternal mortality. Although postpartum tubal ligations were not specifically identified, Hawkins et al. demonstrated a 60% reduction in anesthesia-related maternal mortality rates in the United States when data from 1991 to 2002 were compared to that from 1979 to 1990 (121). The authors also determined no difference in maternal mortality risk between general and neuraxial techniques between 1997 and 2002 (Table 15-7). One tool which has contributed to decreased maternal mortality rates is use of the LMA for failed intubation rescue. In addition, Evans and colleagues reported no occurrences of gastric aspiration with use of the Proseal™ LMA in 90 subjects undergoing postpartum tubal sterilization at least 8 hours after vaginal delivery (122). Despite this promising finding, additional studies identifying the true incidence of

TABLE 15-6 Gastric Antral Cross-sectional Area and Incidence and Volume of Vomiting in Laboring Parturients Randomized to a Light Diet or Water

	Light Diet (n = 26)	Water Only (n = 24)	P Value
Gastric antral cross-sectional area (cm²; mean [SD])	6.35 (1.98)	4.50 (1.64)	0.001
Number vomiting (%)	17 (38)	8 (19)	0.046
Volume vomited (mL; mean [SE])	309 (173)	104 (83)	0.001

SD, standard deviation; SE, standard error.
Modified with permission from: Scrutton MJ, Metcalfe GA, Lowy C, et al. Eating in labour. A randomised controlled trial assessing the risks and benefits. *Anaesthesia* 1999;54:329–334.

TABLE 15-7 Case Fatality Rates and Rate Ratios of Anesthesia-related Deaths During Cesarean Delivery by Type of Anesthesia in the United States, 1979–2002

| Year of Death | Case Fatality Rates[a] | | Rate Ratios |
	General Anesthetic	Neuraxial Anesthetic	
1979–1984	20	8.6	2.3 (95% CI 1.9–2.9)
1985–1990	32.3	1.9	16.7 (95% CI 12.9–21.8)
1991–1996	16.8	2.5	6.7 (95% CI 3.0–14.9)
1997–2002	6.5	3.8	1.7 (95% CI 0.6–4.6)

[a]Deaths per million general or neuraxial anesthetics.
CI, confidence interval.
Modified with permission from: Hawkins JL, Chang J, Palmer SK, et al. Anesthesia-related maternal mortality in the United States: 1979–2002. *Obstet Gynecol* 2011;117:69–74.

gastric aspiration in this population need to be performed before routine use of LMAs can be recommended.

Local Anesthesia

Although neuraxial techniques are the most commonly used anesthetic method for postpartum tubal sterilization in the United States (123), local anesthesia is used for more than 75% of tubal ligations worldwide (124). Benefits of local anesthetic infiltration include: (1) Lower complication rates compared to general anesthesia; (2) decreased morbidity and mortality rates compared to general or neuraxial techniques; (3) significant cost savings; and (4) faster recovery times and less nausea, vomiting, and postoperative pain compared to general anesthesia (125,126). However, as intraoperative sedation is frequently required for such procedures, the risks of hypoventilation and aspiration due to blunted airway reflexes may decrease the safety of local anesthesia compared to other anesthetic modalities.

Several studies have investigated the clinical effectiveness of local anesthesia. Munson and Scott reported favorable outcomes in 138 women undergoing tubal sterilization via the Pomeroy method, after receiving intravenous diazepam and local infiltration of the surgical site with 1% mepivacaine (127). Cruikshank et al. demonstrated similar anesthetic and surgical outcomes in 26 women who received intravenous diazepam, lidocaine 100 mg (20 mL of 0.5% solution) intradermally, and lidocaine 400 mg (80 mL of 0.5% solution) intraperitoneally (128). In a second phase of this study, the authors measured plasma lidocaine concentrations 10, 20, 30, 40, and 60 minutes after intraperitoneal administration of lidocaine 1,000 mg in nine women undergoing general anesthesia for tubal ligation, and found mean peak lidocaine concentrations of 2.92 μg/mL, well within toxicity limits.

Other studies have investigated the use of local anesthesia for laparoscopic tubal ligation. In a retrospective review of more than 2,800 cases, Poindexter et al. describe the ability to perform laparoscopic tubal sterilization with intravenous sedation with fentanyl (50 to 100 μg) and midazolam (5 to 10 mg), 10 mL of 0.5% bupivacaine intradermally, and spraying each tube with 5 mL of 0.5% bupivacaine (129). With this technique, the authors reported a failure rate of 0.14%, with no intraoperative conversions to an open technique. In addition, compared to general anesthesia, they demonstrated decreased surgical times and costs. In another study, Bordahl et al. randomized 150 women undergoing laparoscopic tubal ligation to either general anesthesia (propofol/midazolam/alfentanil/atracurium) or local anesthesia (10 mL 1% lidocaine intradermally and spraying each tube with 5 to 10 mL 0.5% bupivacaine) and sedation (midazolam/alfentanil)

(130). The authors demonstrated that, compared to the general anesthetic group, patients who received local anesthesia had shorter recovery times, less postoperative pain, less operative costs, and higher satisfaction rates.

The safety and cost-effectiveness of local anesthesia for tubal ligation makes this technique a viable option in developing countries, where there may be a lack of availability of anesthesia providers and equipment. A review of the literature concerning the experience with the mini-laparotomy technique under local anesthesia over a 15-year period in Kenya demonstrated acceptable intra- and postoperative pain control, as well as optimal operative conditions and success rates (131).

Neuraxial Anesthesia

Neuraxial anesthesia (spinal or epidural) represents the most common anesthetic technique for postpartum tubal sterilizations in the United States (125). Advantages of a neuraxial technique include superior intraoperative analgesia compared to local techniques, avoidance of airway manipulation, ability to maintain intact airway reflexes to protect against gastric aspiration, avoidance of hypoventilation, and lack of volatile agent-induced uterine atony. For the woman who received labor epidural analgesia, use of the epidural for surgical anesthesia and the ability to provide effective, prolonged postoperative analgesia with neuraxial morphine are additional benefits. Regardless of which neuraxial technique is used, a T4 sensory level is required to block visceral stimulation from manipulation of the fallopian tubes.

Spinal Anesthesia

Spinal anesthesia is preferred over general anesthesia in patients undergoing postpartum tubal ligation who did not receive intrapartum epidural analgesia (81). Despite decreased requirements during pregnancy, spinal anesthesia requirements return to nonpregnant levels by 12 to 36 hours postpartum. Marx found a progressive decrease in block duration during the first 3 days postpartum in women undergoing postpartum tubal ligation (132). Similarly, Abouleish prospectively compared the dose of intrathecal hyperbaric bupivacaine required for elective cesarean delivery versus postpartum tubal ligation, and found that patients required 30% more bupivacaine to achieve a T4 sensory level for postpartum tubal ligations up to 24 hours after delivery (133).

One theory for this change in spinal anesthetic requirements during the postpartum period is a rapid decrease in plasma progesterone levels after placental removal. Datta et al. have performed several in vitro and in vivo investigations into this relationship. In one study, the authors demonstrated shorter time intervals for nerve conduction blockade in phrenic nerves isolated from pregnant rabbits exposed to bupivacaine compared to nonpregnant controls (134). Suspecting changes in progesterone concentrations postpartum, the authors proceeded to investigate plasma and cerebrospinal fluid (CSF) progesterone concentrations in relation to intrathecal lidocaine requirements in nonpregnant, pregnant, and postpartum women 12 to 18 hours after delivery (135). Compared to nonpregnant controls, plasma and CSF progesterone concentrations were 60 and 8 times, respectively, higher in pregnant women, and 7 and 3 times, respectively, higher in the immediate postpartum group. Interestingly, mean intrathecal lidocaine doses were similar for the pregnant and postpartum groups (3.16 ± 0.04 mg/segment and 3.21 ± 0.08 mg/segment), but were still lower than the control group (3.80 ± 0.08 mg/segment; $P < 0.05$). In addition, there was an inverse correlation between intrathecal lidocaine dose and CSF progesterone concentrations (Fig. 15-8). The authors concluded that progesterone is only one of the factors responsible for altered neuronal sensitivity to local anesthetics in pregnancy, and that "a minimum level of progesterone in the CSF and/or plasma is necessary" for this observation.

Due to the relative short duration of tubal ligations compared to other surgical procedures, the use of a relatively short-acting spinal anesthetic agent is ideal. As such, hyperbaric lidocaine has been used effectively for postpartum tubal sterilizations, despite no clear recommendation about dosing requirements. Huffnagle and colleagues investigated the influence of several patient factors (age, height, weight, body mass index, vertebral column length, and time from delivery to initiation of block) on subarachnoid spread of hyperbaric 5% lidocaine 75 mg (136). The authors discovered that only patient height influenced level of spinal blockage, and this positive correlation was so weak ($r^2 = 0.15$) that any dose adjustment would likely not result in any clinically significant benefit. Finally, despite its shorter duration of action, increased concern for TNS after intrathecal usage has dissuaded many providers from using hyperbaric lidocaine for postpartum tubal sterilizations. Although not completely exempt from the risk of TNS, parturients may be at decreased risk compared to nonpregnant patients as discussed previously.

Studies have also investigated the intrathecal use of other local anesthetics for postpartum tubal sterilizations. Huffnagle et al. performed a dose-finding study for intrathecal bupivacaine for postpartum tubal ligation, and found that the 7.5 mg dose produced a higher level of surgical anesthesia than the 5 mg dose, but resulted in quicker motor regression and shorter recovery times compared to the 10 and 12 mg doses (Table 15-8) (137). Panni et al. in two separate studies using up–down sequential allocation, investigated the dose of intrathecal hyperbaric ropivacaine with and without fentanyl 10 μg

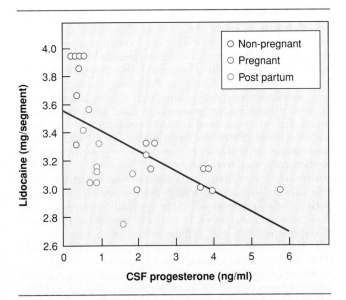

FIGURE 15-8 Correlation between the lidocaine dose requirement (mg/segment) and cerebrospinal fluid progesterone (ng/mL) in nonpregnant patients, term parturients, and postpartum patients. $r = -0.6$, $P = 0.03$. Modified with permission from: Datta S, Hurley RJ, Naulty JS, et al. Plasma and cerebrospinal fluid progesterone concentrations in pregnant and nonpregnant women. *Anesth Analg* 1986;65:950–954.

for postpartum tubal ligation (138). The authors estimated an ED_{95} of 21.9 mg and 21.3 mg for ropivacaine without and with fentanyl, respectively. Finally, Norris et al. randomized 20 patients undergoing postpartum tubal ligation to either hyperbaric 5% lidocaine 70 mg or meperidine 60 mg intrathecally (139). Despite no difference between the groups in terms of hemodynamic changes, inadequate block, or patient satisfaction, patients who received meperidine had longer postoperative analgesia (448 minutes vs. 83 minutes), compared to the lidocaine group, at the expense of increased pruritus.

Epidural Anesthesia

The chief benefit of an epidural anesthetic technique for postpartum tubal ligations is the fact that a functioning labor epidural catheter can be augmented to a surgical level of anesthesia, obviating the need to perform another anesthetic technique. However, the *Practical Guidelines for*

TABLE 15-8 Anesthetic Outcomes in Women Receiving 7.5, 10, or 12.5 mg of Intrathecal Hyperbaric Bupivacaine

Bupivacaine Dose (mg)	Delivery to Spinal Time	Surgery Duration	Mean Motor Regression Time	Mean Spinal to D/C Time	Mean PACU Time
7.5	$1,014 \pm 787$	48.2 ± 12.2	74.4 ± 27.0	101.0 ± 40.8	37.7 ± 39.7
10	657 ± 446	46.8 ± 14.8	117.3 ± 39.6	132.5 ± 48.9	75.3 ± 38.7
12.5	959 ± 778	40.1 ± 15.4	131.3 ± 31.3	144.4 ± 47.2	95.8 ± 53.9
P value	NS	NS	7.5 vs. 10, $P < 0.003$ 7.5 vs. 12.5, $P < 0.001$	NS	7.5 vs. 10, $P < 0.05$ 7.5 vs. 12.5, $P < 0.005$

Times are minutes ± standard deviation.
PACU, postanesthesia care unit; D/C, discharge; NS, not significant.
Reproduced with permission from: Huffnagle SL, Norris MC, Huffnagle HJ, et al. Intrathecal hyperbaric bupivacaine dose response in postpartum tubal ligation patients. *Reg Anesth Pain Med* 2002;27:284–288.

Obstetric Anesthesia suggests that epidural catheters placed for labor may be more likely to fail with longer delivery to reactivation intervals (81). This observation is supported by several studies that have investigated the likelihood of failed augmentation of epidural anesthesia for postpartum tubal ligations in relation to time interval from delivery. Vincent and Reid retrospectively analyzed this relationship in 90 women undergoing postpartum tubal sterilization, and found that women whose epidural catheters were re-dosed within 4 hours of delivery had a higher rate of achieving an appropriate surgical level of anesthesia for postpartum tubal ligation compared to those activated later (95% vs. 67%; $P = 0.029$) (140). In addition, the authors found that the mean interval time between delivery and surgery was shorter in patients who achieved adequate epidural anesthesia versus those who did not (10.6 vs. 14.8 hours). Viscomi and Rathmell also retrospectively analyzed the success of epidural reactivation as a function of delivery-to-surgery time, and reported a 93% success rate in women who underwent tubal ligation 1 to 4 hours after delivery, compared to 70% of women undergoing the procedure 5 or more hours later (Fig. 15-9) (141). Finally, Goodman and Dumas investigated the success rate of epidural reactivation in relation to the following delivery-to-surgery intervals: (1) <8 hours; (2) 8 to <16 hours; (3) 16 to <24 hours; and (4) ≥ 24 hours (142). The authors found that 93% of reactivations were successful in patients undergoing tubal ligation <24 hours after delivery, but only 80% among patients who underwent surgery 24 hours or later. One major limitation of these last two studies is that the reported differences in success rates were not statistically significant, likely due to the studies being not adequately powered to detect a difference. Nevertheless, the evidence suggests that minimizing the delivery-to-tubal ligation time interval greatly decreases the chance of failed epidural anesthesia.

One reason why epidural catheters reactivated at longer delivery-to-surgery times have a higher failure rate is due to a higher rate of catheter migration or dislodgement. In the peripartum period, significant catheter migration occurs in 36% to 54% of patients (143,144). In addition, the position of the epidural catheter may change significantly with patient movement from the sitting-flexed position to the sitting-upright or lateral decubitus position (145). D'Angelo et al. reported that single-orifice epidural catheters had a higher rate of dislodgement when inserted 2 cm within the epidural space, but a higher risk of unilateral block when catheters were inserted 6 to 8 cm (146). Beilin et al. found that insertion of multi-orifice epidural catheters 5 cm in the epidural space was associated with the highest incidence of satisfactory labor analgesia (147). Therefore, to optimize the success rate of epidural catheter reactivation for postpartum tubal ligation, insertion of the epidural catheter 4 to 6 cm within the epidural space is recommended. In addition, securing the epidural catheter to the skin when the patient is in a non-flexed position is recommended, especially in obese parturients (145).

Nevertheless, some patients with functioning labor epidural catheters who undergo catheter reactivation for tubal ligation within a reasonable time interval will still not achieve a surgical level of anesthesia. Anesthetic options after a failed epidural catheter include: replacement of the epidural catheter, spinal anesthesia, a combined spinal–epidural technique, local anesthetic infiltration of the surgical site, or general anesthesia. The employment of a spinal anesthetic technique after epidural catheter failure is controversial. One of the primary concerns with placement of a spinal anesthetic after failed epidural catheter reactivation is the occurrence of high or total spinal anesthesia. Several case reports have described this complication, with a reported incidence of 0.8% to 11% (148,149). Purported mechanisms for this increased risk include decreased size of the intrathecal space due to epidural space distention, passage of epidural medications through a dural hole from the subsequent spinal, and diffusion of epidural medications into the intrathecal space. Several techniques have been proposed to avoid high spinals in this scenario, but none have been demonstrated to decrease the incidence (150,151).

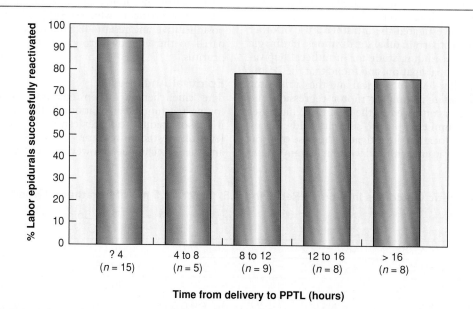

FIGURE 15-9 The percentage of labor epidural catheters successfully reactivated for postpartum tubal ligation versus time interval between delivery and surgery. $P = 0.08$, percentage of success no more than 4 hours versus longer than 4 hours. PPTL, postpartum tubal ligation. Reproduced with permission from: Viscomi CM, Rathmell JP. Labor epidural catheter reactivation or spinal anesthesia for delayed postpartum tubal ligation: a cost comparison. *J Clin Anesth* 1995;7:380–383.

For situations in which reactivation of the epidural catheter has failed, replacement of the epidural catheter is another option. However, two main downsides of this technique are increased risk of local anesthetic toxicity, especially if a large volume of local anesthetic has already been administered, as well as failure of the replaced epidural catheter. A CSE technique utilizing a lower intrathecal dose of local anesthetic will likely decrease the risk of high or total spinal anesthesia, but still allow for additional dosing with local anesthetic if the spinal component is inadequate for surgery or if the procedure lasts longer than expected. Besides decreased risk of high or total spinal anesthesia, use of a lower intrathecal dose of medication has also been demonstrated to reduce the incidence of hypotension and nausea (152,153).

General Anesthesia

As per the *Practice Guidelines for Obstetric Anesthesia*, there is insufficient evidence to compare the benefits of neuraxial anesthesia versus general anesthesia for postpartum tubal ligation (81). However, the guidelines do suggest that a neuraxial technique is preferable, likely due to the higher rate of morbidity and mortality associated with general anesthesia. Nevertheless, there are certain situations (e.g., patient preference, coagulopathy) in which general anesthesia may be superior. If general anesthesia is selected, several considerations must be taken into account. First, pregnancy-induced changes in pharmacokinetics are likely to still be present and impact anesthetic management. Second, changes in cardiopulmonary physiology may not only affect a patient's hemodynamics under general anesthesia, but also the difficulty of mask ventilation and intubation. Third, alterations in gastric physiology (*vide supra*) may increase a postpartum patient's risk of aspiration. As such, providers should treat the patient as a "full stomach" by meeting NPO requirements, administration of gastric acid prophylaxis, and utilization of a rapid sequence induction technique with cricoid pressure. Finally, standard ASA monitors should be used for all patients, especially monitors for oxygenation and ventilation, to help decrease the morbidity and mortality associated with general anesthesia (118–120).

Thiopental has a long history of efficacy and safety as an induction agent in the obstetric patient population (154). However, thiopental's negative inotropic and vasodilatory effects, as well as the recent lack of access in the United States may necessitate the need for alternative induction agents (155). Propofol, with its reliable, fast onset of action, rapid recovery, and lower incidence of nausea and vomiting, is a suitable alternative. In addition, Gin et al. demonstrated that propofol pharmacokinetics were similar in patients undergoing cesarean delivery and those undergoing postpartum tubal ligation (156).

Maintenance of general anesthesia for postpartum tubal ligations can be done either by a total intravenous technique or with volatile halogenated agents. One significant downside of using volatile agents during the immediate postpartum period is their ability to cause uterine relaxation, increasing the risk of postpartum hemorrhage (157). This dose-dependent impact of halogenated agents on uterine contractility has been demonstrated in several studies. Marx et al. evaluated different concentrations of enflurane and halothane on postpartum uterine pressures in 20 women, and found inhibition of spontaneous uterine activity at 0.5 minimum alveolar concentration (MAC) with both agents (158). In addition, the authors reported inhibition of oxytocin-induced uterine contractions at 0.8 MAC for halothane and 0.9 MAC for enflurane. Similar evidence has been demonstrated for isoflurane, desflurane, and sevoflurane (159). Therefore, in order to minimize the risk of postpartum hemorrhage, anesthesia providers using volatile halogenated agents for maintenance of

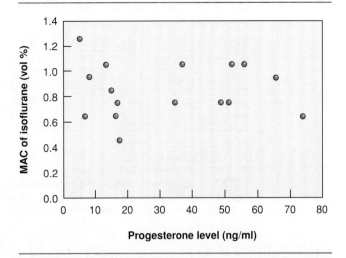

FIGURE 15-10 Linear regression analysis demonstrating no correlation between isoflurane MAC and progesterone concentration in postpartum women undergoing tubal ligation. r = 0.005; *P* = 0.985. *MAC*, minimum alveolar concentration. Modified with permission from: Zhou HH, Norman P, DeLima LG, et al. The minimum alveolar concentration of isoflurane in patients undergoing bilateral tubal ligation in the postpartum period. *Anesthesiology* 1995;82:1364–1368.

general anesthesia for postpartum tubal ligations should use 0.5 MAC, and supplement with intravenous agents as needed to decrease the risk of intraoperative recall.

MAC requirements in pregnant women decrease up to 40%, possibly due to the sedative effects of progesterone and/or endorphins (160). Two studies have investigated the effect of the postpartum period on MAC values. Zhou et al. found a decrease in isoflurane MAC requirements in women undergoing general anesthesia for postpartum tubal ligations, but with a 28% reduction in MAC within the first 12 hours postpartum and a return to normal values 12 to 25 hours after delivery (161). However, decreases in postpartum plasma progesterone levels did not correlate with MAC requirements (Fig. 15-10). Similarly, Chan et al. demonstrated that the MAC value for isoflurane was reduced in women 24 to 36 hours postpartum and gradually increased to nonpregnant values by 72 hours postpartum, but that postpartum changes in progesterone did not fully account for these altered anesthetic requirements (162).

Changes in the response of postpartum patients to depolarizing and nondepolarizing neuromuscular blockers have also been described. Succinylcholine is often used for muscle relaxation for postpartum tubal sterilizations due to its rapid onset and offset of action. Compared to nonpregnant women, pseudocholinesterase activity in parturients decreases by 24% and 33% at delivery and 3 days postpartum, respectively, but return to nonpregnant values 2 to 6 weeks after delivery (163,164). Leighton et al. investigated the significance of this decreased activity during the postpartum period (165). Compared to controls, term parturients and postpartum women had decreased cholinesterase activity, and postpartum women had 25% longer recovery times (Table 15-9). In addition, the preoperative administration of metoclopramide for aspiration prophylaxis may prolong the effects of succinylcholine by as much as 228% due to pseudocholinesterase inhibition (166). This prolonged recovery time may be especially important in "cannot intubate/cannot ventilate" scenarios, when rapid recovery from the effects of succinylcholine is essential.

TABLE 15-9 Recovery and Cholinesterase Data for Succinylcholine 1 mg/kg

	Injection-25% Recovery Time (s)	25–75% Recovery Time (s)	Cholinesterase Activity (U/mL)
Controls (n = 14)	501 ± 21	102 ± 6	5.01 ± 0.33
Oral Contraceptives (n = 7)	499 ± 29	104 ± 8	4.81 ± 0.63
Term Pregnant (n = 5)	470 ± 56	83 ± 6	3.66 ± 0.39[a]
Postpartum (n = 8)	685 ± 22[b]	95 ± 11	2.84 ± 0.35[c]

Values are means ± standard error.
[a]P < 0.05, compared with controls.
[b]P < 0.001, compared with all other groups.
[c]P < 0.05, compared with controls and oral contraceptive patients.
Reproduced with permission from: Leighton BL, Cheek TG, Gross JB, et al. Succinylcholine pharmacodynamics in peripartum patients. *Anesthesiology* 1986;64:202–205.

Conversely, nondepolarizing muscle relaxants exhibit a mixed response in postpartum patients. Compared to its use in nonpregnant controls, vecuronium demonstrates the most pronounced change in duration during the postpartum period, with prolongation of action by more than 50% (167). Proposed mechanisms for this increased sensitivity include decreased hepatic blood flow and decreased hepatic uptake and elimination secondary to increased competition with steroidal sexual hormones at hepatic binding sites. Mivacurium's duration of action is prolonged by 20%, primarily due to decreased pseudocholinesterase activity, which may be further prolonged with metoclopramide administration (168,169). Rocuronium, however, show no change in its duration of action during the postpartum period. Initially, Puhringer et al. reported that the duration of action of rocuronium was prolonged by 25% during the postpartum period (170). However, a subsequent analysis by Gin et al. demonstrated no prolonged duration of action if a patient's lean body mass was used for dosing, instead of total body weight, suggesting that the findings by Puhringer et al. may be due to a relative overdosing of rocuronium in postpartum patients due to their temporary increase in body weight (171). Finally, the duration of cisatracurium was found to be shorter in the postpartum period, primarily due to increased pH- and temperature-dependent Hofmann elimination and renal clearance from physiologic changes of pregnancy (172). Due to the varied response of nondepolarizing muscle relaxants in the postpartum period, as well as the impact of certain medications (e.g., metoclopramide, magnesium) on the duration of these medications, the use of neuromuscular monitoring is recommended.

Postoperative Analgesia

Despite the fact that postoperative pain associated with postpartum tubal sterilization is typically moderate in intensity and of limited duration, patients still require postoperative analgesia. Employment of multimodal analgesia, typically with a combination of oral and/or parental opioids and nonsteroidal anti-inflammatory drugs (NSAIDs), results in improved pain control and patient satisfaction, minimizes opioid-related side effects, and promotes earlier hospital discharge (173). Ketorolac or ibuprofen are commonly used NSAIDs for postoperative analgesia, primarily due to their opioid-sparing effects, although use of other NSAIDs postoperatively may be just as efficacious, when used as part of multimodal analgesia (174,175). One potential concern with ketorolac use after postpartum tubal ligation is the possible adverse effects of prostaglandin synthetase inhibitors on neonates who are breastfeeding. However, the American Academy of Pediatrics has con-

sidered the use of ketorolac during the postpartum to be "compatible with breastfeeding" (176).

Since most postpartum tubal sterilizations are performed with a neuraxial anesthetic, several studies have investigated the postoperative analgesic efficacy of neuraxial morphine administration. Campbell et al. randomized 60 women to receive intrathecal morphine 100 μg or placebo as part of a hyperbaric lidocaine and fentanyl spinal anesthetic for postpartum tubal ligation (177). Not surprisingly, women who received intrathecal morphine had less 24-hour morphine consumption and lower pain scores at rest and with movement; there was no difference between the groups in terms of side effects. However, one limitation of this study was that only intravenous morphine, and not a multimodal approach, was used to treat breakthrough pain postoperatively. Consequently, Habib et al. randomized patients undergoing postpartum tubal ligation to intrathecal morphine 50 μg versus placebo (saline) as part of a hyperbaric bupivacaine/fentanyl spinal anesthetic. In this study, the authors used a multimodal approach for treatment of breakthrough pain during the postpartum period, which included oral naproxen and oxycodone/acetaminophen mixture (178). Despite the lower dose of morphine, the authors still found that, compared to the control group, patients who received intrathecal morphine had longer times to rescue analgesia, less postoperative oxycodone/acetaminophen consumption, lower pain scores at rest at 4 hours postoperatively, and lower pain scores with movement at 4 and 12 hours (Fig. 15-11). However, patients who received morphine also had higher rates of nausea and pruritus. Finally, Marcus et al. randomized women for postpartum tubal ligations to receive placebo, 2 mg, 3 mg, or 4 mg of morphine as part of an epidural anesthetic (179). Utilizing a postoperative multimodal analgesic approach with ibuprofen and hydrocodone/acetaminophen, the authors found that 2 mg of epidural morphine provided better postoperative analgesia compared to saline, but was equally efficacious compared to the 3 mg and 4 mg doses. Moreover, the 2 mg dose was associated with a lower incidence of opioid-induced side effects compared to the other morphine doses. Overall, the evidence supports the postoperative analgesic efficacy of neuraxial morphine in women undergoing postpartum tubal ligation. However, ASA guidelines recommending a minimum 24-hour period of observation for respiratory depression after neuraxial administration of hydrophilic opioid may preclude its routine use, especially in patients who will be discharged to an unmonitored setting before this risk period has expired (180).

Several other postoperative analgesic modalities have been investigated with varying results. Local anesthetic infiltration of the mesosalpinx has been shown to decrease postoperative opioid consumption (181). Van Ee et al. randomized

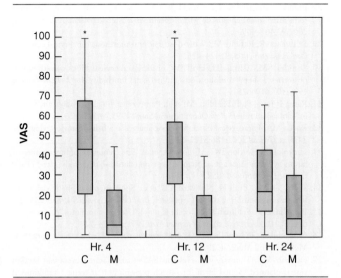

FIGURE 15-11 Pain scores on movement in women receiving placebo versus 50 μg intrathecal morphine for postpartum tubal ligation. Visual analog scale scores (mm) for pain are shown on the y-axis and time (hours) after admission to the postanesthesia care unit on the x-axis. Values are presented in box plot with median and interquartile range; the vertical lines extend to the most extreme point within 1.5 times the interquartile range. *C*, control group; *M*, morphine group; *Hr*, hour; *VAS*, visual analog scale. *P = 0.002 compared with the morphine group at 4 hours and P = 0.0004 compared with the morphine group at 12 hours. Reproduced with permission from: Habib AS, Muir HA, White WD, et al. Intrathecal morphine for analgesia after postpartum bilateral tubal ligation. *Anesth Analg* 2005;100:239–243.

women undergoing laparoscopic tubal ligation under general anesthesia to one of three groups: (1) Preoperative ketoprofen administration with mesosalpinx infiltration with 5 mL 0.9% saline and epinephrine; (2) preoperative ketoprofen with mesosalpinx infiltration with 5 mL bupivacaine 0.5% and epinephrine; or (3) preoperative placebo with mesosalpinx infiltration with 5 mL bupivacaine 0.5% and epinephrine (182). The authors demonstrated improved pain scores, less administration of supplemental analgesics postoperatively, shorter time to discharge, and less emesis in the ketoprofen-infiltration group compared to the other two. Wittels et al. reported similar findings, but in patients who underwent spinal or epidural anesthesia for postpartum tubal ligation (183). Finally, sufentanil infiltration of the mesosalpinx has been demonstrated to result in lower pain scores up to 24 hours after tubal ligation, compared to placebo (184). Besides its analgesic effectiveness, infiltration of the mesosalpinx is a simple, fast technique that can be readily performed intraoperatively by the obstetricians.

KEY POINTS

- Cerclage represents a viable option for the prevention of preterm labor in a subset of women with cervical insufficiency. Cerclage placement can be elective, urgent, or emergent.
- Cerclage placement may be performed transvaginally or transabdominally. The transvaginal cerclage is most commonly used, and is associated with lower risk of perinatal

death and serious complications compared to the transabdominal cerclage.
- Neuraxial anesthetics are the preferred method for transvaginal cerclage placement. A T10 through S4 sensory level is required to ensure perineal, vaginal, and cervical anesthesia. As transabdominal cerclage placements are performed via laparoscopy or laparotomy, general anesthesia is usually required.
- The occurrence of transient neurologic symptoms in parturients is significantly lower than the general population, even if intrathecal lidocaine is used.
- ECV offers a safe, viable option for management of breech fetuses. Several patient factors and interventions affect the likelihood of successful ECV.
- The use of tocolytics has been demonstrated to increase rates of successful ECV. β-adrenergic agonists (e.g., terbutaline) have been associated with higher rates of successful ECV.
- Neuraxial techniques for ECV not only provide superior analgesia and maternal satisfaction, but also increase the rate of successful ECV compared to no or intravenous analgesia. This success rate is likely dose-dependent, with anesthetic levels from neuraxial techniques resulting in higher success rates.
- Several maternal physiologic changes that occur during pregnancy extend into the postpartum period, affecting the anesthetic management of patients undergoing postpartum tubal sterilizations. Cardiovascular changes include increased cardiac output and heart rate. Respiratory changes include increased minute ventilation and oxygen consumption, decreased FRC, and changes in airway anatomy. Gastrointestinal changes include increased risk of gastroesophageal reflux, delayed gastric emptying if intrapartum opioids were administered or solid food was consumed, but no adverse changes in gastric volume or pH.
- Although the true anesthetic risk of performing tubal sterilizations immediately postpartum is unknown, advances in airway management techniques, improvements in intraoperative monitoring of oxygenation and ventilation, and the increased utilization of neuraxial techniques have significantly decreased anesthesia-related maternal mortality rates.
- Local anesthetic infiltration is the most commonly utilized mode of anesthesia for tubal ligations worldwide. Advantages of this technique include lower complication rates compared to general anesthesia, decreased morbidity and mortality rates compared to general or neuraxial techniques, decreased cost, and better quality of recovery.
- Neuraxial techniques are preferred to general anesthesia for postpartum tubal sterilizations. A T_2 to T_4 sensory level is often required to block visceral stimulation due to manipulation of the fallopian tubes.
- Increased intrathecal doses of local anesthetics are often required for postpartum tubal ligation, partially due to decreases in maternal progesterone levels.
- Functioning epidural catheters are more likely to fail with longer delivery to reactivation intervals. Anesthetic management options for failed epidural catheters include replacement of the epidural catheter, spinal anesthesia (increased risk of high or total spinal anesthesia), combined spinal–epidural technique, local anesthetic infiltration, or general anesthesia.
- Pregnancy-induced changes in MAC of volatile anesthetics and pharmacokinetic activity of neuromuscular blockers should be taken into account when using general anesthesia for postpartum tubal ligations.
- Multimodal postoperative analgesia, including opioids and NSAIDs, results in improved pain control and patient satisfaction, decreased opioid side effects, and earlier hospital discharge.

REFERENCES

1. Martin JA, Menacker F. Expanded health data from the new birth certificate, 2004. *Natl Vital Stat Rep* 2007;55:1–22.
2. Anum EA, Brown HL, Strauss JF 3rd. Health disparities in risk for cervical insufficiency. *Hum Reprod* 2010;25:2894–2900.
3. Leduc L, Wasserstrum N. Successful treatment with the Smith-Hodge pessary of cervical incompetence due to defective connective tissue in Ehlers-Danlos syndrome. *Am J Perinatol* 1992;9:25–27.
4. Ludmir J, Landon MB, Gabbe SG, et al. Management of the diethylstilbestrol-exposed pregnant patient: a prospective study. *Am J Obstet Gynecol* 1987;157:665–669.
5. Rahman J, Rahman FZ, Rahman W, et al. Obstetric and gynecologic complications in women with Marfan syndrome. *J Reprod Med* 2003;48:723–728.
6. Warren JE, Silver RM, Dalton J, et al. Collagen 1 Alpha1 and transforming growth factor-beta polymorphisms in women with cervical insufficiency. *Obstet Gynecol* 2007;110:619–624.
7. Romero R, Espinoza J, Erez O, et al. The role of cervical cerclage in obstetric practice: can the patient who could benefit from this procedure be identified? *Am J Obstet Gynecol* 2006;194:1–9.
8. Iams JD, Goldenberg RL, Meis PJ, et al. The length of the cervix and the risk of spontaneous premature delivery. National Institute of Child Health and Human Development Maternal Fetal Medicine Unit Network. *N Engl J Med* 1996;334:567–572.
9. Andrews WW, Copper R, Hauth JC, et al. Second-trimester cervical ultrasound: associations with increased risk for recurrent early spontaneous delivery. *Obstet Gynecol* 2000;95:222–226.
10. Althuisius SM, Dekker GA, Hummel P, et al. Final results of the Cervical Incompetence Prevention Randomized Cerclage Trial (CIPRACT): therapeutic cerclage with bed rest versus bed rest alone. *Am J Obstet Gynecol* 2001;185:1106–1112.
11. Althuisius SM, Dekker GA, Hummel P, et al. Cervical incompetence prevention randomized cerclage trial: emergency cerclage with bed rest versus bed rest alone. *Am J Obstet Gynecol* 2003;189:907–910.
12. Berghella V, Prasertcharoensuk W, Cotter A, et al. Does indomethacin prevent preterm birth in women with cervical dilatation in the second trimester? *Am J Perinatol* 2009;26:13–19.
13. Shiffman RL. Continuous low-dose antibiotics and cerclage for recurrent second-trimester pregnancy loss. *J Reprod Med* 2000;45:323–326.
14. Meis PJ, Klebanoff M, Thom E, et al. Prevention of recurrent preterm delivery by 17 alpha-hydroxyprogesterone caproate. *N Engl J Med* 2003;348:2379–2385.
15. Harger JH. Cerclage and cervical insufficiency: an evidence-based analysis. *Obstet Gynecol* 2002;100:1313–1327.
16. Odibo AO, Berghella V, To MS, et al. Shirodkar versus McDonald cerclage for the prevention of preterm birth in women with short cervical length. *Am J Perinatol* 2007;24:55–60.
17. Abbott D, To M, Shennan A. Cervical cerclage: A review of current evidence. *Aust N Z J Obstet Gynaecol* 2012;52:220–223.
18. Zaveri V, Aghajafari F, Amankwah K, et al. Abdominal versus vaginal cerclage after a failed transvaginal cerclage: a systematic review. *Am J Obstet Gynecol* 2002;187:868–872.
19. Rand L, Norwitz ER. Current controversies in cervical cerclage. *Semin Perinatol* 2003;27:73–85.
20. Alfirevic Z, Stampalija T, Roberts D, et al. Cervical stitch (cerclage) for preventing preterm birth in singleton pregnancy. *Cochrane Database Syst Rev* 2012;4:CD008991.
21. Lee GY, Kim CH, Chung RK, et al. Spread of subarachnoid sensory block with hyperbaric bupivacaine in second trimester of pregnancy. *J Clin Anesth* 2009;21:482–485.
22. Beilin Y, Zahn J, Abramovitz S, et al. Subarachnoid small-dose bupivacaine versus lidocaine for cervical cerclage. *Anesth Analg* 2003;97:56–61, table of contents.
23. Ben-David B, Solomon E, Levin H, et al. Intrathecal fentanyl with small-dose dilute bupivacaine: better anesthesia without prolonging recovery. *Anesth Analg.* 1997;85:560–565.
24. Freedman JM, Li DK, Drasner K, et al. Transient neurologic symptoms after spinal anesthesia: an epidemiologic study of 1,863 patients. *Anesthesiology* 1998;89:633–641.
25. Hampl KF, Schneider MC, Pargger H, et al. A similar incidence of transient neurologic symptoms after spinal anesthesia with 2% and 5% lidocaine. *Anesth Analg* 1996;83:1051–1054.
26. Wong CA, Slavenas P. The incidence of transient radicular irritation after spinal anesthesia in obstetric patients. *Reg Anesth Pain Med* 1999;24:55–58.
27. Aouad MT, Siddik SS, Jalbout MI, et al. Does pregnancy protect against intrathecal lidocaine-induced transient neurologic symptoms? *Anesth Analg* 2001;92:401–404.
28. Philip J, Sharma SK, Gottumukkala VN, et al. Transient neurologic symptoms after spinal anesthesia with lidocaine in obstetric patients. *Anesth Analg* 2001;92:405–409.
29. Schumann R, Rafique MB. Low-dose epidural anesthesia for cervical cerclage. *Can J Anaesth* 2003;50:424–425.
30. Shnider SM, Asling JH, Holl JW, et al. Paracervical block anesthesia in obstetrics. I. Fetal complications and neonatal morbidity. *Am J Obstet Gynecol* 1970;107:619–625.
31. Ranta P, Jouppila P, Spalding M, et al. Paracervical block—a viable alternative for labor pain relief? *Acta Obstet Gynecol Scand* 1995;74:122–126.
32. Rosen MA. Paracervical block for labor analgesia: a brief historic review. *Am J Obstet Gynecol* 2002;186:S127–S130.
33. Hickok DE, Gordon DC, Milberg JA, et al. The frequency of breech presentation by gestational age at birth: a large population-based study. *Am J Obstet Gynecol* 1992;166:851–852.
34. Westgren M, Edvall H, Nordstrom L, et al. Spontaneous cephalic version of breech presentation in the last trimester. *Br J Obstet Gynaecol* 1985;92:19–22.
35. Ben-Rafael Z, Seidman DS, Recabi K, et al. Uterine anomalies. A retrospective, matched-control study. *J Reprod Med* 1991;36:723–727.
36. Cunningham FG, Williams JW. *Williams Obstetrics.* 23rd ed. New York, NY: McGraw-Hill Medical; 2010.
37. Hannah ME, Hannah WJ, Hewson SA, et al. Planned caesarean section versus planned vaginal birth for breech presentation at term: a randomised multicentre trial. Term Breech Trial Collaborative Group. *Lancet* 2000;356:1375–1383.
38. Hehir MP, O'Connor HD, Kent EM, et al. Changes in vaginal breech delivery rates in a single large metropolitan area. *Am J Obstet Gynecol* 2012;206(498):e1–e4.
39. ACOG Committee Opinion No. 340. Mode of term singleton breech delivery. *Obstet Gynecol* 2006;108:235–237.
40. Kotaska A, Menticoglou S, Gagnon R, et al. Vaginal delivery of breech presentation. *J Obstet Gynaecol Can* 2009;31:557–566, 567–578.
41. Shearer EL. Cesarean section: medical benefits and costs. *Soc Sci Med* 1993;37:1223–1231.
42. Cluver C, Hofmeyr GJ, Gyte GM, et al. Interventions for helping to turn term breech babies to head first presentation when using external cephalic version. *Cochrane Database Syst Rev* 2012;1:CD000184.
43. Collaris R, Tan PC. Oral nifedipine versus subcutaneous terbutaline tocolysis for external cephalic version: a double-blind randomised trial. *BJOG* 2009;116:74–80; discussion 80–81.
44. Zhang J, Bowes WA Jr., Fortney JA. Efficacy of external cephalic version: a review. *Obstet Gynecol* 1993;82:306–312.
45. Hofmeyr GJ. Interventions to help external cephalic version for breech presentation at term. *Cochrane Database Syst Rev* 2004;(1):CD000184.
46. Bewley S, Robson SC, Smith M, et al. The introduction of external cephalic version at term into routine clinical practice. *Eur J Obstet Gynecol Reprod Biol* 1993;52:89–93.
47. Hutton EK, Hannah ME, Ross SJ, et al. The Early External Cephalic Version (ECV) 2 Trial: an international multicentre randomised controlled trial of timing of ECV for breech pregnancies. *BJOG* 2011;118:564–577.
48. Yogev Y, Horowitz E, Ben-Haroush A, et al. Changing attitudes toward mode of delivery and external cephalic version in breech presentations. *Int J Gynaecol Obstet* 2002;79:221–224.
49. Caukwell S, Joels LA, Kyle PM, et al. Women's attitudes towards management of breech presentation at term. *J Obstet Gynaecol* 2002;22:486–488.
50. Leung TY, Lau TK, Lo KW, et al. A survey of pregnant women's attitude towards breech delivery and external cephalic version. *Aust N Z J Obstet Gynaecol* 2000;40:253–259.
51. Collaris RJ, Oei SG. External cephalic version: a safe procedure? A systematic review of version-related risks. *Acta Obstet Gynecol Scand* 2004;83:511–518.
52. Grootscholten K, Kok M, Oei SG, et al. External cephalic version-related risks: a meta-analysis. *Obstet Gynecol* 2008;112:1143–1151.
53. Cho LY, Lau WL, Lo TK, et al. Predictors of successful outcomes after external cephalic version in singleton term breech pregnancies: a nine-year historical cohort study. *Hong Kong Med J* 2012;18:11–19.
54. Kok M, Cnossen J, Gravendeel L, et al. Clinical factors to predict the outcome of external cephalic version: a metaanalysis. *Am J Obstet Gynecol* 2008;199:630.e1–630.e7; discussion e1–e5.
55. Kok M, Cnossen J, Gravendeel L, et al. Ultrasound factors to predict the outcome of external cephalic version: a meta-analysis. *Ultrasound Obstet Gynecol* 2009;33:76–84.
56. Kok M, van der Steeg JW, van der Post JA, et al. Prediction of success of external cephalic version after 36 weeks. *Am J Perinatol* 2011;28:103–110.
57. Robertson AW, Kopelman JN, Read JA, et al. External cephalic version at term: is a tocolytic necessary? *Obstet Gynecol* 1987;70:896–899.
58. Tan GW, Jen SW, Tan SL, et al. A prospective randomised controlled trial of external cephalic version comparing two methods of uterine tocolysis with a non-tocolysis group. *Singapore Med J* 1989;30:155–158.

59. Yanny H, Johanson R, Balwin KJ, et al. Double-blind randomised controlled trial of glyceryl trinitrate spray for external cephalic version. *BJOG* 2000;107:562–564.

60. Fernandez CO, Bloom SL, Smulian JC, et al. A randomized placebo-controlled evaluation of terbutaline for external cephalic version. *Obstet Gynecol* 1997;90:775–779.

61. Wilcox CB, Nassar N, Roberts CL. Effectiveness of nifedipine tocolysis to facilitate external cephalic version: a systematic review. *BJOG* 2011;118:423–428.

62. Yoshida M, Matsuda H, Kawakami Y, et al. Effectiveness of epidural anesthesia for external cephalic version (ECV). *J Perinatol* 2010;30:580–583.

63. Goetzinger KR, Harper LM, Tuuli MG, et al. Effect of regional anesthesia on the success rate of external cephalic version: a systematic review and meta-analysis. *Obstet Gynecol* 2011;118:1137–1144.

64. Weiniger CF, Ginosar Y, Elchalal U, et al. Randomized controlled trial of external cephalic version in term multiparae with or without spinal analgesia. *Br J Anaesth* 2010;104:613–618.

65. Weiniger CF, Ginosar Y, Elchalal U, et al. External cephalic version for breech presentation with or without spinal analgesia in nulliparous women at term: a randomized controlled trial. *Obstet Gynecol* 2007;110:1343–1350.

66. Sullivan JT, Grobman WA, Bauchat JR, et al. A randomized controlled trial of the effect of combined spinal-epidural analgesia on the success of external cephalic version for breech presentation. *Int J Obstet Anesth* 2009;18:328–334.

67. Dugoff L, Stamm CA, Jones OW 3rd, et al. The effect of spinal anesthesia on the success rate of external cephalic version: a randomized trial. *Obstet Gynecol* 1999;93:345–349.

68. Schorr SJ, Speights SE, Ross EL, et al. A randomized trial of epidural anesthesia to improve external cephalic version success. *Am J Obstet Gynecol* 1997;177:1133–1137.

69. Mancuso KM, Yancey MK, Murphy JA, et al. Epidural analgesia for cephalic version: a randomized trial. *Obstet Gynecol* 2000;95:648–651.

70. Lavoie A, Guay J. Anesthetic dose neuraxial blockade increases the success rate of external fetal version: a meta-analysis. *Can J Anaesth* 2010;57:408–414.

71. Tan JM, Macario A, Carvalho B, et al. Cost-effectiveness of external cephalic version for term breech presentation. *BMC Pregnancy Childbirth* 2010;10:3.

72. Bolaji I, Alabi-Isama L. Central neuraxial blockade-assisted external cephalic version in reducing caesarean section rate: systematic review and meta-analysis. *Obstet Gynecol Int* 2009;2009:718981.

73. Mosher WD, Jones J. Use of contraception in the United States: 1982–2008. *Vital Health Stat 23* 2010:1–44.

74. Chan LM, Westhoff CL. Tubal sterilization trends in the United States. *Fertil Steril* 2010;94:1–6.

75. Peterson HB, Xia Z, Hughes JM, et al. The risk of pregnancy after tubal sterilization: findings from the U.S. Collaborative Review of Sterilization. *Am J Obstet Gynecol* 1996;174:1161–1168; discussion 1168–1170.

76. Thurman AR, Janecek T. One-year follow-up of women with unfulfilled postpartum sterilization requests. *Obstet Gynecol* 2010;116:1071–1077.

77. Hillis SD, Marchbanks PA, Tylor LR, et al. Poststerilization regret: findings from the United States Collaborative Review of Sterilization. *Obstet Gynecol* 1999;93:889–895.

78. Jamieson DJ, Kaufman SC, Costello C, et al. A comparison of women's regret after vasectomy versus tubal sterilization. *Obstet Gynecol* 2002;99:1073–1079.

79. Peterson HB. Sterilization. *Obstet Gynecol* 2008;111:189–203.

80. Kulier R, Boulvain M, Walker DM, et al. Minilaparotomy and endoscopic techniques for tubal sterilisation. *Cochrane Database Syst Rev* 2004;(3):CD001328.

81. Practice guidelines for obstetric anesthesia: an updated report by the American Society of Anesthesiologists Task Force on Obstetric Anesthesia. *Anesthesiology* 2007;106:843–863.

82. Robson SC, Hunter S, Boys RJ, et al. Serial study of factors influencing changes in cardiac output during human pregnancy. *Am J Physiol* 1989;256:H1060–H1065.

83. Adams JQ, Alexander AM Jr. Alterations in cardiovascular physiology during labor. *Obstet Gynecol* 1958;12:542–549.

84. Robson SC, Dunlop W, Boys RJ, et al. Cardiac output during labour. *Br Med J* 1987;295:1169–1172.

85. Ueland K, Hansen JM. Maternal cardiovascular dynamics. 3. Labor and delivery under local and caudal analgesia. *Am J Obstet Gynecol* 1969;103:8–18.

86. Pyorala T. Cardiovascular response to the upright position during pregnancy. *Acta Obstet Gynecol Scand* 1966;45:Suppl 5:1–116.

87. Robson SC, Hunter S, Moore M, et al. Haemodynamic changes during the puerperium: a Doppler and M-mode echocardiographic study. *Br J Obstet Gynecol* 1987;94:1028–1039.

88. Alaily AB, Carrol KB. Pulmonary ventilation in pregnancy. *Br J Obstet Gynaecol* 1978;85:518–524.

89. Hagerdal M, Morgan CW, Sumner AE, et al. Minute ventilation and oxygen consumption during labor with epidural analgesia. *Anesthesiology* 1983;59:425–427.

90. Spatling L, Fallenstein F, Huch A, et al. The variability of cardiopulmonary adaptation to pregnancy at rest and during exercise. *Br J Obstet Gynaecol* 1992;99(Suppl 8):1–40.

91. Dobb G. Laryngeal oedema complicating obstetric anaesthesia. *Anaesthesia* 1978;33:839–840.

92. Farcon EL, Kim MH, Marx GF. Changing Mallampati score during labour. *Can J Anaesth* 1994;41:50–51.

93. Kodali BS, Chandrasekhar S, Bulich LN, et al. Airway changes during labor and delivery. *Anesthesiology* 2008;108:357–362.

94. Boutonnet M, Faitot V, Katz A, et al. Mallampati class changes during pregnancy, labour, and after delivery: can these be predicted? *Br J Anaesth* 2010;104:67–70.

95. McKeen DM, George RB, O'Connell CM, et al. Difficult and failed intubation: Incident rates and maternal, obstetrical, and anesthetic predictors. *Can J Anaesth* 2011;58:514–524.

96. Mendelson CL. The aspiration of stomach contents into the lungs during obstetric anesthesia. *Am J Obstet Gynecol* 1946;52:191–205.

97. Van Thiel DH, Gavaler JS, Stremple J. Lower esophageal sphincter pressure in women using sequential oral contraceptives. *Gastroenterology* 1976;71:232–234.

98. Llauro JL, Runnebaum B, Zander J. Progesterone in human peripheral blood before, during, and after labor. *Am J Obstet Gynecol* 1968;101:867–873.

99. Vanner RG, Goodman NW. Gastro-oesophageal reflux in pregnancy at term and after delivery. *Anaesthesia* 1989;44:808–811.

100. Whitehead EM, Smith M, Dean Y, et al. An evaluation of gastric emptying times in pregnancy and the puerperium. *Anaesthesia* 1993;48:53–57.

101. Wong CA, Loffredi M, Ganchiff JN, et al. Gastric emptying of water in term pregnancy. *Anesthesiology* 2002;96:1395–1400.

102. Carp H, Jayaram A, Stoll M. Ultrasound examination of the stomach contents of parturients. *Anesth Analg* 1992;74:683–687.

103. La Salvia LA, Steffen EA. Delayed gastric emptying time in labor. *Am J Obstet Gynecol* 1950;59:1075–1081.

104. Kelly MC, Carabine UA, Hill DA, et al. A comparison of the effect of intrathecal and extradural fentanyl on gastric emptying in laboring women. *Anesth Analg* 1997;85:834–838.

105. Murphy DF, Nally B, Gardiner J, et al. Effect of metoclopramide on gastric emptying before elective and emergency caesarean section. *Br J Anaesth* 1984;56:1113–1116.

106. Nimmo WS, Wilson J, Prescott LF. Narcotic analgesics and delayed gastric emptying during labour. *Lancet* 1975;1:890–893.

107. Porter JS, Bonello E, Reynolds F. The influence of epidural administration of fentanyl infusion on gastric emptying in labour. *Anaesthesia* 1997;52:1151–1156.

108. Ewah B, Yau K, King M, et al. Effect of epidural opioids on gastric emptying in labour. *Int J Obstet Anesth* 1993;2:125–128.

109. Wright PM, Allen RW, Moore J, et al. Gastric emptying during lumbar extradural analgesia in labour: effect of fentanyl supplementation. *Br J Anaesth* 1992;68:248–251.

110. O'Sullivan GM, Sutton AJ, Thompson SA, et al. Noninvasive measurement of gastric emptying in obstetric patients. *Anesth Analg* 1987;66:505–511.

111. Lam KK, So HY, Gin T. Gastric pH and volume after oral fluids in the postpartum patient. *Can J Anaesth* 1993;40:218–221.

112. James CF, Gibbs CP, Banner T. Postpartum perioperative risk of aspiration pneumonia. *Anesthesiology* 1984;61:756–759.

113. Kubli M, Scrutton MJ, Seed PT, et al. An evaluation of isotonic "sport drinks" during labor. *Anesth Analg* 2002;94:404–408, table of contents.

114. Kelly KA. Gastric emptying of liquids and solids: roles of proximal and distal stomach. *Am J Physiol* 1980;239:G71–G76.

115. Scrutton MJ, Metcalfe GA, Lowy C, et al. Eating in labour. A randomised controlled trial assessing the risks and benefits. *Anaesthesia* 1999;54:329–334.

116. Jayaram A, Bowen MP, Deshpande S, et al. Ultrasound examination of the stomach contents of women in the postpartum period. *Anesth Analg* 1997;84:522–526.

117. O'Sullivan G, Liu B, Hart D, et al. Effect of food intake during labour on obstetric outcome: randomised controlled trial. *BMJ* 2009;338:b784.

118. Peterson HB, DeStefano F, Rubin GL, et al. Deaths attributable to tubal sterilization in the United States, 1977 to 1981. *Am J Obstet Gynecol* 1983;146:131–136.

119. Destefano F, Greenspan JR, Dicker RC, et al. Complications of interval laparoscopic tubal sterilization. *Obstet Gynecol* 1983;61:153–158.

120. Jamieson DJ, Hillis SD, Duerr A, et al. Complications of interval laparoscopic tubal sterilization: findings from the United States Collaborative Review of Sterilization. *Obstet Gynecol* 2000;96:997–1002.

121. Hawkins JL, Chang J, Palmer SK, et al. Anesthesia-related maternal mortality in the United States: 1979–2002. *Obstet Gynecol* 2011;117:69–74.

122. Evans NR, Skowno JJ, Bennett PJ, et al. A prospective observational study of the use of the Proseal laryngeal mask airway for postpartum tubal ligation. *Int J Obstet Anesth* 2005;14:90–95.

123. Westhoff C, Davis A. Tubal sterilization: focus on the U.S. experience. *Fertil Steril* 2000;73:913–922.

124. Bhiwandiwala PP, Mumford SD, Feldblum PJ. A comparison of different laparoscopic sterilization occlusion techniques in 24,439 procedures. *Am J Obstet Gynecol* 1982;144:319–331.

125. Pati S, Cullins V. Female sterilization. Evidence. *Obstet Gynecol Clin North Am* 2000;27:859–899.

126. Mazdisnian F, Palmieri A, Hakakha B, et al. Office microlaparoscopy for female sterilization under local anesthesia. A cost and clinical analysis. *J Reprod Med* 2002;47:97–100.

127. Munson AK, Scott JR. Postpartum tubal ligation under local anesthesia. *Obstet Gynecol* 1972;39:756–758.

128. Cruikshank DP, Laube DW, De Backer LJ. Intraperitoneal lidocaine anesthesia for postpartum tubal ligation. *Obstet Gynecol* 1973;42:127–130.

129. Poindexter AN 3rd, Abdul-Malak M, Fast JE. Laparoscopic tubal sterilization under local anesthesia. *Obstet Gynecol* 1990;75:5–8.

130. Bordahl PE, Raeder JC, Nordentoft J, et al. Laparoscopic sterilization under local or general anesthesia? A randomized study. *Obstet Gynecol* 1993;81:137–141.

131. Ruminjo JK, Lynam PF. A fifteen-year review of female sterilization by mini-laparotomy under local anesthesia in Kenya. *Contraception* 1997;55:249–260.

132. Marx GF. Regional analgesia in obstetrics. *Anaesthesist* 1972;21:84–91.

133. Abouleish EI. Postpartum tubal ligation requires more bupivacaine for spinal anesthesia than does cesarean section. *Anesth Analg* 1986;65:897–900.

134. Datta S, Lambert DH, Gregus J, et al. Differential sensitivities of mammalian nerve fibers during pregnancy. *Anesth Analg* 1983;62:1070–1072.

135. Datta S, Hurley RJ, Naulty JS, et al. Plasma and cerebrospinal fluid progesterone concentrations in pregnant and nonpregnant women. *Anesth Analg* 1986;65:950–954.

136. Huffnagle SL, Norris MC, Leighton BL, et al. Do patient variables influence the subarachnoid spread of hyperbaric lidocaine in the postpartum patient? *Reg Anesth* 1994;19:330–334.

137. Huffnagle SL, Norris MC, Huffnagle HJ, et al. Intrathecal hyperbaric bupivacaine dose response in postpartum tubal ligation patients. *Reg Anesth Pain Med* 2002;27:284–288.

138. Panni MK, George RB, Allen TK, et al. Minimum effective dose of spinal ropivacaine with and without fentanyl for postpartum tubal ligation. *Int J Obstet Anesth* 2010;19:390–394.

139. Norris MC, Honet JE, Leighton BL, et al. A comparison of meperidine and lidocaine for spinal anesthesia for postpartum tubal ligation. *Reg Anesth* 1996;21:84–88.

140. Vincent RD Jr., Reid RW. Epidural anesthesia for postpartum tubal ligation using epidural catheters placed during labor. *J Clin Anesth* 1993;5:289–291.

141. Viscomi CM, Rathmell JP. Labor epidural catheter reactivation or spinal anesthesia for delayed postpartum tubal ligation: a cost comparison. *J Clin Anesth* 1995;7:380–383.

142. Goodman EJ, Dumas SD. The rate of successful reactivation of labor epidural catheters for postpartum tubal ligation surgery. *Reg Anesth Pain Med* 1998;23:258–261.

143. Bishton IM, Martin PH, Vernon JM, et al. Factors influencing epidural catheter migration. *Anaesthesia* 1992;47:610–612.

144. Phillips DC, Macdonald R. Epidural catheter migration during labour. *Anaesthesia* 1987;42:661–663.

145. Hamilton CL, Riley ET, Cohen SE. Changes in the position of epidural catheters associated with patient movement. *Anesthesiology* 1997;86:778–784; discussion 29A.

146. D'Angelo R, Berkebile BL, Gerancher JC. Prospective examination of epidural catheter insertion. *Anesthesiology* 1996;84:88–93.

147. Beilin Y, Bernstein HH, Zucker-Pinchoff B. The optimal distance that a multiorifice epidural catheter should be threaded into the epidural space. *Anesth Analg* 1995;81:301–304.

148. Visser WA, Dijkstra A, Albayrak M, et al. Spinal anesthesia for intrapartum Cesarean delivery following epidural labor analgesia: a retrospective cohort study. *Can J Anaesth* 2009;56:577–583.

149. Furst SR, Reisner LS. Risk of high spinal anesthesia following failed epidural block for cesarean delivery. *J Clin Anesth* 1995;7:71–74.

150. Portnoy D, Vadhera RB. Mechanisms and management of an incomplete epidural block for cesarean section. *Anesthesiol Clin North America* 2003;21:39–57.

151. Dadarkar P, Philip J, Weidner C, et al. Spinal anesthesia for cesarean section following inadequate labor epidural analgesia: a retrospective audit. *Int J Obstet Anesth* 2004;13:239–243.

152. Lew E, Yeo SW, Thomas E. Combined spinal-epidural anesthesia using epidural volume extension leads to faster motor recovery after elective cesarean delivery: a prospective, randomized, double-blind study. *Anesth Analg* 2004;98:810–814, table of contents.

153. Ben-David B, Miller G, Gavriel R, et al. Low-dose bupivacaine-fentanyl spinal anesthesia for cesarean delivery. *Reg Anesth Pain Med* 2000;25:235–239.

154. Gin T, O'Meara ME, Kan AF, et al. Plasma catecholamines and neonatal condition after induction of anaesthesia with propofol or thiopentone at caesarean section. *Br J Anaesth* 1993;70:311–316.

155. De Oliveira GS Jr., Theilken LS, McCarthy RJ. Shortage of perioperative drugs: implications for anesthesia practice and patient safety. *Anesth Analg* 2011;113:1429–1435.

156. Gin T, Yau G, Jong W, et al. Disposition of propofol at caesarean section and in the postpartum period. *Br J Anaesth* 1991;67:49–53.

157. Chang CC, Wang IT, Chen YH, et al. Anesthetic management as a risk factor for postpartum hemorrhage after cesarean deliveries. *Am J Obstet Gynecol* 2011;205(462):e1–e7.

158. Marx GF, Kim YI, Lin CC, et al. Postpartum uterine pressures under halothane or enflurance anesthesia. *Obstet Gynecol* 1978;51:695–698.

159. Yoo KY, Lee JC, Yoon MH, et al. The effects of volatile anesthetics on spontaneous contractility of isolated human pregnant uterine muscle: a comparison among sevoflurane, desflurane, isoflurane, and halothane. *Anesth Analg* 2006;103:443–447, table of contents.

160. Palahniuk RJ, Shnider SM, Eger EI 2nd. Pregnancy decreases the requirement for inhaled anesthetic agents. *Anesthesiology* 1974;41:82–83.

161. Zhou HH, Norman P, DeLima LG, et al. The minimum alveolar concentration of isoflurane in patients undergoing bilateral tubal ligation in the postpartum period. *Anesthesiology* 1995;82:1364–1368.

162. Chan MT, Gin T. Postpartum changes in the minimum alveolar concentration of isoflurane. *Anesthesiology* 1995;82:1360–1363.

163. Evans RT, Wroe JM. Plasma cholinesterase changes during pregnancy. Their interpretation as a cause of suxamethonium-induced apnoea. *Anaesthesia* 1980;35:651–654.

164. Shnider SM. Serum cholinesterase activity during pregnancy, labor and the puerperium. *Anesthesiology* 1965;26:335–339.

165. Leighton BL, Cheek TG, Gross JB, et al. Succinylcholine pharmacodynamics in peripartum patients. *Anesthesiology* 1986;64:202–205.

166. Kao YJ, Turner DR. Prolongation of succinylcholine block by metoclopramide. *Anesthesiology* 1989;70:905–908.

167. Khuenl-Brady KS, Koller J, Mair P, et al. Comparison of vecuronium- and atracurium-induced neuromuscular blockade in postpartum and nonpregnant patients. *Anesth Analg* 1991;72:110–113.

168. Gin T, Derrick JL, Chan MT, et al. Postpartum patients have slightly prolonged neuromuscular block after mivacurium. *Anesth Analg* 1998;86:82–85.

169. Ward SJ, Rocke DA. Neuromuscular blocking drugs in pregnancy and the puerperium. *Int J Obstet Anesth* 1998;7:251–260.

170. Puhringer FK, Sparr HJ, Mitterschiffthaler G, et al. Extended duration of action of rocuronium in postpartum patients. *Anesth Analg* 1997;84:352–354.

171. Gin T, Chan MT, Chan KL, et al. Prolonged neuromuscular block after rocuronium in postpartum patients. *Anesth Analg* 2002;94:686–689, table of contents.

172. Pan PH, Moore C. Comparison of cisatracurium-induced neuromuscular blockade between immediate postpartum and nonpregnant patients. *J Clin Anesth* 2001;13:112–117.

173. White PF, Kehlet H, Neal JM, et al. The role of the anesthesiologist in fast-track surgery: from multimodal analgesia to perioperative medical care. *Anesth Analg* 2007;104:1380–1396, table of contents.

174. Ng A, Swami A, Smith G, et al. Early analgesic effects of intravenous parecoxib and rectal diclofenac following laparoscopic sterilization: a double-blind, double-dummy randomized controlled trial. *J Opioid Manag* 2008;4:49–53.

175. Ng A, Temple A, Smith G, et al. Early analgesic effects of parecoxib versus ketorolac following laparoscopic sterilization: a randomized controlled trial. *Br J Anaesth* 2004;92:846–849.

176. American Academy of Pediatrics Committee on Drugs. Transfer of drugs and other chemicals into human milk. *Pediatrics* 2001;108:776–789.

177. Campbell DC, Riben CM, Rooney ME, et al. Intrathecal morphine for postpartum tubal ligation postoperative analgesia. *Anesth Analg* 2001;93:1006–1011.

178. Habib AS, Muir HA, White WD, et al. Intrathecal morphine for analgesia after postpartum bilateral tubal ligation. *Anesth Analg* 2005;100:239–243.

179. Marcus RJ, Wong CA, Lehor A, et al. Postoperative epidural morphine for postpartum tubal ligation analgesia. *Anesth Analg* 2005;101:876–881, table of contents.

180. Horlocker TT, Burton AW, Connis RT, et al. Practice guidelines for the prevention, detection, and management of respiratory depression associated with neuraxial opioid administration. *Anesthesiology* 2009;110:218–230.

181. Alexander CD, Wetchler BV, Thompson RE. Bupivacaine infiltration of the mesosalpinx in ambulatory surgical laparoscopic tubal sterilization. *Can J Anaesth* 1987;34:362–365.

182. Van Ee R, Hemrika DJ, De Blok S, et al. Effects of ketoprofen and mesosalpinx infiltration on postoperative pain after laparoscopic sterilization. *Obstet Gynecol* 1996;88:568–572.

183. Wittels B, Faure EA, Chavez R, et al. Effective analgesia after bilateral tubal ligation. *Anesth Analg* 1998;87:619–623.

184. Rorarius M, Suominen P, Baer G, et al. Peripherally administered sufentanil inhibits pain perception after postpartum tubal ligation. *Pain* 1999;79:83–88.

Emily J. Baird • Richard C. Month • Valerie A. Arkoosh

It is estimated that over 100 million babies are born annually worldwide. The successful transition from fetus to neonate hinges on the ability of the newborn to adapt to extrauterine life; this transition is characterized by numerous physiologic changes that must rapidly transpire following delivery. Despite the complexity of this process, only 10% of newborns require assistance with ventilation at birth and 1% require extensive resuscitative measures (Fig. 16-1) (1). Nonetheless, this translates to an estimated 5 to 10 million interventions at birth annually. In order to anticipate the need for resuscitation, and to have both the provisions and knowledge to respond appropriately, it is imperative that all providers in the labor and delivery suite understand neonatal adaptation to extrauterine life, the changes that occur during transition from fetal to adult circulation, and the physiology of fetal asphyxia.

■ NEONATAL ADAPTATIONS TO EXTRAUTERINE LIFE

Fetal Cardiovascular and Pulmonary Physiology

Unlike in the adult, where pulmonary and systemic circulations operate in parallel, the fetal circulation operates in series (Fig. 16-2) (2). In utero, oxygenated blood from the placenta returns via the umbilical vein to the portal vein and is shunted through the ductus venosus into the inferior vena cava (IVC). Nearly 40% of IVC return is directed across the foramen ovale, through the left heart and ascending aorta, to perfuse the heart and brain with maximally oxygenated blood (3). Deoxygenated blood from the head and upper extremities enters the heart through the superior vena cava (SVC). This blood is preferentially directed into the right ventricle, where it mixes with the remainder of the oxygenated IVC return. Due to high pulmonary vascular resistance (PVR), 90% of right ventricular outflow shunts across the ductus arteriosus to the descending aorta to perfuse the abdomen, pelvis, and lower extremities (4). 40% of cardiac output traverses the low-resistance placenta; this contributes to overall low systemic vascular resistance (SVR).

Fetal lung development takes place throughout pregnancy and continues into the neonatal period. In fact, the newborn lung contains only one-third the number of alveoli present in the mature lung, and the process of alveolar development continues through the first 18 months of life (5).

The development of surfactant is also a late occurrence in fetal lung development. Pulmonary surfactant is responsible for reducing alveolar surface tension and allowing for successful ventilation and gas exchange. It is produced by type II pneumocytes in the distal airways, and is typically measurable in fetal lung tissue by 20 weeks of gestation. However, it is not present in the airway lumen until 28 to 32 weeks of gestation, and it is not present in adequate quantity until 34 to 38 weeks of gestation (5).

Normal Peripartum Transition to Extrauterine Life

Parturition leads to rapid and profound changes in neonatal hemodynamics and pulmonary mechanics. During development, the fetal airways contain approximately 30 mL/kg of fluid; during labor, this ultrafiltrate of plasma begins to reabsorb (3). During vaginal delivery, compression of the infant thorax expels further fluid from the mouth and upper airways (2). With the first breath, the lungs fill with air, surfactant is released, and oxygenation is increased (6). This increase in oxygen tension and blood flow has been shown to increase the release of nitric oxide in the pulmonary vasculature, resulting in pulmonary vasodilation and a substantial decrease in PVR (7). Simultaneously, clamping of the umbilical cord removes the low-resistance placenta from the systemic circulation substantially increasing SVR, left atrial pressure increases, and flow through the foramen ovale ceases. Functional closure of the foramen ovale occurs rapidly after birth as left atrial pressures begin to exceed right atrial pressures. The net result is a dramatic reduction, and eventual cessation, of the fetal right-to-left shunt. Right-to-left shunt across the ductus arteriosus reduces substantially within the first few minutes of life. However, anatomic closure of the foramen ovale takes several months; therefore, any circulatory disturbance that elevates right atrial pressure may cause the foramen to remain open, shunting venous flow from right to left and leading to cyanosis.

Prolonged Hypoxia/Acidosis and Failure of Transition: Asphyxia in the Newborn

Transient hypoxemia or acidosis is typically well tolerated by a normal newborn and prompt resuscitation usually prevents permanent physiologic alteration. However, prolonged neonatal

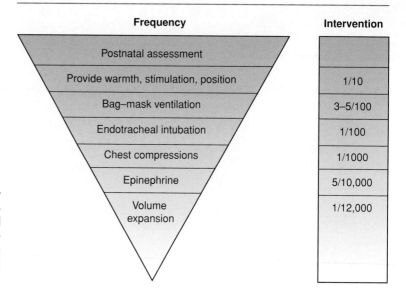

FIGURE 16-1 Type (inverted triangle) and frequency (bar on right) of interventions performed in the delivery room. Modified from: Vento M, Saugstad OD. Resuscitation of the term and preterm infant. *Semin Fetal Neonatal Med* 2010;15(4): 216–222.

hypoxemia or acidosis impedes the transition from fetal to neonatal physiology. Hypoxemia and acidosis promote pulmonary hypertension through hypoxic pulmonary vasoconstriction; this encourages continued flow across the ductus arteriosus. Hypoxia also directly promotes the patency of the ductus arteriosus, as ductal smooth muscle constriction is dependent on arterial oxygen tension. Pulmonary hypertension causes elevated right heart pressures, maintaining right-to-left shunt

across the foramen ovale. Blood flowing through the patent ductus arteriosus (PDA) and foramen ovale is not oxygenated, contributing to increasing hypoxemia (4). Progressive hypoxemia and acidosis ultimately results in myocardial failure and brain damage.

Both the fetus and neonate respond to hypoxemia with a "diving" reflex (known as such due to its similarity to seal physiology during a dive). Blood flow is diverted centrally to

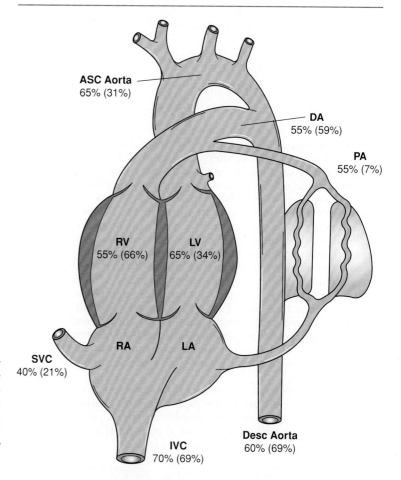

FIGURE 16-2 Oxygen saturation and blood flow through the heart and great vessels in late gestation. Values in the figure are oxygen saturation (percentage of combined ventricular outflow). Adapted from: Rudolph AM, Heyman MA. Fetal and neonatal circulation and respiration. *Annu Rev Physiol* 1974;36:187–207.

the heart, brain, and adrenal glands, and tissue oxygen extraction maximally increases. Although initially a hypertensive response, as oxygen extraction reaches its maximum, myocardial contractility and cardiac output decrease, leading to systemic hypotension (4).

Neonatal ventilation during hypoxia is initially rapid and regular. However, as hypoxia continues, respiration stops in a stage termed *primary apnea*. Stimulation of the neonate during primary apnea will reinitiate respiratory effort. If hypoxia continues, the neonate will begin to attempt irregular, grunting respirations, followed by another cessation of respiration called *secondary* or *terminal apnea*. Stimulation will not reverse secondary apnea, since respiratory drive has been reduced by both central nervous system (CNS) depression and direct diaphragmatic depression (8). The net result of these physiologic responses is a neonate with persistent pulmonary hypertension and little or no ventilatory drive. Ideally, prompt resuscitation prevents these physiologic perturbations.

■ ANTICIPATING THE DEPRESSED NEWBORN

Approximately 80% of neonates requiring resuscitation can be anticipated (1,9). Many of the antepartum and intrapartum factors related to increased likelihood for neonatal resuscitation are listed in Table 16-1.

Antepartum Evaluation

The contraction stress test (CST), originally called the oxytocin challenge test (OCT), was one of the first antepartum tests aimed at assessing fetal well-being (10). Intravenous oxytocin or maternal nipple stimulation is used to induce at least three moderate to strong uterine contractions per 10-minute period for at least 20 minutes. The outcomes of the test are summarized in Table 16-2 (10). Indeterminate or suspicious tests are usually repeated within 24 hours. Positive CST has been shown to correlate well with intrauterine growth restriction, increased incidence of late decelerations in labor, and depressed 5-minute Apgar score (11). The CST has been proven to have a high negative predictive value, with false-negative rates less than 0.4/1,000 patients (12). However, as with most antenatal testing modalities, the false-positive rate remains high at approximately 30% (11).

The biophysical profile (BPP) provides further antepartum evaluation of the fetus. The BPP consists of four ultrasound components and one cardiotocographic component (the nonstress test [NST], which can be used by itself as a screening test) as listed in Table 16-3. Each is scored either zero or two for a final maximum score of ten points (13). A BPP score of 8/10, with normal amniotic fluid volume, is considered reassuring (13), while a BPP score of 6/10 (or 8/10 with abnormal amniotic fluid volume) correlates closely with fetal asphyxia.

The BPP accurately identifies both acute hypoxia (manifested by NST, movement, and breathing) and chronic hypoxia (manifested by reflex movements and amniotic fluid volume) (14). It identifies asphyxiated fetuses in several different high-risk patient populations, including many of those listed in Table 16-1 (15–17). While the test carries a false-negative rate of only 0.7 in 1,000 examinations, the false-positive rate, with a 1-week interval examination period, is approximately 50% (18,19).

The BPP is labor intensive, requiring a continuous 30-minute ultrasound period. In an effort to streamline the test, an indicator of acute hypoxia (NST) and an indicator of chronic hypoxia (amniotic fluid volume) were combined as a first-line test (20). This modified biophysical profile (mBPP) is then

TABLE 16-1 Antepartum and Intrapartum Factors Associated with the Need for Neonatal Resuscitation

Antepartum Factors Associated with Need for Neonatal Resuscitation	
Maternal diabetes	Post-term gestation
Gestational hypertension	Preterm gestation
Previous Rh sensitization	Multiple gestation
Previous stillbirth	Size–dates discrepancy
Vaginal bleeding in the second or third trimester	Polyhydramnios
Maternal infection	Polyhydramnios
Lack of prenatal care	Oligohydramnios
Maternal substance abuse	Known fetal anomalies
Maternal drug therapy including: Reserpine, lithium carbonate, magnesium, adrenergic blockers	

Intrapartum Factors and Events Associated with Need for Neonatal Resuscitation	
Cesarean delivery	General anesthesia
Abnormal fetal presentation	Uterine tetany/hypertonus
Premature labor	Meconium-stained amniotic fluid
Rupture of membranes longer than 24 h	Prolapsed cord
Chorioamnionitis	Placental abruption
Precipitous labor	Uterine rupture
Prolonged labor longer than 24 h	Difficult instrumental delivery
Prolonged second stage longer than 3–4 h	Maternal systemic narcotics within 4 h of delivery
Nonreassuring fetal heart tracing patterns	

followed by a complete BPP if either component is abnormal. This progression of examinations has been a successful compromise for the labor-intensive BPP (12,17).

Intrapartum Evaluation

The primary method of intrapartum evaluation of the fetus continues to be fetal heart rate (FHR) monitoring by cardiotocography. Over time, this has proven to be a consistently reliable method of confirming fetal well-being; a reassuring FHR tracing is more than 90% accurate in identifying a neonate with a 5-minute Apgar score of 8 or higher (21). However, FHR monitoring carries a false-negative rate as high as 50% (21). An abnormal FHR tracing may not be indicative of long-term outcomes; however, it is highly predictive of the need for resuscitative efforts in the delivery room (9).

Intrapartum fetal monitoring utilizes FHR measurement (by external Doppler or by fetal scalp electrode) in concert with measurement of contraction pattern (by external tocodynamometry or intrauterine pressure transducer). These two parameters, together, can suggest fetal well-being; they

TABLE 16-2 Outcomes of the Contraction Stress Test

Test Outcome	Findings
Positive	Late decelerations with *more than half* of uterine contractions, even if uterine activity is less than adequate.
Negative	No late decelerations present on tracing with adequate uterine activity.
Indeterminate— suspicious[a]	Adequate uterine activity present with some late decelerations, not meeting the criteria for a positive test.
Indeterminate— hyperstimulation[a]	Late decelerations present with excessive uterine activity.
Unsatisfactory[a]	Quality of tracing inadequate for accurate interpretation or adequate uterine activity not achieved.

[a]Indeterminate or unsatisfactory tests are usually repeated within 24 h.

can also be a harbinger of fetal asphyxia. Four specific parameters are evaluated when assessing the FHR tracing: **Baseline, variability, accelerations,** and **decelerations** (22). Definitions of each parameter are in Table 16-4.

Utilizing these four parameters, FHR tracings can be placed into three categories, as identified in Table 16-5. *Category I tracings* are classified as *normal*, and are indicative of fetal well-being. *Category II tracings* are classified as *indeterminate*, and are neither indicative of fetal well-being nor predictive of abnormal fetal acid–base status. These tracings require

TABLE 16-3 Biophysical Profile

Biophysical Profile Component	Normal Finding (2 points)
Fetal heart accelerations (nonstress test)	Two or more fetal heart rate accelerations in a 20-min period, each with the following characteristics: • 15 bpm or more • Longer than 15 s in length • Associated with fetal movement
Fetal movement	Two or more discrete limb or body movements in a 30-min period.
Fetal breathing	One or more episodes at least 20 s in length within a 30-min period.
Amniotic fluid volume	One or more pockets of amniotic fluid measuring 2 cm or more in vertical dimension.
Fetal tone/reflex movement	One or more episodes of active extension with return to flexion of the trunk or any limb. Opening and closing of the hand is considered normal tone.

consistent reevaluation and surveillance, taking into account the entire clinical picture. *Category III tracings* are *abnormal* and are highly predictive of *abnormal* fetal acid–base status. *Category III tracings* should be met with prompt evaluation and intervention (22). In addition, the presence of a *sinusoidal FHR pattern*, defined as a tracing with a smooth, sine-wave–like pattern with three to five cycles per minute, persisting 20 minutes or more, necessitates prompt intervention (22).

In the presence of a Category II or III FHR tracing, a confirmatory test of fetal well-being is often prudent. Fetal pH can be measured directly via scalp puncture and can directly confirm or exclude acidosis (23). A scalp pH below 7.20 is considered abnormal and, if confirmed by a second measurement, may indicate the need for expedient delivery. Fetal scalp sampling is not without its challenges; it is an invasive examination for both mother and fetus and requires ruptured membranes to gain access to the fetus. For these reasons, many labor and delivery units have decreased or discontinued the use of fetal scalp sampling and replaced it with digital scalp stimulation (24).

Digital scalp stimulation is administered by gently rubbing the fetal scalp for 15 seconds during a vaginal examination. A FHR acceleration of 10 bpm for 10 seconds or longer after stimulation is highly predictive of a fetal pH greater than 7.20. A lack of acceleration after scalp stimulation, however, is predictive of fetal acidosis with a likelihood ratio greater than 15.

■ EVALUATING THE NEONATE

The Apgar Score

The cornerstone of neonatal evaluation for the past 50 years has been the Apgar score. The score, first published by anesthesiologist Virginia Apgar in 1953, uses five signs: Heart rate, respiratory effort, reflex irritability, muscle tone, and color, each on a 0 to 2 point scale, for a maximum score of 10 (25). These scores are typically measured at 1 minute and 5 minutes postpartum. The individual parameters are listed in Table 16-6.

This simple scoring system, specifically the 5-minute Apgar score, has repeatedly proven useful in predicting neonatal mortality: The term infant with a 5-minute Apgar score of 0 to 3 is 59 to 386 times more likely to die in the neonatal period than the term infant with a score of 7 to 10 (26,27).

However, the Apgar score is not without concerns. There is high inter-observer variation in scoring, both in the total score and in each of the subcategories (28). In addition, the scores have been used incorrectly in an attempt to identify long-term outcomes beyond the increased risk of neonatal death (including long-term neurologic function, cerebral palsy, and even future intelligence). Incorrect Apgar scoring has led to issues of increased medicolegal liability. According to the American Academy of Pediatrics (AAP) and the American College of Obstetricians and Gynecologists (ACOG), the Apgar scoring system, while shown to correlate with neonatal death, is not "[a] conclusive marker ... of an acute intrapartum hypoxic event" (29).

Umbilical Arterial and Venous Blood Gas Analysis

In addition to the Apgar score, umbilical cord blood gas measurements can further elucidate the intrauterine environment of the fetus. Normal umbilical arterial and venous blood gas measurements are found in Table 16-7; however, wide variation can be found in vigorous neonates with Apgar scores between 7 and 10 (30). Cord gas measurements are extracted from umbilical artery and vein samples from a 20 to 30 cm section of cord immediately after cord clamp (30).

TABLE 16-4 Interpretation of Fetal Heart Tracing

Component	Definition
Baseline	The *mean* fetal heart rate in any 10-min window, *disregarding* accelerations or decelerations, and rounded to the nearest 5 bpm. Of the 10-min period, there must be 2 min of identifiable baseline segments (not necessarily contiguous) or the baseline is said to be *indeterminate*. Fetal heart rate baseline is defined as: **Normal:** 110–160 bpm **Tachycardia:** >160 bpm **Bradycardia:** <110 bpm
Variability	Fluctuations in the baseline fetal heart rate that are irregular in both amplitude and frequency. It is also measured over a 10-min window. No distinctions are made between short-term and long-term variability. Variability is classified as: **Absent:** No detectable fluctuation in FHR **Minimal:** Fluctuation detectable, but amplitude less than 5 bpm **Moderate:** Fluctuations of 6–25 bpm from baseline. **Marked:** Fluctuations of greater than 25 bpm from baseline.
Acceleration	A visually apparent *abrupt* (onset to peak <30 s) increase in fetal heart rate. For fetuses 32 wks of gestation and greater, this increase is at least 15 bpm and lasts for at least 15 s. For fetuses less than 32 wks of gestation, this increase is at least 10 bpm and lasts for at least 10 s. **Prolonged acceleration:** Acceleration lasting longer than 2 min, but less than 10. An acceleration longer than 10 min is considered a change in baseline.
Deceleration	A visually apparent *abrupt* decrease in fetal heart rate. This decrease is at least 15 bpm and lasts for at least 15 s. Decelerations are further classified as follows: **Early deceleration:** Visually apparent, usually symmetrical, *gradual* decrease and return of the FHR associated with a uterine contraction. The nadir of the deceleration occurs *at the same time* as the peak of the contraction. **Late deceleration:** Visually apparent usually symmetrical *gradual* decrease and return of the fetal heart rate associated with a uterine contraction. The deceleration is delayed in timing, with the *nadir of the deceleration occurring after the peak of the contraction*. **Variable deceleration:** Visually apparent *abrupt* decrease in FHR. When variable decelerations are associated with uterine contractions, their onset, depth, and duration commonly vary with successive uterine contractions. **Prolonged deceleration:** Deceleration lasting longer than 2 min, but less than 10. A deceleration lasting longer than 10 min is considered a change in baseline. **Intermittent decelerations:** Decelerations occurring with less than 50% of uterine contractions over a 20-min period. **Persistent decelerations:** Decelerations occurring with 50% or more of uterine contractions over a 20-min period.

TABLE 16-5 Categorization of Fetal Heart Rate Tracing

Three-tiered Fetal Heart Rate Interpretation	
Category I	Includes *all* of the following parameters: • **Baseline:** 110–160 bpm • **Variability:** Moderate (6–25 bpm) • **Accelerations:** May be present or absent • **Decelerations:** No *late* or *variable* decelerations
Category II	Includes all tracings which do not fall into Category I or Category III.

Category III	Includes *either*:
	• Absent variability *and* any of the following:
	  • Recurrent late decelerations
	  • Recurrent variable decelerations
	  • Baseline bradycardia
	• Sinusoidal FHR pattern

These two measurements provide different information, and together can provide a picture of the peripartum milieu of the fetus, and may be able to help explain reasons for fetal distress. The umbilical venous sample provides an indication of adequacy of placental transfer, in addition to indirect measurements of maternal and fetal status, as this is blood traveling directly from the placenta. Conversely, the umbilical arterial sample provides a direct measurement of fetal oxygenation and acid–base status, and is analogous to a central venous sample in an adult.

While much information can be gleaned from a solitary umbilical arterial sample, and, should only one of the two samples be collected, it should be an arterial sample, much more data can be extracted from a paired sample (31). First, the two components of a paired sample are always identifiable as arterial and venous, respectively, as a venous cord sample will invariably have a higher pH and higher PO_2 than the coinciding arterial sample. Second, while a solitary arterial sample can identify fetal acidosis and quantify its degree, a paired sample can assist in identifying the etiology of acidosis. Fetal asphyxia due to maternal hypoxia or uteroplacental insufficiency will present as both arterial and venous

TABLE 16-6 Apgar Scoring System

Parameter	Zero Points	One Point	Two Points
		Apgar Scoring System	
Heart rate	No palpable or audible heart rate	<100 bpm	100–160 bpm
Respiratory effort	No respiratory effort	Irregular or gasping respirations	Regular, adequate respirations
Reflex irritability	No response to stimulus	Facial grimace and/or feeble cry with stimulus	Cough, cry, and/or recoil with stimulus
Muscle tone	Flaccid	Some flexion, minimal resistance to extension	Spontaneously flexed arms and legs which resist extension
Color	Cyanotic core and extremities	Centrally pink, with cyanosis of the extremities	Pink core and extremities

hypoxia and acidemia; inadequate oxygenation of placental blood leads to inadequate tissue oxygenation in the fetus. On the other hand, fetal asphyxia due to umbilical cord compression will lead to solitary umbilical arterial acidemia; umbilical venous blood has prolonged gas exchange time (leading to higher PO_2 and pH) and does not reach the fetus, leading to acidosis (31). The cord pH arteriovenous difference can be used as an indication of placental insufficiency versus cord compression as an etiology of fetal acidosis; an arteriovenous pH difference of greater than 0.15 units has been shown to be an effective cutoff between the two etiologies (32).

■ RESUSCITATION OF THE NEWBORN

Although the majority of deliveries are uneventful, approximately 10% of newborns require some assistance in making the transition to extrauterine life. Because of the precarious physical status of the newborn, it is imperative that all providers working within labor and delivery units are familiar with neonatal resuscitation.

Neonatal resuscitation should not only save life but also prevent the sequelae of acute asphyxia, including hypoxic–ischemic encephalopathy, cerebral palsy, cognitive impairment, multiorgan failure, bone marrow depression, disseminated intravascular coagulation, and asphyxial cardiomyopathy. The degree of organ damage and potential for full recovery depends on the severity and duration of the asphyxial event as well as the speed of successful resuscitative efforts.

Steps in Initial Resuscitation

Personnel: Every labor and delivery unit should have a list of both fetal and maternal conditions that require the presence of

TABLE 16-7 Normal Umbilical Arterial and Venous Blood Gas Values

	Umbilical Artery	Umbilical Vein
pH	7.26 ± 0.07[a]	7.34 ± 0.06
PCO_2 (mm Hg)	53 ± 10	41 ± 7
PO_2 (mm Hg)	17 ± 6	29 ± 7
Base excess ($mEq \cdot L^{-1}$)	0.4 ± 3	0.3 ± 3

[a]All values are ± 1 standard deviation.
Adapted from: Helwig JT, Parer JT, Kilpatrick SJ, et al. Umbilical cord blood acid-base state: what is normal? *Am J Obstet Gynecol* 1996;174(6):1807–1812; discussion 1812–1814(30).

a dedicated neonatal resuscitation team at delivery. According to the American Society of Anesthesiologists' practice guidelines, this team should be available for any delivery in which fetal compromise is anticipated (33). On the resuscitation team, each member must be assigned individual tasks including airway management, placement of monitors, insertion of lines, drawing up of medications, and charting. While an anesthesiologist may be invaluable in managing difficult intubation and ventilation, the resuscitation team should *not include the anesthesiologist attending the mother*, though she/he may provide brief assistance if care of the mother is not compromised (34). Additional personnel such as respiratory therapists with newborn resuscitation experience can be a very useful part of the team. Given the urgent nature of neonatal resuscitation, preparation, including practice drills, is an integral aspect of labor floor preparedness.

Equipment: Standard neonatal resuscitation equipment and medications should be organized in a central location, checked frequently for proper functioning and expiration date, and replenished immediately after use (Table 16-8). Suction, oxygen, compressed air, and an air–oxygen blender should be immediately available. In addition, a source of radiant heat should be attached to the resuscitation bed and controlled by a sensor taped to the infant's abdomen.

Neonatal Resuscitation Protocol: The American Heart Association (AHA) and the AAP endorse a neonatal resuscitation protocol based on frequent assessment of the newborn and escalating levels of intervention (Fig. 16-3) (35). The algorithm is organized into 30-second periods in which an intervention is completed, the neonate is reevaluated, and the decision is made whether to progress to the next step. Assessment of the neonate focuses on evaluation of the heart rate and respirations. Successful completion of the previous step is a prerequisite to proceed to the next intervention.

The general condition of the neonate is quickly assessed with three screening questions addressed immediately following delivery: Is the infant full-term? Is the newborn breathing or crying? Does the infant have good muscle tone? Routine care is provided for full-term newborns with good muscle tone and breathing without distress. Neonates with difficulty making the transition to extrauterine life should be warmed, gently stimulated, and placed in the "sniffing position" to open the airway. Suctioning of the pharynx and nose should be brief and gentle. Prolonged or vigorous suctioning may result in breath holding, laryngospasm, and/or bradycardia.

Support of Thermal Stability

Minimizing heat loss is an integral part of neonatal resuscitation. Depressed and asphyxiated infants often have an unstable thermal regulatory system. The large surface area

TABLE 16-8 Essential Supplies for Neonatal Resuscitation

Suction Equipment	Medications
Bulb syringe	Epinephrine 1:10,000
Mechanical suction	Normal saline
Suction catheters 5F–10F	Dextrose 10%
Meconium aspirator	**Vascular Access**
Airway Equipment	Umbilical artery catheterization tray
Neonatal bag with pressure relief valve	Umbilical tape
Newborn face masks	Umbilical catheter 3.5Fr, 5Fr
Oral airways	Syringes and needles
Oxygen with flowmeter	Three-way stopcocks
Intubation Equipment	**Monitoring Devices**
Laryngoscope	Stethoscope
Straight blade #0 and #1	Electrocardiogram
Endotracheal tubes 2.5–4.0 mm	**Miscellaneous**
Stylet	Radiant warmer
Back-up bulbs and batteries	Scissors
Adhesive tape	Gloves

to body mass ratio of the neonate facilitates rapid heat loss by conduction, convection, evaporation, and radiation. The term neonate's primary defense against hypothermia is catecholamine-mediated metabolism of brown fat. Nonshivering thermogenesis, in turn, leads to an increase in oxygen consumption, calorie utilization, and metabolic rate (36). The resulting hypoxemia, hypercarbia, and hypoglycemia promote persistence of the fetal circulation and hinder resuscitation.

Assisted Ventilation

Spontaneously breathing infants generally make their first respiratory efforts seconds after delivery of the thorax. These neonates generate a negative intrathoracic pressure of 60 to 100 cm H_2O and inspire approximately 80 mL of air with their first breath. The majority of air in the first breath is retained within the lungs as part of the developing functional residual capacity (37). Infants who fail to initiate respirations with gentle stimulation, warming, and airway suctioning require further intervention to ensure adequate ventilation.

Assisted ventilation is required in about 3% to 5% of all newborn infants (Fig. 16-1). Positive pressure ventilation is indicated in neonates who remain apneic 30 seconds after delivery, have ineffective or gasping ventilation, and/or a heart rate less than 100 bpm (Fig. 16-3). Assisted ventilation can be initiated with a bag–mask device, a laryngeal mask airway (LMA), or an endotracheal intubation. Traditionally, ventilation is established with a bag–mask device and then converted to an endotracheal tube in the absence of clinical improvement.

Endotracheal Intubation

Endotracheal intubation is indicated in the setting of ineffective or prolonged bag–mask ventilation. Historically, endotracheal intubation was preformed to facilitate tracheal

suction in the setting of meconium-stained amniotic fluid (MSAF) or for the endotracheal administration of drugs. Both of these practices are currently discouraged (35).

For ideal intubating conditions, the infant's head is placed in a neutral "sniffing position" (Fig. 16-4). A small straight blade, such as a Miller 0 or 1, provides the best visualization of the neonatal larynx given its unique anatomic characteristics. Specifically, the newborn larynx is more anterior than the adult and at the level of the third cervical vertebra rather than the sixth. A small air leak with positive pressure ventilation indicates that the uncuffed endotracheal tube is appropriately sized (Table 16-9). An oversized endotracheal tube may cause subglottic stenosis, whereas an undersized endotracheal tube can impede adequate ventilation and may become easily plugged. The endotracheal tube is inserted 2 cm past the vocal cords and tracheal placement is confirmed via detection of end tidal CO_2, bilateral breath sounds, and symmetric chest rise.

Laryngeal Mask Airway

It is important to recognize that both bag–mask and endotracheal ventilation can be accompanied by significant morbidity. Prolonged bag–mask ventilation can result in gaseous distention of the stomach and/or ocular or facial abrasions from pressure applied to the mask. Endotracheal intubation, on the other hand, can be accompanied by a significant hypertensive response contributing to cerebral hemorrhage. In addition, intubation can sometimes be challenging in neonates. A survey of the proficiency of third year pediatric residents at performing neonatal endotracheal intubation (n = 131 observed intubation attempts) found that intubation was successful only 62% of the time on the first or second attempt (38). Given the limitations of bag–mask and endotracheal ventilation, a few investigators have recently advocated for the use of the LMA in neonatal resuscitation (39–41). The size-1 LMA, which fits over the laryngeal inlet, has been used successfully in the resuscitation of both full-term and preterm infants. The advantages of the LMA in neonatal resuscitation include ease of use and decreased hemodynamic stress response. One group reported the successful resuscitation of twenty neonates with the LMA as a conduit for positive pressure ventilation (39). Of note, the investigators had no experience in the use of the LMA in neonates. Another randomized controlled trial found no significant difference between the LMA and endotracheal intubation during resuscitation of infants by experienced providers after cesarean delivery (41).

Although endotracheal intubation is still preferred in situations requiring high peak airway pressures or tracheal suctioning, the LMA can be lifesaving in neonates with difficult airways. Specifically, the LMA has proven particularly useful in neonates with Pierre Robin syndrome or other conditions associated with a hypoplastic mandible where bag–mask ventilation and endotracheal intubation have failed. Of note, there is limited evidence to evaluate the effectiveness of the LMA for newborns weighing <2,000 g, in the setting of MSAF, and during chest compressions (35).

Establishment of Ventilation

The optimal inflation pressure, time, and flow rate to establish ventilation has yet to be determined. With assisted ventilation, pressures of 30 to 40 cm H_2O are often necessary for the first few breaths to establish lung expansion. The use of higher inflation pressures carries the risk of iatrogenic pneumothorax. Once the lungs have been inflated, pressures of 12 to 20 cm H_2O are generally sufficient to deliver adequate tidal volumes of 5 to 7 mL/kg. If positive pressure

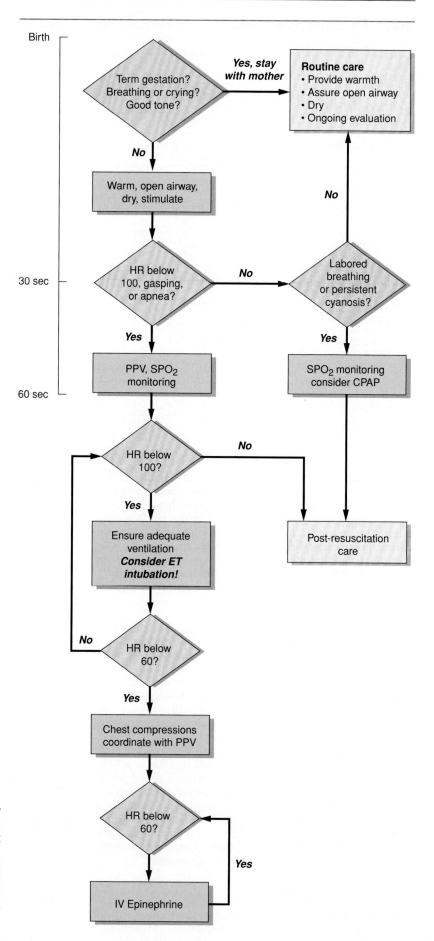

FIGURE 16-3 Flow diagram for neonatal resuscitation based on the American Heart Association guidelines. From: Kattwinkel J, Perlman JM, Aziz K, et al. Neonatal Resuscitation: 2010 American Heart Association guidelines for cardiopulmonary resuscitation and emergency cardiovascular care. *Pediatrics* 2010;126(5):e1400–e1413.

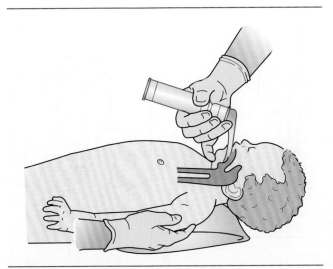

FIGURE 16-4 Technique for laryngoscopy. Left hand holds the laryngoscope and steadies the head and the little finger depresses the hyoid bone to help bring the larynx into view.

ventilation fails to initiate spontaneous respirations, ventilation should be continued at a respiratory rate of 30 breaths per minute. Consideration should be given to the application of positive end–expiratory pressure (PEEP). Some animal studies indicate that when positive pressure ventilation is applied immediately after birth, the application of low-level PEEP (5 cm H_2O) protects against lung injury and improves lung compliance and gas exchange (42). High levels of PEEP (>8 cm H_2O) should be avoided because it may reduce pulmonary blood flow and increase the risk of pneumothorax (35). Regardless of the mode of ventilation, adequate oxygenation is confirmed by an improvement in pulse oximetry, heart rate, and body tone.

Administration of Oxygen

The administration of oxygen historically has been a fundamental aspect of neonatal resuscitation. Recent evidence has challenged the use of 100% oxygen in neonatal resuscitation (43–47) and in the most recent guidelines the AHA and AAP have supported the use of room air in initial resuscitative efforts for the full-term infant (1,35). The growing interest in room air resuscitation was initially sparked by Ramji et al., who showed that room air was as effective as 100% oxygen in neonatal resuscitation (43). Saugstad et al. expanded on these findings, reporting a decrease in neonatal mortality (13.9% vs. 19%) in infants resuscitated with room air instead of 100% oxygen (44). A follow-up study demonstrated no significant difference at 18 to 24 months in neurologic evaluation, somatic growth, or developmental milestones in infants

TABLE 16-9 Recommendation of Endotracheal Tube (ETT) Size

Weight (g)	ETT Size (mm)	Distance from Lip (cm)
<1,000	2.5	7
1,000–2,000	3.0	8
2,000–3,000	3.5	9
>3,500	4.0	10

initially resuscitated with room air as opposed to 100% oxygen (45). A recent report from Spain demonstrated a similar reduction in mortality from 3.5% in the 100% oxygen group to 0.5% in the room air group, suggesting that the reduction in mortality is not exclusive to studies conducted in third world environments (47). The benefits of room air neonatal resuscitation, including a significantly lower neonatal mortality, shorter time to first breath, and higher 5-minute Apgar scores, were recently summarized in a meta-analysis encompassing randomized or pseudorandomized trials of neonatal resuscitation with room air ($n = 881$) versus 100% oxygen ($n = 856$) (46).

Although there is growing evidence that resuscitation with 100% oxygen may be harmful, it is not clear that ventilation with room air is ideal. The recent outpouring of research exploring the effect of oxygen in neonatal resuscitation has revealed that it has a paradoxical contribution to neonatal morbidity and mortality (48–52). Oxygen is clearly an essential component in restoring cellular function following a period of asphyxia. In a neonatal piglet model of intermittent apnea, selective regions of the brain (striatum and hippocampus) were better protected from apoptotic injury when resuscitation was conducted with 100% rather than 21% oxygen (48). Other studies have suggested that resuscitation with 100% oxygen leads to reperfusion injury in the developing brain, lungs, myocardium, and kidneys secondary to excessive production of reactive oxygen species (49–51). In addition, exposure to even brief periods of hyperoxia following delivery has been associated with decreases in cerebral blood flow in term and preterm infants (52). Because of the apparent shifting effect of oxygen in the neonate, resuscitation should be initiated with room air. If, despite effective positive pressure ventilation with room air, there is no increase in heart rate or if oxygenation remains inadequate, use of a higher concentration of oxygen should be considered (35). Increases in oxygen concentration should be guided by preductal values of pulse oximetry (SpO_2) measured on the right hand or wrist.

Chest Compressions

Regardless of the fraction of inspired oxygen used during initial resuscitative efforts, if the heart rate remains less than 60 bpm after 30 seconds of positive pressure ventilation, then chest compressions are indicated (Fig. 16-3). Neonatal cardiac arrest occurs in less than 0.1% of term deliveries (Fig. 16-1) and is most commonly associated with respiratory failure. Hypoxemia and tissue acidosis lead to bradycardia, decreased cardiac contractility, and eventually cardiac arrest. Chest compressions should be initiated at a ratio of 3:1 with 90 compressions and 30 breaths per minute. Two compressive techniques have been described for the neonate (Fig. 16-5). With the "thumb-compression technique," both thumbs are positioned at the lower third of the sternum and the fingers encircle the chest and support the back. Since this method generates higher peak systolic and coronary perfusion pressures, it is recommended over the "two-finger technique" (53). The "two-finger technique" may be preferred in situations where access to the umbilical vessels is necessary. The two-finger technique, with the tips of the middle and index fingers position perpendicular to the chest and a second hand supporting the back, facilitates several simultaneous interventions on the neonate. Regardless of the technique, the sternum is displaced one-third the anterior–posterior chest diameter with each compression. An improvement in the neonate's oximetry and the presence of a palpable pulse confirm the adequacy of cardiac output. Chest compressions may be paused every 2 minutes

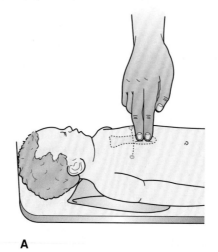
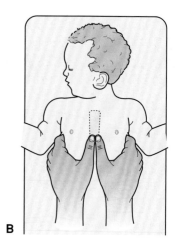

FIGURE 16-5 A: Chest compressions carried out by the preferred thumb compression technique. **B:** Two-finger method.

A

B

for evaluation of the endogenous heart rate. Discontinuation of chest compressions is indicated when the heart rate is greater than 80 bpm and the pulse remains palpable.

Epinephrine

In approximately 0.05% of the deliveries, where the heart rate remains less than 60 bpm despite adequate ventilation and 30 seconds of chest compressions, epinephrine is the vasopressor of choice (Fig. 16-3). Effective administration of epinephrine leads to an increase in myocardial blood flow from α-adrenergically mediated vasoconstriction and a subsequent increase in coronary perfusion pressure. Intravascular epinephrine is currently recommended at doses of 0.01 to 0.03 mg/kg and can be repeated every 3 to 5 minutes until the heart rate is greater than 60 bpm (Table 16-10). It is imperative that adequate ventilation is established prior to its administration, as the α- and β-adrenergic activity of epinephrine increases oxygen consumption and can lead to myocardial damage in the setting of hypoxemia.

There has been some controversy surrounding the administration of endotracheal epinephrine. A recent study revealed only 14 (32%) of 44 neonates experienced a return of spontaneous circulation after administration of endotracheal epinephrine (54). Several factors unique to the neonate may impede alveolar drug absorption. The persistence of the fetal circulation, via a patent foramen ovale and/or ductus arteriosus, may lead to partial bypass of the pulmonary circulation. Alveolar fluid remaining in the lungs after delivery may dilute the epinephrine causing conventional dosing to be inadequate. Finally, pulmonary vasoconstriction from acidosis or epinephrine may lead to pulmonary blood flow insufficient to transport endotracheal administered drugs

from the alveoli into the central circulation. Although there are some animal studies demonstrating a positive result with high-dose endotracheal epinephrine (55), more conventional doses of endotracheal epinephrine fail to show an effect (56). Unfortunately, higher doses of epinephrine are associated with exaggerated hypertension, a decrease in myocardial function, and poor neurologic outcome. Current recommendations support endotracheal administration of epinephrine (0.05 mg/kg to 0.1 mg/kg) only when intravascular access is not available and adequate ventilation and chest compressions have failed to increase the heart rate >60 bpm (35).

Umbilical Vein Catheterization

Cannulation of the umbilical vessels allows for both prompt administration of resuscitative drugs and hemodynamic monitoring. Umbilical vein catheterization provides a reliable conduit for the administration of epinephrine and/or volume. A 3.5 or 5 French catheter is sterilely inserted into the vein at the stump of the umbilical cord. The catheter is advanced 2 to 3 cm, at which point the aspiration of blood should be possible. The catheter must remain *infrahepatic* since hepatic infusion of drugs or hypertonic solutions can cause hepatic necrosis or portal vein thrombosis.

The umbilical artery can be cannulated when it is necessary to frequently assess systemic blood pressure (normal 50 to 70/25 to 45) or arterial blood gases. The tip of the umbilical artery catheter should be positioned above the bifurcation of the aorta and below the celiac, renal, and mesenteric arteries. In a term infant, advancement of the catheter between 9 and 12 cm generally allows for optimal positioning. Radiographic verification of the tip position is indicated if the catheter is to remain in place for an extended period.

TABLE 16-10 Medications for Neonatal Resuscitation

Medication	Concentration	Dosage	Rate
Epinephrine	1:10,000	0.01–0.03 mg/kg	Rapid every 3–5 min
Volume expander	Normal saline	10 mL/kg	Over 5–10 min
	O⁻ blood	10 mL/kg	Over 5–10 min
Naloxone[a]	0.4 mg/mL	0.1 mg/kg	Rapid

[a]Naloxone is not recommended for use in the delivery room during resuscitation.

Treatment of Shock

Although neonatal cardiorespiratory depression is generally secondary to hypoxemia, in rare situations it is the result of significant hypovolemia. The most common cause of neonatal shock is acute compression of the umbilical cord; a tight nuchal cord may result in placental trapping of fetal blood as flow continues through the rigid, muscular umbilical arteries but is inhibited through the compliant umbilical vein. Less frequent causes of neonatal hypovolemia include placental abruption, placenta previa, vasa previa, and fetomaternal hemorrhage. Despite the various potential causes of neonatal blood loss during delivery, volume infusions are rarely indicated and in many situations can be detrimental. In a retrospective study of approximately 38,000 deliveries, only 1:12,000 term infants were in need of volume therapy after birth (57). The current AHA guidelines suggest that volume expansion may be indicated if the infant is not responding to intensive resuscitation and there is evidence of blood loss (1).

In the presence of hypovolemia, volume expansion may be achieved with either isotonic crystalloid, such as normal saline or Ringer's lactate, or O-negative blood. An initial dose of 10 mL/kg over 5 to 10 minutes may be repeated, if necessary (Table 16-10). A randomized controlled trial has shown that there is no benefit of albumin over isotonic crystalloid for the treatment of hypotension in neonates (58).

Although supplementation of blood volume is crucial in the setting of hypovolemia, the inappropriate infusion of fluid may further contribute to cardiac and neurologic compromise. Unfortunately, in the absence of obvious blood loss it is difficult to distinguish a hypovolemic infant from a normovolemic, asphyxiated infant. Both clinical scenarios are characterized by cyanosis, weak pulses, delayed capillary refill, and persistently low heart rate despite adequate ventilation. Given that the neonatal heart has a relatively fixed stroke volume, increased preload can be detrimental in a normovolemic, asphyxiated infant with decreased myocardial function and reduced cardiac output. Furthermore, the cerebral microcirculation of an asphyxiated neonate may be particularly vulnerable to injury with rapid volume expansion. The potential adverse effects of inappropriate volume loading include lower Apgar scores at 10 minutes, lower cord arterial pH, larger base deficits, and longer resuscitation periods in infants receiving volume infusions during cardiopulmonary resuscitation (57).

Correction of Acidosis

Another controversial component of neonatal resuscitation is the administration of sodium bicarbonate for correction of metabolic acidosis. Although acidemia impairs myocardial performance and attenuates the hemodynamic response to catecholamines, the benefit of sodium bicarbonate infusions has been refuted by several studies (59). Among 19 retrospective adult studies examining mortality rates and other outcomes, none demonstrated benefit; 11 showed no difference in outcomes, and 8 suggested a deleterious effect of sodium bicarbonate administration during cardiopulmonary resuscitation (60). The one randomized controlled trial of sodium bicarbonate use in neonatal resuscitation demonstrated no difference in mortality rates or neurologic outcomes (61).

Perhaps more distressing, most studies provide evidence that bicarbonate is detrimental to many organ systems and may reduce the likelihood of a successful resuscitation. AHA guidelines highlight the adverse neurologic and cardiac effects linked to bicarbonate administration (62). Exogenously administered sodium bicarbonate is readily converted into carbon dioxide which, in turn, diffuses into myocardial and cerebral cells and paradoxically contributes to intracellular acidosis and reduced cellular function. The extracellular alkalosis created by sodium bicarbonate shifts the oxyhemoglobin saturation curve, further worsening the intracellular acidosis by impeding oxygen release to the tissues. Sodium bicarbonate infusions also hinder cerebral and coronary perfusion by reducing SVR. The neonate's neurologic status can be further compromised given the strong relationship between intracranial hemorrhage and rapid infusions of hyperosmolar sodium bicarbonate. Therefore, administration of sodium bicarbonate is no longer a component of initial neonatal resuscitation.

Discontinuation of Resuscitative Efforts

In addition to providing guidelines for neonatal resuscitation, the AHA recently released recommendations on when it is appropriate to terminate resuscitation efforts (1,35). Most infants with Apgar scores of zero after 10 minutes of adequate resuscitative measures will expire during the immediate neonatal period from multiorgan failure or will survive with severe hypoxic–ischemic encephalopathy and devastating neurologic sequelae (63). In light of these findings, it is acceptable to withhold or interrupt resuscitation if, after 10 minutes, the infant shows no signs of life.

■ SPECIAL RESUSCITATION CIRCUMSTANCES

Ex utero Intrapartum Treatment

Fetal intrapartum operations on placental support (OOPS), also known as ex utero intrapartum treatment (EXIT), procedures are rare and potentially challenging approaches to the delivery of a fetus at high risk for a difficult airway. The fetus is partially delivered via cesarean section but remains oxygenated via the placenta until the airway is secure. Deep volatile anesthesia, often exceeding 2 MAC, is recommended to anesthetize the mother, provide uterine relaxation, and provide some degree of anesthesia to the fetus. Maintenance of maternal mean arterial pressure and adequate uteroplacental perfusion under these conditions may require maternal administration of both intravenous volume expanders and a sympathomimetic agent, such as dopamine (64).

At delivery if it appears possible to secure the fetal airway with direct laryngoscopy this should be attempted. If endotracheal intubation is not possible, other options include surgical tracheostomy, bronchoscopy, or installation of an extracorporeal membrane oxygenator (ECMO) (65). The partially delivered fetus can be monitored by pulse oximetry with the goal of maintaining fetal oxygen saturation over 40% (66). Although adequate fetal anesthesia is often achieved from the inhalational agent administered to the mother, vecuronium 0.2 µg/kg and fentanyl 15 µg/kg can be given directly to the fetus to facilitate airway management (66). Once the airway, or other means of oxygenation is secure, the fetus is separated from the placenta and care assumed by a neonatology team.

Meconium-stained Amniotic Fluid (MSAF)

Meconium is the breakdown product of swallowed amniotic fluid, gastrointestinal cells, and intestinal secretions. Passage of meconium normally occurs postnatally but intrapartum fetal intolerance of labor can stimulate colonic activity, resulting in MSAF in 10% to 15% of all deliveries (67). Intrapartum hypoxic stress may trigger deep, agonal gasping, leading to meconium aspiration and the development of meconium aspiration syndrome (MAS) in 5% of infants delivered through MSAF (68). The physiologic consequences of severe MAS include inflammation of lung tissue with obstruction of the small airways, the release of vasoactive substances stimulating pulmonary vasoconstriction, and inhibition of surfactant function. MAS may be complicated by the need for prolonged mechanical ventilation, the development of pulmonary air leaks, or persistent pulmonary hypertension. Infants may manifest signs of severe respiratory compromise and the mortality rate among infants with MAS is as high as 5% (68).

The management of infants delivered through MSAF has evolved over the past several decades. In the 1970s, MAS was presumed to be a postnatal event initiated by the aspiration of meconium at the time of the first neonatal breath. Early investigations suggested that meticulous suctioning of the fetal oropharynx and trachea at delivery decreased the rate of MAS (69,70). In 1974, Gregory et al. reported 100% survival in infants born through MSAF who subsequently underwent tracheal intubation and suctioning (69). Two years later, Carson et al. introduced a combined approach involving DeLee suctioning of the upper airway at the perineum followed by tracheal suctioning after delivery (70). Although the clinical significance of these earlier studies was questionable, the combined two-step approach was, until recently, universally adopted.

MAS is no longer considered to be exclusively a postnatal disorder. Recent studies suggest that aspiration of meconium by itself is insufficient to produce the histologic or physiologic changes of severe MAS (71,72). Evidence of long-standing stress in infants with MAS, including pulmonary hypertension and vascular hypertrophy suggests that this is a complex, multifactorial disorder with contributory elements from both the antenatal and intrapartum time periods. It is likely that aspiration of meconium is an event predating labor, and severe MAS is caused by pathologic processes occurring in utero, primarily chronic asphyxia and infection (73).

Therapeutic interventions that have traditionally been advocated, including oropharyngeal and tracheal suctioning, have questionable benefit in altering the outcome of severe MAS. An improved understanding of the etiology of MAS prompted several groups to investigate the utility of routine oropharyngeal and tracheal suctioning of the neonate delivered in the presence of MSAF (74–77). In an international, prospective randomized control trial involving 2,514 infants born through MSAF, Vain et al. demonstrated suctioning of the oro- and nasopharynx prior to delivery of the thorax caused no difference in the incidence of MAS, mechanical ventilation, duration of supplemental oxygen use, or mortality (74). Other investigators have found that vigorous, meconium-stained infants with a heart rate >100 bpm, spontaneous ventilation, and reasonable muscle tone do not benefit from tracheal suctioning (75,76). The benefit of tracheal suctioning in *depressed* infants born through MSAF has yet to be determined. It is imperative to recognize that tracheal suctioning may actually cause complications, including vagal stimulation resulting in bradycardia and apnea; irritation to mucous membranes causing increased mucus production and nasal congestion; and tissue trauma resulting in a break in the natural barrier against infection, therefore, increasing the risk of transmission of infection (78). These findings have led the Neonatal Resuscitation Program (NRP), AHA, and ACOG to modify their guidelines: In the presence of MSAF, intrapartum oropharyngeal and nasopharyngeal suctioning is no longer recommended and tracheal suctioning is advocated only for *depressed* neonates.

Pneumothorax

While pneumothorax during neonatal resuscitation can occur spontaneously, it is most often associated with thick meconium aspiration (secondary to a ball-valve air-trapping effect), or poor lung compliance (as seen in diaphragmatic hernia and pulmonary hypoplasia). Tension pneumothorax, in which high intrathoracic pressure prevents venous return to the heart, is catastrophic and life-threatening. A suspected diagnosis of pneumothorax can be confirmed by transillumination of the chest or an immediate chest x-ray.

Immediate management consists of inserting a 25-gauge needle connected to a three-way stopcock and 20-mL syringe into the thoracic cavity at the second intercostal space. If air is continuously aspirated, then the needle should be replaced with an adequately sized catheter (10 to 16 French) placed in the sixth intercostal space in the midaxillary line and directed anteriorly. The catheter should be connected to continuous suction through an underwater seal.

Premature Infants

Although the survival rate of premature infants has steadily increased over the past few decades (79,80), long-term morbidity and mortality is still prevalent in neonates less than 28 weeks of gestational age (81). Appropriate resuscitation of this subset of newborns requires an understanding of their unique physiologic limitations. Although premature infants are at higher risk for problems with *multiple* organ systems, the pulmonary and cerebral systems deserve special consideration. Fetal lung development during the last trimester is characterized by the saccular development of terminal bronchioli and the formation of surfactant by type II pneumocytes. The reduction in pulmonary surface area and surfactant production characteristic of immature lungs contributes to difficulty in ventilation and increases their vulnerability to barotrauma during positive pressure ventilation. In addition, the antioxidant defense system develops late in gestation and premature neonates may be more susceptible to the adverse effects of excess oxygen. Vento et al. demonstrated that preterm infants resuscitated with 30% oxygen had less oxidative stress, inflammation, and chronic lung disease (82). However, in contrast to full-term infants, room air appears to be insufficient for the resuscitation of neonates at less than 28 weeks of gestation (83–85). Attempts to titrate oxygen concentrations in preterm infants initially receiving room air left several babies with uncertain or dangerously low levels of oxygenation at 9 minutes of life (85). In an attempt to ensure oxygenation while avoiding the complications of hyperoxia, neonates <34 weeks should initially be resuscitated with 30% oxygen (35). If SaO$_2$ is less than 70% at 5 minutes of age or the heart rate is not increasing satisfactorily, additional oxygen should be given (86).

Analogous to the pulmonary system, the cerebral architecture is often insufficiently developed in the premature infant. Although the survival rate of infants weighing less than 1,500 g is approximately 85% (87), a large number of these infants subsequently display neurologic deficits. Specifically, 5% to 10% of these very low birth weight infants develop cerebral palsy and 25% to 50% exhibit behavioral and cognitive deficits (88,89). The fragility of the immature subependymal germinal matrix predisposes these neonates to intraventricular hemorrhage (IVH), which is an early marker for brain injury in preterm infants. Antenatal interventions, such as corticosteroids and magnesium sulfate (90–92), and postnatal management strategies can decrease the risk of IVH and improve neurologic outcome in the premature infant. The establishment of adequate ventilation helps maintain the integrity of the cerebral vasculature. Hypoxemia and hypercarbia have been linked to disruption of cerebrovascular autoregulation and the development of pressure-passive cerebral circulation (89). In addition, the rapid infusion of volume expanders and hypertonic solutions, such as sodium bicarbonate, during neonatal resuscitation has been shown to increase the risk of IVH, and thus neurologic injury (89).

Hypothermia can also cause significant morbidity and mortality in the premature infant. These neonates are prone to thermoregulatory instability. Thin skin and a large body surface area contribute to rapid heat loss while inadequate brown fat stores limit nonshivering thermogenesis. Cold stress in this population leads to increase in oxygen consumption, hypoglycemia, and metabolic acidosis, which hinders resuscitative efforts. Delivery room temperatures >26°C and additional warming techniques, including wrapping in polyethylene bags and radiant warmers, are recommended in preterm, low-birth weight infants to prevent hypothermia (35,93).

Opioid Depression

Fetal exposure to opioid secondary to labor analgesia or maternal addiction may contribute to significant neonatal depression following delivery. The incidence of respiratory depression in the neonate is related to cumulative maternal opioid exposure and the elapsed time from last dosage. Narcotized infants are characterized by hypoventilation and poor response to stimuli. The AAP states naloxone should not be routinely administered to infants exposed to narcotics (94). These neonates should be initially resuscitated with assisted ventilation. Naloxone (0.1 mg/kg) is reserved as an adjunctive therapy in the small subset of infants exposed to opioids who remain significantly depressed with irregular respirations following a period of ventilation (94). There are currently no studies examining the use of naloxone in infants with severe respiratory depression from maternal opioid exposure and there is significant concern about the potential consequences of its administration. In neonates with chronic opioid exposure, naloxone has been reported to cause acute withdrawal symptoms including cardiac arrhythmias, hypertension, noncardiogenic pulmonary edema, and seizures. In addition, there is some suggestion that neonatal administration of naloxone may interfere with critical functions of endogenous opioids and affect behavior long term (95).

Magnesium Intoxication

Hypermagnesemia may be encountered in neonates born to mothers treated with large doses of magnesium for preeclampsia and eclampsia. Magnesium easily crosses the placenta and can influence the neuromuscular and cardiac systems of the newborn. Specifically, hypermagnesemic infants are generally flushed, hypotensive, hypotonic, and peripherally vasodilated. In rare circumstances, hypermagnesemic infants require intubation and mechanical ventilation due to poor respiratory effort. In the presence of adequate renal function, magnesium levels normalize over 24 to 48 hours. If severe hypotension is present, calcium can be used as an antidote; 100 to 200 mg/kg of calcium gluconate given over 5 minutes is usually adequate to increase neonatal blood pressure.

■ RESUSCITATION OF NEONATES WITH HYDROPS FETALIS AND MAJOR ANOMALIES

Hydrops Fetalis

Hydrops fetalis, occurring in approximately 1 in every 3,000 pregnancies, is characterized by excessive fetal fluid accumulation (96). Given that diffuse interstitial edema is a nonspecific, end-stage manifestation of numerous fetal disorders, hydrops fetalis should be viewed as a symptom rather than a specific disorder. Prenatal management focuses on assessment and treatment of the underlying cause.

Although there are over 100 conditions associated with hydrops fetalis, initial classification is based on the involvement of the fetal immune system. Immune-mediated hydrops fetalis results from maternal–fetal antigen incompatibility leading to isoimmunization, fetal hemolysis, and severe anemia. Following the introduction of Rhesus immune globulin prophylaxis, the incidence of immune-mediated hydrops fetalis has dramatically decreased.

Nonimmune-mediated hydrops fetalis (NIHF), which accounts for 90% of hydropic cases, describes a much more heterogeneous group of fetal disorders. The various causes of NIHF include cardiovascular disorders (21.7%), chromosome imbalances (13.4%), hematologic abnormalities (10.4%), infection (6.7%), intrathoracic masses (6.0%), lymph vessel dysplasias (5.7%), twin-to-twin transfusion syndrome and placental causes (5.6%), syndromes (4.4%), urinary tract malformations (2.3%), inborn errors of metabolism (1.1%), extrathoracic tumors (0.7%), gastrointestinal disorders (0.5%), miscellaneous (3.7%), and idiopathic (17.8%). Regardless of the initiating event, the end-stage manifestations of hydrops fetalis are caused by disruption of the normal balance of interstitial fluid formation and removal.

The competing forces of oncotic and hydrostatic pressures between the interstitial and capillary space govern fluid extravasation, capillary reabsorption, and lymphatic return to the central circulation. Many factors contribute to the increased vulnerability of the fetus to interstitial fluid accumulation. Fetal capillaries have increased permeability to plasma proteins, thus colloid oncotic pressure differences are not as effective in encouraging fluid reabsorption into the intravascular space. The fetal interstitial compartment is highly compliant and able to absorb a significant amount of fluid before hydrostatic pressure increases. Finally, the fetus demonstrates increased susceptibility to impaired lymphatic flow; specifically, elevated venous pressure from cardiac failure or obstruction of venous return increases capillary hydrostatic pressure and impairs lymphatic return to the vascular space. The resulting excessive interstitial fluid accumulation leads to pleural effusions, abdominal ascites, pericardial effusions, and/or generalized edema.

Since the mortality rate associated with hydrops fetalis exceeds 50%, neonatal resuscitation should be anticipated for all hydropic cases (96). Following delivery, the infant should be dried and placed under a radiant warmer to prevent cold stress in an already compromised infant. The presence of pleural effusions, ascites, and/or pulmonary hypoplasia may lead to respiratory distress requiring assisted ventilation. Bag–mask ventilation may be difficult given the presence of facial edema and a poor mask fit. Similarly, endotracheal intubation may be complicated by edema of the oropharynx and larynx. Drainage of pleural effusions and/or ascites by needle aspiration may be necessary if adequate ventilation is not achieved after intubation. Paracentesis and/or thoracentesis can be achieved by gently aspirating fluid using an 18- to 20-gauge angiocatheter and a syringe. Cardiocentesis may be required if there is evidence of cardiac tamponade. Umbilical artery and vein catheterization facilitates central access for blood gas determinations, vasopressor infusions, and hemodynamic monitoring. Once the cardiopulmonary status is stabilized, diagnostic evaluation is performed to determine the underlying cause of hydrops fetalis and direct definitive management.

Robin Sequence

Robin sequence (RS), with a prevalence of 1 in 8,500 live births (97), presents a unique challenge in neonatal resuscitation. The micrognathia (small, receded mandible) and glossoptosis (tongue obstructing the posterior pharyngeal space) that characterize RS often results in partial or complete airway obstruction. In addition, cleft palate occurs in up to 90% of neonates with RS (98,99). Respiratory compromise following delivery can quickly lead to hypoxia, pulmonary hypertension, cardiopulmonary arrest, and death. Mortality, which is generally related to airway compromise, ranges from 1.7% to 11.3% and increases to 26% when other anomalies are present (98,100).

Understanding the mechanism of airway obstruction is critical in managing neonates with RS. Disproportionate tongue growth, tongue prolapse into the cleft palate, lack of voluntary control of tongue musculature, and negative pressure pull of the tongue, all potentially contribute to airway occlusion at the level of the epiglottis (101). Although respiratory compromise frequently occurs in RS neonates, the majority of these infants can be successfully managed with nonsurgical airway interventions. Prone positioning displaces the tongue away from the posterior pharyngeal wall and is successful in relieving airway obstruction in >50% of neonates with RS (98,102). When prone positioning alone is inadequate, an oropharyngeal or nasopharyngeal airway may be effective in disrupting the seal between the tongue and the posterior pharynx. For prolonged management, the distal end of a modified endotracheal tube can be placed intranasally and fiberoptically positioned in the distal oropharynx beyond the area of glossoptosis, allowing the neonate to breathe through both the endotracheal tube and contralateral nostril (101). Grasping the tongue with a towel clip and pulling it out is seldom effective and may cause significant harm. This maneuver should only be attempted in life-threatening situations. Endotracheal intubation can be particularly challenging in neonates with RS given the accompanying micrognathia and glossoptosis. Appropriate airway equipment should be readily available. Of note, size-1 LMAs have been successfully used to both deliver positive pressure ventilation and as a conduit for endotracheal intubation (103,104).

Congenital Diaphragmatic Hernia

Congenital diaphragmatic hernia (CDH), a complex condition involving incomplete closure of the diaphragm, affects approximately 1 in 3,000 live births (105). The diaphragmatic defect facilitates herniation of abdominal viscera into the thorax during organogenesis. Although the pathogenesis is incompletely understood, CDH is associated with varying degrees of pulmonary hypoplasia and pulmonary hypertension of *both* lungs. The lung ipsilateral to the diaphragmatic defect is about 20% of its normal size; whereas, the contralateral lung is generally 70% of its usual mass. Respiratory failure at birth is a result of insufficient airway branching, reduced gas exchange surface, abnormal sacculoalveolar maturation, surfactant deficiency, and extensive muscularization of the pulmonary vessels. CDH is also frequently associated with other congenital anomalies involving the cardiac, skeletal, gastrointestinal, and/or CNS, which may further complicate neonatal resuscitation. Despite remarkable advances in antenatal diagnosis and intervention over the past decade, many newborns with CDH continue to experience severe respiratory and cardiac compromise following delivery. Although mortality has traditionally been reported near 50%, new strategies of resuscitation and delayed surgical repair has enabled survival rates of 75% in some centers (106).

The classic clinical presentation of a neonate with CDH includes respiratory distress with reduced breath sounds, scaphoid abdomen with bowel sounds noted in the chest, and displacement of heart sounds to the contralateral side. Significant compromise of oxygenation, ventilation, and cardiac output should be anticipated in the presence of this triad.

Hypoplastic lungs not only impede oxygenation but also encourage right-to-left shunting of blood across the PDA, which further worsens hypoxemia and acidemia. In the setting of suspected CDH, a well-defined protocol of neonatal resuscitation should be promptly implemented.

Bag and mask ventilation should be of limited duration, if not avoided completely. Mask ventilation can lead to gastrointestinal distention further impeding lung expansion and function. Endotracheal intubation with "gentle ventilation" is the definitive management of CDH. Peak airway pressures should be kept low, preferably <25 cm H_2O to avoid barotrauma and volutrauma (107). No attempt should be made to expand the hypoplastic lung because it may lead to a pneumothorax in the contralateral lung. Adequate ventilation is achieved with small, rapid breaths (approximately 60 to 150 breaths per minute). Preductal oxygen saturation should be used to guide oxygen therapy since hypoplastic lungs of CDH are particularly sensitive to toxicity from excessive oxygen delivery (108). Preductal saturation of >80%, PaO_2 of 60 mm Hg, and permissive hypercapnia of up to 55 mm Hg are acceptable goals (109).

In addition to ensuring adequate ventilation, oxygenation can be further improved by optimizing respiratory and cardiac function. Placement of a nasogastric tube and decompression of the gastrointestinal system may improve lung expansion and function. Acidosis, which *both* impedes cardiac function and increases PVR, should be corrected. Blood pressure support may be necessary to discourage right-to-left shunting of blood through the PDA. Hypotension and/or poor perfusion may be initially treated with isotonic fluid therapy (10 to 20 mL/kg). Further blood pressure support may be accomplished with inotropic agents, such as dopamine, epinephrine, norepinephrine, or dobutamine (110). Finally, increased oxygen consumption and exacerbation of pulmonary hypertension caused by hypothermia should be avoided.

Abdominal Wall Defects

Gastroschisis and omphaloceles, the most frequently encountered congenital abdominal wall defects in the neonate, require immediate attention following delivery to minimize morbidity and mortality. Although delivery room management of omphaloceles and gastroschisis are similar, there are important differences in the pathogenesis and clinical presentation that should be appreciated to appropriately manage these neonates.

Omphaloceles, occurring in approximately 1 in 4,000 live births, refer to an anterior abdominal wall defect through which the intestines and other abdominal viscera are extruded (111). During normal organogenesis, the abdominal viscera herniate into the umbilical cord during early gestation and return to the abdominal cavity by the 10th week of gestation. Failure of the abdominal contents to return to the abdominal cavity results in an omphalocele. An omphalocele consists of a sac containing intestines and the variable presence of other abdominal viscera including liver, bladder, and stomach. Following delivery, the omphalocele sac, which consists of the covering layers of the umbilical cord, serves as a protective layer from infection and loss of extracellular fluid. Of note, an omphalocele frequently heralds the presence of other structural or chromosomal abnormalities, most significantly cardiac anomalies, pulmonary hypoplasia, and trisomies 13, 18, and 21.

In contrast, gastroschisis typically occurs as an isolated defect with an incidence of 2.6 in 10,000 live births (112). Gastroschisis develops after the 10th week of gestation following return of the abdominal viscera to the abdominal cavity. Although the exact pathogenesis is not clearly understood, it is generally believed that gastroschisis results from an in utero vascular accident leading to ischemia and atrophy of the various abdominal wall layers at the base of the umbilical cord. The weakened abdominal wall allows evisceration of fetal intestines and other viscera (113). Of significance, the herniated abdominal contents are not covered by any membranes and thus susceptible to massive fluid loss, infection, and trauma following delivery.

Although there are several key differences in the pathogenesis and clinical presentation of omphaloceles and gastroschisis, the initial resuscitative measures are similar. Immediate care involves sterile wrapping of the bowel to preserve heat, minimize insensible fluid loss, and limit physical trauma. Herniated viscera should be wrapped in warm saline-soaked gauze and enclosed in plastic wrap. Gastric decompression with a nasogastric tube prevents further intestinal distension. Appropriate intravenous access should be obtained and fluid resuscitation initiated. In addition, broad-spectrum antibiotics covering maternal vaginal flora (ampicillin and gentamicin) should be considered. Following initial stabilizing measures, the neonate should be thoroughly examined to exclude the coexistence of other anomalies. Specific attention should be directed to the cardiac and pulmonary status of neonates with omphaloceles given the high association of cardiac anomalies and pulmonary hypoplasia.

Myelomeningocele

Myelomeningocele, the most common congenital primary neural tube defect, occurs in approximately 1 out of every 1,000 live births. Failure of neural tube closure during the 4th week of gestation results in aberrant formation of the vertebral arches, meninges, and neural components. Neonates typically present with a lumbosacral cystic mass comprised of nerve tissue, meninges, and cerebrospinal fluid (CSF). The accompanying motor paralysis and sensory loss is a result of not only abnormal development, but also neural damage from prolonged amniotic fluid exposure. In addition, myelomeningoceles are frequently associated with other neurologic anomalies including hydrocephalus, Arnold–Chiari type II malformation, agenesis of the corpus callosum, and/or hypoplasia of cranial nerve nuclei.

Neonatal resuscitation of the setting of a myelomeningocele focuses on protection against further CNS injury, prevention of infection, maintenance of extracellular fluid volume, and screening for accompanying congenital anomalies. The neonate should be placed initially in the prone or lateral decubitus position to avoid direct pressure on the exposed neural placode. Rupture of the posterior cystic mass can lead to ongoing CSF leakage. Covering the neural defect in saline-soaked gauze and a sterile plastic covering provides protection from not only direct injury but also infection and desiccation. Antibiotic therapy can be considered to provide protection against contamination encountered during the delivery. Following initial stabilization, the neonate should be evaluated to determine the level of the CNS lesion and assess for any concomitant life-threatening congenital anomalies. Any further resuscitative efforts should occur in the lateral decubitus position.

■ CONCLUSION

The successful transition from fetus to neonate is characterized by numerous physiologic changes that must rapidly transpire following delivery. Despite the complexity of this process, only 10% of newborns require some intervention at birth. The need for resuscitation is often heralded by fetal and maternal factors present in the antenatal and intranatal period. Prolonged neonatal hypoxemia or acidosis can lead to significant morbidity and mortality, making it imperative that all providers working within labor and delivery suites understand the neonatal adaptions to extrauterine life, recognize the predictors of the need for resuscitation, and have both the provisions and knowledge to respond appropriately.

KEY POINTS

- Transition from fetal to neonatal circulation begins with the neonate's first breath.
- Postpartum maintenance of the intrauterine environment (i.e., acidosis, hypoxia) may impair this transition; this impaired transition can manifest as persistent pulmonary hypertension of the newborn.
- Antepartum testing, including the CST, the NST, the BPP, and others, can be used to ensure fetal well-being. All of these tests, however, have false-positive rates from 30% to 50%.
- Continuous FHR monitoring continues to be the primary method of intrapartum fetal monitoring. Fetal heart tracings are described by four parameters (baseline, variability, accelerations, and decelerations) and are classified into three categories based on these parameters. FHR monitoring is very good at confirming fetal well-being; however, a nonreassuring tracing carries a false-positive rate as high as 50%.
- The Apgar score continues to be the gold standard as a standardized system for evaluating the neonate and identifying the need for resuscitation. However, it is not a conclusive identifier of acute hypoxic event.
- Protecting against hypothermia is an integral part of neonatal resuscitation. The large surface area to body mass ratio of the neonate facilitates rapid heat loss. The resulting nonshivering thermogenesis can lead to hypoxemia, hypercarbia, and hypoglycemia.
- Positive pressure ventilation is indicated in neonates who remain apneic 30 seconds after delivery, have ineffective or gasping ventilation, and/or a heart rate less than 100 bpm. Adequate oxygenation is confirmed by an improvement in heart rate, color, and body tone.
- Chest compressions are indicated if the heart rate remains less than 60 bpm after 30 seconds of positive pressure ventilation. Chest compressions should be initiated at a ratio of 3:1 with 90 compressions and 30 breaths per minute.
- Neonatal cardiorespiratory depression is generally secondary to hypoxemia and rarely a result of significant hypovolemia. Volume infusions are infrequently indicated and may further contribute to cardiac and neurologic compromise in the normovolemic, asphyxiated infant.
- Intrapartum oropharyngeal and nasopharyngeal suctioning is no longer recommended for vigorous, meconium-stained infants with a heart rate >100 bpm, spontaneous ventilation, and reasonable muscle tone. Recent evidence suggests that aspiration of meconium is an event predating labor and severe MAS is caused by pathologic processes occurring in utero.

REFERENCES

1. American Heart Association; American Academy of Pediatrics. 2005 American Heart Association (AHA) guidelines for cardiopulmonary resuscitation (CPR) and emergency cardiovascular care (ECC) of pediatric and neonatal patients: neonatal resuscitation guidelines. *Pediatrics* 2006;117(5):e1029–e1038.
2. Ostheimer GW. Anaesthetists' role in neonatal resuscitation and care of the newborn. *Can J Anaesth* 1993;40(5 Pt 2):R50–R62.
3. Rudolph AM, Heyman MA. Fetal and neonatal circulation and respiration. *Annu Rev Physiol* 1974;36:187–207.
4. Wimmer JE Jr. Neonatal resuscitation. *Pediatr Rev* 1994;15(7):255–265.

5. Schoni-Affolter F, Dubuis-Grieder C, Strauch E. Embryology. *Hum Embryol* 2007. Accessed, 1998.

6. Lawson EE, Birdwell RL, Huang PS, et al. Augmentation of pulmonary surfactant secretion by lung expansion at birth. *Pediatr Res* 1979;13(5 Pt 1):611–614.

7. Lakshminrusimha S, Steinhorn RH. Pulmonary vascular biology during neonatal transition. *Clin Perinatol* 1999;26(3):601–619.

8. Dawes G. *Fetal and Neonatal Physiology: A Comparative Study of the Changes at Birth.* Chicago, IL: Year Book Medical Publishers; 1968.

9. Posen R, Friedlich P, Chan L, et al. Relationship between fetal monitoring and resuscitative needs: fetal distress versus routine cesarean deliveries. *J Perinatol* 2000;20(2):101–104.

10. Ray M, Freeman R, Pine S, et al. Clinical experience with the oxytocin challenge test. *Am J Obstet Gynecol* 1972;114(1):1–9.

11. Lagrew DC Jr. The contraction stress test. *Clin Obstet Gynecol* 1995;38(1):11–25.

12. Freeman RK, Anderson G, Dorchester W. A prospective multi-institutional study of antepartum fetal heart rate monitoring. I. Risk of perinatal mortality and morbidity according to antepartum fetal heart rate test results. *Am J Obstet Gynecol* 1982;143(7):771–777.

13. Manning FA, Platt LD, Sipos L. Antepartum fetal evaluation: development of a fetal biophysical profile. *Am J Obstet Gynecol* 1980;136(6):787–795.

14. Vintzileos AM, Knuppel RA. Multiple parameter biophysical testing in the prediction of fetal acid-base status. *Clin Perinatol* 1994;21(4):823–848.

15. Archibong EI. Biophysical profile score in late pregnancy and timing of delivery. *Int J Gynaecol Obstet* 1999;64(2):129–133.

16. Manning FA, Morrison I, Lange IR, et al. Fetal assessment based on fetal biophysical profile scoring: experience in 12,620 referred high-risk pregnancies. I. Perinatal mortality by frequency and etiology. *Am J Obstet Gynecol* 1985;151(3):343–350.

17. Johnson JM, Harman CR, Lange IR, et al. Biophysical profile scoring in the management of the postterm pregnancy: an analysis of 307 patients. *Am J Obstet Gynecol* 1986;154(2):269–273.

18. Dayal AK, Manning FA, Berck DJ, et al. Fetal death after normal biophysical profile score: An eighteen-year experience. *Am J Obstet Gynecol* 1999;181(5 Pt 1):1231–1236.

19. Manning FA. The fetal biophysical profile score: current status. *Obstet Gynecol Clin North Am* 1990;17(1):147–162.

20. Nageotte MP, Towers CV, Asrat T, et al. Perinatal outcome with the modified biophysical profile. *Am J Obstet Gynecol* 1994;170(6):1672–1676.

21. Schifrin BS, Dame L. Fetal heart rate patterns. Prediction of Apgar score. *JAMA* 1972;219(10):1322–1325.

22. Macones GA, Hankins GD, Spong CY, et al. The 2008 National Institute of Child Health and Human Development workshop report on electronic fetal monitoring: update on definitions, interpretation, and research guidelines. *Obstet Gynecol* 2008;112(3):661–666.

23. Saling E. [A new method for examination of the child during labor. Introduction, technic and principles]. *Arch Gynakol* 1962;197:108–122.

24. Skupski DW, Rosenberg CR, Eglinton GS. Intrapartum fetal stimulation tests: a meta-analysis. *Obstet Gynecol* 2002;99(1):129–134.

25. Apgar V. A proposal for a new method of evaluation of the newborn infant. *Curr Res Anesth Analg* 1953;32(4):260–267.

26. Casey BM, McIntire DD, Leveno KJ. The continuing value of the Apgar score for the assessment of newborn infants. *N Engl J Med* 2001;344(7):467–471.

27. Moster D, Lie RT, Irgens LM, et al. The association of Apgar score with subsequent death and cerebral palsy: A population-based study in term infants. *J Pediatr* 2001;138(6):798–803.

28. O'Donnell CP, Kamlin CO, Davis PG, et al. Interobserver variability of the 5-minute Apgar score. *J Pediatr* 2006;149(4):486–489.

29. American Academy of Pediatrics, Committee on Fetus and Newborn; American College of Obstetricians and Gynecologists and Committee on Obstetric Practice. The Apgar score. *Pediatrics* 2006;117(4):1444–1447.

30. Helwig JT, Parer JT, Kilpatrick SJ, et al. Umbilical cord blood acid-base state: what is normal? *Am J Obstet Gynecol* 1996;174(6):1807–1812; discussion 1812–1814.

31. Thorp JA, Rushing RS. Umbilical cord blood gas analysis. *Obstet Gynecol Clin North Am* 1999;26(4):695–709.

32. Johnson JW, Richards DS. The etiology of fetal acidosis as determined by umbilical cord acid-base studies. *Am J Obstet Gynecol* 1997;177(2):274–280; discussion 280–282.

33. Optimal goals for anesthesia care in obstetrics. *Am Soc Anesthesiol Pract Guidel* 2010.

34. ACOG Committee on Obstetric Practice. ACOG committee opinion No. 433: optimal goals for anesthesia care in obstetrics. *Obstet Gynecol* 2009; 113(5):1197–1199.

35. Perlman JM, Wyllie J, Kattwinkel J, et al. Part 11: Neonatal resuscitation: 2010 International consensus on cardiopulmonary resuscitation and emergency cardiovascular care science with treatment recommendations. *Circulation* 2010;122(16 Suppl 2):S516–S538.

36. Adamson SK Jr, Gandy GM, James LS. The influence of thermal factors upon oxygen consumption of the newborn human infant. *J Pediatr* 1965;66:495–508.

37. Karlberg P. The breaths of life. In: Gluck L, ed. *Modern Perinatal Medicine.* Chicago, IL: Year Book Medical Publishers; 1974:391–408.

38. Falck AJ, Escobedo MB, Baillargeon JG, et al. Proficiency of pediatric residents in performing neonatal endotracheal intubation. *Pediatrics* 2003;112(6 Pt 1):1242–1247.

39. Paterson SJ, Byrne PJ, Molesky MG, et al. Neonatal resuscitation using the laryngeal mask airway. *Anesthesiology.* 1994;80(6):1248–1253; discussion 1227A.

40. Trevisanuto D, Micaglio M, Ferrarese P, et al. The laryngeal mask airway: potential applications in neonates. *Arch Dis Child Fetal Neonatal Ed* 2004;89(6):F485–F489.

41. Esmail N, Saleh M, Ali A. Laryngeal mask airway versus endotracheal intubation for Apgar score improvement in neonatal resuscitation. *Egypt J Anesthesiol* 2002;18:115–121.

42. Probyn ME, Hooper SB, Dargaville PA, et al. Positive end expiratory pressure during resuscitation of premature lambs rapidly improves blood gases without adversely affecting arterial pressure. *Pediatr Res* 2004;56(2):198–204.

43. Ramji S, Ahuja S, Thirupuram S, et al. Resuscitation of asphyxic newborn infants with room air or 100% oxygen. *Pediatr Res* 1993;34(6):809–812.

44. Saugstad OD, Rootwelt T, Aalen O. Resuscitation of asphyxiated newborn infants with room air or oxygen: an international controlled trial: the Resair 2 study. *Pediatrics* 1998;102(1):e1.

45. Saugstad OD, Ramji S, Irani SF, et al. Resuscitation of newborn infants with 21% or 100% oxygen: follow-up at 18 to 24 months. *Pediatrics* 2003;112(2):296–300.

46. Saugstad OD, Ramji S, Vento M. Resuscitation of depressed newborn infants with ambient air or pure oxygen: a meta-analysis. *Biol Neonate* 2005;87(1):27–34.

47. Ramji S, Saugstad OD. Use of 100% oxygen or room air in neonatal resuscitation. *Neoreviews* 2005;6:e172–e196.

48. Mendoza-Paredes A, Liu H, Schears G, et al. Resuscitation with 100%, compared with 21%, oxygen following brief, repeated periods of apnea can protect vulnerable neonatal brain regions from apoptotic injury. *Resuscitation* 2008;76(2):261–270.

49. House JT, Schultetus RR, Gravenstein N. Continuous neonatal evaluation in the delivery room by pulse oximetry. *J Clin Monit* 1987;3(2):96–100.

50. Vento M, Asensi M, Sastre J, et al. Resuscitation with room air instead of 100% oxygen prevents oxidative stress in moderately asphyxiated term neonates. *Pediatrics* 2001;107(4):642–647.

51. Ten VS, Matsiukevich D. Room air or 100% oxygen for resuscitation of infants with perinatal depression. *Curr Opin Pediatr* 2009;21(2):188–193.

52. Niijima S, Shortland DB, Levene MI, et al. Transient hyperoxia and cerebral blood flow velocity in infants born prematurely and at full term. *Arch Dis Child* 1988;63(10 Spec No):1126–1130.

53. Menegazzi JJ, Auble TE, Nicklas KA, et al. Two-thumb versus two-finger chest compression during CRP in a swine infant model of cardiac arrest. *Ann Emerg Med* 1993;22(2):240–243.

54. Barber CA, Wyckoff MH. Use and efficacy of endotracheal versus intravenous epinephrine during neonatal cardiopulmonary resuscitation in the delivery room. *Pediatrics* 2006;118(3):1028–1034.

55. Ralston SH, Voorhees WD, Babbs CF. Intrapulmonary epinephrine during prolonged cardiopulmonary resuscitation: improved regional blood flow and resuscitation in dogs. *Ann Emerg Med* 1984;13(2):79–86.

56. Kleinman ME, Oh W, Stonestreet BS. Comparison of intravenous and endotracheal epinephrine during cardiopulmonary resuscitation in newborn piglets. *Crit Care Med* 1999;27(12):2748–2754.

57. Wyckoff MH, Perlman JM, Laptook AR. Use of volume expansion during delivery room resuscitation in near-term and term infants. *Pediatrics* 2005;115(4):950–955.

58. Oca MJ, Nelson M, Donn SM. Randomized trial of normal saline versus 5% albumin for the treatment of neonatal hypotension. *J Perinatol* 2003;23(6):473–476.

59. Aschner JL, Poland RL. Sodium bicarbonate: basically useless therapy. *Pediatrics* 2008;122(4):831–835.

60. Levy MM. An evidence-based evaluation of the use of sodium bicarbonate during cardiopulmonary resuscitation. *Crit Care Clin* 1998;14(3):457–483.

61. Lokesh L, Kumar P, Murki S, et al. A randomized controlled trial of sodium bicarbonate in neonatal resuscitation-effect on immediate outcome. *Resuscitation* 2004;60(2):219–223.

62. ECC Committee, Subcommittees and Task Forces of the American Heart Association. 2005 American Heart Association guidelines for cardiopulmonary resuscitation and emergency cardiovascular care. *Circulation* 2005;112(24 Suppl):IV1–203.

63. Harrington DJ, Redman CW, Moulden M, et al. The long-term outcome in surviving infants with Apgar zero at 10 minutes: a systematic review of the literature and hospital-based cohort. *Am J Obstet Gynecol* 2007;196(5):463. e1–463.e5.

64. Kuczkowski KM. Advances in obstetric anesthesia: anesthesia for fetal intrapartum operations on placental support. *J Anesth* 2007;21(2):243–251.

65. De Buck F, Deprest J, Van de Velde M. Anesthesia for fetal surgery. *Curr Opin Anaesthesiol* 2008;21(3):293–297.

66. Abraham RJ, Sau A, Maxwell D. A review of the EXIT (Ex utero Intrapartum Treatment) procedure. *J Obstet Gynaecol* 2010;30(1):1–5.

67. Wiswell TE, Bent RC. Meconium staining and the meconium aspiration syndrome. Unresolved issues. *Pediatr Clin North Am* 1993;40(5):955–981.

68. Wiswell TE, Tuggle JM, Turner BS. Meconium aspiration syndrome: have we made a difference? *Pediatrics* 1990;85(5):715–721.

69. Gregory GA, Gooding CA, Phibbs RH, et al. Meconium aspiration in infants– a prospective study. *J Pediatr* 1974;85(6):848–852.

70. Carson BS, Losey RW, Bowes WA Jr, et al. Combined obstetric and pediatric approach to prevent meconium aspiration syndrome. *Am J Obstet Gynecol* 1976;126(6):712–715.

71. Jovanovic R, Nguyen HT. Experimental meconium aspiration in guinea pigs. *Obstet Gynecol* 1989;73(4):652–656.

72. Cornish JD, Dreyer GL, Snyder GE, et al. Failure of acute perinatal asphyxia or meconium aspiration to produce persistent pulmonary hypertension in a neonatal baboon model. *Am J Obstet Gynecol* 1994;171(1):43–49.

73. Ghidini A, Spong CY. Severe meconium aspiration syndrome is not caused by aspiration of meconium. *Am J Obstet Gynecol* 2001;185(4):931–938.

74. Vain NE, Szyld EG, Prudent LM, et al. Oropharyngeal and nasopharyngeal suctioning of meconium-stained neonates before delivery of their shoulders: multicentre, randomised controlled trial. *Lancet* 2004;364(9434):597–602.

75. Wiswell TE, Gannon CM, Jacob J, et al. Delivery room management of the apparently vigorous meconium-stained neonate: results of the multicenter, international collaborative trial. *Pediatrics* 2000;105(1 Pt 1):1–7.

76. Linder N, Aranda JV, Tsur M, et al. Need for endotracheal intubation and suction in meconium-stained neonates. *J Pediatr* 1988;112(4):613–615.

77. Falciglia HS, Henderschott C, Potter P, et al. Does DeLee suction at the perineum prevent meconium aspiration syndrome? *Am J Obstet Gynecol* 1992;167(5):1243–1249.

78. Velaphi S, Vidyasagar D. The pros and cons of suctioning at the perineum (intrapartum) and post-delivery with and without meconium. *Semin Fetal Neonatal Med* 2008;13(6):375–382.

79. Markestad T, Kaaresen PI, Ronnestad A, et al. Early death, morbidity, and need of treatment among extremely premature infants. *Pediatrics* 2005;115(5):1289–1298.

80. Fanaroff AA, Stoll BJ, Wright LL, et al. Trends in neonatal morbidity and mortality for very low birthweight infants. *Am J Obstet Gynecol* 2007;196(2):147.e1–8.

81. Landmann E, Misselwitz B, Steiss JO, et al. Mortality and morbidity of neonates born at <26 weeks of gestation (1998–2003). A population-based study. *J Perinat Med* 2008;36(2):168–174.

82. Vento M, Moro M, Escrig R, et al. Preterm resuscitation with low oxygen causes less oxidative stress, inflammation, and chronic lung disease. *Pediatrics* 2009;124(3):e439–e449.

83. Wang CL, Anderson C, Leone TA, et al. Resuscitation of preterm neonates by using room air or 100% oxygen. *Pediatrics* 2008;121(6):1083–1089.

84. Escrig R, Arruza L, Izquierdo I, et al. Achievement of targeted saturation values in extremely low gestational age neonates resuscitated with low or high oxygen concentrations: a prospective, randomized trial. *Pediatrics* 2008;121(5):875–881.

85. Dawson JA, Kamlin CO, Wong C, et al. Oxygen saturation and heart rate during delivery room resuscitation of infants <30 weeks' gestation with air or 100% oxygen. *Arch Dis Child Fetal Neonatal Ed* 2009;94(2):F87–F91.

86. Vento M, Saugstad OD. Resuscitation of the term and preterm infant. *Semin Fetal Neonatal Med* 2010;15(4):216–222.

87. Hamilton BE, Minino AM, Martin JA, et al. Annual summary of vital statistics: 2005. *Pediatrics* 2007;119(2):345–360.

88. Wolke D, Meyer R. Cognitive status, language attainment, and prereading skills of 6-year-old very preterm children and their peers: the Bavarian longitudinal study. *Dev Med Child Neurol* 1999;41(2):94–109.

89. Volpe JJ. *Neurology of the Newborn*. 5th ed. Philadelphia, PA: Saunders Elsevier; 2008.

90. Moise AA, Wearden ME, Kozinetz CA, et al. Antenatal steroids are associated with less need for blood pressure support in extremely premature infants. *Pediatrics* 1995;95(6):845–850.

91. Nelson KB, Grether JK. Can magnesium sulfate reduce the risk of cerebral palsy in very low birthweight infants? *Pediatrics* 1995;95(2):263–269.

92. Hirtz DG, Nelson K. Magnesium sulfate and cerebral palsy in premature infants. *Curr Opin Pediatr* 1998;10(2):131–137.

93. Watkinson M. Temperature control of premature infants in the delivery room. *Clin Perinatol* 2006;33(1):43–53, vi.

94. American Academy of Pediatrics. Committee on Drugs. Naloxone use in newborns. *Pediatrics* 1980;65(3):667–669.

95. Herschel M, Khoshnood B, Lass NA. Role of naloxone in newborn resuscitation. *Pediatrics* 2000;106(4):831–834.

96. Bukowski R, Saade GR. Hydrops fetalis. *Clin Perinatol* 2000;27(4):1007–1031.

97. Bush PG, Williams AJ. Incidence of the Robin Anomalad (Pierre Robin syndrome). *Br J Plast Surg* 1983;36(4):434–437.

98. Caouette-Laberge L, Bayet B, Larocque Y. The Pierre Robin sequence: review of 125 cases and evolution of treatment modalities. *Plast Reconstr Surg* 1994;93(5):934–942.

99. Marques IL, de Sousa TV, Carneiro AF, et al. [Robin sequence: a single treatment protocol]. *J Pediatr (Rio J)* 2005;81(1):14–22.

100. Holder-Espinasse M, Abadie V, Cormier-Daire V, et al. Pierre Robin sequence: a series of 117 consecutive cases. *J Pediatr* 2001;139(4):588–590.

101. Evans KN, Sie KC, Hopper RA, et al. Robin sequence: from diagnosis to development of an effective management plan. *Pediatrics* 2011;127(5):936–948.

102. Evans AK, Rahbar R, Rogers GF, et al. Robin sequence: a retrospective review of 115 patients. *Int J Pediatr Otorhinolaryngol* 2006;70(6):973–980.

103. Hansen TG, Joensen H, Henneberg SW, et al. Laryngeal mask airway guided tracheal intubation in a neonate with the Pierre Robin syndrome. *Acta Anaesthesiol Scand* 1995;39(1):129–131.

104. Baraka A. Laryngeal mask airway for resuscitation of a newborn with Pierre-Robin syndrome. *Anesthesiology* 1995;83(3):645–646.

105. Langham MR Jr, Kays DW, Ledbetter DJ, et al. Congenital diaphragmatic hernia. Epidemiology and outcome. *Clin Perinatol* 1996;23(4):671–688.

106. Stege G, Fenton A, Jaffray B. Nihilism in the 1990s: the true mortality of congenital diaphragmatic hernia. *Pediatrics* 2003;112(3 Pt 1):532–535.

107. Sakurai Y, Azarow K, Cutz E, et al. Pulmonary barotrauma in congenital diaphragmatic hernia: a clinicopathological correlation. *J Pediatr Surg* 1999;34(12):1813–1817.

108. Keijzer R, Puri P. Congenital diaphragmatic hernia. *Semin Pediatr Surg* 2010;19(3):180–185.

109. Boloker J, Bateman DA, Wung JT, et al. Congenital diaphragmatic hernia in 120 infants treated consecutively with permissive hypercapnea/spontaneous respiration/elective repair. *J Pediatr Surg* 2002;37(3):357–366.

110. van den Hout L, Sluiter I, Gischler S, et al. Can we improve outcome of congenital diaphragmatic hernia? *Pediatr Surg Int* 2009;25(9):733–743.

111. Baird PA, MacDonald EC. An epidemiologic study of congenital malformations of the anterior abdominal wall in more than half a million consecutive live births. *Am J Hum Genet* 1981;33(3):470–478.

112. Vu LT, Nobuhara KK, Laurent C, et al. Increasing prevalence of gastroschisis: population-based study in California. *J Pediatr* 2008;152(6):807–811.

113. Christison-Lagay ER, Kelleher CM, Langer JC. Neonatal abdominal wall defects. *Semin Fetal Neonatal Med* 2011;16(3):164–172.

Management of Neonatal Neurologic Injury: Evidence-based Outcomes

Mihaela Podovei • Bhavani Shankar Kodali

Neonatal neurologic injuries can be due to a variety of perinatal events, such as intrauterine hypoxic–ischemic episodes (cord prolapse, placental abruption, or uterine rupture), birth trauma (shoulder dystocia, instrumental vaginal deliveries), or maternal trauma. However, many of the injuries do not have a recognizable cause. This chapter will focus on the evidence-based management of neonatal neurologic injury.

▪ NEONATAL ENCEPHALOPATHY

Neonatal encephalopathy is a relatively common condition. Nelson and Leviton define it as a clinical syndrome of "disturbed neurologic function in the earliest days of life in the term infant, manifested by difficulty with initiating and maintaining respiration, depression of tone and reflexes, subnormal level of consciousness, and often by seizures" (1). Kurinczuk et al. recently analyzed data on incidence and estimated it to be 3/1,000 live births, with a 95% Confidence Interval (CI) 2.7 to 3.3 (2), with earlier studies placing it between 2 and 6/1,000 live births (1). Neonatal encephalopathy was considered to be the result of an intrapartum event, and different terms were used to define the process: Hypoxic–ischemic encephalopathy, birth asphyxia, postasphyxial encephalopathy, and perinatal asphyxia. In modern thinking, neonatal encephalopathy describes a set of clinical symptoms without assumptions of either etiology or pathogenesis. Hypoxic–ischemic encephalopathy is a subgroup of neonatal encephalopathy, where there is evidence of a recent, usually intrapartum, ischemic event. A recent meta-analysis estimated the incidence of hypoxic–ischemic encephalopathy to be 1.5/1,000 live births (95% CI, 1.3 to 1.7) (2), with previous reports ranging from 1 to 8/1,000 live births.

To differentiate within the spectrum of the clinical syndrome, most investigators use modifications of the criteria Sarnat and Sarnat originally used to characterize 21 cases of neonatal encephalopathy (3):

- Mild/Stage 1: Hyperalertness, hyperreflexia, tachycardia, dilated pupils, absence of seizures;
- Moderate/Stage 2: Lethargy, hyperreflexia, miosis, bradycardia, hypotonia with weak suck and Moro, seizures;
- Severe/Stage 3: Flaccidity, stupor, small to mid-point pupils with poor reaction to light, decreased stretch reflexes, hypothermia, absent Moro.

The presence of neonatal encephalopathy has serious consequences for many infants, including death, cerebral palsy, epilepsy, significant cognitive, developmental, and behavior problems.

Williams et al. studied the extracellular space changes after transient cerebral ischemia in fetal sheep and observed a biphasic distribution of intracellular edema, with early edema resolving slowly and incompletely in (mean +/– SD) 28 +/– 12 minutes and secondary swelling beginning 7 +/– 2 hours later and peaking at 28 +/– 6 hours (4). It is widely accepted today that after a hypoxic–ischemic insult in the newborn, the same biphasic natural course can be identified.

- There is immediate neuronal death due to hypoxia. Neuronal injury results from primary energy failure, acidosis, glutamate release, intracellular calcium accumulation, lipid peroxidation, and nitric oxide neurotoxicity all of which disrupt essential components of the cell resulting in cell death (5–7). The severity and the duration of the insult influence the progression of cellular injury after hypoxia/ischemia.
- After initial resuscitation, oxygenation and circulation are restored. The infant brain goes through a latent period of at least 6 hours, before secondary damage and further neuronal death occurs. There is a window of opportunity between the initial event and the secondary phase of injury, when therapeutic interventions may effectively improve the neurologic outcome.
- Delayed neuronal death occurs due to hyperemia, cytotoxic edema, mitocondrial failure, cytotoxic actions of activated mitochondria, accumulation of excitotoxins, active cell death, nitric oxide synthesis, and free radical damage (4,8–11). Circulating endogenous inflammatory cells and mediators also contribute to ongoing brain injury. Expression of interleukin 1-β and tumor necrosis factor (TNF) α messenger RNA has been demonstrated hours after hypoxia–ischemia, along with induction of α and β chemokines followed by neutrophil invasion of the area of infarction (12,13).

The severity of the secondary stage has been associated with severe neurodevelopmental outcomes at 1 and 4 years (5,14). Significant effort has been concentrated on the identification of interventions that may minimize the neuronal damage and improve the outcome of infants with hypoxic–ischemic encephalopathy (hypothermia, oxygen-free radical inhibitors and scavengers, excitatory amino acid antagonists, growth factors, prevention of nitric oxide formation, and blockage of apoptotic pathways) (5).

Management of infants with hypoxic–ischemic encephalopathy includes (1) identification, (2) supportive care, and (3) interventions against ongoing brain injury. Basic concepts of identification and supportive care, and a summary of interventions designed to lessen further injury are outlined in Table 17-1. Additional discussions of the possible therapeutic interventions are discussed in the sections that follow.

TABLE 17-1 Management of Infants with Hypoxic-ischemic Encephalopathy

Identification

- Evidence of a sentinel event during labor, e.g., fetal heart rate abnormality
- Severely depressed infant (low-extended Apgar score)
- Need for resuscitation in the delivery room
- Evidence of severe fetal acidemia
- Early abnormal neurologic examination (neonatal encephalopathy) and/or abnormal assessment of cerebral function (amplitude-integrated electroencephalogram)
- Amplitude-integrated electroencephalography, head ultrasound, computer tomography, and magnetic resonance imaging can be used to assess the severity and the progression of hypoxic–ischemic encephalopathy (15–18).

Supportive Care

- Maintain adequate ventilation
- Avoid hypotension
- Avoid hypoglycemia. A retrospective review of 185 infants admitted to NICU with acidosis suggests that initial hypoglycemia (BG < 40 mg/dL) is an important predictive factor for perinatal brain injury (19), and may accentuate brain damage (20).
- Treat seizures. Hypoxic–ischemic cerebral injury is the most common cause of early onset neonatal seizures (6). Seizure activity may contribute to ongoing injury: Repetitive seizures disturb the brain growth and development as well as increase the risk for subsequent epilepsy (21,22).

Interventions Against the Ongoing Brain Injury

- Cooling
- Oxygen-free radical inhibitors and scavengers
- Excitatory amino acids antagonists
- Growth factors
- Prevention of nitric oxide formation
- Blockage of apoptotic pathways

■ INTERVENTIONS AGAINST ONGOING BRAIN INJURY

Therapeutic Hypothermia

Over the last decade, significant efforts went into studying the effects of hypothermia on infants with hypoxic–ischemic encephalopathy. Therapeutic hypothermia had been employed in the 1950s and 1960s, but ignored for decades (23–26). Hypothermia re-emerged as a promising intervention in late 1990, and over the last 5 or 6 years, five large randomized-controlled trials (RCTs) with follow-up data at 18 months have been published, all showing some benefit from the intervention (Table 17-2).

Therapeutic hypothermia may improve neurologic outcome after ischemic injury by several mechanisms:

- Inhibition of glutamate release
- Reduction of cerebral metabolism which preserves high-energy phosphates
- Decreasing intracellular acidosis and lactic acid accumulation
- Preservation of endogenous antioxidants
- Reduction of NO production
- Prevention of protein kinase inhibition
- Improving protein synthesis
- Reduction in leukotriene production
- Prevention of blood–brain barrier disruption and brain edema
- Inhibition of apoptosis (5,27,28)

Before instituting hypothermia, several protocol details need to be considered:

1. Time from the insult to the initiation of therapy
2. Method of achieving hypothermia (total body cooling vs. selective head cooling)
3. Degree of hypothermia, site of temperature measurement
4. Duration of hypothermia (48 to 72 hours)

All RCTs of hypothermia in infants with hypoxic–ischemic encephalopathy attempted to initiate the intervention during the latent phase after a hypoxic–ischemic injury, before the onset of the secondary metabolic failure. Universally, the infants were enrolled and cooled within the first 6 hours after birth or an identifiable ischemic event. Most trials belong to one of the two methods of achieving hypothermia—selective head cooling or total body cooling. In selective head cooling, a cap that circulates water at 10°C is placed over the head, while the body is warmed as needed to maintain the rectal temperature at 34°C to 35°C (29–34). In total body cooling, ice or gel packs are used to induce hypothermia, and two cooling blankets above and below the infant are used to maintain the temperature at 33°C to 34°C (35–38).

As noted, the target temperature may vary slightly depending on the cooling method used.

Selective head cooling: The first safety study on therapeutic hypothermia in infants was on selective head cooling (29). The subjects were divided into groups cooled to different target temperatures, as low as 35.5°C, and the study proved hypothermia to be safe and well tolerated (29). Subsequent

TABLE 17-2 Primary Outcome (Death or Severe Disability at 18 Months) in Therapeutic Hypothermia Randomized Controlled Trials

Study	Number of Patients	Primary Outcome in the Intervention Group	Primary Outcome in the Control Group	Odds Ratio	95% CI	P Value
Cool Cap	218	55%	66%	0.61	0.34–1.09	0.1
NICHD	205	44%	62%	0.72	0.54–0.95	0.01
Toby	325	45%	53%	0.86	0.68–1.07	0.17
The China Study	194	31%	49%	0.47	0.26–0.84	0.01
Neo.nEURO. Network	111	51%	83%	0.21	0.09–0.54	0.001

studies of selective head cooling used a target temperature of 34°C to 35°C rectal temperature (17,30–34,39).

Total body cooling: Shankaran et al. published a pilot study to evaluate the reliability and safety of whole body hypothermia to 34°C to 35°C (esophageal temperature), for 72 hours (40). The heart rate decreased with cooling and remained lower than in controls, but was well tolerated; no greater hazards have been identified in the cooled group. Blood pressure, renal failure, persistent pulmonary hypertension, hepatic dysfunction, and need for pressors were similar, and mortality rate was similar between the intervention and the control groups. The same group published a few years later the results of a large RCT using the same cooling methods to an esophageal temperature of 33.5 +/– 0.5°C (41,42). Other RCTs of whole body hypothermia also cooled the infants to 33°C to 34°C rectal temperature and found no major adverse events from the intervention (35–37).

However, Eicher et al. published a safety study of systemic hypothermia, with cooling to a rectal temperature of 33 +/– 0.5°C (38). In this study, the hypothermia group had frequent bradycardia, lower heart rates during the period of hypothermia, longer dependence on pressors, higher prothrombin times, decreased platelet counts, increased plasma and platelet transfusion requirements, and more frequent clinical seizures and electroencephalographic abnormalities.

All observed side effects were considered mild to moderate in severity and manageable with minor interventions.

Between 2005 and 2010, there were five large RCTs and a meta-analysis pertaining to therapeutic hypothermia in infants with hypoxic–ischemic encephalopathy, with over 1,000 infants enrolled. In each trial, the primary outcome was death or severe disability at 18 months.

The Cool Cap Trial was an RCT of selective head cooling with mild systemic hypothermia to a rectal temperature of 34°C to 35°C for 72 hours versus standard treatment. The study enrolled 234 term infants and data was available for 218 infants. Inclusion criteria included amplitude-integrated electroencephalography (aEEG) data in addition to clinical, biochemical, and neurologic criteria of moderate and severe asphyxia. The study reported a 66% prevalence of the primary outcome in the conventional treatment group and 55% in the intervention group, OR 0.61 (0.34 to 1.09), p = 0.1. After adjustment for the severity of aEEG changes the odds ratio for hypothermia treatment was 0.57 (0.32 to 1.01, p = 0.05). A subgroup analysis showed that head cooling had no benefits in infants with the most severe aEEG changes, but was beneficial in infants with less severe aEEG changes (number needed to treat [NNT], 6 [CI, 3 to 27]) (33).

A secondary analysis of the Cool Cap Trial examining factors that may determine the efficacy of treatment found a significant interaction of treatment and birth weight. Larger infants (weight ≥25 percentile) showed a lower frequency of favorable outcomes in the control group but a greater improvement with cooling (34). For larger infants, the NNT was 3.8. Also pyrexia in the control group (≥38°C) was associated with marked increase in adverse outcomes, controlled for the severity of encephalopathy. Out of the 34 control patients that had rectal temperatures above 38°C at any time during the 76 hours monitoring period, 28 had unfavorable outcomes (OR 3.2, 95% CI, 1.2 to 8.4, p = 0.028) (34).

The second large randomized control study was performed by the National Institute of Child Health and Human Development (NICHD) Neonatal Network, referred as **NICHD trial** (41). The study enrolled 208 infants, and data were available for 205. Hypothermia was obtained using cooling blankets to maintain an esophageal temperature of 33°C to 34°C for 72 hours, and the results were compared against the conventional treatment. Unfavorable primary outcome (death or moderate to severe disability at 18 months) was observed in 62% of controls and 44% of the cooled infants, with a risk ratio of 0.72, 95% CI, 0.54 to 0.95, p = 0.01, NNT = 6. Both moderate and severe encephalopathy group had a trend toward decrease for all adverse outcomes in hypothermia group (41).

The third large study—the **TOBY** trial (36) enrolled 325 infants with moderate to severe hypoxic–ischemic encephalopathy at 42 centers worldwide. The intervention was whole body cooling. Gel packs were used to initiate hypothermia, and cooling blankets were used to maintain the temperature at 33°C to 34°C for 72 hours. Unfavorable outcomes were present in 53% of controls and 45% of cooled infants (RR 0.86, 95% CI, 0.68 to 1.07). The difference in primary outcome (death or moderate to severe disability) did not reach statistical significance, but among survivors, infants in the cooled group had increased rate of survival without neurologic abnormality (44% in the cooled group vs. 28% in the standard treatment group, RR 1.57, 95% CI, 1.16 to 2.12, p = 0.003). Also the intervention reduced the risk of cerebral palsy among survivals (RR 0.67, 95% CI, 0.47 to 0.96, p = 0.03), improved scores on the Mental Developmental Index and Psychomotor Index of the Bayley Scales of Infant development II (p = 0.03 for each) and the Gross Motor Classification System (p = 0.01). The study concluded that the induction of moderate hypothermia for 72 hours in infants with perinatal asphyxia did not significantly reduce the combined rate of death or severe disability but resulted in improved neurologic outcomes in survivors (36).

A meta-analysis of the previous randomized control trials of therapeutic hypothermia was published in 2010 (43). The three large trials with 18 months follow-up information, including 767 infants, were analyzed. Seven other trials with mortality information but without appropriate neurodevelopmental data were identified. Therapeutic hypothermia significantly reduced the combined rate of death and severe disability at 18 months: Risk ratio 0.81, 95% CI, 0.71 to 0.93, p = 0.002; risk difference –0.11, 95% CI 0.18 to 0.04, with NNT = 9 (95% CI, 5 to 25).

Hypothermia increased survival with normal neurologic function, reduced the rates of severe disability, cerebral palsy, and mental psychomotor developmental index less than 70 (43).

Since the meta-analysis, two other large RCTs published their results (37,39). A group of investigators from China published the results of a multicenter, randomized control trial of selective head cooling within 6 hours after birth to a nasopharyngeal temperature of 34°C and rectal temperature of 34°C to 35°C for 72 hours. 194 neonates were enrolled. The primary outcome was death and severe disability at 18 months and the prevalence was 31% in the cooling group versus 49% in the control group (OR 0.47, 95% CI, 0.26 to 0.84, p = 0.01). The severe disability prevalence was 14% versus 28%, OR 0.4, 95% CI, 0.17 to 0.92, p = 0.01 (39).

The last published study was a European multicenter study (**Neo.nEURO.network** RCT) of whole body cooling to a rectal temperature of 33°C to 34°C for 72 hours using a cooling blanket. They reported the data from 111 infants. All infants received opioids (morphine or fentanyl) to reduce the discomfort attributable to the encephalopathy and to counteract the stress response induced by hypothermia. The prevalence of the primary outcome was 50.9% in the intervention group and 82.8% in the control group, RR 0.21, 95% CI, 0.09 to 0.54, p = 0.001. The prevalence of cerebral palsy was also lower in the intervention group (12.5% vs. 47.6%, RR 0.15, p = 0.007). The study was terminated early due to ethical concerns regarding the control subjects (37).

In summary, for infants with hypoxic–ischemic encephalopathy, moderate hypothermia is associated with a consistent reduction in death and neurologic impairment at 18 months.

■ OXYGEN-FREE RADICAL INHIBITORS AND SCAVENGERS

Allopurinol

Free radical formation due to conversion of hypoxanthine into xanthine by xanthine-oxidase is an important pathway of brain damage after a hypoxic–ischemic event (44). Administration of the xanthine-oxidase inhibitor allopurinol may reduce the severity of brain damage by several mechanisms including decrease of the free radical production, acting as a direct free radical (hydroxyl) scavenger, and chelation of nonprotein bound iron (44).

Several RCTs and observational studies of allopurinol administration in infants with evidence of ischemic brain injury have been reported. Van Bel et al. enrolled 22 infants admitted to NICU with severe birth asphyxia and randomized them to receiving allopurinol versus controls (45). The study was not blinded, nor placebo controlled. The results suggested a beneficial effect of allopurinol treatment on free radical formation, cerebral blood volume, and electrical brain activity without significant toxic side effects (45). No data on morbidity and mortality was included. This study was followed by a randomized, double blind placebo-controlled trial by Benders et al. (46) that failed to show benefit of allopurinol administration after birth and 12 hours later on mortality and short-term outcome in severely asphyxiated infants. The study concluded that allopurinol treatment started about 4 hours after birth is too late to exert beneficial effects, and, if asphyxia is too severe, postnatal allopurinol does not influence survival or neurodevelopmental outcome (46). On the other hand, early administration of allopurinol (within 2 hours after birth) and continued for 3 days was proven beneficial in a randomized placebo-controlled trial by Gunes et al. (47). The group enrolled 60 neonates with hypoxic–ischemic encephalopathy divided between an intervention group that received allopurinol and a placebo group. Twenty healthy neonates were enrolled in a control group. Severe adverse outcomes (death or severe impairment at 12 or more months) were present in 39.3% of allopurinol-treated and 53.6% of placebo group (*p* < 0.05). Serum nitric oxide levels were measured in all groups, and they correlated with the degree of hypoxic–ischemic encephalopathy. Serum nitric oxide levels decreased significantly within 72 to 96 hours after birth in asphyxiated infants treated with allopurinol (47).

Free radical formation occurs on reperfusion/reoxygenation with maximal formation within 30 minutes after birth. Therefore, the optimal time to start antioxidant treatment is at birth or even before (48). A randomized, double blind placebo-controlled feasibility study of allopurinol administration in pregnant women with signs of fetal asphyxia as indicated by a nonreassuring fetal heart tracing or fetal scalp pH lower than 7.20 showed lower levels of S-100B, a marker of brain injury, in fetuses with therapeutic levels of allopurinol (48). A large randomized double blind placebo-controlled trial (ALLO-Trial) with primary outcomes of S-100B levels and the severity of oxidative stress, and secondary outcomes of neonatal morbidity, mortality, and long-term neurologic status, is underway (44).

Ascorbic Acid

Ascorbic acid at very low concentrations scavenges and neutralizes reactive oxygen species that may contribute to ongoing neuronal damage after hypoxic–ischemic neonatal brain injury. Ascorbic acid also regenerates antioxidants such as α-tocopherol and β-carotene (49). A randomized double blinded controlled study of intravenous ascorbic acid and oral ibuprofen started within 2 hours and continued for 3 days after delivery failed to show an outcome benefit in infants with hypoxic–ischemic encephalopathy (49). Other oxygen-free radical inhibitors and scavengers currently under investigation in animal models include superoxide dismutase and catalase, deferoxamine, and lazaroids (nonglucocorticoid, 21 aminosteroid) (5).

Excitatory Amino Acid Antagonists

Glutamate promotes a cascade of events leading to cellular death (5,6). Accumulation of extra cellular glutamate appears to be important in both neuronal and oligodendroglial death. The N-methyl D-aspartic acid (NMDA) receptor antagonists (dizocilpine [MK-801], magnesium, ketamine, PCP, dextromethorphan) have been extensively studied in various models of ischemic neuronal injury, both in culture and in vivo (animal models) and their neuroprotective effects are well established (6). Magnesium is the NMDA receptor antagonist most extensively studied in humans. Data on magnesium sulfate for the amelioration of neuronal injury emerged from an observational study on premature infants. Cerebral palsy is a nonprogressive disorder of movement and posture and a leading cause of childhood disability. Preterm birth is a major risk factor for the development of cerebral palsy (50). It was observed that maternal use of magnesium as tocolytic agent for preterm labor or as therapy in preeclamptic women with very low birth weight infants (<1,500 g) was associated with lower incidence of cerebral palsy at 3 years as compared with women with very low birth weight infants who did not receive magnesium (51). A subsequent retrospective study found a lower prevalence of cerebral palsy in very low birth weight neonates (<1,500 g) exposed versus not exposed to magnesium sulfate (52). However, evidence has not been consistently positive (6). Mittendorf et al. found an increase in total deaths in the magnesium-treated group (53), but subsequent studies (54,55) failed to show the same result.

To clarify the role of magnesium in the prevention of cerebral palsy, three large randomized placebo-controlled studies have been published (56–58). The primary outcome was death or cerebral palsy by 2 years of age in Crowther et al. (58), death or severe white matter injury before discharge in Marret et al. (56), and death by 1 year or moderate to severe cerebral palsy at or beyond 2 years in Rouse et al. (57). All three studies failed to show a significant difference for the primary outcome in the magnesium-treated group as compared with the placebo group. Secondary analysis, though, demonstrated benefit in the intervention group for all three studies. Crowther et al. showed significantly less frequent substantial motor gross dysfunction (inability to walk without assistance), death, or both in the infants exposed to magnesium sulfate (58). Marret et al. identified significant reductions in death, or gross motor dysfunction, or both; and death, or motor or cognitive dysfunction, or both with magnesium treatment (56). Rouse et al. found a decreased rate of moderate to severe cerebral palsy and less overall cerebral palsy in surviving children born to women treated with magnesium (57).

Several meta-analyses concluded that prenatal administration of magnesium sulfate when given with neuroprotective intent reduces the occurrence of cerebral palsy and the combined outcome of death and cerebral palsy, without affecting fetal or infant death rate (59–61).

The American College of Obstetricians and Gynecologists (ACOG), upon reviewing the data on magnesium and neuroprotection, published in March 2010 a committee opinion on magnesium use before anticipated preterm birth. ACOG recognizes that individual studies failed to find benefit with regard to their primary outcomes. However, the opinion concluded that the available evidence suggests that magnesium sulfate given before anticipated early preterm birth reduces the risk of cerebral palsy in surviving infants (62).

Calcium Channel Blockers

Intracellular calcium accumulation is an important step in the cascade that results in neuronal damage after a hypoxic–ischemic insult. Calcium channel blockers, that would decrease intracellular calcium, seem to be a desirable therapy. Nicardipine has been tested in four severely asphyxiated infants but the positive effects have been contracted by the significant hemodynamic disturbance (63).

Other Agents

Other avenues for potential neuroprotection studied in animal models are xenon, platelet activating factor antagonists, adenosinergic agents, monosialoganglioside, growth factor, insulin-like growth factor-1, and blockage of the apoptotic pathways (minocycline, erythropoietin) (5). Out of the above agents, the one that made it to human trials is erythropoietin.

Erythropoietin was originally used in neonates for its role in erythropoiesis. Clinical trials demonstrated safety and efficacy of human recombinant erythropoietin in the prevention and treatment of anemia of prematurity (64). Systemically administered erythropoietin has been proven neuroprotective in neonatal brain injury models (65). Erythropoietin is believed to prevent neuronal apoptosis, and stimulate vascular endothelial growth factor secretion and angiogenesis. Other effects are mediated through stimulation of the brain derived neurotrophic factor (BDNF) (66).

During a trial of recombinant human erythropoietin for the prevention of anemia of prematurity it was noted that elevated serum erythropoietin concentrations were correlated with higher Mental Developmental Index Scores (67). Other observational studies had similar results (68,69). However, Ohls et al. did not detect a difference in the neurodevelopmental outcome at 18 to 22 months (70).

There is one RCT designed to examine administration of erythropoietin in term infants with moderate to severe hypoxic–ischemic encephalopathy. The primary outcome was death or disability, with neurodevelopmental testing performed at 18 months (64). Outcome data was available in 153 infants. Death or severe disability occurred in 43.8% of the control group and 24.6% of the infants in the erythropoietin group, $p = 0.017$. Subgroup analysis indicates that the intervention improved long-term outcomes only for infants with moderate ($p = 0.001$) but not those with severe hypoxic–ischemic encephalopathy ($p = 0.227$) (64). Erythropoietin was well tolerated; neither allergic reactions nor thrombosis was observed (64).

■ MECHANICAL FETAL AND NEONATAL INJURIES

The mechanical injuries that can result in neonatal neurologic deficits can involve the head (extracranial, cranial, or intracranial) or peripheral nervous system (peripheral nerve palsies).

Some of the risk factors associated with mechanical fetal injury are instrumental vaginal delivery, macrosomia, prematurity, abnormal fetal presentation, prolonged labor, and precipitous delivery (71).

Extracranial injuries. Nearly all infants delivered by vacuum will exhibit scalp effects, most of them transient and without clinical significance.

- **Scalp abrasions and lacerations:** Scalp and face injuries occur in 16% of vacuum deliveries and 17% of forceps deliveries (72). They can be reduced or prevented by the correct placement of the cup, avoidance of cup detachments ("pop-offs") for vacuum deliveries. Facial abrasions and skin bruises can be reduced by the use of protective covers over forceps (72).
- **Facial nerve palsy:** Facial nerve palsies usually are forceps-associated injuries, occurring due to pressure on the stylomastoid foramen or compression of the bone overlying the vertical segment of the facial canal. However, 33% of injuries occur with spontaneous vaginal delivery, probably due to compression against maternal sacral promontory (72). Prognosis is good with recovery expected within 2 weeks (73).
- **Caput succedaneum:** This is an extraperiosteal, serosanguinous collection that extends across the midline and over the suture lines. It is caused by mechanical trauma to the presenting part by pushing against the dilating cervix (71).
- **Chignon:** Vacuum extraction causes a collection of interstitial fluid and microhemorrhages that fill the internal diameter of the vacuum cup. The collection typically resolves in 12 to 18 hours and no treatment is indicated (71).
- **Cephalhematoma:** Cephalhematoma is a subperiosteal collection secondary to rupture of the blood vessels between the skull and the periosteum. It does not cross the suture lines. Rarely this can cause anemia and hypotension. Usually it resolves within a few weeks, and requires no treatment, but it can cause bony swelling for several months. In cases of suspected depressed skull fracture or neurologic symptoms, a skull x-ray and a head computed tomograph (CT) are indicated (72).
- **Subgaleal hemorrhage or subaponeurotic hemorrhage:** Subaponeurotic hemorrhage develops between the periosteum and the galea aponeurotica (a dense layer of fibrous tissue that covers the vault of the skull and is attached to the skin and subcutaneous tissue). Under the galea aponeurotica, there are large emissary veins that connect the dural sinuses with the scalp veins. The potential subgaleal space has a capacity of 260 cc in a term infant and the rupture of the emissary veins can result in life-threatening hemorrhage and anemia. The reported incidence is 4:10,000 vaginal deliveries and ranges from 0% to 21% following vacuum extraction (72). It presents as a diffuse swelling or a fluctuant mass that crosses the suture lines. The blood can shift depending on the fetal head position. Loss of 20% to 40% of the circulating blood volume can cause hypovolemic shock. The mortality in this case approaches 25% (74). A decrease in the hematocrit more than 25% from baseline is associated with severe birth asphyxia (75). Management includes correction of anemia, thrombocytopenia and coagulopathy, and in severe cases surgery to cauterize the bleeding vessels (71).

Cranial Injuries

Skull fractures can result from forceps blades or from pushing against the maternal bony pelvis (71). Other rarer etiologies for fetal skull fracture include maternal trauma, either blunt trauma from motor vehicle accidents and air bag deployment (76,77), or penetrating trauma from stabbing and gunshot wounds (78). Skull fractures due to birth trauma can be linear or depressed (the ping-pong ball-type fracture) (71). The linear fractures are of no clinical significance and require no specific treatment. Depressed skull fractures could be managed nonsurgically but surgical management is indicated if there are neurologic deficits, bone fragments in the cerebrum, signs of intracranial injury, signs of cerebrospinal fluid beneath the galea, and failed closed manipulation. Skull fractures should be suspected in any cephalohematoma or subarachnoid hemorrhage (71,72).

Intracranial Injuries

Intracranial injuries occur in 5 to 6 cases per 10,000 live births and can be potentially fatal or cause lifelong disability (72). Risk factors include forceps or vacuum delivery, prolonged second stage or precipitous delivery, and macrosomia. In addition to birth trauma, other causes of intracranial hemorrhage include birth asphyxia, prematurity, hemorrhagic diathesis, infection, and vascular abnormalities (79). Instrumental delivery is associated with subdural and subarachnoid rather than intraventricular hemorrhage (80). Intraventricular hemorrhage is the most common type of hemorrhage in preterm newborns (infants weighing less than 1,500 g) (80). Epidural, subdural or subarachnoid, intraparenchymal and intraventricular hemorrhage can also occur (72,80). Epidural hemorrhage may present with diffused neurologic symptoms, increased intracranial pressure and bulging fontanels, or localized symptoms such as lateralizing seizures and eye deviation. Subdural hemorrhages present with apnea, unequal pupils, eye deviation, irritability, tense fontanel, seizures, and coma (81). Subarachnoid hemorrhage manifests by seizures, irritability, recurrent apnea, and depressed level of consciousness. Cranial ultrasound is often the first imaging modality for newborns, followed by CT or MRI (80). Treatment depends on the neurologic presentation and the extent of the lesions, and surgical intervention may be required on occasion (71).

Perinatal Peripheral Nerve Injuries

In the newborn, peripheral nerve injuries that affect the upper limb function most consistently involve the brachial plexus (82). Isolated radial nerve palsies have also been described (82,83).

Brachial Plexus Palsies

Obstetrical brachial plexus palsy (OBPP) is the result of injury to one or more cervical and thoracic nerve roots (C5–T1) that occurs before, during, or after the birth process (83). In the majority of cases C5–C6 nerve roots are involved (Erb–Duchenne palsy), but C5–C7, C8–T1 (Klumpke's palsy), total plexopathy or total plexopathy with Horner's syndrome have been described (84). Erb–Duchenne palsy represents 46% of all cases and is associated with the most favorable prognosis (84); it usually resolves within a year, but 5% to 8 % of cases have persistent symptoms. Klumpke's palsy usually persists, with only 40% resolving within a year (85). The incidence of OBPP ranges from 0.42 to 3 per 1,000 live births in western countries, and 1.5/1,000 live births in the United States (83).

The major risk factor for OBPP is shoulder dystocia; however, a significant proportion of cases are secondary to in utero injury. The propulsive forces of labor, intrauterine maladaptation, compression of the posterior shoulder against the sacral promontory, and uterine anomalies are possible intrauterine causes of OBPP (85).

Risk factors for OBPP are shown in Table 17-3.

Preventing obstetric brachial plexus injury is difficult, as the majority of the affected infants do not have identifiable risk factors. Shoulder dystocia is also largely unpredictable. Induction of labor has previously been advocated for suspected fetal macrosomia, but a meta-analysis of two RCTs showed that induction of labor in nondiabetic women suspected of fetal macrosomia does not reduce the risk of maternal or neonatal morbidity (88). Cesarean deliveries have a lower incidence of brachial plexus palsy, so elective cesarean delivery may seem reasonable in cases at risk. Yeo et al. found that an elective cesarean delivery for an estimated

TABLE 17-3 Risk Factors for Obstetric Brachial Plexus Palsy

Maternal
• Diabetes Mellitus • High Body Mass Index or excessive weight gain • Maternal age > 35 • Abnormal maternal pelvic anatomy (flat pelvis) • Nulliparity (85)
Fetal
• Macrosomia • Breech presentation
Obstetrical (85)
• Shoulder dystocia—4–40% of shoulder dystocia cases are complicated by OBPP (86), with 1.6% cases having permanent injury (85,87). Although fetal macrosomia is the most important risk factor for shoulder dystocia, half of the cases occur in infants <4,000 g. • Breech delivery (85) • Cephalopelvic and fetopelvic disproportion • Prolonged second stage, precipitous second stage • Instrumental vaginal delivery • Prior history of OBPP

fetal weight higher than 4 kg would prevent 44% of cases of shoulder dystocia (89). Gilbert et al., studying the risk factors for obstetric brachial plexus injuries in over 1 million parturients, identified diabetic women with macrosomia (over 4.5 kg) undergoing instrumental vaginal delivery to be the highest risk group for the development of neonatal brachial plexus injury. Even in this high risk group, 92% of the infants did not have obstetric nerve palsies, so cesarean delivery would have been unnecessary in a large majority of cases (90). In a review, Doumouchtsis et al. predicted that for diabetic women, 443 cesarean deliveries would be required for the prevention of one permanent OBPP for infants over 4.5 kg, and 489 would be required for the prevention of one OBPP for infants over 4 kg (85).

Appropriate management of shoulder dystocia during labor and delivery may reduce the incidence and severity of neonatal neurologic injury (brachial plexus palsies and hypoxic–ischemic encephalopathy). The obstetrician has a variety of maneuvers at his/her disposal that may help free the shoulder (Table 17-4).

Most cases of neonatal brachial plexus palsy are transient, and recovery with supportive noninterventional care usually results in recovery. Physical therapy conducted at home, supervised by professionals, is the preferred initial treatment (84). The timing of recovery has important prognostic significance: Infants recovering some strength (at least partial antigravity motion) in the first 2 months of life should have complete neurologic recovery within the first 1 to 2 years of life. Conversely, infants who demonstrate return of biceps function later than 3 months rarely have complete recovery. Physiotherapy, microsurgical nerve reconstruction, secondary joint corrections, and muscle transpositions are employed to maximize function in cases of persistent brachial plexus palsy (84).

■ RADIAL NERVE PALSY

Injury of the radial nerve is a rare clinical entity and should be distinguished from the more common brachial plexus injury, especially lower brachial plexus palsy, which affects the wrist and finger

TABLE 17-4 Maneuvers to Manage Shoulder Dystocia

First-line Maneuvers

- McRoberts-acute flexion of the hips in supine position straightens the lumbosacral angle.
- Suprapubic pressure facilitates adduction of the fetal shoulders with reduction of the bisacromial diameter and rotation to an oblique position.

Second-line Maneuvers

- Delivery of the posterior arm.
- Rubin's maneuver: Rotation of the anterior shoulder forward.
- Woods' screw: Pressure is applied on the anterior aspect of the posterior shoulder attempting to rotate the fetus the same direction as Rubin's maneuver.
- Reverse Woods' screw: With two fingers behind the posterior shoulder, attempt is made to rotate opposite to the original Woods'.
- All fours: With the woman on her hands and knees, gentle traction is applied in an attempt to deliver the posterior shoulder, which may descend because of gravity.
- Intentional clavicular fracture performed to deliver the infant has an increased risk of iatrogenic brachial plexus injury, vascular and fetal soft tissue trauma.

Third-line Maneuvers

- Zavanelli maneuver: Reinsertion of the fetus into the pelvis, tocolysis and delivery by cesarean. The maneuver has a success rate of up to 92%, but is associated with severe fetal and maternal morbidity including fetal injuries and deaths, uterine and vaginal rupture.
- Symphysiotomy: Has significant risk of lower urinary tract injury.

Avoid Maneuvers that can Increase the Risk of Brachial Plexus Injuries

- Downward lateral flexion of the head was associated with a 30% increase in brachial plexus stretch as compared with axial positioning of the head (91).
- Fundal pressure can worsen the impaction of the shoulder.
- Traction combined with fundal pressure can cause neurologic complications.

flexors (82). It should be suspected in newborns with absent wrist and digital extension but intact deltoid, biceps, and triceps function (92). It is usually due to intrauterine compression of the radial nerve. Presence of ecchymosis or fat necrosis along the posterolateral arm suggests compression of the nerve in the region of the spiral (radial) groove. Prognosis is good; most infants have complete spontaneous recovery (82,92).

KEY POINTS

- Hypoxic–ischemic encephalopathy is a subgroup of neonatal encephalopathy affecting 1.5/1,000 live births.
- Hypoxic–ischemic insult in the newborn has a biphasic course, with immediate neuronal death, followed by a delayed secondary phase of injury. There is a latent period of at least 6 hours from the initial insult, providing a window of opportunity for neuroprotective interventions that can improve the neurodevelopmental outcome.
- Hypothermia instituted within 6 hours after birth in the term or near term newborn and maintained for 48 to 72 hours is effective in improving the neurodevelopmental outcome at 18 months.
- The xanthine-oxidase inhibitor allopurinol may be beneficial in reducing the severity of secondary ischemic damage if administered within 2 hours and continued for 3 days after birth. The benefits of allopurinol administration to the mothers with signs of fetal ischemia are being investigated.
- Available evidence suggests that magnesium sulfate given before anticipated early preterm birth decreases the risk of cerebral palsy in surviving infants.
- Erythropoietin may improve the neurodevelopmental outcome of infants with moderate hypoxic–ischemic encephalopathy.

- Instrumental vaginal delivery, macrosomia, prematurity, abnormal fetal presentation, prolonged labor, and precipitous deliveries are risk factors for mechanical neurologic neonatal injuries. Some injuries occur in the absence of identifiable risk factors.
- Head injuries—extracranial, cranial, or intracranial—depending on the severity, may cause neurologic deficits. Treatment is either conservative management or surgical intervention.
- Peripheral nerve injuries associated with delivery can involve the facial nerve, the brachial plexus, and rarely the radial nerve. Most of the injuries have good prognosis, with spontaneous recovery within weeks to months. Severe brachial plexus injuries may require surgical intervention.
- Neonatal injuries can be prevented to some extent by appropriate antepartum and intrapartum fetal surveillance and management. However, many injuries may be difficult to prevent.

REFERENCES

1. Nelson KB, Leviton A. How much of neonatal encephalopathy is due to birth asphyxia? *Am J Dis Child* 1991;145(11):1325–1331.
2. Kurinczuk JJ, White-Koning M, Badawi N. Epidemiology of neonatal encephalopathy and hypoxic-ischaemic encephalopathy. *Early Hum Dev* 2010;86(6):329–338.
3. Sarnat HB, Sarnat MS. Neonatal encephalopathy following fetal distress. A clinical and electroencephalographic study. *Arch Neurol* 1976;33(10):696–705.
4. Williams CE, Gunn A, Gluckman PD. Time course of intracellular edema and epileptiform activity following prenatal cerebral ischemia in sheep. *Stroke* 1991;22(4):516–521.
5. Perlman JM. Intervention strategies for neonatal hypoxic-ischemic cerebral injury. *Clin Ther* 2006;28(9):1353–1365.
6. Volpe JJ. Perinatal brain injury: from pathogenesis to neuroprotection. *Ment Retard Dev Disabil Res Rev* 2001;7(1):56–64.
7. Grow J, Barks JD. Pathogenesis of hypoxic-ischemic cerebral injury in the term infant: current concepts. *Clin Perinatol* 2002;29(4):585–602, v.

8. Penrice J, Cady EB, Lorek A, et al. Proton magnetic resonance spectroscopy of the brain in normal preterm and term infants, and early changes after perinatal hypoxia-ischemia. *Pediatr Res* 1996;40(1):6–14.

9. Inder TE, Volpe JJ. Mechanisms of perinatal brain injury. *Semin Neonatol* 2000;5(1):3–16.

10. Gluckman PD, Williams CE. When and why do brain cells die? *Dev Med Child Neurol* 1992;34(11):1010–1014.

11. Lorek A, Takei Y, Cady EB, et al. Delayed ("secondary") cerebral energy failure after acute hypoxia-ischemia in the newborn piglet: continuous 48-hour studies by phosphorus magnetic resonance spectroscopy. *Pediatr Res* 1994;36(6): 699–706.

12. Bona E, Andersson AL, Blomgren K, et al. Chemokine and inflammatory cell response to hypoxia-ischemia in immature rats. *Pediatr Res* 1999;45(4 Pt 1): 500–509.

13. Hagberg H, Gilland E, Bona E, et al. Enhanced expression of interleukin (IL)-1 and IL-6 messenger RNA and bioactive protein after hypoxia-ischemia in neonatal rats. *Pediatr Res* 1996;40(4):603–609.

14. Roth SC, Baudin J, Cady E, et al. Relation of deranged neonatal cerebral oxidative metabolism with neurodevelopmental outcome and head circumference at 4 years. *Dev Med Child Neurol* 1997;39(11):718–725.

15. Rutherford M, Biarge MM, Allsop J, et al. MRI of perinatal brain injury. *Pediatr Radiol* 2010;40(6):819–833.

16. van Wezel-Meijler G, Steggerda SJ, Leijser LM. Cranial ultrasonography in neonates: role and limitations. *Semin Perinatol* 2010;34(1):28–38.

17. Lin ZL, Yu HM, Lin J, et al. Mild hypothermia via selective head cooling as neuroprotective therapy in term neonates with perinatal asphyxia: an experience from a single neonatal intensive care unit. *J Perinatol* 2006;26(3): 180–184.

18. Toet MC, van Rooij LG, de Vries LS. The use of amplitude integrated electroencephalography for assessing neonatal neurologic injury. *Clin Perinatol* 2008;35(4):665–678, v.

19. Salhab WA, Wyckoff MH, Laptook AR, et al. Initial hypoglycemia and neonatal brain injury in term infants with severe fetal acidemia. *Pediatrics* 2004; 114(2):361–366.

20. Payne RS, Tseng MT, Schurr A. The glucose paradox of cerebral ischemia: evidence for corticosterone involvement. *Brain Res* 2003;971(1):9–17.

21. Dzhala V, Ben-Ari Y, Khazipov R. Seizures accelerate anoxia-induced neuronal death in the neonatal rat hippocampus. *Ann Neurol* 2000;48(4):632–640.

22. Holmes GL, Gairsa JL, Chevassus-Au-Louis N, et al. Consequences of neonatal seizures in the rat: morphological and behavioral effects. *Ann Neurol* 1998;44(6):845–857.

23. Gunn AJ, Hoehn T, Hansmann G, et al. Hypothermia: an evolving treatment for neonatal hypoxic ischemic encephalopathy. *Pediatrics* 2008;121(3): 648–649; author reply 649–650.

24. Miller JA Jr., Miller FS, Westin B. Hypothermia in the treatment of asphyxia neonatorum. *Biol Neonat* 1964;6:148–163.

25. Westin B, Miller JA Jr., Nyberg R, et al. Neonatal asphyxia pallida treated with hypothermia alone or with hypothermia and transfusion of oxygenated blood. *Surgery* 1959;45(5):868–879.

26. Cordey R. Hypothermia in resuscitating newborns in white asphyxia; a report of 14 cases. *Obstet Gynecol* 1964;24:760–767.

27. Laptook AR, Corbett RJ. The effects of temperature on hypoxic-ischemic brain injury. *Clin Perinatol* 2002;29(4):623–649, vi.

28. Safar PJ, Kochanek PM. Therapeutic hypothermia after cardiac arrest. *N Engl J Med* 2002;346(8):612–613.

29. Gunn AJ, Gluckman PD, Gunn TR. Selective head cooling in newborn infants after perinatal asphyxia: a safety study. *Pediatrics* 1998;102(4 Pt 1): 885–892.

30. Battin MR, Dezoete JA, Gunn TR, et al. Neurodevelopmental outcome of infants treated with head cooling and mild hypothermia after perinatal asphyxia. *Pediatrics* 2001;107(3):480–484.

31. Battin MR, Penrice J, Gunn TR, et al. Treatment of term infants with head cooling and mild systemic hypothermia (35.0 degrees C and 34.5 degrees C) after perinatal asphyxia. *Pediatrics* 2003;111(2):244–251.

32. Battin MR, Thoresen M, Robinson E, et al. Does head cooling with mild systemic hypothermia affect requirement for blood pressure support? *Pediatrics* 2009;123(3):1031–1036.

33. Gluckman PD, Wyatt JS, Azzopardi D, et al. Selective head cooling with mild systemic hypothermia after neonatal encephalopathy: multicentre randomised trial. *Lancet* 2005;365(9460):663–670.

34. Wyatt JS, Gluckman PD, Liu PY, et al. Determinants of outcomes after head cooling for neonatal encephalopathy. *Pediatrics* 2007;119(5):912–921.

35. Inder TE, Hunt RW, Morley CJ, et al. Randomized trial of systemic hypothermia selectively protects the cortex on MRI in term hypoxic-ischemic encephalopathy. *J Pediatr* 2004;145(6):835–837.

36. Azzopardi DV, Strohm B, Edwards AD, et al. Moderate hypothermia to treat perinatal asphyxial encephalopathy. *N Engl J Med* 2009;361(14):1349–1358.

37. Simbruner G, Mittal RA, Rohlmann F, et al. Systemic hypothermia after neonatal encephalopathy: outcomes of neo.nEURO.network RCT. *Pediatrics* 2010;126(4):e771–e778.

38. Eicher DJ, Wagner CL, Katikaneni LP, et al. Moderate hypothermia in neonatal encephalopathy: safety outcomes. *Pediatr Neurol* 2005;32(1):18–24.

39. Zhou WH, Cheng GQ, Shao XM, et al. Selective head cooling with mild systemic hypothermia after neonatal hypoxic-ischemic encephalopathy: a multicenter randomized controlled trial in China. *J Pediatr* 2010;157(3): 367–372.

40. Shankaran S, Laptook A, Wright LL, et al. Whole-body hypothermia for neonatal encephalopathy: animal observations as a basis for a randomized, controlled pilot study in term infants. *Pediatrics* 2002;110(2 Pt 1):377–385.

41. Shankaran S, Laptook AR, Ehrenkranz RA, et al. Whole-body hypothermia for neonates with hypoxic-ischemic encephalopathy. *N Engl J Med* 2005; 353(15):1574–1584.

42. Shankaran S, Pappas A, Laptook AR, et al. Outcomes of safety and effectiveness in a multicenter randomized, controlled trial of whole-body hypothermia for neonatal hypoxic-ischemic encephalopathy. *Pediatrics* 2008;122(4): e791–e798.

43. Edwards AD, Brocklehurst P, Gunn AJ, et al. Neurological outcomes at 18 months of age after moderate hypothermia for perinatal hypoxic ischaemic encephalopathy: synthesis and meta-analysis of trial data. *BMJ* 2010; 340:c363.

44. Kaandorp JJ, Benders MJ, Rademaker CM, et al. Antenatal allopurinol for reduction of birth asphyxia induced brain damage (ALLO-Trial); a randomized double blind placebo controlled multicenter study. *BMC Pregnancy Childbirth* 2010;10:8.

45. Van Bel F, Shadid M, Moison RM, et al. Effect of allopurinol on postasphyxial free radical formation, cerebral hemodynamics, and electrical brain activity. *Pediatrics* 1998;101(2):185–193.

46. Benders MJ, Bos AF, Rademaker CM, et al. Early postnatal allopurinol does not improve short term outcome after severe birth asphyxia. *Arch Dis Child Fetal Neonatal Ed* 2006;91(3):F163–F165.

47. Gunes T, Ozturk MA, Koklu E, et al. Effect of allopurinol supplementation on nitric oxide levels in asphyxiated newborns. *Pediatr Neurol* 2007;36(1): 17–24.

48. Torrance HL, Benders MJ, Derks JB, et al. Maternal allopurinol during fetal hypoxia lowers cord blood levels of the brain injury marker S-100B. *Pediatrics* 2009;124(1):350–357.

49. Aly H, Abd-Rabboh L, El-Dib M, et al. Ascorbic acid combined with ibuprofen in hypoxic ischemic encephalopathy: a randomized controlled trial. *J Perinatol* 2009;29(6):438–443.

50. Cahill AG, Stout MJ, Caughey AB. Intrapartum magnesium for prevention of cerebral palsy: continuing controversy? *Curr Opin Obstet Gynecol* 2010;22(2):122–127.

51. Nelson KB, Grether JK. Can magnesium sulfate reduce the risk of cerebral palsy in very low birthweight infants? *Pediatrics* 1995;95(2):263–269.

52. Schendel DE, Berg CJ, Yeargin-Allsopp M, et al. Prenatal magnesium sulfate exposure and the risk for cerebral palsy or mental retardation among very low-birth-weight children aged 3 to 5 years. *JAMA* 1996;276(22):1805–1810.

53. Mittendorf R, Covert R, Boman J, et al. Is tocolytic magnesium sulphate associated with increased total paediatric mortality? *Lancet* 1997;350(9090): 1517–1518.

54. Grether JK, Hoogstrate J, Selvin S, et al. Magnesium sulfate tocolysis and risk of neonatal death. *Am J Obstet Gynecol* 1998;178(1 Pt 1):1–6.

55. Hirtz DG, Nelson K. Magnesium sulfate and cerebral palsy in premature infants. *Curr Opin Pediatr* 1998;10(2):131–137.

56. Marret S, Marpeau L, Zupan-Simunek V, et al. Magnesium sulphate given before very-preterm birth to protect infant brain: the randomised controlled PREMAG trial*. *BJOG* 2007;114(3):310–318.

57. Rouse DJ, Hirtz DG, Thom E, et al. A randomized, controlled trial of magnesium sulfate for the prevention of cerebral palsy. *N Engl J Med* 2008;359(9): 895–905.

58. Crowther CA, Hiller JE, Doyle LW, et al. Effect of magnesium sulfate given for neuroprotection before preterm birth: a randomized controlled trial. *JAMA* 2003;290(20):2669–2676.

59. Doyle LW, Crowther CA, Middleton P, et al. Magnesium sulphate for women at risk of preterm birth for neuroprotection of the fetus. *Cochrane Database Syst Rev* 2009;(1):CD004661.

60. Conde-Agudelo A, Romero R. Antenatal magnesium sulfate for the prevention of cerebral palsy in preterm infants less than 34 weeks' gestation: a systematic review and metaanalysis. *Am J Obstet Gynecol* 2009;200(6):595–609.

61. Costantine MM, Weiner SJ. Effects of antenatal exposure to magnesium sulfate on neuroprotection and mortality in preterm infants: a meta-analysis. *Obstet Gynecol* 2009;114(2 Pt 1):354–364.

62. Committee Opinion No. 455: Magnesium sulfate before anticipated preterm birth for neuroprotection. *Obstet Gynecol* 2010;115(3):669–671.

63. Levene MI, Gibson NA, Fenton AC, et al. The use of a calcium-channel blocker, nicardipine, for severely asphyxiated newborn infants. *Dev Med Child Neurol* 1990;32(7):567–574.

64. Zhu C, Kang W, Xu F, et al. Erythropoietin improved neurologic outcomes in newborns with hypoxic-ischemic encephalopathy. *Pediatrics* 2009;124(2):e218–e226.

65. McPherson RJ, Juul SE. Recent trends in erythropoietin-mediated neuroprotection. *Int J Dev Neurosci* 2008;26(1):103–111.

66. McPherson RJ, Juul SE. Erythropoietin for infants with hypoxic-ischemic encephalopathy. *Curr Opin Pediatr* 2010;22(2):139–145.

67. Bierer R, Peceny MC, Hartenberger CH, et al. Erythropoietin concentrations and neurodevelopmental outcome in preterm infants. *Pediatrics* 2006; 118(3):e635–e640.

68. Brown MS, Eichorst D, Lala-Black B, et al. Higher cumulative doses of erythropoietin and developmental outcomes in preterm infants. *Pediatrics* 2009; 124(4):e681–e687.

69. Neubauer AP, Voss W, Wachtendorf M, et al. Erythropoietin improves neurodevelopmental outcome of extremely preterm infants. *Ann Neurol* 2010;67(5): 657–666.

70. Ohls RK, Ehrenkranz RA, Das A, et al. Neurodevelopmental outcome and growth at 18 to 22 months' corrected age in extremely low birth weight infants treated with early erythropoietin and iron. *Pediatrics* 2004;114(5): 1287–1291.

71. Doumouchtsis SK, Arulkumaran S. Head injuries after instrumental vaginal deliveries. *Curr Opin Obstet Gynecol* 2006;18(2):129–134.

72. Doumouchtsis SK, Arulkumaran S. Head trauma after instrumental births. *Clin Perinatol* 2008;35(1):69–83, viii.

73. Towner DR, Ciotti MC. Operative vaginal delivery: a cause of birth injury or is it? *Clin Obstet Gynecol* 2007;50(3):563–581.

74. Amar AP, Aryan HE, Meltzer HS, et al. Neonatal subgaleal hematoma causing brain compression: report of two cases and review of the literature. *Neurosurgery* 2003;52(6):1470–1474; discussion 1474.

75. Ng PC, Siu YK, Lewindon PJ. Subaponeurotic haemorrhage in the 1990s: a 3-year surveillance. *Acta Paediatr* 1995;84(9):1065–1069.

76. Nguyen CS, Chase DM, Wing DA. Severe fetal skull fracture and death subsequent to a motor vehicle crash with frontal airbag deployment. *J Trauma* 2009;67(6):E220–E221.

77. Morgan JA, Marcus PS. Prenatal diagnosis and management of intrauterine fracture. *Obstet Gynecol Surv* 2010;65(4):249–259.

78. Gallo P, Mazza C, Sala F. Intrauterine head stab wound injury resulting in a growing skull fracture: a case report and literature review. *Childs Nerv Syst* 2010;26(3):377–384.

79. Simonson C, Barlow P, Dehennin N, et al. Neonatal complications of vacuum-assisted delivery. *Obstet Gynecol* 2007;109(3):626–633.

80. Gupta SN, Kechli AM, Kanamalla US. Intracranial hemorrhage in term newborns: management and outcomes. *Pediatr Neurol* 2009;40(1):1–12.

81. Uhing MR. Management of birth injuries. *Clin Perinatol* 2005;32(1):19–38, v.

82. Hayman M, Roland EH, Hill A. Newborn radial nerve palsy: report of four cases and review of published reports. *Pediatr Neurol* 1999;21(3): 648–651.

83. Foad SL, Mehlman CT, Ying J. The epidemiology of neonatal brachial plexus palsy in the United States. *J Bone Joint Surg Am* 2008;90(6):1258–1264.

84. Hale HB, Bae DS, Waters PM. Current concepts in the management of brachial plexus birth palsy. *J Hand Surg Am* 2010;35(2):322–331.

85. Doumouchtsis SK, Arulkumaran S. Is it possible to reduce obstetrical brachial plexus palsy by optimal management of shoulder dystocia? *Ann N Y Acad Sci* 2010;1205:135–143.

86. Doumouchtsis SK, Arulkumaran S. Are all brachial plexus injuries caused by shoulder dystocia? *Obstet Gynecol Surv* 2009;64(9):615–623.

87. Gherman RB, Ouzounian JG, Miller DA, et al. Spontaneous vaginal delivery: a risk factor for Erb's palsy? *Am J Obstet Gynecol* 1998;178(3):423–427.

88. Irion O, Boulvain M. Induction of labour for suspected fetal macrosomia. *Cochrane Database Syst Rev* 2000(2):CD000938.

89. Yeo GS, Lim YW, Yeong CT, et al. An analysis of risk factors for the prediction of shoulder dystocia in 16,471 consecutive births. *Ann Acad Med Singapore* 1995;24(6):836–840.

90. Gilbert WM, Nesbitt TS, Danielsen B. Associated factors in 1611 cases of brachial plexus injury. *Obstet Gynecol* 1999;93(4):536–540.

91. Gonik B, Zhang N, Grimm MJ. Prediction of brachial plexus stretching during shoulder dystocia using a computer simulation model. *Am J Obstet Gynecol* 2003;189(4):1168–1172.

92. Monica JT, Waters PM, Bae DS. Radial nerve palsy in the newborn: a report of four cases and literature review. *J Pediatr Orthop* 2008;28(4):460–462.

ANESTHETIC CONSIDERATIONS AND MANAGEMENT OF OBSTETRIC COMPLICATIONS

Abnormal Fetal Positions, Breech Presentations, Shoulder Dystocia, and Multiple Gestation

Thomas A. Gough • Paul Howell

■ INTRODUCTION

Abnormal positions and presentations of the fetus and multiple gestation pregnancies are all associated with an increased risk of complications for both mother and child (1) and their management represents a significant challenge for the obstetrical care providers and anesthesiologist. A team-based approach with clear communication between team members is vital for a successful outcome and as such the anesthesiologist should have a good understanding of the anatomical and physiologic features of these issues.

When describing the orientation of the fetus within the uterus there are three variables to consider: Lie, presentation and position. The *Lie* refers to the long axis of the fetus with regard to the long axis of the uterus. This can be longitudinal, transverse or oblique.

The *Presentation* refers to the part of the fetus that overlies the pelvic inlet and this can normally be palpated through the cervix on vaginal examination. The presentation can be cephalic, breech or shoulder and cephalic is further divided into vertex, brow or face. The normal presentation is vertex and the term *malpresentation* describes any non-vertex presentation.

The *Position* of the fetus describes the relationship between a bony prominence on the presenting part and the maternal pelvis. For vertex presentations this is the occiput, for face the mentum, for breech the sacrum, and for shoulder presentations the acromion.

The majority of singleton deliveries are vertex presentation, occipitoanterior (OA) position, and all other positions or presentations are considered to be abnormal. It is these pregnancies that will be discussed in the following chapter.

■ ABNORMAL FETAL POSITIONS

Occipitoposterior

The incidence of persistent occipitoposterior (OP) is about 5.5% in all women, with it being more common in nulliparas than multiparas (7.2% vs. 4.0%) (2). The mechanism by which it occurs is either by failure to rotate from an initially posterior or transverse position or malrotation from an initially OA position (3,4). The OP position commonly leads to a prolonged labor that is associated with a significantly higher degree of maternal discomfort. Since the fetal head is not ideally fitted to the pelvis, there is slower descent and a delay in cervical dilation. There is increased pressure on the posterior sacral nerves that can result in severe back pain—a common complaint of women undergoing labor with a fetus in the OP position.

Many observational studies have demonstrated an association between the use of epidural analgesia and persistent OP position (2,5,6). However, it was unclear if this association represented a direct causative effect or was a result of an increased request for epidural analgesia in prolonged and more painful labors. Lieberman et al. (7) concluded in a prospective cohort study that epidurals did directly influence position at delivery. In their study of 1,562 women, they examined fetal head position by ultrasound at various stages of labor. While there was no difference in OP position at enrolment between those women who underwent an epidural (92% of study population) and those who did not (23.4% vs. 26.0%), at delivery the epidural group were 4 times more likely to be persistently OP (12.9% vs. 3.3%). From this the authors contended that epidural analgesia was contributing to an increased incidence of persistent OP position at delivery but stopped short of claiming causality. Interestingly, Fitzpatrick et al. (6) concluded the opposite as in their institution the incidence of OP position has declined over a 25-year period in which the epidural rate has risen from 3% to 47%, and intrapartum management has otherwise remained the same. Debate therefore remains as to the precise nature of the association between epidurals and OP position but that it exists is incontrovertible.

Obstetric Management

Persistent OP position can be considered to be a high-risk labor in that the likelihood of cesarean delivery or instrumental delivery is greater than the normal OA position. In fact, while they make up 5.5% of all laboring women, they account for 12% of all cesarean deliveries undertaken for dystocia (6). Persistent posterior positions are also associated with an increased incidence of premature rupture of the membranes, augmentation, episiotomies, vaginal lacerations, hemorrhage, and third or fourth degree tears (2,6). Traditionally, obstetricians attempted to rotate the fetus to an OA position prior to delivery, either manually or using forceps. This technique has become increasingly unpopular as it has been associated with increased maternal and fetal trauma, and more junior obstetricians have less experience and confidence in the use of high rotational forceps (e.g., Kielland's). Instead, the obstetrician now is more likely to allow the labor to progress and deliver the baby in the OP position if rotation to OA does not occur naturally. Spontaneous vaginal delivery in this manner has been shown to be successful in up to a third of nulliparous women and 55% of multiparas (6).

Anesthetic Management

Owing to the often prolonged and exaggerated pain that women undergo and despite the debate noted above, the OP position remains a common indication for regional analgesia in labor. As has previously been noted, low back pain is a particular problem and care should be taken that the block covers the sacral roots. This requires a careful assessment of the dermatomal spread although it should be noted that it may take several top-ups if using an intermittent maintenance technique or several hours if using a continuous infusion. It is generally accepted that the use of a CSE technique results in a faster onset of analgesia than the normal extradural approach and may also give an earlier sacral block. Despite a recent Cochrane review concluding that there was no overall benefit to offering CSE over normal low dose epidurals in labor (8), it might be suggested that its use would be suitable for labor analgesia in OP pregnancies. However, as yet there is no randomized controlled trial to support this view. Some women never gain full relief from the sacral ache and low back pain of the OP position with the usual low dose epidural mixtures of local anesthetic and opioid despite an apparently good sensory block, and these women may need stronger concentrations of local anesthetic agents.

The widespread use of low dose local anesthetic solutions has reduced the amount of motor block seen with modern labor epidurals (9). If the position of the vertex is initially OP, profound relaxation of the pelvic floor muscles and perineum may prevent spontaneous rotation to a normal OA position or allow malrotation of an initially OA fetus to the OP position. However, during an instrumental delivery it may be necessary to assist the obstetrician by intentionally relaxing the pelvic floor to allow for easier placement of forceps or ventouse cup, reducing the risk of vaginal injury (and trauma to the fetal head). This can be achieved by increasing the density of the block with a strong solution of local anesthetic such as 2% or 3% 2-chloroprocaine, 2% lidocaine (with or without adjuvants), 0.5% bupivacaine or levobupivacaine, or 0.75% ropivacaine depending on the urgency and individual preference.

Face and Brow Presentation

In a face presentation, the fetal head and neck are hyperextended with the occiput resting on the upper back. The presenting part is thus the face between the orbital ridges and the mentum. It occurs in approximately 1 in 500 to 600 births and is associated with prematurity, low birth weight, fetal malformations, cephalopelvic disproportion and polyhydramnios (10,11). The mentum can be anterior, transverse, or posterior. A vaginal delivery is generally only possible when the mentum is anterior and this occurs in 60% to 80% of cases. In 10% to 12% of cases the mentum is transverse and these usually rotate to the anterior position spontaneously as labor progresses. In the 20% to 25% of cases that present in the posterior position, about a third convert to anterior on their own. The overall cesarean delivery rate for face presentation is about 15% (12). Attempts to manually rotate the fetus to a more favorable position are rarely successful and are associated with a high perinatal mortality and maternal morbidity; hence this practice has fallen out of favor.

In a brow presentation, the fetal head is midway between full flexion (vertex) and hyperextension (face). The presenting part is the fetal head between the orbital ridge and the anterior fontanelle. It occurs in about 1 in 1,500 deliveries and it is associated with much the same factors as a face presentation. During labor, a brow presentation can progress in one of the three ways. It can convert spontaneously to either a face or vertex presentation, or it can be persistent. Expectant management for labor is therefore reasonable to allow for conversion to a more favorable presentation, but if it remains persistent then dystocia is common and cesarean delivery is the usual outcome.

Shoulder Presentation

This occurs during a transverse lie (when the vertebral column lies perpendicular to that of the mother) or an oblique lie (where there is deviation of the fetal axis toward one or other iliac fossa). It may be successfully converted to a vertex presentation by external cephalic version (ECV) but if this fails then a cesarean delivery is mandatory. The exception to this rule is when a second twin is in a transverse lie following vaginal delivery of the first twin. In this scenario, the obstetrician may attempt internal podalic version, rotating the fetus to a breech presentation and then extracting the fetus manually.

■ BREECH PRESENTATION

The term breech is derived from the Old English word "brec" meaning buttocks or breeches and describes the presenting part in relation to the pelvic inlet, i.e., the buttocks. There are three main types of breech presentation (Fig. 18-1):

1. **Frank:** The fetus' legs are flexed at the hip and extended at the knees. The buttocks are the presenting part.
2. **Complete:** The fetus' legs are flexed at the hip and knees with feet beside the buttocks, which are the presenting part.
3. **Incomplete:** One of both of the fetus' feet (footling breech) or knees (kneeling breech) presents lower than the buttocks (i.e., one or both hips are extended).

The type of breech can typically be determined by ultrasonography (13) that also allows the obstetrician to exclude

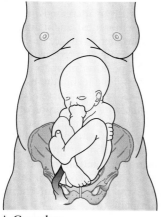
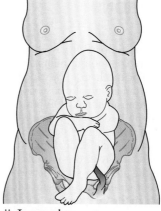
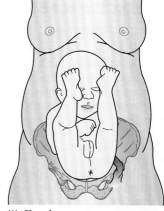

FIGURE 18-1 Types of breech presentation.

i. Complete   ii. Incomplete   iii. Frank

TABLE 18-1 Factors Associated with Breech Presentation

Maternal Factors Associated With Breech Presentation	Fetal Factors Associated With Breech Presentation
Uterine distension or relaxation • Grand multiparity • Multiple gestation • Polyhydramnios Uterine abnormalities • Pelvic tumors (malignant and benign) • Uterine anomalies Obstetric conditions • Previous breech • Oligohydramnios • Placenta previa Non-obstetric conditions • Advanced age • Maternal diabetes • Smoking	Congenital fetal anomalies • Anencephaly • Hydrocephaly Low birth weight • Intrauterine growth retardation • Preterm delivery

Adapted from: references 13–15.

severe congenital abnormalities. This may influence the obstetrician's choice as to mode of delivery. A fetus with a frank breech presentation at term invariably remains so but a complete breech presentation may change to an incomplete breech presentation at any point before or during labor which requires the obstetrician to manage the delivery with the presentation of one or both legs (14).

Epidemiology

The incidence of breech presentation in singleton pregnancies is between 20% and 40% at 28 weeks, decreasing to 3% to 4% at term (15,16). The process by which this occurs appears to be an active one with a normal and mobile fetus adopting a position of best fit within a normal uterus. There are a number of factors that can interfere with this, both maternal and fetal, and they are associated with an increased risk of breech presentation at term. They are summarized in (Table 18-1) (16–18).

Mortality and Morbidity—for Mother and Baby

Fetuses presenting in the breech position have a higher incidence of perinatal mortality and morbidity than those presenting normally, even when adjusted for preterm delivery (1). This is due not only to those factors that predispose to breech delivery but also to the mechanical conditions that may lead to fetal hypoxia and brain injury. Congenital fetal anomalies such as anencephaly or hydrocephaly are a significant cause of immediate fetal death or long-term neurologic sequelae. Maternal conditions such as placenta previa, uterine anomalies or advanced age may also place the newborn at increased risk. With regard to fetal hypoxia during breech delivery there are several ways in which this may occur:

1. Umbilical cord—due to a reduced distance between the umbilical cord insertion point and the fetal body part lowest in the birth canal (when compared to a vertex presentation), breech deliveries are more at risk of pressure on the cord as the fetal pelvis moves downward. This can lead to fetal hypoxia unless there is rapid delivery of the fetal vertex. However, as the vertex is the largest part of

the fetus and often needs time to mould to the shape of the maternal pelvis in order to fit, this can be delayed. This condition is known as **fetal head entrapment** and requires immediate delivery often via cesarean delivery to prevent worsening fetal hypoxia and brain injury. The risk is higher in preterm infants as in these cases the cervix does not always dilate fully and while the legs and shoulders may pass through an incompletely dilated cervix, the head is much more at risk of entrapment (19). Umbilical cord prolapse is another rare but potentially fatal complication, particularly with incomplete breech delivery (20). In this case, the presenting part does not fill the cervix as effectively as in other types of breech presentation (or vertex), which allows the umbilical cord to drop below and prolapse through the cervix into the vagina. Subsequent pressure on the cord or vasospasm can cause fetal hypoxia. This may result in an abnormal fetal heart trace including bradycardia or variable decelerations prompting emergency cesarean delivery.

2. Placenta—owing to an often-protracted second stage of labor (21), there can be a significant reduction in placental perfusion during contractions. During vertex delivery, by the time of delivery of the head and manual extraction, the uterine volume has decreased by one-third (uterine retraction) with concomitant decrease in the uteroplacental exchange unit (22). During breech delivery, a similar stage occurs after delivery of the scapulae (when manual extraction can begin), and by this time the uterine volume has decreased by two-thirds with a correspondingly greater decrease in the uteroplacental exchange unit (23).

The fetus is at risk of complications relating to trauma during delivery. This is not wholly confined to vaginal delivery as access can be more difficult in cesarean delivery for breech delivery. These traumatic complications include general birth trauma (particularly from the use of instruments), hyperextension of head, and spinal cord injuries with deflexion (18).

Maternal morbidity and mortality is also increased with breech presentation. When compared with vertex presentation there are higher rates of perineal trauma particularly if forceps are used, maternal hemorrhage, and infection (19,20,24). The use of forceps may also be associated with direct physical or neurologic injury to the muscles of the pelvic floor resulting in urinary and fecal incontinence, pelvic organ prolapse and dyspareunia (19). These risks are not entirely avoided through abdominal delivery as cesarean delivery is also associated with incontinence, hemorrhage, longer hospital stay and thromboembolic disease (19).

Obstetric Management

There are essentially three avenues of intervention for obstetricians confronted by a breech presentation. Firstly, they may attempt to convert the fetus to a vertex presentation via the process of ECV, which if successful potentially avoids the risk of breech delivery. Secondly, they may attempt to deliver the fetus vaginally, or thirdly they may perform a cesarean delivery to deliver the fetus. This may be either planned or as an emergency.

External Cephalic Version (ECV) for Breech Presentation

ECV involves the manipulation of the fetus through the maternal abdominal wall in order to rotate it from a breech to a vertex presentation. The success rate of ECV is between 30% and 85% (25–28) but there are many factors that influence the outcome. These include race, parity, uterine tone, amniotic fluid volume, engagement of the breech and whether the head is palpable, and the use of tocolysis (27–30). Tocolytics used include terbutaline, ritodrine, and salbutamol.

The aim of ECV is to reduce the adverse outcomes associated with breech delivery. A Cochrane review on ECV at term showed that there was a statistically significant reduction in non-cephalic birth (five trials, 433 women; relative risk (RR) 0.38, 95% confidence interval (CI): 0.18–0.80) and cesarean delivery (five trials, 433 women; RR 0.55, 95% CI: 0.33–0.91) when ECV was attempted (31). The timing of ECV is also a potential factor in outcome. It has been suggested that ECV before term (34 to 35 weeks' gestation) may be associated with a greater reduction in non-cephalic births when compared to ECV at term (32). This was investigated in the Early ECV 2 Trial (33) which determined that while there was an increased reduction in non-cephalic presentation at birth when compared to ECV at term, there was no reduction in the rate of cesarean delivery and that there may be an increase in preterm births (this association did not reach statistical significance).

ECV is a safe procedure with a very low complication rate (34,35). However, there are case reports of placental abruption, uterine rupture and feto-maternal hemorrhage. The incidence of immediate emergency cesarean delivery is estimated at around 0.5% (34,35).

Pain and discomfort can be considerable during ECV and is associated with a lower chance of success (36). However, it has also been considered a marker for potential complications and thus there has been reluctance amongst obstetricians for regional anesthesia to be undertaken for fear of masking warning signs that a complication has occurred. More recently though, there has been increased interest in the use of regional analgesia or anesthesia in order to facilitate ECV. Schorr et al. assigned 35 women to receive an epidural (2% lidocaine with epinephrine) and 34 to no epidural prior to ECV (37). They demonstrated a better success rate in the epidural group (67% vs. 32%, RR 2.1, CI: 1.2–3.6). Mancuso et al. also assigned 108 women equally between epidural (2% lidocaine with fentanyl) and control groups (38). They reported a higher success rate in the epidural group (59% vs. 33%, RR 1.8, CI: 1.2–2.8). In 2010, Weiniger et al. (39) replicated the findings of their own previous study. They demonstrated a higher success rate for regional anesthesia when they assigned 64 women equally between spinal anesthesia (7.5 mg bupivacaine) and control groups (87% vs. 57.5%, P = 0.009; 95% CI: 0.075–0.48). It is interesting to note the relatively high success rate in the control group as this had been a criticism of previous studies, i.e., that a success rate in the control group of 30% to 35% did not adequately reflect normal practice. A number of other studies have also demonstrated that in those women who have previously undergone unsuccessful ECV, the subsequent use of neuraxial anesthesia can result in a successful outcome with success rates ranging from 39.7% to 89% (40–42).

As the published evidence is conflicted with respect to benefit from using neuraxial block for ECV (43–45), a meta-analysis was published in 2010 to review the evidence to date (46). The authors demonstrated that the main difference between the studies was in dose and not technique. They found that if an anesthetic dose was used in the study group the outcome was a statistically significant endorsement of neuraxial block but if an analgesic dose was used then no benefit was found. They also found that apart from maternal hypotension, the incidence of serious adverse events during ECV was unaffected by neuraxial block. It should be noted, however, that given the relatively low incidence of serious adverse events, none of the studies individually were adequately powered to detect statistically significant differences in complication rates.

Currently, there is something of a transatlantic divide in opinion about the use of regional techniques for ECV, being much more common in North America than in the United Kingdom, where neuraxial block is not routinely offered for ECV. However, the increasing body of evidence to support its use suggests another area in which the anesthesiologist may have a role in improving the experience and outcome for women with breech presentations.

Mode of Delivery of Breech Presentation

Probably one of the most contentious areas in the obstetric management of breech presentation is the mode of delivery. In 2000, the TERM breech trial was published in the Lancet (47). A large, multicentre, randomized controlled trial, it compared maternal and fetal outcomes of vaginal breech delivery versus planned cesarean delivery and included data from 2,083 women in 26 countries. The most significant finding was an incidence of neonatal mortality or serious morbidity of 1.6% in the planned cesarean group compared to 5% in the planned vaginal delivery group. This difference was even more marked among countries with a low perinatal mortality rate (UK, USA, Canada). There was no difference in maternal outcomes between the two groups. Following the publication of this study, the rate of cesarean delivery for breech presentation, which had already been rising, increased dramatically. In the United States, the cesarean delivery rate for breech was 11.6% (24) in 1970; by 2001 this had risen to 86.2% (48). A study from the Netherlands directly examined the impact that the TERM breech trial had on the national cesarean delivery rate for breech presentation and found an increase from 50% to 80% in just 2 months following the publication date (49). The American College of Obstetricians and Gynecologists (ACOG) were so moved by the data that in 2001 they amended their recommendation on mode of delivery saying "Patients with a persistent breech presentation at term in a singleton gestation should undergo a planned cesarean delivery" (50).

However, as is common for headline studies, the acclaim was not universal. Many observers felt that flaws in the study, particularly with regard to selection criteria and the conduct of labor, led to a misleading result and that vaginal delivery for breech presentation was still a valid option for a defined group of women (19,51,52). Risk factors for adverse outcomes in vaginal breech delivery include hyperextension of the fetal neck, prolonged labor, the lack of an experienced clinician at delivery and extremes of fetal weight at term (<2,500 g and >4,000 g) (19). Those who favor vaginal delivery believe that by excluding the women who fall into these categories, it is possible to identify patients who are more likely to have a successful outcome and avoid the potential complications of cesarean delivery. It should be noted, however, that clinicians who are experienced in vaginal breech delivery are becoming increasingly rare as training opportunities become more limited in an obstetric climate that favors planned cesarean delivery for these women. Further support for the role of vaginal delivery comes from a 2-year follow-up study of the TERM breech trial. The investigators found that there was no difference in risk of death or neurodevelopmental abnormality at 2 years of age regardless of mode of delivery (53). Potentially this demonstrates that the increased risk of serious morbidity found in the vaginal delivery group in the original study does not lead to any long-term complications.

A rapprochement of sorts has been reached with the 2006 guidelines from ACOG that recommend the decision regarding mode of delivery should depend on the experience of the obstetrician and hospitals should have local protocols in place for the management of vaginal breech delivery (54). The Society of Obstetricians Gynecologists of Canada (SOGC) echoed this and issued a set of guidelines outlining who was suitable for vaginal breech birth and how it should be managed (55). However, it remains to be seen how many obstetricians in the future will be confident in managing vaginal breech delivery and planned cesarean delivery is likely to remain by far the most common mode of delivery.

Anesthetic Management of Breech Presentation

Labor Analgesia

In the past, the use of epidural analgesia in breech delivery has been associated with prolongation of the first stage of labor, as well as an increased operative delivery rate (56–58). This led to a feeling that breech presentation was a relative contraindication to epidural analgesia. However, these were retrospective, observational studies and they may only demonstrate that those women who undergo prolonged and thus more painful labor are more likely to request an epidural. In addition, many are older studies in which epidurals contained stronger local anesthetic solutions than is current practice. Furthermore, some of these studies have demonstrated an improved neonatal outcome associated with epidural use (57–59), effectively making concerns over the duration of labor less persuasive. Currently, most authors consider that breech presentation is a strong indication for a labor epidural as it has a number of benefits:

1. Superior quality of pain relief.
2. Suppression of maternal desire to push early in the first stage of labor. If the patient pushes before the cervix is fully dilated, it increases the risk of both fetal head entrapment and umbilical cord prolapse. However, care must be taken during the second stage to ensure that the mother retains the ability to make adequate expulsive effort.
3. Relaxation of the pelvic floor to facilitate delivery toward the end of the second stage.
4. The option to extend the block to a surgical level. Breech vaginal delivery can rapidly progress to an emergent cesarean delivery and the presence of an anesthesiologist to either top up an epidural or provide general anesthesia for a "crash section" should be considered mandatory.

In the authors' institution, and across the United Kingdom, the commonest solution used to establish and maintain epidural blockade is 0.1% bupivacaine with 2 mcg/mL fentanyl (usually up to a maximum of 20 mL/h administered as bolus "top-ups"). The use of lower dose epidural mixtures or "mobile epidurals" has become well established in the developed world since the landmark Comparative Obstetric Mobile Epidural Trial (COMET) was published in The Lancet in 2001 (9). The authors of COMET demonstrated that when compared to traditional epidural analgesia (0.25% bupivacaine), low dose analgesia (0.1% bupivacaine and 2 mcg/mL fentanyl; either as a combined spinal–epidural [CSE] technique with bolus top-ups or continuous epidural infusion) reduced the number of instrumental deliveries while maintaining analgesic efficacy. The local anesthetic sparing effect of using opioids in epidural solutions had previously been documented (60,61), but the COMET trial demonstrated a clinical benefit as the normal vaginal delivery rate for both mobile epidural techniques was 43% compared to 35% for traditional epidural analgesia ($p = 0.04$). Better preservation of motor function during labor and delivery was thought to be the explanation.

Fetal Head Entrapment

In cases of fetal head entrapment, the experienced obstetrician may attempt Dührssen incisions, which are radial incisions in the cervix at 2, 6, and 10 o'clock. This is often technically difficult and associated with significant maternal hemorrhage. More commonly they may ask the anesthesiologist to provide cervical and uterine relaxation to assist the passage of the aftercoming head. Traditionally, this was achieved with general anesthesia and high concentration of inhalational anesthetic (minimum alveolar concentration of 2 to 3) as all the commonly used volatile agents inhibit uterine contractility in a dose dependent manner (62). However, this exposed the mother to the risks of an emergency general anesthetic.

A less invasive method is to use nitroglycerin, a potent relaxant of smooth muscle, either sublingually or intravenously. There are no large randomized controlled trials to support its use, although case studies have been published (63,64) that demonstrate both safety and efficacy. It has also been suggested that since the cervical tissue consists of only 15% smooth muscle, the role of nitroglycerin in relaxing the cervix is limited at best. Nonetheless, its use is widely accepted. Intravenous doses between 50 and 500 mcg have been suggested, although incremental doses of 50 to 100 mcg are the norm (65). Sublingually, a dose of one or two sprays (400 to 800 mcg) is commonly used. Given the practical aspects of drawing up nitroglycerin for intravenous administration when compared to the simplicity of the sublingual preparation during a potentially challenging period of obstetric management, it might be more practical to opt for the latter route as first line, especially in the absence of evidence to support one over the other. This will however depend on the formulation of nitroglycerin in individual institutions. It should be remembered, however, that the indication for uterine relaxation ends once the baby is delivered and thus uterotonic agents such as oxytocin and ergometrine should be readily at hand and administered as needed to prevent/treat uterine atony.

Cesarean Delivery

Anesthesia for cesarean delivery is covered more extensively elsewhere in this book, and the fundamental principles in breech presentation remain the same. A regional technique is preferable to avoid the risks of general anesthesia, but in some cases this may not be possible. The presence of an existing epidural may speed up the decision-to-incision time in emergency cesarean delivery and is another reason to support its use in parturients with known breech presentation attempting vaginal delivery. The choice of which local anesthetic solution to use for conversion of existing epidural blockade in labor to surgical anesthesia has been the subject of much debate.

When speed is of the essence, a local anesthetic that has a rapid onset of action is preferable. Chloroprocaine 3% has been demonstrated to have a faster onset of action than 1.5% lidocaine (66), although when compared to 2% lidocaine with epinephrine, the onset was similar (67). However, concerns were raised about its potential for neurotoxicity and although some believed that this was a result of the preservative sodium bisulfite, enough doubt remained that its use became less popular (68–70). With the advent of preservative free 3% chloroprocaine, it has become more widely used again, particularly in the United States.

More recently, work has been done comparing lidocaine combined with various adjuvants versus plain racemic bupivacaine or its S-enantiomer—levobupivacaine. A randomized comparison of 0.5% bupivacaine with 2% lidocaine/epinephrine/fentanyl demonstrated that although there was a more rapid median onset time with the lidocaine mixture (13.8 minutes vs. 17.5 minutes), this was not statistically significant and was offset by a longer preparation time (71). Another study demonstrated no difference in the time to surgical anesthesia when comparing plain 0.5% bupivacaine versus a 50:50 mixture of 0.5% bupivacaine/lidocaine 2% with 1:200,000 epinephrine and 2% lidocaine with 1:200,000 epinephrine (72). In contrast, when 2% lidocaine/epinephrine/fentanyl was compared to 0.5% levobupivacaine there was a statistically significant difference to the onset of the block, even with inclusion of the preparation time (73). Levobupivacaine is less cardiotoxic than racemic bupivacaine and therefore more commonly advocated for topping up a labor epidural for cesarean delivery, so this is potentially an important finding. Interestingly, when plain levobupivacaine was compared to a solution containing fentanyl, there was no difference in either speed of block or the quality of analgesia (74). This was attributed to the use of fentanyl-containing solutions for labor analgesia providing a near maximal opioid effect before topping up for section. Clinical experience of the authors also suggests that 15 mL of 0.75% ropivacaine is a rapidly effective solution for topping up a labor epidural in this situation.

Finally, the addition of bicarbonate has been demonstrated to have probably the greatest effect on the rapidity of the onset of the block. When compared to 0.5% levobupivacaine, a solution of lidocaine/bicarbonate/epinephrine halved the time to onset of block (75). Similarly, another group found that alkalinization improved the rapidity of onset when using 2% lidocaine with epinephrine and fentanyl (76), reducing the mean time to surgical anesthesia from 9.7 minutes to 5.2 minutes ($p < 0.001$). Care must be taken when interpreting these results as the definition of the onset of block is not uniform between trials; however, a solution containing 2% lidocaine, epinephrine, and sodium bicarbonate may offer the fastest time of onset even when the time taken to prepare the mixture is taken into consideration. Doubts about the stability of such a solution, especially if exposed to light, suggest it should not be made up in advance (77).

As with vaginal delivery, cesarean delivery for breech presentation is technically more demanding and the surgeon may occasionally request additional uterine relaxation. In the awake patient nitroglycerin can be used, although care must be taken to prevent or rapidly correct hypotension and reverse its tocolytic effects after delivery if necessary. In the patient undergoing general anesthesia, uterine relaxation may be provided by increasing the concentration of inhalational anesthetic to achieve an MAC of 2 to 3 (62). The pediatrician should however be made aware of this as a greater depth of anesthesia can result in a more depressed infant at delivery.

■ SHOULDER DYSTOCIA

ACOG defines shoulder dystocia as a "delivery that requires additional obstetric maneuvers following failure of gentle downward traction on the fetal head to effect delivery of the shoulders" (78). Some obstetricians use their own criteria to diagnose shoulder dystocia including the number of maneuvers required to release the shoulders, and this diagnostic spectrum is reflected in the published incidence which varies from 0.2% to 3% (79). It occurs as a result of disproportion between the bisacromial diameter of the fetus and the antero-posterior diameter of the pelvic inlet, the anterior shoulder of the fetus becoming impacted behind the symphysis pubis. Shoulder dystocia is an obstetric emergency that can result in serious complications for mother and baby. Trauma to the baby can cause lacerations, fractures of the humerus and clavicle and brachial plexus injury with significant neurologic sequelae. A prolonged head to shoulder delivery time can lead to hypoxia with cerebral palsy or death as potential consequences. The incidence of injury is about 20% in babies delivered with shoulder dystocia. For the mother the risks

include cervical lacerations, perineal trauma including third and fourth degree tears, and excessive hemorrhage, either from trauma or uterine atony.

Risk factors include previous shoulder dystocia, macrosomia, diabetes mellitus, maternal body mass index >30 kg/m², induction of labor, prolonged labor (first or second stage), oxytocin augmentation, and assisted vaginal delivery (80). However, although they are statistically associated, these factors have low positive predictive value and in fact the large majority of cases occur in women who have no obvious risk factors. This makes shoulder dystocia difficult to both predict and prevent.

Obstetric Management

Owing to the difficulty in prediction or prevention of shoulder dystocia, management centers around educating all birth attendants how to treat the condition when it arises. Firstly, it is important that the diagnosis is made. Signs include failure to deliver the baby's shoulders with normal maternal effort and traction on the head, or retraction of the baby's head back against the mother's perineum—the "turtle sign." Once diagnosed, help (including the anesthesiologist) should be summoned immediately. Further management utilizes a series of maneuvers that have evolved through clinical practice. They may be facilitated by an episiotomy but this is not mandatory. McRoberts maneuver is the single most successful intervention and should be attempted first (81). This involves flexion and abduction of the maternal hips, positioning the maternal thighs on the abdomen. It is associated with an increase in uterine pressure and amplitude of contractions. Suprapubic pressure may be applied together with McRoberts maneuver to increase the success rate. This reduces the bisacromial diameter and rotates the anterior shoulder into the oblique pelvic diameter, freeing the shoulder to slide under the symphysis pubis (81).

If these maneuvers fail, then a choice is made between internal manipulation and the "all-fours position" that has in one series demonstrated an 83% success rate (82). Internal manipulation is used to rotate the shoulders into an oblique diameter or continued for full rotation to 180 degrees so that the posterior shoulder emerges beneath the pubic symphysis. Alternatively, delivery of the posterior shoulder directly may be attempted by sweeping it across the baby's chest and out. The anterior shoulder should then follow easily. However, if the patient is mobile, rolling her onto all-fours and repeating the original maneuvers may also be effective by altering the angle of the pelvis (82).

For failure of the above methods, several third line procedures are described but are rarely performed. These include cleidotomy (intentional fetal clavicular fracture), symphysiotomy and the Zavanelli maneuver (cephalic replacement of the head), and subsequent cesarean delivery.

Anesthetic Management

Given the unpredictability of shoulder dystocia, the anesthesiologist is usually involved as part of an emergency response although there may be some patients who are identified as high risk, for example, macrosomic fetuses of diabetic mothers, and who can be seen in a calmer environment. However, as has previously been noted, the large majority of cases are unforeseen. In this setting, a preexisting epidural catheter is useful to allow for a top-up with a concentrated, fast-acting local anesthetic such as 3% 2-chloroprocaine, 0.75% ropivacaine, or 2% lidocaine with or without adjuvants as discussed above. This not only ensures adequate analgesia during the painful obstetric maneuvers but also enhances pelvic relaxation to facilitate fetal extraction. If all such maneuvers fail and the decision is made to perform the Zavanelli maneuver, tocolytics such as terbutaline or nitroglycerine (50 to 100 mcg IV) are usually administered and subsequently an anesthetic provided for cesarean delivery. In the patient with a labor epidural in situ, the time required to achieve a full surgical block for cesarean delivery should be similar to the time required to adequately prepare for and administer a general anesthetic (83,84). However, in patients who have no epidural, a general anesthetic will be preferable to a de novo regional anesthetic technique, both for speed and logistical difficulty. It should be noted that in such situations there will likely be a great deal of agitation and anxiety, both for the obstetric team and the parents. The anesthesiologist should endeavor to remain calm and professional, and to provide support to a mother who will be under an immense amount of stress.

■ MULTIPLE GESTATION

Pregnancies with more than one fetus pose significant risks to the mother and her babies. The anesthetic implications include not only the exaggerated physiologic changes when compared to the singleton pregnancy but also specific maternal and fetal co-morbidities associated with multifetal pregnancies. A team-based approach involving clear communication, especially between obstetrician and anesthesia provider, is vital for a successful outcome.

Epidemiology

Monozygotic twins occur when a single fertilized ovum divides into two separate embryos and the incidence is fairly consistent worldwide at about 1 in 250 births. By contrast dizygotic twins, naturally occurring in 1:80 pregnancies, in which two separate eggs are fertilized, show considerable demographic variation. Factors associated with twins include a mother who is herself a twin, ethnicity, increased maternal age and multiparity. The incidence of naturally occurring higher order pregnancies decreases exponentially as compared to twin pregnancies. However, with the advent of assisted fertilization techniques and the delaying of childbirth until later in life, these figures are changing. In the United States, between 1980 and 2001 there was a 77% increase of twin births and a 459% increase in the number of triplets and higher order births (85). The increasing incidence means that all anesthetic providers working in the field of obstetrics should have a thorough understanding of the unique obstetrical and anesthetic challenges presented by multifetal pregnancies.

An important factor in the pregnancy is the configuration of the placentas in multiple gestation—they may be either monochorionic or dichorionic and the amniotic sac in monochorionic twins may be either monoamniotic or diamniotic (Fig. 18-2). All dizygotic twins are dichorionic diamniotic.

Maternal Physiology During Multiple Gestation

The physiologic changes that occur in multiple gestation tend to be an exaggeration of the normal adaptations of pregnancy (86). Maternal blood volume can increase by an additional 500 mL with twin gestation which combined with a lower hematocrit makes anemia more common (87). Cardiac output is increased by a further 20% owing to an increased heart rate and greater contractility (88). This has

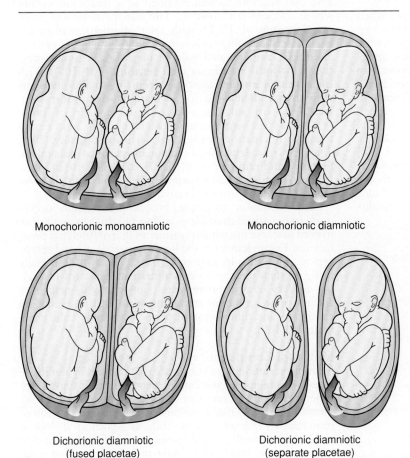

Monochorionic monoamniotic

Monochorionic diamniotic

Dichorionic diamniotic
(fused placetae)

Dichorionic diamniotic
(separate placetae)

FIGURE 18-2 Different configurations of placentas and amniotic sacs in multiple gestation.

been hypothesized to lead to a decreased cardiac reserve at rest as the system is more closely approaching its maximum capacity (88). Aortocaval compression may also be increased due to the larger gravid uterus, which can exert greater pressure on the large veins of the abdomen and lower limbs. This predisposes the mother to the supine hypotension syndrome and epidural venous engorgement.

It is standard teaching that the changes in respiratory function that occur in singleton pregnancies are magnified in multiple gestations. There is little evidence to support this but it seems logical that the greater expansion in uterine size pushes the diaphragm further upward and thus reduces the functional residual capacity (FRC) to a greater extent. This leads to a greater susceptibility to periods of apnea that can result in precipitous desaturation and marked hypoxemia. The larger uterus also increases the risk of aspiration, as it forces the stomach in a cephalad direction and decreases even further the competence of the lower esophageal sphincter (89).

Complications of Multiple Gestation

Twins and higher order pregnancies pose significant risks to both the babies and the mother. The risks are increased with the increasing number of fetuses and maternal mortality is increased three-fold when compared to a singleton pregnancy (90,91). (Table 18-2) shows the complications commonly associated with multiple gestation for both the fetuses and the mother.

Fetal Complications

Preterm labor and delivery is extremely common with the average gestational age decreasing as the number of fetuses increases, and prematurity is the leading cause of perinatal morbidity in this group (48).

Twin-to-twin transfusion syndrome (TTTS) arises when there is uneven flow of blood between fetuses via the vascular anastomoses that exist in monochorionic placentas. It complicates 10% to 15% of all monochorionic pregnancies (92), and while it can occur in monoamniotic twin pregnancies it is far more common in diamniotic twins (93,94). This is felt to be due to the increased presence of arterio-arterial anastomoses in monoamniotic twins which are protective (94). When TTTS occurs, one twin (the recipient) may become overloaded and at risk of cardiac failure while the other (the donor) may suffer from IUGR, hypoperfusion and anemia. There is also an imbalance in amniotic fluid volumes (in diamniotic twins) with the recipient presenting with polyhydramnios and the donor with severe oligohydramnios. This latter finding explains

the "stuck" twin syndrome where the donor twin is adherent to the uterine wall as the reduced amniotic fluid volume affords little room for maneuvering. In severe cases of TTTS, maternal health can also be compromised owing to the development of "Mirror" syndrome (also known as Ballantyne's syndrome). This is a clinical condition affecting the mother which displays many of the features of preeclampsia—widespread edema, proteinuria, hypertension and oliguria—and is associated with severe fetal or placental hydrops (95,96). The outcome for untreated TTTS is poor with mortality for one or both twins between 80% and 90% (97,98). The risk of sudden deterioration is also high with death of the co-twin and neurologic deficit in the survivor (99). The appalling outcomes led to the introduction of techniques to treat the condition including septostomy, making a hole in the dividing membrane to allow the amniotic fluid to equilibrate; amnioreduction, involving serial amniocentesis to reduce the volume of polyhydramnios; and laser photocoagulation, in which a fetoscope is inserted into the uterus and the vascular anastomosis responsible for the condition is cauterized. A recent Cochrane review performed a meta-analysis to determine the treatment with the best perinatal and neonatal outcome (100). They found less overall death in the photocoagulation group when compared with amnioreduction (48% vs. 59%), less perinatal death (26% vs. 44%), and less neonatal death (8% vs. 26%). There was no significant difference in mortality between septostomy and amnioreduction but septostomy was associated with a higher requirement for further interventions. Finally, there was no difference in neurologic outcome postnatally between the laser photocoagulation group and amnioreduction. This led them to conclude that laser photocoagulation should be offered to all patients with TTTS as first line therapy where available and amnioreduction retained as a treatment option where this was not possible. The anesthetic management for treatment of TTTS with laser photocoagulation has been described using various techniques, including general anesthesia with inhaled volatile or TIVA, regional anesthesia, or local anesthesia with sedation (101–105). With the advent of smaller fetoscopes requiring smaller incisions with an attendant reduction in maternal discomfort, local anesthesia with sedation is probably the modality of choice as it causes less hemodynamic instability in the mother and thus less fluctuation in placental perfusion pressure (101). The types of sedation used include intravenous midazolam, fentanyl, and remifentanil (101,103,105). The use of intravenous sedation is also associated with reduced fetal movement that can improve operative conditions (103,106).

Malpresentation including breech presentation occurs more frequently in multiple gestation and this can predispose to cord prolapse in a similar manner to that of singleton pregnancies. Entanglement of the heads (especially when breech-vertex), and difficulty delivering the second twin (especially if bigger than the first twin) are particular hazards of vaginal delivery of twin pregnancies. Congenital abnormalities are also more common and along with cord problems are another major contributor to perinatal mortality and morbidity (91,107).

Maternal Complications

Multiple gestation has a strong association with hypertensive disease of pregnancy, with an incidence of preeclampsia that is between 2 and 3 times that of singleton pregnancies (108). Furthermore, the risk is enhanced via the use of assisted reproductive technologies. A study by Lynch et al. looked at 528 women with multiple gestation and found a two-fold increase in the incidence of mild preeclampsia when using

TABLE 18-2 Complications of Multiple Gestation

Maternal Complications	Fetal Complications
• Preeclampsia	• Preterm delivery
• Preterm labor	• Congenital abnormalities
• Placenta previa/abruption	• Twin-to-twin transfusion syndrome
• Hemorrhage	• Cord entanglement or prolapse
• Anemia	• Intrauterine growth retardation
• Gestational diabetes	• Malpresentation
	• Difficulty in delivering second twin

assisted reproductive technologies compared to spontaneous conception, and a five-fold increase in the incidence of severe preeclampsia (109). This often prompts early delivery with one study demonstrating a rate of delivery by 34 weeks of 70% in quadruplet pregnancies with preeclampsia (110).

The risk of hemorrhage is increased in multiple gestation, both antepartum and postpartum. The rate of placental abruption is 2 to 3 times that seen in singleton pregnancies (111), while placenta previa is 40% more common in twins (112). Blood loss post-delivery is also increased in multiple gestation as uterine atony is more common as a consequence of greater uterine distension. This in turn increases the rate of emergent postpartum hysterectomy—up to six-fold when considering all multiple gestations and an even greater risk is seen in higher order pregnancies (113).

Surgical interventions, either cesarean delivery or operative vaginal deliveries occur in up to 75% of multiple gestations (114) and represent a significant cause of maternal morbidity and mortality.

Obstetric Management

While most triplet and higher order pregnancies are delivered by cesarean delivery, the obstetric management for twins is less clear-cut. A meta-analysis found no difference in maternal morbidity or neonatal outcome when comparing planned cesarean delivery versus planned vaginal delivery for twins, unless the first twin was in a non-vertex presentation (115). It is generally accepted that where the twins are in a vertex–vertex presentation (up to 50% of the time), then vaginal delivery is allowed and the success rate therein is about 70% to 80% (116). Conversely, cesarean delivery is usually recommended when the first twin is in a non-vertex presentation. There is still some disagreement as to the proper course of action when twin A is vertex and twin B is not. If twin A is delivered vaginally then the obstetrician has a number of options:

1. Trial of ECV on twin B and if successful, attempt vaginal delivery.
2. Internal podalic version and total breech extraction as mentioned previously.
3. Cesarean delivery.

Regardless of the choice it is clear that the obstetric anesthesiologist should be present in the room at delivery and able to react quickly to a number of emergent scenarios; hence a flexible approach is called for.

Anesthetic Management

Vaginal Delivery

Traditionally, there were concerns over using epidural analgesia for labor in multiple gestation as one study had demonstrated an association with increased perinatal mortality (117). However, further investigations did not replicate this finding and in fact a later study demonstrated improved umbilical artery pH in second twins when the mother had received epidural analgesia (118). Currently, in the absence of obvious contraindications, most authors recommend using epidural analgesia as it confers several advantages. Adequate analgesia to the perineal region prevents the mother from trying to push too early. Also, the inherent flexibility of an epidural means that the anesthesiologist can rapidly provide deeper analgesia to facilitate internal podalic version or, if required, can extend the block to provide surgical anesthesia for cesarean delivery or operative vaginal delivery. This switch from low dose mixture with the attendant reduction in motor block and preserved maternal expulsive effort to a stronger block for assisted delivery can happen very quickly but good communication with the obstetrician is essential. It should be remembered however that maternal susceptibility to aortocaval compression is exaggerated in multiple gestation and this is exacerbated by the sympathetic block of neuraxial anesthesia. Hence correct positioning of the patient and preparing the means to combat hypotension—large bore IV access, fluids and vasopressor drugs such as ephedrine or phenylephrine—is mandatory. During labor, if the epidural is not entirely satisfactory then it should be re-sited as the rapidly changing analgesic or anesthetic requirements found in vaginal delivery of twins makes a variable or incomplete neuraxial block especially undesirable.

Cesarean Delivery

Where there is a decision to electively deliver the fetuses abdominally, either regional or general anesthesia may be safely administered. Regional anesthesia is usually preferable to mother and also to the clinicians as, apart from the increased risk to the mother associated with general anesthesia (119), the reduction in FRC in multiple gestation means that hypoxemia occurs more quickly during periods of apnea such as in a rapid sequence induction. However, where obvious contraindications to regional techniques exist, a general anesthetic remains a safe alternative.

For regional anesthesia, the choice of technique rests on the preference of the anesthesiologist. There is mixed evidence as to whether a greater cephalad spread of neural blockade with spinal anesthesia (possibly due to increased epidural vein engorgement) occurs with multiple gestations. Jawan et al. demonstrated a higher sensory level in women with multiple gestation when compared to singleton pregnancies (120). Ngan Kee et al. were not able to find a similar association (121). They did however show that there was no difference in the incidence of hypotension or the dose of vasopressors used suggesting that clinically, such concerns are minimal. The authors recommend the administration of a standard dose of spinal agents, but advise close monitoring of the spread of the sensory block and the judicious use of posture to control the spread of the spinal solution (i.e., head up, head down as appropriate). Where concerns exist as to the length of surgery, a combined spinal–epidural technique may represent an ideal approach.

Aside from the choice of anesthetic technique, other considerations include an increased risk of postpartum hemorrhage secondary to uterine atony from the overdistended uterus. Therefore adequate preparation must include large bore IV access, rapid access to cross-matched blood and products, availability of uterotonic agents, and personnel skilled in neonatal resuscitation (of which there should be more than one). Finally, the anesthesiologist should ensure that IV oxytocin is not administered before all the babies have been delivered!

KEY POINTS

- Malpresentations and multiple gestation represent challenging situations for obstetricians and anesthesiologists and good communication is essential.
- Early regional analgesia is useful in controlling pain, reducing maternal desire to push inappropriately, and allowing rapid conversion to anesthesia to facilitate assisted delivery.
- The role of the anesthesiologist extends beyond neuraxial blockade as rapid uterine relaxation may be necessary.
- The anesthesiologist should be present at high-risk deliveries such as vaginal breech birth and multiple gestation.

REFERENCES

1. Albrechtsen S, Rasmussen S, Dalaker K, et al. Perinatal mortality in breech presentation sibships. *Obstet Gynecol* 1998;92(5):775–780.
2. Ponkey SE, Cohen AP, Heffner LJ, et al. Persistent fetal occiput posterior position: obstetric outcomes. *Obstet Gynecol* 2003;101(5 pt 1):915–920.
3. Gardberg M, Laakkonen E, Salevaara M. Intrapartum sonography and persistent occiput posterior position: a study of 408 deliveries. *Obstet Gynecol* 1998; 91(5 pt 1):746–749.
4. Souka AP, Haritos T, Basayiannis K, et al. Intrapartum ultrasound for the examination of the fetal head position in normal and obstructed labor. *J Matern Fetal Neonatal Med* 2003;13(1):59–63.
5. Sizer AR, Nirmal DM. Occipitoposterior position: associated factors and obstetric outcome in nulliparas. *Obstet Gynecol* 2000;96(5 pt 1):749–752.
6. Fitzpatrick M, McQuillan K, O'Herlihy C. Influence of persistent occiput posterior position on delivery outcome. *Obstet Gynecol* 2001;98(6):1027–1031.
7. Lieberman E, Davidson K, Lee-Parritz A, et al. Changes in fetal position during labor and their association with epidural analgesia. *Obstet Gynecol* 2005;105(5 pt 1): 974–982.
8. Simmons SW, Cyna AM, Dennis AT, et al. Combined spinal–epidural versus epidural analgesia in labor. *Cochrane Database Syst Rev* 2007;18(3):CD003401.
9. Comparative Obstetric Mobile Epidural Trial (COMET) Study Group UK. Effect of low-dose mobile versus traditional epidural techniques on mode of delivery: a randomised controlled trial. *Lancet* 2001;358:19–23.
10. Bashiri A, Burstein E, Bar-David J, et al. Face and brow presentation: independent risk factors. *J Matern Fetal Neonatal Med* 2008;21(6):357–360.
11. Shaffer BL, Cheng YW, Vargas JE, et al. Face presentation: predictors and delivery route. *Am J Obstet Gynecol* 2006;194(5):e10–e12.
12. Klatt T, Cruikshank D. Breech, other malpresentations, and umbilical cord complications. In: Gibbs RS, Karlan BY, Haney AF, Nygaard IE, eds. *Danforth's Obstetrics and Gynecology*. 10th ed. Philadelphia, PA: Lippincott Williams & Wilkins; 2008:400–416.
13. Seffah JD, Armah JO. Antenatal ultrasonography for breech delivery. *Int J Gynaecol Obstet* 2000;68(1):7–12.
14. Hartwell BL. Fetal malpresentation and multiple births. In: Norris MC, ed. *Obstetric Anesthesia*. Philadelphia, PA: Lippincott; 1993:689–691.
15. Hickok DE, Gordon DC, Milberg JA, et al. The frequency of breech presentation by gestational age at birth: a large population-based study. *Am J Obstet Gynecol* 1992;166(3):851–852.
16. Albrechtsen S, Rasmussen S, Dalaker K, et al. The occurrence of breech presentation in Norway 1967–1994. *Acta Obstet Gynecol Scand* 1998;77(4):410–415.
17. Rayl J, Gibson PJ, Hickok DE. A population-based case-control study of risk factors for breech presentation. *Am J Obstet Gynecol* 1996;174(1 pt 1):28–32.
18. Lanni SM, Seeds JW. Malpresentations. In: Gabbe SG, Niebyl JR, Simpson JL, eds. *Obstetrics : Normal and Problem Pregnancies*. 5th ed. Edinburgh: Churchill Livingstone; 2007:428–455.
19. Yamamura Y, Ramin KD, Ramin SM. Trial of vaginal breech delivery: current role. *Clin Obstet Gynecol* 2007;50(2):526–536.
20. Cunningham GF, Leveno KJ, Bloom SL, et al. Breech presentation and delivery. In: Cunningham GF, Leveno KJ, Bloom SL, Hauth JC, Gilstrap LC, Wenstrom KD, eds. *Williams Obstetrics*. 22nd ed. New York, NY: McGraw-Hill Medical; 2005:565–586.
21. Herbst A, Wolner-Hanssen P, Ingemarsson I. Risk factors for acidemia at birth. *Obstet Gynecol* 1997;90(1):125–130.
22. Khan R, El-Refaey H. Pathophysiology of postpartum haemorrhage and third stage of labor. In: B-Lynch C, Keith LG, Lalonde AB, Karoshi M, eds. *A Textbook of Postpartum Hemorrhage : a Comprehensive Guide to Evaluation, Management and Surgical Intervention*. Kirkmahoe: Sapiens; 2006:62–69.
23. Moertl MG, Brezinka CA. Multiple gestation and fetal malpresentation. In: Birnbach DJ, Datta S, Gatt SP, eds. *Textbook of Obstetric Anesthesia*. New York, NY: Churchill Livingstone; 2000:356–365.
24. Cheng M, Hannah M. Breech delivery at term: a critical review of the literature. *Obstet Gynecol* 1993;82(4):605–618.
25. American College of Obstetricians and Gynecologists. ACOG Practice Bulletin No. 13: External Cephalic Version. *Obstet Gynecol* 2000;95(2):1–7.
26. Impey L, Lissoni D. Outcome of external cephalic version after 36 weeks' gestation without tocolysis. *J Matern Fetal Med* 1999;8(5):203–207.
27. Lau TK, Lo KW, Wan D, et al. Predictors of successful external cephalic version at term: a prospective study. *Br J Obstet Gynaecol* 1997;104(7):798–802.
28. Zhang J, Bowes WA Jr, Fortney JA. Efficacy of external cephalic version: a review. *Obstet Gynecol* 1993;82(2):306–312.
29. Nor Azlin MI, Haliza H, Mahdy ZA, et al. Tocolysis in term breech external cephalic version. *Int J Gynaecol Obstet* 2005;88(1):5–8.
30. Kok M, Cnossen J, Gravendeel L, et al. Clinical factors to predict the outcome of external cephalic version: a metaanalysis. *Am J Obstet Gynecol* 2008;199(6):630. e1–630.e7.
31. Hofmeyr GJ, Kulier R. External cephalic version for breech presentation at term. *Cochrane Database Syst Rev* 2000;(2):CD000083.
32. Hutton EK, Hofmeyr GJ. External cephalic version for breech presentation before term. *Cochrane Database Syst Rev* 2006;(1):CD000084.
33. Hutton EK, Hannah ME, Ross SJ, et al. The Early External Cephalic Version (ECV) 2 Trial: an international multicentre randomised controlled trial of timing of ECV for breech pregnancies. *BJOG* 2011;118(5):564–577.
34. Collaris RJ, Oei SG. External cephalic version: a safe procedure? A systematic review of version-related risks. *Acta Obstet Gynecol Scand* 2004;83(6):511–518.
35. Nassar N, Roberts CL, Barratt A, et al. Systematic review of adverse outcomes of external cephalic version and persisting breech presentation at term. *Paediatr Perinat Epidemiol* 2006;20(2):163–171.
36. Fok WY, Chan LW, Leung TY, et al. Maternal experience of pain during external cephalic version at term. *Acta Obstet Gynecol Scand* 2005;84(8):748–751.
37. Schorr SJ, Speights SE, Ross EL, et al. A randomized trial of epidural anesthesia to improve external cephalic version success. *Am J Obstet Gynecol* 1997; 177(5):1133–1137.
38. Mancuso KM, Yancey MK, Murphy JA, et al. Epidural analgesia for cephalic version: a randomized trial. *Obstet Gynecol* 2000;95(5):648–651.
39. Weiniger CF, Ginosar Y, Elchalal U, et al. Randomized controlled trial of external cephalic version in term multiparae with or without spinal analgesia. *Br J Anaesth* 2010;104(5):613–618.
40. Rozenberg P, Goffinet F, de Spirlet M, et al. External cephalic version with epidural anaesthesia after failure of a first trial with beta-mimetics. *BJOG* 2000;107(3):406–410.
41. Cherayil G, Feinberg B, Robinson J, et al. Central neuraxial blockade promotes external cephalic version success after a failed attempt. *Anesth Analg* 2002; 94(6):1589–1592.
42. Neiger R, Hennessy MD, Patel M. Reattempting failed external cephalic version under epidural anesthesia. *Am J Obstet Gynecol* 1998;179(5):1136–1139.
43. Dugoff L, Stamm CA, Jones OW 3rd, et al. The effect of spinal anesthesia on the success rate of external cephalic version: a randomized trial. *Obstet Gynecol* 1999;93(3):345–349.
44. Delisle MF, Kamani AA, Douglas MJ, et al. Antepartum external cephalic version under spinal anesthesia: A randomized controlled study. *J Obstet Gynaecol Can* 2003;25(Suppl):S13(abstract).
45. Sullivan JT, Grobman WA, Bauchat JR, et al. A randomized controlled trial of the effect of combined spinal–epidural analgesia on the success of external cephalic version for breech presentation. *Int J Obstet Anesth* 2009;18(4):328–334.
46. Lavoie A, Guay J. Anesthetic dose neuraxial blockade increases the success rate of external fetal version: a meta-analysis. *Can J Anaesth* 2010;57(5):408–414.
47. Hannah ME, Hannah WJ, Hewson SA, et al. Planned caesarean section versus planned vaginal birth for breech presentation at term: a randomised multicentre trial. Term Breech Trial Collaborative Group. *Lancet* 2000;356:1375–1383.
48. Martin JA, Hamilton BE, Ventura SJ, et al. Births: final data for 2001. *Natl Vital Stat Rep* 2002;51(2):1–102.
49. Rietberg CC, Elferink-Stinkens PM, Visser GH. The effect of the Term Breech Trial on medical intervention behaviour and neonatal outcome in The Netherlands: an analysis of 35,453 term breech infants. *Br J Obstet Gynaecol* 2005; 112(2):205–209.
50. ACOG committee opinion: number 265, December 2001. Mode of term single breech delivery. *Obstet Gynecol* 2001;98(6):1189–1190.
51. van Roosmalen J, Rosendaal F. There is still room for disagreement about vaginal delivery of breech infants at term. *Br J Obstet Gynaecol* 2002;109(9):967–969.
52. Glezerman M. Five years to the term breech trial: the rise and fall of a randomized controlled trial. *Am J Obstet Gynecol* 2006;194(1):20–25.
53. Whyte H, Hannah ME, Saigal S, et al. Outcomes of children at 2 years after planned cesarean birth versus planned vaginal birth for breech presentation at term: the International Randomized Term Breech Trial. *Am J Obstet Gynecol* 2004;191(3):864–871.
54. ACOG Committee Opinion No. 340. Mode of term singleton breech delivery. *Obstet Gynecol* 2006;108(1):235–237.
55. Kotaska A, Menticoglou S, Gagnon R, et al. SOGC clinical practice guideline: Vaginal delivery of breech presentation: no. 226, June 2009. *Int J Gynaecol Obstet* 2009;107(2):169–176.
56. Bowen-Simpkins P, Fergusson IL. Lumbar epidural block and the breech presentation. *Br J Anaesth* 1974;46(6):420–424.
57. Darby S, Hunter DJ. Extradural analgesia in labour when the breech presents. *Br J Obstet Gynaecol* 1976;83(1):35–38.
58. Chadha YC, Mahmood TA, Dick MJ, et al. Are breech deliveries an indication for lumbar epidural analgesia? *Br J Obstet Gynaecol* 1992;99(2):96–100.
59. Breeson AJ, Kovacs GT, Pickles BG, et al. Extradural analgesia—the preferred method of analgesia for vaginal breech delivery. *Br J Anaesth* 1978;50(12):1227–1230.
60. Lyons G, Columb M, Hawthorne L, et al. Extradural pain relief in labour: bupivacaine sparing by extradural fentanyl is dose dependent. *Br J Anaesth* 1997;78(5):493–497.
61. Polley LS, Columb MO, Lyons G, et al. The effect of epidural fentanyl on the minimum local analgesic concentration of epidural chloroprocaine in labor. *Anesth Analg* 1996;83(5):987–990.

62. Munson ES, Embro WJ. Enflurane, isoflurane, and halothane and isolated human uterine muscle. *Anesthesiology* 1977;46(1):11–14.

63. Greenspoon JS, Kovacic A. Breech extraction facilitated by glyceryl trinitrate sublingual spray. *Lancet* 1991;338:124–125.

64. Rolbin SH, Hew EM, Bernstein A. Uterine relaxation can be life saving. *Can J Anaesth* 1991;38(7):939–940.

65. Caponas G. Glyceryl trinitrate and acute uterine relaxation: a literature review. *Anaesth Intensive Care* 2001;29(2):163–177.

66. Gaiser RR, Cheek TG, Gutsche BB. Epidural lidocaine versus 2-chloroprocaine for fetal distress requiring urgent cesarean delivery. *Int J Obstet Anesth* 1994;3(4):208–210.

67. Bjornestad E, Iversen OL, Raeder J. Similar onset time of 2-chloroprocaine and lidocaine + epinephrine for epidural anesthesia for elective cesarean delivery. *Acta Anaesthesiol Scand* 2006;50(3):358–363.

68. Barsa J, Batra M, Fink BR, et al. A comparative in vivo study of local neurotoxicity of lidocaine, bupivacaine, 2-chloroprocaine, and a mixture of 2-chloroprocaine and bupivacaine. *Anesth Analg* 1982;61(12):961–967.

69. Wang BC, Hillman DE, Spielholz NI, et al. Chronic neurological deficits and Nesacaine-CE—an effect of the anesthetic, 2-chloroprocaine, or the antioxidant, sodium bisulfite? *Anesth Analg* 1984;63(4):445–447.

70. Taniguchi M, Bollen AW, Drasner K. Sodium bisulfite: scapegoat for chloroprocaine neurotoxicity? *Anesthesiology* 2004;100(1):85–91.

71. Goring-Morris J, Russell IF. A randomised comparison of 0.5% bupivacaine with a lidocaine/epinephrine/fentanyl mixture for epidural top-up for emergency caesarean section after "low dose" epidural for labour. *Int J Obstet Anesth* 2006;15(2):109–114.

72. Lucas DN, Ciccone GK, Yentis SM. Extending low-dose epidural analgesia for emergency caesarean section. A comparison of three solutions. *Anaesthesia* 1999;54(12):1173–1177.

73. Balaji P, Dhillon P, Russell IF. Low-dose epidural top up for emergency caesarean delivery: a randomised comparison of levobupivacaine versus lidocaine/epinephrine/fentanyl. *Int J Obstet Anesth* 2009;18(4):335–341.

74. Malhotra S, Yentis SM. Extending low-dose epidural analgesia in labour for emergency caesarean section—a comparison of levobupivacaine with or without fentanyl. *Anaesthesia* 2007;62(7):667–671.

75. Allam J, Malhotra S, Hemingway C, et al. Epidural lidocaine–bicarbonate–adrenaline vs levobupivacaine for emergency caesarean section: a randomised controlled trial. *Anaesthesia* 2008;63(3):243–249.

76. Lam DT, Ngan Kee WD, Khaw KS. Extension of epidural blockade in labour for emergency caesarean section using 2% lidocaine with epinephrine and fentanyl, with or without alkalinisation. *Anaesthesia* 2001;56(8):790–794.

77. Tuleu C, Allam J, Gill H, et al. Short term stability of pH-adjusted lidocaine–adrenaline epidural solution used for emergency caesarean section. *Int J Obstet Anesth* 2008;17(2):118–122.

78. American College of Obstetricians and Gynecologists. ACOG practice bulletin number 40: shoulder dystocia. *Obstet Gynecol* 2002;100(5):1045–1050.

79. Gherman RB, Chauhan S, Ouzounian JG, et al. Shoulder dystocia: the unpreventable obstetric emergency with empiric management guidelines. *Am J Obstet Gynecol* 2006;195(3):657–672.

80. Royal College of Obstetricians and Gynaecologists. *Shoulder Dystocia. Clinical Green Top Guideline (December) No. 42.* London: RCOG; 2005.

81. Gherman RB, Goodwin TM, Souter I, et al. The McRoberts' maneuver for the alleviation of shoulder dystocia: how successful is it?. *Am J Obstet Gynecol* 1997;176(3):656–661.

82. Bruner JP, Drummond SB, Meenan AL, et al. All-fours maneuver for reducing shoulder dystocia during labor. *J Reprod Med* 1998;43(5):439–443.

83. Popham P, Buettner A, Mendola M. Anaesthesia for emergency caesarean section, 2000–2004, at the Royal women's Hospital, Melbourne. *Anaesth Intensive Care* 2007;35(1):74–79.

84. Lim Y, Shah MK, Tan HM. Evaluation of surgical and anaesthesia response times for crash caesarean sections—an audit of a Singapore hospital. *Ann Acad Med Singapore* 2005;34(10):606–610.

85. Luke B, Martin JA. The rise in multiple births in the United States: who, what, when, where, and why. *Clin Obstet Gynecol* 2004;47(1):118–133.

86. Allsop J, Navaneethan N, Cooper J. Maternal physiology. In: Collis RE, Plaat F, Urquhart J, eds. *Textbook of Obstetric Anaesthesia.* London: Greenwich Medical Media; 2002:23–38.

87. Cunningham FG, Leveno KJ, Bloom SL, et al. Multifetal gestation. In: Cunningham FG, Leveno KJ, Bloom SL, Hauth JC, Gilstrap LC, Wenstrom KD, eds. *Williams Obstetrics.* 22nd ed. New York, NY: McGraw-Hill Medical; 2005:911–948.

88. Veille JC, Morton MJ, Burry KJ. Maternal cardiovascular adaptations to twin pregnancy. *Am J Obstet Gynecol* 1985;153(3):261–263.

89. Craft JB, Levinson G, Shnider SM. Anaesthetic considerations in caesarean section for quadruplets. *Can Anaesth Soc J* 1978;25(3):236–239.

90. Senat MV, Ancel PY, Bouvier-Colle MH, et al. How does multiple pregnancy affect maternal mortality and morbidity? *Clin Obstet Gynecol* 1998;41(1):78–83.

91. Conde-Agudelo A, Belizan JM, Lindmark G. Maternal morbidity and mortality associated with multiple gestations. *Obstet Gynecol* 2000;95(6 Pt 1):899–904.

92. Royal College of Obstetricians and Gynaecologists. Management of monochorionic twin pregnancy. *Clinical Green Top Guideline No. 51.* London: RCOG; 2008.

93. Gallot D, Saulnier JP, Savary D, et al. Ultrasonographic signs of twin–twin transfusion syndrome in a monoamniotic twin pregnancy. *Ultrasound Obstet Gynecol* 2005;25(3):308–309.

94. Umur A, van Gemert MJ, Nikkels PG. Monoamniotic versus diamniotic-monochorionic twin placentas: anastomoses and twin–twin transfusion syndrome. *Am J Obstet Gynecol* 2003;189(5):1325–1329.

95. Carbillon L, Oury JF, Guerin JM, et al. Clinical biological features of Ballantyne syndrome and the role of placental hydrops. *Obstet Gynecol Surv* 1997;52(5):310–314.

96. Braun T, Brauer M, Fuchs I, et al. Mirror syndrome: a systematic review of fetal associated conditions, maternal presentation and perinatal outcome. *Fetal Diagn Ther* 2010;27(4):191–203.

97. Haverkamp F, Lex C, Hanisch C, et al. Neurodevelopmental risks in twin-to-twin transfusion syndrome: preliminary findings. *Eur J Paediatr Neurol* 2001;5(1):21–27.

98. Urig MA, Clewell WH, Elliott JP. Twin–twin transfusion syndrome. *Am J Obstet Gynecol* 1990;163(5):1522–1526.

99. van Heteren CF, Nijhuis JG, Semmekrot BA, et al. Risk for surviving twin after fetal death of co-twin in twin–twin transfusion syndrome. *Obstet Gynecol* 1998;92(2):215–219.

100. Roberts D, Gates S, Kilby M, et al. Interventions for twin–twin transfusion syndrome: a Cochrane review. *Ultrasound Obstet Gynecol* 2008;31(6):701–711.

101. Rossi AC, Kaufman MA, Bornick PW, et al. General vs local anesthesia for the percutaneous laser treatment of twin–twin transfusion syndrome. *Am J Obstet Gynecol* 2008;199(2):137.e1–137.e7.

102. Myers LB, Watcha MF. Epidural versus general anesthesia for twin–twin transfusion syndrome requiring fetal surgery. *Fetal Diagn Ther* 2004;19(3):286–291.

103. Missant C, Van Schoubroeck D, Deprest J, et al. Remifentanil for foetal immobilisation and maternal sedation during endoscopic treatment of twin-to-twin transfusion syndrome : a preliminary dose-finding study. *Acta Anaesthesiol Belg* 2004;55(3):239–244.

104. Cooley S, Walsh J, Mahony R. Successful fetoscopic laser coagulation for twin-to-twin transfusion syndrome under local anaesthesia. *Ir Med J* 2011;104(6):187–190.

105. Morimoto Y, Yoshimura M, Orita H, et al. Anesthesia management for fetoscopic treatment of twin-to-twin transfusion syndrome. *(Japanese) Masui* 2008;57(6):719–724.

106. Gupta R, Kilby M, Cooper G. Fetal surgery and anaesthetic implications. *Contin Educ Anaesth Crit Care Pain* 2008;8:71–75.

107. Ayres A, Johnson TR. Management of multiple pregnancy: prenatal care-part I. *Obstet Gynecol Surv* 2005;60(8):527–537.

108. Sibai BM, Hauth J, Caritis S, et al. Hypertensive disorders in twin versus singleton gestations. *Am J Obstet Gynecol* 2000;182(4):938–942.

109. Lynch A, McDuffie R, Murphy J, et al. Preeclampsia in multiple gestation: the role of assisted reproductive technologies. *Obstet Gynecol* 2002;99(3):445–451.

110. Elliott JP, Radin TG. Quadruplet pregnancy: contemporary management and outcome. *Obstet Gynecol* 1992;80(3):421–424.

111. Ananth CV, Smulian JC, Demissie K, et al. Placental abruption among singleton and twin births in the United States: risk factor profiles. *Am J Epidemiol* 2001;153(8):771–778.

112. Ananth CV, Demissie K, Smulian JC, et al. Placenta previa in singleton and twin births in the United States, 1989 through 1998: a comparison of risk factor profiles and associated conditions. *Am J Obstet Gynecol* 2003;188(1):275–281.

113. Francois K, Ortiz J, Harris C, et al. Is peripartum hysterectomy more common in multiple gestations?. *Obstet Gynecol* 2005;105(6):1369–1372.

114. Walker MC, Murphy KE, Pan S, et al. Adverse maternal outcomes in multifetal pregnancies. *BJOG* 2004;111(11):1294–1296.

115. Hogle KL, Hutton EK, McBrien KA, et al. Cesarean delivery for twins: a systematic review and meta-analysis. *Am J Obstet Gynecol* 2003;188(1):220–227.

116. Stone J, Eddleman K, Patel S. Controversies in the intrapartum management of twin gestations. *Obstet Gynecol Clin North Am* 1999;26(2):327–343.

117. Little WA, Friedman EA. Anesthesia for the twin delivery. *Anesthesiology* 1958;19(4):515–520.

118. Crawford JS. A prospective study of 200 consecutive twin deliveries. *Anaesthesia* 1987;42(1):33–43.

119. Hawkins JL, Koonin LM, Palmer SK, et al. Anesthesia-related deaths during obstetric delivery in the United States, 1979–1990. *Anesthesiology* 1997;86(2):277–284.

120. Jawan B, Lee JH, Chong ZK, et al. Spread of spinal anaesthesia for caesarean section in singleton and twin pregnancies. *Br J Anaesth* 1993;70(6):639–641.

121. Ngan Kee WD, Khaw KS, Ng FF, et al. A prospective comparison of vasopressor requirement and hemodynamic changes during spinal anesthesia for cesarean delivery in patients with multiple gestation versus singleton pregnancy. *Anesth Analg* 2007;104(2):407–411.

Preterm Labor and Delivery

Carlo Pancaro

Preterm delivery, defined as infant birth at less than 37 weeks of gestation, is the leading cause of infant mortality worldwide (1). The United States preterm birth (PTB) rate rose by more than one-third from the early 1980s through 2006, the year it reached its peak. Since that time, PTB rates have declined significantly in 35 states. Only one state, Hawaii, has reported an increase in PTBs (2). Infant mortality rates for preterm infants are lower in the United States than in most European countries; however, infant mortality rates for term infants (born at 37 weeks of gestation or more) are higher in the United States than in most European countries (3). The very high percentage of PTBs in the United States accounts for its comparatively high infant mortality (Fig. 19-1). The increase in PTBs has been associated with a significant increase in the rate of cesarean delivery, thereby increasing the need for anesthesia providers to be immediately available for these deliveries (2).

In 2006, 12.8% of US births occurred preterm with 3.66% occurring at less than 34 weeks of gestation. Approximately 50% of PTBs are idiopathic. Of these 50%, 30% are related to preterm rupture of membranes (PROM) and 20% are attributed to medical indications or performed electively (4).

The major reason for the increase in PTB is a higher occurrence of multiple gestation pregnancies. Between 1996 and 2002, the multiple birth ratio increased more than 20% to 33% per 1,000 live births (twin birth rate: 31/1,000). Pregnancies complicated by multiple gestation are prone to PTB; approximately 50% of twins and 90% of triplets are born preterm compared to less than 10% of singletons.

■ DEFINITIONS

Full-term birth is defined as one occurring from 39 to 41 weeks of gestation. "Early-term birth" occurs from 37 to 38 weeks of gestation. PTB refers to one that occurs before 37 completed weeks of gestation. PTB may be further classified on the basis of gestational age as follows: Late preterm (34 to 36 weeks and 6 days); moderately preterm (32 to 33 weeks and 6 days); very preterm (≤32 weeks); and extremely preterm (≤28 weeks). Since it is more accurate to correlate infant and neonatal outcomes with birth weight than with gestational age, the scientific community has also used birth weight to define PTB such that low birth weight (LBW) is considered less than 2,500 g, very low birth weight (VLBW) is less than 1,500 g, and extremely low birth weight (ELBW) is less than 1,000 g.

■ PATHOGENESIS

Preterm labor may reflect a number of pathogenic processes leading to a final common pathway. The four primary processes are: (1) Premature activation of the maternal or fetal hypothalamic–pituitary–adrenal axis; (2) an exaggerated response to inflammation and infection; (3) decidual hemor-

rhage; and (4) pathologic uterine distention. These processes are not mutually exclusive and may be initiated long before preterm labor or preterm premature rupture of membranes (PPROM) is clinically diagnosed. In addition, these mechanisms share a final common pathway involving the formation of uterotonic agents and proteases that weaken the fetal membranes and cervical stroma.

Activation of the Hypothalamic–Pituitary Axis

The increased placental production of corticotropin-releasing hormone appears to program a "placental clock" which prematurely activates the hypothalamic–pituitary–adrenal axis in the mother (5,6). In addition, there is an increased fetal pituitary adrenocorticotropic hormone secretion which stimulates the production of placental estrogenic compounds thereby activating the myometrium and initiating labor (7).

Major maternal physical or psychological stressors such as depression can activate the maternal hypothalamic–pituitary axis and have been associated with a slightly higher rate of PTB (8). Women with depressive symptoms early in pregnancy have almost twice the PTB risk compared with women without such symptoms (9). Notably, this risk increases with the severity of depression.

In contrast to women with uncomplicated first pregnancies, women whose first pregnancy ends in PTB are at increased risk of PTB, preeclampsia, and fetal growth restriction in their second pregnancy (10).

Exaggerated Response to Inflammation and Infection

There is a link between PTB and systemic or genitourinary tract pathogens (11–17). In a large retrospective study of nearly 200,000 deliveries, 2.5% of patients had asymptomatic bacteriuria which was independently associated with PTB (11). The diagnosis and treatment of asymptomatic bacteriuria appears to reduce the risk of PTB (12).

In a different study of 759 women, those without abnormalities of the vaginal flora during their first trimester had a 75% lower risk of experiencing delivery before 35 weeks than women with abnormal vaginal flora (13). The absence of lactobacilli, the presence of bacterial vaginosis, and the presence of gram-positive coccus aerobic vaginitis are associated with a 2- to 3-fold increased risk of PTB. However, treatment of bacterial vaginosis (BV) does not appear to consistently reduce PTB rates in low-risk patients (18). Similarly, periodontal disease is associated with higher rates of PTB, but treatment does not lower this risk (14,15). Lastly, both clinical and subclinical chorioamnionitis are much more common in preterm than in term deliveries and may account for 50% of PTBs before 30 weeks of gestation (19). These data suggest

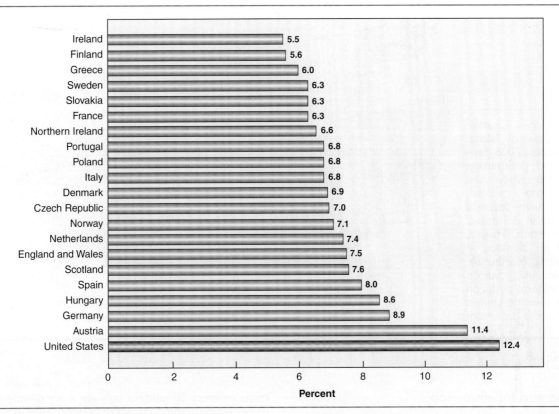

FIGURE 19-1 Percentage of PTB, United States and selected European countries, 2004. From: MacDorman MF, Mathews TJ. Behind international rankings of infant mortality: how the United States compares with Europe. *NCHS Data Brief* 2009;23:1–8.

that disorders of maternal innate or acquired immunity, rather than the mere presence of certain genital tract bacteria, are the primary causes of inflammation-associated PTB.

Bacterial factors trigger a maternal and/or fetal inflammatory response in susceptible individuals that is linked to PTB. This response is characterized by activated neutrophils, activated macrophages, and various pro-inflammatory mediators. Interleukin-1 beta (IL-1 β) and tumor necrosis factor alpha (TNF-α) appear to be the key initial mediators of this response, enhancing prostaglandin production in the amnion and decidua while inhibiting prostaglandin metabolizing enzyme in the chorion (20).

Bacteria also produce phospholipase A2 and endotoxin, substances that stimulate uterine contractions and can cause preterm labor (21).

Furthermore, chorioamnionitis is associated with intense neutrophil recruitment and activation in the decidua. Neutrophils are capable of releasing pro-inflammatory mediators that further enhance decidual and fetal membrane prostaglandin production, thereby recruiting and activating additional neutrophils (22,23). Complement activation also appears to play a role (24). Thus, both maternal and fetal inflammatory responses to infection can lead to preterm labor.

Placental hypoperfusion appears to increase the production of pro-inflammatory mediators (25) justifying the slightly higher rate of spontaneous PTB among growth-restricted infants (26).

Decidual Hemorrhage

Vaginal bleeding from decidual hemorrhage is associated with a high risk of preterm labor and PPROM (27–29). Vaginal bleeding in more than one trimester has been shown to increase the risk of PPROM by 7-fold (27).

The development of PPROM in the setting of abruption may be related to high decidual concentrations of tissue. In laboratory studies, small quantities of thrombin produced during coagulation increased the frequency and intensity of myometrial contractions, an effect that is suppressed by blood containing thrombin inhibitors (30,31).

Pathologic Uterine Distention

Multiple gestation, polyhydramnios, and other causes of excessive uterine distention are risk factors for PTB. Enhanced stretching of the myometrium induces the formation of gap junctions, upregulation of oxytocin receptors, and production of prostaglandins and myosin light chain kinase. All of these are critical events that precede uterine contractions and cervical dilation (32,33).

■ RISK FACTORS

Three types of factors may contribute to spontaneous PTB: Social stress and race, infection and inflammation, and genetics.

Social Stress and Race

Poverty, limited maternal education, young maternal age, unmarried status, and inadequate prenatal care are clearly associated with increased risk of PTB and LBW. Another consistent factor that increases risk is maternal race. In the United States, the rate of PTB among black women is twice as high as the rate among white women (Fig. 19-2); furthermore, the rate of recurrent PTB in black women is 4 times as high as the rate among white women.

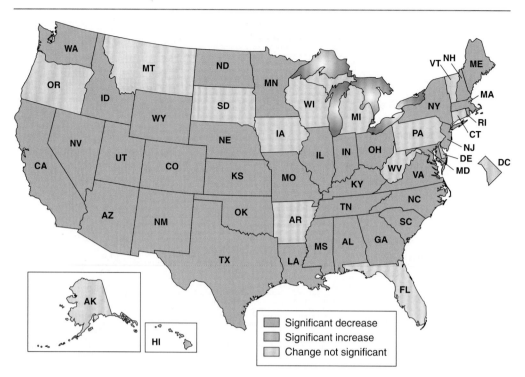

FIGURE 19-2 Change in PTB rates by state: United States 2006 final and 2008 preliminary. Since 2006 when the national rate peaked, PTB rates have declined significantly in 35 states. Only one state, Hawaii, reported an increase in PTBs. From: Martin JA, Osterman MJ, Sutton PD. Are preterm births on the decline in the United States? Recent data from the National Vital Statistics System. *NCHS Data Brief* 2010;1–8.

Infection and Inflammation

Chorioamnionitis is the most obvious example of infection associated with early labor and delivery. Approximately 25% of PTBs are caused by infection, with bacterial colonization ranging from 11% to 79% (34,35). In most cases of preterm labor and delivery, intrauterine infection is not clinically apparent (17). However, histologic evidence of inflammation in the decidua, fetal membranes, or umbilical cord is relatively common.

Genetic Factors

Maternal history of PTB is a strong risk factor for PTB (36). PTB might be considered a common complex disorder that involves gene–gene and gene–environment interactions. Maternal genes, or maternal genes acting in the fetus, largely determine the risk of PTB with a smaller role for paternal genes (37). Common environmental factors influence racial differences in pregnancy outcomes. These influences may overwhelm the effect of what might seem to be small genetic differences. A recent large review of retrospective data (38) as shown that the rate of deaths for infants born during the entire term period has fallen in the past decade. However, the analysis revealed large differences in the decline in the infant death rate between racial and ethnic groups during the early-term period. For example, over the 11-year period of the analysis, the infant death rate for infants born at 37 weeks fell by 35 % and 22 % for Hispanics and non-Hispanic whites respectively, and by 6.8 % for non-Hispanic African-American infants. The rate of deaths within the first month of life for non-Hispanic black infants born at 37 weeks did not decline at all, and in 2006 was the same as the neonatal mortality rate in 1995 for Hispanic and non-Hispanic infants born at 37 weeks.

■ DIAGNOSIS

The diagnosis of preterm labor is clinical. Cervical change or cervical effacement of at least 80%, or cervical dilatation greater than 2 cm together with four regular painful contractions every 20 minutes or eight every 60 minutes commonly establish the diagnosis of preterm labor in a patient at 37 weeks or less of gestational age (39).

The next diagnostic steps commonly performed in women with suspected or diagnosed preterm labor aim at determining whether there is uterine bleeding (possible placenta previa or placental abruption), whether the fetal membranes have ruptured (possible PPROM), and whether there is concomitant chorioamnionitis. In addition, an accurate gestational age and fetal well-being are estimated by ultrasonography and cardiotocography.

In many women, uterine contractions cease spontaneously. In fact, only 20% of women evaluated for preterm labor have preterm delivery (40).

■ THERAPY FOR WOMEN IN PRETERM LABOR

Acute tocolysis and antenatal corticosteroids are the main therapeutic strategies for women in preterm labor (41,42). Except in rare circumstances, there is no way to arrest preterm labor. Physicians can only delay birth by 1 to 7 days with the current therapeutic options available (41). Once the diagnosis has been established, the obstetrician must decide whether to start a short course of tocolytic therapy that aims at delaying the delivery for at least 48 hours (Table 19-1). This time frame is extremely important to allow maternal administration of corticosteroids to accelerate fetal lung maturity (42) and administration of antibiotic therapy to prevent neonatal group B streptococcal infection.

■ ACUTE TOCOLYSIS

Overview of Tocolytic Therapy

Tocolytic therapy for an acute episode of preterm labor often abolishes contractions temporarily, but it does not remove the underlying cause that initiated the process of parturition (Table 19-2). The most important goal of tocolysis is to delay delivery by at least 48 hours so that

TABLE 19-1 Indications and Contraindications for Inhibition of Preterm Labor

Indications
- Gestational age ≤37 wks
- Cervical change or cervical effacement ≥80%, or cervical dilatation >2 cm together with four regular painful contractions every 20 min or eight every 60 min
- Recent intra-abdominal surgery causing preterm labor

Contraindications
- Chorioamnionitis
- Non-reassuring fetal status
- Severe fetal growth restriction
- Severe preeclampsia or eclampsia
- Maternal hemorrhage with hemodynamic instability
- Lethal fetal anomaly
- Intrauterine fetal demise

corticosteroids given to the mother can reach their maximum effect. An additional goal of tocolysis is to allow for more time to transport the mother, if needed, to a hospital that can provide appropriate neonatal care in case she delivers preterm. In addition, tocolytic therapy is beneficial in self-limited conditions that might increase the risk of preterm labor such as pyelonephritis and abdominal surgery (43). The underlying etiology of preterm labor, rather than gestational age, determines when to start acute tocolysis. In fact, there are no definitive data from randomized trials on which to base a recommendation for the lowest gestational age at which inhibition of preterm labor should be considered (44). Many experts choose a gestational age of 15 weeks since early pregnancy loss at that age is less commonly attributable to karyotypic abnormality. Others choose 20 weeks because delivery before this age is considered a spontaneous abortion rather than a PTB. However, inhibiting contractions after intra-abdominal surgery, a self-limited event that can cause preterm labor, may be a reasonable choice regardless of the gestational age (45,46). Inhibition of labor is not attempted after 34 weeks of gestation since this age represents the upper threshold at which perinatal morbidity and mortality are adequately reduced to justify the potential maternal and fetal complications associated with tocolytic therapy (44,47–49).

All of the commonly used tocolytic agents are effective for delaying delivery from 48 hours to 7 days (41). However, pro-

TABLE 19-2 Tocolytic Management of Acute Preterm Labor

Tocolytic Management of Acute Preterm Labor			
Tocolytic Agent	Route of Administration (Dosage)	Maternal Adverse Effects	Fetal Adverse Effects
Magnesium sulfate	IV: 4–6 g bolus, then 2–3 g/h infusion	Cardiorespiratory arrest Pulmonary edema Hypotension Headache Weakness Nausea	Decreased beat-to-beat variability Neonatal drowsiness Hypotonia
β_2-adrenergic Agonists			
Terbutaline sulfate	SQ: 0.25 mg q20 min IV: 2 µg/min to a maximum of 30 µg/min	Tachycardia Cardiac dysrhythmias Palpitations Myocardial ischemia Chest pain Shortness of breath Pulmonary edema Tremor Anxiety and restlessness Nausea and vomiting Rash Hypokalemia Hyperglycemia	Tachycardia Hypotension Ileus Hyperinsulinemia Hypoglycemia
Prostaglandin Inhibitors			
Indomethacin	Oral: 50–100 mg loading dose followed by 25 mg q4–6h Rectal: 100 mg q12h	Interstitial nephritis Platelet dysfunction Gastrointestinal effects (nausea, heartburn)	Premature closure of the neonatal ductus arteriosus Persistent pulmonary hypertension Oligohydramnios
Calcium Channel Blockers			
Nifedipine	Oral: 20–30 mg q4–8h up to a maximum of 180 mg/day	Hypotension Reflex tachycardia Headache Nausea Flushing Hepatotoxicity Respiratory depression	None

longation of pregnancy does not significantly reduce overall rates of respiratory distress syndrome or neonatal death.

Obstetricians use one pharmacologic agent at a time since the concomitant use of different tocolytics offers no additional benefits and adds only side effects (50,51). If the single-agent therapy is not effective, physicians switch to a different agent after ruling out chorioamnionitis. Sixty-five percent of women in whom tocolysis with a single-agent is not successful have positive amniotic fluid cultures (52). In fact, in the absence of clear clinical criteria for infection, some obstetricians might consider amniocentesis to help exclude occult intra-amniotic infection before switching to a second pharmacologic agent.

Contraindications to acute tocolysis include chorioamnionitis, non-reassuring fetal status, severe fetal growth restriction, severe preeclampsia, maternal hemorrhage with hemodynamic instability, lethal fetal anomaly, and intrauterine fetal demise (Table 19-1).

There are two particular situations wherein anesthesia providers may be requested to administer neuraxial analgesia and anesthesia or general anesthesia to preterm labor patients who are receiving tocolytic therapy. The first situation is when tocolysis fails and patients desire labor analgesia or require anesthesia because of a cesarean delivery. The second is when tocolysis is administered before or during the performance of a trans-abdominal or cervical cerclage. Anesthetic management may be easily facilitated when anesthesia providers are familiar with tocolytic pharmacology, side effects, and interaction with anesthetic agents.

Tocolytic Agents

Magnesium Sulfate

Magnesium competes with calcium at the level of the plasma membrane voltage-gated channels. It hyperpolarizes the plasma membrane and inhibits myosin light-chain kinase activity reducing myometrial contractility (53–55). Even though its efficacy is questionable (56), magnesium sulfate is still one of the most common drugs used for the treatment of acute tocolysis in North America. Similarly to β-adrenergic agonists, magnesium sulfate can cause pulmonary edema and chest pain (57). Maternal therapy causes a slight decrease in baseline fetal heart rate and fetal heart rate variability, both of which are not clinically significant (58). Biophysical profile score and non-stress test reactivity are not significantly altered.

Anesthetic Implications of Magnesium Therapy

There are no contraindications to perform a neuraxial block or to administer general anesthesia in a parturient receiving magnesium sulfate. When neuraxial analgesia or anesthesia is given, magnesium decreases maternal blood pressure but not uterine blood flow (UBF) (59). Ephedrine (60) and phenylephrine can be administered to prevent and treat maternal hypotension (61). Even though magnesium sulfate potentiates the neuromuscular blockade induced by non-depolarizing neuromuscular blockers (62,63) and might antagonize the block produced by succinylcholine (64), there is no evidence that the intubating dose of any muscle relaxant should be modified for induction of general anesthesia in a preterm laboring patient.

However, in patients receiving magnesium, the maintenance dose of non-depolarizing neuromuscular blocker must be reduced and carefully titrated with a nerve stimulator to ensure adequate recovery of neuromuscular function at the end of the cesarean delivery. In addition, neostigmine-induced recovery is attenuated in patients treated with magnesium (63). Current evidence suggests that postoperative

analgesic needs are not decreased in patients who receive intravenous magnesium (65). The reader is referred to Chapter 28 for more extensive information on magnesium sulfate dosing regimens, monitoring, toxicity, and interactions with anesthetic drugs. The neuroprotective effects of in utero exposure to magnesium sulfate are addressed in Chapter 17.

β-adrenergic Receptor Agonists

In the United States, terbutaline is the most commonly used β-adrenergic receptor agonist for acute tocolysis. Ritodrine and terbutaline have been studied in several randomized, placebo-controlled trials but ritodrine is no longer available in the United States. Terbutaline can be administered intravenously, subcutaneously, or orally. The desired uterine relaxation following terbutaline is a result of β_2 receptor activity in the uterine smooth muscle. The concomitant stimulation of β_1 receptors results in undesirable maternal and fetal side effects (Table 19-2).

A Cochrane review involving 1,332 patients found that β-adrenergic receptor agonists decreased the number of women giving birth within 48 hours (RR 0.63, 95% CI 0.53–0.75) and possibly within 7 days (RR 0.67, 95% CI 0.48–1.01) (66). There was also a trend toward reduction in respiratory distress syndrome that was not statistically significant. The agonists had no effect on the neonatal death rate.

Although both β_1- and β_2-adrenergic receptors are present in human myometrial tissue at term, uterine relaxation is mediated exclusively by β_2-adrenergic receptors (67). Terbutaline is 60 times more selective for the β_2- than for the β_1-adrenergic receptors (68). It activates the G protein, G_S, which then stimulates intracellular adenylate cyclase. Adenylate cyclase enhances the hydrolysis of adenosine triphosphate (ATP) to cyclic adenosine monophosphate (cAMP) and activates protein kinase, resulting in the phosphorylation of intracellular proteins. This causes a drop in intracellular free calcium resulting in inhibition of the interaction between actin and myosin with the consequential myometrial relaxation.

Recently, a β_3-adrenergic receptor has been found to be the predominant β-adrenergic receptor subtype in the pregnant and non-pregnant human myometrium (69). Its role in the treatment and prevention of preterm labor is currently under investigation (70).

At the author's institution, terbutaline is given subcutaneously by intermittent injection. Usually, 0.25 mg is administered every 20 to 30 minutes up to 4 doses or until tocolysis is achieved. Once labor is inhibited, 0.25 mg can be administered every 3 to 4 hours until the uterus is quiescent. If continuous intravenous infusion is used, terbutaline is usually started at 2.5 to 5 μg/min. This rate can be increased by 2.5 to 5 μg/min every 20 to 30 minutes to a maximum of 30 μg/min, or until the contractions have abated. Once this goal is reached, the infusion can be reduced by decrements of 2.5 to 5 μg/min to the lowest dose that maintains uterine quiescence.

Terbutaline administration can cause significant adverse maternal and fetal side effects in the cardiovascular and central nervous systems as well as in metabolism (Table 19-2). During terbutaline administration, the clinician should monitor fluid intake, urine output, and recognize the occurrence of maternal symptoms, especially shortness of breath, chest pain, and tachycardia. In addition, glucose and potassium concentrations should be monitored every 4 to 6 hours since hyperglycemia and hypokalemia commonly occur. Significant hypokalemia should be treated to minimize risk of arrhythmias, and significant hyperglycemia should be treated with insulin.

Cardiovascular Side Effects

Cardiovascular effects are produced directly by the binding of terbutaline on β_2-adrenergic receptors on adrenergic nerve terminals and indirectly by enhancing norepinephrine release after activation of presynaptic β_2-receptors (71). Increases in heart rate and inotropism induced by terbutaline are mediated almost exclusively by cardiac β_2-adrenergic receptor stimulation (72).

In a study by Jartti et al., a continuous 3-hour intravenous infusion of 10 to 30 μg/min of terbutaline increased the heart rate (from 57 to 109 beats/min) and the minute ventilation (11 to 13 L/min) in healthy volunteers in a dose dependent fashion. In the same experiment, the plasma potassium concentration decreased (from 4 to 2.5 mEq/L) and blood pressure did not change significantly (from 115/65 to 120/64 mm Hg) (73). The cardiovascular response to terbutaline can vary significantly and this phenomenon might be caused by structural differences in the β_2-receptor. β_2-adrenergic receptors are polymorphic, and there are four major coding sequence polymorphisms: Arg19Cys, Arg16Gly, Gln27Glu, and Thr164Ile (74). Some investigators have found that the β_2-adrenergic receptor polymorphism significantly affects the dose–response curves for terbutaline-induced inotropic and chronotropic responses. Subjects with the Thr164Ile receptor show substantial blunting in maximal increase in heart rate and a shortening of the electromechanical systole (75).

It is speculated that the concomitant marked hypokalemia that occurs during terbutaline therapy most likely contributes to the tachycardia by increasing the slope and amplitude of action potentials in the sinoatrial and atrioventricular nodes (73). Similar to cardiac responses, vasodilator responses to β_2-adrenergic stimulation are blunted in subjects carrying one allele of the Ile 164 β_2-adrenergic receptor when compared with subjects homozygous for the Thr164 β_2-adrenergic receptor (76,77). Therefore, stimulation of the β_2-adrenergic receptors on blood vessels can result in various degrees of diastolic hypotension (75,78).

Common cardiovascular symptoms associated with the use of β_2-adrenergic agonists include palpitations (18%), shortness of breath (15%), and chest discomfort (10%) (79). ST-segment depression and T-wave changes can occur and typically resolve once β-adrenergic therapy has been discontinued (80). Myocardial ischemia is also a potential complication of β-adrenergic therapy (80) even though a retrospective study conducted on 8,709 subjects failed to demonstrate any cardiac ischemic event in pregnant patients who received terbutaline therapy (81).

Pulmonary edema has been reported in 0.3% (3/1,000) of patients receiving β-mimetic therapy (81). A study reviewing 62,917 consecutive pregnancies showed pulmonary edema attributable to tocolytic use in 13 patients. All of these patients (whose pulmonary edema was secondary to tocolytic use) received multiple simultaneous tocolytic agents. The most common combination was intravenous magnesium sulfate used in conjunction with subcutaneous terbutaline (82). Multiple gestations, maternal infection, and multiple tocolytic agents seem to be the main risk factors for the development of pulmonary edema (82,83).

Although normal pulmonary capillary wedge pressures have been found in parturients who showed pulmonary edema during β-adrenergic therapy (84), there are two possible factors that play a role in the pathogenesis of tocolytic-induced pulmonary edema: Fluid overload (85) and increased pulmonary capillary permeability (84).

Fluid overload during β-adrenergic therapy is probably the major pathogenic factor during terbutaline tocolysis. It may occur as a combination of fluid and sodium retention secondary to increase in renin and anti-diuretic hormone activity from β-adrenergic receptor stimulation (85).

Some investigators have observed that when β-adrenergic agents are administered, the risk for development of pulmo-

nary edema changes according to which crystalloid solution is used. Isotonic sodium chloride causes more fluid retention than dextrose-containing solutions (86). In pregnant baboons, ritodrine and lactated Ringer's have been associated with more fluid and sodium retention than lactated Ringer's alone (87). In one setting, isotonic solutions cause more sodium and fluid retention; in another setting, dextrose-containing solutions increase the likelihood of hyperglycemia and hypokalemia. Therefore, it seems reasonable to administer the β-adrenergic agent with a hypotonic solution of 0.45% sodium chloride; in addition, it is crucial to carefully monitor the patient's total fluid daily intake.

The administration of β-adrenergic tocolysis in a parturient with preterm labor and infection may increase the risk of developing non-cardiogenic pulmonary edema, probably because of increased pulmonary vascular permeability through the release of endotoxin (88,89).

Pulmonary edema usually develops within 24 to 72 hours after the start of β-adrenergic therapy (90,91) and the clinical presentation is nearly identical to that of other types of pulmonary edema: Dyspnea, tachypnea, tachycardia, hypoxemia, and diffuse crackles. Chest pain and a cough may also be present. A review of 58 case reports and case series found that the following were the most frequent occurrences in tocolytic-related pulmonary edema: Basilar crackles (100%), shortness of breath (76%), chest pain (24%), cough (17%), bilateral air space disease on chest radiograph (81%), and fever (14%) (84). Tocolytic-related pulmonary edema is a diagnosis of exclusion. Mortality is uncommon and treatment is supportive with most patients responding well to discontinuation of the β_2-adrenergic agonist, supplemental oxygen, fluid restriction, and diuresis. Even though mechanical ventilation may be necessary, most cases resolve within 12 to 24 hours. Persistence of symptoms beyond this time period should prompt reconsideration of the diagnosis.

Metabolic Side Effects
β-adrenergic receptor agonist administration is associated with two major metabolic effects: Hyperglycemia (30%) and hypokalemia (39%) (79,92) (Fig. 19-3). By stimulating adenyl cyclase on the membrane of liver cells, β-adrenergic agonists activate hepatic phosphorylase which increases the breakdown of glycogen and results in subsequent production of glucose and development of hyperglycemia. Insulin-dependent diabetics who receive these agents may require more frequent assessment of blood glucose levels and eventually a continuous insulin infusion in order to prevent the development of ketoacidosis (93).

Hypokalemia occurs as a result of the insulin-mediated movement of potassium, together with glucose, from the extracellular to the intracellular space, and to direct stimulation of β_2-receptors in skeletal muscle leading to activation of Na$^+$–K$^+$ ATPase (94). Total body potassium remains unchanged since urinary excretion of potassium is not increased during β-adrenergic therapy. Since serum potassium concentration returns to normal within 3 hours of discontinuing β-adrenergic therapy (95,96), intravenous potassium infusion is usually not needed (93,96,97). In addition, a rebound hyperkalemia might follow potassium infusion in patients undergoing general anesthesia regardless of the use of depolarizing or non-depolarizing muscle relaxants (98–100).

Miscellaneous Maternal Systemic Side Effects
The main central nervous system symptom associated with use of β_2-adrenergic agonists is tremor (79). Cerebral ischemia due to vasospasm has been reported in a patient who had a previous history of migraine (101). There have been four reported cases of terbutaline-associated hepatitis in

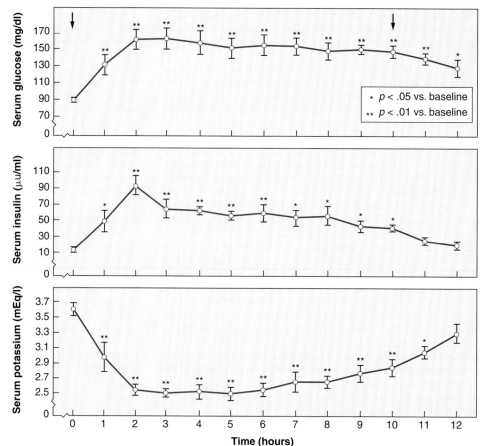

FIGURE 19-3 The levels of mean serum glucose, insulin, and potassium at baseline (*left arrow*), during 10 hours of terbutaline infusion, and 2 hours after the infusion (*right arrow*) in six patients in preterm labor. From: Cotton DB, Strassner HT, Lipson LG, et al. The effects of terbutaline on acid–base, serum electrolytes, and glucose homeostasis during the management of preterm labor. *Am J Obstet Gynecol* 1981;141:617–624, with permission.

pregnancy (102). In each case, discontinuation of terbutaline led to the amelioration of enzymatic markers of liver damage. Muscle weakness and respiratory arrest have been reported in a parturient affected by myasthenia gravis (103).

Fetal Side Effects

β-adrenergic receptor agonists promptly cross the placenta into the fetal compartment causing fetal tachycardia. Neonatal hypoglycemia may result from fetal hyperinsulinemia due to prolonged maternal hyperglycemia.

Contraindications

Labor inhibition with β-adrenergic receptor agonists should be used with caution in women with cardiac disease and in women with poorly controlled hyperthyroidism or diabetes mellitus. In women at risk for massive hemorrhage, β-adrenergic receptor agonists may cause maternal tachycardia and hypotension. The presence of these clinical signs may interfere with the mother's ability to mount a compensatory response to ongoing hemorrhage as well as confuse the clinical presentation.

The final decision of whether or not to administer these agents in these situations requires balancing the perceived benefit of delaying the delivery with potential side effects of treatment.

Anesthetic Implications of β-adrenergic Therapy

Based on published reports of obstetric anesthetic management after administration of β-adrenergic agonists (104–106), there is not enough evidence to suggest delaying neuraxial or general anesthesia when the fetus or the mother is in danger. The main concerns about giving anesthetics during the β-adrenergic therapy involve the tachycardic and hypotensive side effects of terbutaline that might exacerbate the maternal hypotension associated with the use of spinal or general anesthetics. Terbutaline's hemodynamic effects subside within 15 to 30 minutes after the drug is discontinued. The use of phenylephrine, an α_1-adrenergic agonist, counteracts the decrease in systemic vascular resistance associated with terbutaline and may cause a reflex bradycardic effect, which would be beneficial when maternal tachycardia follows terbutaline administration. Chestnut et al. (107) observed that prior administration of ritodrine did not worsen maternal hypotension when epidural lidocaine without epinephrine was administered to gravid ewes (Fig. 19-4). The inotropic and chronotropic effects of ritodrine seemed to preserve cardiac output and Please modify to UBF(Uterine Blood Flow) in that study. It is advisable to avoid aggressive fluid administration prior to or during the induction of regional or general anesthesia in patients who have received β-adrenergic agonists. If hypotension occurs, titration of vasopressors rather than fluids seem the best therapeutic option given these patients' increased propensity to develop pulmonary edema. In gravid animals rendered hypotensive by acute hemorrhage during terbutaline infusion, ephedrine aids restoration of UBF velocity (108) (Fig. 19-5). Some investigators evaluated the prophylactic administration of various vasopressors to normotensive gravid animals pretreated with a ritodrine infusion (109); they have found that while phenylephrine and epinephrine worsened UBF velocity, ephedrine preserved it (Fig. 19-6). However, the doses used to appreciate such a difference (phenylephrine 10 μg/kg and ephedrine 1 mg/kg) in that experiment were nearly 10 times higher than those used for humans in the current

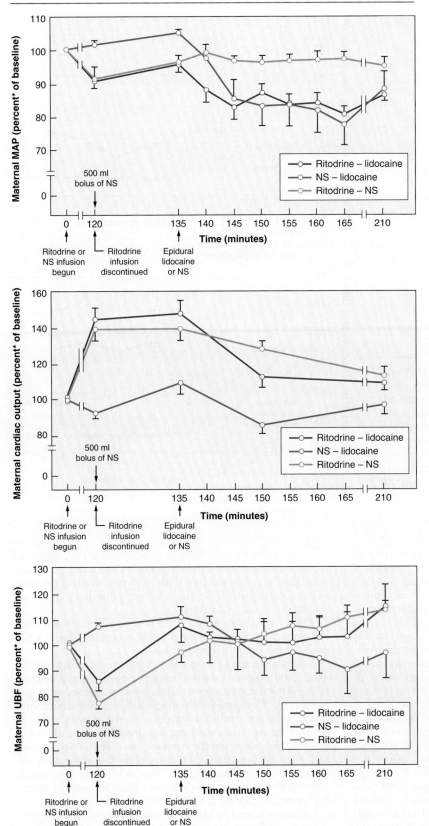

FIGURE 19-4 Response over time of maternal mean arterial pressure (MMAP), cardiac output and UBF after intravenous infusion of ritodrine of normal saline (NS) control for 2 hours, followed by epidural administration of lidocaine or NS control in gravid ewes. From: Chestnut DH, Pollack KL, Thompson CS, et al. Does ritodrine worsen maternal hypotension during epidural anesthesia in gravid ewes? *Anesthesiology* 1990;72:315–321, with permission.

clinical practice. A subsequent study compared the maternal and fetal effects of maternally administered ephedrine to phenylephrine in gravid animals subjected to epidural anesthesia-induced hypotension during ritodrine infusion (110). Ephedrine increased uteroplacental blood flow without changing uterine vascular resistance while phenylephrine administration did not change uteroplacental blood flow but increased uterine vascular resistance (Fig. 19-7). One should be careful in extrapolating laboratory data to clinical practice. To date, the most reasonable approach is to defer to the anesthesia provider's clinical decision as to whether ephedrine or phenylephrine should be used for the treatment and prevention

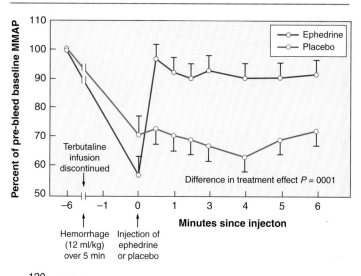

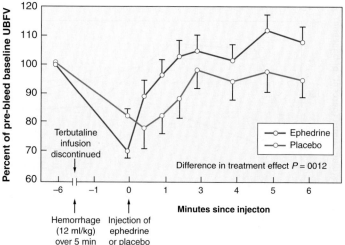

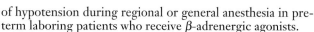

FIGURE 19-5 Response over time of MMAP and uterine artery blood flow velocity (UBFV) after hemorrhage and intravenous administration of ephedrine, 1 mg/kg, or placebo in gravid guinea pigs. All values are expressed as mean (±SEM) percentage of prebleed baseline. From: Chestnut DH, Weiner CP, Wang JP, et al. The effect of ephedrine upon uterine artery blood flow velocity in the pregnant guinea pig subjected to terbutaline infusion and acute hemorrhage. *Anesthesiology* 1987;66:508–512, with permission.

of hypotension during regional or general anesthesia in preterm laboring patients who receive β-adrenergic agonists.

If general anesthesia is required after discontinuation of a β-adrenergic agonist, one should remember that the underlying tachycardia that results from the β-adrenergic therapy makes it difficult to estimate the depth of anesthesia and fluid status. It is useful to monitor anesthesia depth by any of the devices currently available and to communicate closely with the obstetrics team for the estimation of maternal blood loss. Cardiac arrhythmias are associated with the use of β-adrenergic agonists. Shin and Kim (104) reported one case in which ventricular tachycardia and fibrillation developed after administration of ephedrine for treatment of hypotension (during epidural anesthesia for cesarean delivery) 30 minutes after the discontinuation of a ritodrine infusion. When general anesthesia is required, inhalational anesthetics that do not sensitize the myocardium to catecholamine-induced ventricular dysrhythmias (such as sevoflurane or isoflurane) seem to be the anesthetics of choice. Hyperventilation should be avoided as it may increase uterine vascular resistance and induce respiratory alkalosis. Respiratory alkalosis may contribute to the shift of potassium into the intracellular compartment, exacerbating the hypokalemia induced by β-agonist therapy.

Calcium Channel Blockers

Calcium channel blockers directly block the influx of calcium ions through the cell membrane. They also inhibit the release

of intracellular calcium from the sarcoplasmic reticulum and increase calcium efflux from the cell. The ensuing decrease in intracellular free calcium leads to an inhibition of calcium-dependent myosin light-chain kinase phosphorylation and results in myometrial relaxation.

There are no large randomized trials directly examining the efficacy of calcium channel blockers compared with a placebo for treatment of preterm labor.

A meta-analysis of 12 randomized controlled trials involving over 1,000 women compared use of calcium channel blockers to any other tocolytic agent (mainly β-adrenergic receptor agonists) (111). Compared with other tocolytics, calcium channel blockers did not significantly reduce the risk of birth within 48 hours of initiation of treatment, but they did reduce the risk of birth within 7 days. On the contrary, the nine trials comparing use of any calcium channel blockers to any β-adrenergic receptor agonist found that calcium channel blockers significantly decreased the risk of preterm labor within 48 hours of initiating treatment (RR 0.72, 95% CI 0.53–0.97) (111).

Calcium channel blockers also reduce the risk of respiratory distress syndrome, necrotizing enterocolitis (NEC), intraventricular hemorrhage (IVH), and neonatal jaundice. Similar findings were reported from a meta-analysis of nine randomized trials (679 patients) comparing treatment of preterm labor with nifedipine versus terbutaline or ritodrine (112). Nifedipine was more effective than β-adrenergic receptor agonists in delaying delivery for at least 48 hours (OR 1.52, 95% CI 1.03–2.24). A randomized trial comparing nifedipine

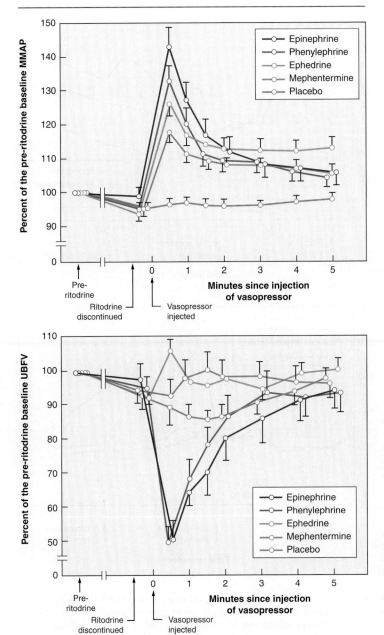

FIGURE 19-6 Response over time of MMAP and uterine artery blood flow velocity (UBFV) after intravenous infusion of ritodrine and subsequent injection of epinephrine (0.001 mg/kg), phenylephrine (0.01 mg/kg), mephentermine (1 mg/kg), ephedrine (1 mg/kg), or placebo (saline, 0.2 mL) in gravid guinea pigs. Each value is expressed as the mean (±SEM) percentage of the pre-ritodrine baseline for that pressor. From: Chestnut DH, Ostman LG, Weiner CP, et al. The effect of vasopressor agents upon uterine artery blood flow velocity in the gravid guinea pig subjected to ritodrine infusion. *Anesthesiology* 1988;68:363–366, with permission.

with magnesium sulfate did not find a significant difference in the rate of delivery within 48 hours (113). A common dosing regimen is to administer an initial loading dose of nifedipine 20 mg orally, followed by another 20 mg orally 90 minutes later. An alternative regimen is to administer 10 mg orally every 20 minutes for up to 4 doses. If contractions persist, 20 mg can be given orally every 3 to 8 hours for up to 72 hours not to exceed a maximum dose of 180 mg/day (Table 19-2).

A single orally administered dose of nifedipine acts for up to 6 hours. Plasma concentrations peak in 30 to 60 minutes. Nifedipine is almost completely metabolized in the liver and excreted by the kidney.

Maternal and Fetal Side Effects
Nifedipine is a peripheral vasodilator and may cause nausea, flushing, headache, vertigo, and palpitations. Nifedipine causes peripheral vasodilation resulting in a decrease in mean arterial pressure with the subsequent activation of baroreceptors, leading to increased peripheral sympathetic nervous system activity that manifest with maternal tachycardia. These

hemodynamic changes are usually mild and less severe than those seen after β-adrenergic agonist treatment (114–116). However, severe hypotension has been described in case reports (117,118) and has been reported in a preeclamptic patient while on a magnesium sulfate infusion (119). There are no data regarding fetal side effects related to oral dosing with the doses commonly used for labor inhibition. Animal studies showed a decrease in UBF and decreased fetal oxygen saturation with the administration of calcium channel blockers; however, in humans, Doppler studies of fetal umbilical and uteroplacental blood flow have been reassuring (120). The fetal acid–base status in the umbilical cord at delivery has not shown any fetal hypoxia or acidosis.

Contraindications
Calcium channel blockers should be used with caution in women with left ventricular dysfunction or congestive heart failure. The concomitant use of a calcium-channel blocker and magnesium sulfate could act synergistically in suppressing muscular contractility and result in respiratory depression

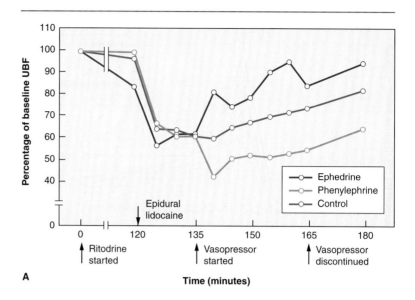

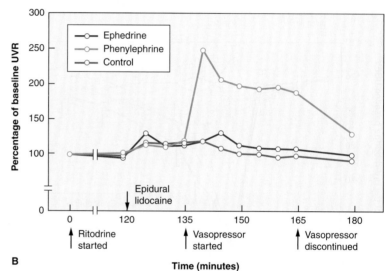

FIGURE 19-7 UBF over time for the ephedrine, phenylephrine and NS control groups. All values are expressed as mean (±SEM) (**A, B**). From: McGrath JM, Chestnut DH, Vincent RD, et al. Ephedrine remains the vasopressor of choice for treatment of hypotension during ritodrine infusion and epidural anesthesia. *Anesthesiology* 1994;80:1073–1081, with permission.

(121). Support of the maternal airway and intravenous calcium administration is the appropriate therapy for such an episode.

Anesthetic Implications of Calcium Channel Blocker Therapy

Calcium channel blockers can be continued until vaginal or cesarean delivery (122). Caution should be used when inhalational anesthetics are administered since calcium channel blockers can depress myocardial contractility and cardiac conduction. Generally speaking, these agents can increase peripheral vasodilation (123) even though nifedipine has fewer cardiovascular effects compared with other drugs of the same class. In addition, if postpartum uterine atony occurs, oxytocin and 15 methyl prostaglandin $F_2\alpha$ may not be effective in the presence of calcium channel blocker therapy thereby leading to an increased risk of postpartum hemorrhage (124).

Cyclooxygenase Inhibitors

Cyclooxygenase is the enzyme responsible for the conversion of arachidonic acid to prostaglandins. Prostaglandins increase available intracellular calcium by raising transmembrane influx and sarcolemmal release of calcium. Cyclooxygenase-1 is constitutively expressed in gestational tissues, while cyclooxygenase-2 is the inducible form that increases in the decidua

and myometrium during term and preterm labor. Cyclooxygenase inhibitors decrease prostaglandin production by either general inhibition of cyclooxygenase or specific inhibition of cyclooxygenase-2, depending upon the agent (125–129).

Indomethacin, a nonspecific cyclooxygenase inhibitor, is the most commonly used tocolytic of this class. A Cochrane review comparing cyclooxygenase inhibitors to a placebo for treatment of preterm labor included two small trials involving 70 patients (130); cyclooxygenase inhibitors were shown to reduce risk of delivery within 48 hours of initiation of treatment and within 7 days compared with the placebo. No differences were detected in perinatal mortality, respiratory distress syndrome, premature closure of the ductus arteriosus, persistent pulmonary hypertension of the newborn, IVH, or neonatal renal failure.

Ten trials compared indomethacin to β-adrenergic receptor agonists and magnesium sulfate (130). When compared with a placebo, indomethacin resulted in fewer births before 37 weeks of gestation as well as an increase in gestational age and birth weight. Compared with any other tocolytic, cyclooxygenase inhibition resulted in fewer births before 37 weeks of gestation and a reduced maternal drug reaction that would require stopping treatment. Based on these data, a decision analysis recommended the use of indomethacin as the first-line therapy for preterm labor before 32 weeks (41).

Even though cyclooxygenase-2 inhibitors have been studied for the treatment of preterm labor (131–135), currently these drugs are not used for treatment of preterm labor in humans. The dose of indomethacin for labor inhibition is given as a 50 to 100 mg loading dose orally or rectally, followed by 25 mg orally every 4 to 6 hours (Table 19-2).

Maternal and Fetal Side Effects

Nausea, esophageal reflux, and gastritis can be seen in patients treated with indomethacin for preterm labor. Maternal interstitial nephritis and platelet dysfunction may also occur. The primary fetal concerns about using indomethacin and other cyclooxygenase inhibitors are constriction of the ductus arteriosus and oligohydramnios.

Premature narrowing or closure of the ductus can cause pulmonary hypertension, tricuspid regurgitation, and persistent fetal circulation. Several cases of premature ductal closure have been reported in pregnancies in which the duration of indomethacin exposure exceeded 48 hours (136,137); however, this complication has not occurred in more than 500 fetuses exposed to shorter-term indomethacin treatment (138–140). Ductal constriction appears to depend upon both gestational age and duration of exposure. It has been described at gestations as early as 24 weeks, but it is most common after 31 to 32 weeks (141). Therefore, indomethacin is not recommended after 32 weeks of gestation and weekly fetal echocardiography should be considered if the duration of therapy exceeds 48 hours. Cyclooxygenase-2 inhibitors may also cause constriction of the ductus arteriosus (142,143).

Indomethacin enhances the action of vasopressin and reduces fetal renal blood flow with a consequential decrease in fetal urine output (144,145). The decrease in fetal urine output causes a reduction in amniotic fluid and oligohydramnios in up to 70% of women with normal amniotic fluid volumes (146).

Contraindications

Maternal contraindications to cyclooxygenase inhibitors include platelet dysfunction or bleeding disorders, hepatic dysfunction, gastrointestinal ulcerative disease, renal dysfunction, and asthma in women with hypersensitivity to aspirin.

Anesthetic Implications of Cyclooxygenase Inhibitors Therapy

As recently reported at the Third Consensus Conference on Neuraxial Anesthesia and Anticoagulation (sponsored by the American Society of Regional Anesthesia and Pain Medicine), cyclooxygenase inhibitors do not increase the risk of developing spinal or epidural hematoma (147). Therefore, if the patient is taking cyclooxygenase inhibitors, it is not necessary to obtain any tests or delay neuraxial analgesia or anesthesia for the preterm laboring patient.

Oxytocin Receptor Antagonists

Oxytocin receptor antagonists compete with oxytocin for binding to oxytocin receptors in the myometrium and decidua, thus preventing the increase in intracellular free calcium and myometrial contraction (148,149). Atosiban is a selective oxytocin receptor antagonist not available in the United States since the Food and Drug Administration declined to approve its use for tocolysis because of a trend toward a higher rate of fetal-infant death when used in patients at less than 28 weeks of gestation (150,151).

A Cochrane review found that atosiban was as effective as β-adrenergic receptor agonists for preventing PTB within 48 hours (RR 0.98, 95% CI 0.68–1.41) to 7 days (RR 0.91, 95% CI 0.69–1.20) of initiating treatment. The use of atosiban was associated with a significantly lower risk of mater-

nal side effects requiring cessation of treatment than were β-adrenergic receptor agonists (RR 0.04, 95% CI 0.02–0.11) (152). Atosiban is available for clinical use in Europe.

Nitric Oxide Donors

Nitric oxide increases the intracellular levels of cyclic guanosine 3′,5′-monophosphate (cGMP) in smooth muscle cells, thereby activating myosin light-chain kinases and relaxing smooth muscle (151). There is not enough evidence at this time to recommend nitric oxide donors for the inhibition of preterm labor (153).

■ ANTENATAL CORTICOSTEROIDS

The reason it is so important to use aggressive acute tocolysis and to delay delivery for at least 48 hours is because the outcome of a premature infant is dramatically improved if corticosteroids are administered to the mother during this time. Premature infants exposed to antenatal glucocorticoids have less incidence of respiratory distress syndrome (154), IVH, NEC, and less mortality compared with infants who have not been exposed to these drugs (155). A significant benefit was observed among infants born between 1 and 7 days after the first treatment dose, but not for those born fewer than 24 hours or more than 7 days after the first dose.

Antenatal glucocorticoid treatment is recommended for women in whom preterm delivery is anticipated within 7 days, between 24 and 34 weeks of gestation (42).

Retreatment can be considered if more than 2 weeks have elapsed since the initial course of antenatal glucocorticoid therapy, the gestational age at administration of the initial course was less than 28 weeks, the current gestational age is less than 33 weeks, and the risk of PTB has increased.

Antenatal glucocorticoid therapy leads to improvement in neonatal lung function via two mechanisms: By enhancing maturational changes in lung architecture and by inducing lung enzymes that favor biochemical maturation (156,157). Two regimens of antenatal glucocorticoid treatment are currently used: Betamethasone (2 doses of 12 mg given intramuscularly 24 hours apart) and dexamethasone (4 doses of 6 mg given intramuscularly 12 hours apart).

One study found betamethasone to be associated with a greater reduction in risk of neonatal death (158) while a trial comparing the two drugs found no significant differences between betamethasone and dexamethasone in the rate of respiratory distress, need for vasopressor therapy, NEC, retinopathy of prematurity, patent ductus arteriosus, neonatal sepsis, or neonatal mortality (159). However, neonates exposed to betamethasone had a significantly higher rate of IVH (17% vs. 6%) and brain lesions (18% vs. 7%); findings in conflict with large studies suggest that dexamethasone is associated with adverse neurologic outcomes (158,160–162).

Since it is not clear whether there is a significant improvement in outcome following antenatal glucocorticoid use after 34 weeks of gestation, the NIH Consensus Development Conference on the Effect of Glucocorticoids for Fetal Maturation on Perinatal Outcomes stated that administration of antenatal glucocorticoids after 34 weeks can be considered if there is evidence of fetal lung immaturity (163).

Even infants who receive 1 dose of betamethasone in utero, but deliver before the second dose can be given, have better outcomes than do infants who do not receive any antenatal glucocorticoids (164).

Side Effects

Antenatal glucocorticoids can be associated with a transient decrease in fetal heart rate variability after 48 to 72 hours from the time of administration (165–167). This clinical effect, therefore, should be kept in mind when assessing a fetus for possible delivery because of a non-reassuring fetal heart rate pattern. Fetal breathing and body movements are also commonly reduced, which may result in a lower biophysical profile score or a nonreactive non-stress test (166,168,169).

Treatment with glucocorticoids does not increase the risk of maternal death, chorioamnionitis, or puerperal sepsis (154). Case reports have described pulmonary edema when corticosteroids were administered in combination with tocolytics in cases of chorioamnionitis or multiple gestation pregnancies (170–172).

Transient hyperglycemia occurs in many women and can be severe in the diabetic patient (173,174); the steroid effect begins approximately 12 hours after the first dose and may last for 5 days.

The total leukocyte count increases by about 30% within 24 hours after betamethasone injection, and the lymphocyte count can decrease by about 50% (175). These changes return to baseline values within 3 days (176).

■ INTRAPARTUM MANAGEMENT OF THE LOW BIRTH WEIGHT FETUS

The goal of intrapartum management of the LBW fetus is to avoid perinatal acidosis and birth trauma (177) since the preterm fetus is not fully physiologically adapted to tolerate the stress of delivery (178). Continuous intrapartum fetal heart rate monitoring of the LBW fetus is essential since a reassuring fetal heart rate pattern correlates well with normal umbilical arterial pH, whereas a non-reassuring tracing is associated with neonatal acidosis at delivery (179–181). However, as compared with a structured program of periodic auscultation, electronic fetal monitoring does not result in improved neurologic development in children born prematurely (181). Preterm fetuses may have decreased variability because of the immaturity of their neurologic and cardiovascular systems and because of the use of maternal corticosteroids.

The place of delivery is extremely important for preterm infants. VLBW infants born in hospitals with level I or II nurseries have higher mortality than those born in hospitals that are also equipped with level III nurseries (36% vs. 21%) (182). The pediatric team must be present at delivery in order to optimize care.

Timing of Birth

When PTB is imminent during early pregnancy (before 34 weeks of gestation), the reasons are either suspected fetal acidosis or maternal conditions where the delivery would be beneficial to the mother's health. The decision becomes much more complicated when timing needs to be decided for late-preterm (34, 35, and 36 weeks) and early-term (37 and 38 weeks) births. Although at less risk than those born before 34 weeks of gestation, infants born late preterm are more likely to have long-term neurodevelopmental problems and infant death than those born at term (183). In addition, neonates born between 34 and 37 weeks account for most admissions to the neonatal intensive care unit and for a large proportion of health care expenditures. In a large study (184), more than one-third of elective (not medically indicated) cesarean deliveries at term occurred before 39 weeks of gestation, with neonates born before 39 weeks being at increased risk for significant complications compared with those born after 39 weeks. The March of Dimes, National Institute of Child Health and Human Development (NICHD), Society for Maternal-Fetal Medicine, and American College of Obstetricians and Gynecologists have since championed the idea of preventing unnecessary PTBs and "early-term births."

Several large health care groups have pushed to decrease the number of non-indicated deliveries before 39 weeks, with demonstrable success (185,186).

Nationally, the percentage of infants born in the late-preterm period declined 3%, from 9.1% in 2006 to 8.8% in 2008, after rising 25% from 7.3% to 9.1% between 1990 and 2006 (187).

After analyzing data from more than 46 million infants born in the United States between 1995 and 2006, Reddy et al. (38) have found that infants born at 37 weeks were twice as likely to die before their first birthday (3.9 deaths for every 1,000 births in 2006) than those born at 40 weeks (1.9 deaths per 1,000 births). Common causes of death included birth defects, sudden infant death syndrome (SIDS), intrauterine and birth hypoxemia, and accidents.

An ongoing clinical evaluation requires balancing the risks of continuing the pregnancy with the risks of delivery before term (Fig. 19-8). In order to simplify the approach to determine the best timing for late preterm and early-term births, three factors dictate the clinical management:

1. Maternal and Obstetric
2. Uteroplacental
3. Fetal

Maternal and Obstetric Factors Influencing Timing of Delivery

Hypertensive disorders, diabetes, and prior stillbirth are the main factors that carry an ongoing risk while preterm labor and PPROM are acute issues.

Hypertensive Disorders and Timing of Delivery

The risks of continued pregnancy in the setting of gestational hypertension or preeclampsia include development of severe preeclampsia and its complications and the additional fetal risk and fetal morbidity (fetal growth restriction, asphyxia after hypertensive crisis and placental abruption, and death). There is evidence-based data from the hypertension and preeclampsia intervention trial at term (HYPITAT) that suggests that delivery is indicated in pregnancies complicated by mild gestational hypertension or mild preeclampsia occurring at 37 or more weeks of gestation (188). By contrast, there are no data to support that expectant monitoring in women with mild gestational hypertension or preeclampsia at 34, 35, and 36 weeks will improve perinatal outcomes or increase maternal and fetal risks. The potential risks from expectant monitoring in such pregnancies are severe hypertension, eclampsia, HELLP syndrome, abruptio placentae, pulmonary edema, fetal growth restriction, and fetal death (189).

In the absence of randomized trials, there are expert opinion recommendations for expectant monitoring in these women in the absence of the following factors: Severe hypertension, preterm labor or rupture of membranes, vaginal bleeding, and abnormal fetal testing (variable or late decelerations, absent or reverse umbilical artery diastolic flow, biophysical score of 6 or less, fetal growth restriction, and oligohydramnios). When the diagnosis of severe preeclampsia is made at or after 34 weeks, imminent delivery is indicated in order to decrease maternal morbidity and mortality (189) (Table 19-3).

Diabetes and Timing of Delivery

The greatest risk associated with diabetes in pregnancy is intrauterine fetal death or stillbirth. Based on a recent report by Reddy et al. (190), there is a 3.1 adjusted absolute risk (per 1,000 births) for stillbirth in women with preexisting diabetes compared with the general population. The risk of stillbirth appears to increase in non-anomalous diabetic pregnancies

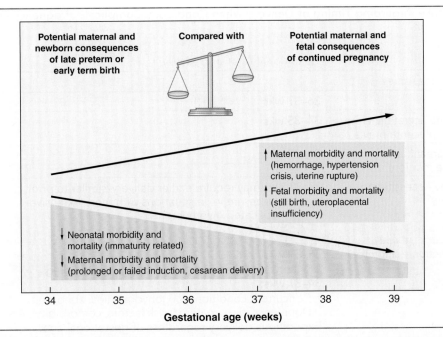

FIGURE 19-8 Conceptual diagram representing the competing risks and benefits of indicated late-preterm or early-term birth compared with pregnancy continuation. The figure does not represent specific magnitudes or rates of changes in risks because these will vary according to the specific pregnancy complication and individual circumstances. Neonatal morbidity and mortality decreases with advancing gestation; these typically are related to prematurity. For these deliveries in the late-preterm or early-term period, maternal morbidity and mortality generally are higher as a result of prolonged or failed induction and resultant cesarean deliveries. Potential maternal consequences of continued pregnancy in the setting of complicated conditions and maternal morbidity and mortality are related to hemorrhage, hypertensive crises, and uterine rupture. Continued pregnancy in these settings also can result in fetal morbidity and stillbirth due to uteroplacental insufficiency. Reprinted with permission from: Spong CY, Mercer BM, D'alton M, et al. Timing of indicated late-preterm and early-term birth. *Obstet Gynecol* 2011;118:323–333.

starting at 34 weeks of gestation (191). Furthermore, at 38 weeks the fetal death rate per 1,000 births actually increases in pregnancies complicated by diabetes. Studies by Cundy et al. (192,193), MacIntosh et al. (193), and Lauenborg et al. (194) reported that from 25% to 38% of all deaths in non-anomalous fetuses of insulin-requiring diabetic women occurred during or after the 37th gestational week. On the basis of factors such as poor maternal glycemic control, at least some of these fetal losses are preventable. However, late fetal deaths have also been reported in diabetic women with good glycemic control and normal antepartum testing (194). Furthermore, beginning in the 37th week, the fetal death rate far exceeded the neonatal death rate (192–194).

This implies that while one cannot exclude neonatal morbidity, there is a real possibility of decreasing perinatal mortality by delivery on or after the beginning of the 37th week.

Even though early delivery in the setting of diabetes may reduce the risks of macrosomia, associated birth trauma, and stillbirth, data from randomized controlled trials are lacking and the optimal timing of delivery in diabetic parturients depends on the severity of the condition, presence of comorbidities, whether treatment with medication is needed, and the occurrence of superimposed obstetric conditions (Table 19-3).

Prior Stillbirth and Timing of Delivery
Women with a history of stillbirth are at increased risk for fetal growth restriction, PTB, preeclampsia and stillbirth. Since delivery before 39 weeks of gestation has not been proven to reduce the risk of recurrent stillbirth or adverse pregnancy outcomes in women with prior stillbirths, in the absence of fetal growth restriction and comorbidities, a

history of an unexplained stillbirth is not an indication for late-preterm or early-term birth (Table 19-3). Given the lack of demonstrable benefit from early delivery in this situation, obstetricians perform amniocentesis for lung maturity if scheduled delivery is intended due to maternal anxiety, preferences, or both before 39 weeks of gestation. Importantly, however, a mature pulmonary profile in the late-preterm or early-term period does not assure the absence of neonatal complications (195).

Preterm Labor, Preterm PROM, and Timing of Delivery
Women presenting with preterm labor or PROM may proceed to deliver spontaneously, but this does not occur in all cases. Expectant management of late-preterm or early-term PROM is associated with increased risks of chorioamnionitis and the potential for fetal death from umbilical cord compression, but the latency until delivery is brief in most cases. Because of brief latency, newborn outcomes are unlikely to be improved with expectant management after late-preterm or early-term PROM, and delivery is recommended with preterm PROM occurring at or after 34 weeks of gestation, or in patients with PROM who have reached 34 weeks (195) (Table 19-3).

Placental and Uterine Factors Influencing Timing of Delivery
The goals of late-preterm and early-term birth for pregnancies complicated by placental and uterine conditions are to avoid acute catastrophic maternal complications and to limit the potential for fetal death or compromise. In addition, early delivery can avert an emergent unscheduled delivery performed under suboptimal circumstances. Relevant conditions include placenta previa; placenta accreta, increta, or percreta

TABLE 19-3 Guidance Regarding Timing of Delivery when Conditions Complicate Pregnancy at or after 34 Weeks of Gestation

Condition	Gestational Age[a] at Delivery	Grade of Recommendation[b]
Placental and Uterine Issues		
Placenta previa[c]	36–37 wks	B
Suspected placenta accreta, increta, or percreta with placenta previa[c]	34–35 wks	B
Prior classical cesarean (upper segment uterine incision)[c]	36–37 wks	B
Prior myomectomy necessitating cesarean delivery[c]	37–38 wks (may require earlier delivery, similar to prior classical cesarean, in situations with more extensive or complicated myomectomy)	B
Fetal Issues		
Fetal growth restriction—singleton	38–39 wks: • Otherwise uncomplicated, no concurrent findings	B
	34–37 wks: • Concurrent conditions (oligohydramnios, abnormal Doppler studies, maternal risk factors, comorbidity)	B
	Expeditious delivery regardless of gestational age: • Persistent abnormal fetal surveillance suggesting imminent fetal jeopardy	
Fetal growth restriction—twin gestation	36–37 wks: • Dichorionic-diamniotic twins with isolated fetal growth restriction	B
	32–34 wks: • Monochorionic-diamniotic twins with isolated fetal growth restriction	B
	• Concurrent conditions (oligohydramnios, abnormal Doppler studies, maternal risk factors, comorbidity)	B
	Expeditious delivery regardless of gestational age: • Persistent abnormal fetal surveillance suggesting imminent fetal jeopardy	
Fetal congenital malformations[c]	34–39 wks: Suspected worsening of fetal organ damage Potential for fetal intracranial hemorrhage (e.g., vein of Galen aneurysm, neonatal alloimmune thrombocytopenia) When delivery prior to labor is preferred (e.g., EXIT procedure) Previous fetal intervention Concurrent maternal disease (e.g., preeclampsia, chronic hypertension) Potential for adverse maternal effect from fetal condition	B
	Expeditious delivery regardless of gestational age: • When intervention is expected to be beneficial • Fetal complications develop (abnormal fetal surveillance, new-onset hydrops fetalis, progressive or new-onset organ injury) • Maternal complications develop (mirror syndrome)	B
Multiple gestations: Dichorionic-diamniotic[c]	38 wks	B
Multiple gestations: Monochorionic-diamniotic[c]	34–37 wks	B
Multiple gestations: Dichorionic-diamniotic or monochorionic-diamniotic with single fetal death[c]	If occurs at or after 34 wks, consider delivery (recommendation limited to pregnancies at or after 34 wks; if occurs before 34 wks, individualize based on concurrent maternal or fetal conditions)	B

TABLE 19-3 Guidance Regarding Timing of Delivery when Conditions Complicate Pregnancy at or after 34 Weeks of Gestation (*Continued*)

Condition	Gestational Age[a] at Delivery	Grade of Recommendation[b]
Multiple gestations: Monochorionic-monoamniotic[c]	32–34 wks	B
Multiple gestations: Monochorionic-monoamniotic with single fetal death[c]	Consider delivery; individualized according to gestational age and concurrent complications	B
Oligohydramnios—isolated and persistent[c]	36–37 wks	B
Maternal Issues		
Chronic hypertension—no medications[c]	38–39 wks	B
Chronic hypertension—controlled on medication[c]	37–39 wks	B
Chronic hypertension—difficult to control (requiring frequent medication adjustments)[c]	36–37 wks	B
Gestational hypertension[d]	37–38 wks	B
Preeclampsia—severe[c]	At diagnosis (recommendation limited to pregnancies at or after 34 wks)	C
Preeclampsia—mild[c]	37 wks	B
Diabetes—pregestational well controlled[c]	LPTB or ETB not recommended	B
Diabetes—pregestational with vascular disease[c]	37–39 wks	B
Diabetes—pregestational, poorly controlled[c]	34–39 wks (individualized to situation)	B
Diabetes—gestational well controlled on diet[c]	LPTB or ETB not recommended	B
Diabetes—gestational well controlled on medication[c]	LPTB or ETB not recommended	B
Diabetes—gestational poorly controlled on medication[c]	34–39 wks (individualized to situation)	B
Obstetric Issues		
Prior stillbirth-unexplained[c]	LPTB or ETB not recommended Consider amniocentesis for fetal pulmonary maturity if delivery planned at less than 39 wks	B C
Spontaneous preterm birth: PPROM[c]	34 wks (recommendation limited to pregnancies at or after 34 wks)	B
Spontaneous preterm birth: Active preterm labor[c]	Delivery if progressive labor or additional maternal or fetal indication	B

[a]Gestational age is in completed weeks; thus, 34 weeks includes 34 0/7 weeks through 34 6/7 weeks.

[b]Grade of recommendations are based on the following: Recommendations or conclusions or both are based on good and consistent scientific evidence (A); limited or inconsistent scientific evidence (B); primarily consensus and expert opinion (C). The recommendations regarding expeditious delivery for imminent fetal jeopardy were not given a grade. The recommendation regarding severe preeclampsia is based largely on expert opinion; however, higher-level evidence is not likely to be forthcoming because this condition is believed to carry significant maternal risk with limited potential fetal benefit from expectant management after 34 weeks.

[c]Uncomplicated, thus no fetal growth restriction, superimposed preeclampsia, etc. If these are present, then the complicating conditions take precedence and earlier delivery may be indicated.

[d]Maintenance antihypertensive therapy should not be used to treat gestational hypertension.

LPTB, late-preterm birth at 34 0/7 weeks through 36 6/7 weeks; ETB, early-term birth at 37 0/7 weeks through 38 6/7 weeks.

(hereafter referred to as "placenta accreta"); chronic abruptio placentae; and conditions that carry a significant risk of uterine rupture such as prior classical cesarean delivery and prior myomectomy (195) (Table 19-3).

Placenta Previa and Timing of Delivery
Placenta previa is likely to result in hemorrhage before delivery of the fetus. For the asymptomatic patient near term, the risk of continuing pregnancy is of an unscheduled delivery due to hemorrhage or labor. Suboptimal timing can result in decreased availability of needed resources (e.g., blood products, dedicated operating room staff and surgical specialists), and in fetal or neonatal hypoxemia or acidemia resulting from maternal hypovolemic shock. Of 230 cases with placenta previa, the risk of an emergent bleed for hemorrhage was 4.7% at 35 weeks, 15% at 36 weeks, 30% at 37 weeks, and 59% at 38 weeks (196,197).

A decision analysis and expert opinion recommended delivery at 36 to 37 weeks of gestation in women with uncomplicated placenta previa (197,198) (Table 19-3).

Placenta Accreta and Timing of Delivery
Forty-four percent of women with placenta accreta will require emergency surgery if delivery is planned after 36 weeks (199). Case-controlled studies of placenta accreta have demonstrated that catastrophic bleeding is common after 36 weeks and planned delivery at 34 to 35 weeks after antenatal steroids resulted in decreased blood loss and blood transfusions (199,200).

A decision analysis came to similar conclusions that in the setting of placenta accreta, delivery without confirmation of fetal lung maturity after 34 weeks results in the highest quality-adjusted life years (201) (Table 19-3).

Chronic Abruptio Placentae and Timing of Delivery
Chronic abruptio placentae is not well defined in the literature but has been described as intermittent or persistent uterine bleeding in the third trimester without other evident cause. Typically, those with abruptio placentae and maternal hemodynamic compromise or non-reassuring fetal testing are delivered rather than managed conservatively. One percent of pregnancies are complicated by abruption placentae, but the incidence of chronic abruption is unknown. Risk factors include trauma, preeclampsia, maternal vascular disease, and substance use. Complications of the condition include uteroplacental insufficiency which in turn can result in fetal growth restriction and stillbirth, as well as complications similar to those noted for placenta previa. Although early delivery potentially could avoid further placental separation with subsequent acute hemorrhage requiring emergent delivery, the lack of a standard definition and limited data regarding the clinical course of this condition preclude recommendations regarding the optimal timing of delivery (195) (Table 19-3).

Prior Classical Cesarean Delivery, Uterine Myomectomy, and Timing of Delivery
Several conditions carry a significant risk of uterine rupture. Prior cesarean delivery with a vertical incision involving the upper muscular portion of the uterus (e.g., classical cesarean) accounted for 9% of indicated repeat cesarean deliveries in one large prospective observational study (202). The prevalence of prior classical cesarean affecting pregnancy is 0.3% to 0.4%, with a risk of uterine rupture in subsequent pregnancies ranging between 1% and 12%. Similarly, myomectomy can involve the muscular portion of the myometrium, but the frequency of this condition complicating pregnancy is unknown. When myomectomy involves the muscular portion of the myometrium, delivery by cesarean is typically recommended (in contrast to myomectomy of a pedunculated myoma where vaginal delivery remains an option). One study found uterine rupture risks of 0.49% to 0.7% after laparoscopic myomectomy and 1.7% after resection at laparotomy; however, it is unknown if any differences in risk relate to the surgical technique or the characteristics of patients selected for one approach over the other (195). Little is known regarding the effect of the location of the leiomyoma (e.g., transmural compared with intramural compared with serosal and upper compared with lower uterine segment), extent of resection (number excised) on uterine rupture risk. After uterine rupture, the fetus is at risk for stillbirth, as well as hypoxia or acidosis and their sequelae.

In women with prior uterine surgery involving the muscular portion, uterine rupture can also occur before the onset of labor (195). Early delivery can avert the risk of uterine rupture and its sequelae. Based on cohort studies and a decision analysis, delivery at 36 to 37 weeks is recommended in the setting of prior classical cesarean, with an estimated trade-off of 22 cases of respiratory distress syndrome to prevent one case of hypoxic ischemic encephalopathy after uterine rupture (195). Although the potential risk for uterine rupture after myomectomy is low, the consequences can be catastrophic. Thus, when cesarean is planned for women with prior myomectomy, the strategy of delivery at 37 to 38 weeks may be considered, with individualization based on the type and extent of the myomectomy surgery (Table 19-3).

Fetal Factors Influencing Timing of Delivery
A number of fetal conditions place the fetus at risk for stillbirth, hypoxia or acidosis, cardiac failure, or all of these. Examples include vasa previa, fetal growth restriction, congenital malformations, multiple gestations, and isolated oligohydramnios. Late-preterm or early-term birth may be beneficial under such circumstances to avoid fetal death and long-term neurologic sequelae secondary to a hostile intrauterine environment.

Vasa Previa and Timing of Delivery
A recent decision analysis suggests that for women with a vasa previa, delivery at 34 to 35 weeks of gestation may balance the risk of perinatal death with the risks of infant mortality, respiratory distress syndrome, mental retardation, and cerebral palsy related to prematurity. At any given gestational age, incorporating amniocentesis for verification of fetal lung maturity does not improve outcomes in parturients with vasa previa (203).

Fetal Growth Restriction and Timing of Delivery
After 34 weeks, intrauterine growth restriction (IUGR) in a singleton or twin pregnancy who develops either oligohydramnios or absent end diastolic flow (AEDF) in the umbilical artery should be delivered proximate to the diagnosis of these complications (204). In singleton pregnancies in which the IUGR fetus has normal amniotic fluid volume, Doppler studies, and biophysical testing, the fetus is likely constitutionally small and may be managed expectantly until 38 to 39 weeks.

If Doppler testing becomes abnormal indicating a placental etiology, delivery by 36 to 37 weeks is reasonable (204) (Table 19-3).

Fetal Anomalies and Timing of Delivery
Many fetal anomalies do not necessitate either late-preterm or early-term birth, and these fetuses are better served by allowing time for growth and maturation in utero. In a few selected circumstances, there are specific maternal risks of continuing pregnancy near term (205). These include maternal risk of uterine rupture for the small number of patients

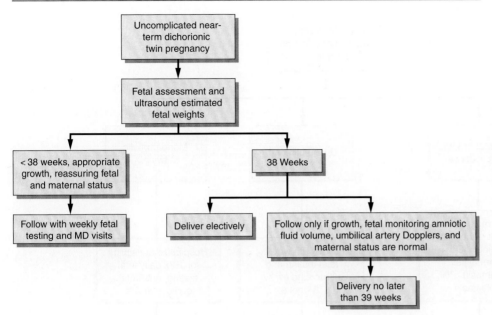

FIGURE 19-9 Algorithm for determining the timing of delivery in uncomplicated, near-term dichorionic twins. Reprinted with permission from: Newman RB, Unal ER. Multiple gestations: timing of indicated late preterm and early-term births in uncomplicated dichorionic, monochorionic, and monoamniotic twins. *Semin Perinatol* 2011;35:277–285.

who undergo invasive fetal intervention during pregnancy. Currently, there are fewer than 25 reported cases of open fetal surgery per year in the United States, and the number is decreasing as interventions shift to endoscopic techniques and limited indications remain. Open fetal surgery involves a hysterotomy; therefore, current recommendations are for delivery at 36 weeks after documentation of fetal lung maturity (206). After endoscopic intervention during pregnancy, timing of delivery is not affected unless there is a need for the ex utero intrapartum technique (EXIT) (207). Delivery is recommended at any point when worsening of fetal organ damage is suspected (Table 19-3).

Multiple Gestations and Timing of Delivery

Multiple gestations carry increased maternal and fetal risks whether uncomplicated or affected by a single fetal death. In addition to PTB, maternal conditions such as gestational diabetes, preeclampsia, abruption placentae, placenta previa, and postpartum hemorrhage are more common in twin pregnancies. Early delivery may reduce the risk of stillbirth and allow timing of delivery to optimize staffing and resources for newborn care in complex cases.

Once the ultrasound shows two placentas (dichorionic) in an uncomplicated twin pregnancy, the obstetrician feels comfortable to wait until 38 weeks when the optimal outcome is expected (Fig. 19-9). When only one placenta (monochorionic) is detected, then it is very important to determine whether one (monoamniotic) or two (diamniotic) amniotic sacs are present. Because of the high risk of cord entanglement resulting in fetal death in monoamniotic twins, delivery at 32 to 34 weeks is recommended. Even uncomplicated diamniotic–monochorionic twins have higher risks of stillbirth; thus, a late-preterm delivery (34 to 37 weeks) is recommended (208) (Fig. 19-10). In the setting of a multiple gestation with one fetal demise, early delivery may prevent a second fetal death. In a dichorionic pregnancy with a single fetal demise, expectant management to 37 weeks with weekly surveillance is generally recommended; however, due to limited data, delivery between 34 and 36 weeks may also be reasonable (208). In monochorionic (mono- and diamniotic) gestations with a single fetal demise, neurologic injury may not be preventable due to the acute cardiovascular effects in the surviving co-twin; however, the risk of stillbirth in the

live fetus versus the risks of early delivery may need to be weighed. Regardless of chorionicity, maternal anxiety in these situations cannot be underestimated and may be a factor in the clinical judgment regarding the timing of delivery. Considerations regarding delivery timing for multiple gestations are summarized in Table 19-3.

Oligohydramnios and Timing of Delivery

Isolated oligohydramnios has been defined by some as a single vertical pocket of 2.0 cm or less and by others as an amniotic fluid index of 5.0 cm or less (195). Oligohydramnios is associated with an increase in nonreactive non-stress tests (NSTs) (1.5-fold), fetal heart rate decelerations (1.8-fold), fetal intolerance in labor, stillbirth (4.5-fold), an Apgar score of 3 at 5 minutes (11-fold), and meconium aspiration (12-fold). Oligohydramnios in the presence of normal fetal growth may be less ominous than when it is associated with abnormal fetal growth. However, ultrasonography is insensitive in the diagnosis of fetal growth restriction when population-based nomograms are used. The advantage of early delivery is the avoidance of stillbirth, but the maternal risks of early delivery are those related to labor induction and cesarean delivery. In the setting of otherwise uncomplicated isolated and persistent oligohydramnios, delivery at 36 to 37 weeks is recommended (Table 19-3). The decision regarding timing of delivery for oligohydramnios is usually made by evaluating the amniotic fluid in concert with fetal testing, evaluation of the fetal growth, and maternal condition (195).

Mode of Delivery and Anesthetic Management

Cesarean Versus Vaginal Delivery

The optimal mode of delivery for women at high risk of delivering a preterm baby is controversial. One might think that routine cesarean delivery of these fetuses would avoid labor and vaginal delivery, thereby reducing hypoxic stress, intracranial trauma, and IVH. However, for the vertex fetus, most studies of routine cesarean versus vaginal delivery have not demonstrated differences in outcome (209–212).

Cesarean deliveries of LBW fetuses, especially those that are in non-vertex presentation, VLBW, or ELBW, may require a vertical or classical hysterotomy incision. The lower uterine segment may not be developed enough to perform a low transverse incision; in addition, if the incision is too

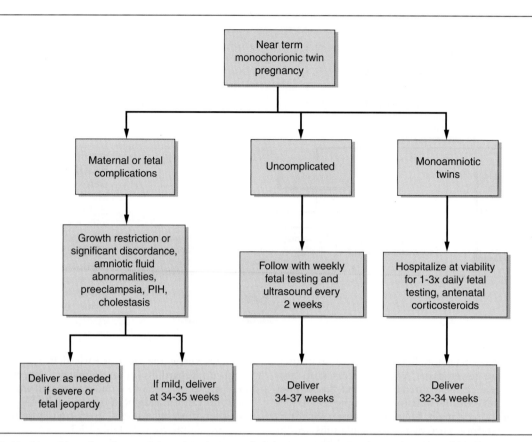

FIGURE 19-10 Algorithm for determining the timing of delivery in uncomplicated, near-term monochorionic twins. Reprinted with permission from: Newman RB, Unal ER. Multiple gestations: timing of indicated late preterm and early-term births in uncomplicated dichorionic, monochorionic, and monoamniotic twins. *Semin Perinatol* 2011;35:277–285.

small, this may not allow for the infant's head to deliver without trauma, thus carrying the additional risk of head compression, head entrapment, and IVH. The vertical uterine incision offers the advantage of an easier surgical approach; however, there is increased risk of postoperative complications such as bleeding and repeat surgery in future pregnancies.

In addition, it is not clear whether the mode of delivery, or whether avoiding fetal head compression, would prevent the development of IVH in fetuses without a bleeding diathesis. A few studies found no correlation between spontaneous vaginal, low forceps vaginal, or cesarean delivery and fetal or neonatal IVH (212,213). However, the three important factors associated with a significantly increased risk of IVH are 1-minute Apgar score of less than 7, birth weight less than 1,250 g, and respiratory distress syndrome (177). In order to decrease perineal resistance and to minimize trauma to the fetal head, episiotomies and instrumental deliveries were recommended in the past. Data available now show no improvement in outcomes for preterm infants who undergo episiotomy and forceps delivery (214,215).

While forceps can be used at any gestational age, experts suggest not using a vacuum in fetuses delivering at less than 34 weeks of gestation due to the risk of fetal IVH. In preterm fetuses, the head is relatively larger than the buttocks and thighs and an eventual breech presentation would be difficult to manage because of the risk of head entrapment. In twin deliveries, when twin B has a non-vertex presentation, total breech extraction might be more complicated if the estimated fetal weight is less than 2,000 g (216), and cesarean delivery might be a better therapeutic option. Many authors have recommended the routine use of cesarean delivery for breech infants weighing less than 1,500 g (153,217–219). At

the author's institution, where preterm twin B vaginal delivery is managed quite often, obstetricians routinely deliver twin B vaginally when the estimated weight is above 1,500 g. However, regardless of twin B's estimated weight, obstetricians at this institution do not attempt breech extractions if twin B's estimated weight is greater than 20% compared with twin A or if twin B is more than 1 lb heavier than twin A.

It is prudent that the obstetric anesthesia provider discuss the plan of action thoroughly with the patient, obstetricians, and neonatologists, especially when the fetus' gestational age puts it at the edge of viability.

As an example, if an emergency cesarean delivery is needed in a morbidly obese patient whose fetus is at the limit of viability, the obstetrician will want to perform skin incision as soon as possible. While anesthesia providers are inherently aware of the potential for a failed maternal airway in this scenario, it is extremely important to raise any issues with the obstetric and neonatology teams well in advance. One might want to attempt a neuraxial block before considering general anesthesia, and all teams should be aware of the anesthesiologists' concerns well in advance. This situation is so dynamic that from 1 day to another the plan might change either because the patient does not want any efforts made to resuscitate the newborn or, alternately, because the fetus' condition is improving. Therefore, the anesthesiologist must be part of the discussion with the teams and the patient.

The American Heart Association and the American Academy of Pediatrics recommend that resuscitation is not indicated if the infant is delivered at less than 23 completed weeks of gestation or if the infant weighs less than 400 g (220). Besides gestational age and weight, exposure to antenatal corticosteroids and female gender (221) also play favorable roles in the infants' outcome as identified in a Neonatal Research Network of the NICHD prospective study involving 4,446 infants born from 22 to 25 weeks of gestational age. These investigators have also posted an online outcome estimator (http://www.nichd.nih.gov/about/org/cdbpm/pp/prog_epbo/epbo_case.cfm) that allows clinicians to have a rough idea of the infant's outcome, keeping in mind that every infant is an individual and that factors beyond those used to formulate standardized assessments may influence an infant's outcome.

Anesthetic Management

The anesthetic options for a patient carrying a preterm fetus are the same as a parturient carrying a fetus at term. Since these patients carry a higher risk of cesarean delivery than do patients close to term, the anesthesiologist should be alert to the possibility of using an early neuraxial block when a non-reassuring fetal heart rate tracing concerns the obstetricians. This decision should be made on a case-by-case basis. If the patient is comfortable but does have a non-reassuring trace, it is not uncommon for the anesthesia provider to be asked to start the neuraxial block at low dose continuous infusion in case a cesarean delivery will be needed shortly. When a non-reassuring tracing occurs, the obstetric team reassesses the patient every 15 minutes. If no fetal heart rate abnormalities are noticed within 30 minutes, the team might decide to let the patient out of bed and allow her to resume her regular activities. In that case, the epidural infusion is stopped and the patient is frequently reassessed to determine whether the infusion needs to be restarted. The non-reassuring trace might change to a reassuring trace and can stay that way a few days. The *nihil per os* (NPO) status, whether the patient should get out of bed, and whether to keep the neuraxial infusion should all be reassessed frequently with the obstetric team. When there is high concern about emergent cesarean delivery and the neuraxial infusion is not desired, the obstetric anesthesia provider may offer the patient the option of having the epidural catheter in place without an infusion. In this situation, the epidural catheter should be flushed every few hours with normal saline to keep it patent and the patient's clinical condition should be frequently reassessed.

The obstetric team does not permit a patient whose cervical dilation is 7 to 8 cm and who is carrying a preterm fetus to get out of bed because that dilation might be enough to allow the delivery of a small preterm infant. In that situation, one may decide to start a continuous infusion of epidural normal saline if the patient is allowed to eat; conversely, one may decide to run an infusion of a low dose local anesthetic (bupivacaine 7.5 mg/h) and opioid (fentanyl 12 μg/h) if the patient is allowed to drink clear fluids only. It is not uncommon to start a local anesthetic and opioid mixture. If the patient is allowed to eat later, the infusion can be stopped, the anesthesia provider can make sure that no motor or sensory blocks are present, and then the patient can be allowed to eat. The previous statements describe how such a situation might be handled in the author's institution. Since other institutions and obstetricians might manage these patients differently, it is mandatory that the anesthesiologist defines the anesthetic plan in concert with all teams involved in the care of the patient and thoroughly discuss all details in advance in case an emergency arises.

If vaginal delivery is expected, the goals of neuraxial analgesia are as follows:

1. Inhibition of inappropriate maternal expulsive efforts before complete cervical dilation
2. Avoidance of precipitous delivery, which may result in fetal head trauma
3. Relaxation of the pelvic floor and perineum which will facilitate a more controlled delivery of the infant's head

This last factor is very important when there is a breech presentation. When vaginal delivery is imminent, combined spinal–epidural analgesia may be preferred over the single-shot spinal technique. Even though both techniques provide quick pain relief and maximal perineal relaxation, if forceps unexpectedly need to be used later or if emergent cesarean delivery is needed, the combined spinal–epidural technique offers the advantage of administering additional medications through the epidural catheter, thereby decreasing the patient's risk of undergoing emergent general anesthesia. Pudendal block and local anesthetic infiltration are not appealing choices since they do not relax the levator ani, bulbocavernosus muscles, and pelvic floor musculature.

When cesarean delivery is indicated in women carrying preterm fetuses, the administration of neuraxial or general anesthesia as well as the anesthetic drugs and doses do not differ from those administered to the parturient carrying a term fetus.

The preterm fetus, in contrast to what was previously thought, is less susceptible to the depressant effects of local anesthetics (222); in fact, the amount of lidocaine necessary to induce seizures in preterm fetal lambs is greater than that required in older fetal lambs. In addition, the cardiovascular response to lidocaine is less severe in younger fetuses.

Pedersen et al. (223) have shown that pharmacokinetics and pharmacodynamics of lidocaine in the maternal and fetal sheep did not differ between term and preterm gestational ages. Overall, pharmacokinetics and pharmacodynamics of lidocaine in the maternal and fetal sheep do not differ between preterm and term gestational ages.

Morishima et al. (224) subjected preterm fetal lambs to modest asphyxia by producing partial umbilical cord occlusion. They then gave the fetuses either intravenous lidocaine or saline-control for 3 hours. At steady state, maternal and fetal plasma lidocaine concentrations were similar to those obtained during epidural anesthesia in humans. Asphyxia and lidocaine resulted in acidosis, a significant decrease in mean arterial pressure, and decreased blood flow to brain, heart, and adrenal glands. These responses differed from the responses to lidocaine in the asphyxiated mature fetal lamb, as observed in an earlier study by the same group of investigators (225). The authors concluded that the preterm, immature fetal lamb "loses its cardiovascular adaptation to asphyxia when exposed to clinically acceptable plasma concentrations of lidocaine obtained transplacentally from the mother." A major limitation of this study is its failure to compare lidocaine with 2-chloroprocaine, which is the local anesthetic most commonly used epidurally in North America when fetal distress occurs. 2-Chloroprocaine is rapidly metabolized in maternal and fetal plasma (226) and its placental transfer is not increased by fetal acidosis (227). In addition, the investigators did not evaluate the potential benefits related to the neuraxial anesthetic, such as reduced maternal catecholamine release and atraumatic delivery of the preterm infant.

Santos et al. (228) reported that bupivacaine abolished the compensatory increase in blood flow to vital organs in asphyxiated preterm fetal lambs but to a lesser extent to what was seen with lidocaine in their earlier study (224).

To date, while animal data show neuronal apoptosis following general anesthetic exposure, there is no substantial evidence that a general anesthetic administered to a human mother of a preterm fetus could have dire consequences for fetal or child brain development (229).

Short-term Complications of the Preterm Infant

The most common complications seen in VLBW infants are respiratory distress, retinopathy of prematurity, patent ductus arteriosus, bronchopulmonary dysplasia, sepsis, NEC, and severe IVH (230). An experienced neonatology team present in the delivery room can reduce the risk of short-term complications in VLBW infants. In fact, approximately half of VLBW infants need intubation at birth (231); in addition, prompt administration of surfactant in very preterm infants can reduce the risk of respiratory distress syndrome, pneumothorax, and pulmonary interstitial emphysema.

Heat loss occurs rapidly in premature infants because of their relatively large body surface area and their inability to produce enough heat. Hypothermia may contribute to hypoglycemia and acidosis, and it is associated with increased mortality in extremely premature infants of less than 26 weeks of gestation (232). Once in the neonatal intensive care unit, premature infants are in an incubator or under a radiant warmer to avoid hypothermia. In developing countries, skin-enhancing emollients such as petroleum jelly ointments or sunflower seed oil provide skin barrier therapy which reduces loss of heat and water, lessens the risk of infections, and even improves survival rates (233).

Respiratory distress syndrome, bronchopulmonary dysplasia, and apnea are the main manifestations of respiratory disease in preterm infants. Premature infants' heart rate and respiration should be continuously monitored beginning immediately after birth. Oxygenation also should be monitored to avoid hypoxia or hyperoxia. If the anesthesiologist is called (due to a lack of additional personnel or resources) to ventilate or intubate a premature infant, it is important to keep in mind that a preductal (right hand) oxygen saturation value of 90% can effectively oxygenate tissues and organs, thereby preventing hyperoxia.

Cardiovascular complications in the premature infant include patent ductus arteriosus and systemic hypotension. Symptomatic patent ductus arteriosus occurs in about 30% of VLBW infants (234). Systemic hypotension in the immediate postnatal period is significantly associated with morbidity and mortality in preterm infants. In one retrospective study of infants born between 23 and 25 weeks of gestation, survivors who had low blood pressure (defined as ≥3 measurements of mean arterial blood pressure ≤25 mm Hg in the first 72 hours of life) were more likely to have poor neurodevelopment at 18 to 22 months' postconceptual age compared with those with normal blood pressure (235).

IVH usually occurs in the fragile germinal matrix and increases in frequency with decreasing birth weight. Severe IVH occurs in about 12% to 15% of VLBW infants (230,234). Blood glucose concentration should be monitored routinely since hypoglycemia and hyperglycemia are common in preterm infants.

NEC occurs in up to 10% of VLBW infants and is associated with an increase in mortality.

Sepsis is a common complication among premature infants, occurring in nearly 20% of VLBW infants (236). ELBW infants who survived after one episode of neonatal infection were more likely to have adverse neurodevelopmental outcomes and poor growth compared with those who were not infected (237).

Retinopathy of prematurity is a vascular proliferative disorder that occurs in the incompletely vascularized retina of premature infants. The disease starts between 30 and 34 weeks postconceptual age, advances irregularly until 40 to 45 weeks, and resolves spontaneously in the majority of infants. However, patients with severe untreated retinopathy of prematurity are at increased risk of vision impairment.

Long-term Complications of the Preterm Infant

The most common chronic conditions associated with PTB are asthma, bronchopulmonary dysplasia, feeding problems, vision and hearing impairment, gastroesophageal reflux, and increased risk of SIDS.

Adults who were born preterm appear to have insulin resistance and higher blood pressure compared with adults born full term (238,239).

The risk of neurodevelopmental impairment is higher in survivors of premature births compared with infants born at full term. ELBV and LBW infants show impaired cognition and neurosensory deficits that persist into childhood and young adulthood (240–245).

KEY POINTS

- PTB is the leading cause of neonatal mortality.
- The goal of tocolytic therapy is to prolong labor by 2 to 7 days in order to allow the following:
  1. Sufficient time for the corticosteroids administered to the patient to accelerate fetal lung maturity, thereby reducing the risk of neonatal respiratory distress syndrome, IVH, NEC, sepsis, and mortality
  2. Transfer of the patient to a facility that can provide an appropriate level of neonatal care if the patient delivers preterm
  3. Prolongation of pregnancy when there are underlying, self-limited conditions (such as pyelonephritis or abdominal surgery) that can cause labor and are unlikely to cause recurrent preterm labor
- Prior therapy with any of the tocolytics currently available does not limit the administration of general or neuraxial anesthesia to the patient.
- Timing of delivery may change suddenly and the obstetric anesthesia provider should actively interact with the obstetric and neonatal teams in order to optimize maternal and neonatal outcomes.
- Anesthetic goals for the vaginal delivery of a preterm infant include:
  1. Inhibition of maternal expulsive efforts
  2. Relaxation of maternal pelvic floor
  3. Prevention of precipitous delivery
- Anesthetic management should be tailored to the patient's most current clinical condition and needs.

REFERENCES

1. Lawn JE, Cousens S, Zupan J. 4 million neonatal deaths: when? Where? Why? *Lancet* 2005;365:891–900.
2. MacDorman MF, Declercq E, Zhang J. Obstetrical intervention and the singleton preterm birth rate in the United States from 1991–2006. *Am J Public Health* 2010;100:2241–2247.
3. MacDorman MF, Mathews TJ. Behind international rankings of infant mortality: how the United States compares with Europe. *NCHS Data Brief* 2009;1–8.
4. Beck S, Wojdyla D, Say L, et al. The worldwide incidence of preterm birth: a systematic review of maternal mortality and morbidity. *Bull World Health Organ* 2010;88:31–38.
5. McLean M, Bisits A, Davies J, et al. A placental clock controlling the length of human pregnancy. *Nat Med* 1995;1:460–463.
6. Korebrits C, Ramirez MM, Watson L, et al. Maternal corticotropin-releasing hormone is increased with impending preterm birth. *J Clin Endocrinol Metab* 1998;83:1585–1591.
7. Challis JR, Hooper S. Birth: outcome of a positive cascade. *Baillieres Clin Endocrinol Metab* 1989;3:781–793.
8. Dole N, Savitz DA, Hertz-Picciotto I, et al. Maternal stress and preterm birth. *Am J Epidemiol* 2003; 157:14–24.
9. Li D, Liu L, Odouli R. Presence of depressive symptoms during early pregnancy and the risk of preterm delivery: a prospective cohort study. *Hum Reprod* 2009;24:146–153.
10. Lykke JA, Paidas MJ, Langhoff-Roos J. Recurring complications in second pregnancy. *Obstet Gynecol* 2009;113:1217–1224.
11. Sheiner E, Mazor-Drey E, Levy A. Asymptomatic bacteriuria during pregnancy. *J Matern Fetal Neonatal Med* 2009;22:423–427.

12. Smaill F. Antibiotics for asymptomatic bacteriuria in pregnancy. *Cochrane Database Syst Rev* 2001;CD000490.

13. Donders GG, Van CK, Bellen G, et al. Predictive value for preterm birth of abnormal vaginal flora, bacterial vaginosis and aerobic vaginitis during the first trimester of pregnancy. *BJOG* 2009;116:1315–1324.

14. Offenbacher S, Lieff S, Boggess KA, et al. Maternal periodontitis and prematurity. Part I: Obstetric outcome of prematurity and growth restriction. *Ann Periodontol* 2001;6:164–174.

15. Khader YS, Ta'ani Q. Periodontal diseases and the risk of preterm birth and low birth weight: a meta-analysis. *J Periodontol* 2005;76:161–165.

16. Lockwood CJ, Kuczynski E. Markers of risk for preterm delivery. *J Perinat Med* 1999;27:5–20.

17. Goldenberg RL, Hauth JC, Andrews WW. Intrauterine infection and preterm delivery. *N Engl J Med* 2000;342:1500–1507.

18. Nygren P, Fu R, Freeman M, et al. Evidence on the benefits and harms of screening and treating pregnant women who are asymptomatic for bacterial vaginosis: an update review for the U.S. Preventive Services Task Force. *Ann Intern Med* 2008;148:220–233.

19. Gravett MG, Novy MJ, Rosenfeld RG, et al. Diagnosis of intra-amniotic infection by proteomic profiling and identification of novel biomarkers. *JAMA* 2004;292:462–469.

20. Challis JR, Lye SJ, Gibb W, et al. Understanding preterm labor. *Ann N Y Acad Sci* 2001;943:225–234.

21. Gibbs RS, Romero R, Hillier SL, et al. A review of premature birth and subclinical infection. *Am J Obstet Gynecol* 1992;166:1515–1528.

22. Lockwood CJ, Arcuri F, Toti P, et al. Tumor necrosis factor-alpha and interleukin-1 beta regulate interleukin-8 expression in third trimester decidual cells: implications for the genesis of chorioamnionitis. *Am J Pathol* 2006;169:1294–1302.

23. Arcuri F, Toti P, Buchwalder L, et al. Mechanisms of leukocyte accumulation and activation in chorioamnionitis: interleukin 1 beta and tumor necrosis factor alpha enhance colony stimulating factor 2 expression in term decidua. *Reprod Sci* 2009;16:453–461.

24. Lynch AM, Gibbs RS, Murphy JR, et al. Complement activation fragment Bb in early pregnancy and spontaneous preterm birth. *Am J Obstet Gynecol* 2008;199:354–358.

25. Pierce BT, Pierce LM, Wagner RK, et al. Hypoperfusion causes increased production of interleukin 6 and tumor necrosis factor alpha in the isolated, dually perfused placental cotyledon. *Am J Obstet Gynecol* 2000;183:863–867.

26. Zeitlin J, Ancel PY, Saurel-Cubizolles MJ, et al. The relationship between intrauterine growth restriction and preterm delivery: an empirical approach using data from a European case-control study. *BJOG* 2000;107:750–758.

27. Harger JH, Hsing AW, Tuomala RE, et al. Risk factors for preterm premature rupture of fetal membranes: a multicenter case-control study. *Am J Obstet Gynecol* 1990;163:130–137.

28. Williams MA, Mittendorf R, Lieberman E, et al. Adverse infant outcomes associated with first-trimester vaginal bleeding. *Obstet Gynecol* 1991;78:14–18.

29. Salafia CM, Lopez-Zeno JA, Sherer DM, et al. Histologic evidence of old intrauterine bleeding is more frequent in prematurity. *Am J Obstet Gynecol* 1995;173:1065–1070.

30. Elovitz MA, Saunders T, Ascher-Landsberg J, et al. Effects of thrombin on myometrial contractions in vitro and in vivo. *Am J Obstet Gynecol* 2000;183:799–804.

31. O'Sullivan CJ, Allen NM, O'Loughlin AJ, et al. Thrombin and PAR1-activating peptide: effects on human uterine contractility in vitro. *Am J Obstet Gynecol* 2004;190:1098–1105.

32. Ou CW, Orsino A, Lye SJ. Expression of connexin-43 and connexin-26 in the rat myometrium during pregnancy and labor is differentially regulated by mechanical and hormonal signals. *Endocrinology* 1997;138:5398–5407.

33. Word RA, Stull JT, Casey ML, et al. Contractile elements and myosin light chain phosphorylation in myometrial tissue from nonpregnant and pregnant women. *J Clin Invest* 1993;92:29–37.

34. Onderdonk AB, Hecht JL, McElrath TF, et al. Colonization of second-trimester placenta parenchyma. *Am J Obstet Gynecol* 2008;199:52.

35. Watts DH, Krohn MA, Hillier SL, et al. The association of occult amniotic fluid infection with gestational age and neonatal outcome among women in preterm labor. *Obstet Gynecol* 1992;79:351–357.

36. Plunkett J, Muglia LJ. Genetic contributions to preterm birth: implications from epidemiological and genetic association studies. *Ann Med* 2008;40:167–195.

37. Plunkett J, Feitosa MF, Trusgnich M, et al. Mother's genome or maternally-inherited genes acting in the fetus influence gestational age in familial preterm birth. *Hum Hered* 2009;68:209–219.

38. Reddy UM, Bettegowda VR, Dias T, et al. Term pregnancy: a period of heterogeneous risk for infant mortality. *Obstet Gynecol* 2011;117:1279–1287.

39. Creasy RK. Preterm birth prevention: where are we? *Am J Obstet Gynecol* 1993;168:1223–1230.

40. Peaceman AM, Andrews WW, Thorp JM, et al. Fetal fibronectin as a predictor of preterm birth in patients with symptoms: a multicenter trial. *Am J Obstet Gynecol* 1997;177:13–18.

41. Haas DM, Imperiale TF, Kirkpatrick PR, et al. Tocolytic therapy: a meta-analysis and decision analysis. *Obstet Gynecol* 2009;113:585–594.

42. ACOG Committee Opinion No. 402: Antenatal corticosteroid therapy for fetal maturation. *Obstet Gynecol* 2008;111:805–807.

43. Simhan HN, Caritis SN. Prevention of preterm delivery. *N Engl J Med* 2007;357:477–487.

44. Goldenberg RL. The management of preterm labor. *Obstet Gynecol* 2002;100:1020–1037.

45. Allen JR, Helling TS, Langenfeld M. Intraabdominal surgery during pregnancy. *Am J Surg* 1989;158:567–569.

46. Hunt MG, Martin JN Jr, Martin RW, et al. Perinatal aspects of abdominal surgery for nonobstetric disease. *Am J Perinatol* 1989;6:412–417.

47. Korenbrot CC, Aalto LH, Laros RK Jr. The cost effectiveness of stopping preterm labor with beta-adrenergic treatment. *N Engl J Med* 1984;310:691–696.

48. Macones GA, Bader TJ, Asch DA. Optimising maternal–fetal outcomes in preterm labour: a decision analysis. *Br J Obstet Gynaecol* 1998;105:541–550.

49. Myers ER, Alvarez JG, Richardson DK, et al. Cost-effectiveness of fetal lung maturity testing in preterm labor. *Obstet Gynecol* 1997;90:824–829.

50. Ingemarsson I. Tocolytic therapy and clinical experience. Combination therapy. *BJOG* 2005;112(Suppl 1):89–93.

51. Ferguson JE, Hensleigh PA, Kredenster D. Adjunctive use of magnesium sulfate with ritodrine for preterm labor tocolysis. *Am J Obstet Gynecol* 1984;148:166–171.

52. Gomez R, Romero R, Edwin SS, et al. Pathogenesis of preterm labor and preterm premature rupture of membranes associated with intraamniotic infection. *Infect Dis Clin North Am* 1997;11:135–176.

53. Lemancewicz A, Laudanska H, Laudanski T, et al. Permeability of fetal membranes to calcium and magnesium: possible role in preterm labour. *Hum Reprod* 2000;15:2018–2022.

54. Cunze T, Rath W, Osmers R, et al. Magnesium and calcium concentration in the pregnant and non-pregnant myometrium. *Int J Gynaecol Obstet* 1995;48:9–13.

55. Mizuki J, Tasaka K, Masumoto N, et al. Magnesium sulfate inhibits oxytocin-induced calcium mobilization in human puerperal myometrial cells: possible involvement of intracellular free magnesium concentration. *Am J Obstet Gynecol* 1993;169:134–139.

56. Mercer BM, Merlino AA. Magnesium sulfate for preterm labor and preterm birth. *Obstet Gynecol* 2009;114:650–668.

57. Macones GA, Sehdev HM, Berlin M, et al. Evidence for magnesium sulfate as a tocolytic agent. *Obstet Gynecol Surv* 1997;52:652–658.

58. Twickler DM, McIntire DD, Alexander JM, et al. Effects of magnesium sulfate on preterm fetal cerebral blood flow using Doppler analysis: a randomized controlled trial. *Obstet Gynecol* 2010;115:21–25.

59. Vincent RD Jr, Chestnut DH, Sipes SL, et al. Magnesium sulfate decreases maternal blood pressure but not uterine blood flow during epidural anesthesia in gravid ewes. *Anesthesiology* 1991;74:77–82.

60. Sipes SL, Chestnut DH, Vincent RD Jr, et al. Which vasopressor should be used to treat hypotension during magnesium sulfate infusion and epidural anesthesia? *Anesthesiology* 1992;77:101–108.

61. ACOG Practice Bulletin. Clinical Management Guidelines for Obstetrician–Gynecologists, Number 70, December 2005 (Replaces Practice Bulletin Number 62, May 2005). Intrapartum fetal heart rate monitoring. *Obstet Gynecol* 2005;106:1453–1460.

62. Fuchs-Buder T, Wilder-Smith OH, Borgeat A, et al. Interaction of magnesium sulphate with vecuronium-induced neuromuscular block. *Br J Anaesth* 1995;74:405–409.

63. Sinatra RS, Philip BK, Naulty JS, et al. Prolonged neuromuscular blockade with vecuronium in a patient treated with magnesium sulfate. *Anesth Analg* 1985;64:1220–1222.

64. Tsai SK, Huang SW, Lee TY. Neuromuscular interactions between suxamethonium and magnesium sulphate in the cat. *Br J Anaesth* 1994;72:674–678.

65. Lysakowski C, Dumont L, Czarnetzki C, et al. Magnesium as an adjuvant to postoperative analgesia: a systematic review of randomized trials. *Anesth Analg* 2007;104:1532–1539, table.

66. Anotayanonth S, Subhedar NV, Garner P, et al. Betamimetics for inhibiting preterm labour. *Cochrane Database Syst Rev* 2004;CD004352.

67. Liu YL, Nwosu UC, Rice PJ. Relaxation of isolated human myometrial muscle by beta2-adrenergic receptors but not beta1-adrenergic receptors. *Am J Obstet Gynecol* 1998;179:895–898.

68. Baker JG. The selectivity of beta-adrenoceptor antagonists at the human beta1, beta2 and beta3 adrenoceptors. *Br J Pharmacol* 2005;144:317–322.

69. Rouget C, Bardou M, Breuiller-Fouche M, et al. Beta3-adrenoceptor is the predominant beta-adrenoceptor subtype in human myometrium and its expression is up-regulated in pregnancy. *J Clin Endocrinol Metab* 2005;90:1644–1650.

70. Bardou M, Rouget C, Breuiller-Fouche M, et al. Is the beta3-adrenoceptor (ADRB3) a potential target for uterorelaxant drugs? *BMC Pregnancy Childbirth* 2007;7(Suppl 1):S14.

71. Johansson LH. Factors behind the functional beta 2-adrenoceptor selectivity of terbutaline. *Pharmacol Toxicol* 1995;77(Suppl 3):21–24.

72. Brodde OE, Michel MC. Adrenergic and muscarinic receptors in the human heart. *Pharmacol Rev* 1999;51:651–690.

73. Jartti TT, Kuusela TA, Kaila TJ, et al. The dose-response effects of terbutaline on the variability, approximate entropy and fractal dimension of heart rate and blood pressure. *Br J Clin Pharmacol* 1998;45:277–285.

74. Leineweber K, Heusch G. Beta 1- and beta 2-adrenoceptor polymorphisms and cardiovascular diseases. *Br J Pharmacol* 2009;158:61–69.

75. Brodde OE, Buscher R, Tellkamp R, et al. Blunted cardiac responses to receptor activation in subjects with Thr164Ile beta(2)-adrenoceptors. *Circulation* 2001;103:1048–1050.

76. Bruck H, Leineweber K, Park J, et al. Human beta2-adrenergic receptor gene haplotypes and venodilation in vivo. *Clin Pharmacol Ther* 2005;78:232–238.

77. Dishy V, Landau R, Sofowora GG, et al. Beta2-adrenoceptor Thr164Ile polymorphism is associated with markedly decreased vasodilator and increased vasoconstrictor sensitivity in vivo. *Pharmacogenetics* 2004;14:517–522.

78. Chruscinski AJ, Rohrer DK, Schauble E, et al. Targeted disruption of the beta2 adrenergic receptor gene. *J Biol Chem* 1999;274:16694–16700.

79. Gyetvai K, Hannah ME, Hodnett ED, et al. Tocolytics for preterm labor: a systematic review. *Obstet Gynecol* 1999;94:869–877.

80. Michalak D, Klein V, Marquette GP. Myocardial ischemia: a complication of ritodrine tocolysis. *Am J Obstet Gynecol* 1983;146:861–862.

81. Perry KG Jr, Morrison JC, Rust OA, et al. Incidence of adverse cardiopulmonary effects with low-dose continuous terbutaline infusion. *Am J Obstet Gynecol* 1995;173:1273–1277.

82. Sciscione AC, Ivester T, Largoza M, et al. Acute pulmonary edema in pregnancy. *Obstet Gynecol* 2003;101:511–515.

83. Lamont RF. The pathophysiology of pulmonary oedema with the use of beta-agonists. *BJOG* 2000;107:439–444.

84. Pisani RJ, Rosenow EC III. Pulmonary edema associated with tocolytic therapy. *Ann Intern Med* 1989;110:714–718.

85. Armson BA, Samuels P, Miller F, et al. Evaluation of maternal fluid dynamics during tocolytic therapy with ritodrine hydrochloride and magnesium sulfate. *Am J Obstet Gynecol* 1992;167:758–765.

86. Philipsen T, Eriksen PS, Lynggard F. Pulmonary edema following ritodrine-saline infusion in premature labor. *Obstet Gynecol* 1981;58:304–308.

87. Hankins GD, Hauth JC, Kuehl TJ, et al. Ritodrine hydrochloride infusion in pregnant baboons. II. Sodium and water compartment alterations. *Am J Obstet Gynecol* 1983;147:254–259.

88. Hatjis CG, Swain M. Systemic tocolysis for premature labor is associated with an increased incidence of pulmonary edema in the presence of maternal infection. *Am J Obstet Gynecol* 1988;159:723–728.

89. Gabel JC, Hansen TN, Drake RE. Effect of endotoxin on lung fluid balance in unanesthetized sheep. *J Appl Physiol* 1984;56:489–494.

90. Benedetti TJ, Hargrove JC, Rosene KA. Maternal pulmonary edema during premature labor inhibition. *Obstet Gynecol* 1982;59:33S-37S.

91. Jacobs MM, Knight AB, Arias F. Maternal pulmonary edema resulting from betamimetic and glucocorticoid therapy. *Obstet Gynecol* 1980;56:56–59.

92. Cotton DB, Strassner HT, Lipson LG, et al. The effects of terbutaline on acid base, serum electrolytes, and glucose homeostasis during the management of preterm labor. *Am J Obstet Gynecol* 1981;141:617–624.

93. Benedetti TJ. Maternal complications of parenteral beta-sympathomimetic therapy for premature labor. *Am J Obstet Gynecol* 1983;145:1–6.

94. Brown MJ, Brown DC, Murphy MB. Hypokalemia from beta2-receptor stimulation by circulating epinephrine. *N Engl J Med* 1983;309:1414–1419.

95. Ying YK, Tejani NA. Angina pectoris as a complication of ritodrine hydrochloride therapy in premature labor. *Obstet Gynecol* 1982;60:385–388.

96. Hurlbert BJ, Edelman JD, David K. Serum potassium levels during and after terbutaline. *Anesth Analg* 1981;60:723–725.

97. Moravec MA, Hurlbert BJ. Hypokalemia associated with terbutaline administration in obstetrical patients. *Anesth Analg* 1980;59:917–920.

98. Kuczkowski KM, Benumof JL. Rebound hyperkalemia after cessation of intravenous tocolytic therapy with terbutaline in the treatment of preterm labor: anesthetic implications. *J Clin Anesth* 2003;15:357–358.

99. Kotani N, Kushikata T, Hashimoto H, et al. Rebound perioperative hyperkalemia in six patients after cessation of ritodrine for premature labor. *Anesth Analg* 2001;93:709–711.

100. Sato K, Nishiwaki K, Kuno N, et al. Unexpected hyperkalemia following succinylcholine administration in prolonged immobilized parturients treated with magnesium and ritodrine. *Anesthesiology* 2000;93:1539–1541.

101. Rosene KA, Featherstone HJ, Benedetti TJ. Cerebral ischemia associated with parenteral terbutaline use in pregnant migraine patients. *Am J Obstet Gynecol* 1982;143:405–407.

102. Quinn PG, Sherman BW, Tavill AS, et al. Terbutaline hepatitis in pregnancy: report of two cases and literature review. *Am J Gastroenterol* 1994;89:781–784.

103. Catanzarite VA, McHargue AM, Sandberg EC, et al. Respiratory arrest during therapy for premature labor in a patient with myasthenia gravis. *Obstet Gynecol* 1984;64:819–822.

104. Shin YK, Kim YD. Ventricular tachyarrhythmias during cesarean section after ritodrine therapy: interaction with anesthetics. *South Med J* 1988;81:528–530.

105. Suppan P. Tocolysis and anaesthesia for caesarean section. *Br J Anaesth* 1982;54:1007.

106. Schoenfeld A, Joel-Cohen SJ, Duparc H, et al. Emergency obstetric anaesthesia and the use of beta2-sympathomimetic drugs. *Br J Anaesth* 1978;50:969–971.

107. Chestnut DH, Pollack KL, Thompson CS, et al. Does ritodrine worsen maternal hypotension during epidural anesthesia in gravid ewes? *Anesthesiology* 1990;72:315–321.

108. Chestnut DH, Weiner CP, Wang JP, et al. The effect of ephedrine upon uterine artery blood flow velocity in the pregnant guinea pig subjected to terbutaline infusion and acute hemorrhage. *Anesthesiology* 1987;66:508–512.

109. Chestnut DH, Ostman LG, Weiner CP, et al. The effect of vasopressor agents upon uterine artery blood flow velocity in the gravid guinea pig subjected to ritodrine infusion. *Anesthesiology* 1988;68:363–366.

110. McGrath JM, Chestnut DH, Vincent RD, et al. Ephedrine remains the vasopressor of choice for treatment of hypotension during ritodrine infusion and epidural anesthesia. *Anesthesiology* 1994;80:1073–1081.

111. King JF, Flenady VJ, Papatsonis DN, et al. Calcium channel blockers for inhibiting preterm labour. *Cochrane Database Syst Rev* 2003;CD002255.

112. Tsatsaris V, Papatsonis D, Goffinet F, et al. Tocolysis with nifedipine or beta-adrenergic agonists: a meta-analysis. *Obstet Gynecol* 2001;97:840–847.

113. Lyell DJ, Pullen K, Campbell L, et al. Magnesium sulfate compared with nifedipine for acute tocolysis of preterm labor: a randomized controlled trial. *Obstet Gynecol* 2007;110:61–67.

114. Bracero LA, Leikin E, Kirshenbaum N, et al. Comparison of nifedipine and ritodrine for the treatment of preterm labor. *Am J Perinatol* 1991;8:365–369.

115. Ferguson JE, Dyson DC, Schutz T, et al. A comparison of tocolysis with nifedipine or ritodrine: analysis of efficacy and maternal, fetal, and neonatal outcome. *Am J Obstet Gynecol* 1990;163:105–111.

116. Ferguson JE, Dyson DC, Holbrook RH Jr, et al. Cardiovascular and metabolic effects associated with nifedipine and ritodrine tocolysis. *Am J Obstet Gynecol* 1989;161:788–795.

117. van Veen AJ, Pelinck MJ, van Pampus MG, et al. Severe hypotension and fetal death due to tocolysis with nifedipine. *BJOG* 2005;112:509–510.

118. Impey L. Severe hypotension and fetal distress following sublingual administration of nifedipine to a patient with severe pregnancy induced hypertension at 33 weeks. *Br J Obstet Gynaecol* 1993;100:959–961.

119. Waisman GD, Mayorga LM, Camera MI, et al. Magnesium plus nifedipine: potentiation of hypotensive effect in preeclampsia? *Am J Obstet Gynecol* 1988;159:308–309.

120. Ray D, Dyson D. Calcium channel blockers. *Clin Obstet Gynecol* 1995;38:713–721.

121. Feldman S, Karalliedde L. Drug interactions with neuromuscular blockers. *Drug Saf* 1996;15:261–273.

122. Reves JG, Kissin I, Lell WA, et al. Calcium entry blockers: uses and implications for anesthesiologists. *Anesthesiology* 1982;57:504–518.

123. Tosone SR, Reves JG, Kissin I, et al. Hemodynamic responses to nifedipine in dogs anesthetized with halothane. *Anesth Analg* 1983;62:903–908.

124. Csapo AI, Puri CP, Tarro S, et al. Deactivation of the uterus during normal and premature labor by the calcium antagonist nicardipine. *Am J Obstet Gynecol* 1982;142:483–491.

125. Doret M, Mellier G, Benchaib M, et al. In vitro study of tocolytic effect of rofecoxib, a specific cyclo-oxygenase 2 inhibitor. Comparison and combination with other tocolytic agents. *BJOG* 2002;109:983–988.

126. Slattery MM, Friel AM, Healy DG, et al. Uterine relaxant effects of cyclooxygenase-2 inhibitors in vitro. *Obstet Gynecol* 2001;98:563–569.

127. Gross G, Imamura T, Vogt SK, et al. Inhibition of cyclooxygenase-2 prevents inflammation-mediated preterm labor in the mouse. *Am J Physiol Regul Integr Comp Physiol* 2000;278:R1415–R1423.

128. Sadovsky Y, Nelson DM, Muglia LJ, et al. Effective diminution of amniotic prostaglandin production by selective inhibitors of cyclooxygenase type 2. *Am J Obstet Gynecol* 2000;182:370–376.

129. Yousif MH, Thulesius O. Tocolytic effect of the cyclooxygenase-2 inhibitor, meloxicam: studies on uterine contractions in the rat. *J Pharm Pharmacol* 1998;50:681–685.

130. King J, Flenady V, Cole S, et al. Cyclo-oxygenase (COX) inhibitors for treating preterm labour. *Cochrane Database Syst Rev* 2005;CD001992.

131. Groom KM, Shennan AH, Jones BA, et al. TOCOX—a randomised, double-blind, placebo-controlled trial of rofecoxib (a COX-2-specific prostaglandin inhibitor) for the prevention of preterm delivery in women at high risk. *BJOG* 2005;112:725–730.

132. McWhorter J, Carlan SJ, OLeary TD, et al. Rofecoxib versus magnesium sulfate to arrest preterm labor: a randomized trial. *Obstet Gynecol* 2004;103:923–930.

133. Stika CS, Gross GA, Leguizamon G, et al. A prospective randomized safety trial of celecoxib for treatment of preterm labor. *Am J Obstet Gynecol* 2002;187:653–660.

134. Locatelli A, Vergani P, Bellini P, et al. Can a cyclo-oxygenase type-2 selective tocolytic agent avoid the fetal side effects of indomethacin? *BJOG* 2001;108:325–326.

135. Sawdy R, Slater D, Fisk N, et al. Use of a cyclo-oxygenase type-2-selective non-steroidal anti-inflammatory agent to prevent preterm delivery. *Lancet* 1997;350:265–266.

136. Moise KJ Jr. Effect of advancing gestational age on the frequency of fetal ductal constriction in association with maternal indomethacin use. *Am J Obstet Gynecol* 1993;168:1350–1353.

137. Moise KJ Jr, Huhta JC, Sharif DS, et al. Indomethacin in the treatment of premature labor. Effects on the fetal ductus arteriosus. *N Engl J Med* 1988;319:327–331.

138. Niebyl JR, Witter FR. Neonatal outcome after indomethacin treatment for preterm labor. *Am J Obstet Gynecol* 1986;155:747–749.

139. Dudley DK, Hardie MJ. Fetal and neonatal effects of indomethacin used as a tocolytic agent. *Am J Obstet Gynecol* 1985;151:181–184.

140. Zuckerman H, Shalev E, Gilad G, et al. Further study of the inhibition of premature labor by indomethacin. Part I. *J Perinat Med* 1984;12:19–23.

141. Vermillion ST, Scardo JA, Lashus AG, et al. The effect of indomethacin tocolysis on fetal ductus arteriosus constriction with advancing gestational age. *Am J Obstet Gynecol* 1997;177:256–259.

142. Sawdy RJ, Lye S, Fisk NM, et al. A double-blind randomized study of fetal side effects during and after the short-term maternal administration of indomethacin, sulindac, and nimesulide for the treatment of preterm labor. *Am J Obstet Gynecol* 2003;188:1046–1051.

143. Takahashi Y, Roman C, Chemtob S, et al. Cyclooxygenase-2 inhibitors constrict the fetal lamb ductus arteriosus both in vitro and in vivo. *Am J Physiol Regul Integr Comp Physiol* 2000;278:R1496–R1505.

144. Gordon MC, Samuels P. Indomethacin. *Clin Obstet Gynecol* 1995;38:697–705.

145. Clive DM, Stoff JS. Renal syndromes associated with nonsteroidal antiinflammatory drugs. *N Engl J Med* 1984;310:563–572.

146. Hendricks SK, Smith JR, Moore DE, et al. Oligohydramnios associated with prostaglandin synthetase inhibitors in preterm labour. *Br J Obstet Gynaecol* 1990;97:312–316.

147. Horlocker TT, Wedel DJ, Rowlingson JC, et al. Regional anesthesia in the patient receiving antithrombotic or thrombolytic therapy: American Society of Regional Anesthesia and Pain Medicine Evidence-Based Guidelines (Third Edition). *Reg Anesth Pain Med* 2010;35:64–101.

148. Goodwin TM, Valenzuela G, Silver H, et al. Treatment of preterm labor with the oxytocin antagonist atosiban. *Am J Perinatol* 1996;13:143–146.

149. Phaneuf S, Asboth G, MacKenzie IZ, et al. Effect of oxytocin antagonists on the activation of human myometrium in vitro: atosiban prevents oxytocin-induced desensitization. *Am J Obstet Gynecol* 1994;171:1627–1634.

150. Wyatt S, Guinn DA. Review: Oxytocin receptor antagonists for preterm labour do not improve infant outcomes more than placebo or other tocolytics. *Evid Based Med* 2006;11:75.

151. Romero R, Sibai BM, Sanchez-Ramos L, et al. An oxytocin receptor antagonist (atosiban) in the treatment of preterm labor: a randomized, double-blind, placebo-controlled trial with tocolytic rescue. *Am J Obstet Gynecol* 2000;182:1173–1183.

152. Papatsonis D, Flenady V, Cole S, et al. Oxytocin receptor antagonists for inhibiting preterm labour. *Cochrane Database Syst Rev* 2005;CD004452.

153. Smith GN, Walker MC, Ohlsson A, et al. Randomized double-blind placebo-controlled trial of transdermal nitroglycerin for preterm labor. *Am J Obstet Gynecol* 2007;196:37–38.

154. Roberts D, Dalziel S. Antenatal corticosteroids for accelerating fetal lung maturation for women at risk of preterm birth. *Cochrane Database Syst Rev* 2006;3:CD004454.

155. Crowley P. Prophylactic corticosteroids for preterm birth. *Cochrane Database Syst Rev* 2000;CD000065.

156. Ballard PL, Ballard RA. Scientific basis and therapeutic regimens for use of antenatal glucocorticoids. *Am J Obstet Gynecol* 1995;173:254–262.

157. Smolders-de HH, Neuvel J, Schmand B, et al. Physical development and medical history of children who were treated antenatally with corticosteroids to prevent respiratory distress syndrome: a 10- to 12-year follow-up. *Pediatrics* 1990;86:65–70.

158. Lee BH, Stoll BJ, McDonald SA, et al. Adverse neonatal outcomes associated with antenatal dexamethasone versus antenatal betamethasone. *Pediatrics* 2006;117:1503–1510.

159. Elimian A, Garry D, Figueroa R, et al. Antenatal betamethasone compared with dexamethasone (betacode trial): a randomized controlled trial. *Obstet Gynecol* 2007;110:26–30.

160. Baud O, Foix-L'Helias L, Kaminski M, et al. Antenatal glucocorticoid treatment and cystic periventricular leukomalacia in very premature infants. *N Engl J Med* 1999;341:1190–1196.

161. Lee BH, Stoll BJ, McDonald SA, et al. Neurodevelopmental outcomes of extremely low birth weight infants exposed prenatally to dexamethasone versus betamethasone. *Pediatrics* 2008;121:289–296.

162. Murphy BP, Inder TE, Huppi PS, et al. Impaired cerebral cortical gray matter growth after treatment with dexamethasone for neonatal chronic lung disease. *Pediatrics* 2001;107:217–221.

163. Effect of corticosteroids for fetal maturation on perinatal outcomes. NIH Consens Statement 1994;12:1–24.

164. Elimian A, Figueroa R, Spitzer AR, et al. Antenatal corticosteroids: are incomplete courses beneficial? *Obstet Gynecol* 2003;102:352–355.

165. Subtil D, Tiberghien P, Devos P, et al. Immediate and delayed effects of antenatal corticosteroids on fetal heart rate: a randomized trial that compares betamethasone acetate and phosphate, betamethasone phosphate, and dexamethasone. *Am J Obstet Gynecol* 2003;188:524–531.

166. Rotmensch S, Liberati M, Celentano C, et al. The effect of betamethasone on fetal biophysical activities and Doppler velocimetry of umbilical and middle cerebral arteries. *Acta Obstet Gynecol Scand* 1999;78:768–773.

167. Mulder EJ, Derks JB, Visser GH. Antenatal corticosteroid therapy and fetal behaviour: a randomised study of the effects of betamethasone and dexamethasone. *Br J Obstet Gynaecol* 1997;104:1239–1247.

168. Rotmensch S, Lev S, Kovo M, et al. Effect of betamethasone administration on fetal heart rate tracing: a blinded longitudinal study. *Fetal Diagn Ther* 2005;20:371–376.

169. Kelly MK, Schneider EP, Petrikovsky BM, et al. Effect of antenatal steroid administration on the fetal biophysical profile. *J Clin Ultrasound* 2000;28:224–226.

170. Ogburn PL Jr, Julian TM, Williams PP, et al. The use of magnesium sulfate for tocolysis in preterm labor complicated by twin gestation and betamimetic-induced pulmonary edema. *Acta Obstet Gynecol Scand* 1986;65:793–794.

171. Ogunyemi D. Risk factors for acute pulmonary edema in preterm delivery. *Eur J Obstet Gynecol Reprod Biol* 2007;133:143–147.

172. Stubblefield PG. Pulmonary edema occurring after therapy with dexamethasone and terbutaline for premature labor: a case report. *Am J Obstet Gynecol* 1978;132:341–342.

173. Bedalov A, Balasubramanyam A. Glucocorticoid-induced ketoacidosis in gestational diabetes: sequela of the acute treatment of preterm labor. A case report. *Diabetes Care* 1997;20:922–924.

174. Fisher JE, Smith RS, Lagrandeur R, et al. Gestational diabetes mellitus in women receiving beta-adrenergics and corticosteroids for threatened preterm delivery. *Obstet Gynecol* 1997;90:880–883.

175. Vaisbuch E, Levy R, Hagay Z. The effect of betamethasone administration to pregnant women on maternal serum indicators of infection. *J Perinat Med* 2002;30:287–291.

176. Kadanali S, Ingec M, Kucukozkan T, et al. Changes in leukocyte, granulocyte and lymphocyte counts following antenatal betamethasone administration to pregnant women. *Int J Gynaecol Obstet* 1997;58:269–274.

177. Welch RA, Bottoms SF. Reconsideration of head compression and intraventricular hemorrhage in the vertex very-low-birth-weight fetus. *Obstet Gynecol* 1986;68:29–34.

178. Bowes WA Jr. Delivery of the very low birth weight infant. *Clin Perinatol* 1980;8:183–195.

179. Bowes WA Jr, Gabre SG, Bowes C. Fetal heart rate monitoring in premature infants weighing 1,500 grams or less. *Am J Obstet Gynecol* 1980;137:791–796.

180. Zanini B, Paul RH, Huey JR. Intrapartum fetal heart rate: correlation with scalp pH in the preterm fetus. *Am J Obstet Gynecol* 1980;136:43–47.

181. Shy KK, Luthy DA, Bennett FC, et al. Effects of electronic fetal-heart-rate monitoring, as compared with periodic auscultation, on the neurologic development of premature infants. *N Engl J Med* 1990;322:588–593.

182. Lasswell SM, Barfield WD, Rochat RW, et al. Perinatal regionalization for very low-birth-weight and very preterm infants: a meta-analysis. *JAMA* 2010;304:992–1000.

183. Mathews TJ, MacDorman MF. Infant mortality statistics from the 2006 period linked birth/infant death data set. *Natl Vital Stat Rep* 2010;58:1–31.

184. Tita AT, Landon MB, Spong CY, et al. Timing of elective repeat cesarean delivery at term and neonatal outcomes. *N Engl J Med* 2009;360:111–120.

185. Donovan EF, Lannon C, Bailit J, et al. A statewide initiative to reduce inappropriate scheduled births at 36(0/7)–38(6/7) weeks' gestation. *Am J Obstet Gynecol* 2010;202:243–248.

186. Oshiro BT, Henry E, Wilson J, et al. Decreasing elective deliveries before 39 weeks of gestation in an integrated health care system. *Obstet Gynecol* 2009;113:804–811.

187. Martin JA, Osterman MJ, Sutton PD. Are preterm births on the decline in the United States? Recent data from the National Vital Statistics System. *NCHS Data Brief* 2010;1–8.

188. Koopmans CM, Bijlenga D, Groen H, et al. Induction of labour versus expectant monitoring for gestational hypertension or mild pre-eclampsia after 36 weeks' gestation (HYPITAT): a multicentre, open-label randomised controlled trial. *Lancet* 2009;374:979–988.

189. Sibai BM. Management of late preterm and early-term pregnancies complicated by mild gestational hypertension/pre-eclampsia. *Semin Perinatol* 2011;35:292–296.

190. Reddy UM, Laughon SK, Sun L, et al. Prepregnancy risk factors for antepartum stillbirth in the United States. *Obstet Gynecol* 2010;116:1119–1126.

191. Mondestin MA, Ananth CV, Smulian JC, et al. Birth weight and fetal death in the United States: the effect of maternal diabetes during pregnancy. *Am J Obstet Gynecol* 2002;187:922–926.

192. Cundy T, Gamble G, Townend K, et al. Perinatal mortality in Type 2 diabetes mellitus. *Diabet Med* 2000;17:33–39.

193. Macintosh MC, Fleming KM, Bailey JA, et al. Perinatal mortality and congenital anomalies in babies of women with type 1 or type 2 diabetes in England, Wales, and Northern Ireland: population based study. *BMJ* 2006;333:177.

194. Lauenborg J, Mathiesen E, Ovesen P, et al. Audit on stillbirths in women with pregestational type 1 diabetes. *Diabetes Care* 2003;26:1385–1389.

195. Spong CY, Mercer BM, D'alton M, et al. Timing of indicated late-preterm and early-term birth. *Obstet Gynecol* 2011;118:323–333.

196. Zlatnik MG, Cheng YW, Norton ME, et al. Placenta previa and the risk of preterm delivery. *J Matern Fetal Neonatal Med* 2007;20:719–723.

197. Zlatnik MG, Little SE, Kohli P, et al. When should women with placenta previa be delivered? A decision analysis. *J Reprod Med* 2010;55:373–381.

198. Oyelese Y, Smulian JC. Placenta previa, placenta accreta, and vasa previa. *Obstet Gynecol* 2006;107:927–941.

199. Warshak CR, Ramos GA, Eskander R, et al. Effect of predelivery diagnosis in 99 consecutive cases of placenta accreta. *Obstet Gynecol* 2010;115:65–69.

200. O'Brien JM, Barton JR, Donaldson ES. The management of placenta percreta: conservative and operative strategies. *Am J Obstet Gynecol* 1996;175:1632–1638.

201. Robinson BK, Grobman WA. Effectiveness of timing strategies for delivery of individuals with placenta previa and accreta. *Obstet Gynecol* 2010;116:835–842.

202. Landon MB, Hauth JC, Leveno KJ, et al. Maternal and perinatal outcomes associated with a trial of labor after prior cesarean delivery. *N Engl J Med* 2004;351:2581–2589.

203. Robinson BK, Grobman WA. Effectiveness of timing strategies for delivery of individuals with vasa previa. *Obstet Gynecol* 2011;117:542–549.

204. Galan HL. Timing delivery of the growth-restricted fetus. *Semin Perinatol* 2011;35:262–269.

205. Craigo SD. Indicated preterm birth for fetal anomalies. *Semin Perinatol* 2011;35:270–276.

206. Adzick NS. Open fetal surgery for life-threatening fetal anomalies. *Semin Fetal Neonatal Med* 2010;15:1–8.

207. Deprest J, Nicolaides K, Done' E, et al. Technical aspects of fetal endoscopic tracheal occlusion for congenital diaphragmatic hernia. *J Pediatr Surg* 2011;46:22–32.

208. Newman RB, Unal ER. Multiple gestations: timing of indicated late preterm and early-term births in uncomplicated dichorionic, monochorionic, and monoamniotic twins. *Semin Perinatol* 2011;35:277–285.

209. Grant A, Glazener CM. Elective caesarean section versus expectant management for delivery of the small baby. *Cochrane Database Syst Rev* 2001; CD000078.

210. Hack M, Fanaroff AA. Outcomes of extremely-low-birth-weight infants between 1982 and 1988. *N Engl J Med* 1989;321:1642–1647.

211. Malloy MH, Rhoads GG, Schramm W, et al. Increasing cesarean section rates in very low-birth weight infants. Effect on outcome. *JAMA* 1989;262:1475–1478.

212. Tejani N, Verma U, Hameed C, et al. Method and route of delivery in the low birth weight vertex presentation correlated with early periventricular/intraventricular hemorrhage. *Obstet Gynecol* 1987;69:1–4.

213. Riskin A, Riskin-Mashiah S, Bader D, et al. Delivery mode and severe intraventricular hemorrhage in single, very low birth weight, vertex infants. *Obstet Gynecol* 2008;112:21–28.

214. Schwartz DB, Miodovnik M, Lavin JP Jr. Neonatal outcome among low birth weight infants delivered spontaneously or by low forceps. *Obstet Gynecol* 1983;62:283–286.

215. The TG. Is routine episiotomy beneficial in the low birth weight delivery? *Int J Gynaecol Obstet* 1990;31:135–140.

216. Chervenak FA, Johnson RE, Youcha S, et al. Intrapartum management of twin gestation. *Obstet Gynecol* 1985;65:119–124.

217. Lewis BV, Seneviratne HR. Vaginal breech delivery or cesarean section. *Am J Obstet Gynecol* 1979;134:615–618.

218. Main DM, Main EK, Maurer MM. Cesarean section versus vaginal delivery for the breech fetus weighing less than 1,500 grams. *Am J Obstet Gynecol* 1983;146:580–584.

219. Sachs BP, McCarthy BJ, Rubin G, et al. Cesarean section. Risk and benefits for mother and fetus. *JAMA* 1983;250:2157–2159.

220. American Heart Association (AHA). Guidelines for cardiopulmonary resuscitation (CPR) and emergency cardiovascular care (ECC) of pediatric and neonatal patients: neonatal resuscitation guidelines. *Pediatrics* 2006; 117:e1029–e1038.

221. Tyson JE, Parikh NA, Langer J, et al. Intensive care for extreme prematurity—moving beyond gestational age. *N Engl J Med* 2008;358:1672–1681.

222. Teramo K, Benowitz N, Heymann MA, et al. Gestational differences in lidocaine toxicity in the fetal lamb. *Anesthesiology* 1976;44:133–138.

223. Pedersen H, Santos AC, Morishima HO, et al. Does gestational age affect the pharmacokinetics and pharmacodynamics of lidocaine in mother and fetus? *Anesthesiology* 1988;68:367–372.

224. Morishima HO, Pedersen H, Santos AC, et al. Adverse effects of maternally administered lidocaine on the asphyxiated preterm fetal lamb. *Anesthesiology* 1989;71:110–115.

225. Morishima HO, Santos AC, Pedersen H, et al. Effect of lidocaine on the asphyxial responses in the mature fetal lamb. *Anesthesiology* 1987;66:502–507.

226. Kuhnert BR, Kuhnert PM, Reese AL, et al. Maternal and neonatal elimination of CABA after epidural anesthesia with 2-chloroprocaine during parturition. *Anesth Analg* 1983;62:1089–1094.

227. Philipson EH, Kuhnert BR, Syracuse CD. Fetal acidosis, 2-chloroprocaine, and epidural anesthesia for cesarean section. *Am J Obstet Gynecol* 1985; 151:322–324.

228. Santos AC, Yun EM, Bobby PD, et al. The effects of bupivacaine, L-nitro-L-arginine-methyl ester, and phenylephrine on cardiovascular adaptations to asphyxia in the preterm fetal lamb. *Anesth Analg* 1997;85:1299–1306.

229. Rappaport B, Mellon RD, Simone A, et al. Defining safe use of anesthesia in children. *N Engl J Med* 2011;364:1387–1390.

230. Stoll BJ, Hansen NI, Bell EF, et al. Neonatal outcomes of extremely preterm infants from the NICHD Neonatal Research Network. *Pediatrics* 2010;126:443–456.

231. Lemons JA, Bauer CR, Oh W, et al. Very low birth weight outcomes of the National Institute of Child health and human development neonatal research network, January 1995 through December 1996. NICHD Neonatal Research Network. *Pediatrics* 2001;107:E1.

232. Costeloe K, Hennessy E, Gibson AT, et al. The EPICure study: outcomes to discharge from hospital for infants born at the threshold of viability. *Pediatrics* 2000;106:659–671.

233. Darmstadt GL, Saha SK, Ahmed AS, et al. Effect of skin barrier therapy on neonatal mortality rates in preterm infants in Bangladesh: a randomized, controlled, clinical trial. *Pediatrics* 2008;121:522–529.

234. Fanaroff AA, Stoll BJ, Wright LL, et al. Trends in neonatal morbidity and mortality for very low birthweight infants. *Am J Obstet Gynecol* 2007;196:147–148.

235. Batton B, Zhu X, Fanaroff J, et al. Blood pressure, anti-hypotensive therapy, and neurodevelopment in extremely preterm infants. *J Pediatr* 2009;154:351–357, 357.e1.

236. Stoll BJ, Hansen N, Fanaroff AA, et al. Late-onset sepsis in very low birth weight neonates: the experience of the NICHD Neonatal Research Network. *Pediatrics* 2002;110:285–291.

237. Stoll BJ, Hansen NI, Adams-Chapman I, et al. Neurodevelopmental and growth impairment among extremely low-birth-weight infants with neonatal infection. *JAMA* 2004;292:2357–2365.

238. Hovi P, Andersson S, Eriksson JG, et al. Glucose regulation in young adults with very low birth weight. *N Engl J Med* 2007;356:2053–2063.

239. Rotteveel J, van Weissenbruch MM, Twisk JW, et al. Infant and childhood growth patterns, insulin sensitivity, and blood pressure in prematurely born young adults. *Pediatrics* 2008;122:313–321.

240. De G I, Vanhaesebrouck P, Bruneel E, et al. Outcome at 3 years of age in a population-based cohort of extremely preterm infants. *Obstet Gynecol* 2007; 110:855–864.

241. Hack M, Klein N. Young adult attainments of preterm infants. *JAMA* 2006;295:695–696.

242. Johnson S, Fawke J, Hennessy E, et al. Neurodevelopmental disability through 11 years of age in children born before 26 weeks of gestation. *Pediatrics* 2009;124:e249–e257.

243. Marlow N, Wolke D, Bracewell MA, et al. Neurologic and developmental disability at six years of age after extremely preterm birth. *N Engl J Med* 2005;352:9–19.

244. Mikkola K, Ritari N, Tommiska V, et al. Neurodevelopmental outcome at 5 years of age of a national cohort of extremely low birth weight infants who were born in 1996–1997. *Pediatrics* 2005;116:1391–1400.

245. Wood NS, Marlow N, Costeloe K, et al. Neurologic and developmental disability after extremely preterm birth. EPICure Study Group. *N Engl J Med* 2000;343:378–384.

Intrapartum Fever, Infection, and Sepsis

Laura Goetzl

■ EPIDEMIOLOGY OF INTRAPARTUM INFECTION AND SEPSIS

Rates and causes of maternal sepsis vary widely between developed and developing countries. In developing countries, infectious agents such as HIV and malaria account for a significant proportion of infection coincident with pregnancy while in developed countries these agents are much less common. The incidence of early pregnancy complications such as septic abortion vary with access to care and use of antibiotic prophylaxis, and again are far more common in developing countries. Although the obstetric anesthesiologist may be called upon to participate in the care of women with serious postpartum infection such as intraabdominal abcesses, infected episiotomies, and wound debridement, these infections have much in common with typical polymicrobial postsurgical deep tissue infections. Therefore, this chapter will focus on unique features of intrapartum fever (maternal temperature >38°C) and maternal infection related to obstetric causes. In addition, the chapter will discuss the treatment of maternal sepsis, which remains a leading cause of maternal death (1), and how maternal physiologic changes may alter the typical classification, triage, and treatment.

■ ETIOLOGIES OF INTRAPARTUM FEVER

Rates of intrapartum fever vary widely with patient risk factors for infection, parity, and use of epidural analgesia. The lowest rates of intrapartum fever are seen in low risk, predominantly parous populations with lower rates of epidural analgesia. Traditionally, chorioamnionitis is diagnosed based on the three following criteria (2):

■ Maternal temperature >38°C
■ Fundal (uterine) tenderness to palpation
■ Foul vaginal discharge

Epidural analgesia is often established relatively early in labor prior to the onset of maternal fever; therefore, uterine tenderness is not a particularly helpful clinical sign. Vaginal discharge has always been subjectively defined and is imprecise. Other ancillary signs such as maternal or fetal tachycardia are closely correlated to maternal and fetal hyperthermia and can be present whenever maternal fever occurs (3). It is well recognized that epidurals are associated with an increase in core temperature in labor, though the reason for this remains unknown. This is discussed in greater detail in a following section. Maternal white blood cell counts increase with duration of labor and can be markedly elevated without any evidence of infection (4). Further, white blood cell counts cannot be used to reliably distinguish between chorioamnionitis and epidural associated fever, although significant shift toward immature forms (bandemia) is concerning at

any absolute white cell count. Ultimately, there is no reliable way to distinguish between infectious and non-infectious (epidural related) fever; intrapartum fever likely represents a combination of both of these types (5). Due to the potential neonatal sepsis risk, a conservative approach, where all maternal intrapartum fever is an indication to administer maternal antibiotics, is recommended.

■ CHORIOAMNIONITIS

Chorioamnionitis is defined as inflammation of the placenta, membranes, amniotic fluid, maternal decidua and in many cases, the fetus, usually due to bacterial infection. Risk factors for chorioamnionitis are largely associated with longer labors or prolonged rupture of membranes (6,7). Maternal bacterial vaginosis and colonization with Group B streptococcus are also weak risk factors (8–10). In addition, labor at <37 weeks' gestation itself is a significant risk factor, with a rate of intrauterine infection estimated at 25% to 45% (11). Although the number of vaginal examinations during labor had been thought to be associated with infection, more recent investigations suggest that this is not an independent risk factor when the length of labor is scrupulously controlled for in multivariable analysis (12). The risk of neonatal sepsis rises with increasing maternal temperature: Approximately 2% with maternal temperatures <38.6°C and 6% with temperatures ≥38.6°C (13). Neonatal sepsis evaluations are recommended in infants born to women diagnosed with chorioamnionitis; however, the scope of sepsis evaluation and treatment varies locally.

Maternal treatment for chorioamnionitis should include broad spectrum coverage. Prior to maternal screening and treatment for maternal Group B Streptococcus carriage, maternal intrapartum antibiotic treatment reduced the risk of neonatal sepsis by up to 86% (14,15). Changes in screening practices and antibiotic prophylaxis may have altered the efficacy of treatment of suspected maternal chorioamnionitis in the prevention of neonatal sepsis; little modern data is available. Group B streptococcus and other organisms associated with obstetric infections are shown in Table 20-1. Standard therapy includes a combination of ampicillin and gentamicin. While 8-hour dosing of gentamicin is most common, there is some evidence to support daily dosing as being equally effective (16). Alternate antibiotic regimens include clindamycin or cefoxitin. Labor should be managed routinely and cesarean delivery reserved for the usual indications. Truncating fetal exposure to infection has not been associated with improved outcomes and maternal antibiotic treatment should result in therapeutic fetal levels of antibiotics. Further, cesarean delivery in the setting of chorioamnionitis is associated with increased maternal morbidity. Chorioamnionitis is a risk factor for maternal uterine atony (RR 2.5; 95% CI 2.2–2.8,17).

TABLE 20-1 Common Organisms Associated with Obstetric Infection

Group B streptococcus
Enterococcus
Escherichia coli
Staphylococcus aureus
Streptococcus pneumoniae
Gardnerella vaginalis
Group A streptococcus
Mycoplasma and ureaplasma species
Other streptococcus species
Klebsiella pneumoniae
Other enterobacteria
Pseudomona aeruginosa
Group A streptococci
Bacteroides species
Clostridia perfringens
Other anaerobes

Therefore, it is prudent to have uterotonic agents immediately available prior to delivery in these women.

There is little definitive evidence to guide anesthetic management of women with suspected chorioamnionitis. While known sepsis is generally suggested as a contraindication to regional analgesia, the rate of maternal bacteremia is estimated at 5.2% to 9.2% in the setting of clinical chorioamnionitis (18). Two retrospective cohort studies describe a total of 850 women with chorionamnionitis who received epidural analgesia without infectious complications (19,20). Further, only 19% (166/850) received antibiotic treatment prior to epidural analgesia. Therefore, while there is a theoretical risk of seeding the epidural or intrathecal space during the placement of regional anesthesia, the actual risks are exceedingly low. There is no data from obstetric populations to guide a recommendation of the relative safety of epidural versus spinal anesthesia. Overall it seems reasonable to perform regional analgesia in women with a clinical diagnosis of chorioamnionitis in the absence of overt signs of sepsis. Ideally, antibiotics should be initiated prior to regional analgesia.

■ EPIDURAL ASSOCIATED FEVER

The association between epidural analgesia and progressive increase in maternal temperature was first described in 1989 (3). Since then, an increased risk of intrapartum fever in women receiving epidural analgesia has been consistently confirmed in randomized studies (21–24). The primary clinical risk factor for developing fever after epidural analgesia is duration of exposure; therefore, multiparous patients are rarely at increased risk. The widespread introduction of epidural analgesia may be an important influence on the temporal incidence rates of intrapartum fever. Historical rates of intrapartum fever were generally reported to be 1% to 5% (2). Current rates of intrapartum fever in nulliparas have been reported between 13% and 33% (Table 20-2) while rates in multiparous patients are generally not increased (27).

The rate of increase in maternal temperature in women with epidural analgesia is controversial. Initial studies (3,28) presented mean rises in temperature on the assumption that the mechanism for epidural related hyperthermia was thermoregulatory and therefore logically would affect all women equally. However, more recent studies have suggested that temperature response to epidural analgesia may not be uniform. Nulliparous women who ultimately remain afebrile over the entire course of labor have no increase in temperature in the first 4 hours following epidural analgesia while women who ultimately become febrile have an immediate response that is significantly within 1 hour (Fig. 20-1). In women with a predisposition to hyperthermia, temperature increases can be rapid, averaging 0.33°F/h (29). This is consistent with observational studies that demonstrate a significant increased risk of maternal fever >38°C after 4 to 6 hours of exposure to epidural analgesia (25).

The etiology of epidural related fever also remains controversial. Proposed etiologies include a perturbation of maternal thermoregulation, acquired intrapartum infection, and non-infectious inflammation (30,31). Since the majority of women with epidural analgesia do not experience any increase in temperature with epidural analgesia (29), it is difficult to support a thermoregulatory mechanism based on the physiologic effects of epidural analgesia. In contrast, several studies have identified pre-epidural maternal inflammation, measured by maternal serum interleukin-6 (IL-6) levels, as a significant risk factor for subsequent fever (32,33). Women with early labor IL-6 levels in the highest quartile have a markedly increased rate of subsequent fever (Fig. 20-2). There is no evidence that underlying maternal serum IL-6 levels are higher in women choosing epidural analgesia (33). Therefore, there does not appear to be a selection bias for an increased risk of inflammation/fever in women selecting epidural analgesia. Women with the tumor necrosis factor (TNFα) Δ308 polymorphism, which increases

TABLE 20-2 Risk of Intrapartum Fever in Nulliparous Patients

Study	Type of Study	Rate of Fever Epidural Arm (%)	Rate of Fever Control Arm (%)	Relative Risk (95% CI)
25	Observational	15	1	14.5 (6.3–33.2)
26	Observational	20	2	9.8 (2.4–39.7)
Yancy (2001)	Observational	13	1.1	11.3 (1.6–79.4)
22	Randomized	33	7	4.8 (2.9–8.0)
21[a]	Randomized	24	5	5.0 (2.5–9.9)
23	Randomized	Not stratified by parity		
24	Randomized	Not stratified by parity		

[a]Results from this trial stratified by parity presented in (Philip J, Alexander JM, Sharma SK, et al. Epidural analgesia during labor and maternal fever. *Anesthesiology* 1999;90:1271–1275).

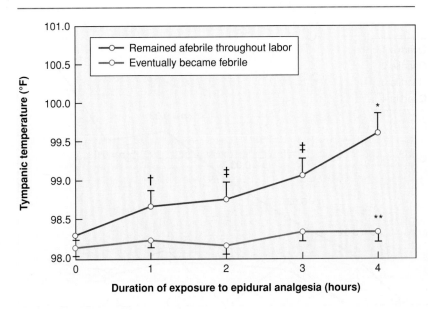

FIGURE 20-1 Maternal tympanic temperature in the 4 hours immediately following initiation of epidural analgesia, stratified by ultimate intrapartum fever status. Temperature points that are significantly different between the two curves are marked (repeated measures analysis †, $p < 0.05$; ‡, $p \le 0.01$; *, $p < 0.0001$). Repeated measures analysis was used to evaluate changes in temperature over time in the afebrile group. No significant increase was observed (**, $p = 0.26$). Goetzl L, Zighelboim I, Badell M, et al. Maternal corticosteroids to prevent intrauterine exposure to hyperthermia and inflammation; a randomized, double-blind, placebo-controlled trial. *Am J Obstet Gynecol* 2006;195:1031–1037. Reprinted with permission from: Goetzl L, Rivers J, Zighelboim I, et al. Intrapartum epidural analgesia and maternal temperature regulation. *Obstet Gynecol* 2007;109:687–690.

levels of this pro-inflammatory cytokine, have an increased risk of intrapartum fever (24.4%) compared with controls (RR 3.3; 95% CI 1.3–7.1,34). Perhaps the most compelling evidence for an inflammatory etiology is that prophylactic administration of maternal corticosteroids immediately prior to placement of epidural analgesia reduces the risk of subsequent fever by more than 90% (35). The source of the maternal inflammation is not well understood although an increase in placental inflammation has been observed in women with fever following epidural analgesia (36) and placental inflammation may account, in part, for the unique temperature response to epidural analgesia observed in pregnancy.

While acquired infection undoubtedly accounts for a small portion of observed intrapartum fever at term, epidural analgesia itself should not be associated with a significant increased risk of acquired maternal infection. Placentas of women receiving epidural analgesia do not show significant rates of infection, whether associated with fever or not (33). Critically, epidural analgesia should have a minimal effect on the risk of prolonged labor, the most powerful risk factor for infectious fever. In most summary analyses, the effect of epidural analgesia on the duration of labor is small (37), although an increased rate of oxytocin use is also required.. Again, while vaginal examinations may occur more often in women with superior pain control, this is not associated with increased risk of infection (38). Finally, antibiotic prophylaxis for group B streptococcus is not associated with decreased rates of fever following epidural analgesia, again arguing against an infectious etiology.

Cytokines can cause fever directly through stimulation of prostaglandin synthesis in the preoptic area of the hypothalamus. Several other factors likely modulate the degree of temperature elevation in women following epidural analgesia. Epidural analgesia has been associated with maternal shivering and rigors and in turn maternal shivering has been associated with fever following epidural analgesia (39,40). Shivering and shaking rigors are common in systemic infection and likely to be cytokine mediated. The administration of IL-6 to healthy volunteers induced shivering that was dose dependent (41). Therefore, one alternate pathway through which elevated levels of maternal inflammation may result in subsequent hyperthermia is through heat generating rigors. However, rigors are unlikely to be the sole pathway to hyperthermia as paralysis only slightly reduces the febrile response to interleukin-2 (IL-2) in non-pregnant subjects (Fig. 20-3) (42). Maternal opioids have also been associated with a small decrease in maternal temperature following epidural analgesia in some but not all studies (28,43,44). This effect may be mediated through a decrease in shivering (45) and/or a direct inhibition of cytokine release (46). Finally, alterations in sweating and hyperventilation with epidural analgesia may have minor effects on maternal temperature regulation.

At this time, there is no effective preventative strategy for reducing the risk of maternal hyperthermia following epidural analgesia. Maternal steroid administration, while effective, is associated with an increased risk of asymptomatic neonatal bacteremia (35). Acetaminophen does not alter the maternal temperature curve following epidural analgesia (47). In a small randomized trial, epidural dexamethasone attenuated the rise in maternal IL-6 and temperature, but the rate of clinical fever was unusually low and did not differ between groups (48). Effective strategies will depend on both

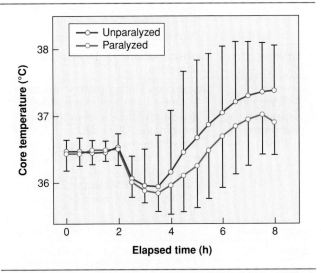

FIGURE 20-2 Fever rate by duration of epidural analgesia and maternal IL-6 quartile. Reprinted with permission from: Goetzl L, Hill EG, Brown JL, et al. Maternal temperature response to epidural analgesia and pro-inflammatory activation. *Reprod Sci* 2010;17:177A.

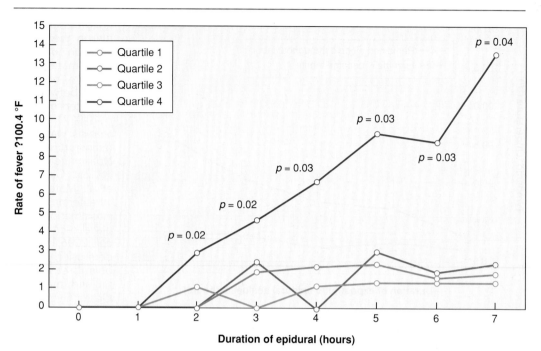

FIGURE 20-3 Change in core temperature in response to IL-2 challenge by paralysis status. Reprinted with permission from: Lenhardt R, Negishi C, Sessler DI, et al. Paralysis only slightly reduces the febrile response to IL-2 during isoflurane anesthesia. *Anesthesiology* 1998;89:648–656.

accurate prediction of subsets of women at risk and more targeted mechanism-based interventions.

■ TREATMENT OF SERIOUS MATERNAL INFECTION

While maternal survival following puerperal sepsis has improved steadily, infection remains a significant cause of maternal morbidity and mortality (1,38). Common maternal conditions associated with antepartum and peripartum sepsis are listed in Table 20-3. Serious maternal infection can result in various degrees of systemic involvement: Systemic inflammatory response syndrome (SIRS), sepsis, severe sepsis, or septic shock (Table 20-4) (49). Some diagnostic criteria may be difficult to interpret in the setting of maternal labor as (a) maternal leukocytosis results from the normal labor process (4), (b) physiologic respiratory alkalosis is seen in normal pregnancy and may not represent compensation for acidosis, and (c) maternal tachycardia often results from labor or postoperative pain. Therefore it is unsurprising that recent data demonstrate a lack of predictive value of both the SIRS and the Modified Early Warning Score (MEWS) in obstetric patients (50). Scoring systems have been adapted for use in pregnant women, with thresholds altered to accommodate normal physiologic changes of pregnancy. These

Modified Early Obstetric Warning Scores (MEOWS) may enable sick parturients to be more easily identified; however, only one validation study has been performed to date and only 40 patients (20%) in the cohort had infection (51). Maternal outcome depends on the etiologic agent and the balance between a physiologic immune response and an excess inflammatory response. Maternal mortality with documented bacteremia has previously been estimated at 6.8% (52). While this is much lower than in non-obstetric

TABLE 20-3 Maternal Conditions Associated with Septic Shock

Pyelonephritis
Septic abortion
Chorioamnionitis
Endometritis
Toxic shock syndrome
Necrotizing fasciitis
Septic pelvic thrombophlebitis
Surgical site infections (obstetric or non-obstetric)
Appendicitis
Pneumonia
Cholecystitis
Meningitis

TABLE 20-4 Definition of Key Terms

Infection	Invasion of normally sterile host tissue by microorganisms and/or the inflammatory response to these microorganisms
Bacteremia	Presence of viable bacteria in the blood; with or without clinical significance
Sepsis	Systemic inflammatory response to infection
Systemic inflammatory response syndrome (SIRS)	Widespread inflammatory response defined by two or more of the following (outside of pregnancy) Temperature >38 or <36°C Pulse <90 beats/min Respiratory rate >20/min or $PaCO_2$ <32 mm Hg White blood cell count >12,000 or <4,000 or >10% band (immature forms)
Severe sepsis	Sepsis with associated organ failure
Septic shock	Sepsis with hypotension refractory to fluid resuscitation

Adapted from: Bone RC, Balk RA, Cerra FB, et al. American College of Chest Physicians/Society of Critical Care Medicine Consensus Conference: Definitions for sepsis and organ failure and guidelines for the use of innovative therapy in sepsis. *Crit Care Med* 1992;20:864–874.

patients, more recent estimates are not available. In cases of antepartum maternal infection, elective delivery has not been shown to improve maternal survival, except those involving maternal cardiac arrest, when perimortem cesarean may improve maternal resuscitation (53). Transfer to an intensive care setting and use of higher level nursing care should be based on the level of care that can be provided safely in the labor and delivery suite as this varies widely by individual site.

Antibiotic Choice

Initial antibiotic therapy should be broad spectrum based on the most likely etiologic agents and should include coverage for group A strep. In cases of pregnancy termination or post-amniocentesis pregnancy loss, antibiotic treatment should include coverage for Clostridia species. Ideally, two maternal blood cultures should be obtained prior to the start of antibiotic treatment. If central access is present, one set of cultures should be drawn peripherally and one from the central access port. In antepartum patients prior to active labor, amniocentesis should be considered for Gram stain and culture if the source of the infection is suspected to be intrauterine. Gram stain is the most specific rapid test for intrauterine infection, while culture confirms the final diagnosis and organisms (5). Endometrial and vaginal cultures usually reveal polymicrobial growth that may not accurately reflect the primary etiologic agent(s).

Additional Therapies and Considerations

Maternal acidosis and hypotension should be treated aggressively both to improve maternal outcome and, in the antepartum setting, to minimize adverse fetal exposures. It is reasonable to adjust therapy with the goal of maintaining mean arterial pressures ≥65 mm Hg and urine output >0.5 mL/kg/h (54), although there is little research examining the correlation between the use of goal-directed therapy and outcomes during pregnancy. Additional invasive maternal cardiovascular monitoring can be considered in selected cases. Endotoxin-mediated hypotension may be especially profound in the setting of Staphylococcal, Clostridia, or Group A Streptococcal infection. The optimal choice of inotropes in pregnancy is not known. Ephedrine bolus treatment can be used for transient hypotension due to its mixed α-1 and β-2 adrenergic receptor actions and positive effect on uterine perfusion and fetal acidosis (55). For continuous infusion, various agents have been used, most commonly dopamine and norepinephrine (56). Clinical trials have decreased theoretical concerns regarding the excess fetal acidosis with phenylephrine that had been observed in some animal models (57). Oxygen saturation (SaO_2) of >93% is generally desirable both to prevent fetal hypoxia and to improve maternal outcomes (58). Maternal left lateral positioning should be maintained with a hip or flank roll to prevent decreased preload from aorto-caval compression by the uterus. Feedback from fetal heart rate monitoring can be helpful if recurrent late decelerations are noted, to increase efforts toward intrauterine resuscitation. Fluid resuscitation should be given as needed, but with the understanding that the combination of pregnancy and endothelial inflammation is a potent risk factor for pulmonary edema. Acute respiratory distress syndrome (ARDS) may complicate cases of sepsis and is associated with maternal mortality rates of 20% to 40% (59,60). If maternal mechanical ventilation is required and a degree of permissive hypercapnia thought necessary, consideration should be given to the normal pregnancy related reduced normal baseline of CO_2 and bicarbonate levels. If initial response

to crystalloid is suboptimal, it is reasonable to transfuse with CMV-negative, Kell-negative matched packed red cells (if available) to achieve a minimum initial hematocrit of 30%. Cytokine-mediated induction of nitric oxide production and resulting underperfusion is associated with an increased risk of sepsis-induced renal failure which is potentially both a cofactor and a marker for increased mortality (61).

In the setting of infection following delivery or pregnancy termination, the uterus should be evaluated for retained products of conception (62). Dilation and evacuation should be considered if retained products are identified as they may contribute to sustained infection. The use of steroid therapy to improve maternal survival has not been well studied in the setting of pregnancy but is not contraindicated. If clinically indicated for adjunctive treatment of sepsis, corticosteroids should not be withheld because of pregnancy concerns. If fetal lung maturity is desired, additional treatment with steroids with known placental passage (i.e., betamethasone or dexamethasone) should be given in addition at the usual obstetric doses. The use of intensive insulin therapy has not been evaluated in the setting of intrapartum sepsis. However, the use of insulin infusions is common in the intrapartum setting and is unlikely to be harmful if maternal hypoglycemia is avoided. Disseminated intravascular coagulation should be treated with clotting factors and blood component replacement as appropriate. The use of novel therapies such as activated protein C has not been formally evaluated in pregnant patients, although a few case reports have been published. Due to the increased risk of hemorrhage following either cesarean or vaginal delivery, the individual risks and benefits must be weighed, as in the perioperative non-pregnant patient. The risk of maternal thromboembolic complications are increased in the setting of maternal infection. Although this specific risk factor is not addressed in the most current guidelines (63), in patients without signs of DIC or active hemorrhage, thromboprophylaxis with serial compression devices and prophylactic doses of unfractionated heparin is reasonable.

■ PREVENTION OF OTHER PERIPARTUM INFECTIOUS MORBIDITY

Although maternal bacteremia is estimated to occur in 2 to 7.5 per 1,000 admissions (52,64), maternal complications including infectious endocarditis and sepsis are uncommon. The current American College of Obstetricians and Gynecologists (ACOG) guidelines state that antibiotics for endocarditis prophylaxis should be given only to those women with the highest risk cardiac conditions including prosthetic heart valves or other indwelling prosthetic material, known history of infective endocarditis, unrepaired cyanotic heart disease or repaired congenital heart disease with residual defects (65,66). Prophylactic antibiotics for other indications are given commonly in obstetric practice. It is standard of care to culture pregnant women for Group B Streptococcus (GBS) between 35 and 37 weeks' gestation (67). Women who present in labor at <37 weeks with unknown GBS status are generally treated as positive due to the increased risk of infection in preterm neonates.

Finally, there are multiple clinical trials suggesting a benefit of antibiotic treatment given prior to skin incision for preventing post-cesarean endometritis and wound infection. A recent Cochrane review (68) suggested that the average risk ratio was 0.45 (95% CI 0.39–0.51) for febrile morbidity, 0.39 (95% CI 0.32–0.48) for wound infection, and 0.38 (95% CI 0.19–0.48) for endometritis. Short-term adverse effects center on allergic reactions while unknown adverse effects may include selection of antibiotic resistant bacterial strains. ACOG currently recommends antibiotic prophylaxis within the 60 minutes prior to skin incision (69) rather than after cord clamping as was previously commonplace. Cefazolin (1 to 2 g) is recommended except in women with a known history of immediate type sensitivity reactions to cephalosporins and perhaps severe such reactions to penicillins. Some recent evidence has raised concerns that even a 2 g dose may be insufficient in pregnant women with a body mass index exceeding 40 kg/m² (70). Research is ongoing to optimize dosing strategies. Peripartum/perioperative tight glycemic control (glucose <110 mg/dL) in diabetic patients is recommended to reduce rates of neonatal hypoglycemia (71). Some studies also suggest that tight glycemic control in the first 24 to 48 hours post cesarean decreases the rate of wound infection. Oxygen supplementation has not been shown to decrease perioperative wound infection following cesarean (72).

■ MATERNAL SEQUELAE OF INTRAPARTUM FEVER

Since epidural analgesia increases the clinical diagnosis of chorioamnionitis through the increased incidence of maternal fever, it is not surprising that epidural analgesia has been associated with an increase in maternal intrapartum antibiotic treatment (26,73). In addition, mothers who develop an intrapartum temperature >99.5°F have a two-fold increased risk of cesarean delivery (95% CI 1.5–3.4) even after controlling length of labor (74). The reason for this increased cesarean rate is not certain but one potential mechanism is the decreased contractility in uterine muscle exposed to inflammation (75). Alternatively, the presence of maternal fever may alter obstetrical decision making regarding the mode of delivery, in order to avoid potential harm to the fetus (31). The risk of postpartum infection is also increased including wound infection and endomyometritis (17,76). Long-term sequelae are uncommon. The increased risk of postpartum hemorrhage has already been reviewed above.

■ NEONATAL SEQUELAE OF INTRAPARTUM FEVER

Short-term complications of chorioamnionitis include significant increases in neonatal infection. At term, treated chorioamnionitis is associated with an increased risk of sepsis (1.3% absolute risk) but not of neonatal death (17). Risk of infectious complications are significantly higher in preterm infants. Maternal fever is also associated with fetal exposure to significant hyperthermia. Oral temperature is the best indicator of intrauterine temperature but underestimates it by an average of 0.8°C (77). In turn, fetal core temperature is approximately 0.75°C higher than fetal skin/intrauterine temperature (McCauley 1992). Therefore a maternal temperature of 38°C is generally associated with fetal core/brain temperatures of 39.5°C or higher. Maternal fever is also associated with intrauterine fetal exposure to inflammation (32,78). Both increased brain temperature and fetal inflammatory activation may be directly neurotoxic and the combination, even in the absence of infection, may be particularly injurious. In 16 infants with encephalopathy born to febrile mothers, only one (6.4%) had documented sepsis as a contributing factor to the brain injury (79). Clinical chorioamnionitis at term is associated with a more than four-fold increased risk of neonatal hypoxic ischemic encephalopathy (HIE) and a four- to nine-fold increased risk of cerebral palsy (79–81). Supporting a partly inflammatory mechanism, term infants with cerebral palsy are more likely to carry a functional polymorphism in the IL-6 gene (82). IL-6 and IL-8 are also elevated in the amniotic fluid of gestations resulting in cerebral palsy, compared to controls

TABLE 20-5 Absolute Risk of Neonatal Encephalopathy Based on Intrapartum Factors (84,89)

	No Maternal Fever (%)	Maternal Fever (%)
No fetal acidosis	0.12	1.13
Fetal acidosis	1.58	12.50

(83). In addition, intrapartum fever may lower the threshold for fetal hypoxic injury. In a recent study, the risk of neonatal encephalopathy with either maternal fever or fetal acidosis alone was approximately 1%. However, when both maternal fever and fetal acidosis are present, the risk of neonatal encephalopathy was 12.5% Table 20-5 (84). This relationship is not mediated through an increase in fetal oxidative stress in the setting of maternal fever (85). Even in the absence of severe injury, exposure of preterm fetuses to intrapartum fever has been linked to an increased trend in the likelihood (OR 3.4; 95% CI 0.94–12) of non-verbal intelligence scores <70 (excluding cases of cerebral palsy) (86). Finally, the newborn is more likely to undergo sepsis evaluation and antibiotic treatment, though largely as a consequence of the central role of maternal fever in accepted criteria for such workup (25,87). This risk varies among institutions, however, underscoring the importance of neonatology practice style (Kaul 2011, 88). Defining the risks of exposure to intrapartum hyperthermia and inflammation is an active area of research, as is work investigating potential neuroprotectants. N-Acetyl Cysteine (NAC), an anti-oxidant with anti-inflammatory properties, is currently being investigated in women with clinical chorioamnionitis (clinicaltrials.gov).

KEY POINTS

- Maternal fever at term is due to a combination of infectious chorioamnionitis and non-infectious fever; both are associated with fetal exposure to hyperthermia and inflammation.
- Maternal fever in preterm gestations is associated with higher rates of frank intrauterine infection than fever at term.
- Maternal intrapartum fever should be treated as infectious chorioamnionitis and maternal antibiotics administered; common regimens include ampicillin and gentamicin.
- Chorioamnionitis is a risk factor for maternal uterine atony; therefore, it is prudent to have uterotonic agents readily available prior to delivery.
- Maternal sepsis is a rare but serious condition with significant rates of maternal mortality.
- In the setting of maternal sepsis, protocols for goal-directed therapy should be followed with adjustments for known changes in maternal physiology.
- Prophylactic antibiotics should be given shortly prior to skin incision for cesarean delivery to reduce the risk of postoperative infectious complications. Dose should be adjusted for maternal body mass index.
- Prophylactic antibiotics to prevent endocarditis in laboring women should be reserved for prosthetic heart valves or other indwelling prosthetic material, known history of infective endocarditis, unrepaired cyanotic heart disease, or repaired congenital heart disease with residual defects.
- Further research is needed to understand and prevent intrauterine fetal injury associated with inflammation and hyperthermia.

REFERENCES

1. Centre for Maternal and Child Enquiries (CMACE). Saving Mothers' Lives: reviewing maternal deaths to make motherhood safer: 2006–2008. The Eighth Report on Confidential Enquiries into Maternal Deaths in the United Kingdom. *BJOG* 2011;118(Suppl 1):1–203.
2. Newton ER. Chorioamnionitis and intraamniotic infection. *Clin Obstet Gynecol* 1993;36:795–808.
3. Fusi L, Steer PJ, Maresh MJ, et al. Maternal pyrexia associated with the use of epidural analgesia in labour. *Lancet* 1989;1:1250–1252.
4. Acker DB, Johnson MP, Sachs BP, et al. The leukocyte count in labor. *Am J Obstet Gynecol* 1985;153:737–739.
5. Tita ATN, Andrews WW. Diagnosis and management of clinical chorioamnionitis. *Clin Perinatol* 2010;37:339–354.
6. Herbst A, Kallen K. Time between membrane rupture and delivery and septicemia in term neonates. *Obstet Gynecol* 2007;110:612–618.
7. Soper DE, Mayhall CG, Froggatt JW. Characterization and control of intraamniotic infection in an urban teaching hospital. *Am J Obstet Gynecol* 1996;175:304–309.
8. Newton ER, Piper J, Peairs W. Bacterial vaginosis and intraamniotic infection. *Am J Obstet Gynecol* 1997;176:672–677.
9. Yancey MK, Duff P, Clark P, et al. Peripartum infection associated with vaginal group B streptococcal colonization. *Obstet Gynecol* 1994;84:816–819.
10. Anderson BL, Simhan HN, Simons KM, et al. Untreated asymptomatic group B streptococcal bacteriuria early in pregnancy and chorioamnionitis at delivery. *Am J Obstet Gynecol* 2007;196:524.e1–524.e5.
11. Goldenberg RL, Hauth JC, Andrews WW. Intrauterine infection and preterm delivery. *N Engl J Med* 2000;342:1500–1507.
12. Cahill AG, Odibo AO, Roehl KA, et al. How many cervical exams are to many in management of labor at term? *Am J Obstet Gynecol* 2011;204:S52.
13. Escobar GJ, Li DK, Armstrong MA, et al. Neonatal sepsis workups in infants ≥2000 grams at birth: a population based study. *Pediatrics* 2000:106:256–263.
14. Sperling RS, Ramamurthy RS, Gibbs RS. A comparison of intrapartum versus immediate postpartum treatment of intra-amniotic infection. *Obstet Gynecol* 1987;70:861–865.
15. Gilstrap LC, Leveno KJ, Cox SM, et al. Intrapartum treatment of acute chorioamnionitis: impact on neonatal sepsis. *Am J Obstet Gynecol* 1988;159:579–583.
16. Lyell DJ, Pullen K, Fuh K, et al. Daily compared with 8-hour gentamicin for the treatment of intrapartum chorioamnionitis: a randomized controlled trial. *Obstet Gynecol* 2010;115:344–349.
17. Rouse DJ, Landon M, Leveno KJ, et al. The maternal-fetal medicine units cesarean registry: Chorioamnionitis at term and its duration—relationship to outcomes. *Am J Obstet Gynecol* 2004;191:211–216.
18. Locksmith GJ, Duff P. Assessment of the value of routine blood cultures in the evaluation and treatment of patients with chorioamnionitis. *Infect Dis Obstet Gynecol* 1994;2:111–114.
19. Bader AM, Gilbertson L, Kirz L, et al. Regional anesthesia in women with chorioamnionitis. *Reg Anesth* 1992;17(2):84–86.
20. Goodman EJ, DeHorta E, Taguiam JM. Safety of spinal and epidural anesthesia in parturients with chorioamnionitis. *Reg Anesth* 1996;21(5):436–441.
21. Sharma SK, Sidawi JE, Ramin SM, et al. Cesarean delivery: a randomized trial of epidural versus patient-controlled meperidine analgesia during labor. *Anesthesiology* 1997;87:487–494.
22. Sharma SK, Alexander JM, Messick G, et al. Cesarean delivery: a randomized trial of epidural analgesia versus intravenous meperidine analgesia during labor in nulliparous women. *Anesthesiology* 2002;96:546–551.
23. Ramin SM, Gambling DR, Lucas MJ, et al. Randomized trial of epidural versus intravenous analgesia during labor. *Obstet Gynecol* 1995;86:783–789.
24. Lucas MJ, Sharma SK, McIntire DD, et al. A randomized trial of labor analgesia in women with pregnancy-induced hypertension. *Am J Obstet Gynecol* 2001;185:970–975.
25. Lieberman E, Lang JM, Frigoletto F, et al. Epidural analgesia, intrapartum fever, and neonatal sepsis evaluation. *Pediatrics* 1997;99:415–419.
26. Mayer DC, Chescheir NC, Spielman FJ. Increased intrapartum antibiotic administration associated with epidural analgesia in labor. *Am J Perinat* 1997;14:83–86.
27. Philip J, Alexander JM, Sharma SK, et al. Epidural analgesia during labor and maternal fever. *Anesthesiology* 1999;90:1271–1275.
28. Camann WR, Hortvet LA, Hughes N, et al. Maternal temperature regulation during extradural analgesia for labour. *Br J Anaesth* 1991;67:565–568.
29. Goetzl L, Rivers J, Zighelboim I, et al. Intrapartum epidural analgesia and maternal temperature regulation. *Obstet Gynecol* 2007;109:687–690.
30. Eltzschig HK, Lieberman ES, Camann WR. Regional anesthesia and analgesia for labor and delivery. *New Engl J Med* 2003;348:319–332.
31. Segal S. Labor epidural analgesia and maternal fever. *Anesth Analg* 2010;111:1467–1475.
32. Goetzl L, Evans T, Rivers J, et al. Elevated maternal and fetal serum interleukin-6 levels are associated with epidural fever. *Am J Obstet Gynecol* 2002;187:834–838.
33. Riley LE, Celi AC, Onderdonk AB, et al. Association of epidural-related fever and noninfectious inflammation in term labor. *Obstet Gynecol.* 2011;117(3):588–595.
34. Simhan HN, Krohn MA, Zeevi A, et al. Tumor necrosis factor-alpha promoter gene polymorphism-308 and chorioamnionitis. *Obstet Gynecol* 2003;102:162–166.
35. Goetzl L, Zighelboim I, Badell M, et al. Maternal corticosteroids to prevent intrauterine exposure to hyperthermia and inflammation; a randomized, double-blind, placebo-controlled trial. *Am J Obstet Gynecol* 2006;195:1031–1037.
36. Dashe JS, Rogers BB, McIntire DD, et al. Epidural analgesia and intrapartum fever: placental findings. *Obstet Gynecol* 1999;93:341–344.
37. Halpern SH, Leighton BL, Ohlsson A, et al. Effect of epidural vs parental opioid analgesia on the progress of labor. *JAMA* 1998;280:2105–2110.
38. Dolea C, Stein C. *Global burden of maternal sepsis in the year 2000. Evidence and Information for policy.* Geneva, Switzerland: World Health Organization; 2006: 1–18.
39. Gleeson NC, Nolan KM, Ford MR. Temperature, labour, and epidural analgesia. *Lancet* 1989;2:861–862.
40. Benson MD, Haney E, Dinsmoor M, et al. Shaking rigors in parturients. *J Repro Med* 2008;53:685–690.
41. Steensberg A, Fischer CP, Sacchetti M, et al. Acute interleukin-6 administration does not impair muscle glucose uptake or whole-body glucose disposal in healthy humans. *J Physiol* 2003;548:631–638.
42. Lenhardt R, Negishi C, Sessler DI, et al. Paralysis only slightly reduces the febrile response to interleukin-2 during isoflurane anesthesia. *Anesthesiology* 1998;89:648–656.
43. Negishi C, Lenhardt R, Ozaki M, et al. Opioids inhibit febrile responses in humans, whereas epidural analgesia does not; an explanation for hyperthermia during epidural analgesia. *Anesthesiology* 2001;94:218–222.
44. Gross JB, Cohen AP, Lang JM, et al. Differences in systemic opioid use do not explain increased fever incidence in parturients receiving epidural analgesia. *Anesthesiology* 2002;97:157–161.
45. Negishi C, Kim JS, Lenhardt R, et al. Alfentanil reduces the febrile response to interleukin-2 in humans. *Critical Care Med* 2000;28:1295–1300.
46. McCarthy DO, Murray S, Galagan D, et al. Meperidine attenuates the secretion but not the transcription of interleukin 1(beta) in human mononuclear leukocytes. *Nurs Res* 1998;47:19–24.
47. Goetzl L, Rivers J, Evans T, et al. Prophylactic acetaminophen does not prevent epidural fever in nulliparous women: a double-blind placebo-controlled trial. *J Perinatol* 2004;24:471–475.
48. Wang LZ, Hu XX, Liu X, et al. Influence of epidural dexamethasone on maternal temperature and serum cytokine concentration after labor epidural analgesia. *Int J Gynaecol Obstet.* 2011;113(1):40–43.
49. Bone RC, Balk RA, Cerra FB, et al. American College of Chest Physicians/Society of Critical Care Medicine Consensus Conference: Definitions for sepsis and organ failure and guidelines for the use of innovative therapy in sepsis. *Crit Care Med* 1992;20:864–874.
50. Lappen JR, Keen M, Lore M, et al. Existing models fail to predict sepsis in an obstetric population with intrauterine infection. *Am J Obstet Gynecol* 2010;203:573.e1–573.e5.
51. Singh S, McGlennan A, England A, et al. A validation study of the CEMACH recommended modified early obstetric warning system (MEOWS). *Anaesthesia* 2012;67:12–18.
52. Bryan CS, Reynolds KL, Moore EE. Bacteremia in obstetrics and gynecology. *Obstet Gynecol* 1984;64:155–158.
53. Dijkman A, Huisman CM, Smit M, et al. Cardiac arrest in pregnancy; increasing use of perimortem caesarean section due to emergency skills training? *BJOG* 2010;117:282–287.
54. Rivers E, Nguyen B, Havstad S, et al. Early goal-directed therapy in the treatment of severe sepsis and septic shock. *N Engl J Med* 2001;345:1368–1377.
55. Ko R, Mazur JE, Pastis NJ, et al. Common problems in critically ill obstetric patients, with an emphasis on pharmacotherapy. *Am J Med Sci* 2008;335:65–70.
56. Dellinger RP, Carlet JM, Masur H, et al. Surviving sepsis campaign guidelines for management of severe sepsis and septic shock. *Crit Care Med* 2004;32:858–873.
57. Lee A, Kee N, Gin T. A quantitative, systematic review of randomized controlled trials of ephedrine versus phenylephrine for the management of hypotension during spinal anesthesia for cesarean delivery. *Anesth Analg* 2002;94:920–926.
58. Guinn D, Abel D, Tomlinson M. Early goal directed therapy for sepsis during pregnancy. *Obstet Gynecol Clin North Am* 2007;34:459–479.
59. Catanzarite V, Willms D, Wong KG, et al. Acute respiratory distress syndrome in pregnancy and puerperium: causes, courses and outcomes. *Obstet Gynecol* 2001;97:760–764.
60. Chen CY, Chen CP, Wang KG, et al. Factors implicated in outcome of pregnancies complicated by acute respiratory failure. *J Reprod Med* 2003;48:641–648.

61. Schrier RW, Wang W. Acute renal failure and sepsis. *N Engl J Med* 2004;351:159–169.
62. Rahangdale L. Infectious complications of pregnancy termination. *Clin Obstet Gynecol* 2009;52:198–204.
63. Bates SM, Greer IA, Pabinger I, et al. Venous thromboembolism, thrombophilia, antithrombotic therapy, and pregnancy: American College of Chest Physicians Evidence-Based Clinical Practice Guidelines (8th Ed.). *Chest* 2008;133(6 Suppl):844S–886S.
64. Blanco JD, Gibbs RS, Castaneda YS, et al. Bacteremia in obstetrics: clinical course. *Obstet Gynecol* 1981;58:621–625.
65. American College of Obstetricians and Gynecologists. Antibiotic prophylaxis for infective endocarditis. ACOG Committee Opinion No.421. *Obstet Gynecol* 2008;112:1193–1194.
66. Wilson W, Taubert KA, Gewitz M, et al. Prevention of infective endocarditis: guidelines from the American Heart Association: a guideline from the American Heart Association Rheumatic Fever, Endocarditis, and Kawasaki Disease Committee, Council on Cardiovascular Disease in the Young, and the Council on Clinical Cardiology, Council on Cardiovascular Surgery and Anesthesia, and the Quality of Care and Outcomes Research Interdisciplinary Working Group [published erratum appears in Circulation 2007;116:e376–e377]. *Circulation* 2007;116:1736–1754.
67. Prevention of perinatal group B streptococcal disease. Revised guidelines from CDC, 2010. *MMWR.* 2010;59 (RR-10):1–32.
68. Smaill FM, Gyte GM. Antibiotic prophylaxis versus no prophylaxis for preventing infection after cesarean section. *Cochrane Database Syst Rev* 2010:1:CD007482.
69. American College of Obstetricians and Gynecologists. Antimicrobial prophylaxis for cesarean delivery: timing of administration. Committee Opinion No. 465. *Obstet Gynecol* 2010;116:791–792.
70. Pevzner L, Swank M, Krepel C, et al. Effects of maternal obesity on tissue concentrations of prophylactic cefazolin during cesarean delivery. *Am J Obstet Gynecol* 2011;104:S24.
71. American College of Obstetricians and Gynecologists. Pregestational diabetes mellitus. ACOG Practice Bulletin No. 60. *Obstet Gynecol* 2005;105:675–685.
72. Gardella C, Goltra LB, Laschansky E, et al. High-concentration supplemental perioperative oxygen to reduce the incidence of postcesarean surgical site infection: a randomized controlled trial. *Obstet Gynecol* 2008;112:545–552.
73. Goetzl L, Cohen A, Frigoletto F Jr., et al. Maternal epidural analgesia and rates of maternal antibiotic treatment in a low-risk nulliparous population. *J Perinatol* 2003;23:457–461.
74. Lieberman E, Cohen A, Lang J, et al. Maternal intrapartum temperature elevation as a risk factor for cesarean delivery and assisted vaginal delivery. *Am J Public Health* 1999;89:506–510.
75. Mark SP, Croughan-Minihane MS, Kilpatrick SJ. Chorioamnionitis and uterine function. *Obstet Gynecol* 2000;95:909–912.
76. Hauth JC, Gilstrap LC, Hankins GD, et al. Term maternal and neonatal complications of acute chorioamnionitis. *Obstet Gynecol* 1985;66:59.
77. Banerjee S, Cashman P, Yentis SM, et al. Maternal temperature monitoring during labor: concordance and variability among monitoring sites. *Obstet Gynecol* 2004;103:287–293.
78. Shalak LF, Laptook AR, Jafri HS, et al. Clinical chorioamnionitis, elevated cytokines, and brain injury in term infants. *Pediatrics* 2002;110:673–680.
79. Impey LWM, Greenwood C, MacQuillan K, et al. Fever in labour and neonatal encephalopathy: a prospective cohort study. *BJOG* 2001;108:594–597.
80. Wu YW, Escobar GJ, Grether JK, et al. Chorioamnionitis and cerebral palsy in term and near term infants. *JAMA* 2003;290:2677–2684.
81. Grether JK, Nelson KB. Maternal infection and cerebral palsy in infants of normal birth weight. *JAMA* 1997;278:207–211.
82. Wu YW, Croen LA, Torres AR, et al. Interleukin-6 genotype and risk for cerebral palsy in term and near-term infants. *Ann Neurol* 2009;66:663–670.
83. Yoon BH, Romero R, Park JS, et al. Fetal exposure to an intra-amniotic inflammation and the development of cerebral palsy at the age of three years. *Am J Obstet Gynecol* 2000;182:675–681.
84. Impey LWM, Greenwood CEL, Black RS, et al. The relationship between intrapartum maternal fever and neonatal acidosis as risk factors for neonatal encephalopathy. *Am J Obstet Gynecol* 2008;198:49.e1–49.e6.
85. Goetzl L, Hill EG, Brown JL, et al. Maternal temperature response to epidural analgesia and pro inflammatory activation. *Reprod Sci* 2010;17:177A.
86. Dammann O, Drescher J, Veelken N. Maternal fever at birth and nonverbal intelligence at age 9 years in preterm infants. *Dev Med Child Neurol* 2003;45:148–151.
87. Yancey MK, Zhang J, Schwarz J, et al. Labor epidural analgesia and intrapartum maternal hyperthermia. *Obstet Gynecol* 2001;98:763–770.
88. Goetzl L, Cohen A, Frigoletto F Jr., et al. Maternal epidural use and neonatal sepsis evaluation in afebrile mothers. *Pediatrics* 2001;108:1099–10102.
89. Goetzl L, Korte JE. Interaction between intrapartum maternal fever and fetal acidosis increases risk for neonatal encephalopathy. *Am J Obstet Gynecol* 2008;199(2):e9.
90. Kaul B, Vallejo M, Ramanathan S, et al. Epidural labor analgesia and neonatal sepsis evaluation rate: a quality improvement study. *Anesth Analg* 2001;93:986–990.
91. Goetzl L, Manevich Y, Roedner C, et al. Maternal and fetal oxidative stress and intrapartum term fever. *Am J Obstet Gynecol* 2010;202:363.e1–363.e5.
92. Macaulay JH, Bond K, Steer PJ. Epidural analgesia in labor and fetal hyperthermia. *Obstet Gynecol* 1992;80:665–669.
93. Mantha VR, Vallejo MC, Ramesh V, et al. The incidence of maternal fever during labor is less with intermittent than with continuous epidural analgesia: a randomized controlled trial. *Int J Obstet Anesth* 2008;17:123–129.
94. Morales WJ, Washington SR 3rd, Lazar AJ. The effect of chorioamnionitis on perinatal outcome in preterm gestation. *J Perinatol* 1987;7:105–110.
95. Shatrov JG, Birch SC, Lam LT, et al. Chorioamnionitis and cerebral palsy: a meta-analysis. *Obstet Gynecol* 2010;116:387–392.

CHAPTER

21

Obstetric Hemorrhage, Novel Pharmacologic Interventions, Blood Conservation Techniques, and Hemorrhage Protocols

Ashutosh Wali • Jonathan H. Waters

■ DEFINITION OF HEMORRHAGE

Several definitions of hemorrhage have been proposed such as blood loss that leads to a 10% drop in hematocrit, hemorrhage significant enough to cause hemodynamic instability, or hemorrhage significant enough to result in transfusion (1). While a 10% drop in hematocrit seems like a significant drop, a drop from a predelivery hematocrit of 35% to 25% can be clinically inconsequential in healthy, young parturients. Hemorrhage significant enough to cause hemodynamic instability starts to identify factors which separate normal from abnormal postpartum bleeding. To retrospectively decide whether hemodynamic instability is related to bleeding or the effect of anesthesia is often difficult.

Definition and Classification of Obstetric Hemorrhage

Obstetrical hemorrhage, also known as peripartum hemorrhage, is defined as hemorrhage during pregnancy (antepartum), during labor (intrapartum), or during puerperium (postpartum hemorrhage [PPH]). Antepartum hemorrhage is further subdivided into the early and late antepartum subperiods based on a cut-off at 20 weeks of gestation; intrapartum hemorrhage is the end result of blood loss during the typical delivery process; and PPH is further subdivided into the early and late postpartum subgroups based on hemorrhage occurring before or after 24 hours following delivery. Clinically, such distinct delineation may not be possible due to the potential for sequential blood loss throughout pregnancy, beginning from the antepartum period through the intrapartum phase and ending in the postpartum period. The term peripartum hemorrhage is typically associated with abnormal or excessive blood loss greater than 1,000 mL (2).

Incidence of Obstetric Hemorrhage

Obstetric hemorrhage continues to be a leading cause of maternal morbidity and mortality worldwide even though the incidence has decreased over the years. In the United States, there has been a dramatic decrease in hemorrhage-related maternal mortality from 25.8% in the time period 1986 to 1990 (3), to 18.2% in the time period 1991 to 1997 (4). The decline has been attributed to two factors: The ability to diagnose and treat ectopic pregnancy early leading to a decrease in ectopic pregnancy-related mortality from 10.7% (3) to 5.6% (4) over the same time periods and the advancements in the management of obstetric hemorrhage including the use of prostaglandins and new surgical techniques,

such as embolization (5). In the United Kingdom, similar decline in hemorrhage-related maternal mortality has been observed over the last decade. Hemorrhage was the second leading cause of maternal mortality in the time period, 2000 to 2002, with 17 deaths and a rate of 0.85/100,000 deliveries (6), dropped to being the fifth leading cause during the time period, 2003 to 2005, with 14 deaths and a rate of 0.66/100,000 deliveries (7), and has stayed as the fifth leading cause during the time period, 2006 to 2008, with 9 deaths and a rate of 0.39/100,000 deliveries (8) (Table 21-1).

Compensation for Obstetric (Peripartum) Hemorrhage

A major problem associated with obstetric (peripartum) hemorrhage is differentiating normal peripartum blood loss from clinically significant peripartum hemorrhage. Over the course of gestation, many physiologic changes occur. Of these changes, one of the most dramatic is that of the expansion of the blood volume. Typically, there is an increase in plasma volume of up to 55% above the prepregnancy state (9), that reaches its peak around 30 weeks of gestation (10,11). Associated with this plasma volume increase is an increased red cell mass up to 30% above the prepregnancy state (9). The red cell mass expansion is surpassed by a plasma volume expansion resulting in a physiologic anemia of pregnancy. These changes provide a compensatory reserve in the event of acute blood loss during and after delivery. The greatest threat of hemorrhage during pregnancy is not to the mother, but to the fetus (12). Under most circumstances, blood loss up to 1,000 mL is easily compensated by the gestational plasma volume expansion. Over the years, the incidence of severe obstetric hemorrhage has decreased from 4.5/1,000 deliveries in 2003 to 2005 (7) to 3.7 in 2006 to 2008 (8) in the United Kingdom.

Pregnancy results in an increase in blood volume from 76 mL/kg to 94 mL/kg (9), leading to a total blood volume of approximately 6,600 mL in a 70 kg parturient. The traditional categorization of hemorrhage, into four classes, is based on percentage blood volume loss and the typical physiologic response to the blood loss (13). Class 1 hemorrhage is characterized by a 15% blood volume deficit (990 mL) resulting in a mild physiologic response of dizziness and palpitations (13). Class 2 hemorrhage correlates with a 20% to 25% blood volume deficit (1,320 to 1,650 mL) leading to tachycardia, tachypnea, sweating, orthostatic hypotension, and a narrow pulse pressure. Narrowing of pulse pressure occurs due to the activation of the sympathoadrenal system, leading to systemic vasoconstriction and increase in the diastolic blood pressure. As a consequence, there is redistribution of blood from the

TABLE 21-1 Numbers and Rates of Hemorrhage-related Maternal Mortality in the United Kingdom: 2000–2008

Numbers			Rates per 100,000 Maternities		
2000–2002	2003–2005	2006–2008	2000–2002	2003–2005	2006–2008
17	14	9	0.85	0.66	0.39

Modified from: Cantwell R, Clutton-Brock T, Cooper G, et al. Saving mothers' lives: Reviewing maternal deaths to make motherhood safer: 2006–2008. The eighth report of the confidential enquiries into maternal deaths in the United Kingdom. *BJOG* 2011;118 Suppl 1.

nonvital organs, such as skin and muscle, to vital organs, such as the brain and heart (13). Class 3 hemorrhage corresponds to a 30% to 35% blood volume deficit (1,980 to 2,310 mL) and manifests as restlessness, worsening tachycardia (120 to 160 beats/min), worsening tachypnea (30 to 50 breaths/min), overt hypotension, pallor, and cool extremities (13). Class 4 hemorrhage correlates with a 40% blood volume deficit or more resulting in absent distal pulses, air hunger, shock, and oliguria/anuria (13).

Antepartum Hemorrhage

Antepartum hemorrhage is theoretically subclassified into an early antepartum hemorrhage period before 20 weeks of gestation, the commonest causes being threatened abortion and ectopic pregnancy, and the late antepartum hemorrhage period after 20 weeks of gestation, the commonest causes being placental abruption and placenta previa. However, for practical and clinical purposes, the gestational age cut-off between early and late antepartum hemorrhage should be at the age of viability of 24 weeks.

Early Antepartum Hemorrhage
Threatened Abortion
The World Health Organization defines abortion as spontaneous or induced termination of pregnancy, before 20 weeks of gestation. Vaginal bleeding before 20 weeks of gestation is thus termed as threatened abortion. The incidence of threatened abortion is about 20% of all pregnancies and 50% of them abort spontaneously (14).

Ectopic Pregnancy
Ectopic pregnancy is defined as an extrauterine pregnancy that is usually not viable and occurs in about 3% of pregnancies. Commonest causes are inflammation, infection, or surgery of the fallopian tubes resulting in unsuccessful passage of the fertilized egg from the fallopian tube to the uterus. Risk factors include advanced maternal age more than 35 years, in vitro fertilization, and use of multiple sexual partners. Clinical presentation includes abdominal pain, vaginal bleeding, and amenorrhea. Diagnosis is based on clinical signs and symptoms, serum human chorionic gonadotropin levels, serum progesterone levels, hematocrit, and transvaginal ultrasonography. Since the ectopic pregnancy is not viable, due to rupture and hemorrhage, it may become a life-threatening emergency, requiring laparoscopic surgical intervention.

Late Antepartum Hemorrhage
Placental Abruption
Placental abruption is essentially a problem with the disruption of the union between the placenta and the endometrial lining and is defined as the premature (after 20 weeks of gestation) (15,16), predelivery severance of the placenta from the decidua basalis of the endometrium (17). Based on the extent of separation, placental abruption is classified as marginal,

partial, or complete (18) (Fig. 21-1) and is responsible for direct fetal compromise due to loss of placental surface area for maternal–fetal exchange of oxygen (19).

Epidemiology. Risk factors (17,20) for placental abruption include physical forces such as trauma and membrane rupture; exposures such as amphetamine, cocaine, methadone, and tobacco; comorbid conditions such as hypertension with superimposed preeclampsia, severe preeclampsia, uterine fibroids, chorioamnionitis, acute/chronic respiratory illnesses (21), advanced maternal age/parity (12), multiple gestation, and previous history of placental abruption (16). Preeclampsia is the commonest risk factor for placental abruption, accounting for 50% of patients (22).

The overall incidence for placental abruption is 5.9 to 6.5 per 1,000 singleton births and 12.2 per twin births (23,24). However, the incidence of placental abruption related to gestational age was found to be 60% for preterm gestation (20% before 34 weeks and 40% between 34 and 37 weeks) and 40% for after 37 weeks of gestation. This incidence was causally related to the low birth weight newborns seen in parturients with placental abruption as compared to parturients without placental abruption (25). The relative risk for delivering a low birth weight newborn in placental abruption is shown in Table 21-2. Recent data show that perinatal mortality rates have dropped from almost 80% several decades ago to 12% (19).

Diagnosis. The typical clinical presentation of placental abruption is usually impressive and includes abdominal pain, vaginal bleeding, uterine tenderness, uterine irritability,

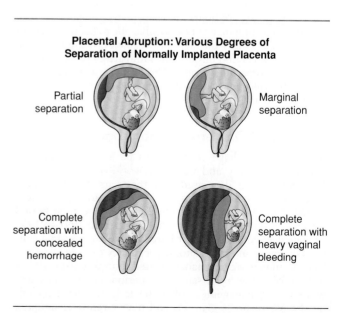

Placental Abruption: Various Degrees of Separation of Normally Implanted Placenta

Partial separation

Marginal separation

Complete separation with concealed hemorrhage

Complete separation with heavy vaginal bleeding

FIGURE 21-1 Classification of placental abruption.

TABLE 21-2 Relative Risk for Delivering a Low Birth Weight Newborn in Placental Abruption

Weight of Newborn in Grams (g)	Adjusted Relative Risk (ARR)	ARR Range
>2,500 g	4.6	4–5.3
1,500–2,499 g	4.1	3.4–4.8
<1,500 g	11.4	8.6–15

Modified from: Ananth CV, Berkowitz GS, Savitz DA, et al. Placental abruption and adverse perinatal outcomes. *JAMA* 1999;282(17): 1646–1651.

coagulopathy, preterm labor, and nonreassuring fetal heart rate. Vaginal bleeding may be profuse and is termed "revealed" or may be absent, if a sequestered retroplacental clot is formed, and is termed "concealed". Unexplained maternal hypotension, in the absence of vaginal bleeding, may be the presenting feature in concealed placental abruption. In contrast to placenta previa where diagnosis is largely based on imaging, placental abruption has to be diagnosed clinically since Kleihauer–Betke assay and ultrasonography have a limited role (19,26).

However, ultrasonography may aid confirmation in the event of clinical suspicion of placental abruption (27), help determine the age of the hematoma (28), and rule out placenta previa (29). Normal placental thickness is up to 5 cm and if the placenta is more than 8 to 9 cm, one should consider placental abruption as part of the differential diagnosis (30).

Differential diagnosis for revealed vaginal hemorrhage should include placenta previa, genital tract trauma, marginal sinus rupture, hematuria, and vasa previa (17). Differential diagnosis for concealed hemorrhage should include acute appendicitis, chorioamnionitis, uterine fibroid degeneration, ovarian rupture and torsion, pyelonephritis, retroplacental abruption, and uterine rupture (17).

Pathophysiology. Placental abruption is also classified as mild, moderate, or severe (Table 21-3). Complications of severe placental abruption include hemorrhagic shock, disseminated intravascular coagulopathy (DIC), anemia, acute renal failure, uterine atony, pituitary necrosis, and fetal distress/demise (12,17).

DIC, in placental abruption, occurs in 20% of patients (31), increases with fetal demise, and is due to release of thromboplastin, a thrombogenic substance. Thromboplastin activates the extrinsic coagulation cascade and releases thrombin, converting fibrinogen to fibrin, and sets off massive intravascular coagulation resulting in consumption of clotting factors I,

II, V, VIII, and platelets (17). Laboratory confirmation is in the form of elevated levels of prothrombin time (PT), partial thromboplastin time (PTT), thrombin time (TT), fibrin split products (FSP), thrombocytopenia, hypofibrinogenemia, and a typical thromboelastography (TEG) profile (17). Fibrin and thrombin plug the microcirculation and disrupt essential blood flow to critical organs. Simultaneously, secondary fibrinolysis occurs to break down the excessive fibrin (17). Rotational thromboelastometry (ROTEM) is being recommended to help with early diagnosis of fibrinolytic activity and to initiate intervention.

Uterine atony, in placental abruption, is due to the increased levels of FSP in maternal serum and lochia (32). FSP reduce myometrial contractility in vitro (32) and may predispose to ongoing hemorrhage in vivo (17). Also, antifibrinolytics have been shown to enhance myometrial contractility in placental abruption (33).

Obstetric Management. Obstetric management of placental abruption is best accomplished by delivery of the fetus and placenta. However, clinical considerations for route and timing of delivery should include the severity of placental abruption, gestational age, cardiovascular stability, coagulation profile, and fetal status (15,17). Electronic fetal heart rate monitoring (EFHR) and continuous tocodynamometry, with an intrauterine pressure catheter, are the mainstay of obstetric management.

■ If the fetus is nonviable or not alive, vaginal delivery is preferred.
■ If the fetus is viable and alive, EFHR is reassuring, abruption is mild, and gestation is *full term*, vaginal delivery is preferred and labor may have to be induced. However, oxytocin augmentation may not be necessary due to the inherent uterine hyperactivity in placental abruption (34).
■ If the fetus is viable and alive, EFHR is reassuring, abruption is mild, but gestation is *preterm*, delivery is postponed and the pregnancy is permitted to carry on to ensure fetal lung maturation.
■ If the fetus is viable and alive, EFHR is nonreassuring (usually secondary to severe abruption irrespective of gestational age), immediate cesarean delivery is performed to minimize perinatal morbidity and mortality (35).

Anesthetic Management. Anesthetic management for placental abruption should involve early patient evaluation and preparation, including large-bore intravenous access; type and cross-match for 4 to 6 units of packed erythrocytes; laboratory analysis for complete blood count (with platelet count), coagulation profile (PT, PTT, and fibrinogen), arterial blood gas, and TEG (if available). Acute blood loss and the consequent hemodynamic response warrants

TABLE 21-3 Grading of Placental Abruption

	Class 0	Class 1	Class 2	Class 3
Vaginal bleeding	None	None–mild	None–moderate	None–severe
Uterine tenderness	None	Slight	Moderate	Severe
Maternal hemodynamics	Stable	Normal HR Normal BP	Tachycardia Orthostatic hypotension	Hypovolemic shock HR > 120/min SBP < 80 mm Hg
Hypofibrinogenemia	None	None	Hypofibrinogenemia, mild (>150 mg/dL)	Hypofibrinogenemia, severe (<150 mg/dL)
Coagulation profile	Normal	Normal	Mild abnormality	Frank coagulopathy
Fetal status	Reassuring	Reassuring	Fetal stress/distress	Fetal distress

aggressive volume resuscitation; left uterine displacement; urinary catheterization; oxygen therapy based on pulse oximetry; and gastrointestinal prophylaxis in preparation for a general anesthetic (12,17).

An easy, inexpensive, and rapid bedside test for coagulation status is to monitor a red top glass test tube, filled with blood, to clot within 6 to 7 minutes or for the clot to break down within 60 minutes; if either does not occur, it suggests the presence of a coagulation abnormality (20). Obviously, the red top test tube examination is a crude surrogate to more specific coagulation tests such as PT, PTT, fibrinogen, platelet count, and TEG. Even though it may not be very reliable, the red top test tube examination may be of some value in situations and facilities where access to coagulation tests is not readily available.

An ominous and not so uncommon consumptive coagulopathy in placental abruption is hypofibrinogenemia, usually below 150 mg/dL (36), and is directly related to degree of placental separation (36). The TEG may show an increase in the K time (normal range, 2 to 4 minutes) and a decrease in the alpha angle (normal range, 50° to 75°). Both these parameters on the TEG are predominantly affected by fibrinogen levels and reflect the speed of clotting. Hypofibrinogenemia responds extremely well to cryoprecipitate transfusion, which is a rich source of fibrinogen, and contains three to ten times more fibrinogen per unit volume as compared to fresh frozen plasma (FFP) (17). Typically, a unit (10 to 15 mL) of cryoprecipitate raises the serum fibrinogen level by 6 to 7 mg/dL (37), so that 13 to 16 units of cryoprecipitate would be needed to raise the serum fibrinogen level by 100 mg/dL (17), in the event FFP is not used to correct the hypofibrinogenemia.

Invasive arterial blood pressure and central venous pressure monitoring is indicated in patients presenting with significant hemodynamic instability and class 3 to 4 hemorrhage to assess and guide fluid and blood management, to maintain urine output at 0.5 to 1 mL/kg/h, and to keep hemoglobin above 6 gm% (38) or 7 gm% (39) respectively.

Anesthetic care should be guided by the necessity for delivery of fetus and degree of placental abruption (12). Neuraxial anesthetic techniques such as continuous epidural analgesia and combined spinal–epidural analgesia may be used for labor and vaginal delivery provided there are no contraindications such as nonreassuring fetal status (NRFS), hypovolemia, or DIC (17). The appropriateness of regional anesthesia, the risk for further extension of abruption and further hemorrhage with an adverse impact on uteroplacental perfusion, is a major concern. Epidural anesthesia significantly worsened maternal hypotension, uterine blood flow, fetal PaO_2 and pH during *untreated* hemorrhage (20 mL/kg blood loss) in gravid ewes (40). However, with prompt recognition and adequate intravascular volume replacement, there were no differences between the cardiac output, mean arterial pressure, and fetal PaO_2 in the study and control groups. The authors concluded that epidural anesthesia and the associated sympathetic block may adversely affect the compensatory responses in untreated hemorrhage in pregnant patients.

Therefore, close supervision and observation is necessary since new onset hemorrhage or coagulopathy may set in after neuraxial analgesia is started requiring cessation of neuraxial technique; institution of appropriate hemodynamic and neurologic monitoring; and institution of appropriate hemodynamic and neurosurgical intervention.

Cesarean delivery for placental abruption is usually reserved for ongoing hemorrhage, DIC, or NRFS. General anesthesia, using rapid sequence induction/intubation technique

and cricoid pressure, is favored. Ketamine, up to 1 mg/kg, is preferred if uterine tone is low or normal. Higher doses of ketamine may increase uterine tone in early pregnancy, but not at term (41). Etomidate, 0.3 mg/kg, should be used in situations such as increased uterine tone or hemodynamic instability (42). Propofol and sodium thiopental are relatively contraindicated in parturients with ongoing hemorrhage or hemodynamic instability because of the potential for exaggerating maternal hypotension and worsening fetal status. Maintenance of general anesthesia with low-dose inhalational agent is recommended to prevent awareness, but may worsen uterine atony, requiring uterotonics after delivery, and may worsen hypotension requiring vasopressor use to maintain hemodynamic stability.

Placenta Previa

Placenta previa is essentially a problem with placental implantation; placenta previa is present when the placenta implants in advance of the fetal presenting part. Normally, in early pregnancy, the placenta is located in the lower uterine segment near the internal cervical os. However, as the pregnancy advances, the placenta seems to seek the more vascularized part of the uterus (for nutrition and oxygen) and migrates to a more cephalad location to the body of the uterus or the fundus, allowing the fetal presenting part to occupy the lower uterine segment. Based on the final location of the placenta in relation to the internal cervical os, placenta previa is subclassified as low-lying (placenta is in the lower uterine segment), marginal (placenta encroaches, but does not cover the internal cervical os), partial (placenta covers the internal cervical os partially), and total (placenta covers the internal cervical os completely) (Fig. 21-2).

Epidemiology. Risk factors for placenta previa include conditions that prevent the upward migration of the placenta, within the uterus, such as previous uterine surgery (cesarean delivery, myomectomy, and dilation/curettage), previous history of placenta previa, advanced maternal age, and multiparity.

The incidence of placenta previa is 3.6/1,000 pregnancies (43), the distribution being 40% total previa, 30% partial placenta previa, and 30% marginal and low-lying placenta previa. Reported perinatal mortality rate is 2.3% (44).

Diagnosis. The classic clinical hallmark of placenta previa is painless vaginal bleeding, that may be very subtle at times, and occurs especially during the second or third trimester. The absence of abdominal pain and abnormal uterine tone does not exclude placental abruption, because as many

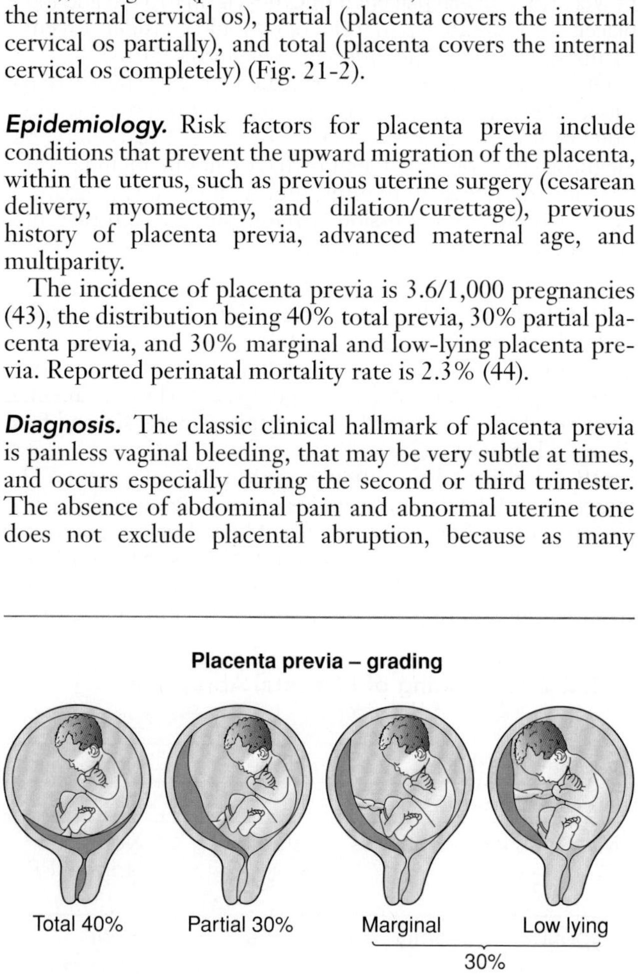

Placenta previa – grading

Total 40%   Partial 30%   Marginal   Low lying

30%

FIGURE 21-2 Classification of placenta previa.

as 10% of patients with placenta previa have coexisting placental abruption (45). The fetal presenting part is usually not palpable on cervical examination, since the placenta occupies the lower uterine segment, and consequently, a breech or transverse position is observed in 33% of parturients with placenta previa (46,47). The initial bleed usually stops spontaneously and seldom leads to maternal or fetal morbidity/mortality (12). Torrential hemorrhage may be precipitated on cervical examination in an undiagnosed placenta previa.

In contrast to placental abruption where diagnosis is largely clinical, placenta previa is diagnosed by ultrasonography, with 93% to 97% accuracy (48,49), in patients with a full urinary bladder. Transvaginal ultrasonography has 100% sensitivity and permits finer clarity of the placental–uterine border (50), but has the potential for trauma and hemorrhage provoked by vaginal probe placement. Magnetic resonance imaging provides an excellent resolution of the cervical–placental interface and is a useful and more accurate modality for diagnosing placenta previa (51); however, it can be cost prohibitive (17).

Obstetric Management. Obstetric management of placenta previa depends on the acuity of vaginal bleeding and degree of fetal lung maturity (12). However, if vaginal bleeding is minimal, fetal lungs are not mature, or patient is not in active labor, patients are hospitalized and managed conservatively (17). If vaginal bleeding has stopped for more than 48 hours and the patient has easy, quick access to a tertiary care hospital with facilities such as obstetrics, anesthesiology, neonatology, and blood banking the patients are sent home with clear instructions to return in the event of vaginal bleeding or onset of labor (17). Vaginal delivery may be chosen if the placenta is low-lying and more than 2 cm proximal to the internal cervical os (52) provided the fetal status is stable, maternal hemodynamics are stable, there is no ongoing vaginal hemorrhage, and facilities for cesarean delivery are readily available (53). However, cesarean delivery is indicated for a marginal or complete placenta previa (52,53). Cesarean delivery is also indicated if there is ongoing excessive hemorrhage, fetal lungs are mature, or the parturient is in active labor (17).

Tocolytic therapy is essential, especially before 32 weeks of gestation to allow fetal lung maturity, reduce neonatal morbidity and mortality (54), and provide fetal neuroprotection (55). However, most tocolytic agents have cardiovascular side effects that should be weighed against the benefit of improving fetal lung maturity (17). Similarly, blood transfusion therapy becomes essential for extending the pregnancy and for allowing fetal lungs to mature, but the risk of blood and blood product transfusion-related side effects must be constantly evaluated and compared (17).

Anesthetic Management. Preanesthetic assessment is essential in all parturients presenting to labor and delivery with antepartum hemorrhage (56). Special emphasis should be placed on previous history of cesarean delivery, location of placenta in the current gestation, a thorough airway evaluation, assessment of intravascular volume status, and evaluation of any anticipated ongoing hemorrhage (12,17). Rapid placement of at least two short, but wide-bore peripheral intravenous catheters (16G), blood draw for blood type and screen and complete blood count, and assessment of fetal heart tones are essential (17). Intravascular volume may be replaced with a nondextrose crystalloid solution if hematocrit is acceptable and patient is hemodynamically stable, nonheme colloid solution if

hematocrit is acceptable and patient is unstable, or packed erythrocytes if hematocrit is unacceptably low and patient is unstable. In the event of ongoing excessive hemorrhage in a hemodynamically stable patient or if the parturient is hemodynamically unstable, blood type and cross-match for 4 units of packed erythrocytes should be ordered and made available.

The choice of anesthetic management has to be individualized for each patient based on hemodynamic stability and preoperative airway assessment. Similar results, in terms of estimated blood loss, urine output, and neonatal Apgar scores have been observed in hemodynamically stable patients administered general anesthesia or epidural anesthesia for placenta previa requiring elective cesarean delivery (57). However, neuraxial anesthesia remains the preferred choice of anesthesia amongst anesthesiologists and anesthetists taking care of patients with placenta previa with no known placenta accreta, hemodynamic instability, or maternal hypovolemia (1,58). The choices within neuraxial anesthesia range from single-shot spinal anesthesia, continuous epidural anesthesia, and combined spinal–epidural anesthesia; and all three choices have been used successfully. However, the risk of excessive intraoperative hemorrhage in placenta previa patients is fairly high due to the direct surgical incision through an anteriorly located placenta previa, inability of the distended lower uterine segment to contract adequately after delivery, and the increased risk of placenta accreta in patients with previous uterine surgery including cesarean delivery (17). As a general rule, parturients with placenta previa undergoing cesarean delivery, under neuraxial anesthesia, should be made aware that intraoperative induction of general anesthesia, electively or emergently, may be necessary usually after delivery in the event of ongoing excessive hemorrhage requiring cesarean hysterectomy (12). Such ongoing hemorrhage is usually from placenta accreta. Securing the airway early allows the anesthesia care team to focus exclusively on maternal volume resuscitation.

General anesthesia should be chosen as the initial anesthetic in the bleeding placenta previa patient. Since the source of bleeding is the placenta itself, removal of the placenta following delivery of the fetus is essential. Typically, due to the emergent nature of these cases, adequate preoperative evaluation may not occur. However, one has to concurrently assess, resuscitate, and get the patient ready for cesarean delivery (12). Preoperative packed erythrocyte transfusion may be necessary emergently without a blood cross-match being available. In such situations, type specific blood or type O, Rh-negative blood should be administered. At Baylor College of Medicine (Ashutosh Wali), we have immediate access to 4 units of type O, Rh-negative erythrocytes, at all times in the labor and delivery refrigerator, for emergency use.

Invasive hemodynamic monitoring, including an intra-arterial catheter for beat to beat blood pressure recording and frequent blood sampling; and central venous catheter for intravascular volume status and volume replacement, is required for the patient with ongoing excessive hemorrhage (17). In addition, patient temperature should be monitored. Hypothermia should be avoided to prevent coagulopathy and shivering by using a rapid infuser, fluid warming device, warming mattress, and warming blanket.

If airway evaluation is not reassuring, one may either secure the airway awake or proceed with rapid sequence induction. However, in the event of rapid sequence induction, the difficult airway cart with advanced airway equipment must be available in the operating room, adequate backup personnel readily accessible, and an in-house surgeon informed and available to provide surgical airway access, if necessary (see chapter on Difficult Airway Management for further details).

However, if the airway assessment is reassuring, one should proceed with rapid sequence induction of general anesthesia using appropriate gastrointestinal prophylaxis, adequate preoxygenation to allow effective denitrogenation of lungs, left uterine displacement, and efficacious cricoid pressure application to prevent regurgitation of gastric contents (17). The selection of the intravenous induction agent depends on the level of hemodynamic stability. Etomidate (0.3 mg/kg) has a good track record of safety in obstetric anesthesia (59) and is recommended if uterine tone is increased or the patient is hemodynamically unstable (42). Side effects of etomidate include pain at venous injection site, hiccups, nausea, vomiting, and myoclonus. Ketamine (0.75 to 1 mg/kg) is easy to administer and ideal for the bleeding parturient if uterine tone is normal or decreased (17). Ketamine stimulates the central sympathetic nervous system and inhibits the reuptake of norepinephrine resulting in indirect increase in heart rate, cardiac output, and arterial blood pressure. In patients with severe hemorrhagic shock where catecholamine stores may be exhausted, ketamine may cause direct myocardial depression, due to inhibition of calcium transients, and exaggerate the hypotension (60). Side effects include intraoperative increase in uterine tone compromising the already stressed fetus and postoperative nightmares/hallucinations in doses exceeding 2 mg/kg.

Choice of the maintenance anesthetic agent also depends on hemodynamic stability. Volatile halogenated agents result in uterine muscular relaxation and increased bleeding during cesarean delivery (61), but help to prevent maternal awareness. A combination of oxygen, nitrous oxide as tolerated to keep oxygen saturation within normal range, and low concentration volatile halogenated anesthetic are used until delivery of the fetus. After delivery, small doses of short-acting opioids and short-acting benzodiazepines are administered intravenously to supplement the anesthetic, thereby allowing a reduction in the concentration of the volatile agent and nitrous oxide as necessary (17).

After delivery of the fetus and placenta, because of the previous implantation of the placenta, the lower uterine segment may not contract and result in continued bleeding that may require discontinuing the volatile halogenated agent, administering intravenous oxytocin, intramuscular methylergonovine, intramuscular and/or intramyometrial 15-methyl prostaglandin F2£, and rectal misoprostol. Coagulopathy, in placenta previa, is unusual and may manifest as a dilutional thrombocytopenia from the use of crystalloids/colloids and packed erythrocytes (12,17).

Uterine Rupture

Epidemiology. Uterine rupture is essentially a problem leading to parting of the uterine muscle, either in the presence of a previous uterine scar or in the absence of one, and the commonest cause is due to the disruption of a previous cesarean hysterotomy scar (36).

The etiology of uterine rupture can be subdivided into two groups, pregestational and gestational. Pregestational causes include surgical (previous cesarean delivery, previous myomectomy scar (62), previous repair of uterine rupture, and dilation and curettage (63)), traumatic (blunt, penetrating, sharp trauma), and congenital anomalies (bicornuate uterus (64), and undeveloped uterine horn (36)). Gestational causes reflect causes in the current pregnancy and include antepartum (spontaneous and intense uterine hyperstimulation, augmented stimulation of labor with oxytocin or prostaglandins (64), external cephalic version, uterine overdistension from multiple gestation or polyhydramnios, intra-amniotic instillation of saline or prostaglandins), intrapartum (dif-

ficult forceps delivery, tumultuous breech extraction) (65), and acquired (placenta percreta, gestational trophoblastic neoplasia) (36). A recent study (2001) drew attention to the increased risk of uterine rupture associated with the use of prostaglandin induction and advised against its use in patients with previous cesarean delivery (66). The overall risk of real uterine rupture in an unscarred uterus is almost nonexistent (67) and in parturients with a scarred uterus, it is still low at 1% (64). However, the relative risk of uterine rupture during spontaneous labor compared to nonlaboring patients is 3.3 (95% C.I., 1.8 to 6), is considerably higher at 15.6 (95% C.I., 8.1 to 30) when prostaglandins are used for induction of labor, but is unclear for oxytocin use (68).

Most uterine rupture, during labor, occurs in the lower anterior uterine segment leading to increased maternal morbidity and mortality (7), because the anterior uterine wall is highly vascular and may include the site for placental implantation (12); whereas uterine rupture, before labor, occurs at the fundus (69). Fetal mortality rate of 35% has been reported in a review of 23 parturients with severe uterine rupture; no maternal mortality occurred in that series (65). Neonatal mortality rises 60 times in uterine rupture (67).

Risk factors include previous cesarean delivery, congenital uterine anomalies, fetal malpresentation, grand multiparity, labor induction with oxytocin or prostaglandins, and previous myomectomy (12).

Diagnosis. Uterine rupture can be catastrophic to both, the mother and her fetus. Fortunately, it is very uncommon. However, when it occurs, maternal and fetal morbidity and mortality are dependent on its severity that in turn, relies on whether the rupture is complete or is merely a uterine scar dehiscence. Complete uterine rupture causes an extensive uterine wall deficiency, leading to fetal compromise and maternal hemorrhage, requiring surgical intervention (12). On the other hand, uterine scar dehiscence leads to a minimal uterine wall deficiency that may be asymptomatic or does not cause fetal compromise or maternal hemorrhage requiring surgical intervention (12).

The commonest and most reliable clinical sign of uterine rupture, in labor, is sudden onset of a nonreassuring fetal heart rate and is reported in 81% of patients (70). Other clinical findings include vaginal bleeding, hypotension, hematuria, and absence of uterine contraction (12). Abdominal pain may not be a consistent symptom of uterine rupture (71).

Obstetric Management. Obstetric management of uterine rupture has to be individualized and depends on the severity of signs and symptoms. If a uterine rent is noted during a postpartum examination following a vaginal birth after cesarean delivery, and the patient is hemodynamically stable without evidence of vaginal bleeding, parturients should be carefully monitored under close observation and concealed hemorrhage should be excluded (17). On the other hand, if there is ongoing excessive maternal hemorrhage and/or fetal distress, cesarean delivery with surgical repair of uterine rupture site may be undertaken, especially if future fertility is desired. If surgical repair is performed, elective cesarean delivery may be indicated in future pregnancies (24). However, surgical repair carries the risk of recurrence of uterine rupture, and may be fatal (24). Definitive management is proceeded with a hysterectomy, and subtotal hysterectomy has been shown to have decreased operating time, lower morbidity, lower mortality, and shorter hospital stay than surgical repair (72). Evidence shows that blood transfusion is required for patients with rupture of unscarred uterus as opposed to patients with scarred uterus. The fibrous and scarred edges of a scar bleed less than the edges of a newly ruptured, unscarred uterus.

Anesthetic Management. Anesthetic management includes caring for any bleeding parturient requiring a cesarean hysterectomy with particular emphasis on the airway, hemodynamics, hematologic system, and status of the fetus. Aggressive volume replacement with blood and blood products, general anesthesia, invasive hemodynamic monitoring, rapid infusion systems, warming devices should be employed for the hemodynamically unstable patient as has been addressed in the earlier section on placental abruption in this chapter. However, if the patient is hematologically and hemodynamically well compensated, a pre-existing labor epidural catheter may be activated for surgical anesthesia with the understanding that intraoperative induction of general anesthesia may be necessary, at any point during surgery to secure the airway and concentrate on volume resuscitation (73).

Vasa Previa

Vasa previa is essentially a problem where fetal vessels go across the fetal membranes in front of the fetal presenting part, at or near the internal cervical os, thereby, affording no protection to the fetal vessels, normally provided by the placenta or the umbilical cord, and may lead to fetal hypoxia and ischemia from direct compression of the fetal vessels by the fetal presenting part (52). Also, during artificial or spontaneous rupture of fetal membranes, fetal vessels may undergo shearing stresses, tears, and rupture leading to fetal exsanguination (12).

Epidemiology. Fetal mortality is reported to be as high as 50% to 75% (12). Maternal hemodynamics and hematologic profile are usually not affected.

The only known risk factor is multiple gestation, so that the incidence of velamentous insertion of umbilical cord is directly proportional to the number of fetuses. However, the overall incidence is quite low at 0.0004% (52).

Diagnosis. Diagnosis is commonly ultrasonographic (12), confirmed with color Doppler imaging (17), and made antenatally with good perinatal results (74). Sometimes, the diagnosis is based on the association between onset of vaginal bleeding and rupture of fetal membranes, followed by NRFS (12). At other times, diagnosis may be made by palpation of the pulsation in the fetal membranes during routine cervical examination of parturients (17). Chemical tests, such as the Apt test (resistance to denaturation of fetal hemoglobin under alkaline conditions) or the Wright stain (detection of nucleated erythrocytes in fetal blood), have been used to aid diagnosis in the setting of vaginal bleeding associated with fetal membrane rupture (17).

Obstetric Management. Obstetric management is focused toward optimizing fetal outcomes, especially in parturients with bleeding vasa previa where cesarean delivery is the norm. Elective cesarean delivery may have to be performed for preterm parturients at 36 weeks of gestation (52), and emergency cesarean delivery may have to be performed for a ruptured vasa previa. Emergency cesarean delivery has been associated with poor fetal outcomes (75), despite proceeding within minutes of vaginal bleeding (76) due to a small fetal blood volume reserve of 80 to 100 mL/kg (12), and commonly requires neonatal volume resuscitation with packed erythrocytes (12).

Anesthetic Management. Anesthetic management should cater to the ongoing needs of both the mother and her fetus at risk, and has been addressed in the earlier section on placenta previa in this chapter.

Postpartum Hemorrhage
Significance of Postpartum Hemorrhage
PPH is further subdivided into the early and late postpartum hemorrhage subgroups based on hemorrhage occurring before or after 24 hours following delivery. PPH is the leading cause of death in pregnancy (4,77). In the developing world, death from PPH occurs in approximately 1 out of 1,000 deliveries (78). Though not as common in the United States, PPH accounts for 11% to 13% of maternal mortalities, making it a significant public health care concern (79). In addition to death, PPH results in significant morbidity. This morbidity can result in hypovolemic shock, DIC, renal and hepatic failure, acute respiratory distress syndrome (ARDS), and neurologic injury such as Sheehan's syndrome.

Though less life altering, PPH can reduce iron stores leading to postpartum iron deficiency and iron deficiency anemia. The prevalence of postpartum iron deficiency and iron deficiency anemia is high even in women who have not suffered a PPH (80). Anemia is associated with decreased work capacity, impaired cognitive function, and a heightened incidence of postpartum depression (81). The following discussion highlights the most common causes of PPH.

Uterine Atony
Epidemiology. Uterine atony is defined as inability of the uterine smooth muscle to contract satisfactorily after delivery of the fetus. PPH results from the dilated arterioles and veins in the placental bed (17) that would ordinarily be constricted by the contracting uterine smooth muscle and may be unresponsive to vasoconstrictors (82). Parturients with obstetric hemorrhage may have uterine arteries that are relatively unresponsive to vasoconstrictors (82). It is the commonest cause of PPH, accounting for almost 80% of the cases (1), and the commonest indication for postpartum blood transfusion (83,84). Uterine contraction and involution, mediated by endogenous oxytocin and prostaglandins, helps control PPH and acts as the primary hemostasis after delivery (12).

Risk factors for uterine atony are best divided into labor-related (arrested active phase of labor requiring oxytocin augmentation, precipitous labor, protracted labor); fetus-related (fetal macrosomia, multiple gestation, placental abruption, placenta previa, polyhydramnios); or mother-related (chorioamnionitis, family history, grand multiparity, laceration during cesarean delivery, use of tocolytics, high concentration of volatile anesthetic) causes (17).

Diagnosis. Diagnosis is usually simple and is based on palpation of a soft postpartum uterus in the setting of vaginal bleeding (12). However, uterine atony may coexist with other causes of PPH and such causes should be excluded before initiating pharmacologic treatment. Inspection must be performed for placental fragmentation, uterine retained placental products, cervical laceration, and vaginal lacerations (17). A high index of suspicion for placenta accreta is warranted if the uterus feels gritty to palpation during manual exploration (17).

Obstetric Management. Obstetric management should consider early pharmacologic therapy (oxytocin, methylergonovine, 15-methyl prostaglandin F2 alpha, and misoprostol) (1); direct uterine manipulation (bimanual compression, uterine massage); or surgical intervention (B-Lynch procedure, hysterectomy) (17). Frequently, pharmacologic therapy and uterine manipulation are applied concurrently and failure to respond to such treatment should be readily communicated between the anesthesiologist and the obstetrician before proceeding with surgical intervention (17). Early administration of oxytocin after delivery is essential in preventing uterine atony (1) and to prevent severe maternal morbidity/mortality (85,86). Evidence suggests that alternative uterotonics may not confer any benefit (87).

Anesthetic Management. Anesthetic management is guided by the patient's airway examination, hemodynamic stability, and hematologic status. Calcium chloride, administered intravenously, may augment uterine contractility in the setting of refractory uterine atony, especially when the patient has received magnesium sulfate. In addition to using uterotonic agents, essential principles are similar to any other case of PPH and are discussed, in detail, later in this chapter.

Uterine Inversion

Uterine inversion is essentially a problem where reversal of the uterine cavity occurs so that it is turned inside-out. Uterine inversion may be incomplete or complete (36) and acute or chronic (12).

Epidemiology. The incidence of uterine inversion is variable and is reported as 1 in 3,000 from a pooled sample of three studies over a 25-year period (88–90). Maternal mortality is rare in developed countries and there were no cases reported in the Confidential Enquiry into Maternal and Child Health (CEMACH) 2007 (7) and one case reported in the Center for Maternal and Child Enquiries (CMACE) 2010 reports (8).

Risk factors include extreme umbilical cord traction, undue fundal pressure, uterine atony, fundal location of placenta, and a short umbilical cord (12,24).

Diagnosis. Diagnosis is straightforward in the presence of a vaginal mass, severe vaginal hemorrhage, and absence of uterus on abdominal palpation and is classified as complete inversion (91); whereas in the absence of an apparent vaginal mass, the diagnosis may be delayed with catastrophic outcome and is known as incomplete inversion (92).

Clinical presentation is one of intense shock that may be both hemorrhagic and neurogenic in nature (24), the hemorrhagic component is usually severe (24), is observed in 90% of the patients (88), and is from placental separation in the setting of uterine atony (24) while the neurogenic component is from the traction on the uterine ligaments (24).

Obstetric Management. Obstetric management should involve calling for help and immediate replacement/eversion of the uterus manually, to prevent catastrophic hemorrhage (92) without removing the placenta (93) to minimize blood loss (93).

Uterine relaxation is usually required to manually evert and replace the uterus. A wide variety of tocolytics are available, including intravenous terbutaline, intravenous nitroglycerin (94), and intravenous magnesium sulfate. Intravaginal hydrostatic replacement, with or without a ventouse cup—a vacuum extractor normally used to deliver fetuses during prolonged second stage of labor, has had good results (94,95,96). Rapid diagnosis and immediate uterine replacement help prevent a surgical intervention (24). If all the above measures are tried and are found to be unsuccessful, an exploratory laparotomy may have to be performed immediately by the obstetrician, using either the Huntingdon or the Haultain procedure, to replace the uterus. The Huntingdon procedure entails sustained pull on the inverted uterine cone or the round ligaments, by means of Allis forceps

gradually, as the uterine fundus surfaces (97). If the Huntingdon procedure is unsuccessful, the Haultain procedure may be attempted whereby the posterior cervical ring is slit longitudinally to relieve the cervical constriction and permit gradual uterine restoration (97).

After uterine replacement, it is critical to add ecbolic agents such as oxytocin, carboprost, and methyl ergonovine to maintain good uterine contractility (92).

Anesthetic Management. Anesthetic priorities should include instantaneous uterine relaxation to facilitate eversion of the inverted uterus to restore back its normal configuration, return of uterine tone after the maneuver, and profound analgesia (12). Uterine relaxant, such as nitroglycerin, is ideal with its rapid onset and offset of action (98,99) and analgesia may be achieved with intravenous fentanyl. Nitroglycerin is administered sublingually, as two doses of 400 µg/spray, or intravenously as a 50 to 100 µg bolus, and helps relax the uterus even after delivery of placenta, suggesting a nitric oxide (NO)-independent mechanism for its action (98) in contrast to the earlier belief that nitroglycerin acts only via a NO-dependent mechanism and requires the presence of placental tissue (100). A suitable alternative is to administer general anesthesia using a halogenated hydrocarbon, such as sevoflurane, to provide uterine relaxation and prevent awareness with the stipulation of tracheal intubation to secure the airway. Administration of general anesthesia, especially in an emergency situation precluding an airway assessment preoperatively, is fraught with dangers such as difficult/failed tracheal intubation, pulmonary aspiration of gastric contents, and difficult extubation.

Placenta Accreta/Increta/Percreta

Placenta accreta is essentially a problem with abnormal adherence of the placental villi directly on the myometrium, due to the absence of the spongy layer of the decidua basalis that normally separates the placenta from the myometrium (36). Three subtypes have been described (Fig. 21-3).

- ■ *Placenta accreta vera* is abnormal placental villous adherence to the myometrium, without invasion;
- ■ *Placenta increta* is abnormal placental villous adherence to the myometrium, with invasion;
- ■ *Placenta percreta* is abnormal placental villous adherence through the myometrium and beyond into other pelvic organs (12,36).

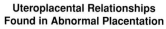
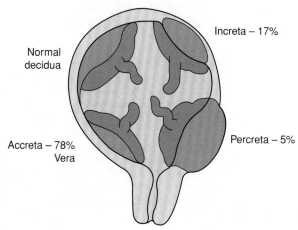

Uteroplacental Relationships Found in Abnormal Placentation

Increta – 17%

Normal decidua

Accreta – 78%
Vera

Percreta – 5%

FIGURE 21-3 Classification of placenta accreta.

TABLE 21-4 Risk of Having a Placenta Accreta Relative to Prior Cesarean Deliveries

Number of Prior Cesarean Deliveries	% of Patients with Placenta Accreta[a]	% of Patients with Placenta Accreta[b]
0	5	3
1	24	11
2	47	40
3	40	61
4 or more	67	67

Modified from:
[a]Clark SL, Koonings PP, Phelan JP. Placenta previa/accreta and prior cesarean section. *Obstet Gynecol* 1985;66(1):89–92.
[b]Silver RM, Landon MB, Rouse DJ, et al. Maternal morbidity associated with multiple repeat cesarean deliveries. *Obstet Gynecol* 2006; 107(6):1226–1232.

Epidemiology. Major risk factors for placenta accreta include previous history of lower uterine segment surgery (low transverse cesarean delivery scar, uterine curettage, and myomectomy). Risk stratification for placenta accreta has shown association with presence of placenta previa (54-fold increased risk), maternal serum alpha-fetoprotein (MSAFP) greater than 2.5 MoM (8-fold increased risk), maternal free HCG greater than 2.5 MoM (4-fold increased risk), and advanced maternal age greater than 35 years (3-fold increased risk) (36,101). MoM is defined as the multiple of the median, when the median is calculated for an appropriate reference population.

Incidence of placenta accreta has been on the rise over the last few decades due to the increasing cesarean delivery rate (36,52,102) rising from 1:2,500 in the 1980s, to 1:535 in 2002, and to 1:210 in 2006 (103). The risk of having a placenta accreta in a parturient presenting with a current placenta previa and no previous cesarean deliveries has been reported as 3% (104) and 5% (105) rising to 11% (104) and 24% (105) in patients with one previous cesarean scar and a current placenta previa. The risk increases further as the number of previous cesarean deliveries increases and is reported as 40% (104) and 47% (105) in patients with two prior cesarean deliveries; 61% (104) and 40% (105) in parturients with three previous cesarean deliveries; and 67% (104,105) in patients with four prior cesarean deliveries (Table 21-4).

Diagnosis. Clinical diagnosis is uncommon antepartum, bleeding is usually due to the presence of a contemporaneous placenta previa, and may be about 500 mL (36). Diagnosis is usually suspected postpartum, with difficulty encountered in removal of placenta, and estimated blood loss may be up to 4 to 5 L. Clinical suspicion for placenta accreta include a retained placenta, massive hemorrhage after removal of placenta, hematuria, uterine inversion, and a uterine cavity that is rough to palpation after manual removal of placenta indicating an eroded myometrium (17). Confirmatory diagnosis is really made at laparotomy (12).

Antepartum ultrasonography has a reported sensitivity of only 33% for diagnosing placenta accreta (106). Addition of color Doppler flow mapping, during ultrasonography, helps better diagnose placenta accreta (reported sensitivity of 100% and a positive predictive value of 78%) by identifying two highly predictive factors for myometrial invasion by the placenta such as the presence of large intraplacental lakes and a reduced distance (less than 1 mm) between the retroplacental vessels and the uterine serosa–urinary bladder interface (107).

MRI may be necessary for confirming placenta accreta, if ultrasonography results are equivocal or suspicious, and may actually help in assessment of uterine wall invasion (108). A two-step MRI protocol has been suggested with excellent results in a cohort of 40 patients, where 14 out of 14 patients were accurately ruled out and 23 out of 26 patients were correctly predicted (109). Three highly predictive MRI findings for diagnosing placenta accreta have been proposed and include heterogenous signal intensity within the placenta, presence of dark intraplacental bands on T2 weighted imaging, and uterine bulging (110). However, MRI has disadvantages such as increased expense, lack of universal availability, and lack of better sensitivity than ultrasonography (12).

Antepartum diagnosis, clinical and/or radiologic, of placenta accreta is desirable in assisting with successful preparation, but may not always be available. The American College of Obstetricians and Gynecologists (ACOG) (1) recommends the following:

1. Preoperative counseling of patients with known placenta accreta for hysterectomy
2. Availability of blood/blood product transfusion
3. Optimization of location and timing of delivery to make certain the accessibility to appropriate obstetric personnel and equipment
4. Preoperative anesthesiology consult
5. Blood bank notification to ensure availability of adequate blood and blood products and
6. Use of intraoperative blood salvage (12).

Obstetric Management. Obstetric management of placenta accreta should ideally be considered within two subgroups, the *anticipated* placenta accreta and the *unanticipated* placenta accreta (111). If placenta accreta is identified in the prelabor phase, there is usually time for planning a well-organized delivery process and managing prospective hemorrhage (112).

Antenatal diagnosis allows for adequate preparation and conservative management, for example in select cases, internal iliac artery balloon placement has been advocated as a means to decrease blood loss, use less blood transfusion, and to provide a better surgical field and shorter operation time (113). However, if placenta accreta is not recognized in the prelabor period, excessive hemorrhage may be ongoing at detection and maternal mortality may be as high as 7% (114). Unplanned and unanticipated hysterectomy is an emergency with an incidence of 0.3 to 0.8 per 1,000 births (115,116). Multidisciplinary teamwork cannot be emphasized enough in successfully managing a cesarean hysterectomy for placenta accreta and includes services such as obstetrical, anesthesiology, laboratory, blood banking, operating rooms, radiologic, urologic, gynecologic, oncologic, surgical, vascular surgical, neonatal, and nursing teams (112). Obviously, it is easier to coordinate all the services that might be involved if the procedure is anticipated and planned in advance. A vast majority (81%) of cesarean hysterectomies for placenta accreta follow repeat cesarean delivery (117). The risk of having a cesarean hysterectomy, in a patient presenting with a placenta previa and a prior history of two or more cesarean deliveries, is 30% to 50% (111).

In the event of an unanticipated placenta accreta, early identification and rapid resuscitation help prevent maternal and fetal morbidity/mortality. If the lower uterine segment seems highly vascular at repeat cesarean delivery, a classical uterine incision or a fundal incision should be made to prevent going through a low-lying placenta and avoiding massive hemorrhage. If the placenta is not easy to remove and is morbidly adherent, no attempt should be made to force its removal (111). Instead, the hysterotomy incision should be closed, oxytocin infusion should not be administered, baseline laboratory samples (complete blood count, coagulation profile, TEG, red top test tube of blood, and arterial blood gases) and blood/blood products ordered, appropriate personnel organized, and decision should be made to proceed with hysterectomy (111). Point-of-care testing with TEG has been used to determine the coagulation profile in healthy and high-risk parturients (118) and to manage peripartum coagulopathy (119). In the exsanguinating patient if the coagulation profile and TEG are not readily accessible, a red top tube of blood may be collected and examined. If the red top tube does not form a firm clot within 7 minutes, a coagulopathy may be likely and an empiric transfusion of cryoprecipitate, fresh frozen plasma, and platelets is suggested (20). Even though the red top test tube examination is an antiquated method for checking the coagulation status of patients, it may offer a starting point for decision making, especially in clinical facilities and clinical situations where coagulation tests are not promptly obtainable.

During a cesarean hysterectomy, vigilant vital sign monitoring is critical. Normal or near normal blood pressure can mislead the practitioner in to believing that maternal hemorrhage has slowed down or stopped. Maternal heart rate changes, in the absence of vasopressors and uterotonics, may act as a better surrogate for ongoing hemorrhage. Maternal heart rate above 120/min and respiratory rate above 20/min may be associated with a loss of 30% to 40% of total blood volume (120), which is a class 3 obstetric hemorrhage, and may be a better proxy for compensated reversible hemorrhagic shock (111). *In addition, a low pulse pressure, especially in the presence of maternal tachycardia, is a subtle indicator of impending decompensated hemorrhagic shock* (111,121). The decrease in pulse pressure is due to an increase in the diastolic pressure, mediated by the catecholamine-induced vasoconstriction (37), as a compensatory mechanism in impending hemorrhagic shock.

Complications include higher peripartum maternal morbidity; longer duration of surgery; increased hemorrhage; organ injury; increased blood and blood product usage; higher transfusion-related problems, such as dilutional thrombocytopenia, DIC, and transfusion-related acute lung injury (TRALI); and infection (111). The morbidity and mortality is high in patients with placenta percreta and the incidence of blood transfusion is high (114). Serious consideration must be given to the use of prophylactic internal iliac artery balloon catheter placement and availability of cell salvage in patients with placenta percreta (122,123).

Anesthetic Management. Anesthetic management has to be individualized to best suit each patient's needs and general principles regarding induction of anesthesia, maintenance, and emergence from anesthesia should follow the description in the earlier section on anesthetic management of placenta previa.

Intraoperative monitoring should include serial assessment of arterial blood gases, complete blood count, coagulation profile, TEG, and electrolytes (17). Additional modalities have been suggested for the unanticipated placenta accreta at cesarean delivery, without adequate scientific evidence. These modalities include activation of a massive transfusion protocol; empirical use of fresh frozen plasma and packed erythrocytes in a 1:1 ratio in order to reduce maternal mortality, correct coagulopathy earlier, and to reduce usage of packed erythrocytes in ICU (124–126); and use of recombinant factor VIIa (rFVIIa), in a dose of approximately 70 μg/kg, to decrease bleeding in a majority (90%) of the patients as reported in a paper reviewing 118 cases of massive PPH (127). A recent study showed that the use of rFVIIa in patients with amniotic

fluid embolism, had worse outcomes than cohorts who did not receive rVIIa. It is recommended that rVIIa be used in AFE patients only when hemorrhage cannot be stopped by massive blood component replacement (128).

Postoperatively, patients with placenta accreta should be monitored and recovered in an intensive care unit setting. Frequently, they require elective ventilation for up to a few hours to a couple of days to allow for intravascular and interstitial fluids to equilibrate, airway swelling to dissipate, and pain control to become easier and more manageable. Patients are sedated and provided intravenous analgesia as needed; laboratory values and chest radiographs assessed serially; normothermia maintained; and when there is evidence of no ongoing hemorrhage and tracheal extubation criteria are met, the patient's trachea is extubated.

Postoperative complications can be life-threatening and include persistent intra-abdominal bleeding, pelvic thromboembolism, renal and bowel ischemia, noncardiogenic pulmonary edema, TRALI, transfusion associated circulatory overload (TACO), myocardial depression, and Sheehan's syndrome (111).

Retained Placenta

Retained placenta is defined as the inability of the placenta to deliver, within 30 minutes (129) or 60 minutes (130), after the birth of the newborn. The reported worldwide incidence varies from 0.01% to 6.3% of vaginal deliveries (131), and depends on the study population and diagnostic criteria. The incidence is higher in women with uterine scarring and a history of retained placenta. Other risk factors include age, early labor, and small or low-lying placenta.

Retained placenta does not allow the uterus to contract, leading to PPH. Various types of retained placenta have been described: Trapped placenta, where the placenta is trapped behind a partially closed cervix; placenta adherens, where the placenta is adherent to the endometrial lining of the uterus, but manually separable; and placenta accreta, where the placenta is abnormally adherent to the myometrium.

The ideal time to intervene and treat the patient with a retained placenta is variable and should balance the risks of manually removing the placenta, such as hemorrhage, infection, and trauma, against the risks of leaving the placenta in place, such as hemorrhage and infection, compared to waiting for the placenta to deliver spontaneously with expectant management (132).

Obstetric Management. Studies have shown that the risk of hemorrhage increases when the duration of placental retention exceeds 30 minutes (133) versus 18 minutes (134). Obstetric management includes manual removal of the placenta, use of ecbolic drugs, such as oxytocin, to rapidly increase uterine tone, and monitoring for any signs of persistent bleeding (12).

Anesthetic Management. Anesthetic management should include provision of patient comfort and uterine relaxation. If the patient does not have ongoing hemorrhage, patient comfort can be provided with a spinal anesthetic covering from T10 to S4 dermatomal level, allowing for manual exploration of the uterus and removal of the placenta; otherwise, a pre-existing epidural catheter should be dosed up with local anesthetic and opioids. In the presence of ongoing hemorrhage, it is safer to proceed with rapid sequence induction of general anesthesia followed by tracheal intubation, taking necessary precautions such as preoperative airway assessment, gastrointestinal prophylaxis, good intravenous access, and availability of packed erythrocytes.

Uterine relaxation may be provided with volatile agents such as sevoflurane or desflurane, provided that the patient is under general anesthesia and has the airway secured with a tracheal tube. The degree of uterine relaxation is similar between volatile agents provided equipotent doses are used (135). If the patient is not under general anesthesia, nitroglycerin is administered either sublingually, as 2 doses of 400 μg/spray, or intravenously as a 50 to 100 μg bolus (136). The advantages of nitroglycerin include its rapid onset, rapid offset, uterine relaxation, and avoidance of volatile anesthetic agents. Its main disadvantage is the potential for hypotension that may get exaggerated in the presence of ongoing hemorrhage; however, the hypotension is usually short lived, due to short plasma half-life of nitroglycerin (1 to 3 minutes) (137).

■ PHARMACOLOGIC MANAGEMENT OF HEMORRHAGE

Uterotonics

Uterotonic agents increase uterine tone and are also known as ecbolic agents. Three classes of drugs are in use and include oxytocin, ergot alkaloids, and prostaglandins.

Oxytocin

Oxytocin, administered intravenously, has an immediate onset of action on the uterine high-affinity oxytocin receptors (138), a mean plasma half-life of 3 minutes (24), a rapid offset of action, and requires a continuous intravenous infusion for a lasting effect on uterine contractility (24). Typically, after umbilical cord clamping at cesarean fetal delivery or after placental removal at vaginal delivery, the usual infusion of 20 to 40 units per liter of crystalloid is administered rapidly to clamp down the uterus, followed by slowing down of the infusion rate to maintain uterine contractility. Further titration of infusion rate is regulated based on the response, has fewer side effects when used alone, reduces the need for manual removal of placenta, and decreases the need for any other medication (139). Metabolism is rapid and is mediated through the liver, kidneys, and the enzyme oxytocinase resulting in a short half-life (24,12). Oxytocin is stable up to 25°C (24). However, refrigeration may prolong its shelf life.

Side effects include relaxation of vascular smooth muscle, resulting in vasodilation, hypotension, and a reflex tachycardia (24). A bolus injection of 3 to 5 units may cause chest pain in addition to other side effects mentioned above, but has been shown to not reduce the estimated blood loss compared to the infusion (140). In the triennial report, Why Mothers Die, 1997 to 1999, from the Confidential Enquiries into Maternal Deaths (CEMD) in the United Kingdom, published in 2001, it was recommended that the practice of administering bolus doses of 10 IU of oxytocin was responsible for two maternal deaths in cardiovascularly unstable patients (141). They also recommended that only 5 IU of oxytocin be administered slowly after cesarean delivery (141). The practice of bolus administration of oxytocin has lost favor due to its side effect profile and has now been replaced by oxytocin infusion, as described above. In addition, patients undergoing cesarean delivery for arrest of labor, after prolonged oxytocin augmentation, have been shown to require 3 IU rapid infusion of oxytocin to achieve effective uterine contraction after delivery (142), a dose that is 9 times more than the dose required after elective cesarean delivery in nonlaboring parturients (143). The authors concluded that oxytocin receptor desensitization, from exogenous oxytocin administration during labor, may be responsible for the higher dose requirements (142) and suggested the use of alternative uterotonic agents, rather than additional oxytocin, to achieve better uterine contraction

and control of hemorrhage during cesarean delivery for arrest of labor (142).

Methylergonovine

Methylergonovine, a semisynthetic ergot alkaloid, produces an instantaneous and lasting uterine smooth muscle contraction by stimulating the alpha-adrenergic receptors (138). The dose is 0.2 mg, onset of action is 2 to 4 minutes, and duration of action is 2 to 4 hours after the recommended intramuscular administration. Methylergonovine undergoes extensive hepatic metabolism and its plasma half-life is 30 minutes. The drug is heat and light sensitive and should be stored below 8°C and clear of light (24).

Side effects include nausea, vomiting, and severe alpha-mediated vasoconstriction, leading to elevation of central venous pressure, pulmonary arterial pressure, and arterial blood pressure. Severe side effects such as pulmonary edema (144), hypertensive crises (145), myocardial infarction (146,147), and stroke (148) have been reported and patients with pre-existing hypertension and preeclampsia are particularly at extreme risk. Vasodilator therapy may be needed to control the vasoconstrictive effects of methylergonovine in such patients (12). However, a large meta-analysis comparing oxytocin therapy along with the combination of oxytocin and ergometrine (parent compound of methylergonovine) found no significant difference in blood loss between the two groups when blood loss was greater than 1,000 mL (149). Intravenous administration exacerbates the side effects such as discussed above, makes the risk immediate and more severe, and should be avoided.

Carboprost

Carboprost (15-methyl prostaglandin F2 alpha) is a well-recognized secondary therapy, in intractable uterine atony, causing uterine smooth muscle contraction (138,150,151). It is approved for intramuscular or intramyometrial injection and the recommended dose is 0.25 mg. The intramyometrial route is preferable during hemorrhagic shock as intramuscular absorption may be limited (150). Repeat doses may be administered, every 15 to 20 minutes, up to a maximum of 8 doses (2 mg). In the awake patient, under regional anesthesia, it may be prudent to place the intramuscular injection in the thigh versus the deltoid, since the thigh is numb and has better absorption due to regional anesthesia-related vasodilation.

Side effects are due to an exaggerated response to smooth muscle contraction throughout the body, leading to broncho-constriction, venoconstriction, and gastrointestinal smooth muscle spasm (nausea, vomiting, and diarrhea). Hypotension, ventilation–perfusion mismatch, intrapulmonary shunting, and hypoxemia have also been reported (152,153). No significant difference in postpartum blood loss was observed between parturients receiving intramuscular carboprost compared to intramuscular methylergonovine (139).

Misoprostol

Misoprostol (15-deoxy-16-hydroxy-16-methyl PGE1), a synthetic analog of prostaglandin E1, helps ripen the cervix and increases uterine tone. The cervical softening has been attributed to a primary effect on the cervix directly and a secondary effect from the uterine contractions (154). The increase in uterine contractility occurs within 30 minutes by all routes and lasts up to 4 hours. However, for a sustained effect, repeated doses are necessary (155,156). Advantages of misoprostol include stability at room temperature, availability for oral administration, availability in developing countries, minimal side effects, and being inexpensive. Besides the oral route, it can be administered via the sublingual, buccal, vaginal, and rectal routes (154). Clinical indications in obstetrics include cervical softening before induction of labor (157), medical abortion, before surgical evacuation of uterus (158), and prophylaxis/therapy for PPH (154).

The major concern with misoprostol is the possible risk of uterine rupture in the third trimester in patients with a previous history of cesarean delivery, especially during induction of labor (159,160). The risk seems to increase as gestation progresses. Other side effects are uncommon and self-limiting, but include diarrhea, nausea, and vomiting (154). Other side effects reported are fever and chills, especially in the setting of PPH prevention or treatment (154).

Novel Pharmacologic Interventions and Coagulation Enhancing Drugs

Two different and novel classes of drugs have been advocated to enhance clotting function in the bleeding patient and are discussed below.

Recombinant Factor VIIa

The FDA labeling of rFVIIa restricts its use to patients with acquired or inherited factor VII, VIII, or IX deficiencies. All other uses of the drug are considered off-label. There is growing interest in using recombinant activated factor VII for treatment of PPH (161). Evidence for doing so is limited to anecdote and case reports. No randomized control trials have been performed with the use of rFVIIa in obstetrical hemorrhage. In a systematic review of case reports of hemorrhage associated with amniotic fluid embolism, Leighton et al. compared outcomes in 16 cases where rFVIIa was used against 28 cases where it was not. They concluded that the death and permanent disability were significantly greater in patients who had received rFVIIa and that rFVIIa should be used only in the most desperate of cases of amniotic fluid embolism (128).

Recently, Franchini and colleagues (162) summarized available case series, which in total, included 272 women suffering from PPH. With median doses of 81.5 μg/kg being administered, they reported on stopping or reducing bleeding in 85% of the patients. The problem with case series is that significant biasing results due to investigator tendency to report positive results more frequently than negative ones. Franchini also reported a 2.5% incidence of thromboembolic events. Thromboembolic events have been the source of extensive scrutiny with the off-label use of this drug. In a meta-analysis evaluating 36 placebo-controlled trials, Levi et al. (163) found a significant increase in arterial thromboembolic events with the use of rFVIIa. A similar meta-analysis on the treatment of bleeding in patients without hemophilia concluded that only modest benefit was gained through its use while sizeable thromboembolic risk existed. Because of this risk, the authors concluded that, until better evidence was available, rFVIIa should only be used in clinical trials (164). In addition to sizeable thromboembolic risk, caution is advised when thinking about use of this drug because of the very high cost ($4,500.00).

Antifibrinolytics

Lysine analogues, such as tranexamic acid (50 to 100 mg/kg) or epsilon aminocaproic acid (10 to 15 g), administered after the induction of anesthesia are indicated to enhance hemostasis when fibrinolysis contributes to bleeding. Both lysine analogues attenuate fibrinolysis by inhibiting lysis of plasminogen to plasmin and, to a lesser degree, by directly inhibiting plasmin activity. Scant data is available on the use of these drugs in the treatment of obstetrical hemorrhage. Two reviews have recently been published on the use of tranexamic acid given prophylactically (165,166). Both concluded that

minor reductions in blood loss occurred; however, they both commented that available studies are weak in design and that no study has evaluated thromboembolic complications.

■ OBSTETRICAL INVASIVE MANAGEMENT OF HEMORRHAGE

B-Lynch Technique

B-Lynch technique is used for uterine atony and involves application of a single, long, absorbable suture to vertically compress the body of the uterus on itself, thus obliterating the uterine cavity while compressing the blood vessels traversing from the cornual region of the uterus (17), and preventing the need for hysterectomy (167). Efficacy of this uterine brace suture can be predicted by application of bimanual uterine compression to stop bleeding; if hemorrhage stops, the B-Lynch suture should be effective (24). Moderate success has been reported with this technique (168) and follow-up has shown resumption of normal anatomy and physiology (169). A modified B-Lynch suture, consisting of two fundal sutures, tied laterally to apply greater tension and prevent slippage, has been reported and seems promising (170).

Uterine Balloon Tamponade

Uterine balloon tamponade has been used to treat PPH from uterine atony, has received widespread attention recently (171,172), and works by direct compression of uterine vasculature (173). The technique is easy and simple, hemostasis is achieved rapidly, and evaluation of its effect is quick and reliable (111). The "tamponade test" is used to assess the efficacy of balloon tamponading. In this test, the tamponade balloon is placed in the uterus transcervically via the vagina. The balloon is inflated until it becomes visible at the cervical canal. In order to maintain uterine contraction over the balloon, an oxytocin infusion is administered continuously during the test. The balloon is left inflated with constant monitoring for bleeding around the balloon or through the lumen of the attached catheter. In addition, hemoglobin levels, platelet count, and coagulation profile are checked periodically. If the patient continues to show evidence of on-going hemorrhage, then the patient is declared to have failed the "tamponade test" and requires definitive therapy such as hysterectomy. In most reports of successful tamponade, the balloon is left in situ for 12 to 24 hours, at which time, it is deflated gradually over an hour or so under constant monitoring for bleeding.

Devascularization of the Uterus

Uterine devascularization techniques have been used prophylactically, in parturients with placenta accreta diagnosed during cesarean delivery in the operating room, as preparation before proceeding with hysterectomy (24). They have also been used therapeutically for managing PPH from uterine atony, placenta previa, placental abruption, and trauma (24).

Ligation of Uterine Arteries

Uterine arteries supply the bulk (90%) of the uterus during pregnancy and ligation of bilateral uterine arteries is an easy, secure, and successful substitute for hysterectomy (174). A large case series, over 30 years, reported a 96% success rate in 265 patients with postcesarean delivery hemorrhage, using conventional uterine artery ligation, while preserving fertility and menstrual cycles (175). Conventional uterine artery ligation is performed, with an absorbable suture placed laterally, through an avascular window in the broad ligament bilaterally. However, in patients with placenta previa, with or without accreta, a step-wise devascularization technique has been described allowing uterine preservation for further pregnancies (176). Since the lower uterine segment may not contract effectively, in placenta previa, an additional lower suture is placed, 3 to 5 cm below the original suture, to cut off the ascending branches of the cervicovaginal artery and the uterine artery branches supplying the lower uterine segment and the upper part of cervix; 100% success with hemorrhage control was reported (176).

Ligation of Ovarian Arteries
In addition, bilateral ovarian artery ligation is performed, medial to the ovary to preserve ovarian blood supply, and cut off the remaining 10% blood supply to the uterus as part of the step-wise devascularization technique (176).

Hypogastric Artery Balloon Catheters

Even though some have proposed preoperative placement of hypogastric artery balloon catheters in the interventional radiology suite and intraoperative inflation following cesarean delivery in parturients with placenta accreta (177), others have questioned its clinical use due to opening up of deeper pelvic collaterals, making hemorrhage control more difficult (178). Other potential drawbacks include possibility of infection at insertion site, hematoma formation, abscess formation, and lower limb ischemia (111). A case control study found no differences in blood loss, duration of surgery, duration of hospital stay, or amount of blood and blood product usage in parturients undergoing cesarean hysterectomy for placenta accreta with or without prophylactic intravascular balloon catheters (113). However, theoretical advantages include ability to deflate the catheters following surgery if hemorrhage is well controlled, ability to leave the catheters in situ for 24 hours or more, and ability to reinflate them if necessary (24).

Radiologic Embolization of Uterine and Ovarian Arteries

Uterine arterial embolization is gaining acceptance in hospitals with proficiency in interventional radiology. Temporary blockage of uterine arteries, for up to 10 days, is achieved selectively using absorbable gelatin sponge (179). Success rates are shown to be higher for uterine atony and pelvic trauma (180) and lower for placenta accreta (181). Advantages include direct visualization of arterial bleeders, ability to occlude distal arterial bleeders, ability to assess efficacy of the procedure simultaneously, and ability to repeat the procedure, if required (179). Disadvantages include prolonged length of procedure, availability of interventional radiology personnel and suite at short notice, and the necessity of transferring a hemorrhaging patient to a remote location from the operating room or intensive care unit (24).

Cesarean or Postpartum Hysterectomy

Definitive therapy for obstetrical hemorrhage is hysterectomy. The commonest indication for cesarean hysterectomy is uterine atony. While the decision to perform a hysterectomy can be difficult, especially in primiparous women, delay in performing a hysterectomy may be fatal. The management of hysterectomy has been described under earlier sections on placental abruption, placenta previa, uterine rupture, uterine atony, and placenta accreta.

■ POINT-OF-CARE TESTING

Point-of-care or near care laboratory testing places laboratory analysis devices near or at the patient bedside. By doing so, patient management decisions are enhanced by having data in real time, rather than sending a blood sample to a central laboratory where results can take 30 to 45 minutes to be reported. Point-of-care devices can measure a wide variety of parameters including arterial blood gas endpoint, hemoglobin, PT/PTT, and coagulation function via whole blood viscosity parameters (TEG and ROTEM). Within the realm of cardiac surgery, several studies have demonstrated 70% reductions in transfusion; fewer operating room take-backs; and, less postoperative chest tube drainage when point-of-care testing and an algorithm driven transfusion strategy is applied (182,183). Similar point-of-care, bedside assessment of coagulation function has been advocated during obstetrical hemorrhage (184,185). Point-of-care testing allows microliter samples to be used to obtain hemoglobin, prothrombin time, PTT, INR, and to assess platelet number and function.

The value of point-of-care testing extends beyond giving laboratory data at the bedside. The use of point-of-care devices can reduce blood loss through microsampling. Microsampling is a key component to point-of-care testing in that it involves microliter blood samples rather than 10 to 20 mL samples as is normally drawn for routine laboratory blood work. Iatrogenic blood loss from phlebotomy due to frequent sampling can lead to sizeable blood loss (186).

■ HEMORRHAGE AND BLOOD TRANSFUSION

Hemorrhage frequently results in packed red cell and blood product transfusion. Transfusion therapy has a list of morbidities which may be of greater significance for the young woman when compared to the vast majority of patients that receive transfusions who are elderly and, on average, are within 2 years of death. One of the consequences of transfusion which may be of greater consequence in the young is that of transfusion-associated microchimerism (187). Transfusion-associated microchimerism is the transfer of components of cellular immunity from donor to recipient. Some investigators have suggested that a patient who receives a transfusion at a young age develop blood-borne cancers (188) and autoimmune disease (187) at rates which are higher than a nontransfused patient.

More recognized complications of transfusion and, foremost on most people's minds when they think about allogeneic transfusion, is the risk of infectious complications. Modern blood banking and screening has markedly reduced the risk of disease transmission to a level where the risk is extremely small. The infectious viral risk per unit of blood transfusion in the United States is estimated at 1 in 2.993 million for HTLV, 1 in 1.467 million for HIV, 1 in 1.149 million for HCV, 1 in 1 million for HAV, and 1 in 280,000 for HBV (189). Bacterial contamination, most prominently in units of platelets, is the most common infectious risk of transfusion (190). Recently, TRALI has been recognized to be the leading cause of morbidity and mortality following allogeneic transfusion (191). TRALI occurs within 1 to 2 hours following transfusion and results in severe hypoxemia, bilateral pulmonary edema, hypotension and fever, and is indistinguishable from ARDS. The incidence of TRALI appears to have dramatically decreased due to elimination of multiparous females from donating plasma (192). Several experts have suggested that TACO is now of greater significance.

The risk of transfusion-related immunosuppression (TRIM) following allogeneic blood transfusion is less often mentioned, but is of greater importance to short and long-term patient outcome than are the risks of viral transmission (193). An increased incidence of postoperative infection and cancer recurrence is thought to occur from TRIM, following allogeneic transfusion. Studies evaluating postoperative infection following allogeneic transfusions have demonstrated as much as a 10-fold greater rate of infection in patients receiving allogeneic blood (194–196). In obstetrics, postcesarean infection rates range from 5% to 25% (197,198). Thus, increases in infection rate due to TRIM offers a profound effect on patient morbidity.

In addition to being associated with the risks of TRALI, TACO, TRIM, and viral exposure, blood is altered by storage. The most significant of these storage-related decline is the decreased levels of 2, 3-diphosphoglycerate (2, 3 DPG) in red blood cells (RBCs). Decreased levels of 2, 3-DPG shift the oxyhemoglobin dissociation curve to the left, making it more difficult for oxygen to bind with hemoglobin as its carrier. Restoration of normal levels of 2, 3-DPG can take up to a day to occur following reinfusion of stored blood which means that the oxygen delivery of transfused blood is not initially comparable to in vivo blood. In recent studies, there has been a suggestion that the reduction in 2, 3-DPG along with an associated red cell shape change may lead to a worsening of tissue oxygen levels and worsened outcome (199).

■ TRANSFUSION TRIGGERS IN THE PERIPARTUM PERIOD

Debate regarding the appropriate trigger for transfusion is on-going for all patients. The debate has focused on appropriate transfusion of RBCs but is evolving to include plasma and platelet transfusion.

Red Cell Transfusion

No data exist that specifically addresses transfusion of red cells in the peripartum patient. Inferences can be drawn from studies done in other patient populations and probably be used as an appropriate transfusion guideline. The most recent ASA guidelines (38), published in 2006, state that "red blood cells should usually be administered when the hemoglobin level is less than 6 g/dL and...that red blood cells are usually unnecessary when the level is more than 10 g/dL". This recommendation is based on little evidence other than ASA member and expert opinion. The only prospective, randomized control trial currently in the literature is the Transfusion Requirements in Critical Care (TRICC) trial (39) which suggests that a reasonable guideline for transfusion of RBCs in a critically ill patient is a hemoglobin of 7 g/dL or less. It is important to recognize that this number is a guideline and should be used in conjunction with the patient's clinical condition. Indications for transfusion can be varied. Transfusion should not take place based solely on a number in an asymptomatic patient, regardless of the hemoglobin level. Transfusion of blood products should be considered in light of the complications which were previously discussed. The young peripartum women being transfused incur risks of complications which can take place decades after the transfusion. Some of this risk relates to prior disease as well as an immunomodulatory effect of getting an allogeneic transfusion.

In a patient who has suffered a peripartum hemorrhage and falls within close approximation of a transfusion guideline, it is important to remember that in the days following delivery, hemoconcentration occurs through decreases in plasma volume. The hemoconcentration results in quick amelioration of the postpartum anemia without necessitating transfusion. In the borderline case, thought should also be given to iron therapy.

Plasma

Once again, plasma transfusion trigger is poorly defined in the obstetric population. A rational approach would be to transfuse plasma when INR levels increase beyond 1.6 in association with clinical evidence of bleeding (200,201). For the nonpregnant patient, INR levels greater than 1.6 are associated with coagulation factor concentrations of less than 30%. Whether this is true for pregnancy has not been elucidated. Plasma transfusion carries the greatest risk of TRALI, so serious thought needs to be given prior to administration in a young, healthy peripartum female. Plasma transfusion should never be considered for reversal of coumadin except when active bleeding is occurring.

Platelets

While guidelines for transfusion of platelets in hematologic malignancy and bone marrow transplantation are well established, guidelines for the peripartum and surgical patient are based on consensus, rather than evidence-based outcome data. The guideline proposed by the ASA calls for platelet transfusion when evidence of bleeding is accompanied by platelet count less than 50,000/μL.

Cryoprecipitate

Cryoprecipitate, the thawed by-product of plasma, is a rich source of fibrinogen, factor VIII, von Willebrand factor, factor XIII, and fibronectin. Cryoprecipitate is indicated for hypofibrinogenemia during obstetric hemorrhage, is available for intravenous use in a plasma suspension of 10 to 15 mL, and is transfused in a 4 to 6 unit prepooled concentrate. Each unit of cryoprecipitate raises the serum fibrinogen level by 6 to 7 mg/dL (17,37).

Prothrombin Complex Concentrates

Prothrombin complex concentrates (PCC), a rich source of factors II, VII, IX, and X, are used in Europe for rapidly reversing vitamin K antagonism and congenital factor deficiencies. PCC has been suggested as an experimental strategy for treating dilutional coagulopathy following massive blood transfusion (202,203), but has not gained universal acceptance due to lack of scientific clinical evidence.

Blood Conservation Therapy and Blood Management

"Patient blood management" involves the appropriate provision and use of blood, its components and derivatives, and strategies to reduce and avoid the need for a blood transfusion. Ideally, blood conservation therapy is approached as a multimodal technique (204). Multimodal strategies that can be applied to conserve the need for a transfusion in the antepartum period include optimization of the hematocrit, predelivery autologous blood donation, and acute normovolemic hemodilution (ANH) while the modality of choice in the postpartum period is blood salvage.

Iron and Erythropoietin

Iron and erythropoietin are widely advocated in blood management. In pregnancy, erythropoietin levels normally increase by over 2-fold which is one of the drivers of the increased red cell mass associated with pregnancy (205). Thus, exogenous sources of erythropoietin are typically unnecessary. If pregnancy is complicated by chronic renal insufficiency, normal increases in erythropoietin will be inhibited necessitating erythropoietin (206).

During pregnancy, iron deficiency anemia arises because fetal growth coupled with expansion of maternal blood volume exhausts available maternal iron stores. Iron deficiency is the most common cause of anemia in pregnancy (207). Even in the industrial world, anemia in pregnancy affects 18% of the population (208). As such, it is routinely recommended that a pregnant woman take iron supplements. The most common oral preparation is a ferrous salt (ferrous sulfate) which is inexpensive and available without a prescription.

Adverse gastrointestinal effects are a substantial challenge to effective therapy with oral iron agents. When administered a ferrous iron agent daily for up to 12 weeks, up to 76% of women experience abdominal pain, dyspepsia, or constipation (209). In 33% of women given oral iron, GI symptoms are sufficiently severe to interfere with taking medication as prescribed. Not surprisingly, nonadherence to oral iron administration among women is high.

Intravenous iron therapy is an alternative to oral iron; however, it has not been widely used in the treatment of iron deficiency in pregnancy because of cost and a fear of anaphylaxis. Current IV iron agents include iron dextran and the nondextran containing agents, iron sucrose and sodium ferric gluconate complex (SFGC). Iron dextran administration risks sudden and sometimes fatal anaphylaxis (210) even if a test dose has been given successfully, so nondextran containing agents should be used preferentially. With this complication, it seems reasonable to avoid iron dextran in pregnancy. Nondextran containing IV iron agents must be administered in multiple small doses to avert hypotension, cramping, and chest pain (211). Due to these constraints, IV iron agents should be reserved for patients who may have significant risk of peripartum hemorrhage, patients with rare antibodies, or patients who do not accept blood.

Predelivery Autologous Blood Donation
Predelivery autologous blood donation, which is more commonly called preoperative autologous donation (PAD), is the practice of the patient donating their own blood prior to an expected surgical procedure. This practice was propagated in the 1980s as a way of minimizing the risk associated with contracting HIV from an allogeneic blood product. Since then, the risk of HIV transmission via blood has been virtually eliminated. As such, the risk of allogeneic blood is similar to that of PAD blood; however, PAD blood is wasted in 50% to 60% of the procedures making it cost prohibitive (212). In four studies in pregnant patients with placenta previa or other high risk factors, 40 of 297 (13%) of the patients received their blood back (213–216) making the cost even more prohibitive than it is in the general nonpregnant population (217). In addition, timing of the donation can be problematic in that delivery dates are frequently unpredictable. With blood storage times being limited, this can restrict the effectiveness of the strategy. In addition, most blood donor centers will not allow donation when hemoglobin values are less than 11 g/dL. Since this level is close to normal levels of hemoglobin in pregnancy, many women become ineligible for this strategy. Lastly, the rate for vasovagal attacks in pregnant women is higher than it is for nonpregnant women, making it potentially unsafe.

Acute Normovolemic Hemodilution
ANH was originally used in cardiac surgery as a blood conservation technique in 1957 (218) and became popular in orthopedics (219) and urology (220) later. ANH use in obstetrical patients has been limited due to the concern of worsening the physiologic anemia of pregnancy and producing peripartum fluid shifts (17). The first report of ANH use in obstetrics was from Baylor College of Medicine (Ashutosh Wali) in 1997 (221).

The ANH technique involves preoperative and preanesthetic withdrawal of a fixed volume of whole blood, under continuous monitoring of arterial blood pressure and central venous pressure, in the operating room (17). In addition, for the obstetric patient, continuous fetal heart rate monitoring should be employed (17). Whole blood is withdrawn into blood bags containing citrate phosphate dextrose adenine (CPDA), an anticoagulant, over 15 to 20 minutes while simultaneously infusing an appropriate volume of crystalloid or nonheme colloid to maintain normovolemia (221). Based on Gross' formula (222), the allowable amount of blood to be withdrawn is precalculated as follows (17):

$$V = EBV \times \frac{H_i - H_f}{H_{av}}$$

where,

V is the volume of blood to be removed
EBV is the estimated blood volume of the patient (average, 85 mL/kg in pregnant adults; range 76 to 94 mL/kg) (223)
H_i is the initial hematocrit at time of whole blood withdrawal
H_f is the final or target hematocrit
H_{av} is the average hematocrit (average of H_i and H_f)
In an 80-kg parturient, the EBV = 6,800 mL. If the H_i = 35% and H_f = 25%, the H_{av} = 30% and the allowable amount of whole blood to be removed would be

$$6800 \times \frac{0.35 - 0.25}{0.30} = 2267 \text{ mL}$$

The whole blood that is removed in the beginning has the richest concentration of erythrocytes, coagulation factors, and platelets and accordingly, the whole blood that is withdrawn last has the lowest concentration (17). At the end of surgery, collected whole blood is transfused back to the patient in the reverse order so that the bag containing the highest concentration of erythrocytes, coagulation factors, and platelets is administered at the end (17).

Common indications for ANH (17) include Jehovah's witnesses that accept closed circuit ANH (221), patients with rare antibodies in blood, patients with unusual blood types, patients with a hematocrit greater than 35% with an expected blood loss of more than 2 L, and in institutions with poor blood banking resources. Common contraindications to ANH (17) include anemia, cardiac compromise, coagulation disturbance, and renal insufficiency.

Common benefits of ANH use include lessening allogeneic blood transfusion requirement; enhancing oxygen delivery and tissue perfusion; permitting dispensation of fresh whole blood with near normal concentration of erythrocytes, coagulation factors, platelets, ATP, p50, and 2,3-DPG; avoiding blood transfusion-related reactions; preventing blood-borne disease transmission; precluding blood compatibility issues; and averting clerical errors (17,204).

The process of ANH involves the removal of a patient's whole blood, preferably in the operating room under strict monitoring, prior to the start of a surgical procedure while simultaneously maintaining normovolemia with crystalloid or colloid as appropriate. The idea is that the shed blood, during the procedure, is less concentrated with packed erythrocytes, clotting factors, and platelets. The sequestered blood is then returned to the patient at the end of the procedure at which point, a transfusion is potentially avoided. An example is helpful in illustrating this technique. If a patient were to lose 1,000 mL of blood during a cesarean delivery and their hematocrit was 35%, then they will have lost 350 mL of RBCs. If the patient were hemodiluted to a hematocrit of 25% and the same 1,000 mL of RBCs is lost, then 250 mL of RBCs are lost. As a result, the sequestered blood has saved 100 mL of RBCs from being lost. An additional benefit to performing this technique is that plasma and platelets are sequestered.

Safety data regarding this technique in pregnancy is limited. In one study in 38 women with placental abnormalities, a limited amount of blood was sequestered (<1,000 mL) (224). No impact was seen on the fetus, in utero, and all umbilical cord gases were within normal range and APGAR scores were acceptable. This study had no control group in order to compare outcomes.

Blood Salvage

Blood salvage is a unique strategy of using intraoperative or postoperative blood collection and readministration in women suffering from PPH. The collection, processing, and reinfusion of shed blood have been termed "blood salvage." Many practitioners refer to the technique and the device as "cell saving" and "cell saver"; however, the term "cell saver" is the brand name of a device manufactured by Haemonetics, Inc. (Braintree, MA). A more generic term for the technology is simply "blood salvage" (Fig. 21-4). Blood salvage can take place intraoperatively or postoperatively. Typically, intraoperative salvage involves the collection, concentration, washing, and readministration of the blood, whereas, postoperative salvage is performed with a wound drain, which most commonly, is not washed when reinfused.

Classically, intraoperative blood salvage during obstetrical hemorrhage has been considered contraindicated. This contraindication primarily relates to the FDA labeling for the device. The original reason for the labeling contraindication was due to a fear of entraining amniotic fluid from the surgical field, readministering the salvaged blood with this amniotic fluid, and causing an iatrogenic amniotic fluid embolus. However, no clinical evidence is available which supports this fear. In fact, the use of blood recovery in obstetric hemorrhage now encompasses close to 400 reported cases in which blood contaminated with amniotic fluid has been washed and readministered without clinical harm. Due to the lack of evidence to support an obstetrical contraindication, the ACOG (225), the Obstetric Anesthetists Association of Great Britain (226), and the British CEMACH (6) have advocated the use of blood salvage in obstetrics. In fact, the National Institute for Health and Clinical Excellence (NICE) in England, Wales, Scotland, and Northern Ireland has issued a guidance document on intraoperative blood cell salvage in obstetrics, which states that adequate safety evidence is available to support its use (227). Because of the endorsement of blood salvage in obstetrics from these major organizations, it was reported that 38% of United Kingdom obstetrical units used blood salvage (228).

Intraoperative blood salvage has been associated with a number of adverse events including air embolism, renal failure, and the cell salvage syndrome. All are preventable which

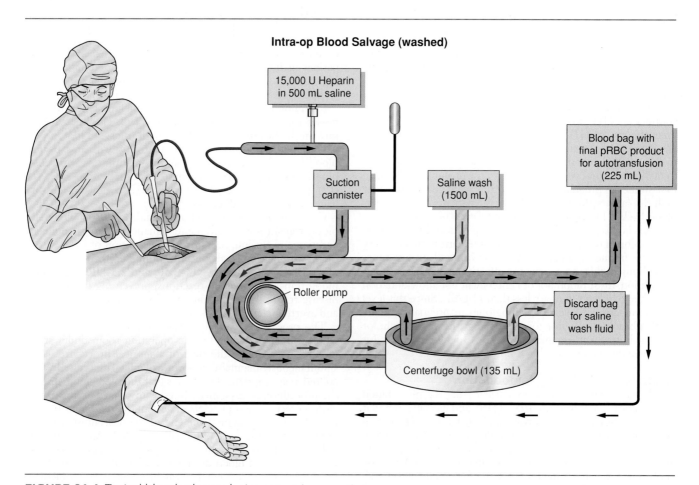

Intra-op Blood Salvage (washed)

15,000 U Heparin in 500 mL saline

Suction cannister

Saline wash (1500 mL)

Blood bag with final pRBC product for autotransfusion (225 mL)

Roller pump

Discard bag for saline wash fluid

Centerfuge bowl (135 mL)

FIGURE 21-4 Typical blood salvage device set-up in operation.

emphasizes the need for knowledge and understanding in the technology's application. The AABB (formerly known as the American Association of Blood Banks), Standards for Perioperative Autologous Blood Collection and Administration (229), and the associated Guidelines for Blood Recovery and Reinfusion in Surgery and Trauma (230) outline quality systems that should accompany the safe use of this technology. If the practitioner is considering implementing a blood salvage program, it is strongly recommended that these documents be studied.

In the obstetrical patient, amniotic fluid is known to contain lanugo, hair, vernix caseosa, meconium, fetal cellular debris, and tissue factor. Blood salvage combined with leukocyte reduction filtration (Pall RS leukocyte depletion filter, Pall Corporation, Port Washington, NY) has been shown to remove fetal squamous cells, bacterial contamination, and lamellar bodies to a level similar to circulating levels of these materials in the mother (231). By way of simple washing, laboratory studies have demonstrated the complete removal of biologic markers of amniotic fluid (alpha-fetal protein and tissue factor) from washed recovered red cells (232). While the cause of amniotic fluid embolism is unknown, the use of these filters may garner additional safety during blood salvage application.

In the obstetrical patient undergoing cesarean delivery, it is important to recognize that much of the lost blood is contained within laparotomy sponges. By rinsing the sponges in a wash basin filled with normal saline prior to discard, approximately 75% of the red cells can be recovered. The rinse solution can then be suctioned into the blood salvage reservoir for later processing. Since a fully soaked laparotomy sponge can contain as much as 100 mL of blood, rinsing of sponges can serve as a rich source of salvaged blood. Lastly, suction should be downregulated in order to minimize mechanical shear stress on the red cells. Typical wall suction is −300 mm Hg. Downregulation to −80 to −120 will decrease the mechanical shear and lead to sizeable increases in red cell return (233).

Hemorrhage Protocols

The incidence of major PPH is increasing worldwide (234–236). Associated with this increased hemorrhage rate is an increase in the rate of maternal death (237). The California Maternal Quality Care Collaborative (CMQCC) has identified several common errors which occur that can lead to hemorrhagic death (238). Underestimation of blood loss, delay in administration of blood, lack of working equipment, delay in response from obstetrical team members and a lack of an organized standardized team approach are several of the errors that the CMQCC has identified.

In order to address the first of these errors, that is, underestimation of blood loss, several groups have recommended training in visually identifying blood loss (239,240). This generally takes the form of pictures with specified amounts of blood on sheets, towels, laparotomy sponges, surgeon's gowns, and the delivery room floor. By doing so, it is hoped that labor and delivery staff will more readily identify patients that are suffering from blood loss greater than the routine.

Delay in response of obstetrical team members has led to the development of rapid response teams with specific expertise in peripartum emergencies (241). At the Magee Womens Hospital in Pittsburgh (Jonathan H. Waters), a "Condition O" was created to bring additional manpower resources to a patient's bedside anytime that a health care provider feels that a life-threatening event might be occurring (242). Intuitively, it makes sense to have the same level if not greater level of rapid response for a peripartum mother undergoing a life-threatening event as we do when we have a cardiac arrest in a 90-year old. This Condition O is a rapid response team that emergently mobilizes an obstetrician, a senior obstetrical resident, an intensivist, several nurses, a respiratory therapist, and an anesthesiologist to the patient's bedside.

Crew resource management is another tool that has been used to address poor communication between providers. Health care providers are trained in isolated silos with contrasting perspectives and differing priorities. Crew resource management training, which is a tool utilized in the airline industry, has been advocated to address these silos. Pettker et al. demonstrated a 2.5- to 4-fold increase in their unit's perception of a good teamwork climate through the use of crew resource management (243). In conjunction, they saw a statistically significant reduction in adverse outcomes as measured by the Adverse Outcomes Index (AOI).

Massive Transfusion Protocols

Over the last 3 years, multiple reports have arisen out of the Iraq and Afghanistan conflicts regarding the appropriate ratios of blood products (RBC:plasma:platelets) (244–246). Within these reports is a consensus that the ratio in massive hemorrhage, defined as transfusion of greater than 10 units of PRBCs, should be in 1:1:1 ratio. None of the data that advocates aggressive plasma and platelet use has been generated in an obstetrical population.

While there is sizeable retrospective, observational data in the trauma patients to advocate this strategy, it is important to recognize that this data suffers from significant survivor bias, which would suggest caution before following the recommendations. In addition, the data referenced is predominantly military injury, which is significantly different from the obstetrical population.

Survivor bias is illustrated in the referenced articles in that the patients who survived ultimately received more blood products than those who died. Over the course of the survivor's care, they received total blood products that tallied up to equal the 1:1:1 ratio, which is the supporting evidence for this recommendation. Those patients who died from injuries may very well have received the same blood products, but they did not survive long enough to receive the products, especially plasma. When survivor bias is corrected for, Snyder et al. found that the aggressive plasma transfusion led to no added benefit in outcome (247). Sperry et al. concluded that patients who received high plasma ratios had a 2-fold increase in postoperative adult respiratory distress syndrome (248). Further, Johnson et al. found that trauma patients treated with aggressive plasma use were more likely to suffer from multiorgan failure (249). Thus, caution should be used before translating this trauma data to the obstetrical patient.

Another problem with transfusion based on a 1:1:1 recommendation is that it is advocating a cookbook approach to the transfusion of patients that will result in an unnecessary volume of blood products transfused in some. Recent evidence suggests that a *goal-directed strategy by using point-of-care testing would provide an equal level of care but avoid unnecessary transfusion* (250). Several prospective trials in the cardiac surgery population have demonstrated an improvement in outcome when point-of-care testing is implemented (183,251). While allogeneic transfusion may be lifesaving, like all therapies, it comes with risks. Blind acceptance of the 1:1:1 ratio in the hemorrhaging obstetric patient, without convincing evidence, completely ignores the risks of allogeneic blood transfusion.

KEY POINTS

- Obstetrical hemorrhage incidence is rising worldwide and continues to be a leading source of maternal morbidity and mortality.
- Underestimation of peripartum blood loss is a key error, masked by the physiologic increase in blood volume and cardiac output during pregnancy, and may contribute to hemorrhagic death in obstetrics.
- Placental abruption is a prominent cause of fetal growth restriction, preterm delivery, and a high perinatal mortality rate.
- Hypofibrinogenemia is not an uncommon consumptive coagulopathy following placental abruption and responds well to cryoprecipitate transfusion.
- Uterine atony is the most common cause of obstetrical hemorrhage, usually responds well to multidrug therapy, and warrants a trial of uterine compression sutures and intrauterine balloon catheter inflation, before proceeding with peripartum hysterectomy for refractory uterine atony.
- Placenta accreta incidence is rising due to an increasing cesarean delivery rate, and has the potential for life-threatening PPH and the need for postpartum hysterectomy.
- Point-of-care testing should be used to help guide transfusion of blood products.
- An understanding of the risks of transfusion needs to be weighed against the benefits when considering a transfusion in a young woman.
- Intraoperative blood salvage can be safely used in obstetrical hemorrhage.
- The use of TEG, internal iliac balloon catheter inflation, rFVIIa, and massive transfusion protocol has been suggested as efficacious and safe in multiple case reports of peripartum hemorrhage, but has not been validated in clinical trials in obstetrics.

REFERENCES

1. American College of Obstetricians and Gynecologists. ACOG practice bulletin: Clinical management guidelines for obstetrician-gynecologists number 76, October 2006: Postpartum hemorrhage. *Obstet Gynecol* 2006;108(4): 1039–1047.
2. Oyelese Y, Scorza WE, Mastrolia R, et al. Postpartum hemorrhage. *Obstet Gynecol Clin North Am* 2007;34(3):421–441, x.
3. Berg CJ, Atrash HK, Koonin LM, et al. Pregnancy-related mortality in the united states, 1987–1990. *Obstet Gynecol* 1996;88(2):161–167.
4. Berg CJ, Chang J, Callaghan WM, et al. Pregnancy-related mortality in the United States, 1991–1997. *Obstet Gynecol* 2003;101(2):289–296.
5. ACOG educational bulletin. Postpartum hemorrhage. Number 243, January 1998 (replaces no. 143, July 1990). American college of obstetricians and gynecologists. *Int J Gynaecol Obstet* 1998;61(1):79–86.
6. Hall M. Why mothers die 2000–2002—the sixth report on confidential enquiries into maternal deaths in the United Kingdom. *Haemorrhage.* UK: RCOG Press at the Royal College of Obstetricians and Gynaecologists; 2004:91.
7. Liston W. The seventh report of the confidential enquiries into maternal deaths in the United Kingdom. In: Lewis G, ed. *The Confidential Enquiry into Maternal and Child Health (CEMACH): Saving Mothers' Lives: Reviewing Maternal Deaths to Make Motherhood Safer—2003–2005.*2007:78–85.
8. Norman J. Haemorrhage. *Saving Mothers' Lives: Reviewing maternal deaths to make motherhood safer: 2006–2008 The Eighth Report of the Confidential Enquiries into Maternal Deaths in the United Kingdom. Centre for Maternal and Child Enquiries (CMACE).* 8th ed. New York: Wiley-Blackwell, 2011:71.
9. Gaiser R. Physiologic changes of pregnancy, Chapter 2. *Chestnut* 4th ed. 2009.
10. Scott DE. Anemia in pregnancy. *Obstet Gynecol Annu* 1972;1:219–244.
11. Conklin KA. Maternal physiological adaptations during gestation, labor, and the puerperium. *Semin Anesth* 1991;10:221–234.
12. Mayer DC, Smith K. Antepartum and postartum hemorrhage. *Chestnut's Obstetric Anesthesia Principles and Practice.* 4th ed. Philadelphia, PA: Mosby Elsevier; 2009:811.

13. Francois K, Foley MR. Antepartum and postpartum hemorrhage. In: Gabbe SG, Niebyl JR, Simpson JL, et al., eds. *Obstetrics: Normal and Problem Pregnancies.* 6th ed. Philadelphia, PA: Elsevier Saunders, 2007:457.
14. Everett C. Incidence and outcome of bleeding before the 20th week of pregnancy: Prospective study from general practice. *BMJ* 1997;315(7099):32–34.
15. Camann W, Biehl D. Antepartum and postartum hemorrhage. In: Hughes SC, ed. *Shnider and Levinson's Anesthesia for Obstetrics.* Philadelphia, PA: Lippincott Williams & Wilkins; 2002:361.
16. Wilson R. Bleeding during late pregnancy. In: Wilson R, Carrinton E, Ledger W, eds. *Obstetrics and Gynecology.* 7th ed. St. Louis: CV Mosby; 1983:356.
17. Wali A, Suresh MS, Gregg A. Antepartum hemorrhage. *Anesthetic and Obstetric Management of High-Risk Pregnancy.* 3rd ed. New York, NY: Springer; 2004:87.
18. Ananth CV, Berkowitz GS, Savitz DA, et al. Placental abruption and adverse perinatal outcomes. *JAMA* 1999;282(17):1646–1651.
19. Oyelese Y, Ananth CV. Placental abruption. *Obstet Gynecol* 2006;108(4): 1005–1016.
20. Hiippala S. Replacement of massive blood loss. *Vox Sang* 1998;74(Suppl 2):399–407.
21. Getahun D, Ananth CV, Peltier MR, et al. Acute and chronic respiratory diseases in pregnancy: Associations with placental abruption. *Am J Obstet Gynecol* 2006;195(4):1180–1184.
22. Lowe TW, Cunningham FG. Placental abruption. *Clin Obstet Gynecol* 1990;33(3):406–413.
23. Ananth CV, Smulian JC, Demissie K, et al. Placental abruption among singleton and twin births in the United States: Risk factor profiles. *Am J Epidemiol* 2001;153(8):771–778.
24. Stafford I, Belfort M, Dildy GA 3rd. Etiology and management of hemorrhage. In: Belfort M, Saade G, Foley M, Phelan J, Dildy GA 3rd, eds. *Critical Care Obstetrics.* 5th ed. UK: Wiley-Blackwell (A John Wiley & Sons, Ltd.,Publication); 2010:308.
25. Paterson ME. The aetiology and outcome of abruptio placentae. *Acta Obstet Gynecol Scand* 1979;58(1):31–35.
26. Baron F, Hill WC. Placenta previa, placenta abruptio. *Clin Obstet Gynecol* 1998;41(3):527–532.
27. Glantz C, Purnell L. Clinical utility of sonography in the diagnosis and treatment of placental abruption. *J Ultrasound Med* 2002;21(8):837–840.
28. Nyberg DA, Cyr DR, Mack LA, et al. Sonographic spectrum of placental abruption. *AJR Am J Roentgenol* 1987;148(1):161–164.
29. Spirt BA, Kagan EH, Rozanski RM. Abruptio placenta: Sonographic and pathologic correlation. *AJR Am J Roentgenol* 1979;133(5):877–881.
30. Jaffe MH, Schoen WC, Silver TM, et al. Sonography of abruptio placentae. *AJR Am J Roentgenol* 1981;137(5):1049–1054.
31. Douglas RG, Buchman MI, Macdonald FA. Premature separation of the normally implanted placenta. *J Obstet Gynaecol Br Emp* 1955;62(5):710–722; discussion, 722–736.
32. Basu HK. Fibrinolysis and abruptio placentae. *J Obstet Gynaecol Br Commonw* 1969;76(6):481–496.
33. Sher G. Pathogenesis and management of uterine inertia complicating abruptio placentae with consumption coagulopathy. *Am J Obstet Gynecol* 1977; 129(2):164–170.
34. Hibbard BM, Jeffcoate TN. Abruptio placentae. *Obstet Gynecol* 1966;27(2): 155–167.
35. Kayani SI, Walkinshaw SA, Preston C. Pregnancy outcome in severe placental abruption. *BJOG* 2003;110(7):679–683.
36. Williams Obstetrics. Obstetrical hemorrhage. In: Cunningham FG, Leveno KJ, Bloom SL, Hauth JC, Rouse DJ, Spong CY, eds. *Williams Obstetrics.* 23rd ed. USA: The McGraw-Hill Companies, Inc.; 2010:757.
37. Santoso JT, Saunders BA, Grosshart K. Massive blood loss and transfusion in obstetrics and gynecology. *Obstet Gynecol Surv* 2005;60(12):827–837.
38. American Society of Anesthesiologists Task Force on Perioperative Blood Transfusion and Adjuvant Therapies. Practice guidelines for perioperative blood transfusion and adjuvant therapies: An updated report by the American society of anesthesiologists task force on perioperative blood transfusion and adjuvant therapies. *Anesthesiology* 2006;105(1):198–208.
39. Hebert PC, Wells G, Blajchman MA, et al. A multicenter, randomized, controlled clinical trial of transfusion requirements in critical care. Transfusion requirements in critical care investigators, Canadian critical care trials group. *N Engl J Med* 1999;340(6):409–417.
40. Vincent RD Jr, Chestnut DH, Sipes SL, et al. Epidural anesthesia worsens uterine blood flow and fetal oxygenation during hemorrhage in gravid ewes. *Anesthesiology* 1992;76(5):799–806.
41. Oats JN, Vasey DP, Waldron BA. Effects of ketamine on the pregnant uterus. *Br J Anaesth* 1979;51(12):1163–1166.
42. Suresh M. Comparison of etomidate with thiopental for induction of anesthesia at cesarean section. *Anesthesiology* 1986;65(3A):A400.
43. Ananth CV, Savitz DA, Luther ER. Maternal cigarette smoking as a risk factor for placental abruption, placenta previa, and uterine bleeding in pregnancy. *Am J Epidemiol* 1996;144(9):881–889.

44. Crane JM, van den Hof MC, Dodds L, et al. Neonatal outcomes with placenta previa. *Obstet Gynecol* 1999;93(4):541–544.

45. Ramin SM. Placental abnormalities: Previa, abruption, and accreta. In: Plauche WC, Morrison JC, O'Sullivan MJ, eds. *Surgical Obstetrics*. Philadelphia, PA: WB Saunders; 1999:203.

46. Cotton DB, Read JA, Paul RH, et al. The conservative aggressive management of placenta previa. *Am J Obstet Gynecol* 1980;137(6):687–695.

47. Silver R, Depp R, Sabbagha RE, et al. Placenta previa: Aggressive expectant management. *Am J Obstet Gynecol* 1984;150(1):15–22.

48. Wexler P, Gottesfeld KR. Second trimester placenta previa. An apparently normal placentation. *Obstet Gynecol* 1977;50(6):706–709.

49. Wexler P, Gottesfeld KR. Early diagnosis of placenta previa. *Obstet Gynecol* 1979;54(2):231–234.

50. Farine D, Peisner DB, Timor-Tritsch IE. Placenta previa—is the traditional diagnostic approach satisfactory? *J Clin Ultrasound* 1990;18(4):328–330.

51. Powell MC, Buckley J, Price H, et al. Magnetic resonance imaging and placenta previa. *Am J Obstet Gynecol* 1986;154(3):565–569.

52. Oyelese Y, Smulian JC. Placenta previa, placenta accreta, and vasa previa. *Obstet Gynecol* 2006;107(4):927–941.

53. Rehman K, Johnson T. Bleeding after 20 weeks' gestation: Maternal and fetal assessment. In: Andrea Seils, Regina Y, Brown, eds. *Obstetric & Gynecologic Emergencies Diagnosis and Management*. New York: The McGraw-Hill Companies, Inc., 2004:114.

54. Brenner WE, Edelman DA, Hendricks CH. Characteristics of patients with placenta previa and results of "expectant management". *Am J Obstet Gynecol* 1978;132(2):180–191.

55. Nelson KB, Grether JK. Can magnesium sulfate reduce the risk of cerebral palsy in very low birthweight infants? *Pediatrics* 1995;95(2):263–269.

56. American Society of Anesthesiologists Task Force on Obstetric Anesthesia. Practice guidelines for obstetric anesthesia: An updated report by the American society of anesthesiologists task force on obstetric anesthesia. *Anesthesiology* 2007;106(4):843–863.

57. Hong JY, Jee YS, Yoon HJ, et al. Comparison of general and epidural anesthesia in elective cesarean section for placenta previa totalis: Maternal hemodynamics, blood loss and neonatal outcome. *Int J Obstet Anesth* 2003;12(1):12–16.

58. Bonner SM, Haynes SR, Ryall D. The anaesthetic management of caesarean section for placenta praevia: A questionnaire survey. *Anaesthesia* 1995; 50(11):992–994.

59. Downing JW, Buley RJ, Brock-Utne JG, et al. Etomidate for induction of anaesthesia at caesarean section: Comparison with thiopentone. *Br J Anaesth* 1979;51(2):135–140.

60. Morgan GE, Mikhail MS, Murray MJ. Nonvolatile anesthetic agents. *Clinical Anesthesiology*. 4th ed. USA: Lange Medical Books/McGraw-Hill Medical Publishing Division; 2006:179.

61. Andrews WW, Ramin SM, Maberry MC, et al. Effect of type of anesthesia on blood loss at elective repeat cesarean section. *Am J Perinatol* 1992;9(3):197–200.

62. Pelosi MA 3rd, Pelosi MA. Spontaneous uterine rupture at thirty-three weeks subsequent to previous superficial laparoscopic myomectomy. *Am J Obstet Gynecol* 1997;177(6):1547–1549.

63. Kieser KE, Baskett TF. A 10-year population-based study of uterine rupture. *Obstet Gynecol* 2002;100(4):749–753.

64. Walsh CA, Baxi LV. Rupture of the primigravid uterus: A review of the literature. *Obstet Gynecol Surv* 2007;62(5):327–334; quiz 353–354.

65. Plauche WC, Von Almen W, Muller R. Catastrophic uterine rupture. *Obstet Gynecol* 1984;64(6):792–797.

66. Lydon-Rochelle M, Holt VL, Easterling TR, et al. Risk of uterine rupture during labor among women with a prior cesarean delivery. *N Engl J Med* 2001;345(1):3–8.

67. Kaczmarczyk M, Sparen P, Terry P, et al. Risk factors for uterine rupture and neonatal consequences of uterine rupture: A population-based study of successive pregnancies in Sweden. *BJOG* 2007;114(10):1208–1214.

68. Zelop CM, Shipp TD, Repke JT, et al. Uterine rupture during induced or augmented labor in gravid women with one prior cesarean delivery. *Am J Obstet Gynecol* 1999;181(4):882–886.

69. Schrinsky DC, Benson RC. Rupture of the pregnant uterus: A review. *Obstet Gynecol Surv* 1978;33(4):217–232.

70. Phelan JP. Uterine rupture. *Clin Obstet Gynecol* 1990;33(3):432–437.

71. Farmer RM, Kirschbaum T, Potter D, et al. Uterine rupture during trial of labor after previous cesarean section. *Am J Obstet Gynecol* 1991;165(4 Pt 1):996–1001.

72. Thakur A, Heer MS, Thakur V, et al. Subtotal hysterectomy for uterine rupture. *Int J Gynaecol Obstet* 2001;74(1):29–33.

73. Mayer DC, Spielman FJ. Antepartum and postpartum hemorrhage. In: Chestnut DH, ed. *Obstetric Anesthesia Principles and Practice*. 1st ed. St. Louis, MO: Mosby-Year Book, Inc.; 1994:699.

74. Catanzarite V, Maida C, Thomas W, et al. Prenatal sonographic diagnosis of vasa previa: Ultrasound findings and obstetric outcome in ten cases. *Ultrasound Obstet Gynecol* 2001;18(2):109–115.

75. Antoine C, Young BK, Silverman F, et al. Sinusoidal fetal heart rate pattern with vasa previa in twin pregnancy. *J Reprod Med* 1982;27(5):295–300.

76. Benirschke K, Kaufman P. *The Pathology of the Human Placenta*. New York, NY: Springer-Verlag; 1995.

77. Chang J, Elam-Evans LD, Berg CJ, et al. Pregnancy-related mortality surveillance—United States, 1991–1999. *MMWR Surveill Summ* 2003;52(2):1–8.

78. Abou Zahr C, Royston E. Global mortality. In: *Global Factbook*. Bethesda, MD: WHO; 1991.

79. Rochat RW, Koonin LM, Atrash HK, et al. Maternal mortality in the United States: Report from the maternal mortality collaborative. *Obstet Gynecol* 1988;72(1):91–97.

80. Bodnar LM, Cogswell ME, Scanlon KS. Low income postpartum women are at risk of iron deficiency. *J Nutr* 2002;132(8):2298–2302.

81. Meyer JW, Eichhorn KH, Vetter K, et al. Does recombinant human erythropoietin not only treat anemia but reduce postpartum (emotional) distress as well? *J Perinat Med* 1995;23(1–2):99–109.

82. Nelson SH, Suresh MS. Lack of reactivity of uterine arteries from patients with obstetric hemorrhage. *Am J Obstet Gynecol* 1992;166(5):1436–1443.

83. World Health Organization. Making pregnancy safer reducing the global burden: Postpartum haemorrhage. *World Health Organization Hot Topics Issue*. 2007(4):1.

84. Bouwmeester FW, Bolte AC, van Geijn HP. Pharmacological and surgical therapy for primary postpartum hemorrhage. *Curr Pharm Des* 2005;11(6): 759–773.

85. Knight M, UKOSS. Peripartum hysterectomy in the UK: Management and outcomes of the associated haemorrhage. *BJOG* 2007;114(11):1380–1387.

86. Saito K, Haruki A, Ishikawa H, et al. Prospective study of intramuscular ergometrine compared with intramuscular oxytocin for prevention of postpartum haemorrhage. *J Obstet Gynaecol Res* 2007;33(3):254–258.

87. Gulmezoglu AM, Forna F, Villar J, et al. Prostaglandins for preventing postpartum haemorrhage. *Cochrane Database Syst Rev* 2007;3(3):CD000494.

88. Platt LD, Druzin ML. Acute puerperal inversion of the uterus. *Am J Obstet Gynecol* 1981;141(2):187–190.

89. Baskett TF. Acute uterine inversion: A review of 40 cases. *J Obstet Gynaecol Can* 2002;24(12):953–956.

90. Achanna S, Mohamed Z, Krishnan M. Puerperal uterine inversion: A report of four cases. *J Obstet Gynaecol Res* 2006;32(3):341–345.

91. Kitchin JD 3rd, Thiagarajah S, May HV Jr, et al. Puerperal inversion of the uterus. *Am J Obstet Gynecol* 1975;123(1):51–58.

92. You WB, Zahn CM. Postpartum hemorrhage: Abnormally adherent placenta, uterine inversion, and puerperal hematomas. *Clin Obstet Gynecol* 2006; 49(1):184–197.

93. Brar HS, Greenspoon JS, Platt LD, et al. Acute puerperal uterine inversion. New approaches to management. *J Reprod Med* 1989;34(2):173–177.

94. Dayan SS, Schwalbe SS. The use of small-dose intravenous nitroglycerin in a case of uterine inversion. *Anesth Analg* 1996;82(5):1091–1093.

95. O'Sullivan J. A simple method of correcting puerperal uterine inversion. *BMJ* 1945;2.282.

96. Ogueh O, Ayida G. Acute uterine inversion: A new technique of hydrostatic replacement. *Br J Obstet Gynaecol* 1997;104(8):951–952.

97. Burton R, Belfort MA. Etiology and management of hemorrhage. In: Dildy GA III, Belfort MA, Saade G, Phelan JP, Hankins GD, Clark SL, eds. *Critical Care Obstetrics*. 4th ed. USA: Blackwell Publishing Company; 2004:298.

98. Hong RW, Greenfield ML, Polley LS. Nitroglycerin for uterine inversion in the absence of placental fragments. *Anesth Analg* 2006;103(2):511–512.

99. Dufour P, Vinatier D, Puech F. The use of intravenous nitroglycerin for cervico-uterine relaxation: A review of the literature. *Arch Gynecol Obstet* 1997; 261(1):1–7.

100. Harnett MJ, Segal S. Presence of placental tissue is necessary for TNG to provide uterine relaxation. *Anesth Analg* 2000;91(4):1043–1044.

101. Hung TH, Shau WY, Hsieh CC, et al. Risk factors for placenta accreta. *Obstet Gynecol* 1999;93(4):545–550.

102. Wu S, Kocherginsky M, Hibbard JU. Abnormal placentation: Twenty-year analysis. *Am J Obstet Gynecol* 2005;192(5):1458–1461.

103. Stafford I, Belfort MA. Placenta accreta, increta, and percreta: A team-based approach starts with prevention (part 1). *Contemporary OB/Gyn* 2008;53(5):48.

104. Silver RM, Landon MB, Rouse DJ, et al. Maternal morbidity associated with multiple repeat cesarean deliveries. *Obstet Gynecol* 2006;107(6):1226–1232.

105. Clark SL, Koonings PP, Phelan JP. Placenta previa/accreta and prior cesarean section. *Obstet Gynecol* 1985;66(1):89–92.

106. Lam H, Pun TC, Lam PW. Successful conservative management of placenta previa accreta during cesarean section. *Int J Gynaecol Obstet* 2004;86(1):31–32.

107. Twickler DM, Lucas MJ, Balis AB, et al. Color flow mapping for myometrial invasion in women with a prior cesarean delivery. *J Matern Fetal Med* 2000;9(6):330–335.

108. Palacios Jaraquemada JM, Bruno CH. Magnetic resonance imaging in 300 cases of placenta accreta: Surgical correlation of new findings. *Acta Obstet Gynecol Scand* 2005;84(8):716–724.

109. Warshak CR, Eskander R, Hull AD, et al. Accuracy of ultrasonography and magnetic resonance imaging in the diagnosis of placenta accreta. *Obstet Gynecol* 2006;108(3 Pt 1):573–581.

110. Lax A, Prince MR, Mennitt KW, et al. The value of specific MRI features in the evaluation of suspected placental invasion. *Magn Reson Imaging* 2007;25(1):87–93.

111. Belfort MA. Pregnancy-related hemorrhage. *Precis: An Update in Obstetrics and Gynecology*. 4th ed. Washington, DC: The American College of Obstetricians and Gynecologists; 2010:61.

112. Hudon L, Belfort MA, Broome DR. Diagnosis and management of placenta percreta: A review. *Obstet Gynecol Surv* 1998;53(8):509–517.

113. Shrivastava V, Nageotte M, Major C, et al. Case-control comparison of cesarean hysterectomy with and without prophylactic placement of intravascular balloon catheters for placenta accreta. *Am J Obstet Gynecol* 2007;197(4):402.e1–402.e5.

114. O'Brien JM, Barton JR, Donaldson ES. The management of placenta percreta: Conservative and operative strategies. *Am J Obstet Gynecol* 1996;175(6):1632–1638.

115. Kastner ES, Figueroa R, Garry D, et al. Emergency peripartum hysterectomy: Experience at a community teaching hospital. *Obstet Gynecol*. 2002;99(6):971–975.

116. Kwee A, Bots ML, Visser GH, et al. Emergency peripartum hysterectomy: A prospective study in the Netherlands. *Eur J Obstet Gynecol Reprod Biol* 2006;124(2):187–192.

117. Shellhaas CS, Gilbert S, Landon MB, et al. The frequency and complication rates of hysterectomy accompanying cesarean delivery. *Obstet Gynecol* 2009;114(2 Pt 1):224–229.

118. Sharma SK, Philip J, Whitten CW, et al. Assessment of changes in coagulation in parturients with preeclampsia using thromboelastography. *Anesthesiology* 1999;90(2):385–390.

119. Sharma SK, Vera RL, Stegall WC, et al. Management of a postpartum coagulopathy using thrombelastography. *J Clin Anesth* 1997;9(3):243–247.

120. American College of Surgeons. ATLS, advanced trauma life support program for doctors. *ACS.* 7th ed. Chicago, IL; 2004.

121. Ardagh MW, Hodgson T, Shaw L, et al. Pulse rate over pressure evaluation (ROPE) is useful in the assessment of compensated haemorrhagic shock. *Emerg Med (Fremantle)* 2001;13(1):43–46.

122. Dubois J, Garel L, Grignon A, et al. Placenta percreta: Balloon occlusion and embolization of the internal iliac arteries to reduce intraoperative blood losses. *Am J Obstet Gynecol* 1997;176(3):723–726.

123. Allam J, Cox M, Yentis SM. Cell salvage in obstetrics. *Int J Obstet Anesth* 2008;17(1):37–45.

124. Holcomb JB, Wade CE, Michalek JE, et al. Increased plasma and platelet to red blood cell ratios improves outcome in 466 massively transfused civilian trauma patients. *Ann Surg* 2008;248(3):447–458.

125. Gonzalez EA, Moore FA, Holcomb JB, et al. Fresh frozen plasma should be given earlier to patients requiring massive transfusion. *J Trauma* 2007;62(1):112–119.

126. Gunter OL Jr, Au BK, Isbell JM, et al. Optimizing outcomes in damage control resuscitation: Identifying blood product ratios associated with improved survival. *J Trauma* 2008;65(3):527–534.

127. Franchini M, Franchi M, Bergamini V, et al. A critical review on the use of recombinant factor VIIa in life-threatening obstetric postpartum hemorrhage. *Semin Thromb Hemost* 2008;34(1):104–112.

128. Leighton BL, Wall MH, Lockhart EM, et al. Use of recombinant factor VIIa in patients with amniotic fluid embolism: A systematic review of case reports. *Anesthesiology* 2011;115(6):1201–1208.

129. National Collaborating Centre for Women's and Children's Health (UK). 2007.

130. World Health Organization (WHO). *Pregnancy, Childbirth, Postpartum and Newborn Care: A Guide for Essential Practice.* 2nd ed. Geneva: WHO; 2006. Report No.: B11.

131. Cheung WM, Hawkes A, Ibish S, et al. The retained placenta: Historical and geographical rate variations. *J Obstet Gynaecol* 2011;31(1):37–42.

132. Hidar S, Jennane TM, Bouguizane S, et al. The effect of placental removal method at cesarean delivery on perioperative hemorrhage: A randomized clinical trial ISRCTN 49779257. *Eur J Obstet Gynecol Reprod Biol* 2004;117(2):179–182.

133. Combs CA, Laros RK Jr. Prolonged third stage of labor: Morbidity and risk factors. *Obstet Gynecol* 1991;77(6):863–867.

134. Magann EF, Evans S, Chauhan SP, et al. The length of the third stage of labor and the risk of postpartum hemorrhage. *Obstet Gynecol* 2005;105(2):290–293.

135. Turner RJ, Lambros M, Kenway L, et al. The in-vitro effects of sevoflurane and desflurane on the contractility of pregnant human uterine muscle. *Int J Obstet Anesth* 2002;11(4):246–251.

136. DeSimone CA, Norris MC, Leighton BL. Intravenous nitroglycerin aids manual extraction of a retained placenta. *Anesthesiology* 1990;73(4):787.

137. Caponas G. Glyceryl trinitrate and acute uterine relaxation: A literature review. *Anaesth Intensive Care* 2001;29(2):163–177.

138. Dollery CE. *Therapeutic Drugs.* 2nd ed. Edinburgh: Churchill Livingstone; 1999.

139. Chelmow D, O'Brien B. Postpartum haemorrhage: Prevention. *Clin Evid* 2006;(15):1932–1950.

140. Thomas JS, Koh SH, Cooper GM. Haemodynamic effects of oxytocin given as i.v. bolus or infusion on women undergoing caesarean section. *Br J Anaesth* 2007;98(1):116–119.

141. CEMD. *Why Mothers die. Report on Confidential Enquiries into Maternal deaths, 1997–1999. Royal London: College of Obstetricians and Gynaecologists, 2001.* Royal London: College of Obstetricians and Gynaecologists; 2001.

142. Balki M, Ronayne M, Davies S, et al. Minimum oxytocin dose requirement after cesarean delivery for labor arrest. *Obstet Gynecol* 2006;107(1):45–50.

143. Carvalho JC, Balki M, Kingdom J, et al. Oxytocin requirements at elective cesarean delivery: A dose-finding study. *Obstet Gynecol* 2004;104(5 Pt 1):1005–1010.

144. Sanders-Bush E, Mayer SE. 5-hydroxytryptamine (serotonin): Receptor agonists and antagonists. In: Hardman JG, Limbird LE, Gilman AG, eds. *Goodman & Gillman's The Pharmacological Basis of Therapeutics.* 10th ed. New York, NY: McGraw-Hill; 2001:269.

145. Casady GN, Moore DC, Bridenbaugh LD. Postpartum hypertension after use of vasoconstrictor and oxytocic drugs. Etiology, incidence, complications, and treatment. *J Am Med Assoc* 1960;172:1011–1015.

146. Lin YH, Seow KM, Hwang JL, et al. Myocardial infarction and mortality caused by methylergonovine. *Acta Obstet Gynecol Scand* 2005;84(10):1022.

147. Hayashi Y, Ibe T, Kawato H, et al. Postpartum acute myocardial infarction induced by ergonovine administration. *Intern Med* 2003;42(10):983–986.

148. Abouleish E. Postpartum hypertension and convulsion after oxytocic drugs. *Anesth Analg* 1976;55(6):813–815.

149. McDonald S, Abbott JM, Higgins SP. Prophylactic ergometrine-oxytocin versus oxytocin for the third stage of labour. *Cochrane Database Syst Rev* 2004;1(1):CD000201.

150. Hayashi RH, Castillo MS, Noah ML. Management of severe postpartum hemorrhage with a prostaglandin F2 alpha analogue. *Obstet Gynecol* 1984;63(6):806–808.

151. Bigrigg A, Chissell S, Read MD. Use of intra myometrial 15-methyl prostaglandin F2 alpha to control atonic postpartum haemorrhage following vaginal delivery and failure of conventional therapy. *Br J Obstet Gynaecol* 1991;98(7):734–736.

152. Andersen LH, Secher NJ. Pattern of total and regional lung function in subjects with bronchoconstriction induced by 15-me PGF2 alpha. *Thorax* 1976;31(6):685–692.

153. O'Leary AM. Severe bronchospasm and hypotension after 15-methyl prostaglandin F(2alpha) in atonic post partum haemorrhage. *Int J Obstet Anesth* 1994;3(1):42–44.

154. Tang OS, Gemzell-Danielsson K, Ho PC. Misoprostol: Pharmacokinetic profiles, effects on the uterus and side-effects. *Int J Gynaecol Obstet* 2007;99(Suppl 2):S160–S167.

155. Danielsson KG, Marions L, Rodriguez A, et al. Comparison between oral and vaginal administration of misoprostol on uterine contractility. *Obstet Gynecol* 1999;93(2):275–280.

156. Aronsson A, Bygdeman M, Gemzell-Danielsson K. Effects of misoprostol on uterine contractility following different routes of administration. *Hum Reprod* 2004;19(1):81–84.

157. el-Refaey H, Calder L, Wheatley DN, et al. Cervical priming with prostaglandin E1 analogues, misoprostol and gemeprost. *Lancet* 1994;343(8907):1207–1209.

158. Ngai SW, Tang OS, Lao T, et al. Oral misoprostol versus placebo for cervical dilatation before vacuum aspiration in first trimester pregnancy. *Hum Reprod* 1995;10(5):1220–1222.

159. Plaut MM, Schwartz ML, Lubarsky SL. Uterine rupture associated with the use of misoprostol in the gravid patient with a previous cesarean section. *Am J Obstet Gynecol* 1999;180(6 Pt 1):1535–1542.

160. Weeks A, Alfirevic Z, Faundes A, et al. Misoprostol for induction of labor with a live fetus. *Int J Gynaecol Obstet* 2007;99(Suppl 2):S194–S197.

161. Moscardo F, Perez F, de la Rubia J, et al. Successful treatment of severe intra-abdominal bleeding associated with disseminated intravascular coagulation using recombinant activated factor VII. *Br J Haematol* 2001;114(1):174–176.

162. Franchini M, Franchi M, Bergamini V, et al. The use of recombinant activated FVII in postpartum hemorrhage. *Clin Obstet Gynecol* 2010;53(1):219–227.

163. Levi M, Levy JH, Andersen HF, et al. Safety of recombinant activated factor VII in randomized clinical trials. *N Engl J Med* 2010;363(19):1791–1800.

164. Lin Y, Stanworth S, Birchall J, et al. Use of recombinant factor VIIa for the prevention and treatment of bleeding in patients without hemophilia: A systematic review and meta-analysis. *CMAJ* 2011;183(1):E9–E19.

165. Novikova N, Hofmeyr GJ. Tranexamic acid for preventing postpartum haemorrhage. *Cochrane Database Syst Rev* 2010;(7):CD007872.

166. Ferrer P, Roberts I, Sydenham E, et al. Anti-fibrinolytic agents in post partum haemorrhage: A systematic review. *BMC Pregnancy Childbirth* 2009;9:29.

167. B-Lynch C, Coker A, Lawal AH, et al. The B-lynch surgical technique for the control of massive postpartum haemorrhage: An alternative to hysterectomy? Five cases reported. *Br J Obstet Gynaecol* 1997;104(3):372–375.

168. Ferguson JE, Bourgeois FJ, Underwood PB. B-lynch suture for postpartum hemorrhage. *Obstet Gynecol* 2000;95(6 Pt 2):1020–1022.

169. Habek D, Kulas T, Bobic-Vukovic M, et al. Successful of the B-lynch compression suture in the management of massive postpartum hemorrhage: Case reports and review. *Arch Gynecol Obstet* 2006;273(5):307–309.

170. Tamizian O, Arulkumaran S. The surgical management of postpartum haemorrhage. *Curr Opin Obstet Gynecol* 2001;13(2):127–131.

171. Bakri YN, Amri A, Abdul Jabbar F. Tamponade-balloon for obstetrical bleeding. *Int J Gynaecol Obstet* 2001;74(2):139–142.

172. Johanson R, Kumar M, Obhrai M, et al. Management of massive postpartum haemorrhage: Use of a hydrostatic balloon catheter to avoid laparotomy. *BJOG* 2001;108(4):420–422.

173. Cho Y, Rizvi C, Uppal T, et al. Ultrasonographic visualization of balloon placement for uterine tamponade in massive primary postpartum hemorrhage. *Ultrasound Obstet Gynecol* 2008;32(5):711–713.

174. O'Leary JL, O'Leary JA. Uterine artery ligation for control of postcesarean section hemorrhage. *Obstet Gynecol* 1974;43(6):849–853.

175. O'Leary JA. Uterine artery ligation in the control of postcesarean hemorrhage. *J Reprod Med* 1995;40(3):189–193.

176. AbdRabbo SA. Stepwise uterine devascularization: A novel technique for management of uncontrolled postpartum hemorrhage with preservation of the uterus. *Am J Obstet Gynecol* 1994;171(3):694–700.

177. Bodner LJ, Nosher JL, Gribbin C, et al. Balloon-assisted occlusion of the internal iliac arteries in patients with placenta accreta/percreta. *Cardiovasc Intervent Radiol* 2006;29(3):354–361.

178. Mok M, Heidemann B, Dundas K, et al. Interventional radiology in women with suspected placenta accreta undergoing caesarean section. *Int J Obstet Anesth* 2008;17(3):255–261.

179. Vedantham S, Goodwin SC, McLucas B, et al. Uterine artery embolization: An underused method of controlling pelvic hemorrhage. *Am J Obstet Gynecol* 1997;176(4):938–948.

180. Hansch E, Chitkara U, McAlpine J, et al. Pelvic arterial embolization for control of obstetric hemorrhage: A five-year experience. *Am J Obstet Gynecol* 1999;180(6 Pt 1):1454–1460.

181. Pelage JP, Le Dref O, Mateo J, et al. Life-threatening primary postpartum hemorrhage: Treatment with emergency selective arterial embolization. *Radiology* 1998;208(2):359–362.

182. Nuttall GA, Oliver WC, Santrach PJ, et al. Efficacy of a simple intraoperative transfusion algorithm for nonerythrocyte component utilization after cardiopulmonary bypass. *Anesthesiology* 2001;94(5):773–781; discussion 5A–6A.

183. Shore-Lesserson L, Manspeizer HE, DePerio M, et al. Thromboelastography-guided transfusion algorithm reduces transfusions in complex cardiac surgery. *Anesth Analg* 1999;88(2):312–319.

184. Annecke T, Geisenberger T, Kurzl R, et al. Algorithm-based coagulation management of catastrophic amniotic fluid embolism. *Blood Coagul Fibrinolysis* 2010;21(1):95–100.

185. Huissoud C, Carrabin N, Audibert F, et al. Bedside assessment of fibrinogen level in postpartum haemorrhage by thromboelastometry. *BJOG* 2009;116(8):1097–1102.

186. Smoller BR, Kruskall MS. Phlebotomy for diagnostic laboratory tests in adults. Pattern of use and effect on transfusion requirements. *N Engl J Med* 1986;314(19):1233–1235.

187. Utter GH, Reed WF, Lee TH, et al. Transfusion-associated microchimerism. *Vox Sang* 2007;93(3):188–195.

188. Chang CM, Quinlan SC, Warren JL, et al. Blood transfusions and the subsequent risk of hematologic malignancies. *Transfusion* 2010;50(10):2249–2257.

189. AABB (American association of blood banks) technical manual. In: Grossman BJ, Harris T, Hillyer CD, eds. 17th ed. Bethesda, MD: AABB, 2011.

190. Eder AF, Kennedy JM, Dy BA, et al. Bacterial screening of apheresis platelets and the residual risk of septic transfusion reactions: The American red cross experience (2004–2006). *Transfusion* 2007;47(7):1134–1142.

191. Whitaker BI, Sullivan M. *The 2005 Nationwide Blood Collection and Utilization Survey Report.* Department of Health and Human Services; 2006.

192. Eder AF, Herron RM Jr, Strupp A, et al. Effective reduction of transfusion-related acute lung injury risk with male-predominant plasma strategy in the American red cross (2006–2008). *Transfusion* 2010;50(8):1732–1742.

193. Perkins HA. Transfusion-induced immunologic unresponsiveness. *Transfus Med Rev* 1988;2(4):196–203.

194. Murphy P, Heal JM, Blumberg N. Infection or suspected infection after hip replacement surgery with autologous or homologous blood transfusions. *Transfusion* 1991;31(3):212–217.

195. Mezrow CK, Bergstein I, Tartter PI. Postoperative infections following autologous and homologous blood transfusions. *Transfusion* 1992;32(1):27–30.

196. Tartter PI, Quintero S, Barron DM. Perioperative blood transfusion associated with infectious complications after colorectal cancer operations. *Am J Surg* 1986;152(5):479–482.

197. Mathelier AC. A comparison of postoperative morbidity following prophylactic antibiotic administration by combined irrigation and intravenous route or by intravenous route alone during cesarean section. *J Perinat Med* 1992;20(3):177–182.

198. Di Lieto A, Albano G, Cimmino E, et al. Retrospective study of postoperative infectious morbidity following cesarean section. *Minerva Ginecol* 1996;48(3):85–92.

199. Tsai AG, Cabrales P, Intaglietta M. Microvascular perfusion upon exchange transfusion with stored red blood cells in normovolemic anemic conditions. *Transfusion* 2004;44(11):1626–1634.

200. O'Shaughnessy DF, Atterbury C, Bolton Maggs P, et al. Guidelines for the use of fresh-frozen plasma, cryoprecipitate and cryosupernatant. *Br J Haematol* 2004;126(1):11–28.

201. Rossaint R, Bouillon B, Cerny V, et al. Management of bleeding following major trauma: An updated European guideline. *Crit Care* 2010;14(2):R52.

202. Dickneite G, Pragst I. Prothrombin complex concentrate vs fresh frozen plasma for reversal of dilutional coagulopathy in a porcine trauma model. *Br J Anaesth* 2009;102(3):345–354.

203. Dickneite G, Dorr B, Kaspereit F, et al. Prothrombin complex concentrate versus recombinant factor VIIa for reversal of hemodilutional coagulopathy in a porcine trauma model. *J Trauma* 2010;68(5):1151–1157.

204. Baker BW. Blood conservation, obstetrics, and jehova's witnesses. *Anesthesiol Clin N Am* 1998:375.

205. Barton DP, Joy MT, Lappin TR, et al. Maternal erythropoietin in singleton pregnancies: A randomized trial on the effect of oral hematinic supplementation. *Am J Obstet Gynecol* 1994;170(3):896–901.

206. Vora M, Gruslin A. Erythropoietin in obstetrics. *Obstet Gynecol Surv* 1998;53(8):500–508.

207. Rouse DJ, MacPherson C, Landon M, et al. Blood transfusion and cesarean delivery. *Obstet Gynecol* 2006;108(4):891–897.

208. Blot I, Diallo D, Tchernia G. Iron deficiency in pregnancy: Effects on the newborn. *Curr Opin Hematol* 1999;6(2):65–70.

209. Patterson AJ, Brown WJ, Roberts DC. Dietary and supplement treatment of iron deficiency results in improvements in general health and fatigue in Australian women of childbearing age. *J Am Coll Nutr* 2001;20(4):337–342.

210. Walters BA, Van Wyck DB. Benchmarking iron dextran sensitivity: Reactions requiring resuscitative medication in incident and prevalent patients. *Nephrol Dial Transplant* 2005;20(7):1438–1442.

211. Van Wyck DB. Labile iron: Manifestations and clinical implications. *J Am Soc Nephrol* 2004;15(Suppl 2):S107–S111.

212. Brecher ME, Goodnough LT. The rise and fall of preoperative autologous blood donation. *Transfusion* 2001;41(12):1459–1462.

213. Kruskall MS, Leonard S, Klapholz H. Autologous blood donation during pregnancy: Analysis of safety and blood use. *Obstet Gynecol* 1987;70(6):938–941.

214. Druzin ML, Wolf CF, Edersheim TG, et al. Donation of blood by the pregnant patient for autologous transfusion. *Am J Obstet Gynecol* 1988;159(5):1023–1027.

215. McVay PA, Hoag RW, Hoag MS, et al. Safety and use of autologous blood donation during the third trimester of pregnancy. *Am J Obstet Gynecol* 1989;160(6):1479–1486; discussion 1486–1488.

216. Kuromaki K, Takeda S, Seki H, et al. Clinical study of autologous blood transfusion in pregnant women. *Nihon Sanka Fujinka Gakkai Zasshi* 1994;46(11):1213–1220.

217. Combs CA, Murphy EL, Laros RK Jr. Cost-benefit analysis of autologous blood donation in obstetrics. *Obstet Gynecol* 1992;80(4):621–625.

218. Dodril FD. The use of the heart-lung apparatus in human cardiac surgery. *J Thorac Cardiovasc Surg* 1957;33:60.

219. Stehling L, Zauder HL. Controversies in transfusion medicine. Perioperative hemodilution: Pro. *Transfusion* 1994;34(3):265–268.

220. Monk TG, Goodnough LT. Blood conservation strategies to minimize allogeneic blood use in urologic surgery. *Am J Surg* 1995;170(6A Suppl):69S–73S.

221. Estella NM, Berry DL, Baker BW, et al. Normovolemic hemodilution before cesarean hysterectomy for placenta percreta. *Obstet Gynecol* 1997;90(4 Pt 2):669–670.

222. Gross JB. Estimating allowable blood loss: Corrected for dilution. *Anesthesiology* 1983;58(3):277–280.

223. Lund CJ, Donovan JC. Blood volume during pregnancy. Significance of plasma and red cell volumes. *Am J Obstet Gynecol* 1967;98(3):394–403.

224. Grange CS, Douglas MJ, Adams TJ, et al. The use of acute hemodilution in parturients undergoing cesarean section. *Am J Obstet Gynecol* 1998;178(1 Pt 1):156–160.

225. Committee on Obstetric Practice. ACOG Committee opinion. Placenta accreta. American college of obstetricians and gynecologists. *Int J Gynaecol Obstet* 2002;77(1):77–78.

226. OAA/AAGBI guidelines for obstetric anaesthetic services. Revised edition: OAA/AAGBI. 2005:25.

227. Intraoperative blood salvage in obstetrics. Interventional procedure guidance 144. [Internet]. London WC1V 6NA: National Institute for Health and Clinical Excellence; 2005.

228. Teig M, Harkness M, Catling S, et al. Survey of cell-salvage use in obstetrics in the UK. *Int J Obstet Anesth* 2007;16:S30.

229. Ilstrup SE. *Standards For Perioperative Autologous Blood Collection And Administration.* 4th ed. Bethesda, MD, American Association of Blood Banks: 2009.

230. Waters JH, Dyga RM, Yazer MH. *Guidelines for Blood Recovery and Reinfusion in Surgery and Trauma.* Bethesda, MD: American Association of Blood Banks, 2010.

231. Waters JH, Biscotti C, Potter PS, et al. Amniotic fluid removal during cell salvage in the cesarean section patient. *Anesthesiology* 2000;92(6):1531–1536.

232. Bernstein HH, Rosenblatt MA, Gettes M, et al. The ability of the haemonetics 4 cell saver system to remove tissue factor from blood contaminated with amniotic fluid. *Anesth Analg* 1997;85(4):831–833.

233. Waters JH, Williams B, Yazer MH, et al. Modification of suction-induced hemolysis during cell salvage. *Anesth Analg* 2007;104(3):684–687.

234. Haynes K, Stone C, King J. *Major Morbidities Associated with Childbirth in Victoria: Obstetric Heamorrhage and Associated Hysterectomy.* Bethesda, MD: Public Health Group, Department of Human Services; 2004.

235. Cameron CA, Roberts CL, Olive EC, et al. Trends in postpartum haemorrhage. *Aust N Z J Public Health* 2006;30(2):151–156.

236. Joseph KS, Rouleau J, Kramer MS, et al. Investigation of an increase in postpartum haemorrhage in Canada. *BJOG* 2007;114(6):751–759.

237. Healthy people 2010 [Internet].

238. [Internet]. Available from: http://www.cmqcc.org/resources/1484.

239. Bose P, Regan F, Paterson-Brown S. Improving the accuracy of estimated blood loss at obstetric haemorrhage using clinical reconstructions. *BJOG* 2006;113(8):919–924.

240. Toledo P, McCarthy RJ, Hewlett BJ, et al. The accuracy of blood loss estimation after simulated vaginal delivery. *Anesth Analg* 2007;105(6):1736–1740, table of contents.

241. Fuchs KM, Miller RS, Berkowitz RL. Optimizing outcomes through protocols, multidisciplinary drills, and simulation. *Semin Perinatol* 2009;33(2):104–108.

242. Gosman GG, Baldisseri MR, Stein KL, et al. Introduction of an obstetric-specific medical emergency team for obstetric crises: Implementation and experience. *Am J Obstet Gynecol* 2008;198(4):367.e1–367.e7.

243. Pettker CM, Thung SF, Norwitz ER, et al. Impact of a comprehensive patient safety strategy on obstetric adverse events. *Am J Obstet Gynecol* 2009; 200(5):492.e1–492.e8.

244. Borgman MA, Spinella PC, Perkins JG, et al. The ratio of blood products transfused affects mortality in patients receiving massive transfusions at a combat support hospital. *J Trauma* 2007;63(4):805–813.

245. Murad MH, Stubbs JR, Gandhi MJ, et al. The effect of plasma transfusion on morbidity and mortality: A systematic review and meta-analysis. *Transfusion* 2010;50(6):1370–1383.

246. Duchesne JC, Kimonis K, Marr AB, et al. Damage control resuscitation in combination with damage control laparotomy: A survival advantage. *J Trauma* 2010;69(1):46–52.

247. Snyder CW, Weinberg JA, McGwin G Jr, et al. The relationship of blood product ratio to mortality: Survival benefit or survival bias? *J Trauma* 2009;66(2):358–362; discussion 362–364.

248. Sperry JL, Ochoa JB, Gunn SR, et al. An FFP:PRBC transfusion ratio >/=1:1.5 is associated with a lower risk of mortality after massive transfusion. *J Trauma* 2008;65(5):986–993.

249. Johnson JL, Moore EE, Kashuk JL, et al. Effect of blood products transfusion on the development of postinjury multiple organ failure. *Arch Surg* 2010; 145(10):973–977.

250. Kashuk JL, Moore EE, Sawyer M, et al. Postinjury coagulopathy management: Goal directed resuscitation via POC thrombelastography. *Ann Surg* 2010;251(4):604–614.

251. Nuttall GA, Oliver WC, Ereth MH, et al. Coagulation tests predict bleeding after cardiopulmonary bypass. *J Cardiothorac Vasc Anesth* 1997;11(7):815–823.

CHAPTER

22

Amniotic Fluid Embolism

Quisqueya T. Palacios

■ INTRODUCTION

In 1987, maternal mortality rates were reported to be 6.6 deaths per 100,000 live births by the Health Resources and Services Administration and held for a period of more than 10 years (1). In 2010, the World Health Organization (WHO) estimated maternal mortality rate to be approximately 17/100,000 pregnancies in the United States. This was significantly higher than the goal of 3.3/100,000 live births set by the US Department of Health and Human Services in healthy people for 2010. In the triennium 2003 to 2005, the Centre for Maternal and Child Enquiries (CMACE) reported that the maternal mortality rate was 13.95/100,000 maternities. In 2011, CMACE reported that the maternal mortality rate for the most recent triennium 2006 to 2008 was 11.39/100,000 maternities.

According to a study by the Centers for Disease Control and Prevention (CDC) of pregnancy-related mortality in the United States between 1991 and 1998, the leading causes of maternal deaths are hemorrhage, pregnancy-related hypertensive disorders, pulmonary embolism, amniotic fluid embolism (AFE), infection, and pre-existing chronic conditions, such as, cardiovascular disease (2). Clark confirmed that AFE is one of the leading causes of maternal death in addition to preeclampsia, pulmonary thromboembolism, obstetric hemorrhage, and cardiac disease (3). Combined AFE and pulmonary thromboembolism account for approximately 25% of maternal deaths (Table 22-1). An estimated 5% to 15% of all maternal deaths in Western countries are due to AFE. In the triennium 2006 to 2008, CMACE reported AFE, the fourth leading cause of direct maternal deaths in the United Kingdom. Although the majority of deaths from AFE are not preventable, it is up to the anesthesia care provider to have a thorough understanding of the anesthetic implications of AFE in order to immediately diagnose and treat AFE during pregnancy and delivery.

AFE is thought to be a rare but often fatal complication of pregnancy whose onset can neither be predicted nor prevented (4). However, early diagnosis, expeditious resuscitation and delivery, and management of sequelae by a team approach including anesthesiologist, obstetrician, and intensivist may improve maternal and fetal outcomes. Despite aggressive and early management, maternal and fetal morbidity and mortality remained unacceptably high between 60% and 80% through the mid-1990s (5). However, new strategies and innovative approaches to management and treatment of AFE, including the use of an intra-aortic balloon pump with extracorporeal membrane oxygenation (ECMO) (6–8), cardiopulmonary bypass (9), inhaled nitric oxide (10), right ventricular assist devices (8), recombinant factor VIIa (rFVIIa) (7,11), have been reported with success and should be considered when all established, "standard of care" management approaches have failed. Although manifestations of AFE may be along a continuum from mild and transient to severe and fulminant cardiopulmonary collapse, prompt diagnosis and aggressive management improve maternal outcomes (12).

Although Meyer first reported a case of stillbirth associated with maternal death and AFE to the lungs in 1926 (13), Steiner and Lushbaugh first described the AFE syndrome in a case report of eight women who died unexpectedly from obstetric shock associated with pathologic evidence of AFE of fetal material in maternal lung blood vessels in 1941 (14). They theorized that amniotic fluid was forced into the maternal circulation during contractions. Steiner and Lushbaugh also described experimental evidence of the syndrome in dogs and rabbits following intravenous injection of human amniotic fluid rich in vernix or meconium which leads to a similar clinical presentation as described in the autopsies of eight parturients associated with plugging of the pulmonary vessels by squamous cells, presumably of fetal origin. On the basis of experimental animal studies supporting detailed pathologic findings in eight cases of unexpected maternal death resulting from a physical obstruction of the pulmonary vasculature by fetal material, Steiner and Lushbaugh proposed a new obstetrical disease, AFE.

Although the diagnosis of AFE is clinically based, the presence of sequelae including but not limited to respiratory arrest, cardiac shock, coagulopathy and DIC, and nonreassuring fetal heart tones in association with the presence of anucleated squamous cells in the pulmonary artery blood are not pathognomonic of AFE. In 1995, Clark confirmed that fetal squamous cells were found in the pulmonary circulation in 73% of fatal cases of AFE (5). In addition, fetal squamous cells were detected in only 50% of patients with a diagnosis of AFE during aspiration of pulmonary arterial blood. Also, the presence of squamous cells in the circulation during the peripartum period is not always associated with AFE (15). Contamination of the maternal blood by fetal squames may occur during pulmonary artery insertion and may be minimized by following the method suggested by Masson (16). However, the demonstration of fetal debris is highly significant and consistent with the diagnosis of AFE. However, the high variability in symptoms, the lack of characteristic findings on radiologic examination, the absence of a dose–response effect

TABLE 22-1 Leading Causes of Maternal Death

Cause of Death	Number	(%)
Complications of preeclampsia	15	(16)
Amniotic fluid embolism	13	(14)
Obstetric hemorrhage	11	(12)
Cardiac disease	10	(11)
Pulmonary thromboembolism	9	(9)
Obstetric infection	7	(7)

Adapted from: Clark SL, Belfort MA, Dildy GA, et al. Maternal death in the 21st century: causes, prevention, and relationship to cesarean delivery. *Am J Obstet Gynecol* 2008;199(1):36.e1–36.e5; discussion 91–92.e7–e11.

on symptoms, and the occurrence of coagulopathies are not entirely consistent with a physical block to the circulation as the main mechanism of disease. Alternatively, it might be the result of complement activation initiated by fetal antigen leaking into the maternal circulation. The rare immune response may be initiated by a rare pathologic antigen, or by common antigens presented uncommonly (17).

In 1995, Clark established a National Registry of AFE cases with 46 entries and in 2005, Tuffnell established a UK registry of AFE cases with 44 entries, both depended on self-reporting and had similar established entry criteria (5,18) (Table 22-2). Although the majority of cases of AFE occurred during labor, Clark confirmed that 19% of cases of AFE in their registry women became symptomatic during cesarean delivery when not in labor. In an analysis of the National Registry of cases of AFE, Clark reports a history of allergies in 41% of patients. Clark also reported a similarity between the clinical course, biphasic response, and hemodynamic changes of AFE to patients with anaphylactic shock and proposed that AFE was immunologic versus nonimmunologic and supported changing the name from AFE to anaphylactoid syndrome of pregnancy. Although Clark used the term anaphylactoid versus anaphylactic syndrome of pregnancy suggesting that the process associated with mast cell degranulation was not associated with an antigen and antibody, Benson suggested that placenta, fetus, and meconium-stained amniotic fluid could potentially be either sources of foreign antigens or lead to exposure to large quantities of nonantigenic materials and a fatal nonimmune anaphylaxis (19–21).

TABLE 22-2 Amniotic Fluid Embolism National and UK Registries' Entry Criteria

Acute hypoxia
Acute hypotension/cardiac arrest
Coagulopathy
Onset of symptoms During labor Cesarean delivery Dilation and evacuation Within 30 min postpartum
Other possible diagnosis have been excluded
Occurrence within 5 yr of registry opening

Adapted from: Clark SL, Hankins GVD, Dudley DA, et al. Amniotic fluid embolism: analysis of the national registry. *Am J Obstet Gynecol* 1995;172(4 Pt 1):1158–1167; discussion 1167–1169.

There are many unanswered questions regarding the etiology and mechanism of AFE if an "all or nothing" mechanism is considered in the presence of conflicting results of animal models and the pathologic absence of mechanical obstruction from fetal debris. Alternatively, one may consider "a response continuum" to AFE in pregnant women with increased immunologic reactivity, many of whom may have an associated underlying subclinical sepsis, trauma, or other risk factors during labor and the immediate postpartum period as the possible etiology and mechanisms of AFE. Romero describes two such cases of maternal deaths associated with subclinical intra-amniotic infection. He proposes that the mechanism of peripartum cardiovascular collapse may be infection and systemic inflammation instead of AFE. On the other hand, I propose that infection and systemic inflammation may lead to lowering of the threshold for cardiovascular collapse seen with AFE. Therefore, in these cases laboratory tests should include specific immunologic testing, multiple blood cultures, and specifically directed antibiotic therapy in addition to following the management protocols of AFE. Further improvements in maternal outcomes may be seen if recombinant human-activated protein C is included in the management of the subset of patients with clinical evidence of sepsis, prolonged rupture of membranes, prolonged labor, meconium staining of amniotic fluid, and fever associated with cardiovascular collapse at delivery (22).

Perhaps once a certain threshold is reached, especially in the presence of other immunologic factors, such as an intrauterine infection, an early first response is respiratory with clinical dyspnea and hypoxia, associated with pulmonary arterial hypertension and severe transient vasospasm. This usually leads to right ventricular failure and cardiac arrest. If the patient survives, left ventricular failure develops. However, in patients with an associated patent foramen ovale, ASD, VSD, or PDA, perhaps this initial phase may be more transient or absent and instead replaced by an immediate, sustained, and severe left heart failure and/or DIC. Alternatively, left ventricular dysfunction may be the direct effect of endogenous mediators causing cardiac depression and coagulopathy. This might explain the presence or lack of commonly presenting clinical symptoms, such as dyspnea, hypotension, seizures, DIC, and nonreassuring fetal status. Immune tolerance may explain why all mothers do not develop an immune response to their fetus as seen in Rh-negative mothers who do not develop isoimmunization on subsequent pregnancies or why all mothers do not reject the fetus (17). In addition, a better understanding of immune tolerance may help elucidate the pathophysiology of AFE and other diseases such as, preeclampsia and recurrent miscarriage.

■ INCIDENCE AND MORTALITY

Historically, the incidence of AFE in the United States is estimated to occur between 1 in 8,000 and 1 in 80,000 deliveries. However, more recently in 2008, Abenhaim in a retrospective population-based study on 3 million birth records in the United States from 1999 to 2003 estimated an incidence of approximately 7.7/100,000 deliveries or 1:13,000 deliveries (23).

In 2006, Kramer in a retrospective population-based hospital database in Canada estimated the incidence of AFE in 6.1 cases per 100,000 births (24). In a prospective national cohort study which included data from 3 million hospital deliveries from 1991 to 2002 and utilized information from the UK Obstetric Surveillance System (UKOSS) in the United Kingdom, Knight estimated a significantly lower incidence of 2/100,000 deliveries (25). Recently in the UKOSS, Dawson reported an incidence of AFE of 2 cases per 100,000 maternities for the 4-year period, 2005 to 2009 (26). In 2010, Roberts reported the AFE incidence rate of 3.3/100,000, maternal mortality rate of 35%, and perinatal mortality rate of 32%

in an Australian population-based cohort study (27). Newly identified risk factors included induction with vaginal prostaglandin and manual removal of the placenta.

In 1979, Morgan reviewed 272 documented cases of AFE in UK medical literature and reported a mortality rate of 86%. Of those, 25% of the deaths occurred within the first hour of the onset of symptoms. In 1995, Clark published the national registry of AFE and reviewed 46 cases of AFE and reported the maternal mortality rate of 61% (5). In Clark's study, more than 50% of patients died within the first hour and two-thirds of these deaths occurred within 5 hours of the AFE and only 15% of survivors remain neurologically intact. However, more recently, Gilbert reported a lower mortality rate of 27% in a population-based study in 1999 (28).

In 2005, Tuffnell also suggested a lower mortality rate of 37% in UK Registry (18,25). In 2011, CMACE confirmed AFE is the fourth leading cause of maternal mortality in the triennium 2006 to 2008 in the United Kingdom (29). CMACE reported on the deaths of 13 out of 261 women in the United Kingdom who died directly or indirectly related to pregnancy giving a maternal death rate of 0.57/100,000 directly associated with AFE. Although this represents a decline in maternal mortality, consistent with the report of the latest morbidity study from the UKOSS, it is not statistically significant. In addition, substandard care was implicated in 62% (major 15%, minor 46%) of these cases as the cause of deaths (30). Implicated in substandard care were poor organization of transfers, communication breakdowns, poor documentation, ineffective resuscitation, and avoidable delays in performing perimortem cesarean delivery within 5 minutes of collapse, which may have contributed to poor outcomes and deaths. In addition, mortality was associated increasingly with minority ethnicities and the Black African group. In 2006, Kramer reported a maternal mortality rate of 13% in a Canadian population-based cohort study (24).

In 2008, Abenhaim estimated a case mortality rate of 21.6% (23). He also found that AFE was associated with maternal age greater than 35, placenta previa, cesarean delivery in addition to preeclampsia, abruptio placenta, and the use of forceps. Abenhaim recommends the continuation of the National Registry of AFE to collect and review differences in management practices and outcomes in order to develop evidence-based algorithms for the treatment of AFE. In addition to newer management strategies and better outcomes, perhaps some of these patients did not present with all of the classic features of AFE and the wide range of maternal mortality and morbidity may describe a response continuum to AFE.

In 1995, Clark reported a neonatal mortality rate of 20% to 25% and only 50% of survivors remain neurologically intact. As maternal resuscitation and maternal outcomes improve, neonatal outcomes should also improve.

■ ETIOLOGY

Usually throughout pregnancy, intact membranes separate the maternal circulation from the amniotic fluid. For AFE to occur amniotic fluid must find a mode of entry into the maternal circulation. This is usually associated with rupture of membranes in 78% of cases. Symptoms of AFE occur in 14% of patients within 3 minutes of rupture of membranes (5). Potential modes of entry include the intrauterine pressure catheter, uterine trauma, small tears in the lower uterine segment, and the endocervix during placental abruption at the placental implantation site (Fig. 22-1). In addition, it has been

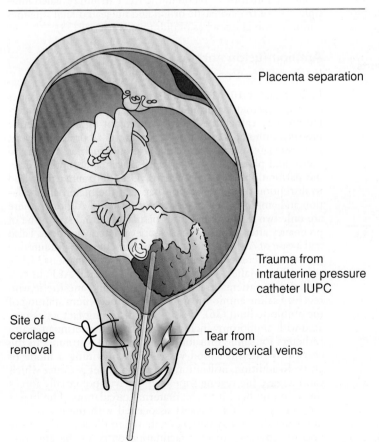

FIGURE 22-1 Possible sites of AFE into the maternal circulation.

assumed that there is a bulk movement of amniotic fluid due to a pressure gradient which facilitates the easy entry of amniotic fluid into blood vessels in the uterus. Karetzky suggests that chemical mediators of AFE move largely down an electrochemical gradient (31). Although some describe induction of labor with oxytocin and strong contractions as possible risk factors of AFE, tetanic contractions would actually impede the entry of amniotic fluid into the maternal circulation. Perhaps, strong and hypertonic contractions are the result of vasospasm of the uterus, myometrium, and vasculature following the previous entry of amniotic fluid.

Typically AFE occurs during labor and delivery or in the immediate postpartum period. Approximately 70% of cases occur before delivery and the remainder can occur as late as 48 hours postpartum. In 13% of cases, AFE occurs prior to the onset of labor. However, there are reported cases of AFE following induced abortion, transabdominal amniocentesis, abdominal and surgical trauma, and cerclage removal.

■ RISK FACTORS

Although predisposing factors, such as advanced maternal age, multiparity, and tumultuous labor, were initially considered predisposing to AFE by Steiner, others could not confirm any direct correlation. However, macrosomia, advanced gestational age, amnioinfusion, induction of labor were considered predisposing factors to AFE by Morgan. However, more recently, Abenheim identified only advanced maternal age and cesarean delivery as risk factors in a large population-based cohort study (23). In 1995, Clark published the analysis of the AFE Registry and only confirmed ruptured membranes as a predisposing risk factor to AFE; he included the demographic characteristics of patients with AFE (Table 22-3). Although Clark suggests only one predisposing risk factor associated with AFE, others continue to refer to additional risk factors. However, Knight described a possible increased risk of dying from AFE in older, ethnic-minority women for reasons related to underlying medical problems and/or access to care. Oi suggests fatal factors of clinical manifestations and laboratory testing in patients with fatal AFE: Multiparity, cardiac arrest, dyspnea, or loss of consciousness; higher sialyl levels were also seen in cases of fatal AFE (32).

Advanced Maternal Age and Multiple Pregnancies

However, Knight showed evidence of an association of AFE with multiple pregnancies, and older, ethnic-minority women in addition to induction of labor. In addition, Knight found an association of Cesarean delivery with postnatal AFE. Knight carried out a prospective population-based cohort study with case-control analysis, using the UKOSS from which 60 women having AFE in the United Kingdom were identified between February, 2005 and February, 2009. Knight estimated an incidence of AFE of 2/100,000 deliveries. Maternal mortality was estimated 20% and perinatal mortality was estimated 135/1,000 live births (25). Women who died were significantly more likely to be older and from ethnic-minority groups. Twenty-six of sixty women had AFE after delivery; nineteen of twenty-six women or 73% of these had AFE after cesarean delivery. Ten of the nineteen women who had AFE after cesarean delivery were not in labor at the time of cesarean. Fifty-five of sixty women or 92% developed AFE within 45 minutes of ruptured membranes. Women with AFE presented with premonitory symptoms as the first sign of AFE in 30% of cases, followed by shortness of breath in 20% and fetal bradycardia or other nonreassuring fetal heart tones in 20% of cases. Mulder described a case of a 44-year old Mexican multigravid woman who developed fetal bradycardia associated painful contractions following artificial amniotomy with meconium-stained fluid seen. Patient arrested and resuscitation was not successful and male infant subsequently died following cesarean delivery under general anesthesia. Microscopic examination of blood in the right atrium revealed multiple cells of trophoblastic origin and nucleated fetal squames within terminal branches of pulmonary arteries (33).

Amnioinfusion and Insertion of Intrauterine Pressure Catheter

In 2008 and 2010, Matsuo and Harbison described two cases of anaphylactoid syndrome after placement of an intrauterine pressure catheter. Although placement of an intrauterine pressure catheter is a routine procedure in labor and delivery, it is associated with a few complications, such as, trauma to uterus and placenta associated with placental abruption, uterine perforation, and endometritis. Uterine trauma may lead to disruption of the separation between the maternal circulation and amniotic fluid, a risk factor for AFE. Although there are only two documented cases of anaphylactoid syndrome of pregnancy after intrauterine pressure catheter placement, I also had a case of AFE associated with placement of an intrauterine pressure catheter confirmed by pathologic examination (34,35).

In 1994, Maher describes two cases of fatal AFE in two nulliparous patients in labor with an epidural anesthetic who received saline amnioinfusion for thick meconium staining of the amniotic fluid (36). Possible predisposing factors associated with amniotomy include the use of intrauterine pressure catheters for saline infusion which can lead to trauma to the cervical or uterine blood vessels thus providing a mode of entry. In addition, utilization of a pump under pressure which can increase the resting tone of the uterus potentially forces the amniotic fluid into the maternal circulation. The hypotension and possible toxicity associated with the use of epidural anesthesia may have contributed to the lowering of the pressure gradient further facilitating entry of the amniotic fluid into the maternal circulation. In addition, meconium

TABLE 22-3 Demographic Characteristics of Patients with Amniotic Fluid Embolism

Factor	Mean (+/−SD)
Maternal age	27 (+/−9)
Gravidity	3 (+/−2)
Parity	2 (+/−2)
Maternal weight (kg)	73 (+/−11)
Gestational age (wk)	39 (+/−2)
Birth weight (g)	3519 (+/−732)

Race
  White
  Hispanic
  Black
  Asian
	Number of patients (%)
	29 (63)
	8 (17)
	7 (15)
	2 (4)

Male fetus	35/37 (67)
Twin gestation	1 (2)
Prior elective abortion	9 (20)
Prior spontaneous abortion	8 (17)
History of drug allergy or atopy	19 (41)

Adapted from Clark SL, Hankins GVD, Dudley DA, et al. Amniotic fluid embolism: analysis of the national registry. *Am J Obstet Gynecol* 1995;172(4 Pt 1):1158–1167; discussion 1167–1169.

staining of the amniotic fluid potentially contains leukotrienes and may lead to an anaphylactic reaction.

■ AMNIOTOMY AND AMNIOCENTESIS

Mato describes a case of a 40-year-old patient at 41 weeks of gestation admitted for induction of labor for postdates who arrested immediately following amniotomy and an uneventful combined spinal–epidural 3 hours previously (37). Resuscitation was successful following emergency cesarean delivery, and hysterectomy for severe uterine atony and DIC with massive transfusion of 12 units of packed red blood cells, 24 units of pooled platelets, 8 units of cryoprecipitate, and 8 units of fresh frozen plasma. Although surgical hemostasis was achieved following ligation of uterine vessels and hysterectomy, moderate to severe oozing consistent with DIC continued. Resuscitation also included the use of recombinant coagulation factor VIIa 200 μg/kg over 30 minutes which was associated with improvement of hemostasis. Pathologic examination of peripheral blood revealed few fetal squames cells. Other possible differential diagnoses were ruled out. AFE following amniocentesis is very rare.

■ ATOPY AND MALE FETUS

Clark showed that 41% of the patients had a history of atopy or known drug allergies (5). In the analysis of the national registry, Clark showed that 67% of the pregnant patients with AFE had male fetuses.

■ BLUNT ABDOMINAL TRAUMA

Trauma is a leading nonobstetric cause of maternal death in the United States. The primary causes of trauma in pregnancy include motor vehicle accidents, falls, assaults, homicides, domestic violence, and penetrating wounds. Not only is trauma associated with increased risk of abruption but also fatal hemorrhage and AFE (38). Rainio describes a case AFE in a patient at 38 weeks of gestation who sustained blunt abdominal trauma associated with improper use of a seat belt in a motor vehicle accident. Pathologic examination revealed hematoxylin–eosin staining, phloxine–tartrazine red staining of squamous material in the pulmonary blood vessels. In addition, there was positive immunohistochemical staining for cytokeratins and positive monoclonal antibody staining specific for tryptase-positive granules. The baby also did not survive and died later of anoxic brain damage and pneumonia (39). Ellingsen also describes a case of minor blunt abdominal trauma in a patient whose injuries would not have been associated with AFE had she not been pregnant, although there were no signs of abruption or uterine tear with presumed entry of amniotic fluid into the maternal circulation. Pathologic examination of the lungs revealed blood vessels with mucus and epithelial squames and the lower uterine segment revealed blood vessel with mucus (40). Pluymakers describes a case of blunt abdominal trauma due to a blow in the stomach requiring laparotomy for torsion of the left adnexa in a patient who developed tachypnea and hypotension requiring intubation and hemodynamic support. Pathologic examination of blood drawn from the pulmonary artery and bronchoalveolar lavage demonstrated fetal squames cells (41).

Cervical Suture Removal

Although AFE is most commonly seen in a laboring patient, AFE can have many presentations. Haines described a case of presumed nonfatal AFE associated with pulmonary edema, hypoxemia and oxygen desaturation, and hypotension in a multiparous patient with a history cerclage or cervical suture removal under general anesthesia complicated by placental abruption and required emergency cesarean delivery. Patient had a history of cerclage placement in three prior successful pregnancies followed by six previous recurrent spontaneous abortions (42). This patient had several possible risk factors: Multiparity, premature separation of placenta, and presumed cervical tear during removal of the cervical suture which allowed a mode of entry of the amniotic fluid into the maternal circulation, right side of the heart, and into the pulmonary vasculature. Pluymakers describes a case of AFE in a patient with a history of cervicouterine suture at 14 weeks who was admitted with spontaneous rupture of membranes with meconium-stained fluid, fetal demise, and suspected intrauterine infection for removal of cervicouterine suture and curettage. Patient developed signs and symptoms of AFE requiring intubation, pressure-controlled ventilation with high PEEP, 100% oxygen, up to 20 ppm nitric oxide by inhalation, and hemodynamic support. Pathologic examination of blood aspirated from the pulmonary artery and bronchoalveolar lavage revealed fetal squamous cells and mucin (41).

■ CESAREAN DELIVERY

McDougall describes a case in which a patient developed AFE during a cesarean delivery under general anesthesia following delivery of the placenta (43). Although resuscitation was initially successful, the patient developed sepsis, acute respiratory distress syndrome, and acute renal failure and died on the seventh day. Postmortem examination was suggestive of AFE with evidence of diffuse alveolar damage, DIC, foci of fetal squames in the pulmonary vessels. There was no evidence consistent with a thromboembolism (44).

■ EPIDURAL AND SPINAL BLOCKADE

Sprung describes a case of a 27-year-old patient who had a cesarean delivery of a healthy baby for previous cesarean and failed induction under an uneventful epidural anesthesia. The patient first complained about a funny sensation in her head, became unresponsive, and developed tonic–clonic seizures immediately after delivery of the placenta and exteriorization of the uterus. Patient became hemodynamically unstable with severe hypotension, bradycardia, DIC, and respiratory arrest and desaturation. Resuscitation was successful. The epidural catheter was removed atraumatically prior to the patient receiving blood products, 4 units of FFP, 4 units of PRBCs, and 8 units of cryoprecipitate to treat the coagulopathy. If there is bleeding around the epidural insertion site, correction of coagulopathy is recommended before catheter removal. Spontaneous epidural hematomas rarely develop, but may require surgical laminectomy (45).

Pang suggests that a favorable gradient for amniotic fluid to enter maternal circulation occurred following the sympathetic block during cesarean delivery under spinal anesthesia. This contributed to dilated uterine vessels and effective pooling of fetal debris which were mobilized into the maternal circulation during treatment with vasopressors and return of sympathetic tone. Therefore, avoidance of hypotension with effective coloading of fluids and prophylactic vasopressors during cesarean delivery is recommended to avoid the possibility of circulation of amniotic fluid and debris into the maternal circulation (46).

Bastien describes a case of AFE with the presenting sign of DIC following a forceps-assisted vaginal delivery under epidural anesthesia. Patient developed epistaxis, bleeding from the epidural site, and postpartum hemorrhage associated with uterine atony. Despite aggressive resuscitation and transfusion of multiple blood products including 10 units of PRBCs, 6 packed platelets, 6 units of FFP, patient did not survive.

During coagulopathy and evidence of bleeding, removal of an in situ epidural catheter should not be attempted until the coagulopathy is treated and corrected and the patient survives (47).

Fetal Demise and Second Trimester Abortion

In 1995 Clark found three cases of AFE during second trimester abortions (5). Ray describes a case of AFE in a woman with an intrauterine fetal demise at 18 weeks of gestation. Patient also had a history of asthma and had several allergies to antibiotics. In addition, the fetus was male. Following placement of cervical osmotic dilators and aspiration of amniotic fluid, the patient had a dilation and extraction (D & E) with acute onset of paroxysmal coughing, restlessness, and peripheral cyanosis. The patient developed hypotension, shock, respiratory arrest, pulseless electrical activity, hemorrhage, and DIC. The patient was successfully resuscitated after cardiopulmonary resuscitation, fluid resuscitation, vasopressors, blood products, and uterotonics (48).

Price describes a case of a patient at 24.5 weeks with fetal demise who became profoundly hypotensive and developed severe peripheral cyanosis and DIC during dilation and suction curettage. She was successfully resuscitated and received packed red blood cells, fresh frozen plasma, and cryoprecipitate (49).

The risk of maternal mortality increases with increasing gestational age at time of abortion. The risk is 24 times greater when the abortion is at 20 weeks as compared to at 15 weeks of gestation.

Induction of Labor

Caughey, in a recent cochrane systematic review of randomized controlled trials comparing elective induction of labor versus expectant management of labor, found a decreased risk for cesarean delivery and meconium-stained amniotic fluid with elective induction of labor (50). Although Kramer found medical induction of labor nearly doubled the risk of overall cases of AFE, an association which was stronger for fatal cases, multiple factors, such as, maternal age of 35 years or older, cesarean or instrumented delivery, polyhydramnios, cervical laceration or uterine rupture, placenta previa or abruption, eclampsia, and fetal distress were also associated with an increased risk of AFE (24). Albeit a relative low risk of AFE and a need for standardization in epidemiologic studies of AFE, obstetricians should be aware of this risk when making decisions about elective induction of labor. Price describes a case of a morbidly obese patient who arrested approximately 15 hours after spontaneous rupture of membranes, 6.5 hours after a scalp electrode and an internal pressure catheter were placed and pitocin augmentation started. Resuscitation was not successful (49). Fletcher describes a case of a 41-year-old primigravida at 41 weeks of gestation who presented for induction of labor with prostin and oxytocin infusion and artificial rupture of membranes with meconium-stained fluid and developed fetal late decelerations requiring emergency cesarean delivery under general anesthesia. The patient developed respiratory and renal failure requiring mechanical ventilation and hemodialysis, hemodynamic instability, and coagulopathy requiring hysterectomy. Transthoracic echocardiography did not reveal any obstruction to blood flow and showed mild dilation of the right ventricle and atriums and normal-sized left ventricle (51). Knight also suggests that induction of labor is associated with an increased risk factor of 35%, in addition to cesarean section, multiple pregnancies, and in older ethnic-minority groups in the occurrence of AFE (25). However, many of these cases of AFE are not associated with only one potential risk factor but are multifactorial in their presentation and a direct causal relationship between induction of labor and AFE has not been established.

Multiple Gestations

In a retrospective, Canadian population-based cohort study, Kramer estimated the incidence of AFE was 6/100,000 deliveries for singleton deliveries and 14.8/100,000 for multiple-birth delivery (24). Mortality rate for women with singleton deliveries who had AFE was 13%. Papaioannou reports a possible case of nonfatal AFE in a twin pregnancy associated with premature rupture of membranes and acute respiratory failure following tocolysis with ritodrine. Patient developed severe hypoxemia, hypotension, fever, and coagulopathy 2 hours following a cesarean delivery with spinal anesthesia which required intubation and intensive care (52).

Meconium Staining of Amniotic Fluid

In experimental animal studies, amniotic fluid containing meconium was associated with a higher risk of developing AFE syndrome than filtered amniotic fluid. It was thought that the particulate matter seen in meconium was responsible for the emboli in the maternal lung. In cases of intra-amniotic infection, meconium-stained amniotic fluid is seen more frequently than clear amniotic fluid. Romero reported that immunogenic endotoxins can be detected more frequently in meconium-stained amniotic fluid as compared to clear amniotic fluid (22).

Preeclampsia, Placental Abruption, and Placenta Previa

Ratten describes two cases of AFE associated with cesarean delivery under general for placenta previa. Resuscitation was successful in one patient despite the use of epinephrine, hydrocortisone, defibrillation, and internal cardiac massage. Pathologic examination revealed the presence of amniotic fluid debris in pulmonary arterioles (53).

Ruptured Membranes

Morgan found only two risk factors in his review of AFE in 1979 (54). Multiparity was found in 78% of cases in addition to ruptured membranes. Clark analyzed 121 different risk factors and identified ruptured membranes as the only consistent predisposing maternal risk factor for AFE. Rupture of membranes, either spontaneous or following amniotomy, was seen in 88% of patients with AFE. Onset of symptoms was also temporally related to rupture of membranes, with symptoms occurring within 3 minutes of rupture. Price also describes a case of a patient who developed worsening of shortness of breath associated with an acute sharp back pain and fetal bradycardia following amniotomy with meconium-stained fluid, placement of fetal scalp electrode and an internal pressure catheter. Patient arrested and developed DIC and resuscitation was not successful. The uterus did not reveal a gross tear to account for the portal of entry of amniotic fluid (49).

Uterine Rupture

Greene describes a case of cardiovascular collapse following vaginal delivery with epidural anesthesia in a patient at term with spontaneous contractions and a history of previous low transverse cesarean delivery, resection of a leiomyoma, as well as three spontaneous abortions (55). Immediately following delivery, the patient was found to have a uterine rupture associated with significant bleeding of 1 L, hypotension, and cyanosis. Patient had a cardiopulmonary arrest which was managed with intubation, cardiopulmonary resuscitation, transfusion of PRBCs and fresh frozen plasma, and hysterectomy. Attempts at resuscitation were not successful.

Clinical Presentation

A typical, classic, clinical form of AFE is seen with three phases: Phase 1, respiratory and cardiovascular dysfunction; Phase 2, coagulopathy; Phase 3, acute respiratory distress syndrome and acute renal failure. However, a second, atypical presentation also is seen: Coagulopathy associated with postpartum hemorrhage or acute respiratory distress syndrome or acute renal failure develops without the initial phase of respiratory and cardiovascular dysfunction (56). Clark confirmed that AFE usually occurred during labor and vaginal delivery or in the immediate postpartum period in 19% of cases. He found the most common presenting signs and symptoms were hypotension and signs of nonreassuring fetal status in all cases of AFE. Respiratory symptoms were present in 93%, cardiac arrest in 87%, and cyanosis and coagulopathy in 83% of cases. Seizures occur in 50% of patients with AFE. Typically, AFE may include any or all of the following symptoms (Table 22-4).

Premonitory symptoms include restlessness, agitation, anxiety, numbness, tingling, shivering, and feeling of impending doom.

Pulmonary

Dyspnea, tachypnea, cough, cyanosis, sudden desaturation on pulse oximetry, decrease and loss of end-tidal carbon dioxide may be seen in intubated patients.

Cardiac

Parturients with AFE may develop tachycardia, hypotension, cardiac arrest, and pulmonary edema.

Coagulopathy

Postpartum hemorrhage, uterine atony, and DIC may be the only sign of AFE.

Neurologic

A presenting sign of AFE may include seizures and coma.

Fetal

Fetal bradycardia may be the first sign of AFE and may precede the onset of symptoms of AFE or follow shortly thereafter (Fig. 22-2).

Pathogenesis: Animal Model

Early animal studies were inconsistent and the pathophysiology of AFE was thought to be associated with pulmonary vasospasm, pulmonary hypertension, and right heart failure. Variability in factors such as, the use of heterologous versus homogenous, filtered versus meconium-stained amniotic fluid of varying amounts in nonpregnant versus pregnant animals, etc. contributed to variable responses ranging from transient hemodynamic and pulmonary changes in sheep, dogs, and calves to death in rabbits. Steiner and Lushbaugh demonstrated that injection of human amniotic fluid and meconium into rabbits and dogs led to death in most cases (57). Attwood et al. demonstrated that injection of human amniotic fluid and meconium in dogs caused a significant but inconsistent increase in pulmonary vascular resistance, central venous pressure, and pulmonary artery pressures. Neither Spence nor Stolte could reproduce the syndrome associated with AFE

TABLE 22-4 Comparative Table of Signs and Symptoms of Amniotic Fluid Embolism

Signs and Symptoms	Knight Number of Patients (%)	Morgan Numbers of Patients (%)	Clark Number of Patients (%)
Maternal premonitory symptoms	28 (47)		
Respiratory		(51)	
Pulmonary edema/ARDS		65 (24)	28 (93)
Cyanosis			38 (83)
Dyspnea	37 (62)		22 (49)
Bronchospasm			7 (15)
Cough			3 (7)
Cardiac			
Hypotension	38 (63)	(27)	43 (100)
Cardiopulmonary arrest	24 (43)		40 (87)
Dysrhythmias	16 (27)		
Other			
Coagulopathy	37 (62)	(12)	38 (83)
Hemorrhage	39/60 (65)		11 (23)
Seizures	9 (15)	(10)	22 (48)
Fetal			
Fetal bradycardia	26 (43)		30 (100)

Adapted from: Knight M, Tuffnell D, Brocklehurst P, et al. UK Obstetric Surveillance System. Incidence and risk factors for amniotic-fluid embolism. *Obstet Gynecol* 2010;115(5):910–917.

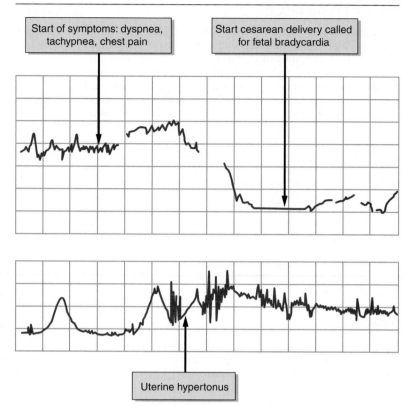

FIGURE 22-2 Fetal heart rate tracing in a patient with amniotic fluid embolism with clinical presentation and symptoms occurring during labor requiring aggressive resuscitation for shock and DIC.

when homologous amniotic fluid was injected into pregnant rabbits and when amniotic fluid containing meconium was infused into monkeys (58,59). Hankins injected pregnant goats with 2.5 mL/kg of autologous amniotic fluid and reported an acute and transient but marked increase in both systemic and pulmonary vascular resistance associated with right heart failure, in addition to a minimal increase in cardiac output. However, injection of amniotic fluid containing meconium produced left heart failure and hypoxia associated with a greater and significant decrease in the cardiac output and the increase in systemic and pulmonary vascular resistance was significantly greater. Therefore, Hankins was able to confirm in the goat model, that severe pulmonary hypertension develops acutely following AFE especially in meconium-stained amniotic fluid. In addition, a transient left ventricular dysfunction was also seen (60,61). Maternal outcomes appear to be worse in Clark's analysis of cases in the registry of AFE associated with meconium-stained amniotic fluid. However, it is difficult to say whether the meconium staining was caused by a sign of AFE, fetal stress, or meconium-stained AFE caused the syndrome associated with AFE (Table 22-5).

Pathophysiology

Air, thromboembolism, as well as AFE were thought to cause a mechanical obstruction which lead to severe pulmonary hypertension, decreased left-sided filling, and consequently hypotension. This could cause an increase in pulmonary artery pressure, pulmonary capillary wedge pressure (PCWP), and consequently right-sided filling pressure and elevated central venous pressure. This mechanical obstruction could cause V/Q mismatch and hypoxemia and obstruction to venous drainage and may lead to superior vena cava syndrome and facial edema.

The proposed pathophysiology associated with AFE is multifactorial and includes immunoglobulin E, endotoxins associated with sepsis, and direct physiologic effects of the amniotic fluid (62). The most current theory of how AFE

impacts the maternal circulation leading to the anaphylactoid syndrome of pregnancy, AFE syndrome is that the amniotic fluid contains a complex mixture of maternal extracellular fluid, fetal urine, fetal squamous cells, lanugo hairs, vernix caseosa, mucin and meconium, in addition to fetal antigens and potent vasoactive components, such as, thromboplastin, plasmin activator, vasoconstrictor endothelin, platelet-activating factor, and prostaglandin F2 alpha, a potent pulmonary vasoconstrictor. Endogenous mediators include histamine, bradykinins, endothelin, leukotriene, and arachidonic acid metabolites. These immune immunoglobulin IgE-mediated anaphylactic or nonimmune non-IgE anaphylactoid reactions to amniotic fluid both involve mast cell and basophil stimulation, cause activation of complement, thrombin and coagulation cascade and are potentially fatal and may require emergency treatment (63). Leukotrienes in the amniotic fluid are thought to cause a localized or generalized anaphylactoid reaction, which leads to alveolar capillary leak and pulmonary edema. This anaphylactoid reaction is usually associated with a clinical presentation of rash, bronchospasm, cardiovascular arrest. Elevation in serum tryptase, a serine protease, and specific and sensitive enzyme marker of mast cells degranulation and anaphylactoid or anaphylactic reactions may be seen in laboratory tests (19). The presence of these immunologic factors is suggested by a higher incidence of AFE with male fetus and in patients with a history of drug allergy. In addition, the presence of intravascular macrophages suggests a nonspecific immune mechanism to reactive foreign substances. Depending on the insult and injury, there are cases in which patients develop eosinophilic myocarditis, focal eosinophilic pneumonitis, and focal portal eosinophilic hepatitis. Definitive diagnosis is confirmed by the immunohistologic demonstration of amniotic fluid-derived mucin, detection of fetal keratin squames, and careful and systematic examination of the cervix at autopsy or hysterectomy (64,65).

The mechanisms for myocardial dysfunction that lead to early hypotension are multifactorial. Proposed explanations

TABLE 22-5 Effects of Amniotic Fluid Embolism in Whole Animal Models

Principal Investigator	Year	Animal (#)[a] Animaldied	Anesthetized	Pregnant	Filtered AF	Meconium AF	AF Species (autologous[b])
Steiner & Luschbaugh	1941	Rabbit[a] (9)/ Dog (11)	No/No	No	No effect/Not examined	Yes/Yes	Human/ Human
Cron et al.	1952	Rabbit[a] (14)	Variable	No	Not examined	Yes	Human
Schneider	1955	Dog[a] (10)	No	No	Not examined	Yes	Human
Jacques et al.	1960	Dog (9)	Yes	No	Not examined	Not examined	Human/ Dog[b]
Halmagyi et al.	1962	Sheep (7)	Yes	No	No effect	Not examined	Human
Atwood & Downing	1965	Dog (44)	Yes	No	Yes	Yes	Human
Stolte et al.	1967	Rhesus Monkey (12)	Yes	Yes	Not examined	Yes	Human/ Monkey[b]
MacMillan	1968	Rabbit[a] (12)	No	No	Not examined	Not examined	Human
Reis et al.	1969	Sheep (10)	Yes	Yes	Yes	Not examined	Sheep[b]
Dutta et al.	1970	Rabbit[a] (34)	Yes	No	No examined	Not examined	Human
Adamsons et al.	1971	Rhesus Monkey (9)	Yes	Yes	Not examined	Not examined	Monkey[b]
Kitzmeller & Lucas	1972	Cat	Yes	No	No effect	No effect	Human
Spence & Mason	1974	Rabbit (26)	No	Yes	No effect	Not examined	Rabbit[b]
Reeves et al.	1974	Calf (14)	No	No	Not examined	Not examined	Calf[b]
Azegami & Mori	1986	Rabbit[a] (36)	No	No	No effect	Not examined	Human
Richards et al.	1988	Rat	Yes	No	Yes		Human
Hankins et al.	1993	Goat	Yes	Yes	Yes		Goat[b]
Petroianu et al.	1999	Mini Pigs	Yes	Yes	Yes		Mini Pig[b]

[a]Death of animal.
[b]Autologous amniotic fluid.
AF, amniotic fluid.
Adapted from: Dildy GA, Belfort MA, Clark SL. Anaphylactoid syndrome of pregnancy (amniotic fluid embolism). In: Belfort MA, Saade G, Foley MR, Phelan JP, Dildy GA, eds. *Critical Care Obstetrics*. 5th ed. Wiley-Blackwell; 2010:466–474.

include myocardial failure in response to sudden pulmonary hypertension, a direct myocardial depressant effect of vasoconstrictive mediators in amniotic fluid, deviation of the intraventricular septum due to right ventricular dilation, and possibly ischemic myocardial injury from hypoxemia (66).

In addition to cardiopulmonary instability and shock, and seizures, disseminated intravascular coagulopathy is a complication of AFE. The etiology of coagulopathy is thought to be multifactorial. Dolak showed that meconium staining of amniotic fluid in maternal blood activates the procoagulopathic effects of amniotic fluid. Meconium-stained amniotic fluid was shown to result in a significant decrease in activating clotting time and an increase in rate of clot formation in an in vitro model (67). In 2004, Dolak showed that a dose-dependent effect of amniotic fluid on decreasing ACT and time to peak clot in a highly sensitive model of AF-induced coagulation using the sonoclot analyzer (68). In addition, tissue factor found in amniotic fluid which increases with gestation may facilitate the initiation of clot formation. Thrombin stimulates the release of vascular endothelin which may depress myocardial and myometrial contractility and lead to hemodynamic instability and uterine atony. In Matsuda's review of nine patients, four of whom did not survive, 50% of nonsurvivors had a twin pregnancy which increases the risk of postpartum atony also developed significant shock and uterine atony (69).

Diagnosis

The diagnosis of AFE is clinical and a diagnosis of exclusion, and should be suspected when a pregnant woman suddenly develops significant hypotension, coagulopathy, and respiratory and fetal distress during labor, cesarean delivery, dilatation and evacuation or immediately after delivery. In addition, continuous pulse oximetry and arterial blood gas measurements should evaluate extent of hypoxemia and acidosis. Serial complete blood counts and coagulation studies and TEG may identify early coagulopathy.

Nonspecific and Specific Laboratory Tests

Identification of squamous cells in the maternal pulmonary arterial circulation is not pathognomonic of AFE, since contamination of squamous cells during insertion of PA catheters may occur in pregnant as well as nonpregnant patients. Therefore, blood from the distal port of PA catheter should be aspirated as described by Masson's technique (16), heparinized and analyzed utilizing Papanicolaou's method. Squamous cells coated with neutrophils or thrombocytes, accompanied by fetal debris, or eosinophilic granular material with adherent leukocytes is more suggestive of AFE. Routine staining, with alcian blue, hematoxylin, and eosin, of maternal lung sections may not identify fetal mucin in the maternal lung sections. Proposed biochemical markers of AFE include zinc coproporphyrin, sialyl Tn antigen, and compliment C3 and C4. Kobayashi describes the immunohistochemical staining with the sensitive monoclonal antibody TKH-2 against fetal antigen (sialyl Tn) which is a more sensitive method to detect AF-derived mucin in lung sections (64). Measuring zinc coproporphyrin I, a characteristic fetal-gut component of meconium, in maternal plasma may also be a sensitive method to diagnose AFE (70) (Table 22-6).

Transesophageal Echocardiography

Both transthoracic and transesophageal echocardiography has been used in the early diagnosis and management of AFE. The efficacy of echocardiography is a sensitive tool to evaluate cardiac function, intravascular volume status, and identification of the embolism by confirming acute pulmonary vasoconstriction, right ventricular dilation, and a failing left ventricle with deviation of the intraventricular septum is well documented (9,71). The use of echocardiography led to the early diagnosis and treatment with the successful use of cardiopulmonary bypass. Utilizing TEE, Stanten confirmed the development of severe pulmonary vasoconstriction and right heart failure within 10 minutes of onset of symptoms. Therefore, an acute phase of severe pulmonary vasoconstriction is transient which may either resolve spontaneously or lead to left ventricular failure. In 1999, Shechtman confirmed the diagnosis of fatal AFE associated with occurrence of severe pulmonary artery hypertension and right heart failure by transesophageal echocardiography within 15 minutes of the onset of symptoms. In 2009, Vellayappan described a case of cardiac arrest and suspected AFE following rupture of membranes in a woman in labor who was delivered by emergency cesarean under general anesthesia. A TEE performed during the cesarean delivery confirmed a large mobile mass, thrombus, which extended from the right atrium through a patent foramen ovale into the left atrium. This thrombus-like embolus could have initially been formed from amniotic fluid and because of the procoagulant activity of amniotic fluid converted to a thrombus. Therefore, the use of TEE not only confirmed a transseptal paradoxical AFE, but also facilitated the therapeutic treatment of AFE by its removal (72).

National and United Kingdom AFE Registries

The criteria for entry into the National AFE Registry and United Kingdom AFE Registry have been standardized. Table 22-2 describes the inclusion criteria for AFE.

Differential Diagnosis

The differential diagnosis of AFE includes obstetric, nonobstetric, and possible complications of anesthesia as possible etiologies of symptoms associated with AFE. The diagnosis of AFE is based on presenting symptoms and clinical course

TABLE 22-6 Nonspecific and Specific Laboratory Tests

Nonspecific
ECG
Tachycardia
Dysrhythmias
Ischemia
CBC
Decreased hemoglobin and hematocrit
Coagulation profile
Prolonged PT and PTT
Decreased fibrinogen
CHEST X-RAY
Pulmonary edema
ARDS
ABG
Respiratory acidosis
Hypoxemia
Intrapulmonary shunting
ECHOCARDIOGRAPHY
Acute left heart failure
V/Q scan
Pulmonary angiogram or spiral CT scan
Specific Biochemical Markers
Maternal zinc coproporphyrin, a component of meconium
Serum tryptase (normal <1 ng/mL)
Histologic examination: Squamous cells in the cervix, lungs, and other organs
A sensitive antimucin monocloncal antibody, TKH-2, immune-staining test detects AFE, by reacting with meconium and mucin-type glycoprotein, Sialyl Tn antigen, derived from AF, to stain the lung tissue
Identify amniotic debris in pulmonary edema fluid

and is one of exclusion. Laboratory and pathologic findings only support the diagnosis of AFE (Table 22-7).

Anaphylactic Response During Pregnancy

The incidence and severity of anaphylactic reactions in obstetric patients is increased due to greater reactivity of the immunologic response (73). Progesterone, depressed T-cell response, and cytokine signaling may all play a role in the heightened response in pregnant patients. In response to an antigen, histamine, produced by basophils and mast cells primarily in skin, lungs, blood vessels, and gastrointestinal tract, in addition to cytokines, serine proteases and prostaglandins are released producing constriction of smooth muscles, increased permeability of blood vessels, and direct-acting H-2 receptor-mediated relaxing effect and indirect-acting of H-1 receptor release of NO and prostanoids. This response may range from a subclinical reaction, allergic reaction (atopy), anaphylactoid reaction (a nonimmunologic mast cell activation, and non-IgE-mediated

TABLE 22-7 Differential Diagnosis of Amniotic Fluid Embolism

Obstetric Causes
Peripartum cardiomyopathy
Eclampsia
Placental abruption
Intrauterine infection or septic shock
Ruptured uterus
Postpartum hemorrhage

Anesthetic complications
    Total spinal or high epidural block
    Local anesthetic toxicity
    Pulmonary aspiration

Medication error
Nonobstetric causes

Pulmonary thromboembolism
    Air embolism
    Acute myocardial infarction
    Aortic dissection
    Adverse drug reaction or anaphylactic reaction
    Seizure
    Cerebral hemorrhage or cerebrovascular accident

response) to true anaphylaxis (an immediate type 1 response or delayed type 4 hypersensitivity and IgE-mediated response). Common antigens include antibiotics, oxytocin, muscle relaxants, local anesthetics, ranitidine, insulin, latex, blood and blood products, colloid solutions, laminaria, contrast media, snake antivenom, seminal plasma, and chlorhexidine. The anaphylaxis response varies from grade I, associated with skin symptoms and possible mild fever reactions, such as, itching, burning, flushing, swelling hives, and rash; grade II, associated with a nonlife-threatening, respiratory and gastrointestinal disturbances, such as, tachycardia, hypotension, and palpitations; grade III, associated with shock, life-threatening smooth muscle spasm, such as, laryngeal edema, bronchospasm, pulmonary edema, characterized by wheezing, coughing; and grade IV, associated with cardiac or respiratory arrest. In a few cases, a biphasic presentation is characterized by a recurrence of symptoms without a repeat exposure to the antigen. Management includes establishing an airway and providing ventilatory support with 100% oxygenation; cardiovascular support and correction of hypotension with aggressive fluid resuscitation; use of vasopressors, such as, phenylephrine, a pure alpha-1 agonist and vasoconstrictor, helps maintain blood pressure and correct systemic vasodilation, and epinephrine, norepinephrine, and dopamine should be considered for inotropic support. Epinephrine, a beta-2 receptor agonist stimulant, causes an anti-inflammatory response, inhibiting release of mediators from mast cells and basophils. Vasopressin may also be used and causes minimal vasoconstriction of the pulmonary vasculature and milrinone or other phosphodiesterase inhibitors in patients with heart failure should be considered. General support is provided with H-1 receptor blockers, diphenhydramine, H-2 receptor blockers, ranitidine, and corticosteroids, such as, methylprednisolone.

Immunologic Response

Plasma tryptase levels, a mast cell enzyme, may be elevated and is helpful in the diagnosis of AFE (17). Also, C3 and C4 levels are significantly decreased in women with AFE and

may suggest complement activation plays a greater role in AFE compared to mast cell degranulation (74).

Anaphylactoid Syndrome During Pregnancy

The clinical presentation and pathophysiology of AFE are similar to type 1 hypersensitivity reactions which vary in a continuum from a mild reaction to anaphylaxis and shock. Clark suggests that AFE variability in severity is due to variation of the antigenic exposure and the individual response. Although anaphylactic response results from re-exposure to an antigen, AFE occurs in nulliparas as well as multiparas.

Arterial Blood Gases

Arterial blood gases may show changes consistent with hypoxemia and metabolic acidosis.

CBC with Platelets

Coagulopathy is associated with AFE in 83% of patients. The onset can occur as quickly as 10 to 30 minutes from onset of symptoms or may be delayed by as many as 4 hours. There are various factors which may be associated with coagulopathy. Amniotic fluid may have a procoagulant effect. Tissue factor contained in amniotic fluid binds factor VII and activates the extrinsic coagulation pathway. In addition, increased levels of plasminogen activation inhibitor 1 also seen in amniotic fluid may cause fibrinolysis and be a factor in coagulopathy. Circulating myometrial depressant factor and uterine hypoperfusion may lead to uterine atony and postpartum hemorrhage contributing to a consumptive coagulopathy.

Prothrombin Time, Partial Thromboplastin, Fibrinogen

There may be evidence of DIC with prolonged PT, low fibrinogen, low hematocrit, and decreased platelets. Increased fibrinolysis is associated with increased fibrin split products and D-dimers.

Thromboelastography

Thromboelastography (TEG) provides real time assessment of hemostasis including platelet function and fibrinolysis during management of coagulopathy and postpartum hemorrhage associated with AFE. Annecke describes an algorithm-based approach in the management of coagulopathy and hemorrhage in a fatal case of AFE (75). Perhaps in the future, rotational thromboelastometry will provide real time assessment of hemostasis as reference values are validated during pregnancy, nonhemorrhagic deliveries, and postpartum hemorrhage.

Chest X-ray

This may be normal or show an enlarged heart or pulmonary edema.

12-lead ECG

An ECG may show tachycardia, nonspecific ST–T changes, or a right heart strain pattern.

Monitoring

In addition to basic routine monitoring including ECG, pulse oximetry, end-tidal carbon dioxide, continuous fetal monitoring until delivery, invasive monitoring with intra-arterial catheter, central venous catheterization, pulmonary artery catheterization, transesophageal echocardiography (TEE) may show evidence of acute right ventricular pressure overload with enlargement of the right ventricle and main pulmonary trunk. Acute pulmonary hypertension and vasospasm may be transient and a cause of sudden death. Patients with intrinsic pulmonary disease may have elevated pulmonary artery pressures with diastolic pressures greater than 6 to 10 mm Hg greater than the PCWP. However, of the patients who survive, some may develop left ventricular failure with left ventricular dysfunction associated with elevated pulmonary artery diastolic pressures and a gradient between pulmonary artery diastolic pressure and PCWP of less than 6 mm Hg. Echocardiography may also reveal left atrial enlargement (LAE), decreased ejection fraction, and hypokinesis consistent with left ventricular failure. The timeline of the development of symptoms and signs of AFE and the exclusion of peripartum cardiomyopathy lead to the diagnosis consistent with AFE.

Initial Cardiopulmonary Resuscitation

Recently Lipman evaluated the quality of obstetric advanced cardiac life support (ACLS) performed during the management of 18 videotaped simulations of maternal AFE and resultant cardiac arrest for suboptimal cardiopulmonary resuscitation (76). A checklist containing ten current American Heart Association (AHA) recommendations for ACLS in obstetric patients was utilized. Lipman found multiple deficits in the provision of CPR to parturients during simulated arrests: Left uterine displacement and placement of a firm back support prior to compressions were not provided in 44% and 22% of cases, respectively, resulting in improper delivery of compressions and ventilations 44% and 50% of the time, respectively. There was a delay of 1 minute and 42 seconds in calling the neonatal team and 83% of neonatal teams were called only after the simulated patient was completely unresponsive. Also, basic information to facilitate neonatal resuscitation was not provided to the neonatal teams in 50% of cases as required by neonatal resuscitation provider guidelines. Lipman suggested frequent simulation training, clinical multidisciplinary obstetric team drills, and recertification or development of an AHA obstetric life support course certification, and inclusion of didactic modules specific to resuscitation of pregnant women in ACLS courses (77).

Management

Early recognition of AFE and aggressive pulmonary and cardiovascular resuscitation, and preemptive management of known sequelae is essential for improving the possibility of a successful outcome. Recent studies report a decrease in mortality rate from 61% to 86% before the mid-1990s to 13.3% to 44% since the mid-2000s (23–25,28). The team approach with early intervention by the obstetrician and anesthesiologist, and intensivist improves maternal resuscitation and maternal and neonatal outcomes. In addition, invasive monitoring with intra-arterial, central venous access and pulmonary artery catheter, TEE, and urinary catheterization facilitates management of volume status and blood product resuscitation, vasopressor therapy and pulmonary, myocardial and renal dysfunction. More invasive approaches to resuscitation have been reported, including exchange transfusion, ECMO, cardiopulmonary bypass, a right ventricular assist device, and uterine artery embolization (8,78). Both aerosolized prostacyclin and inhaled nitric oxide (NO) act as direct pulmonary vasodilators and have been successfully used to treat acute pulmonary vasoconstriction (10,47,66,79).

ANESTHETIC CONSIDERATIONS
Oxygenation and Ventilatory Support

Maintain oxygenation with intubation, mechanical ventilation with 100% oxygen, $PaCO_2$ between 28 and 32 mm Hg, mean pH of 7.42, and mean bicarbonate level 18 mmol/L. Pregnant patients typically have a respiratory alkalosis with compensatory metabolic acidosis. $PaCO_2$ greater than 32 to 34 mm Hg may indicate hypoventilation and lead to respiratory acidosis.

Cardiovascular Support and Resuscitation

Follow AHA guidelines for CPR in pregnancy and ACLS protocols with patient in the supine position with left uterine displacement (77). In the majority of cases of AFE presenting prior to delivery, immediate delivery of fetus is essential to improve venous return to the heart and cardiac output, facilitate maternal resuscitation and minimize fetal morbidity and mortality by limiting fetal exposure to hypoxia during maternal hypotension, and resuscitation. Perimortem delivery within 5 to 15 minutes correlates with neonatal outcomes of 67% intact survival (Table 22-8). Alon highlights the importance of left uterine displacement during resuscitation and immediate cesarean delivery to facilitate maternal resuscitation (80).

Establish intravenous access with several large bore catheters or a central venous catheter. Optimize cardiac preload with fluid resuscitation with crystalloid, colloid, and blood products to maintain circulating volume (81). Invasive monitoring with pulmonary artery catheter and TEE facilitates correction of pulmonary edema and treatment of left heart failure with inotropes, diuretics, and vasopressors. Although not always successful, pulmonary embolectomy, cardiopulmonary bypass, and the use of extracorporeal circulatory support may be considered (9,78). Afterload reduction may be beneficial in restoring cardiac output in some cases. Hemodialysis may treat fluid overload, improve cardiac function, and help remove immunologic mediators in anuric patients.

Restore Uterine Tone

Postpartum hemorrhage contributes significantly to increased morbidity and mortality. The primary treatment of postpartum hemorrhage includes strategies and measures to improve uterine tone, blood and fluid resuscitation, and replacement

TABLE 22-8 Maternal Cardiac Arrest to Delivery Time and Neonatal Outcome Following Amniotic Fluid Embolism Predelivery in 16 Patients with Cardiac Arrest while Fetus was in Utero with Known Interval

Interval (min)	Neonatal Survival (16 total number of patients)	Neurologically Intact Neonatal Survival (%)
<5	3/3	2/3 (67)
5–15	3/3	2/3 (67)
16–25	2/5	2/5 (40)
26–35	3/4	1/4 (25)
36–54	0/1	0/1 (0%)

Reproduced with permission from: Clark SL, Hankins GVD, Dudley DA, et al. Amniotic fluid embolism: analysis of the national registry. *Am J Obstet Gynecol* 1995;172(4 Pt 1):1158–1167; discussion 1167–1169.

of coagulation factors in addition to surgical and invasive procedures. The following uterotonics should be considered including oxytocin (pitocin) 40 to 80 IU in 500 mL to 1,000 mL of lactated ringers solution or 0.9% saline solution intravenous infusion over 4 to 8 hours, methylergonovine (methergine) 0.2 mg intramuscular may repeat dose in 30 minutes. Carboprost (15 methyl prostaglandin F2 alpha, hemabate) 250 μg intramuscular or intramyometrial may be given every 15 minutes with a maximum dose of 2 mg. Misoprostol (cytotec) 800 to 1,000 mg per rectum or 400 mg buccal, and calcium chloride up to 1 g intravenous may also be considered to improve uterine tone. Calcium is helpful in patients previously receiving magnesium sulfate or patients receiving multiple blood products during hysterectomy for postpartum hemorrhage.

In 2010, Knight reported the survival of 13 of 14 women treated with human rFVIIa for coagulopathy (25). In 2010, Franchini also reports in a large case series including international registries of 272 cases of postpartum hemorrhage the successful "off-label" use of rFVIIa in the management of postpartum hemorrhage unresponsive to medical and surgical procedures which may include cases of AFE (82). The dose of 81.5 μg/kg rFVIIa is effective in reducing or stopping postpartum hemorrhage in 85% of the cases. Franchini recommends correction of acidosis, thrombocytopenia, hypofibrinogenemia, hypothermia, and hypocalcemia prior to administration of initial dose of rFVIIa 90 μg/kg. A second dose of rFVIIa may be given 20 minutes following the first dose if there is no response. Hysterectomy should be considered if postpartum hemorrhage continues despite two dose of rFVIIa and correction of all factors which may negatively impact the efficacy of rFVIIa (82).

Correction of Coagulopathy

Clark found the development of coagulopathy in 83% of cases of AFE in the triad of symptoms presenting with AFE in addition to respiratory distress and cardiac arrest. Coagulopathy may develop as early as 10 to 30 minutes from onset of symptoms, may be the only initial presenting sign, or may be delayed in hours in presentation. Although the coagulopathy may be multifactorial, associated with the presence of procoagulant and tissue factor, activation of the extrinsic coagulation pathway, fibrinolysis, hypothermia, etc. management requires basic resuscitation and "all hands on deck". Treatment of DIC may require massive transfusion of fresh frozen plasma, packed RBCs, platelets, and cryoprecipitate utilizing a rapid volume infuser. Activation of a massive transfusion protocol with notification of the blood bank facilitates the prompt delivery of needed blood products in a timely manner. Use of blood warmers, heating blankets help prevent hypothermia and associated coagulopathy, thrombocytopenia, dysrhythmias, and peripheral tissue ischemia. In addition, hypocalcemia, hyperkalemia, and pulmonary edema should be avoided. Cryoprecipitate restores low fibronectin levels in addition to fibrinogen, clotting factors and facilitates the removal of antigenic substances.

Annecke describes an algorithm-based approach in managing coagulopathy and hemorrhage in a fatal case of AFE which included the use of thromboelastometry during administration of tranexamic acid, high-dose fibrinogen and platelets, 1:1 transfusion regimen of packed red blood cells and fresh frozen plasma, in addition to the use of prothrombin complex concentrate (75).

The goal of transfusion of blood products to correct coagulopathy with platelets, fresh frozen plasma, and cryoprecipitate should be to maintain a platelet count greater than 50,000/mm^3 and a fibrinogen level greater than 100,000 mg/dL. Continued

coagulopathy despite adequate transfusion of blood products may require the use of rFVIIa to prevent fatal exsanguination (3,7). Recently, Huber evaluated the effectiveness of rFVIIa in avoiding hysterectomy postpartum in the management of severe postpartum hemorrhage due to uterine atony (32%), placenta increta (9%), and one case of AFE was included in a large single center study (83). Huber found that the administration of rFVIIa was effective in stopping the postpartum hemorrhage and avoiding postpartum hysterectomy after conservative medical and surgical measures had failed in 20/22 women (91%). Two patients with persistent hemorrhage despite rFVIIa treatment, who required postpartum hysterectomy, had placenta increta. No thromboembolic event was described (83).

However, major organ thrombosis is a potential, very serious complication of rFVIIa administration. A recent retrospective systematic review of AFE patients with massive hemorrhage who had surgery to control bleeding confirms negative significantly worse outcomes including death and permanent disability in 88% of patients receiving rFVIIa compared with 39% of patients who did not receive rFVIIa. In addition among survivors, 75% of patients receiving rFVIIa had permanent disability as compared with 19% of patients who did not receive rFVIIa. Permanent disability includes coma, stroke, memory loss, pulmonary hypertension, and new systemic hypertension in patients receiving rFVIIa may have been caused by organ thrombosis (84). Therefore, Leighton recommends the initial therapy of AFE-associated consumptive coagulopathy should consist of blood component replacement, including PRBC, FFP, platelets, cryoprecipitate, and possibly fibrinogen concentrate. rFVIIa should be considered in AFE patients only when the hemorrhage cannot be stopped by massive blood component replacement and surgery after consultation with the hematologist.

Obstetric and Surgical Control Hemorrhage

Conservative surgical procedures including B-Lynch suture, internal iliac or uterine artery ligation, internal uterine tamponade with Bakri balloon, and uterine artery radiologic embolization may be considered initially in patients wanting additional children (82). Although early embolization or ligation of uterine artery may preserve fertility, hysterectomy may be lifesaving (85). Goldszmidt reported two cases of AFE associated with hemorrhage with successful uterine artery embolization to control hemorrhage in lieu of hysterectomy (86). However, cesarean hysterectomy may be required to establish surgical hemostasis if less invasive measures have been unsuccessful.

Managing an in situ Epidural Catheter

If hemorrhage and DIC occurs in association with AFE in a patient with an in situ epidural catheter, confirm correction of coagulopathy before removing the epidural catheter. The patient should be monitored and neurologic function should be assessed frequently for the development of spinal or epidural hematoma with an in situ catheter and after its removal.

Other Additional Considerations

Epinephrine is an alpha- and beta-adrenergic agonist which mediates cyclic adenosine monophosphate and results in vasoconstriction, bronchodilation, and decreased mediators release from mast cells and basophils. Although a Cochrane systematic review was unable to make any recommendations regarding the use of epinephrine for the treatment of anaphylaxis, epinephrine is the treatment of choice for anaphylaxis (87). In addition to epinephrine, inhaled beta 2-agonists are used in the case of respiratory compromise (87).

As adjuvant therapies, **H1–H2-antihistamines** and steroids may also be used although there is little data to support their use. During an acute allergic reaction, mediators including tryptase, mast cell carboxypeptidase, platelet-activating factor, prostaglandins, leukotrienes, and cytokines are released. Antihistamines are used to downregulate this allergic response by combining with and stabilizing the histamine receptor. H1-antihistamines, such as diphenhydramine, decrease itching, flushing, hives, sneezing, rhinorrhea. H-2 antihistamines, such as ranitidine, decrease vascular permeability, flushing, gastric acid secretion, hypotension, tachycardia, mucous production. There is a mild additive effect when both H1- and H2-antihistamines are given to decrease vascular permeability, flushing, and hypotension. However, a Cochrane systematic review of the use of H1-antihistamines for the treatment of anaphylaxis could not make any recommendations for clinical practice (88).

High-dose corticosteroids have an anti-inflammatory effect by down-regulating the late-phase eosinophilic inflammatory response. Action requires time for protein synthesis and should be given early after initial resuscitation. Short term use of glucocorticoids may prevent or lessen the biphasic response seen in anaphylactic reactions. Glucocorticoids, such as, hydrocortisone 200 mg, may be given intravenously or intramuscularly followed by a course of several days. However, a Cochrane systematic review could not make any recommendations for clinical practice (73,89).

Anecdotal cases involving the use of various alternative treatments with successful outcomes are well documented but should not be considered as the standard of care at this time. McDonnell reported the successful use of inhaled nitric oxide to treat right heart failure and hypoxemia (10).

Plasma exchange transfusion should be considered as an extension of supportive care. Knight described the use of exchange transfusion in seven women with AFE, all of whom survived (25).

Newer Strategies in the Management of AFE

Cardiopulmonary bypass and pulmonary artery thromboembolectomy have been used successfully in the treatment of AFE (90). ECMO and intra-aortic balloon counterpulsation (IABP) have been used successfully in patients with left ventricular failure unresponsive to medical treatment (4,6).

■ MATERNAL AND FETAL OUTCOMES

Can Outcomes be Predicted and Affected?

In 2010, Oi identified several fatal factors associated with maternal death in patients with AFE (32). These included multiparity, noncesarean delivery at full term, and three clinical manifestations: Cardiac arrest, dyspnea, and loss of consciousness. In addition, serum sialyl Tn levels were significantly higher in patient with fatal AFE than nonfatal AFE and may be prognostic of poor outcome.

In 1995, Clark reported an overall maternal mortality rate of 61%. Death occurred within 2 hours of onset of symptoms in 36% of cases and within 5 hours in 63% of cases. Of patients who were successfully resuscitated and survived cardiac arrest, only 8% survived neurologically intact (5). In 2009, Matsuda reviewed the clinical records of nine patients who had died from AFE in a tertiary care center between 1989 and 2000. A mortality rate of 44.4% was reported. Matsuda found a difference in the mean interval between the

onset of clinical symptoms and treatment was significantly shorter for survivors than for nonsurvivors, 48 minutes (range 10 to 90 minutes) and 137.5 minutes (range 75 to 180 minutes) respectively. Also, the number of failed organs was significantly fewer for the survivors compared to nonsurvivors. Therefore, early diagnosis and treatment of AFE is critical for survival. For long-term survival, patients who survive the initial phases of AFE require a multidisciplinary approach to the intensive care of failed organs which may include lungs, heart, liver, kidney, and GI tract (69).

The time interval to delivery following maternal arrest associated with the best neonatal outcomes is 5 to 15 minutes (91). Stehr describes a case of AFE of successful resuscitation of mother and newborn following maternal cardiac arrest prior to delivery complicated by coagulopathy, severe hemorrhage, and a subcapsular hepatic hematoma. A short interval of 9 minutes to decision to proceed with a perimortem section contributed to the successful outcome. Development of an interdisciplinary alerting system for emergency cesarean delivery including perimortem cesarcan delivery is critical to successful resuscitation and good outcome (92,91).

For cases of AFE at time of cesarean delivery, immediate initiation of resuscitative measures while still in the operating room may facilitate a successful outcome.

Knight reported successful outcomes associated with management techniques which included hysterectomy, exchange transfusion, plasma exchange, and rFVIIa as compared to supportive treatment alone (25).

Use of Hypothermia

Hosono describes a case of successful recovery from delayed AFE with prolonged cardiac resuscitation with permissive hypothermia during rapid transfusion of multiple blood products. Although hypothermia may protect the brain and other vital organs during hemorrhagic shock, hypothermia may lead to coagulopathy and dysrhythmias (93).

Fetal Outcomes

Although perinatal outcome is reported to be only 21%, 50% of these infants had permanent neurologic injury. Clark reported 60% of patients developed AFE while the fetus was alive in utero. Although a 79% fetal survival rate has been reported, only 39% of these infants survived neurologically intact (5). In 2010, perinatal mortality rate is 135/1,000 births (25). An arrest to delivery time between 5 and 15 minutes might not only improve fetal outcome, but may also facilitate maternal resuscitation and surgeons should be prepared to perform an immediate perimortem cesarean delivery (5) (Table 22-8).

Recurrence

In 1992, Clark described successful pregnancy outcomes of two women after AFE in previous pregnancies (94). In 1998, Collier reported one case of successful pregnancy following previous AFE. The patient arrested following delivery of her baby with an epidural and during delivery of the placenta in her first pregnancy, with a massive hemorrhage and DIC, requiring 40 units of blood and blood products. The epidural catheter was left in situ until the coagulopathy was corrected. The patient had a normal vaginal delivery 15 months later (95). In 1998 and 2000, Duffy and Stiller provided case reports of successful pregnancies and uncomplicated deliveries in women with a previous history of AFE in a previous pregnancy (96,79).

KEY POINTS

- AFE contributes significantly to maternal morbidity and mortality.
- Early diagnosis and aggressive management improve maternal and neonatal outcomes.
- AFE is nonpreventable, unpredictable, and a diagnosis of exclusion.
- AFE should be suspected in pregnant patients with a sudden onset of respiratory distress, cardiac arrest, seizures, abnormal bleeding, and/or unexplained fetal bradycardia associated with an anaphylactoid-type response.
- AFE may occur at any time during labor, vaginal delivery, cesarean delivery, and in the postpartum period.
- A multidisciplinary team approach with early recognition, effective communication and resuscitation, and expeditious perimortem delivery is critical regardless of the underlying cause of collapse and improves maternal and fetal prognosis and outcomes.

REFERENCES

1. Health resources and services administration. Maternal mortality. Child health USA 2008–2009 [Internet]. Available from: http://mchb.hrsa.gov/chusa08/hstat/hsi/pages/204mm.html.
2. Berg CJ, Callaghan WM, Syverson C, et al. Pregnancy-related mortality in the United States, 1998 to 2005. *Obstet Gynecol* 2010;116(6):1302–1309.
3. Conde-Agudelo A, Romero R. Amniotic fluid embolism: an evidence-based review. *Am J Obstet Gynecol* 2009;201(5):445.e1–445.e13.
4. Gist RS, Stafford IP, Leibowitz AB, et al. Amniotic fluid embolism. *Anesth Analg* 2009;108(5):1599–1602.
5. Clark SL, Hankins GD, Dudley DA, et al. Amniotic fluid embolism: analysis of the national registry. *Am J Obstet Gynecol* 1995;172(4 Pt 1):1158–1167; discussion 1167–1169.
6. Hsieh YY, Chang CC, Li PC, et al. Successful application of extracorporeal membrane oxygenation and intra-aortic balloon counterpulsation as lifesaving therapy for a patient with amniotic fluid embolism. *Am J Obstet Gynecol* 2000;183(2):496–497.
7. Prosper SC, Goudge CS, Lupo VR. Recombinant factor VIIa to successfully manage disseminated intravascular coagulation from amniotic fluid embolism. *Obstet Gynecol* 2007;109(2 Pt 2):524–525.
8. Nagarsheth NP, Pinney S, Bassily-Marcus A, et al. Successful placement of a right ventricular assist device for treatment of a presumed amniotic fluid embolism. *Anesth Analg* 2008;107(3):962–964.
9. Stanten RD, Iverson LI, Daugharty TM, et al. Amniotic fluid embolism causing catastrophic pulmonary vasoconstriction: Diagnosis by transesophageal echocardiogram and treatment by cardiopulmonary bypass. *Obstet Gynecol* 2003;102(3):496–498.
10. McDonnell NJ, Chan BO, Frengley RW. Rapid reversal of critical haemodynamic compromise with nitric oxide in a parturient with amniotic fluid embolism. *Int J Obstet Anesth* 2007;16(3):269–273.
11. Leighton BL, Wall MH, Lockhart EM, et al. Use of recombinant factor VIIa in patients with amniotic fluid embolism: a systematic review of case reports. *Anesthesiology* 2011;115(6):1201–1208.
12. Dildy GA, Belfort MA, Clark SL. Anaphylactoid syndrome of pregnancy (amniotic fluid embolism). In: Belfort MA, Saade G, Foley MR, Phelan JP, Dildy GA, eds. *Critical Care Obstetrics*. 5th ed. Wiley-Blackwell; 2010:466–474.
13. Meyer J. Embolia pulmonar amniocaseosa. *Bras/Med* 1926;2:301–303.
14. Steiner PE, Lushbaugh CC. Maternal pulmonary embolism by amniotic fluid. *JAMA* 1941;117:1245.
15. Lee W, Ginsburg KA, Cotton DB, et al. Squamous and trophoblastic cells in the maternal pulmonary circulation identified by invasive hemodynamic monitoring during the peripartum period. *Am J Obstet Gynecol* 1986;155(5):999–1001.
16. Masson RG. Amniotic fluid embolism. *Clin Chest Med* 1992;13(4):657–665.
17. Benson MD. A hypothesis regarding complement activation and amniotic fluid embolism. *Med Hypotheses* 2007;68(5):1019–1025.
18. Tuffnell DJ. United Kingdom amniotic fluid embolism register. *BJOG* 2005;112(12):1625–1629.
19. Benson MD. Anaphylactoid syndrome of pregnancy. *Am J Obstet Gynecol* 1996;175(3 Pt 1):749.
20. Benson MD, Lindberg RE. Amniotic fluid embolism, anaphylaxis, and tryptase. *Am J Obstet Gynecol* 1996;175(3 Pt 1):737.
21. Benson MD, Kobayashi H, Silver RK, et al. Immunologic studies in presumed amniotic fluid embolism. *Obstet Gynecol* 2001;97(4):510–514.
22. Romero R, Kadar N, Vaisbuch E, et al. Maternal death following cardiopulmonary collapse after delivery: Amniotic fluid embolism or septic shock due to intrauterine infection? *Am J Reprod Immunol* 2010;64(2):113–125.
23. Abenhaim HA, Azoulay L, Kramer MS, et al. Incidence and risk factors of amniotic fluid embolisms: a population-based study on 3 million births in the United States. *Am J Obstet Gynecol* 2008;199(1):49.e1–49.e8.
24. Kramer MS, Rouleau J, Baskett TF, et al. Amniotic-fluid embolism and medical induction of labour: a retrospective, population-based cohort study. *Lancet* 2006;368(9545):1444–1448.
25. Knight M, Tuffnell D, Brocklehurst P, et al. Incidence and risk factors for amniotic-fluid embolism. *Obstet Gynecol* 2010;115(5):910–917.
26. Dawson A. Chapter 5: Amniotic fluid embolism. In: Cantwell Rea, ed. *Saving Mothers' Lives: Reviewing Maternal Deaths to Make Motherhood Safer: 2006–2008. The Eighth Report of the Confidential Enquiries into Maternal Deaths in the United Kingdom*. 8th ed. London: Wiley-Blackwell; 2011:77.
27. Roberts CL, Algert CS, Knight M, et al. Amniotic fluid embolism in an Australian population-based cohort. *BJOG* 2010;117(11):1417–1421.
28. Gilbert WM, Danielsen B. Amniotic fluid embolism: Decreased mortality in a population-based study. *Obstet Gynecol* 1999;93(6):973–977.
29. Cantwell R, Clutton-Brock T, Cooper G, et al. Saving Mothers' Lives: Reviewing maternal deaths to make motherhood safer: 2006–2008. The Eighth Report of the Confidential Enquiries into Maternal Deaths in the United Kingdom. *BJOG* 2011;118 suppl 1:1–203.
30. Lewis G. Chapter 1: The women who died 2006–2008. In: Cantwell Rea, ed. *Saving Mothers' Lives: Reviewing Maternal Deaths To Make Motherhood Safer: 2006–2008. The Eighth Report of the Confidential Enquiries into Maternal Deaths in the United Kingdom*. 8th ed. London: Wiley-Blackwell; 2011:30.
31. Karetzky M, Ramirez M. Acute respiratory failure in pregnancy. An analysis of 19 cases. *Medicine (Baltimore)* 1998;77(1):41–49.
32. Oi H, Naruse K, Noguchi T, et al. Fatal factors of clinical manifestations and laboratory testing in patients with amniotic fluid embolism. *Gynecol Obstet Invest* 2010;70(2):138–144.
33. Mulder JI. Amniotic fluid embolism: an overview and case report. *Am J Obstet Gynecol* 1985;152(4):430–435.
34. Matsuo K, Lynch MA, Kopelman JN, et al. Anaphylactoid syndrome of pregnancy immediately after intrauterine pressure catheter placement. *Am J Obstet Gynecol* 2008;198(2):e8–e9.
35. Harbison L, Bell L. Anaphylactoid syndrome after intrauterine pressure catheter placement. *Obstet Gynecol* 2010;115(2 Pt 2):407–408.
36. Maher JE, Wenstrom KD, Hauth JC, et al. Amniotic fluid embolism after saline amnioinfusion: Two cases and review of the literature. *Obstet Gynecol* 1994;83(5 Pt 2):851–854.
37. Mato J. Suspected amniotic fluid embolism following amniotomy: A case report. *AANA J* 2008;76(1):53–59.
38. Oxford CM, Ludmir J. Trauma in pregnancy. *Clin Obstet Gynecol* 2009;52(4):611–629.
39. Rainio J, Penttila A. Amniotic fluid embolism as cause of death in a car accident—a case report. *Forensic Sci Int* 2003;137(2–3):231–234.
40. Ellingsen CL, Eggebo TM, Lexow K. Amniotic fluid embolism after blunt abdominal trauma. *Resuscitation* 2007;75(1):180–183.
41. Pluymakers C, De Weerdt A, Jacquemyn Y, et al. Amniotic fluid embolism after surgical trauma: Two case reports and review of the literature. *Resuscitation* 2007;72(2):324–332.
42. Haines J, Wilkes RG. Non-fatal amniotic fluid embolism after cervical suture removal. *Br J Anaesth* 2003;90(2):244–247.
43. McDougall RJ, Duke GJ. Amniotic fluid embolism syndrome: case report and review. *Anaesth Intensive Care* 1995;23(6):735–740.
44. Hardin L, Fox LS, O'Quinn AG. Amniotic fluid embolism. *South Med J* 1991;84(8):1046–1048.
45. Sprung J, Rakic M, Patel S. Amniotic fluid embolism during epidural anesthesia for cesarean section. *Acta Anaesthesiol Belg* 1991;42(4):225–231.
46. Pang AL, Watts RW. Amniotic fluid embolism during Caesarean section under spinal anaesthesia. Is sympathetic blockade a risk factor? *Aust N Z J Obstet Gynaecol* 2001;41(3):342–343.
47. Bastien JL, Graves JR, Bailey S. Atypical presentation of amniotic fluid embolism. *Anesth Analg* 1998;87(1):124–126.
48. Ray BK, Vallejo MC, Creinin MD, et al. Amniotic fluid embolism with second trimester pregnancy termination: A case report. *Can J Anaesth* 2004;51(2):139–144.
49. Price TM, Baker VV, Cefalo RC. Amniotic fluid embolism. Three case reports with a review of the literature. *Obstet Gynecol Surv* 1985;40(7):462–475.
50. Caughey AB, Sundaram V, Kaimal AJ, et al. Systematic review: elective induction of labor versus expectant management of pregnancy. *Ann Intern Med* 2009;151(4):252–263, W53–W63.
51. Fletcher SJ, Parr MJ. Amniotic fluid embolism: A case report and review. *Resuscitation* 2000;43(2):141–146.
52. Papaioannou VE, Dragoumanis C, Theodorou V, et al. A step-by-step diagnosis of exclusion in a twin pregnancy with acute respiratory failure

due to non-fatal amniotic fluid embolism: a case report. *J Med Case Rep* 2008;2:177.

53. Ratten GJ. Amniotic fluid embolism—2 case reports and a review of maternal deaths from this cause in Australia. *Aust N Z J Obstet Gynaecol* 1988;28(1):33–35.

54. Morgan M. Amniotic fluid embolism. *Anaesthesia.* 1979;34(1):20–32.

55. Greene M, Roberts D, Mark E. Case records of the Massachusetts General Hospital. Weekly clinicopathological exercises. Case 9–1998. Cardiovascular collapse after vaginal delivery in a patient with a history of cesarean section. *N Engl J Med* 1998;338(12):821–826.

56. Uszynski M. Amniotic fluid embolism: Literature review and an integrated concept of pathomechanism. *Open J Obstet Gynecol* 2011;1:178–183.

57. Steiner PE, Lushbaugh CC. Landmark article, Oct. 1941: Maternal pulmonary embolism by amniotic fluid as a cause of obstetric shock and unexpected deaths in obstetrics. By Paul E. Steiner and C. C. Lushbaugh. *JAMA* 1986;;255(16):2187–2203.

58. Spence M, Mason KG. Experimental amniotic fluid embolism in rabbits. *Am J Obstet Gynecol* 1974;119(8):1073–1078.

59. Stolte L, van Kessel H, Seelen J, et al. Failure to produce the syndrome of amniotic fluid embolism by infusion of amniotic fluid and meconium into monkeys. *Am J Obstet Gynecol* 1967;98(5):694–697.

60. Hankins GD, Snyder RR, Clark SL, et al. Acute hemodynamic and respiratory effects of amniotic fluid embolism in the pregnant goat model. *Am J Obstet Gynecol* 1993;168(4):1113–1129; discussion 1129–1130.

61. Petroianu GA, Altmannsberger SH, Maleck WH, et al. Meconium and amniotic fluid embolism: Effects on coagulation in pregnant mini-pigs. *Crit Care Med* 1999;27(2):348–355.

62. Clark SL, Montz FJ, Phelan JP. Hemodynamic alterations associated with amniotic fluid embolism: A reappraisal. *Am J Obstet Gynecol* 1985;151(5):617–621.

63. El-Shanawany T, Williams PE, Jolles S. Clinical immunology review series: An approach to the patient with anaphylaxis. *Clin Exp Immunol* 2008;153(1):1–9.

64. Kobayashi H, Ohi H, Terao T. A simple, noninvasive, sensitive method for diagnosis of amniotic fluid embolism by monoclonal antibody TKH-2 that recognizes NeuAc alpha 2–6GalNAc. *Am J Obstet Gynecol* 1993;168(3 Pt 1):848–853.

65. Cheung AN, Luk SC. The importance of extensive sampling and examination of cervix in suspected cases of amniotic fluid embolism. *Arch Gynecol Obstet* 1994;255(2):101–105.

66. Dean LS, Rogers RP 3rd., Harley RA, et al. Case scenario: Amniotic fluid embolism. *Anesthesiology* 2012;116(1):186–192.

67. Dolak JA, Waters JH. Meconium accelerates the procoagulopathic effects of amniotic fluid. *Anesthesiology* 2005;102(supp 1):SOAP A-29.

68. Dolak JA, Dubsky JA, Waters JH. A novel in vitro model of amniotic fluid-induced hypercoagulability. *Anesthesiology* 2004;100(supp 1).

69. Matsuda Y, Kamitomo M. Amniotic fluid embolism: a comparison between patients who survived and those who died. *J Int Med Res* 2009;37(5):1515–1521.

70. Kanayama N, Yamazaki T, Naruse H, et al. Determining zinc coproporphyrin in maternal plasma—a new method for diagnosing amniotic fluid embolism. *Clin Chem* 1992;38(4):526–529.

71. Shechtman M, Ziser A, Markovits R, et al. Amniotic fluid embolism: Early findings of transesophageal echocardiography. *Anesth Analg* 1999;89(6):1456–1458.

72. Vellayappan U, Attias MD, Shulman MS. Paradoxical embolization by amniotic fluid seen on the transesophageal echocardiography. *Anesth Analg* 2009;108(4):1110–1112.

73. Simons FE. Anaphylaxis. *J Allergy Clin Immunol* 2010;125(2 Suppl 2):S161–S181.

74. Tuffnell DJ. Amniotic fluid embolism. *Curr Opin Obstet Gynecol* 2003;15(2):119–122.

75. Annecke T, Geisenberger T, Kurzl R, et al. Algorithm-based coagulation management of catastrophic amniotic fluid embolism. *Blood Coagul Fibrinolysis* 2010;21(1):95–100.

76. Lipman SS, Daniels KI, Carvalho B, et al. Deficits in the provision of cardiopulmonary resuscitation during simulated obstetric crises. *Am J Obstet Gynecol* 2010;203(2):179.e1,179.e5.

77. American Heart Association. Part 10.8: Cardiac arrest associated with pregnancy. *Circulation* 2005;112(24):IV-150–IV-153.

78. Firstenberg MS, Abel E, Blais D, et al. Temporary extracorporeal circulatory support and pulmonary embolectomy for catastrophic amniotic fluid embolism. *Heart Surg Forum* 2011;14(3):E157–E159.

79. Stiller RJ, Siddiqui D, Laifer SA, et al. Successful pregnancy after suspected anaphylactoid syndrome of pregnancy (amniotic fluid embolus). A case report. *J Reprod Med* 2000;45(12):1007–1009.

80. Alon E, Atanassoff PG. Successful cardiopulmonary resuscitation of a parturient with amniotic fluid embolism. *Int J Obstet Anesth* 1992;1(4):205–207.

81. Vercauteren MP, Coppejans HC, Sermeus L. Anaphylactoid reaction to hydroxyethylstarch during cesarean delivery in a patient with HELLP syndrome. *Anesth Analg* 2003;96(3):859–861, table of contents.

82. Franchini M, Franchi M, Bergamini V, et al. The use of recombinant activated FVII in postpartum hemorrhage. *Clin Obstet Gynecol* 2010;53(1):219–227.

83. Huber AW, Raio L, Alberio L, et al. Recombinant human factor VIIa prevents hysterectomy in severe postpartum hemorrhage: single center study. *J Perinat Med* 2011;40(1):43–49.

84. Leighton BL, Wall MH, Lockhart EM, et al. Use of recombinant factor VIIa in patients with amniotic fluid embolism: A systematic review of case reports. *Anesthesiology* 2011;115(6):1201–1208.

85. Peitsidou A, Peitsidis P, Tsekoura V, et al. Amniotic fluid embolism managed with success during labour: Report of a severe clinical case and review of literature. *Arch Gynecol Obstet* 2008;277(3):271–275.

86. Goldszmidt E, Davies S. Two cases of hemorrhage secondary to amniotic fluid embolism managed with uterine artery embolization. *Can J Anaesth* 2003;50(9):917–921.

87. Sheikh A, Shehata YA, Brown SG, et al. Adrenaline for the treatment of anaphylaxis: Cochrane systematic review. *Allergy* 2009;64(2):204–212.

88. Sheikh A, Ten Broek V, Brown SG, et al. H1-antihistamines for the treatment of anaphylaxis: Cochrane systematic review. *Allergy* 2007;62(8):830–837.

89. Choo KJ, Simons E, Sheikh A. Glucocorticoids for the treatment of anaphylaxis: Cochrane systematic review. *Allergy* 2010;65(10):1205–1211.

90. Esposito RA, Grossi EA, Coppa G, et al. Successful treatment of postpartum shock caused by amniotic fluid embolism with cardiopulmonary bypass and pulmonary artery thromboembolectomy. *Am J Obstet Gynecol* 1990;163(2):572–574.

91. Katz V, Balderston K, DeFreest M. Perimortem cesarean delivery: were our assumptions correct? *Am J Obstet Gynecol* 2005;192(6):1916–1920; discussion 1920–1921.

92. Stehr SN, Liebich I, Kamin G, et al. Closing the gap between decision and delivery–amniotic fluid embolism with severe cardiopulmonary and haemostatic complications with a good outcome. *Resuscitation* 2007;74(2):377–381.

93. Hosono K, Matsumura N, Matsuda N, et al. Successful recovery from delayed amniotic fluid embolism with prolonged cardiac resuscitation. *J Obstet Gynaecol Res* 2011;37(8):1122–1125.

94. Clark SL. Successful pregnancy outcomes after amniotic fluid embolism. *Am J Obstet Gynecol* 1992;167(2):511–512.

95. Collier C. Recurring amniotic fluid embolism. *Anaesth Intensive Care* 1998;26(5):599–600.

96. Duffy BL. Does amniotic fluid embolism recur? *Anaesth Intensive Care* 1998;26(3):333.

CHAPTER 23

Venous Thromboembolism in Pregnancy and Guidelines for Neuraxial Anesthesia Following Anticoagulant and Antithrombotic Drugs

Quisqueya T. Palacios

◾ INTRODUCTION

In 2010, the World Health Organization (WHO) estimated maternal mortality rate to be approximately 17/100,000 pregnancies in the United States (1). The maternal mortality rate for the triennium, 2006 to 2008, was 11.39/100,000 maternities compared with the 13.95/100,000 maternities reported for the previous triennium, 2003 to 2005 in the United Kingdom (2). The Centre for Maternal and Child Enquiries (CMACE) reported maternal mortality rate from thromboembolism, the leading cause of death in the United Kingdom since 1985, was 32/100,000 maternities in the triennium 1985 to 1988 compared to 1.94 and 0.79 per 100,000 maternities in the trienniums, 2003 to 2005 and 2006 to 2008, respectively. In the summary section of the UK Obstetric Surveillance System (UKOSS) report on near-miss studies, Knight reported an estimated incidence of antenatal pulmonary embolism of 1.3/10,000 maternities (3). The main risk factors identified for pulmonary embolism were multiparity, increasing maternal age, and obesity. The overall increased prevalence of obesity among pregnant women reflects the increased prevalence in the general population. The prevalence of obesity in the UK women 16 years old or more was estimated 24% in 2007 compared to 16% in 1993 (2). Maternal weight was found to most significantly impact mortality from thromboembolism compared to any other cause of death and 78% of the mothers who died from thromboembolism were overweight or obese. Despite a significant decrease in the maternal mortality rate from thromboembolism following the publication of the 2004 Royal College of Obstetricians and Gynecologists' guideline "Thromboprophylaxis during pregnancy, labour, and after normal vaginal delivery" risk assessment during all the three trimesters and the postpartum period continues to be a key factor in reducing maternal mortality (4–6). In addition, the guideline for thromboprophylaxis was updated and revised in 2009 to include weight specific dosage recommendations in morbidly obese patients (7). In 2012, Schoenbeck reported on the successful use of a scoring system of individual risk factors for the development of venous thromboembolism (VTE) in pregnancy to guide the administration of dalteparin for thromboprophylaxis in high-risk pregnant patients (8). The scoring system improved clinical management of women at risk for VTE without an increase in obstetric or anesthetic morbidity.

According to a study by the Centers for Disease Control and Prevention (CDC) of pregnancy-related mortality in the United States between 1991 and 1998, pulmonary embolism was a leading cause of maternal deaths (9). In 2008, a retrospective study of medical records from all maternal deaths in a series of 1.5 million deliveries within 124 Hospital Corporation of America (HCA) hospitals in the previous 6 years reviewed individual causes of maternal deaths (10). Clark et al. confirmed pulmonary thromboembolism as a leading cause of maternal death in addition to preeclampsia, AFE, obstetric hemorrhage, and cardiac disease, accounting for 10% of maternal deaths. See Table 23-1. Clark et al. concluded that a nationwide systematic and universal adoption of VTE prophylaxis measures would essentially eliminate thrombus as a preventable cause of maternal death from pulmonary embolism. In 2010, The Joint Commission released Sentinel Event Alert, Issue 44, which recommended the use of pneumatic compression devices for women at high risk for pulmonary embolism undergoing cesarean delivery (11). In addition, their National Patient Safety Goal 16 was elevated to one of the 2010 standards for hospitals, which requires the development of written criteria describing early warning signs of a change or deterioration in a patient's condition and when to seek further assistance. Furthermore, The Joint Commission established a call to action for hospitals to develop effective strategies for preventing pregnancy-related mortality and severe morbidity. Despite increased awareness of the risks of VTE and the use of prophylaxis, pulmonary embolism continues to be a leading cause of maternal mortality. Therefore, a thorough understanding of the anesthetic implications of the risk factors, diagnosis, prevention, and management of pulmonary thromboembolism during pregnancy and anticoagulation during neuraxial anesthesia for vaginal and cesarean delivery is essential.

Pregnant women are at increased risk of thromboembolism compared with nonpregnant women especially during cesarean delivery. Pregnant women have a two- to fivefold increase of deep venous thrombosis (DVT) and PE compared with nonpregnant women of childbearing age (12). In the retrospective review in 2008, Clark et al. confirmed pulmonary thromboembolism was associated with a maternal mortality rate of 2/100,000 deliveries following cesarean delivery which was 10 times the maternal mortality rate following vaginal delivery of 0.2/100,000 deliveries (10). The majority of these deaths, 77% (7 of 9) patients died from pulmonary thromboembolism following primary and repeat cesarean delivery compared to 22% (2 of 9) patients following vaginal delivery. None of the nine women had received peripartum thromboembolism prophylaxis with either fractionated or unfractionated heparin or pneumatic compression devices. See Table 23-2. Regardless of the mode of delivery and risk

349

TABLE 23-1 Leading Causes of Maternal Death

Cause of Death	Number	%
Complications of preeclampsia	15	16
Amniotic fluid embolism	13	14
Obstetric hemorrhage	11	12
Cardiac disease	10	11
Pulmonary thromboembolism	9	9
Obstetric infection	7	7

Adapted from: Clark SL, Belfort MA, Dildy GA, et al. Maternal death in the 21st century: Causes, prevention, and relationship to cesarean delivery. *Am J Obstet Gynecol* 2008;199(1):36.e1–e5.

of major surgery associated with thromboembolism, maternal mortality rate of women undergoing vaginal and cesarean delivery exceeded expectations. Furthermore, one expects to also see a similar 70% to 80% reduction in VTE in pregnant women undergoing cesarean delivery as seen in surgical patients if a universal use of medical or mechanical thromboprophylaxis been in place. This universal practice alone would reduce the maternal mortality rate attributed causally to cesarean delivery from 2 to 0.9 per 100,000 (10).

In a 5-year retrospective, population-based, case-control study from 1996 to 2000 in France, Deneux-Tharaux et al. also confirmed an increased risk of postpartum death of 3.6 times following cesarean compared to after vaginal delivery (13) (Table 23-3). Deneux-Tharaux et al. found that cesarean delivery was associated with a significantly increased risk of maternal death from complications of general anesthesia, infection, hemorrhage, and VTE.

■ INCIDENCE

VTE, which refers to both DVT and pulmonary embolism (PE), is associated with significant morbidity and mortality. Berg et al. found that 11% of maternal deaths during pregnancy were related to PE (9). DVT accounts for 75% to 80% of pregnancy-related VTE and pulmonary embolism accounts for 20% to 25%. The incidence of VTE is 0.025% to 0.1% or 0.5 to 3 per 1,000 deliveries. Approximately, 66% of all DVTs occur antepartum and 50% of these occur before the third trimester. In comparison, PE occurs

TABLE 23-2 Causal Relationship Between Maternal Death and Mode of Delivery

Mode of Delivery	Number of Cases	Number of Deaths	Death (per 100,000) Cases
Vaginal	1,003,173	2	0.20
Primary cesarean	282,632	7	2.5
Repeat cesarean	175,465	2	1.1
Total cesarean	458,097	9	2
Total	1,461,270	11	0.75

Adapted from: Clark SL, Belfort MA, Dildy GA, et al. Maternal death in the 21st century: Causes, prevention, and relationship to cesarean delivery. *Am J Obstet Gynecol* 2008;199(1):36.e1–e5.

TABLE 23-3 Risk Factors for Venous Thromboembolism During Pregnancy

History of Previous VTE	Venous Stasis Disease
Family history of VTE	Surgery
Pregnancy and postpartum	Oral contraceptives
Prolonged bed rest or immobility	Smoking
Age greater than 35–40 yrs	Inflammatory bowel disease
Obesity	Indwelling central venous catheters
Trauma	Malignancy
Multiparity	Multiple gestation
Postcesarean hysterectomy	Inherited or acquired thrombophilias
Presence of antiphospholipid antibodies	

less frequently during pregnancy but more often than DVT postpartum. Approximately 25% of patients with DVTs will develop PE if untreated. Therefore, the goal of treatment of DVT is the prevention of PE. When DVT occurs during pregnancy, it is more likely to be proximal, massive, and in the left iliac vein of the lower extremity. Distal thrombosis can occur either on the right or the left. Pelvic vein thrombosis is usually associated with pregnancy or pelvic surgery, and accounts for 10% to 12% of DVT during pregnancy and the postpartum period. DVT of the upper extremities or neck is very rare and usually associated with pregnancies with assisted reproductive technologies or complicated by the ovarian hyperstimulation syndrome. DVT and PE are often preventable and usually treatable. Approximately 30% of patients will develop a recurrent DVT. When untreated, approximately 25% of patients with DVT will develop PE. Acute PE is a common and often fatal disease. As the cesarean rate now exceeds 30% in the United States, and maternal mortality rate due to pulmonary thromboembolism is higher with cesarean deliveries, it is the responsibility of the anesthesia care providers to understand the additional risk factors, anesthetic implications, and management of pulmonary thromboembolism.

■ MORBIDITY AND MORTALITY

The mortality rate of PE is approximately 15%. Mortality can be reduced by prompt diagnosis and treatment. The risk of pulmonary thromboembolism is decreased to 4.5% and mortality is decreased to less than 1% in pregnant patients with DVT who receive anticoagulation.

■ ETIOLOGY

Pregnancy is a hypercoagulable state which is associated with changes in the coagulation pathways. Factors II, VII, VIII, and X, and fibrinogen are increased and protein S levels are decreased which may lead to clot formation. Also, fibrinolysis is inhibited during the third trimester of pregnancy. Venous stasis from swelling of the lower extremity veins due to edema formation and bed rest during pregnancy leads to VTE. Venous stasis due to the gravid uterus compressing the inferior vena cava (IVC) and venous outflow of the internal iliac, femoral, and popliteal veins from the lower extremities and pelvis, also leads to venous thrombosis. This occurs on the left side to a greater extent. During pregnancy, the site of thrombosis is usually proximal in the iliofemoral vein. However, the popliteal area is more often affected in the postpartum period. Furthermore, hormonally induced, increased venous capacitance and vascular injury increase the risk of pregnancy-associated VTE. Pregnant patients who require prolonged bed rest, smoke, are obese, or have a thrombophilia are at increased risk of DVT and PE. Maternal age, multiparity, sepsis, instrumented or cesarean delivery, hemorrhage, and cardiac disease, including the presence of atrial fibrillation and mechanical valves also increase the risk of VTE. Although the risk of VTE may be higher during the third trimester than in the first or second trimester, the risk of VTE is still increased during the first 12 weeks, clearly before the anatomic changes of pregnancy produce increased venous stasis. However, the postpartum period is also associated with an increased risk of thrombosis of the ovarian veins, which is typically related to infection and cesarean delivery. Approximately 80% of thromboembolic events are venous and 20% are arterial. Compared to pregnancy, the risk of VTE is 20 to 80 times higher during the first 6 weeks postpartum and 100 times higher during the first week postpartum.

RECURRENCE

Approximately 15% to 25% of thromboembolic events during pregnancy are recurrent during pregnancy and subsequent pregnancies, and VTE is the cause of 10% of all maternal deaths. The most important risk factor for VTE during pregnancy is a history of thrombosis. The risk of recurrence VTE during pregnancy is increased 3 to 4 times. The rate of recurrence of VTE in women not receiving prophylaxis anticoagulation was reported to be 2.4% to 12.2%. However, in women receiving prophylaxis anticoagulation, the rate of recurrence of VTE was reported to be below 2.4%. Also, patients with a history of VTE during pregnancy have a recurrence rate 4% to 15% of VTE in a subsequent pregnancy. Women with a known thrombophilia associated with a hypercoagulable state are also at increased risk of VTE during pregnancy and should receive prophylaxis. Effective prophylaxis with unfractionated heparin is usually achieved with a twice-daily average daily dose of 16,400 IU/day or 225 IU/kg of body weight per 24 hours. It is not unusual for the prophylactic daily dose to increase through the second and third trimesters.

RISK FACTORS

Risk factors include a history of prior VTE, inherited or acquired thrombophilia, a maternal age greater than 35, pregnancy related and delivery complications, multiparity, obesity, surgical procedures during pregnancy including cesarean delivery, and previous history of pulmonary thromboembolism (Table 23-4).

However, most women do not require anticoagulation despite the increased risk of VTE during pregnancy and the postpartum period. Indications for anticoagulation include women with current VTE, a history of VTE, thrombophilia and a history of poor outcome during pregnancy, or presence of risk factors during the postpartum period. The indications for prophylactic or level of therapeutic anticoagulation will depend on the risk factors and require a VTE risk assessment (14). Pregnant and postpartum patients are considered low risk if less than 35 years and following vaginal delivery. The risk of DVT without thromboprophylaxis is less than 10% in nonpregnant patients. Early ambulation and hydration are recommended. Patients at bed rest and following cesarean delivery and having one to two risk factors are at moderate risk. SCDs

TABLE 23-4 Estimates of Fetal Exposure and Type of Radiographic Study Used in the Diagnosis of Maternal Venous Thromboembolism

Type of Radiography	Estimate of Radiation Fetal Exposure	Relative Radiation Ratio
Chest radiograph	<0.001 rad	<1
Ventilation/ perfusion scan	0.001–0.035/0.006– 0.018 rad	1–5/6–12
Pulmonary angiogram	0.221–0.405 rad	<50
Chest CT scan	0.016 rad	15
Spiral CT Scan	0.00033–0.01 rad	<0.3

Adapted from: Mclintock C, Brighton T, Chunilal S. Recommendations for the diagnosis and treatment of deep venous thrombosis and pulmonary embolism in pregnancy and the postpartum period. *Aust N Z J Obstet Gynaecol* 2012; 52(1);14–22. Copyright 2011.

are recommended and prophylactic anticoagulation should be considered. However, pregnant or postpartum patients with three or more risk factors in addition to one or more of the following: Prior history of VTE, or thrombophilia are at high risk. These patients have a risk of DVT without thromboprophylaxis between 40% and 80%. Prophylactic anticoagulation is recommended and SCDs may be considered. The goal at delivery is to weigh the benefit of anticoagulation while continuing to minimize the risk of VTE and bleeding.

COMPLICATIONS OF VTE

Approximately 30% of patients develop recurrent DVTs and approximately 20% to 30% will develop long-term complications, including venous insufficiency, right-sided heart failure, post-thrombotic syndrome, and pulmonary hypertension. Post-thrombotic syndrome is a long-term complication of DVT characterized by venous stasis chronic swelling, redness, ulcerations, persistent leg pain, and increased risk of future VTE (15,16). Hospitals have taken the initiative and adapted the use of performance measures and compliance with the Joint Commission's 2012 Hospital National Patient Safety Goal 03.05.01 to decrease the likelihood of patient harm and complications associated with the use of anticoagulant therapy and treatment of VTE, and to improve the maternal mortality rates.

DIAGNOSIS OF DVT AND PE

Early diagnosis utilizing imaging techniques and treatment decrease the risk of pulmonary embolism. However, diagnosis in pregnant patients can be challenging since symptoms associated with pulmonary embolism can also be seen throughout normal pregnancy. Shortness of breath, tachypnea, tachycardia, palpitations, and leg swelling are seen during normal pregnancy. Patients with acute pulmonary embolism typically develop symptoms and signs immediately after obstruction of the pulmonary artery or one of its branches by a thrombus usually originating in the lower extremity. Although symptoms may be absent in 70% of patients with documented PE, symptoms may include sudden onset of dyspnea, tachypnea, pleuritic chest pain, a nonproductive cough, hemoptysis, and tachycardia. Due to the nonspecificity of these symptoms, radiographic evaluation is important to the prompt diagnosis of PE.

The diagnosis of VTE is made by clinical examination and correlation with clinical presentation in addition to laboratory studies and radiographic studies. Accurate diagnostic testing to confirm or exclude DVT or PE is necessary because the diagnosis of either requires prolonged treatment during pregnancy, prophylaxis during future pregnancies, and the use of oral contraceptives should be avoided. Unfortunately, clinical presentation of pulmonary embolism is variable and nonspecific especially during pregnancy, making accurate diagnosis difficult. When pulmonary embolism is suspected and the clinical suspicion is high for PE, anticoagulation should be considered until the evaluation is completed and the diagnosis of PE is excluded.

Each diagnostic test presents advantages and disadvantages for the pregnant patient. Chest x-ray may be abnormal in 80% of patients with PE; however, the findings are usually nonspecific. In addition, ECG may also have nonspecific findings. In 70% of patients with PE, arterial oxygen tension is low. The efficacy of compression ultrasound, ventilation/perfusion (V/Q) scanning, pulmonary angiography, and spiral computerized tomography (CT) scanning in pregnant patients has not been thoroughly evaluated.

Contrast venography requires injection of radiopaque dye into the vein below the site of the suspected thrombus. A filling defect seen during imaging has been considered the gold standard in the diagnosis of DVT in nonpregnant patients. However, compression ultrasound and impedance plethysmography have replaced contrast venography in pregnant patients (17). Compression ultrasonography utilizes color flow Doppler imaging while applying firm compression to the ultrasound transducer to detect intraluminal filling defects of the major venous systems of the legs, including the common femoral, superficial femoral, greater saphenous, and popliteal veins (16). Noncompressibility of the venous lumen is the most accurate ultrasound criteria for thrombosis. Compression ultrasound is the least invasive test, can be repeated if necessary, and does not expose the mother or fetus to radiation. Therefore, ACOG recently made a level 1A recommendation for compression ultrasound as the initial diagnostic test for new onset of DVT during pregnancy (18). If a DVT is identified, then PE can be assumed, and treatment should be started without further testing. Sensitivity and specificity of compression ultrasound are 95% and 96%, respectively in the detection of proximal DVT. However, compression ultrasound is not effective in the diagnosis of isolated calf DVT or isolated iliac vein thrombosis. Additional testing is warranted when compression ultrasound scans are negative because these proximal DVTs are associated with a high risk for embolization. However, compression ultrasound is the diagnostic test of choice in women with clinical suspicion of DVT (19). Impedance plethysmography is noninvasive and safe during pregnancy and measures the impedance to blood flow. Impedance plethysmography utilizes the application of high-frequency continuous current to the affected lower extremity and a decrease in impedance of blood flow corresponds to an increased venous outflow resistance in the deep veins of the proximal lower extremity. It is not as useful as compression ultrasound in diagnosis of DVT in the femoral, superficial femoral, or popliteal veins, most isolated calf thrombi or nonobstructive proximal thrombi.

V/Q scanning, spiral CT scanning, and pulmonary angiography are associated with dose-dependent radiation exposure, generally 10 to 37 mrad and 6 mrad for the first two, respectively. The fetus is exposed to 30% of the maternal radiation dose. Shielding reduces fetal radiation dose by 30%. However, radiation exposure greater than 5 rads are thought to potentially cause radiation-induced central nervous system fetal damage, especially during the 8 to 15 weeks of organogenesis. Although fetal exposure to radiation is minimal during V/Q scans, an initial diagnostic perfusion scan further reduces fetal exposure (20). V/Q scans are categorized into low, intermediate, high, normal, and indeterminate diagnostic probability categories according to comparative images produced by inhaled radioactive aerosol gases and radiolabeled markers injected intravenously, such as technetium-99m (21,22). A low probability refers to either no perfusion defects or nonsegmental defects, matched V/A defects of subsegmental perfusion defects. A high probability refers to either two or more mismatched segmental defects, or defects much larger than chest radiograph abnormality. See Figure 23-1. A perfusion scan is considered diagnostic if a defect of pulmonary arterial blood flow is seen in symptomatic patients. A ventilation scan will differentiate matched defects from unmatched defects in perfusion scans with defects not attributable to PE. A low, intermediate, or indeterminate result may require additional testing. Prior V/Q scan results should be reviewed since defects from prior thromboembolism may not have resolved completely. Chest radiographs should also be reviewed for atelectasis, effusions, and consolidations. Technetium-99m, the intravenous contrast media used during perfusion scan, is excreted by the kidneys and in breast milk, and fetal exposure may be decreased by increased fluid intake for 4 to 6 hours in the pregnant patient and substituting breast milk with formula for 2 days following a test. A perfusion scan should be ordered before a ventilation scan since a normal perfusion scan rules out a PE. Xe-133 is the radioactive agent utilized for ventilation scan in addition to technetium-99m. Therefore, maternal and fetal radiation exposure may be decreased by utilizing a ventilation scan when the perfusion scan is abnormal. V/S scan is the preferred diagnostic testing in pregnant women with suspected PE who have a normal chest x-ray.

If the V/Q scan is normal, no additional testing is required. However, in a large study of pregnant patients, only 3.3% of the V/Q scans were interpreted as high probability as compared to nonpregnant patients (20). In pregnant patients with a moderate to high clinical suspicion for PE, treatment should be started without additional testing when the V/Q scan has a high probability. In the same study, only 25% of V/Q scans were considered nondiagnostic in pregnant patients as compared to 47% to 57% in nonpregnant patients and required additional testing. Pregnant patients tend to be both younger and healthier than most patients requiring chest imaging and have normal ventilation and perfusion scans more frequently as compared to nonpregnant patients, 72.5% versus 27% to 36%, respectively.

D-dimers are produced from the breakdown of fibrin and levels are increased with pulmonary embolism. Therefore, a negative D-dimer test reliably excludes the diagnosis of PE in nonpregnant patients with a low clinical probability of PE. During pregnancy, D-dimers increase during gestation, after surgery, during preterm labor, preeclampsia, and placental abruption. Therefore, pregnancy decreases the accuracy of D-dimer testing and limits the efficacy in the diagnosis of VTE during pregnancy. Therefore, D-dimer testing is **not recommended** for the diagnostic testing of suspected DVT or PE in pregnancy or early postpartum period (19).

In a recent review of the literature, spiral CT was reported to be equivalent to pulmonary angiography in excluding PE in nonpregnant patients and has been shown to be cost effective and safe in all trimesters during the evaluation of suspected PE in pregnant patients (23). Fetal exposure to radiation with the use of intravenous contrast is minimal during spiral CT and less than during V/Q scanning (20). The use of contrast may lead to allergic reactions and renal dysfunction, and patients should be well-hydrated postspiral CT using contrast. Spiral CT scan is highly predictive of PE with a sensitivity and specificity range between 57% to

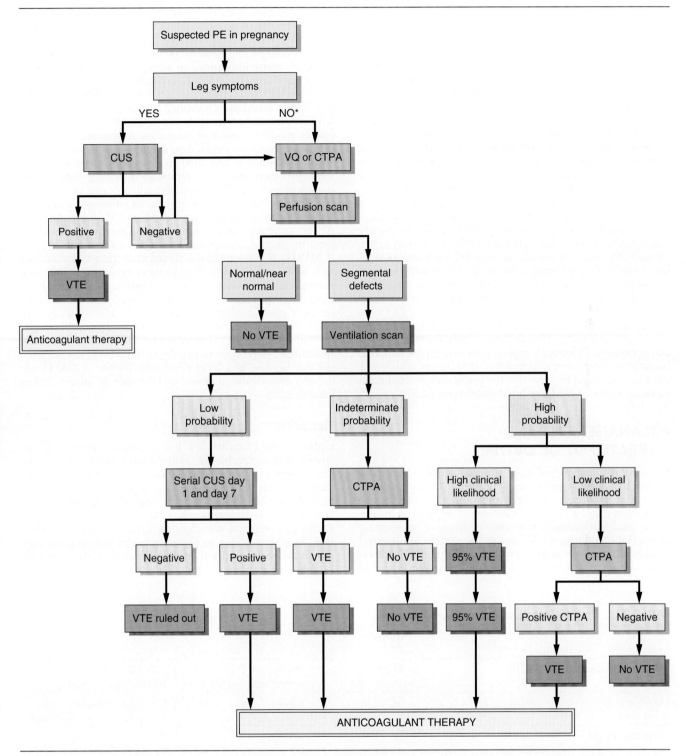

FIGURE 23-1 Algorithm for VTE workup in pregnancy. CUS, compression ultrasonography; VQ, ventilation/perfusion scan; CTPA, computerized tomography pulmonary angiography; VTE, venous thromboembolism. *Some experts recommend using compression ultrasonography as a first-line test irrespective of the presence of symptoms of deep vein thrombosis. Adapted from: Bourjeily G, Paidas M, Khalil H, et al. Pulmonary embolism in pregnancy. *Lancet* 2010;375(9713): 500–512.

94% and 64% to 100%, respectively. However, during pregnancy, spiral CT scans have a higher nondiagnostic rate of 36% as compared to a nondiagnostic rate of 25% associated with V/Q scan. Other differential diagnoses of PE such as pulmonary infiltrate, pneumonia, and effusions may also be excluded by a spiral CT scan. Spiral CT scans are considered safe during pregnancy and have greater diagnostic value of pulmonary embolism in main and lobar arteries compared to segmental pulmonary arteries. Therefore, spiral CT scan is just as highly diagnostic of a PE as is pulmonary angiography. Spiral CT is recommended in women with an abnormal chest x-ray or when V/Q scan is inconclusive (19).

Magnetic resonance imaging (MRI) is another alternative to V/Q scan and spiral CT scan. MRI imaging utilizes gadolinium injection to visualize the pulmonary vasculature (20). MRI has a similar sensitivity and specificity to spiral CT scan for the diagnosis of PE and the fetus is not exposed to either intravenous contrast or radiation. However, during pregnancy studies done with gadolinium enhancement should be avoided because of fetal exposure. Fetal exposure may be prolonged because gadolinium crosses the placenta, is seen in the fetal bladder which is excreted into amniotic fluid and swallowed by the fetus. Although, MRI is effective in the diagnosis of isolated iliac vein thrombosis in pregnancy, gadolinium has not been proved to be safe in pregnancy and is considered a Class C drug during pregnancy (17,20).

However, if V/Q or spiral CT scans are nondiagnostic, the gold standard for diagnosing PE is pulmonary angiography. Specificity is approximately 100% (16). Pulmonary angiography involves catheterization of the pulmonary artery through the internal jugular or femoral vein and observing a filling defect during fluoroscopy. Although the fetal exposure to radiation with the use of intravenous contrast is lower than spiral CT scan, it is considered very invasive and associated with an increased risk of complications (0.3% to 1% and a mortality rate of 0.5%). Complications include a risk of allergy to contrast, perforation, renal and pulmonary failure, and hematoma. Pulmonary angiography may expose maternal breast tissue to relatively high doses of radiation, which may carry an increased lifetime risk for breast cancer. Radiation exposure to breast can be reduced with breast shields.

■ MANAGEMENT AND TREATMENT OF DVT/PE

In addition to supportive care, anticoagulation is the main treatment for acute pulmonary embolism. Oxygen supplementation by face mask or intubation with mechanical ventilation may be required. Circulatory support with inotropes and vasopressors may require invasive monitoring of arterial blood gases, CVP or cardiac output with central venous catheter, or pulmonary artery catheter. The incidence of mortality in untreated patients due to recurrence of

pulmonary embolism is approximately 30%. This risk outweighs the risk of major bleeding which is less than 3%. Initial management of suspected VTE depends upon the degree of clinical suspicion for acute pulmonary embolism, whether there are contraindications to anticoagulation, and whether pulmonary embolism, DVT, or both are suspected. When there is a high index of suspicion for acute pulmonary embolism, anticoagulation is indicated before diagnostic testing. If VTE is excluded anticoagulation is discontinued. In cases of low or moderate index of suspicion, anticoagulation before diagnostic testing is decided on an individual basis.

An IVC filter is indicated in cases of suspected pulmonary embolism and VTE confirmed with diagnostic testing but anticoagulation is contraindicated. In cases of suspected DVT alone without any evidence of acute pulmonary embolism, anticoagulation is usually not started until VTE is confirmed. Acute anticoagulation with intravenous unfractionated heparin or (subcutaneous) low–molecular-weight heparin (LMWH) is recommended throughout pregnancy and up to 6 to 8 weeks postpartum. If anticoagulation is indicated throughout pregnancy, there are advantages and disadvantages of prophylactic and therapeutic anticoagulation based on their pharmacology. See Table 23-5. The advantages of LMWH are a lower risk of heparin-induced thrombocytopenia and osteoporosis as compared to unfractionated heparin. In addition, only—one to two doses of LMWH are required per day because of a longer half-life. Neither LMWH nor heparin crosses the placenta, and are safe in infants during breastfeeding.

Heparin

Unfractionated heparin is a heterogeneous mixture of sulfated mucopolysaccharides isolated from porcine or bovine gut or lung with a molecular weight of 5,000 to 30,000 Da. Heparin binds antithrombin III and potentiates the inhibition of thrombin, IXa, Xa, XIa, and XIIa. Unfractionated heparin's bioavailability is only 30% because of its high affinity for proteins and therefore its action is very unpredictable. In addition, due to physiologic changes of pregnancy associated with increased protein binding, plasma volume, and glomerular filtration rate, a higher dosing schedule may

TABLE 23-5 Pharmacology of Anticoagulant Drugs

Drug	Mode of Action	Route of Administration	Onset of Action	Elimination Half-Life
Unfractionated heparin	Bind ATIII	SC; IV	Within 2 h (SC); immediate (IV)	30, 60, 150 min (25 IU/kg, 100 IU/kg, 400 IU/kg)
LMWH	Bind ATIII	SC	±3–4 h	3–6 h; dose independent; prolonged in renal failure
Fondaparinux	Selective inhibition of factor Xa	SC	Within 2 h	17 h
Aspirin	Irreversible inhibition of COX-1	Oral	Within 5 h	7.5 h (of main metabolite)
Ticlodipine	Inhibit ADP-induced platelet aggregation	Oral	1–8 h	20–50 h
Warfarin	Inhibit γ-carboxylation of factors II, VII, IX, X	Oral	Within 90 min	36–42 h

A summary of pharmacologic data (based on non-obstetric patients) for unfractionated heparin, LMWH, Fondaparinux, aspirin, clopidogrel, triclopidine, and warfarin.

AT, antithrombin; COX, cyclooxygenase; IV, intravenous; IU, international units; LMWH, low–molecular-weight heparin; SC, subcutaneous.

Reprinted by permission from: Butwick AJ, Carvalho B. Anticoagulant and antithrombotic drugs in pregnancy: What are the anesthetic implications for labor and cesarean delivery?. *J Perinat* 2011;31:73–84. Copyright 2011.

be required to maintain therapeutic efficacy, especially with pregnancy-induced heparin resistance (24). Heparin does not dissolve the thrombi or emboli already formed. However, it does prevent new formation of clots or growth of existing clots, thereby decreasing the morbidity and mortality from pulmonary embolism (25).

Heparin has been studied extensively and is considered very safe during pregnancy. Heparin is usually administered during the first and third trimesters of pregnancy. Heparin 5,000 to 7,500 units subcutaneously every 12 hours during the first trimester, 7,500 to 10,000 units subcutaneously every 12 hours during the second trimester, and 10,000 units subcutaneously every 12 hours during the third trimester may be given for thromboprophylaxis during pregnancy. An initial loading dose of 5,000 to 10,000 units of intravenous unfractionated heparin should be started immediately following the diagnosis of acute pulmonary embolism. Following the initial loading, an infusion of 18 U/kg should be started for maintenance. The activated partial thromboplastin time (aPTT) should be monitored 6 hours after injection and maintained in the therapeutic range of 1.5 to 2.5 times baseline. For maintenance, subcutaneous injections of 10,000 IU may be given two times daily throughout pregnancy until just prior to delivery. Following delivery, warfarin can be started to achieve an International Normalized Ratio (INR) of —two to three for at least 6 to 8 weeks postpartum. Heparin-induced thrombocytopenia is seen in approximately 3% of patients receiving unfractionated heparin (16). Type I thrombocytopenia, believed to be caused by platelet aggregation, occurs quickly usually within 3 to 4 days of starting treatment, and is usually reversible. Heparin treatment may be continued and the thrombocytopenia is usually self-limiting. Type II thrombocytopenia usually occurs within 5 to 14 days after starting treatment and is immunoglobulin mediated and occurs in 1% to 3% of nonpregnant patients. Significant morbidity from arterial thrombosis and venous thrombosis may occur in untreated heparin-induced thrombocytopenia (17). Therefore, platelet count should be monitored closely during the first 2 weeks of treatment. Heparin prophylaxis should be discontinued and an alternative treatment should be started if platelet counts decrease significantly after the first seven7 to 10 days of use. However, unfractionated heparin may be preferred to other anticoagulants in patients who are hemodynamically unstable, at significant risk for hemorrhage, or near term and delivery, and requiring regional anesthesia. The effects of heparin are easily reversed with protamine if necessary and its half-life is dose dependent ranging between 30, 60, and 150 minutes (26). Osteopenia has been reported with the use of unfractionated heparin for greater than 6 months and pregnant patients should receive calcium and vitamin D supplementation. Heparin is safe in lactating women. LMWH is recommended as an alternative treatment to minimize frequent monitoring of platelets and aPTT and in cases of heparin-induced thrombocytopenia and osteoporosis.

Low–molecular-weight Heparin

LMWH is a shorter polysaccharide produced by an enzymatic depolymerization of unfractionated heparin and has a molecular weight of 4,000 to 6,000 Da. This leads to lower protein binding and higher bioavailability (90%), greater predictability, peak onset of 3 to 4 hours, dose-dependent elimination half time, and prolonged duration of action of 12 hours. LMWH binds to antithrombin III and has similar inhibition of factor Xa as unfractionated heparin and lower antithrombin, factor II activity. The peak LMWH antifactor Xa activity occurs approximately 4 hours after subcutaneous injection, and at 12 hours, antifactor Xa activity is approximately 50% of peak levels (27). Anti-Xa levels for thrombo-

prophylaxis should be 0.1 to 0.2 U/mL and 0.5 to 0.8 for anticoagulation treatment. However, monitoring anti-Xa level is not predictive of neuraxial bleeding and is therefore not recommended during neuraxial blockade. Enoxaparin 40 mg may be given once or twice daily for intermediate thromboprophylaxis during pregnancy (28). However, twice-daily weight specific dosing over once-daily dosing of enoxaparin 1 mg/kg subcutaneously may be the preferred treatment for acute VTE in pregnancy (18). Therapeutic anticoagulation should continue for 20 weeks followed by prophylactic anticoagulation for 6 weeks. At 36 weeks, LMWH is discontinued and prophylactic heparin started until the onset of labor. Dalteparin 5,000 units may be given once or twice daily for intermediate thromboprophylaxis during pregnancy and a weight specific dose of 100 units/kg twice daily or 200 units once daily for therapeutic anticoagulation (28). Regional anesthesia is contraindicated within 24 hours of the last therapeutic LMWH dose. Recommendations for neuraxial anesthesia during labor and delivery when LMWHs are used for prophylaxis and treatment of VTE in the antenatal and postpartum periods are presented in Table 23-6.

LMWH is considered relatively safe during pregnancy. Successful pregnancy was reported over 96% of the time when LMWH was used for VTE prophylaxis or treatment. The advantages of LMWH is that it has improved bioavailability and can be given once a day, does not cross the placenta and is not be associated with teratogenicity. LMWH has a more predictable

TABLE 23-6 American Society of Regional Anesthesia and Pain Medicine (ASRA) Guidelines Regarding Anticoagulation with LMWH and Neuraxial Anesthesia and Analgesia

1. Weigh risk of spinal hematoma versus benefits of regional anesthesia or analgesia for pregnant patients on LMWH when deciding to place a neuraxial block
2. The concomitant use of antiplatelet or oral anticoagulation medications increase risk of spinal hematoma
3. Patients receiving prophylactic LMWH, neuraxial block should be placed 10–12 h after the last dose of LMWH
4. Patients receiving high dose or therapeutic dose of LMWH, such as enoxaparin 1 mg/kg twice per day, or enoxaparin 1.5 mg/kg daily, neuraxial block should be placed no earlier than 24 h after the last dose.
5. The first dose of LMWH postoperatively depends on the prescribed dosing schedule
   a. Twice-daily dosing: The first dose of LMWH should be given no earlier than 24 h postoperatively. First dose of LMWH should be held for 2 h after indwelling epidural catheters are removed.
   b. Single-daily dosing: The first dose of LMWH should be given 6–8 h postoperatively. The second dose should be given no earlier than 24 h after first dose. Indwelling epidural catheters may be maintained and should not be removed less than 10–12 h after last dose of LMWH. Subsequent dose of LMWH should be held for 2 h after in situ catheters are removed.
6. If blood is seen during needle or catheter placement, the first dose of LMWH should be delayed 24 h postoperatively.

Adapted with permission from: Beilin Y. Thrombocytopenia and low molecular weight heparin in the parturient: Implications for neuraxial anesthesia. ASA Refresher Course in Anesthesiology. 2010;Course 202:1–7.

anticoagulant response and does not require monitoring, does not increase the risk of bleeding during cesarean deliveries and other surgical procedures, and is associated with a lower risk of platelet activation and heparin-induced thrombocytopenia and osteoporosis. LMWH is not secreted in breast milk and is safe in lactating women. LMWH is excreted by the kidneys and care is advised with use in pregnant women with kidney dysfunction. Potential adverse effects include arterial thrombosis 0.50% and significant bleeding 1.98% (27). The American College of Chest Physicians (ACCP) guidelines for the management of VTE during pregnancy include a Grade 1A recommendation to weight-adjusted dose of LMWH or unfractionated heparin for at least 5 days of therapy (29). Pregnant patients with mechanical heart valves or mitral stenosis also have a significant risk of thromboembolism. Prophylactic anticoagulation is indicated in cardiac patients with mitral stenosis with atrial fibrillation or a prior history of VTE (30). The use of LMWH over unfractionated heparin received a Grade 2C recommendation for the prevention and treatment of VTE. The ACCP also made a Grade 2C recommendation for the use of subcutaneous LMWH or unfractionated heparin for at least 6 weeks postpartum. It is also suggested that pregnant patients with acute VTE should receive anticoagulants for at least 6 weeks postpartum for a minimum of total 6 months duration of therapy (29).

Warfarin

A 13-member thrombosis working group developed a consensus report and recommendations for prevention and treatment of VTE during pregnancy (31). This review made recommendations regarding measuring antithrombin levels and appropriate use of regional anesthesia. Also, they recommended that maternal anticoagulation with warfarin prior to delivery should be avoided where possible. Warfarin should be avoided during early pregnancy and is contraindicated in the first trimester. Warfarin blocks the vitamin K-dependent glutamate carboxylation of factors II, VII, IX, and X. Onset of action is within 90 minutes of oral administration of warfarin. However, it requires 2 to 3 days to achieve adequate prophylactic effect. The therapeutic range is narrow and monitoring of effectiveness is necessary and desired INR is between —two and three. Warfarin has a long elimination half-life of 36 to 42 hours. Warfarin crosses the placenta and is associated with teratogenicity such as cleft lip, cleft palate, and cataracts. In addition, warfarin is associated with spontaneous abortions, maternal bleeding, neonatal and fetal hemorrhage, and placental abruption. Otherwise, warfarin is relatively safe during the second trimester until 2 to 4 weeks prior to anticipated delivery, and in lactating women. Also, warfarin is indicated in pregnant patient with mechanical heart valves to further decrease the risk of thrombosis seen with therapeutic anticoagulation with heparin or LMWH (18,29).

Aspirin produces fast irreversible inhibition of platelet cyclooxygenase, COX-1, and decreased thromboxane A2 after low-dose oral administration of 160 mg. The elimination half-life is 30 minutes and long duration of action 7 to 10 days. The ACCP provided a Grade 1 recommendation and recommended against the use of aspirin alone as thromboprophylaxis for any patient group (29). Aspirin did not provide protection against DVT and provided inferior protection against VTE. Aspirin is effective in preventing arterial thrombosis. US guidelines do not include any contraindications for the timing of neuraxial anesthesia in patients receiving aspirin (24).

Fondaparinux, a synthetic heparin pentasaccharide that selectively binds to antithrombin III to selectively inhibit factor Xa, may be the preferred anticoagulant in cases of severe allergies or heparin-induced thrombocytopenia in pregnancy. The onset of action is within 2 hours. Fondaparinux

is primarily eliminated through the kidney and has a dose-dependent elimination half-life of 17 hours. However, there is insufficient data regarding use during pregnancy, monitoring of anticoagulation activity is more frequent (24).

Thienopyridines indirectly and irreversibly inhibit ADP-induced platelet aggregation and is effective in the prevention of arterial thrombosis (24). Clopidogrel produces maximum inhibition of ADP-induced platelet aggregation within 5 hours after oral administration of Ticlopidine. Inactive metabolites of Clopidogrel are eliminated through the kidneys and the elimination half-life is 7.5 hours. Normal platelet function is seen in 7 days following discontinuation of Clopidogrel treatment. Following oral administration of Ticlopidine, platelet inhibition begins within 1 hour due to its 90% bioavailability. Maximum inhibition of platelet function occurs after 3 to 5 days of oral administration. The elimination half-life is 24 to 36 hours. Platelet function recovers slowly over 3 to 8 days (26).

Other options include thrombolysis, embolectomy, and IVC filters. Treatment guidelines by the ACCP include recommendations for thrombolysis in hemodynamically compromised patients or in high-risk patients without hypotension following risk stratification and assessment of severity and prognosis of pulmonary embolism and risk of bleeding. Several case reports confirm the efficacy of thrombolysis during pregnancy and should be considered in a patient with recurrence of thromboembolism despite adequate anticoagulation. Thrombolysis during pregnancy is associated with a maternal mortality rate of 1%, a fetal loss rate of 6%, and a prematurity rate of 6%. In contrast, embolectomy and cardiopulmonary bypass are associated with a much higher rate of fetal loss of 20% to 40%. The use of recombinant tissue plasminogen activator (rtPA) appears to be the preferred thrombolytic because of its high molecular weight and inability to readily cross the placenta, shorter administration time, and lower risk of allergic reaction and hemorrhage than streptokinase or urokinase. rtPA, a large polypeptide activates plasminogen to form plasmin, the fibrinolytic enzyme which cleaves fibrin, fibrinogen, factor V, and factor VIII. rtPA is also nonantigenic (17). The ACCP guideline recommends that the use of thrombolysis be reserved to treat PE in the unstable pregnant patient or in life-threatening situations (19,29). Streptokinase also does not readily cross the placenta. However, it has a high antigenic effect and should not be given for 6 months after the initial dose. Urokinase readily crosses the placenta and is associated with a higher incidence of fetal coagulopathy and should be avoided during pregnancy. Neuraxial anesthesia is absolutely contraindicated in patients requiring thrombolytics (14).

Treatment guidelines by the ACCP include recommendations for catheter embolectomy and surgical embolectomy in selected highly compromised patients at high risk from bleeding for thrombolysis or insufficient time for systemic thrombolysis to be effective. However, embolectomy is rarely indicated during pregnancy. Embolectomy is reserved in cases in which the parturient's life is in jeopardy and when hemodynamically unstable patients remain unresponsive to anticoagulation and vasopressors (25,29).

The indications for IVC filters in pregnant and nonpregnant patients are patients with an acute VTE in whom anticoagulation is contraindicated, stable patients with recurrence of VTE despite adequate anticoagulation, and or hemodynamically unstable patients in whom a recurrence would be likely fatal (19). IVC filters block migration of venous emboli from the lower extremities to the heart and lungs, thereby preventing PE. The risk of complications is relatively low. However, potential complications associated with IVC filters are IVC occlusion, filter migration, filter breakage and embolization, perforation of vena cava, and trauma to nearby structures and retroperitoneal hematoma (17).

■ COMPLICATIONS OF ANTICOAGULATION DURING PREGNANCY

Although pregnancy is a hypercoagulable state, anticoagulation may be required in parturients with a history of high risk of thromboembolism, mechanical heart valves, fetal loss associated with antithrombin III deficiency, antiphospholipid syndrome, protein S and C deficiencies, and other thrombophilias and hypercoagulable states.

In addition to increased risk of bleeding, thrombocytopenia, and spinal and epidural hematoma, anticoagulation during pregnancy is of great concern to anesthesia care providers. Anticoagulation should be discontinued with active nonsurgical bleeding until laboratory test correctly assesses abnormalities which may be corrected with blood products including fresh frozen plasma, platelets, cryoprecipitate, factors, and packed red blood cells (24). The effects of anticoagulation with unfractionated heparin may be successfully reversed with protamine. Partial reversal of the effects of LMWH may be seen with protamine. Reversal of warfarin may require fresh frozen plasma, prothrombin concentrates, or activated recombinant factor VIIa. A spinal or epidural hematoma can lead to permanent paralysis. The risk of epidural or spinal hematoma after regional anesthesia is 1:150,000 and 1:220,000, respectively during normal pregnancy. The greater risk of epidural hematoma is associated in anticoagulated patients during insertion and removal of epidural catheters. Spinal hematoma may cause severe radicular backache associated with radiculopathy, neurologic deficits including bowel and bladder dysfunction, tenderness over the spinous or paraspinous areas, and unexplained fever. MRI or CT scan may confirm the diagnosis and spinal cord decompression during laminectomy by neurosurgeons within 8 hours improve return of neurologic function (10,32).

Horlocker et al. reported an incidence of spinal or epidural hematoma in nonpregnant patients who received LMWH may be as high as 1 in 3,000 for continuous epidural anesthesia and 1 in 100,000 for spinal anesthesia (33). However, Forsnes et al. reported a case of spontaneous spinal–epidural hematoma during pregnancy associated with LMWH (34). Of 61 cases of anesthesia-related spinal hematoma, Beilin et al. showed in 1997 that most (68%) occurred in patients with coagulopathies and 75% were associated with epidural anesthesia and epidural catheter insertion versus spinal anesthesia. Almost 50% of the patients (15 of 30 parturients) developed an epidural hematoma after epidural catheter removal (35). However, anesthesia-related maternal mortality is significantly higher during general anesthesia for cesarean delivery versus regional anesthesia. Therefore, patient safety is of upmost importance in the decision-making process of weighing the risk benefit of general anesthesia and regional anesthesia. In addition, platelet counts decrease by approximately 20% during pregnancy. Platelet counts less than 150,000/mm^3 and platelet counts less than 100,000/mm^3 are seen in approximately 7% and 0.5% to 1%, respectively of all parturients. Based on Beilin's survey showing the relative safety of epidural anesthesia in noncoagulated parturients with platelet counts below 100,000/mm^3, most anesthesia care providers perform epidural anesthesia when platelet count is stable and between 80,000 and 100,000/mm^3 (35).

Anesthesia care providers may safely provide epidural and spinal anesthesia if American Society of Regional Anesthesia and Pain Medicine (ASRA) guidelines and recommendations are followed regarding anticoagulation with LMWH and neuraxial analgesia and anesthesia (36) (Table 23-7). In addition, epidural anesthesia should be avoided in patients with a significant history of easy bruising and rapidly decreasing platelet counts associated with disorders such as, severe preeclampsia and HELLP syndrome. In such cases, a platelet count should be obtained immediately before placement and removal of an epidural catheter for parturients for labor analgesia. Motor function should be evaluated frequently throughout labor until resolution of sensory and motor blockade. If a parturient develops a coagulopathy or hemorrhage requiring multiple blood products during labor or cesarean delivery, a coagulation profile should be obtained to determine coagulation status prior to removal of an epidural catheter. A spinal anesthetic utilizing a small gauge spinal needle is preferable to an epidural anesthetic requiring an epidural catheter insertion for cesarean delivery (36). An MRI should be done if a parturient develops a pronounced motor block to assess the possibility of an epidural hematoma, which requires emergency laminectomy and decompression within 6 to 12 hours for preservation of neurologic function (14,37).

■ PREVENTION AND THROMBOPROPHYLAXIS

The indications for thromboprophylaxis differ in the antepartum and postpartum period. There is a lower threshold to initiate pharmacoprophylaxis in the postpartum period because the risk of VTE is higher in postpartum than antepartum. In addition, the duration of anticoagulation is usually shorter and there are no longer concerns regarding fetal complications. Conservative prophylaxis includes ambulation, compression devices such as graduated compression stockings and intermittent pneumatic compression devices. Graduated compression stockings reduce venous stasis in the lower extremities and are effective in reducing the risk of venous thrombosis. Graduated compression stockings are more commonly known as thromboembolic deterrent (TED) hose. Prophylactic mechanical devices include intermittent pneumatic compression and sequential compression devices. Intermittent pneumatic compression devices prevent venous thrombosis by increasing venous flow rates and venous return from the lower extremities. Intermittent pneumatic compression device utilizes a single bladder sleeve to provide intermittent nonuniform inflation, which is available in calf and full lengths. Both the graduated compression stockings and the intermittent pneumatic compression devices should be properly fitted especially in morbidly obese surgical patients and initiated prior to any surgical procedures and used intraoperatively and postoperatively. Graduated compression stockings are more effective when used in combination with a second prophylactic method. ACOG makes a level C recommendation for the placement of pneumatic compression devices before cesarean delivery for all women not already receiving thromboprophylaxis (28). In addition, pneumatic compression devices should be left in place until the patient is ambulatory and anticoagulation is restarted. Compression devices do not increase risk of bleeding and may be used in combination of pharmacologic prophylaxis. Sequential compression device utilizes multichamber sleeves with sequential inflation with different pressures, is available in calf and full length sleeves.

However, pharmacologic prophylaxis may be required in patients at high risk for VTE (28). Thromboprophylaxis may be indicated in pregnant patient with a history of antiphospholipiid syndrome, DVT in a prior pregnancy, unexplained or recurrent DVT or VTE, or while on oral contraceptives. Therapeutic anticoagulation 4 to 6 months followed by

TABLE 23-7 US Guidelines for Timing of Neuraxial Anesthesia in Patients Receiving Anticoagulation

Drug	Timing of Anticoagulation
Unfractionated Heparin Subcutaneous	
Before neuraxial blockade/after catheter withdrawal	No time interval for 5,000 U twice daily Greater than 4 d, check platelet count
After neuraxial blockade/after catheter withdrawal	1 h
Unfractionated Heparin Intravenous	
Before neuraxial blockade/after catheter withdrawal	None recommended/2–4 h
After neuraxial blockade/after catheter withdrawal	1 h
Low–molecular-weight Heparin (LMWH) (prophylactic dose)	
Before neuraxial blockade/after catheter withdrawal	10–12 h
After neuraxial blockade/after catheter withdrawal	6–8 h first postoperative dose (single dosing) Second postoperative dose 24 h after first dose Regardless dosing schedule, wait 2 h after catheter removal
Low–molecular-weight Heparin (LMWH) (therapeutic dose)	
Before neuraxial blockade/after catheter withdrawal	24 h
After neuraxial blockade/after catheter withdrawal	24 h/>2 h
Fondaparinux Subcutaneous	
Before neuraxial blockade/catheter withdrawal	Recommended with single-shot spinal, atraumatic blocks, no in situ catheter
After neuraxial blockade/catheter withdrawal	Recommended with single-shot spinal, atraumatic blocks, no in situ catheters
Aspirin	**No Contraindications**
Clopidogrel/before neuraxial blockade/catheter withdrawal	7 d
Ticlopidine/before neuraxial blockade/catheter withdrawal	14 d
Warfarin	
Before neuraxial blockade/catheter withdrawal	Recommend normal/INR ≤ 1.5
After neuraxial blockade/catheter withdrawal	May restart after catheter withdrawal

Adapted with permission from: Butwick AJ, Carvalho B. Neuraxial anesthesia with anticoagulant drugs. *Int J Obstet Anesth* 2010;19(2):193–201. Copyright 2011.

prophylactic anticoagulation for 6 to 12 weeks postpartum is indicated with DVT or VTE during a current pregnancy or history of VTE in a prior pregnancy.

Past idiopathic VTE and known thrombophilia increase the risk of recurrent VTE during pregnancy. In 2011, Knight reported the incidence of recurrent pulmonary thromboembolism of 1.4% and a maternal mortality rate of 3.5% in the UKOSS report on near-miss studies (3). In the United States, the ACCP recommends clinical antepartum surveillance and postpartum prophylaxis for parturients without a history of thrombophilia and single prior incidence of VTE during pregnancy (29). However, prophylactic LMWH may be recommended with history of inherited thrombophilia or factor V Leiden, or antithrombin deficiency, without prior VTE, presence of acquired thrombophilias, such as antiphospholipid antibody syndrome and adverse pregnancy outcomes. Intermediate dose of LMWH is recommended with a history of inherited thrombophilia, factor V Leiden, or antithrombin deficiency and a history of VTE. A weight specific dose is recommended in patients with a history of multiple thromboemboli, for those receiving long-term anticoagulation prior to pregnancy, receiving treatment of VTE during pregnancy, with acquired thrombophilia antiphospholipid antibodies syndrome and history of VTE.

Guidelines for Neuraxial Techniques in the Anticoagulated Pregnant Patient

Neuraxial anesthetic techniques including epidural, spinal, and combined spinal–epidural not only provide effective pain relief during labor and cesarean delivery but also post-cesarean analgesia. Adverse neurologic complications are rare and neuraxial anesthetic techniques are associated with reduced maternal morbidity and mortality. The FDA issued an advisory in 1997 for LMWHs following an increase in reported spinal hematoma with the use of LMWH for surgical thromboprophylaxis after neuraxial anesthesia (33). However, recent large retrospective reviews suggest that the risk of spinal hematoma after neuraxial blockade in obstetric patients is very low; reported rates of spinal hematoma following epidural and spinal blocks for cesarean delivery were 1:200,000 and 1:50,000, respectively (27,38). Although anticoagulants and antithrombotic drugs can increase the incidence of spinal hematoma in obstetric patients after neuraxial anesthesia, the exact incidence of spinal hematoma in obstetric patients receiving anticoagulation is unknown. The ASRA consensus committee established guidelines for performing neuraxial anesthesia in patients receiving anticoagulation (14,33). Epidural or spinal needle placement should be delayed at least 12 hours following preoperative LMWH thromboprophylaxis and 24 hours following preoperative therapeutic LMWH. LMWH prophylaxis should be withheld for 24 hours postoperatively if bleeding is seen during epidural needle or catheter placement. Following prophylactic postoperative twice-daily dosing, the initial dose of LMWH should be given no earlier than 24 hours postoperatively, regardless of the technique. Following postoperative single-daily dosing, the initial dose of LMWH may be given 6 to 8 hours postpartum. Also, indwelling epidural catheters should not be removed less than 12 hours following the last dose of LMWH. Following epidural catheter removal, LMWH may be restarted after 2 hours. During neuraxial blockade in anticoagulated patients, ASRA Consensus statement recommends the use of dilute concentrations of local anesthetics or opioid for infusion to facilitate frequent monitoring of neurologic function. These guidelines are included in Table 23-8 (14,24).

TABLE 23-8 **Summary of Guidelines for Neuraxial Anesthesia Following Anticoagulants and Thrombotic Drugs**

	ACOG	ACCP	ASRA
General	Initial diagnostic test for acute DVT is CUS. Therapeutic anticoagulation with acute thromboembolism during current pregnancy or with mechanical heart valves Place PCD before cesarean delivery for all women and maintain in place until patient is ambulatory and anticoagulation is restarted Resume anticoagulation therapy no sooner than 4–6 h after vaginal delivery or 6–12 h after cesarean delivery	The use of antithrombotic agents is not recommended in patients without thrombophilia or women with thrombophilia in the absence of thromboembolism or poor pregnancy outcome Avoid or limit epidural analgesia to < 48 h, withdraw catheter when INR < 1.5 with warfarin Spinal safe, avoid epidural analgesia with fondaparinux Use of direct thrombin inhibitors, thrombolytics not addressed	Normal INR before neuraxial technique and withdraw catheter when INR < 1.5 with warfarin Delay needle placement 36–42 h after last fondaparinux dose, wait 6–12 h after catheter withdrawal for subsequent fondaparinux dose Avoid neuraxial techniques with direct thrombin inhibitors Absolute CI with thrombolytics
Following antiplatelet drugs		NSAIDs: no CI Discontinue clopidogrel 7 d before neuraxial blockade	NSAIDs: No CI Discontinue ticlopidine 14 d and clopidogrel 7 d
Following subcutaneous UFH	Women receiving either therapeutic or prophylactic oral anticoagulation may be converted to LMWH with similar dosing no later than 36 wks of pregnancy until 36 h before induction of labor or cesarean delivery, Convert to SC or IV UFH until 4–6 h before delivery	Needle placement 8–12 h after SC UFH dose; subsequent dose 2 h after block or epidural catheter withdrawal	No CI with twice-daily SC dosing and total daily dose < 10,000 U Consider holding SC UFH if neuraxial blockade is anticipated to be technically difficult Start IV UFH 1 h after neuraxial technique, remove catheter 2–4 h after last UFH dose, no delay required if traumatic Resume prophylaxis 12 h after cesarean or catheter withdrawal with twice-daily dose of 5,000 U of UFH Delay prophylaxis for 24 h with weight adjusted UFH dosing regardless of mode of delivery
Following subcutaneous LMWH	At least 36 h before and Withhold neuraxial blockade for 12 h after the last prophylactic dose of LMWH or 24 h after the last therapeutic dose of LMWH	Needle placement 8–12 h after LMWH dose; subsequent LMWH dose 2 h after block or catheter withdrawal. Indwelling catheter safe with twice-daily LMWH prophylactic dosing	Twice-daily prophylactic dosing: LMWH 24 h after surgery, regardless of technique; Remove neuraxial catheter 2 h before first LMWH dose Therapeutic dose: Delay block for >18 h Resume prophylaxis 12 h after cesarean delivery or catheter withdrawal with 40 mg enoxaparin once daily Delay prophylaxis for 24 h with LMWH 1 mg/kg every 12 h regardless of mode of delivery

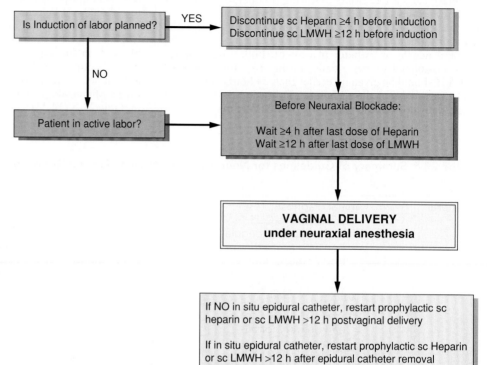

FIGURE 23-2 Vaginal delivery management: Prophylactic subcutaneous heparin or subcutaneous LMWH. Adapted with permission from: Butwick AJ Carvalho B. Algorithm for the timing of prophylactic subcutaneous heparin or LMWH administration before and after vaginal delivery. *J Perinat* 2011:31:73–84. Copyright 2011.

Management of patient receiving prophylactic anticoagulation with unfractionated heparin and LMWH for vaginal and cesarean delivery. See Figures 23-2 and 23-3.

Management of patient receiving therapeutic anticoagulation with unfractionated heparin and LMWH for vaginal and cesarean delivery. See Figures 23-4 and 23-5.

To decrease spinal hematoma, the Royal College of Obstetricians and Gynecologists' recommendation for thromboprophylaxis guidelines after cesarean delivery states the first weight specific dose of LMWH should be given 4 hours following spinal or epidural anesthesia or removal of epidural catheter. In situ epidural catheters should not be removed less

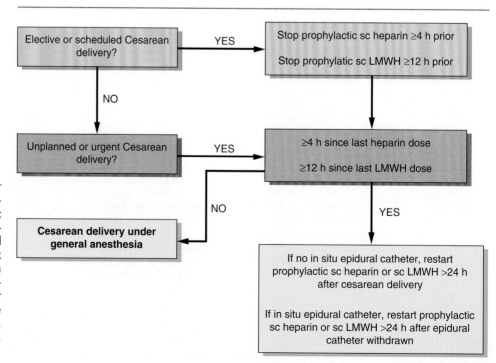

FIGURE 23-3 Cesarean delivery management: Prophylactic subcutaneous heparin or subcutaneous LMWH. Adapted with permission from: Butwick AJ, Carvalho B. Algorithm for the timing of prophylactic subcutaneous heparin or LMWH administration before and after cesarean delivery. *J Perinat* 2011;31:73–84. Copyright 2011.

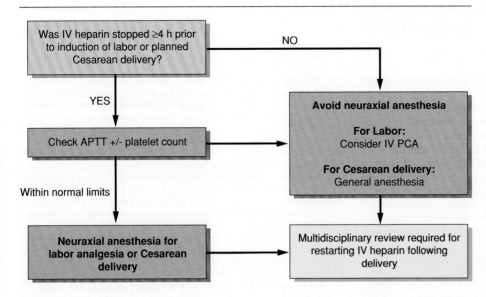

FIGURE 23-4 Peripartum management: Therapeutic intravenous heparin for vaginal or cesarean delivery. IV, intravenous; SC, subcutaneous; LMWH, low–molecular-weight heparin; PCA, patient controlled analgesia. Reprinted with permission from: Butwick AJ, Carvalho B. Algorithm for the timing of therapeutic low molecular weight heparin administration before and after vaginal or cesarean delivery. *J Perinat* 2011;31:73–84. Copyright 2011.

than 12 hours after the last dose of LMWH and not less than 4 hours before the next dose (39). See Figures 23-4 and 23-5.

■ POSTPARTUM THROMBOPROPHYLAXIS

Postpartum prophylaxis is recommended for women with prior VTE or thrombophilia and a family history of VTE (12). Postpartum patients are still at risk for pulmonary thromboembolism regardless of the mode of delivery. Prophylactic anticoagulation should be restarted 3 to 6 hours after vaginal delivery and 6 to 8 hours after uncomplicated cesarean delivery (16). Morbidly obese patients with a BMI greater than 40 should continue thromboprophylaxis with LMWH for 6 weeks regardless of the mode of delivery or the presence of other risk factors according to the updated RCOG guidelines of 2009 and the CMACE guidelines (5). BMI should be accurately calculated and weight specific prophylactic dosing started. In addition, patients should be alerted to report calf pain, breathlessness, and chest symptoms.

For summary of guidelines for neuraxial anesthesia following prophylactic and therapeutic anticoagulant and antithrombotic drugs and management of VTE in pregnancy, see Table 23-8.

Guidelines for Anticoagulation in Pregnant Patients with Prosthetic Heart Valves The 2008 American College of Cardiology and American Heart Association published recommendations for continuous therapeutic anticoagulation during pregnancy in all patients with mechanical prosthetic heart valves (40). Recommendations included early pregnancy testing for women receiving warfarin to ensure continued anticoagulation with continuous intravenous unfractionated heparin, weight specific dosing of unfractionated heparin, or weight specific dosing of subcutaneous LMWH when warfarin is discontinued between 6 and 12 weeks of gestation. Anticoagulation with continuous intravenous unfractionated heparin, weight specific dosing of unfractionated heparin, or weight specific dosing of subcutaneous LMWH may continue until 36 weeks. Otherwise, warfarin may be restarted between 12 weeks and 36 weeks gestation to maintain the INR 3. LMWH should be given twice daily subcutaneously to maintain therapeutic anti-XA levels between 0.7 and 1.2 units/mL 4 hours following dosing. In patients receiving unfractionated heparin, the aPTT should be twice control levels. Please see the Cardiac Disease chapter for additional recommendations in pregnant patients with mechanical prosthetic heart valves.

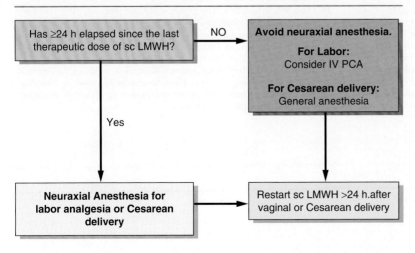

FIGURE 23-5 Peripartum management: Therapeutic SC LMWH for vaginal or cesarean delivery. IV, intravenous; SC, subcutaneous; LMWH, low–molecular-weight heparin; PCA, patient controlled analgesia. Reproduced with permission from: Butwick AJ, Carvalho B. Algorithm for the timing of therapeutic low molecular weight heparin administration before and after vaginal or cesarean delivery. *J Perinat* 2011;31:73–84. Copyright 2011.

KEY POINTS

- Pulmonary thromboembolism contributes significantly to maternal morbidity and mortality.
- Early diagnosis and aggressive management improve maternal and neonatal outcomes.
- Pulmonary thromboembolism is an essentially preventable obstructive and embolic phenomenon. The goal of management of deep vein thrombosis and pulmonary embolus is to prevent pulmonary embolism and recurrence.
- Regional anesthesia may be used safely in pregnant patients receiving prophylactic or therapeutic anticoagulation prior to or following vaginal and cesarean delivery if American Society of Regional Anesthesia Guidelines are followed.
- A multidisciplinary team approach with early recognition and immediate resuscitation improves maternal and fetal prognosis and outcomes.

REFERENCES

1. WHO. Trends in maternal mortality: 1990 to 2008 estimates developed by WHO, UNICEF, UNFPA, and the World Bank, World Health Organization 2010, Annex 1. [Internet]. Available from: http://whqlibdoc.who.int/publications/2010/9789241500265_eng.pdf.
2. Lewis G. Chapter 1: The women who died 2006–2008. In: Cantwell R, ed. *Saving Mothers' Lives: Reviewing Maternal Deaths to Make Motherhood Safer: 2006–2008.* 8th ed. London: Wiley-Blackwell; 2011:30.
3. Knight M. Appendix 2A: Summary of United Kingdom obstetric surveillance system (UKOSS) report on near-miss studies. In: Cantwell R, ed. *Saving Mothers' Lives: Reviewing Maternal Deaths to Make Motherhood Safer: 2006–2008.* 8th ed. London: Wiley-Blackwell; 2011:191.
4. Cantwell R, Clutton-Brock T, Cooper G, et al. Saving mothers' lives: Reviewing maternal deaths to make motherhood safer: 2006–2008. The Eighth Report of the Confidential Enquiries into Maternal Deaths in the United Kingdom. *BJOG* 2011;118(suppl 1):1–203.
5. Drife J. Chapter 2: Thrombosis and thromboembolism. In: Cantwell R, ed. *Saving Mothers' Lives: Reviewing Maternal Deaths to Make Motherhood Safer: 2006–2008.* 8th ed. London: Wiley-Blackwell; 2011:57.
6. Royal College of Anaesthetists. Initial assessment of competency. CCT in anaesthesia II: Competency based basic level training and assessment. 2007.
7. Royal College of Obstetricians and Gynaecologists. Reducing the risk of thrombosis and embolism during pregnancy and puerperium. Green-top Guideline No. 37. 2009.
8. Schoenbeck D, Nicolle A, Newbegin K, et al. The use of a scoring system to guide thromboprophylaxis in a high-risk pregnant population. *Thrombosis* 2011;2011:652796.
9. Berg CJ, Callaghan WM, Syverson C, et al. Pregnancy-related mortality in the United States, 1998 to 2005. *Obstet Gynecol* 2010;116(6):1302–1309.
10. Clark SL, Belfort MA, Dildy GA, et al. Maternal death in the 21st century: Causes, prevention, and relationship to cesarean delivery. *Am J Obstet Gynecol* 2008;199(1):36.e1–e5; discussion 91–92. e7–e11.
11. Joint Commission on Accreditation of Healthcare Organizations, USA. Preventing maternal death. *Sentinel Event Alert* 2010;(44):1–4.
12. Chunilal SD, Bates SM. Venous thromboembolism in pregnancy: Diagnosis, management, and prevention. *Thromb Haemost* 2009;101(3):428–438.
13. Deneux-Tharaux C, Carmona E, Bouvier-Colle MH, et al. Postpartum maternal mortality and cesarean delivery. *Obstet Gynecol* 2006;108(3 pt 1):541–548.
14. Horlocker TT, Wedel DJ, Rowlingson JC, et al. Regional anesthesia in the patient receiving antithrombotic or thrombolytic therapy: American Society of Regional Anesthesia and Pain Medicine Evidence-Based Guidelines (Third Edition). *Reg Anesth Pain Med* 2010;35(1):64–101.
15. Krivak TC, Zorn KK. Venous thromboembolism in obstetrics and gynecology. *Obstet Gynecol* 2007;109(3):761–777.
16. Rosenberg VA, Lockwood CJ. Thromboembolism in pregnancy. *Obstet Gynecol Clin North Am* 2007;34(3):481–500.
17. Stone SE, Morris TA. Pulmonary embolism and pregnancy. *Crit Care Clin* 2004;20(4):661–677.
18. James A, Committee on Practice Bulletins—Obstetrics. Practice bulletin no. 123: Thromboembolism in pregnancy. *Obstet Gynecol* 2011;118(3):718–729.
19. McLintock C, Brighton T, Chunilal S, et al. Recommendations for the diagnosis and treatment of deep venous thrombosis and pulmonary embolism in pregnancy and the postpartum period. *Aust N Z J Obstet Gynaecol* 2012;52(1):14–22.
20. Chan WS, Ray JG, Murray S, et al. Suspected pulmonary embolism in pregnancy: Clinical presentation, results of lung scanning, and subsequent maternal and pediatric outcomes. *Arch Intern Med* 2002;162(10):1170–1175.
21. Parker JA, Coleman RE, Grady E, et al. SNM practice guideline for lung scintigraphy 4.0. *J Nucl Med Technol* 2012;40(1):57–65.
22. Bourjeily G, Paidas M, Khalil H, et al. Pulmonary embolism in pregnancy. *Lancet* 2010;375(9713):500–512.
23. Quiroz R, Kucher N, Zou KH, et al. Clinical validity of a negative computed tomography scan in patients with suspected pulmonary embolism: A systematic review. *JAMA* 2005;293(16):2012–2017.
24. Butwick AJ, Carvalho B. Anticoagulant and antithrombotic drugs in pregnancy: What are the anesthetic implications for labor and cesarean delivery? *J Perinatol* 2011;31(2):73–84.
25. Gei AF, Vadhera RB, Hankins GD. Embolism during pregnancy: Thrombus, air, and amniotic fluid. *Anesthesiol Clin North America* 2003;21(1):165–182.
26. Butwick AJ, Carvalho B. Neuraxial anesthesia in obstetric patients receiving anticoagulant and antithrombotic drugs. *Int J Obstet Anesth* 2010;19(2):193–201.
27. Greer IA, Nelson-Piercy C. Low-molecular-weight heparins for thromboprophylaxis and treatment of venous thromboembolism in pregnancy: A systematic review of safety and efficacy. *Blood* 2005;106(2):401–407.
28. Committee on Practice Bulletins—Gynecology, American College of Obstetricians and Gynecologists. ACOG practice bulletin no. 84: Prevention of deep vein thrombosis and pulmonary embolism. *Obstet Gynecol* 2007;110(2 pt 1):429–440.
29. Bates SM, Greer IA, Pabinger I, et al. Venous thromboembolism, thrombophilia, antithrombotic therapy, and pregnancy: American College of Chest Physicians Evidence-Based Clinical Practice Guidelines (8th Edition). *Chest* 2008;133(6 suppl):844S–886S.
30. Goland S, Elkayam U. Anticoagulation in pregnancy. *Cardiol Clin* 2012;30(3):395–405.
31. Duhl AJ, Paidas MJ, Ural SH, et al. Antithrombotic therapy and pregnancy: Consensus report and recommendations for prevention and treatment of venous thromboembolism and adverse pregnancy outcomes. *Am J Obstet Gynecol* 2007;197(5):457.e1–e21.
32. Vandermeulen EP, Van Aken H, Vermylen J. Anticoagulants and spinal–epidural anesthesia. *Anesth Analg* 1994;79(6):1165–1177.
33. Horlocker TT, Wedel DJ. Neuraxial block and low-molecular-weight heparin: Balancing perioperative analgesia and thromboprophylaxis. *Reg Anesth Pain Med* 1998;23(6 suppl 2):164–177.
34. Forsnes E, Occhino A, Acosta R. Spontaneous spinal epidural hematoma in pregnancy associated with using low molecular weight heparin. *Obstet Gynecol* 2009;113(2 pt 2):532–533.
35. Beilin Y, Zahn J, Comerford M. Safe epidural analgesia in thirty parturients with platelet counts between 69,000 and 98,000 mm(-3). *Anesth Analg* 1997;85(2):385–388.
36. Beilin Y. Thrombocytopenia and low molecular weight heparin in the parturient: Implications for neuraxial anesthesia. ASA Refresher Course in Anesthesiology. 2010;Course 202:1–7.
37. Abramovitz S, Beilin Y. Thrombocytopenia, low molecular weight heparin, and obstetric anesthesia. *Anesthesiol Clin North America* 2003;21(1):99–109.
38. Davis SM, Branch DW. Thromboprophylaxis in pregnancy: Who and how? *Obstet Gynecol Clin North Am* 2010;37(2):333–343.
39. McClure J, Cooper G. Chapter 8: Anaesthesia. In: Cantwell R, ed. *Saving Mothers' Lives: Reviewing Maternal Deaths to Make Motherhood Safer: 2006–2008.* 8th ed. London: Wiley-Blackwell; 2011:102.
40. Bonow RO, Carabello BA, Chatterjee K, et al. A report of the American College of Cardiology/American Heart Association Task Force on 2008 Practice Guidelines for the management of patients with valvular heart disease). *J Am Coll Cardiol* 2008;52(13):e1–e142.

Difficult and Failed Intubation: Strategies, Prevention and Management of Airway-related Catastrophes in Obstetrical Patients

Maya S. Suresh • Ashutosh Wali • Edward T. Crosby

■ BACKGROUND

Complications of airway management, that is, difficult laryngoscopy, failed tracheal intubation, and inability to ventilate or oxygenate following induction of general anesthesia (GA) for cesarean delivery (CD) are major contributory factors leading to maternal morbidity and mortality in the United States (1). The trend in clinical practice of obstetric anesthesia has shifted toward enhanced use of regional anesthesia (RA) thus resulting in a dramatic decline in GA even in large tertiary centers with high volume deliveries (2). The enthusiasm for providing GA in obstetrics has been severely diminished as reflected by the serial reports from the Confidential Enquiries into Maternal Deaths in the United Kingdom, from 1976 to 2005, detailing the all too frequent deaths of mothers resulting from a failure to establish an airway.

The decreased use of GA in obstetrics raises several concerns:

Clinical Concern: Obstetric patients that do receive GA have the following characteristics: (a) Majority are high-risk patients with additional comorbidities and (b) Obesity during pregnancy has increased exponentially, thus these patients pose increased risks and challenges in providing GA.

Patient Safety Concern: The incidence of difficult intubation (DI) in pregnant patients has not changed significantly and continues to be a problem. Since GA for cesarean delivery is frequently reserved for true emergencies, these high level stress situations may lead to an inadequate airway assessment, inadequate preparation, or inadequate experience of the anesthesia practitioner to manage the difficult airway in the obstetric patient. These high stress situations, thus, can contribute to the risk of difficult or failed tracheal intubation, leading to the possibility of 200% morbidity and mortality, that is, in mother and baby.

Educational Concern: The declining GA experience of anesthesia trainees necessitates academic obstetric anesthesiologists to search for alternative educational modalities to enhance the advanced airway experience.

There have been tremendous advances in airway management in recent years: (1) Introduction and revision of the American Society of Anesthesiologists' (ASA) Task Force Recommendations for Management of the Difficult Airway (3), (2) vast increase in the body of knowledge in advanced airway management, (3) availability of numerous airway devices as adjuncts to airway management, and (4) exponential increase in publications worldwide in advanced airway management. These improvements have led to a documented decline in the incidence of airway-related perioperative morbidity in the general surgical population (4). In obstetrical patients, because of increased use of regional anesthesia

and the experience with the laryngeal mask airway (LMA) in managing the difficult airway, the incidence of brain death and mortality has decreased (5); however, the incidence of difficult tracheal intubation has not declined.

■ GOALS AND STEPS IN OBSTETRIC ANESTHESIA WITH RELATION TO AIRWAY MANAGEMENT

Since the impact of maternal death due to failed tracheal intubation is enormous in terms of its devastating effect on the family and the financial liability in obstetric-related claims, the following goals are important to implement (Table 24-1):

1. Ensuring safe and optimal outcomes for both mother and fetus
2. Establishing oxygenation and ventilation should take a priority requiring the use of alternative rescue airway devices in these emergent situations in an obstetric patient
3. Balancing the urgency of delivering the baby while keeping maternal safety in mind
4. Preventing pulmonary aspiration particularly with the use of supraglottic airways in a patient with full stomach
5. The ultimate goal should be to eliminate entirely the airway-related maternal and neonatal adverse outcomes.

With these goals in mind, it is prudent for the obstetric anesthesia practitioner to follow these steps:

(1) Determine the predictors of the difficult airway; (2) assess risk factors that predispose to airway-related complications; (3) have a pre-formulated airway rescue plan, within the framework of a well thought out algorithm, for managing the difficult airway which should be worked out ahead of time; (4) have airway devices/equipment/difficult airway cart immediately available in the labor and delivery suite and the operating rooms to manage the difficult airway. When tracheal intubation has failed, ventilation with mask and cricoid pressure, or with a supraglottic airway device (e.g., intubating laryngeal mask airway; (Fastrach™) Combitube® should be considered for maintaining an airway and ventilating the lungs; (5) understand balancing the urgency of delivering the baby and also preventing pulmonary aspiration with the use of supraglottic airways for oxygenation and ventilation; (6) acquire and maintain advanced airway management skills, including cricothyroidotomy skills. If it is not possible to ventilate or awaken the patient, an airway should be created surgically.

The ASA task force on obstetric anesthesia published the *Practice Guidelines for Obstetric Anesthesia* in 2007 (6). The

TABLE 24-1 Goals and Steps for Difficult Airway Management in Obstetric Anesthesia

Goals	Steps to Achieve Goals
Ensure safe outcomes for mother and baby	Be cognizant of predictors of the difficult airway
Establish oxygenation and ventilation; a priority which may require the use of alternative airway device	Assess risk factors that predispose to airway-related complications
Balance urgency of delivering the baby while keeping maternal safety in mind	Have an airway rescue plan, within the framework of a well thought out algorithm, for managing the difficult airway
Prevent regurgitation and pulmonary aspiration	Have airway devices/equipment/difficult airway cart *immediately* available in the labor and delivery suite and the operating rooms to manage the difficult airway
Eliminate airway-related maternal and neonatal adverse outcomes entirely	Acquire and maintain advanced airway management skills, including cricothyroidotomy skills

guidelines clearly state that labor and delivery suites should have personnel and equipment readily available to manage airway emergencies, including a pulse oximeter and qualitative carbon dioxide detector, consistent with the ASA Practice Guidelines for Management of the Difficult Airway (3).

■ EPIDEMIOLOGY OF AIRWAY-RELATED MORBIDITY AND MORTALITY

Anesthesia-related mortality ranks seventh among the leading causes of maternal deaths in the United States (7) and United Kingdom (8). Even in developing countries, anesthesia is emerging as an additional risk for maternal mortality (9) and remains largely under-reported. The inability to maintain a patent airway and effectively oxygenate after failed intubation and ventilation remains a major concern and a significant source of malpractice claims in obstetric anesthesia (5).

Epidemiology of General Anesthesia-related Morbidity and Mortality

United States of America (USA) Data

Overall anesthesia-related complications have progressively declined and currently account for 1.6% of total pregnancy-related deaths in the USA (10). In the last three decades, GA-related complications, specifically airway-related complications leading to maternal deaths, have declined significantly (10). The shift away from GA to regional anesthesia (RA) in obstetrical care was accelerated in 1997, when Hawkins et al. published the first national study in the United States, reporting a 16.7 relative risk increase in mortality in mothers provided GA compared with those who had received RA (1). The majority of the anesthesia-related deaths (82%) took place during CD and these deaths were due to difficult or failed intubation, pulmonary aspiration, and respiratory-related complications. Death rates during CD increased from 20 per million (1979–1984) to 32.3 per million (1985–1990) for GA (Table 24-2). Conversely, the death rate for RA during the same time periods declined from 8.6 to 1.9 per million. The relative risk ratio of GA mortality was 2.3 times that of RA (1).

In a follow-up study, Hawkins et al. examined and estimated the trends in 12 years of anesthesia-related maternal deaths from 1991 to 2002 and compared it to previous data of anesthesia-related maternal mortality from 1979 to 1990 (10). The case fatality risk ratio between the two techniques for 1997–2002 was 1.7 compared with 16.7 for the previous study period from 1985 to 1990. Anesthetic-related maternal mortality decreased nearly 60% when comparing the 1979–1990 epoch with that of 1991–2002. Although the data is encouraging, the follow-up study shows that complications related to anesthesia continue to occur. The results showed that of the 86 pregnancy deaths, with the exclusion of 30 deaths (27 due to early losses—abortion and ectopic pregnancies and 3 deaths whose pregnancy outcome was not known); the remaining 56 maternal deaths were associated with mainly airway-related complications of anesthesia and accounted for 1.6% of total pregnancy-related deaths. Case fatality rates for GA continued to decline from 16.8 per million in 1991–1996 to 6.5 per million in 1997–2002 (Table 24-2). Almost all women who died from complications of anesthesia, between the periods of 1991 and 2002, were undergoing cesarean delivery (86%), similar to the previous report (82%) (1,10). Overall, the leading causes of anesthesia-related maternal mortality in pregnancy, during 1991–2002, were tracheal intubation failure or induction problems (23%), respiratory failure (20%), and high spinal or epidural block (16%) which was also followed by respiratory failure.

TABLE 24-2 Case Fatality Rates and Rate Ratios of Anesthesia-related Deaths During Cesarean Delivery by Type of Anesthesia in the United States, 1979–2002

Year of Death	Case Fatality Rates[a]		Rate Ratios
	General Anesthetic	Regional Anesthetic	
1979–1984	20.0	8.6	2.3 (95% CI 1.9–2.9)
1985–1990	32.3	1.9	16.7 (95% CI 12.9–21.8)
1991–1996	16.8	2.5	6.7 (95% CI 3.0–14.9)
1997–2002	6.5	3.8	1.7 (95% C 0.6–4.6)

CI, confidence interval.
[a]Deaths per million general or regional anesthetics.
Reprinted with permission from: Hawkins JL, Chang J, Palmer SK, et al. Anesthesia-related maternal mortality in the united states: 1979–2002. *Obstet Gynecol* 2011;117(1):69–74.

Improvements in case fatality rate for GA are especially notable, given the fact that recent reports indicate that GA in obstetrical patients is reserved for high-risk parturients with comorbidities and in cases where there is a perceived lack of time for RA techniques (11). These findings were corroborated by Bloom et al. in 2005, who reported that GA is increasingly reserved for cases when the decision-to-incision interval is less than 15 minutes or when ASA status is greater than 4, that is, for the most emergent cases and the sickest patients (12). These findings are further supported by those of Palanisamy et al. in 2011 who found that GA was used for less than 1% of CD in a major USA center and was administered predominantly for emergency indications where there is perceived lack of time for neuraxial techniques, and in high-risk parturients with associated significant hematologic, neurologic, infectious or cardiac diseases (2).

Data suggests that the anesthetic death rate has stabilized at about 1 per million live births (10). The elements of care which have led to a reduction in maternal mortality associated with GA have not been identified, but changing patterns of anesthesia practice, greater use of protocols and algorithms for the management of difficult airway, and the increased availability and application of alternate airway technologies are likely relevant in this regard (10).

The increased utilization of neuraxial techniques for providing labor analgesia and anesthesia for CD has been prompted by a number of benefits and concerns, with the most prominent reason being to avoid the potentially difficult airway and the risk of pulmonary aspiration in obstetric patients. Although case fatality rates for GA are falling, there is a new emerging problem, the rate for RA case fatality has increased from 2.5 per million in 1991–1996 to 3.8 per million in 1997–2002 with a slight increase in deaths associated with RA- and airway-related issues (10). The exact causes for RA-related mortality during the latest study period is not substantiated; it could be due to undetected intrathecal catheters during epidural placement, high spinal, followed by respiratory arrest and unavailability of trained personnel and airway equipment for timely intervention (5).

United Kingdom (UK) Data

The Confidential Enquiries into Maternal Death in England and Wales reports are comprehensive and have provided continuous information since 1952. In the United Kingdom, despite the decline in the total number of maternal deaths, from 1968 to 1984, anesthetic deaths consistently accounted for approximately 10% of the total direct deaths. The pregnancy-related mortality ratios from anesthesia are very similar in the United States and in the United Kingdom (Table 24-3) (10). Similar to the United States, the anesthesia-related maternal mortality changes in anesthesia practice in the United Kingdom have been associated with a decline in anesthesia-related maternal mortality (13) from 8.7 in 1979–1981 to 1.4 maternal deaths per million live births in 1997–1999 followed by an increase to 3.0 maternal deaths per million maternities in 2000–2002 (10).

During the triennium, 1982 to 1984, anesthesia was the third leading cause of death resulting in 19 of 243 deaths, of which 15 deaths were due to airway-related difficulties (14).

The confidential enquiry spanning 1994 to 1996 showed that anesthesia was responsible for only one out of 268 maternal deaths. In the Confidential Enquiry into Maternal and Child Health (CEMACH) 2000–2002 study, there were six direct deaths due to anesthesia; of the six deaths there were two deaths and one *direct late death* that resulted from esophageal intubation. In two of the cases, anesthesia was being administered for urgent CD by trainees without senior backup. The anesthesia care that was rendered was considered substandard (8).

TABLE 24-3 Pregnancy-related Mortality Ratio Due to Anesthesia in the United States and United Kingdom, 1979–2002

Triennium	United States[a]	United Kingdom[b]
1979–1981	4.3	8.7
1982–1984	3.3	7.2
1985–1987	2.3	1.9
1988–1990	1.7	1.7
1991–1993	1.4	3.5
1994–1996	1.1	0.5
1997–1999	1.2	1.4
2000–2002	1.0	3.0

[a]Maternal deaths per million live births.
[b]Maternal deaths per million maternities (live births, stillbirths, pregnancy terminations, ectopic pregnancies, and abortions).
From: Hawkins JL, Chang J, Palmer SK, et al. Anesthesia-related maternal mortality in the United States: 1979–2002. *Obstet Gynecol* 2011;117(1):71.

The estimated risk of death due to GA was calculated as one death per 20,000 general anesthetics (8).

Maternal Deaths and Airway-related Issues Following Emergence

USA Data

Where once airway-attributed maternal death was most likely to be a result of failed ventilation or pulmonary aspiration associated with difficult intubation at the *induction of anesthesia*, now it seems to be increasingly associated with *extubation or respiratory difficulties arising in the early postoperative period*. Following a review of records for pregnancy-associated deaths in the state of Michigan between 1985 and 2003, Mhyre et al. reported that 8 of 855 pregnancy-associated deaths (15) that occurred during emergence. Of these eight deaths, five deaths resulted from hypoventilation or airway obstruction during emergence, extubation, or recovery. This study highlighted the importance of airway-related problems, during emergence, particularly in the morbidly obese and Africa-American population, the lack of proper supervision and the importance of vigilance in monitoring and management in the postoperative period so as to prevent airway-related complications. The strategies and recommendations for avoiding hypoventilation or airway obstruction and airway catastrophes in the postoperative are explained later in the chapter.

UK Data

Concurrent with the reduction in the use of GA in obstetrics, there has also been a change in the etiology of anesthesia-attributable maternal deaths when they do occur (16). In the CEMACH study, spanning the period from 2003 to 2005, there were six maternal deaths directly related to anesthesia similar to 2000–2002. Of the six direct deaths attributable to anesthesia care in the 2003–2005 Confidential Enquiries report, one resulted from respiratory distress on extubation and two from postoperative respiratory insufficiency, one occurring immediately postoperatively and the other some hours later (17). No deaths resulted from airway management at the induction of GA. The reasons for the maternal deaths were due to inadequate close supervision of inexperienced trainees by consultants; the two deaths were due

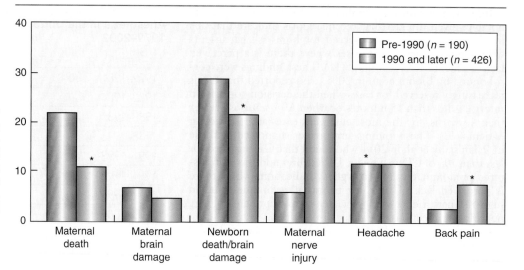

FIGURE 24-1 Comparison of injuries in obstetric anesthesia claims before and after 1990. Reprinted with permission from: Davies JM, Posner KL, Lee LA, et al. Liability Associated with obstetric anesthesia: A closed claims analysis. *Anesthesiology* 2009;110: 131–139.

to postoperative hypoventilation and failure to monitor adequately; and failure to adequately manage the airway and ventilation. Morbid obesity was also a contributory factor in four out of six maternal deaths. Further, of the seven anesthesia-attributable deaths detailed in the Eighth Report (2006–2008), accounting for 6.5% of direct maternal deaths, only two were airway related (18). One was due to persistent attempts to intubate the trachea despite adequate ventilation through a laryngeal mask, and the other was the result of pulmonary aspiration following extubation of the trachea after emergency cesarean delivery in a woman recognized to have a full stomach.

Canadian Data

Finally, the only anesthesia-attributed direct maternal death reported in Canada from 1992 to 2000 was attributed to issues arising out of the extubation of the trachea postoperatively (19).

Obstetric Anesthesia Closed Claims Analysis

The practice of obstetrics carries a high medical liability risk; the 2006 American College of Obstetricians and Gynecologists (ACOG) on professional liability reported a "continuing negative trend" that professional liability was having on the practice of obstetrics and gynecology. The survey data showed that 89.2% obstetricians who responded had at least one professional liability claim during their career or an average of 2.62 claims per OB/GYN doctor (20). Similarly, obstetric anesthesia also carries high liability (5). The trend continues, similarly in the 2012 ACOG Survey on professional liability also showed that 77.3% OB/GYN practitioners experienced at least one professional liability claim filed against them during their professional careers with an average of 2.69 claims per OB/GYN (21).

The ASA Closed Claims Project is a structured evaluation of adverse events from the closed claim files of 35 United States professional liability insurance companies. Maternal death and newborn death/brain damage were the most common obstetric anesthesia malpractice claims in ASA closed database before 1990 (5). The liability profile changed, as the trends in obstetric anesthesia have changed dramatically in the last three decades. Obstetric anesthesia claims for injuries from 1990 to 2003 were compared to obstetric anesthesia claims for injuries before 1990. Compared to pre-1990 claims, the proportion of obstetric anesthesia claims from

1990 or later associated with cesarean delivery decreased; the claims associated with GA decreased ($p < 0.01$), the proportion of maternal death/brain damage and newborn death/brain damage decreased (Fig. 24-1). Malpractice claims from 1990 or later related to respiratory causes of injuries decreased from 24% (*pre-1990*) to 4%; claims (*1990 or later claims*) related to inadequate oxygenation/ventilation and pulmonary aspiration of gastric contents and esophageal intubation also decreased. *However, despite the decrease in claims, the most common anesthetic causes of maternal death/brain damage in claims associated with general anesthesia were difficult intubation and maternal hemorrhage. The seven difficult intubation injuries occurred between 1991 and 1998, mostly upon induction (six of seven cases).* The airway-related claims involved multiple attempts at tracheal intubation leading to progressive difficulty with ventilation. In two of the claims, tracheal intubation was assessed to be difficult preoperatively, with a backup plan to awaken the patient and perform fiberoptic intubation. However, progressive airway difficulties occurred while attempting to awaken the patients, thus resulting in adverse outcomes. The claims related to DI after 1990, as compared to claims pre-1990 have not changed (5) (Table 24-4). The overall improvement in the closed claims statistics and decline in anesthesia-related maternal mortality in the past few years and overall risk ratio between GA and RA can be attributed to the practice guidelines introduced by ASA including the ASA Practice Guidelines in Obstetric anesthesia. These initiatives include implementation of minimum standard of care requiring the use of respiratory system monitors (pulse oximetry and capnography) during anesthesia; enhanced awareness of the risk of pulmonary aspiration of gastric contents in the obstetric patient (22); decreased utilization of GA in obstetric practice and the heightened awareness of the ASA difficult airway algorithm (10). During the past two decades, anesthesiologists have focused on improving their management of difficult/failed intubation management and gaining experience with the laryngeal mask airway and other airway devices (10).

Similarly, the Doctors Insurance Company reported on 22 anesthesia malpractice closed claims between 1998 and 2006, filed after maternal cardiac arrests in the labor and delivery suites (23). Adverse events resulted in 10 maternal deaths; 11 had anoxic brain damage with only one patient surviving neurologically intact. Of the 22 malpractice claims, only one case involved GA and failed intubation. Thirteen cases were regional anesthesia-related respiratory arrests after epidurals

TABLE 24-4 Comparison of Injuries in Obstetric Anesthesia Claims Before and After 1990

	Pre-1990*	1990 or Later	P Value
Respiratory damaging event	46 (24%)	17 (4%)	<0.001
Aspiration of gastric contents	8 (4%)	2 (<1%)	0.012
Difficult intubation	10 (5%)	11 (3%)	NS
Esophageal intubation	7 (4%)	0 (0%)	0.007
Inadequate oxygenation/ventilation	10 (5%)	3 (1%)	0.006
Standard of care			
Substandard care	74 (39%)	92 (22%)	<0.001
Appropriate	87 (46%)	293 (69%)	<0.001

*Data from pre-1990 previously published and used with permission of author and publisher.
NS, not statistically significant ($p > 0.05$); SD, standard deviation.
Modified with permission from: Davies JM, Posner KL, Lee LA, et al. Liability associated with obstetric anesthesia: A closed claims analysis. *Anesthesiology* 2009;110: 131–139.

with unintentional intrathecal injections and five high spinals during cesarean delivery. Seven patients were moved to the operating room for resuscitation due to lack of airway equipment in the labor and delivery suite. Five arrests occurred during spinal anesthesia for cesarean delivery in the operating room. However, none of the operating rooms had audible alarms on the monitors at the time of arrest (23). The details of airway management were not outlined.

■ DEFINITIONS OF DIFFICULT AIRWAY

One of the difficulties with a review of the literature evaluating the incidence and epidemiology of the difficult airway in obstetrics is that there are no consistent and agreed upon definitions for the difficult maternal airway. For the purpose of this chapter, the definitions used by the ASA Task Force on Difficult Airway Management will be assumed (3):

Difficult Airway: It is defined as the clinical situation in which the anesthesia practitioner experiences difficulty with facemask ventilation, difficulty with tracheal intubation, or both leading to hypoxemia or soiling of the tracheobronchial tree.

Difficult Tracheal Intubation (DI): DI is defined as when intubation requires multiple attempts.
  Time taken to achieve intubation: The original ASA description of DI included a time limit of 10 minutes or requiring multiple attempts. The wisdom of this definition must be questioned in obstetrics, especially, given the fact that GA is generally reserved for emergency CD where delivery of the baby is of the utmost urgency. One definition of difficult or failed intubation, which may be used in obstetrics, incorporates a differently defined time limit. The common practice in obstetrical anesthesia is to accomplish the intubation using a single dose of succinylcholine when anesthetizing for cesarean delivery under GA. In the obstetrical situation, *difficult intubation* could be defined as the inability of an experienced anesthesia practitioner to intubate within the time provided by one dose of succinylcholine (24).

Failed Intubation: In surgical patients, it is defined as when placement of the tracheal tube fails even after multiple attempts. However, in obstetrical patients, failed intubation should be considered as the inability to secure the airway with two attempts (25), which includes the best attempt at intubation using the conventional laryngoscope or the use of an alternative airway device to assist with tracheal intubation.

Difficult Laryngoscopy: There is probably the least agreement in the literature regarding the definition of difficult laryngoscopy with many authors defining it as a poor view (grade 3 or 4) of the glottis. The ASA Practice Guidelines in 2003 described it as when it is not possible to visualize any portion of the vocal cords even after multiple attempts at conventional laryngoscopy (3). Considering the four grades of laryngeal exposure as described by Cormack and Lehane (26), a Grade 3 (view of epiglottis only) or Grade 4 (no view of the larynx) view at laryngoscopy indicates difficult direct laryngoscopy.

Difficult Facemask Ventilation (MV): It is defined as the inability to maintain oxygen saturation >90%, with 100% oxygen via face mask, or to reverse the signs of inadequate ventilation.

Difficult Laryngeal Mask Ventilation: It has not been defined by the ASA or any other major difficult airway society guidelines. However, the definition of difficult laryngeal mask ventilation utilized in research studies is the inability to place the LMA in a satisfactory position to allow clinically adequate ventilation and airway patency. Indices of clinically adequate ventilation are expired tidal volume >7 mL/kg and leak pressure >15–20 cm H_2O. In a study of more than 11,000 patients using this definition, the failure rate was 0.16% (27).

■ INCIDENCE OF DIFFICULT AIRWAY, FAILED INTUBATION, AND CANNOT INTUBATE CANNOT VENTILATE IN OBSTETRICS

The incidence of difficult laryngoscopy or tracheal intubation in the nonobstetric population is reported as 0.1% to 13% (28). In the obstetric population, the incidence of difficult tracheal intubation is typically reported as between 1:249 and 1:300 (29–32). It is worth noting that countries that have a high rate of general anesthetic usage, such as South Africa, report a low failed intubation rate at 1:750 (33). Furthermore, in the United States, where obstetric anesthesia is supervised by attending anesthesiologists in teaching hospitals, the rate of failed tracheal intubation is also low (2,34,35). A number of authors have compared the incidence of difficult or failed intubation in obstetric and nonobstetric airways, and although the definitions have varied somewhat from study to study, similar incidences were reported across the studies (36–39). These authors concluded that the incidence of DI ranged from 1% to 6% and the incidence of failed tracheal intubation ranged from 0.1% to 0.6%. Others have described the occurrence of difficult or failed intubation in series of obstetrical patients in a noncomparative fashion (29,33,34,40). Again, these studies reported incidences of DI ranging from 1.5% to 8.5% and an incidence of failed tracheal intubation ranging from 0.13% to 0.3%; these incidences are consistent with the ranges reported for general surgical patients (41–44).

A review of general anesthesia for cesarean deliveries at an academic practice in a tertiary hospital from 1990 to 1995 showed the incidence of DI ranged from as high as 16.3% (1994) to as low as 1.3% (1992) with only one failed intubation (34). There was one sentinel incident of cannot intubate cannot ventilate (CICV) situation for an overall incidence of one CICV per 536 general anesthetics. In this case, there were multiple attempts at intubation, unsuccessful mask ventilation, failed Combitube™ placement and an unsuccessful cricothyroidotomy, resulting in cardiopulmonary arrest, followed by surgical tracheostomy. Resuscitation was accomplished, however, mother remained in coma until death and the baby suffered significant neurologic injury (34). In a follow-up review of GA for cesarean deliveries covering the period 2000–2005, the same authors reported an even lower rate of GA and again one failed intubation, resulting in an incidence of CICV of 1:98 (2). Since a difficult airway was suspected in this emergent cesarean delivery, a surgeon was immediately available on standby. The CICV incident occurred following failed tracheal intubation, unsuccessful LMA placement, and hypoxemia followed by a successful cricothyroidotomy by the surgeon, resulting in a good outcome for both mother and baby (2). The excellent reporting system of details in the two studies helps the anesthesia practitioner in formulating the rescue plan, thus averting maternal mortality.

Recently, McDonnell et al. conducted a prospective observational study in 13 Australian maternity hospitals (49,500 deliveries per annum) during 2005–2006 and obtained data from 1,095 women receiving general anesthesia for CD (45). DI occurred in 3.3% of patients and there were four failed tracheal intubations (0.4%).

Similarly, McKeen et al., after reviewing the data extracted from a provincial database, from 1984 to 2003, on 102,587 pregnant and immediate postpartum (within 3 days of delivery) women who were administered GA at a regional tertiary Canadian center, concluded that DI was encountered in 60 of 1,052 (5.7%) women who had CD and failed intubation occurred in none (46). The rate of DI remained stable over the 20 years of the review. These findings are consistent with other reports that have concluded that the incidence of difficult maternal airway is low, albeit variable, and has remained relatively unchanged over the last several decades and is similar in magnitude to that seen in the general surgical population. A composite of the incidence of difficult airway and CICV in obstetrical patients is outlined in Table 24-5.

■ FACTORS CONTRIBUTING TO THE DIFFICULT MATERNAL AIRWAY

Anatomical and physiologic factors alter the airway during pregnancy, placing the parturient at risk for difficult laryngoscopy, difficult tracheal intubation, and difficult mask ventilation. There is no single factor for the high incidence of failed tracheal intubation and respiratory-related injury in obstetrics. The following factors have been incriminated: Difficult laryngoscopy or difficult mask ventilation due to excessive weight gain, upper airway edema during pregnancy

TABLE 24-5 Difficult Airway Incidence

Surgical Patients	Obstetrical Patients
Difficult intubation occurs relatively commonly in association with GA Estimated incidence 1–3%	Cormack et al. Difficult laryngoscopy Grade III view 1:2,000
Difficult mask ventilation Estimated incidence 0.9–5% in general surgery patients	Hawthorne et al. Failed intubation 1:250
Cannot intubate cannot ventilate (CICV) Estimated incidence CICV— 0.01% to 2 per 10,000	Lyons Failed intubation 1:300 Samsoon & Young Failed intubation 1:283 Rocke et al. Failed intubation 1:750 Tsen et al. *CICV 1:536 Palanisamy et al. *CICV 1:98

*CICV, Cannot intubate cannot ventilate.
Cormack RS, Lehane GR, Adams AP, et al. Laryngoscopy grades and percentage glottic opening. *Anesthesia* 2000;55(2):184; Hawthorne L, Wilson R, Lyons G, et al. Failed intubation revisited: 17-yr experience in a teaching maternity unit. *Brit J Anaesth* 1996;76(5):680–684. Lyons G. Failed intubation. six years' experience in a teaching maternity unit. *Anaesthesia* 1985;40(8):759-762. Samsoon GL, Young JR. Difficult tracheal intubation: A retrospective study. *Anaesthesia* 1987;42(5):487-490. Rocke DA, Murray WB, Rout CC, et al. Relative risk analysis of factors associated with difficult intubation in obstetric anesthesia. *Anesthesiology* 1992;77(1):67–73. Tsen LC, Pitner R, Camann WR. General anesthesia for cesarean section at a tertiary care hospital 1990–1995: Indications and implications. *Int J Obstet Anesth* 1998;7(3):147–152. Palanisamy A, Mitani AA, Tsen LC. General anesthesia for cesarean delivery at a tertiary care hospital from 2000 to 2005: A retrospective analysis and 10-year update. *Int J Obstet Anesth* 2011;20(1):10–16.

compounded by additional changes in preeclampsia, and breast enlargement. Rapid onset of hypoxemia associated with difficult airway occurs due to respiratory changes of pregnancy, cardiovascular impairment from aorto-caval compression, gastrointestinal changes placing the parturient at risk for pulmonary aspiration and respiratory-related complications.

Airway Changes

The hormonal influences of pregnancy and, in particular, the effects of estrogen resulting in an increase in the ground substance of the airway connective tissue, increased blood volume, an increase in total body water, and an increase in interstitial fluid, result in hypervascularity and edema of oropharynx, nasopharynx, and respiratory tract thus contributing to soft tissue airway edema. Airway changes with an increase in the Mallampati (MP) scores have been shown to occur during pregnancy, labor, and delivery (47). Further, the incidence of MP classes III and IV increases during labor compared to the prelabor period, and these changes are not reversed by 48 hours after delivery (48). Therefore, it is absolutely necessary to examine the airway of a parturient in labor prior to administering anesthesia for a CD (48). Excessive weight gain during pregnancy, preeclampsia, iatrogenic fluid overload, bearing-down efforts during labor with increases in venous pressure, all may lead to an increase in upper airway mucosal edema. Additional upper airway change includes tongue engorement during pregnancy leading to decreased mobility of the floor of the mouth (49) and changes in the MP score (50). Several published reports describe difficulties in intubation secondary to development of airway edema during labor and delivery, preeclampsia, and status-post massive fluid and blood transfusion resuscitation following postpartum hemorrhage all resulting in higher MP scores (51).

Difficulties with tracheal intubation due to facial and laryngeal edema in patients with preeclampsia and eclampsia have also been described, including instances of rapid development of airway edema (52). Due to the increased vascularity, engorgement of the mucosa and swelling of the airway, the parturient is not only at increased risk for epistaxis following manipulation of nasopharynx with nasotracheal intubation, but also vulnerable to increased trauma with repeated attempts at intubation (53). Avoiding manipulation of nasopharynx, using smaller-sized tracheal tube, and *strict adherence to no more than two attempts at orotracheal intubation, are important to avoid airway management–related trauma, bleeding, edema and further complications, and catastrophes* (53).

Respiratory Changes

The gravid uterus displaces the diaphragm cephalad with progression of the pregnancy and leads to a 20% decrease in functional residual capacity (FRC); this decrease will be exacerbated to a significant degree in the supine position. In the supine position, the FRC is 70% of its normal capacity measured in the upright position. In an obese parturient, the supine position can result in airway closure and an increase in alveolar–arterial gradient during normal tidal respiration, predisposing the parturient to lower partial pressure of oxygen (54). At the same time, oxygen consumption is increased by 20% secondary to the metabolic needs of the growing fetus, uterus, and placenta. Chest wall compliance is decreased and the effect of the anatomical changes imposed by the pregnancy is a 50% increase in the oxygen cost of breathing. Ventilatory drive is increased by progesterone during pregnancy, giving rise to hyperventilation to meet the increased oxygen demands of the pregnant mother. Both the oxygen consumption and carbon dioxide production are increased by 20% to 40% at term. The decrease in FRC coupled with increased oxygen utilization shortens the safe apnea time after induction of anesthesia (55). The time to desaturation and hypoxemia is much faster, than the recovery from the time needed to recover from the apnea produced by the succinylcholine (56).

Preoxygenation also plays a critical role in maximizing the safe duration of apnea. The purpose of preoxygenating a patient before induction of general anesthesia is to provide the maximum duration that a patient can safely tolerate apnea so that airway interventions may be undertaken at the lowest threat to the patient, even in situations where unanticipated difficulties arise. This issue on preoxygenation is discussed in the section on preoxygenation.

Cardiovascular Changes and Resuscitation Implications

The gravid uterus compresses the inferior vena cava in the supine position resulting in a decrease in venous return and cardiac output. The reduction in cardiac output and elevated oxygen consumption can further decrease the oxygen saturation. The decrease in cardiac output, and the ensuing

hypoxemia, during a difficult intubation, failed intubation, or CICV situation predisposes the mother to the risk for myocardial hypoxia, cardiovascular arrest, and compromised uteroplacental perfusion, which can also place the fetus' well-being at risk. Maintaining left uterine tilt, establishing an airway with adequate ventilation and oxygenation in a timely manner, maintaining adequate perfusion in mother and baby, and cardiovascular stability become extremely important in order to ensure safe outcome for both.

Gastrointestinal Changes

Gastrointestinal changes which include hormonal, anatomical, and physiologic changes during pregnancy are recognized risk factors for gastric regurgitation and pulmonary aspiration during a general anesthetic. The decrease in gastric pH and an increase in intragastric pressure associated with an increasingly incompetent gastroesophageal sphincter raise a concern about a "full stomach" in obstetrical patients; further, with the onset of labor there is also a delay in gastric emptying. Aspiration-related deaths during pregnancy occur from complications associated with induction problems such as difficult intubation, esophageal intubation, and inadequate attempts at ventilation (1,8,57).

Obesity

During the last two decades, obesity has become a global epidemic with more than one billion overweight adults worldwide (58). In the United States, the Centers for Disease Control (CDC) trends by states, from 1985 to 2009, show that during the past 20 years, there has been a dramatic increase in obesity with 33 states, having a prevalence equal to or greater than 25%, and in 9 states with a prevalence of obesity greater than 30% (59). Obesity in pregnancy has increased in accordance with the increased prevalence of obesity in the general population, with the prevalence of obesity during pregnancy varying from 6% to 28% (60).

A body mass index (BMI) greater than 25 kg/m^2 is considered overweight and a BMI greater than 30 kg/m^2 is considered obese. In the nonobstetric population, a BMI greater than 26 kg/m^2 results in a three-fold increase in the incidence of difficult mask ventilation (61). Several review articles support an association between obesity and DI in the obstetric and nonobstetric patients (62).

On the basis of an analysis of 20 years of data from a large tertiary Canadian maternity center, McKeen has recently reported that maternal age >35 years, weight 90 to 99 kg, and the absence of active labor were associated with an increased risk for DI (46). Although these findings are concerning, due to the increasing prevalence of obesity in the maternal population and the larger number of women delaying conception, they are also difficult to apply clinically.

Both prepregnancy obesity and excessive weight gain during pregnancy are associated with comorbidities such as hypertension or preeclampsia with intrauterine growth retardation, diabetes and macrosomia, and dysfunctional labor, thus increasing the incidence of operative CD. The incidence of postpartum hemorrhage is also higher in these obese patients leading to an increased likelihood of a general anesthetic intervention.

Weight gain during pregnancy results from the increasing size of the uterus and fetus, increased blood and interstitial fluid volumes, and deposition of new fat. *There is a correlation between weight gain and an increase in the Mallampati score* (63). The weight gain and obesity are associated with an increase in the Mallampati score; the incidence of partially obliterated oropharyngeal space in an obese parturient is doubled compared to nonpregnant patients (64). Obesity compounds the effects of pregnancy on the increase in breast size and engorgement. In the supine position, the enlarged breasts can encroach into the neck area impeding effective application of cricoid pressure and cause difficulty with laryngoscope blade insertion. An increase in neck circumference is an added risk factor for DI and difficult MV (65). These aforementioned changes, the breast engorgement, along with anthropometrical difference between patients, create a risk for difficult laryngoscopy, difficult tracheal intubation, and difficult mask ventilation (33). DI is encountered more frequently in morbidly obese parturients weighing more than 130 kg (62). In obesity, the respiratory-related changes of pregnancy are even more significant, with marked decrease in FRC such that the closing capacity exceeds FRC during tidal breathing, thus leading to a decrease in arterial oxygen tension and predisposing the parturient to a much higher risk of hypoxemia during a difficult tracheal intubation or difficult mask ventilation encounter (66).

In the obese parturient, a thorough preoperative assessment, review of comorbidities, and previous anesthetic history for difficulty with tracheal intubation is essential so as to allow for proper preparation and appropriate interventions. The "ramped position" in obese parturients prior to induction of general anesthesia becomes critical so as to facilitate ventilation and improve the laryngoscopic visualization of the glottis for tracheal intubation. The aim is to achieve the "best alignment" of the three axes, (oral, pharyngeal, and laryngeal) in the obese patient.

■ PREDICTION OF DIFFICULT AIRWAY

Strategies for prevention of airway problems in the obstetrical patient require adequate preoperative airway assessment, proper planning, and implementation of safe, best anesthesia practices, in order to ensure safe outcomes for both mother and baby.

The ASA Difficult Airway Task Force guidelines recommend an airway-related history to detect medical, surgical, and anesthetic factors that might indicate the presence of difficult airway. Similarly, the Practice Guidelines in Obstetric Anesthesia (2007) also recommend a focused history and physical examination, including an airway examination (6). The ASA Closed Claims analysis (2005) showed that 8% of patients did not have a preoperative history or airway physical examination (67). An audit for failed tracheal intubation in obstetrics, a 6-year review, showed that of the 36 failed tracheal intubations in 8,970 obstetric general anesthetics (incidence 1/249) only 26 records were available for examination. Examination of data on the 26 patients showed that preoperative airway assessment was found in less than half the cases (39). Lack of preoperative airway assessment is a contributory factor in anesthesia-related mortality (68). In a retrospective audit of 5,802 cesarean deliveries, done under GA, there were 23 failed intubations, an incidence of 1:250; although all patients had a preoperative assessment, difficulty in tracheal intubation was anticipated in only one-third of the cases, and two had documented records of prior difficulties (29). A follow-up postoperative examination showed the commonest findings to be; receding jaw, limited mouth opening, prominent or awkward teeth, and limited neck mobility (29). A multivariate analysis of risk factors for difficult tracheal intubation in obstetrics demonstrates that the risk dramatically increases as the number of abnormal airway findings increases (33). A meta-analysis of the diagnostic accuracy of bedside tests for predicting difficult tracheal intubation in nonobstetric and obstetric patients shows that a combination of tests add incremental diagnostic value to predicting

difficult tracheal intubation rather than the value of each test alone (69).

Importance of Assessment and Prediction of Difficult Airway in Obstetrical Patients

The cornerstone in prevention of airway catastrophes in obstetric patients is firstly, to attempt to predict which obstetric patients are at risk for difficult laryngoscopy, DI, and difficult mask ventilation.

Numerous investigators have attempted to predict the difficult airway by using simple bedside physical examination. There are numerous publications using univariate or multivariate predictors of difficult intubation in the nonobstetric patients and a handful of publications utilizing multivariate predictors in predicting the difficult airway in obstetric patients (70). Yentis (70) describes the problems with many studies examining the prediction of difficult airway; therefore, it is appropriate to delineate the terms used to describe the accuracy or predictive power of the tests. The various tests used to predict a difficult airway in the general population as well as the obstetric population will also be described in this section.

Descriptive Terms Analyzing Predictive Tests

A test to predict difficult intubation should have high *sensitivity*, so that it will identify most patients in whom intubation will be truly difficult. It should also have a high *positive predictability value*, so that only few patients with airways actually easy to intubate are subjected to the protocol for difficult airway management (64).

Preoperative Assessment
History and Evaluation

Assessment of difficult airway begins with a comprehensive history and physical examination. The ASA Task Force on Difficult Airway Management Guidelines and the ASA Practice Guidelines on Obstetric Anesthesia (6) recommend that an airway history should be conducted, whenever feasible, prior to the initiation of anesthetic care and airway management in all patients. There is suggestive evidence that some features of a patient's medical history or prior medical records may be related to the likelihood of encountering a difficult airway. The evidence is based on association between a difficult airway and a variety of congenital, acquired, or traumatic disease conditions. Examination of previous medical, surgical, and anesthetic records, if available (particularly in patients with high airway risk) in a timely manner, may yield useful information on airway management. A history of difficult airway management should be considered a strong predictor of problems unless the history was related to a specific reversible disease process. The history may be available from verbal recollections from the patient, previous anesthetic records, hospital notes, and a letter of difficult airway management, or a Medic-Alert bracelet. The introduction of anesthesia information management systems along with the introduction of mandatory electronic medical records will be tremendously helpful in readily accessing critical information.

Physical Examination

The guidelines also recommend an airway physical examination using multiple airway features assessment (3) and 6D method of airway assessment (71) prior to initiation of anesthetic care and airway management in all patients (Table 24-6).

TABLE 24-6 Preoperative Tests for Predicting DI in Obstetrical Patients

Sign of Difficulty	Description	Acceptable Findings not Usually Associated with Difficulty	Quantitative or Qualitative Findings Reported to be Associated with Difficulty
Disproportion	Increased size of tongue in relation to pharyngeal size	Mallampati class I or II	Mallampati class III or IV
Distortion	Airway swelling (preeclampsia) Airway trauma (blunt or penetrating) Neck mass (Thyroid enlargement)	Midline trachea Mobile laryngeal anatomy Easily palpated thyroid cartilage Easily palpated cricoid cartilage	Possibly difficult to assess Blunt or penetrating airway trauma Tracheal deviation Neck asymmetry Voice changes Laryngeal immobility Nonpalpable thyroid cartilage Nonpalpable cricoid cartilage
Decreased thyromental distance	Anterior larynx and decreased mandibular space	Thyromental distance ≥6.5 (3 fb) No receding chin	Thyromental distance <6.5 cm (<3 fb) measured from the superior aspect of the thyroid cartilage to the tip of the chin Receding chin
Decreased interincisor gap	Reduced mouth opening	Interincisor gap >3 cm (2 fb)	Distance between upper and lower incisors (i.e., interincisor gap) <3 cm (<2 fb)
Decreased range of motion in any or all of the joints of the airway (i.e., atlanto-occipital joint, temporo-mandibular joints, cervical spine); atlanto-occipital range of motion is critical for assuming the sniffing position	Limited head extension secondary to arthritis, diabetes, or other diseases Neck contractures secondary to burns or trauma	Head extension ≥35-degree atlanto-occipital extension Cervical spine flexion ≥35 degrees Long, thin neck	Head extension <35 degrees Neck flexion <35 degrees Long, thin neck
Dental overbite (upper lip bite test)	Protruding incisors disrupting the alignment of the airway axes and possibly decreasing the interincisor gap	No dental overbite	Dental overbite

The 6-D method of airway assessment helps practitioners remember to assess for each of the six signs that can be associated with a difficult intubation. Each sign begins with the letter D like the word difficult. The potential for difficult intubation is generally proportional to the number of signs observed.
Modified with permission from: Rich JM. Recognition and management of the difficult airway with special emphasis on the intubating LMA-Fastrach/whistle technique: A brief review with case reports. *Proc (Bayl Univ Med Cent)* 2005;18(3):220–227.

Predictors for Difficult Mask Ventilation

It is also of paramount importance to recognize the predictors for "*difficult to mask ventilate*" in obstetric patients. Successful mask ventilation (MV) provides anesthesia practitioner with a rescue technique during unsuccessful attempts at laryngoscopy and unanticipated difficult airway management situations. Pregnant women become hypoxemic more rapidly during episodes of apnea as detailed in the section on respiratory changes during pregnancy. Computer modeling of the rate of arterial oxyhemoglobin desaturation in fully oxygenated patients suggests that this process occurs significantly more rapidly in moderately ill and obese patients compared to healthy individuals (56) (Fig. 24-2). Similarly, utilizing a computer model, it is observed that there is reduced tolerance

for apnea in pregnant patients particularly in the Trendelenberg position (54). These studies emphasize the importance of recognizing early that one is in a difficult intubation scenario, and strategizing how to oxygenate and ventilate the mother.

Although there is an extensive body of literature addressing predictive factors for difficult laryngoscopy and grading its view, investigations that focus on difficult MV are limited (69). A four-point scale to grade difficulty in MV has been identified (Table 24-7). Encountering a clinical situation with either a grade 3 MV (inadequate, unstable, or requiring two providers) or a grade 4 MV (impossible to ventilate) with a difficult intubation (DI) represents the most feared airway outcomes; a patient in whom establishing tracheal intubation is difficult and the primary rescue technique of conventional

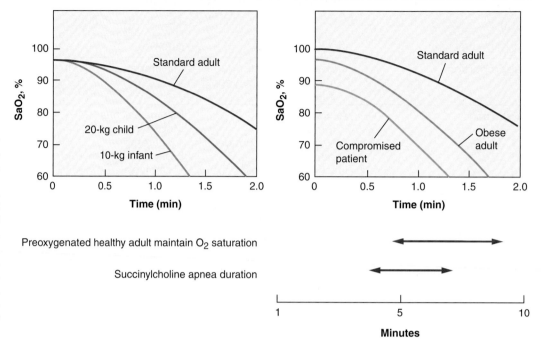

FIGURE 24-2 Oxyhemoglobin desaturation during apnea. Reprinted with permission from: Benumof JL, Dagg R, Benumof R. Critical hemoglobin desaturation will occur before return to an unparalyzed state following 1 mg/kg intravenous succinylcholine. *Anesthesiology* 1997;87(4):979–982.

MV is also challenging. Therefore, it is important to predict this situation thus allowing the practitioner to be prepared with alternative tools, that is, laryngeal mask airway, video laryngoscopes, and so forth.

In an observational study of 22,660 attempts at MV in nonobstetric patients, the criteria that correlated with grade 3 or 4 MV and DI may be applicable to the obstetric population, include independent risk factors, such as (1) limited or severely limited mandibular protrusion, thick or obese neck anatomy, (2) a history of sleep apnea, (3) a history of snoring, and BMI of 30 kg/m² or greater (72). This study supported and was able to demonstrate the value of the mandibular protrusion test in predicting difficult MV and DI as suggested by Takenaka et al. (73).

Specific Individual Tests for Assessment of Difficult Tracheal Intubation

Interincisor distance (limited mouth opening): The interincisor distance (IID) is the distance between the upper and lower incisors. The normal IID is >4.6 cm; while an IID <3 cm or <2 fingerbreadths (fb) is nonreassuring and may predict difficult laryngoscopy and <1 fb will impair insertion of a laryngeal mask. An IID of less than 5 cm or 2 to

TABLE 24-7 Mask Ventilation Difficulty Scale

Grade	Description
1	Ventilated by mask
2	Ventilated by mask with oral airway/ adjuvant with or without muscle relaxant
3	Difficult ventilation (inadequate, unstable, or requiring two providers) with or without muscle relaxant
4	Unable to mask ventilate with or without muscle relaxant

Reprinted with permission from: Kheterpal S, Han R, Tremper KK, et al. Incidence and predictors of difficult and impossible mask ventilation. *Anesthesiology* 2006;105(5):885-891.

3 fb may be indicative of difficult laryngoscopy and less than 1 fb or 1.5 cm will impair insertion of an LMA and laryngoscope. A distance of 2 cm is required to insert an intubating LMA. Maximal mouth opening is influenced by atlanto-occipital joint extension and is not a reliable predictor of difficult tracheal intubation in either general or obstetric patents.

The IID by itself is not a reliable predictor of difficult tracheal intubation in either general or obstetric patents (74). The maximal mouth opening is influenced by the degree of atlanto-occipitatl joint extension (75). Even though Savva et al. found that the IID was not a useful independent test in identifying difficult tracheal intubation (74), in the Australian Critical Incident Monitoring Study (76), the four variables associated with difficult intubation were limited mouth opening, obesity, limited neck extension, and lack of a trained assistant. Limited mouth opening along with limited jaw protrusion often ranks high in composite scores such as the Wilson Risk Sum (77) (weight, head and neck movement, interincisor gap, mandibular jaw protrusion, receding mandible, buck teeth), and the Arne Risk Index scores (28) (history of DI, pathologies associated with DI, clinical symptoms, TMD <6.5 cm, restricted head and neck movement, Mallampati scores 2 to 4, IID <5 cm, jaw protrusion class B or C) are used to predict difficult tracheal intubation.

Jaw Protrusion or Mandibular Protrusion test: The ability to slide the lower incisors in front of the upper ones may be classified as A, B, or C (Fig. 24-3) (73). Based on the classification, Class C protrusion is associated with difficult laryngoscopy and difficult mask ventilation, whereas Class A protrusion rarely produced any difficulty (78). In obstetric patients using the Wilson risk sum along with the Mallampati score showed high sensitivity, specificity, and positive predictive value (79).

Upper lip bite test (ULBT): The ULBT assesses the degree to which the lower incisors can advance over the upper lip and includes three classes (Fig. 24-4). This test has the ability to assess jaw protrusion movement and protruding incisors simultaneously. A recent study, in nonobstetric patients, showed that Class III ULBT along with IID <4.5 cm,

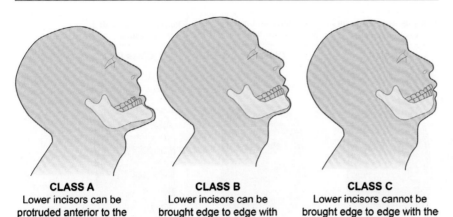

FIGURE 24-3 Mandibular protrusion test for prediction of difficult mask ventilation. Reprinted with permission from: Takenaka I, Aoyama K, Kadoya T. Mandibular protrusion test for prediction of difficult mask ventilation. *Anesthesiology* 2001;94(5):935.

thyromental distance (TMD) <6.5 cm and sternomental distance (SMD) <13 cm were defined as predictors of difficult tracheal intubation. Specificity and accuracy of the ULBT were significantly higher than TMD, SMD, or IID individually (specificity was 91.69%, 82.27%, and 82.27%, respectively). The combination of the ULBT with SMD tests provided the highest sensitivity. The recommendation is to use ULBT in conjunction with other tests to more reliably predict ease of laryngoscopy or tracheal intubation (80).

Modified Mallampati Test

In 1985, Mallampati et al. first described the relationship of the base of the tongue to the oropharyngeal structures—uvula, tonsillar pillars, and faucial pillars (50). Mallampati hypothesized that when the base of the tongue is disproportionately large in relation to the oropharyngeal cavity, the enlarged base of the tongue can obscure the visibility of the tonsillar pillars and uvula resulting in difficult laryngoscopy and tracheal intubation. Originally, Mallampati described three classes; Samsoon and Young later modified the classification and added a fourth class (30). Classification is assigned according to the extent the base of the tongue is able to mask the visibility of the pharyngeal structures (Fig. 24-5). The test is performed with the patient in the sitting position,

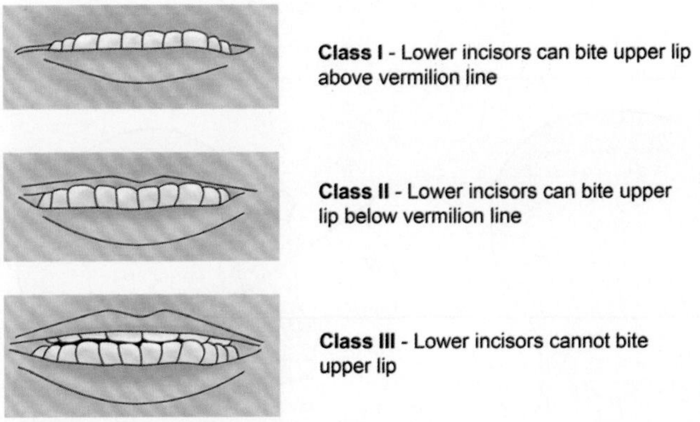

Class I - Lower incisors can bite upper lip above vermilion line

Class II - Lower incisors can bite upper lip below vermilion line

Class III - Lower incisors cannot bite upper lip

FIGURE 24-4 Upper lip bite test. Reprinted with permission from: Khan ZH, Mohammadi M, Rasouli MR, et al. The diagnostic value of the upper lip bite test combined with SMD, TMD, and interincisor distance for prediction of easy laryngoscopy and intubation: A prospective study. *Anesth Analg* 2009;109(3):822–824. SMD, Sternomental distance; TMD, Thyromental distance.

head in the neutral position, the mouth wide open, and the tongue protruding to its maximum. Patient should not be encouraged to actively phonate as it can cause contraction of the soft palate leading to false positive results. To avoid false positive or false negative, this test should be repeated twice.

The Mallampati classification has been used either as a single univariate predictor or as a part of multivariate analysis to predict difficult tracheal intubation. In obstetrical patients, the MP classification test has been used as a single parameter to illustrate the dramatic airway changes in pregnancy and to highlight the importance of preoperative assessment of the airway. Pilkington et al. evaluated the MP class at 12 weeks and 38 weeks gestation by photographs taken at the two time periods and demonstrated that the increase in MP class in the same patient. As gestation advanced, it correlated with an increase in body weight and increase in airway connective tissue and vascularity resulting in the oropharyngeal edema and was responsible for the increase in the MP scores (63).

More recently, Kodali et al. performed a two-part study to evaluate the changes during labor and delivery (47). In part 1 of the study, they used conventional Samsoon modification of the MP airway classification. The airway was photographed at the onset and at end of labor. Pregnant women with MP class IV airways were excluded from the initial part 1 study. In part 2 of the study, upper airway volumes were measured using acoustic reflectometry at the onset and conclusion of labor. In part 1 ($n = 61$), there was a significant increase in the MP class from prelabor to postlabor ($p < 0.0001$). The airway increased one MP class higher in 20 (33%) and two grades higher in 3 (5%) patients after labor. At the end of labor, there were eight parturients with MP class IV ($p < 0.01$) and 30 parturients with MP class III or IV ($p < 0.0001$). In part 2 ($n = 21$), there were significant decreases in oral volume ($p < 0.05$) and pharyngeal volume area ($p < 0.05$), and volume ($p < 0.001$) after labor and delivery.

Boutonnet et al. methodically evaluated the changes in MP class at four time intervals in 87 pregnant patients, during the 8th month of pregnancy (T_1), placement of epidural catheter (T_2), 20 minutes after delivery (T_3), and 48 hours after delivery (T_4) (48). MP class did not change for 37% of patients. The proportions of patients falling into MP III and IV at various times of assessment were as follows: T_1 10.3%, T_2 36.8%, T_3 51%, and T_4 20.7%. The differences in the percentages were all significant ($p < 0.01$). The incidence of MP class III and IV increased during labor compared with prelabor period and these changes were not reversed by 48 hours after delivery.

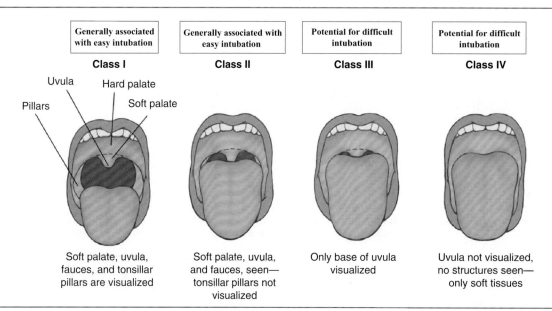

Generally associated with easy intubation	Generally associated with easy intubation	Potential for difficult intubation	Potential for difficult intubation
Class I	**Class II**	**Class III**	**Class IV**
Soft palate, uvula, fauces, and tonsillar pillars are visualized	Soft palate, uvula, and fauces, seen—tonsillar pillars not visualized	Only base of uvula visualized	Uvula not visualized, no structures seen—only soft tissues

FIGURE 24-5 Difficulty of intubation. Modified from: Mallampati Classification. Samsoon GL, Young Jr. Difficult tracheal intubation: A retrospective study. *Anaesthesia* 1987;42:487–90; Mallampati SR, Gatt SP, Gugino LD, et al. A clinical sign to predict difficult tracheal intubation: A prospective study. *Can Anaesth Soc J* 1985;32 (4):429–434.

These studies confirm the frequent increase in MP scores during pregnancy and particularly during the course of labor. These findings suggest that it is imperative to evaluate the airway in early labor and to re-evaluate before the anesthetic management for operative delivery for prediction of possible difficult mask ventilation and difficult tracheal intubation.

Atlanto-occipital (AO) joint extension: The sniffing or Magill position is considered the optimal "classical" position of the head and neck for facilitating tracheal intubation. The patient is asked to hold the head erect, face directly to the front, is asked to extend the head maximally, and the examiner estimates the angle traversed by the occlusal surface of the upper teeth. Measurement can be by simple visual estimate or more accurately with a goniometer. Normal AO joint extension is a 35-degree extension of the head over the neck (Fig. 24-6) (81). The extension of the AO joint on the upper cervical spine allows the alignment of the three axes (oral, pharyngeal, and laryngeal)

into a straight line during laryngoscopy, thus enhancing the ease of laryngoscopy and tracheal intubation (Fig. 24-7).

Any reduction in extension is expressed in grades:

Grade I: >35 degrees
Grade II: 22 to 34 degrees
Grade III: 12 to 21 degrees
Grade IV: <12 degrees

A reduction in the extension of the joint can cause difficulty with laryngoscopic view and intubation. Complete AO joint immobility can compromise the view of the glottis during laryngoscopy (75). Mouth opening and cranio-cervical mobility, which is synonymous with AO joint extension; have long been identified as crucial to successful airway management. Extension at the cranio-cervical junction is integral to basic airway maintenance maneuvers and direct laryngoscopy (82). Calder et al. hypothesized, in an observational study in volunteers, that cranio-cervical extension occurs during normal

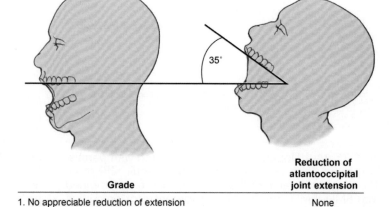

FIGURE 24-6 Clinical method for quantitating atlanto-occipital joint extension. Reprinted with permission from: Bellhouse CP, Dore C. Criteria for estimating likelihood of difficulty of endotracheal intubation with the Macintosh laryngoscope. *Anaesth Intensive Care* 1988;16(3):329–337.

Grade	Reduction of atlantooccipital joint extension
1. No appreciable reduction of extension	None
2. Approximately 1/3 reduction	1/3
3. Approximately 2/3 reduction	2/3
4. No appreciable extension	Complete

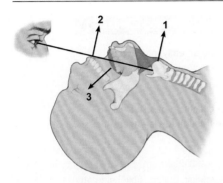

A direct line of sight to the vocal cords
may be blocked by:

1. A relatively anterior larynx
2. Prominent upper incisors
3. A large and posteriorly located tongue

FIGURE 24-7 Visualizing the vocal cords. Reprinted with permission from: Cormack RS, Lehane J. Difficult tracheal intubation in obstetrics. *Anaesthesia* 1984;39:1105–1111.

mouth opening (75). The investigators demonstrated that maximal mouth opening was achieved with 26 degrees of cervical extension from neutral; and that mandibular movement, mouth opening, and cranio-cervical flexion/extension are all interrelated. Patients with restricted cranio-cervical movement may have reduced mouth opening ability. This phenomenon may contribute to the difficulties with airway management that can occur in patients with reduced cranio-cervical extension (75).

Thyromental distance (TMD) (Patil's Test): TMD is defined as the distance from the chin (mentum) to the top of the notch of the thyroid cartilage with the head fully extended and can be measured with a ruler for accuracy. The TMD gives an estimate of the mandibular space and helps in determining how readily the laryngeal axis will align with the pharyngeal axis when the atlanto-occipital joint is extended (Fig. 24-8).

- **TMD measurement of >6.5 cm:** With no other abnormalities, indicates the likelihood of easy intubation.
- **TMD measurement of 6.0 to 6.5 cm:** This indicates that the alignment of the pharyngeal and laryngeal axes is difficult, thus resulting in difficulty with laryngoscopy and intubation. However, intubation is possible with the use of adjuncts to intubation such as gum elastic bougie or optical stylet.
- **TMD measurement of <6cm:** This indicates laryngoscopy and specifically, tracheal intubation may be impossible (83). TMD, in conjunction with other parameters

like Mallampati classification, has been used to predict difficult tracheal intubation; a patient with an MP class III or IV and a decreased TMD is likely to prove difficult to intubate (84).

Sternomental distance (SMD): SMD is measured from the sternum to the tip of the mandible with the head fully extended and the mouth closed. The normal SMD measurement is 13.5 cm. Savva et al. evaluated 355 consecutive patients (322 non-obstetric and 28 obstetric; 185 female) using the following parameters to assess for difficult intubation: TMD, SMD, protrusion of mandible, and IID (74). Tracheal intubation was difficult in 17 (4.9%), of whom four had Cormack–Lehane grade 3 or 4 laryngoscopic view. Savva et al. did not indicate how many of the four were obstetric patients and it is possible that increased weight gain associated with pregnancy resulted in reduced ability to see the larynx (40). An SMD of 12.5 cm or less with the head fully extended on the neck and the mouth closed predicted 14 of the 17 patients in whom tracheal intubation was difficult (74). The results of this study showed that SMD had a sensitivity of 82.4% and a specificity of 88.6% and was the best predictor for difficult tracheal intubation amongst all the tests including SMD, TMD, modified MP, jaw protrusion test, and IID.

SMD and view on laryngoscopy were documented in 523 parturients undergoing elective or emergency cesarean delivery under general anesthesia (40). An SMD of 13.5 cm or less had a sensitivity of 66.7%, specificity of 71%, and PPV of only 7.6%. Eighteen (3.5%) had a Cormack–Lehane grade 3 or 4 laryngoscopic view and were classified as potential difficult tracheal intubations. The SMD, while on its own was not useful as a sole predictor of difficult laryngoscopy or difficult tracheal intubation in obstetric patients; it could be part of the preoperative airway examination along with other quick simple tests (40).

Mandibulo-hyoid distance: Measurement of the mandibular length from the chin (mentum) to hyoid should be at least 4 cm or 3 fb (85). If the vertical distance between the mandible and the hyoid bone is increased, it might pose a problem with difficult laryngoscopy. A relatively short mandibular ramus or a relatively caudal larynx may be unfavorable anatomic factors in difficult laryngoscopy (85).

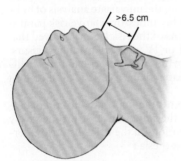

>6.5 cm

≥6.5 cm - Normal, easy intubation

6.0-6.5 cm - Laryngoscopy/ intubation difficult but may be possible

<6.0 cm - Laryngoscopy/ intubation impossible

FIGURE 24-8 Mandibular space. Based on Patil Vijayalakshmi U, Stehling Linda C, Zauder Howard L. Fiberoptic endoscopy in anaesthesia. Chicago: Year Book Medical Publishers; 1983; Bellhouse CP, Dore C. Criteria for estimating likelihood of difficulty of endotracheal intubation with the macintosh laryngoscope. *Anaesth Intensive Care* 1988;16(3):329–337; Frerk CM. Predicting difficult intubation. *Anaesthesia* 1991;46(12):1005–1008.

■ PREDICTORS OF THE DIFFICULT AIRWAY IN OBSTETRICS

The decreasing use of GA makes the study of difficult laryngoscopy and difficult tracheal intubation in the obstetrical population difficult. However, GA is still required in many cases and therefore, makes it imperative for the anesthesia practitioner to methodically assess the patient preoperatively

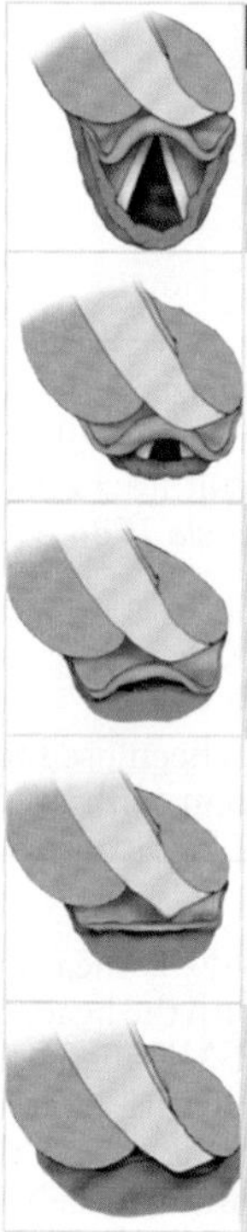

Grade	Visualized Oral Anatomy	Potentional Intubation Implications
1	Entire glottic opening from the anterior to posterior commissure	Should facilitate an easy intubation
2	Just the posterior portion of glottis	Normally not difficult to pass a styleted tracheal tube through the laryngeal aperture
3a*	Epiglottis only (epiglottis can be lifted using a laryngoscope blade)	Intubation is difficult, but possible using an Eschmann bougie introducer or flexible fiberoptic scope
3b*	Epiglottis only (but epiglottis cannot be lifted from the posterior pharyx using a laryngoscope blade)	Intubation can be difficult, because insertion of an Eschmann bougie introducer may be impeded. Successful tracheal intubation can be accomplished with optical stylet or a flexible fiberoptic scope
4	Only soft tissue, with no identifiable airway anatomy	Difficult intubation, requiring advanced techniques to intubate the trachea

Tracheal intubation normally requires an advanced airway technique beyond direct larynoscopy.

FIGURE 24-9 Cormack and Lehane's laryngeal grades of the airway. Reprinted with permission from: Cormack RS, Lehane JR, Adams AP, et al. Laryngoscopy grades and percentage glottic opening. *Anaesthesia* 2000;55(2):184.

and make an informed decision of the potential risk for difficult tracheal intubation.

Rocke et al. were the first to use multivariate analysis to predict difficult tracheal intubation. Preoperative airway assessment and potential risk factors were evaluated and recorded in 1,500 patients undergoing emergency and elective CD (33). Airway assessment, using the MP test, evaluated the oropharyngeal structures visible on maximal mouth opening. Other potential risk factors evaluated included obesity, short neck, and missing, protruding, or single maxillary incisors. Short neck equates with decreased atlanto-occipital joint extension, receding mandible equates with decreased TMD; protruding maxillary incisors equate with a significant overbite or Class III ULBT. Subsequent to induction of GA, the Cormack–Lehane laryngoscopic view and difficulty in tracheal intubation were graded.

The ease or difficulty of tracheal intubation was made according to the following scale (Fig. 24-9):

Grade 1: Easy, intubation at first attempt, no difficulty;
Grade 2: Some difficulty, insertion of tracheal tube not achieved at first attempt, no difficulty but successful after adjustment of laryngoscope blade and/or adjustment of head position, but not requiring additional equipment, removal and reinsertion of the laryngoscope or senior assistance;
Grade 3: Very difficult, requiring removal of the laryngoscope, further oxygenation by mask ventilation and subsequent intubation with or without the use of airway adjuncts. Grade 3 is further divided into 3A and 3B.
3A Epiglottis is only visualized (epiglottis can be lifted using a straight laryngoscope blade). Intubation is difficult but possible using a bougie introducer or flexible fiberoptic scope.

3B Epiglottis is only visualized (but epiglottis cannot be lifted from the posterior pharynx using a laryngoscope blade). Successful intubation is accomplished using optical stylet or flexible fiberoptic scope.
Grade 4: Failed intubation, several attempts at tracheal intubation or unrecognized esophageal intubation by resident, followed by subsequent tube placement by senior anesthesiologist.

The relative risk of experiencing difficult tracheal intubation in comparison to an uncomplicated MP class I airway assessment was as follows: MP class II 3.23; class III 7.58; class IV, 11.3: short neck, 5.01; receding mandible, 9.71; and protruding incisors, 8.0. Using the univariate analysis of individual risk factors, a probability index/or relative risk parameters for various combinations of the risk factors showed that a patient with MP class III or IV, plus protruding incisors, short neck, and receding mandible, the probability of difficult laryngoscopy was greater than 90% (52) as shown in Figure 24-10.

Rocke et al.'s study highlights the importance of preoperative airway assessment and the importance of prospectively preparing for airway interventions in the true obstetric emergency CD under general anesthesia (33).

Combining Tests to Better Predict Difficult Intubation in Obstetrics

1. *Using MP classification and Wilson Risk Sum*
   Gupta et al. (79) used a combination of MP classification and the Wilson risk sum (77) to predict difficult intubation in 372 obstetric patients undergoing elective and emergency cesarean delivery (79). The Wilson risk sum score is calculated by adding scores of five factors,

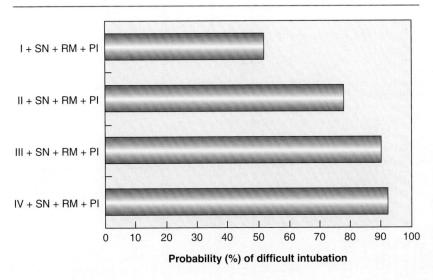

FIGURE 24-10 Probability of experiencing difficult intubation for varying combinations of risk factors. Modified with permission from: Rocke DA, Murray WB, Rout CC, et al. Relative risk analysis of factors associated with difficult intubation in obstetric anesthesia. *Anesthesiology* 1992;77(1): 67–73.

three objective and two subjective criteria (weight, head and neck movement, jaw movement/jaw protrusion along with IDD, receding mandible, and buck teeth). Combining the MP classification and Wilson risk sum has been shown to improve the sensitivity, specificity, and positive predictive value for prediction of difficult airway in obstetric patients (79). The subjective assessment of ease or difficulty in tracheal intubation was documented as described by Rocke et al. (33). In this study, 25 patients (6.7%) out of 372 patients had difficult laryngoscopy. Even though MP was found to be more sensitive test for prediction of difficult laryngoscopy in comparison to the Wilson risk sum, either test when used alone showed the sensitivity of the tests to be low and yielded many false negatives and false positive results. However, the combination of the MP and Wilson risk sum improved sensitivity to 100% while specificity was 96.2%. The study concluded that the two tests should be routinely performed during preoperative assessment of the obstetric patients. If these two tests are positive, difficult laryngoscopy/tracheal intubation can be predicted and adequate measures can be taken to plan the anesthetic so as to avoid airway-related catastrophes.

2. *Using MP classification, TMD, SMD, Mandibulo-hyoid distance and IID*

Merah et al. evaluated 80 consecutive obstetric patients, over a 1-year period who required GA for CD (64). The investigators studied the potential of five airway measurements to predict a difficult direct laryngoscopy in these 80 obstetric patients of West African descent which included the MP score, TMD, SMD, horizontal length of mandible, and IID. Out of the 80 patients, eight patients (10%) had difficult laryngoscopy. The investigators calculated the sensitivity, specificity, and positive predictive value of the test parameters. The MP test (MPT) had the highest values: Sensitivity 87.5%, specificity 95.8%, and positive predictive value 70%. The combined sensitivity of all tests was 100%, the specificity 36.1%, and the positive predictive value 14.8%. However, when the MP and TMD were combined 100% sensitivity was achieved but the specificity dropped to 93.1% and the positive predictive value dropped to 61.5% from 70% as compared to using MP alone. Perhaps a larger sample would have made a difference in the results obtained. The investigators concluded that there was a strong correlation

between modified MPT and prediction of difficult laryngoscopy.

3. *Meta-analysis of Bedside Screening Test Performance*

Shiga et al. performed a meta-analysis of studies on the diagnostic accuracy of bedside tests for predicting difficult tracheal intubation in patients with no airway pathology (69). Thirty five studies (50,760 patients) including both surgical and obstetrical patients were selected from an electronic database; details are shown in Table 24-8. The overall incidence of difficult tracheal intubation was 5.8% (95% confidence interval (CI), 4.5% to 7.5%). Screening tests included the MP classification, TMD, SMD, mouth opening, and Wilson risk score. Each test yielded poor to moderate sensitivity (20% to 62%) and moderate to fair specificity (2% to 97%). The meta-analysis found that the most useful bedside test for prediction was found to be a combination of the MP classification and TMD (positive likelihood ratio, 9.9; 95% CI, 3.1 to 31.9). The study concluded that in the surgical patients, a combination of tests adds some incremental diagnostic value in comparison to the value of each test alone.

In the obstetric cases (2,155 patients), the prevalence of difficult tracheal intubation was 3.1% (95% CI, 1.7–5.5). The result of the meta-analysis was that the diagnostic performance of the Mallampati classification in obstetric and obese populations is similar to that in the overall surgical population. The diagnostic odd ratios in these populations are similar, and the trend toward poor sensitivity and fair specificity remained. In the obstetric patients, the MP classification score yielded a sensitivity of 56%, specificity of 81%, and likelihood ratio of 0.6%. However, for obstetrical patients the meta-analysis remains inconclusive because of the small number of studies and issues with heterogeneity.

In obese patients (BMI >30 kg/m^2), the incidence of difficult tracheal intubation was 15.8% or three times higher than normal patients. Obese patients with a 15% pretest probability of difficult tracheal intubation had a 34% risk of difficult intubation with higher MP scores, which is twice the risk of the normal population with a 5% pretest probability. Excessive soft tissue in the velopalate, retropharynx, and submandibular regions in obese patients may cause difficulty in laryngoscopy. *Similarly, obese pregnant patients also had a higher incidence of difficult intubation.* Because of the higher incidence of difficult tracheal intubation, the MP classification score may yield

TABLE 24-8 **Pooled Estimates of Bayesian Statistics of Six Different Bedside Tests for Difficult Intubation**

Diagnostic Test	No. of Studies Included	No. of Patients	Prevalence of Difficult Intubation (95% CI), %	Pooled Sensitivity (95% CI), %	Pooled Specificity (95% CI), %	Pooled Likelihood Ratio Pos.	Pooled Likelihood Ratio Neg.	Pooled Log Diagnostic Odds Ratio (95% CI)
Overall Population								
Mallampati classification	31	41,193	5.7 (4.4–7.3)[a]	49 (41–57)[a]	86 (81–90)*	3.7 (3.0–4.6)*	0.5 (0.5–0.6)*	2.0 (1.7–2.3)*
Thyromental distance	17	29,32	6.5 (4.6–9.1)[a]	20 (11–29)[a]	94 (89–99)*	3.4 (2.3–4.9)*	0.8 (0.8–0.9)*	1.7 (1.2–2.1)*
Sternomental distance	3	1,085	5.4 (3.1–9.2)[a]	62 (37–86)[a]	82 (67–97)*	5.7 (2.1–15.1)*	0.5 (0.3–0.8)	2.7 (1.4–3.9)*
Mouth opening	3	20,614	5.6 (2.2–14.5)[a]	22 (9–35)[a]	97 (93–100)*	4.0 (2.0–8.2)*	0.8 (0.7–1.0)*	1.7 (1.2–2.3)*
Wilson risk score	5	6,076	4.0 (1.8–9.0)[a]	46 (36–56)	89 (85–92)	5.8 (3.9–8.6)*	0.6 (0.5–0.9)	2.3 (1.8–2.8)*
Combination of Mallampati classification and thyromental distance	5	1,498	6.6 (2.8–15.6)[a]	36 (14–59)[a]	87 (74–100)*	9.9 (3.1–31.9)*	0.6 (0.5–0.9)*	3.3 (1.5–5.0)*
Obstetric Subgroup								
Mallampati classification	3	2,155	3.1 (1.7–5.5)[a]*	56 (41–72)	81 (67–95)*	6.4 (1.1–36.5)*	0.6 (0.4–0.8)	2.5 (0.6–4.4)*
Obese Subgroup (BMI >30)								
Mallampati classification	4	378	15.8 (14.3–17.5)	74 (51–97)*	74 (62–87)*	2.9 (1.6–5.3)*	0.4 (0.2–0.8)	2.1 (0.8–3.3)*

Posttest probability = [(pretest odds) *likelihood ratio]/[1 + (pretest odds) *likelihood ratio], where pretest odds = pretest probability/(1 − pretest probability).

DerSimonian–Laird random effects model was used throughout.

[a]Significant heterogeneity ($p < 0.1$) was found.

BMI, body mass index; CI, confidence interval; Neg., negative; Pos., positive; ROC, receiver operating characteristic curve.

Reprinted with permission from: Shiga T, Wajima Z, Inoue T, et al. Predicting difficult intubation in apparently normal patients: A meta-analysis of bedside screening test performance. Anesthesiology 2005;103(2):429–437.

TABLE 24-9 LEMON: Airway Assessment Method

L = Look externally for anatomic feature that may make intubation difficult
E = Evaluate the 3-3-2 rule – Mouth opening (3 fb) – Hyoid–chin distance (3 fb) – Thyroid cartilage-floor of mouth distance (2 fb)
M = Mallampati score – Class 1: Soft palate, uvula, pillars visible – Class II: Soft palate, uvula visible – Class III: Soft palate, base of uvula visible – Class IV: Hard palate visible
O = Obstruction: Examine for partial or complete upper airway obstruction.
N = Neck mobility

fb, finger breadths.
Reprinted with permission from: Reed MJ, Dunn MJ, McKeown DW. Can an airway assessment score predict difficulty at intubation in the emergency department? *Emerg Med J* 2005;22(2):99–102.

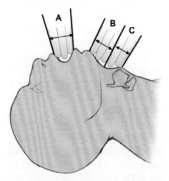

A. Inter-incisor distance in fingers (3 fb)

B. Hyoid mental distance in fingers (3 fb)

C. Thyroid to floor of mouth in fingers (2 fb)

FIGURE 24-11 LEMON airway assessment method. Murphy MF, Wall RM. The difficult and failed airway. Reprinted with permission from: Murphy MF, Walls RM. The difficult and failed airway. Manual of Emergency Airway Management. Chicago, Illinois: Lippincott Williams & Wilkins; 2000: 31–39, fb, finger breadths.

higher posttest probability of difficult tracheal intubation in obese patients than in normal patients (69).

4. *Quantitative Evaluation of Difficult Intubation*—**Lemon Test** Multiple external features are associated with difficult laryngoscopy and intubation. In an urgent or emergent obstetric situation, a practical, systematic and rapid evaluation of the airway is necessary and important to predict a potentially difficult laryngoscopic view and difficult mask ventilation, before initiation of rapid sequence induction for GA for CD. The evaluation should dictate the management plan and the availability of airway rescue devices.

The "LEMON" mnemonic represents one such assessment that is simple, quick, and can be performed on any emergency patient and has proven to have high predictive value (86). The LEMON mnemonic represents five elements for preanesthetic assessment, shown in Table 24-9 and Figure 24-11.

In the future, with the declining use of GA in obstetric patients, it will be increasingly difficult to conduct meaningful, prospective studies to predict difficult tracheal intubation. In light of the current state of knowledge, and until scientific validation of evidence from multicenter trials is available in the obstetric population with respect to prediction of difficult airway, the aforementioned type of multivariate analysis is as good as it gets in predicting a difficult laryngoscopy and difficult tracheal intubation (87). However, it requires continued education of future trainees on proper assessment of the airway for difficult laryngoscopy, difficult tracheal intubation, difficult mask ventilation, difficult supraglottic device placement, and difficult surgical airway. In parturients suspected of having a difficult airway, it warrants proper planning of anesthetic management of the patient while in labor and prior to operative delivery. It also requires timely decision on strategies and techniques to rescue the difficult airway by providing ventilation and oxygenation to the mother so as to avert airway catastrophes; while also being cognizant of how vitally important it is to balance the importance of the obstetrician delivering the baby.

■ ANESTHETIC MANAGEMENT IN OBSTETRIC PATIENTS WITH A DIFFICULT AIRWAY

The planning of the anesthetic management of parturients with predicted difficult airways undergoing labor or operative deliveries and the management of the anticipated and the unanticipated difficult airway in the obstetric patients during CD should be based within the framework of the ASA Practice Guidelines for Obstetric Anesthesia (6) and the ASA Practice Guidelines for Management of the Difficult Airway (3).

Management of the difficult airway has emerged as one of the most important safety issues in both the nonobstetric and obstetric population. Therefore, guidelines and strategies for management of the adult surgical difficult airway have been published by the ASA (3), the Difficult Airway Society in United Kingdom (88), the Canadian Difficult Airway Management Guidelines (41), the French (89), Italian (90), and more recently by the Australian (91) National Societies' work groups on Difficult Airway Management.

The strengths of the ASA Practice Guidelines for Obstetric Anesthesia published in 2007 are that it provides specific recommendations to decrease the maternal, fetal, and neonatal complications and includes the following:

Based on the recognition of anesthetic or obstetric risk, that is, morbid obesity and difficult airway, it should warrant consultation between the anesthesia and obstetric provider. A strategy to avoid instrumentation of the airway in patients who are at risk for DI or difficult mask ventilation is to plan ahead while the patient is in labor. The strategy requires prophylactically placing an epidural catheter early in labor in high-risk cases (e.g., obesity, difficult airway, preeclampsia, high-risk obstetric complications, and patients attempting vaginal birth after CD, which is in keeping with the recommendations of the ASA Practice Guidelines for obstetric anesthesia (6).

Early placement of a functioning neuraxial catheter for obstetric or anesthetic indications (difficult airway or obesity) should be considered to reduce the need for general anesthesia, if an emergent procedure becomes necessary.

Planning is also required for the immediate availability of personnel and equipment to manage airway emergencies and a means to provide oxygenation and ventilation to oxygenate or to manage a critical airway which means creating a surgical airway, if it becomes necessary (6).

A key point of the ASA Difficult Airway Algorithm (DAA) and its strength is the recommendation for management of both the ASA DAA for management of both the anticipated and the unanticipated DA in adult surgical patients (3). The ASA task force on difficult airway management also strongly recommends the use of strategies to maintain oxygenation throughout the process of airway management. Oxygenation is the cornerstone of airway management in situations including the nonemergency pathway, emergency pathway, and the CICV critical airway situation (3). Unfortunately, the ASA DAA also does not address the management of an airway emergency following rapid sequence induction in a patient with full stomach and studies show that it is difficult to recall the ASA DAA in an emergency.

Recent publications have prospectively validated that by simplifying the DAA, adhering strictly to a DAA, and using airway devices as gum elastic bougie, intubating LMA and the new video laryngoscope leads to a higher success rate of tracheal intubation in patients with difficult airways (92). The UK Difficult Airway Society has developed simple, clear, and definitive flow charts for three different scenarios of difficult intubation: Routine induction; unanticipated difficult tracheal intubation during rapid sequence induction of anesthesia (with succinylcholine) in a nonobstetric patient rapid sequence induction; and failed intubation/CICV situation with increasing hypoxemia in the paralyzed, anesthetized patients (88).

However, none of the DAA guidelines address the strategies for management of an obstetrical patient with predicted difficult airway undergoing labor, or the management of the difficult airway following rapid sequence induction, especially in the context of the urgency to deliver the baby. Therefore, the following section provides recommendations for:

A. Management of the parturient with a predicted difficult airway undergoing (i) labor or (ii) operative delivery, where airway management is not necessary;
B. Management of anticipated difficult airway in a parturient undergoing CD, where airway management is necessary;
C. Management of unanticipated difficult airway following rapid sequence induction;
D. Management of a CICV (cannot-intubate/cannot-ventilate) situation using (i) noninvasive airway rescue devices and (ii) invasive airway rescue devices during increasing hypoxemia, in the context of an emergency cesarean delivery and urgency to deliver the baby.

The recommendations have been formulated and based on the ASA Practice Guidelines for Obstetric Anesthesia, the ASA Practice Guidelines for Difficult Airway Management and the UK Difficult Airway Society Guideline for Management of Difficult Airway specifically following rapid sequence induction (3,6,88).

Anesthetic Management of the Parturient with a Predicted Difficult Airway

Labor

In order to provide safe maternal and fetal outcomes and to eliminate airway-related maternal mortality, it is important to incorporate "Best Practices" in the anesthetic management plan of the parturient. This means, first, evaluating high-risk obstetric patients antenatally and initiating multidisciplinary discussions for a cogent plan of action to manage the high-risk parturient in labor (93). In France, an antenatal anesthetic visit has been mandatory for all pregnant women (94). Since mandatory evaluation may not be cost effective, clear indications for selective antenatal anesthesiology evaluation, for example, patients with morbid obesity, known difficult airway, or significant comorbidities should be established.

Second, as part of "Best Practice," one should create the availability of anesthesia services to evaluate and provide consultation services to all parturients on the labor floor,

thus preventing being caught off guard in anesthetizing a patient with a predicted difficult airway. A collegial and collaborative approach between obstetricians and anesthesiologists when dealing with high-risk parturients facilitates optimum care.

According to the American College of Obstetricians and Gynecologists Committee opinion 1992, the obstetrical team should alert the anesthesiologists to the presence of risk factors that place the parturient at risk for complications from general anesthesia (95). Consideration should be given to early placement of a functioning epidural catheter in these patients (95). In the event of an urgent or emergent CD, establishing surgical anesthesia with a functioning epidural is much quicker as compared to attempting an awake, tracheal intubation especially in a patient with difficult airway; or, even worse, securing an airway after failed intubation under suboptimal conditions (96).

Educating and training obstetrical residents in evaluation of the airway, and risks of failed intubation is also important because it has been shown to change their approach toward labor analgesia (97). In this study, the obstetricians requested prophylactic placement of epidural catheters in patients who were thought to have a difficult airway thus providing one more step toward improving patient safety.(97).

Having a policy of incorporating the practice of placing neuraxial catheters such as continuous epidural analgesia or continuous spinal analgesia "prophylactically" early in labor in the laboring parturient who is considered to be high risk from an anesthetic perspective and who is at risk for CD reduces the risk of an unanticipated GA (6). This practice has been validated in large population studies (2,98). A functioning epidural catheter usually avoids the need for GA and the associated potential airway complications, especially during emergency surgery (6). It has also been suggested that in these high-risk patients, the epidural or spinal catheter may be placed before the onset of labor or at the patient's request for labor analgesia early in labor (6). Morbidly obese parturients have an initial high failure rate (62); therefore, the epidural catheter should be placed early in labor, to ensure adequate function (99).

Another option of providing labor analgesia is the use of combined spinal epidural (CSE) analgesia. However, its utility in patients with a predicted difficult airway, morbid obesity, or patients with high probability of operative delivery, is debatable. During the initial phase of analgesia provided by intrathecal medications, the functionality of the epidural catheter is not known and therefore there is no guarantee that surgical anesthesia will be achieved for an urgent or emergent CD posted during the initial CSE placement (100). However, Bloom et al. reported that failed regional anesthesia requiring conversion to GA occurred more commonly with an epidural than spinal or combined spinal–epidural (4.3% vs. 2.1% and1.7%, respectively) (12).

Finally, as part of best practice, there should be an aggressive approach toward management of an inadequate neuraxial block, for example, prompt replacement of nonfunctioning or poorly functioning epidural catheters (2).

Operative Delivery

Neuraxial techniques for CD are safe and predictable (1); therefore, for the patient undergoing elective or emergent CD, if airway intervention is deemed not necessary, one may proceed with a neuraxial anesthetic such as single-shot spinal anesthesia, continuous epidural anesthesia, combined spinal–epidural anesthesia, or continuous spinal anesthesia (101). While it may seem obvious, it is vital that all essential monitoring with functioning monitor alarms, drugs, and checked equipment be ready prior to any major neuraxial

TABLE 24-10 Factors Associated with Difficult Airway

Previous history of difficult airway
Morbid obesity
Diabetes, acromegaly, rheumatoid arthritis, obstructive sleep apnea, osteogenesis imperfecta
Trauma, facial burn injuries, swelling, head and neck infection, hematoma of the mouth, tongue, pharynx, larynx, trachea, or neck
Large tongue, receding jaw, high arched palate, prominent upper incisors, short thick neck, large breasts, microstomia, fixed or "high" larynx
Mouth opening, 2–3 cm, jaw protrusion class C, Mallampati class 3 or 4, thyromental distance <6 cm, reduced head/neck mobility
Voice change, shortness of breath, difficulty swallowing, choking stridor, inability to lie flat, drooling of saliva, lingular tonsillar hyperplasia

block. Emergency airway devices along with a difficult airway cart should be readily available. Needless to say, the regional technique should be performed in the operating room.

Management of Predicted Difficult Airway in A Parturient Undergoing Cesarean Delivery, where Airway Management is Necessary

Awake Tracheal Intubation
The patient undergoing CD where airway intervention is deemed necessary, one should proceed with an awake tracheal intubation. Indications for awake tracheal intubation in patients undergoing CD include previously documented history of difficult/failed intubation, osteogenesis imperfecta, severe rheumatoid arthritis, severe facial burn injuries, abnormal upper airway pathology, acromegaly, lingular tonsillar hyperplasia, morbid obesity with obstructive sleep apnea, and predicted difficult or impossible mask ventilation (72,102) (Table 24-10). In such patients, although neuraxial anesthesia may be a consideration, albeit challenging, it may be prudent to secure the airway awake so as to have a safe outcome for mother and baby.

Anesthetic management of a parturient with a predicted difficult airway presenting for CD is not a straightforward decision because following induction of anesthesia, intubation of the trachea may be impossible and a CICV situation may ensue. Conversely, regional techniques can be unsuccessful or though rarely complications arise that require emergency intubation (5,12,23,103).

The basic component steps for a successful awake tracheal intubation are as follows:

- Patient counseling
- Patient consent
- Use of an anti-sialagogue
- Judicious sedation
- Airway topicalization with local anesthetic
- Clinical pearls to successful fiberoptic technique

Patient counseling: Providing all options, discussing risks and benefits, obtaining informed consent cannot be emphasized enough. It requires spending enough time with the

patient and the family. Glycopyrrolate, 0.2 mg intravenously, should be administered 15 minutes before applying local anesthetic to the upper airway. It helps dry oropharyngeal secretions, thereby facilitating quick absorption of undiluted local anesthetic by the oropharyngeal mucosa and improves fiberoptic visualization of the glottic opening (104). An additional advantage in the parturient is that glycopyrrolate, a quarternary ammonium compound, does not cross the placental barrier and thus, has no effect on the fetus.

Sedation: Careful titration of sedatives such as midazolam 15 to 30 µg/kg intravenously to allay anxiety and fentanyl 1.5 µg/kg administered intravenously (ideal body weight) to provide analgesia, depress airway reflexes, facilitate airway instrumentation, improve patient comfort and cooperation during the procedure without risking respiratory depression in the mother or the newborn (105).

Dexmedetomidine is another choice to consider for sedation as it does not cross the placenta, and has been used successfully for sedation during fiberoptic intubation. Dexmedetomidine 1.0 µg/kg infusion, over 10 minutes, provides good to excellent tolerance to the procedure; more stable hemodynamics; and preserves a patent airway without causing respiratory depression (106).

Topicalization: Traditionally, the oral route is used for airway access; the nasotracheal intubation is avoided in pregnant women, due to the risk of initiating epistaxis from the hyperemic nasal mucosa. The aim of airway topicalization with local anesthetic such as lidocaine is to depress pharyngeal, laryngeal, and tracheobronchial reflexes and to facilitate smooth tracheal intubation (105). A needleless approach to local anesthetic topicalization of the airway may be achieved in the following manner: (1) Combined pharyngeal, periglottic anesthesia: Have an assistant pull tongue gently anterior with gauze padded finger and thumb while lidocaine gel 2% is applied with a tongue blade to the both sides of the tongue, tip of the tongue and to the base of the tongue. Place 1 inch of 5% lidocaine ointment on the tongue blade and place it like a lollipop midline as far as posterior on the tongue as tolerated; (2) glossopharyngeal nerve block: (a) Employ a tongue depressor on the lateral surface to shift the tongue medially and, spray 4% lidocaine on the palate, base of the tongue, uvula, posterior pharyngeal wall, and the anterior/posterior tonsillar pillars, (b) The MADgic® atomizer (Wolfe Tory Medical, Inc., Salt Lake City, Utah) works well for the local anesthetic spray since the droplet size is very small (107); the atomized particles are gently dispersed across a broad area of the mucosa for optimal coverage and absorption of local anesthetic is rapid, especially if the mucosa is dry (108,105), (c) apply gauze pledget balls soaked with 4% lidocaine with a curved clamp to the pyriform fossa for ≤5 min. *Eliminating the gag reflex is critical for a successful awake intubation, which means applying topical local anesthetic to the base of the tongue and the peritonsillar pillars liberally to block the* **glossopharyngeal nerve** *(via applying local anesthetic to the base of the tongue, uvula and spraying the peritonsillar fossae) is important.* Use Yankauer or soft suction to clear the secretions and test for reaction (gag, cough); (3) Superior laryngeal and Recurrent laryngeal nerve blocks: The "Spray As You Go" technique—the side port of the fiberoptic bronchoscope preloaded with a 5 mL Luer slip syringe containing 2% to 4% lidocaine, is then used to spray 2 to 3 cc on the anterior and superior aspects of the epiglottis in order to block the **superior laryngeal nerve**; and the posterior and inferior aspects of the epiglottis, the vocal cords, and upper trachea to block the ***recurrent laryngeal nerve*** (109).

Since it is essential that gagging, coughing, and laryngeal spasm are prevented with adequate airway topicalization prior to an awake tracheal intubation, there has been concern that the depression of laryngeal and gag reflexes in patients at risk for regurgitation of gastric contents may place the patient at risk for pulmonary aspiration. However, those fears have been allayed and found to have no merit in a study in a similar subset of patients at high risk for aspiration (110). Regardless of the extent of airway topicalization with local anesthetic, lower esophageal tone seems to be preserved, provided sedation is used judiciously.

Following topicalization of the upper airway and elimination of the gag reflex, tracheal intubation may be achieved by either flexible fiberoptic bronchoscopy or as recent reports suggest the use of video laryngoscopy-aided awake tracheal intubation (103,111–113).

Clinical Pearls to Successful Fiberoptic Technique

1. Before advancing the fiberscope, measure the distance from the corner of the mouth to the ear; that is, the distance from the mouth opening to the glottis. Place an intubating oral airway in the mouth (Ovassapian, Berman, Patil–Syracuse, Williams, or MAD)
2. Keep the fiberscope straight and follow the midline of the hard palate. Dominant hand performs finer, complex movement of aiming the tip in the correct direction.
3. Advance the fiberscope to 10 cm and look at the video monitor to visualize identifiable airway structures.
4. Make small movements with the lever as you advance the bronchoscope.
5. If the beveled tip of the tracheal tube impinges on the right arytenoid cartilage, try pulling back the tracheal tube, over the fiberoptic bronchoscope by 2 cm, and then rotating it by 90 degrees clockwise or counterclockwise so that the right beveled tip is either at the 6 o'clock or 12 o'clock position, respectively
6. Identify the carina, advance the fiberscope to three rings above carina, note do not touch the carina because it provokes coughing. Ask the patient to inhale deeply, before advancing the tube to its final position and removing the scope. If the TT meets resistance while trying to advance it into the larynx, withdraw 1 to 2 cm, rotate 90 degrees counterclockwise and advance the TT.
7. Stabilize the TT with one hand and inflate the cuff. Confirm the tube placement with ETCO$_2$ while hand ventilating and the presence of bilateral breath sounds before inducing GA.

Awake Glidescope intubation: In a difficult airway requiring awake intubation, the same approach for an awake fiberoptic intubation including antisialogogue administration, judicious sedation, and excellent topicalization can be used with a Glidescope in the same fashion as a fiberoptic scope. The skill level for the awake Glidescope appears to be less, making it a useful tool for awake intubation. Intubation by fiberoptic bronchoscope is a safe and gold standard of care technique for awake intubation due to direct control under direct vision. Advancement of the TT is not always easy in a traumatized airway following several attempts at intubation. The Glidescope allows for direct visualization of the vocal cords and passage of the TT.

A study compared fiberoptic intubation to Glidescope videolaryngoscope (VL) for awake intubation following mild

sedation. The results showed shorter intubation times and lesser stress response with the Glidescope VL (114). There are other studies to show the usefulness of awake Glidescope VL intubation as an alternative to awake fiberoptic intubation and the skills required are less with Glidescope (113,115). Refer to the section on clinical pearls to successful video laryngoscope/Glidescope intubation.

Management of the Unanticipated Difficult Airway Following Rapid Sequence Induction of Anesthesia

The anesthesia care provider must follow an organized strategy to effectively manage an unanticipated difficult airway that declares itself emergently during a stat cesarean delivery. We provide a simple, **logical and linear 5-step approach** to address the clinical scenarios outlined in Figure 24-12, of which the first 3 steps belong to this section. Our recommendations are based on the ASA Difficult Airway Algorithm (ASA DAA) and the United Kingdom Difficult Airway Society (DAS) guidelines. *Each step is time limited to not more than 30 to 45 seconds, so that the decision to provide emergency invasive airway access in the "Emergency Pathway, Critical Airway" scenario should occur within 5 minutes of initial presentation.*

Prior to the first attempt at tracheal intubation, proper planning is required and includes aspiration prophylaxis, proper positioning, left uterine displacement, and optimal preoxygenation.

Pulmonary Aspiration Prophylaxis

Parturients are at risk for gastric regurgitation and pulmonary aspiration of gastric contents, due to the anatomical and physiologic changes of pregnancy, despite prolonged fasting. This risk can be minimized by administering appropriate gastrointestinal prophylaxis using oral sodium citrate, 30 ml, 15 to 20 minutes before induction of GA to neutralize gastric acidity (116); intravenous famotidine, 20 mg, 45 to 60 minutes prior to induction of GA, to reduce gastric hydrochloric acid secretion (117); an option is to administer intravenous metoclopramide, 10 mg, 60 to 90 minutes before induction of GA, to increase lower esophageal sphincter tone and hasten emptying of the stomach (118).

Proper Positioning
Head Elevated Laryngoscopy Position (HELP)
Positioning in parturients is really aided by using the Head Elevated Laryngoscopy Position (HELP) using a preformed elevation pillow, such as the Troop Elevation Pillow (Mercury Medical, Clearwater, Florida) or using a set of folded blankets and sheets to create a ramp. The aim of HELP is to ensure that an imaginary horizontal line connects the external auditory meatus to the sternal notch, so that the position of the patient's head is above the level of the chest to facilitate optimal laryngoscopy, tracheal intubation, and facemask ventilation (119). Laryngeal exposure has been shown to be superior at 25-degree elevated positions when compared to the supine position (120).

Preoxygenation
Term parturients are at risk for rapid arterial desaturation during a period of apnea as mentioned earlier in the physiologic changes during pregnancy. In addition, room air is

Unanticipated difficult tracheal intubation, during rapid sequence induction of anesthesia, in the obstetric patient

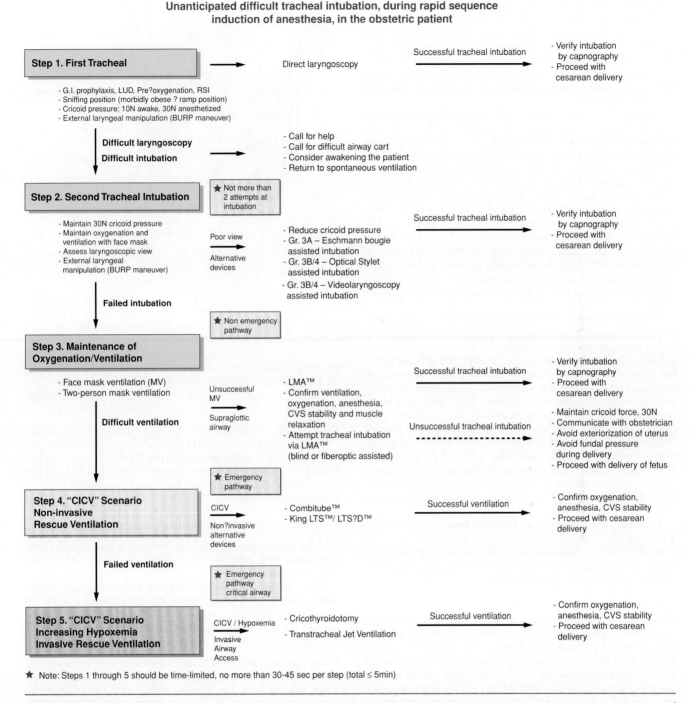

FIGURE 24-12 Comprehensive plan for unanticipated difficult tracheal intubation, during rapid sequence induction of anesthesia, in the obstetric patient.

continually entrained into the alveoli to replace the effects of constant uptake of alveolar oxygen by the pulmonary vasculature, thereby worsening arterial oxygen desaturation.

During periods of apnea associated with rapid sequence induction of GA, the PaO_2 falls at more than twice the rate in pregnant than in nonpregnant women (139 mm Hg/min vs. 58 mm Hg/min) (55). After complete denitrogenation via inhalation of 100% oxygen, nonpregnant patients tolerate 9 minutes of apnea before oxygen saturation is less than 90%, whereas parturients tolerate only 2 to 3 minutes of

apnea (55). There is no evidence that would support the once-conventional pattern of practice to refrain from bag–mask ventilation of the lungs in the interval from induction of anesthesia until laryngoscopy and tracheal intubation is performed and, in fact, there is evidence that would encourage it (121). In order to maximize the safe apnea time, consideration should be given to providing oxygen and allowing tidal volume ventilation for at least 3 minutes or providing for eight deep breaths, in 60 seconds, to maximize the duration of safe apnea time. Preoxygenation of obese patients, in the head-up position compared with the supine position, has been shown to provide a prolonged safe apnea time after induction and its use should be considered in obstetrical anesthesia (122). Therefore, adequate preoxygenation, in an optimal position, and limiting not only the number but also the duration of intubation attempts during the period of apnea from succinylcholine, becomes critical to avoid the onset of maternal oxygen desaturation, hypoxemia, and subsequent adverse neurologic maternal and fetal outcomes.

Effective de-nitrogenation of the lungs requires maximal oxygen storage in the pulmonary, vascular, and tissue compartments of the body (117). Some have argued that effective preoxygenation may be achieved by breathing with FiO_2 of 1 for 3 to 5 minutes or with four deep breaths of FiO_2 1.0 over 30 seconds (4DB/30 s) (123). However, the 4DB/30 s technique was later shown to predispose to rapid oxygen desaturation, especially during a period of apnea (124). Oxygen desaturation occurs quicker and worsens faster in children, obese individuals, and parturients (117). Later studies have shown that 8 deep breaths over 1 minute are comparable to 3 minutes of tidal volume breaths in obese patients (125) and term pregnant patients (126) and much superior to the 4DB/30 s technique in preventing desaturation during apnea (127).

Apneic Oxygenation (AO): AO has been used for many years to provide oxygenation through the process of diffusion (128). Using pharyngeal oxygen insufflation, this concept has been validated by studies in nonobese, healthy patients undergoing general anesthesia, who tolerated a period of apnea up to 10 minutes (129) and 6 minutes (130), without dropping arterial oxygen saturation level below 95%. A similar study was conducted in obese patients, undergoing simulated difficult laryngoscopy, using oxygen insufflation via nasal prongs. Nasal oxygen administration was associated with prolongation of duration of oxygen saturation >95% (5.29 minutes vs. 3.49 minutes); a significant increase in the number of patients with oxygen saturation >95% after 6 minutes of apnea (8 vs. 1); and significantly higher minimum arterial oxygen saturation (94.3% vs. 87.7%) (131).

Step One: First Attempt at Tracheal Intubation (see Step 1 Fig. 24-12)

Rapid sequence induction of anesthesia and tracheal intubation with cricoid pressure is the norm for providing general anesthesia for cesarean delivery.

Cricoid Pressure

The aim of cricoid pressure is to avoid gastric regurgitation into the hypopharynx (132); excessive or improper application of cricoid pressure may displace the vocal cords anteriorly or laterally, thus preventing a good view of the larynx during direct laryngoscopy (133). Sellick first introduced the use of pressure on the cricoid cartilage, during rapid sequence induction of anesthesia, in 1961, in order to prevent gastric inflation and regurgitation of gastric contents by compressing the esophagus between the cricoid cartilage anteriorly and the body of the sixth cervical vertebra posteriorly (134). The assistant applies a force of 10 Newton (N) with the thumb and index finger, in the awake patient, and increases the force to 30 N, with the index finger, as the patient becomes unconscious with induction of GA to seal the esophagus without obstructing the airway (134–137). Despite very little other clinical evidence to support this hypothesis, the practice is widespread. Properly applied cricoid pressure may also impair laryngoscopy by directly causing flexion of the head on the neck in contrast to the extension of the head on the neck required for maintaining the sniffing position or the head elevated laryngoscopy position. This problem can be circumvented by using bimanual cricoid pressure with one hand applying

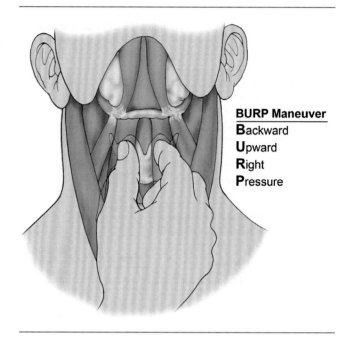

BURP Maneuver
Backward
Upward
Right
Pressure

FIGURE 24-13 External laryngeal manipulation.

cricoid pressure and the other hand supporting the back of the neck to prevent head flexion on the neck (138).

The considerations to improve and obtain the best view at laryngoscopy and best attempt at intubation require the following:

■ Optimum position of head and neck (sniff position): External laryngeal manipulation (BURP maneuver—**b**ackward, **u**pward, **r**ight-sided **p**ressure) (Fig. 24-13)
■ Single change in laryngoscope blade/handle: Miller straight blade, Macintosh 4 blade, or short handle)
■ Eschmann bougie
■ Easing up on the cricoid pressure, as excess or inexpertly applied cricoid pressure could obscure the glottic view

If the first attempt at tracheal intubation is *successful*, verify intubation with capnography and proceed with CD or else proceed to step 2.

Step Two: Second Tracheal Intubation/Best Attempt—Difficult Laryngoscopy/Difficult Intubation (see Step 2 Fig. 24-12)

Following difficult laryngoscopy/difficult intubation during the first attempt, one needs to focus on ensuring adequate oxygenation and ventilation. These are the recommended steps:

■ Call for help and the DA cart while mentally assessing the laryngoscopic view of the first attempt. It is prudent to call for help early in the process, either help for individual/s with expertise in DA management or a surgeon, in the eventuality that surgical airway is required.
■ Maintain cricoid pressure, at 30 N, but consider releasing transiently during the second attempt (25).
■ Attempt bag/mask ventilation.
■ Maintain/reinforce the head elevated laryngoscopy position.
■ Change laryngoscope blade type and size, use a smaller diameter tracheal tube.
■ Consider using Eschmann bougie, optical stylet, or videolaryngoscope depending upon the laryngoscopic view at first attempt (grade 3A, 3B, 4, respectively).
■ Have the most experienced person available make the second attempt; use external laryngeal manipulation/BURP maneuver.
■ Consider awakening the patient and returning to spontaneous ventilation.

TABLE 24-11 Difficult Airway Cart Contents

Location	Contents
Top shelf	Prep items for awake intubation Eschmann bougie Optical Stylet
Side slot	Fiberoptic bronchoscope
Drawer A	Supraglottic airway sizes 3 and 4: LMA Classic™, LMA Fastrach™, LMA Proseal™, LMA Supreme™
Drawer B	Specialized supraglottic airways: Combi-tube™ SA 37 Fr, King LTS-D™
Drawer C	Invasive airway equipment: Cricothyroid-otomy kit, transtracheal jet cannula with adapter, retrograde intubation kit

LMA, Laryngeal mask airway; SA, Small adult.
A Videolaryngoscope is readily available at all times in the obstetric operating suite.

Based on the recommendations of the ASA-DAA(3) and the ASA Practice Guidelines for Obstetric Anesthesia (6), we (authors MSS and AW) have a dedicated difficult airway (DA) cart immediately available in our obstetric operating suite that has proved to be invaluable during obstetric airway emergencies (Table 24-11) (139–141).

The second attempt should be well optimized and should be the ***best attempt*** at intubation. It is equally important to realize that repeated attempts during emergency tracheal intubation have an increased incidence of airway-related complications, as the number of laryngoscopic attempts increase from (<2 vs. >2 attempts), resulting in hypoxemia (11.8% vs. 70%), regurgitation of gastric contents (1.9% vs. 22%), aspiration of gastric contents (0.8% vs. 13%, bradycardia [1.6% vs. 21%], and cardiac arrest [0.7% vs. 11%] $p < 0.001$) (Fig. 24-14) (53). It is recommended that the tracheal intubation attempts should be limited to two in an emergency CD (25,49). The relative efficacy of the old and new airway devices in the management of difficult laryngoscopy/tracheal intubation in obstetrics has not been studied.

In the event of difficult laryngoscopy, clinical judgment becomes crucial and one has to weigh the risk of continuing cricoid pressure without being able to see the glottic opening versus reducing or transiently eliminating cricoid pressure and being able to improve the laryngeal view to expedite tracheal intubation despite the potential risk for gastric regurgitation and possible pulmonary aspiration (142,143). It is important to realize in this setting that pulmonary aspiration can be effectively treated, whereas, if the patient suffers cerebral hypoxia from inability to oxygenate, irreversible cerebral damage may occur.

Sellick allowed for lungs to be ventilated during rapid sequence induction with cricoid pressure without the risk for gastric distension and regurgitation (134). However, over the years, there were reports of esophageal rupture and pulmonary aspiration in patients during induction (144) and emergence from general anesthesia (145). As a result, perhaps, the practice of continuing ventilation during rapid sequence of anesthesia was dropped and has over time been accepted as the norm. More recently, questions have been raised regarding discontinuation of ventilation during rapid sequence of anesthesia and some anesthesiologists routinely use low-pressure manual ventilation, with peak airway pressure below 15 mm Hg, during the period of apnea following RSI using cricoid pressure to prevent arterial oxygen desaturation (146). In addition to providing oxygenation (hopefully) in a patient who is often not optimally oxygenated/denitrogenated, it also provides information early about ease of MV before the first attempt at DL.

Backward Upper Right Pressure (BURP)

In contrast to cricoid pressure, application of **b**ackward, **u**pward, and **r**ightward **p**ressure (BURP) maneuver on the thyroid cartilage (147) improves the glottic view during a difficult direct laryngoscopy, because the thyroid cartilage is the anatomical surface marking for glottis in the anterior neck, with the right hand while performing direct laryngoscopy with the left hand; the maneuver is also known as optimal external laryngeal manipulation (OELM). The BURP maneuver improved the laryngoscopic view by one grade or higher in patients with class 2, 3, or 4 Cormack and Lehane views and reduced the failure rate from 9.2% to 1.6% in a study comparing laryngoscopic views with or without application of the BURP maneuvers (147).

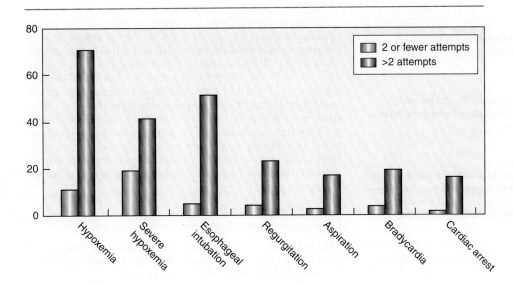

FIGURE 24-14 Graphic display of complications by intubation attempts. Reprinted with permission from: Mort TC. Tracheal Intubation: Complications associated with repeated laryngoscopic attempts. *Anesth Analg* 2004; 99: 607–613.

Eschmann Bougie

The Eschmann bougie is a useful airway device, commonly used to assist with tracheal intubation during difficult direct laryngoscopy, especially in grade 2 or grade 3A laryngoscopic views. In the original Cormack and Lehane classification, just the posterior portion of the glottic opening is visualized in a grade 2 view, whereas in a grade 3 view, only the epiglottis is seen (26). This classification was modified by Cook, who stated that grade 3 should be subdivided into grade 3A, where the epiglottis only is seen but can be elevated slightly with the laryngoscope blade away from the posterior pharyngeal wall, and grade 3B where only the epiglottis is seen but cannot be elevated away from the posterior pharyngeal wall by the laryngoscope blade (Fig. 24-9) (148).

During advancement of the Eschmann bougie into the trachea, tracheal clicks are readily appreciated, as the 35-degree angulated distal tip slides against the anterior tracheal rings (Fig. 24-15). These tracheal clicks have been demonstrated successfully in 78% patients with simulated and genuine grade 3 laryngoscopy (149). On the other hand, no clicks were appreciated in the other 22% patients resulting in esophageal intubation. A second test to confirm tracheal placement is to advance the Eschmann bougie gently deeper into the trachea until it "holds up" at the carina or in a smaller peripheral airway (149). With the laryngoscope blade in place in the oral cavity, the TT is railroaded over the Eschmann bougie. The commonest reason for inability to railroad the TT is the impingement of the distal beveled right tip of the tracheal tube on the right arytenoid cartilage, right vocal cord, or the right aryepiglottic fold. This can be taken care of by withdrawing the tracheal tube by 2 to 3 cm, rotating it 90 degrees counterclockwise, and then advancing it into the trachea (149). A maneuver known as the *Cossham twist* has been described where the TT is preemptively rotated 90 degrees counterclockwise on the Eschmann stylet before advancing into the trachea in order to avoid this delay in successful intubation (150). Alternatively, optical stylets may also be used in patients with grade 3A laryngoscopy (31 seconds intubation time) with no particular advantage over the Eschmann bougie (29.2 seconds intubation time) and has been demonstrated to have similar success rates (151).

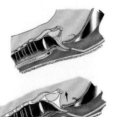
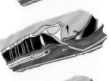
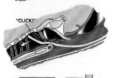
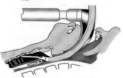

- Distal 3 cm is angulated 35°, tip should be introduced pointing anteriorly

- Tip of Eschmann Bougie passes under the epiglottis

- When passing through the trachea, the tip vibrates or tracheal ring clicks are felt

- TT railroaded over the bougie - When correctly placed in trachea, the bougie gets held at approx. 45 cm, making further advancement impossible

FIGURE 24-15 Eschmann Bougie-guided tracheal intubation.

Optical Stylets

In contrast, with either grade 3B or 4 laryngoscopic view, an optical stylet can be placed around the corner, below and behind the epiglottis, as a useful guide to visualize the glottic opening (151). With this technique, alignment of the three airway axes is not critical as tracheal intubation is achieved without establishing a "line of sight." The time to tracheal intubation and the success rates with optical stylets are far superior (31 seconds) than with the Eschmann stylet (45.6 seconds) during grade 3B laryngoscopy, but with grade 3A views they offer no advantage (31 seconds vs. 29.2 seconds, respectively) (151). The Levitan optical stylet has been used successfully following a failed tracheal intubation for a stat cesarean delivery (140).

Video laryngoscopy

Video laryngoscopy has become very popular in airway management due to its superior online display of anatomical details, allowing simultaneous clinical and educational input and value. It is an invaluable device to effectively teach both direct and indirect laryngoscopy (152). Some institutions have already incorporated the use of video laryngoscopes as their device of choice for the first attempt at tracheal intubation for stat cesarean delivery under GA, or in situations where tracheal intubation is anticipated to be difficult. Many video laryngoscopes are commercially available and include the nonchanneled ones such as the Berci Kaplan DCI, McGrath scope, Glidescope, and CMAC Storz scope, or the channeled video laryngoscopes such as the Pentax, AirTraq, and the King Vision. Their portability (153) allows for use anywhere in the hospital including the emergency room, operating room, intensive care unit, radiology suite, and endoscopy suite; and outside the hospital, in the prehospital setting.

Achieving Laryngeal View and Defining the View Axis (see Fig. 24-16: (154))

McGrath, Glidescope, and Storz C-Mac Video laryngoscopes

- Compared to direct laryngoscopy, these video laryngoscopes (VL) provide a look around the curve from 0 degrees to a **visual axis of approximately 270 to 300 degrees**.
- The distal tips of these video laryngoscopes point toward the 290 degrees.
- The cameras have a wide field of view: Both up and down; left to right; including the distal tip of their blades.
- Result is **supraepiglottic panoramic view of the larynx**, from above the epiglottis and posterior to the base of the tongue.

These devices provide an excellent view of the glottic opening without having to align the three airway axes in contrast to that need during traditional direct laryngoscopy. Most of the clinical studies and case reports in the literature are related to the use of Glidescope, McGrath, C-Mac, and Air Traq (112,153,155,156). Glidescope use is facilitated by using a preformed Glidescope-specific rigid stylet or a standard malleable stylet to shape the tracheal tube and assist with tracheal intubation (157). Airtraq, the disposable channeled videolaryngoscope, was successfully used in two morbidly obese pregnant patients undergoing emergency cesarean delivery after failed tracheal intubation attempts with direct laryngoscopy (156).

Clinical Pearls for Successful Video Laryngoscopy Include the Following Steps

1. Look in the mouth to introduce the scope in **midline**.
2. Look at the video screen to obtain the best optimal glottic view (top 1/3 of the video screen).

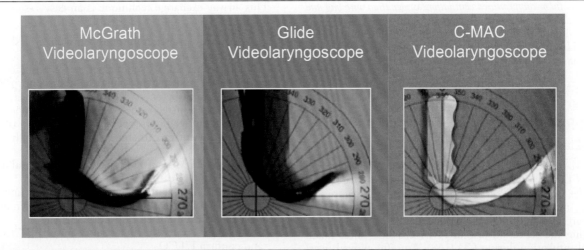

FIGURE 24-16 Achieving laryngeal view and defining the view axis. Reprinted with permission from: Levitan RM, Heitz JW, Sweeney M, et al. The complexities of tracheal intubation with direct laryngoscopy and alternative intubation devices. *Ann Emerg Med* 2011;57(3):240–247.

3. Back to the mouth to introduce TT:
   Use the Glide Rite 70-degree angled stylet reinforced TT, bent into a 90-degree angle.
   Insert the TT sideways in a horizontal plane through the mouth; **along the blade**.
4. Look at the screen to intubate the trachea. Rotate the TT into a vertical plane. Withdraw the stylet slightly as the tip of the TT enters the trachea to facilitate tracheal entry and prevent mucosal injury.

The commonest problem with the Glidescope is the inability to intubate the trachea, despite a good laryngoscopic view, and the TT seems to head posteriorly toward the arytenoids. To solve this problem, withdraw the Glidescope slightly until only the bottom 75% of the larynx comes into view, rotate the TT slightly toward the left arytenoid cartilage, gently twist the TT into the upper trachea, and then withdraw the stylet simultaneously over the patient's chest as the TT enters the trachea.

Complications with the Glidescope: Laryngoscopy with the Glidescope requires less upward lifting force (35 to 47.6 N). Needless to say that oropharyngeal injuries are less likely to be caused if decreased force is applied to the soft tissues. However, some injuries such as perforation of the palatopharyngeal arch, the palatoglossal arch, tonsillar pillar, and the soft palate (158–163) have been reported with the Glidescope VL. Tonsillar injury has been reported with the Airtraq optical laryngoscope as well (164).

Precautions that should be used include the following recommendations:

- Visualize the TT go into the mouth and around the tongue to avoid injury to the lips, teeth, and tongue.
- As the VL is advanced to achieve laryngeal visualization, upward force stretches the tonsillar pillars making them taut and susceptible to perforation by an advancing TT.
  - Glidescope requires less upward lifting force (35 to 47.6 N).
- To avoid injury, insertion of the TT parallel to and as close as possible to the laryngoscope blade attempting to reproduce its course to avoid injury to the right palaglossal arch and the right tonsillar pillar.
- Introduce TT in midline, with proximal end oriented toward the right and then rotate counterclockwise 90 degrees in a horizontal plane bringing it parallel to the blade to avoid soft tissue trauma.
- If slightest resistance is encountered, STOP, do not use force.

If second attempt at tracheal intubation is successful, verify with ETCO$_2$ and proceed with CD. If second attempt at tracheal intubation is unsuccessful (failed intubation), then it is important to focus on maintaining effective oxygenation and ventilation.

***Step Three: Maintenance of Oxygenation/Ventilation— Failed Intubation* (see Step 3 of** Fig. 24-12**)**

Airway management strategies from this point onward critical to avoiding adverse respiratory, cardiac, or neurologic complications are: (1) Providing maternal oxygenation, (2) preserving airway protection, (3) prevention of gastric regurgitation and pulmonary aspiration, (4) while simultaneously allowing for delivery of the fetus.

If tracheal intubation fails, only one well-optimized attempt should be undertaken, so that the anesthesia caregiver can instead proceed with providing oxygenation to the parturient and her fetus by other means. Early acceptance of failure to intubate the trachea is paramount in arriving at this decision. If the fetal heart tones are reassuring despite failed tracheal intubation, plans should be made to wake the parturient. If CD is still necessary, neuraxial anesthesia may be considered. If CD is not necessary at this point, no anesthetic would be required. However, if the fetal heart tones are nonreassuring after failed tracheal intubation, the anesthesia care provider must rely on a preformulated strategy and approach (6) including "Tunstall's failed intubation drill" where one of the options is to have the CD proceed under facemask anesthesia after return of spontaneous respiratory effort in the mother (165). However, cricoid pressure should be maintained (165,166) and the anesthetic deepened with an inhalation anesthetic.

Facemask Ventilation: In the event of unsuccessful ventilation with bag and mask, repositioning of the patient's head and chest, placement of an oropharyngeal airway, use of the airway strap around the facemask, and using a two-person technique are critical next steps (25). Two-person mask ventilation can be achieved by either the primary provider holding the mask with two hands while simultaneously providing chin elevation/jaw lift and the assistant compressing the reservoir bag, or the primary provider holds the mask in the left hand while simultaneously compressing the reservoir bag with the right hand and the assistant helps with chin elevation and jaw lift on the right side (25). The risk with this technique is gastric insufflation and regurgitation/aspiration.

Unsuccessful or compromised ventilation/oxygenation with bag and mask mandates the placement of a supraglottic device to maintain oxygenation. There are many commercially available supraglottic devices. However, most case series and case reports in obstetric anesthesia are with the laryngeal mask airway (LMA™).

■ DIFFICULT VENTILATION/ OXYGENATION: USE OF A SUPRAGLOTTIC AIRWAY

LMA Classic™

The LMA Classic™ has been used successfully in a large series of 1,067 patients scheduled for elective cesarean delivery under GA (167). No complications such as gastric regurgitation, pulmonary aspiration, or hypoxia were reported. There are also multiple case reports in the literature demonstrating the successful use of LMA Classic™ after failed tracheal intubation during CD (168). A useful clinical pearl for successful placement of the LMA Classic™ is to use the Archie Maneuver or the "Up–Down" Maneuver to relieve airway obstruction from the LMA™ tip either down folding the epiglottis or folding back on itself. It involves withdrawing the LMA™ by 6 cm followed by reinsertion without deflating the cuff; it has a high success rate (169).

Maintaining cricoid pressure during LMA insertion may prevent proper placement of the LMA™ tip behind the cricoid and arytenoid cartilages (see Fig. 24-17). LMA insertion has been shown to be more successful without cricoid pressure (94%) versus with cricoid pressure (79%) (142). Therefore, it may be necessary to transiently release cricoid pressure to allow proper placement of the LMA (see Fig. 24-17) (25). Communication with the obstetric team cannot be overemphasized enough: Avoid fundal pressures to minimize reflux of gastric contents and avoid uterine exteriorization to prevent retching, nausea, and vomiting.

In addition, the LMA Classic™ has been used as a conduit for blind or fiberoptic-guided tracheal intubation, but a longer tracheal tube may be required. This problem can be circumvented by using an airway exchange catheter (AEC) such as the Aintree catheter (Cook Medical, Bloomington, Illinois) preloaded over a fiberoptic bronchoscope, to guide passage of the tracheal tube (see Fig. 24-18) (170,171). This is an adaptation of the Cook Airway Exchange Catheter®. The 56 cm long, 4.8 mm inner diameter Aintree catheter should be preloaded on a 4 mm fiberoptic bronchoscope, allowing the distal 3 to 4 cm of the fiberscope to be available for maneuvering and passage through the LMA Classic™ into the trachea. The 6.5 mm external diameter of the Aintree catheter requires that the inner diameter of the tracheal tube be at least 7 mm or more.

This airway exchange technique is an easy 7-step process involving:

1. LMA Classic insertion in the recommended fashion, followed by cuff inflation
2. Capnographic $ETCO_2$ confirmation for ventilation
3. With visual guidance introduce the fiberscope, preloaded with Aintree catheter, via LMA into the trachea
4. Railroad the Aintree catheter over the fiberscope into the trachea. Remove fiberscope after visualization of carina, leaving the Aintree catheter in the trachea, with LMA in situ
5. Deflation of LMA cuff, followed by the removal of LMA over the Aintree catheter
6. Load the TT over the Aintree catheter. Passage of tracheal tube of at least 7 mm internal diameter or more over the Aintree catheter into the trachea
7. Remove the Aintree catheter and connect TT to circuit and confirm $ETCO_2$

The catheter also has a removable Rapi-fit connector which is removable and allows for oxygen insufflation, if necessary, during the airway exchange process (172).

Clearly, a larger tracheal tube can be inserted without being impeded by the LMA. The risk of accidental extubation, if the LMA is removed, is also eliminated as the LMA is removed before the tracheal tube is actually inserted. In summary, the Aintree Intubation Catheter offers an elegant solution to the problems associated with fibreoptic-guided endotracheal intubation using a laryngeal mask airway as a conduit.

LMA Fastrach™

Sometimes, there is difficulty with blind tracheal intubation via the LMA Classic™ (173) and the LMA Fastrach™ (referred to as the intubating LMA) was designed to circumvent that issue. It has been used successfully in patients with known difficult airways (174) and following failed tracheal intubation during emergency cesarean delivery (141).

A useful clinical pearl for insertion of the LMA Fastrach™ is the *Chandy Maneuver* which significantly improves the success rate of its placement (175). It is a 2-step sequential technique that optimizes the success of lung ventilation and blind tracheal intubation via the LMA Fastrach™ by aligning the internal aperture of the device with the glottic opening. The first step is to grasp the Fastrach™ handle and rotate it in a sagittal plane until least resistance to bag ventilation is achieved. The second step involves lifting, but not tilting, the device away from the posterior pharyngeal wall thereby preventing the TT from colliding with the arytenoids and facilitating its smooth passage into the trachea (see Fig. 24-19) (169).

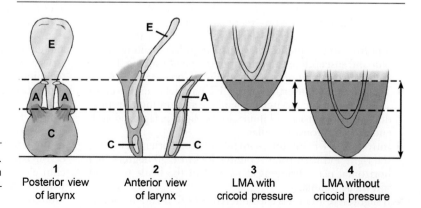

FIGURE 24-17 LMA and cricoid pressure. Reprinted with permission from: Asai T, Vaughan RS. Misuse of the laryngeal mask airway. *Anaesthesia* 1994;49:467–469.

1 Posterior view of larynx
2 Anterior view of larynx
3 LMA with cricoid pressure
4 LMA without cricoid pressure

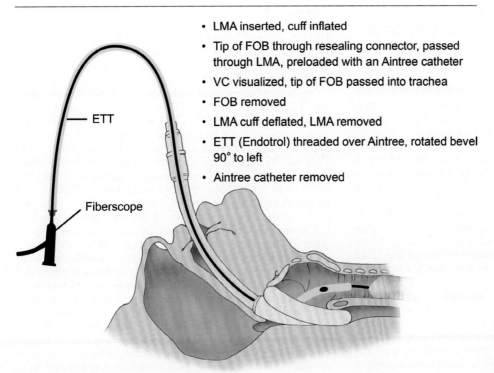

- LMA inserted, cuff inflated
- Tip of FOB through resealing connector, passed through LMA, preloaded with an Aintree catheter
- VC visualized, tip of FOB passed into trachea
- FOB removed
- LMA cuff deflated, LMA removed
- ETT (Endotrol) threaded over Aintree, rotated bevel 90° to left
- Aintree catheter removed

FIGURE 24-18 Fiberscope/Aintree-guided intubation via LMA.

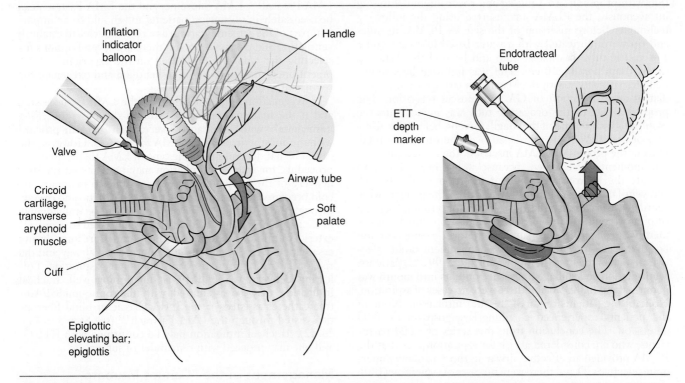

FIGURE 24-19 The two steps of the Chandy maneuver. **A:** After insertion of the LMA-Fastrach, optimal ventilation is established by slightly rotating the device in the sagittal plane, using the metal handle, until the least resistance to bag ventilation is achieved. This helps to align the internal aperture of the device with the glottic opening. **B:** Just before blind intubation, the LMA-Fastrach is slightly lifted (but not tilted) away from the posterior pharyngeal wall using the metal handle. This prevents the endotracheal tube (ETT) from colliding with the arytenoids and facilitates the smooth passage of the ETT into the trachea. Reprinted with permission from: Verghese C. Laryngeal mask airway devices: Three maneuvers for any clinical situation. *Anesthesiology News* 2010;36:8 (15–16).

■ DIFFICULT VENTILATION AND PREVENTION OF ASPIRATION: USE OF A SPECIALIZED SUPRAGLOTTIC AIRWAY

LMA Proseal™

The Proseal™ LMA (PLMA)™, a double lumen LMA, is specifically designed to prevent pulmonary aspiration if regurgitation of gastric contents occurs and provides several advantages over the LMA Classic™. It is particularly useful for failed tracheal intubation in obstetrics because it (1) enables correct positioning, isolating the larynx from the esophagus, and therefore may provide airway protection and protection against pulmonary aspiration (176); (2) provides a conduit for passive venting of gastric contents; (3) allows passage of a 14 Fr orogastric tube to empty the stomach; (4) provides better ventilation due to its higher seal pressure of greater than 10 cm H_2O compared to the LMA Classic™ (177). There are multiple case reports of the successful use of the LMA Proseal™ after failed tracheal intubation during emergency cesarean delivery (176).

Although the PLMA has been reported to be a successful rescue device for failed tracheal intubation in obstetrics (178,179), it was not until recently that it has been evaluated as a routine airway for patients undergoing elective CD. A prospective study (180) reported their experience with the PLMA in 3,000 elective CD from a single center using a method that involves rapid establishment of a patent airway plus gastric drainage. All patients were fasted for at least 8 hours and were given ranitidine 50 mg intravenously. Following preoxygenation and a modified rapid sequence induction with propofol 2 to 3 mg/kg and rocuronium 0.9 mg/kg intravenously, the PLMA was inserted using the following technique: Before insertion of the size #4 PLMA, its sides and tip were lubricated with a water-based lubricant and a 14# gastric tube was loaded into and beyond the distal tip of the drain port by 10 cm. This was followed by a modified pharyngoscopy with the Macintosh laryngoscope immediately after induction of GA and muscle relaxation The protruded part of the orogastric tube was guided into the esophagus with the aid of the Magill forceps, before the insertion of the PLMA was railroaded over the orogastric tube. During the process of PLMA insertion, the cricoid pressure was momentarily released, because it has been shown to impede the appropriate depth of insertion of the PLMA and ventilation through the PLMA (181). The patients were ventilated with an inspired tidal volume of 6 to 8 ml/kg at a respiratory rate of 10 to 14 per minute. Appropriate placement was confirmed with square waveform capnogram and positive $ETCO_2$. The successful establishment of an effective airway on the first attempt was in 2,992 (99.7%) patients; regurgitation and spillage of gastric contents into mouth was in one patient (0.003%) and there were no cases of aspiration. None of the patients required "rescue" intubation. None of the patients experienced coughing/laryngospasm or ICU admission. The conclusion from this series of 3,000 parturients, who are considered at risk for aspiration, was that the PLMA provided an effective airway in those patients undergoing elective CD and there were no cases of aspiration (180).

LMA Supreme™

The LMA Supreme™ is a single-use, supraglottic device created as an alternative to conventional, tracheal intubation. It has some features that are similar to the Fastrach™ and some to the Proseal™; it has a shorter stem and handle to allow manipulation as per the Fastrach™ (but not designed as a conduit for a TT) and similar to the Proseal™; it features a built-in drain tube designed to channel fluids and gas away from the airway. The elliptical shape and integrated bite block facilitates proper placement and prevents kinking. The LMA Supreme™ provides a good seal for positive pressure ventilation. The new LMA Supreme ™, a disposable version of the LMA Proseal™, may be useful as a rescue device in a similar obstetrical situation.

In a large observational study, Yao et al. (182) describe their use of LMA Supreme™ for 700 nonemergent cesarean deliveries. A total of 700 ASA 1 to 2 (576 elective, 124 urgent) term parturients, with the application of stringent criteria, were applied to exclude those at higher risk for aspiration. Mean BMI was 25.6 kg/m²; parturients had fasted at least 6 hours in elective cases or at least 4 hours in urgent cases and had received antacid prophylaxis. The success rate of first attempt insertion of LMA Supreme™ insertion was 98% (686 parturients) and time to establishing effective airway was 19.5 (±3.9) seconds with maintenance of ventilation and oxygenation in all parturients and there was no evidence of aspiration. It should be noted that a rapid sequence induction technique was performed with rocuronium as the neuromuscular blocking agent. This study is of interest for several reasons: It gives further evidence that the Supreme LMA™ allows effective ventilation even with pregnancy-related gastrointestinal changes. The uneventful use of the LMA Supreme in 700 parturients undergoing CD is reassuring. There is an important caveat: These patients were carefully selected, they were nonobese, fasted, had no gastroesophageal reflux and were low-risk parturients. Therefore, its usefulness in parturients with difficult airways, obese individuals is not known.

The aforementioned studies have demonstrated, in large series of patients and in case reports, that the LMA Classic, LMA Proseal™, LMA Supreme, and the LMA Fastrach can be used safely in obstetrical patients and should be an important part of the armamentarium as a rescue device to establish ventilation and oxygenation and there are several options for selecting the type of LMA based on the experience of the practitioner, that can be used to ventilate and oxygenate the parturient in an emergent situation.

If oxygenation and ventilation via the LMA is successful, and if the maternal or fetal condition dictates proceeding immediately with cesarean delivery, then one can proceed with the anesthetic using the LMA for the CD. However, the caveat is that depending on the type of LMA that is used, the procedure for tracheal intubation may be deferred till after delivery of the baby. One should continue to maintain cricoid pressure and provide inhalational anesthetic and oxygen through the LMA; the obstetric team should be immediately made aware of the unprotected airway and asked to avoid: (1) exteriorization of the uterus, and (2) fundal pressure during cesarean delivery, because of the unprotected airway and the risk of gastric regurgitation and pulmonary aspiration. Following delivery, if the LMA is functioning well, tracheal intubation may be attempted with fiberoptic-guided/Aintree catheter assisted via the LMA Classic or blind/fiberoptic assisted through the LMA Fastrach™ (see Step 3 of Fig. 24-12). Tracheal intubation may be confirmed with $ETCO_2$ and one may proceed with remainder of surgery.

Management of the "Cannot Intubate Cannot Ventilate" Situation

Use of Noninvasive Rescue Devices (Step 4 Fig. 24-12)

According to the ASA DAA, following failed intubation and if both facemask ventilation and LMA ventilation are ineffective in maintaining oxygenation (difficult ventilation), the patient is considered to be on the *Emergency* pathway (*"Cannot Intubate Cannot Ventilate"*) and should receive immediate rescue ventilation with other noninvasive devices such as Combitube™ or King LTS™/LTS-D™ (3,88).

Combitube™

The Combitube™ has been recommended for the emergency airway pathway, especially when tracheal intubation has failed, an LMA is not functional, and patient is at risk for pulmonary aspiration (183,184). Combitube™ continues to be a part of the ASA DAA, the American Heart Association guidelines, and the European Resuscitation Council guidelines. However, it has become obsolete in Canada and the United Kingdom due to its complication profile from years past, especially in the prehospital setting (185). The original Combitube™ was 41 Fr in size and is larger than the latest smaller version, the SA (small adult) size, that is 37 Fr. The Combitube SA™ is recommended for individuals between 4 and 6 ft tall (186). The ASA DAA task force suggests using Combitube™ after failed pulmonary ventilation with conventional face mask and LMA (3).

The Combitube™ has been successfully used after failed tracheal intubation in an emergency CD (183), in a morbidly obese patient with a bull neck (187), after a failed LMA (188), and in the CICV situation (189). It has also been reported and shown to prevent pulmonary aspiration of gastric contents when used during cardiopulmonary resuscitation (190) and during cesarean delivery (191). Advantages of the Combitube™ over the LMA™ in the pregnant patient, who is prone to rapid arterial oxygen desaturation, include minimal preparation for use, rapid oxygenation capability, isolation of the larynx from the esophagus, protection from gastric regurgitation (183), minimal risk for pulmonary aspiration (192), and higher seal pressures of up to 50 cm H_2O for pulmonary ventilation (193). In addition, airway exchange can be accomplished with the Combitube™ in situ, by partially deflating the latex hypopharyngeal balloon, and passing a fiberoptic bronchoscope preloaded with a TT along the side of the Combitube ™ (191).

Clinical pearls for successful Combitube™ use include: (1) Insert the Combitube™ in warm saline or water immediately prior to use, (2) hold the device just above the yellow latex balloon in the right hand, and pressing the tongue out of the way and lifting the jaw with the left hand, (3) insert the Combitube™ along the surface of the tongue following the natural curve from the mouth to the esophagus, (4) stop when the black ring straddles the teeth, (5) use the minimal volume inflation technique to prevent pharyngeal mucosal injury (194), and

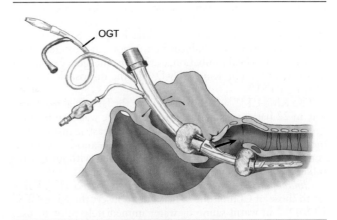

FIGURE 24-20 Correct position of the King LTS-D in the esophagus with OGT in situ.

(6) use everything marked in blue first, including the pilot balloon for cuff inflation/deflation and lumen for pulmonary ventilation (186). The most current recommendation is to use a laryngoscope for adequate exposure and to facilitate esophageal placement of the Combitube™ (194).

King LTS™/LTS-D™

The King LTS™ is the double lumen version of the King LT™; it is similar to the Combitube™ but is smaller, shorter, and softer; it has a nonlatex oropharyngeal cuff, and dedicated channels for ventilation and esophageal/gastric access. It is designed for easy placement (195), uses low-pressure cuffs (196), and has minimal complications reported (197). The King LTS™ simultaneously isolates the esophagus from the airway by allowing passage of an 18 Fr orogastric tube via the posteriorly placed gastric drainage lumen to aspirate any stomach contents (Fig. 24-20). King LTS™ allows passage of an AEC over a fiberoptic bronchoscope to facilitate intubation with a tracheal tube so as to establish a definitive airway (see Fig. 24-21) (198). It is a useful airway device that can be

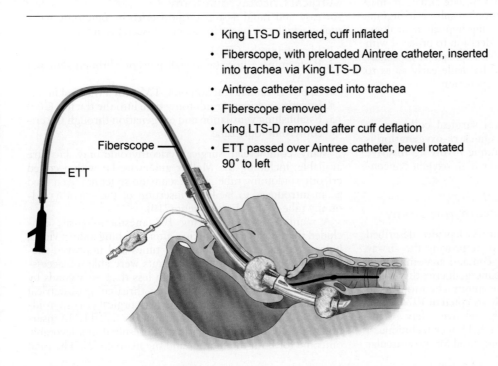

- King LTS-D inserted, cuff inflated
- Fiberscope, with preloaded Aintree catheter, inserted into trachea via King LTS-D
- Aintree catheter passed into trachea
- Fiberscope removed
- King LTS-D removed after cuff deflation
- ETT passed over Aintree catheter, bevel rotated 90° to left

FIGURE 24-21 Tracheal intubation via King LTS-D using Aintree catheter and fberscope.

used in elective, emergent or difficult airway scenarios and has been used in spontaneously breathing patients (195) and during controlled ventilation (199). The King LTS™ has been successfully used to establish ventilation and oxygenation, after failed tracheal intubation, during an emergency cesarean delivery (200). The King LTS-D™ is the disposable version of King LTS™.

The King LT™ was compared with the laryngeal mask airway in 22 patients. The mean leak pressure was significantly greater for King LT™ versus LMA™ and gastric insufflation did not occur with the King LT™ (196). In another study, a ventilatory seal of 40 cm H_2O was achieved without gastric inflation in 30 patients with the King LT™ (197).

Clinical pearls for successful use of King LTS™/LTS-D™: Similar to those of Combitube™ placement, insert the King LTS/LTS-D™ in warm saline or water immediately prior to use, holding the device just above the upper oropharyngeal balloon in the right hand, pressing the tongue out of the way and lifting the jaw with the left hand, inserting the King LTS/LTS-D™ along the surface of the tongue following the natural curve from the mouth to the esophagus, and using the minimal volume inflation technique to prevent pharyngeal mucosal injury.

On the *Emergency* pathway (*"Cannot Intubate Cannot Ventilate"*), if oxygenation and ventilation with the noninvasive devices Combitube™ or King LTS™ are successful, one should maintain anesthesia, cardiovascular stability, and proceed with CD.

If oxygenation and ventilation are not possible despite using the Combitube™ or King LTS™/LTS-D™ and the patient condition worsens due to increasing hypoxemia associated with bradycardia (CICV with increasing hypoxemia), the patient is considered to be on the *Emergency Pathway— Critical Airway Situation*, which is a life-threatening emergency requiring **immediate invasive intervention and rescue ventilation** using either surgical cricothyroidotomy, needle cricothyroidotomy with transtracheal jet ventilation, or surgical tracheostomy (see Step 5 of Fig. 24-12) (3,88).

Emergency Pathway Critical Airway Situation: Use of Invasive Rescue Airway Techniques with CICV and Increasing Hypoxemia (Step 5 of Fig. 24-12)

Failed tracheal intubation, with increasing hypoxemia and difficult ventilation situation, is usually due to multiple unsuccessful attempts when a 'Can Ventilate situation' may hastily develop into a "CICV situation" resulting in significant maternal/fetal morbidity, including hypoxic neurologic injury, and maternal mortality. The decision to proceed with invasive airway access for progressive hypoxemia, especially associated with bradycardia, should be made early so as to establish effective ventilation and oxygenation.

Invasive Airway Techniques

Involvement and assistance from a surgical colleague is mandatory and may be lifesaving. Quick re-oxygenation is vital and is achieved with a technique involving invasive airway access and a means to deliver high oxygen concentration.

Emergency Percutaneous Cricothyroidotomy

In 100 BCE, the Persian physician Asclepiades described in detail a tracheostomy incision for improving the airway (201,3). Vicq d'Azyr, a French surgeon and anatomist, first described cricothyrotomy in 1805. Emergent cricothyroidotomy (also known as cricothyrotomy, minitracheostomy, and "high tracheostomy") became widely accepted in 1976, when Brantigan and Grow confirmed the relative safety of the procedure (202). A decade later, the Seldinger technique, a wire-over-needle technique commonly used for intravascular

cannulation, was adapted for use in obtaining both emergent and nonemergent surgical airways.

Invasive airway access techniques via the cricothyroid membrane (CTM) are fraught with complications and the possible risks should be continually balanced against the risks of hypoxic brain damage and maternal death (203). Once the decision is made to perform an emergent surgical airway, no absolute contraindications remain; it is a last-resort, lifesaving measure especially in an obstetrical situation to save the mother and the baby.

Successful outcome requires a thorough understanding of the anatomy of the CTM (204), the invasive airway access technique (205), and the nuances of the ventilation devices.

Any practitioner who performs intubations must know and review the structures of the neck and structures that support the airway (thyroid cartilage, cricoid cartilage, and tracheal rings). The vocal cords are located a short distance (approximately 0.7 cm) above the thyroid notch. An attempt to place a surgical airway here would be harmful. Cricoid cartilage is a complete ring that can be felt in most individuals, except in obese patients. The CTM, which has a vertical height of 8 to 19 mm and a width of 9 to 19 mm, is located between the thyroid and cricoid cartilages. Branches of the thyroid arteries pierce the CTM in its upper third; it is advisable to approach the access to its lower third. Identifying the midline of the structure is important, as roughly 30% of the population has large–caliber veins within 1 cm of the midline, whereas only 10% have veins greater than 2 mm in diameter that cross the midline. *In patients in whom the landmarks are difficult to identify, the membrane is usually 4 fb from the sternal notch.*

Emergent cricothyroidotomy is not a procedure that is easily practiced for "real-life" situations. Exposure to the procedure and skills can be improved through simulation (206,207).

The three procedures that might be considered in an emergency airway setting include: (1) Surgical cricothyroidotomy (traditional four steps or percutaneous tracheostomy), (2) needle cricothyroidotomy with or without transtracheal jet ventilation (TTJV), or (3) a formal tracheostomy in the CICV situation. The complication rate for emergent cricothyrotomy ranges from 10% to 40% of cases (208).

Surgical Cricothyroidotomy

An easy and rapid 4-step surgical cricothyroidotomy technique, which can be performed in 30 seconds, involves:

1. Identifying the CTM
2. Performing a horizontal stab incision through skin and CTM
3. Applying caudad traction on CTM with a tracheal hook
4. Inserting a cricothyroidotomy tube into the trachea (209)
5. Establishing ventilation and oxygenation through the cricothyroidotomy tube

Many commercial surgical cricothyroidotomy kits are available, including the Melker guidewire kit with a cuffed cricothyroidotomy tube. The Eschmann stylet has been used as an introducer to facilitate insertion of the cricothyroidotomy tube in the obese patient (210).

A manikin study, involving 102 anesthesiologists, concluded that practice in manikins, after watching a short video, helped reduce cricothyroidotomy times and improved success rates so that 96% of participants were able to successfully perform cricothyroidotomy in less than 40 seconds by their fifth attempt (206). In a real-life–threatening obstetrical situation, a rapid decision to perform a surgical cricothyroidotomy following failed tracheal intubation, failed LMA insertion, and CICV situation during CD resulted in a favorable outcome for both the mother and the neonate (2). The total time taken from rapid sequence induction of GA to completion of surgical cricothyroidotomy was less than 5 minutes, thus averting adverse respiratory-related events (2).

Needle Cricothyroidotomy with Percutaneous Transtracheal Jet Ventilation (TTJV)

This technique is associated with a low success rate (211), a high complication rate (212,213), and is not necessarily recommended because of the potential for associated barotrauma. A combination of a 14-gauge needle/cannula insertion through the CTM and connection to a high-pressure source for jet ventilation is used (214). A few suggestions (215) for successful outcome include use of preformed needle cricothyroidotomy kits; insertion of the needle through the CTM in a caudad direction, aspiration of air freely from the 14-gauge needle and subsequently the 14-gauge cannula; a designated individual holding the 14-gauge cannula firmly to prevent dislodgement or kinking; tightly attaching the cannula to a high-pressure oxygen source (up to 50 psi); use of an in-line pressure regulator to reduce pressure to 15 to 20 psi or lower; short inspiratory time of less than 1 second; longer expiratory time greater than 1 second; and maintenance of upper airway patency using oropharyngeal airway, nasal trumpets, and jaw thrust/chin lift to prevent potential air trapping in the lungs/subcutaneous tissues and pulmonary barotrauma/subcutaneous emphysema (117).

Needle Cricothyroidotomy Using Seldinger Technique

- Assemble and prepare equipment.
- Patient should be placed in the supine position and the neck in a neutral position.
- Clean the patient's neck in a sterile fashion using antiseptic swabs.
- Assemble a 12- or 14-gauge, 8.5 cm over-the-needle catheter, to a 10 mL syringe.
- Locate the CTM anteriorly between the thyroid and cricoid cartilages.
- Stabilize the trachea with the thumb and forefinger of one hand.
- Using the other hand, puncture the skin in the midline with the catheter over the CTM.
- Direct the needle at a 45-degree angle caudally while applying negative pressure to the syringe.
- Maintain needle aspiration as the needle is inserted through the lower half of the CTM. Aspiration of air signifies entry into the tracheal lumen.
- Remove the syringe and needle while advancing the catheter to the hub.
- Confirm aspiration of air from the catheter.
- Advance the guidewire through the catheter. (A small incision with a No. 11 blade may be made first to facilitate passage of the dilator over the wire.)
- Remove the catheter.
- Insert dilator and airway tube combination over the guidewire. Once the airway device is in place, the dilator and guidewire are removed.
- Attach the oxygen catheter and secure the airway.

Following invasive airway access and establishing successful ventilation and oxygenation, and averting a crisis, one should proceed with CD while maintaining anesthesia, oxygenation, and cardiovascular stability.

Thorough and extensive documentation, communication with the patient and family, establishing airway alert identifiers, and enrollment in difficult airway registry should follow (see Airway Alerts section).

■ EXTUBATION AND PACU AIRWAY ISSUES

Maternal Mortality Following Extubation and Emergence

A new problem that is emerging in obstetric patients is *deaths following emergence from GA*. Maternal mortality surveillance of anesthesia-related maternal deaths in Michigan from 1985 to 2003, reviewed retrospectively, indicates that there were no deaths during induction of GA (15). However, there were 15 either anesthesia-related or anesthesia-associated maternal deaths that occurred during emergence, after extubation, and in recovery (15). Similarly, the Confidential Enquiries into Maternal Deaths, reported a new problem and that is deaths following extubation and on emergence from anesthesia; of the six direct deaths attributable to anesthesia care in the 2003–2005 Confidential Enquiries report, one resulted from respiratory distress on extubation and two from postoperative respiratory insufficiency, one occurring immediately postoperatively and the other some hours later (17). Furthermore, of the seven anesthesia-attributable deaths detailed in the Eighth Report (2006–2008) (18), one death was from aspiration following extubation of the trachea after emergency cesarean delivery in a woman recognized to have a full stomach. In the Canadian special report on Maternal Mortality, from 1992 to 2000, the only anesthesia-attributed direct maternal death was postoperatively following extubation of the trachea (19). Although airway disaster during induction of GA remains one of the leading causes of maternal mortality, Mhyre et al. (15) did not find a single case of airway disaster or failed intubation during induction of GA. In contrast, during this retrospective review of 855 pregnancy-associated deaths, there were eight anesthesia-related and seven anesthesia contributing maternal deaths, all of which occurred following extubation/emergence from anesthesia. The data from these deaths during emergence illustrated three key issues: 1) All anesthesia-related deaths from airway obstruction or hypoventilation took place during emergence and recovery, not during induction of GA; (2) systems error (one of the major ACGME core competencies includes systems-based practice) with specific lapses including inadequate postoperative monitoring and inadequate supervision by an anesthesiologist, seemed to contribute to more than half the cases and played a role in the majority of cases; (3) obesity and African-American ethnicity were also important risk factors for anesthesia-related maternal mortality (15).

Although tracheal intubation receives much attention, especially with regard to management of the difficult airway, there has been very little emphasis and research on complications following tracheal extubation and emergence issues in PACU, both in the general and obstetrical patients. The ASA Task Force on the Management of the Difficult Airway regards the concept of extubation strategy as a logical extension of the intubation process (3) in order to avoid airway catastrophes in the emergence period.

■ STRATEGIES AND RECOMMENDATION FOR AVOIDING POSTOPERATIVE AIRWAY CATASTROPHES

It is incumbent on each anesthesia practice to establish protocols that not only reduces anesthetic risks during labor, and during induction of GA, but also to reduce risks associated with extubation, emergence from GA, and it must be applied to the obstetrical patients recovering from both regional and GA anesthesia following CD.

Firstly, airway management needs to be considered as a continuum of patient care from intubation, maintenance of anesthesia, and extubation, with continued control of the airway into the postextubation period. As per the 2005 Closed Claims Analysis of difficult airway management, developing strategies to cover emergence and the recovery phases after extubation may improve patient safety (67). There is insufficient literature to support the merits of a specific extubation strategy either in the general surgical population or in obstetrical patients (3). Yet, it seems logical that maintaining a conduit within the trachea to allow the feasibility of re-securing the airway would add to patient safety particularly in the high-risk patient such as the morbidly obese, those with obstructive sleep apnea, and African-American women with severe preeclampsia who have edematous airways.

Airway exchange catheters (AECs) have been used successfully to either safely change a TT or to maintain access to the airway after extubation, thus allowing re-intubation should extubation fail (216).

An arbitrary recommendation is to maintain continuous access via an AEC and to extend the duration of the indwelling AEC, for 60 to 120 minutes, in particularly high-risk patients such as those with periglottic edema (216). The same principles of using an indwelling AEC to allow re-securing of airway is applicable to the high-risk obstetric patient (i.e., the morbidly obese, those with obstructive sleep apnea, and preeclampsia with periglottic edema) and if used, may enhance patient safety given the latest morbidity/mortality data.

Secondly, adequate supervision by appropriate anesthesia personnel and appropriate equipment is required in the postoperative period to avert adverse airway-related catastrophes (217). The 2009 ACOG guideline on Optimal Goals for Anesthesia Care in Obstetrics (218) state that there should be: "Availability of equipment, facilities, and support personnel equal to that provided in the surgical suite. This should include the availability of a properly equipped and staffed recovery room capable of receiving and caring for all patients recovering from major RA or GA. Birthing facilities, when used for analgesia or anesthesia must be appropriate to provide safe anesthetic care during labor and delivery or postanesthesia recovery care."

Thirdly, implementation of monitoring measures that specifically address the perioperative risks associated with obesity and obstructive sleep apnea, with special focus on reducing the risks of airway obstruction and hypoventilation should be the standard of care. The ASA standard of care for monitoring for postoperative care suggests that pulse oximetry monitoring is associated with early detection of hypoxemia during emergence and recovery particularly in the African-American population in whom cyanosis may not be detected visually (217).

Effective respiratory monitoring is critical to patient safety in clinical situations where hypoventilation, respiratory obstruction and respiratory depression, and arrest are not only a potential complication, but a common theme in preventable deaths. While pulse oximetry provides an excellent measure of oxygenation, studies demonstrate its inadequacy in monitoring ventilation.

During apnea, oxygen desaturation may not occur for several minutes, especially in patients receiving supplemental oxygen. Technologies such as Microstream® Capnography with Integrated Pulmonary Index provides a complete picture of the patient's respiratory status which includes: (1) Accurate physiologic respiratory rate, (2) adequacy of ventilation represented by a numeric value for end-tidal CO_2, (3) a breath-to-breath waveform that indicates any respiratory conditions such as hypoventilation, apnea, or airway obstruction, whereas respiratory rate monitoring alone by itself does not provide complete factual information. As an O_2 nasal cannula is often already part of patient care in the PACU, the Microstream® capnography integrates oxygen delivery and CO_2 sampling into a single line, and eliminates the need for another device. Capnography is becoming recognized as a standard of care for monitoring ventilation in nonintubated patients. A growing body of clinical studies has validated capnography's superiority over pulse oximetry and respiratory rate monitoring to detect respiratory depression; as a result, a number of organizations are endorsing enhanced monitoring for ventilation in the high-risk population, which perhaps will become a standard of care in the future (219).

■ AIRWAY ALERTS

Attention should be paid to the importance of follow-up after encountering a difficult airway. It is important to document and communicate an episode of DA for patient care and legal reasons (220). Although a significant body of literature is dedicated to identifying and managing the DA, relatively little has been published on the aftercare of these patients. The ASA Task Force on Difficult Airway (3) recommends that the anesthesiologist document in the medical record the nature of the difficult airway and the management techniques. The documentation and communication of airway problems provide knowledge and prior warning to future anesthesia providers, thus allowing for the safe and effective anesthetic management of the patient with difficult airway. Guidance is provided by the ASA Task force (3) and the Canadian Airway Focus Group (41) with recommendations regarding documentation and communication of airway problems.

A patient whose airway management was demonstrably difficult is at risk in future; therefore, developing a uniform airway alert system comprising a combination of methods to convey vital information regarding a difficult airway is crucial in reducing future risks and in enhancing patient safety (221). Barron et al. developed an airway alert form which aims at not only documenting in the medical record, but it also allows concise quick documentation and communication of an episode of difficulty which serves as a prompt for action (221).

An airway alert system should include the following:
Documentation of the following items:

- Documentation of the preanesthetic airway assessment findings in the medical record
- Documentation of the presence and nature of airway difficulties in medical records with description of airway difficulties encountered
- Ease of mask ventilation (easy, difficult, two-person MV, impossible MV)
- Difficult ventilation with LMA™
- Description of airway difficulties encountered with tracheal intubation
- Grade of laryngoscopic view
- Equipment/maneuvers that failed to achieve the intubation
- Description of alternative airway devices, equipment maneuvers that were successful in achieving ventilation or intubation (supraglottic airway devices, Eschmann bougie, optical stylet, type of laryngoscope, videolaryngoscope, BURP maneuver)
- If a CICV situation ensued, steps taken to establish an airway

- Documentation of informing patient or a responsible person
- Evaluation and documentation of follow-up with the patient for potential complications of the difficult airway management
- Documentation of *notification systems:* Letter to the patient, medical records, communication with the surgeon or primary care, airway alert form completion, Medic Alert® bracelet

The details of the recommended documentation are shown in Figure 24-22 (222). There are drawbacks with this system: Documentation in medical records may not be available and the at-risk patient may fail to inform; however, the notification system with multiple layers of documentation and methods adds to the error reduction system. The utility of a postoperative letter informing the patient of a difficult airway was examined (223). The results showed that of the 142 patients that participated, majority of the patients who were sent "Difficult Airway" letter did not obtain a Medic Alert® bracelet, although it was recommended. However, majority of the patients who had subsequent surgery informed their anesthesiologists or surgeons of their airway history (223).

■ DIFFICULT AIRWAY REGISTRIES

Many institutions and countries such as Denmark (224) and Austria (225) have difficult airway registries with extensive standardized documentation. This is an effective system, provided the patient receives care within the same system. Making such information universally available is not easy,

---

Difficult Airway Letter

Date_____

_____has a difficult airway,

During your recent anesthetic and surgery, your anesthesia providers noted that you have a difficult airway.

Specifically: __ difficult mask ventilation, ___difficult laryngoscopy,

__difficult intubation, or ___failed intubation.

An unexpected difficult airway is a known potential concern with general anesthesia and can be dangerous. If you should need anesthesia or mechanical ventilation in the future, it is important that you inform you anesthesiologist and surgeon of the potential for a difficult airway. Ideally you would give them this letter to review.

Physical Exam:

Body mass index (BMI) <25_____ 25–30_____ >30_____

Mallampati airway classification: ___I- soft palate, uvula, pillars ___ II- soft palate, pillars,

___III-soft palate ___IV-hard palate

Mouth opening: _____cm

Dentition: Native __prominent incisors__edentulous__jaw protrusion (can protrude lower incisors beyond upper incisors)

Thyromental distance: ___>6 cm___<6 cm

Neck extension: _____full (35°) _____limited (<15°)

Details of what actually took place during airway management:

Intubation: _____emergency _____elective

Bag and mask ventilation was _____Easy _____Difficult _____Not possible

Muscle relaxants were ___administered ___not administered

Cormack/Lehane Laryngoscopic view:

___I - full view ofthe glottis opening ___II - epiglottis and arytenoids

___III - tip ofepiglottis ___IV - only soft palate

Intubation ___Successful ___Not successful

____An LMA was placed and anesthesia proceeded without further difficulties

____Intubation was performed _____through a Fast track laryngeal mask airway

_____with video assisted laryngoscopy

_____with fiberoptic bronchoscope guidance

____An emergency tracheostomy was performed

____Your surgery and anesthetic was rescheduled

____Dexamethasone was administered to prevent swelling postoperatively

____You were admitted postoperatively for_____

____Other_____

Extubation was ____routine _____over a stylet

Complications_____

Although minor sore throat is common after general anesthesia, if you experience a persistent severe sore throat, difficulty swallowing or fever, immediately contact your surgeon and the anesthesiologist on call at the facility.

Sincerely,

FIGURE 24-22 Sample standardized patient notification of a difficult airway. Reprinted with permission from: Koenig HM. No more difficult airway, Again! Time for Standardized Written Patient Notification of a Difficult Airway. APSF Summer Newsletter 2010.

because of the USA Health Insurance Portability and Accountability Act (HIPPA) regulations. The patient or her healthcare advocate should be empowered to deliver the complete template as a letter or better still as a wallet card to future providers (226).

As travelling within the country and abroad has increased, so has the incidence of receiving healthcare in facilities that have no access to medical records from previous surgeries. Using standardized notification and perhaps registering into the Medic Alert registry will facilitate global reporting and management strategies (222) and staying in compliance with HIPPA regulations. Possession of a Medic Alert® bracelet and entering the patient into a National Airway Registry Database further permits identification of an airway problem and thus adds to patient safety. In 1992, the Anesthesia Advisory Council with Medic Alert foundation created a National Difficult Airway/Intubation Registry, from 1992 to 1994, which initially enrolled 111 patients and since then, the registry has grown exponentially. Between 1992 and 2010, over 11,000 patients with difficult airway have been enrolled in the registry (227). Similarly, in obstetric anesthesia, difficult airway complications can also be reported; the Society of Obstetric Anesthesia and Perinatology Severe Complications Repository (SCORE) project is a reporting system established through its research committee led by Robert D' Angelo. The ultimate goal of the repository is (1) to capture reliable information on serious obstetric anesthesia complications, (2) to identify any associated factors, and (3) to improve patient safety (228).

ADDRESSING THE DECLINE IN THE USE OF GA IN OBSTETRICS AND TRAINEES' EXPERIENCE IN AIRWAY SKILLS

Anesthesia Trainees' Experience in GA for Cesarean Delivery

In the United States, the trends in obstetric anesthesia have drastically changed and the use of RA has increased from 55% in 1981 to 99.3% in 2005, whereas the use of GA has declined from 45% to 0.7% (1) (Fig. 24-23). Johnson et al., similarly, found a marked decline in GA for CD from 79% to fewer than 10% over the same period in the United Kingdom (Fig. 24-24) (229). NHS maternity statistics have shown that the number of obstetric GA for CD, administered in the United Kingdom, has fallen from 50% to as low as 4.6% (230).

A number of authors have reported significant reductions in both experience and training opportunities as the use of GA in obstetrics has diminished. Palanisamy et al. reported the deliveries at their institution, from 2000 to 2005, were >9,000 per year; the average number of general anesthetics for CD were only16 per year, and with 12 to 15 anesthesia residents on the obstetric anesthesia rotation per month they noted that the rate of GA would imply 1 to 1.5 cases per month (2). They concluded that the lack of GA for CD resulted in a severe lack of exposure amongst trainees. *Further, many residents graduated without having performed a GA*

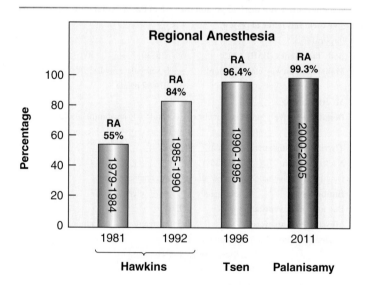

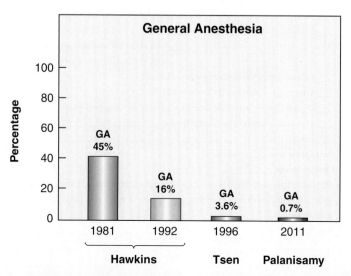

FIGURE 24-23 Trends in anesthesia in the United States. Reprinted with permission from: Hawkins JL, Koonin LM, Palmer SK, et al. Anesthesia-related deaths during obstetric delivery in the United States, 1979–1990. *Anesthesiology* 1997;86(2):277–284.

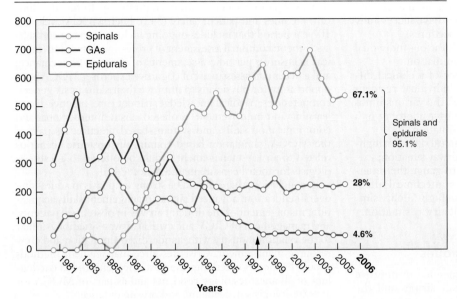

FIGURE 24-24 Trends in anesthesia for caesarean deliveries at St. James University Hospital in the United Kingdom: 1982–2006. Reprinted with permission from: Searle RD, Lyons G. Vanishing experience in training for obstetric general anesthesia: An observational study. *Int J Obstet Anesth* 2008;17(3):233–237.

in an obstetric patient (2). Panni et al. reported that the use of GA for CD was less common in institutions with a 24-hour obstetric anesthesia staffing pattern and was not correlated to the number of deliveries at an institution (35).

Searle and Lyons reviewed audit data collected within annual reviews in a single UK teaching hospital from 1998 to 2006 and reported that the mean number of obstetric general anesthetics given per trainee fell to one per annum in 2006; it had been 15 to 20 through the 1990s (230). Smith et al. reported that, in a large Australian metropolitan teaching hospital, the total caseload per trainee remained stable from 1998 to 2008, but that GA for CD fell from an average of nine cases to six cases per trainee per year (231). Guidelines containing recommendations for anesthesia training are updated and published in the United States and the United Kingdom. The USA educational governing body, the Accreditation Council for Graduate Medical Education (ACGME) Resident Review Committee, requires that the trainees should have involvement in at least 20 CDs, but does not offer specific recommendations for providing GA for CD. The ACGME requirement, Section IV.A.5.(a).(1).(0) states the following for resident training: For patients who require specialized techniques for their perioperative care; there must be significant experience with a broad spectrum of airway management techniques (e.g., performance of fiberoptic intubation and lung isolation technique such as double lumen endotracheal tube placement and endobronchial blockers) (232).

Approaches to Airway Management Training in Obstetrical Situations

Simulation-based training has been advocated for teaching of residents especially for procedures that are less common; or for critical scenarios that the residents may not gain adequate experience during their training. Educators have advocated the increased use of simulation-based training for GA in obstetrical cases. In an academic institution, using a modified Delphi technique, educators developed a standardized scoring system, for evaluating resident performance of GA for an emergency CD situation on a human patient simulator. The scoring system was found to be reliable and the senior residents scored better than the junior residents (233). The same investigators conducted a randomized controlled trial of the impact of simulation-based training on resident performance during a simulated obstetric anesthesia emergency (234). Residents assigned to the CD group or a control group trained on

the simulator using a different GA scenario. The anesthesiology residents in the CD group had higher scores in the preoperative assessment, equipment availability check, and intraoperative management subset categories than the residents in the sham group. Simulator-based training not only helped in the improvement of the performance as well as efficiency. Further, the residents who underwent focused training on a simulator, that included performance of a GA for emergency CD, exhibited improved performance during a subsequent simulated anesthetic scenario compared with trainees who did not undergo such training, indicating that there was retention of cognitive, noncognitive, and performance skills (234).

Simulation Training in Advanced Airway Management (AAM) Skills

Lastly, the ultimate goal in obstetric anesthesia should be to *entirely eliminate* airway-related adverse events and maternal mortality. Advanced airway management with emphasis on difficult airway management and mastering critical airway skills (invasive techniques/cricothyroidotomy) must be a mandatory and a critical aspect of anesthesiology training. The US residency programs were surveyed, with a response rate of 79%, and showed that two-thirds of the responding programs acknowledged their lack of a difficult airway teaching rotation. Further, less than 20% of residency programs that have a formal airway teaching rotation do not have a requirement that a resident be evaluated to have successfully performed a "required number" of procedures to demonstrate competence (235). The USA Anesthesiology residency program ACGME requirements in difficult airway management are limited to nonspecific statements such as "significant experience with specialized techniques for airway management needed." Kiyama and colleagues (236) documented an informal approach to difficult airway teaching in Japan and the United Kingdom. A Danish study evaluated the anesthesiology residents' knowledge and skills in difficult airway management and they documented deficiencies that needed to be addressed by standardized educational effort (237).

An airway training course should start with educational tools to improve advanced airway management skills which should include:

1. Develop a curriculum with a set of educational goals and objectives that address the learning of three skill domains: Cognitive, psychomotor, and affective

2. A dedicated structured airway rotation in the general operating room (a prerequisite that they have successfully performed a "required number" of procedures)
3. Systematic practice and repetition with various individual airway devices and tools to facilitate intubation
4. High-fidelity simulation-based practice of a clinical difficult airway situation in which the individual resident must attempt to manage in "real time" the various limbs of the ASA algorithm including cricothyroidotomy in a "Cannot Intubate Cannot Ventilate" situation
5. An assessment of technical and nontechnical skills in a high-fidelity–simulated obstetrical difficult airway situation;
6. Reassessment in 6 months to 1 year, to gauge the retention of cognitive, psychomotor, and nontechnical affective skills by the anesthesia trainee with high-fidelity simulation of the same obstetrical difficult airway situation.

Simulation Training in Critical Airway Management and Invasive Techniques

Simulation-based training is also recommended to improve the management of unanticipated difficult airway and the CICV situation. Not only is there a lack of training in airway management skills, it has been demonstrated that although guidelines for difficult airway management have been published in the United States and United Kingdom, there is lack of adherence to these guidelines and majority of anesthetists in practice are not prepared for a CICV situation (238). High-fidelity simulation was used to assess how anesthesia practitioners use the ASA guidelines to deal with an unanticipated CICV airway situation (239). The results showed that consultant anesthesiologists did not lack the knowledge of the ASA guidelines; however, they did not routinely adhere to the guidelines, but adapted the guidelines based on their own clinical experience, airway skills in the use of the devices, and their own interpretation of the guidelines (239).

Simulator-based airway management course have been shown to have significant impact on self-reported accuracy and confidence in evaluation of airways, use of alternative devices, and changes in the practitioner's toward difficult airway situations (240). A prospective study using medium-fidelity simulator examined the management of unanticipated difficult airway in two scenarios: "Cannot intubate Can Ventilate" and "Cannot Intubate Cannot Ventilate" situation. The volunteer anesthesia practitioners participating in the study first underwent training in the "Difficult Airway Society" Algorithm and were then tested on the two scenarios. The participants demonstrated a more structured approach following training ($p < 0.05$) which was sustained at 6 to 8 months. And in both scenarios, there was a reduced incidence of misuse of equipment. The conclusion was that simulation based training significantly improved performance; and training should be repeated at intervals of 6 months or less (241).

■ FUTURE RECOMMENDATIONS FOR AIRWAY MANAGEMENT IN OBSTETRICS

Ideally, anesthesia trainees should train with obstetrical clinical scenarios and should be able to apply their knowledge, judgment, technical and nontechnical skills in real-time simulation. Simulation-based training should be a mandatory part of the obstetric anesthesia curriculum and training.

Maintenance of Certification in Anesthesiology (MOCA)

MOCA has become mandatory in the United States. The American Board of Anesthesiology (ABA) has been charged with implementing MOCA activities that will assure the public that its diplomates demonstrate commitment to quality clinical outcomes and patient safety (242). Each MOCA cycle is a 10-year period that includes ongoing lifelong learning and self-assessment; continual assessment of professional standing (medical licensure); periodic assessments of practice performance; and a decennial assessment of cognitive expertise. MOCA is an opportunity for physicians to improve their skills in six general competencies: Medical knowledge, patient care, practice-based learning and improvement, professionalism, interpersonal and communication skills, and systems-based practice. As part of the MOCA, simulation-based training in obstetric scenarios related to airway management should be offered to anesthesiologists for their licensure maintenance (242).

In conclusion, there should be strong emphasis in addressing overall education, advanced airway management skills acquisition, management of the difficult airway in obstetrical patients, and management of CICV and critical airway situation, similar to the aviation industry with standardized simulation and crew resource management. Crisis resource management methods should be incorporated into the obstetrical anesthesia curriculum of all anesthesiology residents and as part of MOCA for anesthesiologists in academic and private practice.

KEY POINTS

- Anesthesia-related maternal mortality ranks seventh among the leading causes of maternal mortality. Difficult laryngoscopy, failed tracheal intubation, and inability to ventilate or oxygenate following induction of GA for CD are major contributory factors leading to maternal morbidity and mortality.
- The necessity of a focused history, physical examination, and airway evaluation for predictors of difficult intubation and difficult ventilation allows the anesthesia practitioner to develop appropriate strategies for management of the obstetrical patient.
- The heightened awareness of GA-related maternal mortality has led to the widespread adoption of neuraxial techniques for labor analgesia and CD and improvements in management of the difficult airway has led to significant decrease in airway-related deaths in the last 20 years.
- The emergency airway management, following failed tracheal intubation in obstetrics is challenging for the anesthesia practitioner.
- The dictum of having preformulated strategies for airway management, prior to induction of GA, is important.
- Keys to successful outcome for both mother and baby include: (a) Seeking help sooner rather than later; (b) decision to restrict the number of attempts to no more than two following failed tracheal intubation; (c) use of alternative devices to assist tracheal intubation; (d) use of supraglottic airways; (e) maintenance of oxygenation throughout the execution of the plan; (f) invasive techniques such as cricothyroidotomy in a CICV situation.
- Anesthesia-related deaths from airway obstruction or hypoventilation during postoperative period are emerging as new airway-related problems.
- Each anesthesia practice must establish protocols to not only reduce anesthetic risks during labor and during induction of GA, but also reduce risks associated with extubation, emergence from GA, and in PACU.
- The declining use of GA in obstetrics is concerning because of the diminished airway management skills of the anesthesia trainees in obstetrics.
- Solutions to the problem include: (1) A dedicated and structured advanced airway management (AAM) rotation for anesthesia trainees; (2) formal curriculum and teaching

of DAA; (3) systematic practice and repetition of AAM clinical skills in the operating room in surgical patients (4) high-fidelity simulation training with formal instruction in the management of scenarios such as failed tracheal intubation, difficult ventilation; and 5) cricothyroidotomy skills in obstetrical emergency situation should be taught and practiced in the mannikin.

REFERENCES

1. Hawkins JL, Koonin LM, Palmer SK, et al. Anesthesia-related deaths during obstetric delivery in the united states, 1979–1990. *Anesthesiology* 1997;86(2):277–284.
2. Palanisamy A, Mitani AA, Tsen LC. General anesthesia for cesarean delivery at a tertiary care hospital from 2000 to 2005: A retrospective analysis and 10-year update. *Int J Obstet Anesth* 2011;20(1):10–16.
3. American Society of Anesthesiologists Task Force on Management of the Difficult Airway. Practice guidelines for management of the difficult airway: An updated report by the American society of anesthesiologists task force on management of the difficult airway. *Anesthesiology* 2003;98(5):1269–1277.
4. Cheney FW. The American society of anesthesiologists closed claims project: What have we learned, how has it affected practice, and how will it affect practice in the future? *Anesthesiology* 1999;91(2):552–556.
5. Davies JM, Posner KL, Lee LA, et al. Liability associated with obstetric anesthesia: A closed claims analysis. *Anesthesiology* 2009;110(1):131–139.
6. American Society of Anesthesiologists Task Force on Obstetric Anesthesia. Practice guidelines for obstetric anesthesia: An updated report by the American society of anesthesiologists task force on obstetric anesthesia. *Anesthesiology* 2007;106(4):843–863.
7. Berg CJ, Callaghan WM, Syverson C, et al. Pregnancy-related mortality in the united states, 1998 to 2005. *Obstet Gynecol* 2010;116(6):1302–1309.
8. Cooper GM, McClure JH. Maternal deaths from anaesthesia. an extract from why mothers die 2000–2002, the confidential enquiries into maternal deaths in the united kingdom: Chapter 9: Anaesthesia. *Br J Anaesth* 2005;94(4):417–423.
9. Onwuhafua PI, Onwuhafua A, Adze J. The challenge of reducing maternal mortality in Nigeria. *Int J Gynaecol Obstet* 2000;71(3):211–213.
10. Hawkins JL, Chang J, Palmer SK, et al. Anesthesia-related maternal mortality in the United States: 1979–2002. *Obstet Gynecol* 2011;117(1):69–74.
11. Tsen LC, Camann W. Training in obstetric general anaesthesia: A vanishing art? *Anaesthesia* 2000;55(7):712–713.
12. Bloom SL, Spong CY, Weiner SJ, et al. Complications of anesthesia for cesarean delivery. *Obstet Gynecol* 2005;106(2):281–287.
13. Jenkins JG, Khan MM. Anaesthesia for caesarean section: A survey in a UK region from 1992 to 2002. *Anaesthesia* 2003;58(11):1114–1118.
14. Turnbull A, Tindall VR, Beard RW, et al. Report on confidential enquiries into maternal deaths in england and wales 1982–1984. *Rep Health Soc Subj (Lond)* 1989;34:1–166.
15. Mhyre JM, Riesner MN, Polley LS, et al. A series of anesthesia-related maternal deaths in michigan, 1985–2003. *Anesthesiology* 2007;106(6):1096–1104.
16. Wong CA. Saving mothers' lives: The 2006–8 anaesthesia perspective. *Br J Anaesth* 2011;107(2):119–122.
17. Cooper GM, McClure JH. Anaesthesia chapter from saving mothers' lives; reviewing maternal deaths to make pregnancy safer. *Br J Anaesth* 2008;100(1):17–22.
18. McClure JH, Cooper GM, Clutton-Brock TH, et al. Saving mothers' lives: Reviewing maternal deaths to make motherhood safer: 2006–8: A review. *Br J Anaesth* 2011;107(2):127–132.
19. Health Canada. *Special report on maternal mortality and severe morbidity in canada—enhanced surveillance: The path to prevention.* Ottawa: Minister of Public Works and Government Services Canada; 2004.
20. Overview of the 2006 ACOG survey on professional liability. [Internet]. Available from: www.acog.org/departments/professionalliability/2006surveyNatl.pdf.
21. Klagholz J, Strunk AL. Overview of the 2012 ACOG survey on professional liability. American Congress of Obstetricians and Gynecologists (ACOG); 2012.
22. D'Angelo R. Anesthesia-related maternal mortality: A pat on the back or a call to arms? *Anesthesiology* 2007;106(6):1082–1084.
23. Lofsky AS. Doctors company reviews maternal arrests cases. 2007. In press.
24. Pearce A. Evaluation of the airway and preparation for difficulty. *Best Pract Res Clin Anaesthesiol* 2005;19(4):559–579.
25. Suresh MS, Wali A. Failed intubation in obstetrics—airway management strategies. In The High-Risk Obstetric Patient; June 1998;16(2): 477–498.
26. Cormack RS, Lehane JR, Adams AP, et al. Laryngoscopy grades and percentage glottic opening. *Anaesthesia* 2000;55(2):184.
27. Verghese C, Brimacombe JR. Survey of laryngeal mask airway usage in 11,910 patients: Safety and efficacy for conventional and nonconventional usage. *Anesth Analg* 1996;82(1):129–133.
28. Arne J, Descoins P, Fusciardi J, et al. Preoperative assessment for difficult intubation in general and ENT surgery: Predictive value of a clinical multivariate risk index. *Br J Anaesth* 1998;80(2):140–146.
29. Hawthorne L, Wilson R, Lyons G, et al. Failed intubation revisited: 17-yr experience in a teaching maternity unit. *Br J Anaesth* 1996;76(5):680–684.
30. Samsoon GL, Young JR. Difficult tracheal intubation: A retrospective study. *Anaesthesia* 1987;42(5):487–490.
31. Macintosh R, Richards H. Illuminated introducer for endotracheal tubes. *Anaesthesia* 1957;12(2):223–225.
32. Lyons G. Failed intubation. six years' experience in a teaching maternity unit. *Anaesthesia* 1985;40(8):759–762.
33. Rocke DA, Murray WB, Rout CC, et al. Relative risk analysis of factors associated with difficult intubation in obstetric anesthesia. *Anesthesiology* 1992;77(1):67–73.
34. Tsen LC, Pitner R, Camann WR. General anesthesia for cesarean section at a tertiary care hospital 1990–1995: Indications and implications. *Int J Obstet Anesth* 1998;7(3):147–152.
35. Panni MK, Camann WR, Tsen LC. Resident training in obstetric anesthesia in the united states. *Int J Obstet Anesth* 2006;15(4):284–289.
36. Wong SH, Hung CT. Prevalence and prediction of difficult intubation in Chinese women. *Anaesth Intensive Care* 1999;27(1):49–52.
37. Yeo SW, Chong JL, Thomas E. Difficult intubation: A prospective study. *Singapore Med J* 1992;33(4):362–364.
38. Dhaliwal A, Tinnell C, Palmer S. Difficulties encountered in airway management: A review of 15,616 general anesthetics at a university medical center. *Anesth Analg* 1996;82:S92.
39. Barnardo PD, Jenkins JG. Failed tracheal intubation in obstetrics: A 6-year review in a UK region. *Anaesthesia* 2000;55(7):690–694.
40. Al Ramadhani S, Mohamed LA, Rocke DA, et al. Sternomental distance as the sole predictor of difficult laryngoscopy in obstetric anaesthesia. *Br J Anaesth* 1996;77(3):312–316.
41. Crosby ET, Cooper RM, Douglas MJ, et al. The unanticipated difficult airway with recommendations for management. *Can J Anaesth* 1998;45(8):757–776.
42. Yamamoto K, Tsubokawa T, Shibata K, et al. Predicting difficult intubation with indirect laryngoscopy. *Anesthesiology* 1997;86(2):316–321.
43. El-Ganzouri AR, McCarthy RJ, Tuman KJ, et al. Preoperative airway assessment: Predictive value of a multivariate risk index. *Anesth Analg* 1996;82(6):1197–1204.
44. Rose DK, Cohen MM. The airway: Problems and predictions in 18,500 patients. *Can J Anaesth* 1994;41(5 pt 1):372–383.
45. McDonnell NJ, Paech MJ, Clavisi OM, et al. Difficult and failed intubation in obstetric anaesthesia: An observational study of airway management and complications associated with general anaesthesia for caesarean section. *Int J Obstet Anesth* 2008;17(4):292–297.
46. McKeen DM, George RB, O'Connell CM, et al. Difficult and failed intubation: Incident rates and maternal, obstetrical, and anesthetic predictors. *Can J Anaesth* 2011;58(6):514–524.
47. Kodali BS, Chandrasekhar S, Bulich LN, et al. Airway changes during labor and delivery. *Anesthesiology* 2008;108(3):357–362.
48. Boutonnet M, Faitot V, Katz A, et al. Mallampati class changes during pregnancy, labour, and after delivery: Can these be predicted? *Br J Anaesth* 2010;104(1):67–70.
49. Wali A, Suresh MS. Maternal morbidity, mortality, and risk assessment. *Anesthesiol Clin* 2008;26(1):197–230, ix.
50. Mallampati SR, Gatt SP, Gugino LD, et al. A clinical sign to predict difficult tracheal intubation: A prospective study. *Can Anaesth Soc J* 1985;32(4):429–434.
51. Jouppila R, Jouppila P, Hollmen A. Laryngeal oedema as an obstetric anaesthesia complication: Case reports. *Acta Anaesthesiol Scand* 1980;24(2):97–98.
52. Rocke DA, Scoones GP. Rapidly progressive laryngeal oedema associated with pregnancy-aggravated hypertension. *Anaesthesia* 1992;47(2):141–143.
53. Mort TC. Emergency tracheal intubation: Complications associated with repeated laryngoscopic attempts. *Anesth Analg* 2004;99(2):607–613, table of contents.
54. McClelland SH, Bogod DG, Hardman JG. Apnoea in pregnancy: An investigation using physiological modelling. *Anaesthesia* 2008;63(3):264–269.
55. Archer GW Jr., Marx GF. Arterial oxygen tension during apnoea in parturient women. *Br J Anaesth* 1974;46(5):358–360.
56. Benumof JL, Dagg R, Benumof R. Critical hemoglobin desaturation will occur before return to an unparalyzed state following 1 mg/kg intravenous succinylcholine. *Anesthesiology* 1997;87(4):979–982.
57. Hawkins JL. Anesthesia-related maternal mortality. *Clin Obstet Gynecol* 2003;46(3):679–687.
58. Seidell JC. Epidemiology of obesity. *Semin Vasc Med* 2005;5(1):3–14.
59. United states obesity trends by states 1985 –2010 [Internet]; 2011.
60. Usha Kiran TS, Hemmadi S, Bethel J, et al. Outcome of pregnancy in a woman with an increased body mass index. *BJOG* 2005;112(6):768–772.
61. Langeron O, Masso E, Huraux C, et al. Prediction of difficult mask ventilation. *Anesthesiology* 2000;92(5):1229–1236.

62. Hood DD, Dewan DM. Anesthetic and obstetric outcome in morbidly obese parturients. *Anesthesiology* 1993;79(6):1210–1218.

63. Pilkington S, Carli F, Dakin MJ, et al. Increase in mallampati score during pregnancy. *Br J Anaesth* 1995;74(6):638–642.

64. Merah NA, Foulkes-Crabbe DJ, Kushimo OT, et al. Prediction of difficult laryngoscopy in a population of Nigerian obstetric patients. *West Afr J Med* 2004;23(1):38–41.

65. Brodsky JB, Lemmens HJ, Brock-Utne JG, et al. Morbid obesity and tracheal intubation. *Anesth Analg* 2002;94(3):732,6; table of contents.

66. Juvin P, Lavaut E, Dupont H, et al. Difficult tracheal intubation is more common in obese than in lean patients. *Anesth Analg* 2003;97(2):595–600, table of contents.

67. Peterson GN, Domino KB, Caplan RA, et al. Management of the difficult airway: A closed claims analysis. *Anesthesiology* 2005;103(1):33–39.

68. Gannon K. Mortality associated with anaesthesia. A case review study. *Anaesthesia* 1991;46(11):962–966.

69. Shiga T, Wajima Z, Inoue T, et al. Predicting difficult intubation in apparently normal patients: A meta-analysis of bedside screening test performance. *Anesthesiology* 2005;103(2):429–437.

70. Yentis SM. Predicting difficult intubation–worthwhile exercise or pointless ritual? *Anaesthesia* 2002;57(2):105–109.

71. Rich JM. Recognition and management of the difficult airway with special emphasis on the intubating LMA-Fastrach/whistle technique: A brief review with case reports. *Proc (Bayl Univ Med Cent)* 2005;18(3):220–227.

72. Kheterpal S, Han R, Tremper KK, et al. Incidence and predictors of difficult and impossible mask ventilation. *Anesthesiology* 2006;105(5):885–891.

73. Takenaka I, Aoyama K, Kadoya T. Mandibular protrusion test for prediction of difficult mask ventilation. *Anesthesiology* 2001;94(5):935; author reply 937.

74. Savva D. Prediction of difficult tracheal intubation. *Br J Anaesth* 1994;73(2):149–153.

75. Calder I, Picard J, Chapman M, et al. Mouth opening: A new angle. *Anesthesiology* 2003;99(4):799–801.

76. Williamson JA, Webb RK, Szekely S, et al. The Australian incident monitoring study. difficult intubation: An analysis of 2000 incident reports. *Anaesth Intensive Care* 1993;21(5):602–607.

77. Wilson ME, Spiegelhalter D, Robertson JA, et al. Predicting difficult intubation. *Br J Anaesth* 1988;61(2):211–216.

78. Calder I, Calder J, Crockard HA. Difficult direct laryngoscopy in patients with cervical spine disease. *Anaesthesia* 1995;50(9):756–763.

79. Gupta S, Pareek S, Dulara SC. Comparison of two methods for predicting difficult intubation in obstetric patients. *Middle East J Anesthesiol* 2003;17(2):275–285.

80. Khan ZH, Mohammadi M, Rasouli MR, et al. The diagnostic value of the upper lip bite test combined with sternomental distance, thyromental distance, and interincisor distance for prediction of easy laryngoscopy and intubation: A prospective study. *Anesth Analg* 2009;109(3):822–824.

81. Bellhouse CP, Dore C. Criteria for estimating likelihood of difficulty of endotracheal intubation with the macintosh laryngoscope. *Anaesth Intensive Care* 1988;16(3):329–337.

82. Sawin PD, Todd MM, Traynelis VC, et al. Cervical spine motion with direct laryngoscopy and orotracheal intubation. an in vivo cinefluoroscopic study of subjects without cervical abnormality. *Anesthesiology* 1996;85(1):26–36.

83. Patil Vijayalakshmi U, Stehling Linda C, Zauder Howard L. Fiberoptic endoscopy in anesthesia. Chicago: Year Book Medical Publishers; 1983.

84. Frerk CM. Predicting difficult intubation. *Anaesthesia* 1991;46(12):1005–1008.

85. Chou HC, Wu TL. Mandibulohyoid distance in difficult laryngoscopy. *Br J Anaesth* 1993;71(3):335–339.

86. Murphy MF, Walls RM. The difficult and failed airway. Manual of Emergency Airway Management. Chicago, IL: Lippincott Williams & Wilkins; 2000:31–39.

87. Murphy M, Hung O, Launcelott G, et al. Predicting the difficult laryngoscopic intubation: Are we on the right track? *Can J Anaesth* 2005;52(3):231–235.

88. Henderson JJ, Popat MT, Latto IP, et al. Difficult airway society guidelines for management of the unanticipated difficult intubation. *Anaesthesia* 2004;59(7):675–694.

89. Boisson-Bertrand D, Bourgain JL, Camboulives J, et al. Difficult intubation. French society of anesthesia and intensive care. A collective expertise. *Ann Fr Anesth Reanim* 1996;15(2):207–214.

90. Frova G. The difficult intubation and the problem of monitoring the adult airway. Italian society of anesthesia, resuscitation, and intensive therapy (SIAARTI). *Minerva Anestesiol* 1998;64(9):361–371.

91. Baker PA, Flanagan BT, Greenland KB, et al. Equipment to manage a difficult airway during anaesthesia. *Anaesth Intensive Care* 2011;39(1):16–34.

92. Combes X, Le Roux B, Suen P, et al. Unanticipated difficult airway in anesthetized patients: Prospective validation of a management algorithm. *Anesthesiology* 2004;100(5):1146–1150.

93. Rosaeg OP, Yarnell RW, Lindsay MP. The obstetrical anaesthesia assessment clinic: A review of six years experience. *Can J Anaesth* 1993;40(4):346–356.

94. Ministere de la sante et des solidarites: Decret n 98–900 du 9 octobre 1998 relatif aux conditions techniques de fonctionnement auxquelles doivent satisfaire les etablissments de sante pour etre autorises a pratiquer les activities d'obstetrique, de neonatologie ou de reanimation neonatale et modifiant le code de la sante publique. Bulletin Officiel Sante. 1998.

95. Anesthesia for emergency deliveries. ACOG committee opinion: Committee on obstetrics: Maternal and fetal medicine. number 104–March 1992. *Int J Gynaecol Obstet* 1992;39(2):148.

96. Munnur U, de Boisblanc B, Suresh MS. Airway problems in pregnancy. *Crit Care Med* 2005;33(10 suppl):S259–S268.

97. Gaiser RR, McGonigal ET, Litts P, et al. Obstetricians' ability to assess the airway. *Obstet Gynecol* 1999;93(5 pt 1):648–652.

98. Tsen LC, Datta S. Nitrous oxide inhalation: Effects on the maternal and fetal circulations at term. *Obstet Gynecol* 1996;88(5):899–900.

99. Saravanakumar K, Rao SG, Cooper GM. Obesity and obstetric anaesthesia. *Anaesthesia* 2006;61(1):36–48.

100. Vallejo MC. Anesthetic management of the morbidly obese parturient. *Curr Opin Anaesthesiol* 2007;20(3):175–180.

101. Wong CA. Epidural and spinal Analgesia/Anesthesia for labor and vaginal delivery. In: Chestnut DH, ed. *Chestnut's Obstetric Anesthesia Principles and Practice.* 4th ed. Philadelphia, PA: Mosby Elsevier; 2009:429.

102. Langeron O, Semjen F, Bourgain JL, et al. Comparison of the intubating laryngeal mask airway with the fiberoptic intubation in anticipated difficult airway management. *Anesthesiology* 2001;94(6):968–972.

103. Trevisan P. Fibre-optic awake intubation for caesarean section in a parturient with predicted difficult airway. *Minerva Anestesiol* 2002;68(10):775–781.

104. Benumof JL. Management of the difficult adult airway. With special emphasis on awake tracheal intubation. *Anesthesiology* 1991;75(6):1087–1110.

105. Wheeler M, Ovassapian A. Fiberoptic endoscopy-aided techniques. In: Hagberg C, ed. *Benumof's Airway Management.* 2nd ed. Philadelphia, PA: Mosby Elsevier; 2007:399–438.

106. Tsai CJ, Chu KS, Chen TI, et al. A comparison of the effectiveness of dexmedetomidine versus propofol target-controlled infusion for sedation during fibreoptic nasotracheal intubation. *Anaesthesia* 2010;65(3):254–259.

107. Xue FS, Yang QY, Liao X, et al. Topical anesthesia of the airway using fibreoptic bronchoscope and the MADgic atomizer in patients with predicted difficult intubation. *Can J Anaesth* 2007;54(11):951–952.

108. Ovassapian A, Wheeler M. Fiberoptic endoscopy-aided techniques. In: Benumof JL, ed. *Airway Management: Principles and Practice.* St. Louis: Mosbyp; 282.

109. Webb AR, Fernando SS, Dalton HR, et al. Local anaesthesia for fibreoptic bronchoscopy: Transcricoid injection or the "spray as you go" technique? *Thorax* 1990;45(6):474–477.

110. Ovassapian A, Krejcie TC, Yelich SJ, et al. Awake fibreoptic intubation in the patient at high risk of aspiration. *Br J Anaesth* 1989;62(1):13–16.

111. Suresh MS, Krasuski P, Shukla N, Wali A, Lim Y, Vadhera R. Fiberoptic intubation in patients undergoing cesarean section. Abstract presentation at Society for Obstetric Anesthesia and Perinatology Annual Meeting 2002.

112. Doyle DJ. Awake intubation using the GlideScope video laryngoscope: Initial experience in four cases. *Can J Anaesth* 2004;51(5):520–521.

113. Sinofsky AH, Milo SP, Scher C. The awake glidescope intubation: An additional alternative to the difficult intubation. *Middle East J Anesthesiol* 2010;20(5):743–746.

114. Jakushenko N, Kopeika U, Nagobade D. Comparison of awake endotracheal intubation with glidescope videolaryngoscope and fiberoptic bronchoscope in patients with difficult airway. *Eur J Anaesth* 2010;27(47):264.

115. Jones PM, Harle CC. Avoiding awake intubation by performing awake GlideScope laryngoscopy in the preoperative holding area. *Can J Anaesth* 2006;53(12):1264–1265.

116. Gibbs CP, Banner TC. Effectiveness of bicitra as a preoperative antacid. *Anesthesiology* 1984;61(1):97–99.

117. Thomas J, Hagberg C. The difficult airway: Risks, prophylaxis, and management. In: Chestnut DH, ed. *Chestnut's Obstetric and Anesthesia Principles and Practice.* 4th ed. Philadelphia, PA: Mosby Elsevier; 2009:651.

118. Cohen SE, Jasson J, Talafre ML, et al. Does metoclopramide decrease the volume of gastric contents in patients undergoing cesarean section? *Anesthesiology* 1984;61(5):604–607.

119. Levitan RM. Patient safety in emergency airway management and rapid sequence intubation: Metaphorical lessons from skydiving. *Ann Emerg Med* 2003;42(1):81–87.

120. Lee BJ, Kang JM, Kim DO. Laryngeal exposure during laryngoscopy is better in the 25 degrees back-up position than in the supine position. *Br J Anaesth* 2007;99(4):581–586.

121. Neilipovitz DT, Crosby ET. No evidence for decreased incidence of aspiration after rapid sequence induction. *Can J Anaesth* 2007;54(9):748–764.

122. Dixon BJ, Dixon JB, Carden JR, et al. Preoxygenation is more effective in the 25 degrees head-up position than in the supine position in severely obese patients: A randomized controlled study. *Anesthesiology* 2005;102(6):1110–1115; discussion 5A.

123. Norris MC, Dewan DM. Preoxygenation for cesarean section: A comparison of two techniques. *Anesthesiology* 1985;62(6):827–829.
124. Gambee AM, Hertzka RE, Fisher DM. Preoxygenation techniques: Comparison of three minutes and four breaths. *Anesth Analg* 1987;66(5):468–470.
125. Rapaport S, Joannes-Boyau O, Bazin R, et al. Comparison of eight deep breaths and tidal volume breathing preoxygenation techniques in morbid obese patients. *Ann Fr Anesth Reanim* 2004;23(12):1155–1159.
126. Chiron B, Laffon M, Ferrandiere M, et al. Standard preoxygenation technique versus two rapid techniques in pregnant patients. *Int J Obstet Anesth* 2004;13(1):11–14.
127. Soro Domingo M, Belda Nacher FJ, Aguilar Aguilar G, et al. Preoxygenation for anesthesia. *Rev Esp Anestesiol Reanim* 2004;51(6):322–327.
128. Frumin MJ, Epstein RM, Cohen G. Apneic oxygenation in man. *Anesthesiology* 1959;20:789–798.
129. Teller LE, Alexander CM, Frumin MJ, et al. Pharyngeal insufflation of oxygen prevents arterial desaturation during apnea. *Anesthesiology* 1988;69(6):980–982.
130. Taha SK, Siddik-Sayyid SM, El-Khatib MF, et al. Nasopharyngeal oxygen insufflation following pre-oxygenation using the four deep breath technique. *Anaesthesia* 2006;61(5):427–430.
131. Ramachandran SK, Cosnowski A, Shanks A, et al. Apneic oxygenation during prolonged laryngoscopy in obese patients: A randomized, controlled trial of nasal oxygen administration. *J Clin Anesth* 2010;22(3):164–168.
132. Fanning GL. The efficacy of cricoid pressure in preventing regurgitation of gastric contents. *Anesthesiology* 1970;32(6):553–555.
133. Allman KG. The effect of cricoid pressure application on airway patency. *J Clin Anesth* 1995;7(3):197–199.
134. SELLICK BA. Cricoid pressure to control regurgitation of stomach contents during induction of anaesthesia. *Lancet* 1961;2(7199):404–406.
135. Vanner RG, O'Dwyer JP, Pryle BJ, et al. Upper oesophageal sphincter pressure and the effect of cricoid pressure. *Anaesthesia* 1992;47(2):95–100.
136. Herman NL, Carter B, Van Decar TK. Cricoid pressure: Teaching the recommended level. *Anesth Analg* 1996;83(4):859–863.
137. Wraight WJ, Chamney AR, Howells TH. The determination of an effective cricoid pressure. *Anaesthesia* 1983;38(5):461–466.
138. Crowley DS, Giesecke AH. Bimanual cricoid pressure. *Anaesthesia* 1990;45(7):588–589.
139. Suresh MS, Gardner M, Key E. Intubating laryngeal mask airway (ILMA): A life saving rescue device following failed tracheal intubation during cesarean section. Ft. Myers, FL. *Anesthesiology*; 2004:A135.
140. Suresh MS, Mason LaToya. Airway management using the levitan optical stylet in an emergency cesarean section. Abstract presentation at Society for Obstetric Anesthesia and Perinatology Annual Meeting. New Orleans; 2009.
141. Chandrasekhar S, Munnur U, Suresh MS. Management of unanticipated difficult intubation with intubating LMA (fastrach LMA) and review of literature with comparison to classic LMA, Abstract presentation at Society for Obstetric Anesthesia and Perinatology Annual Meeting. 2010.
142. Aoyama K, Takenaka I, Sata T, et al. Cricoid pressure impedes positioning and ventilation through the laryngeal mask airway. *Can J Anaesth* 1996;43(10):1035–1040.
143. Brimacombe J, White A, Berry A. Effect of cricoid pressure on ease of insertion of the laryngeal mask airway. *Br J Anaesth* 1993;71(6):800–802.
144. Forrester P. Active vomiting during cricoid pressure. *Anaesthesia* 1985;40(4):388.
145. Whittington RM, Robinson JS, Thompson JM. Prevention of fatal aspiration syndrome. *Lancet* 1979;2(8143):630–631.
146. Ruben H, Knudsen Ej, Carugati G. Gastric inflation in relation to airway pressure. *Acta Anaesthesiol Scand* 1961;5:107–114.
147. Knill RL. Difficult laryngoscopy made easy with a "BURP". *Can J Anaesth* 1993;40(3):279–282.
148. Cook TM. A new practical classification of laryngeal view. *Anaesthesia* 2000;55(3):274–279.
149. Kidd JF, Dyson A, Latto IP. Successful difficult intubation. Use of the gum elastic bougie. *Anaesthesia* 1988;43(6):437–438.
150. Cossham PS. The anticlockwise twist. *Anaesthesia* 2002;57(8):824–825.
151. Kovacs G, Law JA, McCrossin C, et al. A comparison of a fiberoptic stylet and a bougie as adjuncts to direct laryngoscopy in a manikin-simulated difficult airway. *Ann Emerg Med* 2007;50(6):676–685.
152. Kaplan MB, Ward D, Hagberg CA, et al. Seeing is believing: The importance of video laryngoscopy in teaching and in managing the difficult airway. *Surg Endosc* 2006;20 (suppl 2):S479–S483.
153. Doyle DJ. Miniaturizing the GlideScope video laryngoscope system: A new design for enhanced portability. *Can J Anaesth* 2004;51(6):642–643.
154. Levitan RM, Heitz JW, Sweeney M, et al. The complexities of tracheal intubation with direct laryngoscopy and alternative intubation devices. *Ann Emerg Med* 2011;57(3):240–247.
155. Piepho T, Fortmueller K, Heid FM, et al. Performance of the C-MAC video laryngoscope in patients after a limited glottic view using macintosh laryngoscopy. *Anaesthesia* 2011;66(12):1101–1105.
156. Dhonneur G, Ndoko S, Amathieu R, et al. Tracheal intubation using the airtraq in morbid obese patients undergoing emergency cesarean delivery. *Anesthesiology* 2007;106(3):629–630.
157. Turkstra TP, Harle CC, Armstrong KP, et al. The GlideScope-specific rigid stylet and standard malleable stylet are equally effective for GlideScope use. *Can J Anaesth* 2007;54(11):891–896.
158. Cooper RM. Complications associated with the use of the GlideScope videolaryngoscope. *Can J Anaesth* 2007;54(1):54–57.
159. Leong WL, Lim Y, Sia AT. Palatopharyngeal wall perforation during glidescope intubation. *Anaesth Intensive Care* 2008;36(6):870–874.
160. Hirabayashi Y. Pharyngeal injury related to GlideScope videolaryngoscope. *Otolaryngol Head Neck Surg* 2007;137(1):175–176.
161. Cross P, Cytryn J, Cheng KK. Perforation of the soft palate using the GlideScope videolaryngoscope. *Can J Anaesth* 2007;54(7):588–589.
162. Hsu WT, Hsu SC, Lee YL, et al. Penetrating injury of the soft palate during GlideScope intubation. *Anesth Analg* 2007;104(6):1609–10; discussion 1611.
163. Kim YH, Jeon SY, Choe JH. Faucial pillar perforation by glidescope intubation with incorrectly placed stylet. *Hong Kong J Emerg Med* 2012;19(1):62–64.
164. Shimada N, Hirabayashi Y. Tonsillar injury caused by the airtraq optical laryngoscope in children. *J Clin Anesth* 2011;23(4):344–345.
165. Tunstall M. Failed intubation drill. *Anaesthesia* 1976;31:850.
166. Tunstall ME, Sheikh A. Failed intubation protocol: Oxygenation without aspiration. *Clin Anaesthesiol* 1986;4:171.
167. Han TH, Brimacombe J, Lee EJ, et al. The laryngeal mask airway is effective (and probably safe) in selected healthy parturients for elective cesarean section: A prospective study of 1067 cases. *Can J Anaesth* 2001;48(11):1117–1121.
168. Chadwick IS, Vohra A. Anaesthesia for emergency caesarean section using the Brain laryngeal airway. *Anaesthesia* 1989;44(3):261–262.
169. Verghese C. Laryngeal mask airway devices: Three maneuvers for any clinical situation. *Anesthesiology News* 2010;36:8 (15–16).
170. Higgs A, Clark E, Premraj K. Low-skill fibreoptic intubation: Use of the aintree catheter with the classic LMA. *Anaesthesia* 2005;60(9):915–920.
171. Atherton DP, O'Sullivan E, Lowe D, et al. A ventilation-exchange bougie for fibreoptic intubations with the laryngeal mask airway. *Anaesthesia* 1996;51(12):1123–1126.
172. Ferson DZ, Brain A. Laryngeal mask airway. In: Hagberg C, ed. *Benumof's Airway Management*. 2nd ed. Philadelphia, PA: Mosby Elsevier; 2007:476–501.
173. Lim CL, Hawthorne L, Ip-Yam PC. The intubating laryngeal mask airway (ILMA) in failed and difficult intubation. *Anaesthesia* 1998;53(9):929–930.
174. Parr MJ, Gregory M, Baskett PJ. The intubating laryngeal mask. Use in failed and difficult intubation. *Anaesthesia* 1998;53(4):343–348.
175. Ferson DZ, Rosenblatt WH, Johansen MJ, et al. Use of the intubating LMA-fastrach in 254 patients with difficult-to-manage airways. *Anesthesiology* 2001;95(5):1175–1181.
176. Keller C, Brimacombe J, Lirk P, et al. Failed obstetric tracheal intubation and postoperative respiratory support with the ProSeal laryngeal mask airway. *Anesth Analg* 2004;98(5):1467–1470, table of contents.
177. Lu PP, Brimacombe J, Yang C, et al. ProSeal versus the classic laryngeal mask airway for positive pressure ventilation during laparoscopic cholecystectomy. *Br J Anaesth* 2002;88(6):824–827.
178. Awan R, Nolan JP, Cook TM. Use of a ProSeal laryngeal mask airway for airway maintenance during emergency caesarean section after failed tracheal intubation. *Br J Anaesth* 2004;92(1):144–146.
179. Sharma B, Sahai C, Sood J, et al. The ProSeal laryngeal mask airway in two failed obstetric tracheal intubation scenarios. *Int J Obstet Anesth* 2006;15(4):338–339.
180. Halaseh BK, Sukkar ZF, Hassan LH, et al. The use of ProSeal laryngeal mask airway in caesarean section–experience in 3000 cases. *Anaesth Intensive Care* 2010;38(6):1023–1028.
181. Brimacombe J, Berry A. Cricoid pressure and the LMA: Efficacy and interpretation. *Br J Anaesth* 1994;73(6):862–865.
182. Yao WY, Li SY, Sng BL, et al. The LMA supreme in 700 parturients undergoing cesarean delivery: An observational study. *Can J Anaesth* 2012;59(7):648–654.
183. Baraka A, Salem R. The combitube oesophageal-tracheal double lumen airway for difficult intubation. *Can J Anaesth* 1993;40(12):1222–1223.
184. Eichinger S, Schreiber W, Heinz T, et al. Airway management in a case of neck impalement: Use of the oesophageal tracheal combitube airway. *Br J Anaesth* 1992;68(5):534–535.
185. Vezina MC, Trepanier CA, Nicole PC, et al. Complications associated with the esophageal-tracheal combitube in the pre-hospital setting. *Can J Anaesth* 2007;54(2):124–128.
186. Frass M, Urtubia R, Hagberg C. The combitube: Esophageal-tracheal double-lumen airway. In: Hagberg C, ed. *Benumof's Airway Management*. 2nd ed. Philadelphia, PA: Mosby Elsevier; 2007:594–615.
187. Banyai M, Falger S, Roggla M, et al. Emergency intubation with the combitube in a grossly obese patient with bull neck. *Resuscitation* 1993;26(3):271–276.

188. Mercer M. Respiratory failure after tracheal extubation in a patient with halo frame cervical spine immobilization–rescue therapy using the combitube airway. *Br J Anaesth* 2001;86(6):886–891.

189. Tunstall ME, Geddes C. "Failed intubation" in obstetric anaesthesia. an indication for use of the "esophageal gastric tube airway." *Br J Anaesth* 1984; 56(6):659–661.

190. Frass M, Frenzer R, Rauscha F, et al. Evaluation of esophageal tracheal combitube in cardiopulmonary resuscitation. *Crit Care Med* 1987;15(6):609–611.

191. Urtubia RM, Aguila CM, Cumsille MA. Combitube: A study for proper use. *Anesth Analg* 2000;90(4):958–962.

192. Hagberg CA, Vartazarian TN, Chelly JE, et al. The incidence of gastroesophageal reflux and tracheal aspiration detected with pH electrodes is similar with the laryngeal mask airway and esophageal tracheal combitube–a pilot study. *Can J Anaesth* 2004;51(3):243–249.

193. Frass M, Rodler S, Frenzer R, et al. Esophageal tracheal combitube, endotracheal airway, and mask: Comparison of ventilatory pressure curves. *J Trauma* 1989;29(11):1476–1479.

194. Agro F, Frass M, Benumof JL, et al. Current status of the combitube: A review of the literature. *J Clin Anesth* 2002;14(4):307–314.

195. Hagberg C, Bogomolny Y, Gilmore C, et al. An evaluation of the insertion and function of a new supraglottic airway device, the king LT, during spontaneous ventilation. *Anesth Analg* 2006;102(2):621–625.

196. Asai T, Shingu K. The laryngeal tube. *Br J Anaesth* 2005;95(6):729–736.

197. Dorges V, Ocker H, Wenzel V, et al. The laryngeal tube: A new simple airway device. *Anesth Analg* 2000;90(5):1220–1222.

198. Genzwuerker HV, Vollmer T, Ellinger K. Fibreoptic tracheal intubation after placement of the laryngeal tube. *Br J Anaesth* 2002;89(5):733–738.

199. Gaitini LA, Vaida SJ, Somri M, et al. An evaluation of the laryngeal tube during general anesthesia using mechanical ventilation. *Anesth Analg* 2003; 96(6):1750–1755, table of contents.

200. Zand F, Amini A. Use of the laryngeal tube-S for airway management and prevention of aspiration after a failed tracheal intubation in a parturient. *Anesthesiology* 2005;102(2):481–483.

201. Pahor AL. Ear, nose and throat in ancient Egypt. Part III. *J Laryngol Otol* 1992;106(10):863–873.

202. Brantigan CO, Grow JB S. Cricothyroidotomy: Elective use in respiratory problems requiring tracheotomy. *J Thorac Cardiovasc Surg* 1976;71(1):72–81.

203. Tighe SQ. Failed tracheal intubation. *Anaesthesia* 1992;47(4):356.

204. Bennett JD, Guha SC, Sankar AB. Cricothyrotomy: The anatomical basis. *J R Coll Surg Edinb* 1996;41(1):57–60.

205. Burkey B, Esclamado R, Morganroth M. The role of cricothyroidotomy in airway management. *Clin Chest Med* 1991;12(3):561–571.

206. Wong DT, Prabhu AJ, Coloma M, et al. What is the minimum training required for successful cricothyroidotomy?: A study in mannequins. *Anesthesiology* 2003;98(2):349–353.

207. Vadodaria BS, Gandhi SD, McIndoe AK. Comparison of four different emergency airway access equipment sets on a human patient simulator. *Anaesthesia* 2004;59(1):73–79.

208. DeLaurier GA, Hawkins ML, Treat RC, et al. Acute airway management. role of cricothyroidotomy. *Am Surg* 1990;56(1):12–15.

209. Brofeldt BT, Panacek EA, Richards JR. An easy cricothyrotomy approach: The rapid four-step technique. *Acad Emerg Med* 1996;3(11):1060–1063.

210. Morris A, Lockey D, Coats T. Fat necks: Modification of a standard surgical airway protocol in the pre-hospital environmental. *Resuscitation* 1997;35(3):253–254.

211. Metz S, Parmet JL, Levitt JD. Failed emergency transtracheal ventilation through a 14-gauge intravenous catheter. *J Clin Anesth* 1996;8(1):58–62.

212. Egol A, Culpepper JA, Snyder JV. Barotrauma and hypotension resulting from jet ventilation in critically ill patients. *Chest* 1985;88(1):98–102.

213. Benumof JL, Gaughan SD. Concerns regarding barotrauma during jet ventilation. *Anesthesiology* 1992;76(6):1072–1073.

214. Patel RG. Percutaneous transtracheal jet ventilation: A safe, quick, and temporary way to provide oxygenation and ventilation when conventional methods are unsuccessful. *Chest* 1999;116(6):1689–1694.

215. Rosenblatt W, Benumof J. Transtracheal jet ventilation via percutaneous catheter and high-pressure source. In: Hagberg C, ed. *Benumof's Airway Management*. 2nd ed. Philadelphia, PA: Mosby Elsevier; 2007:616–630.

216. Mort TC. Continuous airway access for the difficult extubation: The efficacy of the airway exchange catheter. *Anesth Analg* 2007;105(5):1357–1362, table of contents.

217. Standards for postanesthesia care [Internet]; 2009 [updated October 21, 2009]. Available from: www.asahq.org.

218. ACOG Committee on Obstetric Practice. ACOG committee opinion no. 433: Optimal goals for anesthesia care in obstetrics. *Obstet Gynecol* 2009;113(5):1197–1199.

219. Stoelting R, Weinger M. Dangers of postoperative opioids – is there A cure? *APSF Newsletter.* 2009. In press.

220. Latto IP. Management of difficult intubation. In: Latto IP, Vaughn RS, eds. *Difficulties in Tracheal Intubation*. London: WB Saunders; 1997:107–160.

221. Barron FA, Ball DR, Jefferson P, et al. 'Airway alerts'. How UK anaesthetists organise, document and communicate difficult airway management. *Anaesthesia* 2003;58(1):73–77.

222. No more difficult airway, again! time for consistent standardized written patient notification of a difficult airway [Internet]: Journal of Anesthesia Patient Safety Foundation; 2010. Available from: www.apsf.org/newsletter/html/2010/summer/06_diffairway.htm.

223. Trentman TL, Frasco PE, Milde LN. Utility of letters sent to patients after difficult airway management. *J Clin Anesth* 2004;16(4):257–261.

224. Rosenstock C, Rasmussen LS. The danish difficult airway registry and preoperative respiratory airway assessment. *Ugeskr Laeger* 2005;167(23):2543–2544; author reply 2544.

225. ADAIR: Austrian difficult Airway/Intubation registry [Internet]; 1999. Available from: www.adair.at/. Accessed May 20, 2010.

226. Mark LJ, Beattie C, Ferrell CL, et al. The difficult airway: Mechanisms for effective dissemination of critical information. *J Clin Anesth* 1992;4(3):247–251.

227. Dahab, Roman, Herzer, Medic Alert Anesthesia Advisory Council. Medic alert national registry for difficult Airway/Intubation 1992–2010. Chicago, IL: Society for Airway Management; 2010.

228. D'Angelo R. SOAP SCOREsBig with new adverse complications tracking project. American Society of Anesthesiologists Newsletter. April 2005;69(No. 4).

229. Johnson RV, Lyons GR, Wilson RC, et al. Training in obstetric general anaesthesia: A vanishing art? *Anaesthesia* 2000;55(2):179–183.

230. Searle RD, Lyons G. Vanishing experience in training for obstetric general anaesthesia: An observational study. *Int J Obstet Anesth* 2008;17(3):233–237.

231. Smith NA, Tandel A, Morris RW. Changing patterns in endotracheal intubation for anaesthesia trainees: A retrospective analysis of 80,000 cases over 10 years. *Anaesth Intensive Care* 2011;39(4):585–589.

232. Program requirements for residency education in anesthesiology [Internet]. Accreditation Council for Graduate Medical Education; 2011. Available from: www.acgme.org.

233. Scavone BM, Sproviero MT, McCarthy RJ, et al. Development of an objective scoring system for measurement of resident performance on the human patient simulator. *Anesthesiology* 2006;105(2):260–266.

234. Scavone BM, Toledo P, Higgins N, et al. A randomized controlled trial of the impact of simulation-based training on resident performance during a simulated obstetric anesthesia emergency. *Simul Healthc* 2010;5(6):320–324.

235. Hagberg CA, Greger J, Chelly JE, et al. Instruction of airway management skills during anesthesiology residency training. *J Clin Anesth* 2003;15(2):149–153.

236. Kiyama S, Muthuswamy D, Latto IP, et al. Prevalence of a training module for difficult airway management: A comparison between Japan and the United Kingdom. *Anaesthesia* 2003;58(6):571–574.

237. Rosenstock C, Ostergaard D, Kristensen MS, et al. Residents lack knowledge and practical skills in handling the difficult airway. *Acta Anaesthesiol Scand* 2004;48(8):1014–1018.

238. Green L. Can't intubate, can't ventilate! A survey of knowledge and skills in a large teaching hospital. *Eur J Anaesthesiol* 2009;26(6):480–483.

239. Borges BC, Boet S, Siu LW, et al. Incomplete adherence to the ASA difficult airway algorithm is unchanged after a high-fidelity simulation session. *Can J Anaesth* 2010;57(7):644–649.

240. Russo SG, Eich C, Barwing J, et al. *J Clin Anesth* 2007;19(7):517–522.

241. Kuduvalli PM, Jervis A, Tighe SQ, et al. Unanticipated difficult airway management in anaesthetised patients: A prospective study of the effect of mannequin training on management strategies and skill retention. *Anaesthesia* 2008;63(4):364–369.

242. Maintenance of certification in anesthesiology (MOCA) [Internet]. American Board of Anesthesiology; 2011. Available from: http://www.the aba.org/Home/ anesthesiology_ maintenance.

NPO Controversies—Pulmonary Aspiration: Risks and Management

Geraldine O'Sullivan • Scott Segal

■ INTRODUCTION

The first reported anesthesia-related death was likely due to aspiration of gastric contents. James Simpson, an obstetrician, reported it in 1848, just 2 years after the first public demonstration of anesthesia. The patient, a teenage girl anesthetized for a minor (nonobstetric) procedure, aspirated either gastric contents or brandy administered by her physician, and likely died of this complication. A century later, Curtis Mendelson highlighted the risk among obstetric patients and also demonstrated in seminal animal experiments that acidic and particulate aspirates were particularly dangerous (1). Subsequently, he recommended parturients not eat or drink in labor, more frequent use of antacids and regional anesthesia, and administration of general anesthesia by competent and experienced practitioners. His recommendations became an established dogma in obstetric anesthesia for decades.

Today the incidence of pulmonary aspiration in obstetrics, and in particular at the time of induction of anesthesia for emergency surgery during labor, is vanishingly rare. Figure 25-1 shows the death rate from aspiration in the United Kingdom since the introduction of the Confidential Enquires into Maternal Deaths in the 1950s (2). An increasing cause of maternal death and the commonest in the United Kingdom in the period 2005 to 2007 was sepsis, an issue now so important that it should put the rare incidence of aspiration into perspective. Current evidence suggests that the incidence of aspiration in the United States is not dissimilar to that in the United Kingdom (3). The main difference between the United States and the United Kingdom (and other European countries) is that NPO policies are still more widely practiced in the United States than in the United Kingdom and the rest of Europe. Although maternal mortality may be slightly higher in the United States than in the United Kingdom (4), intrapartum deaths from aspiration are very rare in both countries.

While few present-day practitioners would disagree with the prudence of competent administration of regional anesthesia as the preferred technique for laboring patients, the suggestion that all pregnant women are at increased risk of aspiration is far more controversial, as are fasting guidelines for pregnant patients, particularly those in labor. In this chapter, we review the evidence surrounding this issue and rationale for present guidelines for oral intake in labor and aspiration prophylaxis for labor, delivery, and obstetric surgical procedures.

■ PATHOPHYSIOLOGY OF PULMONARY ASPIRATION OF GASTRIC CONTENTS

Pulmonary aspiration of gastric contents can be caused by solid or liquid material. Aspiration of solid material may cause death by asphyxiation, whereas in pulmonary injury caused by liquid aspiration a distinction needs to be made between aspiration pneumonitis and aspiration pneumonia (5). Aspiration pneumonia is an infection of the respiratory tract caused by the inhalation of oropharyngeal material colonized by organisms such as gram-positive, gram-negative, and anaerobic bacteria. It is most often seen in the elderly and is often associated with dysphagia and/or abnormal gastric motility. Usually, patients first present with the typical signs and symptoms of pneumonia.

Aspiration pneumonitis is usually an acute lung injury (ALI) caused by the inhalation of acidic and/or particulate gastric contents. It is usually associated with a depressed level of consciousness due to anesthesia, sedation, seizures, or drug overdose. Aspiration injury models indicate that the inflammatory response is similar and most pronounced after aspiration of acidic aspirates and aspirates containing small particulate matter (6,7). Clinically, the most severe lung injury is observed in patients who aspirate acidic gastric contents with particulate matter (8). The aspirate induces a chemical burn, often associated with bronchospasm, which results in an alveolar exudate composed of edema, albumin, fibrin, cellular debris, and red blood cells. Ultimately there is an increase in intra-alveolar water and protein with a loss of lung volume leading to a reduction in lung compliance with intrapulmonary shunting of blood. This results in hypoxemia and an increase in pulmonary vascular resistance. After the initial injury there is an intense inflammatory response with the release of cytokines, interleukins, and tumor necrosis factor. Further amplification of the inflammatory process may result in ALI or acute respiratory distress syndrome (ARDS) (9,10). Most patients will have an abnormal chest x-ray but this may take several hours before it becomes apparent (Fig. 25-2) (11). Several detailed reviews of the physiology of pulmonary aspiration of gastric contents in the setting of anesthesia have been published (12–15).

Classically aspiration in obstetrics was described as occurring at the time of induction of anesthesia, with the anesthetist observing the passage of gastric contents into the tracheobronchial tree. In particular, aspiration in obstetrics was often associated with repeated attempts at intubation in women with a difficult airway or in women in whom the airway had become distorted due to misplaced cricoid pressure. Such events are now rarer and aspiration seems to be as or more likely to occur at the end of surgery when the woman is being extubated (16). In a review of 183 cases of aspiration in the perianesthetic period, 85% presented as observed regurgitation, but the remainder was first manifest by respiratory problems observed later (17).

■ MANAGEMENT OF ASPIRATION

If pulmonary aspiration is observed, the tracheobronchial tree should be suctioned and bronchoscopy may be required

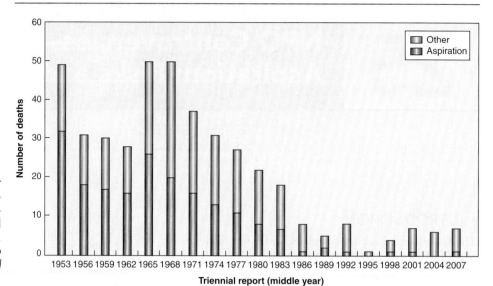

FIGURE 25-1 Maternal anesthetic deaths in the United Kingdom 1952 to 2008. Adapted from: UK Department of Health, *Confidential Enquiries into Maternal Deaths in the United Kingdom. 1952–2008.*

to remove large particles of food. Bronchospasm should be treated as indicated. Bronchial or bronchoalveolar lavage is not recommended due to the possibility of further spreading particulate matter deeper into the lung. Prophylactic antibiotic therapy is not indicated in aspiration unless/until the clinical course suggests infection (clinical deterioration, fever, leukocytosis, deterioration of chest x-ray). However, antibiotics may be indicated if bacterial colonization of the gastric aspirate is suspected (rarely in obstetrics) or if the clinical condition is not improving at 48 hours (12–15).

Exudation of fluid into the alveoli, alteration of surfactant, and intrapulmonary shunting can all lead to hypoxemia. CPAP or protective ventilation strategies may be required while the lung injury resolves. The routine use of corticosteroids was, for many years, a standard practice in the management of aspiration. Thereafter, their use became controversial and current evidence no longer supports their use in aspiration syndromes (5).

In severe cases pulmonary aspiration can ultimately cause an ALI or ARDS. In such cases protective ventilatory strategies

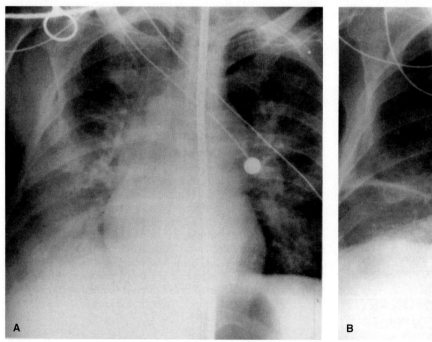
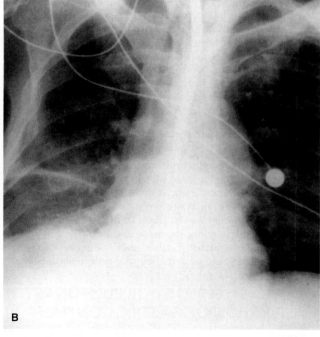

FIGURE 25-2 Chest x-ray taken immediately and 2 hours after pulmonary aspiration. Reprinted with permission from: Goodman LR. Postoperative chest radiograph: I. Alterations after abdominal surgery. *Am J Roentgenol* 1980;134(3): 533–541.

have been shown to improve outcome; a tidal volume of 6 mL/kg with a plateau pressure less than 30 cm H_2O has been shown to reduce mortality when compared to the use of a tidal volume of 12 mL/kg and a plateau pressure of 50 cm H_2O (18,19). In a randomized controlled trial of 1,000 patients with ARDS, it has been demonstrated that the patients who received conservative as opposed to liberal fluid management, guided by central venous pressure and/or pulmonary capillary wedge pressure measurements, had better lung function and a shorter duration of mechanical ventilation (20). As in uncomplicated aspiration syndromes the use of corticosteroids also does not appear to improve lung function or recovery in patients with ALI and ARDS (21,22). Minimizing the risk of sepsis and the use of prophylaxis against gastrointestinal bleeding and thromboembolic events are considered a basic standard of care in any critically ill patient; adequate thromboprophylaxis is particularly important in the higher-risk obstetric patient.

INCIDENCE OF PULMONARY ASPIRATION

Despite being one of the most feared and debated complications of general anesthesia, pulmonary aspiration in anesthetic practice is actually quite rare. Several observational studies based on quality assurance data or electronic medical records have estimated the overall risk in the general surgical population to be 3 to 5 per 10,000, or 1:2,000 to 1:3,500. In 1986, Olsson et al. analyzed 185,358 computerized anesthetic records at the Karolinska Hospital and concluded that the incidence of aspiration was 4.7 in 10,000 anesthetics, or 1:2,131 (23). Similarly, Warner et al. analyzed 215,488 anesthetics at the Mayo Clinic taking place in the late 1980s. They found the incidence of aspiration to be 1:3,216, or 3.1/10,000 (24). Two large studies from the United Kingdom and France each concluded the risk of aspiration was approximately 1:14,000 (25,26), while a Canadian report found a higher incidence of 1:1,116 among 112,000 patients treated in the 1970s at a single teaching hospital (27). Sakai et al. more recently reported results from analysis of 99,441 anesthetics at the University of Pittsburgh between 2001 and 2004; they found an incidence of 1:7,103 (or 1.4/10,000) (28). Nearly every study has demonstrated considerably higher incidence in emergency surgery, as well as trauma surgery and upper gastrointestinal, thoracic, and esophageal procedures (15).

The incidence of aspiration in pregnant patients is likely higher than in general surgical patients, but some caution is in order in interpreting the statistics. Mendelson, who first characterized the acid aspiration syndrome in laboring patients, found an overall incidence of 15/10,000 (1), though this was in the 1940s and in an era of frequent use of mask inhalation anesthesia, limited use of regional analgesia, and before any limitations on oral intake or use of antacids. Krantz and Edwards (29) reported an overall incidence of 1.6/10,000 among vaginal deliveries between 1962 and 1965. Nurses with no formal anesthesia training administered inhalation mask anesthesia. The incidence fell to 0.9/10,000 in the period from 1965 to 1972. Conversely, the incidence in cesarean delivery was higher, 1:430 (23.3/10,000). Dindelli et al. evaluated 12,380 cesarean deliveries under general anesthesia in an Italian hospital between 1977 and 1992. They found the incidence of aspiration to be 1:1,547, or 6.4/10,000 (30). Nearly all cases were associated with emergency surgery or difficult intubation. Soreide et al. studied cases in two Norwegian hospitals over 4 years and found an incidence of aspiration during cesarean delivery of 11/10,000 (31), but all cases were felt to have other risk factors.

Most recently, several investigators have reported general anesthesia without tracheal intubation in peripartum

patients with low incidence of aspiration. Ezri et al. studied 1,870 patients undergoing general anesthesia without antacid therapy, cricoid pressure, or tracheal intubation. No cesarean deliveries were included, and most patients underwent procedures in the immediate postpartum period for conditions such as laceration repair and extraction of retained placenta. One case of mild aspiration was reported (1:1,870, or 5.3/10,000) (32). Han et al. reported 1,067 elective cesarean deliveries performed with the laryngeal mask airway (LMA) in fasted patients with no other risk factors for aspiration. Antacid and ranitidine premedication was used, and cricoid pressure was maintained until delivery. There were no cases of aspiration or regurgitation, and no surrogate indicators such as broncho- or laryngospasm, bile-stained LMA, or unexplained hypoxemia (33). Finally, Halaseh et al. (34) and Yao et al. (35) each reported series of 3,000 and 700 cesarean deliveries (some of which were urgent) in fasted patients with the Proseal® LMA and LMA Supreme® respectively. These devices allow gastric suctioning through an integrated port, and the stomach contents were aspirated after securing the airway. No cases of aspiration were reported in either study.

In summary, some older series of pregnant patients undergoing general anesthesia demonstrated an increased risk of aspiration, but many were characterized by outdated anesthetic techniques and studied patients with other risk factors besides pregnancy. In particular, emergency surgery is a known risk factor for aspiration and this likely increased the risk, even in contemporary series. In properly fasted pregnant patients undergoing elective cesarean delivery, and even in peripartum surgery following vaginal delivery, the risk of aspiration appears extremely low.

RISK FACTORS FOR PULMONARY ASPIRATION

"At-risk" Criteria for Pulmonary Aspiration

Traditional teaching holds that a parturient is considered "full stomach" and therefore at risk for aspiration if she has gastric material >25 mL at a pH <2.5. Because actual aspiration is so rare, these values have been widely cited as physiologic surrogates by studies examining the effect of various maneuvers on being clinically at risk. The data supporting these limits, however, are astonishingly limited.

Mendelson's seminal work in the 1940s suggested that it was the acidic pH of gastric contents that was primarily responsible for lung injury. Subsequent work in other animal models confirmed that pH <2.5 was injurious, whereas liquid material of pH >3 caused little damage (36). In another seminal study in 1974, Roberts and Shirley extrapolated animal data to adult humans (37). The investigators cited "preliminary work in the rhesus monkey" suggesting that aspiration of 0.4 mL/kg of material with pH <2.5 led to significant lung injury. In a remarkably candid statement, they then stated: "As this translates to approximately 25 mL in the adult human female, we have arbitrarily defined the patient at risk as that patient with at least 25 mL of gastric juice of pH below 2.5 in the stomach at delivery." They measured gastric volume and pH in parturients and found that 14 of 52 (27%) met their criteria. They concluded, "a high gastric content volume or a low pH cannot be excluded in any patient irrespective of the time between the last meal and either onset of labor or delivery." This idea rapidly became an established dogma and was cited in major textbooks and reviews for decades.

However, the work cited "in the rhesus monkey" was apparently meant literally. Their study was confined to an experiment in a *single monkey*, the details of which were later reported (38). Gastric juice alkalinized with THAM to pH

7.45 (0.4 mL/kg) was injected into the left mainstem bronchus and produced transient tachypnea and a slight increase in blood pressure. Conversely, when gastric juice acidified with HCl to pH 1.26 was injected in the right mainstem bronchus, tachycardia, hypotension, and cardiac arrest ensued the monkey was successfully resuscitated.

Subsequent work has challenged the validity of the at-risk criteria. Experiments in other species suggest larger volumes are required, on the order of 1 to 2 mL/kg (39,40). More importantly, all animal models involve direct instillation of acidic material into the tracheobronchial tree, rather than aspiration from the stomach itself. It is likely that much higher gastric volumes are required to lead to clinically significant aspiration, but the exact volume so required is unknown. In an anesthetized cat model, 20.8 mL/kg were required to produce spontaneous regurgitation under ketamine anesthesia (41). In humans, there appears to be little direct relationship between gastric volume and aspiration risk. For example, in critically ill patients receiving enteral feedings, there is no consistent relationship between residual volume and aspiration (42). Finally, though 30% to 70% of pregnant women meet the Roberts and Shirley criteria (43–47), other groups of surgical patients not usually treated clinically as "full stomach" also meet such criteria. These include fasted nonpregnant inpatients and outpatients (45% to 60%) (48,49), and fasted children (64% to 77%) (50), who are routinely induced by mask inhalation.

Gastrointestinal Physiology During Pregnancy

There are three physiologic changes of pregnancy commonly claimed to increase the risk of aspiration among pregnant patients: Increased gastric acid production, decreased gastric emptying, and increased gastroesophageal reflux. In fact, pregnant patients likely have normal or decreased acid production and normal gastric emptying until labor commences. The issue of gastroesophageal reflux is more complex.

Immunoreactive gastrin probably increases in pregnancy (51), in part due to placental production, although this observation is not consistent (52,53). Total gastric acid production, however, is actually *decreased* in first and second trimester pregnancies, though it may increase to nonpregnant values closer to term (54,55). Peptic ulcer disease is less common in pregnancy, perhaps due in part to decreased acid secretion (56). Hong et al. (57) compared pregnant women presenting for elective cesarean delivery to nonpregnant controls undergoing gynecologic surgery. Serum gastrin levels did not differ between groups (which was notable since the placenta produces gastrin). Gastric pH was lower in the pregnant group (median 1.8 vs. 2.1, *p* <0.05) although preoperative anxiety levels were also higher in the pregnant group. Pyrosis (heartburn) increases progressively through normal pregnancy, approaching 80% at term (see below), but this is likely due to factors other than gastric acid production.

One of the most common misconceptions about gastrointestinal physiology in pregnant patients concerns gastric emptying time. Traditional teaching holds that gastric emptying is impaired by 12 weeks' gestation, requiring rapid sequence induction of anesthesia for virtually all pregnant patients. The data from a variety of modalities, however, does not support increased gastric emptying time. Gastric emptying time may be measured by the absorption of acetaminophen after oral ingestion (because it is absorbed rapidly and only from the small bowel, not from the stomach). Acetaminophen is ingested orally and then serial blood levels are determined over time. The peak level, time to peak, and area under the concentration–time curve are measures of gastric emptying. Several investigations utilizing this methodology have demonstrated no difference during any trimester of pregnancy

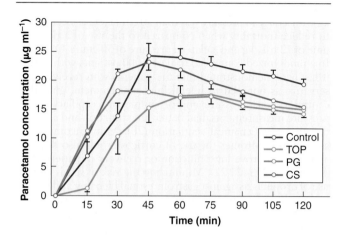

FIGURE 25-3 Acetaminophen absorption method of measuring gastric emptying. Concentration of acetaminophen over time is shown for nonpregnant women undergoing minor gynecologic delivery (open squares), first trimester pregnant women undergoing suction termination (filled circles), second trimester pregnant women undergoing prostaglandin-induced termination (open circles), and cesarean delivery at term (filled squares). There was no difference in peak concentration or time-to-peak, and area under the concentration–time curve differed only in the first trimester group, which was lower than the other groups. Redrawn with permission from: Macfie AG, Magides AD, Richmond MN, et al. Gastric emptying in pregnancy. *Br J Anaesth* 1991;67:54–57.

prior to labor, compared to nonpregnant controls (58,59) (Fig. 25-3). Other methods find the same result, including ultrasound (60,61), dye dilution (62), epigastric impedance (63), and applied potential tomography (64). Interestingly, one study found delayed acetaminophen absorption at 8 to 12 weeks' gestation, a time when nearly all anesthesiologists feel comfortable managing pregnant patients without aspiration prophylaxis (65). These studies may be biased because they studied anxious patients in the preoperative period for pregnancy termination. Importantly, all of these methods generally have studied emptying of liquids rather than solids. However, Carp et al. using ultrasound, found no food in the stomach 4 hours after a substantial standardized meal (fruit juice, muffin, roll, butter, jam, cereal with milk) in either nonpregnant or near-term pregnant women. Conversely, they found delayed gastric emptying in laboring women, with up to two-third of women showing food in the stomach up to 24 hours after ingestion (66).

Gastroesophageal reflux disease (GERD), resulting in heartburn, is a common complication of late pregnancy. Pregnancy compromises the integrity of the lower esophageal sphincter. It alters the anatomic relationship of the esophagus to the diaphragm and stomach, increases intragastric pressure, and in some women limits the ability of the lower esophageal sphincter to increase its tone (53,67–69). Progesterone, which relaxes smooth muscle, probably accounts for the reduced tone of the lower esophageal sphincter (70). Lower esophageal pH monitoring in pregnant women at term has shown an increased incidence of reflux compared to nonpregnant controls, even in women who are asymptomatic. A pregnant woman at term, requiring anesthesia, should therefore be regarded as having an incompetent lower esophageal sphincter. These physiologic changes return to their prepregnant level by 48 hours after

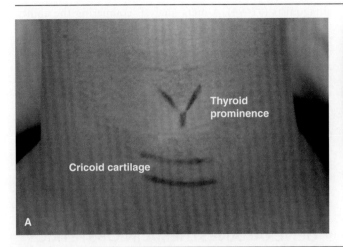
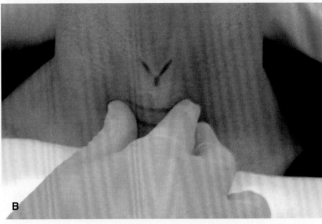

FIGURE 25-4 **(A)** The cricoid cartilage and the upper edge of the thyroid cartilage. **(B)** The application of cricoid pressure.

delivery (69). Interpreting these findings as putting every pregnant woman at risk of aspiration is, however, controversial. Although logical, there is no experimental or epidemiologic evidence that a history of reflux increases the risk of pulmonary aspiration under general anesthesia (71,72). Certainly, many anesthesiologists willingly anesthetize nonpregnant patients with GERD without treating them as full stomachs. Moreover, the overall risk of aspiration is several orders of magnitude lower than the incidence of GERD. Thus, GERD is unlikely to be a statistically significant risk factor for aspiration. Furthermore, lower esophageal sphincter (LES) tone decreases in all patients after usual general anesthesia induction agents (12).

Gastrointestinal Physiology During Labor and Postpartum

Labor significantly alters gastrointestinal physiology, particularly gastric emptying. Though the mechanism is unclear, gastric emptying appears to be delayed, perhaps by the pain and stress of labor (66,73,74). In addition, opioids given by any route further reduce gastric emptying (73,75–78). However, epidural analgesia without opioids or with fentanyl given in low-dose infusions rather than epidural boluses does not impair gastric emptying (79,80). Conversely, studies demonstrate that modest amounts of clear liquids, including isotonic sports drinks and clear juices, may be consumed in labor without increasing gastric volume, and presumably aspiration risk (81).

There is considerable controversy regarding when the altered physiology in labor returns to normal. Gastric emptying appears to be impaired for solids in the first day postpartum (82) but may be normal within 18 hours or on the second day (59,64). Many postpartum women demonstrate "at-risk" pH and volume (83,84).

■ STRATEGIES FOR PREVENTING PULMONARY ASPIRATION DURING OBSTETRIC SURGERY

The ultimate aim is that aspiration syndromes should never occur. It is important therefore to identify risk and in obstetrics the risk of aspiration is greatest when emergency surgery is performed under general anesthesia during labor. Loss of consciousness with depression of reflexes means that a patient cannot protect their airway should gastric contents

reflux into the oropharynx. Therefore the single most effective strategy for the prevention of pulmonary aspiration is the avoidance of general anesthesia. The ethos that regional anesthesia is the optimal form of anesthesia for parturients, with obvious exceptions, should be paramount on all delivery units. This inevitably has training implications for young anesthesiologists, and means that skills in rapid sequence induction of anesthesia will need to be acquired in simulation units or in the general operating theatres. Most obstetric emergencies are encountered during labor but hemorrhage, fetal compromise, maternal collapse, and trauma, can occur at any time. General anesthesia will often be required in these instances and a rapid sequence induction of anesthesia with cricoid pressure must be employed (Fig. 25-4) (85). Preoperative fasting and pharmacologic prophylaxis play an important role in the prevention of perioperative aspiration.

Preoperative Fasting

The purpose of fasting is to ensure a relatively empty stomach whilst at the same time minimizing thirst and dehydration. Preoperative fasting guidelines have been liberalized, for both pregnant and nonpregnant patients, in recent years. A Cochrane review compared perioperative complications in groups who either had shortened or traditional preoperative fasting regimens and noted that the volume or pH of gastric contents at the time of intubation did not differ significantly between the groups (86). In addition, patients with preoperative water intake had a smaller gastric volume of higher pH. Gastric emptying in nonlaboring parturients at term is not delayed and therefore preoperative fasting times prior to cesarean delivery should be the same as for nonobstetric surgery (Table 25-1).

Pharmacologic Prophylaxis

There is no direct evidence to link the reduction in the incidence of pulmonary aspiration in obstetrics to the use of antacids, H_2-receptor antagonists, or to proton pump inhibitors (PPIs). Deaths from aspiration were already declining at the time of these drugs' introduction as a result of the more widespread use of regional anesthesia. However, logic would support the concept that increasing gastric pH and decreasing gastric volume should help prevent aspiration or at least mitigate against an adverse outcome. As the risk of aspiration appears to be as great during emergence as during induction of anesthesia, the chosen prophylactic regimen should

TABLE 25-1 Fasting Recommendations for Healthy Patients Undergoing Elective Procedures. The Fasting Periods Apply to Patients of all Ages Including Women Undergoing Elective Cesarean Delivery, But not to Women in Labor

Summary of Fasting	Recommendations
Clear liquids	2 h
Breast milk	4 h
Infant formula	6 h
Nonhuman milk	6 h
Light meal	6 h
Heavy meal	8 h (possibly longer) (fried/fatty foods, meat)

provide protection during both induction of—and emergence from—general anesthesia (16,24).

The ASA practice guidelines (87) for obstetric anesthesia state *"Before surgical procedures (i.e., cesarean delivery, postpartum tubal ligation) practitioners should consider the timely administration of non-particulate antacids, H$_2$-receptor antagonists, and/ or metoclopramide for aspiration prophylaxis."* The role of oral antacid solutions is probably small. Nonparticulate antacids (e.g., 0.3 M sodium citrate, Bicitra, Alka-Seltzer effervescent) should be used. However, their duration of action is variable (55,80) and therefore they should be administered within 20 minutes of the induction of general anesthesia. The principal role of oral antacid solutions is when emergency surgery is required and there is insufficient time for a coadministered H$_2$-receptor antagonist to be effective. There is no place for the routine use of oral antacids prior to elective or even semi-elective surgery under regional anesthesia as their duration of action is too short should conversion to general anesthesia be required and in addition they cause nausea in some women. Particulate antacids should not be used as when aspirated they have been shown to cause an aspiration syndrome similar to that seen after acid aspiration (88).

H$_2$-receptor antagonists block histamine receptors on the oxyntic cell and thus decrease gastric acid production; this also results in a slight reduction in gastric volume in the fasting patient (89). When given intravenously, an H$_2$-receptor antagonist begins to take effect in as little as 30 minutes, but 60 to 90 minutes are required for maximal effect. After oral administration, gastric pH is greater than 2.5 in approximately 60% of patients at 60 minutes and in 90% at 90 minutes. The duration of action is sufficiently long to cover emergence from general anesthesia for a cesarean delivery (89–91). PPIs such as omeprazole and lansoprazole inhibit the hydrogen ion pump on the gastric surface of the oxyntic cell and have a similar profile of effect to H$_2$-receptor

antagonists (92–94). A meta-analysis comparing the ability of PPIs and H$_2$-receptor to achieve therapeutic targets suggests that premedication with ranitidine is more effective than PPIs in reducing the volume of gastric secretions (by an average of 0.22 mL/kg; 95% confidence interval 0.04 to 0.41) and increasing gastric pH (by an average of 0.85 pH units; 95% confidence interval −1.14 to −0.28) (95). These conclusions were based on nine randomized controlled trials, of which seven were suitable for meta-analysis. In these trials a total of 223 patients received ranitidine, which was the sole H$_2$ blocker used in the included trials, and 222 patients received different PPIs (omeprazole, lansoprazole, pantoprazole, and rabeprazole). Suitable preoperative antacid regimens for both elective and emergency surgery are shown in Table 25-2.

■ GENERAL ANESTHESIA IN OBSTETRICS

Inevitably some women will require obstetric surgery under general anesthesia, and this will often be required in difficult and emergency situations. In cases of elective general anesthesia, ordinary fasting precautions and induction procedures are reasonable. In the case of the much more likely emergency operation, especially for a laboring patient, careful preparation is essential prior to induction of anesthesia. A pillow should be placed under the parturient's shoulder and the head should be fully extended. The woman should be positioned with a left lateral tilt and possible also in a slightly head-up position. It has been shown that in a 20° head-up position the pressure of refluxed gastric contents in the upper esophagus would be reduced by an amount (in cm H$_2$O) equal to the height of the cricoid cartilage above the stomach. The apneic time before hypoxemia develops is longer in the 20° head-up position than in the supine position following preoxygenation in nonpregnant patients (96) and functional residual capacity is greater at term in the 30° head-up position than supine (97). In addition, the view at laryngoscopy may be improved in the head-up position (98). After careful preoxygenation a rapid sequence induction of anesthesia with cricoid pressure should be employed. The aim of cricoid pressure is to compress the esophagus, or perhaps more accurately the cricopharyngeus muscle against the body of C6 and thereby prevent gastric contents from passing into the oropharynx (99). The anesthetic assistant should place the thumb and middle finger on either side of the cricoid cartilage and downward pressure should be applied as loss of consciousness occurs (Fig. 25-4). A force of 30 N is recommended as being sufficient to prevent passive regurgitation of esophageal contents during induction of anesthesia, though this is not routinely achieved in practice (100,101). The pressure should be maintained until successful tracheal intubation has been confirmed by the detection of end-tidal CO$_2$. Cricoid pressure has never been subjected to a randomized controlled trial nor has it been definitively shown to reduce

TABLE 25-2 Pharmacologic Prophylaxis Prior to Elective and Emergency Caesarean Delivery

	Oral Antacid	H$_2$-receptor Antagonist (Ranitidine)	Prokinetic Agents, e.g., Metoclopramide
Elective CS	No	150 mg on the night prior to and on the morning of surgery	10 mg on the night prior to and on the morning of surgery
Emergency CS	0.3 M Sodium citrate (30 mL) Prior to induction of general anesthesia *only*	Prior to surgery 50 mg IV	
High-risk labor	No	150 mg 6 hourly during labor	

the incidence of aspiration (85,102). Conversely its misapplication has probably contributed to maternal airway deaths. In an analysis of nearly 5,000 emergency cesarean deliveries performed under general anesthesia in Malawi, the incidence of regurgitation was lower, though not significantly, in those who *did not* have cricoid pressure applied (103). However, it may not be valid to compare clinical situations in Sub-Saharan Africa to those in the developed world.

Nevertheless rapid sequence induction with cricoid pressure remains the standard of care for emergency obstetric surgery under general anesthesia. High-risk women can be given oral ranitidine 150 mg during labor. 30 mL of oral 0.3 M sodium citrate and intravenous (IV) ranitidine 50 mg should be administered prior to surgery. This strategy will ensure that gastric pH is high at both intubation and extubation. Any woman requiring surgery during labor should be considered as having a relatively full stomach; in such women consideration should be given to emptying the stomach intraoperatively through a large-bore orogastric tube, the aim being to ensure an empty stomach at extubation. The parturient should not be extubated until the gag and cough reflex have returned. In women with a known difficult airway an awake fiber optic intubation should be considered.

■ THE ROLE OF NPO POLICIES IN LABOR IN MODERN OBSTETRIC PRACTICE

The proponents of natural childbirth have long argued that denying women food during labor can cause an adverse obstetric outcome. This issue has been addressed in a randomized controlled trial in 2,443 low-risk nulliparae in labor who were assigned to an "eating" or a "water only" group. The study demonstrated that eating during labor did not improve obstetric outcome, that is, the rate of spontaneous vaginal delivery was not increased, the duration of labor was not shorter, and fetal outcomes (Apgar scores and NICU admissions) were not altered. Equally this study did not show that eating in labor is safe as the study was underpowered to demonstrate safety (104).

Current evidence suggests that the risk of aspiration is greatest if the woman is critically ill, obese, or has a difficult airway; and such women should remain NPO (apart from water) during labor. The American Society of Anesthesiology (ASA) recommends that low-risk women be allowed to consume moderate amounts of clear liquids during labor (87). Therefore women should be advised to alleviate thirst during labor by consuming ice chips and clear fluids (isotonic sports drinks, fruit juices, tea and coffee, water). Women should be discouraged from eating *solid* food during labor as eating confers no benefit to obstetric outcome and gastric emptying of solids is impaired in active labor. Arguably, however, low-risk women could be allowed to consume low-residue foods (e.g., soups, yogurt, ice cream) during labor, especially in view of the almost negligible incidence of deaths from aspiration (81,105). When deciding whether or not to allow women to eat during labor, the use of parenteral opioids, because of their profound delay on the rate of gastric emptying, must be considered. In addition, units which perform a significant volume of their emergency obstetric surgery under general anesthesia should also probably not allow women to eat during labor.

Maternal death from aspiration of regurgitated gastric content is now extremely rare, and its decline probably owes more to the widespread use of regional anesthesia for operative obstetrics than to fasting policies. Thus, while there is no objective benefit to eating in labor, the decision to eat during labor becomes a risk/benefit analysis. For many women and their caregivers it is likely that this risk/benefit analysis favors drinking and perhaps eating during labor.

KEY POINTS

- Aspiration of gastric contents has remained a feared complication of anesthesia in pregnant women since its recognition in the earliest days of anesthesia practice and its scientific characterization in the mid-20th century.
- Pulmonary aspiration of gastric contents is rare, and only slightly more common in pregnant patients than in the general surgical population. The emergency nature of many general anesthetics in obstetrics is likely the most important additional risk factor.
- The scientific basis of at-risk criteria for aspiration is quite limited.
- Pregnant, nonlaboring patients are not at increased risk of aspiration compared to nonpregnant patients. Labor significantly delays gastric emptying of solids but not limited amounts of clear liquids. Postpartum patients return to normal risk by the second postpartum day.
- Nonlaboring patients should observe unmodified fasting guidelines prior to elective operations.
- The ideal pharmacologic regimen to lower the risk of pulmonary aspiration remains somewhat controversial. When considering physiologic surrogates, H_2-receptor antagonists are more effective than PPIs, and both are superior to nonparticulate antacids except in emergency surgery. However, no outcome data supports the use of any pharmacologic prophylaxis in fasted patients undergoing elective procedures.
- General anesthesia for pregnant patients is best reserved for emergencies, and maneuvers to reduce the risk of aspiration include nonparticulate antacids (e.g., 30 mL sodium citrate), H_2 blockers (e.g., ranitidine 50 mg), raising the head of the bed 20° to 30°, and consideration of cricoid pressure. The latter has never been shown to reduce the risk of aspiration, and indeed evidence suggests otherwise, but is considered standard of care in many venues nonetheless.
- Oral intake in labor does not improve maternal or fetal outcomes, though consumption of modest amounts of water or other clear liquids is recommended. The liberal use of regional anesthesia is the best strategy for reducing the risk of aspiration.

REFERENCES

1. Mendelson CL. The aspiration of stomach contents into the lungs during obstetric anesthesia. *Am J Obstet Gynecol* 1946;52:191–205.
2. Wilkinson H. Saving mothers' lives. Reviewing maternal deaths to make motherhood safer: 2006-2008. *BJOG* 2011;118:1402–1403; discussion 3–4.
3. Hawkins JL, Chang J, Palmer SK, et al. Anesthesia-related maternal mortality in the United States: 1979-2002. *Obstet Gynecol* 2011;117:69–74.
4. Berg CJ, Callaghan WM, Henderson Z, et al. Pregnancy-related mortality in the United States, 1998 to 2005. *Obstet Gynecol* 2011;117:1230.
5. Marik PE. Aspiration pneumonitis and aspiration pneumonia. *N Engl J Med* 2001;344:665–671.
6. Knight PR, Rutter T, Tait AR, et al. Pathogenesis of gastric particulate lung injury: a comparison and interaction with acidic pneumonitis. *Anesth Analg* 1993;77:754–760.
7. Knight PR, Davidson BA, Nader ND, et al. Progressive, severe lung injury secondary to the interaction of insults in gastric aspiration. *Exp Lung Res* 2004;30:535–557.
8. Fowler AA, Hamman RF, Good JT, et al. Adult respiratory distress syndrome: risk with common predispositions. *Ann Intern Med* 1983;98:593–597.
9. Günther A, Ruppert C, Schmidt R, et al. Surfactant alteration and replacement in acute respiratory distress syndrome. *Respir Res* 2001;2:353–364.
10. Matthay MA. Conference summary: Acute lung injury. *Chest* 1999;116:119S–126S.
11. Aspiration http://www.learningradiology.com/archives06/COW 211-Aspiration pneumonia/aspirationcorrect.htm
12. Ng A, Smith G. Gastroesophageal reflux and aspiration of gastric contents in anesthetic practice. *Anesth Analg* 2001;93:494–513.

13. Engelhardt T, Webster NR. Pulmonary aspiration of gastric contents in anaesthesia. *Br J Anaesth* 1999;83:453–460.
14. Janda M, Scheeren TW, Noldge-Schomburg GF. Management of pulmonary aspiration. *Best Pract Res Clin Anaesthesiol* 2006;20:409–427.
15. Beck-Schimmer B, Bonvini JM. Bronchoaspiration: Incidence, consequences and management. *Eur J Anaesthesiol* 2011;28:78–84.
16. McDonnell NJ, Paech MJ, Clavisi OM, et al. Difficult and failed intubation in obstetric anaesthesia: an observational study of airway management and complications associated with general anaesthesia for caesarean section. *Int J Obstet Anesth* 2008;17:292–297.
17. Kluger MT, Visvanathan T, Myburgh JA, et al. Crisis management during anaesthesia: regurgitation, vomiting, and aspiration. *Qual Saf Health Care* 2005;14:e4.
18. The Acute Respiratory Distress Syndrome Network. Ventilation with lower tidal volumes as compared with traditional tidal volumes for acute lung injury and the acute respiratory distress syndrome. *N Engl J Med* 2000;342:1301–1308.
19. Fessler HE, Brower RG. Protocols for lung protective ventilation. *Crit Care Med* 2005;33:S223–S227.
20. Wiedemann HP, Wheeler AP, Bernard GR, et al. Comparison of two fluid-management strategies in acute lung injury. *N Engl J Med* 2006;354:2564–2575.
21. Steinberg KP, Hudson LD, Goodman RB, et al. Efficacy and safety of corticosteroids for persistent acute respiratory distress syndrome. *N Engl J Med* 2006;354:1671–1684.
22. Bernard GR, Luce JM, Sprung CL, et al. High-dose corticosteroids in patients with the adult respiratory distress syndrome. *N Engl J Med* 1987;317:1565–1570.
23. Olsson GL, Hallen B, Hambraeus-Jonzon K. Aspiration during anaesthesia: A computer-aided study of 185,358 anaesthetics. *Acta Anaesthesiol Scand* 1986;30:84–92.
24. Warner MA, Warner ME, Weber JG. Clinical significance of pulmonary aspiration during the perioperative period. *Anesthesiology* 1993;78:56–62.
25. Tiret L, Desmonts JM, Hatton F, et al. Complications associated with anaesthesia–a prospective survey in France. *Can Anaesth Soc J* 1986;33:336–344.
26. Leigh JM, Tytler JA. Admissions to the intensive care unit after complications of anaesthetic techniques over 10 years. 2. The second 5 years. *Anaesthesia* 1990;45:814–820.
27. Cohen MM, Duncan PG, Pope WD, et al. A survey of 112,000 anaesthetics at one teaching hospital (1975-83). *Can Anaesth Soc J* 1986;33:22–31.
28. Sakai T, Planinsic RM, Quinlan JJ, et al. The incidence and outcome of perioperative pulmonary aspiration in a university hospital: A 4-year retrospective analysis. *Anesth Analg* 2006;103:941–947.
29. Krantz ML, Edwards WL. The incidence of nonfatal aspiration in obstetric patients. *Anesthesiology* 1973;39:359.
30. Dindelli M, La Rosa M, Rossi R, et al. [Incidence and complications of the aspiration of gastric contents syndrome during cesarean section in general anesthesia]. *Ann Ostet Ginecol Med Perinat* 1991;112:376–384.
31. Soreide E. Prevention of aspiration pneumonitis in the obstetric patient. *Acta Anaesthesiol Scand Suppl* 1997;110:23–24.
32. Ezri T, Szmuk P, Stein A, et al. Peripartum general anasthesia without tracheal intubation: incidence of aspiration pneumonia. *Anaesthesia* 2000;55:421–426.
33. Han TH, Brimacombe J, Lee EJ, et al. The laryngeal mask airway is effective (and probably safe) in selected healthy parturients for elective Cesarean section: A prospective study of 1067 cases. *Can J Anaesth* 2001;48:1117–1121.
34. Halaseh BK, Sukkar ZF, Hassan LH, et al. The use of ProSeal laryngeal mask airway in caesarean section–experience in 3000 cases. *Anaesth Intensive Care* 2010;38:1023–1028.
35. Yao WY, Li SY, Sng BL, et al. The LMA Supreme in 700 parturients undergoing Cesarean delivery: An observational study. *Can J Anaesth* 2012;59:648–654.
36. Awe WC, Fletcher WS, Jacob SW. The pathophysiology of aspiration pneumonitis. *Surg* 1966;60:232–239.
37. Roberts RB, Shirley MA. Reducing the risk of acid aspiration during cesarean section. *Anesth Analg* 1974;53:859–868.
38. Roberts RB, Shirley MA. Antacid therapy in obstetrics. *Anesthesiology* 1980;53:83.
39. James CF, Modell JH, Gibbs CP, et al. Pulmonary aspiration–effects of volume and pH in the rat. *Anesth Analg* 1984;63:665–668.
40. Raidoo DM, Rocke DA, Brock-Utne JG, et al. Critical volume for pulmonary acid aspiration: reappraisal in a primate model. *Br J Anaesth* 1990;65:248–250.
41. Plourde G, Hardy JF. Aspiration pneumonia: assessing the risk of regurgitation in the cat. *Can Anaesth Soc J* 1986;33:345–348.
42. McClave SA, Lukan JK, Stefater JA, et al. Poor validity of residual volumes as a marker for risk of aspiration in critically ill patients. *Crit Care Med* 2005;33:324–330.
43. Okasha AS, Motaweh MM, Bali A. Cimetidine—antacid combination as premedication for elective Caesarean section. *Can Anaesth Soc J* 1983;30:593–597.
44. Dewan DM, Floyd HM, Thistlewood JM, et al. Sodium citrate pretreatment in elective cesarean section patients. *Anesth Analg* 1985;64:34–37.
45. Cohen SE, Jasson J, Talafre ML, et al. Does metoclopramide decrease the volume of gastric contents in patients undergoing cesarean section? *Anesthesiology* 1984;61:604–607.
46. Wyner J, Cohen SE. Gastric volume in early pregnancy: effect of metoclopramide. *Anesthesiology* 1982;57:209–212.
47. McCaughey W, Howe JP, Moore J, et al. Cimetidine in elective Caesarean section. Effect on gastric acidity. *Anaesthesia* 1981;36:167–172.
48. Manchikanti L, Colliver JA, Marrero TC, et al. Ranitidine and metoclopramide for prophylaxis of aspiration pneumonitis in elective surgery. *Anesth Analg* 1984;63:903–910.
49. Manchikanti L, Marrero TC, Roush JR. Preanesthetic cimetidine and metoclopramide for acid aspiration prophylaxis in elective surgery. *Anesthesiology* 1984;61:48–54.
50. Cote CJ, Goudsouzian NG, Liu LM, et al. Assessment of risk factors related to the acid aspiration syndrome in pediatric patients-gastric ph and residual volume. *Anesthesiology* 1982;56:70–72.
51. Rooney PJ, Dow TG, Brooks PM, et al. Immunoreactive gastrin and gestation. *Am J Obstet Gynecol* 1975;122:834–836.
52. Chiloiro M, Darconza G, Piccioli E, et al. Gastric emptying and orocecal transit time in pregnancy. *J Gastroenterol* 2001;36:538–543.
53. Van Thiel DH, Gavaler JS, Joshi SN, et al. Heartburn of pregnancy. *Gastroenterology* 1977;72:666–668.
54. Murray FA, Erskine JP, Fielding J. Gastric secretion in pregnancy. *J Obstet Gynaecol Br Emp* 1957;64:373–381.
55. O'Sullivan GM, Bullingham RE. The assessment of gastric acidity and antacid effect in pregnant women by a non-invasive radiotelemetry technique. *Br J Obstet Gynaecol* 1984;91:973–978.
56. Cappell MS. Gastric and duodenal ulcers during pregnancy. *Gastroenterol Clin North Am* 2003;32:263–308.
57. Hong JY, Park JW, Oh JI. Comparison of preoperative gastric contents and serum gastrin concentrations in pregnant and nonpregnant women. *J Clin Anesth* 2005;17:451–455.
58. Macfie AG, Magides AD, Richmond MN, et al. Gastric emptying in pregnancy. *Br J Anaesth* 1991;67:54–57.
59. Whitehead EM, Smith M, Dean Y, et al. An evaluation of gastric emptying times in pregnancy and the puerperium. *Anaesthesia* 1993;48:53–57.
60. Rådberg G, Asztély M, Cantor P, et al. Gastric and gallbladder emptying in relation to the secretion of cholecystokinin after a meal in late pregnancy. *Digestion* 1989;42:174–180.
61. Wong CA, Loffredi M, Ganchiff JN, et al. Gastric emptying of water in term pregnancy. *Anesthesiology* 2002;96:1395–1400.
62. Davison JS, Davison MC, Hay DM. Gastric emptying time in late pregnancy and labour. *J Obstet Gynaecol Br Commonw* 1970;77:37–41.
63. O'Sullivan GM, Sutton AJ, Thompson SA, et al. Noninvasive measurement of gastric emptying in obstetric patients. *Anesth Analg* 1987;66:505–511.
64. Sandhar BK, Elliott RH, Windram I, et al. Peripartum changes in gastric emptying. *Anaesthesia* 1992;47:196–198.
65. Levy DM, Williams OA, Magides AD, et al. Gastric emptying is delayed at 8-12 weeks' gestation. *Br J Anaesth* 1994;73:237–238.
66. Carp H, Jayaram A, Stoll M. Ultrasound examination of the stomach contents of parturients. *Anesth Analg* 1992;74:683–687.
67. Lind JF, Smith AM, McIver DK, et al. Heartburn in pregnancy—a manometric study. *Can Med Assoc J* 1968;98:571–574.
68. Hey VM, Cowley DJ, Ganguli PC, et al. Gastro–oesophageal reflux in late pregnancy. *Anaesthesia* 1977;32:372–377.
69. Vanner RG, Goodman NW. Gastro-oesophageal reflux in pregnancy at term and after delivery. *Anaesthesia* 1989;44:808–811.
70. Van Thiel DH, Gavaler JS, Stremple J. Lower esophageal sphincter pressure in women using sequential oral contraceptives. *Gastroenterology* 1976;71:232–234.
71. Kozlow JH, Berenholtz SM, Garrett E, et al. Epidemiology and impact of aspiration pneumonia in patients undergoing surgery in Maryland, 1999-2000. *Crit Care Med* 2003;31:1930–1937.
72. Hardy JF, Lepage Y, Bonneville-Chouinard N. Occurrence of gastroesophageal reflux on induction of anaesthesia does not correlate with the volume of gastric contents. *Can J Anaesth* 1990;37:502–508.
73. Nimmo WS, Wilson J, Prescott LF. Narcotic analgesics and delayed gastric emptying during labour. *Lancet* 1975;1:890–893.
74. Nimmo WS. The measurement of gastric emptying during labour. *J Int Med Res* 1978;6 (suppl 1):52–53.
75. Kelly MC, Carabine UA, Hill DA, et al. A comparison of the effect of intrathecal and extradural fentanyl on gastric emptying in laboring women. *Anesth Analg* 1997;85:834–838.

76. Porter JS, Bonello E, Reynolds F. The influence of epidural administration of fentanyl infusion on gastric emptying in labour. *Anaesthesia* 1997;52:1151–1156.
77. Wright PM, Allen RW, Moore J, et al. Gastric emptying during lumbar extradural analgesia in labour: effect of fentanyl supplementation. *Br J Anaesth* 1992;68:248–251.
78. Ewah B, Yau K, King M, et al. Effect of epidural opioids on gastric emptying in labour. *Int J Obstet Anesth* 1993;2:125–128.
79. Zimmermann DL, Breen TW, Fick G. Adding fentanyl 0.0002% to epidural bupivacaine 0.125% does not delay gastric emptying in laboring parturients. *Anesth Analg* 1996;82:612–616.
80. O'Sullivan GM, Bullingham RE. Noninvasive assessment by radiotelemetry of antacid effect during labor. *Anesth Analg* 1985;64:95–100.
81. Kubli M, Scrutton MJ, Seed PT, et al. An evaluation of isotonic "sport drinks" during labor. *Anesth Analg* 2002;94:404–408, table of contents.
82. Jayaram A, Bowen MP, Deshpande S, et al. Ultrasound examination of the stomach contents of women in the postpartum period. *Anesth Analg* 1997;84:522–526.
83. Blouw R, Scatliff J, Craig DB, et al. Gastric volume and pH in postpartum patients. *Anesthesiology* 1976;45:456–457.
84. James CF, Gibbs CP, Banner T. Postpartum perioperative risk of aspiration pneumonia. *Anesthesiology* 1984;61:756–759.
85. Holmes N, Martin D, Begley AM. Cricoid pressure: a review of the literature. *J Perioper Pract* 2011;21:234–238.
86. Brady M, Kinn S, Stuart P. Preoperative fasting for adults to prevent perioperative complications. *Cochrane Database Syst Rev* 2003:CD004423.
87. American Society of Anesthesiologists Task Force on Obstetric Anesthesia. Practice guidelines for obstetric anesthesia: an updated report by the American Society of Anesthesiologists Task Force on Obstetric Anesthesia. *Anesthesiology* 2007;106:843–863.
88. Gibbs CP, Schwartz DJ, Wynne JW, et al. Antacid pulmonary aspiration in the dog. *Anesthesiology* 1979;51:380–385.
89. Maile CJ, Francis RN. Pre-operative ranitidine. Effect of a single intravenous dose on pH and volume of gastric aspirate. *Anaesthesia* 1983;38:324–326.
90. Dammann HG, Muller P, Simon B. Parenteral ranitidine: onset and duration of action. *Br J Anesth* 1982;54:1235–1236.
91. Francis RN, Kwik RS. Oral ranitidine for prophylaxis against Mendelson's syndrome. *Anesth Analg* 1982;61:130–132.
92. Ewart MC, Yau G, Gin T, et al. A comparison of the effects of omeprazole and ranitidine on gastric secretion in women undergoing elective caesarean section. *Anaesthesia* 1990;45:527–530.
93. Yau G, Kan AF, Gin T, et al. A comparison of omeprazole and ranitidine for prophylaxis against aspiration pneumonitis in emergency caesarean section. *Anaesthesia* 1992;47:101–104.
94. Levack ID, Bowie RA, Braid DP, et al. Comparison of the effect of two dose schedules of oral omeprazole with oral ranitidine on gastric aspirate pH and volume in patients undergoing elective surgery. *Br J Anesth* 1996;76:567–569.
95. Clark K, Lam LT, Gibson S, et al. The effect of ranitidine versus proton pump inhibitors on gastric secretions: A meta-analysis of randomised control trials. *Anaesthesia* 2009;64:652–657.
96. Lane S, Saunders D, Schofield A, et al. A prospective, randomised controlled trial comparing the efficacy of pre-oxygenation in the 20 degrees head-up vs supine position. *Anaesthesia* 2005;60:1064–1067.
97. Hignett R, Fernando R, McGlennan A, et al. A randomized crossover study to determine the effect of a 30 degrees head-up versus a supine position on the functional residual capacity of term parturients. *Anesth Analg* 2011;113:1098–1102.
98. Lee BJ, Kang JM, Kim DO. Laryngeal exposure during laryngoscopy is better in the 25 degrees back-up position than in the supine position. *Br J Anesth* 2007;99:581–586.
99. Vanner R. Cricoid pressure. *Int J Obstet Anesth* 2009;18:103–105.
100. Vanner RG, Pryle BJ, O'Dwyer JP, et al. Upper oesophageal sphincter pressure and the intravenous induction of anaesthesia. *Anaesthesia* 1992;47:371–375.
101. Vanner RG, O'Dwyer JP, Pryle BJ, et al. Upper oesophageal sphincter pressure and the effect of cricoid pressure. *Anaesthesia* 1992;47:95–100.
102. El-Orbany M, Connolly LA. Rapid sequence induction and intubation: current controversy. *Anesth Analg* 2010;110:1318–1325.
103. Fenton PM, Reynolds F. Life-saving or ineffective? An observational study of the use of cricoid pressure and maternal outcome in an African setting. *Int J Obstet Anesth* 2009;18:106–110.
104. O'Sullivan G, Liu B, Hart D, et al. Effect of food intake during labour on obstetric outcome: randomised controlled trial. *BMJ* 2009;338:b784.
105. Scrutton MJ, Metcalfe GA, Lowy C, et al. Eating in labour. A randomised controlled trial assessing the risks and benefits. *Anaesthesia* 1999;54:329–334.

26

Neurologic Complications of Regional Anesthesia in Obstetrics

David Wlody

The increasing use of neuraxial anesthesia for labor and both vaginal and cesarean deliveries has unquestionably led to decreases in maternal morbidity and mortality associated with general anesthesia, particularly complications of airway management such as aspiration of gastric contents and failed intubation. Equally apparent, however, is a subsequent increase in the number of complications of regional anesthesia in the obstetric population (Table 26-1). Some of these complications, such as transient neurologic symptoms (TNS) after lidocaine spinal anesthesia, may be mild and self-limited; others, such as epidural abscess or bacterial meningitis, may lead to permanent neurologic injury or even death. A thorough understanding of the risk factors and underlying pathophysiology of the common and most serious complications of regional anesthesia will permit the anesthesiologist to quantitate the risk of neurologic injury in patients receiving spinal or epidural anesthesia, and will enable them to modify their anesthetic technique to decrease the risk of those complications. An understanding of the obstetric nerve palsies will enable the practitioner to distinguish those nerve deficits due to pregnancy itself from those due to regional anesthesia. And finally, a review of diagnostic studies for evaluating neurologic deficits will enable the anesthesiologist to choose a tool that can identify lesions requiring urgent intervention, those in which intervention is not indicated, and to utilize these tools to determine the prognosis of a neurologic deficit.

■ INCIDENCE

Extrapolation from studies of neurologic complications after neuraxial anesthesia in non-obstetric patients to the obstetric population is fraught with difficulty. It is likely that the young, typically healthy parturient is protected from neurologic injury for a number of reasons. First, few of these patients are receiving medications affecting coagulation, unlike elderly orthopedic patients who may be disproportionately represented in studies of regional anesthesia in the non-obstetric population. Such patients may be receiving antiplatelet medications for pre-existing cardiac disease and oral anticoagulants for venous thromboembolism prophylaxis after total joint replacement. Second, the incidence of atherosclerotic vascular disease is lower in the obstetric population, and if there is a vascular component to certain neurologic deficits then it is likely that the absence of pre-existing disease will be protective. Finally, osteoarthritic changes in the vertebral column of the elderly patient limit the patency of the intervertebral foramina; thus, egress of blood accumulating within the epidural space is limited. The patency of the intervertebral foramina in the obstetric population is maintained, allowing blood within the epidural space to dissipate, minimizing the increases in epidural pressure that can lead to spinal cord compression.

Studies in the obstetric population have demonstrated a consistently low risk of significant neurologic injury after neuraxial anesthesia. In a prospective study over a 10-month period, 8,150 French anesthesiologists reported two peripheral neuropathies and no serious sequelae in 5,640 obstetric spinal anesthetics. In almost 30,000 epidurals, there were no neurologic sequelae (1). Moen et al. reported the results of a retrospective postal survey and national registry search of complications of central neuraxial blockade in Sweden from 1990 to 1999. In 200,000 lumbar epidural anesthetics performed for labor, there were eight serious complications (1:25,000). There were two serious complications described in 50,000 spinal anesthetics performed for cesarean delivery (1:25,000) (2). Cook et al. reported the results of the Third National Audit of the Royal College of Anaesthetists. Data were interpreted "pessimistically," that is, when causation was unclear it was attributed to regional anesthesia, or "optimistically," in which causation was attributed to the anesthetic only when evidence was strongly suggestive of such a relationship. The incidence of permanent neurologic injury caused by obstetric neuraxial anesthesia was estimated to range from 0.3/100,000 anesthetics (optimistic) to 1.2/100,000 anesthetics (pessimistic) (3).

■ INFECTIOUS COMPLICATIONS

Infection after neuraxial anesthesia is typically seen in elderly, immunocompromised patients, and is rarely seen in the obstetric population. Nevertheless, analysis of data from the American Society of Anesthesiologists (ASA) Closed Claims Project revealed that 46% of all claims filed from 1980 to 1999 secondary to complications of obstetric neuraxial anesthesia involved infectious complications, either epidural abscess or bacterial meningitis (4). There is growing concern that by inserting an epidural catheter in close proximity to a dural puncture, as occurs routinely with combined spinal–epidural anesthesia (CSEA) for labor, anesthesiologists are providing a direct route from a potentially contaminated external environment to the central nervous system. And finally, there is clear evidence that some common anesthetic practices, as well as technical lapses that are not infrequently observed, can play a direct role in the development of infectious complications after spinal and epidural anesthesia.

Risk Factors for and Prevention of Neuraxial Infectious Complications

In a 2008 review of neurologic infection after neuraxial anesthesia, Reynolds illustrated the difficulty of identifying risk factors for infection in the obstetric population. In a summation of studies comprising over 1 million obstetric anesthetics, the incidence of meningitis after spinal anesthesia was

TABLE 26-1 Closed Claims in Obstetric Anesthesia

Category of Claimed Injury	Pre-1990	1990 and Later
Maternal death[a]	22%	11%
Maternal brain damage	7%	5%
Newborn death/brain damage[a]	29%	21%
Maternal nerve injury[a]	8%	21%
Headache	12%	12%
Backache[a]	5%	10%

Percentage of claims in each category of injury.
[a]$p < 0.05$ comparing two time periods.
Adapted with permission from: Davies JM, Posner KL, Lee LA, et al. Liability associated with obstetric anesthesia: A closed claims analysis. *Anesthesiology* 2009;110:131–139.

1:39,000, and that of epidural abscess after epidural anesthesia was 1:303,000. The total number of infections was small enough that it was difficult to identify causative factors in the OB population (5). In the surgical literature, however, there is a clear relationship between epidural abscess and patient age, immunocompromise, and prolonged epidural catheterization (6). The possibility of spontaneous epidural abscess in the absence of epidural anesthesia should be considered (7), as should coincidental community-acquired meningitis; the causative organism, however, may be very helpful in determining the time of acquisition of infection (Table 26-2).

Hand hygiene has been recognized for well over a century and a half as an integral part of infection control in the health care setting. The integrity of sterile gloves worn during neuraxial anesthesia can never be guaranteed, and appropriate hand hygiene will decrease the bacterial inoculum should a glove be punctured or torn during the procedure. Rings and wristwatches should be removed before hand washing, which is the most effective when an antimicrobial cleanser containing alcohol is used.

Since the most common causative agent for epidural abscess is *Staphylococcus aureus* (8), appropriate skin preparation is

TABLE 26-2 Risk Factors: Neurologic Infectious Complications

Advanced Age
Prolonged epidural catheterization
Cancer
Diabetes
Immunosupression
Substance abuse
Pancreatitis, GI bleeding

Reprinted with permission from: Wang LP, Hauerberg J, Schmidt JF. Incidence of spinal epidural abscess after epidural analgesia: A national 1-year survey. *Anesthesiology* 1999;91:1928–1936; American Society of Anesthesiologists Task Force on infectious complications associated with neuraxial techniques. Practice advisory for the prevention, diagnosis, and management of infectious complications associated with neuraxial techniques: A report by the American Society of Anesthesiologists Task Force on infectious complications associated with neuraxial techniques. *Anesthesiology* 2010;112:530–545.

essential. Numerous studies have shown the superiority of chlorhexidine–alcohol to povidone–iodine in reducing growth of *S. aureus*, and in the prevention of central line associated infections (9–11). Iodophor–alcohol solutions are similarly superior to povidone–iodine alone in both immediate skin disinfection as well as epidural catheter colonization (12). Chlorhexidine is not inactivated in the presence of organic material such as blood, and its penetration of the stratum corneum of the skin gives it a prolonged duration of action, and effectively kills bacteria within hair follicles and sebaceous glands (13). While the package insert for the most commonly used chlorhexidine–alcohol preparation specifically states that it is not to be used prior to lumbar puncture (14), both the ASA in its practice advisory for the prevention of infectious complications in neuraxial anesthesia (15) and the American Society of Regional Anesthesia and Pain Medicine (ASRA) (16) have recommended the routine use of chlorhexidine–alcohol solutions for skin preparation prior to neuraxial anesthesia. The failure to demonstrate any increase in the incidence of neurologic deficits above baseline after the use of chlorhexidine for skin preparation in spinal anesthesia provides further evidence of its safety (17). And while chlorhexidine has been shown to be more cytotoxic than povidone–iodine at low concentrations in an in vitro model, there is no difference in toxicity at clinically relevant concentrations. Following the manufacturer's instructions to allow the solution to dry for 2 to 3 minutes after application can further minimize any risk of toxicity of chlorhexidine (18).

In 2012, it is frankly astonishing that masks are not always worn during neuraxial anesthesia. It has been demonstrated that wearing a face mask results in a marked reduction in the bacterial contamination of a surface in close proximity to the upper airway (19). Both ASA and ASRA recommend the routine use of a face mask during neuraxial anesthesia, (15,16) and this is in fact a requirement of the United States Centers for Disease Control and Prevention (CDC) (20).

Further, there are numerous reports of cases of meningitis after spinal anesthesia in which a mask was not worn during the procedure (21–23). In a noteworthy report from the CDC, two separate outbreaks of meningitis in five obstetric patients receiving neuraxial anesthesia were described (24). Three women in New York State who received CSEA from the same anesthesiologist were found to have the identical strain of *Streptococcus salivarius*, a common nasopharyngeal organism. While the anesthesiologist reported wearing a mask during the procedures, the hospital permitted unmasked visitors to freely enter labor rooms during neuraxial procedures. In Ohio, two women received single-shot spinal anesthetics from the same anesthesiologist, who was determined to have routinely performed neuraxial procedures without a mask; one of these women died. The causative organism in both cases was a strain of *S. salivarius* that was genetically identical to an organism cultured from the anesthesiologist's nasopharynx. **The need for the operator to wear a mask during neuraxial procedures cannot be overemphasized.** Requiring any other personnel in the labor room during the neuraxial procedure to wear a mask, including family members, should be considered as well.

While the ASA has recommended that a gown be worn during invasive procedures performed in immunosuppressed patients, there is no evidence that this is beneficial or necessary in routine neuraxial anesthesia. It should be noted, however, that while the ASA makes no recommendations regarding the use of sterile gowns, a substantial minority (33%) of the participating consultants agreed or strongly agreed that gowns should in fact be worn during neuraxial anesthesia (15), and this practice is fairly common in the United Kingdom.

The integrity of the epidural infusion system must be maintained at all times; this is of particular importance in patients receiving postoperative analgesia on the postpartum ward, where the level of surveillance for breaks in sterility may not be as great as in a labor and delivery unit. Disconnections and reconnections should be minimized, and catheter removal should be seriously considered in the setting of an unwitnessed disconnection.

In-line antibacterial filters are commonly used in the United Kingdom (25) and the ASA suggests consideration of their use in the setting of long-term epidural catheterization (15). While there is in vitro evidence that these filters are effective in eliminating passage of bacteria contained within even highly contaminated solutions (26), clinical studies suggest that the use of filters does not decrease the incidence of catheter tip colonization (27), and CNS infections have been reported even when filters were used (28–30).

Bacterial contamination can occur at the time that epidural local anesthetic infusions are prepared, and while local anesthetics are weakly bacteriostatic (31–34), microbial growth can occur during prolonged infusion. It should be noted that the newer single-enantiomer agents, ropivacaine and levobupivacaine, have lower antimicrobial activity than the older racemic mixtures (35–37).

In 2004, the United States Pharmacopeia formulated regulations, USP Chapter 797, regarding the compounding of pharmaceutical preparations, including local anesthetic infusions for epidural administration. These regulations, which represent a national standard enforceable by the U.S. Food and Drug Administration (FDA), state boards of medicine, and the Joint Commission, mandate that local anesthetic infusions intended to be infused over several days be prepared under a laminar flow workbench (38–40). Unfortunately, these guidelines do not specifically address infusions administered over a shorter time frame. Nevertheless, a close reading of the regulations suggest that multidrug infusions (e.g., local anesthetic and opioid +/– epinephrine) are considered medium-risk preparations, and as such should be prepared under a laminar flow hood in a pharmacy (Table 26-3).

Clinical Aspects of Infectious Complications

The two major infectious complications of neuraxial anesthesia are meningitis and epidural abscess. While there may be some overlap in their clinical presentations, they differ significantly in their incidence, risk factors, microbial etiology, pathophysiology, and treatment. An excellent review of these complications is provided by Reynolds (5).

Meningitis

The frequent clustering of cases of meningitis after neuraxial anesthesia, which suggests a unique causation (e.g., a practitioner using poor sterile technique), makes the task of estimating the incidence of infection a difficult one. Older surveys and case reports may reflect practices that are no longer commonly used; multi-institutional surveys may reflect a wide range of practices that influence the risk for infection. Nevertheless, a review of some of the large-scale, nationwide surveys may be useful in determining the risk of meningitis. For example, in Moen's survey of neurologic complications after neuraxial anesthesia in Sweden, the overall incidence of meningitis after spinal block was 1:53,000; again, however, a cluster of four cases in a single institution (yielding an incidence of 1:3,000 at that site) clearly skewed the results (2). In 50,000 spinal anesthetics performed for cesarean delivery, there were no cases of meningitis. The Third National Audit

TABLE 26-3 Prevention of Infectious Complications in Neuraxial Anesthesia

Consider use of pre-procedural antibiotics in patients with suspected bacteremia
Hand washing
Remove wristwatches and jewelry
Always wear a cap and face mask
Consider a gown in immunocompromised patients
Utilize single-use packets of skin preparation solutions
Prepare skin with chlorhexidine (preferably with alcohol) or iodophor–alcohol solutions in preference to povidone–iodine
Consider use of bacterial filters during extended epidural catheterization
Limit disconnection and reconnection of infusion systems
Consider removal of catheter after unwitnessed disconnections

Reprinted with permission from: American Society of Anesthesiologists Task Force on infectious complications associated with neuraxial techniques. Practice advisory for the prevention, diagnosis, and management of infectious complications associated with neuraxial techniques: a report by the American Society of Anesthesiologists Task Force on infectious complications associated with neuraxial techniques. *Anesthesiology* 2010;112:530–545.

Project of the Royal College of Anaesthetists identified three cases of meningitis in some 707,000 central neuraxial blocks, performed for obstetric, surgical, and chronic pain indications; none suffered permanent sequelae (3).

In view of the low incidence of meningitis after neuraxial anesthesia, much of our knowledge of the clinical presentation of the disease is based on case reports. Reynolds identified 38 cases of meningitis in obstetric patients that received neuraxial anesthesia; in all but two cases (one viral, one community-acquired) the anesthetic was determined to be the causative factor (5). The clinical presentation is like that of meningitis seen in other settings, with headache, nausea, fever, meningeal signs, and alterations in consciousness appearing hours to several days after anesthesia. Notably, meningitis has been confused with post-dural puncture headache (PDPH), one of these patients having received two epidural blood patches.

When faced with a patient developing meningitis after neuraxial anesthesia, it is understandable that those involved in the anesthetic care of the patient would consider the possibility that the infectious process was unrelated to the anesthetic procedure, and that the development of meningitis was coincidental. However, the organisms responsible for community-acquired meningitis (*Neisseria meningitidis, Streptococcus pneumoniae, Haemophilus influenzae*) are only rarely found in obstetric patients. Most often, meningitis seen in the setting of neuraxial anesthesia is caused by alpha-hemolytic streptococcus, typically *S. salivarius*, an organism found in both the nasopharynx and the vagina. As mentioned previously, the frequency with which this organism is seen in cases of meningitis after spinal anesthesia makes the use of a mask during preparation for and performance of spinal anesthesia mandatory.

Of the 36 cases of anesthesia-related meningitis identified by Reynolds, 30 were associated with a recognized dural puncture, two were likely to have been complicated by unrecognized dural puncture, and two probably represented epidural infection (5). Thus, dural puncture appears to be a prerequisite for anesthesia-related meningitis. Again, this may represent introduction of bacteria into the subarachnoid space via contaminated equipment or medications. It may also represent introduction of bacteria from the bloodstream; animal studies have demonstrated lumbar puncture in the setting of bacteremia may lead to meningitis (41). The ASA has recommended that in the setting of suspected bacteremia, a full consideration of the risks and benefits of neuraxial anesthesia should occur, and that the use of pre-procedural antibiotics should be strongly considered (15). ASRA has recommended that in the setting of systemic infection, if antibiotic therapy is initiated prior to neuraxial anesthesia, an effective response to that therapy should be demonstrated, for example, decrease in fever, before the neuraxial procedure is attempted (42). The use of regional anesthesia in the patient with chorioamnionitis appears to be safe (43,44).

Epidural Abscess

Almost 95% of epidural abscesses are unrelated to neuraxial anesthesia, the great majority of cases being a result of hematogenous seeding of the epidural space from a distant infection, or local spread from a cutaneous infection. The most common risk factors are diabetes, trauma, intravenous drug abuse, and alcoholism, that is, conditions that predispose to immune suppression (45). Reynolds identified 16 cases of epidural abscess after obstetric neuraxial anesthesia, and all occurred after epidural or CSEA; none occurred after spinal anesthesia alone (5). Similarly, in Moen's study of complications after neuraxial anesthesia in Sweden, 12 of 13 cases of epidural abscess occurred after epidural anesthesia (2). Given the rarity of reported cases of abscess after epidural anesthesia, bacterial colonization of epidural catheters is surprisingly common; in one study, 5.8% of patients receiving postoperative epidural analgesia for an average of 5 days had positive catheter tip cultures, 75% of which were *Staphylococcus epidermidis*. None of these patients developed an epidural abscess (46). Again, while it is difficult to describe a true incidence of epidural abscess in the obstetric population, it appears to be extremely low; in Moen's study, one case of epidural abscess was identified in 200,000 obstetric epidurals (2), and in the Royal College survey, one case of epidural abscess was identified in 161,000 obstetric patients receiving epidurals (3).

Kindler reviewed and published 42 cases of epidural abscess after epidural anesthesia in both surgical and obstetric patients (8). Back pain and fever were seen in over 90% of patients. Leukocytosis was common, and the erythrocyte sedimentation rate and C-reactive protein levels were elevated in all patients in whom those studies were obtained. Thirty-six percent of patients had a risk factor, including diabetes, corticosteroid therapy, and alcoholism. The mean duration of catheterization was 4 days, and symptoms developed in 5 days or less in 48% of cases. Staphylococcus species were the causative organism in 70% of cases. Troublingly, only 45% of patients had a full recovery; these patients had a shorter interval from symptom onset to surgical intervention than the 48% of patients with permanent sequelae.

The clinical presentation of epidural abscess in obstetric patients identified by Reynolds largely mirrors Kindler's findings (5). The median duration of catheterization was 1 day, and the median time to onset of symptoms was 6 days. In the majority of cases, staphylococcus species were identified as the causative organism; streptococcal infection was also identified in several patients. Patients were typically healthy, with few comorbidities predisposing the patient to epidural abscess.

A consistent pattern in case reports of epidural abscess is the poor outcome seen when definitive therapy is delayed. **In the setting of fever, back pain, and leukocytosis, prompt imaging of the spine is essential, especially when lower extremity neurologic changes are present.** MRI is the imaging technique of choice (47).

Laminectomy is generally accepted as the most effective technique for ensuring that areas of infection are completely eradicated. However, medical treatment with antibiotics alone has been utilized in cases of epidural abscess in which significant neurologic deficit has not yet developed (48,49). There are also numerous case reports of percutaneous drainage of epidural abscess (50–52). Should neurologic deficits develop or progress at any time during conservative treatment, however, surgical intervention is indicated.

■ EPIDURAL HEMATOMA

Other than the absence of signs of infection such as fever and leukocytosis, the presentation of epidural hematoma is similar to that of epidural abscess, that is, back pain, sometimes severe, eventually followed by weakness and sensory alterations in the lower extremities. Unlike epidural abscess, however, which may take days to manifest itself, the signs and symptoms of epidural hematoma may develop within 12 hours of the initial neuraxial procedure. Herein lies a diagnostic challenge, since an epidural hematoma may develop during the time period in which motor and sensory blockade might be expected to persist after an uncomplicated neuraxial anesthetic. **Recurrence of motor block after partial recovery, or prolonged block in patients at risk for an epidural hematoma, should serve as a red flag to initiate diagnostic studies to rule out possible spinal cord compression.** Optimal results of surgical intervention are seen when decompression occurs within 8 hours of onset of paraplegia; outcomes markedly worsen when the 8 hour limit is exceeded (53).

The incidence of epidural hematoma is extraordinarily low in the obstetric population. In the Royal College survey, there was not a single incidence of epidural hematoma in 295,000 neuraxial anesthetics (3). A retrospective study of 505,000 obstetric epidurals administered over a 5-year period revealed one epidural hematoma (54); in a 2-year prospective study by the same author, there were no hematomas identified in over 122,000 patients that received neuraxial anesthesia (55). In Moen's study, two patients with HELLP syndrome developed an epidural hematoma, one after subarachnoid block and one after epidural block, yielding an incidence of epidural hematoma after spinal and epidural anesthesia of 1:50,000 and 1:200,000, respectively (2). In contrast, the incidence of epidural hematoma in female patients undergoing knee arthroplasty was 1:3,600. This difference is likely due to combination of the greater use of anticoagulants in this population, as well as a less compliant epidural space secondary to anatomic changes in the osteoporotic spine (56). Finally, the possibility that an epidural hematoma is unrelated to a neuraxial anesthetic cannot be discounted; four such cases have been identified since 1966 (7,57).

A detailed description of the many coagulation disturbances that predispose to the development of epidural hematoma in the parturient is beyond the scope of this review. These disturbances can be divided into two groups: Coagulopathy due to underlying disease and iatrogenic disturbances due to therapeutic anticoagulation.

Coagulopathy Due to Underlying Disease

The most common disturbance of coagulation seen in pregnancy is thrombocytopenia, which can be due to gestational thrombocytopenia (82.3%), preeclampsia (14.1%), or immune disorders (2.5%) (58). For many years, a platelet count of 100×10^9/L was considered the minimum acceptable level for performing neuraxial anesthesia. This practice was supported by the prolongation of bleeding time seen in severely preeclamptic patients with platelet counts less than 100×10^9/L (59), and alterations in coagulation as measured by thromboelastography in patients with platelet counts below that level (60). However, the utility of bleeding time in predicting hemorrhagic complications, particularly complications in a single patient with an abnormal bleeding time, has been questioned (61). In addition, there is a large and growing experience in the administration of neuraxial anesthesia to obstetric patients with platelet counts lower than the traditional threshold. Beilin reported 80 patients with a platelet count less than 100×10^9/L at the time of epidural placement, or whose platelet count dropped below that level subsequent to epidural placement. None of these patients had a postpartum neurologic deficit (62). Rasmus described 14 parturients who received epidural anesthesia with platelet counts between 15×10^9/L and 99×10^9/L with no complications (63). In a retrospective review of 119 deliveries in patients with idiopathic thrombocytopenic purpura (ITP), 19 epidurals were placed with platelet counts of 76×10^9/L to 100×10^9/L, 6 with platelet counts of 50×10^9/L to 75×10^9/L, and 1 with a platelet count of less than 50×10^9/L; no complications were noted (64). Thus, there is growing support for the use of regional anesthesia in patient with platelet counts of greater than 75×10^9/L to 80×10^9/L (65,66).

Nevertheless, patients with thrombocytopenia should be approached with caution before undertaking regional anesthesia. Preeclampsia is a dynamic process; the preeclamptic parturient with a rapidly dropping platelet count is likely at higher risk than a patient with chronic, stable ITP and an identical platelet count. The presence of clinical markers of coagulopathy such as widespread petechiae should give one pause prior to regional anesthesia. Identification of additional risk factors, such as an abnormality of platelet function, another disorder affecting coagulation (e.g., hepatic dysfunction), or concomitant antiplatelet therapy (see later), will influence the decision to perform a regional anesthetic. In patients with ITP who are not already receiving corticosteroid therapy, this should be considered as there is usually a significant response to such treatment (67). There may also be a benefit to corticosteroid therapy in the patient with HELLP syndrome (68,69). Ultimately, the decision to perform a regional anesthetic in a patient with significant thrombocytopenia will be based on an assessment of the risks and benefits in that patient; a morbidly obese patient with an anticipated difficult airway and a platelet count of 60×10^9/L about to undergo an urgent cesarean delivery may be a better candidate for regional anesthesia than a fully dilated grand multipara with a platelet count of 80×10^9/L requesting epidural labor analgesia.

Coagulopathy Due to Drug Therapy

Pregnant patients can receive a variety of medications that affect coagulation. ASRA has published guidelines for the use of regional anesthesia in patients receiving antithrombotic or thrombolytic therapy (70). A complete discussion of these guidelines is beyond the scope of this review, but a brief summary of management recommendations for the most common antithrombotic agents seen in pregnant patients follows (Table 26-4) **(for additional details, see Chapter 34).**

TABLE 26-4 ASRA Recommendations Anticoagulant Therapy

Drug	Recommendation
Nonsteroidal anti-inflammatory agents	No additional precautions
Unfractionated heparin 5,000 U SC q12h	No additional precautions
Heparin 5,000 U SC q8h	No additional precautions
LMWH once daily (prophylactic) dosing	Needle placement 12 h after last dose
LMWH twice daily (therapeutic) dosing	Needle placement 24 h after last dose
Warfarin	Needle placement delayed until INR in normal range

Reprinted with permission from: Horlocker TT, Wedel DJ, Rowlingson JC, et al. Regional anesthesia in the patient receiving antithrombotic or thrombolytic therapy: American Society of Regional Anesthesia and Pain Medicine Evidence-Based Guidelines (Third Edition). *Reg Anesth Pain Med* 2010;35:64–101.

Nonsteroidal anti-inflammatory agents (NSAIDs) are widely used during pregnancy, perhaps most notably in the form of low-dose aspirin administered for the prevention of severe preeclampsia in patients thought to be at high risk of developing the disease (71). The paucity of reports of epidural hematoma in patients receiving NSAIDs, and the lack of neurologic sequelae in a series of 1,422 women who underwent epidural analgesia while receiving 60 mg/day of aspirin (72), led ASRA to conclude that the use of NSAIDs added no significant risk for the development of spinal hematoma. It was recommended, however, that regional anesthesia be avoided if the patient was receiving any additional medications affecting coagulation.

Subcutaneous unfractionated heparin is commonly administered to pregnant patients at high risk of developing deep venous thrombosis. Administration of 5,000 units subcutaneously every 12 hours does not increase the risk of spinal hematoma after neuraxial anesthesia (73), and ASRA concluded that this dosing regimen was not a contraindication to regional techniques. The guidelines, however, noted the increasingly widespread utilization of 5,000 unit dosing three times a day, and indicated that the risk of hematoma in this setting could not be estimated; they recommended enhanced monitoring for the development of neurologic deficits in patients on this treatment regimen.

Low-molecular-weight heparins (LMWH) are increasingly used for thromboprophylaxis during pregnancy in high-risk patients. As effective as unfractionated heparin in preventing DVT, they have the added advantage of a predictable response without the need for routine monitoring of activated PTT. However, the anticoagulant effect of LMWH is not easily quantitated, making it difficult to determine when the effect has waned to a level at which neuraxial anesthesia is safe; further, reversal of anticoagulant effect with protamine is unpredictable. The initial European experience with LMWH and regional anesthesia suggested that the risk of spinal hematoma was quite low (74); neuraxial anesthesia was administered to 9,013 patients receiving LMWH without evidence of neurologic injury (75). However, the experience after the introduction of LMWH into the United States in 1993 was quite different; nearly 60 cases of neuraxial hematoma were reported to the FDA between 1993 and 1998 (70). Notably, European administration practices were quite different from those utilized in the United States at that time; once daily dosing was standard in Europe, while twice daily dosing was commonly used in the United States. ASRA now recommends that in patients receiving preoperative, once daily thromboprophylaxis with LMWH, needle placement should be delayed at least 10 to 12 hours after a dose; that regional anesthesia be delayed at least 24 hours after LMWH administration in patients receiving therapeutic dosing twice daily; that epidural catheters be removed at least 2 hours prior to the first postoperative dose when twice daily dosing is planned; and that an epidural catheter can be maintained during once once daily postoperative dosing, but that catheter removal should not occur any sooner than 12 hours after a dose.

ASRA recommends that patients chronically anticoagulated with **warfarin** should not undergo neuraxial anesthesia until the INR is within normal range; this can be expected to take 4 to 5 days after warfarin therapy is discontinued. If warfarin therapy is restarted after delivery, epidural catheters should be removed when the INR is still less than 1.5, and enhanced surveillance of neurologic function should occur for at least 24 hours after catheter removal.

■ CHEMICAL INJURY

A wide variety of drugs have been accidentally injected into the epidural space, including neuromuscular blockers (76–79), ondansetron (80), thiopental (81), acetaminophen (82), and potassium chloride (83). Permanent neurologic injury is rare, but has been reported, as in the case of a parturient who received an accidental injection of chlorhexidine through an epidural catheter and was rendered paraplegic (84). The causes for such errors are numerous, including "look-alike" drug ampoules, incorrect labeling of syringes, and the accidental attachment of intravenous lines to epidural catheters. The compatibility of connectors for systems designed for either intravenous or neuraxial administration is clearly a source of error; it has been strongly argued that epidural and spinal infusion systems be redesigned in a way that would prevent them from being connected to syringes and infusion pumps designed for intravenous drug delivery (85). Drug administration errors can never be eliminated, but appropriate vigilance should minimize their occurrence. Ampoules should be identified by their labeling, and not by color; syringes should be carefully labeled, preferably with preprinted labels; hospital pharmacies should be notified if a potentially neurotoxic agent has labeling similar to commonly used local anesthetics.

In vitro and animal studies demonstrate that commonly used local anesthetics, when administered in sufficiently high doses, can be neurotoxic (86,87). Toxicity may be enhanced in the setting of pre-existing neurologic injury, such as diabetic neuropathy (88). Of the agents that are currently in common use in obstetric anesthesia, hyperbaric lidocaine for subarachnoid block and 2-chloroprocaine (2-CP) are most commonly associated with such injury.

■ HYPERBARIC LIDOCAINE: CAUDA EQUINA SYNDROME AND TRANSIENT NEUROLOGIC SYMPTOMS

In 1991, Rigler et al. reported four cases (89), and Schell et al. reported two cases (90) of persistent neurologic injury consistent with the cauda equina syndrome in patients who received continuous spinal anesthesia for a variety of surgical procedures. In five of these cases, hyperbaric lidocaine was administered via a 28-gauge spinal microcatheter. An initial

failure to achieve adequate levels of surgical anesthesia led to the administration of additional doses of local anesthetic, one patient receiving 285 mg over 30 minutes. Both publications suggested that the limited extent of sensory blockade reflected a limited spread of local anesthetic within the subarachnoid space, due to the difficulty of injecting fluid rapidly through a long, small-diameter catheter. It was hypothesized that the limited spread of lidocaine within the subarachnoid space produced localized drug concentrations that exceeded the level necessary to produce neurotoxicity. This hypothesis was supported by a study of the distribution of methylene blue in a "glass spine" model, which demonstrated consistently greater maldistribution of drug when 28-gauge catheters were used compared to 20-gauge catheters (91). In 1992, spinal catheters were withdrawn from the US market by the FDA (92). However, cauda equina syndrome has been reported after a single-injection spinal anesthetic (1); should limited spread of sensory block occur after attempted subarachnoid anesthesia, the risk of producing toxic drug levels in the CSF should be considered before repeating the block.

In 1993, Schneider et al. described four patients who reported transient neurologic dysfunction after spinal anesthesia with 5% lidocaine (93). The patients received 50 to 75 mg of lidocaine, and all underwent procedures performed in the lithotomy position. They all developed postoperative pain in the buttocks radiating to the thighs and calves. There were no motor or sensory disturbances, and symptoms resolved within several days. **TNS**, as this phenomenon has been named, is significantly more common with lidocaine than bupivacaine (RR 5.1, 95% C.I. 2.5 to 10.2). (94). In patients receiving lidocaine, procedures performed in the lithotomy position were more likely to be complicated by TNS (RR. 2.6, 95% C.I. 1.5 to 4.5), than procedures performed in other positions, and outpatients receiving lidocaine were more likely to develop TNS than inpatients (RR 3.6, 95% C.I. 1.9 to 6.8). Age, gender, and lidocaine dose and concentration did not influence risk. Pregnancy, however, appears to have a protective effect; the incidence of TNS after postpartum tubal ligation performed under lidocaine spinal anesthesia was 3% (95), and the incidence after cesarean delivery with lidocaine spinal anesthesia was 0% (95% C.I. 0% to 3%), identical to bupivacaine (96). It is tempting to identify TNS as one end of a spectrum of neuronal injury that culminates in the cauda equina syndrome, but further study is needed before that conclusion can be reached (97). Indeed, Pollock et al. (98) found no evidence of neurologic dysfunction by electromyography (EMG) or nerve conduction velocity studies in volunteers who developed TNS after lidocaine spinal anesthesia.

The range of neurologic complications that can follow the use of intrathecal lidocaine has called the continuing usefulness of that agent into question. Some have suggested that the use of lidocaine in obstetric spinal anesthesia is no longer justified and it should not be used (99). Unfortunately, there are few alternative agents that have a similar clinical profile and less toxicity. Procaine and mepivacaine have a similarly short duration, and are less toxic (100,101), but are not readily available. Removal of glucose from the commercial preparation of lidocaine does not appear to offer any advantages with respect to neurotoxicity (102). In an editorial concerning the safety of lidocaine, Drasner made several recommendations, including limiting the total dose of drug to 60 mg and avoiding the use of epinephrine to prolong the duration of the block (103). This author would add that although pregnancy is protective against TNS, the use of lidocaine for cervical cerclage, which is performed in the lithotomy position, often on an outpatient basis, should be avoided.

■ LOCAL ANESTHETIC NEUROTOXICITY: 2-CHLOROPROCAINE

The ester local anesthetic, 2-CP, is unique in its rapid onset, short duration, and minimal systemic toxicity due to rapid hydrolysis by plasma cholinesterase. However, 2-CP can produce significant, prolonged neurotoxicity when large volumes are accidentally injected into the subarachnoid space (104–106). An in vitro study by Gissen et al. suggested that the cause of neural injury was a combination of low pH and the antioxidant sodium metabisulfite, and not 2-CP itself (107). Subsequent to this study, 2-CP was reformulated in a less acidic solution without sodium metabisulfite. Since that reformulation occurred, there have been no case reports of 2-CP neurotoxicity, although other factors, such as the more widespread use of fractionated dosing, cannot be excluded as a possible cause for this. However, more recent work suggests that the role of bisulfite in producing neuronal injury has been overstated, and that 2-CP in fact does have intrinsic neurotoxicity (108), although this conclusion has been challenged (109). To further complicate the issue, there is a growing experience in the use of preservative-free 2-CP as a spinal anesthetic without any evidence of neurotoxicity (110–113). **Nevertheless, one cannot assume that the accidental intrathecal injection of large volumes and large doses of drugs meant for epidural anesthesia will be as benign as small doses of 2-CP intended for subarachnoid use.** It thus remains critically important that an epidural catheter should be demonstrated to be within the epidural space before large doses of local anesthetics are injected, and that fractionated dosing be utilized unless there is an extremely compelling argument to do otherwise.

■ DIRECT INJURY TO THE SPINAL CORD

Inevitably, neuraxial anesthesia carries the risk of injury to the spinal cord. The ASA Closed Claims Project reported two cases in which spinal cord injury was felt to be related to direct injury to the spinal cord (4). Auroy reported three patients who reported paresthesias during spinal anesthesia who had residual neurologic injury 6 months later (1). Reynolds reported six patients who underwent spinal or CSEA for cesarean delivery or vaginal delivery and were found to have deficits consistent with injury to the conus medullaris (114). In all cases, injection was reported to be no more cephalad than the L2 to L3 interspace. Pain during needle insertion occurred in all cases, but free flow of CSF was noted, and spinal anesthesia was adequate in most cases. All patients were found to have residual unilateral sensory loss involving several dermatomes, most

TABLE 26-5 Factors Contributing to Direct Spinal Cord Injury During Neuraxial Anesthesia

Extension of conus medullaris below L1–L2 interspace
Unreliability of Tuffier's line as marker for L4–L5 interspace
Inability of physician to identify interspace level by landmark alone
Increasing willingness to perform lumbar puncture at levels above L2–L3

Reprinted with permission from: Reynolds F. Damage to the conus medullaris following spinal anaesthesia. *Anaesthesia* 2001;56:238–247.

had residual foot drop, and three had urinary symptoms. MRI usually revealed a syrinx on the side corresponding to both the initial paresthesia as well as the residual deficit. It was concluded that these injuries were in large part due to puncture at a level higher than the actual termination of the spinal cord.

Reynolds noted a number of possible predisposing factors that may have led to these injuries (114). An MRI study has shown that the conus medullaris extends below the L1 to L2 interspace in over 21% of subjects (115), rendering lumbar puncture at that interspace potentially hazardous. Tuffier's line, the imaginary landmark connecting the posterior superior iliac spines and which is widely thought to indicate the L4 to L5 interspace, may indicate a level ranging up to one interspace higher (116,117). Pregnancy may render the usefulness of Tuffier's line even less reliable (118,119). Finally, anesthesiologists are remarkably unsuccessful at identifying lumbar interspaces by external landmarks alone. One radiologic study demonstrated that the level of lumbar puncture was misidentified in 59% of cases (120). Broadbent utilized MRI to compare the actual spinal interspace corresponding to a skin marker with anesthesiologists' estimates of that level. The correct level was identified only 29% of the time. 15% of the time the actual spinal level was two interspaces higher than the physician's estimate, and in 1.5% of observations the actual interspace was three or four levels higher than the estimated level (121). Given the uncertainties in determining the site of injection, the L3 to L4 interspace should remain the level of choice for spinal and CSEA (122,123). In addition, while injury may have already occurred at the time of a painful subarachnoid needle placement, injection should be avoided and the needle be repositioned before administration of medication (114) (Table 26-5) (Figs. 26-1 and 26-2).

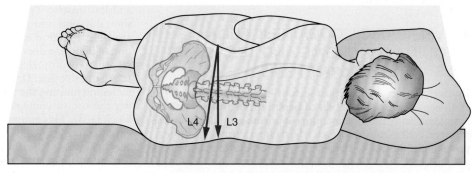

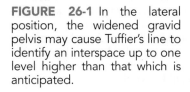

FIGURE 26-1 In the lateral position, the widened gravid pelvis may cause Tuffier's line to identify an interspace up to one level higher than that which is anticipated.

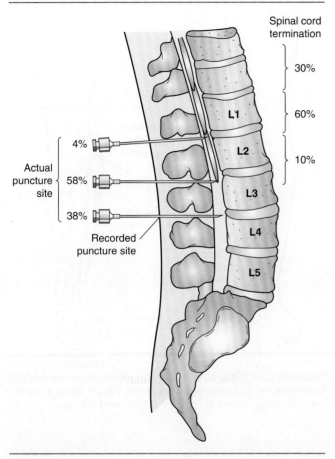

FIGURE 26-2 Left, actual site of dural puncture when recorded puncture site was L3 to L4. More often than not the actual puncture site was at least one interspace higher than anticipated. Right, termination of spinal cord may extend as caudad as L2 to L3 interspace.

■ OBSTETRIC NERVE PALSIES

From the perspective of a new mother, her obstetric provider, and perhaps her anesthesiologist, any postpartum neurologic deficit will be attributed to neuraxial anesthesia. In reality, neurologic deficit after childbirth is most often secondary to compression or stretching of a peripheral nerve as a consequence of pregnancy or delivery itself. Wong et al. asked over 6,200 women on the first postpartum day if they had leg weakness or numbness. Positive responses led to formal evaluation by a physiatrist. 0.92% of women were diagnosed with a peripheral nerve injury consistent with obstetric nerve palsy (124). The most significant risk factors for injury were nulliparity and prolonged second stage. Dar et al. found the incidence of obstetric nerve palsy to be 0.58%; a significant number of women did not spontaneously report these deficits until they were specifically questioned regarding the presence of sensory or motor disturbances (125). Familiarity with and the ability to diagnose the common obstetric nerve palsies is important, both for medicolegal reasons as well as to be able to provide the patient with a more accurate prognosis for recovery. A summary of the most common obstetric nerve palsies follows (119,126,127) (Table 26-6 and Fig. 26-3):

Lumbosacral trunk injury is caused by compression of this structure, consisting of fibers derived from the L4 and L5 roots, by the fetal head at the sacral ala. Patients present with weakness of ankle dorsiflexion and eversion (foot drop), and decreased sensation along the lateral aspect of the lower leg and the dorsal surface of the foot. These findings are almost always seen on the side opposite the fetal occiput. Risk factors include prolonged labor, a large fetus, and a flattened, wide posterior pelvis with pronounced sacroiliac joints (126). Historically, it often presented after midforceps rotation, and the abandonment of that obstetric maneuver has undoubtedly led to a decreased incidence of this injury; in Wong's study, the incidence was less than 0.05% (124). Like the other obstetric nerve palsies, recovery can be expected over a period of weeks to several months.

Common peroneal nerve palsy results secondary to compression of the nerve against the fibular head, usually due

TABLE 26-6 Clinical Characteristics: Obstetric Nerve Palsies

Lesion	Presentation	Pathophysiology and Risk Factors
Lumbosacral trunk	Weakness of ankle dorsiflexion and eversion (foot drop), decreased sensation lateral aspect of the lower leg and dorsal surface of the foot.	Compression of lumbosacral trunk by fetal head at sacral ala, seen after prolonged labor with macrosomic fetus.
Common peroneal nerve	Similar to lumbosacral trunk, ankle inversion may be preserved.	Compression of nerve against fibular head due to poorly positioned stirrups in lithotomy position.
Meralgia paresthetica	Pure sensory loss in superior portion of anterolateral thigh.	Compression of lateral femoral cutaneous nerve under inguinal ligament following prolonged hyperflexion of hips in second stage of labor.
Femoral nerve	Quadriceps weakness (impaired stair climbing) and decreased sensation medial calf and foot.	Compression of femoral nerve by fetal head or by retractor during pelvic surgery.
Obturator nerve	Weakness of hip adduction and rotation, decreased sensation upper inner thigh.	Compression of nerve within obturator canal due to exaggerated hip flexion in lithotomy position, compression by fetal head at pelvic brim.

From: Wong CA. Nerve injuries after neuraxial anesthesia and their medicolegal implications. *Best Pract Res Clin Obstet Gynaecol* 2010;24:367–381; Donaldson JO. Neuropathy. In *Neurology of Pregnancy.* 2nd ed. Philadelphia, PA: WB Saunders, 1989:23–59.

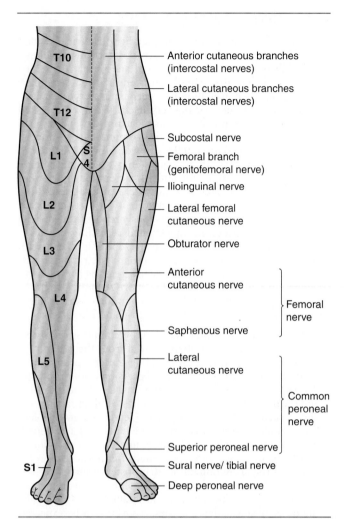

FIGURE 26-3 Innervation arising from spinal nerve roots (right leg) and peripheral nerves (left leg). Sensory loss limited to the area supplied by a peripheral nerve is strongly suggestive of obstetric nerve palsy unrelated to neuraxial anesthesia.

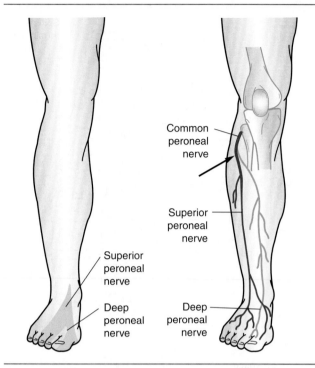

FIGURE 26-4 Course of common peroneal nerve and its branches. Note proximity of nerve to fibular head where it can be compressed by poorly positioned stirrups.

noticeably during stair climbing. There is commonly a loss of sensation on the medial calf and foot.

Obturator nerve palsy is rare, seen in 0.05% of postpartum patients (124). It can be caused by compression of the nerve within the obturator canal due to exaggerated lithotomy position, and can also be secondary to compression by the fetal head at the pelvic brim (127). It is associated with diminished sensation on the upper inner thigh, and weakness of hip adduction and rotation (Fig. 26-5).

■ PRE-EXISTING DISEASE AND THE RISK OF NEUROLOGIC INJURY

Pregnant patients may have any of a variety of pre-existing disorders that may increase the risk of neurologic complications after neuraxial anesthesia. Hebl et al. reviewed the experience with 937 patients at the Mayo Clinic who carried a diagnosis of **spinal stenosis** or **lumbar disk disease** and received neuraxial anesthesia over a 15-year period (128). New neurologic deficits or worsening of pre-existing deficits were seen in 1.1% of patients, higher than the rate reported in previous studies of the general population (1,2). The presence of preoperative compressive radiculopathy or multiple neurologic diagnoses were risk factors for postoperative injury; previous spinal surgery, however, did not increase risk. It is not clear that this study is directly applicable to the obstetric population, however, as 8 of 10 patients with new or worsened deficits were greater than 70 years of age. The most common vertebral column abnormalities seen in the obstetric population are corrected or uncorrected **scoliosis**; while success rates for neuraxial anesthesia are lower and complication rates are higher, these techniques are a viable option. Spinal anesthesia appears to have a higher success rate than epidural anesthesia in these patients, due to adhesions within

to poorly positioned stirrups when patients are placed in the lithotomy position. It may be difficult to distinguish this lesion from lumbosacral trunk injury, but normal ankle inversion and normal ankle jerk suggest the more peripheral lesion (127) (Fig. 26-4).

Meralgia paresthetica is the most common of the obstetric nerve palsies, seen in 0.4% of patients studied by Wong et al (124). This injury is secondary to compression of the lateral femoral cutaneous nerve under the inguinal ligament. There is a unique pattern of decreased sensation in the superior portion of the anterolateral thigh; motor impairment is absent. The major risk factor is prolonged hyperflexion of the hips, as in the lithotomy position or when a McRoberts maneuver is performed.

Femoral nerve palsy is the second most common injury seen in Wong's study (124). It can result from compression of the nerve within the pelvis by the fetal head or by retraction during pelvic surgery. It can also be compressed more peripherally under the inguinal ligament due to exaggerated hip flexion, but this mechanism is less common. This lesion presents with quadriceps weakness, perhaps most

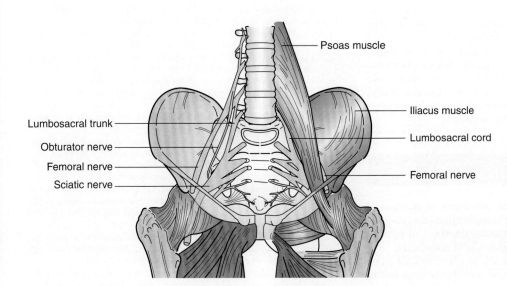

FIGURE 26-5 Pelvic branches of lumbosacral nerve roots. Note proximity of lumbosacral trunk to sacral ala, where it can be compressed by fetal head. The femoral nerve and obturator nerve can also be compressed by the fetus in their intrapelvic course.

the epidural space and restricted spread of local anesthetic within the space. Ultrasound guidance may improve success rates (129,130).

Parturients with **multiple sclerosis** clearly have an increased rate of relapse in the first three postpartum months (131,132), and there are some who would argue that a neuraxial anesthetic will be implicated should such a relapse occur, and should therefore be avoided. However, Bader et al. demonstrated that the rate of relapse was no higher in women who received epidural analgesia than in those who received local anesthetic infiltration alone (133). Hebl et al. showed a similar lack of effect of neuraxial anesthesia in patients with multiple sclerosis as well as a wide variety of other chronic neurologic diseases (134).

Reynolds points out that patients with **diabetes** may be vulnerable to neurologic complications of neuraxial anesthesia on several grounds: They are susceptible to infection, they may have vascular disease, and they may have a peripheral neuropathy (118). Hebl et al. retrospectively investigated 567 patients with pre-existing peripheral sensorimotor neuropathy or diabetic polyneuropathy who underwent neuraxial anesthesia. Two patients suffered a new or worsening deficit in the postoperative period (135). While low, this still represented a higher level of postoperative neurologic deficit than that reported in the general population (1,2).

Vascular abnormalities may predispose the parturient to neurologic injury in the postpartum period. An arteriovenous malformation of the spinal cord can decrease cord perfusion through a steal effect, rupture and production of an epidural hematoma, or compression of the cord via mass effect. In patients with a so-called "high take-off" of the artery of Adamkiewicz, perfusion of the lower spinal cord will be dependent upon lumbar branches arising from the iliac arteries. These vessels can be compressed by the fetal head, resulting in spinal cord ischemia (118) (Fig. 26-6).

■ EVALUATION OF NEUROLOGIC DEFICIT AFTER REGIONAL ANESTHESIA

The most important step in evaluating a post-anesthetic neurologic deficit is to rule out a rapidly expanding mass lesion, such as an epidural hematoma or epidural abscess. As this cannot be overemphasized, the prognosis for recovery

decreases dramatically if relief of compression is delayed for more than 8 hours; urgent radiologic investigation should not be delayed if there is any suggestion of spinal cord compression.

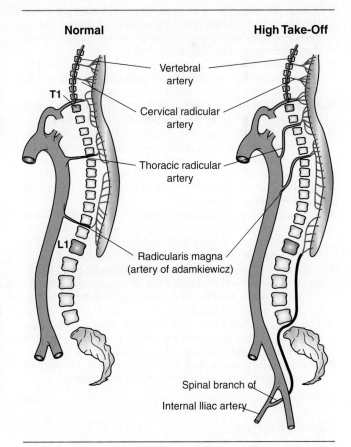

FIGURE 26-6 Variant arterial supply to spinal cord. Left, normal take-off of Artery of Adamkiewicz. Right, high take-off of artery. Note that arterial supply of lower spinal cord arises from spinal branch of iliac artery that can be compressed by fetus.

With a nonprogressive deficit, investigation can occur at a more leisurely pace. History and physical examination alone may be sufficient to make the diagnosis of obstetric nerve palsy. The use of both routine lumbosacral films and more advanced imaging techniques can be helpful in delineating the anatomic location of an injury. EMG can be helpful in defining both the anatomic and temporal locations of a lesion, as denervation potentials do not develop until 2 weeks after a nerve injury; the presence of such potentials soon after a regional anesthetic suggests that the injury preceded the anesthetic.

KEY POINTS

- The increasing use of neuraxial anesthesia in obstetrics, while decreasing the number of complications due to general anesthesia, has led to increasing numbers of neurologic complications of spinal and epidural anesthesia.
- Nevertheless, pregnant women are at lower risk of neurologic complications of neuraxial anesthesia than is the general population, due to their younger age, their lack of comorbidities, and the decreased use of anticoagulants.
- Careful attention to aseptic technique is essential to the prevention of infectious complications of neuraxial anesthesia. Face masks are essential during neuraxial anesthesia.
- Chlorhexidine–alcohol skin preparation solutions provide more effective and more prolonged skin antisepsis than povidone–iodine solutions, with no greater risk of neurologic injury.
- The great majority of cases of bacterial meningitis seen after spinal anesthesia is not community-acquired, but is due to streptococcal species that are often cultured from the oropharynx of the anesthesiologist.
- Neurologic deficit due to compression of the spinal cord by epidural abscess or epidural hematoma must be definitively addressed within 8 hours if full recovery is to occur.
- Neuraxial anesthesia is safe in patients with a platelet count as low as $75 \times 10^9/L$ in the absence of other risk factors.
- Guidelines of the American Society of Regional Anesthesia for patients receiving medications affecting coagulation will minimize the risk of neuraxial hematoma.
- Reinjection of lidocaine after failed spinal anesthesia should be undertaken with great caution due to the risk of cauda equina syndrome.
- Estimation of spinal interspace level is difficult to perform accurately based on anatomic landmarks alone. Therefore, dural puncture should preferentially be performed at the L3 to L4 interspace to minimize the risk of direct spinal cord injury.
- It is essential for the obstetric anesthesiologist to be familiar with the clinical characteristics of the common obstetric nerve palsies in order to distinguish them from deficits related to neuraxial anesthesia.
- Pre-existing conditions such as spinal stenosis, diabetes, and vascular malformations may predispose the parturient to neurologic complications of neuraxial anesthesia.
- EMG can be a useful tool in determining the etiology of neurologic deficits seen after neuraxial anesthesia.

REFERENCES

1. Auroy Y, Benhamou D, Barques L, et al. Major complications of regional anesthesia in France: The SOS Regional Anesthesia Hotline Service. *Anesthesiology* 2002;97:1274–1280.
2. Moen V, Dahlgren N, Irestedt L. Severe neurological complications after central neuraxial blockades in Sweden, 1990–1999. *Anesthesiology* 2004;101:950–959.
3. Cook TM, Counsell D, Wildsmith JAW. Major complications of central neuraxial block. Report on the Third National Audit Project of the Royal College of Anaesthetists. *Br J Anaesth* 2009;102:179–190.
4. Davies JM, Posner KL, Lee LA, et al. Liability associated with obstetric anesthesia: A closed claims analysis. *Anesthesiology* 2009;110:131–139.
5. Reynolds F. Neurological infections after neuraxial anesthesia. *Anesthesiol Clin* 2008;26:23–52.
6. Wang LP, Hauerberg J, Schmidt JF. Incidence of spinal epidural abscess after epidural analgesia: A national 1-year survey. *Anesthesiology* 1999;91:1928–1936.
7. Loo CC, Dahlgren G, Irestedt L. Neurological complications in obstetric regional anaesthesia. *Int J Obstet Anesth* 2000;9:99–124.
8. Kindler CH, Seeberger MD, Staender SE. Epidural abscess complicating epidural anesthesia and analgesia. *Acta Anaesthesiol Scand* 1998;42:614–620.
9. Sakuragi T, Yanagisawa K, Dan K. Bactericidal activity of skin disinfectants on methicillin-resistant Staphylococcus aureus. *Anesth Analg* 1995;81:555–558.
10. Mimoz O, Pieroni L, Lawrence C, et al. Prospective, randomized trial of two antiseptic solutions for prevention of central venous or arterial catheter colonization and infection in intensive care unit patients. *Crit Care Med* 1996;24:1818–1823.
11. Maki DG, Ringer M, Alvarado CJ. Prospective randomised trial of povidone-iodine, alcohol, and chlorhexidine for prevention of infection associated with central venous and arterial catheters. *Lancet* 1991;338:339–343.
12. Birnbach DJ, Meadows W, Stein DJ, et al. Comparison of povidone iodine and DuraPrep, an iodophor-in-isopropyl alcohol solution, for skin disinfection prior to epidural catheter insertion in parturients. *Anesthesiology* 2003;98:164–169.
13. Hebl JR, Niesen AD. Infectious complications of regional anesthesia. *Curr Opin Anaesthesiol* 2011;573–580.
14. ChloraPrep: Labeled warnings. http://www.carefusion.com/medical-products/infection-prevention/skin-preparation/labeled-warnings.aspx. Accessed July 28, 2012.
15. American Society of Anesthesiologists Task Force on infectious complications associated with neuraxial techniques. Practice advisory for the prevention, diagnosis, and management of infectious complications associated with neuraxial techniques. *Anesthesiology* 2010;112:530–545.
16. Hebl JR. The importance and implications of aseptic techniques during regional anesthesia. *Reg Anesth Pain Med* 2006;31:311–323.
17. Sviggum HP, Jacob AK, Arendt KW, et al. Neurologic complications after chlorhexidine antisepsis for spinal anesthesia. *Reg Anesth Pain Med* 2012;37:139–144.
18. Doan L, Piskoun B, Rosenberg AD, et al. In vitro antiseptic effects on viability of neuronal and Schwann cells. *Reg Anesth Pain Med* 2012;37:131–138.
19. Philips BJ, Fergusson S, Armstrong P, et al. Surgical face masks are effective in reducing bacterial contamination caused by dispersal from the upper airway. *Br J Anaesth* 1992;69:407–408.
20. CDC Clinical reminder: Spinal injection procedures performed without a facemask pose risk for bacterial meningitis. http://www.cdc.gov/injectionsafety/PDF/Clinical_Reminder_Spinal-Infection_Meningitis.pdf. Accessed July 28, 2012.
21. Lee JJ, Parry H. Bacterial meningitis following spinal anaesthesia for caesarean section. *Br J Anaesth* 1991;66:383–386.
22. Davis L, Hargreaves C, Robinson PN. Postpartum meningitis. *Anaesthesia* 1993;48:788–789.
23. Lurie S, Feinstein M, Heifetz C, et al. Iatrogenic bacterial meningitis after spinal anesthesia for pain relief in labor. *J Clin Anesth* 1999;11:438–439.
24. Centers for Disease Control and Prevention. Bacterial meningitis after intrapartum spinal anesthesia. *MMWR Morb Mortal Wkly Rep* 2010;59:65–69.
25. McKenzie AG, Darragh K. A national survey of prevention of infection in obstetric central neuraxial blockade in the UK. *Anaesthesia* 2011;66:497–502.
26. Morris W, Simon L, Pineiro A. Evaluation of antibacterial filters for peridural obstetrical anesthesia. *Ann Fr Anesth Reanim* 2001;20:600–603 [French].
27. Abouleish E, Amortegui AJ, Taylor FH. Are bacterial filters needed in continuous epidural analgesia for obstetrics? *Anesthesiology* 1977;46:351–354.
28. Bevacqua BK, Slucky AV, Cleary WF. Is postoperative intrathecal catheter use associated with central nervous system infection? *Anesthesiology* 1994;80:1234–1240.
29. Seth N, Macqueen S, Howard RF. Clinical signs of infection during continuous postoperative epidural analgesia in children: The value of catheter tip culture. *Paediatr Anaesth* 2004;14:996–1000.
30. James FM, George RH, Raiem H, et al. Bacteriologic aspects of epidural analgesia. *Anesth Analg* 1976;55:187–190.
31. Rosenberg PH, Renkonen OV. The antimicrobial activity of bupivacaine and morphine. *Anesthesiology* 1985;62:178–179.
32. Sakuragi T, Ishino H, Dan K. Bactericidal activity of preservative-free bupivacaine on microorganisms in the human skin flora. *Acta Anaesthesiol Scand* 1998;42:1096–1099.

33. Feldman JM, Chapin-Robertson K, Turner J. Do agents used for epidural analgesia have antimicrobial properties? *Reg Anesth* 1994;19:43–47.

34. Zaidi S, Healy TEJ. A comparison of the antibacterial properties of six local analgesic agents. *Anaesthesia* 1977;32:69–70.

35. Hodson M, Gajraj R, Scott NB. A comparison of the antibacterial activity of levobupivacaine vs. bupivacaine: An in vitro study with bacteria implicated in epidural infection. *Anaesthesia* 1999;54:683–702.

36. Pere P, Lindgren L, Vaara M. Poor antibacterial effect of ropivacaine: Comparison with bupivacaine. *Anesthesiology* 1999;91:884–886.

37. Aydin ON, Eyigor M, Aydin N. Antimicrobial activity of ropivacaine and other local anaesthctics. *Eur J Anaesthiol* 2001;18:687–694.

38. Kastango ES, Bradshaw BD. USP chapter 797: Establishing a practice standard for compounding sterile preparations in pharmacy. *Am J Health Syst Pharm* 2004;61:1928–1938.

39. The ASHP Discussion Guide on USP Chapter 797. www.ashp.org/s_ashp/docs/files/discguide797-2008.pdf. Accessed July 28, 2012.

40. Head S, Enneking FK. Infusate contamination in regional anesthesia: What every anesthesiologist should know. *Anesth Analg* 2008;107:1412–1418.

41. Carp H, Bailey S. The association between meningitis and dural puncture in bacteremic rats. *Anesthesiology* 1992;76:667–669.

42. Wedel DJ, Horlocker TT. Regional anesthesia in the febrile or infected patient. *Reg Anesth Pain Med* 2006;31:324–333

43. Bader AM, Gilbertson L, Kirz L, et al. Regional anesthesia in women with chorioamnionitis. *Reg Anesth* 1992;17:84–86.

44. Goodman EJ, DeHorta E, Taguiam JM. Safety of spinal and epidural anesthesia in parturients with chorioamnionitis. *Reg Anesth* 1996;21:436–441.

45. Reihsaus E, Waldbaur H, Seeling W. Spinal epidural abscess: A meta-analysis of 915 patients. *Neurosurg Rev* 2000;232:175–204.

46. Steffen P, Seeling W, Esig A, et al. Bacterial contamination of epidural catheters: Microbiological examination of 502 epidural catheters used for postoperative analgesia. *J Clin Anesth* 2004;16:92–97.

47. Diehn FE. Imaging of spine infection. *Radiol Clin N Am* 2012;50: 777–798.

48. Veiga Sanchez AR. Vertebral osteomyelitis and epidural abscess after epidural anesthesia for a cesarean section. *Rev Esp Anestesiol Reanim* 2004;51:44–46 [Spanish].

49. Chiang HL, Chia YY, Chen YS, et al. Epidural abscess in an obstetric patient with patient-controlled epidural analgesia: A case report. *Int J Obstet Anesth* 2005;14:242–245.

50. Perez-Toro MR, Burton AW, Hamid B, et al. Two-tuohy needle and catheter technique for fluoroscopically guided percutaneous drainage of spinal epidural abscess: A case report. *Pain Med* 2009;10:501–505.

51. Siddiq F, Malik AR, Smego RA. Percutaneous computed tomography-guided needle aspiration drainage of spinal epidural abscess. *South Med J* 2006; 99:1406–1407.

52. Siddiq F, Chowfin A, Tight R, et al. Medical vs. surgical management of spinal epidural abscess. *Arch Intern Med* 2004;164:2409–2412.

53. Vandermeulen EP, Van Aken H, Vermylen J. Anticoagulants and spinal-epidural anesthesia. *Anesth Analg* 1994;79:1165–1177.

54. Scott DB, Hibbard BM. Serious non-fatal complications associated with extradural block in obstetric practice. *Br J Anaesth* 1990;64:537–541.

55. Scott DB, Tunstall ME. Serious complications associated with epidural/spinal blockade in obstetrics: A two-year prospective study. *Int J Obstet Anesth* 1995;4:133–139.

56. Usubiaga JE, Wikinski JA, Usubiaga LE. Epidural pressure and its relation to the spread of anesthetic solutions in the epidural space. *Anesth Analg* 1967;46:440–446.

57. Bose S, Ali Z, Rath GP, et al. Spontaneous spinal epidural haematoma: A rare cause of quadriplegia in the post-partum period. *Br J Anaesth* 2007;99: 855–857.

58. Kadir RA, McLintock C. Thrombocytopenia and disorders of platelet function in pregnancy. *Semin Thromb Hemost* 2011;37:640–652.

59. Ramanathan J, Sibai BM, Vu T, et al. Correlation between bleeding times and platelet counts in women with preeclampsia undergoing cesarean section. *Anesthesiology* 1989;71:188–191.

60. Sharma SK, Philip J, Whitten CW, et al. Assessment of changes in coagulation in parturients with preeclampsia using thromboelastography. *Anesthesiology* 1999;90:385–390.

61. Channing Rodgers RP, Levin J. A critical reappraisal of the bleeding time. *Semin Thromb Hemost* 1990;16:1–30.

62. Beilin Y, Zahn J, Comerford M. Safe epidural analgesia in thirty parturients with platelet counts between 69,000 and 98,000 mm^{-3}. *Anesth Analg* 1997;85:385–388.

63. Rasmus KT, Rottman RL, Kotelko DM, et al. Unrecognized thrombocytopenia and regional anesthesia in parturients: A retrospective review. *Obstet Gynecol* 1989;73:943–946.

64. Webert KE, Mittal R, Sigouin C, et al. A retrospective 11-year analysis of obstetric patients with idiopathic thrombocytopenic purpura. *Blood* 2003; 102:4306–4311.

65. Dennis AT. Management of pre-eclampsia: Issues for anaesthetists. *Anaesthesia*; Epub ahead of print 26 June 2012; http://dx.doi.org/10.1111/j.1365-2044.2012.07195.x, accessed August 2, 2012.

66. Van Veen JJ, Nokes TJ, Makris M. The risk of spinal haematoma following neuraxial anesthesia or lumbar puncture in thrombocytopenic individuals. *Br J Haematol* 2010;148:15–25.

67. Fujita A, Sakai R, Matsuura S, et al. A retrospective analysis of obstetric patients with idiopathic thrombocytopenic purpura: A single center study. *Int J Hematol* 2010;92:463–467.

68. Basaran A, Basaran M, Sen C. Choice of glucocorticoid in HELLP syndrome-dexamethasone vs. betamethasone: Revisiting the dilemma. *J Matern Fetal Neonatal Med*; Epub ahead of print 30 July 2012. http://informahealthcare.com/doi/abs/10.3109/14767058.2012.712571, accessed August 2, 2012.

69. Woudstra DM, Chandra S, Hofmeyr GJ, et al. Corticosteroids for HELLP (hemolysis, elevated liver enzymes, low platelets) syndrome in pregnancy. *Cochrane Database of Syst Rev* 2010;Issue 9. Art. No: CD008148. doi:10.1002/14651858.

70. Horlocker TT, Wedel DJ, Rowlingson JC. Regional anesthesia in the patient receiving antithrombotic or thrombolytic therapy. American Society of Regional Anesthesia and Pain Medicine Evidence-Based Guidelines (Third Edition). *Reg Anesth Pain Med* 2010;35:64–101.

71. Roberge S, Giguere Y, Villa P, et al. Early administration of low-dose aspirin for the prevention of severe and mild preeclampsia: A systematic review and meta-analysis. *Am J Perinatol* 2012;29:551–556.

72. CLASP: A randomised trial of low-dose aspirin for the prevention and treatment of pre-eclampsia among 9364 pregnant women. CLASP (Collaborative Low-dose Aspirin Study in Pregnancy) Collaborative Group. *Lancet* 1994;343:619–629.

73. Liu SS, Mulroy MF. Neuraxial anesthesia and analgesia in the presence of standard heparin. *Reg Anesth Pain Med* 1998;23:157–163.

74. Bergqvist D, Lindblad B, Mätzsch T. Risk of combining low molecular weight heparin for thromboprophylaxis and epidural or spinal anesthesia. *Semin Thromb Hemost* 1993;19(suppl 1):147–151.

75. Tryba M. Hemostatic requirements for the performance of regional anesthesia. Workshop on hemostatic problems in regional anesthesia. *Reg Anaesth* 1989;12:127–131 [German].

76. Shin SW, Yoon JU, Baik SW, et al. Accidental epidural injection of rocuronium. *J Anesth* 2011;25:753–755.

77. Sofianou A, Chatzieleftheriou A, Mavrommati P, et al. Accidental epidural administration of succinylcholine. *Anesth Analg* 2006;102:1139–1140.

78. Krataijan J, Laeni N. Accidental epidural injection of pancuronium. *Anesth Analg* 2005;100:1546–1547.

79. Furuya T, Suzuki T, Yokotsuka S, et al. Prolonged neuromuscular block after an accidental epidural injection of vecuronium. *J Clin Anesth* 2011;23:673.

80. Huang JJ. Inadvertent epidural injection of ondansetron. *J Clin Anesth* 2006; 18:216–217.

81. Weigert A, Lawton G. Accidental injection of thiopental into the epidural space. *Eur J Anaesthesiol* 2000;17:69–70.

82. Courrèges P. Inadvertent epidural infusion of paracetamol in a child. *Paediatr Anaesth* 2005;15:1128–1130.

83. Peduto VA, Mezzetti D, Gori F. A clinical diagnosis of inadvertent epidural administration of potassium chloride. *Eur J Anaesthesiol* 1999;16:410–412.

84. O'Connor M. Responsiveness to the chlorhexidine epidural tragedy: A mental block? *J Law Med* 2012;19:436–443.

85. Birnbach DJ, Vincent CA. A matter of conscience: A call to action for system improvements involving epidural and spinal catheters. *Anesth Analg* 2012;114:494–496.

86. Ready LB, Plumer MH, Haschke RH, et al. Neurotoxicity of intrathecal local anesthetics in rabbits. *Anesthesiology* 1985;63:364–370.

87. Myers RR, Sommer C. Methodology for spinal neurotoxicity studies. *Reg Anesth* 1993;18:439–447.

88. Kalichman MW, Calcutt NA. Local anesthetic-induced conduction block and nerve fiber injury in streptozotocin-diabetic rats. *Anesthesiology* 1992;77:941–947.

89. Rigler ML, Drasner K, Krejcie TC, et al. Cauda equina syndrome after continuous spinal anesthesia. *Anesth Analg* 1991;72:275–281.

90. Schell RM, Brauer FS, Cole DJ, et al. Persistent sacral nerve root deficits after continuous spinal anesthesia. *Can J Anaesth* 1991;38:908–911.

91. Rigler ML, Drasner K. Distribution of catheter-injected local anesthetic in a model of the subarachnoid space. *Anesthesiology* 1991;75:684–692.

92. FDA Safety Alert: Cauda equina syndrome associated with use of small-bore catheters in continuous spinal anesthesia. http://www.fda.gov/MedicalDevices/Safety/AlertsandNotices/PublicHealthNotifications/ucm242746.htm. Accessed August 4, 2012.

93. Schneider M, Ettlin T, Kaufmann M, et al. Transient neurologic toxicity after hyperbaric subarachnoid anesthesia with 5% lidocaine. *Anesth Analg* 1993;76:1154–1157.

94. Freedman JM, Li DK, Drasner K, et al. Transient neurologic symptoms after spinal anesthesia: An epidemiologic study of 1,863 patients. *Anesthesiology* 1998;89:633–641.

95. Philip J, Sharma SK, Gottumukkala VNR, et al. Transient neurologic symptoms after spinal anesthesia with lidocaine in obstetric patients. *Anesth Analg* 2001;92:405–409.

96. Aouad MT, Siddik SS, Jalbout MI, et al. Does pregnancy protect against intrathecal lidocaine-induced transient neurologic symptoms? *Anesth Analg* 2001;92:401–404.

97. Johnson ME, Uhl CB, Spittler KH, et al. Mitochondrial injury and caspase activation by the local anesthetic lidocaine. *Anesthesiology* 2004;101:1184–1194.

98. Pollock JE, Burkhead D, Neal JM, et al. Spinal nerve function in five volunteers experiencing transient neurologic symptoms after lidocaine subarachnoid anesthesia. *Anesth Analg* 2000;90:658–65.

99. Schneider MC, Birnbach DJ. Lidocaine neurotoxicity in the obstetric patient: Is the water safe?. *Anesth Analg* 2001;92:287–290.

100. Forster JG, Rosenberg PH. Revival of old local anesthetics for spinal anesthesia in ambulatory surgery. *Curr Opin Anaesthesiol* 2011;24:633–637.

101. Kasaba T, Onizuka S, Takasaki M. Procaine and mepivacaine have less toxicity in vitro than other clinically used local anesthetics. *Anesth Analg* 2003;97:85–90.

102. Hashimoto K, Sakura S, Bollen AW, et al. Comparative toxicity of glucose and lidocaine administered intrathecally in the rat. *Reg Anesth Pain Med* 1998;23:444–450.

103. Drasner K. Lidocaine spinal anesthesia: A vanishing therapeutic index? *Anesthesiology* 1997;87:469–472.

104. Covino BG, Marx GF, Finster M, Zsigmond EK. Prolonged sensory/motor deficits following inadvertent spinal anesthesia. *Anesth Analg* 1980;59:399–400.

105. Ravindran RS, Bond VK, Tasch MD, et al. Prolonged neural blockade following regional analgesia with 2-chloroprocaine. *Anesth Analg* 1980;59:447–451.

106. Reisner LS, Hochman BN, Plumer MH. Persistent neurologic deficit and adhesive arachnoiditis following intrathecal 2-chloroprocaine injection. *Anesth Analg* 1980;59:452–454.

107. Gissen A, Datta S, Lambert D. The chloroprocaine controversy: II. Is chloroprocaine neurotoxic? *Reg Anesth* 1984;9:135–144.

108. Taniguchi M, Bollen AW, Drasner K. Sodium bisulfite: Scapegoat for chloroprocaine neurotoxicity? *Anesthesiology* 2004;100:85–91.

109. Lambert DH, Strichartz GR. In defense of in vitro findings. *Anesthesiology* 2004;101:1246–1247.

110. Gonter AF, Kopacz DJ. Spinal 2-chloroprocaine: A comparison with procaine in volunteers. *Anesth Analg* 2005;100:573–579.

111. Kouri ME, Kopacz DJ. Spinal 2-chloroprocaine: A comparison with lidocaine in volunteers. *Anesth Analg* 2004;98:75–80.

112. Yoos JR, Kopacz DJ. Spinal 2-chloroprocaine: A comparison with small-dose bupivacaine in volunteers. *Anesth Analg* 2005;100:566–572.

113. Sell A, Tein T, Pitkanen M. Spinal 2-chloroprocaine: Effective dose for ambulatory surgery. *Acta Anaesthesiol Scand* 2008;52:695–699.

114. Reynolds F. Case report: Damage to the conus medullaris following spinal anaesthesia. *Anaesthesia* 2001;56:238–247.

115. Saifuddin A, Burnett SJ, White J. The variation of position of the conus medullaris in an adult population. A magnetic resonance imaging study. *Spine* 1998;23:1452–1456.

116. Hogan QH. Tuffier's line: The normal distribution of anatomic parameters. *Anesth Analg* 1994;78:194–195.

117. Margarido CB, Mikhael R, Arzola C, et al. The intercristal line determined by palpation is not a reliable anatomical landmark for neuraxial anesthesia. *Can J Anaesth* 2011;58:262–266.

118. Reynolds F. Neurologic complications of pregnancy and regional anesthesia. In: Chestnut DH, Polley LS, Tsen LC, Wong CA, eds. *Obstetric Anesthesia: Principles and Practice.* 4th ed. Philadelphia, PA: Elsevier Mosby; 2009:701–726.

119. Wong CA. Nerve injuries after neuraxial anesthesia and their medicolegal implications. *Best Pract Res Clin Obstet Gynaecol* 2010;24:367–381.

120. Van Gessel EF, Forster A, Gamulin Z. Continuous spinal anesthesia: Where do spinal catheters go? *Anesth Analg* 1993;76:1004–1007.

121. Broadbent CR, Maxwell WB, Ferrie R, et al. Ability of anaesthetists to identify a marked lumbar interspace. *Anaesthesia* 2000;55:1122–1126.

122. Reynolds F. Logic in the safe practice of spinal anesthesia. *Anaesthesia* 2000;55:1045–1046.

123. Horlocker T. Complications of regional anesthesia and acute pain management. *Anesthesiol Clin* 2011;29:257–278.

124. Wong CA, Scavone BM, Dugan S, et al. Incidence of postpartum lumbosacral spine and lower extremity nerve injuries.*Obstet Gynecol* 2003;101:279–288.

125. Dar AQ, Robinson APC, Lyons G. Postpartum neurological symptoms following regional blockade: A prospective study with case controls. *Int J Obstet Anesth* 2002;11:85–90.

126. Donaldson JO. Neuropathy. In: *Neurology of Pregnancy.* 2nd ed. London: W.B. Saunders; 1989:23–59.

127. Wong CA. Neurologic deficits and labor analgesia. *Reg Anesth Pain Med* 2004;29:341–351.

128. Hebl JR, Horlocker TT, Kopp SL, et al. Neuraxial blockade in patients with preexisting spinal stenosis, lumbar disk disease, or prior spine surgery: Efficacy and neurologic complications. *Anesth Analg* 2010;111:1511–1519.

129. Ko JY, Leffert LR. Clinical implications of neuraxial anesthesia in the parturient with scoliosis. *Anesth Analg* 2009;109:1930–1934.

130. Vercauteren M, Waets P, Pitkanen M, et al. Neuraxial techniques in patients with pre-existing back impairment or prior spine interventions: A topical review with special reference to obstetrics. *Acta Anaesthesiol Scand* 2011;55:910–917.

131. Confavreux C, Hutchinson M, Hours MM, et al. Rate of pregnancy-related relapse in multiple sclerosis. Pregnancy in Multiple Sclerosis Group. *N Engl J Med* 1998;339:285–291.

132. Vukusic S, Hutchinson M, Hours M, et al. Pregnancy and multiple sclerosis (the PRIMS study): Clinical predictors of post-partum relapse. *Brain* 2004;127:1353–1360.

133. Bader AM, Hunt CO, Datta S, et al. Anesthesia for the obstetric patient with multiple sclerosis. *J Clin Anesth* 1988;1:21–24.

134. Hebl JR, Horlocker TT, Schroeder DR. Neuraxial anesthesia and analgesia in patients with preexisting central nervous system disorders. *Anesth Analg* 2006;103:223–228.

135. Hebl JR, Kopp SL, Schroeder DR, et al. Neurologic complications after neuraxial anesthesia or analgesia in patients with preexisting peripheral sensorimotor neuropathy or diabetic polyneuropathy. *Anesth Analg* 2006;103:1294–1299.

CHAPTER
27

Postdural Puncture Headache

Alice L. Oswald

■ INTRODUCTION

Postdural puncture headache (PDPH) is a frequent complication of dural puncture, whether it is performed for diagnostic or therapeutic purposes, or occurs during placement of neuraxial blockade. It is also known as a spinal or post-spinal headache. Prophylaxis and treatment of this subject has been studied and discussed for more than 100 years, but for the most part, a clear consensus is lacking. The headache can be incapacitating for a postpartum patient since these women have to care for a newborn and recover from delivery while dealing with the headache. As a result, this patient population is frequently studied in regards to PDPH. Labor epidural analgesia is frequently an elective procedure, so morbidity from possible iatrogenic injury is quite unfortunate.

The headache is usually described as a severe frontal or occipital pain that is exacerbated by sitting up or standing and partially relieved in the supine position (see Fig. 27-1). Accompanying symptoms may consist of tinnitus and hyperacusis, diplopia, nausea and vomiting, or neck pain (1,2). The International Classification of Headache Disorders (ICHD) published by the International Headache Society is considered the official classification of headache-related disorders by the World Health Organization. Their diagnostic criteria, first published in 1998 and revised in 2003 (ICHD-2), is used in the International Classification of Diseases (ICD-10). The criteria for PDPH is outlined in Table 27-1. Auditory symptoms result from dysfunction of the VIII cranial nerve and may occur because the circulation of endolymph in the cochleae and semicircular canals is dependent on cerebrospinal fluid (CSF) pressure (3). The visual disturbances may occur because the VI cranial nerve has a long intracranial course. Symptoms will usually present within 48 hours after dural puncture, but can take up to 7 days to appear (4). PDPH is usually a self-limiting condition and will resolve within 2 to 14 days. If the headache persists, it may be secondary to a CSF fistula, but other serious causes also need to be considered (5).

■ HISTORY

German physician Heinrich Quincke introduced needle lumbar puncture in 1891 as a treatment to lower intracranial pressure in patients with tuberculosis meningitis and hydrocephalus. Around the same time, London physician Walter Wynter was also establishing this as a procedure by inserting a catheter into his patients with the purpose of removing CSF to treat meningitis (6–8). In 1895, a New York neurologist, Corning, is credited as performing the first spinal anesthetic when he tried using spinal cocaine as a local anesthetic to treat a man of habitual masturbation. He reported injecting cocaine at the T11/T12 interspace to decrease sensation of the lower limbs and groin (9,10) and observed a transient paralysis of the lower limbs. Corning recognized the potential use of the spinal anesthetic for surgery, so he worked on developing a spinal needle and introducer, and published his design in the New York Journal of Medicine. A couple of years later, a German surgeon Karl August Bier wrote about PDPH in 1898 after he injected 10 to 15 mg of spinal cocaine into himself, his assistant, and seven of his patients. Four of the nine people, including him, developed PDPH (11). Spinal anesthesia with large gauge needles soon became more frequently reported in the literature in the early 1900s and the headache that was associated with it seemed to affect about half the patients and was noted to last for about 24 hours (12). Around 1920, technologic advances from the introduction of stainless steel allowed a fine gauge needle to be sharpened to a point without deformation or breakage. Whitacre and Hart were not the first to develop the pencil-point spinal needle but are commonly associated with this advancement in design, and in 1951 they reported significant decrease in the incidence of PDPH using this modification. Since then, there have been some minor modifications to the pencil-point spinal needle, but the basic design has remained the same (12).

■ PATHOPHYSIOLOGY

Anatomy

The spinal dura mater extends from the foramen magnum to the second sacral spinal segment. It contains CSF and encases the spinal nerves after they leave the spinal cord. The pia mater and arachnoid fuse with the connective tissue of the spinal nerves, making up the lateral borders of the dural sac (see Fig. 27-2). The dura is a dense, connective tissue layer created by longitudinal lamella of collagen and elastin fibers. It was believed that these fibers ran in a longitudinal direction and this thought was initially supported by microscopic studies (13). However, more recent light and electron microscopic studies describe the dura mater as consisting of collagen fibers arranged in several layers parallel to the surface of the medulla spinalis. The direction of the fibers in each sub-lamina do not demonstrate any specific orientation (14). The outer layer may be arranged in a longitudinal direction but this is not necessarily repeated through the more interior dural layers.

CSF

Over 100 years ago, Bier attributed persistent leakage of CSF through the dural puncture as the cause of the headache, but today the exact mechanism is not still entirely clear. One theory is that when the patient's position changes

425

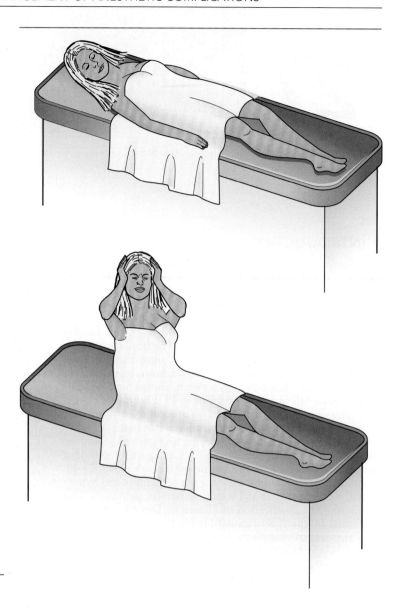

FIGURE 27-1 The postural component of PDPH.

from supine to an upright position, there is a downward traction on pain-sensitive nerves, intracranial veins, and meninges, which causes the pain. This sagging of intracranial structures has been demonstrated on magnetic resonance imaging (MRI) (15). If the leakage of CSF exceeds the rate of production, the cushioning effect on the brain is lost (16). The average production rate of CSF is 0.3 mL/kg/h, 0.3 to 0.4 mL/min, or about 500 mL/day for a 70 kg person. The total volume of CSF is about 150 mL at a given time, distributed half in the intracranial space and the other half cushioning the spinal cord. The choroid plexus secretes the majority of the CSF, and the rest is secreted by the brain (interstitial space of the brain, the ependymal lining of the ventricles, and the dura of the nerve root sleeves), as a byproduct of oxidative metabolism (17). Reabsorption of CSF is primarily by the arachnoid granulations in the venous sinuses.

Headache usually develops when more than 10% of CSF volume is lost (18). In a series of experiments, PDPH was induced in volunteers by draining 15 to 20 mL CSF uniformly and rapidly. Replacement of the CSF volume with

a sterile crystalloid relieved the headache completely and in less than a few minutes (18). Another cause of the headache could be from intracranial hypotension after leakage of CSF. This may explain why injection of the crystalloid into the epidural or subarachnoid space, or insertion of blood into the epidural space in an attempt to increase the epidural and subarachnoid pressure, can relieve a headache rapidly. Normal lumbar CSF pressure in the supine position is about 5 to 15 cm H_2O and can increase to about 40 cm H_2O in the sitting position (19).

In addition to the CSF, the arachnoid space contains veins that may dilate as a result of loss of CSF in order to maintain constant intracranial volume. This concept is defined by the Monro–Kellie doctrine, which states that the total intracranial volume is fixed because of the inelastic nature of the skull (20). The intracranial volume is equal to the sum of its components: Brain, CSF, and blood. When there is a decrease in one component, such as loss of CSF, the compensatory action to maintain constant intracranial volume may be vasodilation. Meningeal vessels may be pain sensitive and vasodilation can lead to increased cerebral blood flow. Also, when there is a

TABLE 27-1 Postdural (Post-Lumbar) Puncture Headache The International Headache Society's International Classification of Headache Disorders (ICHD-2)

Diagnostic Criteria
A. Headache that worsens within 15 min after sitting or standing and improves within 15 min after lying, with at least one of the following and fulfilling criteria C and D: 　1. Neck stiffness 　2. Tinnitus 　3. Hypacusia 　4. Photophobia 　5. Nausea B. Dural puncture has been performed C. Headache develops within 5 days after dural puncture D. Headache resolves either[a]: 　1. Spontaneously within 1 wk 　2. Within 48 h after effective treatment of the spinal fluid leak (usually by epidural blood patch)

[a]In 95% of cases this is so. When headache persists, causation is in doubt.

sudden decrease in CSF volume, adenosine receptors may be activated to compensate by producing arterial and venous vasodilation. The relief of headache with caffeine supports the vascular theory of PDPH from vasodilation since caffeine inhibits adenosine receptors to act as a cerebral vasoconstrictor (21).

■ INCIDENCE

Reported frequency rates of headache after intentional dural puncture range from 6% to 36% of patients depending on the needle size and type of needle used (see Table 27-2) (22). The frequency of accidental dural puncture (ADP) after attempted epidural placement ranges from 0.19% to 3.6% (23–28). The injury could be from obvious perforation of the dura by the epidural needle, or a nick in the dura that either leads to an unrecognized dural puncture or subsequent perforation of the dura by the epidural catheter. The number of previous epidural anesthetics placed may affect the incidence of ADP (27). In a series of 4,600 women who received an epidural, there were 74 occurrences of ADP. Anesthesiologists who had placed less than 10 prior epidurals had an ADP rate of 2.5%, which was almost twice the rate of 1.3% in those practitioners who had placed more than 90 epidurals (29,30). If there was an ADP during attempted epidural with a large-bore needle, most studies report the incidence of PDPH being 16% to 86% (4,31–34), with the meta-analysis done by Choi et al. in 2003 finding the overall incidence to be about 50% to 55% (4).

The frequency of ADP or PDPH does not appear increased with combined spinal–epidural (CSE) blocks compared to epidural blocks, even though there is an intentional dural puncture with the former (35,36). van de Velde et al. reported a low incidence of PDPH with CSEs using 27 or 29 G spinal needles in a 10-year single-institution prospective study (37). When CSEs were compared to single shot spinals, there was also not an increased risk of PDPH (37). His study confirmed previous reports that the incidence of ADP does not decrease when performing CSEs compared to performing epidural blocks (37,38). He hypothesized that the reason for the low

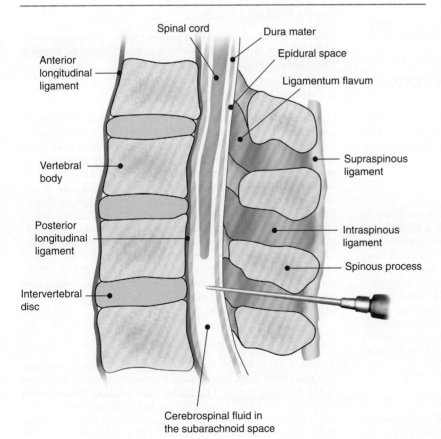

Spinal cord
Dura mater
Epidural space
Ligamentum flavum
Anterior longitudinal ligament
Vertebral body
Posterior longitudinal ligament
Intervertebral disc
Supraspinous ligament
Intraspinous ligament
Spinous process
Cerebrospinal fluid in the subarachnoid space

FIGURE 27-2 Anatomy of the lumbar spine.

TABLE 27-2 Frequency of PDPH with Different Spinal Needles

Needle Type	Needle Gauge	Frequency of PDPH (%)
Quincke	22	36
Quincke	24	11.2
Quincke	25	3–25
Quincke	26	0.3–20
Quincke	27	1.5–5.6
Quincke	29	0–2
Quincke	32	0.4
Sprotte	22	12.2
Sprotte	24	0–9.6
Pencan (Sprotte)	27	0.98
Whitacre	20	2–5
Whitacre	22	0.63–4
Whitacre	25	0–14.5
Whitacre	27	0–1.7
Atraucan	26	2.5–4.6
Tuohy	16	70

Adapted from: Turnbull DK, Shepherd DB. Post-dural puncture headache: Pathogenesis, prevention and treatment. *Br J Anaesth* 2003;91(5):718–729; and Bezov D, Ashina S, Lipton R. Post-dural puncture headache: Part II—prevention, management, and prognosis. *Headache* 2010;50(9):1482–1498.

incidence of PDPH with CSEs may be that there is decreased CSF leak from increased pressure of having volume in the epidural space.

■ PATIENT-DEPENDENT RISK FACTORS

Not every person that has a dural puncture will develop a headache afterward and the reasons for this are multifactorial. The obstetric population is particularly at risk since young, pregnant women are at an increased risk of developing PDPH.

Age

Patients between the ages of 20 and 30 are more likely to develop PDPH after a dural puncture (39,40). Children and patients who are older than 60 years do not commonly report the headache (40,41). This may be due to older people having lower CSF pressures (42,43) and decreased elasticity of the dura, so dural perforations may not stay patent as compared to dural punctures in younger people (16,44). Vandem and Dripps studied over 9,000 patients who had received a spinal anesthetic and found the incidence of PDPH in the 20- to 29-year-old age group to be 16%. This was significantly higher than the 40- to 49-year-old (8%) and 50- to 59-year-old (4%) age group (45).

Female Gender

Most large studies find that there is a significantly higher incidence of PDPH in women compared to men (45–47).

This may be a reporting error due to differences in pain perception or that women may be more likely to report a headache. Another explanation for this could be due to hormone-mediated cerebrovascular changes, similar to what might occur in migraine headaches. A large study of spinal anesthetics by Lybecker et al. found no significant association between gender and incidence of PDPH (40).

BMI

The incidence of PDPH is higher in people with a low BMI (31,48–50). One reason could be that there may be increased intra-abdominal pressure from obesity raising CSF pressure, so that even with a CSF leak, these patients do not develop headache. Another is that in attempted epidural placement, the epidural space may be unexpectedly shallow, resulting in an ADP. The incidence of ADP may be higher in the morbidly obese; however, there are not many studies that support this theory (37).

Pregnancy

It is unclear whether this is a risk factor by itself, published studies showing the opposite finding (51,52). Laboring patients may be at an increased risk because many of them receive epidural analgesia with a large-bore needle and good positioning may be challenging due to the gravid abdomen as well as influence of contraction pain.

Varying Dural Thickness

Recent studies have demonstrated that the dura has varying thickness. One reason that some people do not develop a PDPH may be that if the dural puncture occurs in a thicker area, a headache may not develop (12,14).

Other Possible Factors

Many studies have found that patients with a previous history of PDPH or chronic headache are more likely to develop PDPH (40,53,54).

■ DIFFERENTIAL DIAGNOSIS

Headache in the postpartum period is not an infrequent complaint, but this section will concentrate on headaches that have a postural component to them. Patients may present with a positional headache after experiencing intentional, inadvertent, or unrecognized dural puncture. About 40% of women will have a postpartum headache or neck pain in the week after delivery (55). Postpartum headache can be due to relatively benign reasons such as tension or migraine related, caffeine withdrawal, hunger, or sleep deprivation (56). Headaches that present immediately postpartum or more than 72 hours after delivery are not as likely to be PDPH, and other causes should be explored (55,56). The rare but potentially life-threatening diagnoses that are in the following discussion will usually need neuro-imaging and the assistance of a neurologic consultation.

Subdural Hemorrhage

This is a rare, but serious consequence of dural puncture that can occur from intracranial hypotension causing tearing of the bridging veins. The patient can initially present with symptoms of a PDPH, but then the headache becomes severe, non-postural, and associated with neurologic deficits. Zeidan et al. reported a patient who received spinal anesthesia with a 26 gauge (G) needle for cesarean section who postoperatively developed a severe non-postural headache associated with right eye tearing, V cranial nerve palsy, and left hemiparesis. A cranial subdural hematoma was confirmed with a computed tomography (CT) scan (57). He then performed a literature review and studied 46 patients who received spinal or epidural anesthesia and developed PDPH complicated by subdural hematoma. Most had associated neurologic deficits in addition to the severe headache. Sharma reported a case of a 31-year-old primigravid term woman who had a dural puncture during attempted epidural analgesia for labor and an intrathecal catheter was placed. Twenty-three hours later she had sudden loss of consciousness, her CT scan showed a large subdural hematoma, and craniotomy revealed active bleeding from a ruptured temporal bridging vein (58). Intracranial hypotension occurred while an intrathecal catheter was present demonstrating that the hypothetical plug that a large-bore catheter provides does not necessarily prevent efflux of CSF. Amorin reviewed 35 case reports of intracranial subdural hematoma that occurred after spinal anesthesia. These patients experienced headache (74%), changes in the level of consciousness (40%), vomiting (31%), hemiplegia or hemiparesis (23%), diplopia or VI cranial nerve paresis (14%), and language disorders (11%) (59). After this review, he recommended neuro-imaging evaluation in patients whose headache persisted for more than a week and with disappearance of the postural component. He determined contributing factors to include pregnancy, multiple attempts, use of anticoagulants, intracranial vascular abnormalities, and brain atrophy. In his review of 35 case reports, four patients (11.4%) did not survive (59). Subdural hematomas usually need to be surgically evacuated and time to evacuation is important depending on the size of the hematoma and how rapidly it is expanding (see Fig. 27-3).

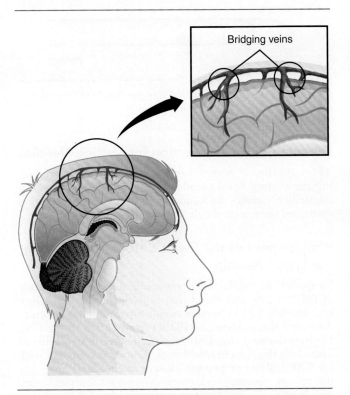

FIGURE 27-3 Bridging veins run between the surface of the brain and the dura mater of the skull.

Severe Preeclampsia or Eclampsia

If the patient had a headache and high blood pressure prior to or after a neuraxial block was placed, the diagnosis of preeclampsia would have to be considered. New seizure activity in this setting would also lead to increased suspicion of eclampsia or an intracranial vascular injury.

Venous Sinus Thrombosis/Cortical Vein Thrombosis

This predominantly occurs in females, the headache is acute in onset, there are focal neurologic signs, there can be a postural component, and it frequently presents during pregnancy and after delivery. Vasodilation that occurs as a result of CSF leakage has a role in the formation of thrombus. A stroke of venous origin is greater in pregnancy because of the prothrombotic state, and hypercoagulability is increased after delivery due to volume depletion and vascular trauma. MRI or angiography may be superior to CT in diagnosis in visualizing venous thrombosis (60). Therapy to prevent seizures and ischemia consists of heparin, oral anticoagulants, and possibly antibiotics for a favorable outcome.

Posterior Reversible (leuko) Encephalopathy Syndrome (PRES)

The symptoms of PRES include headache, focal neurologic deficits, seizures, acute changes in blood pressure, and altered mental status. The pathophysiology of PRES is severe hypertension or vasoconstriction leading to brain hypoperfusion that results in altered cerebrovascular regulation and vasogenic edema. PRES is associated with preeclampsia/eclampsia occurring postpartum, and the presence of a coincidental dural puncture may confuse or delay the diagnosis.

Meningitis

There is not usually a postural component to this, but meningitis is always of concern whenever a postpartum patient that has received a neuraxial block develops headache along with neck stiffness and fever. The white blood count is not as helpful in diagnosis because it is usually elevated after delivery. If meningitis is suspected, it would be sensible to obtain blood and CSF cultures and start prophylactic antibiotics immediately.

Pneumocephalus

If air is unintentionally injected into the subarachnoid space, usually occurring during epidural placement with loss-of-resistance to air technique, pneumocephalus may result. This air or gas may enter into the subarachnoid space and migrate intracranially resulting in meningeal irritation. The symptoms consist of pain in the neck and shoulder that may occur quickly after the neuraxial block was placed. This could also occur if there is a small, unrecognized dural puncture or nick that occurred during attempted epidural placement. Fortunately, it is usually a self-limited process and will resolve on its own within days.

■ IMAGING

When patients do not improve with treatment for presumed PDPH, develop focal neurologic signs, or new seizures, neuro-imaging should be used to diagnose or exclude more concerning causes of headache. Non-contrast CT is the initial

TABLE 27-3 Possible MRI Findings in Intracranial Hypotension (Gadolinium Enhanced)

- Diffuse non-nodular pachymeningeal enhancement due to dilation of men in seal vessels
- Descent of the cerebellar tonsils and/or medulla
- Obliteration of basilar cisterns
- Decreased ventricular size
- Enlargement of the pituitary gland
- Subdural fluid collections

study of choice to evaluate for hemorrhage or infarction, followed by MRI if needed. MRI may be helpful to show signs of intracranial hypotension (see Table 27-3) (61).

■ PREVENTION

Atraumatic Pencil-point Spinal Needles

The pencil-point spinal needle was introduced in 1951. It was believed that the pencil-point would stretch and separate the dural fibers instead of cutting them so that when the needle was removed, the dural fibers would return, decreasing the chance of leakage of CSF. Electron microscopy showed that lesions with a cutting type needle resulted in clean-cut openings while a pencil-point needle produced a more traumatic opening with tearing and severe disruption of the collagen fibers (14). A different study with electron microscopy also showed that atraumatic needles result in two to three times less CSF leakage compared to cutting needles of the same corresponding size (62). An older study done by Keener et al. stated that repair of the dural hole is facilitated by fibroblastic proliferation of the surrounding tissues and that the repair is better in the presence of a blood clot along with damage to the pia arachnoid and underlying brain (63,64). This may mean that if the perforation made by the spinal needle is too atraumatic, the dura may not heal as quickly. Introduction of the atraumatic needle has been the most significant development for the last 60 years in preventing PDPH. There are numerous large studies that have provided overwhelming evidence to support using atraumatic needles over cutting needles to decrease incidence of PDPH. Table 27-2 shows the frequency of PDPH with different types and gauges of commonly used spinal needles (65).

Use of atraumatic needles is recommended in the 2007 American Society of Anesthesiologists practice guideline for obstetric anesthesia. Also the most recent guideline published by the American Academy of Neurology (AAN) in 2005 supports the use of atraumatic pencil-point needles for diagnostic lumbar puncture to reduce the frequency of PDPH (66). The reason that some practitioners continue to use cutting needles may be because of the learning curve associated with use of atraumatic needles. The Whitacre and Sprotte needles frequently require an introducer to pass the needle through the skin, and the feel is different as the needle passes through the different muscles and ligaments (see Fig. 27-4 for images of the various needle type tips) (67,68). Another reason is delay by manufacturers to include atraumatic needles instead of cutting needles into spinal and diagnostic lumbar puncture trays (67). The flow rate may be thought to be less in atraumatic needles; however, this has been disproven (69). In addition, neurologists have been slow to make the switch from using cutting needles. Opening pressure measurements and flow rates with 20 G atraumatic needles were found to be adequate in a study that compared needles of comparable sizes (70). In a 2001 survey of AAN members, only 2% of neurologists surveyed reported using atraumatic needles frequently (71).

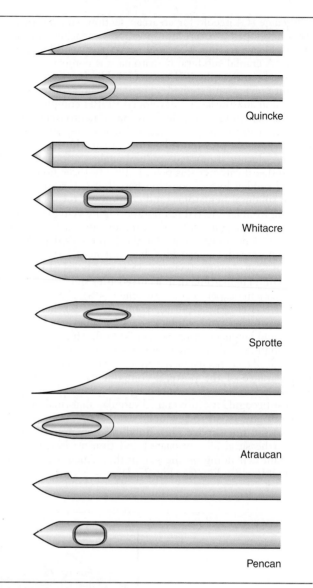

FIGURE 27-4 Types of spinal needle tips (not to scale).

(labels in figure, top to bottom:) Quincke / Whitacre / Sprotte / Atraucan / Pencan

Direction of Bevel Insertion for Cutting Needles

There are clinical studies that support the belief that orienting the cutting bevel parallel to the believed longitudinal dural fibers reduces the frequency of PDPH because there is decreased tension on the dural hole (40,72,73).

Replacement of the Stylet Before Withdrawing the Spinal Needle

Strupp et al. conducted a randomized prospective study of 600 patients and found that replacing the stylet before withdrawing a 21 G Sprotte needle after a lumbar puncture decreased the incidence of PDPH from 16.3% to 5% (74). He hypothesized that leakage of CSF may drag arachnoid mater into the open needle that on removal may act as a wick for CSF leakage or prevent closure of the dural hole. For this reason, neurologists commonly replace the stylet before withdrawing the needle when performing lumbar punctures. This has not been recommended in anesthesiology because medication is injected through the spinal needle that makes pulling arachnoid mater through the dural hole less likely.

There is one case report of transection and withdrawal of a nerve filament due to replacement of the stylet following a lumbar myelogram (75).

Smaller Needle Size

A smaller needle size is associated with reduced frequency of PDPH. However, if there is unrecognized dural puncture due to a slower flow from very small gauge needles, there could be multiple dural punctures, a greater failure rate, and this could increase the incidence of PDPH (65).

Ultrasound Guided Neuraxial Blocks

Schnabel et al. reviewed six clinical trials published between 2001 and 2009. This review of 659 patients made comparisons between the conventional loss-of-resistance technique and neuraxial blocks placed after prepuncture ultrasound scanning. His review found a 71% success rate with the first attempt in hypothetically difficult patients after ultrasound guidance versus a 20% rate using a conventional technique (76). His conclusions were that ultrasound-facilitated neuraxial blocks required a lower number of puncture attempts and fewer puncture levels (76). Prepuncture ultrasound scanning was used to identify the site, depth, and angle of the spinal processes (77). There was also a lower rate of ADP, PDPH, and injury to surrounding vasculature (76).

Other Techniques that May Affect the Incidence of PDPH

Seeberger et al. did a prospective analysis on 8,034 spinal anesthetics performed in one institution over 5 years and found that repeated dural punctures will increase the risk of PDPH significantly (78). There are studies that have found a decreased incidence of PDPH when the Tuohy needle was inserted with the bevel parallel to the long axis of the spine and other studies where no difference is found (79,80). There are some studies that evaluate insertion of the spinal needle at an acute angle or via a paramedian approach; however, there is not enough evidence to support these practices with respect to decreasing the PDPH rate (81,82). Some practitioners have adopted using saline for loss-of-resistance instead of air because there may be a decrease in frequency of PDPH from pneumocephalus-related headaches in the case of an ADP. Other techniques that have been evaluated in the past include placing patient supine or prone after ADP, evaluating the type of antiseptic used for the skin, and restricting maternal pushing for vaginal delivery (83). None of these methods have strong convincing clinical evidence or are applicable to modern clinical practice (26,28,51,84).

■ MEASURES TO DECREASE PDPH AFTER ACCIDENTAL DURAL PUNCTURE (ADP)

Apfel et al. published a very thorough quantitative systematic review of the prevention of PDPH after ADP. Seventeen studies were reviewed that included 1,264 patients. Prophylactic measures included threading an intrathecal catheter, prophylactic epidural blood patch (EBP), prophylactic epidural or intrathecal saline prior to removal of the catheter, and epidural morphine (85). This review found a limited number of randomized controlled trials (RCTs) and could not find clear evidence of the efficacy of any specific treatment. There was a favorable relative risk for two measures: Prophylactic EBP and use of epidural morphine (however, this was based on one study) (85). The other interventions mentioned were based on non-RCTs and failed statistical significance including those evaluating intrathecal catheters with a relative risk of 0.21 (0.02 to 2.65) (85).

Intrathecal Catheters

Some studies have shown that if ADP occurs with an epidural needle, there is a decrease in PDPH if the epidural catheter is threaded into the subdural space and left as an intrathecal catheter. There may be irritation/inflammation of the dura around the catheter to help the dural hole close after the catheter is removed. This is further supported by other studies that have shown that there is a larger decrease in the incidence of PDPH if the catheter is left in for more than 24 hours (86,87). However, this is not a consistent finding as shown by Kaul et al.'s published 5 year experience (88). Leaving an intrathecal catheter in place for more than 24 hours can be difficult if you are worried about an increased risk of infection or the possibility of unintended injection into the intrathecal catheter. One way to decrease the danger would be to ensure that the dressing is intact on the patient's back after delivery, and secure the epidural injection port by putting many knots in the epidural catheter and taping the injection port closed.

There was a multicenter trial published by Arkoosh in 2008 that used 28 G spinal catheters for labor analgesia (89). There was no difference found in PDPH, but there were more catheter failures compared to continuous epidural catheters and the continuous spinal catheters were more difficult to remove. Spinal catheters were originally introduced in 1989 as a way to decrease PDPH; however, in 1992 they were quickly banned in the United States due to reports of spinal cord toxicity from the concentrated local anesthetic (5% lidocaine) and reports of cauda equina syndrome. Baysinger et al. sent out a survey in 2008 to members of the Society of Obstetric Anesthesiology and Perinatology (SOAP); 160 (19%) out of 843 responses were received stating that after ADP, 25% of the respondents placed an intrathecal catheter and 75% of them would reattempt epidural placement. Out of those that would place an intrathecal catheter, 76% of them would leave it in place for 24 hours in an attempt to reduce the incidence of PDPH (90). In 2006, Harrington and Schmitt sent a survey to practicing members of the American Society of Regional Anesthesia and Pain Medicine (ASRA) in the United States, of which 1,024 (29.4%) surveys were returned. If an ADP occurred during epidural placement for labor analgesia, 73.4% respondents would attempt the epidural at another level and 19% would place an intrathecal catheter (91). If the anesthesiologist chose to place an intrathecal catheter, 56.5% of them would remove the catheter immediately after delivery (91). Marcus et al. also published results of a questionnaire that was sent to 709 anesthesiology departments in Germany with obstetric units, of which 360 of them were returned (50.8%), accounting for 330,000 births per year. After ADP, 69.9% responded that they would reattempt epidural placement at another level and 2.6% stated that they would place an intrathecal catheter (92).

Baraz and Collis sent out a questionnaire to all maternity units in the United Kingdom and received a 71% response. Of those that were returned, 144 units (85%) had written guidelines for the management of ADP. In 47 units (28%), an intrathecal catheter is threaded, and in 69 units (41%), a repeat epidural block is attempted at a different level. The top two reasons why an intrathecal catheter is threaded after an ADP are because the respondents wanted to avoid another dural puncture (76%) and to provide very quick labor analgesia (93).

Prophylactic Epidural Injection of Saline or Blood

Another maneuver to restore CSF volume or to increase intracranial pressure is to prophylactically inject saline or blood prior to catheter removal. There have been studies evaluating single and multiple epidural saline injections of 40 to 60 mL, or prophylactic epidural injections of 5 to 20 mL blood prior to removal of the epidural catheter. In the Apfel literature review, the relative risk for headache after prophylactic blood patch was 0.48 in five non-randomized controlled trials (non-RCTs) and 0.32 in four RCTs although there was no statistical significance (0.10 to 1.03) in the four RCTs (85). In a 2006 survey of ASRA members, 12% to 25% used epidural saline and 10% to 31% performed prophylactic EBPs to prevent PDPH (91). Apfel et al. noted that the failure of a prophylactic blood patch may be due to timing of administration, but there is limited evidence that this is the case.

Intrathecal Saline

One study by Charsley and Abram evaluated prophylactic intrathecal saline. Twenty-eight patients received 10 mL of intrathecal saline, either administered immediately after ADP through the epidural needle (22 patients), or through an intrathecal catheter prior to removal (6 patients) (94). Thirty-two percent of the patients who received intrathecal saline through the epidural needle developed headache compared with 62% of controls. No patients in the intrathecal catheter saline injection group developed headaches compared with three patients in the control group of five (94). This study was included in the review by Apfel et al. but failed to reach statistical significance (RR = 0.51, 0.26 to 1.03) (85).

Epidural Morphine

Al-metwalli et al. conducted a prospective randomized double-blind trial of 25 patients who all received two injections 24 hours apart of either epidural morphine 3 mg in 10 mL saline, or 10 mL of plain saline. In this study, 12% (3/25) of the morphine patients experienced severe headache versus 48% (12/25) of the patients who received plain saline. Six of the patients in the saline group required EBP compared to none in the morphine group (95). While this study shows promise, it would require prolonged monitoring for respiratory depression, which is not ideal for outpatients. There were no incidents of respiratory depression in his study, and the most common side effect noted was nausea (95). In the survey by Baraz and Collis, mentioned earlier, 26% of the respondents would treat PDPH with an EBP as soon as it was diagnosed, whereas in 71% of the units the EBP is performed only after conservative therapy fails.

Prophylactic Bedrest

A 2002 Cochrane review of eleven trials among 1,723 patients by Sudlow and Warlow showed no difference in the incidence of PDPH when comparing either bedrest versus immediate ambulation, or a shorter period of bedrest versus a longer period (96). Thoennisen et al. conducted a systematic review of 16 RCTs (with some overlap of trials in the above mentioned Cochrane review) and also found no benefit to routine bedrest. He encouraged early mobilization for thromboprophylaxis (97). Prophylactic bedrest is not recommended for prevention of PDPH as it does not decrease the incidence of PDPH. Those that end up with PDPH will naturally tend toward a supine position to lessen the severity of their headache.

Prophylactic Hydration

Many practitioners believe that adequate hydration may help a patient with PDPH ensure that they are able to make adequate CSF. As long as the patient is able to drink adequate amounts of fluid, there may not be a need to give them intravenous fluids. There is a prospective study by Dieterich and Brandt of 100 neurologic patients in which half the patients were asked to drink 1.5 L of fluids per day for 5 days following a lumbar puncture and the other half was asked to do the same but with 3 L of fluids. There was no difference in incidence of headache found between the two groups (98).

■ TREATMENT

Patients who develop PDPH need to be monitored closely. The author recommends that patients who have received neuraxial analgesia be evaluated the next day by a member of the anesthetic care team for presence of headache, ambulation, fever, and neurologic deficits. This may help with early detection of serious complications and provide feedback for improved patient satisfaction. Patients with PDPH need to receive reassurance and be presented with the options of conservative and invasive treatment. Communication is important and even if this complication was discussed at length when consent was obtained or at the time of recognized ADP, it may be important to readdress the reason for the headache, how long the symptoms may last with and without treatment, and what options are available. Conservative treatment will not provide complete relief in most patients who have had a large gauge ADP. Analgesics, bedrest, and hydration may be enough supportive therapy to avoid invasive treatment until the dura is able to heal. There are some studies that suggest that when some severe headaches are left untreated, the headache may become chronic and can last for months to years (16,30).

Non-opioid Oral Analgesics

These are the first line of therapy in conservative treatment. Common regimens include acetaminophen/paracetamol, ibuprofen, naproxen, and other non-steroidal anti-inflammatory drugs (NSAIDs). These can be written as scheduled dosing for 24 to 48 hours instead of "as needed" dosing so the patient receives them without waiting for the headache to return.

Opioid Analgesics

For moderate or severe headaches non-opioid oral analgesics may not be adequate, and oral or intravenous narcotics may be necessary as needed.

Caffeine, ACTH and Other Pharmacologic Therapies

In a letter to the editor of JAMA in 1944, H.G. Holder recommended a slow intravenous infusion of 500 mg caffeine sodium benzoate (CSB) that could be repeated 6 hours later for the treatment of PDPH (99). Many studies followed evaluating oral and intravenous caffeine in different regimens and it became recognized that while treatment with caffeine may provide analgesia, its duration of action was temporary and ongoing relief required re-dosing. Drip coffee contains between 85 and 250 mg of caffeine per cup. Oral and intravenous infusions are commonly prescribed as 300 to 500 mg caffeine per treatment. In dosages of approximately 5 to 10 g, caffeine can lead to seizures from central nervous system stimulation. There have been some case reports of postpartum seizures associated with intravenous CSB therapy. The cause of these seizures are unclear given that eclampsia can also be a reason, but intravenous CSB is usually described as being given several hours prior to the seizure with and without an EBP to complicate the picture. Oral and intravenous theophylline has been studied as a treatment because its vasoconstrictive effects last longer than oral caffeine, and it is a stronger cerebral vasoconstrictor, but it is not commonly used in clinical practice.

A Cochrane review of RCTs conducted by Basurto Ona et al. in 2011 assessed the effectiveness of pharmacologic drugs in treating PDPH. Seven RCTs with 200 participants were included and the drugs assessed were oral and intravenous caffeine, subcutaneous sumatriptan, oral gabapentin, oral theophylline, intravenous hydrocortisone, and intramuscular adrenocorticotropic hormone (ACTH) (100). The authors concluded that caffeine has shown effectiveness for treating PDPH compared with placebo (100). Gabapentin, theophylline, and hydrocortisone also showed a decrease in pain severity scores compared with placebo. ACTH has been used and there are many theories on the mechanism by which it could decrease the severity of PDPH. One thought is that ACTH may increase production of aldosterone and increase intravascular volume or dural edema (101). A second theory is that ACTH may increase CSF production, and a third theory is that it could increase the pain threshold by increasing production of beta endorphins in the central nervous system (102,103). Despite all these theories, ACTH has not been shown beyond one case series to be efficacious in treating PDPH (100). Sumatriptan is a 5-HT receptor agonist that is used primarily in the treatment of migraine headaches. With the cerebral vasodilation that may take place during PDPH a migraine-like headache occurs, so vasoconstrictive agents like sumatriptan were evaluated and used successfully in few case reports; however, a RCT found no relevant effectiveness (104). Intravenous hydrocortisone and the anticonvulsant gabapentin (a structural analog of GABA) have both been used in some case reports and small non-RCTs to reduce the severity of PDPH but the mechanism for the success is unknown (100,105).

Hydration, Bedrest, and Abdominal Binders

Hydration and bedrest were previously mentioned in the section for prophylaxis against PDPH after ADP with no real benefit. There has also been no evidence that hydration and bedrest are effective treatments after the headache occurs (96). Abdominal binders and the prone position were thought to help increase the abdominal subarachnoid CSF pressure so that more CSF would be displaced to the cranium to help relieve the intracranial hypotension (106). Both of these measures are not used widely because they can be uncomfortable for a postpartum patient.

■ INVASIVE THERAPEUTIC OPTIONS
Epidural Blood Patch

EBP was first described by Gormley after he noticed that there were fewer headaches in those patients who had a "bloody tap" (107). The mechanisms of relief are theorized to be, first, from an increase in intracranial pressure from the blood in the epidural space compressing the thecal sac, therefore displacing CSF from the spinal cord area cephalad toward the brain. Second, that the injected blood forms a fibrin clot around the dural puncture, sealing the hole until the dura heals, which is why injection of blood into the epidural space is more effective than injection with crystalloids

or colloids. However, the actual mechanism of action is still unknown (1). Another theory suggests that EBP quickly raises intrathecal pressures thus deactivating adenosine receptors and reversing vasodilatation. The decrease in cerebral blood flow results in reduction of the headache (108). If patients have symptoms of PDPH after ADP, about two-thirds of them receive an EBP (25,37,51). Overall, the success rate of EBP is about 70% to 98% if it is performed at least 24 hours after the dural perforation (12) (109). There appears to be better success when an EBP is performed at least 24 hours after the initial puncture. If this is done, reported success rate of the first EBP approaches 93% and increases to 97% with repeated second EBP (1,110,111). In a 2006 survey of practicing members of the ASRA, Harrington and Schmitt noted that there was a wide variation on how the EBP was performed except for amount of blood volume (16 to 20 mL) injected (91). The authors also noted that injection of other substances into the epidural space besides blood was rare in clinical practice (91).

Recently, Paech conducted a multicenter, multicountry RCT evaluating the injection of 15, 20, or 30 mL of blood for EBP in 121 patients, following them for 5 days (112). After EBP, there was partial or permanent relief in the 15, 20, and 30 mL group of 61%, 73%, and 67% and complete relief of the headache in 10%, 32%, and 26% (112). All of these patients received their EBP more than 24 hours after the dural puncture. This study supported the practice of administering 20 mL of blood at least 24 hours after the ADP (112).

A Cochrane Database systemic review by Boonmak in 2010, completed prior to the important Paech study mentioned above, was unable to draw unequivocal conclusions about the efficacy of EBP because there are an inadequate number of RCT studies comparing EBP to no EBP in the treatment or prevention of PDPH (113). However, EBPs have been accepted clinically as the gold standard of treatment for severe PDPH (114,115). Most practitioners would advocate for patients to remain supine for at least 30 minutes after placing the EBP. There are case reports of patients who required three EBP procedures following ADP with an epidural needle for labor analgesia (116). However, most practitioners would think about further neurologic workup including neuro-imaging if the patient's symptoms did not resolve after the second EBP.

With the increased use of ultrasound imaging in anesthesiology, there have been some case reports using ultrasound to help estimate the optimal blood volume during EBP. In one case, the dura mater was seen to expand while the subarachnoid space became compressed during injection of the blood in the epidural space. In another case, the area of the epidural space was unchanged, but the contrast of the space was altered in a mosaic pattern by injection of 17 mL of blood (117). Another study discussed performing EBP under fluoroscopy in prone position (118). The investigators injected a 4:1 mixture of autologous blood and contrast medium with enough volume to cover the dural puncture. The success rate in the six patients with PDPH was 100% with a mean blood volume of 7.2 mL. The only complication that was associated with this was a mild backache, which is a common symptom after EBP performed without contrast. They concluded that fluoroscopy guided EBP may be safe to treat persistent PDPH with a relatively small volume of blood. Given the rates of false loss-of-resistance reported (17% to 30%), the use of real time imaging to ensure proper placement of the EBP should be considered if the patient has failed the initial EBP (119).

EBP rarely has significant complications, but is contraindicated in the presence of fever, cellulitis at the puncture site, and any coagulation abnormalities. About 35% of patients who receive an EBP complain of back pain, either at the time of injection, or shortly afterward. Another complication is the chance of a repeated ADP at the time of placing an EBP. There are many case reports in the literature about complications during EBP that include neck pain, leg pain, paresthesias, paraparesis, cauda equine syndrome, radicular pain, meningeal irritation, elevated intracranial pressures, infection, subdural hematoma, and temporary cranial nerve palsies (12,109,120–123). Recommended monitoring include having intravenous access and non-invasive blood pressure; it would also be reasonable to monitor basic vital signs.

Other Invasive Therapeutic Options

There are reports of other invasive strategies to decrease PDPH including injecting normal saline as epidural or caudal boluses or as an infusion. There are case reports of using low molecular weight dextran, gelatin powder, and fibrin glue (124–126). It is unknown what the long-term effects of injecting autologous blood or other substances may be.

■ CONCLUSIONS

PDPH can be a very distressing complication for both the patient and the anesthesia provider. Although it is a well-known complication, an analysis of the American Society of Anesthesiologists 1990 closed claims database show that in obstetric claims, headache is the second most common reason for litigation, behind nerve damage and ahead of maternal death. It is unknown what the actual mechanism of the headache is, only that it is most likely due to leakage of CSF through the dural puncture as first postulated by Bier more than a century ago. There is a large variation on prophylactic and conservative therapeutic treatments because of the lack of enough large randomized controlled clinical trials to provide satisfactory evidence-based recommendations. Since PDPH has a relatively low prevalence, a prospective large RCT would be difficult. Also, because the symptoms usually resolve on their own in 1 or 2 weeks (12), there would also need to be a large control group to adequately interpret the results. Further study is certainly needed and warranted. PDPH interferes with initial mother–infant bonding and may lead to chronic headaches if untreated. This complication may also decrease satisfaction of our specialty, increase the anesthetic workload, prolong the patient's hospital stay, and contribute to ever-increasing healthcare costs (37).

KEY POINTS

- The estimated incidence of ADP is about 1% in obstetric patients during epidural attempt and more than half of those patients will develop PDPH.
- Obstetric patients have an increased risk of developing a PDPH as they have the risk factors of being young, female, and pregnant.
- EBP is the gold standard for treating severe PDPH.
- Neurologic imaging is recommended after EBP treatment has been twice unsuccessful to evaluate for other serious causes of persistent postpartum headache.

REFERENCES

1. Gaiser R. Postdural puncture headache. *Curr Opin Anaesthesiol* 2006;19(3):249–253.
2. Lybecker H, Andersen T. Repetitive hearing loss following dural puncture treated with autologous epidural blood patch. *Acta Anaesthesiol Scand* 1995;39(7):987–989.
3. Gentili ME. Are postdural puncture symptoms immediate in elderly patients? *Anesth Analg* 2000;91(5):1311.
4. Choi PT, Galinski SE, Takeuchi L, et al. PDPH is a common complication of neuraxial blockade in parturients: A meta-analysis of obstetrical studies. *Can J Anesth* 2003;50(5):460–469.
5. Olesen J, Bousser MG, Diener HC, et al. The International Classification of Headache Disorders. Cephalalgia: an International Journal of Headache 2004; 24(Suppl 1):1.
6. Pearce JM. Walter Essex Wynter, Quincke, and lumbar puncture. *J Neurol Neurosurg Psychiatry* 1994;57(2):179.
7. Pearce JM. Nicolaus Petreus Tulpius (1593–1674) on headaches. *J Neurol Neurosurg Psychiatry* 1994;57(5):625.
8. Frederiks JA, Koehler PJ. The first lumbar puncture. *J Hist Neurosci* 1997;6(2):147–153.
9. Gorelick PB, Zych D. James Leonard Corning and the early history of spinal puncture. *Neurology* 1987;37(4):672–674.
10. Marx GF. The first spinal anesthesia. who deserves the laurels? *Reg Anesth* 1994;19(6):429–430.
11. Wulf HF. The centennial of spinal anesthesia. *Anesthesiology* 1998;89(2):500–506.
12. Turnbull DK, Shepherd DB. Post-dural puncture headache: Pathogenesis, prevention and treatment. *Br J Anaesth* 2003;91(5):718–729.
13. Patin DJ, Eckstein EC, Harum K, et al. Anatomic and biomechanical properties of human lumbar dura mater. *Anesth Analg* 1993;76(3):535–540.
14. Reina MA, de Leon-Casasola OA, Lopez A, et al. An in vitro study of dural lesions produced by 25-gauge Quincke and Whitacre needles evaluated by scanning electron microscopy. *Reg Anesth Pain Med* 2000;25(4):393–402.
15. Rozen T, Swidan S, Hamel R, et al. Trendelenburg position: A tool to screen for the presence of a low CSF pressure syndrome in daily headache patients. *Headache* 2008;48(9):1366–1371.
16. Evans RW. Complications of lumbar puncture. *Neurol Clin* 1998;16(1):83–105.
17. Kuczkowski KM, Benumof JL. Decrease in the incidence of post-dural puncture headache: Maintaining CSF volume. *Acta Anaesthesiol Scand* 2003; 47(1):98–100.
18. Kunkle EC, Ray BS, Wolff HG. Experimental studies on headache: Analysis of the headache associated with changes in intracranial pressure. *AMA Arch Neurol Psychiatry* 1943;49:323.
19. Brownridge P. The management of headache following accidental dural puncture in obstetric patients. *Anaesth Intensive Care* 1983;11(1):4–15.
20. Mokri B. The Monro–Kellie hypothesis: Applications in CSF volume depletion. *Neurology* 2001;56(12):1746–1748.
21. Camann WR, Murray RS, Mushlin PS, et al. Effects of oral caffeine on postdural puncture headache. A double-blind, placebo-controlled trial. *Anesth Analg* 1990;70(2):181–184.
22. Evans RW, Armon C, Frohman EM, et al. Assessment: Prevention of postlumbar puncture headaches: Report of the therapeutics and technology assessment subcommittee of the American Academy of Neurology. *Neurology* 2000;55(7):909–914.
23. Darvish B, Gupta A, Alahuhta S, et al. Management of accidental dural puncture and post-dural puncture headache after labour: A Nordic survey. *Acta Anaesthesiol Scand* 2011;55(1):46–53.
24. Berger CW, Crosby ET, Grodecki W. North American survey of the management of dural puncture occurring during labour epidural analgesia. *Can J Anaesth* 1998;45(2):110–114.
25. Sprigge JS, Harper SJ. Accidental dural puncture and post dural puncture headache in obstetric anaesthesia: Presentation and management: A 23-year survey in a district general hospital. *Anaesthesia* 2008;63(1):36–43.
26. Khan KJ, Stride PC, Cooper GM. Does a bloody tap prevent postdural puncture headache? *Anaesthesia* 1993;48(7):628–629.
27. Dittmann M, Schaefer HG, Renkl F, et al. Spinal anaesthesia with 29 gauge Quincke point needles and post dural puncture headache in 2,378 patients. *Acta Anaesthesiol Scand* 1994;38(7):691–693.
28. Gleeson CM, Reynolds F. Accidental dural puncture rates in UK obstetric practice. *Int J Obstet Anesth* 1998;7(4):242–246.
29. MacArthur C, Lewis M, Knox EG. Accidental dural puncture in obstetric patients and long term symptoms. *BMJ* 1993;306(6882):883–885.
30. Reynolds F. Dural puncture and headache. *BMJ* 1993;306(6882):874–876.
31. Liu S, Kopacz DJ, Carpenter RL. Quantitative assessment of differential sensory nerve block after lidocaine spinal anesthesia. *Anesthesiology* 1995;82(1):60–63.
32. Sharma SK, Gambling DR, Joshi GP, et al. Comparison of 26-gauge Atraucan and 25-gauge Whitacre needles: Insertion characteristics and complications. *Can J Anaesth* 1995;42(8):706–710.
33. Pan PH, Fragneto R, Moore C, et al. Incidence of postdural puncture headache and backache, and success rate of dural puncture: Comparison of two spinal needle designs. *South Med J* 2004;97(4):359–363.

34. Vallejo MC, Mandell GL, Sabo DP, et al. Postdural puncture headache: A randomized comparison of five spinal needles in obstetric patients. *Anesth Analg* 2000;91(4):916–920.

35. Miro M, Guasch E, Gilsanz F. Comparison of epidural analgesia with combined spinal–epidural analgesia for labor: A retrospective study of 6497 cases. *Int J Obstet Anesth* 2008;17(1):15–19.

36. Hartopp R, Hamlyn L, Stocks G. Ten years of experience with accidental dural puncture and post-dural-puncture headache in a tertiary obstetric anaesthesia department. *Int J Obstet Anesth* 2010;19(1):118.

37. van de Velde M, Schepers R, Berends N, et al. Ten years of experience with accidental dural puncture and post-dural puncture headache in a tertiary obstetric anaesthesia department. *Int J Obstet Anesth* 2008;17(4):329–335.

38. van de Velde M, Teunkens A, Hanssens M, et al. Post dural puncture headache following combined spinal–epidural or epidural anaesthesia in obstetric patients. *Anaesth Intensive Care* 2001;29(6):595–599.

39. Wadud R, Laiq N, Qureshi FA, et al. The frequency of postdural puncture headache in different age groups. *J Coll Physicians Surg Pak* 2006;16(6):389–392.

40. Lybecker H, Moller JT, May O, et al. Incidence and prediction of postdural puncture headache. A prospective study of 1021 spinal anesthesias. *Anesth Analg* 1990;70(4):389–394.

41. Carbajal R, Simon N, Olivier-Martin M. Post-lumbar puncture headache in children. Treatment with epidural autologous blood (blood patch). *Arch Pediatr* 1998;5(2):149–152.

42. Tourtellotte WW, Henderson WG, Tucker RP, et al. A randomized, double-blind clinical trial comparing the 22 versus 26 gauge needle in the production of the post-lumbar puncture syndrome in normal individuals. *Headache* 1972;12(2):73–78.

43. Bezov D, Ashina S, Lipton R. Post-dural puncture headache: Part II—prevention, management, and prognosis. *Headache* 2010;50(9):1482–1498.

44. Ghaleb A. Postdural puncture headache. *Anesthesiol Res Pract* 2010: Epub 2010 Aug 11; doi: 10.1155/2010/102967

45. Vandam LD, Dripps RD. Long-term follow-up of patients who received 10,098 spinal anesthetics; syndrome of decreased intracranial pressure (headache and ocular and auditory difficulties). *J Am Med Assoc* 1956;161(7):586–591.

46. Vilming ST, Schrader H, Monstad I. The significance of age, sex, and cerebrospinal fluid pressure in post-lumbar-puncture headache. *Cephalalgia* 1989;9(2):99–106.

47. Flaatten H, Rodt SA, Vamnes J, et al. Postdural puncture headache. A comparison between 26- and 29-gauge needles in young patients. *Anaesthesia* 1989;44(2):147–149.

48. Kuntz KM, Kokmen E, Stevens JC, et al. Post-lumbar puncture headaches: Experience in 501 consecutive procedures. *Neurology* 1992;42(10):1884–1887.

49. Lavi R, Yarnitsky D, Rowe JM, et al. Standard vs atraumatic Whitacre needle for diagnostic lumbar puncture: A randomized trial. *Neurology* 2006;67(8):1492–1494.

50. Faure E, Moreno R, Thisted R. Incidence of postdural puncture headache in morbidly obese parturients. *Reg Anesth* 1994;19(5):361–363.

51. Paech M, Banks S, Gurrin L. An audit of accidental dural puncture during epidural insertion of a tuohy needle in obstetric patients. *Int J Obstet Anesth* 2001;10(3):162–167.

52. Kuczkowski KM. Post-dural puncture headache in the obstetric patient: An old problem. New solutions. *Minerva Anestesiol* 2004;70(12):823–830.

53. Amorim JA, Valenca MM. Postdural puncture headache is a risk factor for new postdural puncture headache. *Cephalalgia* 2008;28(1):5–8.

54. Clark JW, Solomon GD, Senanayake PD, et al. Substance P concentration and history of headache in relation to postlumbar puncture headache: Towards prevention. *J Neurol Neurosurg Psychiatry* 1996;60(6):681–683.

55. Eede HV, Hoffmann VL, Vercauteren MP. Post-delivery postural headache: Not always a classical post-dural puncture headache. *Acta Anaesthesiol Scand* 2007;51(6):763–765.

56. Stella CL, Jodicke CD, How HY, et al. Postpartum headache: Is your work-up complete? *Am J Obstet Gynecol* 2007;196(4):318.e1–318.e7.

57. Zeidan A, Farhat O, Maaliki H, et al. Does postdural puncture headache left untreated lead to subdural hematoma? Case report and review of the literature. *Int J Obstet Anesth* 2006;15(1):50–58.

58. Sharma S, Halliwell R, Dexter M, et al. Acute subdural haematoma in the presence of an intrathecal catheter placed for the prevention of post-dural puncture headache. *Anaesth Intensive Care* 2010;38(5):939–941.

59. Amorim JA, Remigio DS, Damazio Filho O, et al. Intracranial subdural hematoma post-spinal anesthesia: Report of two cases and review of 33 cases in the literature. *Rev Bras Anestesiol* 2010;60(6):620–629, 344–349.

60. Bousser MG. Cerebral venous thrombosis: Diagnosis and management. *J Neurol* 2000;247(4):252–258.

61. Vaghela V, Hingwala DR, Kapilamoorthy TR, et al. Spontaneous intracranial hypo and hypertensions: An imaging review. *Neurol India* 2011;59(4):506–512.

62. Holst D, Mollmann M, Ebel C, et al. In vitro investigation of cerebrospinal fluid leakage after dural puncture with various spinal needles. *Anesth Analg* 1998;87(6):1331–1335.

63. Keener EB. An experimental study of reactions of the dura mater to wounding and loss of substance. *J Neurosurg* 1959;16(4):424–447.

64. Keener EB. Regeneration of dural defects; a review. *J Neurosurg* 1959;16(4):415–423.

65. Halpern S, Preston R. Postdural puncture headache and spinal needle design. Metaanalyses. *Anesthesiology* 1994;81(6):1376–1383.

66. Strupp M, Schueler O, Straube A, et al. "Atraumatic" Sprotte needle reduces the incidence of post-lumbar puncture headaches. *Neurology* 2001;57(12):2310–2312.

67. Arendt K, Demaerschalk BM, Wingerchuk DM, et al. Atraumatic lumbar puncture needles: After all these years, are we still missing the point? *Neurologist* 2009;15(1):17–20.

68. Armon C, Evans RW, Therapeutics and Technology Assessment Subcommittee of the American Academy of Neurology. Addendum to assessment: Prevention of post-lumbar puncture headaches: Report of the Therapeutics and Technology Assessment Subcommittee of the American Academy of Neurology. *Neurology* 2005;65(4):510–512.

69. Abouleish E, Mitchell M, Taylor G, et al. Comparative flow rates of saline in commonly used spinal needles including pencil-tip needles. *Reg Anesth* 1994;19(1):34–42.

70. Carson D, Serpell M. Choosing the best needle for diagnostic lumbar puncture. *Neurology* 1996;47(1):33–37.

71. Birnbach DJ, Kuroda MM, Sternman D, et al. Use of atraumatic spinal needles among neurologists in the United States. *Headache* 2001;41(4):385–390.

72. Flaatten H, Thorsen T, Askeland B, et al. Puncture technique and postural postdural puncture headache. A randomised, double-blind study comparing transverse and parallel puncture. *Acta Anaesthesiol Scand* 1998;42(10):1209–1214.

73. Richman JM, Joe EM, Cohen SR, et al. Bevel direction and postdural puncture headache: A meta-analysis. *Neurologist* 2006;12(4):224–248.

74. Strupp M, Brandt T, Muller A. Incidence of post-lumbar puncture syndrome reduced by reinserting the stylet: A randomized prospective study of 600 patients. *J Neurol* 1998;245(9):589–592.

75. Young DA, Burney RE 2nd. Complication of myelography—transection and withdrawal of a nerve filament by the needle. *N Engl J Med* 1971;285(3):156–157.

76. Schnabel A, Schuster F, Ermert T, et al. Ultrasound guidance for neuraxial analgesia and anesthesia in obstetrics: A quantitative systematic review. *Ultraschall Med* 2010 epub ahead of print Nov 15.

77. Liu SS, Ngeow JE, Yadeau JT. Ultrasound-guided regional anesthesia and analgesia: A qualitative systematic review. *Reg Anesth Pain Med* 2009;34(1):47–59.

78. Seeberger MD, Kaufmann M, Staender S, et al. Repeated dural punctures increase the incidence of postdural puncture headache. *Anesth Analg* 1996;82(2):302–305.

79. Norris MC, Leighton BL, DeSimone CA. Needle bevel direction and headache after inadvertent dural puncture. *Anesthesiology* 1989;70(5):729–731.

80. Richardson MG, Wissler RN. The effects of needle bevel orientation during epidural catheter insertion in laboring parturients. *Anesth Analg* 1999;88(2):352–356.

81. Ready LB, Cuplin S, Haschke RH, et al. Spinal needle determinants of rate of transdural fluid leak. *Anesth Analg* 1989;69(4):457–460.

82. Hatfalvi BI. Postulated mechanisms for postdural puncture headache and review of laboratory models. Clinical experience. *Reg Anesth* 1995;20(4):329–336.

83. Raskin NH. Lumbar puncture headache: A review. *Headache* 1990;30(4):197–200.

84. Russell R. Loss of resistance to saline is better than air for obstetric epidurals. *Int J Obstet Anesth* 2001;10(4):302–304.

85. Apfel CC, Saxena A, Cakmakkaya OS, et al. Prevention of postdural puncture headache after accidental dural puncture: A quantitative systematic review. *Br J Anaesth* 2010;105(3):255–263.

86. Ayad S, Demian Y, Narouze SN, et al. Subarachnoid catheter placement after wet tap for analgesia in labor: Influence on the risk of headache in obstetric patients. *Reg Anesth Pain Med* 2003;28(6):512–515.

87. Cohen S, Amar D, Pantuck EJ, et al. Decreased incidence of headache after accidental dural puncture in caesarean delivery patients receiving continuous postoperative intrathecal analgesia. *Acta Anaesthesiol Scand* 1994;38(7):716–718.

88. Kaul B, Sines D, Vallejo M, et al. A five-year experience with post dural puncture headaches. *Anesthesiology* 2007;107:A1762.

89. Arkoosh VA, Palmer CM, Yun EM, et al. A randomized, double-masked, multicenter comparison of the safety of continuous intrathecal labor analgesia using a 28-gauge catheter versus continuous epidural labor analgesia. *Anesthesiology* 2008;108(2):286–298.

90. Baysinger CL, Pope JE, Lockhart EM, et al. The management of accidental dural puncture and postdural puncture headache: A North American survey. *J Clin Anesth* 2011;23(5):349–360.

91. Harrington BE, Schmitt AM. Meningeal (postdural) puncture headache, unintentional dural puncture, and the epidural blood patch: A national survey of United States practice. *Reg Anesth Pain Med* 2009;34(5):430–437.

92. Marcus HE, Fabian A, Dagtekin O, et al. Pain, postdural puncture headache, nausea, and pruritus after cesarean delivery: A survey of prophylaxis and treatment. *Minerva Anestesiol* 2011;77(11):1043–1049.

93. Baraz R, Collis RE. The management of accidental dural puncture during labour epidural analgesia: A survey of UK practice. *Anaesthesia* 2005;60(7):673–679.

94. Charsley MM, Abram SE. The injection of intrathecal normal saline reduces the severity of postdural puncture headache. *Reg Anesth Pain Med* 2001;26(4):301–305.

95. Al-metwalli RR. Epidural morphine injections for prevention of post dural puncture headache. *Anaesthesia* 2008;63(8):847–850.

96. Sudlow C, Warlow C. Posture and fluids for preventing post-dural puncture headache. *Cochrane Database Syst Rev* 2002;(2):CD001790.

97. Thoennissen J, Herkner H, Lang W, et al. Does bed rest after cervical or lumbar puncture prevent headache? A systematic review and meta-analysis. *CMAJ* 2001;165(10):1311–1316.

98. Dieterich M, Brandt T. Incidence of post-lumbar puncture headache is independent of daily fluid intake. *Eur Arch Psychiatry Neurol Sci* 1988;237(4):194–196.

99. Holder HG. Reactions after spinal anesthesia. *JAMA* 1944;124(1):56.

100. Basurto Ona X, Martinez Garcia L, Sola I, et al. Drug therapy for treating post-dural puncture headache. *Cochrane Database Syst Rev* 2011;(8):CD007887.

101. Baysinger CL, Menk EJ, Harte E, et al. The successful treatment of dural puncture headache after failed epidural blood patch. *Anesth Analg* 1986;65(11):1242–1244.

102. Carter BL, Pasupuleti R. Use of intravenous cosyntropin in the treatment of postdural puncture headache. *Anesthesiology* 2000;92(1):272–274.

103. Collier BB. Treatment for post dural puncture headache. *Br J Anaesth* 1994;72(3):366–367.

104. Connelly NR, Parker RK, Rahimi A, et al. Sumatriptan in patients with post-dural puncture headache. *Headache* 2000;40(4):316–319.

105. Neves JF, Vieira VL, Saldanha RM, et al. Hydrocortisone treatment and prevent post-dural puncture headache: Case reports. *Rev Bras Anestesiol* 2005;55(3):343–349.

106. Handler CE, Perkin GD. Post lumbar puncture headache. *J R Soc Med* 1982;75(10):829.

107. Gormley J. Treatment of post spinal headache. *Anesthesiology* 1960;21:565.

108. Desai MJ, Dave AP, Martin MB. Delayed radicular pain following two large volume epidural blood patches for post-lumbar puncture headache: A case report. *Pain Physician* 2010;13(3):257–262.

109. Abouleish E, Vega S, Blendinger I, et al. Long-term follow-up of epidural blood patch. *Anesth Analg* 1975;54(4):459–463.

110. Safa-Tisseront V, Thormann F, Malassine P, et al. Effectiveness of epidural blood patch in the management of post-dural puncture headache. *Anesthesiology* 2001;95(2):334–339.

111. Berrettini WH, Simmons-Alling S, Nurnberger JI Jr. Epidural blood patch does not prevent headache after lumbar puncture. *Lancet* 1987;1(8537):856–857.

112. Paech MJ, Doherty DA, Christmas T, et al. The volume of blood for epidural blood patch in obstetrics: A randomized, blinded clinical trial. *Anesth Analg* 2011;113(1):126–133.

113. Boonmak P, Boonmak S. Epidural blood patching for preventing and treating post-dural puncture headache. *Cochrane Database Syst Rev* 2010;(1):CD001791.

114. Sudlow C, Warlow C. Epidural blood patching for preventing and treating post-dural puncture headache. *Cochrane Database Syst Rev* 2002;(2):CD001791.

115. Paech M. Epidural blood patch myths and legends. *Can J Anaesth* 2005;52(6):R1–R5.

116. Villevieille T, Pasquier P, Muller V, et al. Obstetrical epidural analgesia during labour: One dural puncture, repeated postural headaches, three blood patches. *Ann Fr Anesth Reanim* 2010;29(11):803–836.

117. Masui. *Ultrasound Obstet Gynecol* 2011;38(1).

118. Kawaguchi M, Hashizume K, Watanabe K, et al. Fluoroscopically guided epidural blood patch in patients with postdural puncture headache after spinal and epidural anesthesia. *J Anesth* 2011;25(3):450–453.

119. Bartynski WS, Grahovac SZ, Rothfus WE. Incorrect needle position during lumbar epidural steroid administration: Inaccuracy of loss of air pressure resistance and requirement of fluoroscopy and epidurography during needle insertion. *AJNR Am J Neuroradiol* 2005;26(3):502–505.

120. Oh J, Camann W. Severe, acute meningeal irritative reaction after epidural blood patch. *Anesth Analg* 1998;87(5):1139–1140.

121. Sperry RJ, Gartrell A, Johnson JO. Epidural blood patch can cause acute neurologic deterioration. *Anesthesiology* 1995;82(1):303–305.

122. Diaz JH. Permanent paraparesis and cauda equina syndrome after epidural blood patch for postdural puncture headache. *Anesthesiology* 2002;96(6):1515–1517.

123. Simopoulos TT, Kraemer JJ, Glazer P, et al. Vertebral osteomyelitis: A potentially catastrophic outcome after lumbar epidural steroid injection. *Pain Physician* 2008;11(5):693–697.

124. Schick U, Musahl C, Papke K. Diagnostics and treatment of spontaneous intracranial hypotension. *Minim Invasive Neurosurg* 2010;53(1):15–20.

125. Aldrete JA. Persistent post-dural-puncture headache treated with epidural infusion of dextran. *Headache* 1994;34(5):265–267.

126. Ambesh SP, Kumar A, Bajaj A. Epidural gelatin (gelfoam) patch treatment for post dural puncture headache. *Anaesth Intensive Care* 1991;19(3):444–447.

CHAPTER

28

Hypertensive Disorders of Pregnancy

Jaya Ramanathan • Ravpreet Singh Gill • Baha Sibai

Hypertension is the most common medical disorder during pregnancy (1). Hypertension complicates 5% to 10% of all pregnancies and is a major cause of maternal morbidity and mortality worldwide particularly in developing countries. Approximately 70% of women diagnosed with hypertension during pregnancy will have gestational hypertension—preeclampsia. The term hypertensive disorders of pregnancy encompasses a wide spectrum of disorders including preeclampsia, a condition in which patients who may have only mild elevation in blood pressure or, severe hypertension with various organ dysfunctions, atypical preeclampsia. It also includes disorders such as acute gestational hypertension, eclampsia and the syndrome of hemolysis, elevated liver enzymes, and low platelet count (HELLP syndrome) (1,2).

While preeclampsia is considered a disease of the young primigravida, it also seems to affect older age group. In general, maternal and fetal outcomes are better in previously healthy women who develop preeclampsia after 36 weeks of gestation, and less favorable in those women who develop the symptoms earlier than 32 weeks of gestation and in those with any of the abovementioned risk factors. Long-term morbidity and outcome are related to onset of acute complications such as cerebrovascular accidents, acute renal and cardiac failure and these mothers are at increased risk for developing related problems later in life. Neonatal outcome is related to factors such as the presence of intrauterine growth retardation and prematurity.

■ DEFINITIONS AND CLASSIFICATIONS

Hypertension is defined as a systolic blood pressure ≥140 mm Hg or a diastolic blood pressure ≥90 mm Hg (3). These measurements must be made on at least two occasions, no less than 4 hours and no more than a week apart. *Proteinuria* in pregnancy that is considered abnormal is defined as the excretion of ≥300 mg of protein in 24 hours. The most accurate measurement of total urinary excretion of protein is with the use of a 24-hour urine collection (4). However, in certain instances the use of semi-quantitative dipstick analysis may be the only measurement available to assess urinary protein (2). Table 28-1 lists the classification of hypertensive disorders in pregnancy.

Gestational Hypertension

Gestational hypertension is the elevation of blood pressure during the second half of pregnancy or in the first 24 hours postpartum, without proteinuria and without symptoms. Treatment is generally not warranted since most patients will have only mild hypertension. Gestational hypertension at term in and of itself, has little effect on maternal or perinatal morbidity or mortality. However, approximately 40% to 50% of patients diagnosed with preterm mild gestational hypertension will develop preeclampsia (5). Parturients with severe gestational hypertension are at risk for adverse maternal and perinatal outcomes and management of these patients should be similar to those with severe preeclampsia (5). If a woman with gestational hypertension is considered to have a severe disease, she should receive antihypertensive therapy. Therefore, antihypertensive drugs should not be used during ambulatory management of these women (1,5,6).

Preeclampsia

Preeclampsia is defined as gestational hypertension plus proteinuria developing after 20 weeks of gestation. Preeclampsia can be mild or severe (Table 28-1). If a 24-hour urine collection is not possible, then proteinuria is defined as a concentration of at least 30 mg/dL (1+ on dipstick) on two occasions at least 4 hours apart.

Eclampsia

Another severe form of preeclampsia is eclampsia, which is the occurrence of seizures not attributable to other causes.

Atypical Preeclampsia

The traditional criteria to confirm a diagnosis of preeclampsia are the presence of *proteinuric hypertension* (new onset of hypertension and new onset of proteinuria after 20 weeks of gestation). However, recent data suggest that in some women, preeclampsia and even eclampsia may develop in the absence of either hypertension *or* proteinuria (7). In many of these women, there are usually other manifestations of preeclampsia such as the presence of signs and symptoms or laboratory abnormalities. Criteria for atypical preeclampsia are described below:

- Gestational hypertension plus one or more of the following
  - Symptoms of preeclampsia
  - Hemolysis
  - Thrombocytopenia (<100,000/mm³)
  - Elevated liver enzymes (2× the upper limit of the normal value for AST/ALT)
- Early signs and symptoms of preeclampsia–eclampsia at <20 weeks
- Late postpartum preeclampsia–eclampsia (>48 hours postpartum)

437

TABLE 28-1 Classification of Hypertensive Disorders of Pregnancy

1. Gestational hypertension[a]

   Mild
   - Systolic BP ≥140–160 mm Hg
   - Diastolic BP ≥90–110 mm Hg

   Severe
   - Systolic BP ≥160 mm Hg
   - Diastolic BP ≥110 mm Hg

2. Preeclampsia (Hypertension and proteinuria, onset >20 weeks)

   Mild preeclampsia
   - Systolic BP ≥140–160 mm Hg, OR
   - Diastolic BP ≥90–110 mm Hg
   - Mild proteinuria ≥1+ on dipstick and <5 g/24 h[b]

   Severe preeclampsia
   - (A) Severe hypertension and severe proteinuria
     - Systolic BP ≥160 mm Hg, OR
     - Diastolic BP ≥110 mm Hg
     - Severe proteinuria ≥5 g/24 h[b]
   - (B) Mild hypertension (defined above) with severe proteinuria (defined above)
   - (C) Preeclampsia plus oliguria, cerebral/visual disturbances, pulmonary edema, right upper quadrant pain, thrombocytopenia, impaired liver function, IUGR

3. Chronic hypertension
4. Chronic hypertension with superimposed preeclampsia

[a]Hypertension documented on at least two occasions 4 hours apart.
[b]Dipstick documented on at least two occasions.

In the absence of proteinuria, the syndrome of preeclampsia should be considered when gestational hypertension is present in association with persistent symptoms, or with abnormal laboratory tests. It is also important to note that 25% to 50% of women with mild gestational hypertension will progress to preeclampsia (5,7). The rate of progression depends on gestational age at onset of hypertension, that is, the rate approaches 50% when gestational hypertension develops before 32 weeks of gestation (4,5). In these women, the majority will result in preterm delivery and/or fetal growth restriction (5,7). Therefore, such women require close observation with frequent prenatal visits and serial evaluation of platelets and liver enzymes) and/or fetal growth (serial ultrasound).

HELLP Syndrome

A particularly severe form of preeclampsia is HELLP syndrome, which is an acronym for *hemolysis* (H), *elevated liver enzymes* (EL), and *low platelet count* (LP). The diagnosis may be deceptive because blood pressure may be only marginally elevated (8). A patient diagnosed with HELLP syndrome is automatically classified as having severe preeclampsia.

Capillary Leak Syndrome: Facial Edema, Ascites and Pulmonary Edema, or Gestational Proteinuria

Hypertension is considered to be the hallmark for the diagnosis of preeclampsia; however, recent evidence suggests that in some patients with preeclampsia, the disease may manifest itself in the form of a capillary leak with proteinuria, ascites, pulmonary edema, generalized edema and excessive weight gain, or a spectrum of abnormal hemostasis with multiple organ dysfunction. Therefore, women with capillary leak syndrome with or without hypertension should be evaluated for platelet, liver enzyme, or renal abnormalities (7,9).

Chronic Hypertension

Hypertension complicating pregnancy is considered chronic if a patient is diagnosed with hypertension before pregnancy, if hypertension is present prior to 20 weeks of gestation, or if it persists longer than 6 weeks after delivery (10). Women with chronic hypertension are at risk of developing superimposed preeclampsia. Superimposed preeclampsia is defined as an exacerbation of hypertension and new onset of proteinuria (10).

■ ETIOLOGY

The etiology of preeclampsia remains an obstetric enigma. Several theories have been proposed but most have not withstood the test of time. Some of the suggested causes include abnormal trophoblast invasion of uterine vessels, immunologic intolerance between fetoplacental and maternal tissues, maladaptation to cardiovascular changes, inflammatory changes of pregnancy, abnormal angiogenesis, and genetic abnormalities (11,12). Some reported abnormalities of preeclampsia include placental ischemia, generalized vasospasm, abnormal hemostasis with activation of the coagulation system, vascular endothelial dysfunction, abnormal nitric oxide and lipid metabolism, leukocyte activation, and changes in various cytokines and growth factors. Recently, there is substantial evidence suggesting that the pathophysiologic abnormalities of preeclampsia are caused by *abnormal angiogenesis*, particularly an imbalance in soluble fms like tyrosine kinase 1:Placental growth factor ratio (sFlt-1:PlGF ratio) as well as in soluble endoglin (13–17) and serum levels of these markers have been suggested for the prediction of preeclampsia Figure 28-1 (16,18–20).

■ PREDICTION OF PREECLAMPSIA

A review of the literature reveals that more than 100 clinical, biophysical, and biochemical tests have been recommended to predict or identify the patient at risk for the future development of the disease (21–30). The results of

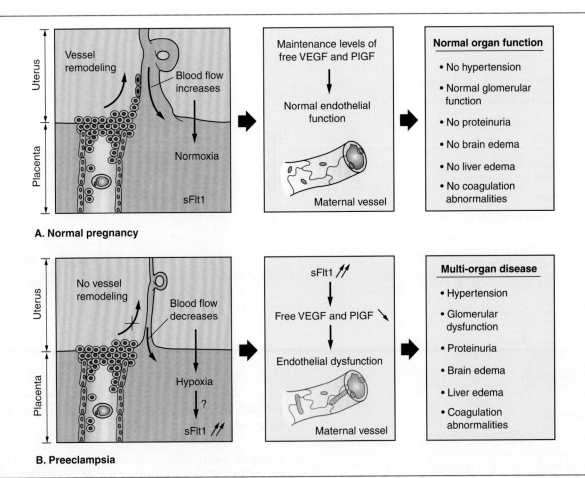

FIGURE 28-1 Hypothesis on the role of sFlt1 in preeclampsia. **A:** During normal pregnancy, the uterine spiral arteries are infiltrated and remodeled by endovascular invasive trophoblasts, thereby increasing blood flow significantly in order to meet the oxygen and nutrient demands of the fetus. **B:** In the placenta of preeclamptic women, trophoblast invasion does not occur and blood flow is reduced, resulting in placental hypoxia. In addition, increased amounts of soluble Flt1 (sFlt1) are produced by the placenta and scavenge VEGF and PlGF, thereby lowering circulating levels of unbound VEGF and PlGF. This altered balance causes generalized endothelial dysfunction, resulting in multiorgan disease. It remains unknown whether hypoxia is the trigger for stimulating sFlt1 secretion in the placenta of preeclamptic mothers and whether the higher sFlt1 levels interfere with trophoblast invasion and spiral artery remodeling. From: Luttun A, Carmeliet P. Soluble VEGF receptor Flt1: The elusive preeclampsia factor discovered? *J Clin Invest* 2003;111:600–602.

the pooled data for the various tests and the lack of agreement between serial tests suggest that none of these clinical tests is sufficiently reliable for use as a screening test in clinical practice (21–31).

Numerous biochemical markers have been proposed to predict which women are destined to develop preeclampsia. These biochemical markers were generally chosen on the basis of specific pathophysiologic abnormalities that have been reported in association with preeclampsia. Thus, these markers have included markers of placental dysfunction, endothelial and coagulation activation, angiogenesis, and markers of systemic inflammation. However, the results of various studies evaluating the reliability of these markers in predicting preeclampsia have been inconsistent, and many of these markers suffer from poor specificity and predictive values for routine use in clinical practice.

■ EPIDEMIOLOGY AND RISK FACTORS

The incidence of preeclampsia is approximately 3% to 10% of all pregnancies in the United States. Other industrialized nations estimate 3% to 5% incidence in studies based on the Swedish, Norwegian, and Danish Medical Birth Reg-

isters (32). In fact, in the United States, the incidence preeclampsia has steadily increased from 2.4% between 1987 and 1988 to 2.9% in 2003 and 2004 (33) while the rate of eclampsia has declined. The rise in the rate of preeclampsia, gestational hypertension, and chronic hypertension may be related to the changing trends in maternal characteristics such as increases in maternal age and prepregnancy weight whereas the decline in the rate of eclampsia is presumably due to better antenatal care and the use of prophylactic measures such as prompt treatment with magnesium sulfate and antihypertensives (32). Women under the age of 20 years and women in the south of the United States were at significantly higher risk for developing both gestational hypertension and preeclampsia compared to those living in the Northeast USA. Worldwide, maternal hypertension is a leading cause of maternal mortality contributing to 9% of maternal deaths in Asia and Africa and 20% in Latin America and the Caribbean countries (32).

There are several risk factors for the development of preeclampsia. Among the pre conceptional risk factors, preexisting diseases, familial factors, lifestyle, and partner-related factors play a major role (5,11). Women with chronic hypertension, diabetes mellitus, endoglin, and morbid obesity are at

TABLE 28-2 **Risk Factors**

Risk Factors	% Risks
Preconceptional Factors	
Chronic hypertension/renal disease	15–40
Pregestational diabetes mellitus	10–35
Connective tissue diseases	10–20
Thrombophilia	10–40
Obesity/insulin resistance	10–15
Older age >40 yr	10–20
Family history of preeclampsia	10–15
Woman born as small for gestational age one- to five-fold	
Adverse outcome in a previous pregnancy two- to three-fold	
Partner-related Factors	
Limited sperm exposure	10–35
(Donor insemination, oocyte donation)	
Partner who fathered preeclamptic-two-fold pregnancy in another woman	
Pregnancy-related Factors	
Hydrops	
Multifetal gestation	
Unexplained fetal growth restriction	
Urinary tract and periodontal infection	

Modified from: Barton JR, Sibai BM. Prediction and prevention of recurrent preeclampsia. *Obstet Gynecol* 2008;112(2)(Pt.1):359–372.

higher risk for preeclampsia. Other factors include extremes of age and chronic cigarette smoking. A familial history of preeclampsia increases the risk in subsequent pregnancies. In addition, recent evidence shows that partner-related factors also play a role. For example, men who fathered a pregnancy with preeclampsia are more likely to father another pregnancy with the same problem. Nulliparous women have higher incidence compared with multiparous women. Limited exposure to partner's sperm is a contributing factor. For example, women who receive donor insemination, women who change partners, and women who use barrier contraception are at higher risk for developing preeclampsia. Pregnancy-related factors include multifetal gestation, infections, and hydrops. The preconceptional and pregnancy-related risk factors for preeclampsia are listed in Table 28-2 (5).

■ PATHOPHYSIOLOGY

Pathophysiologic changes of preeclampsia involve all the major organ systems and these changes are described in the following paragraphs (Fig. 28-2).

Hemodynamic Changes

Since the early 1980s, there have been several studies attempting to define the hemodynamic changes associated with severe preeclampsia. Almost all were prospective observational studies that used invasive hemodynamic monitoring with pulmonary artery (PA) catheters. These studies have provided valuable insight into the hemodynamic profiles in severe preeclampsia before and after the initiation of

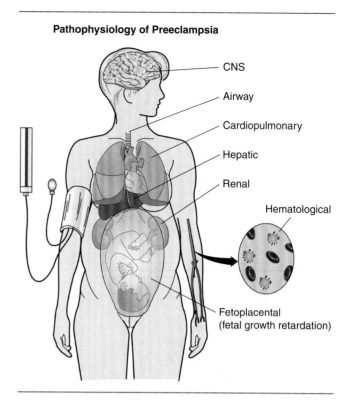

Pathophysiology of Preeclampsia

- CNS
- Airway
- Cardiopulmonary
- Hepatic
- Renal
- Hematological
- Fetoplacental (fetal growth retardation)

FIGURE 28-2 Pathophysiology of preeclampsia showing widespread multiorgan involvement.

treatment with antihypertensives and fluids. Furthermore, the various etiologic factors and pathophysiologic changes contributing to the development of pulmonary edema in severe preeclampsia had been identified, thus facilitating the appropriate choice of treatment of this severe life-threatening complication.

In normotensive pregnant women, the limited data available from earlier studies show that cardiac output (CO), heart rate (HR), and stroke volume (SV) are significantly higher compared with nonpregnant values with no appreciable changes in central venous pressure (CVP) and pulmonary capillary wedge pressure (PCWP) (34). Systemic and pulmonary vascular resistances (SVR and PVR) decrease (Table 28-3). In addition, plasma oncotic pressure (POP) drops

TABLE 28-3 **Hemodynamic Changes in Nonpregnant and Healthy-term Pregnant Women**

	Nonpregnant (n = 10)	Healthy pregnant (n = 10)
MAP (mm Hg)	86 ± 7.5	99 ± 5.8
Heart rate (beats/min)	71 ± 10	83 ± 10
Cardiac output (L/min)	4.3 ± 0.9	6.2 ± 1.0
SVR (dyn s cm⁻⁵)	1530 ± 520	1210 ± 265
PCWP (mm Hg)	6.3 ± 2.1	7.5 ± 1.8
CVP (mm Hg)	3.7 ± 2.6	3.6 ± 2.5
LVSWI (g mm²)	41 ± 8	48 ± 6
COP (mm Hg)	21 ± 1	18 ± 1.5

Data from: Clark S, Cotton DB, Lee W. Central hemodynamic assessment of normal term pregnancy. *Am J Obstet Gynecol* 1989;161:1439–1442.

TABLE 28-4 Hemodynamic Changes in Severe Preeclampsia

Hemodynamic Variables	Untreated Patients[37] (n = 87)	Treated Patients[38] (n = 45)	Treated Patients[39] (n = 41)	Pulmonary Edema[39] (n = 8)
MAP (mm Hg)	—	138 ± 3	130 ± 2	136 ± 3
CVP (mm Hg)	2	4 ± 1	4.8 ± 0.4	11 ± 1
PCWP (mm Hg)	7	10 ± 1	8.3 ± 0.3	18 ± 1
Cardiac index (1 min^{-1} m^{-2})	3.3	—	—	—
Cardiac output (L/min)	—	7.5 ± 0.2	8.4 ± 0.2	10.5 ± 0.6
SVR (dyn s cm^{-5})	3003	1496 ± 64	1226 ± 37	964 ± 50
PVR (dyn s cm^{-5})	131	70 ± 5	65 ± 3	71 ± 9
LVSWI (g mm^2)	—	81 ± 2	84 ± 4	87 ± 10

Data from: Visser W, Wallenburg HC. Central hemodynamic observations in untreated preeclampsia patients. *Hypertension* 1991;17:1072–1077; Cotton DB, Lee W, Huhta JC, et al. Hemodynamic profile of severe pregnancy-induced hypertension. *Am J Obstet Gynecol* 1988;158:523–529; and Mabie WC, Ratts TE, Sibai BM. The central hemodynamics of severe preeclampsia. *Am J Obstet Gynecol* 1989;161:1443–1448.

with narrowing of POP–PCWP gradients. Left ventricular function remains within normal limits with no evidence of hyperdynamic changes. These changes are outlined in detail in Chapter 1.

In patients with severe preeclampsia, the findings vary based on whether or not they had received any treatment with fluids or antihypertensives. Untreated preeclamptic patients almost always have the classic, uniform pattern consisting of low CVP, low PCWP, and CO, and a significantly elevated SVR indicating widespread vasoconstriction, decreased intravascular volume, and low filling pressures (35) (Table 28-4). Interestingly, pooled data from five different studies indicate that 86% of these untreated patients have the ventricular function curve shifted to the left indicating hyperdynamic left ventricular function (Fig. 28-3) (36).

Preeclamptic patients, who had received treatment with fluids and antihypertensive drugs, have no uniform hemodynamic pattern; they have either abnormally high or low values thus making the hemodynamic pathophysiology less clear. In most studies, CO, SV, HR, and PCWP are in the normal to high range with significantly elevated SVR (37,38,39) (Table 28-4). Furthermore, pooled data from various studies involving 89 treated preeclamptic patients show that 65 (73%) had hyperdynamic circulatory pattern, 18 patients (20%) had normal function, and 6 patients (7%) had depressed left ventricular function (Fig. 28-4) (36).

In untreated preeclamptic patients, there is a modest correlation between CVP and PCWP whereas in treated patients the situation is different. In patients receiving treatment, for any given CVP value, there is a wide variation in PCWP. This discrepancy had been well demonstrated by prior studies (40,41,42). The normal difference between PCWP and CVP is 4 and 5 mm Hg. In treated preeclamptic patients this value may vary widely between –1.6 and 17 mm Hg. In the majority of patients, PCWP–CVP differences tend to be significantly higher than normal limits (Table 28-5). A small increase in CVP may lead to a significant and disproportionate rise in PCWP and pulmonary edema. The etiology for this discrepancy and lack of correlation between CVP and wedge pressures is unclear, presumably related to factors such as slow equilibration of volume between the left and the right ventricles, "stiff" left ventricle with high left ventricular filling pressures (diastolic dysfunction), and the markedly elevated SVR (40,41,42).

Given the abovementioned hemodynamic changes, until a decade ago, invasive monitoring with PA catheters was considered crucial for the peripartum management of patients with severe preeclampsia. However, PA catheter placement is asso-

ciated with significant risks including, life-threatening complications such as pneumothorax and pulmonary artery rupture. There is no evidence that invasive monitoring improves patient outcome in severe preeclampsia (43,44). Furthermore, most obstetric units lack the obstetric intensive care units (ICUs) and trained ICU nurses to monitor the patients. At present, the use of invasive techniques with PA catheters is recommended only for specific indications such as pulmonary edema, persistent oliguria, and massive hemorrhage (2).

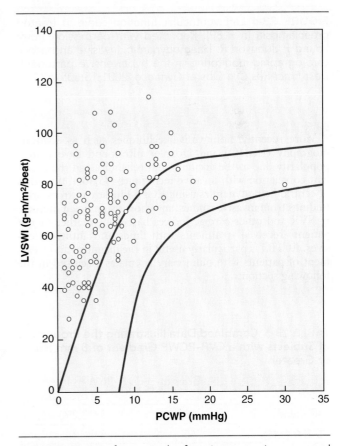

FIGURE 28-3 Left ventricular function curve in untreated preeclampsia (n = 109). Reprinted with permission from: Young P, Johnson R. Haemodynamic, invasive and echocardiographic monitoring in the hypertensive parturient. *Best Pract Res Clin Obstet Gynaecol* 2001;15:605–622.

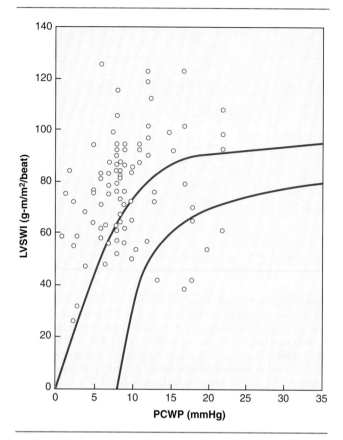

FIGURE 28-4 Left ventricular function curve in treated preeclampsia (n = 89). Reprinted with permission from: Young P, Johnson R. Haemodynamic, invasive and echocardiographic monitoring in the hypertensive parturient. *Best Pract Res Clin Obstet Gynaecol* 2001;15:605–622.

More recently, noninvasive techniques such as echocardiography (ECHO) and Doppler ultrasound have gained popularity due to the accuracy and reliability and the excellent correlation with invasive techniques (45,46,47). Studies of central hemodynamics using ECHO mostly mirrors prior findings from invasive studies, and show a significant increase in SVR and other cardiac indices based on whether or not patients received treatments with fluids and antihypertensives. ECHO is particularly useful in the diagnosis and treatment of patients with pulmonary edema as discussed in the following section.

TABLE 28-5 Combined Data Illustrating the Proportion of Subjects with a CVP–PCWP Gradient of 8 mm Hg or Greater

CVP	Number of Subjects	CVP–PCWP Gradient 8 mm Hg or Greater
All values	98	13 (13.2%)
5–8 mm Hg	65	8 (8.1%)
4 mm Hg or less	41	4 (10.3%)

Adapted from: Young P, Johanson R. Haemodynamic, invasive and echocardiographic monitoring in the hypertensive parturient. *Best Pract Res Clin Obstet Gynaecol* 2001;15:605–622.

Pulmonary Edema in Severe Preeclampsia

Pulmonary edema is one of the most serious complications of severe preeclampsia and is associated with high maternal and fetal morbidity and mortality. The incidence is 3% and the condition is largely preventable. Pulmonary edema in preeclampsia can be noncardiogenic or cardiogenic (45,47).

Noncardiogenic pulmonary edema is caused by increased capillary permeability due to the widespread endothelial damage of all vascular beds including the pulmonary vasculature. In addition, POP is significantly lower in preeclampsia with values of 17 mm Hg or less (compared to 18 to 21 mm Hg in healthy pregnant women), presumably due to hypoalbuminemia from hepatic dysfunction and ongoing renal loss. After delivery, POP can decrease to values as low as 13 mm Hg or less, possibly from iatrogenic fluid overload. This causes further narrowing of POP–PCWP difference leading to pulmonary edema. Noncardiac pulmonary edema is often self-limiting and responds well to standard treatment with no need for long-term interventions.

Cardiogenic pulmonary edema is caused by left ventricular systolic or diastolic dysfunction. In a landmark study, Mabie et al. (47) studied a group of 45 patients with pulmonary edema admitted to the obstetric ICU in our institution. The authors performed two-dimensional and M-Mode ECHO and continuous pulsed color Doppler ECHO in all patients. They identified three therapeutically and prognostically distinct groups: Those with systolic dysfunction; those with normal systolic function, but increased left ventricular mass and diastolic dysfunction; and the third group with normal hearts.

Those with *systolic dysfunction*, have severely depressed left ventricular contractile function. Such patients tend to be older, multiparous, and may have pre-existing cardiac diseases such as chronic hypertension and dilated cardiomyopathy. Pulmonary edema may occur in the antepartum or postpartum period. These patients should be admitted to the ICU and treatment with furosemide, digoxin, and oxygen should be initiated. Early and aggressive treatment is needed to stop the progression of the disease and worsening of the condition. The long-term prognosis in such patients is poor (47).

Patients with *isolated diastolic dysfunction* have a different hemodynamic profile. Typically, such patients have a normal left ventricular stroke volume and cardiac output. They have a significant left ventricular hypertrophy and normal SVR. The "stiffness" of the left ventricle results in high filling pressures, that is, even a small increase in filling volume, causes disproportionately large increases in left ventricular end-diastolic pressure and PCWP leading to pulmonary edema. These patients are usually obese and multiparous, with a history of chronic hypertension. They are overly sensitive to intravascular volume shifts. Treatment options include: Diuretics, antihypertensives, β-adrenergic blockers, and calcium channel antagonists. The long-term survival is better, compared to those with systolic dysfunction.

Not uncommonly, patients with pulmonary edema may have *both systolic and diastolic dysfunction*. Patients with normal hearts have noncardiogenic pulmonary edema as discussed earlier. Thus, patients with pulmonary edema pose a challenge and the accurate diagnosis of the different subtypes of cardiac dysfunction as well as the differentiation of cardiac and non cardiogenic pulmonary edema is difficult with routine clinical examination and chest x-rays (47). In such patients, it is imperative that the ECHO is performed to aid the management.

Respiratory System

Generalized edema of preeclampsia involves the upper airway and a difficult tracheal intubation should be anticipated. Any incidental upper respiratory infection can also cause severe airway obstruction and shortness of breath in these patients.

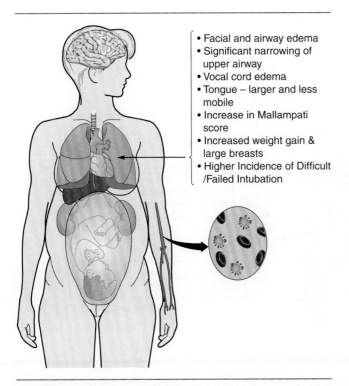

FIGURE 28-5 Airway changes in severe preeclampsia.

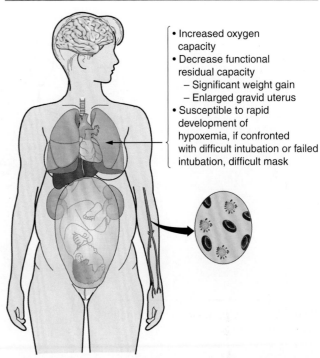

FIGURE 28-6 Changes in respiratory system in severe preeclampsia.

Earlier studies showed that maternal oxygen dissociation curve is shifted to the left due to a decrease in 2,3-diphosphoglycerate level and increased carboxyhemoglobin derived from increased catabolism of red blood cells (Figs. 28-5 and 28-6) (48,49).

Central Nervous System

Central nervous system manifestations include severe headache, blurred vision, hyper-reflexia, and the most serious of all, eclamptic seizures (Fig. 28-7). Eclampsia is one of the major causes of maternal mortality, especially in the developing world. The exact etiology of eclampsia remains an enigma just as it is for preeclampsia. Available data suggest two opposing factors namely, the syndrome of hypertensive encephalopathy or alternatively, cerebral vasospasm causing areas of cerebral ischemia (50). In preeclampsia, the larger proximal cerebral blood vessels autoregulate blood flow in the distal smaller vessels. Episodes of high systemic blood pressures overwhelm the autoregulatory capacity causing hyperperfusion and forced overdistension of cerebral blood vessels. Failure of autoregulation results in vasogenic edema. Cerebral blood flow velocity is significantly elevated and shows a positive correlation with high systemic blood pressures (50). On the other hand, hypoperfusion and areas of ischemia from cerebral vasoconstriction can also contribute to the CNS symptoms. Other findings include a differential vascular sensitivity in the occipital lobes, especially in eclampsia leading to visual disturbances and even transient blindness.

Syndrome of posterior reversible encephalopathy (PRES) is worth mentioning because it is being recognized now as a syndrome, which involves headache, confusion, seizures, and visual disturbances, very similar to eclampsia but can occur in the absence of high blood pressures (51). Visual loss is the major finding. Retinal hemorrhages, disc edema, and macular exudates may be present. An MRI is crucial for the correct diagnosis. Correction of the etiologic factors is the only treatment for this condition (51).

Pathophysiology: CNS

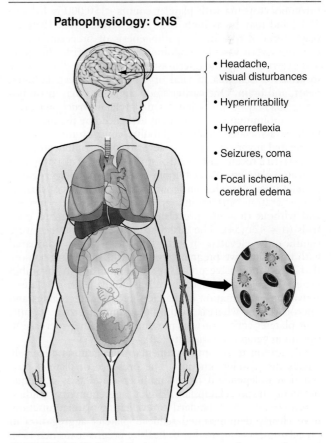

FIGURE 28-7 Central nervous system changes in preeclampsia.

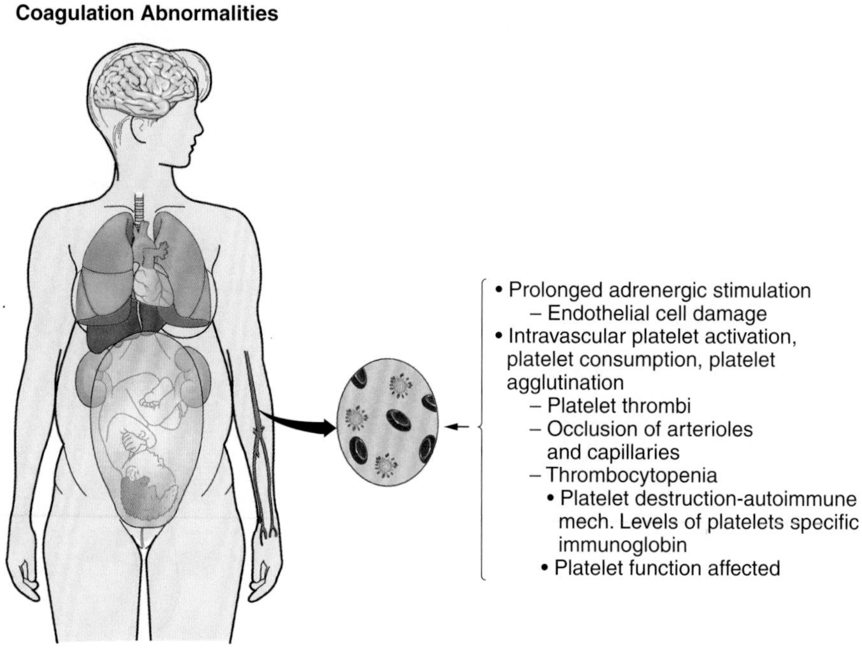

Coagulation Abnormalities

FIGURE 28-8 Coagulation abnormalities in preeclampsia.

Coagulation Abnormalities

Preeclampsia is associated with microvascular endothelial damage and enhanced clotting. The most common hematologic abnormality is thrombocytopenia. Platelet activation, increased platelet consumption, and decreased platelet lifespan are common features (Fig. 28-8). The incidence of thrombocytopenia with platelet counts <150,000 is 15% to 20%, and may be as high as 50% in severe cases. Platelets play a crucial role in the pathogenesis of preeclampsia by causing severe vascular endothelial damage with clumping and obstruction in the microvasculature (52,53). This results in areas of ischemia in vital organs such as liver, kidneys, heart, and brain. One earlier study suggested that thrombocytopenia may be due to increased platelet destruction caused by an autoimmune mechanism as evidenced by the increased platelet associated immunoglobulin concentrations which correlated inversely with the severity of thrombocytopenia (52,53). In a recent case-control study, Macey et al. compared activated platelets, platelet–monocyte/neutrophil aggregates, platelet microparticles, and four different markers of thrombin generation capacity in a group of patients with (n = 46) and without (n = 46) preeclampsia and nonpregnant controls (n = 42) (54). The authors found that all values were significantly elevated in preeclamptic patients compared with normotensive pregnant women. It is important to note that in normotensive pregnant women, although thrombin generation was increased, there was no evidence of platelet activation or formation of platelet leucocyte aggregates and microparticles, whereas in the preeclampsia group, significant platelet activation was present with further increase in thrombin generation capacity (54).

In addition to thrombocytopenia, preeclampsia adversely affects the platelet function. The presence of platelet dysfunction independent of the number platelets is a unique problem in preeclampsia. Platelet aggregometry studies, considered the gold standard for evaluating platelet function, have clearly demonstrated reduced platelet aggregation in preeclamptics compared with healthy pregnant women (55). However, aggregometry studies are time-consuming and not available at bedside. Other tests such as the template bleeding

time, an in vivo platelet function test also showed prolongation despite the presence of adequate platelet counts (56) and is no longer used clinically.

Recently, the use of thromboelastography (TEG) (Hemoscope, Skokie, IL) and platelet function analyzer (PFA-100) has become popular. These tests are used to assess the platelet function in severe preeclampsia. The use of TEG parameters and platelet count in 52 healthy pregnant women, 140 patients with mild preeclampsia, and 114 patients with severe preeclampsia (57) showed that the incidence of thrombocytopenia with platelet count <1,000,000 mm^3 was 3% in mild preeclamptic group and 30% in severely preeclamptic patients. The authors concluded that "severe preeclamptic women with platelet counts <100,000 mm^3 are hypocoagulable, when compared to healthy pregnant women and other preeclamptic women" (57). TEG measures whole blood coagulation providing an assessment of all clotting factors including platelets but, not specific for platelet dysfunction, because the maximum amplitude (MA) values, one of the parameters of TEG is a composite of platelet activity and fibrinogen, and a relatively high fibrinogen level can compensate for the deficiencies in other clotting factors including platelets. Since the platelet dysfunction is the primary defect in preeclampsia, some authors question the use of TEG as the assessment tool for hemostasis before obstetric regional anesthesia (58). Yet there are some institutions that routinely use TEG prior to regional techniques in severe preeclamptic patients.

The platelet function analyzer (PFA-100) (Dade-Behring, Marburg, Germany) is a point-of-care device for platelet function assessment (59). The derived parameter closure time (CT) indicates platelet function. The PFA-100 device has been found to be as sensitive and specific as platelet aggregometry and is independent of fibrinogen levels. In a prospective observational study comparing hemostatic function in healthy pregnant women and preeclamptic patients using the PFA-100 and TEG devices, Davies and colleagues found that increasing severity of preeclampsia was associated with increasing prolongation of CT even in the presence of normal platelet counts. In the severe preeclampsia group, the CT was 155 ± 65 seconds, which far exceeded the 95% reference interval of the control group 70 to 139 seconds.

In contrast, TEG maximum amplitude (MA) values in the severe preeclampsia group 71 ± 8 mm remained within the 95% reference interval of 64 to 82 mm for MA values in the control group. In a post hoc analysis to determine the effect of low platelet count in lengthening CT, the data was analyzed after excluding patients with platelet counts less than 100,000 mm³. The mean CT was 105 ± 18 seconds in the control group (n = 92), while in mild preeclamptics (n = 22) the CT was 114 ± 22 seconds whereas it was significantly prolonged in the severe preeclampsia group (n = 22) with the CT value 135 ± 48 seconds (p < 0001) (59). The findings from this report unequivocally confirm, the presence of a primary hemostatic dysfunction in patients with severe preeclampsia, which is independent of the number of platelets. Other studies using the PFA-100 have shown similar findings (60,61).

Platelet count, liver enzymes, and serum creatinine are the required laboratory tests in patients with preeclampsia. Other coagulation tests are not needed in the presence of normal platelet count and liver enzymes or in the absence of placental abruption (62). Prolonged PT, aPTT, and decreased fibrinogen may be present in patients with platelet counts <100,000 mm³ (63) and therefore, these tests are recommended to evaluate hemostasis in such patients specifically, if regional anesthesia is planned. Thrombocytopenia persists after delivery and spontaneous resolution occurs within 67 ± 25 hours after delivery and 44 ± 17 hours after platelet nadir (64). In this study, the platelet counts were >100,000 mm³ by 111 hours after delivery and by 88 hours after platelet nadir in all patients in this study (64).

Hepatic Changes

Hepatic damage in patients with severe preeclampsia is caused by vasospasm resulting in mid-zonal necrosis and multiple areas of infarctions. Subcapsular hemorrhages cause right upper quadrant pain (Fig. 28-9). Formation of a large subcap-

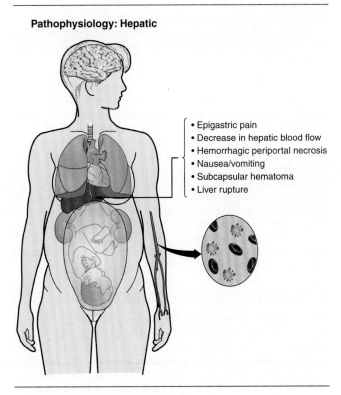

Pathophysiology: Hepatic

- Epigastric pain
- Decrease in hepatic blood flow
- Hemorrhagic periportal necrosis
- Nausea/vomiting
- Subcapsular hematoma
- Liver rupture

FIGURE 28-9 Hepatic changes in severe preeclampsia.

Pathophysiology: Renal

- Renal endotheliosis
  - Renal vasospasm, capillary endothelial swelling
- Increases in serum creatinine and uric acid
- Proteinuria
  - > 300 gms/24 hrs
- Sodium retention
- Oliguria

FIGURE 28-10 Changes in renal function.

sular hematoma and rupture can sometimes occur in patients with HELLP syndrome. Lesions seen in liver biopsy and at autopsy show periportal hemorrhages, ischemic lesions, and fibrin depositions (Fig. 28-10). Elevated liver enzymes and serum bilirubin and decreased albumin levels are commonly present (8). Plasma pseudocholinesterase levels are found to be lower in severe preeclampsia although clinically, this does not seem to significantly affect the metabolism and duration of action of drugs such as succinylcholine (65).

Changes in Renal Function

In normotensive pregnant women, renal plasma flow and glomerular filtration rate increase by 30% to 50% and serum creatinine levels rarely rises above normal and often less than normal (0.9 mg/dL). In patients with preeclampsia, renal perfusion decreases significantly, due to intense vasoconstriction. Other changes include swelling of glomerular endothelial cells, narrowing of the capillary lumen and fibrin deposition. Significant renal protein loss is common (9,66,67). Renal insufficiency leads to oliguria (<500 mL/24 h) and increased serum creatinine levels. Profound renal insufficiency can deteriorate into acute tubular necrosis. Although rare, may occur in placental abruption, HELLP syndrome, and severe uncorrected blood loss (9).

■ PREVENTION OF PREECLAMPSIA

There are numerous clinical trials describing the use of various methods to prevent or reduce the incidence of preeclampsia (5,31). Since the etiology of the disease is unknown, these interventions have been used in an attempt to correct theoretical abnormalities in preeclampsia. Previous randomized trials have evaluated protein or salt restriction; zinc, magnesium, fish oil, or vitamins C and E supplementation; the use of diuretics and other antihypertensive agents; as well as low-dose aspirin and heparin to prevent preeclampsia in women with various risk factors.

Calcium Supplementation

The relationship between dietary calcium intake and hypertension has been the subject of several experimental and observational studies. Epidemiologic studies have documented an inverse association between calcium intake and maternal BP, and the incidences of preeclampsia and eclampsia (68). The BP-lowering effect of calcium is thought to be mediated by alterations in plasma renin activity and parathyroid hormone (68).

There are 13 clinical studies (15,730 women) comparing the use of calcium versus no treatment or a placebo in pregnancy (68). These trials differ in the populations studied (low-risk or high-risk for hypertensive disorders of pregnancy), study design (randomization, double-blind, or use of a placebo), gestational age at enrollment (20 to 32 weeks of gestation), sample size in each group (range 22 to 588), dose of elemental calcium used (156 to 2,000 mg/d), and the definition of hypertensive disorders of pregnancy used. In the Cochrane review, calcium supplementation was associated with reduced hypertension; (relative risk [RR] 0.65, 95% CI 0.53 to 0.81) reduced preeclampsia, (RR 0.45; 95% CI 0.31 to 0.65) particularly for those at high risk and with low baseline dietary calcium intake (for those with adequate calcium intake, the difference was not statistically significant) (68). No side effects of calcium supplementation have been recorded in the trials reviewed. In contrast, a recent evidence-based review by the U.S. Food and Drug Administration concluded that "the relationship between low calcium and risk of hypertension in pregnancy is inconsistent and inconclusive, and the relationship between calcium and the risk of pregnancy-induced hypertension and preeclampsia is highly unlikely" (69). At present, the benefit of calcium supplementation for preeclampsia prevention in women with low dietary calcium intake remains unclear. It is also important to note that none of the published randomized trials included women with high-risk factors, such as previous preeclampsia, chronic hypertension, twins, or pregestational diabetes mellitus.

Antithrombic Agents

Preeclampsia is associated with vasospasm and activation of the coagulation–hemostasis systems. Enhanced platelet activation plays a central role in the abovementioned process and reflects abnormalities in the thromboxane/prostacyclin balance. Hence, several authors have used pharmacologic manipulation to alter the abovementioned ratio in an attempt to prevent or ameliorate the course of preeclampsia.

Earlier studies for the rationale of recommending aspirin prophylaxis, is the theory that the vasospasm and coagulation abnormalities in preeclampsia are caused partly by an imbalance in the thromboxane A_2 to prostacyclin ratio. Aspirin inhibits the synthesis of prostaglandins by irreversibly acetylating and inactivating cyclooxygenase. In vitro, platelet cyclooxygenase is more sensitive to inhibition by low doses of aspirin (<80 mg) than vascular endothelial cyclooxygenase. This biochemical selectivity of low-dose aspirin appears to be related to its unusual kinetics that result in presystemic acetylation of platelets exposed to higher concentrations of aspirin in the portal circulation. Recently, the Perinatal Antiplatelet Review of International Studies (PARIS) Collaborate Group performed a meta-analysis of the effectiveness and safety of antiplatelet agents, predominantly aspirin, for the prevention of preeclampsia (70). Thirty-one trials involving 32,217 women were included in this review. There was a 10% reduction in the risk of preeclampsia associated with the use

of antiplatelet agents (RR 0.90, 95% CI 0.84 to 0.96). For women with previous history of hypertension or preeclampsia (n = 6,107), who were assigned to antiplatelet agents, the RR for developing preeclampsia was 0.86 (95% CI 0.77 to 0.97). There were no significant differences between treatment and control groups in any other measures of outcome. The reviewers concluded that antiplatelet agents, largely low-dose aspirin, have small to moderate benefits when used for prevention of preeclampsia (70). However, more information is clearly required to assess which women are most likely to benefit from this therapy as well as when the treatment is optimally started, and what dose to use (5). Several studies evaluated the efficacy of aspirin in the prevention of preeclampsia in high-risk pregnancies as determined by Doppler ultrasound or other risk factors when aspirin was used early in pregnancy (71,72). A large multicenter National Institute of Child Health and Human Development-sponsored study that included 2,539 women with pregestational insulin-treated diabetes mellitus, chronic hypertension, multifetal gestation, or preeclampsia in a previous pregnancy showed no beneficial effect from low-dose aspirin in such high-risk women (72).

Recommendations

The 2002 American College of Obstetricians and Gynecologists Practice Bulletin states that low-dose aspirin in women at low risk has not been shown to prevent preeclampsia and therefore is not recommended. They make no specific statement regarding the use of low-dose aspirin in moderate- to high-risk pregnancies (1,73).

The Australasian Society for the Study of Hypertension in Pregnancy concludes that low-dose aspirin for prevention of preeclampsia is reasonable for the following conditions: (1) Prior fetal loss after first trimester due to placental insufficiency or severe fetal growth retardation, and (2) women with severe early onset preeclampsia in previous pregnancy necessitating delivery ≤32 weeks of gestation. Despite difficulties in predicting who will deliver preterm, consider women who have had severe early-onset preeclampsia in a previous pregnancy for low-dose aspirin therapy (2,74).

The Canadian Hypertension Society Consensus Panel concludes low-dose aspirin therapy is effective in decreasing the incidence of preterm delivery and early-onset preeclampsia among women at risk of developing the syndrome (3,75).

Vitamin C and E reduced antioxidant capacity, increased oxidative stress, or both in the maternal circulation and in the placenta have been proposed to play a major role in the pathogenesis of preeclampsia. Consequently, several trials were designed using vitamins C and E for the prevention of preeclampsia. The first trial suggested a beneficial effect from pharmacologic doses of vitamins E and C in women identified as being at risk for preeclampsia by means of abnormal uterine Doppler flow velocimetry (76). However, the study had limited sample size and must be confirmed in other populations. In contrast, several randomized trials with large sample size in women at low risk and very high risk for preeclampsia found no reduction in the rate of preeclampsia with vitamin C and E supplementation (77,78).

■ OBSTETRIC MANAGEMENT

The objective of management in women with gestational hypertension–preeclampsia, must always be safety of the mother, and then delivery of a mature newborn who will not require intensive and prolonged neonatal care. This objective can only be achieved by a plan that takes into consideration one or more of the following: The severity of the disease process, fetal gestational age, maternal and fetal status at time of

TABLE 28-6 Adverse Outcomes in Severe Hypertensive Disorders of Pregnancy

Maternal Complications

- Abruptio placentae
- Disseminated intravascular coagulopathy
- Eclampsia
- Renal failure
- Liver hemorrhage or failure
- Intracerebral hemorrhage
- Hypertensive encephalopathy
- Pulmonary edema
- Death

Fetal-neonatal Complications

- Severe intrauterine growth retardation
- Oligohydramnios
- Preterm delivery
- Hypoxia-acidosis
- Neurologic injury

the initial evaluation, presence of labor, and the consent of the mother. Pregnancies complicated by hypertensive disorders, are associated with increased maternal and perinatal complications (Table 28-6). Therefore, optimal management of these pregnancies is important to reduce or prevent some of these complications.

Management of Mild Preeclampsia >37 Weeks

Once the diagnosis of mild gestational hypertension or mild preeclampsia is made, subsequent therapy will depend on the results of maternal and fetal evaluation. In general, women with mild disease developing at 37 weeks of gestation or longer have a pregnancy outcome similar to that found in normotensive pregnancy; therefore, only patients who are at or greater than 37 weeks of gestation should undergo induction of labor for delivery.

Mild Preeclampsia <37 Weeks

All patients with mild preeclampsia should receive maternal and fetal evaluation at the time of their diagnosis. Maternal evaluation includes measurements of blood pressure, weight, and urine protein, and questioning about symptoms of head-

ache, visual disturbances, and epigastric pain. Laboratory evaluation includes determinations of hematocrit, platelet counts, liver enzyme levels, and a 24-hour urine collection once a week. This evaluation is important because patients may develop thrombocytopenia and abnormal liver enzyme levels with minimal blood pressure elevation.

Fetal evaluation should include ultrasonography to determine fetal growth and amniotic fluid volume every 3 weeks, daily fetal movement count, and nonstress testing at least once weekly.

Diuretics, antihypertensive drugs, and sedatives are not used because these agents are shown to improve pregnancy outcome, and may conversely increase the incidence of fetal growth restriction (1). With expectant management, patients are instructed to be on restricted but not complete bed rest, to have BP checked daily and to report symptoms of severe disease. Any evidence of disease progression or development of severe hypertension is an indication for prompt hospitalization.

Obstetric Management of Severe Preeclampsia

Patients with severe preeclampsia should be admitted and initially observed in a labor and delivery unit. Initial workup should include assessment for fetal well-being, monitoring of maternal blood pressure and symptomatology, as well as laboratory evaluation (79). Laboratory assessment should include hematocrit, platelet count, serum creatinine, and aspartate aminotransferase (AST). An ultrasound for fetal growth and amniotic fluid index should also be obtained. Candidates for expectant management should be carefully selected. They should also be counseled regarding the risks and benefits of expectant management. Guidelines for expectant management are outlined in Table 28-7. Fetal well-being should be assessed on a daily basis by nonstress testing and weekly amniotic fluid index determination. The patient should also be instructed on fetal movement assessment. An ultrasound for fetal growth should be performed every 2 to 3 weeks. Maternal laboratory evaluation should be done daily or every other day. If the patient maintains a stable maternal and fetal course, she may be expectantly managed until 34 weeks.

Worsening maternal or fetal status warrants delivery, regardless of gestational age. Women with a nonviable fetus (<24 weeks) should be presented with the option of pregnancy termination (79,80). Patients with severe fetal growth restriction (estimated fetal weight [EFW] <5th percentile) and those with HELLP syndrome should be delivered after completion of a course of corticosteroids (79,80). A trial of

TABLE 28-7 Guidelines for Management of Severe Preeclampsia

	Maternal	Fetal
Expeditious delivery (within 72 h)	One or more of the following: • Uncontrolled severe hypertension • Eclampsia • Platelet count <100,000/mm³ • AST or ALT >2× upper limit of normal with RUQ or epigastric pain • Pulmonary edema • Compromised renal function • Abruptio placentae • Persistent, severe headache or visual changes	One or more of the following: • Repetitive late or severe variable heart rate decelerations • Biophysical profile ≤4 on two occasions, 4 h apart • Ultrasound EFW <5th percentile • Reverse umbilical artery diastolic flow
Consider expectant management	One or more of the following: • Controlled hypertension • Urinary protein of any amount • Oliguria (<0.5 mL/kg/h) which resolves with hydration • AST/ALT >2× upper limit of normal without RUQ or epigastric pain	One or more of the following: • Biophysical profile >6 • Ultrasound EFW >5th percentile • Reassuring fetal heart rate

labor is indicated in patients with severe preeclampsia, if gestational age is >30 weeks and/or if cervical Bishop score is ≥6. However, an appropriate time frame should be established regarding the achievement of active labor (3).

■ TREATMENT

The goals of treatment are prevention of convulsions, control of blood pressures, and optimization of intravascular volume.

Prevention and Control of Seizures

Magnesium Sulfate

Intravenous magnesium sulfate has become the cornerstone of seizure prophylaxis and considered the standard of care in the United States. Many randomized clinical trials have compared magnesium with other anticonvulsants such as phenytoin, diazepam, lytic cocktails, etc. and the results show that magnesium treatment was associated with a significantly lower rate of recurrent seizures and maternal death. In addition to reducing the rate of eclampsia and its complications, magnesium also reduced the rate of progression to severe disease in those with mild preeclampsia (81). The recent MAG-PIE trial, the largest so far, involving 10,141 patients showed that magnesium significantly lowered the risk of eclampsia and reduced the risk of maternal death (82). The mechanism of action of magnesium includes direct cerebral vasodilatation and relief of vasospasm by N-methyl-D-aspartate antagonism and improvement of cerebral blood flow (83). Other effects include general CNS depression and a mild antihypertensive effect. Magnesium impairs peripheral neuromuscular transmission by competitively inhibiting calcium at the neuromuscular junction (84). Magnesium potentiates and prolongs the actions of all muscle relaxants (85). Magnesium also transiently affects pulmonary functions causing restrictive type of changes (86).

Placental Transfer and Effects on the Fetus and Neonate

Following maternal administration, magnesium levels rise in the fetal blood within an hour and in the amniotic fluid within 2 to 3 hours with equilibration of maternal and fetal serum levels within 2 hours. The fetal levels correlate significantly with the total maternal dose and the duration of infusion. Magnesium has a mild vasodilatory effect on uterine vessels and placental blood flow.

Neuroprotective Effects of Magnesium on the Fetus and Neonate

In one of the earlier case-control studies, Nelson and colleagues reported that in utero exposure to magnesium was associated with a lower prevalence of cerebral palsy in infants born weighing less than 1,500 g (87). This was subsequently followed by other similar observational studies with conflicting results (88). In order to specifically assess and delineate the neuroprotective effects of magnesium specifically in women at risk for preterm delivery, a number of prospective randomized controlled trials were performed. The Cochrane review (89) and meta-analysis of five such trials show that in the subgroup where the trials are specifically conducted examining the neuroprotective effects of magnesium, there was significant reduction in death or cerebral palsy (RR 0.85; 95% CI 0.74 to 0.98) in the in utero magnesium-exposed infants. The overall risk of cerebral palsy was 3.7% for fetuses exposed to magnesium in utero versus 5.4% for fetuses not exposed to magnesium and an absolute risk reduction of 1.7%. Furthermore, there was a significant reduction in the risk of substantial motor dysfunction (89).

Currently, there are no guidelines for the use of magnesium for fetal neuroprotection, and ACOG has issued a statement encouraging the development of such guidelines (90).

Magnesium is administered by intravenous route (IV) but can be given intramuscularly. The standard regime consists of IV bolus of 6 g over 20 minutes followed by an infusion of 2 g per hour. The therapeutic goal is to maintain serum levels at 5 to 7 mg/dL.

Magnesium is eliminated almost entirely by the kidneys. With judicious administration, toxic effects are uncommon, but can occur in the presence of renal dysfunction or from iatrogenic overdose. Monitoring patients for potential signs of magnesium toxicity should be done throughout the course of its administration, which includes eliciting deep tendon reflexes, assessing mental status, and checking respiratory rate.

The clinical findings associated with increasing serum magnesium levels are listed in Table 28-8. If a patient develops signs of magnesium toxicity, the infusion should be stopped immediately and the patient should be evaluated for respiratory compromise. Administration of oxygen, close observation

TABLE 28-8 Magnesium Sulfate Dosages, Serum Levels, and Associated Findings

Magnesium Doses	
Loading dose:	6 g IV over 20–30 min (6 g of 50% solution diluted in 150 mL D$_5$W)
Maintenance dose:	2–3 g IV per h (40 g in 1 L D$_5$LR at 50 mL/h)
Recurrent seizures:	Reload with 2 g over 5–10 min. Other drugs such as benzodiazepam or barbiturates may be given.
Magnesium Levels and Associated Findings	
Loss of patellar reflexes	8–12 mg/dL
Feeling of warmth, flushing, double vision	9–12 mg/dL
Somnolence	10–12 mg/dL
Slurred speech	10–12 mg/dL
Muscular paralysis	15–17 mg/dL
Respiratory difficulty	15–17 mg/dL
Cardiac arrest	20–35 mg/dL

of patient for magnesium toxicity, and assessment of serum magnesium level are all equally important. If magnesium toxicity is diagnosed simple discontinuation may be sufficient. Otherwise, the patient should be treated with 10 mL of 10% calcium gluconate or calcium chloride (which has more ionic availability of calcium) solution, infused over 3 minutes. Calcium competitively inhibits magnesium at the neuromuscular junction and decreases the toxic effects. The impact of calcium is transient and the patient should be closely monitored for continued magnesium toxicity. Should respiratory or cardiac arrest occur, immediate resuscitation including intubation and mechanical ventilation should be initiated. Patients receiving magnesium are at increased risk for postpartum hemorrhage due to uterine atony. Therefore these steps should be taken to ensure availability of cross-matched blood and blood products especially prior to cesarean deliveries.

Although magnesium has been in use for several decades as the drug of choice for seizure prevention and treatment for severe preeclampsia, recent studies suggest alternatives. For example, Belfort et al. (91) found that labetalol decreased maternal systemic blood pressure and the cerebral perfusion pressure without affecting cerebral blood flow (91). Furthermore, labetalol decreased the cerebral perfusion pressure more reliably compared to magnesium (92). In a recent review, Belfort et al. discussed in detail the pathophysiologic changes in the cerebral blood flow associated with severe hypertension in preeclamptic women (50) and proposed labetalol as an effective antihypertensive as well an alternative drug for seizure prophylaxis instead of magnesium sulfate.

However, magnesium has been in use for the last several decades and has been consistently proven to be reliable in prevention and treatment of convulsion and, needless to say, large scale randomized trials are needed before adopting any new regime for this purpose.

■ CONTROL OF HYPERTENSION

Maternal blood pressure control is essential with expectant management or during delivery. Medications can be given orally or intravenously as necessary to maintain blood pressure between 140 and 155 mm Hg systolic and 90 and 105 mm Hg diastolic. Care should be taken not to decrease the blood pressure too rapidly so as to avoid reduced renal and placental perfusion. Patients with generalized swelling and/or hemoconcentration (hematocrit ≥40%) usually have a marked reduction in plasma volume. The acute use of rapid-acting vasodilators in such patients can result in an excessive hypotensive response with secondary reduction in tissue perfusion and uteroplacental blood flow.

Many pharmacotherapeutic options are available for blood pressure control. There is a general agreement that maternal and fetal risks are significantly reduced by the control of blood pressures. The choice of an antihypertensive agent is based on the severity of preeclampsia, gestational age, and the presence of concurrent medical problems. Ideally, the drug should be effective, easy to titrate with no danger of overshoot hypotension. In addition, the drug should have minimal placental transfer, few drug interactions, lactation safety, and absence of teratogenic effects in the fetus. The commonly used antihypertensives are classified as direct-acting vasodilators, β-adrenergic blocking agents, and calcium channel blockers (Table 28-9).

Direct-acting Vasodilators

Hydralazine

Hydralazine is the most commonly used antihypertensive agent in pregnant women. Hydralazine lowers blood pressure by direct relaxation of arteriolar smooth muscle causing a decrease in SVR. The effects on precapillary resistance vessels are more pronounced than postcapillary capacitance vessels and the effects on coronary, cerebral, and splanchnic vessels are more than in other vascular beds. The decrease in blood pressure is accompanied by reflex tachycardia, and an increase in CO, left ventricular EF and SV with no changes in PCWP (93). The drug is more effective when used in combination with a β-adrenergic blocking agent. The decrease in blood pressure with hydralazine treatment does not affect the placental or maternal renal blood flow. Hydralazine readily crosses the

TABLE 28-9 Treatment of Hypertension

Medication	Onset of Action (min)	Dose	Comments
Hydralazine	10–20	5–10 mg IV every 20 min up to a maximum of 40 mg.	Slow onset, delayed peak effect, causes a reflex tachycardia. Effects last 2–4 h.
Labetalol	5–10	20 mg IV, then 40–80 mg IV every 10–15 min up to a maximum dose of 300 mg IV. Can also be used for blunting hypertensive response to tracheal intubation.	Avoid in patients with bradycardia or asthma. Effects last 2–6 h.
Sodium nitroprusside	0.5–1	Start infusion at 0.3–0.5 μg/kg/min. Increase in increments of 0.5 μg/kg/min. Maximum dose 5 μg/kg/min.	When treatment lasts for ≥24–48 h, or if there is renal insufficiency, the risk of maternal and fetal cyanide toxicity increases. Risk is also increased when needing more than 2 μg/kg/min. Treatment: Stop the infusion. Effects last 2–3 min.
Nitroglycerin	1–2	Start infusion at 5 μg/min. Increase by 5–10 μg/min every 2–3 min up to a maximum dose of 200 μg/min.	Tolerance may develop. Excellent uterine smooth muscle relaxant.
Nicardipine	5–15	Start infusion at 2.5 mg/h. Increase rate by 2.5 mg/h up to a maximum dose of 15 mg/h.	Can cause reflex tachycardia. Does increase ICP. Contraindicated in heart blocks.

placental barrier, and, the fetal serum levels are shown to be equal to or greater than maternal levels. Hydralazine is excreted in the breast milk, with a milk:plasma ratio of 1:4, 2 hours after the last dose. Nevertheless, hydralazine is considered safe for the infant and compatible with breast-feeding (94). Hydralazine can be given in doses of 5 mg IV every 20 minutes and titrated to decrease the diastolic pressures below 110 mm Hg. The slow onset, delayed peak effect (20 minutes) and reflex tachycardia makes hydralazine a less than an ideal agent to prevent hypertensive response during tracheal intubation.

Sodium Nitroprusside

Being an extremely potent arteriolar vasodilator, sodium nitroprusside (SNP) is a useful drug for patients with severe intractable hypertension not responding to standard treatment and also for life-threatening hypertensive emergencies. Needless to say, such patients should be monitored in the ICU with invasive central hemodynamic monitoring. SNP is administered as continuous infusion and the recommended dose is 0.5 to 5 μg/kg/min. SNP has a rapid onset of action and lowers the mean arterial pressure (MAP) and PCWP promptly (95). SNP and its metabolic products thiocyanate and cyanide cross the placenta and the potential for fetal cyanide toxicity is a major concern. In an earlier study, Naulty et al. investigated placental transfer and fetal toxicity in a pregnant ewe model. In this model, SNP was administered in doses sufficient to reduce MAP by 20% for 1 hour. Maternal fetal levels of SNP reached equilibrium in 20 minutes and more importantly, fetal death from cyanide toxicity occurred in five of the eight animals (96). However, SNP has been safely used for intractable hypertension with pulmonary edema with no evidence of adverse fetal effects. Limiting the dose and duration of infusion minimizes the risk of cyanide toxicity (95) (Table 28-9).

Nitroglycerine

Unlike SNP, nitroglycerine (NTG) is a venodilator and expands the venous capacitance vessels. Similar to SNP, NTG can be used for the treatment of intractable hypertension (Table 28-9). NTG lowers the MAP but does not increase the heart rate significantly. Transcranial Doppler and single-photon emission computed tomography studies have shown that 1 mg of NTG administered sublingually caused a significant decrease in mean blood flow velocities of maternal middle cerebral artery without changes in the regional cerebral blood flow. NTG also lowers cardiac index and PCWP, but has no effect on CVP and SV (97,98). Pretreatment with NTG is effective in blunting the hypertensive response to tracheal intubation in preeclamptic patients receiving general anesthesia for cesarean deliveries (99). However, the response to NTG is less pronounced in patients who had received volume expansion before cesarean section (100).

β-Adrenergic Blocking Agents

Labetalol

Labetalol is a unique drug with $\beta 1$, $\beta 2$, as well as postsynaptic $\alpha 1$-adrenergic receptor blocking effects. The β-blockade is more potent than the α-blockade and varies with the route of administration. When given intravenously, the $\beta{:}\alpha$ blocking ratio is 7:1 and with oral administration, 3:1. The liver rapidly metabolizes the drug and the plasma half-life ranges from 1.7 to 5.8 hours. Labetalol crosses the placental barrier with the fetal:maternal ratio of 1. There are no adverse effects on fetal blood flow as measured by umbilical and fetal middle cerebral artery flow velocities. An earlier

study in near-term pregnant ewes showed that intravenous bolus administration of labetalol ameliorated the effects of norepinephrine on maternal blood pressures, uterine blood flow, fetal pH, and fetal arterial O_2 tension and produced less adrenergic blockade in the fetus than in the mother (101). In one of the earliest comparative clinical trials, Mabie et al. randomized a group of patients with severe preeclampsia to receive either intravenous labetalol or hydralazine for the acute management of hypertension (Fig. 28-11). (102) The important findings in this study, were that while both drugs reduced the blood pressures, labetalol had a more rapid onset of action; and hydralazine lowered the blood pressure to a greater degree. The major drawback with labetalol, was the significant inter-patient variability, in the dose response that could not be predicted by any clinical characteristics. In this study, labetalol was well-tolerated by the mothers and there were no bradycardia or hypoglycemic events in the labetalol-exposed infants. In a more recent large clinical trial, Vigil-De Garcia et al. compared the safety and efficacy of intravenous labetalol and hydralazine for acutely lowering blood pressures in pregnancy (103). Two hundred patients with severe pregnancy-induced hypertension were randomized to receive either hydralazine 5 mg boluses every 20 minutes up to a maximum of 5 doses or labetalol 20 mg, 40 mg, and 80 mg every 20 minutes up to a maximum of 300 mg. Both drugs lowered blood pressures to target levels. Maternal tachycardia and palpitations were present only in the mothers who received hydralazine. The number of patients with persistent hypertension and overshoot hypotension was

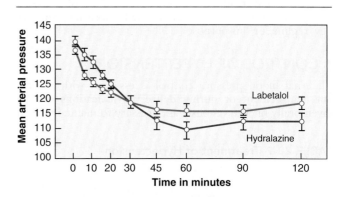

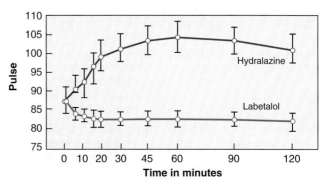

Changes in MAP and HR with repeated boluses of IV labetalol (20-80 mg) or IV hydralazine (5 mg) given at 10 min. intervals.

FIGURE 28-11 Labetalol versus hydralazine. From: Mabie WC, Gonzalez AR, Sibai BM, et al. A comparative trial of labetalol and hydralazine in the acute management of severe hypertension complicating pregnancy. *Obstet Gynecol* 1987;70:328–333.

similar in the two groups. However, the incidence of hypotension and bradycardia was significantly higher in the labetalol-exposed infants. In patients with severe preeclampsia, undergoing general anesthesia, pretreatment with intravenous labetalol in 5 to 10 mg boluses up to a total of 1 mg/kg, is shown to effectively blunt the hypertensive response to tracheal intubation (104) (Table 28-9). Labetalol can also be used to treat malignant ventricular arrhythmias associated with eclampsia.

Calcium Channel Blocking Agents

Nifedipine
Nifedipine is a calcium channel blocker with a selective renal arteriolar vasodilator action. In patients with severe preeclampsia, nifedipine causes a significant decrease in MAP with no effect on the uteroplacental circulation. Cardiac index increases significantly and SVR decreases. Nifedipine is administered sublingually as liquid-filled capsules. There have been several reports of the drug causing precipitous drop in blood pressures with ischemic cardiac changes (105). In addition, nifedipine interacts with magnesium sulfate causing severe hypotension and neuromuscular blockade (105,106). Nifedipine is no longer considered safe for use to treat hypertension in pregnant patients.

Nicardipine
Nicardipine is a calcium channel blocking agent. It is a dihydropyridine derivative that inhibits calcium ion influx in cardiac and vascular smooth muscles. Nicardipine is more selective for vascular smooth muscles than cardiac smooth muscles and therefore, has a less negative inotropic effect compared with other calcium channel blockers.

Nicardipine decreases systolic, diastolic, and mean blood pressures and SVR. Cardiac output and ejection fraction may increase. The drug is highly protein bound and has a half-life of 2 to 5 minutes after an IV bolus and 1 to 2 hours after prolonged continuous infusion. Placental transfer is 9% with maternal:fetal levels of 54.6 ng/mL and 4.18 ng/mL. The recommended dose regimen is to begin infusion at 2.5 mg/h and increase the infusion by 2.5 mg/h every 5 to 10 minutes to a maximum of 15 mg/h until the target blood pressures are achieved.

In a prospective study, Elatrous et al. studied 60 preeclamptics randomly assigned to receive either intravenous labetalol (n = 30) or nicardipine (n = 30) to lower the blood pressures by 20% from baseline (107). The primary outcome endpoints were the success rate and the time to achieve the target blood pressures. The authors found that both drugs achieved the 20% lowering of blood pressures (63% of patients in the labetalol group and 70% in the nicardipine group). Nicardipine caused greater decrease in pressures, but no patient had hypotension. The length of time to achieve the goal was similar (12 minutes for labetalol vs. 11 minutes for nicardipine). The authors concluded that both labetalol and nicardipine are effective and safe in the initial treatment of severe hypertension of pregnancy (107). Maternal side effects of nicardipine include tachycardia and palpitation, fatigue, dry mouth, and nasal congestion. Hypotensive overshoot episodes are uncommon. Drug interactions include increased plasma levels of nicardipine by H_2 blocker cimetidine, in patients receiving the two drugs concomitantly. Nicardipine being a calcium channel blocking agent may have a synergistic effect with magnesium, but so far reports indicate no adverse effects with the combination therapy. Fetal complications include transient loss of beat-to-beat variability, that resolves spontaneously on discontinuation of the drug. In patients with cardiac compromise nicardipine should be used with extreme

caution. Overall, when used appropriately, nicardipine has proven to be an excellent choice for the treatment of severe hypertension in pregnant patients (107,108) (Table 28-9).

■ FLUID MANAGEMENT

In patients with severe preeclampsia, preoperative intravenous hydration is often a challenge, but necessary for several reasons. Patients with severe preeclampsia have decreased circulating plasma volume. They also may have oliguria with urine output <500 mL/24h. It is not always possible to distinguish whether the low urine output is due to prerenal causes or intrinsic renal pathology, and both may be present in any given patient. Use of a diuretic can worsen the condition due to the presence of underfilling of vascular beds. A fluid challenge with 250 mL of crystalloid should be considered. Improved urine output is a good sign and allows for further fluid administration. Persistent oliguria not responding to IV fluid challenge is an indication for central hemodynamic monitoring. In the majority of such cases, a central line placement (CVP) alone is adequate as this provides a baseline value for reference followed by a trend of changes from baseline with fluid administration. Crystalloids may be administered to increase the CVP to values not exceeding 4 to 5 mm Hg. Any increase above 4 to 5 mm Hg should be avoided. The normal difference of PCWP–CVP is 3 to 4 mm Hg and in severe preeclampsia PCWP–CVP difference can be twice as normal, up to 8 to 10 mm Hg or more (36). Therefore, administration of fluids to increase the CVP to a normal value of 6 to 8 mm Hg may correspond to a rise in PCWP of 14 to 16 mm Hg. This causes volume overload and pulmonary edema. In a study involving 50 patients with severe preeclampsia, Wallenberg et al. showed that none of the patients with a CVP of 4 mm Hg or less had PCWP values exceeding 12 mm (35). As previously noted, the indications for the insertion of PA catheter lines are limited to patients with intractable pulmonary edema not responding to standard treatment.

As for the type of fluids for hydration, there is a hypothetical case for plasma volume expansion with colloids. However, prior studies have shown no benefit with colloid regimen. Besides, using colloids for volume expansion carries a serious risk of volume overload with pulmonary and cerebral edema (109). If colloids are used for volume loading, central hemodynamic monitoring is required.

■ ANESTHETIC MANAGEMENT
Preoperative Evaluation and Monitoring

Anesthetic management of patients with preeclampsia poses a challenge because in addition to the pathophysiologic changes of the disease itself, the presence of concurrent obstetric and medical problems such as prematurity, diabetes, morbid obesity, extremes of age, chronic hypertension, etc. can add to the complexity of the problem. Besides, the condition can suddenly deteriorate into hypertensive crisis, pulmonary edema, placental abruption, and eclampsia or HELLP syndrome. Therefore, the anesthetic plan should be flexible to include strategies to manage all of the aforementioned complications. It is important to ensure that hypertension is well controlled, seizure prophylaxis is initiated, and volume status is optimized. A complete physical examination including proper airway evaluation is important and equipment to manage a difficult airway should be immediately available.

For those with mild preeclampsia, automatic blood pressure cuff, continuous EKG, and other standard monitoring should be initiated. Placement of a radial arterial catheter for continuous and beat-to-beat monitoring is recommended specifically in acute hypertensive crisis, patients receiving potent vasodilators or calcium channel blockers, and in morbidly obese women in whom the blood pressures measured by the cuff may not be accurate. Two free-flowing IV lines are necessary. Blood and blood products must be cross-matched and made available as needed.

Laboratory investigations should include complete blood count, hemoglobin levels, platelet count, liver function tests, serum BUN and creatinine, and urine analysis. Estimation of PT, PTT, fibrinogen levels, and INR are needed only in the presence of admission platelet counts <100,000 mm³, abnormal liver enzyme levels, placental abruption, and HELLP syndrome (1,63).

A platelet count of 100,000 mm³ is considered adequate for the safe administration of the block. In a patient with severe preeclampsia and thrombocytopenia, a major concern regarding the administration of a neuraxial block is the potential for epidural bleeding and hematoma formation. This is a rare but devastating complication. There have been reports of healthy parturients with platelet counts far less than 100,000 mm³, receiving epidural anesthesia safely with no evidence of any neurologic deficits (110). However, no assessment of platelet function had been done in these studies, and abnormal platelet function is quite rare in healthy women. In contrast, in patients with severe preeclampsia, thrombocytopenia and abnormal platelet aggregation are frequently present. When the platelet count decreases below 75,000/mm³, other tests such as PT, PTT and fibrinogen levels, and TEG also tend to become abnormal (62,63). Currently, no data exists to show the lowest platelet count considered safe enough to perform a neuraxial block. A recent review suggests a platelet count of 75,000 mm³ or above may be acceptable (111). Others suggest higher numbers of 80,000/mm³ or above as the safe lower limit (112). Fortunately, epidural hematomas are rare in obstetric population. A recent report from Sweden showed that the incidence of spinal–epidural hematoma is 1:200,000 in obstetrical patients, far less than the incidence of 1:5,400 in orthopedic patients (113). Similarly, an audit from the United Kingdom showed five cases of epidural hematomas among 700,000 patients who received neuraxial blocks, confirming the rarity nonetheless a devastating complication (114) if not recognized immediately and managed appropriately.

As such, the decision to proceed with a neuraxial block in preeclamptic patients with thrombocytopenia should be undertaken with caution. This should not be based on a single admission platelet count, but rather, on the changing trends with serial estimation of platelet counts (significant change/decrease since admission), platelet function (which is directly related to the severity of preeclampsia), and the presence of comorbidities and complications of severe preeclampsia such as placental abruption, disseminated intravascular coagulation, HELLP syndrome, etc.

Analgesia for Labor and Vaginal Delivery
Epidural analgesia is eminently suitable for providing pain relief for labor and delivery. There is a wealth of scientific evidence available with documentation of many beneficial effects (115). Chief among them is the provision of excellent pain relief without any untoward maternal or fetal side effects. The careful and meticulous technique minimizes the incidence of hypotension. Some of the beneficial effects include: Decrease in maternal basal metabolic rate, oxygen consumption, and the circulating catecholamines. Furthermore, when MAP is maintained, the intervillous blood flow improves significantly after epidural placement, a beneficial effect in these patients with vasospasm of placental circulation. With careful fluid administration and slow induction of

the block, the hemodynamics remains stable with little if any changes in CI, CVP, and PCWP (116). In terms of choice of local anesthetics, there are no contraindications for the use of any one of the commonly available local anesthetics.

Technique of Labor Epidural Analgesia
Standard monitoring should include continuous maternal EKG, FHR, and BP measurements using an automatic cuff. Oxygen administration via a facemask or nasal cannula is beneficial. After placing the epidural catheter in the routine manner, 10 mL of bupivacaine 0.125% mixed with fentanyl 2 μg/mL, or 0.2% plain ropivacaine can be used as a loading dose followed by 10 to 12 mL/h of the same mixture as epidural infusion. This will provide excellent analgesia with minimal motor block. Alternatively, patient-controlled epidural anesthesia (PCEA) can be used. Epinephrine-containing local anesthetics are preferably avoided in patients with preeclampsia.

Prophylactic Epidural Catheter Placement
Most obstetric anesthesiologists are familiar with the concept of prophylactic epidurals and would agree that epidural catheters should be placed early in labor in all high-risk patients including those with severe preeclampsia. The placement of epidural catheters in early labor is not necessarily for providing labor analgesia, rather, a precautionary prophylactic measure. The goal is to avoid a general anesthetic if an urgent cesarean section becomes necessary for maternal or fetal indications. Patients with severe preeclampsia are at a significantly greater risk for developing complications during labor such as placental abruption, HELLP syndrome, eclampsia, etc. and a rapid abdominal delivery may become necessary. There is ample evidence that the incidence of airway disasters is significantly higher during general anesthesia for urgent cesarean section. In such cases, the prophylactically placed epidurals can be easily activated with the use of a rapid-acting local anesthetic to provide adequate block for cesarean deliveries. Results from a recent retrospective review suggest that early prophylactic placement epidurals in high-risk patients decreased the need for general anesthesia for urgent cesarean sections (117). Furthermore, practice guidelines for obstetric anesthesia from ASA Taskforce on Obstetric Anesthesia recommends prophylactic epidural catheter placements in all high-risk parturients (118). The technique is as described previously. It is important to test the catheter with a small dose of local anesthetic to ensure that the catheter is functioning appropriately.

Anesthesia for Cesarean Delivery
Regional anesthesia is the method of choice for cesarean delivery on account of the overwhelming evidence of maternal and fetal safety and efficacy. Needless to say, the major advantage is the avoidance of general anesthesia and the risks of difficult airway management. There are other advantages for using epidural anesthesia. For example, while the stress-related hormones such as ACTH, cortisol and catecholamine levels remain stable or decrease in those receiving epidural block, they increase significantly during cesarean deliveries in patients receiving general anesthesia (119). Anesthetic options include conventional epidurals, single shot spinal and combined spinal–epidural anesthesia.

With a conventional epidural anesthetic, the advantages are the superior hemodynamic stability, highly desirable in patients with severe preeclampsia. The disadvantages are the slow onset and less intense block compared to spinal.

One of the concerns with the use of spinal anesthesia in patients with severe preeclampsia used to be the anticipated profound hypotension from sympathetic blockade in the presence of pre-existing intravascular volume depletion. Recent studies show that, curiously enough, the incidence of

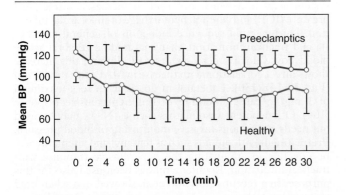

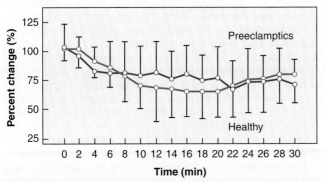

FIGURE 28-12 Changes in mean blood pressures after spinal anesthesia in preeclamptic patients (n = 30) and healthy parturients (n = 30). The incidence of hypotension was significantly less in the preeclamptic group (16.6%) compared with normotensive parturients (53.3%) (p < 0.006). From: Aya, AGM, Mangin R, Vialles N et al. Patients with severe preeclampsia has less hypotension during spinal anesthesia for elective cesarean delivery than healthy parturients: A cohort comparison. *Anesth Analg* 2003;97(3):867–872.

hypotension is significantly less in patients with preeclampsia compared to normotensive women (120,121,122). Notably, the decreased incidence of hypotension was not related to the smaller uterine mass due to IUGR or prematurity and therefore less aortocaval compression (Fig. 28-12).

Another option is the use of sequential low dose combined spinal–epidural anesthetic (CSE). This technique provides remarkable hemodynamic stability, intense motor and sensory block and the ability to maintain the level of the block with epidural top-up doses. In an earlier study, the safety and efficacy of low dose CSE was evaluated in a total of 85 patients with severe preeclampsia (120). The study groups consisted of 46 patients who underwent cesarean sections and 39 delivered vaginally. Patients in the cesarean group received intrathecal doses hyperbaric bupivacaine 7.5 mg with fentanyl 25 μg and the group delivering vaginally received 1.25 mg of plain bupivacaine with 25 μg fentanyl followed by epidural infusion of 0.0625% bupivacaine with fentanyl 2 μg/mL at a rate of 10 to 12 mL/h for labor analgesia. All except four patients in the cesarean group had adequate block levels extending to T4 dermatome and these four patients received epidural top-up doses. No required conversions to general anesthesia. The vaginal delivery group had satisfactory levels. The maximum decrease in the MAP was 15% ± 8% in the cesarean group and 16% ± 9% in the vaginal delivery group. Neonatal outcome were similar in both groups (120). In a recent prospective randomized study, Van de Velde et al. also showed that CSE is a safe alternative

to conventional epidural anesthesia in severe preeclamptic women with excellent maternal fetal outcome (123).

Hypotension and the Use of Vasopressors

In general, in patients receiving neuraxial blocks, maternal MAP is maintained within 20% to 30% of baseline values with IV fluids and vasopressors. However, blood pressure may be a poor indicator of cardiac output in patients with abnormally high SVR. It is crucial to maintain cardiac output, in such patients since placental blood flow, is directly related to maternal CO (124,125). Until recently, there was a paucity of data on the effects of spinal anesthesia and vasopressors (ephedrine and phenylephrine) on maternal CO in patients with severe preeclampsia. Recently, in an observational study, Dyer et al. measured SV, CO and SVR in 15 patients with severe preeclampsia receiving spinal anesthesia for cesarean delivery using a noninvasive pulse waveform analysis cardiac monitor (126). The findings from this important study revealed that spinal anesthesia was associated with minimal changes in CO and a modest decrease in the afterload. Oxytocin caused a transient and marked hypotension and tachycardia while CO increased significantly. Interestingly, while phenylephrine caused restoration of blood pressures, CO remained unchanged or even decreased in several of their patients. The mean change in CO after phenylephrine was not significant but the authors contend that this may be due to problems with statistical power. The authors concluded that in patients with severe preeclampsia, further studies are necessary to evaluate the effects of phenylephrine. In a follow-up study in 43 normotensive patients receiving spinal anesthesia for cesarean delivery, the authors compared the effects of phenylephrine and ephedrine on maternal CO, SVR and SV using the pulse waveform analysis and transthoracic bioimpedance technique (127). The patients were randomly assigned to receive either 10 mg ephedrine or 50 μg of phenylephrine. As in their previous study, the authors found that the bolus phenylephrine reduced CO when compared to ephedrine, and CO correlated with heart rates emphasizing the importance of heart rate as a surrogate indicator of CO. Dyer et al. did not measure the placental blood flow in their patients in the above studies (126,127). However, based on their findings, the use of phenylephrine is associated with a significant decrease in CO and this may indirectly and adversely affect the placental blood flow. Further studies are needed to define the effects of phenylephrine on placental blood flow in patients with severe preeclampsia.

Technique

After the initiation of all monitoring including FHR, patient should receive hydration with crystalloids preferably as a co-load. Epidural, spinal, or CSE anesthetic may be used. CSE is the preferred method for all scheduled cesarean deliveries at our institution. Hyperbaric bupivacaine 7.5 mg mixed with 25 μg of fentanyl can be used for the intrathecal dose. Any decrease in BP 30% from baseline requires treatment with a vasopressor, such as ephedrine in 5 mg boluses. Phenylephrine may be administered cautiously only if the patient develops severe tachycardia with heart rate >120 minutes. After delivery of the infant, oxytocin should be added to the IV infusion. Blood loss should be carefully monitored as uterine atony may be present from the tocolytic effects of magnesium sulfate infusion. Epidural dosing may be initiated if the surgery outlasts the duration of spinal anesthesia. Epidural morphine 3 to 4 mg can be used for post-cesarean delivery pain relief.

General Anesthesia

The indications for general anesthesia are: Patient refusal of regional anesthesia, emergency cesarean delivery for fetal bradycardia, coagulopathy, hypovolemia from severe hemorrhage, and inability to site the epidural due to anatomic problems such as scoliosis, or back surgeries in the lumbar area. There are two major risks associated with the induction of general anesthesia and rapid sequence tracheal intubation, namely, reflex tachycardia and severe hypertension as well as the possibility of a very difficult tracheal intubation. Generalized edema of preeclampsia also involves the structures in the upper airway causing severe upper airway swelling. A difficult airway should be anticipated in all patients with severe preeclampsia (128,129). Preparations should include immediate access to a difficult airway cart with equipment to manage the airway such as different laryngoscope blades and tracheal tubes of various sizes, laryngeal mask airways, bronchoscope, etc. Repeated attempts at tracheal intubation leads to significant swelling of the soft tissues, secretions, and bleeding which further worsens the situation. In addition, this can also result in a significant increase in both systolic–diastolic pressures and PCWP leading to pulmonary edema (Fig. 28-13) (45).

With rapid sequence induction, severe hypertension and tachycardia can occur triggered by the sympathetic nervous system activation which can lead to increased intracranial pressure (ICP) and cerebral hemorrhage or myocardial infarction. During rapid sequence induction of general anesthesia and tracheal intubation, maternal middle cerebral artery blood flow velocity increases dramatically and this increase shows direct correlation with the rise in MAP with intubation (Fig. 28-14) (130). Labetalol in doses of up to a maximum of 1 mg/kg causes blunting of this hypertensive response (104). Other potent vasodilators such as NTG may be used but needs continuous invasive monitoring of blood pressure. Pretreatment with opioids such as fentanyl and alfentanil may be effective in attenuating the hypertensive response with tracheal intubation. Remifentanil has been used also for this purpose. In a recent study, Yoo et al. showed that when used in doses of 1 µg/kg as a bolus prior to tracheal intubation, remifentanil effectively blunts the hypertensive response to tracheal intubation. However, in this study, remifentanil use was associated with neonatal respiratory depression requiring resuscitation (131). This is the major disadvantage of using opioids prior to delivery. As magnesium prolongs the actions of all muscle relaxants, judicious use of nondepolarizing muscle relaxants, monitoring of neuromuscular block, and full reversal of muscle relaxant effects should be accomplished prior to extubation of trachea. As in the beginning of surgery, extubation can also trigger a severe hypertensive response that can be managed with IV labetalol.

Postoperatively, all patients should be in a monitored area for 12 to 24 hours while they continue to receive magnesium infusion to prevent eclampsia. Antihypertensive treatment should be continued. Patients should be monitored for other serious complications such as pulmonary edema.

HELLP Syndrome

HELLP syndrome is one of the most serious complications of severe preeclampsia. The specific laboratory abnormalities demonstrating hemolysis elevated liver enzymes and low platelets are shown in Table 28-10. The clinical presentation of patients with HELLP syndrome is highly variable. However, HELLP patients generally are multiparous, white females who present at less than 35 weeks of gestation. In fact, hypertension may be absent (20%), mild (30%), or severe (50%) in women diagnosed with HELLP syndrome. Therefore, the diagnosis of HELLP syndrome cannot necessarily be ruled out in the normotensive patient who has other signs and symptoms that are consistent with preeclampsia (8).

Differential Diagnosis of HELLP Syndrome

HELLP may be confused with other medical conditions, particularly in the face of normotension. HELLP can be confused with two other specific medical conditions, acute fatty liver of pregnancy (FLP) and thrombotic thrombocytopenic purpura/hemolytic uremic syndrome (TTP/HUS) (132). The differentiation among the three entities is based on specific laboratory findings (Table 28-11).

Management

The initial evaluation in women diagnosed with HELLP syndrome should be the same as that for severe preeclampsia. The patient should be cared for at a tertiary care center. Management initially should include maternal and fetal assessment, control of severe hypertension (if present), initiation of magnesium sulfate infusion, correction of coagulopathy, and maternal stabilization. Immediate delivery should be performed in patients more than 34 weeks. In patients less than 34 weeks without proven lung maturity, corticosteroids

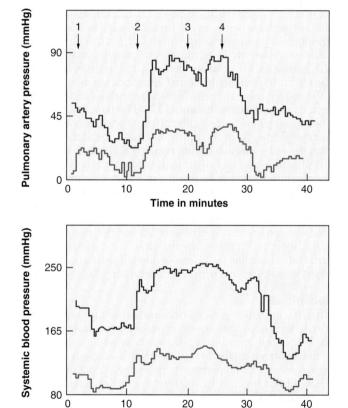

FIGURE 28-13 Continuous recording of pulmonary arterial and systemic arterial blood pressure during difficult intubation. Note hypoxic pulmonary vasoconstriction. 1: 100 mcg bolus of IV nitroprusside given to lower blood pressure; 2: Start of intubation; 3: Onset of pulmonary edema; 4: Successful awake intubation. Reprinted with permission from: Mabie WC, Ratts TE, Ramanathan KB, et al. Circulatory congestion in obese hypertensive parturients: A subset of pulmonary edema in pregnancy. *Obstet Gynecol* 1988;72:553–558.

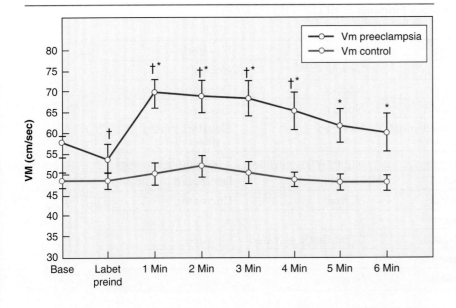

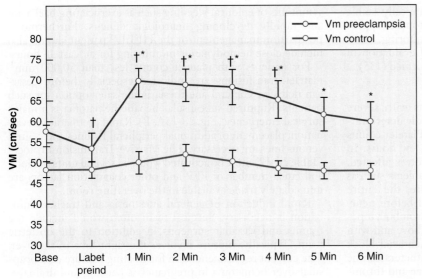

FIGURE 28-14 Changes in mean arterial pressures (MAP) and mean middle cerebral artery blood flow velocity (VM) with induction of general anesthesia and tracheal intubation. Reprinted with permission from: Ramanathan J, Angel JJ, Bush AJ, et al. Maternal middle cerebral artery blood flow velocity associated with general anesthesia in severe preeclampsia. *Anesth Analg* 1999;88:357–361.

should be given and delivery planned in 48 hours, provided there is no worsening of maternal or fetal status in the meantime. The use of steroids, volume expanders, plasmapheresis, and antithrombotic agents in patients with HELLP have produced only marginal results, although some evidences suggest a benefit of steroid therapy for improvement in maternal condition. However, two recent multicenter placebo-controlled trials revealed that high-dose dexamethasone does not improve maternal outcome in patients with HELLP syndrome in the antepartum or postpartum period (133). In addition, a Cochrane review found no benefits from corticosteroids in women with HELLP syndrome (134). Conserva-

tive management of HELLP syndrome poses a significant risk of abruptio placentae, pulmonary edema, adult respiratory distress syndrome (ARDS), ruptured liver hematoma, acute renal failure, disseminated intravascular coagulation, eclampsia, intracerebral hemorrhage, and maternal death. Therefore, expectant management past 48 hours is not warranted for the potential minimal fetal benefits when weighed against the profound maternal risk (8).

Patients with a favorable cervix and a diagnosis of HELLP syndrome should undergo a trial of labor, particularly if they present in labor. An operative delivery in some situations may even be harmful. However, elective cesarean delivery should be considered in patients at very early gestational ages with unfavorable cervices. Intraoperative considerations should include drain placement (subfascial, subcutaneous, or both) due to generalized oozing.

A potential life-threatening complication of HELLP syndrome is subcapsular liver hematoma. Clinical findings consistent with this complication include phrenic nerve pain. Referred pain from phrenic nerve such as pericardium, peritoneum, pleura, shoulder, and esophagus are consistent with this condition and commonly present. Confirmation of the diagnosis can be obtained via the CT scan, ultrasonography, or MRI.

TABLE 28-10 Criteria for HELLP Syndrome

Hemolysis	• Abnormal peripheral smear
Elevated liver enzymes	• Total bilirubin ≥1.2 mg/dL
Low platelets	• Reduced serum haptoglobin
	• Serum AST >70 U/L
	• Lactate dehydrogenase 2× upper limit of normal
	• <100,000/mm³

TABLE 28-11 Clinical/Laboratory Findings in HELLP/TTP/HUS/AFLP

	HELLP	TTP/HUS	AFLP
Ammonia	Normal	Normal	Elevated
Anemia	±	Severe	Normal
Antithrombin III	±	Normal	Decreased
AST	Elevated	Normal	Elevated
Bilirubin	Elevated, mostly indirect	Elevated	Elevated, mostly direct
Creatinine	±	Significantly elevated	Significantly elevated
Fibrinogen	Normal	Normal	Decreased in all cases
Glucose	Normal	Normal	Decreased
Hypertension	Present	±	±
LDH	Elevated	Significantly elevated	Elevated
Proteinuria	Present	±	±
Thrombocytopenia	Present	Severe	±

Conservative management in a hemodynamically stable patient with an unruptured subcapsular hematoma is appropriate, provided that close hemodynamic monitoring, serial evaluations of coagulation profiles, and serial evaluation of the hematoma with radiologic studies are performed (135).

Anesthesia Management

Anesthesia management is similar to patients with severe preeclampsia. The major difference is the rapidly deteriorating coagulation status in HELLP syndrome. Platelet counts can decrease dramatically in the course of a few hours. In addition to thrombocytopenia, platelet function is affected. It is important to keep in mind additional problems such as placental abruption might develop. Therefore, the entire coagulation panel of tests should be obtained before neuraxial anesthesia. For those with a moderate thrombocytopenia with a platelet count of 80,000 mm³ and above and with normal aPTT, PT, and fibrinogen levels, a neuraxial block may be considered. After delivery, epidural catheters can be safely removed after coagulation tests normalize and thrombocytopenia is resolved. Most patients should show reversal of laboratory parameters within 48 hours after delivery (8). However, patients should be closely monitored for signs and symptoms of epidural bleeding such as excruciating back pain and rapidly developing neurologic deficits. Furthermore, postpartum management of the HELLP patient should also include close hemodynamic monitoring for at least 48 hours.

For patients with platelet counts less than 50,000 mm³, platelet transfusions are indicated especially before cesarean delivery. General anesthesia is the safer option for such patients. Ruptured subcapsular hepatic hematoma is a major surgical emergency (Fig. 28-15A, B). Rapid preoperative evaluation, placement of additional peripheral IV lines and central venous lines are necessary. The Massive Transfusion Protocol (Table 28-12) must be activated whereby several units of blood and equal number of FFP and other coagulation factors are immediately made available in the operating room.

Rapid induction of general anesthesia and tracheal intubation is necessary. Surgical team often would include the trauma and vascular surgeons in addition to the obstetric team. Typically, rupture involves the right lobe of the liver. The current recommendation for treating rupture of subcapsular liver hematoma in pregnancy is packing and drainage. Maternal and fetal mortality is over 50%, even with immediate intervention. Postpartum, the patient should be monitored in the ICU.

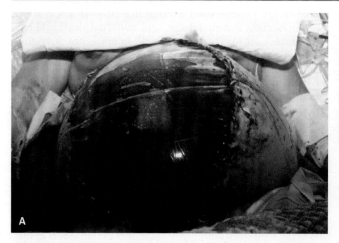
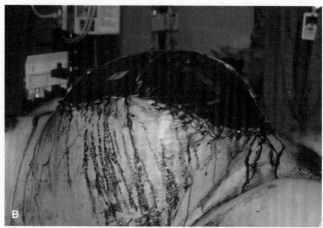

FIGURE 28-15 A and **B:** Rupture of liver in a patient with HELLP syndrome and severe preeclampsia. Patient required multiple units of blood and blood products. Patient underwent laparotomy, abdomen was packed. She eventually succumbed.

TABLE 28-12 Massive Transfusion Protocol

- During massive blood loss
- Goal is to approximate whole blood
  - Concept is FFP and platelets relative to RBC
- Many protocols exist
  - Red blood cells: 6 units
  - FFP: 6 units
  - Platelets: 1 apheresis unit (6 units platelets)
  - Cryoprecipitate: 1 pooled unit (5 units cryo)

From: Duschesne JC, Islam TM, Stuke L, et al. Hemostatic resuscitation during surgery improves survival in patients with traumatic-induced coagulopathy. *J Trauma* 2009;67:33–39.

Eclampsia

Eclampsia is defined as the new onset of seizures *and/or* unexplained coma during pregnancy or postpartum in patients with signs and symptoms of preeclampsia, but without a pre-existing neurologic disorder (2). In the Western world, the incidence ranges from 1 in 2,000 to 1 in 3,448 pregnancies. Incidence is higher in tertiary referral centers, in the developing countries, and in patients with no prenatal care. Eclampsia continues to be a major cause of maternal and perinatal morbidity and mortality worldwide. The maternal mortality rate is approximately 4.2%. The perinatal mortality rate ranges from 13% to 30%. Eclampsia can occur antepartum (50%), intrapartum (25%), or postpartum (25%) (9). In the postpartum period, eclampsia can develop as late as 2 weeks after delivery (136). Postpartum eclampsia is a diagnostic dilemma. Any woman seizing in the postpartum period should be considered to have eclampsia; however, other disorders must be ruled out. Patients who develop postpartum eclampsia usually will have symptoms prior to seizure activity including severe, persistent headache, blurred vision, photophobia, epigastric pain, nausea and vomiting, and transient mental status changes. Therefore, it is important to educate patients to immediately report these symptoms to health care providers so as to initiate preeclampsia evaluation.

Clinical Presentation

Signs and symptoms include persistent headache, blurry vision, scotomata, altered mental status, hyperreflexia, and epigastric or right upper quadrant pain. There can even be rare cases of temporary blindness, lasting from a few hours to up to a week (136,137). These signs and symptoms can occur before or after the seizure.

Eclamptic seizures typically occur suddenly. They begin with facial twitching that is followed by a tonic phase lasting for 15 to 20 seconds. This progresses to a generalized clonic phase and apnea lasting approximately 60 seconds followed by a postictal phase. Seizures are self-limiting but can recur. Seizures can be severe enough to cause respiratory arrest and cardiovascular collapse, but this is very rare. The mechanism of the seizures is not clearly understood. It is presumably due to loss of cerebral autoregulation, forced vasodilation, and hyperperfusion resulting in vasogenic edema. Other theories include development of focal areas of hypoperfusion caused by cerebral vasoconstriction and ischemia (83,138). The differential diagnosis for seizures is broad; however, all seizures in the peripartum period should be considered eclampsia until proven otherwise, and treatment should be initiated immediately. Although hypertension is considered the hallmark for the diagnosis of eclampsia, it can be absent in 15% to 20% prior to seizures. In these cases, the patient usually has proteinuria and associated central nervous system symptoms or epigastric pain with nausea and vomiting.

Management of Eclampsia

The principles to management of an eclamptic seizure include support and protection of the airway, providing supplemental oxygenation, support of the circulation, and prevention of injury. The steps unique to a seizure in a parturient include left uterine displacement (manual or by applying a wedge) to prevent aorto-venacaval compression, control of blood pressure with IV labetalol, administration of a magnesium sulfate as 6 g as IV bolus and 2 to 3 g infusion to treat and prevent further seizures, and facilitation of delivery of the fetus within 24 hours. Magnesium sulfate is the drug of choice for eclampsia (139,140). Drugs such as benzodiazepines and barbiturates although effective in seizure control are potent sedatives and should be used with caution to avoid the risk respiratory depression and aspiration. Guidelines for the management of eclamptic seizures are given in Table 28-13.

During and immediately after the seizure, it not uncommon to find FHR abnormalities such as prolonged deceleration or bradycardia, tachycardia, decreased beat-to-beat variability, and transient late decelerations. In addition, uterine contraction monitoring shows increases in both uterine tone and frequency. These usually last from 3 to 15 minutes. It may take longer for the heart rate pattern to return to baseline in an eclamptic woman whose fetus is preterm with growth restriction. It is important not to proceed directly to cesarean delivery after a seizure. Vaginal delivery is preferred and cesarean deliveries are performed for obstetric indications only. Labor may be induced and magnesium infusion should be continued.

Anesthetic Management

Anesthetic management principles are the same as those for severe preeclampsia, as outlined earlier in this chapter. The key addition for eclamptic women is assessment of seizure control and neurologic status, with particular attention to signs of increased ICP and focal deficits (140,141).

TABLE 28-13 Management of an Eclamptic Seizure

Airway
- Apply jaw thrust
- Tilt the patient to the left or manually displace the uterus to the left with wedge
- Protect the head and body from injury

Breathing
- Attempt ventilation using a bag–valve–mask with 100% oxygen.
- Do *not* attempt to insert the oral airway. If necessary, insert a soft and well-lubricated nasal airway.
- Apply pulse oximeter and continuously monitor SpO$_2$

Circulation
- Secure intravenous access
- Continuously monitor the electrocardiogram
- Check blood pressure frequently and treat hypertension

Drugs
- Magnesium sulfate
  - 4–6 g IV over 15–20 min as a loading dose
  - 1–2 g/h IV for maintenance
  - 2 g IV over 5–10 min for recurrent seizures
- Antihypertensive medications
  - Labetalol 20–40 mg IV every 5–10 min or Hydralazine 5–10 mg IV every 15–20 min as needed

All coagulation studies such as platelet count, PT, PTT, and fibrinogen should be obtained. Intracranial imaging is typically not warranted unless focal neurologic signs persist, or the diagnosis is uncertain. Patients with eclampsia may have profound volume depletion and hemoconcentration. On the other hand, these patients can also exhibit capillary leakage syndrome and therefore are predisposed to developing pulmonary edema. Fluid management is a challenge and close hemodynamic monitoring is indicated.

ICP in the eclamptic patient may be elevated and should be taken into consideration when planning anesthesia management (141). However, eclampsia is *not* an absolute contraindication to neuraxial anesthesia. In fact, neuraxial anesthesia is the method of choice in patients with no focal signs of neurologic deficits, alert mental status, and normal coagulation parameters. Advantages of neuraxial anesthesia include ability to monitor mental status, blunting of the sympathetic responses, improved blood pressure control, and improvements in uteroplacental perfusion. As discussed earlier, prophylactic placement of epidural is necessary in such patients as the catheter can be used to provide adequate block for urgent cesarean deliveries and avoid all the complications associated with the general anesthetics as described below.

The concerns regarding a difficult airway management are magnified in a patient with eclampsia. A difficult airway cart with various sizes of tracheal tubes, laryngeal mask airways, etc. should be immediately available (see Chapter 23). There have been several instances where the swollen tongue (from patient biting her tongue during seizures) completely obscuring the laryngeal view making tracheal intubation impossible via regular route. An increase in the ground substance of the airway connective tissue, due to elevated levels of estrogen during pregnancy, an increase in total body water, and an increase in interstitial fluid and blood volume results in hypervascularity and edema of oropharynx, nasopharynx, and respiratory tract. Excessive weight gain during pregnancy, preeclampsia, iatrogenic fluid overload, excessive bearing-down efforts during labor, and increase in venous pressure, all lead to an increase in mucosal upper airway edema. Additional upper airway changes include, tongue engorgement during pregnancy leading to decreased mobility of the floor of the mouth and changes in the Mallampati score. Several published reports describe development of airway edema during labor and delivery. In some of these reports, the associated difficulties in tracheal intubation were secondary to changes in the Mallampati score. If time permits an awake oral fiber optic intubation via the should be considered as option in such cases. (See Chapter 23 for the technique of awake fiber optic intubation.) Tracheal intubation may be associated with severe hypertensive response. Needless to say, antihypertensive drugs such as labetalol should be administered as prophylaxis before intubation attempts. Intraoperative management is similar to that described for preeclampsia earlier in this chapter.

Postpartum eclampsia can occur even in patients receiving magnesium. Pulmonary edema is an ever-present danger. Patients should be monitored closely for the signs and symptoms of seizures and pulmonary edema. Magnesium and antihypertensive drugs should be continued. Finally, once the laboratory values return to normal and hypertension is controlled the patient may be discharged.

Postpartum instructions should include educating her to the occurrence of symptoms such as blurred vision, persistent headache, etc. that herald the onset of a seizure and to return immediately. In the absence of such symptoms, the patient should be instructed to return in a week for outpatient follow-up.

Postpartum Long-term Follow-up

Patients with severe preeclampsia have three- to four-fold higher incidence of chronic hypertension (5,11). They also have two-fold increased risk of stroke and maternal death. Furthermore, the risks of venous thrombosis and massive pulmonary embolism are significantly higher. Recurrent preeclampsia in subsequent pregnancies is common. The incidence of cardiac complications such as peripartum cardiomyopathy and myocardial infarction are significantly higher. Therefore, long-term follow-up and appropriate management are essential in such patients (11).

■ SUMMARY

Hypertensive disorders of pregnancy are the major contributory and leading causes of maternal and fetal morbidity and mortality worldwide. Etiology is unknown and delivery of the infant is the only effective cure. The goals of treatment are prevention of seizures, control of hypertension and optimization of intravascular volume status. Anesthetic management is a challenge because of the presence of concurrent medical and obstetric problems such as morbid obesity, diabetes, prematurity, chronic hypertension, etc. In addition, complications of preeclampsia such as pulmonary edema, eclampsia, HELLP syndrome, and placental abruption may occur, adding to the complexity of the problem. Regional anesthesia is the method of choice for labor pain relief and cesarean delivery due to the overwhelming evidence of maternal and fetal safety compared with other anesthetic techniques. Recent studies using the noninvasive cardiac monitors show new information on the effects of neuraxial blocks and vasopressors on maternal cardiac output and other cardiac indices in severe preeclampsia, and stress the importance of maintaining maternal cardiac output during cesarean delivery. General anesthesia may be needed in some instances and difficult tracheal intubation should be anticipated in such cases. The risk of eclampsia and pulmonary edema persists in the postpartum period and patients should be closely monitored to prevent and treat such complications.

KEY POINTS

- Hypertension is the most common medical disorder during pregnancy and severe preeclampsia is one of the leading causes of maternal morbidity and mortality.
- The etiology remains an obstetric enigma and delivery of the fetus is the only cure for this disease.
- The pathophysiology involves the early occurrence of placental ischemia, abnormal placental angiogenesis and widespread endothelial dysfunction involving all major vascular beds.
- Development of seizures signals the onset of eclampsia, a major complication that may occur before or during labor or in the immediate postpartum period.
- Magnesium sulfate is considered the drug of choice for prophylaxis and treatment of seizures.
- Onset of HELLP syndrome leads to rapid deterioration of platelet function. Placental abruption further complicates the management. Although rare, rupture of liver is another serious life-threatening complication.
- The goals of therapy include treatment of hypertension, prevention of seizures and optimization of fluid status.
- For monitoring, PA catheters are no longer used. A central line may be necessary in selected patients for fluid management to assess the changes in trends from baseline measurements. A radial arterial line is recommended for

those receiving nicardipine or powerful vasodilators such as nitroprusside or nitroglycerine for hypertension.

- Uncontrolled hypertension in the presence of diastolic or systolic dysfunction can lead to pulmonary edema. Serial ECHO evaluation of cardiac function should be considered.
- Neuraxial blocks are excellent choices for both labor analgesia and cesarean delivery.
- If general anesthesia is chosen, airway edema and difficulties in airway management should be anticipated. Prophylactic measures are necessary to avoid reflex hypertensive response to tracheal intubation.
- Blood and blood products should be immediately available.
- Postpartum management includes observation in a step down unit for 12 to 24 hours.
- Long-term maternal morbidity and outcome are related to complications such as cardiac failure or renal failure and cerebrovascular accidents.

REFERENCES

1. Sibai BM. Diagnosis and management of gestational hypertension and pre-eclampsia. *Obstet Gynecol* 2003;102:181–192.
2. ACOG Committee on Practice Bulletins–Obstetrics. ACOG practice bulletin. Diagnosis and management of preeclampsia and eclampsia. Number 33, January 2002. *Obstet Gynecol* 2002;99:159–167.
3. Report of the National High Blood Pressure Education program working group on high blood pressure in pregnancy. *Am J Obstet Gynecol* 2000;183:S1–S22.
4. Lindheimer MD, Kanter D. Interpreting abnormal proteinuria in pregnancy. The need for a more pathophysiological approach. *Obstet Gynecol* 2010;115:365–375.
5. Barton JR, Sibai BM. Prediction and prevention of recurrent preeclampsia. *Obstet Gynecol* 2008;112(2)(Pt.1):359–372.
6. Buchbinder A, Sibai BM, Caritis S, et al. Adverse perinatal outcomes are significantly higher in severe gestational hypertension than in mild preeclampsia. *Am J Obstet Gynecol* 2002;186:66–71.
7. Sibai BM, Stella CL. Diagnosis and management of atypical preeclampsia-eclampsia. *Am J Obstet Gynecol* 2009;200:481.e1–481.e7.
8. Sibai BM. Diagnosis, controversies, and management of the syndrome of hemolysis, elevated liver enzymes, and low platelet count. *Obstet Gynecol* 2004;105:981–991.
9. Sibai BM. Diagnosis, prevention, and management of eclampsia. *Obstet Gynecol* 2005;105:402–410.
10. Sibai BM. Chronic hypertension in pregnancy. *Obstet Gynecol* 2002;100:369–377.
11. Sibai B, Dekker G, Kupferminc M. Pre-eclampsia. *Lancet* 2005;365:785–799.
12. Steegers EA, Von Dadelszen P, Duvekot JJ, et al. Pre-eclampsia. *Lancet* 2010;376:631–644.
13. Khankin EV, Royle C, Karumanchi SA. Placental vasculature in health and disease. *Semin Thromb Hemost* 2010;36:309–320.
14. Chaiworapongsa T, Romero R, Kusanovic JP, et al. Plasma soluble endoglin concentration in pre-eclampsia associated with an increased impedance to flow in the maternal and fetal circulations. *Ultrasound Obstet Gynecol* 2010;35:155–162.
15. Lapaire O, Shennan A, Stepan H. The preeclampsia biomarker soluble fms-like tyrosine kinase-1 and placental growth factor: current knowledge, clinical implications and future application. *Eur J Obstet Gynecol Reprod Biol* 2010;151:122–129.
16. Rana S, Karumanchi A, Levine FJ, et al. Sequential changes in antiangiogenic factors in early pregnancy and risk of developing preeclampsia. *Hypertension* 2007;50:137–142.
17. Moore Simas TA, Crawford SL, Solitro MJ, et al. Angiogenic factors for the prediction of preeclampsia in high-risk women. *Am J Obstet Gynecol* 2007;197:244.e1–244.e8.
18. Espinoza J, Romero R, Nien JK, et al. Identification of patients at risk for early onset and/or severe preeclampsia with the use of uterine artery Doppler velocimetry and placental growth factor. *Am J Obstet Gynecol* 2007;196:326.e1–326.e13.
19. Maynard SE, Jiang-Yong Min, Merchan J, et al. Excess placental soluble fms-like tyrosine kinase 1 (sFlt1) may contribute to endothelial dysfunction, hypertension and proteinuria in preeclampsia. *J Clin Invest* 2003;111:649–658.
20. Luttun A, Carmeliet P. Soluble VEGF receptor Flt1: The elusive preeclampsia factor discovered? *J Clin Invest* 2003;111:600–602.
21. Conde-Agudelo A, Romero R, Lindheimer MD. Tests to predict pre-eclampsia. In: Lindheimer MD, Roberts JM, Cunningham FG, eds. *Chesley's*

Hypertensive Disorders In Pregnancy. Amsterdam: Academic Press, Elsevier; 2009:189–211.
22. Papageorghiou AT, Leslie K. Uterine artery Doppler in the prediction of adverse pregnancy outcome. *Curr Opin Obstet Gynecol* 2007;19:103–109.
23. Pilalis A, Souka AP, Antsaklis P, et al. Screening for pre-eclampsia and small for gestational age fetuses at the 11-14 weeks scan by uterine artery dopplers. *Acta Obstet Gynecol Scand* 2007;86:530–534.
24. DePaco C, Kametas N, Renceret G, et al. Maternal cardiac output between 11 and 12 weeks of gestation in the prediction of preeclampsia and small for gestational age. *Obstet Gynecol* 2008;111:292–300.
25. Cnossen JS, Vollebregt KC, de Vrieze N, et al. Accuracy of mean arterial pressure and blood pressure measurements in predicting preeclampsia: Systematic review. *BMJ* 2008;336:1117–1120.
26. Cnossen JS, Morris RK, Ter Riet G, et al. Use of uterine artery Doppler ultrasonography to predict pre-eclampsia and intrauterine growth restriction. A systemic review and bivariable meta-analysis. *CMAJ* 2008;178:701–711.
27. Poon LC, Kametas NA, Maiz N, et al. First trimester prediction of hypertensive disorders in pregnancy. *Hypertension* 2009;53:812–818.
28. Poon LCY, Strateiva V, Piras S, et al. Hypertensive disorders in pregnancy: Combined screening by uterine artery Doppler, blood pressure and serum PAPP-A at 11-13 weeks. *Ultrasound Obstet Gynecol* 2009;34:497–502.
29. Dugoff L, Society for Maternal-Fetal Medicine. First- and second-trimester maternal serum markers for aneuploidy and adverse obstetric outcomes. *Obstet Gynecol* 2010;115:1052–1061.
30. Akolekar R, Syngelaki A, Sarguis R, et al. Prediction of early, intermediate and late preeclampsia from maternal factors, biophysical and biochemical markers at 11-13 wks. *Prenat Diagn* 2011;31:66–74.
31. Briceño-Pérez C, Briceño-Sanabria L, Vigil-De Gracia P. Prediction and prevention of preeclampsia. *Hypertens Pregnancy* 2009;28:138–155.
32. Hutcheon JA, Lisonkova S, Joseph KS. Epidemiology of pre-eclampsia and other hypertensive disorders of pregnancy. *Best Pract Res Clin Obstet Gynaecol* 2011;25:391–403.
33. Wallis AB, Saftlas AF, Hsia J, et al. Secular trends in the rates of preeclampsia, eclampsia, and gestational hypertension, United States,1987-2004. *Am J Hypertens* 2008;21:521–526.
34. Clark S, Cotton DB, Lee W. Central hemodynamic assessment of normal term pregnancy. *Am J Obstet Gynecol* 1989;161:1439–1442.
35. Wallenburg HCS. Hemodynamics in hypertensive pregnancy. In: Rubin PCV, ed. *Handbook of Hypertension.* Amsterdam: Elsevier; 1988:66–101.
36. Young P, Johanson R. Haemodynamic, invasive and echocardiographic monitoring in the hypertensive parturient. *Best Pract Res Clin Obstet Gynaecol* 2001;15:605–622.
37. Visser W, Wallenburg HC. Central hemodynamic observations in untreated preeclampsia patients. *Hypertension* 1991;17:1072–1077.
38. Cotton DB, Lee W, Huhta JC, et al. Hemodynamic profile of severe pregnancy-induced hypertension. *Am J Obstet Gynecol* 1988;158:523–529.
39. Mabie WC, Ratts TE, Sibai BM. The central hemodynamics of severe preeclampsia. *Am J Obstet Gynecol* 1989;161:1443–1448.
40. Tellez R, Curiel R. Relationship between central venous pressure and pulmonary capillary wedge pressure in severely toxemic patients. *Am J Obstet Gynecol* 1991;165:487.
41. Bolte AC, Dekker GA, van Eyck J, et al. Lack of agreement between central venous pressure and pulmonary capillary wedge pressure in preeclampsia. *Hypertens Pregnancy* 2000;19:261–271.
42. Cotton DB, Gonik B, Dorman K. Cardiovascular alterations in severe pregnancy-induced hypertension: Relationship of central venous pressure to pulmonary capillary wedge pressure. *Am J Obstet Gynecol* 1985;151:762–764.
43. Gilbert WM, Towner DR, Field NT, et al. The safety and utility of pulmonary artery catheterization in severe preeclampsia and eclampsia. *Am J Obstet Gynecol* 2000;182:1397–1403.
44. Practice Guidelines for pulmonary artery catheterization: An updated report by the American society of anesthesiologists task force of pulmonary artery catheterization. *Anesthesiology* 2003;99:988–1014.
45. Mabie WC, Ratts TE, Ramanathan KB, et al. Circulatory congestion in obese hypertensive parturients: a subset of pulmonary edema in pregnancy. *Obstet Gynecol* 1988;72:553–558.
46. Belfort MA, Rocky R, Saade GR, et al. Rapid echocardiographic assessment of left and right heart hemodynamics in critically ill obstetric patients. *Obstet Gynecol* 1994;171:884–892.
47. Mabie WC, Hackman BB, Sibai BM. Pulmonary edema associated with pregnancy: echocardiographic insights and implications for treatment. *Obstet Gynecol* 1993;81:227–234.
48. Kambam J, Handt R, Brown W. Effects of normal and preeclamptic pregnancies on oxyhemoglobin dissociation. *Anesthesiology* 1986;65:426–427.
49. Kambam JR, Entman S, Mouton S, et al. Effect of preeclampsia on carboxyhemoglobin levels: a mechanism for a decrease in P50. *Anesthesiology* 1988;68:433–434.

50. Belfort MA, Clark SL, Sibai B. Cerebral hemodynamics in preeclampsia: Cerebral perfusion and the rationale for an alternative to magnesium sulfate. *Obstet Gynecol Surv* 2006;61:655–665.

51. Pula JH, Eggenberger E. Posterior reversible encephalopathy syndrome. *Curr Opin Ophthalmol* 2008;19:479–484.

52. Zemel MB, Zemel PC, Berry S, et al. Altered platelet calcium metabolism as an early predictor of increased peripheral vascular resistance and preeclampsia in urban black women. *N Engl J Med* 1990;323:434–438.

53. Burrows RF, Hunter DJS, Andrew M, et al. A prospective study investigating the mechanism of thrombocytopenia in preeclampsia. *Obstet Gynecol* 1987; 70:334–338.

54. Macey MG, Bevan S, Alam S, et al. Platelet activation and endogenous thrombin potential in pre-eclampsia. *Thromb Res* 2010;125:e76–e81.

55. Norris LA, Gleeson N, Sheperd BL, et al. Whole blood platelet aggregation in moderate and severe pre-eclampsia. *Br J Obstet Gynaecol* 1993;100:684–688.

56. Ramanathan J, Sibai BM, Vu T, et al. Correlation between bleeding times and platelet counts in women with preeclampsia undergoing cesarean section. *Anesthesiology* 1989;71:188–191.

57. Sharma SK, Phillip J, Whitten CW, et al. Assessment of changes in coagulation in parturients with preeclampsia using thromboelastography. *Anesthesiology* 1999;90:385–390.

58. Samama CM. Should a normal thromboelastogram allow us to perform a neuraxial block? A strong word of warning. *Can J Anaesth* 2003;50:761–763.

59. Davies JR, Fernando R, Hallworth SP. Hemostatic function in healthy pregnant and preeclamptic women: An assessment using the platelet function analyzer (PFA-100®) and Thromboelastograph®. *Anesth Analg* 2007;104:416–420.

60. Marietta M, Castelli I, Piccinini F, et al. The PFA-100 system for the assessment of platelet function in normotensive and hypertensive pregnancies. *Clin Lab Haematol* 2001;23:131–134.

61. Vincelot A, Nathan N, Collet D, et al. Platelet function during pregnancy: An evaluation using the PFA-100 analyser. *Br J Anaesth* 2001;87:890–893.

62. Barron WM, Heckerling P, Hibbard JU, et al. Reducing unnecessary coagulation testing in hypertensive disorders of pregnancy. *Obstet Gynecol* 1999; 94:364–370.

63. Leduc L, Wheeler JM, Kirshon B, et al. Coagulation profile in severe preeclampsia. *Obstet Gynecol* 1992;79:14–18.

64. Chandran R, Serra-Serra V, Redman C. Spontaneous resolution of preeclampsia-related thrombocytopenia. *Br J Obstet Gynaecol* 1992;99:887–890.

65. Kambam J, Mouton S, Entman S, et al. Effects of pre-eclampsia on plasma cholinesterase activity. *Can J Anaesth* 1987;34:509–511.

66. Moran P, Baylis PH, Lindheimer MD, et al. Glomerular ultrafiltration in normal and preeclamptic pregnancies. *J Am Soc Nephrol* 2003;14:648–652.

67. Lindheimer M, Katz A. The kidney in pregnancy. In: Brenner B, Rector F, eds. *The Kidney*. Philadelphia, PA: WB Saunders; 1986:1253.

68. Hofmeyr GJ, Lawrie TA, Atallah A, et al. Calcium supplementation during pregnancy for preventing hypertensive disorders and related problems. *Cochrane Database Syst Rev* 2010;(8):CD001059. DOI:10.R1002/14651858.

69. Trumbo PR, Ellwood KC. Supplemental calcium and risk reduction of hypertension, pregnancy-induced hypertension, and preeclampsia: an evidence-based review by the US food and drug administration. *Nutr Rev* 2007;65:78–87.

70. Askie LM, Duley L, Henderson-Smart DJ, et al. PARIS Collaborative Group. Antiplatelet agents for prevention of pre-eclampsia: A meta-analysis of individual patient data. *Lancet* 2007;369:1791–1798.

71. Bujold E, Roberge S, Lacasse Y, et al. Prevention of preeclampsia and intrauterine growth restriction with aspirin started in early pregnancy: A meta-analysis. *Obstet Gynecol* 2010;116:402–414.

72. Chappell LC, Seed PT, Briely AL, et al. Effect of antioxidants on the occurrence of pre-eclampsia in women at increased risk: a randomized trial. *Lancet* 1999;354:810–816.

73. ACOG Committee on Obstetric Practice. Diagnosis and management of preeclampsia and eclampsia. ACOG Practice Bulletin, no 33. *Int J Gynaecol Obstet* 2002;77:67–75.

74. Brown MA, Brennecke SP, Crowther CA, et al. Aspirin and prevention of preeclampsia. *Aust N Z J Obstet Gynaecol* 1995;35:38–41.

75. Moutquin JM, Garner PR, Burrows RF, et al. Report of the Canadian Hypertension Society Consensus Conference: 2. Nonpharmacologic management and prevention of hypertensive disorders in pregnancy. *Can Med Assoc J* 1997; 57:907–919.

76. Rumbold AR, Cowther CA, Haslam RR, et al. Vitamins C and E and the risks of pre-eclampsia and perinatal complications. *N Engl J Med* 2006;354:1796–1802.

77. Poston L, Briley AL, Seed PT, et al. Vitamin C and E in pregnant women at risk for pre-eclampsia (VIP trial): randomised placebo-controlled trial. *Lancet* 2006;367:1145–1154.

78. Spinnato JA 2nd, Freire S, Pinto E Silva JL, et al. Antioxidant therapy to prevent pre-eclampsia: A randomised controlled trial. *Obstet Gynecol* 2007; 110:1311–1318.

79. Sibai BM, Barton JR. Expectant management of severe preeclampsia remote from term: Patient selection, treatment, and delivery indications. *Am J Obstet Gynecol* 2007;196:514.e1–514.e9.

80. Bombrys AE, Barton JR, Nowacki E, et al. Expectant management of severe preeclampsia at <27 weeks gestation: maternal and perinatal outcomes according to gestational age by weeks at onset of expectant management. *Am J Obstet Gynecol* 2008;199:247.e1–247.e6.

81. Sibai BM. Magnesium sulfate prophylaxis in preeclampsia. Lessons learned from recent trials. *Am J Obstet Gynecol* 2004;190:1520–1526.

82. Altman D, Carroli G, Duley L, et al., The Magpie Trial Collaborative Group. Do women with pre-eclampsia, and their babies benefit from magnesium sulphate? The magpie trial: A randomized placebo-controlled trial. *Lancet* 2002; 359:1877–1890.

83. Zeeman GG, Fleckenstein JL, Twickler DM, et al. Cerebral infarction in eclampsia. *Am J Obstet Gynecol* 2004;190:714–720.

84. Ramanathan J, Sibai BM, Pillai R, et al. Neuromuscular transmission studies in preeclamptic women receiving magnesium sulfate. *Am J Obset Gynecol* 1998; 158:40–46.

85. Gaiser RR, Seem EH. Use of rocuronium in a pregnant patient with an open eye injury receiving magnesium medication for preterm labour. *Br J Anaesth* 1996;66:669.

86. Ramanathan J, Sibai BM, Duggirala V, et al. Pulmonary function in preeclamptic women receiving magnesium sulfate. *J Reprod Med* 1988;33:432–435.

87. Nelson KB, Grether JK. Can magnesium sulfate reduce the risk of cerebral palsy in very low birthweight infants? *Pediatrics* 1995;95:263–269.

88. Schendel DE, Berg CJ, Yeargin-Allsopp M, et al. Prenatal magnesium sulfate exposure and the risk of cerebral palsy or mental retardation among very low-birth-weight children aged 3 to 5 years. *JAMA* 1996;276:1805–1810.

89. Simhan HN, Hines KP. Neuroprotective effects of in-utero exposure to magnesium sulfate. *UpToDate*, 2012.

90. American College of Obstetricians and Gynecologists Committee on Obstetric Practice, Society for maternal-fetal medicine. Committee Opinion No. 455: Magnesium sulfate before anticipated preterm birth for neuroprotection. *Obstet Gynecol* 2010;115:669.

91. Belfort MA, Tooke-Miller C, Allen JC Jr, et al. Labetalol decreases cerebral perfusion pressure without negatively affecting cerebral blood flow in hypertensive gravidas. *Hypertens Pregnancy* 2002;21:185–197.

92. Frias A, Aagaard-Tillery K, Holmgren C, et al. Labetalol, but not MgSO4, lowers cerebral perfusion pressure (CPP) in preeclamptic patients. *J Soc Gynecol Investig* 2005;12:218.

93. Cotton DB, Gonik B, Dorman KF. Cardiovascular alterations in severe pregnancy-induced hypertension seen with an intravenously given hydralazine bolus. *Hypertens* 1985;161:240–243.

94. American Academy of Pediatrics Committee on Drugs. The transfer of drugs and other chemicals into the breast milk. *Pediatrics* 1994;93:137–150.

95. Stempel JE, O'Grady JP, Morton JP, et al. Use of sodium nitroprusside in complications of gestational hypertension. *Obstet Gynecol* 1982;60:533–538.

96. Naulty J, Cefalo RC, Lewis PE. Fetal toxicity of nitroprusside in the pregnant ewe. *Am J Obstet Gynecol* 1981;139:708–711.

97. Cotton DB, Jones MM, Longmire S, et al. Role of intravenous nitroglycerin in the treatment of severe pregnancy-induced hypertension complicated by pulmonary edema. *Am J Obstet Gynecol* 1986;154:91–93.

98. Cotton DB, Longmire S, Jones MM, et al. Cardiovascular alterations in severe pregnancy-induced hypertension: Effects of intravenous nitroglycerin coupled with blood volume expansion. *Am J Obstet Gynecol* 1986;154:1053–1059.

99. Hood DD, Dewan DM, James FM 3rd, et al. The use of nitroglycerin in preventing the hypertensive response to tracheal intubation in severe preeclampsia. *Anesthesiology* 1985;63:329–332.

100. Longmire S, Leduc L, Jones MM, et al. The hemodynamic effects of intubation during nitroglycerin infusion in severe preeclampsia. *Am J Obstet Gynecol* 1991;164:551–556.

101. Eisenach JC, Mandell G, Dewan DM. Maternal and fetal effects of labetalol in pregnant ewes. *Anesthesiology* 1991;74:292–297.

102. Mabie WC, Gonzalez AR, Sibai BM, et al. A comparative trial of labetalol and hydralazine in the acute management of severe hypertension complicating pregnancy. *Obstet Gynecol* 1987;70:328–333.

103. Vigil-De Gracia P, Lasso M, Ruiz E, et al. Severe hypertension in pregnancy: Hydralazine or labetalol. A randomized clinical trial. *Eur J Obstet Gynecol Reprod Biol* 2006;128:157–162.

104. Ramanathan J, Sibai BM, Mabie WC, et al. The use of labetalol for attenuation of the hypertensive response to endotracheal intubation in preeclampsia. *Am J Obstet Gynecol* 1988;159:650–654.

105. Scardo JA, Vermillion ST, Newman RB, et al. A randomized, double-blind, hemodynamic evaluation of nifedipine and labetalol in preeclamptic hypertensive emergencies. *Am J Obstet Gynecol* 1999;181:862–866.

106. Ben-Ami M, Giladi Y, Shalve E. The combination of magnesium sulfate and nifedipine: A cause for neuromuscular blockade. *Br J Obstet Gynaecol* 1994; 101:262–263.

107. Elatrous S, Nouira S, Ouanes B, et al. Short term treatment of severe hypertension of pregnancy: Prospective comparison of nicardipine and labetalol. *Intensive Care Med* 2002;28:1281–1286.

108. Nij Bijvank SW, Duvekot JJ. Nicardipine treatment of severe hypertension in pregnancy. A review of literature. *Obstet Gynecol Surv* 2010;65:341–347.

109. Duley L, Williams J, Henderson-Smart DJ. Plasma volume expansion for treatment of women with pre-eclampsia. *Cochrane Database Syst Rev* 2000;124: CD001805.

110. Beilin Y, Zahn J, Comerford M. Safe epidural analgesia in thirty parturients with platelet counts between 69,000 and 98,000 mm³. *Anesth Analg* 1997;85: 385–388.

111. Douglas MJ. Platelets, the parturient and regional anesthesia. *Int J Obstet Anesth* 2001;10:113–120.

112. Douglas M. The use of neuraxial anesthesia in parturients with thrombocytopenia: What is an adequate platelet count? In: Halpern S, Douglas M, eds. *Evidence-Based Obstetric Anesthesia*. Oxford: Blackwell Publishing; 2005:165–177.

113. Moen V, Dahlgren N, Irestedt L. Severe neurological complications after central neuraxial blockades in Sweden. *Anesthesiology* 2004;101:950–959.

114. Cook TM, Counsell D, Wildsmith JA. Major complications of central neuraxial block: Report on the third national audit project of the Royal College of Anaesthetists. *Br J Anaesth* 2009;102:179–190.

115. Ramanathan J, Bennett K. Pre-eclampsia: Fluids, drugs, and anesthetic management. *Anesthesiol Clin North America* 2003;21:145–163.

116. Newsome LR, Bramwell RS, Curly PE. Severe preeclampsia: Hemodynamic effects of lumbar epidural anesthesia. *Anesth Analg* 1986;65:31–36.

117. Palanisamy A, Mitani AA, Tsen LC. General anesthesia for cesarean delivery at a teritiary care hospital from 2000–2005: A retrospective analysis and 10-year update. *Int J Obstet Anesth* 2011;20:10–16.

118. American Society of Anesthesiologists Task Force on Obstetric Anesthesia. Practice Guidelines for Obstetric Anesthesia: an updated report by The American Society of Anesthesiologists Task Force on Obstetric Anesthesia. *Anesthesiology*. 2007;106:843–863.

119. Ramanathan J, Coleman P, Sibai BM. Anesthetic modification of hemodynamic and neuroendocrine stress responses to cesarean delivery in women with severe preeclampsa. *Anesth Analg* 1991;73:772–779.

120. Ramanathan J, Vaddadi AK, Arheart KL. Combined spinal and epidural anesthesia with low doses of intrathecal bupivacaine in women with severe preeclampsia: A preliminary report. *Reg Anesth Pain Med* 2001;26:46–51.

121. Aya AG, Mangin R, Vialles N, et al. Patients with severe preeclampsia has less hypotension during spinal anesthesia for elective cesarean delivery than healthy parturients: A cohort comparison. *Anesth Analg* 2003;97(3): 867–872.

122. Visalyaputra S, Rodanant O, Somboonviboon W, et al. Spinal versus epidural anesthesia for cesarean delivery in severe preeclampsia: A prospective, randomized, multicenter study. *Anesth Analg* 2005;101:862–868.

123. Van De Velde M, Berends N, Spitz B et al. Low-dose combined spinal-epidural anesthesia vs. conventional epidural anesthesia for Caesarean section in preeclampsia: A retrospective analysis. *Eur J Anaesthesiol* 2004;21:454–459.

124. Clark VA, Sherwood-Smith GH, Stewart AV. Ephedrine requirements are reduced during spinal anesthesia for cesarean section in preeclampsia. *Int J Obstet Anesth* 2005;14:9–13.

125. Valensise H, Vasapollo B, Novelli GP, et al. Maternal and fetal hemodynamic effects induced by nitric oxide donors and plasma volume expansion in pregnancies with gestational hypertension complicated by intrauterine growth restriction with absent end- diastolic flow in the umbilical artery. *Ultrasound Obstet Gynecol* 2008;31:55–64.

126. Dyer RA, Piercy JL, Reed AR, et al. Hemodynamic changes associated with spinal anesthesia for cesarean delivery in severe preeclampsia. *Anesthesiology* 2008;108:802–811.

127. Dyer RA, Reed AR, van Dyk D, et al. Hemodynamic effects of ephedrine, phenylephrine, and the coadministration of phenylephrine with oxytocin during spinal anesthesia for elective cesarean delivery. *Anesthesiology* 2009; 111:753–765.

128. Kodali BS, Chandrasekhar S, Bulich LN, et al. Airway changes during labor and delivery. *Anesthesiology* 2008;108:357–362.

129. Munnur U, de Boisblanc B, Suresh MS. Airway problems in pregnancy. *Crit Care Med* 2005;33:S259–S268.

130. Ramanathan J, Angel JJ, Bush AJ, et al. Changes in maternal middle cerebral artery blood flow velocity associated with general anesthesia in severe preeclampsia. *Anesth Analg* 1999;88:357–361.

131. Yoo KY, Jeong CW, Park BY, et al. Effects of remifentanil on cardiovascular and bispectral index responses to endotracheal intubation in severe preeclamptic patients undergoing caesarean delivery under general anesthesia. *Br J Anaesth* 2009;102:812–819.

132. Sibai BM. Imitators of severe pre-eclampsia. *Semin Perinatol* 2009;33:196–205.

133. Fonseca JE, Mendez F, Catano C, et al. Dexamethasone treatment does not improve the outcome of women with HELLP syndrome: a double-blind, placebo-controlled, randomized clinical trial. *Am J Obstet Gynecol* 2005; 193:1591–1598.

134. Wondstra DM, Chandra S, Hofmeyr GJ, et al. Corticosteroids for HELLP syndrome in pregnancy. *Cochrane Database Syst Rev* 2010;9:CD008148.

135. Barton JR, Sibai BM. Gastro intestinal complications of preeclampsia. *Semin Perinatol* 2009;33:179–188.

136. Chames MC, Livingston JC, Ivester T, et al. Late postpartum eclampsia: A preventable disease? *Am J Obstet Gynecol* 2002;186:1174–1177.

137. Cunningham FG, Fernandez CO, Hernandez C. Blindness associated with preeclampsia and eclampsia. *Am J Obstet Gynecol* 1995;172:1291–1298.

138. Shah AK, Rajamani K, Whitty JE. Eclampsia: A neurological perspective. *J Neurol Sci* 2008;271:158–167.

139. Duley L, Gülmezoglu AM, Henderson-Smart DJ, et al. Magnesium sulphate and other anticonvulsants for women with pre-eclampsia. *Cochrane Database Syst Rev* 2010;(11):CD000025.

140. Suresh M. HELLP syndrome: An Anesthesiologist's Perspective. *Anesthesiol Clin North America* 1998;16:331–348.

141. Cipolla MJ. Cerebrovascular function in pregnancy and eclampsia. *Hypertension* 2007;50:14–24.

CHAPTER 29

Anesthesia for Pregnant Patients with Endocrine Disorders

Peter H. Pan • Ashley M. Tonidandel

■ GENERAL CONSIDERATIONS

The maternal hormonal milieu has become a subject of keen research interest with significant societal health implications. Recent evidence suggests that placental transfer and in utero exposure may lead to obesity and autoimmune conditions years later (1–4). The most common endocrine disorders associated with pregnancy are diabetes mellitus (DM) and thyroid disease, both of which can have substantial impact on fetal outcomes if poorly managed. Other pathologies, particularly those associated with the hypothalamic–pituitary–ovarian axis, are seen less frequently due to concomitant infertility issues. Although rare, endocrinopathies, such as pheochromocytoma, can complicate maternal course and fetal growth and development with devastating consequences. Continued research and close collaboration between obstetricians, endocrinologists, neonatologists, and anesthesiologists are necessary to ensure optimal outcomes for both mother and child.

Pregnancy induces several physiologic changes specific to the endocrine system, starting early in the first trimester. These changes are initially necessary to sustain the lining of the uterus and later promote uteroplacental blood flow, provide for the increased metabolic demands of a growing fetus, and prepare the mother for labor and delivery. The placenta itself also becomes an endocrine organ, serving as a primary source for many hormones during pregnancy, including but not limited to growth hormone, human chorionic gonadotropin (hCG), and progesterone. These hormones have complex interactions with native endocrine pathways, sometimes becoming the driving force, to sustain the pregnant state and provide optimal conditions for fetal survival. These complex hormonal adjustments also prepare the mother for the demands of labor and delivery. However, these same adaptations can exacerbate or unmask symptoms of coexisting disease. Careful monitoring throughout the gestation and into the postpartum period is necessary to prevent acute crises that put both mother and baby at risk.

■ DIABETES MELLITUS

Definition and Screening

Gestational diabetes mellitus (GDM) is typically defined as glucose intolerance of variable severity with onset or first recognition during the second or third trimester of pregnancy (5). In contrast, overt or pregestational diabetes is defined by the American Diabetes Association (ADA) by a random glucose >200 mg/dL with classic signs and symptoms or a fasting glucose >125 mg/dL (see Table 29-1). Women with fasting hyperglycemia before 24 weeks probably have overt diabetes, as their pregnancy outcomes are similar to those with overt diabetes (6). Depending on the criteria, GDM complicates an estimated 2% to 9% of pregnancies, with the prevalence increasing over the past 20 years, most likely due to the obesity epidemic (7). The United States Preventive Services Task Force published summary recommendations in 2003 regarding population screening for GDM (8). While the task force found fair to good evidence that screening combined with diet and insulin therapy reduces fetal macrosomia, routine screening for low-risk individuals is not mandated due to insufficient evidence that it reduces important adverse health outcomes (9). Other than obesity, known risk factors for GDM include advanced maternal age, family history, glucose intolerance with prior pregnancy, and ethnicity, with women of color being at higher risk in the United States (10). Despite the lack of a mandate, survey results suggest that 96% of obstetricians universally screen during all pregnancies with an overwhelming majority (95.2%) using a 50 g glucose 1-hour oral test (11). Figure 29-1 shows a flowchart summarizing a screening and diagnostic strategy specific to GDM based on underlying risk factors. The most common diagnostic criteria used for GDM are the Carpenter–Coustan revised criteria recommended by the ADA (used by 38% of obstetricians surveyed) and the National Diabetes Data Group criteria (used by 59%) (11) (see Table 29-2). The Carpenter–Coustan criteria is more inclusive and sensitive, while still identifying patients with a higher risk for cesarean or operative vaginal delivery, macrosomia, and shoulder dystocia (12). This increased sensitivity is potentially very important beyond the perinatal period as GDM likely represents a stage in the evolution of diabetes with most, but not all, women going on to develop diabetes outside of pregnancy (13,14).

An additional 1% of pregnancies are complicated by pregestational or preexisting DM, with type 2 DM being more common than type 1 (15). As caloric and insulin needs increase during pregnancy, these women need careful monitoring to prevent both fetal morbidity and worsening of end-organ disease. Perinatal outcomes have improved markedly in recent years and are optimal when vascular disease is not present and glucose control is achieved before conception (15). Historically, White's classification system was used to predict perinatal risk, such as prematurity or hypertensive disorders, based primarily on age of onset of diabetes and end-organ involvement. Variations of this classification scheme labeled individuals with a letter, with category A representing gestational diabetes and B–H indicating increasing duration of disease (B less than 10 years, C greater than 10 years) and presence of benign retinopathy (D), nephropathy (F), proliferative retinopathy (R), and cardiac disease (H). White's system was used extensively from 1978 through approximately 1994 when the American College/Congress of Obstetricians and Gynecologists (ACOG) decided to shift clinical focus on whether diabetes existed before pregnancy and the adequacy of metabolic control (16).

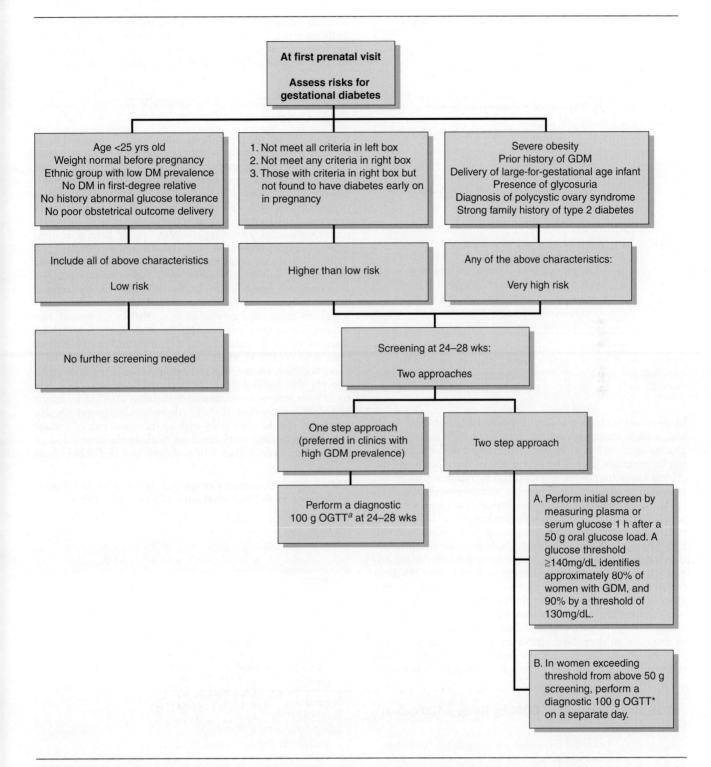

FIGURE 29-1 Screening and diagnosis of GDM. ([a]Diagnostic criteria for 100 g OGTT is shown in Table 29-2.) Copyright 2008 American Diabetes Association. From: *Diabetes Care* 2008;31:S12–S54. Modified and reproduced by permission of: The American Diabetes Association.

Pathophysiology

Normal pregnancy is characterized by diurnal changes in plasma glucose and insulin with mild fasting hypoglycemia and postprandial hyperglycemia. This normal pregnancy physiology has been described as a diabetogenic state marked overall by increased insulin resistance and reduced sensitivity to insulin action (16,17). This resistance begins midway through pregnancy and peaks in the third trimester to approximate type 2 diabetes (13). The exact mechanism of insulin resistance is not fully known, but the effect is likely mediated by progesterone and estrogen, either directly or indirectly. Placental hormones, such as human placental lactogen, may also increase lipolysis, thus increasing circulating free fatty acids, and worsening tissue insulin resistance (18,19). The resultant prolonged postprandial hyperglycemia from peripheral insulin resistance likely serves to ensure a glucose supply to the fetus. Other changes to maternal glucose

TABLE 29-1 Criteria for the Diagnosis of Diabetes

Criteria 1	Fasting plasma glucose ≥126 mg/dL (7.0 mmol/L). Fasting is defined as no caloric intake for at least 8 h[a].
	OR
Criteria 2	Symptoms of hyperglycemia and a casual plasma glucose ≥200 mg/dL (11.1 mmol/L). Casual is defined as any time of day without regard to time since last meal. The classic symptoms of hyperglycemia include polyuria, polydipsia, and unexplained weight loss.
	OR
Criteria 1	2 h plasma glucose ≥200 mg/dL (11.1 mmol/L) during an oral glucose tolerance test. (The test should be performed as described by the World Health Organization, using a glucose load containing the equivalent of 75 g anhydrous glucose dissolved in water. [a])

[a]In the absence of unequivocal hyperglycemia, these criteria should be confirmed by repeat-testing on a different day. (Copyright 2008 American Diabetes Association. From: *Diabetes Care* 2008;31:S12–S54. Reproduced by permission of the American Diabetes Association.)

homeostasis include transient hypoglycemia between meals and at night due to continuous fetal draw with mean fasting glucose levels as low as 56 mg/dL in healthy patients 28 to 38 weeks' gestation (20). The hypothesis of the placenta as the critical endocrine organ is supported by rapid improvement in insulin resistance after delivery in normal pregnancies (13).

Women with GDM have an inadequate endogenous insulin supply to meet tissue demands during the period of increased resistance associated with pregnancy. For these women, hyperglycemia is a result of both inadequate insulin production combined with a more chronic form of insulin resistance exacerbated by physiologic changes of pregnancy (21). Beta cell dysfunction is apparent prior to conception and does not abate after delivery as in normal pregnancies, reinforcing the idea of chronic glucose intolerance unmasked by gestational changes. Women with GDM still increase insulin production in response to decreased sensitivity. However, they secrete 40% to 70% less insulin for any degree of insulin resistance, reflecting progressive loss of beta cell compensation due to

TABLE 29-2 Diagnosis of GDM by Using a 100 g Oral Glucose Load

	National Diabetes Data Group (mg/dL)	Carpenter/Coustan Conversion (mg/dL)
Fasting	105	95
1 h	190	180
2 h	165	155
3 h	145	140

A diagnosis of gestational diabetes mellitus requires at least two or more of the venous plasma concentrations meeting or exceeding the threshold. The 100 g Oral Glucose Tolerance Test should be performed the morning after an overnight fast of at least 8 h. (Reprinted with permission from: Gabbe SG, Gregory RP, Power ML, et al. Management of diabetes mellitus by obstetrician-gynecologists. *Obstet Gynecol* 2004;103:1229–1234.)

a variety of mechanisms such as obesity, genetics, and autoimmune changes (13). Variations in the etiology of glucose intolerance may explain differences in severity, responses to medication, and progression of disease after pregnancy.

Effects of Diabetes on Pregnancy: Fetal Outcomes

Glucose crosses the placenta by facilitated diffusion and leads to fetal hyperglycemia in poorly controlled diabetic states (15). If this hyperglycemia occurs early in gestation, as in pregestational diabetes, fetal anomalies (rather than chromosomal) are possible. Significant hyperglycemia during organogenesis of 5 to 8 weeks' gestation may cause severe congenital malformations and subsequent potential for spontaneous abortion, including complex cardiac defects, central nervous system anomalies, and skeletal malformations (22). Table 29-3 shows common congenital anomalies and their incidence in infants of women with overt diabetes (22,23). Glycosylated hemoglobin levels are consistently related to the frequency of anomalies (24). The mechanism causing these congenital anomalies is not fully understood, but hyperglycemia may induce oxidative stress in the fetus which disrupts the cardiac neural crest migration and causes outflow tract defects (25). Women with preexisting DM should have preconception counseling and optimized glucose control to prevent this leading cause of perinatal mortality, with 6% to 12% of infants of women with diabetes affected by major congenital anomalies (15). Furthermore, maternal obesity itself may also be associated with an increased risk of certain types of congenital malformations, making the overall risk of an anomaly even higher when obesity and diabetes coexist

TABLE 29-3 Common Congenital Anomalies in Infants of Women with Pregestational Diabetes Mellitus

Types of Congenital Anomalies in Infants of Women with Overt Diabetes	Relative Incidence (Ratio of Incidence as Compared with the General Population)
Skeletal:	
Caudal regression	252
Cardiac:	
Situs inversus	84
Transposition of great vessels, ventricular septal defect, atrial septal defect	4
Neural:	
Anencephaly	3
Spina bifida, hydrocephaly, and other central nervous system defects	2
Gastrointestinal:	
Anal/rectal atresia	3
Renal:	
Duplex ureter	23
Agenesis	4
Cystic kidney	4
Other renal anomalies	5

Copyright 1979 American Diabetes Association. From: *Diabetes* 1979;28:292–293; and Copyright 2009 American Diabetes Association. From: Medical Management of Pregnancy Complicated by Diabetes. 4th ed. Modified with permission from: The American Diabetes Association.

(25,26). Women with GDM alone do not appear to be at risk for fetal congenital anomalies, as hyperglycemia is probably not severe enough to impair organogenesis during that time period (27).

If the fetus survives this initial period of organogenesis, the fetal pancreatic beta cells secrete insulin in response to the abnormally high glucose load. Insulin is a potent growth hormone–stimulating excessive fetal growth, particularly in adipose tissue (15). The concept of hyperglycemia leading to fetal hyperinsulinemia and adiposity is often referred to as the Pederson hypothesis (28). Macrosomia, often defined as birth weight greater than 4,500 g, is the most commonly encountered adverse outcome in term infants of pregnancy complicated by diabetes, with a large-for-gestational-age rate of 45.2% compared with 12.6% in one population-based study (22,29). The significant increase in adipose tissue is disproportionately concentrated around the shoulders and chest, more than doubling the risk of shoulder dystocia or birth trauma at vaginal delivery, as well as increasing the rate of cesarean delivery (29,30). Figure 29-2 illustrates the excessive fetal growth that can occur with poorly controlled diabetes. The multicenter prospective Hyperglycemia and Adverse Pregnancy Outcomes (HAPO) study demonstrated continuous linear relationships between increasing maternal glucose measures and birth weight, primary cesarean delivery, clinical neonatal hypoglycemia, premature delivery, shoulder dystocia or birth injury, and preeclampsia (31). Maternal prepregnancy weight is a confounding factor in diagnosing gestational diabetes and likely is an independent risk factor for macrosomia. Unfortunately, diabetes and maternal weight are not sufficient predictors of shoulder dystocia to warrant the risk of planned cesarean delivery in all cases. Shoulder dystocia can also occur unpredictably in infants of normal birth weight.

Pregnancies complicated by diabetes are also more likely to result in prematurity or growth-restricted infants. For example, spontaneous preterm labor occurs up to 2 to 5 times more often in women with pregestational diabetes as compared to non-diabetic pregnant patients, perhaps related to increased incidence of hydramnios from poor glycemic control, fetal hyperglycemia, and polyuria (15,22). Preexisting renal dysfunction (creatinine >1.5 mg/dL) has been associated with delivery before 32 weeks' gestation, very low birth weight, and increased incidence of neonatal hypoglycemia, independent of degree of proteinuria and glycemic control during any trimester (32). Vasculopathy, either from chronic diabetes or preeclampsia, can result in uteroplacental insufficiency and fetal growth restriction. Ultimately, these infants may be delivered early for fetal or maternal reasons, such as preeclampsia.

In addition to gestational size differences, infants of diabetic mothers are more at risk for perinatal death and stillbirth, typically associated with large-for-gestational age fetuses during the last 4 to 6 weeks of gestation (22,23). Hypothetically, fetal demise may result from villous edema, induced osmotically by hyperglycemia, leading to poor fetal oxygen transport and placental dysfunction (33). Unfortunately, early delivery is not an acceptable strategy to prevent intrauterine fetal death as these infants are also at higher risk for respiratory distress (14). After delivery, infants must be monitored carefully to avoid profound hypoglycemia. Hyperplasia of the fetal beta-islet cells in response to the maternal glucose load during gestation leads to increased circulating fetal insulin and subsequent hypoglycemia in newborn. The hypoglycemia after delivery may be related more to maternal hyperglycemia during labor, rather than reflecting chronic levels as measured by HbA_{1c}. Various fetal and neonatal consequences of maternal diabetes are summarized in Table 29-4.

The effects of maternal hyperglycemia do not end in the peripartum period. Prospective studies have examined the role of diabetes exposure on childhood obesity and offspring risk for type 2 diabetes. Close and long-term follow-up of the offspring of two populations, a Chicago cohort and a Pima Indian group, demonstrated increased weight and impaired glucose tolerance or prevalence of type 2 diabetes (4). This predisposition to glucose intolerance exists even after adjusting for presence of diabetes in the father and obesity in the offspring, implicating the non-genetic effect of intrauterine environment. These long-term effects appear to be similar regardless of maternal diabetes type (4). Future research in this area will need to focus on whether glycemic control can prevent the vicious cycle of obesity and diabetes.

Effects of Diabetes on Pregnancy: Maternal Outcomes

Many maternal consequences of diabetic pregnancies are likely related to severity of preexisting disease and degree of glycemic control (15). Excessive fetal growth clearly puts the mother at higher risk for birth trauma and operative delivery and potential for associated wound infections. Infections during pregnancy, including wound infections after cesarean delivery, are more common in women with pregestational diabetes when compared to non-diabetic controls (34,35). Fortunately, the current practice of routine antimicrobial prophylaxis has resulted in low rates of wound infection and endometritis, reportedly only 0.7% and 3% in an analysis of over 200 nulliparous women with type 1 diabetes (36). Other,

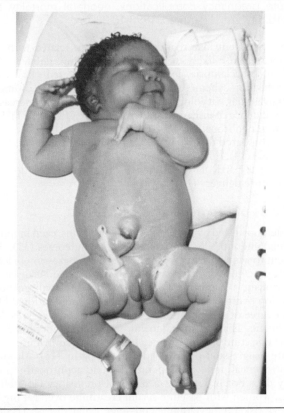

FIGURE 29-2 A macrocosmic infant of 6,060 g born to a woman with gestational diabetes. Reprinted with permission from: Cunningham FG, Leveno KJ, Bloom SL, et al. Diabetes. In: Cunningham FG, Leveno KJ, Bloom SL, Hauth JC, Rouse DJ, Spong CY, eds. *Williams Obstetrics.* 23rd ed. New York, NY: McGraw-Hill Companies, Inc. 2010.

TABLE 29-4 Potential Fetal and Neonatal Complications with Maternal Diabetes Mellitus

Demises:
First trimester miscarriage
Unexplained fetal demise
Increased perinatal mortality

In utero development:
Hydramnios
Large-for-gestation fetus
Small-for-gestation fetus
Macrosomia
Congenital anomalies (see Table 29-3)

Delivery process:
Preterm delivery
Shoulder dystocia, brachial plexus injury, clavicular fracture
birth injury and/or trauma with vaginal delivery
Operative delivery

Neonatal abnormal laboratory findings:
Neonatal hypoglycemia and hyperinsulinemia
Hypocalcemia
Hyperbilirubinemia
Polycythemia

Neonatal pathologic syndrome:
Neonatal respiratory distress syndrome
Organomegaly
Hypertrophic cardiomyopathy

Long-term impact:
Adolescent obesity
Impaired glucose tolerance
Inheritance of diabetes

Adapted from: Dabelea D. The predisposition to obesity and diabetes in offspring of diabetic mothers. *Diabetes Care* 2007;30(Suppl 2):S169–S174; Brody SC, Harris R, Lohr K. Screening for gestational diabetes: a summary of the evidence for the U.S. Preventive Services Task Force. *Obstet Gynecol* 2003;101:380–392; Eriksson UJ. Congenital anomalies in diabetic pregnancy. *Semin Fetal Neonatal Med* 2009;14:85–93; Yang J, Cummings EA, O'connell C, et al. Fetal and neonatal outcomes of diabetic pregnancies. *Obstet Gynecol* 2006;108:644–650; Daskalakis G, Marinopoulos S, Krielesi V, et al. Placental pathology in women with gestational diabetes. *Acta Obstet Gynecol Scand* 2008;87:403–407.

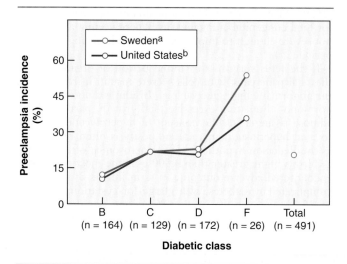

FIGURE 29-3 Incidence of Preeclampsia in 491 diabetics according to White's classification. Reprinted with permission from: Cunningham FG, Leveno KJ, Bloom SL, et al. Diabetes. In: Cunningham FG, Leveno KJ, Bloom SL, Hauth JC, Rouse DJ, Spong CY, eds. *Williams Obstetrics.* 23rd ed. New York, NY: McGraw-Hill Companies, Inc. 2010. Original data adapted from: [a]Sibai BM, Caritis S, Hauth J, et al. Risks of preeclampsia and adverse neonatal outcomes among women with pregestational diabetes mellitus. *Am J Obstet Gynecol* 2000;182:364; and [b]Hanson U, Persson B. Outcome of pregnancies complicated by type 1 insulin-dependent diabetes in Sweden: Acute pregnancy complications, neonatal mortality and morbidity. *Am J Perinatol* 1993;10:330.

pressure associated with pregnancy, exacerbation of hypertension from preeclampsia, increased incidence of urinary tract infections, or inability to use angiotensin-converting enzyme (ACE) inhibitors during gestation (37). Preeclampsia and preterm births in pregestational diabetes may also predict a long-term increased risk of ESRD and death, perhaps representing a marker for severity of disease or vasculopathy (38). Cardiovascular disease in pregestational diabetics, previously referred to as Class H, is not well studied due to limited sample sizes. These patients do appear to be at risk for myocardial infarction and death associated with the hemodynamic changes of pregnancy and the peripartum period. This mortality may be decreased in women who have undergone coronary artery bypass grafting prior to pregnancy, but definitive conclusions are not possible given limited data (39). ACOG recommends early comprehensive eye examinations and baseline evaluation of renal function by serum creatinine and urinary protein excretion for women with pregestational DM (15). Electrocardiogram and echocardiography should be considered in women with signs or symptoms of coronary artery disease (14). Information on the interaction between

more prevalent maternal complications associated with diabetes are more likely to result in a premature delivery. The risk of preeclampsia, for example, varies based on White's classification scheme, with progressive indications of underlying vascular pathology and hypertension greatly increasing the incidence of disease as shown in Figure 29-3 (15,31). Preexisting nephropathy is associated with preeclampsia rates of 50% compared to 15% to 20% in women without renal dysfunction (14). The combination of nephropathy and hypertension is particularly predictive of growth restriction and premature delivery (15).

Effects of Pregnancy on Diabetes

As demonstrated by the HAPO study, diabetes, even in milder forms, undoubtedly impacts pregnancy outcomes (31). The extent to which pregnancy influences the progression of long-term outcomes of diabetes is less clearly defined. As discussed previously, a majority of women with GDM will go on to develop overt diabetes. For women with pregestational DM, the degree of deterioration of end-organ disease as a result of pregnancy changes may depend on baseline function. Strict glycemic control in pregnancy may actually contribute to the acute progression of preexisting retinopathy (15). Although controversial, mild to moderate diabetic nephropathy probably does not progress as a result of pregnancy (15). However, women with baseline serum creatinine over 1.4 mg/dL are at risk for developing end-stage renal disease (ESRD) postpartum. In a retrospective analysis of diabetic parturients with moderate-to-severe renal dysfunction at pregnancy onset, 45% required dialysis approximately 36 months earlier than predicted by prepregnancy estimates based on linear decline in glomerular filtration rates (37). This accelerated rate of progression may be due to increased intraglomerular pregnancy and somatic or autonomic neuropathy in diabetes is limited, but the natural course of existing neuropathy is likely not substantially changed (39). Nausea and vomiting during pregnancy might be worsened in the setting of gastroparesis from autonomic neuropathy, further complicating diet and glycemic control (14).

Treatment of Diabetes during Pregnancy

Intensive treatment of severe hyperglycemia during pregnancy results in a reduction in the incidence of macrosomia based on summary of evidences from randomized controlled trials (9). The benefit for tight treatment of milder hyperglycemia is less clear. However, a recent randomized trial showed definite significant benefit for women with mild to moderate GDM randomized to interventions of individualized dietary changes, daily monitoring of glucose levels, and insulin therapy as needed compared to a routine-care group (40). Specifically, significant differences were found in percent with any serious perinatal complication (1% vs. 4%), birth weight, and percent with macrosomia (10% vs. 21%) (40). The benefit of treatment for mild hyperglycemia was confirmed in a subsequent randomized multicenter trial for women with mild GDM comparing outcomes of birth weight, cesarean delivery, shoulder dystocia, and rates of preeclampsia (41).

The goals of glycemic control in diabetic parturients have not been well studied and are typically based on normative values for non-diabetics during pregnancy. "Upper boundary" treatment targets are probably sufficient given that observational studies have shown an increased likelihood of small-for-gestational age infants with low mean capillary glucose levels (<87 mg/dL) (21). For example, ACOG recommends a glucose target of ≤95 mg/dL during fasting, ≤100 mg/dL preprandial, ≤140 mg/dL 1 hour after eating, and ≤120 mg/dL 2 hours after a meal (15). Trials specifically addressing whether these glycemic-control targets are appropriate for diabetics in pregnancy are needed.

With pregestational diabetes, obstetric management begins with preconception counseling, education and evaluation on diet, exercise, and insulin therapy, and nutrition and folate supplementation (15). Ideally, women who anticipate pregnancy should also have optimized control, including monitoring of pre and postprandial glucose with subsequent adjustments of insulin requirements. The adequacy of chronic metabolic control should be assessed with an HbA_{1c}. Select women with longstanding diabetes may need even fur-

ther evaluation, including retinal examination, 24-hour urine collection for protein excretion and creatinine clearance, and electrocardiography. Thyroid function studies are also recommended in type 1 diabetics due to the high percentage of women with concomitant disease (40%) (15). The primary goal of this preconception optimization is to reduce risk of neural tube defects and congenital anomalies. Parturients without prenatal counseling have been shown to have 4 times as many fetal and neonatal death or congenital abnormalities compared to individuals with counseling (42,43).

After conception and during the first trimester, clinicians should encourage frequent self-monitoring of glucose levels with appropriate adjustments in insulin and diet. Insulin requirements may actually decrease by 10% to 20% in the first trimester, including a risk of hypoglycemia at night after prolonged fasting due to continuous fetal uptake of glucose (44). If glycemic control is poor, then hospitalization may be needed to achieve better glycemic control during this critical period of organogenesis. Historically, insulin is the mainstay of treatment for pregestational DM or poorly controlled GDM (15,21). Biosynthetic human insulin is most commonly used during pregnancy in an effort to decrease fetal antibody response to the small amount of maternal insulin that crosses the placenta bound to the IgG antibody (15,21). The pharmacologic profiles of commonly used insulins are listed in Table 29-5 (45). Insulin demands increase throughout pregnancy, so careful monitoring is a necessity to prevent negative effects of hypoglycemia. Gabbe and Graves described one strategy for initiating insulin therapy based on patient weight. The total insulin dose can be approximated as 0.8 Units per kilogram per day (U/kg/day) in the first trimester, 1.0 U/Kg/day in the second trimester, and 1.2 U/kg/day for the third trimester. Two-thirds of the total dose should be intermediate-acting (NPH or Lente, half given before breakfast the other half before bedtime), and one-third should be short-acting administered with each meal (lispro or regular, 15 or 30 minutes before eating) (14). Alternatively, subcutaneous insulin infusion therapy may be used to closely mimic physiologic insulin secretion, with approximately 50% administered basally and 50% divided before meals and snacks. Retrospective review and survey data suggests high maternal satisfaction based on continued pump use after pregnancy, but potentially higher costs of care compared to multiple insulin injections (46).

In the second and third trimesters, euglycemia remains the goal, and insulin requirements often increase along with

TABLE 29-5 Pharmacologic Profiles of Commonly Used Insulin

		Source	Onset (h)	Peak (h)	Duration (h)
Short-acting:	Humulin R (Lilly)	Human	0.5	2–4	5–7
	Velosulin-H (Novo Nordisk)	Human	0.5	1–3	8
	Novolin R (Novo Nordisk)	Human	0.5	2.5–5	6–8
	Lispro	Analog	0.25	0.5–1.5	6–8
	Aspart	Analog	0.25	1–3	3–5
	Glulisine	Analog	0.25	1	4
Intermediate-acting:	Humulin Lente (Lilly)	Human	1–3	6–12	18–24
	Humulin NPH (Neutral protamine Hagedorn) (Lilly)	Human	1–2	6–12	18–24
	Novolin L (Novo Nordisk)	Human	2.5	7–15	22
	Novolin N (Novo Nordisk)	Human	1.5	4–12	24
Long-acting:	Humulin Ultralente (Lilly)	Human	4–6	8–20	>36
	Glargine	Analog	1.1	5	24
	Detemir	Analog	1–2	5	24

Reprinted with permission from: Gabbe SG, Carpenter LB, Garrison EA. New strategies for glucose control in patients with type 1 and type 2 diabetes mellitus in pregnancy. *Clin Obstet Gynecol* 2007;50:1014–1024.

insulin resistance from hormonal changes. Ultrasound and alpha fetal protein can be obtained during this time period to further evaluate for potential neural tube defects and other anomalies. Ultrasound assessment of fetal abdominal circumference (AC) in the second and third trimesters for women with GDM may aid in selecting targets and intensity of therapy. Compared to conventional therapy, multiple studies have shown a reduction in large-for-gestational age infants when insulin and stricter glucose control was instituted for women with "high-risk" fetal AC above the seventy-fifth percentile (47). Other measures of glucose control, such as glycosylated hemoglobin, have not yet demonstrated value in influencing management decisions and predicting macrosomia (48).

For GDM patients, the cornerstone of treatment is medical nutrition therapy and lifestyle interventions. The food plan, ideally prescribed by a registered dietician, should meet nutrient requirements for pregnancy and restrict carbohydrate load while avoiding starvation ketosis associated with severe calorie restrictions (21,49). Nutrition practice guidelines have been shown to reduce the need for insulin compared to usual nutrition care (49). Nutrition therapy is likely to be particularly important for obese women who are prone to larger infants irrespective of diabetic status. Maternal weight gain in the first trimester has been shown to be more predictive of infant weight than gain later in pregnancy (50). The ADA Clinical Practice Recommendations suggest a moderate 30% calorie restriction for obese women (BMI >30 kg/m^2) with GDM to control weight gain and glucose levels while avoiding ketosis (50).

Patients who are not adequately controlled with nutritional management or who exhibit excessive fetal growth should receive pharmacologic intervention, most commonly insulin, but more recently with oral antidiabetic agents. The three main classifications of oral pharmacologic interventions for diabetes are insulin secretagogues, insulin sensitizers, and alpha-glucosidase inhibitors. Insulin secretagogues stimulate beta cells to secrete insulin, so residual beta cell function is necessary. This class includes sulfonylureas and meglitinide, of which only glyburide has been demonstrated to have minimal placental transfer without excess neonatal hypoglycemia (21,51). Its onset of action is approximately 4 hours with a duration of 10 hours (14). Glyburide may be more beneficial in women with normal or slightly increased body weight (51). Metformin is the most commonly used insulin sensitizer, although the majority of its use in pregnancy is in women with polycystic ovarian syndrome (PCOS) (15). Metformin does cross the placenta, and at this time, beneficial or deleterious effects to the fetus are not fully known. In a prospective randomized trial comparing metformin with insulin therapy, the rate of neonatal complications based on a composite measure was not different, although severe hypoglycemia occurred more often in the insulin group. Women in the metformin group were much more likely to prefer that regimen for a subsequent pregnancy compared to insulin, but 46.3% in that group required supplemental insulin to meet glycemic targets (52). Acarbose, the alpha-glucosidase inhibitor, has also not been studied extensively, but preliminary results suggest reduced postprandial glucose in GDM with expected abdominal cramping (21). In a recent systematic review of the literature comparing insulin with all oral hypoglycemic agents, only four randomized controlled trials and five cohort studies were identified that had appropriate diagnostic criteria and comparison groups for maternal and fetal outcomes (53). No significant differences were found in maternal glycemic control or cesarean delivery rates with similar infant birth weights among women treated with either insulin or glyburide. Neonatal hypoglycemia was more

common (8.1%) with insulin when compared with metformin (3.3%). Rates of congenital malformations did not differ in infants of women treated with oral agents versus insulin, suggesting that if placental transfer occurs, the impact on the fetus is neutral or at least not harmful (53).

Acute Management of Diabetic Manifestations during Pregnancy

Despite aggressive therapy, the physiologic changes associated with pregnancy may contribute to the development of diabetic ketoacidosis (DKA) in 5% to 10% of pregnancies with pregestational DM. DKA is more common in type 1 diabetics and occurs with more frequency during pregnancy due to worsening insulin resistance (15). The pathophysiology of DKA is summarized in Figure 29-4 (54). This life-threatening emergency can develop rapidly during pregnancy and with less extreme hyperglycemia (55). Case reports have even described "euglycemic" DKA during pregnancy with initial presentation of nausea, abdominal pain, ketonuria and high anion gap metabolic acidosis but with a normal glucose of 77 mg/dL. The parturient improved appropriately with insulin and dextrose infusions (55). Risk factors for the development of DKA include new onset during pregnancy, infections, poor patient compliance, insulin pump malfunction, and treatment with beta-mimetic tocolytic medications or antenatal corticosteroids (15). DKA can occur during pregnancy without precipitating events other than emesis. In a small case series of 37 parturients with DKA, 42% had emesis with rapidly evolving starvation ketosis and no known precipitating factors (56). The management strategy for DKA during pregnancy is described in Table 29-6 and typically involves intensive care unit monitoring for aggressive hydration, insulin infusion, and frequent assessment of glucose and potassium concentrations (15). Continuous fetal monitoring may show recurrent late decelerations that improve with maternal condition. The fetal mortality rate has improved recently from 35% to approximately 10% of cases (39).

Rather than DKA often associated with type I diabetes, pregnant patients with pregestational type 2 diabetes may be more prone to develop a hyperosmolar hyperglycemic non-ketotic state (HHNS) (57). HHNS is characterized by hyperglycemia, hyperosmolality (often >360 mOsm/L), and extreme hypovolemia without ketonemia. Patients may have mental status changes including confusion, somnolence, and possible coma or seizure activity as hyperosmolarity increases. At least initially, the syndrome occurs without ketosis or acidosis, unless superimposed with other metabolic acidoses, such as infection, sepsis, dehydration-related renal failure, or lactic acidosis. At this time, HHNS outcomes in pregnancy are limited to case reports but the incidence may increase along with the prevalence of type 2 diabetes associated with the obesity epidemic. The hallmark of treatment is volume resuscitation with metabolic derangements corrected as appropriate (57,58). The average fluid deficit in non-pregnant patients is approximately 9 L. Relatively small-dose insulin infusions are usually used to correct hyperglycemia after volume replacement has been initiated. Metabolic, electrolyte, and fluid abnormalities may put the parturient at risk for intrauterine fetal demise (IUFD), as occurred in at least two published cases (57,58). Overly rapid correction of maternal glucose can also cause adverse fluid and osmotic events in the placenta. Placental perfusion may also be compromised by the overall dehydration and blood volume reduction caused by osmotic diuresis from sustained glycosuria (57). Finally, HHNS heightens the risk for thromboembolic events during pregnancy, presumably due to stasis

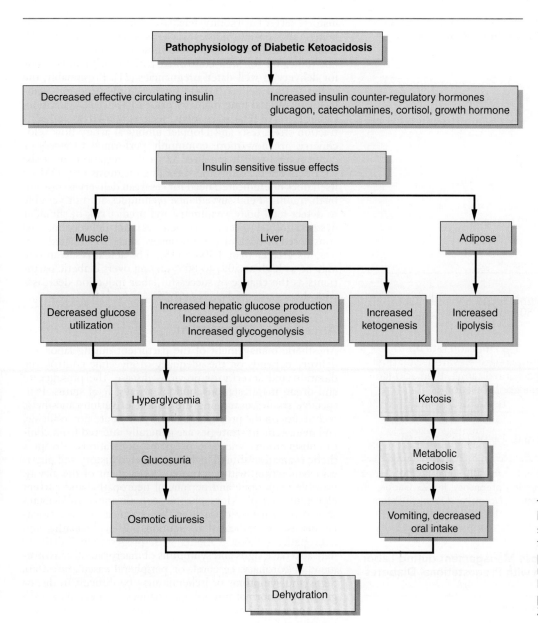

FIGURE 29-4 Pathophysiologic process leading to DKA. Reprinted with permission from: Carroll MA, Yeomans ER. Diabetic ketoacidosis in pregnancy. *Crit Care Med* 2005;33(10):S347–353.

from the low blood volume state. Prophylactic heparin may be indicated in situations where the patient is remote from delivery (57).

In addition to the increased incidence of hyperglycemic crises, women with pregnancies complicated by diabetes are also prone to hypoglycemia. Patients and families should be taught how to respond quickly and appropriately to signs and symptoms of hypoglycemia (often defined as glucose less than 60 mg/dL), with ACOG recommending a glass of milk over fruit juice. Type I diabetics may also need glucagon on hand for severe hypoglycemia and loss of consciousness (15). During labor and delivery, maternal glucose should be kept in the high-normal range (approximately 100 mg/dL) to prevent the extremes. ACOG's recommendations for insulin management during labor and delivery are shown in Table 29-7 (15). Hypoglycemia should be managed with the understanding that overshooting maternal targets may increase the incidence of fetal hypoglycemia after delivery. If glucose levels are less than 70 mg/dL and oral intake is not possible as in the case of scheduled elective cesarean delivery, 2 to 5 g of glucose can be administered intravenously, with appropriate

communication to the neonatal team regarding need for maternal glucose administration (59).

Obstetric Management during Labor and Delivery

Preterm labor in diabetic parturients should be managed carefully with close monitoring of maternal glucose levels. Beta-adrenergic agents, such as terbutaline, may cause hyperglycemia, making magnesium the tocolytic of choice. Antenatal corticosteroids to promote fetal lung maturity will also complicate management, with increased insulin requirements expected over the next 5 days after administration (15). A consideration of fetal and maternal conditions is necessary to determine optimal timing of delivery (15).

Published recommendations from the Fifth International Workshop-Conference on GDM held in 2005 do not support routine delivery before 38 weeks' gestation without evidence of specific maternal or fetal compromise (21). Mode and time of delivery has to be assessed based on multiple factors such as severity and control of diabetes, previous obstetric

TABLE 29-6 Protocol Recommended by the ACOG (2005) for Management of Diabetic Ketoacidosis during Pregnancy

Laboratory assessment
Obtain arterial blood gasses to document degree of acidosis present; measure <u>glucose</u>, ketones, and electrolyte levels at 1- to 2-h intervals

Insulin
Low-dose, intravenous
Loading dose: 0.2–0.4 U/kg
Maintenance: 2–10 U/h

Fluids
Isotonic sodium chloride
Total replacement in first 12 h of 4–6 L
1 L in first hour
500–1,000 mL/h for 2–4 h
250 mL/h until 80% replaced

Glucose
Begin 5% <u>dextrose</u> in <u>normal saline</u> when <u>glucose</u> plasma level reaches 250 mg/dL (14 mmol/L)

Potassium
If initially normal or reduced, an infusion rate up to 15–20 mEq/h may be required; if elevated, wait until levels decrease into the normal range, then add to intravenous solution in a concentration of 20–30 mEq/L

Bicarbonate
Add one ampule (44 mEq) to 1 L of 0.45% <u>normal saline</u> if pH is <7.1

Reprinted with permission from: Landon MB, Catalano PM, Gabbe SG. Diabetes mellitus complicating pregnancy. In: SG Gabbe, JR Niebyl, JL Simpson, eds. *Obstetrics: Normal and Problem Pregnancies.* 5th ed. Elsevier, Inc.; 2007:977–1011.

TABLE 29-7 Blood Glucose Management during Labor and Delivery for Women with Pregestational Diabetes Mellitus

- At bedtime: Usual dose of intermediate-acting insulin.
- In the morning: Insulin is withheld.
- Before active labor onset: Start intravenous normal saline infusion.
- Once active labor begins or glucose levels <70 mg/dL:
  - Start 5% dextrose solution for intravenous infusion.
  - Set at rate of approximately 100–150 mL/h (or 2.5 mg/kg/min).
  - Goal of blood glucose level around 100 mg/dL.
  - Monitor frequent blood glucose level (hourly or as appropriate) to titrate for dextrose infusion rate or to determine the need of insulin.
  - If blood glucose level >100 mg/dL, use short-acting regular insulin administered by intravenous infusion at a rate of 1.25 U/h.

Adapted from: ACOG Committee on Practice Bulletins. ACOG Practice Bulletin. Clinical Management Guidelines for Obstetrician-Gynecologists. Number 60, March 2005. Pregestational diabetes mellitus. *Obstet Gynecol* 2005;105:675–685; Coustan DR. Delivery: timing, mode, and management. In: Reece EA, Coustan DR, Gabbe SG, eds. *Diabetes in Women: Adolescence, Pregnancy, and Menopause.* 3rd ed. Philadelphia, PA: Lippincott Williams & Wilkins, 2004; and Jovanovic L, Peterson CM. Management of the pregnant, insulin-dependent diabetic woman. *Diabetes Care* 1980;3:63–68.)

history, cervix favorability, fetal size, fetal and maternal well-being, and co-morbidities such as preeclampsia (60,61). Similarly, amniocentesis to determine fetal lung maturity is not indicated for well-controlled patients with indications for delivery in well-dated pregnancies (21). Presumably, the indication for delivery would supercede the need for establishment of fetal lung maturity prior to 38 weeks' gestation. Other types of fetal assessment, such as non-stress and contraction stress tests and Doppler umbilical artery flow velocimetry, are now more commonly performed to assess or confirm fetal well-being after 32 weeks' gestation and assist with delivery decisions (62–64). The diagnosis of GDM by itself does not indicate a need for cesarean delivery to prevent birth trauma. Fetal surveillance techniques are not yet able to detect fetal body asymmetry and predict risk of shoulder dystocia (60). However, planned cesarean delivery may be considered in extreme circumstances, such as estimated fetal weights greater than 4,500 g (15). The actual cesarean rate may be as high as 50% to 80% among overt diabetic parturients as the chance of successful labor induction decreases with the severity of diabetes (61,65).

Anesthetic Management

Anesthetic management of the parturient during labor and delivery depends on the adequacy of glycemic control, the duration and severity of previous disease, the presence of end-organ manifestations, and, as always, fetal status. Prospective studies examining the impact of various anesthetic techniques on the pregnant diabetic patient are not available, and management strategies are generally inferred from clinical observations and non-pregnant populations. Preanesthetic evaluation should include a targeted history and physical examination, with appropriate assessment of the airway, possible autonomic and peripheral neuropathy, and current glycemic control. More chronic complications of diabetes should be considered, such as the presence of microvascular disease, as indicated by retinopathy, nephropathy, and neuropathy (59,66). Patients with pregestational diabetes may also have signs and symptoms of macrovascular involvement in coronary, cerebral, or peripheral vasculature (66). Signs and symptoms of ischemia may be difficult to distinguish from normal physiologic changes of pregnancy, such as dyspnea with exertion. Patients with chronic disease and questionable symptoms should undergo further diagnostic testing, including possible cardiac testing to identify risk and prevent myocardial stress during labor and delivery (15,59).

Difficult tracheal intubation is 7 to 10 times higher in pregnant women, with diabetes likely increasing the magnitude of this problem (59). In particular, preexisting diabetes and subsequent glycosylation of collagen in small joints may lead to the development of limited joint mobility (66). This stiffness may be present in the cervical spine and atlanto-occipital joint, limiting neck extension (59). The stiff joint syndrome, also called diabetic scleroderma, is also associated with non-familial short stature, thick skin, and the "hallmark" prayer sign where individuals are unable to approximate the palmar surfaces of the interphalangeal joints. The clinical significance of this constellation of symptoms is unknown, and the true incidence of difficult airway resulting from collagen glycosylation may be very small (67). More commonly, diabetic parturients may be more difficult to intubate due to their often concurrent disease processes, mainly preeclampsia and obesity.

In addition to risk factors for difficult intubation, the physical examination should include documentation of existing sensory and motor deficits from peripheral neuropathy so as to avoid wrongful implication of regional anesthesia. Proper attention to padding in the lithotomy position will be necessary to prevent further superficial nerve damage for patients with longstanding microvascular disease (59). The presence of autonomic neuropathy as suggested by postural hypotension or gastroparesis may predict responses to various anesthetic techniques (68). Patients with pregestational diabetes and cardiovascular autonomic neuropathy may have hampered physiologic adaptations to pregnancy, such as inadequate increase in heart rate, stroke volume, and cardiac output to tolerate exercise or prevent supine hypotension from aortocaval compression (39). In addition to uterine displacement, these women may require more aggressive hydration or vasopressors after regional anesthesia to prevent hypotension caused by sympathetic blockade. Response to vasopressors may be blunted, suggesting a need for frequent monitoring and early correction of blood pressure lability. Presence of gastroparesis may increase risk of aspiration but is unlikely in gestational diabetes. Hong found no difference in aspirated gastric pH and volumes in parturients with gestational diabetes compared to controls undergoing elective cesarean delivery (69).

Virginia Hartridge, an anesthesiologist from Rochester, Minnesota, detailed the anesthetic concerns for the diabetic parturient in an eloquent paper published in 1962 (70). While the morbidity and mortality has improved drastically since that time for this population, her statement that "There is no single 'best way' to manage the anesthesia for delivery of the pregnant diabetic patient" still rings true (70). For labor analgesia, neuraxial techniques are preferred to optimize pain control, indirectly improving placental perfusion through a variety of mechanisms. Maternal response to labor pain has been well documented with increases in stress markers of cortisol, catecholamines, and beta endorphins (71). These elevated stress markers may prolong labor and impair placental blood flow via uterine artery vasoconstriction (71). Epidural local anesthetics have been shown to decrease this stress response, reduce maternal hyperventilation that leads to uterine vasoconstriction, and promote direct uterine vasodilation through sympathetic blockade (71). Scull and colleagues demonstrated a decrease in plasma beta-endorphin and cortisol concentrations after initiation of epidural analgesia for women in early labor (72). Combined spinal–epidural (CSE) techniques are also effective at reducing circulating catecholamines. For example, Cascio found that 25 μg of intrathecal fentanyl reduced maternal plasma epinephrine levels at least to the same extent and more rapidly compared to 10 mL of 1.5% lidocaine (73). Reduction of the maternal stress response to labor is probably particularly important for pregestational diabetics with the potential for macrovascular coronary artery involvement. In short, advantages of neuraxial catheter techniques in diabetic parturients include reduced maternal stress hormones, decreased hyperventilation, uterine vasodilation due to sympathetic blockade, analgesia with minimal placental transfer, and ability to extend analgesia for forceps or cesarean delivery (71).

Neuraxial techniques for labor may also improve glycemic control through the modification of the neuroendocrine stress response. In non-pregnant surgical populations, epidural analgesia initiated prior to incision can prevent hyperglycemia, presumably by blockade of afferent pathways of the adrenal gland (T11-L1) (74). Therefore, initiation of neuraxial analgesia to T11-L1 levels early in labor could theoretically decrease the need for insulin during labor. However, while combinations of lower concentration local anesthetic with opioid reduce motor blockade and total analgesic consumption, the resulting block may not be dense enough to fully suppress the stress response and lead to clinically significant changes (74). No randomized studies have compared neuraxial techniques specifically in a diabetic parturient population, and this type of study is unlikely to be done as the overwhelming majority of patients and infants do well with both epidural and CSE strategies. Catheter-based strategies seem more prudent than single shot approaches as they allow for extension of analgesia for instrumental or cesarean delivery. Regardless of the technique chosen or the combination of drugs used, careful monitoring of glucose and hemodynamics throughout labor is necessary. One case report described hypoglycemia to 57 mg/dL after a CSE technique in a patient with gestational diabetes, presumably due to rapid onset of analgesia and abrupt decrease in catecholamine and cortisol levels, again highlighting the need for frequent monitoring of glucose to prevent maternal and fetal morbidity (75).

For elective or emergent cesarean delivery, the presence of diabetes by itself should not dictate any particular strategy. General anesthesia should be avoided unless dictated by fetal circumstances, maternal coagulation issues, or other specific regional anesthesia contraindications. Anesthesia providers should be aware of the potential for difficult airway, possible gastroparesis and increased aspiration risk, increased hemodynamic response to intubation, and impaired hormonal compensation to hypoglycemia. Administration of a nonparticulate antacid prior to surgery can minimize risk of complications from aspiration. Similarly, metoclopramide (10 mg) can be given to promote gastric emptying 30 to 40 minutes before surgery in patients with known or suspected autonomic neuropathy or gastroparesis (76).

The choice of regional anesthesia should be based on individual patient circumstances. Glucose levels should be monitored prior to surgery if at all possible, with adjustments made and communicated to the neonatal team. Historically, Datta and colleagues published a series of studies examining acid–base status of diabetic mothers and their infants undergoing elective cesarean delivery using general, spinal, or epidural anesthesia. They discovered an increased incidence of neonatal acidosis as demonstrated by significantly lower average pH values in umbilical artery and vein samples in the diabetic patients who received spinals and developed subsequent hypotension compared to general anesthesia (77). Neonatal acidosis was also predicted by the combination of hypotension and severity or chronicity of diabetes after epidural anesthesia for cesarean delivery (78). In subsequent studies, dextrose-containing solutions were eliminated, and parturients were given at least 1,500 mL preload prior to induction of spinal anesthesia. Maternal hypotension was also aggressively treated with ephedrine and standard left lateral tilt to avoid aortocaval compression. Using these conditions, Datta found no differences between infants in the diabetic and control groups, suggesting that spinal anesthesia can be used safely for diabetic mothers undergoing cesarean delivery (79). Ramanathan confirmed these results of normal acid–base fetal status with epidural analgesia for cesarean delivery (80). Either spinal anesthesia or slower onset epidural blockade can be used safely and successfully without fear of neonatal acidosis in diabetic patients undergoing cesarean delivery. Following regional anesthesia, providers should be aware of the potential for infectious complications. Although very rare, diabetes is considered a common risk factor for the development of epidural or spinal abscess, and severe back pain with associated fever should prompt consideration of diagnostic imaging (81,82).

Postnatal Management

Following delivery, insulin requirements drop precipitously, and pregestational diabetic women may only need half of their predelivery dose to maintain normoglycemia (14). For this reason, long-acting insulins should be avoided around the time of delivery. For women with only GDM, the majority return to normal glucose tolerance immediately after delivery but remain at risk for development of type 2 diabetes within 10 years (21). A fasting or random plasma glucose is often done 1 to 3 days postdelivery to detect persistent, overt diabetes, with subsequent assessments occurring 6 to 12 weeks after delivery, 1-year postpartum, annually, and prior to conception with subsequent pregnancies. All types of insulin, as well as glyburide and glipizide, and probably metformin, are safe for breastfeeding women if glucose tolerance persists. Limited studies suggest that breast feeding may actually have a protective effect on subsequent risk of diabetes and should be encouraged (21).

■ THYROID DISORDERS

Under normal physiologic conditions of pregnancy, the thyroid gland increases production by 40% to 100% to meet maternal and fetal metabolic needs. While mild enlargement of thyroid volume occurs due to glandular hyperplasia and hypervascularity, palpable goiters are not normally associated with pregnancy and should be further evaluated (83). hCG, made by the placenta, is structurally similar to thyroid-stimulating hormone (TSH) and slightly upregulates thyroid hormone production by the gland. This upregulation can lead to normal suppression of TSH, especially during weeks 8 to 14 when hCG levels peak, causing a misdiagnosis of subclinical hyperthyroidism (84). In patients with real hypothyroidism, the expected elevations in TSH may be suppressed from pregnancy, leading to a failure to identify early hypothyroidism (83). This clinical scenario is more problematic as the fetus is completely dependent on the mother for thyroid hormone production during the early period of brain and nervous system development (85). Gestational age-specific TSH nomograms are available to assist with diagnostic decisions (83). The diagnostic picture is also complicated by estrogen-driven increases in thyroid hormone-binding proteins with increased levels of total triiodothyronine (T3) and thyroxine (T4) expected throughout pregnancy. However, the unbound active free T3 and T4 measurements should remain relatively normal (86). Figure 29-5 illustrates relative changes in maternal thyroid function during pregnancy (83).

The incidence of thyroid dysfunction during pregnancy has been estimated at 4% to 5%, confirming that thyroid disease is the second most common endocrine disease affecting women of reproductive age (86–88). This data is based on prospective analyses of over 25,000 parturients (87,88). Table 29-8 shows overall changes in thyroid function tests in normal pregnancy compared to thyroid disease states (86). Given the potential for adverse pregnancy outcomes, considerable controversy exists over whether parturients should be screened routinely for thyroid dysfunction. Multiple endocrine societies recommend routine TSH screening preconceptually or as soon as pregnancy is identified due to evidence of impaired brain development in children of mothers with abnormal thyroid function (89). Specifically, several

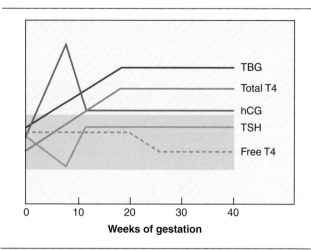

FIGURE 29-5 Pattern of changes in serum concentrations of thyroid function study results and hCG during pregnancy. The shaded area represents the normal range of normal thyroid laboratory values in non-pregnant patients. (TBG, thyroid-binding globulin; T4, thyroxine; TSH, thyroid-stimulating hormone.) Reprinted with permission from: Casey BM, Leveno KJ. Thyroid disease in pregnancy. *Obstet Gynecol* 2006;108(5):1283–1292.

studies have found a relationship between hypothyroidism and lower intelligence quotient (IQ) scores, as well as preterm delivery (85,90). Maternal hypothyroidism is suspected to cause a range of cognitive and developmental abnormalities, likely dependent on the severity of the disease. However, ACOG does not support routine screening due to lack of evidence that identification and treatment of subclinical disease actually improves maternal or fetal outcomes (85). A multicenter, randomized trial to address whether screening and treatment of subclinical hypothyroidism or hypothyroxinemia (low free T4 levels) impacts pediatric neurodevelopment is currently underway and will likely determine standard of care for obstetrics in the United States (89). ACOG does recommend appropriate evaluation of significant goiter or thyroid nodules and testing of thyroid function in women with a personal history or symptoms of disease or other medical conditions associated with thyroid disease, such as DM (85,86).

Pathophysiology

The normal progression of pregnancy requires an increased hormonal output by the maternal thyroid gland. This demand for increased production is the result of several factors, such as increased thyroxine-binding globulin (TBG) (leading to diminished free hormone concentrations), stim-

TABLE 29-8 Changes in Thyroid Function Test Results in Normal Pregnancy and in Thyroid Diseases

Maternal Status	TSH	FT₄	FTI	TT₄	TT₃	RT₃U
Normal Pregnancy	No Change	No Change	No Change	↑	↑	↓
With Hyperthyroidism	↓	↑	↑	↑	↑ or No Change	↑
With Hypothyroidism	↑	↓	↓	↓	↓ or No Change	↓

TSH, thyroid-stimulating hormone; FT4, free thyroxine; FTI, free thyroxine index;
TT₄, total thyroxine; TT₃, total tri-iodothyroxine; RT₃U, resin; T₃, uptake; ↑, increase; ↓, decrease.
Modified with permission from ACOG Committee on Practice Bulletins. ACOG Bulletin. Clinical Management Guidelines for Obstetrician-Gynecologists, Number 37, August 2002. Thyroid Disease in Pregnancy. *Obstet Gynecol* 2002;2:387–396.

TABLE 29-9 Signs, Symptoms and Possible Etiologies of Thyroid Dysfunction

	Increased Thyroid Hormone Production	Decreased Thyroid Hormone Production
Etiology	Graves' disease (autoimmune) (85–90%) Excess TSH production Gestational trophoblastic neoplasia Hyperfunctioning thyroid adenoma Toxic multinodular goiter Subacute thyroiditis Ectopic thyroid tissue Hyperemesis gravidarum Struma ovarii Amiodarone-induced	Hashimoto's (chronic thyroiditis or autoimmune) Subacute thyroiditis Previous radioactive iodine treatment Previous thyroidectomy Iodine deficiency Amiodarone-induced (structurally related to thyroid hormone and has 39% iodine by weight and can result in hypothyroidism or thyrotoxicosis)
Signs and Symptoms General Cardiovascular	Weight loss with ↑ appetite Heat intolerance & sweating Muscle weakness Proximal myopathy Diarrhea, polyuria Hyperreflexia Oligomenorrhea, loss of libido Insomnia, hyperactivity Irritability and dysphoria Warm moist skin Nervousness Fine tremor Exophthalmos Goiter Sinus tachycardia Atrial fibrillation Palpitation Hypertension High-output heart failure Intravascular hypovolemia	Weight gain Cold intolerance Muscle cramp, fatigue Constipation Hyporeflexia Dry coarse skin, hair loss Menorrhea, (later oligo/amenorrhea) Intellectual slowing, insomnia Puffy hand/feet/face—myxedema Flat facial expression Voice change Carpel tunnel syndrome Serous cavity effusion Paresthesia, impaired hearing Decreased heart rate, Myocardial contractility, Stroke volume, and Cardiac output Low-output heart failure Peripheral vasoconstriction (cool extremities)
Extreme presentation	Thyroid storm: Altered consciousness (coma, restlessness, delirium, seizure) Tachycardia to Arrhythmia—commonly atrial fibrillation Hyperpyrexia Hypotension to shock/heart Failure	Myxedema coma: Impaired mentation Myxedema Hypoventilation Hypothermia Hyponatremia (from SIADH) Congestive heart failure

Adapted from ACOG Committee on Practice Bulletins. ACOG Bulletin. Clinical Management Guidelines for Obstetrician-Gynecologists, Number 37, August 2002. Thyroid Disease in pregnancy. *Obstet Gynecol* 2002;100:387–396.

ulatory effect of hCG on the TSH receptor as discussed above, and decreased iodine supply to the maternal thyroid gland due to fetal consumption and increased maternal renal clearance (91). With a normally functioning thyroid gland in an iodine-sufficient environment, the increased hormonal demands associated with pregnancy are not a problem. However, if the functional capacity of the thyroid is limited, physiologic adaptation may not be sufficient to meet maternal and fetal demands. Functional capacity can be limited due to a variety of causes, including iodine deficiency or autoimmune disorders. Iodine deficiency is known to lead to glandular stimulation and goiter formation in both mother and fetus, with volume of the goiter directly correlated with the degree of iodine restriction (91). The World Health Organization recommends 250 μg of daily iodine intake for pregnant and lactating women to prevent goiter formation and impaired mental development of offspring (92). Iodine deficiency is not generally a problem in countries such as the United States with national programs for dietary sup-

plementation, typically using the strategy of universal salt iodization (92).

More commonly in developed countries, functional capacity of the thyroid is altered by the presence of autoantibodies to various cell components, resulting in either stimulation or inhibition of thyroid functions (93). Alterations in thyroid function due to autoimmune disease are often associated with infertility and early spontaneous abortion. However, pregnancies do occur in the setting of coexisting or new-onset thyroid disease. Thyrotoxicosis can be due to hyperfunctioning of the thyroid gland (hyperthyroidism) or any other stimulation of the hypothalamic–pituitary–thyroid axis. Signs, symptoms, and etiologies of thyrotoxicosis are listed in Table 29-9 (86,94). Overt hyperthyroidism occurs in approximately 0.2% of pregnancies with Graves' disease accounting for 95% of these cases (86). In Graves' disease, the body produces an antibody, sometimes called thyroid-stimulating immunoglobulin or TSH receptor antibody, which mimics TSH and causes increased thyroid hormone production (86). More rarely, hyperthyroidism in pregnancy can be caused by high levels of hCG, causing stimulation of the TSH receptors due to structural similarities. In addition to signs and symptoms of transient hyperthyroidism, women with extremely high levels of hCG more often develop hyperemesis gravidarum with nausea and vomiting so severe that dehydration or weight loss are possible. This rare cause of hyperthyroidism typically abates in the second half of pregnancy as the placenta decreases production of hCG (86).

In developed countries, hypothyroidism during pregnancy is also most commonly due to an autoimmune process, namely Hashimoto's disease also called chronic autoimmune thyroiditis. In Hashimoto's disease, the body produces antithyroid antibodies such as thyroid antimicrosomal and antithyroglobulin antibodies that block thyroid hormone production. As with iodine deficiency, compensatory TSH production in Hashimoto's disease results in increased thyroid volume or goiter. Signs and symptoms of inadequate thyroid hormone production and common etiologies are listed in Table 29-9 (86,94). The generalized immunosuppression of pregnancy may actually decrease the severity of autoimmune thyroid disorders during some pregnancies, only to have potential rebound effects after delivery (95).

Effects of Thyroid Disease on Pregnancy: Maternal and Fetal Outcomes

Untreated or inadequately treated thyroid disease can be associated with a number of adverse maternal and fetal outcomes. Thyrotoxicosis has been associated with miscarriage, placental abruption, preeclampsia, and preterm delivery (86,96). In extreme cases (1% of hyperthyroid pregnant patients), thyroid storm and possible congestive heart failure can occur, with a maternal mortality rate reported as high as 25% (86). The incidence of fetal death in patients with hyperthyroidism is also slightly higher than expected at 5.6%. These fetal losses may be related to teratogenicity of treatment or to the disease process itself (97). Medically indicated preterm deliveries with resultant prematurity and low birth weight probably account for the majority of the fetal complications of thyrotoxicosis. Due to these known associations, clinically overactive thyroid disease should be treated preconceptually and throughout pregnancy. However, unlike subclinical hypothyroidism, subclinical hyperthyroidism (defined by low TSH and normal free T4 levels) does not appear to be associated with adverse maternal or fetal/neonatal outcomes. For example, in a prospective study of over 25,000 pregnant women screened for thyroid disease, subclinical hyperthyroidism was not related to premature delivery, placental abruption, low birth weight, or any other pregnancy or neonatal outcomes (88).

Poorly controlled hypothyroidism can have similar effects as hyperthyroidism during pregnancy, including low birth weight or fetal demise from preterm delivery, preeclampsia, or placental abruption (86,87). In addition, women with iodine-deficient hypothyroidism are at risk for delivery of infants with congenital cretinism, characterized by growth failure, mental retardation, and other neuropsychologic deficits (86,87). In iodine-sufficient areas, overt hypothyroidism with low thyroid hormone concentrations in early gestation may have similar consequences, as the fetus is completely dependent on maternal thyroid function until the fetal thyroid gland begins concentrating iodine at 10 to 12 weeks of gestation (86). Haddow et al. found that 19% of 7-year-old children of women with untreated hypothyroidism had intelligence quotient (IQ) scores less than 85% compared to only

5% of carefully matched controls (90). Unfortunately, in contrast to hyperthyroidism, even subclinical hypothyroidism may also have a significant impact on pregnancy outcomes and neurodevelopment of infants. Children whose mothers had normal TSH and low T4 levels (subclinical hypothyroidism) have also been shown to have decrements in IQ scores compared to controls (98). Casey and colleagues found an increased incidence of placental abruption and preterm birth in women with subclinical hypothyroidism based on prospective screening data, suggesting that IQ deficits may be related to prematurity rather than organogenesis effects (87).

Thyroid disease that is attributed to an autoimmune process can also cause fetal and neonatal effects through placental transfer of antibodies. Graves' and Hashimoto's disease both place the newborn at risk for hyper- or hypofunctioning glands and goiter, depending on the ratio of blocking and stimulating antibodies, degree of maternal control, and presence of drug therapy. For example, women who are on antithyroid drug therapy for Graves' disease during pregnancy may be less likely to have an infant with hyperthyroidism as those drugs will also cross the placenta. In contrast, women previously treated with radioactive iodine or surgery prior to pregnancy still have placental transfer of antibodies without counteractive drug effects, placing their infants more at risk. Neonatal providers should be aware of the maternal history of thyroid disease, management strategies, and potential for fetal thyroid dysfunction and enlargement (86). In the United States, all infants are screened for congenital hypothyroidism to prevent delay in diagnosis and allow for early initiation of thyroid hormone replacement. If identified early, infants can expect near-normal growth and intelligence (86).

Treatment of Thyroid Disease during Pregnancy

Mild hyperthyroidism with low TSH and normal free T4 levels probably does not need to be treated during pregnancy. Overt hyperthyroidism can and should be treated with thioamides, specifically propylthiouracil (PTU) or methimazole, both of which cross the placenta. These drugs decrease thyroid hormone synthesis by blocking the organification of iodide, and, for PTU, by also blocking peripheral conversion of T4 to T3 (86). Historically, PTU was preferred in pregnancy as it was thought to cross the placenta to a lesser extent and is not present in as high of a concentration in breast milk (96). Earlier concerns about methimazole and development of congenital scalp defects (fetal aplasia cutis) may not be warranted based on comparison studies (86). The most common side effects of thionamide therapy are nausea, rash, and arthralgias, and the most serious complication is agranulocytosis necessitating immediate cessation (96). The goal of drug therapy is to maintain the free T4 in the high-normal range using the lowest possible dosage to minimize fetal exposure and risk of fetal hypothyroidism. Figure 29-6 illustrates the potential for neonatal goiter formation in parturients treated with thionamide therapy. Frequent monitoring of thyroid hormone levels may initially be necessary until a euthyroid state is obtained (86). Anti-thyroid drugs and their mechanisms of action are summarized in Table 29-10 (95,99). Surgery (partial or total thyroidectomy) should be considered during pregnancy for women who cannot tolerate drug therapy, have poor control despite medication, demonstrate malignant potential, or display pressure symptoms from large goiters (96). Radioactive iodine 131 is contraindicated during pregnancy due to risk of fetal thyroid ablation. Women should also avoid conception until at least 4 months after treatment with iodine (86).

Hypothyroidism in pregnant women, either from previous ablation, surgery, or thyroid dysfunction, can be treated

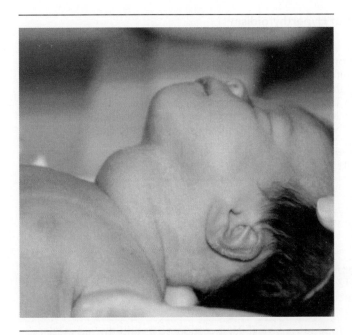

FIGURE 29-6 Term neonate delivered of a woman with a 3-year history of thyrotoxicosis that recurred at 26 weeks' gestation. The mother was given methimazole, 30 mg orally daily, and she was euthyroid at delivery. Laboratory studies showed that the infant was hypothyroid. Reprinted with permission from: Cunningham FG, Leveno KJ, Bloom SL, et al. Medical and Surgical Complications. In: Cunningham FG, Leveno KJ, Bloom SL, Hauth JC, Rouse DJ, Spong CY, eds. *Williams Obstetrics*. 23rd ed. New York, NY: McGraw-Hill Companies, Inc. 2010.

similarly to non-pregnant patients, namely using levothyroxine in sufficient dosages to normalize TSH levels (86). Increases in levothyroxine requirements associated with pregnancy occur as early as the fifth week of gestation. In a prospective study with frequent evaluation of thyroid function, mean requirements increased 47% during the first half of pregnancy and plateaued by week 16. Recommendations from this data included increasing baseline doses of levothyroxine by 30% as soon as pregnancy was confirmed to prevent negative neuro-developmental consequences (100). Women should be aware of the potential for decreased absorption of levothyroxine when taken with prenatal vitamins that contain iron and calcium. Adjustments in dosing are not required if prenatal vitamins are taken 4 hours after levothyroxine ingestion (101). Frequent monitoring of TSH levels at least every trimester should be performed to ensure euthyroid state with labs redrawn every 4 weeks after an adjustment in medication (86).

Acute Management of Thyroid Disease Manifestations during Pregnancy

Rarely, thyroid disease during pregnancy can result in severe symptoms requiring emergency medical treatment. Thyroid storm occurs in approximately 1% of pregnant patients with hyperthyroidism but carries a high mortality rate of up to 25% (86). Thyroid storm represents extreme thyrotoxicosis, with the transition point not clearly defined. Precipitating events may ignite this transition from thyrotoxicosis to storm, including infection, surgery, labor and delivery, trauma, thromboembolism, DKA, and even possible pseudoephedrine or salicylate use (84,86,102). Common signs and

symptoms of thyroid storm are described in Table 29-9 (86). Burch and Wartofsky developed a point system to standardize the definition of thyroid storm by assessing degrees of thermoregulatory dysfunction, central nervous system effects, gastrointestinal or hepatic complications, tachycardia, congestive heart failure, and atrial fibrillation (103). However, rather than focusing on specific diagnostic criteria, patients with severe thyrotoxicosis should be assumed to have impending storm and receive aggressive treatment to prevent heart failure, shock, stupor, and coma (84,102). Treatment should not be withheld for laboratory confirmation if the diagnosis is suspected.

Treatment of thyroid storm includes maternal supportive measures such as oxygen, intravenous fluids and electrolyte replacement, and antipyretic therapy, as well as pharmacologic agents to suppress thyroid function (84). Assessment of intravascular volume status may require invasive central monitoring. Pharmacologic therapy includes PTU, potassium iodide, dexamethasone, propranolol, and phenobarbital, with each agent chosen for its synergistic effect at suppression of thyroid function (84). Table 29-11 summarizes the management of thyroid storm in pregnant patients. The order of drug therapy is important, as iodine may stimulate new hormone synthesis if given initially (102). Frequent fetal assessment is also recommended using ultrasound, biophysical profile, or non-stress test depending on the gestational age with delivery reserved only for fetal indications that outweigh risks to the mother (84). Treatment of precipitating events and the thyroid storm itself will hopefully eliminate the need for delivery and its associated hemodynamic consequences.

Anesthetic Management

Preanesthetic evaluation of the parturient with thyroid disease should focus on presence of goiter, current symptoms, adequacy of treatment, and cardiovascular manifestations. Signs and symptoms of heart failure should prompt further diagnostic work-up, such as echocardiography. Cardiomyopathy from excessive T4 occurs more commonly during pregnancy in patients with uncontrolled hyperthyroidism (104). Physical examination may reveal a palpable goiter with potential partial airway obstruction in patients with hyper-, hypo-, and even euthyroid glands. In a non-pregnant population, patients with goiters and radiographic evidence of tracheal deviation were at increased risk for difficult intubation using conventional laryngoscopy (105). While subsequent studies were not able to confirm this association, the presence of an enlarged thyroid with concomitant symptoms of airway obstruction, such as orthopnea or stridor, may prompt further imaging (106). Nandwani and colleagues described a case report of dyspnea and coughing in pregnancy. While a chest x-ray was unremarkable, soft tissue x-ray and CT scan of the neck eventually showed tracheal compression at the level of C7/8 and retrosternal extension of the goiter. Respiratory symptoms including stridor and orthopnea occurred intermittently until cesarean delivery of the infant using an epidural technique. The stridor resolved rapidly after delivery, presumably due to improvement in respiratory mechanics, and mother and baby were discharged after 5 days. The mother returned for an uneventful subtotal thyroidectomy 3 weeks later (107).

As with elective procedures, patients with thyroid disease should be optimized with the goal of euthyroid functioning prior to labor and/or delivery for both maternal and fetal reasons. If the euthyroid state is not possible prior to delivery, anesthesia providers should be prepared to treat the extremes of thyroid function, including thyroid storm or myxedema hypothyroid coma. Myxedema coma is extraordinarily rare in pregnancy due to anovulation with severe hypothyroidism;

TABLE 29-10 Drugs and their Mechanisms for Treatment of Hyperthyroidism

Drugs	Mechanism	Other Concerns or Side Effects
Propylthiouracil (PTU) and methimazole (Goal—titrating regimen to maintain the high normal thyroxine level with the lowest dose possible)	Decrease thyroid hormone synthesis by blocking organification/iodination of thyroglobulin Blocks peripheral T4 to T3 conversion (i.e., blocks deiodination of thyroxine to tri-iodothyroxine)	Crosses placenta, potential fetal hypothyroidism Nausea, rash, arthralgias Agranulocytosis (Fetal aplasia cutis and choanal atresia associated with methimazole—not shown in later studies)
Radioactive iodine 131 (Absolute contraindication during pregnancy because of risk of fetal thyroid ablation)	Ablation/destruction of thyroid	Fetal thyroid destruction Maternal hypothyroidism
Potassium iodide, sodium iodide (use for thyroid storm)	Prevents release of thyroxine	Only give 1–2 h after PTU administration as iodine by itself may stimulate new thyroid hormone synthesis
Dexamethasone	Decreases release and blocks conversion of T4 to T3 Also for relative adrenocorticoid deficiency	
Lithium carbonate (use instead of iodide if allergic to iodide)	Increases intrathyroidal iodine Inhibit formation and release of T3 and T4	(First investigated as anti-thyroid medication when noted high incidence of hypothyroidism among psychiatric patients receiving lithium.) Monitor for electrolyte abnormalities
Beta blocker (Propranolol, esmolol)	Control/reduce tachycardia and hyperdynamic adrenergic over activity Blocks peripheral conversion of T4 to T3 (Propranolol)	Potential transient neonatal hypoglycemia, apnea and bradycardia; Long-term use may be associated with intrauterine growth restriction; Potential negative ionotropic effect on ongoing heart failure
Phenobarbital (for extreme agitation)	Increases catabolism of thyroid hormone	

however, at least one case report has described altered mental status initially attributed to preeclampsia, later recognized as myxedema coma and treated with acute intravenous thyroid hormone replacement and glucocorticoid supplementation (108). Thyroid storm or thyrotoxicosis typically has a precipitating event, such as infection, DKA, preeclampsia, hypoglycemia, parturition, or pulmonary embolism (109). Thyroid storm with severe symptoms can be treated as explained previously in Table 29-11. Treatment should not be withheld awaiting laboratory confirmation. Clinical similarities with other conditions, such as pheochromocytoma and malignant hyperthermia, may complicate the diagnostic picture. Anxiety, tachycardia, and hyperthermia, as well as tachyarrhythmias, are features of all three conditions. However, malignant hyperthermia requires anesthetic triggers and should also be characterized by muscle rigidity, whereas pheochromocytoma may present with more paroxysmal symptoms (110). In urgent settings for thyroid storm, propranolol can be used intravenously in incremental doses of 1 mg given over 5 minutes with continuous cardiac monitoring (usually around 5 to 6 mg total), titrated based on maternal and fetal heart rate (109,111). Esmolol can also be used perioperatively and may be chosen for its short half-life, beta-selectivity, and minimal neonatal effects (109,111). However, esmolol is not likely to have any peripheral blocking effects on conversion of T4 to T3 (112). Perioperative steroid use, such as dexamethasone or hydrocortisone (100 mg iv), is recommended due to potential relative adrenocorticoid deficiency, possibly due to increased destruction in a hypercatabolic state (109,111).

Prospective studies examining the impact of various anesthetic techniques on the pregnant patient with thyroid disease are not available. Given the potential for stress and catecholamines to elicit or intensify symptoms of thyrotoxicosis, labor analgesia with a neuraxial technique is probably warranted in patients with poor hormonal control. Anesthesia providers should be aware of an association between thyroid dysfunction and effects on coagulation and fibrinolysis. Specifically, a comprehensive review of all published case-control or interventional cohort studies suggested that non-pregnant patients with hyper or hypothyroidism appear to have an increased risk of thrombosis or bleeding, respectively, with degree of coagulation test abnormalities possibly dependent on severity of disease (113). Clinical history and laboratory coagulation studies, if warranted for uncontrolled disease, should guide placement of regional anesthesia. Subclinical disease does not appear to affect coagulation studies (113). Despite this potential for bleeding tendency in patients with hypothyroidism, there are no known published reports of spinal or epidural hematoma attributed to thyroid dysfunction in the parturient following regional anesthesia. Halpern (111) described the use of an epidural catheter for cesarean delivery in a patient with thyrotoxic symptoms. He avoided the use of epinephrine in test and induction doses of local anesthesia to prevent potential for stimulation of adrenergic receptors (111). However, some studies have reported normal hemodynamic responses to epinephrine, norepinephrine, phenylephrine, and clonidine in the setting of hyperthyroidism (114,115).

TABLE 29-11 Management of Thyroid Storm (Severe Thyrotoxicosis) in Pregnant Patients

A. General support:
   a. Supportive care with intensive care monitoring
   b. Protect airway, breathing, circulation—100% oxygen, supportive ventilation, and aggressive fluid replacement as needed
   c. Identify and treat precipitating factor such as infection, DKA
   d. Active and passive cooling—IV fluid, force air cooling or cooling blanket, nasogastric/bladder lavage, cool environment
B. Drug treatment:
   a. Propylthiouracil (PTU)—to inhibit T4 to T3 conversion makes this the first choice of drug for acute treatment. Start with large loading dose of PTU—600–800 mg orally or per nasal gastric tube (NGT), STAT, then 150–200 mg orally/NGT every 4–6 h.
   b. Start stable iodide treatment 1–2 h after PTU administration to block hormone synthesis via Wolff–Chaikoff effect (the delay prevents excessive iodide being incorporated into thyroid hormone):
      – Potassium Iodide (SSKI, Lugol's Solution)—6–8 drops every 6 h orally/NGT; or
      – Sodium Iodide (but may not always be available)—0.25–1.0 g IV every 6–8 h; or
      – Lithium carbonate, 300 mg orally every 6 h.
   c. Beta blocker to reduce tachycardia and adrenergic overactivity.
      Propranolol, 20–80 mg orally every 4–6 h, or propranolol 1–2 mg intravenously every 5 min for a total of 6 mg, then 1–10 mg every 4 h. (Other beta blockers can be titrated to effect, but high-dose propranolol has ability to block conversion of T4 to T3.)
      – If beta blocker is contraindicated (e.g., severe bronchospastic disease), consider:
         – Reserpine, 1–5 mg intramuscularly every 4–6 h
         – Guanethidine, 1 mg/kg orally every 12 h
         – Diltiazem, 60 mg orally every 6–8 h
   d. Dexamethasone, 2 mg intravenously or intramuscularly every 6 h for 4 doses.
   e. Phenobarbital, 30–60 mg orally every 6–8 h as needed for extreme restlessness
   f. Acetaminophen antipyretics as needed—(avoid aspirin which may displace T4 from its carrier protein)
C. Other treatments if necessary:
   Consider removal of circulating thyroid hormones by plasmapheresis or cholestyramine-binding therapy if other treatments not successful.

Adapted from ACOG Committee on Practice Bulletins. ACOG Practice Bulletin. Clinical Management Guidelines for Obstetrician-Gynecologists, Number 37, August 2002. Thyroid disease in pregnancy. *Obstet Gynecol* 2002;2:387–396; Ecker JL, Musci TJ. Thyroid function and disease in pregnancy. *Curr Probl Obstet Gynecol Fertil* 2000;23:109–122; Molitch ME. Endocrine emergencies in pregnancy. *Balliere's Clin Endocrinol Metab* 1992;6:167–191; and Graham GW, Unger B, Coursin DB. Perioperative management of selected endocrine disorders. *Int Anesthesiol Clin* 2000;38:31–67.

For cesarean delivery, regional or general anesthesia can be safe alternatives depending on clinical status. General anesthesia may be necessary in emergencies or in the presence of coagulopathy or high-output cardiac failure. The airway may need to be secured with awake/spontaneous ventilation techniques rather than the more typical rapid sequence induction, in the setting of an enlarged gland or clinical stridor. Epidural or spinal techniques can also be used to obtain surgical anesthesia. Epidural strategies have been advocated in patients with dyspnea or goiter to allow for titration and better control over block height. Excessively high thoracic blockade may result in respiratory compromise for patients with limited reserve (107). In euthyroid patients without orthopnea, spinal anesthesia can be administered safely. Interestingly and historically, Knight in 1945 described the use of spinal anesthesia to control sympathetic and adrenal overactivity in patients with overt hyperthyroidism undergoing surgery (116). While not a current strategy for suppressing sympathetic activity, medications that elicit tachycardia, such as ketamine, glycopyrrolate, atropine, pancuronium, and beta-mimetics for tocolysis, are probably best avoided when possible for thyrotoxic patients (111). Additional anesthetic considerations include careful eye protection to prevent corneal abrasion for exophthalmic patients, multiple ECG leads to readily diagnose supraventricular tachycardias, and temperature monitoring to detect thyroid storm under anesthesia (admittedly an unlikely initial symptom) (111).

Postnatal Management

In patients with normal thyroid function, the increased gland size associated with pregnancy returns to normal in the postpartum period (86). Patients with autoimmune-induced disease may experience an exacerbation due to resurgence of antibodies following relief of the immunosuppressive state of pregnancy (93). TSH levels should be checked routinely to ensure appropriate dosing; levothyroxine may need to be decreased gradually if increases were made during pregnancy (95). Treatment of thyroid dysfunction should continue postpartum, with levothyroxine, PTU, and propranolol all considered compatible with breast feeding (84,95). Approximately 6% to 9% of women without thyroid disease during pregnancy may develop postpartum thyroiditis, or inflammation of the thyroid gland caused by an autoimmune process (84). This diagnosis is made by documenting new-onset abnormal levels of TSH, free T4, or both (86). Postpartum thyroiditis is more common in women with high thyroid autoantibody titers in early pregnancy or in women with other autoimmune conditions, such as insulin-dependent DM (104). 44% of patients present in a hypothyroid state, with the remaining 56% exhibiting thyrotoxicosis or thyrotoxicosis followed by hypothyroidism. Thyroiditis may mimic postpartum depression. Women with goiter, fatigue, weight change, dry skin, temperature intolerance, depression, or palpitations should have their thyroid function evaluated in the postpartum period (86).

■ DISORDERS OF THE HYPOTHALAMIC–PITUITARY AXIS

The hypothalamic–pituitary–adrenal axis is dramatically altered during normal pregnancy to regulate maternal fertility, parturition, blood pressure control, and sodium balance (117). The overall result is increased circulating cortisol and ACTH during gestation to values that can be seen in pathologic Cushing's syndrome. Adrenal aldosterone secretion is also stimulated to four- to six-fold times the upper limits seen in euvolemic non-pregnant adults. The aldosterone may serve to counteract the natriuretic effect of progesterone and atrial natriuretic peptide and help to maintain sodium balance (83). Placental hormones may help to regulate the production of pituitary and adrenal hormones in a manner similar to the hypothalamic-releasing hormones (117). Like the thyroid gland, the pituitary gland also enlarges during pregnancy, although not typically enough to compress the optic chiasm and cause impaired vision (83). From the anterior pituitary, prolactin concentrations increase throughout pregnancy to prepare the breast tissue for lactation, with lactotrophs accounting for a majority of the enlargement (118,119). The posterior pituitary stores antidiuretic hormone (ADH or vasopressin), which helps to regulate plasma osmolality, and oxytocin that is released continuously across gestation and is intricately involved in labor and the "let down" response during lactation (119). Despite the normal increase in size, the pituitary gland is not necessary for successful pregnancy assuming glucocorticoids and thyroid hormone are replaced (83). Similarly, women with known adrenal insufficiency can have uneventful pregnancies if adequately treated with glucocorticoid and mineralocorticoid therapy. Fetal/placental sources of cortisol may also help to achieve necessary stress responses during crisis periods of gestation (117). However, unrecognized pituitary or adrenal insufficiency, or excessive production of catecholamines as in pheochromocytoma, can have devastating maternal and fetal consequences.

Hypopituitarism and Sheehan's Syndrome

In 1937, Sheehan described a syndrome of hypopituitarism resulting from pituitary necrosis following severe obstetric hemorrhage. Acutely, women may exhibit persistent hypotension or circulatory collapse, tachycardia, hypoglycemia, and failure of lactation (93). More chronically, reduced secretion of pituitary hormones, including growth hormone, luteinizing hormone, follicle-stimulating hormone, TSH, ACTH, and prolactin leads to a range of clinical manifestations including amenorrhea, failure of lactation, weakness, dry skin, loss of axillary and pubic hair, breast atrophy, and psychiatric disturbance (120). Latency between hemorrhage and clinical disease varies from immediate to 40 years according to published case series (93,120,121). Based on laboratory data from patients with postpartum hypopituitarism, this latency in the development of symptoms may be partially due to autoimmunity rather than the direct impact of ischemia. 63% of patients with Sheehan's syndrome had autoantibodies against the pituitary, perhaps as a result of antigens released during tissue necrosis (122). Anesthesia providers should consider hypopituitarism acutely and in subsequent encounters with patients that have experienced significant postpartum hemorrhage. Treatment of shock in those patients would be aided by glucocorticoid therapy in the short-term and subsequent endocrinology follow-up. Fortunately, this complication of pregnancy has likely decreased in incidence in industrialized countries due to improvements in medical care and the availability of blood products and fluid replacement alternatives (120).

Diabetes Insipidus

Diabetes insipidus (DI) is a rare condition during pregnancy, occurring in only 4 out of 100,000 pregnancies and characterized by polyuria, polydipsia, excessive thirst, and dehydration (123). These symptoms of polyuria and polydipsia may be difficult to distinguish from normal pregnancy as the normal thirst threshold in pregnancy is reduced to 287 mOsm/kg from the non-pregnant 298 mOsm/kg (124). Diagnosis is usually confirmed with a high volume of urine output, high serum osmolality (>290 mOsm/kg H_2O), and decreased urine osmolality (<275 mOsm/kg H_2O) (125). In non-pregnant populations, DI is usually categorized as either central (neurogenic) or nephrogenic. Symptoms of central DI are due to decreased production of vasopressin from destruction or dysfunction of the posterior pituitary gland. For example, DI has been described in conjunction with Sheehan's syndrome (126). Central DI responds readily to exogenous synthetic 1-deamino-8-D-arginine vasopressin (dDAVP) through the reduction of urine output and concentration of urine by the kidney (125). In contrast, nephrogenic DI is due to the inability of the kidney to respond to the normal antidiuretic effects of vasopressin, typically as a result of drugs, kidney disease, or certain inheritable conditions (127). In pregnant women, a third type of DI has been described, often termed gestational DI. This syndrome is transient and has been associated with preeclampsia and fatty liver of pregnancy. The cause of gestational DI is thought to be increased vasopressinase activity and decreased renal responsiveness to arginine-vasopressin (AVP) (128). Vasopressinase is a placental enzyme that breaks down endogenous AVP but not synthetic dDAVP, making the condition often readily amenable to drug therapy (123). The liver is at least partially responsible for normal degradation of vasopressinase, explaining the numerous case reports showing associations of gestational DI with fatty liver and HELLP syndrome (123). From an anesthetic perspective, the use of spinal, epidural, and CSE techniques have been described depending on clinical condition in pregnant women with DI. Careful attention should be paid to volume status and electrolyte abnormalities, including the potential for extreme hypernatremia (123,128,129). While not routinely necessary, Passannante and colleagues described the use of central venous pressure monitoring to assist with volume resuscitation for epidural placement in the setting of suspected dehydration in a parturient with extreme thirst (129). Careful consideration should be given to limiting oral intake during the labor process. Parturients with DI should be allowed access to water for as long as practically possible with appropriate fluid and electrolyte replacement during periods of restriction (129).

Pheochromocytoma

Pheochromocytoma is a catecholamine-secreting tumor thought to be rare in pregnancy, with fewer than 300 cases reported and a prevalence estimated at 1 in 54,000 (130). The classic triad of paroxysmal hypertension with paroxysmal headache, sweating, and palpitations predicts the diagnosis with a sensitivity of 91% and specificity of 94% in the non-pregnant population (131). Other associated signs and symptoms can occur, including cardiomyopathy and dependent edema (see Table 29-12), often making the diagnosis difficult to distinguish from preeclampsia (131,132). In contrast to preeclampsia, pheochromocytoma may cause hypertension throughout pregnancy and is not typically associated with proteinuria. The common "rule of 10s" seems likely to apply to pregnant women with the disease, including 10% occurrence outside the adrenal medulla, 10% malignancy rate, 10% bilateral or multiple, and 10% (or even more) with

TABLE 29-12 Common Signs and Symptoms of Pheochromocytoma

Signs	Symptoms
Hypertension ++++	Headaches ++++
Sustained hypertension ++	Palpitations ++++
Paroxysmal hypertension ++	Anxiety/nervousness +++
Postural hypotension +	
Tachycardia or reflex brady-cardia +++	Tremulousness ++
	Weakness, fatigue ++
Excessive sweating ++++	Nausea/vomiting +
Pallor ++	Pain in chest/abdo-men +
Flushing +	
Weight loss +	Dizziness or faintness +
Fasting hyperglycemia ++	Paresthesias +
Decreased gastrointestinal motility +	Constipation (rarely diarrhea) +
Increased respiratory rate +	Visual disturbances +

Reprinted with permission from: Pacak K. Preoperative management of the pheochromocytoma patient. *J Clin Endocrinol Metab* 2007;92:4069–4079. Copyright 2007, The Endocrine Society. Adapted from: Eisenhofer G, et al. *Drug Saf* 2007;30:1031–1062.

familial links, such as the autosomal dominant multiple endocrine neoplasia (MEN) type 2 (131,132). MEN type 2A has been described rarely in pregnancy but should be suspected in patients with a history of medullary thyroid carcinoma and/or hyperparathyroidism (132). Pregnancy may reveal previously undetected tumors due to increased vascularity or mechanical factors from an enlarging uterus-stimulating catecholamine release (133). After biochemical confirmation with elevated urinary and plasma catecholamines and their metabolites (e.g., vanillylmandelic acid, metanephrine, and normetanephrine), ultrasound and magnetic resonance imaging are considered safe modalities to attempt tumor localization during pregnancy (133). Diagnosis prior to delivery is critical; Harper reports an overall maternal mortality of 17% and fetal loss of 26%, improved to 0% and 15%, respectively with antenatal diagnosis (134).

Obstetric Management

Overall catecholamine production from the chromaffin cells of the tumor does not generally increase during pregnancy. However, paroxysms can be precipitated by stress, increased abdominal pressure, medications such as metoclopramide, fetal movements, and vaginal delivery (130). Hypertensive crises can lead to uteroplacental insufficiency with resultant intrauterine growth restriction, fetal hypoxia, abruption, and possibly death. On the maternal side, potential complications include hemorrhage and infarction of vital organs, congestive heart failure, cardiac dysrhythmias, and death (133). Uterine contractions and maternal expulsive efforts likely increase mechanical pressure and catecholamine release (133). Vaginal delivery should typically be avoided as a potential trigger of a hypertensive crisis with documented higher maternal mortality compared to cesarean delivery (31% vs. 19%) (133). Surgical resection is the definitive treatment following localization of the tumor. The optimal timing of tumor resection is controversial and dependent on gestation at the time of diagnosis as well as success of treatment of maternal symptoms (130,133). If gestational age is less than 24 weeks, the tumor should be resected immediately and pregnancy continued or terminated based on clinical circumstances (133). The laparoscopic approach has been established as the preferred technique for tumors less than 6 cm due to lower postoperative morbidity and shorter hospital stays (130).

Laparoscopy has also been associated with less cardiovascular instability, presumably as a result of decreased tumor manipulation and release of catecholamines (133). For pregnancies past 24 weeks' gestation, the uterine size makes surgical approaches more difficult. Medical management, including adrenergic blockade, should be attempted until fetal maturity can be reached if possible with the goals of controlling maternal symptoms and preparing for surgery (133). The tumor resection can occur in conjunction with the cesarean delivery or staged with laparoscopy at a later date (131,133).

Anesthetic Management

Medical optimization prior to surgery or delivery likely contributes to more recent improved outcomes with pregnancy. To blunt catecholamine-induced changes, patients have typically received 7 to 14 days of alpha blockade in preparation for surgery (135). A number of alpha-blocking agents are available, including prazosin, doxazosin, alpha methyl tyrosine, and intravenous phentolamine, but oral phenoxybenzamine has been most commonly used preoperatively during pregnancy to provide irreversible alpha receptor antagonism (130,135). Phenoxybenzamine does cross the placenta with select reports of neonatal hypotension with drug use prior to delivery (130). Despite the lack of formal testing, these drugs are generally considered safe in pregnancy (131). Alpha blockade should be started before beta blockade to avoid the possibility of extreme hypertension from unopposed alpha-vasoconstriction (130). Beta blockers can be added to the regimen, with options including labetalol (both alpha and beta effects in a 1:7 ratio), atenolol, metoprolol, and propranolol (130). Beta blockers should be considered in the setting of persistent hypertension, tachycardia, or tachyarrhythmias, including premature ventricular contractions (133). As suggested in Table 29-13, overall goals for medical optimization include normalizing blood pressure, heart rate, and organ function, restoring volume depletion, and preventing catecholamine-induced storm.

Patients with pheochromocytoma are probably at greatest risk of hemodynamic instability during intubation of the trachea, tumor manipulation, and after ligation of venous drainage of the tumor (133). Intraoperative anesthetic goals during cesarean and/or tumor resection include avoidance of events or drugs that trigger catecholamine release and activation of the sympathetic nervous system (133). Invasive monitoring with an arterial line probably assists with early detection of cardiovascular changes, and pulmonary artery catheterization can also be considered (133). Regional

TABLE 29-13 Criteria to Determine Preoperative Optimization for Patients with Pheochromocytoma

1. No in-hospital BP reading higher than 165/90 mm Hg should be evident for 48 h before surgery. Arterial BP measured every min for 1 h in a stressful environment (postanesthesia care unit). If no BP reading is greater than 165/90, this criterion is considered satisfied.
2. Orthostatic hypotension should be present, but BP on standing should not be lower than 80/50 mm Hg.
3. ECG should be free of ST–T changes that are not permanent.
4. No more than one premature ventricular contraction (PVC) should occur every 5 min.

Data from: Ronald D. Miller, Lars I. Eriksson, Lee A. Sleisher, Jeanine P. Wiener-Kronish, William L. Young, eds. *Miller's Anesthesia*. 7th ed. Elsevier, Inc. Churchill Livingstone; 2010, Volume 1: 1085.

TABLE 29-14 Strategies for Preoperative Hypertensive Control and Prevention of Catecholamines Release during Anesthesia in Patients with Pheochromocytoma

Epidural anesthesia Magnesium	
Alpha-receptor antagonism	Phenoxybenzamine (oral) Phentolamine (intravenous)
Beta blockers	Labetalol (1:7 alpha:beta)
Other anti-hypertensives	Metoprolol Esmolol
Anesthetic drugs	Calcium-channel blockers Nitroglycerin Nitroprusside Lidocaine Volatile agent Remifentanil Sufentanil

Adapted from: Grodski S, Jung C, Kertes P, et al. Pheochromocytoma in pregnancy. *Intern Med J* 2006;36:604–606; Hamilton A, Sirrs S, Schmidt N, et al. Anaesthesia for pheochromocytoma in pregnancy. *Can J Anaesth* 1997;44(6):654–657; and Dugas G, Fuller J, Singh S, et al. Pheochromocytoma and pregnancy: A case report and review of anesthetic management. *Can J Anaesth* 2004;51(2):134–138.

and general techniques have been used for preferred cesarean delivery in pregnant patients with pheochromocytoma (131,133,135). While spinal or CSE techniques have been described without mortality, epidural anesthesia likely provides more opportunity for careful titration and avoidance of abrupt hemodynamic changes. If tumor resection is planned early in gestation, with laparoscopy, or in conjunction with cesarean delivery, general anesthesia is probably the most common technique. Table 29-14 lists strategies that have been used perioperatively to control hypertension and prevent catecholamine release during anesthesia for patients with pheochromocytoma (131,133,135). The variety in this list highlights the importance of adequate depth of anesthesia and hemodynamic control before stimulating events, rather than any one particular agent. These agents are considered reasonably safe for intraoperative use during pregnancy, although the newborn should be followed closely for possible hypotension and need for vasopressors after delivery (133). Interestingly, magnesium is used frequently in pregnancy for a number of other indications with known fetal effects and may be an excellent choice if cesarean is planned in conjunction with tumor resection. Its advantages include direct vasodilation, inhibition of catecholamine release from the adrenal medulla, reduction in sensitivity of alpha receptors, and potent antiarrhythmic effects (135). In a review of 17 anesthetics for pheochromocytoma, magnesium sulfate produced satisfactory hemodynamic stability during induction and intubation for most patients, but additional antihypertensives were required in at least five of the cases (136). Drugs that should probably be avoided if possible due to catecholamine-stimulating effects include ketamine, halothane, desflurane at high concentrations, and non-depolarizing muscle relaxants with vagolytic or histamine-releasing properties (130,133). Following tumor resection, hypotension may need to be treated aggressively with volume resuscitation and vasopressors if necessary. If medical optimization with alpha blockade cannot occur prior to delivery due to late diagnosis, case reports have described successful outcomes with close monitoring of hemodynamics, epidural analgesia for labor, and a short second stage without active pushing (137). Regardless of the specific anesthetic technique chosen,

pheochromocytoma in pregnancy, as with all endocrine disorders, requires close collaboration with obstetricians, medical optimization, and careful monitoring to achieve the best outcomes for both mother and fetus.

KEY POINTS

- The most common endocrine disorders associated with pregnancy are diabetes mellitus (DM) and thyroid disease, both of which can have substantial impact on fetal outcomes if poorly managed.
- Women with GDM have an inadequate endogenous insulin supply to meet tissue demands during the period of increased resistance associated with pregnancy. For these women, hyperglycemia is a result of both inadequate insulin production combined with a more chronic form of insulin resistance exacerbated by physiologic changes of pregnancy.
- For women with preexisting DM, significant hyperglycemia during organogenesis of 5 to 8 weeks' gestation may cause severe congenital malformations and subsequent potential for spontaneous abortion.
- Macrosomia, often defined as birth weight greater than 4,500 g, is the most commonly encountered adverse outcome in term infants of pregnancy complicated by diabetes.
- The multicenter prospective HAPO study showed continuous linear relationships between increasing maternal glucose measures and birth weight, primary cesarean delivery, clinical neonatal hypoglycemia, premature delivery, shoulder dystocia or birth injury, and preeclampsia.
- When the maternal source of glucose is gone, newborns are at risk to drop glucose levels below 45 mg/dL. This fetal hypoglycemia after delivery may be related more to maternal hyperglycemia during labor, rather than reflecting chronic levels as measured by HbA$_{1c}$.
- The effects of maternal hyperglycemia do not end in the peripartum period. Close and long-term follow-up of offspring has demonstrated increased weight and impaired glucose tolerance or prevalence of type 2 diabetes. These long-term effects appear to be similar regardless of maternal diabetes type. Future research in this area will need to focus on whether glycemic control can prevent the vicious cycle of obesity and diabetes.
- Despite aggressive therapy, the physiologic changes associated with pregnancy may contribute to the development of DKA in 5% to 10% of pregnancies with pregestational DM. The management strategy for DKA during pregnancy typically involves intensive care unit monitoring for aggressive hydration, insulin infusion, and frequent assessment of glucose and potassium concentrations.
- Published recommendations from the Fifth International Workshop-Conference on GDM held in 2005 do not support routine delivery before 38 weeks' gestation without evidence of specific maternal or fetal compromise. Mode and time of delivery has to be assessed based on multiple factors such as severity and control of diabetes, previous obstetric history, cervix favorability, fetal size, fetal and maternal well-being, and co-morbidities such as preeclampsia.
- Anesthetic management of the parturient during labor and delivery depends on the adequacy of glycemic control, the duration and severity of previous disease, the presence of end-organ manifestations, and, as always, fetal status.
- Advantages of neuraxial catheter techniques in laboring diabetic parturients include reduced maternal stress hormones, decreased hyperventilation, uterine vasodilation due to sympathetic blockade, analgesia with minimal

placental transfer, and ability to extend analgesia for forceps or cesarean delivery.

■ During regional anesthesia, diabetic parturients should receive left lateral tilt, appropriate volume resuscitation with non–dextrose-containing solutions, and aggressive treatment of hypotension. Under these conditions, either spinal anesthesia or slower onset epidural blockade can be used safely and successfully without fear of neonatal acidosis in diabetic patients undergoing cesarean delivery.

■ Several studies have found a relationship between hypothyroidism and lower intelligence quotient (IQ) scores, as well as preterm delivery.

■ The normal progression of pregnancy requires an increased hormonal output by the maternal thyroid gland. With a normally functioning thyroid gland in an iodine-sufficient environment, the increased hormonal demands associated with pregnancy are not a problem. However, if the functional capacity of the thyroid is limited, physiologic adaptation may not be sufficient to meet maternal and fetal demands. Functional capacity can be limited due to a variety of causes, including iodine deficiency or autoimmune disorders.

■ Thyrotoxicosis has been associated with miscarriage, placental abruption, preeclampsia, and preterm delivery. In extreme cases (1% of hyperthyroid pregnant patients), thyroid storm and possible congestive heart failure can occur, with a maternal mortality rate reported as high as 25%. Treatment of thyroid storm includes maternal supportive measures such as oxygen, intravenous fluids and electrolyte replacement, and antipyretic therapy, as well as pharmacologic agents to suppress thyroid function.

■ Preanesthetic evaluation of the parturient with thyroid disease should focus on presence of goiter, current symptoms, adequacy of treatment, and cardiovascular manifestations. As with elective procedures, patients with thyroid disease should be optimized with the goal of euthyroid functioning prior to labor and/or delivery for both maternal and fetal reasons. For cesarean delivery, regional or general anesthesia can be safe alternatives depending on clinical status. General anesthesia may be necessary in emergencies or in the presence of coagulopathy or high-output cardiac failure.

■ The classic triad of symptoms of pheochromocytoma is paroxysmal hypertension with paroxysmal headache, sweating, and palpitations. Other associated signs and symptoms can occur, including cardiomyopathy and dependent edema, often making the diagnosis difficult to distinguish from preeclampsia. Diagnosis prior to delivery is critical to reduce the likelihood of maternal and fetal mortality.

■ Uterine contractions and maternal expulsive efforts likely increase mechanical pressure and catecholamine release in patients with pheochromocytoma. Vaginal delivery should typically be avoided as a potential trigger of a hypertensive crisis with documented higher maternal mortality compared to cesarean delivery.

■ Anesthesia for patients with endocrine disorders has not been well studied with randomized trials. The choice of general versus regional anesthesia should be based on current clinical status of the mother and fetus. Continued research and close collaboration between obstetricians, endocrinologists, neonatologists, and anesthesiologists are necessary to ensure optimal outcomes for both mother and child.

REFERENCES

1. Feig DS, Palda VA. Type 2 diabetes in pregnancy: a growing concern. *Lancet* 2002;359:1690–1692.
2. Muraji T, Hosaka N, Irie N, et al. Maternal microchimerism in underlying pathogenesis of biliary atresia: quantification and phenotypes of maternal cells in the liver. *Pediatrics* 2008;121:517–521.
3. Silverman BL, Rizzo TA, Cho NH, et al. Long-term effects of the intrauterine environment. The Northwestern University Diabetes in Pregnancy Center. *Diabetes Care* 1998;21(Suppl 2):B142–B149.
4. Dabelea D. The predisposition to obesity and diabetes in offspring of diabetic mothers. *Diabetes Care* 2007;30(Suppl 2):S169–S174.
5. Hedderson MM, Gunderson EP, Ferrara A. Gestational weight gain and risk of gestational diabetes mellitus. *Obstet Gynecol* 2010;115:597–604.
6. Most OL, Kim JH, Arslan AA, et al. Maternal and neonatal outcomes in early glucose tolerance testing in an obstetric population in New York City. *J Perinat Med* 2009;37:114–117.
7. King H. Epidemiology of glucose intolerance and gestational diabetes in women of childbearing age. *Diabetes Care* 1998;21(Suppl 2):B9–B13.
8. U.S. Preventive Services Task Force. Screening for gestational diabetes mellitus: recommendations and rationale. *Obstet Gynecol* 2003;101:393–395.
9. Brody SC, Harris R, Lohr K. Screening for gestational diabetes: a summary of the evidence for the U.S. Preventive Services Task Force. *Obstet Gynecol* 2003;101:380–392.
10. Ferrara A. Increasing prevalence of gestational diabetes mellitus: a public health perspective. *Diabetes Care* 2007;30(Suppl 2):S141–S146.
11. Gabbe SG, Gregory RP, Power ML, et al. Management of diabetes mellitus by obstetrician–gynecologists. *Obstet Gynecol* 2004;103:1229–1234.
12. Cheng YW, Block-Kurbisch I, Caughey AB. Carpenter–Coustan criteria compared with the national diabetes data group thresholds for gestational diabetes mellitus. *Obstet Gynecol* 2009;114:326–332.
13. Buchanan TA, Xiang A, Kjos SL, et al. What is gestational diabetes? *Diabetes Care* 2007;30(Suppl 2):S105–S111.
14. Gabbe SG, Graves CR. Management of diabetes mellitus complication pregnancy. *Obstet Gynecol* 2003;102:857–868.
15. ACOG Committee on Practice Bulletins. ACOG Practice Bulletin. Clinical Management Guidelines for Obstetrician–Gynecologists. Number 60, March 2005. Pregestational diabetes mellitus. *Obstet Gynecol* 2005;105:675–685.
16. Cunningham FG, Leveno KJ, Bloom SL, et al. Diabetes. In: Cunningham FG, Leveno KJ, Bloom SL, Hauth JC, Rouse DJ, Spong CY, eds. *Williams Obstetrics*. 23rd ed. New York, NY: The McGraw-Hill Companies, Inc; 2010:1104–1125.
17. Phelps RL, Metzger BE, Freinkel N. Carbohydrate metabolism in pregnancy. XVII. Diurnal profiles of plasma glucose, insulin, free fatty acids, triglycerides, cholesterol, and individual amino acids in late normal pregnancy. *Am J Obstet Gynecol* 1981;140:730–736.
18. Freinkel N. Banting Lecture 1980. Of pregnancy and progeny. *Diabetes* 1980;29:1023–1035.
19. Freemark M. Regulation of maternal metabolism by pituitary and placental hormones: roles in fetal development and metabolic programming. *Horm Res* 2006;65(Suppl 3):41–49.
20. Parretti E, Mecacci F, Papini M, et al. Third-trimester maternal glucose levels from diurnal profiles in nondiabetic pregnancies: correlation with sonographic parameters of fetal growth. *Diabetes Care* 2001;24:1319–1323.
21. Metzger BE, Buchanan TA, Coustan DR, et al. Summary and recommendations of the Fifth International Workshop-Conference on Gestational Diabetes Mellitus. *Diabetes Care* 2007;30(Suppl 2):S251–S260.
22. Yang J, Cummings EA, O'connell C, et al. Fetal and neonatal outcomes of diabetic pregnancies. *Obstet Gynecol* 2006;108:644–650.
23. Eriksson UJ. Congenital anomalies in diabetic pregnancy. *Semin Fetal Neonatal Med* 2009;14:85–93.
24. Guerin A, Nisenbaum R, Ray JG. Use of maternal GHb concentration to estimate the risk of congenital anomalies in the offspring of women with pre-pregnancy diabetes. *Diabetes Care* 2007;30:1920–1925.
25. Morgan SC, Relaix F, Sandell LL, et al. Oxidative stress during diabetic pregnancy disrupts cardiac neural crest migration and causes outflow tract defects. *Birth Defects Res A Clin Mol Teratol* 2008;82:453–463.
26. Watkins ML, Rasmussen SA, Honein MA, et al. Maternal obesity and risk for birth defects. *Pediatrics* 2003;111:1152–1158.
27. Sheffield JS, Butler-Koster EL, Casey BM, et al. Maternal diabetes mellitus and infant malformations. *Obstet Gynecol* 2002;100:925–930.
28. Pederson J. Hyperglycemia–hyperinsulinism theory and birthweight. In: Pederson J, ed. *The Pregnant Diabetic and Her Newborn: Problems and Management*. 2nd ed. Baltimore, MD: Williams & Wilkins; 1977:211–220.
29. ACOG Committee on Practice Bulletins. Clinical Management Guidelines for Obstetrician–Gynecologists. ACOG Practice Bulletin No. 22. Fetal macrosomia. American College of Obstetricians and Gynecologists, Washington, DC: November 2000.
30. Gherman RB, Chauhan S, Ouzounian JG, et al. Shoulder dystocia: the unpreventable obstetric emergency with empiric management guidelines. *Am J Obstet Gynecol* 2006;195:657–672.
31. HAPO Study Cooperative Research Group, Metzger BE, Lowe LP, et al. Hyperglycemia and adverse pregnancy outcomes. *N Engl J Med* 2008;358:1991–2002.
32. Khoury JC, Miodovnik M, LeMasters G, et al. Pregnancy outcome and progression of diabetic nephropathy. What's next? *J Matern Fetal Neonatal Med* 2002;11:238–244.

33. Daskalakis G, Marinopoulos S, Krielesi V, et al. Placental pathology in women with gestational diabetes. *Acta Obstet Gynecol Scand* 2008;87:403–407.

34. Takoudes TC, Weitzen S, Slocum J, et al. Risk of cesarean wound complications in diabetic gestations. *Am J Obstet Gynecol* 2004;191:958–963.

35. Stamler EF, Cruz ML, Mimouni F, et al. High infectious morbidity in pregnant women with insulin-dependent diabetes: an understated complication. *Am J Obstet Gynecol* 1990;163:1217–1221.

36. Lepercq J, Le Meaux JP, Agman A, et al. Factors associated with cesarean delivery in nulliparous women with type 1 diabetes. *Obstet Gynecol* 2010;115:1014–1020.

37. Purdy LP, Hantsch CE, Molitch ME, et al. Effect of pregnancy on renal function in patients with moderate-to-severe diabetic renal insufficiency. *Diabetes Care* 1996;19:1067–1074.

38. Sandvik MK, Iversen BM, Irgens LM, et al. Are adverse pregnancy outcomes risk factors for development of end-stage renal disease in women with diabetes? *Nephrol Dial Transplant* 2010;25:3600–3607.

39. Reece EA, Coustan DR, Gabbe SC. *Diabetes Mellitus in Women: Adolescence Through Pregnancy and Menopause*. 3rd ed. Philadelphia, PA: Lippincott Williams & Wilkins; 2004.

40. Crowther CA, Hiller JE, Moss JR, et al. Effect of treatment of gestational diabetes mellitus on pregnancy outcomes. *N Engl J Med* 2005;352:2477–2486.

41. Landon MB, Spong CY, Thom E, et al. A multicenter, randomized trial of treatment for mild gestational diabetes. *N Engl J Med* 2009;361:1339–1348.

42. Reece EA, Homko CJ. Why do diabetic women deliver malformed infants? *Clin Obstet Gynecol* 2000;43:32–45.

43. Holing EV, Beyer CS, Brown ZA, et al. Why don't women with diabetes plan their pregnancies? *Diabetes Care* 1998;21:889–895.

44. Jovanovic L, Knopp RH, Brown Z, et al. Declining insulin requirement in the late first trimester of diabetic pregnancy. *Diabetes Care* 2001;24:1130–1136.

45. Gabbe SG, Carpenter LB, Garrison EA. New strategies for glucose control in patients with type 1 and type 2 diabetes mellitus in pregnancy. *Clin Obstet Gynecol* 2007;50:1014–1024.

46. Gabbe SG, Holing E, Temple P, et al. Benefits, risks, costs, and patient satisfaction associated with insulin pump therapy for the pregnancy complicated by type 1 diabetes mellitus. *Am J Obstet Gynecol* 2000;182:1283–1291.

47. Kjos SL, Schaefer-Graf UM. Modified therapy for gestational diabetes using high-risk and low-risk fetal abdominal circumference growth to select strict versus relaxed maternal glycemic targets. *Diabetes Care* 2007;30(Suppl 2):S200–S205.

48. Hod M, Yogev Y. Goals of metabolic management of gestational diabetes: is it all about the sugar? *Diabetes Care* 2007;30(Suppl 2):S180–S187.

49. Reader D, Splett P, Gunderson EP, et al. Impact of gestational diabetes mellitus nutrition practice guidelines implemented by registered dietitians on pregnancy outcomes. *J Am Diet Assoc* 2006;106:1426–1433.

50. Reader DM. Medical nutrition therapy and lifestyle interventions. *Diabetes Care* 2007;30(Suppl 2):S188–S193.

51. Coustan DR. Pharmacological management of gestational diabetes: an overview. *Diabetes Care* 2007;30(Suppl 2):S206–S208.

52. Rowan JA, Hague WM, Gao W, et al. Metformin versus insulin for the treatment of gestational diabetes. *N Engl J Med* 2008;358:2003–2015.

53. Nicholson W, Bolen S, Witkop CT, et al. Benefits and risks of oral diabetes agents compared with insulin in women with gestational diabetes: a systematic review. *Obstet Gynecol* 2009;113:193–205.

54. Carroll MA, Yeomans ER. Diabetic ketoacidosis in pregnancy. *Crit Care Med* 2005;33(10 Suppl):S347–S353.

55. Tarif N, Al Badr W. Euglycemic diabetic ketoacidosis in pregnancy. *Saudi J Kidney Dis Transpl* 2007;18:590–593.

56. Rodgers BD, Rodgers DE. Clinical variables associated with diabetic ketoacidosis during pregnancy. *J Reprod Med* 1991;36:797–800.

57. Nayak S, Lippes HA, Lee RV. Hyperglycemic hyperosmolar syndrome (HHS) during pregnancy. *J Obstet Gynaecol* 2005;25:599–601.

58. Gonzalez JM, Edlow AG, Silber A, et al. Hyperosmolar hyperglycemic state of pregnancy with intrauterine fetal demise and preeclampsia. *Am J Perinatol* 2007;24:541–543.

59. Ramanathan J, Ivester T. Diabetes mellitus in pregnancy: pathophysiology and obstetric and anesthetic management. *Semin Anesth Perio M* 2002;21:26–34.

60. Conway DL. Obstetric management in gestational diabetes. *Diabetes Care* 2007;30(Suppl 2):S175–S179.

61. Martin FI, Heath P, Mountain KR. Pregnancy in women with diabetes mellitus. Fifteen years' experience: 1970–1985. *Med J Aust* 1987;146:187–190.

62. Landon MB, Gabbe SG, Sachs L. Management of diabetes mellitus and pregnancy: a survey of obstetricians and maternal-fetal specialists. *Obstet Gynecol* 1990;75:635–640.

63. Johnstone FD, Steel JM, Haddad NG, et al. Doppler umbilical artery flow velocity waveforms in diabetic pregnancy. *Br J Obstet Gynaecol* 1992;99:135–140.

64. Tamura RK, Dooley SL. The role of ultrasonography in the management of diabetic pregnancy. *Clin Obstet Gynecol* 1991;34:526–534.

65. Schneider JM, Curet LB, Olson RW, et al. Ambulatory care of the pregnant diabetic. *Obstet Gynecol* 1980;56:144–149.

66. McAnulty GR, Robertshaw HJ, Hall GM. Anaesthetic management of patients with diabetes mellitus. *Br J Anaesth* 2000;85:80–90.

67. Kadoi Y. Anesthetic considerations in diabetic patients. Part I: preoperative considerations of patients with diabetes mellitus. *J Anesth* 2010;24:739–747.

68. Burgos LG, Ebert TJ, Asiddao C, et al. Increased intraoperative cardiovascular morbidity in diabetics with autonomic neuropathy. *Anesthesiology* 1989;70:591–597.

69. Hong JY. Comparison of preoperative gastric contents between gestational diabetic and normal pregnant women undergoing elective cesarean delivery. *Korean J Anesthesiol* 2006;50:S25–S27.

70. Hartridge VB. Anesthesia for the delivery of the diabetic patient. *Clin Obstet Gynecol* 1962;5:438–449.

71. Reynolds F. The effects of maternal labour analgesia on the fetus. *Best Pract Res Clin Obstet Gynaecol* 2010;24:289–302.

72. Scull TJ, Hemmings GT, Carli F, et al. Epidural analgesia in early labour blocks the stress response but uterine contractions remain unchanged. *Can J Anaesth* 1998;45:626–630.

73. Cascio M, Pygon B, Bernett C, et al. Labour analgesia with intrathecal fentanyl decreases maternal stress. *Can J Anaesth* 1997;44:605–609.

74. Velickovic I, Yan J, Grass JA. Modifying the neuroendocrine stress response. *Semin Anesth Perio M* 2002;21:16–25.

75. Crites J, Ramanathan J. Acute hypoglycemia following combined spinal-epidural anesthesia (CSE) in a parturient with diabetes mellitus. *Anesthesiology* 2000;93:591–592.

76. Pani N, Mishra SB, Rath SK. Diabetic parturient—Anaesthetic implications. *Indian J Anaesth* 2010;54:387–393.

77. Datta S, Brown WU Jr. Acid-base status in diabetic mothers and their infants following general or spinal anesthesia for cesarean section. *Anesthesiology* 1977;47:272–276.

78. Datta S, Brown WU Jr, Ostheimer GW, et al. Epidural anesthesia for cesarean section in diabetic parturients: maternal and neonatal acid-base status and bupivacaine concentration. *Anesth Analg* 1981;60:574–578.

79. Datta S, Kitzmiller JL, Naulty JS, et al. Acid-base status of diabetic mothers and their infants following spinal anesthesia for cesarean section. *Anesth Analg* 1982;61:662–665.

80. Ramanathan S, Khoo P, Arismendy J. Perioperative maternal and neonatal acid-base status and glucose metabolism in patients with insulin-dependent diabetes mellitus. *Anesth Analg* 1991;73:105–111.

81. Kindler CH, Seeberger MD, Staender SE. Epidural abscess complicating epidural anesthesia and analgesia. An analysis of the literature. *Acta Anaesthesiol Scand* 1998;42:614–620.

82. Reihsaus E, Waldbaur H, Seeling W. Spinal epidural abscess: a meta-analysis of 915 patients. *Neurosurg Rev* 2000;23:175–204.

83. Cunningham FG, Leveno KJ, Bloom SL, et al. Maternal physiology. In: Cunningham FG, Leveno KJ, Bloom SL, Hauth JC, Rouse DJ, Spong CY, eds. *Williams Obstetrics.* 23rd ed. New York, NY: The McGraw-Hill Companies, Inc; 2010:107–135.

84. Neale DM, Cootauco AC, Burrow G. Thyroid disease in pregnancy. *Clin Perinatol* 2007;34:543–557.

85. Committee on Patient Safety and Quality Improvement; Committee on Professional Liability. ACOG Committee Opinion No. 381: Subclinical hypothyroidism in pregnancy. *Obstet Gynecol* 2007;110:959–960.

86. ACOG Committee on Practice Bulletins. ACOG Practice Bulletin. Clinical Management Guidelines for Obstetrician-Gynecologists. Number 37, August 2002. (Replaces Practice Bulletin Number 32, November 2001). Thyroid disease in pregnancy. *Obstet Gynecol* 2002;100:387–396.

87. Casey BM, Dashe JS, Wells CE, et al. Subclinical hypothyroidism and pregnancy outcomes. *Obstet Gynecol* 2005;105:239–245.

88. Casey BM, Dashe JS, Wells CE, et al. Subclinical hyperthyroidism and pregnancy outcomes. *Obstet Gynecol* 2006;107:337–341.

89. Gyamfi C, Wapner RJ, D'Alton ME. Thyroid dysfunction in pregnancy: the basic science and clinical evidence surrounding the controversy in management. *Obstet Gynecol* 2009;113:702–707.

90. Haddow JE, Palomaki GE, Allan WC, et al. Maternal thyroid deficiency during pregnancy and subsequent neuropsychological development of the child. *N Engl J Med* 1999;341:549–555.

91. Glinoer D. What happens to the normal thyroid during pregnancy? *Thyroid* 1999;9:631–635.

92. International Council for Control of Iodine Deficiency Disorders. Iodine requirements in pregnancy and infancy. IDD Newsletter 2007;23:1–2. Available at: http://www.iccidd.org/media/IDD%20Newsletter/2007-present/feb2007.pdf. Accessed January 14, 2011.

93. Cunningham FG, Leveno KJ, Bloom SL, et al. Thyroid and other endocrine disorders. In: Cunningham FG, Leveno KJ, Bloom SL, Hauth JC, Rouse DJ, Spong CY, eds. *Williams Obstetrics.* 23rd ed. New York, NY: The McGraw-Hill Companies, Inc.; 2010:1126–1144.

94. Jameson JL, Weetman Anthony P. "Chapter 335. Disorders of the Thyroid Gland" (Chapter). Fauci AS, Braunwald E, Kasper DL, Hauser SL, Longo DL, Jameson JL, Loscalzo J: Harrison's Principles of Internal Medicine, 17e. Available at: http://www.accessmedicine.com/content.aspx?aID=2877285. Accessed January 14, 2011.

95. Abalovich M, Amino N, Barbour LA, et al. Management of thyroid dysfunction during pregnancy and postpartum: an Endocrine Society Clinical Practice Guideline. *J Clin Endocrinol Metab* 2007;92(8 Suppl):S1–S47.

96. Lazarus JH, Kokandi A. Thyroid disease in relation to pregnancy: a decade of change. *Clin Endocrinol (Oxf)* 2000;53:265–278.

97. Hamburger JI. Diagnosis and management of Graves' disease in pregnancy. *Thyroid* 1992;2:219–224.

98. Pop VJ, Brouwers EP, Vader HL, et al. Maternal hypothyroxinaemia during early pregnancy and subsequent child development: a 3-year follow-up study. *Clin Endocrinol (Oxf)* 2003;59:282–288.

99. Cooper DS. Antithyroid drugs. *N Engl J Med* 2005;352:905–917.

100. Alexander EK, Marqusee E, Lawrence J, et al. Timing and magnitude of increases in levothyroxine requirements during pregnancy in women with hypothyroidism. *N Engl J Med* 2004;351:241–249.

101. Chopra IJ, Baber K. Treatment of primary hypothyroidism during pregnancy: is there an increase in thyroxine dose requirement in pregnancy? *Metabolism* 2003;52:122–128.

102. Nayak B, Burman K. Thyrotoxicosis and thyroid storm. *Endocrinol Metab Clin North Am* 2006;35:663–686.

103. Burch HB, Wartofsky L. Life-threatening thyrotoxicosis. Thyroid storm. *Endocrinol Metab Clin North Am* 1993;22:263–277.

104. Casey BM, Leveno KJ. Thyroid disease in pregnancy. *Obstet Gynecol* 2006; 108:1283–1292.

105. Voyagis GS, Kyriakos KP. The effect of goiter on endotracheal intubation. *Anesth Analg* 1997;84:611–612.

106. Amathieu R, Smail N, Catineau J, et al. Difficult intubation in thyroid surgery: myth or reality? *Anesth Analg* 2006;103:965–968.

107. Nandwani N, Tidmarsh M, May AE. Retrosternal goitre: a cause of dyspnoea in pregnancy. *Int J Obstet Anesth* 1998;7:46–49.

108. Turhan NO, Koçkar MC, Inegöl I. Myxedematous coma in a laboring woman suggested a pre-eclamptic coma: a case report. *Acta Obstet Gynecol Scand* 2004;83:1089–1091.

109. Sarlis NJ, Gourgiotis L. Thyroid emergencies. *Rev Endocr Metab Disord* 2003;4:129–136.

110. Pugh S, Lalwani K, Awal A. Thyroid storm as a cause of loss of consciousness following anaesthesia for emergency caesarean section. *Anaesthesia* 1994;49:35–37.

111. Halpern SH. Anesthesia for caesarean section in patients with uncontrolled hyperthyroidism. *Can J Anaesth* 1989;36:454–459.

112. Sherman SC. Thyroid emergencies. In: Wolfson AB, Hendey GW, eds. *Harwood-Nuss' Clinical Practice of Emergency Medicine*. 5th ed. Philadelphia, PA: Lippincott Williams & Wilkins; 2009:1021–1029.

113. Squizzato A, Romualdi E, Büller HR, et al. Clinical review: Thyroid dysfunction and effects on coagulation and fibrinolysis: a systematic review. *J Clin Endocrinol Metab* 2007;92:2415–2420.

114. Aoki VS, Wilson WR, Theilen EO. Studies of the reputed augmentation of the cardiovascular effects of catecholamines in patients with spontaneous hyperthyroidism. *J Pharmacol Exp Ther* 1972;181:362–368.

115. Del Rio G, Zizzo G, Marrama P, et al. Alpha 2-adrenergic activity is normal in patients with thyroid disease. *Clin Endocrinol (Oxf)* 1994;40:235–239.

116. Knight RT. The use of spinal anesthesia to control sympathetic overactivity in hyperthyroidism. *Anesthesiology* 1945;6:225–230.

117. Lindsay JR, Nieman LK. The hypothalamic-pituitary-adrenal axis in pregnancy: challenges in disease detection and treatment. *Endocr Rev* 2005;26:775–799.

118. Dinç H, Esen F, Demirci A, et al. Pituitary dimensions and volume measurements in pregnancy and post partum. MR assessment. *Acta Radiol* 1998;39: 64–69.

119. Foyouzi N, Frisbaek Y, Norwitz ER. Pituitary gland and pregnancy. *Obstet Gynecol Clin North Am* 2004;31:873–892.

120. Feinberg EC, Molitch ME, Endres LK, et al. The incidence of Sheehan's syndrome after obstetric hemorrhage. *Fertil Steril* 2005;84:975–979.

121. Dökmeta HS, Kilicli F, Korkmaz S, et al. Characteristic features of 20 patients with Sheehan's syndrome. *Gynecol Endocrinol* 2006;22:279–283.

122. Goswami R, Kochupillai N, Crock PA, et al. Pituitary autoimmunity in patients with Sheehan's syndrome. *J Clin Endocrinol Metab* 2002;87:4137–4141.

123. Kalelioglu I, Kubat Uzum A, Yildirim A, et al. Transient gestational diabetes insipidus diagnosed in successive pregnancies: review of pathophysiology, diagnosis, treatment, and management of delivery. *Pituitary* 2007;10: 87–93.

124. Davison JM, Gilmore EA, Dürr J, et al. Altered osmotic thresholds for vasopressin secretion and thirst in human pregnancy. *Am J Physiol* 1984;246: F105–F109.

125. Kumar A, Thirumavalavan VS, Kumari V. Diabetes insipidus in pregnancy. *Hospital Phys* 2001;37:47–49.

126. Briet JW. Diabetes insipidus, Sheehan's syndrome and pregnancy. *Eur J Obstet Gynecol Reprod Biol* 1998;77:201–203.

127. Baylis PH, Cheetham T. Diabetes insipidus. *Arch Dis Child* 1998;79:84–89.

128. Lacassie HJ, Muir HA, Millar S, et al. Perioperative anesthetic management for cesarean section of a parturient with gestational diabetes insipidus. *Can J Anaesth* 2005;52:733–736.

129. Passannante AN, Kopp VJ, Mayer DC. Diabetes insipidus and epidural analgesia for labor. *Anesth Analg* 1995;80:837–838.

130. George J, Tan JYL. Pheochromocytoma in pregnancy: a case report and review of literature. *Obstetric Medicine* 2010;3:83–85.

131. Grodski S, Jung C, Kertes P, et al. Pheochromocytoma in pregnancy. *Intern Med J* 2006;36:604–606.

132. Wattanachanya L, Bunworasate U, Plengpanich W, et al. Bilateral pheochromocytoma during the postpartum period. *Arch Gynecol Obstet* 2009;280:1055–1058.

133. Dugas G, Fuller J, Singh S, et al. Pheochromocytoma and pregnancy: a case report and review of anesthetic management. *Can J Anaesth* 2004;51:134–138.

134. Harper MA, Murnaghan GA, Kennedy L, et al. Pheochromocytoma in pregnancy. Five cases and a review of the literature. *Br J Obstet Gynaecol* 1989;96:594–606.

135. Hamilton A, Sirrs S, Schmidt N, et al. Anaesthesia for pheochromocytoma in pregnancy. *Can J Anaesth* 1997;44:654–657.

136. James MF. Use of magnesium sulphate in the anaesthetic management of pheochromocytoma: a review of 17 anaesthetics. *Br J Anaesth* 1989;62:616–623.

137. Junglee N, Harries SE, Davies N, et al. Pheochromocytoma in Pregnancy: When is Operative Intervention Indicated? *J Womens Health (Larchmt)* 2007;16:1362–1365.

Anesthetic Management of the Pregnant Cardiac Patient

Shobana Chandrasekhar • Daniel A. Tolpin • Dennis T. Mangano

■ INTRODUCTION

The pregnant parturient with cardiac disease continues to challenge the anesthesiologist's skills. Pregnancy, labor, and delivery impose unique stresses on the circulation. In fact, the induction and delivery of anesthesia may further destabilize these patients if not approached cautiously and comprehensively. To avoid cardiac decompensation, the anesthesiologist must be thoroughly aware of the normal physiology of labor, delivery, and the puerperium (1); the nature and progression of heart disease during pregnancy (2); the cardiovascular effects of various anesthetic regimens (3); and the therapies available to manage acute complications (4). In the first section of this chapter, we review the incidence, risks, morbidity, and mortality of cardiovascular diseases that are known to occur in these patients. We review expected changes to the cardiovascular system that occur during all phases of pregnancy, and make recommendations for the choice of anesthetic and the mode of delivery. The second, third, and fourth sections review significant cardiovascular diseases that anesthesiologists encounter in parturients. The final section addresses the less common, but important issue of surgical treatment of cardiac disease during pregnancy and cardiac transplantation, with particular attention to the effects on the fetus.

■ BACKGROUND

Epidemiology

The incidence of heart disease among pregnant patients varies by age, country, and socioeconomic status from less than 0.1% to 3.9% and has decreased over the past 4 decades (1–11). In particular, among patients in developing countries, the incidence appears highest with rheumatic heart disease (RHD) being the most prevalent type of cardiac disease in parturients (12–14). Among developed countries, despite advances in the prophylaxis for, and treatment of, cardiac disease, challenges continue given the increasing age of parturients and the attendant risks regarding disease progression (15–17). Notably, several diseases appear most challenging, including right-sided lesions, right-to-left congenital shunts, aortic stenosis, and heart failure (12,13,17–21).

Cardiovascular Changes Associated with Pregnancy and Delivery

Cardiovascular changes, associated with pregnancy and delivery, induce progressive stress on both mother and fetus. During labor, stress, pain, and compensatory changes trigger increases in stroke volume and cardiac output by 50% over prelabor values. Additionally, other stresses can impose acute increases in central blood volume and lead to

cardiac decompensation, such as acute uterine contraction (increasing central blood volume and cardiac output by 10% to 25%), and, following delivery, relief of vena cava obstruction (increasing central blood volume and cardiac output by 50% to 100%). These acute changes are well tolerated by the normal heart; however, such preload stress may be intolerable to a diseased heart that has become increasingly compromised throughout pregnancy and labor. When combined with postdelivery cardiovascular changes and those induced by hemorrhage or administration of oxytocic drugs, rapid decompensation may occur (Figs. 30-1 and 30-2).

Overview of Anesthetic Considerations

Anesthetic management involves an understanding of the type, severity, and progression of the disease in the context of the normal cardiovascular adaptations to pregnancy. Preanesthetic assessment in each trimester of pregnancy is of paramount importance as the presence or worsening of symptoms correlate directly with morbidity and mortality. Physical examination and consultation with the primary physician and the cardiologist are necessary to define the severity of the disease.

There are very few controlled studies addressing the effects of anesthetics and therapeutics on pregnant patients with cardiac disease. However, the physiologic changes occurring during pregnancy, the pathophysiology of cardiac disease processes, and the effects of anesthetics on pregnant patients without cardiac disease are well documented. Anesthetic management of pregnant patients with cardiac disease involves a firm understanding of the above complex issues.

Cardiovascular maternal morbidity and mortality during pregnancy correlate strongly with maternal functional status (22–24). Women with NYHA class I and II (no or minor symptoms) are likely to tolerate pregnancy without major deterioration, whereas risk progressively increases among those with NYHA III and IV (25). See Table 30-1.

Choice of Technique

Analgesic techniques and anesthetic management for vaginal delivery or cesarean delivery of pregnant cardiac patients are largely determined by the nature of the presenting illness. The primary concern of the anesthesiologist is to avoid and/or treat specific pathophysiologic changes that can exacerbate the disease process. Of note are auto transfusion during uterine contractions, effects of oxytocic agents, and degree of hemorrhage. The risks of each anesthetic technique must be balanced against the possible benefits to both the mother and the fetus, in the context of the presenting cardiac disease. In general, no one anesthetic approach is exclusively indicated or contraindicated.

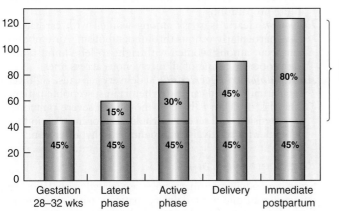

FIGURE 30-1 Cardiac output changes during labor and delivery.

Monitoring

In addition to routine monitoring (continuous electrocardiography, pulse oximetry, and noninvasive blood pressure assessment), the use of more invasive monitoring (intra-arterial, central venous, pulmonary artery, echocardiography [ECG]) during labor and delivery depends on the severity and progression of the cardiovascular disease prior to, and during, pregnancy (26–29). Asymptomatic patients without any evidence of disease progression most likely will experience an uneventful course and will not require invasive monitoring. However, exceptions do exist and must be considered even among asymptomatic patients who present with primary pulmonary hypertension, right-to-left shunt, dissecting aortic aneurysm, severe aortic stenosis, or coarctation of the aorta. Such patients, as well as those manifesting signs and/or symptoms of cardiovascular compromise, should undergo thorough hemodynamic profiling including measurement of cardiac output, vascular resistance, and central pressure, and function (surface ECG). Based on these measurements, a therapeutic plan should be designed for

handling each of the acute complications that may occur with the specific disease.

Perioperative use of pulmonary artery catheters (PACs) remains controversial (30); however, under certain conditions where central pressure and peripheral resistance measurements are critical, we continue to recommend its use. For example, we believe that PAC placement is indicated in patients with decompensated cardiac disease, pulmonary hypertension, severe mitral/aortic stenosis, patients with NYHA IV heart disease, ARDS, and preeclampsia with refractory oliguria or pulmonary edema (23,31,32).

Both transthoracic echocardiography (TTE) and trans-esophageal echocardiography (TEE) can provide critical information regarding risk assessment and disease progression (33). Among our population, use of these techniques is highly recommended, certainly for those undergoing general anesthesia (TEE) and those undergoing regional anesthesia (TTE).

A review by Armstrong et al. highlights newer technologies that are available and maybe integrated in routine practice in the future management of severely ill,

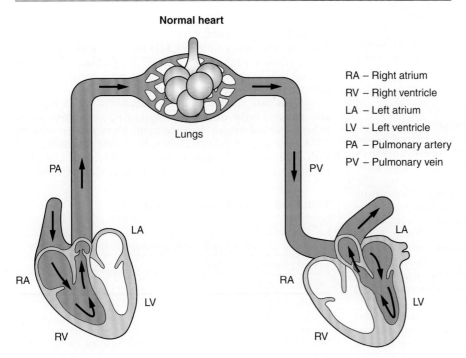

RA – Right atrium
RV – Right ventricle
LA – Left atrium
LV – Left ventricle
PA – Pulmonary artery
PV – Pulmonary vein

FIGURE 30-2 Normal heart.

TABLE 30-1 NYHA Classification System for Heart Failure

Class	Symptoms
1	No limitation of activities
2	Slight limitation of activities
3	Marked limitation of activities
4	Symptoms at rest. Unable to carry out any physical activity without symptoms

NYHA, New York Heart Association.

pregnant cardiac patients (34). Apart from TTE that has been validated and proven useful for pregnancy, there are other noninvasive or minimally invasive monitors used in current obstetric practice. TTE is precisely accurate and informative, but is highly specialized and needs training and expertise on a routine basis, which is hard to acquire by the obstetric anesthesiologist in everyday practice. The normal structural and functional changes that occur during pregnancy have to be understood when interpreting these studies.

TEE provides clearer images due to signal attenuation by the chest wall. It also provides better views of the atria, septum, and detection of thrombi. However, it will not be tolerated in an awake obstetric patient. Hence, this device is most useful in parturients undergoing delivery under general anesthesia. Recent National Institute for Health and Clinical Excellence (NICE) guidelines have recommended the use of esophageal Doppler in major or high risk surgery to reduce the need for central venous catheterization and postsurgical morbidity (35).

The suprasternal Doppler ultrasound is a completely noninvasive method for measuring hemodynamic variables. They could be ideal for use in pregnant patients; however, there are interobserver variabilities and naturally there is a learning curve. More research is needed into this technology.

There are also minimally invasive techniques based on analysis of the arterial waveform (LiDCO, PiCCO, and FloTrac-Vigileo). These are the pulse contour devices that seem promising based on their ease of use and calibration, measurement of fluid responsiveness, and their precision when compared to PAC derived measures of cardiac output (34,35). The latter group measures the electrical resistance changes induced by vascular flow (bioimpedance and bioreactance techniques).

Potential Problems at Delivery

Hemorrhage is not well tolerated in patients with coexisting cardiac disease since they may be unable to compensate given limitations in heart rate and stroke volume responses. Bleeding may be increased due to concurrent anticoagulation.

Pulmonary edema is more likely to occur in the peripartum period in patients with depressed cardiac function due to fluid shifts and as a consequence of additional intravenous (IV) fluids to replace intravascular volume losses. Careful fluid balance is essential; urine output and blood loss should be closely monitored and care should be taken in administering fluids. This may be aided by running drug infusions in smaller volumes of increased concentration to reduce excess IV fluid administration.

Dysrhythmias and tachycardia are poorly tolerated in most patients with significant cardiac disease. Pharmacologic agents causing tachycardia should be avoided or limited.

Oxytocin after delivery should be used in slower and more dilute preparations.

Embolism clearly is a risk among women with cardiac disease, particularly venous thromboembolism. Air embolism can occur among women with right-to-left shunt, requiring proper de-airing of all intravenous access lines.

Acute pulmonary hypertension at delivery can cause right ventricular failure and cardiac ischemia in susceptible patients. The risk of death is high in those with severe pulmonary hypertension, and severe morbidity can occur even in those patients with relatively mild pulmonary hypertension.

Postoperative Care

Since hemodynamic aberrations associated with labor and delivery continue after delivery, patients with symptomatic heart disease who have had a complicated peripartum course should be managed in a multidisciplinary intensive care unit.

■ CONGENITAL HEART DISEASE

The overall incidence of congenital heart disease (CHD) has remained stable over the last 5 decades with most studies reporting *incidences* of 4/1,000 to 12/1,000 live births (36–38). However, the *prevalence* of CHD in the adult population has increased in this same time period due to improvement in therapies aimed at increasing the survival of infants born with CHD (36–39). Cardiac disease in the parturient is increasingly attributable to CHD as opposed to acquired disease. Management of the parturient with CHD requires an understanding of underlying physiology associated with different CHD defects as well as the cardiovascular changes of pregnancy. In addition, cardiac function, coexisting cardiac disease, and type of surgical repair all affect the care of the parturient with CHD.

We will address CHD separately among three groups based on lesion physiology: left-to-right shunts (atrial septal defect [ASD], ventricular septal defect [VSD], patent ductus arteriosus [PDA]), right-to-left shunts (tetralogy of Fallot [TOF], Eisenmenger's syndrome), and congenital valvular and vascular lesions (coarctation of the aorta, aortic stenosis [AS], pulmonary stenosis [PS]).

Left-To-right Shunt

Atrial Septal Defect

ASDs are the most common CHD found in adults occurring in up to 21% of adults with CHD (37,40) (Table 30-2). Symptomatic ASDs are typically corrected early in life; patients with small- or moderate-sized ASDs usually do not develop symptoms until the fourth or fifth decade of life. Symptomatic patients may display dysrhythmias, congestive heart failure, and pulmonary hypertension. Most women with an ASD (corrected or uncorrected) will tolerate pregnancy well with little increased risk of maternal morbidity or mortality. Women with uncorrected ASDs may be at increased risk for

TABLE 30-2 Atrial Septal Defect

Hemodynamic Goals
Prevent or immediately treat supraventricular arrhythmias
Avoid increases in SVR
Avoid decreases in PVR
With pulmonary hypertension present avoid further increases in PVR

SVR, Systemic Vascular Resistance; PVR, Pulmonary Vascular Resistance.

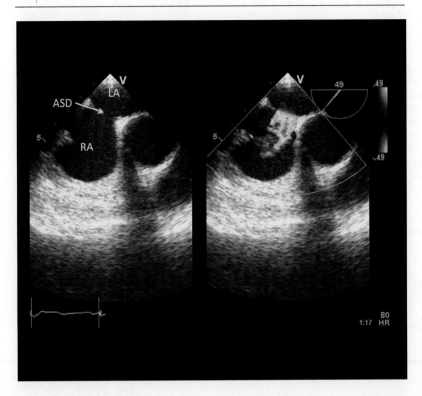

FIGURE 30-3 Modified mid-esophageal aortic valve short-axis view demonstrating a large ASD (left-to-right blood flow). LA, Left atrium; RA, Right atrium; ASD, Atrial septal defect.

delivering small-for-gestational-age infants (41). The most common maternal complications associated with pregnancy in patients with an ASD are cardiac dysrhythmias, endocarditis, heart failure, and cerebrovascular events (19,41). Fetal and perinatal mortality are increased and occur in up to 2.4% of pregnancies (19,41,42).

Clinical Manifestations

Signs and Symptoms: Physical examination findings include fixed expiratory splitting of the second heart sound and a systolic ejection murmur at the left upper sternal border, whose intensity varies with the degree of left-to-right shunting (43).

Test Indicators: Chest x-ray may reveal cardiomegaly, pulmonary artery prominence, and increased pulmonary vascular markings. Electrocardiography usually demonstrates signs of increased right-sided pressures (right ventricular hypertrophy, right atrial enlargement, right axis deviation) (44). ECG can be utilized to visualize and classify the ASD (primum, secundum, and sinus venosus). RV function and size, LV function and size, PA pressure and shunt fraction can all be assessed with ECG (Figs. 30-3 and 30-4). Cardiac catheterization usually reveals normal RA, RV, and PA pressures, even in the presence of cardiac chamber dilation.

Pathophysiology: Left-to-right shunting increases the amount of volume delivered to the right ventricle. The resultant rise in RV preload increases RV volume work and pulmonary blood flow. Compensatory changes in the capacitance of the pulmonary vascular system maintain normal PA pressures until the fourth or fifth decade of life. Chronic volume overload of the right and left atria leads to biatrial enlargement, and the onset of supraventricular dysrhythmias, particularly atrial fibrillation. Eventually, the pulmonary vasculature can no longer manage the increased pulmonary blood flow leading to increased pulmonary vascular resistance (PVR) and pulmonary hypertension. Right ventricular failure secondary to the chronic increased volume workload may occur, particularly when pressure work increases or in the presence of pulmonary hypertension.

Cardiovascular changes of pregnancy augment the physiologic derangements of left-to-right shunts. Normal increases in cardiac output and blood volume during pregnancy may increase the amount of left-to-right shunting, leading to increased work of the ventricles and increased pulmonary blood flow. Depending on the severity of the underlying disease, may precipitate left or right ventricular failure and pulmonary hypertension. Supraventricular dysrhythmias are of particular concern because incomplete left atrial emptying leads to volume and pressure increases in the left atrium worsening any left-to-right shunt.

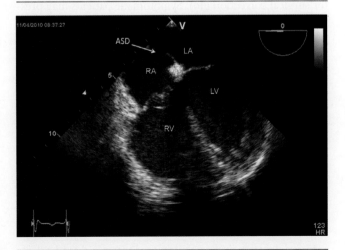

FIGURE 30-4 Mid-esophageal four chamber view demonstrating a large ASD (secundum). Also note enlarged right ventricle secondary to chronic volume overload. RA, Right atrium; RV, Right ventricle; LA, Left atrium; LV, Left ventricle.

Anesthetic Considerations: Asymptomatic patients who have no evidence of pulmonary hypertension or RV compromise can go through labor without special care. Patients with symptoms of RV compromise or pulmonary hypertension should have arterial, central venous, or pulmonary arterial catheter monitoring depending on the severity of their symptoms. The following key points should be noted.

Supraventricular dysrhythmias are poorly tolerated and may increase left-to-right shunt. Generally, antiarrhythmic medications should be continued throughout the pregnancy and the peripartum period. New onset dysrhythmias associated with hypotension or RV failure should be treated immediately with direct current cardioversion or use of pharmacologic rate control (β-blockers, calcium channel blockers, amiodarone, etc.).

Increases in systemic vascular resistance (SVR) may worsen a left-to-right shunt. Increases in vascular resistance increase the impedance to left ventricular emptying, increasing pressure in the left-sided heart chambers and worsening a left-to-right shunt.

Decreases in PVR may worsen a left-to-right shunt. Decreases in PVR may decrease the pressures in the right side of the heart thus increasing the pressure difference between the left and right sides of the heart. This worsens a left-to-right shunt and may lead to hypotension.

Increases in PVR exacerbate pre-existing pulmonary hypertension, which may lead to right ventricular failure.

Anesthesia for Vaginal Delivery and Cesarean Delivery

Lumbar epidural anesthesia for either vaginal delivery or cesarean delivery avoids the harmful increases in SVR that may worsen left-to-right shunting across an ASD. General anesthesia that keeps the above goals in mind can also be safely used.

Ventricular Septal Defect

VSDs are the most common congenital heart defect present at birth. However, about two-thirds resolve (close) after birth with three-quarters resolving spontaneously by age 70 (36) (Table 30-3). Among adults with CHD, about 20% present with VSDs (37,40,45). Small defects typically require no medical or surgical intervention and most of these will eventually close on their own. Larger VSDs require medical management for heart failure symptoms and are usually referred for surgical correction (46). Symptomatic patients may present in heart failure, with dysrhythmias or in severe cases with Eisenmenger's syndrome.

Women with small isolated VSDs usually tolerate pregnancy and delivery without any problems. Women with repaired VSDs can also undergo pregnancy and delivery safely though they may be at higher risk for preterm delivery and for delivering small-for-gestational age infants (47). The most serious complications occur in pregnancies (CHF, dysrhythmia, major cardiovascular events) complicated by reversal of their left-to-right

shunt (Eisenmenger's syndrome discussed in right-to-left section), and in those patients with other congenital heart defects in addition to their VSD (19,42,48). Neonatal mortality is slightly increased at 1.4% in women with a VSD (19).

Clinical Manifestations

Signs and Symptoms: Physical examination features of VSDs depend on the size and location of the lesion. Auscultation typically reveals a pansystolic murmur. Smaller defects may have the loudest murmur associated with them along with a thrill. The murmur may be loudest at different locations along the precordium depending if the VSD is in the muscular and membranous septum. Larger lesions that cause elevations in the pulmonary artery pressure may cause splitting of the second heart sound. However, as ventricular pressure equalizes, the flow murmur diminishes (46).

Test Indicators: Most asymptomatic VSD patients will present with a normal electrocardiogram and chest x-ray. The ECG and chest x-ray will reflect the changes that occur in the heart as the shunt increases. Left ventricular hypertrophy (LVH) and left atrial enlargement may be present in predominantly left-to-right shunts with normal PAP; a slight increase in pulmonary vasculature may be present on chest x-ray. As the shunt increases more, and the PAP rises, the ECG will show signs of right axis deviation and right ventricular hypertrophy. The chest x-ray shows increased vascularity and signs of right heart enlargement (46). ECG will identify lesion anatomy, associated lesions, shunt direction, and the shunt ratio (Qp/Qs) (Fig. 30-5).

Pathophysiology: Similar to ASDs, most VSDs result in small left-to-right shunts that are usually well tolerated with PVR decreasing to accommodate the increase in pulmonary blood flow and maintain normal PAP. With larger VSDs, left-to-right shunting of blood increases, eventually limiting PVR compensation, and resulting in increases in PAP. Left ventricular volume work increases, leading to dysfunction, elevated PCWPs, and progressive worsening of pulmonary hypertension. Consequent is right ventricular

TABLE 30-3 Ventricular Septal Defect

Hemodynamic Goals
Avoid marked increases in heart rate
Avoid increases in SVR
With pulmonary hypertension present, avoid marked decreases in SVR
With pulmonary hypertension present, avoid further increases in PVR

SVR, Systemic Vascular Resistance; PVR, Pulmonary Vascular Resistance.

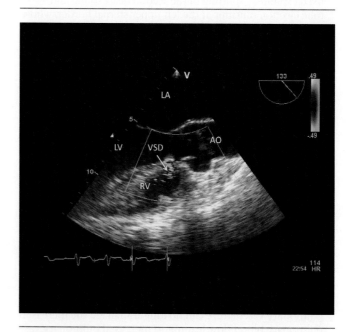

FIGURE 30-5 Mid-esophageal long-axis view demonstrating a VSD with left-to-right ventricular flow. LA, Left atrium; LV, Left ventricle; RV, Right ventricle; AO, Ascending aorta; VSD, Ventricular septal defect.

failure, equalization of right and left ventricular pressures, bidirectional shunting, cyanosis, and clubbing.

Increases in cardiac output, intravascular volume, and heart rate which occur with pregnancy may worsen the existing left-to-right shunt and lead to right or left ventricular heart failure. Increases in stress as seen in labor or from surgical stimulation may produce intolerable increases in SVR and PVR resulting in left or right ventricular failure.

Anesthetic Considerations: Pregnant woman with small, asymptomatic VSDs may undergo pregnancy and delivery without the use of extra monitors or special care. Women with symptomatic, large VSDs, or signs of heart failure should have invasive monitoring during labor and delivery proportionate to the degree of their symptoms. Invasive arterial monitoring, central venous access, PAC use, and ECG may be used in the care of these patients. Important anesthetic considerations are summarized below.

Increases in SVR may not be tolerated. Increases in SVR may worsen a left-to-right shunt and lead to right or left ventricular dysfunction. Afterload-reducing agents such as nicardipine or nitroglycerine may be useful. If there is evidence of ventricular dysfunction, vasodilators such as dobutamine or phosphodiesterase inhibitors may be useful.

Marked increases in heart rate are poorly tolerated. In addition to increases in SVR worsening left-to-right shunting, increases in heart rate may also worsen left-to-right shunting. β-blockers or calcium channel blockers should be continued, and/or started if indicated. Adequate pain control for the different stages of labor and delivery is needed to prevent tachycardia and increases in SVR.

With pulmonary hypertension and right ventricular compromise, marked decreases in SVR may not be well tolerated. Patient with pulmonary hypertension and right ventricular dysfunction are susceptible to bidirectional shunting or reversal of a left-to-right shunt with marked decreases in SVR. Right-to-left shunting and systemic hypoxia may ensue. Vasoconstrictors such as phenylephrine are useful to help reverse large decreases in SVR as seen with the onset of a lumbar epidural sympathetic blockade. In addition, patients with increased right-sided pressures are at risk for ischemia if the systemic blood pressure is low enough to critically reduce coronary perfusion pressure to the right side of the heart.

Factors that increase PVR should be avoided in patients with pulmonary hypertension and evidence of right ventricular compromise. In patients who already have evidence of pulmonary hypertension and RV compromise, any further increases (hypercarbia, hypoxia, sympathetic stimulation) can result in right ventricular failure.

Anesthesia for Vaginal Delivery and Cesarean Delivery

Continuous lumbar epidural anesthesia provides excellent anesthesia for both labor and delivery, either via vaginal delivery or cesarean delivery. In addition, the afterload reduction associated with continuous lumbar epidural anesthesia reduces the impedance to left ventricular emptying, reducing intraventricular pressure and thus decreasing the amount of blood shunted from left to right. Spinal anesthesia should be used with caution, as large decreases in SVR may not be tolerated. Vasopressors should be titrated as needed to offset the rapid sympathectomy that accompanies spinal anesthesia with local anesthetics. General anesthesia may be used safely if the above goals are kept in mind. Inhaled anesthetics combined with intravenous opioids provide a balance of blunting the sympathetic response to surgery and minimizing any increases in SVR with minimal cardiac depression. Additional vasodilators may be necessary.

TABLE 30-4 Patent Ductus Arteriosus

Hemodynamic Goals
Avoid marked increases in blood volume
Avoid increases in SVR
With pulmonary hypertension present, avoid marked decreases in SVR
With pulmonary hypertension present, avoid further increases in PVR

SVR, Systemic Vascular Resistance; PVR, Pulmonary Vascular Resistance.

Potential Complications: Cyanosis or hypoxia in the presence of an increased cardiac output likely represents an imbalance between the pulmonary and SVRs with resultant right-to-left shunting. Treatment includes switching to 100% oxygen, and increasing the SVR by and the addition of a vasopressor such as phenylephrine. If the cardiac output is depressed, 100% oxygen should be administered along with a reduction in anesthesia and the addition of inotropes or vasodilators (depending on SVR).

Patent Ductus Arteriosus

The reported incidence of PDA ranges from 1/500 to1/2,000 (37,49,50) (Table 30-4). Up to 23% of PDAs may resolve spontaneously (51). Similar to other causes of left-to-right shunt, the timing and severity of the symptoms is dependent on the degree of shunt. Small PDAs may not develop symptoms until the fourth or fifth decade of life. Larger PDAs develop symptoms earlier in life including reactive airway disease, dyspnea on exertion, dysrhythmias, pulmonary hypertension and/or heart failure (50). Infrequent complications include aneurysm of the ductus, recurrent laryngeal nerve injury, and infective endarteritis (50). Little evidence is available as to the outcomes of pregnancy with PDAs; however, outcomes appear to be dependent on the severity of symptoms. Complications associated with pregnancy include dysrhythmias, heart failure, and pulmonary artery rupture (along with small-for-gestational-age fetuses) (42,52).

Clinical Manifestations

Signs and Symptoms: Small, asymptomatic PDAs may have no physical examination findings. Classically, the murmur associated with PDAs is a continuous murmur heard best at the left sternal border ending in late or mid-diastole. The murmur may radiate around to the back. Large PDAs may cause widening of the pulse pressure and signs of heart failure (50).

Test Indicators: Patients with a small PDA may have a normal ECG and chest x-ray. Larger PDAs may show evidence of LV or RV hypertrophy or dysrhythmias (commonly atrial fibrillation). Chest x-ray in patients with larger PDAs may display signs of pulmonary vascular congestion or cardiomegaly (50).

Pathophysiology: Shunting of blood across a PDA results in a left-to-right shunt, increasing blood flow through pulmonary vasculature at the expense of flow through the systemic circulation. The amount of blood shunted from left-to-right depends on the resistance to flow across the PDA. The resistance is determined by the size and length of the ductus as well as the pressure difference between the aortic and pulmonary blood pressure. Small PDAs (<1 cm) impart a large resistance to flow and result in minimal shunting of blood that is well tolerated. Moderately sized PDAs (1 to 2 cm) and large PDAs (>2 cm) result in significantly more blood flow through the pulmonary vasculature.

When the pulmonary vasculature can no longer compensate, pulmonary hypertension ensues. Left ventricular work is increased to compensate for the left-to-right shunt, eventually left ventricular failure develops worsening any existing pulmonary hypertension and leading to biventricular failure. Large shunts can eventually result in reversal leading to a right-to-left shunt (Eisenmenger's syndrome).

With pregnancy, the increased intravascular volume can increase shunting across the PDA worsening pulmonary hypertension and left ventricular work. In addition, the increased heart rate and stroke volume will increase myocardial oxygen demand and may compromise left ventricular function during stressful periods, such as uterine contractions. The decrease in SVR seen throughout pregnancy and the postpartum period may lead to shunt reversal and cyanosis in patients with large PDAs.

Anesthetic Considerations: Asymptomatic patients with small shunts and no evidence of ventricular dysfunction may undergo labor and delivery without special considerations. Women with symptomatic, large PDAs, pulmonary hypertension, or signs of ventricular dysfunction should have invasive monitoring during labor and delivery proportionate to the degree of their symptoms. Invasive arterial monitoring, central venous access, PAC, and ECG may be used in the care of these patients. Important anesthetic considerations are summarized below.

Increases in SVR may not be tolerated. Increases in SVR may worsen left-to-right shunting and pulmonary hypertension.

Marked increases in blood volume may be poorly tolerated. Increases in blood volume may lead to ventricular failure by increasing ventricular work and oxygen demand.

Marked decreases in SVR or increases in pulmonary resistance may lead to reverse shunting in patients with pre-existing pulmonary hypertension and right ventricular compromise. See section on Eisenmenger's syndrome.

Patients with left ventricular failure may not tolerate additional myocardial depression.

Anesthesia for Vaginal Delivery and Cesarean Delivery

The decrease in afterload associated with continuous lumbar epidural anesthesia makes it an excellent choice for pain control during labor and delivery. Lumbar epidural anesthesia is also excellent for cesarean delivery as it will prevent increases in SVR associated with painful stimulation. Spinal anesthesia with narcotics alone or combined with local anesthetics may be used. However, care should be taken not to severely decrease SVR as this may cause a reversal of flow through a PDA. Spinal anesthesia should be used with particular caution if at all, in patients with large PDAs. General anesthesia can safely be administered to patients with a PDA undergoing cesarean delivery; supplementation with additional vasodilators may be needed to prevent increases in SVR.

Monitoring Concerns: Monitoring extremities with pulse oximetry has been shown to be useful (53). The right hand blood flow is predominantly preductal; blood flow to the feet is postductal. When the oxygen saturation of the right hand is constant, the oxygen saturation of the foot will change inversely with the amount of right-to-left shunting through the PDA.

Right-To-left Shunt
Tetrology of Fallot

TOF is the most common of the cyanotic congenital heart defects and comprises 5% to 10% of all congenital heart defects, with TOF occurring in 3/100,000 to 4.7/100,000 live births (49,54–56) (Table 30-5). TOF is characterized by right ventricular outflow obstruction, VSD, right ventricular

TABLE 30-5 Tetralogy of Fallot

Hemodynamic Goals
Avoid decreases in blood volume and decreases in venous return
Avoid decrease in SVR
Avoid increase in PVR
Avoid myocardial depressants

SVR, Systemic Vascular Resistance; PVR, Pulmonary Vascular Resistance.

hypertrophy, and an overriding aorta (an aortic valve with biventricular connection, which is situated above the VSD and connected to both the right and the left ventricle). The degree to which the aorta is attached to the right ventricle is referred to as its degree of "override." Medical and surgical advances in the last 5 decades have led to the long-term survival of females born with this CHD allowing these women to lead normal lives including going through pregnancy and childbirth. Multiple centers have a 30-year long-term survival after TOF repair of up to 86% (57–59).

Pregnancy in patients with uncorrected TOF is usually counseled against and is associated with worsened maternal and fetal outcomes (55,60). Risk factors for increased morbidity and mortality include syncope, polycythemia, low arterial oxygen saturation (< 80%), and right ventricular hypertension (1,4,5,28,29,61–64). As discussed above, most women reaching childbearing age will have had surgical corrective or palliative procedures. Women with corrected TOF are not at increased risk for mortality during pregnancy; however, they are at higher risk for maternal and neonatal morbidity. Women with corrected TOF are at higher risk for ventricular/supraventricular dysrhythmias (up to 7%) and heart failure (2.4%) (19,42,55,65–67). Risk factors for cardiovascular complications include severe pulmonary regurgitation, pulmonary hypertension, and right ventricular dilation. In addition, women with uncorrected or corrected TOF are at increased risk for delivering small-for-gestational-age infants (up to 30% and 35% respectively). Fetal mortality is not increased in women with corrected TOF (19,55,60,65).

Clinical Manifestations

Signs and Symptoms: TOF results in right-to-left shunting of blood leading to cyanosis, clubbing, and pulmonary hypertension. S_2 in TOF patients is exaggerated and a systolic ejection murmur is present at the left sternal border near the second or third intercostal space. Severely obstructed patients have little flow through the pulmonary outflow tract and will subsequently have a softer murmur. ECG typically demonstrates right axis deviation and right ventricular hypertrophy. Chest x-ray displays cardiomegaly, classically in a "boot" shape. ECG can be used to differentiate the different anatomical varieties of TOF, assess the degree of pulmonic outflow obstruction, and identify any other coexisting lesions (54).

Pathophysiology: Right ventricular outflow obstruction increases intraventricular pressure in the right ventricle promoting right-to-left shunting through the VSD. The degree of shunting depends on the following: The size of the VSD, the obstruction to outflow from the right ventricle, and the ability of the right ventricle to overcome that obstruction. Right ventricular outflow obstruction often has two components: A fixed obstruction from pulmonic stenosis and a dynamic component from infundibular hypertrophy. Obstruction as a result of infundibular hypertrophy is worsened by hypovolemia, catecholamines, or other hyperdynamic states (see section on asymmetric septal hypertrophy) (54). If the dynamic component is absent, maintenance of right ventricular contractility is important for pulmonary blood flow and peripheral oxygenation. Regardless of the type of right ventricular outflow obstruction, decreases in SVR may exacerbate right-to-left shunting and produce cyanosis.

Pregnancy-induced Changes: The physiologic changes associated with labor and delivery can compromise parturients with TOF. The stress and pain associated with labor and delivery can increase PVR, thereby worsening right-to-left shunting. SVR is reduced throughout pregnancy and may lead to worsening of a right-to-left shunt. Dynamic obstruction may particularly worsen during delivery when contractility is the highest.

Anesthetic Considerations: As a result of the success of surgical correction of TOF, most pregnant patients presenting with TOF will have already been surgically corrected. In the rare event that an uncorrected TOF patient arrives for labor and delivery, invasive monitoring is in order (arterial line and central venous pressure monitoring). In addition, a TTE or TEE may help to characterize the cardiac function. Corrected TOF patients may have varying levels of residual right ventricular failure and pulmonary hypertension (see section on pulmonary hypertension). Careful review of the patient's history and medical records as well as consultation with the primary care physician, will help delineate the type of correction performed and the residual cardiac function. The following important considerations should be noted.

Decreases in vascular resistance, blood volume, or venous return are not well tolerated. A reduction in SVR increases right-to-left shunt, while a decline in blood volume or in venous return compromises right ventricular perfusion of the lungs. High central blood volumes are essential to maintain right ventricular output when this ventricle is compromised.

Myocardial depression may not be well tolerated. If right ventricular compromise is present, inotropic support (epinephrine/dopamine) may be necessary to offset the effects of even small amounts of myocardial depression.

Anesthesia for Vaginal Delivery and Cesarean Delivery

Vaginal Delivery: Decreases in SVR as associated with lumbar epidural or spinal anesthesia will worsen right-to-left shunts and therefore epidural/spinal anesthesia should be used with extreme caution. Injection of only narcotics (other than meperidine) into the epidural/spinal space may decrease the sympathectomy associated with local anesthetic use, but may not be effective. To blunt decreases in SVR and venous return, volume infusion and continuous left uterine displacement are recommended. Ephedrine should be administered cautiously because it may produce a marked increase in PVR. Vasopressin may be useful if the SVR is low. Labor and vaginal delivery in parturients with TOF is best managed with systemic medications, paracervical, or pudendal nerve block.

Cesarean Delivery: Continuous epidural or spinal anesthesia for cesarean delivery in patients with TOF may exacerbate right-to-left shunting as mentioned above. However, in corrected TOF patients with good functional status, slow, careful titration of an epidural or spinal anesthetic is reasonable and effective. Invasive monitoring with the use of an arterial line and central venous catheter is helpful to closely monitor fluid status and SVR. For patients with poor residual cardiac function or uncorrected TOF, general anesthesia using a combination of narcotics and low levels of inhalational anesthetics may provide the most

TABLE 30-6 Eisenmenger's Syndrome

Hemodynamic Goals
Avoid decreases in venous return
Avoid decrease in SVR
Avoid increase in PVR (hypercarbia, hypoxia, acidosis)
Avoid myocardial depressants

SVR, Systemic Vascular Resistance; PVR, Pulmonary Vascular Resistance.

stable hemodynamics. Invasive monitors and TEE are helpful adjuncts in assessing cardiac function, fluid status, and SVR. Vasopressin may be helpful when increases in SVR are needed with pre-existing pulmonary hypertension. PACs should not be used in patients with artificial pulmonic valves and/or pulmonary outflow grafts.

Complications: The presence of an increasing peripheral cyanosis in patients with uncorrected TOF but without infundibular obstruction usually indicates a decrease in SVR or increased right ventricular compromise. Treatment consists of delivering the maximum concentration of oxygen and decreasing the anesthetic depth.

In patients with a history of significant infundibular obstruction, an increase in peripheral cyanosis is typically precipitated by tachycardia, increased myocardial contractility, and/or decreased right ventricular volume. Treatment consists of increasing the depth of inhalational anesthesia, increasing venous return and central blood volume, and decreasing contractility and heart rate with the use of β-blockers (titration of esmolol, either bolus or infusion).

Eisenmenger's Syndrome

Eisenmenger's syndrome consists of pulmonary hypertension and a right-to-left or bidirectional shunt with peripheral cyanosis (68,69) (Table 30-6, Fig. 30-6). The shunt may be atrial, ventricular, or aortopulmonary. A left-to-right shunt reversal commonly occurs during the later stages of a PDA, VSD, and ASD (69). Approximately 3% of all patients with CHD are reported to have Eisenmenger's syndrome; prognosis is poor for most of these patients, with survival beyond the age of 40 unlikely. Unfortunately, the condition of high pulmonary artery pressures with a fixed vascular resistance is not reversible by surgical intervention (51,68,70).

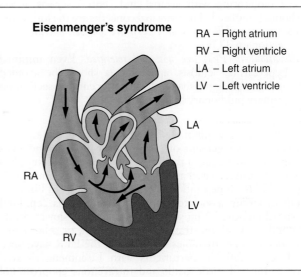

FIGURE 30-6 Eisenmenger's syndrome.

Maternal outcomes in patients with Eisenmenger's syndrome are poor. Major cardiovascular mortality including heart failure and death occur in up to 33.3% of parturients with Eisenmenger's syndrome (19,51,53,61–63,71–76). Neonatal outcomes are poor as well, with almost two-thirds of deliveries occurring prematurely and elevated rates of fetal and perinatal mortality (9.5% and 18.2% mortality, respectively) (19).

Clinical Manifestations

Signs and Symptoms: Clinical manifestations of Eisenmenger's syndrome depend on the degree of pulmonary hypertension and right-to-left shunt (2,43,53,69,73,77). The underlying defect directly influences the type of heart murmur that will be present (e.g., a systolic ejection murmur with ASD or a holosystolic murmur with VSD).

Test Indicators: ECG usually demonstrates right ventricular hypertrophy with right axis deviation. Chest x-ray typically reveals increased pulmonary artery markings with a prominent right ventricle. TEE usually displays signs of right-sided volume and work overload. Right atrial/ventricular enlargement is typically present. Decreased right and left ventricular contractility may be present. The underlying structural defect (ASD, VSD, etc.) may also be visualized on TEE.

Pathophysiology: The degree of right-to-left shunt depends on three factors: (a) The severity of the pulmonary hypertension and size of the right-to-left communication; (b) the relationship between the pulmonic and SVR, that is, increases in PVR or decreases in SVR exacerbate the right-to-left shunt, producing peripheral cyanosis; and (c) the contractile state of the right ventricle (progressive right ventricular dysfunction decreases pulmonary blood flow and increases right-to-left shunt).

Pregnancy-induced Changes: In Eisenmenger's syndrome, PVR is fixed and is not altered with pregnancy. However, the SVR decreases as usual in pregnancy, markedly increasing the right-to-left shunt (5,61,78). Other cardiovascular changes associated with pregnancy including increases in heart rate, stroke volume, and blood volume, all contribute to increasing right ventricular oxygen consumption which in the presence of desaturated blood may lead to right ventricular compromise (43,78).

Anesthetic Considerations: All patients with Eisenmenger's syndrome should be considered high risk and their care should be approached in a multidisciplinary fashion. Invasive monitoring with arterial and central venous access should be utilized. The principal concerns are the following.

Decreases in SVR or venous return are not well tolerated (see section on TOF).

Elevations in PVR are not well tolerated. Even minimal hypercarbia, acidosis, and hypoxia should be avoided and treated aggressively when they occur (see section on primary pulmonary hypertension).

Anesthesia for Vaginal Delivery and Cesarean Delivery

Anesthetic management of parturients with Eisenmenger's syndrome is identical to that of patients with TOF. Regional anesthesia can be used in parturients with Eisenmenger's, but should be done cautiously (79,80). Attempts to limit the sympathectomy associated with local anesthesia (epidural or spinal anesthesia) must be considered (i.e., slowly titrate epidural level, administration of vasopressin, or other vasopressor). Adjunct therapies for lowering the PVR have been used successfully in parturients with Eisenmenger's syndrome. Inhaled nitric oxide and intravenous epoprostenol have both been utilized to assist in the care of parturients

TABLE 30-7 Coarctation of Aorta

Hemodynamic Goals
Avoid bradycardia
Avoid decrease in SVR
Avoid hypertension
Maintain left ventricular filling

SVR, Systemic Vascular Resistance.

with Eisenmenger's syndrome. However, their availability and experience in parturients is limited (81–83).

Other Congenital Heart Diseases

Coarctation of the Aorta

Coarctation of the aorta occurs in 4 to 4.4 per 10,000 of live births and represents approximately 8% of all CHD in adults (49,51,56) (Table 30-7). Most cases are surgically corrected in early childhood, decreasing the incidence of coarctation in the pregnant population. Parturients with corrected isolated coarctation of the aorta are not at increased risk for morbidity and mortality (5,19,84–87). Previous reports indicated that parturients with uncorrected coarctation had maternal mortality rates as high as 9%; however, recently published data report that these patients can undergo labor and delivery safely with no increase in maternal mortality (5,19,84–94).

Clinical Manifestations

Signs and Symptoms: Physical examination usually reveals a significant difference in blood pressures in the upper and lower extremities, or in the right and left upper extremities. Other signs include an increase in intensity of the aortic component of the second heart sound, a medium-pitched systolic blowing murmur (heard best between the scapulae), a ventricular heave, and a laterally displaced apical impulse. In pregnancy, aortic coarctation may present as unexplained hypertension during pregnancy (91,95).

Test Indicators: Late in the course of the disease, an ECG will demonstrate signs of LVH. A chest x-ray will demonstrate left ventricular enlargement and a characteristic "three" sign in the aortic knob. TEE may be used to evaluate the aorta as well as any coexisting cardiac disease (Fig. 30-7).

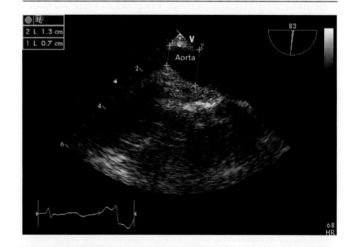

FIGURE 30-7 Descending aorta long-axis view demonstrating a narrowing of the descending aorta as seen in a patient with aortic coarctation.

Cardiac catheterization is indicated for complicated cases and is useful in assessing the severity of the disease.

Pathophysiology: Coarctation, like aortic stenosis, represents a fixed obstruction to left ventricular ejection. Stroke volume tends to be limited, and increases in cardiac output are achieved primarily through increases in heart rate. Due to increased left ventricular afterload, ventricular pressure work increases and concentric hypertrophy occurs. Patients with mild coarctation tolerate this well, and progression to ventricular dilation and failure occurs late in the course. With severe coarctation, ventricular changes occur earlier, along with pathologic changes in the arterial wall at the site of coarctation that serve as the nidus for dissection and rupture.

Pregnancy-induced Changes: Pregnancy may exacerbate both left ventricular compromise and vascular wall damage. Because stroke volume is limited, the increase in intravascular volume and metabolic demand associated with pregnancy is accommodated by increase in the heart rate. During labor and delivery, heart rate compensation may not be adequate, and left ventricular failure may occur. Pregnancy can also precipitate changes in the media and intima of the aorta, resulting in catastrophic complications (84,85). Aortic dissection, pseudoaneurysm formation, and aortic rupture may occur as a result of the physiologic alterations and vascular changes during pregnancy in patients with coarctation (86,96). Depending on the severity of aortic coarctation, the vasodilation associated with pregnancy may be poorly tolerated in patients with pre-existing hypotension below the level of coarctation resulting in decreased uterine blood flow. Finally, these patients have increased blood flow proximal to the aortic narrowing, and should be monitored for signs of intracranial hypertension, especially if preeclampsia is also present.

Anesthetic Considerations: Previously corrected patients and asymptomatic patients without evidence of cardiac enlargement or dysfunction can safely undergo labor and delivery without special considerations. Patients with coexisting cardiac disease or symptomatic lesions should have additional monitoring proportional to the level of their disease (radial and/or femoral artery monitoring, PA catheter, TEE). The following summarizes the anesthetic considerations for these patients.

Decreases in SVR are not well tolerated. Stroke volume is relatively fixed and therefore there is limited capacity to compensate for decreases in SVR. In addition, while blood flow proximal to the coarctation may be adequate, distal flow may be severely limited, and any further decreases may lead to critically low uterine/placental blood flow. Vasoconstrictors may be needed to offset any decreases of SVR associated with anesthetic use. It is important to monitor for awareness using devices such as the bispectral index monitor (BIS).

Decreases in heart rate are not well tolerated. When stroke volume is fixed, cardiac output becomes dependent on heart rate. Vagal stimulations, medications, or anesthetics which result in decreases in heart rate may be poorly tolerated and should be avoided. Decreases in heart rate should be treated by removing the causative stimulus and/or pharmacologic treatment with ephedrine or glycopyrrolate.

Decreases in left ventricular filling are not well tolerated. As stroke volume is relatively restricted by stenosis in the aorta, adequate end-diastolic volumes are critical in maintaining stroke volume. Avoid hypovolemia or other causes of decreased preload. Maintain sinus rhythm. Atrial fibrillation is particularly deleterious as it can cause loss of the atrial ("kick") component of ventricular filling, which can seriously compromise cardiac output.

Anesthesia for Vaginal and Cesarean Delivery

Anesthetic management of patients with aortic coarctation is similar to the management of patients with aortic stenosis. Vaginal delivery can be safely achieved with the use of intravenous pain medications or local nerve blocks. Spinal anesthesia with only narcotic may also be used. A lumbar epidural anesthetic using a combination of low dose local anesthetic with a narcotic can be used, but should be titrated slowly with careful monitoring of maternal blood pressure and fetal heart rate. Fluid administration and vasopressors should be used if SVR is decreased.

Cesarean delivery can be accomplished with a balanced general anesthetic technique (nitrous oxide/inhalational agent/opioid/muscle relaxant) that maintains the anesthetic goals discussed above (94). Neuraxial techniques have been used for cesarean delivery but we recommend general anesthesia for patients with moderate-to-severe aortic coarctation (97). Invasive monitoring should be used in proportion to the patient's disease severity. Patients with severe stenotic lesions may benefit from pre- and poststenotic blood pressure monitoring. If aortic dissection is present, consult the anesthetic considerations listed in the aortic dissection section.

Congenital Aortic Stenosis

Congenital aortic stenosis comprises lesions that may occur at the aortic, subvalvular, or supravalvular location (98–101). The supravalvular lesion has been described in the maternal rubella syndrome (102), where the narrowing occurs just distal to the coronary artery orifices. Subvalvular stenosis may be fibrous (subaortic membrane) or muscular (hypertrophic obstructive cardiomyopathy [HOCM]) in nature (101). The most common cause of congenital aortic stenosis is the bicuspid aortic valve, which occurs in 1% to 2% of the general population (103–105). Patients with bicuspid aortic valves often do not become symptomatic until later in life (105).

Effects on Pregnancy: Historically, the literature regarding pregnancy and aortic stenosis has been limited. However, several recent publications help to shed light on the effects of aortic stenosis on maternal and neonatal outcomes (19,106–108). Although mild-to-moderate aortic stenosis was not reported to be associated with increased mortality, it was associated with increased rates of maternal dysrhythmia, pulmonary edema, and worsening heart failure (up to 7.3%, 10%, and 7.3% respectively) (19,106–108). Additionally, one-in-seven deliveries among patients with aortic stenosis are associated with small-for-gestational-age infants (19,106–108).

Anesthetic Considerations: The anesthetic considerations for congenital cases of aortic stenosis are similar to those for acquired causes of aortic stenosis and are described in this chapter in the next section (Table 30-8).

Pulmonic Stenosis

The incidence of congenital pulmonic stenosis is 7.3/10,000 live births and comprises 10% to 12% of CHD in adults

TABLE 30-8 Aortic Stenosis

Hemodynamic Goals
Avoid bradycardia
Avoid myocardial depressants
Avoid decreases in SVR
Maintain venous return and left ventricular filling

SVR, Systemic Vascular Resistance.

TABLE 30-9 Congenital Pulmonic Stenosis

Hemodynamic Goals
Avoid bradycardia
Avoid decrease in SVR
Maintain intravascular volume
Avoid myocardial depressants

SVR, Systemic Vascular Resistance.

(49,109) (Table 30-9). The region of stenosis is typically at the valve (90% of cases) (109). Most patients with isolated pulmonic stenosis do not develop symptoms until later in adult life (109). However, the subvalvular lesion that has a different pathophysiology can be progressive.

Effects on Pregnancy: The literature on the effects of pulmonic stenosis on pregnancy is limited. One large review of 81 pregnancies found no increased risk of maternal mortality, but did find increased rates of thromboembolic events (3.7%), hypertensive disorders of pregnancy (14.8%), premature delivery (16%), and increased infant mortality (4.8%) (110).

Clinical Manifestations

Signs and Symptoms: Severe right ventricular failure decreases left ventricular output, producing symptoms of fatigue and syncope. Auscultation reveals a normal first heart sound and a widely split second sound; a systolic ejection murmur is also present. As the degree of pulmonic stenosis worsens, the murmur increases in duration and has a late systolic accentuation.

Test Indicators: ECG usually demonstrates right axis deviation and right ventricular hypertrophy. With severe stenosis, a predominant R wave occurs in lead V1 that usually exceeds 20 mm in height (111), and correlates with a right ventricular systolic pressure of at least 80 mm Hg (112). Right ventricular strain manifested by negative T waves in the right precordial leads also may occur. Chest x-ray reveals dilation of the main pulmonary artery and reduced peripheral pulmonary vascular markings (109).

Pathophysiology: With progressive stenosis of the right ventricular outflow tract, pressure work increases and concentric hypertrophy occurs. The right ventricle compensates until late in the disease when systolic pressure exceeds 80 mm Hg (113). As right ventricular output decreases, so does left ventricular preload and thus cardiac output. SVR increases in an effort to compensate for decreased left ventricular output. However, as right ventricular failure progresses, further decreases in cardiac output are uncompensated, and symptoms of low cardiac output, such as fatigue and syncope, occur with exercise and later at rest.

Pregnancy-induced Changes: Many patients with isolated pulmonic stenosis will not develop symptoms until after childbearing age; however, patients with advanced disease are susceptible to the stresses involved in pregnancy and delivery. Increases in intravascular volume and heart rate associated with pregnancy can precipitate right ventricular failure. Decreases in SVR seen with pregnancy may counteract compensatory mechanisms triggered by during low ventricular output states.

Anesthetic Considerations: Patients with asymptomatic disease and no symptoms of right ventricular compromise can be managed in the standard fashion. Patients with advanced disease or signs of compromise should have invasive monitoring including arterial monitoring and central venous access in proportion to their disease level. The following considerations should be noted.

Marked increases or decreases in right ventricular filling pressure are not well tolerated. Right ventricular filling pressures must be maintained to ensure adequate stroke volume. Excessive preload can overdistend the right ventricle leading to right ventricular failure. Too little volume in the right ventricle may lead to ineffective contraction and decreased preload to the left ventricle.

Decreases in heart rate are not well tolerated. Because of the presence of right ventricular outflow stenosis, stroke volume is relatively fixed. Therefore, cardiac output is reliant on maintaining an adequate heart rate. Decreases in heart rate should be treated quickly with positive chronotropic drugs. Anesthetic agents and levels should be chosen to limit decreases in heart rate.

Marked decreases in SVR may not be tolerated. In patients with severe pulmonic stenosis, cardiac output is limited and systemic blood pressure is preserved by compensatory increases in SVR. Maintaining SVR by the use of vasoconstrictors such as ephedrine is necessary.

Negative inotropes may not be well tolerated. Any agents that decrease the contractile function of the right ventricle may be poorly tolerated and lead to ventricular failure. Use of medications or techniques with positive inotropic action is therefore recommended.

Anesthesia for Vaginal Delivery and Cesarean Delivery

Vaginal Delivery: Patients with mild disease can be managed in the normal fashion while those with more severe disease should be managed with techniques that optimize the anesthetic considerations discussed previously. Systemic medications or local blocks (pudendal, paracervical) should be used for vaginal delivery. Spinal anesthesia utilizing only opioids (other than meperidine) satisfies many of the criteria listed above. Epidural or spinal anesthesia using a combination of local anesthetic and narcotics can be utilized; however, care should be taken to maintain the physiologic parameters mentioned above. Preload should be maintained with volume loading prior to the onset of the sympathectomy; vasoconstrictors should be readily available to maintain system vascular resistance.

Cesarean Delivery: Careful titration of epidural anesthesia with the use in invasive arterial monitoring (central venous access should be considered) can be safely used (114). The level of anesthesia should be slowly titrated with careful following of the heart rate, preload, and systemic blood pressure. General anesthesia using predominantly nitrous oxide/narcotic/muscle relaxant combination may help maintain adequate heart rate, preload, and myocardial contractility. If right ventricular failure develops, anesthetic concentration should be reduced and inotropes administered.

Asymmetric Septal Hypertrophy

Also known as idiopathic hypertrophic subaortic stenosis, this condition typically manifests in the third or fourth decade (See Table 30-10 and Fig. 30-8). It is characterized by marked

TABLE 30-10 Asymmetric Septal Hypertrophy

Hemodynamic Goals
Avoid or correct arrhythmias
Avoid decrease in SVR
Maintain blood volume and venous return
Avoid increases myocardial contractility
Treat ventricular compromise/hypotension with phenylephrine, intravenous fluids, and propranolol

SVR, Systemic Vascular Resistance.

Asymmetric septal hypertrophy

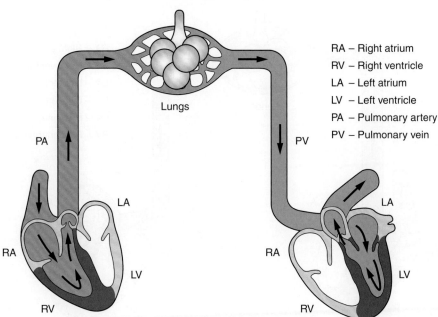

RA – Right atrium
RV – Right ventricle
LA – Left atrium
LV – Left ventricle
PA – Pulmonary artery
PV – Pulmonary vein

FIGURE 30-8 Asymmetric septal hypertrophy.

hypertrophy of the ventricle, involving the interventricular septum and outflow tract. During ventricular systole, constriction of the outflow tract occurs, producing obstruction to ventricular ejection.

Clinical Manifestations
Patient develops exertional dyspnea, angina pectoris, and syncope. Late in the course of the disease, left ventricular failure occurs. Physical examination reveals a double apical impulse and a systolic murmer best heard at the apex.

Test Indicators: Chest x-ray shows cardiomegaly and ECG evidence of LVH and a Wolff–Parkinson–White syndrome or abnormal Q waves in inferior or left precordial leads are seen. ECG will reveal a ventricular septum that is disproportionately hypertrophied compared with the posterobasal left ventricular free wall.

Pathophysiology: Patients with asymmetric septal hypertrophy (ASH) involving the left ventricle (LV) exhibit a marked hypertrophy of the entire LV, with bulging of the ventricular myocardium in the septal region several centimeters below the aortic valve. The ventricular cavity is relatively small. With each systolic contraction, the muscle around the outflow tract constricts and left ventricular ejection is obstructed. Progression of LVH eventually leads to ventricular failure.

Anesthetic Considerations: *Decreases in preload are not well tolerated.* Maintaining slight hypervolemia is recommended because the increase in ventricular volume tends to decrease the amount of outflow obstruction.

Tachycardia and dysrhythmias are not well tolerated. There is decreased time for ventricular filling and immediate treatment with β-blockers to slow heart rate or direct cardioversion is advocated.

Increases in contractility and decreases in SVR are not well tolerated as it may markedly increase outflow obstruction.

Treatment of ventricular failure in patients with ASH is to increase preload and afterload, and slow heart rate and contractility, which is different from the treatment of other types of heart failure.

Management of Labor and Delivery
Pregnancy and delivery are usually well tolerated in patients with ASH despite decrease in SVR and the risk of impaired venous return owing to uterine compression of the inferior vena cava. They present a major anesthetic challenge at term, as bearing down (Valsalva maneuver) may increase LVOT obstruction. Although general anesthesia is preferred in these patients, there are case reports where epidural anesthesia has been successfully used with CVP monitoring (115). Oxytocin must be administered carefully because of its vasodilating properties and compensatory tachycardia. Pulmonary edema has been observed in parturients with HCM after delivery, emphasizing the judicious fluid management in these patients (116).

■ ACQUIRED HEART DISEASE

Rheumatic Heart Disease

Rheumatic fever is a diffuse inflammatory disease affecting the heart, joints, and subcutaneous tissues following group A β-hemolytic streptococcal infection. Acute rheumatic fever is evidenced by a history of streptococcal infection and subsequent clinical picture that usually includes recurrent migratory polyarthritis with or without carditis, which can progressively and permanently damage the valves or heart muscle. Although the prophylactic administration of antibiotics generally prevents the sequelae of rheumatic fever; RHD continues to be a common cause of death in the United States and in many other countries (43,117–122).

Left or right ventricular failure, atrial dysrhythmias, systemic or pulmonary embolism, and infective endocarditis may complicate RHD during pregnancy. The most common sequelae in parturients are mitral valve stenosis, regurgitation or prolapse, and/or aortic valve stenosis or regurgitation.

Mitral Stenosis
Rheumatic mitral valve stenosis is the most frequent RHD encountered in the pregnant population worldwide (Figs. 30-9 and 30-10) (Table 30-11). Mitral stenosis is the lesion

Mitral stenosis

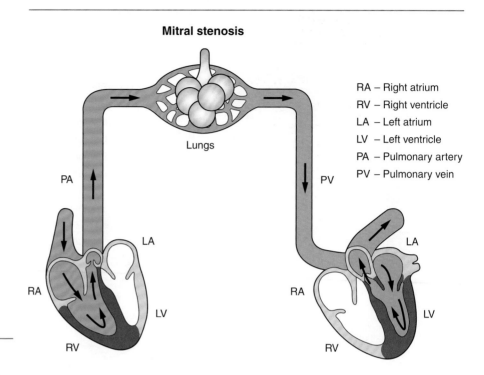

RA – Right atrium
RV – Right ventricle
LA – Left atrium
LV – Left ventricle
PA – Pulmonary artery
PV – Pulmonary vein

FIGURE 30-9 Mitral stenosis.

that most frequently requires therapeutic intervention during pregnancy.

Clinical Manifestations

Signs and Symptoms: The initial symptoms are fatigue and dyspnea progressing to paroxysmal nocturnal dyspnea, orthopnea, and dyspnea at rest. Hemoptysis with rupture

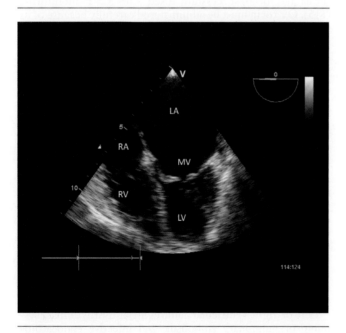

FIGURE 30-10 Mid-esophageal four chamber view demonstrating an enlarged left atrium and thickened, restricted mitral valve leaflets in a patient with RHD. Note the thickening of the mitral valve leaflets is primarily at the leaflet tips resulting in the characteristic "hockey stick" deformation of the mitral valve leaflets classically seen with RHD. LA, Left atrium; MV, Mitral valve; LV, Left ventricle; RA, Right atrium; RV, Right ventricle.

of bronchopulmonary varices can occur. In severe mitral stenosis, superimposition of atrial fibrillation, pulmonary embolism, infection, or pregnancy can cause rapid decompensation.

Physical examination may reveal a presystolic or middiastolic murmur. In addition to the murmur, an opening snap may be heard at the base of the heart along the left sternal border. Approximately, one-third of patients with mitral stenosis develop atrial fibrillation.

Test Indicators: Radiologic studies that may be normal early in the disease will show left atrial and right ventricular enlargement as the disease progresses. Severe mitral stenosis will result in pulmonary edema on chest x-ray. The ECG typically indicates broad P waves in lead V1, signifying left atrial enlargement. Right axis deviation signifies right atrial enlargement. Cardiac catheterization shows elevated pulmonary capillary wedge pressures of 25 to 30 mm Hg (normally 0 to 12 mm Hg) occurring when the mitral valve orifice is less than 2 cm². There is an associated increase in PVR (117,123,124).

Echocardiographic Examination for Mitral Stenosis: Normally, the area of the mitral valve is between 4 and 6 cm². When the area is reduced to less than 2 cm², the transvalvular pressure gradient is increased. Continuous wave Doppler ultrasound should be used to measure the velocity of blood flow across the mitral valve (the use of pulse wave Doppler may result in "aliasing" at high-velocity blood flow). After

TABLE 30-11 Mitral Stenosis

Hemodynamic Goals
Prevent rapid ventricular rates
Minimize increase in central blood volume
Avoid marked decreases in SVR
Prevent increases in pulmonary artery pressure

SVR, Systemic Vascular Resistance.

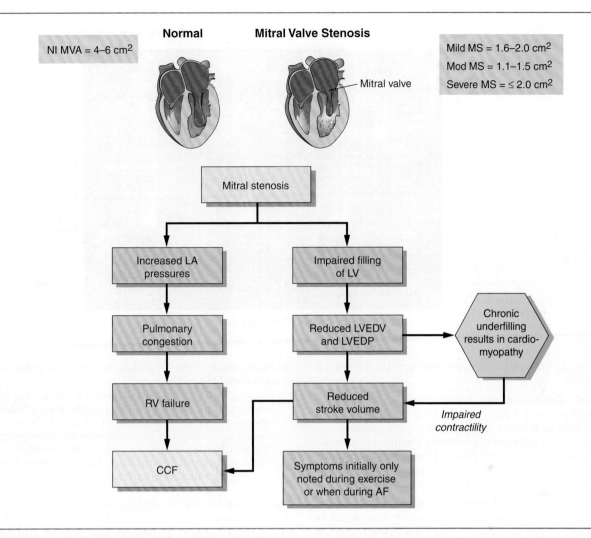

FIGURE 30-11 Pathophysiology of mitral stenosis.

measuring the velocity, the transvalvular pressure gradient can be estimated by using the modified Bernoulli equation. Mean gradient is more precise and clinically relevant. Mean gradients in the range of 5 to 10 mm Hg are consistent with moderate mitral stenosis; mean gradients above 10 mm Hg are consistent with severe mitral stenosis (125).

Two other echocardiographic evaluations are useful in estimating the severity of mitral stenosis.

1. The measurement of mitral valve pressure half time (i.e., the time it takes for the transvalvular pressure gradient to decrease to 50% of its maximum value). Mitral valve area of 1 to 1.5 cm^2 is consistent with moderate mitral stenosis and an area less than 1 cm^2 is consistent with severe mitral stenosis.
2. The area of the mitral valve orifice also can be estimated using planimetry. The opening of the mitral valve can be visualized and the area traced to provide an estimation of the MVA. Severe calcification of the mitral valve may interfere with a determination of its area by planimetry, and in patients with significant subvalvular stenosis, the degree of hemodynamic compromise may be underestimated.

Pathophysiology: The decrease in mitral valve orifice area impairs left ventricular filling, which will cause left atrial enlargement and increases in left atrial volume and pressures. This causes increased pressure in the pulmonary circulation, increased pulmonary capillary wedge pressures, and pulmonary edema. Compensatory RV hypertrophy

leads to right heart failure. Factors aggravating this situation are tachycardia, atrial fibrillation, and increased preload (Figs. 30-11 and 30-12).

Pregnancy-induced Changes: Prognosis depends on the severity of the valve stenosis, heart rate and rhythm, atrial compliance, circulating blood volume, and pulmonary vascular response. A narrowed mitral valve orifice allows a relatively fixed amount of blood to move across during diastole. Thus, when cardiac output and blood volume increase during pregnancy and the mitral valve stenotic, left atrial pressure is markedly increased. Additionally, increased cardiac output increases the transmitral pressure gradient, which worsens symptoms of congestive heart failure and eventually leads to pulmonary edema and respiratory distress.

With pregnancy, an anatomically moderate stenosis can become functionally severe. Pregnant patients with mitral stenosis can have an increased incidence of pulmonary congestion (25%), atrial fibrillation (7%), and paroxysmal atrial tachycardia (3%) (88). Left ventricular dysfunction is very uncommon in pure mitral stenosis and its presence suggests coexisting mitral or aortic insufficiency.

During pregnancy and labor, the increased heart rate, increased cardiac output and demand, and decreased ventricular filling causes back pressure in the pulmonary circulation and risk for pulmonary edema. Immediately after delivery is the most likely time for decompensation and pulmonary

Pressure gradient

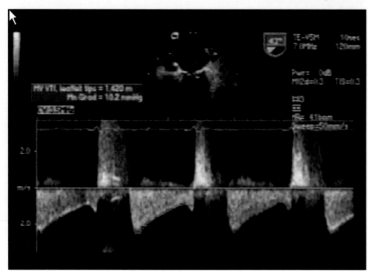

NL
Mild < 6 mm Hg
Moderate 6–12 mm Hg
Severe > 12 mm Hg

FIGURE 30-12 Pressure gradient across the stenotic mitral valve.

Mean PG 10.2 mm Hg

edema due to tachycardia and increased preload from autotransfusion.

Anesthetic Considerations: Patients with a mitral orifice area of less than 1.5 cm² can be treated medically, whereas parturients with severe stenosis may require percutaneous mitral balloon valvotomy, a procedure with a low complication rate in experienced hands. Closed and open mitral commissurotomy have been performed with low maternal risk and a fetal survival of greater than 90% (126).

Closed or open mitral commissurotomy, balloon valvuloplasty, and valve replacement are usually considered in patients with a valve area greater than 1.2 cm², poor response to medical therapy, and the absence of valve calcification. Percutaneous balloon valvuloplasty of the mitral valve is the preferred method when intervention is needed during pregnancy (12,123).

Kasab et al. (123) have shown that pregnant patients with symptomatic mitral stenosis can be safely treated with β-blockade and this significantly reduces the incidence of pulmonary edema. It has also been shown that those with severe symptoms who undergo valvuloplasty before pregnancy have fewer complications than those treated medically.

See table for anesthetic considerations and monitoring (Table 30-11):

1. *Neither sinus tachycardia nor atrial fibrillation with a rapid ventricular response is tolerated well.*
   Sinus tachycardia should be corrected immediately by reversing the precipitating event (pain, anxiety, light general anesthesia, hypovolemia, hypercarbia, and acidosis) or by administering β-blockers intravenously.
2. *Marked increases in central blood volume are poorly tolerated.*
   Over transfusion, Trendelenburg position, or autotransfusion via uterine contraction can precipitate right ventricular failure, pulmonary hypertension, pulmonary edema, or atrial fibrillation. Monitoring and watching CVP and PCWP trends are helpful in managing volume overload.
3. *Marked decreases in SVR may not be tolerated.*
   With severe mitral stenosis, decreases in SVR are compensated for by increases in heart rate (stroke volume is fixed). This tachycardia may lead to decompensation. Phenylephrine is the drug of choice in this situation.

4. *Pulmonary hypertension and right ventricular failure can be exacerbated by multiple factors.*
   Any degree of hypercarbia, hypoxia, acidosis, lung hyperinflation, or increased lung water can increase PVR. Prostaglandins used to treat uterine atony should be used with caution since they may have effects on the pulmonary vasculature. Inotropic support, pulmonary vasodilators, and mechanical ventilation may be required if hemodynamic or pulmonary decompensation occurs.

Anesthesia for Vaginal and Cesarean Delivery
There are no evidence based guidelines about the superiority of any one technique for management of labor analgesia or cesarean delivery in patients with mitral stenosis.

Vaginal Delivery: Labor epidural analgesia has been used with success for labor and vaginal delivery (123,124,127). This prevents the pain and tachycardia, and the perineal analgesia avoids the urge to push and thereby prevents exertion, fatigue, and the deleterious effects of a Valsalva maneuver. Fetal descent is accomplished by the uterine contractions per se, and delivery is facilitated with vacuum extraction or outlet forceps. Judicious fluid administration and left uterine displacement can prevent hypotension. Phenylephrine is the vasopressor of choice to treat hypotension. Another advantage of epidural analgesia is the increased venous capacitance caused by sympathetic blockade. This helps to accommodate the autotransfused fluid during uterine contractions and after delivery, mitigating the preload and development of pulmonary edema.

Combined spinal–epidural for labor analgesia with a lipophilic narcotic (fentanyl) given intrathecally with a low dose local anesthetic solution (0.125% bupivacaine) can be used with success in these patients (128).

Cesarean Delivery (Regional Anesthesia): A controlled lumbar epidural block is preferred to spinal anesthesia because epidural anesthesia produces more controllable hemodynamic changes. A review by Gomar et al. (129) on neuraxial anesthesia for pregnant patients with cardiac disease shows that a single-shot spinal technique is not recommended for patients with significant mitral stenosis. The anesthetic level should be titrated slowly. Epinephrine is omitted from the local anesthetic solution because of the potential for tachycardia and peripheral vasodilation. Again, hypotension should be prevented and treated with judicious fluid administration and phenylephrine bolus or infusion. Central venous pressure monitoring will help guide management.

Cesarean Delivery (General Anesthesia): NYHA Class III and IV patients are better managed under general anesthesia. General anesthesia should avoid drugs that cause tachycardia and lower SVR. A balanced anesthetic with a high dose titrated opioid induction with β-blockade has been used with success. General anesthesia also provides the advantage of continuous TEE monitoring. Avoidance of the hemodynamic response to laryngoscopy and intubation is imperative. Adequate depth of anesthesia to avoid tachycardia and hypertension is needed. Numerous case reports have indicated good maternal and fetal outcomes with use of general anesthesia. Remifentanil, a short-acting synthetic opioid, has been used as it provides intraoperative hemodynamic stability and rapid emergence due to its extremely short half-life. It also avoids prolonged neonatal depression. Other opioids administered before delivery of the baby can cause neonatal respiratory depression, and the neonatal care team should be informed.

In moderate-to-severe stenosis, pulmonary artery catheterization is helpful for management. Fluid restriction, use of diuretics and β-blockers, and supplemental oxygen are all advocated. After delivery, oxytocin infusions should be administered carefully avoiding any bolus administration as it may precipitate systemic hypotension and pulmonary hypertension. Phenylephrine can be used to restore hemodynamics, but if hypotension persists, norepinephrine maybe used to provide additional inotropic support without causing excessive tachycardia.

If atrial fibrillation occurs it should be promptly managed. β-blockers, digoxin, and cardioversion have all been used in recent onset (<24 hours atrial fibrillation). Anticoagulation

TABLE 30-12 Mitral Regurgitation

Hemodynamic Goals
Maintain normal to slightly elevated heart rates
Avoid myocardial depressants
Avoid marked increase in SVR
Prevent increases in pulmonary artery pressures
Higher central blood volumes are usually well tolerated

SVR, Systemic Vascular Resistance.

should be initiated as soon as possible to prevent thromboembolism.

Mitral Regurgitation

Mitral valve insufficiency is the second most common valve disease in pregnancy (88) (Table 30-12 and Fig. 30-13). Left ventricular volume load is chronically increased but patients can remain asymptomatic for 30 to 40 years. However, congestive heart failure follows and with symptoms a rapid downhill course occurs with a 5-year mortality of 50%.

Other complications occurring in the fourth or fifth decade are atrial fibrillation, systemic embolization, and bacterial endocarditis (130).

Clinical Manifestations

Signs and Symptoms: The principal symptoms of advanced mitral regurgitation (MR) are those of left ventricular failure. The cardinal sign is a pansystolic murmur at the cardiac apex, referred to the left axilla or infrascapular area. Atrial fibrillation occurs in approximately one-third of patients. Late sequelae include pulmonary congestion, pulmonary hypertension, and right ventricular enlargement.

Test Indicators: ECG may be normal if mild, but can show LVH or RVH if severe. Similarly, chest x-ray reveals left ventricle enlargement. Two-dimensional or Doppler ECG is indicated in all suspected cases of mitral valve insufficiency

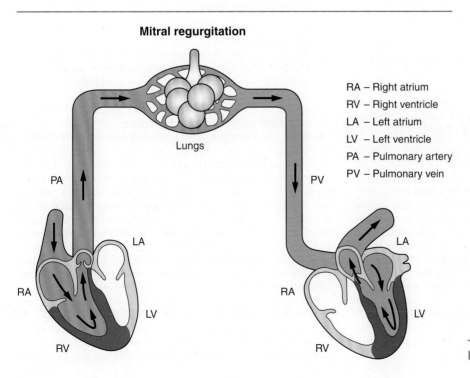

Mitral regurgitation

RA – Right atrium
RV – Right ventricle
LA – Left atrium
LV – Left ventricle
PA – Pulmonary artery
PV – Pulmonary vein

Lungs

PA   PV

LA   LA

RA   RA

LV   LV

RV   RV

FIGURE 30-13 Mitral regurgitation.

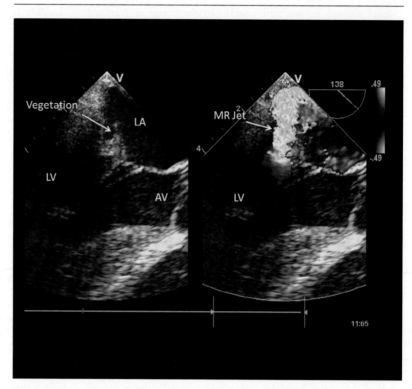

FIGURE 30-14 Mid-esophageal long-axis view demonstrating a large vegetation on the anterior leaflet of the mitral valve. Note the large eccentric posterior directed regurgitant jet into the left atrium resulting in severe mitral regurgitation. LA, Left atrium; LV, Left ventricle; AV, Aortic valve; MR, Mitral regurgitation.

to confirm its presence and determine the severity of the disease. Left atrial enlargement may also be visualized as well as signs of right ventricular failure in cases of severe MR. Left ventricular function and pulmonary artery pressures can also be accessed via intraoperative TEE. Two-dimensional ECG usually reveals the cause (e.g., the presence of myxomatous mitral valve disease and leaflet prolapse or evidence of underlying dilated cardiomyopathy) (Fig. 30-14). Evaluation of the severity of mitral regurgitation on ECG requires an integrated assessment of several parameters, including regurgitant jet size by color Doppler, regurgitant jet density by continuous-wave (CW) Doppler, and pulmonary vein and mitral valve inflow by pulse-wave (PW) Doppler (131).

Newer applications of Doppler ECG allow quantitative measurement of mitral regurgitation, including the regurgitant volume and the regurgitant orifice area (ROA)—that is, the area through which the valve leaks in systole. In asymptomatic patients with significant mitral regurgitation, serial ECG every 6 to 12 months to assess LV size and systolic function is important for optimal timing of surgery (132).

Pathophysiology: Mitral insufficiency causes regurgitation of blood from the left ventricle through the incompetent mitral valve into the left atrium. With chronic mitral insufficiency, the left atrium adapts to the increased blood volume by dilating. When left atrial pressure rises, pulmonary venous and PCW pressures also rise, causing pulmonary congestion and edema. With progressive left ventricular failure, pulmonary hypertension and right ventricular compromise will occur. Left atrial pressure does not increase until late in the course of the disease; thus the left atrium protects the pulmonary venous, capillary, and arterial bed from pressure overload. Left ventricular dilation also occurs. Reduction of vascular resistance and thereby left ventricular afterload can play an important role in decreasing the amount of regurgitant blood flow and increasing forward cardiac output.

Pregnancy-induced Changes: Mitral regurgitation is typically well tolerated in pregnancy. The decrease in SVR associated with pregnancy may improve forward flow. However, the increased volume load of pregnancy may not be well tolerated by a chronically compromised left ventricle, resulting in pulmonary congestion. During labor and delivery, pain, uterine contractions, and anxiety may increase ventricular rate by augmenting sympathetic activity. The resultant decrease in forward flow and increase in regurgitant flow may precipitate left ventricular failure and pulmonary congestion.

Anesthetic considerations:

1. *Avoid bradycardia. Maintenance of normal to elevated heart rate is advocated.*
2. *Avoid myocardial depression. As left ventricular impairment usually accompanies mitral insufficiency, even minimal myocardial depression may cause significant compromise.*
3. *Avoid increases in vascular resistance as it will increase the regurgitant flow and decrease forward flow. Ephedrine is the vasopressor of choice for mild hypotension.*
4. *Atrial fibrillation can cause left ventricular decompensation.*

Anesthesia for Vaginal and Cesarean Delivery
Asymptomatic patients with unchanged status after echocardiographic evaluation may be approached in a routine but cautious fashion. Standard monitoring is likely to be sufficient, including continuous electrocardiography, pulse oximetry, NIBP, and supplemental oxygen during labor and delivery. Early epidural placement to prevent increases in SVR from pain and anxiety likely will be helpful. Most patients tolerate vaginal delivery with good maternal and fetal outcomes.

Patients with severe regurgitation and symptoms of left ventricular failure will need diuretic and afterload reduction. As ACE inhibitors are contraindicated, nitrates and calcium channel blockers may be administered. Invasive hemodynamic monitoring including arterial and pulmonary catheter may be needed

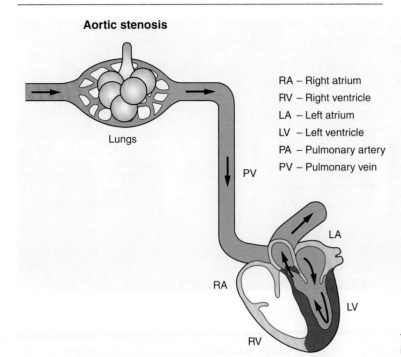

Aortic stenosis

Lungs

PV

LA

RA

RV

LV

RA – Right atrium
RV – Right ventricle
LA – Left atrium
LV – Left ventricle
PA – Pulmonary artery
PV – Pulmonary vein

FIGURE 30-15 Aortic stenosis.

in patients with left ventricular dysfunction. General anesthesia with TEE will help manage these patients for cesarean delivery.

The principles of anesthetic management are the same as for vaginal delivery; maintain a higher heart rate (sinus rhythm), lower SVR, and avoid myocardial depression.

Aortic Stenosis

Rheumatic aortic stenosis as the dominant lesion in pregnancy is relatively rare (Table 30-13 and Fig. 30-15). This is because of the 35- to 40-year latent period between rheumatic fever and the development of significant aortic stenosis. Most patients with this etiology become symptomatic in the fifth or sixth decade.

Asymptomatic pregnant patients with aortic stenosis are not at risk for developing left ventricular decompensation even though they have reduced hemodynamic compensation to the demands of pregnancy and labor and delivery.

If symptoms like syncope, angina and dysrhythmias, and heart failure are present prior to pregnancy, maternal morbidity and mortality are high (133).

Clinical Manifestations

Signs and Symptoms: The cross-sectional area of the aortic valve in adults is 2.6 to 3.5 cm². A 25% to 50 % decrease in area results in a loud aortic systolic murmur. Narrowing to less than 1 cm² markedly increases left ventricular-end diastolic pressures. Areas below 0.75 cm² produce exertional dyspnea, angina pectoris, and syncope. A systolic ejection

murmur loudest in the second right intercostal space adjacent to the sternum and radiating to the neck is heard.

The ECG usually demonstrates LVH and occasionally a left bundle branch block. Chest x-ray usually reveals a left ventricular enlargement and poststenotic dilatation of aorta. ECG shows calcified, restricted aortic valve leaflets. Planimetry of the aortic valve will demonstrate the restricted aortic valve opening. Doppler examination in severe aortic stenosis will demonstrate a peak velocity greater than 4 m/s and mean pressure through the aortic valve greater than 50 mm Hg (Fig. 30-16). However, when correlated with symptoms, ECG estimation of the valve area, rather than the pressure gradient is superior in detecting the severity of the disease in pregnancy as the hyperdynamic flow in pregnancy can overestimate the valve gradient (134). Isolated reports have suggested utility of exercise Doppler ECG for assessment of cardiac function and velocity gradients (135).

Cardiac catheterization commonly indicates substantive pressure gradient (left ventricle to aorta) when the aortic valve area is less than 1 cm². A pressure gradient exceeding 50 mm Hg typically indicates severe stenosis except among patients with congestive heart failure, where reduced left ventricular stroke volume may produce only 30 mm Hg gradient, even with severe aortic stenosis.

Anesthetic Considerations: The general principles of managing patients with aortic stenosis are to avoid fluid depletion, hypotension, and maintain sinus rhythm. The presence of symptoms, evidence of left ventricular failure, or progression of stenosis requires radial artery and possibly pulmonary artery monitoring.

Decreases in SVR are poorly tolerated. Blood pressure maintenance is the key to ensure adequate coronary perfusion. Coronary perfusion pressure is dependent on the difference between aortic root pressure and left ventricular end-diastolic pressure. Hence, a drop in aortic pressure can precipitate coronary ischemia. In healthy parturients, decreases in SVR are compensated by increases in stroke volume and heart rate. However, in pregnant patients with aortic stenosis, SVR must be maintained since stroke

TABLE 30-13 Aortic Insufficiency

Hemodynamic Goals
Maintain a normal or slightly elevated heart rate
Avoid myocardial depressants
Avoid marked increase in SVR
Higher central blood volumes are usually well tolerated

SVR, Systemic Vascular Resistance.

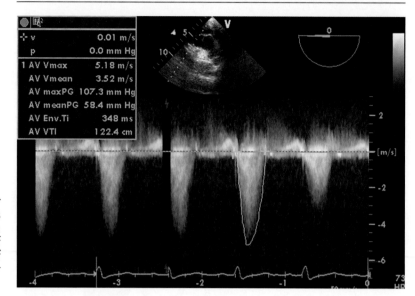

FIGURE 30-16 Deep transgastric long-axis view with continuous wave Doppler through the aortic valve. Note the peak velocity of 5.18 m/s and mean pressure gradient of 58.4 mm Hg which both meet the criteria for severe aortic stenosis.

volume is limited, making cardiac output primarily driven by heart rate. As well, decreases in SVR will increase the aortic valve gradient. Vascular resistance should be maintained with $\alpha2$-agonists like phenylephrine.

Avoid tachycardia. Heart rates should be maintained between 60 and 80 beats per minute. Tachycardia decreases the diastolic time, resulting in lower end-diastolic volumes and decreased stroke volume. In addition, tachycardia increases the myocardial oxygen demand and may lead to ischemia, even in patients without evidence of coronary atherosclerotic disease.

Decreased venous return (preload) and left ventricular filling are poorly tolerated. Due to the increased and fixed afterload, left ventricular stroke volume will be maintained only if the end-diastolic volume is adequate. Marked decreases in ventricular filling will decrease stroke volume and cardiac output. Maintenance of adequate preload and time for left ventricular filling (avoid tachycardia) are paramount in the care of patients with aortic stenosis. In addition, since the left ventricle is noncompliant, small changes in fluid loading will result in large changes in filling pressure.

Maintain sinus rhythm. Patients with severe aortic stenosis inevitably develop LVH and diastolic dysfunction. Adequate preload is necessary to maintain cardiac output; however, as a result of LVH, the left ventricle becomes more dependent on the active atrial contribution for filling. Loss of sinus rhythm may result in a decrease in cardiac output and sinus rhythm should be restored as quickly as possible.

Anesthesia for Vaginal and Cesarean Delivery

Vaginal Delivery: Asymptomatic patients during pregnancy tolerate labor and delivery well with noninvasive close monitoring and titrated gradual epidural analgesia with low concentration local anesthetic and narcotics. Reducing the duration of the second stage of labor will mitigate effects of Valsalva. This can be facilitated with an early epidural. At a minimum, monitoring should include continuous electrocardiography, pulse oximetry, and NIBP. A reasonable approach is the combined spinal–epidural technique using intrathecal opioids and epidural infusions of low dose local anesthetics.

Cesarean Delivery: In patients with more severe disease, cesarean delivery has been managed with a gradually titrated block with regional analgesia using an epidural

approach (136,137) and a subarachnoid approach (138) with invasive arterial monitoring. Postoperative pain management can be instituted with neuraxial administration of preservative free morphine.

General Anesthesia: A balanced anesthetic with a high dose titrated opioid induction with β-blockade has been used with success. General anesthesia also provides the advantage of using continuous TEE monitoring. Avoidance of the hemodynamic response to laryngoscopy and intubation is imperative. Adequate depth of anesthesia to avoid tachycardia and hypertension is needed.

Arterial monitoring along with TEE is useful in patients with more severe disease who are symptomatic. Maintenance of left uterine displacement, judicious fluid administration, and hemodynamic management can be associated with good maternal and fetal outcomes (139).

Oxytocin use should be considered very carefully and if necessary very low dose infusions should be administered to avoid hypotension (140). Phenylephrine for maintenance of blood pressure has been used successfully in patients with aortic stenosis undergoing cesarean delivery under general anesthesia with no adverse effects on left ventricular function (141,142).

Postoperative multidisciplinary management for 24 to 48 hours usually is indicated.

Aortic Regurgitation

A 7- to 10-year latent period after rheumatic fever usually precedes the development of aortic regurgitation with associated widened pulse pressure, decreased systemic diastolic pressure, and bounding peripheral pulses (Table 30-14 and

TABLE 30-14 Criteria for Peripartum Cardiomyopathy

Heart Failure in the Last Month of Pregnancy or Within 5 m
Absence of identifiable causes
Absence of prior heart disease
Echocardiographic evidence of LV dysfunction with EF < dysfunction of EF <45% and or fractional shortening <30% and end-diastolic dimension 2.7 cm/m² BSA

LV, Left Ventricle; EF, Ejection Fraction; BSA, Body Surface Area.

Aortic Regurgitation

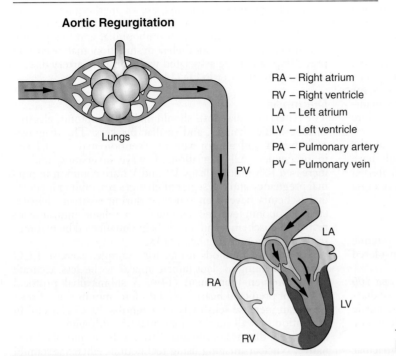

RA – Right atrium
RV – Right ventricle
LA – Left atrium
LV – Left ventricle
PA – Pulmonary artery
PV – Pulmonary vein

FIGURE 30-17 Aortic regurgitation.

Fig. 30-17). The disease usually remains asymptomatic for another 7 to 10 years. Patients presenting with left ventricular enlargement, ECG evidence of ventricular hypertrophy, and a large peripheral pulse pressure have a 33% chance of developing heart failure, angina, or death within 1 year; a 50% chance within 2 years; a 65% chance within 3 years; and an 87% chance within 6 years (130).

As symptoms develop during the fourth or fifth decade of life, most patients with dominant aortic insufficiency have uneventful pregnancies. However, heart failure complicates 3% to 9% of such cases during pregnancy (1,5,88).

Clinical Manifestations

Signs and Symptoms: The symptoms of aortic regurgitation relate to left ventricular failure. The signs include widened pulse pressure, low diastolic pressures, and an early blowing diastolic murmur heard along the left sternal border in the second, third, or fourth intercostal space.

Test Indicators: Commonly, the chest x-ray will reveal left ventricular enlargement, and the ECG indicates LVH, with increased QRS amplitude, depressed ST segments and inverted T waves, and a horizontal axis. ECG will reveal either malcoaptation of the aortic leaflets, restricted motion of the aortic valve leaflets, prolapse of a leaflet, dilated aortic valve annulus, or a combination of the aforementioned. A large left ventricle with eccentric hypertrophy may be seen. Color flow Doppler will reveal blood regurgitating back into the left ventricle during diastole (Fig. 30-18). If pulse wave Doppler of the descending aorta demonstrates reversal of flow during diastole, this is highly specific for severe aortic regurgitation.

Pathophysiology: Left ventricular volume overload is common among patients with aortic insufficiency, leading to progressive distension and LVH. However, increased volume usually is readily accommodated for multiple years, during which left ventricular end-diastolic pressure

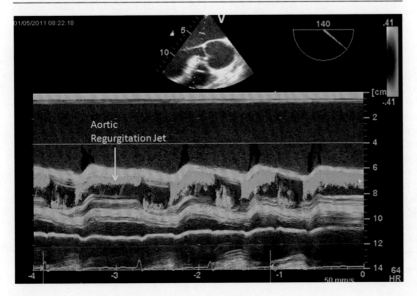

FIGURE 30-18 M-mode with color Doppler through the left ventricular outflow tract utilizing the mid-esophageal aortic valve long-axis view. Note the continuous color flow during diastole indicative of aortic regurgitation.

remains relatively normal. If uncorrected, eventually left ventricular failure results, causing an elevation of left ventricular end-diastolic pressure. Pulmonary capillary congestion and pulmonary edema follow.

Pregnancy-induced changes such as increased heart rate, and decreased SVR and increased circulating volume during pregnancy are usually well tolerated by parturients with aortic insufficiency. However, once symptoms manifest, risks increase precipitously, and left ventricular failure worsens as pregnancy advances.

Anesthetic Considerations: Asymptomatic patients in the NYHA class I and II are at minimal risk and usually have an uneventful pregnancy and delivery with good maternal and fetal outcome. Symptomatic patients will require close monitoring and multidisciplinary management.

Principles include

Avoid increases in SVR. Afterload reduction with systemic vasodilators and regional anesthesia should be considered in symptomatic aortic regurgitation.

Avoid bradycardia and maintain heart rate between 80 and 100 beats per minute. Bradycardia increases the duration of diastole and consequent regurgitant fraction across the aortic valve. Ephedrine or indirect-acting vasopressors should be used for maintaining blood pressure.

Avoid myocardial depressants. Some degree of left ventricular impairment must be expected among patients with aortic insufficiency. Decreased diastolic pressure, increased arterial pulse pressure, or increased intensity or duration of the aortic murmur indicates left ventricular compromise. Elevation of left ventricular end-diastolic or pulmonary capillary wedge pressure is a late sign, and suggests significant left ventricular impairment.

Anesthesia for Vaginal Delivery and Cesarean Delivery

Anesthetic management of parturient with aortic regurgitation is similar to that for patients with mitral insufficiency (see section under Mitral Regurgitation). Continuous epidural analgesia for labor and delivery and even cesarean delivery with appropriate monitoring is recommended for most of these patients. Diuretics and vasodilators to reduce afterload are helpful unless the blood pressure is low. Angiotensin receptor antagonists and ACE inhibitors are contraindicated and hydralazine is avoided in the first and second trimester of pregnancy. Other vasodilators (nitroprusside, calcium channel blockers) may be considered as well.

■ ISCHEMIC/MYOPATHIC/ ARTERIAL DISEASES

Ischemic Heart Disease

The incidence of acute myocardial infarction (MI) is estimated at 0.6 to 1 per 10,000 pregnancies (143,144). Most maternal deaths occur at the time of infarction or within 2 weeks of the event. The risk of MI is three times higher than nonpregnant women of reproductive age (144) and is increased with advancing maternal age and in multigravid patients (144,145).

Acute myocardial infarction occurs more commonly in multigravidas and all stages of pregnancy. The majority of patients are greater than 30 years and most of the time (78%) it occurs in the anterior wall. Risk factors include family history of atherosclerotic disease, dyslipidemias (146), previous use of oral contraceptives, cigarette smoking, cocaine use, and diabetes mellitus.

Although underlying atherosclerotic disease may be the leading cause, other causes include thrombosis, coronary artery spasm, coronary artery dissection, vasculitis, embolism, pheochromocytoma, and use of methergine (methylergonovine maleate). Comorbidities include hypertension, preeclampsia, smoking and thrombophilia, and postpartum infections. Vascular endothelial dysfunction that occurs in preeclampsia may be associated with coronary artery disease in these patients later in life (144).

Diagnosis

The criteria for diagnosis should include symptoms, electrocardiographic changes, and cardiac markers. The diagnosis of ischemia and appropriate intervention may be delayed in pregnancy. Axis deviation, T wave inversions, and an increased R/S ratio in leads V1 and V2 are common in normal pregnancy and ST segment changes resembling myocardial ischemia have been reported during cesarean delivery (147). Troponin level measurements are reliable indicators of myocardial ischemia and injury, being unaffected by myometrial contraction during labor (148).

Noninvasive methods using, for example, exercise ECG provide meaningful data (albeit appear to be less accurate among women than men) (149). A submaximal protocol (<70% of predicted heart rate) with fetal monitoring, if possible, can increase sensitivity of diagnosis. ECG is useful in evaluation of wall motion abnormalities although it cannot definitively diagnose ischemia. Stress echo is another alternative. Nuclear imaging using technetium-labeled sestamibi or thallium 20 is best avoided especially during the first trimester during organogenesis. Even in the other trimesters, it carries the risk of fetal growth retardation and malignancy.

During cardiac catheterization, abdominal shielding and short fluoroscopy times will decrease radiation exposure. Exposure greater than 15 rad carries a risk of harm to the fetus (150). Cardiac catheterization carries the increased risk of coronary dissection and hence a noninvasive method of diagnosis should be attempted in stable patients (145).

Spontaneous Coronary Dissection

In a recent review of pregnant patients presenting with myocardial infarction during pregnancy, coronary dissection accounted for 35% of cases followed by stenosis (30%), thrombus (15%), and spasm (less than 5%). The coronary arteries are normal in about 10% of cases (145). Most of the cases of spontaneous coronary dissection occurred in the last 4 weeks of pregnancy. Risk factors include multiparity, advancing age and association of coronary dissection with menstruation, oral contraceptive use, and hepatic cirrhosis that suggests a case of altered estrogen and progesterone levels as risk factors (151–154). The majority of the cases occurs in the left coronary vessels and involves multiple vessels in 40% of cases.

Management of Myocardial Ischemia and Acute Myocardial Infarction in Pregnancy

Medical management includes aspirin, β-blockers, nitroglycerin, and heparin, but these are anecdotal data and the optimal combination in pregnancy has not been investigated. High dose aspirin causes mortality, IUGR, bleeding, acidosis, and premature ductal closure in the fetus. In addition, maternal anemia, hemorrhage, prolonged gestation, and labor have been reported with aspirin use. However, low dose aspirin (40 to 150 mg/d) is recommended in pregnant patients with known coronary artery disease. Heparin is the anticoagulant of choice before elective delivery. It should be discontinued 24 hours prior to delivery and restarted postpartum after adequate hemostasis is confirmed. Antiplatelet agents like clopidogrel, ticlodipine, and glycoprotein IIb/IIIa have been used with limited published information. Use of statins during pregnancy is contraindicated—ACE inhibitors, angiotensin II receptor blockers, and direct renin inhibitors are also contraindicated due to risk of teratogenicity and death.

Revascularization During Pregnancy

No comparative studies exist contrasting thrombolysis versus revascularization among pregnant patients. Case series reported serious safety concerns when such techniques are used in the parturient, including maternal hemorrhage, preterm delivery, and fetal loss (155,156). Thus, unless critical, thrombolysis should be approached cautiously among parturients (156). Generally, there is a reluctance to intervene even though percutaneous intervention has been used with some success (144).

Percutaneous coronary intervention using bare metal stents may be preferred over drug-eluting stents, given that the safety of prolonged antiplatelet therapy is unknown among parturients. Clearly, medical therapy for ischemia/infarction should be the mainstay among parturients with myocardial ischemia. Invasive treatment should be reserved for progressive disease not responsive to medical therapy.

Surgical correction of coronary obstruction with coronay artery bypass grafting (CABG) has been reported for 5 decades, and carries risk (maternal mortality at 1.7% to 3%; fetal mortality at 9.5% to 19%) (157–159). More problematic is open heart surgery (160), with maternal mortality associated with aortic or arterial dissection and pulmonary embolism. An important consideration is the timing of surgery. Surgery is best performed in the early second trimester. First trimester surgery (during organogenesis) is associated with impaired fetal outcome, and late second trimester or early third trimester surgery risks preterm labor.

Cardiopulmonary bypass (CPB) may have deleterious effects on the uteroplacental vasculature and fetus (158,161). If the fetus is viable, uterine tone and fetal heart rate should be monitored, and a dedicated perinatologist or obstetrician should be in attendance. Fetal bradycardia, sinusoidal patterns, and late decelerations are all indicators of fetal asphyxia and may occur during CPB initiation or emergence (162). Potential reasons for fetal asphyxia include low uteroplacental blood flow (UBF), hemodilution, hypothermia, particulate or air embolism, obstruction of venous drainage during inferior vena cava cannulation, prolonged CPB, or maternal narcotic administration.

Although conventional coronary artery revascularization using CPB has evolved due to advances in pharmacologic management and monitoring, other approaches to surgical revascularization should be considered, including off-pump surgery. Data, however, suggest greater safety, but comparison studies are lacking.

Management of Labor and Delivery in Pregnant Patients with Ischemic Heart Disease

The hemodynamic strain placed on the heart during labor and delivery suggests that delivery should be delayed for at least 2 weeks after a myocardial infarction if possible. Cesarean delivery is indicated for obstetric reasons, as it is well known that vaginal delivery is less stressful. However, recent reviews have not supported one method of delivery over the other. During vaginal delivery, assistance with the second stage of labor and good epidural anesthesia facilitates good outcomes (163). The labor and delivery team should be ready for an operative delivery if maternal or fetal decompensation occurs.

During labor, use of supplemental oxygen, use of left lateral decubitus positioning, and monitoring with continuous electrocardiography and pulse oximetry (mother) as well as fetal monitoring are recommended. When impaired

TABLE 30-15 Primary Pulmonary Hypertension

Hemodynamic Goals
Avoid increase in PVR
Avoid decrease in SVR
Maintain intravascular volume
Avoid myocardial depressants

SVR, Systemic Vascular Resistance; PVR, Pulmonary Vascular Resistance.

left ventricular function is suspected, an arterial and PAC/TEE monitoring is recommended. Early epidural, prevention of tachycardia and hypertension, and prompt treatment of hypotension with ephedrine or phenylephrine are important. Methergine should be avoided and close monitoring continued for 48 hours after delivery. Patients who have had an infarction recently or revascularization should be advised to avoid pregnancy for at least a year as there is potential risk for further ischemia and LV (left ventricular) dysfunction.

Peripartum Cardiomyopathy

Peripartum cardiomyopathy (PPCM) is a rare form of heart failure, which presents with symptoms of left ventricular dysfunction in the last month of pregnancy and up to 5 months after delivery (Table 30-15). It was originally described by Demakis and Rahimtoola in 1971. The echocardiographic features were added later by the PPCM workshop committee of the National Institute of Health (NIH).

The clinical presentation is very similar to nonischemic dilated cardiomyopathy except for its relationship to pregnancy and the higher chances of full recovery in almost half of the patients. It has a tendency to recur in subsequent pregnancies and can result in chronic disability and fatality in young women in their reproductive years (164,165). There is strong evidence to suggest inflammation, viral infection, 16 kDa prolactin induced apoptosis and autoimmunity. Myocardial biopsy is not routinely recommended and shows myocarditis, progressive death of cardiac myocytes, and destruction of the cytoskeleton of the heart (166,167). The risk factors include advanced maternal age, multiparity, African-American race, twin gestation, preeclampsia, and gestational hypertension and use of tocolytics.

Clinical Manifestations

Signs and Symptoms: The clinical symptoms and signs are those of biventricular failure including orthopnea, dyspnea on exertion, palpitations, chest pain, cough, and malaise. Supraventricular and ventricular dysrhythmias, thrombosis, and pulmonary and systemic embolism can all occur as complications. Electrocardiography shows LV hypertrophy, diffuse ST wave abnormalities, or LV conduction defects. CXR is consistent with cardiomegaly and pulmonary congestion. ECG shows dilated cardiomyopathy with LV hypokinesis and dilated chambers with regurgitation across the valves (Fig. 30-19). Intracardiac thrombus may be present.

Pathophysiology: As pregnancy advances, the increased preload associated with uterine contractions, increased blood volume and later delivery can increase cardiac demand (heart rate, stroke volume and contractility) and will increase stress on myocardial function. With progressive ventricular failure, end-diastolic volume increases (decreasing subendocardial blood flow), cardiac output decreases (decreasing coronary perfusion), and myocardial oxygen demand

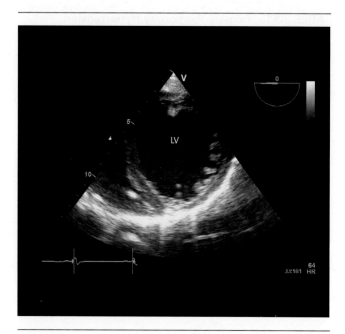

FIGURE 30-19 Transgastic mid-papillary short-axis view demonstrating a severely enlarged left ventricle as accompanies severe heart failure. LV, Left ventricle.

increases. The result is a myocardial oxygen supply demand imbalance, leading to further ventricular compromise.

General Management Principles: The treatment of PPCM, particularly in patients with severe systolic dysfunction, involves the use of diuretics, salt restriction, and afterload reduction with vasodilators. Hydralazine, nitrates, or calcium channel blockers like amlodipine are some of the drugs that have been recommended for afterload reduction. ACE (angiotensin-converting inhibitors) inhibitors are generally contraindicated in the antepartum period due to the risk of teratogenicity, neonatal anuria and renal failure, and neonatal death (168). These drugs may be used after delivery of the baby or on a case-to-case basis as mandated by the maternal condition. This clearly involves a clear informed consent discussion. ACE inhibitors are used effectively postpartum even if the mother is breast-feeding. Newer therapy includes pooled polyclonal antibodies which have been shown to improve overall survival in pregnant patients with dilated cardiomyopathy (169). Atrial dysrhythmias can be treated with digoxin and other indicated antiarrhythmic drugs as required. Drug choice in such patients is best made in consultation with a cardiologist.

Anticoagulation with unfractionated or low-molecular-weight heparin (LMWH) should be considered in patients with very low ejection fraction due to the risk of thromboembolism. Oral anticoagulation with warfarin is useful in the postpartum period. Heparin, warfarin, β-blockers, digoxin, and some ACE inhibitors (captopril and enalapril) are safe during breastfeeding.

Anesthesia for Vaginal Delivery and Cesarean Delivery

The mode of delivery in patients with PPCM is usually determined by obstetric indications and the maternal functional status. At the time of delivery, oxygen supplementation, continuous electrocardiography, pulse oximetry, and radial and pulmonary artery catheterization are recommended. If heart failure is well controlled with good response to medical treatment, pregnancy can be allowed to go to term (37 weeks) and labor induced for vaginal delivery with close monitoring in the peripartum period. Epidural analgesia helps reduce the sympathetic stress of pain and decreases afterload.

A multidisciplinary approach helps with delivery planning, and in most cases, vaginal delivery is appropriate in a well-compensated and medically optimized mother. The advantages of vaginal delivery are greater hemodynamic stability, decreased blood loss, minimal surgical stress, and lower risk of postoperative infection. Epidural analgesia with slow titration of low concentrations of local anesthetic has the advantages of decreasing preload and afterload, and helps in accommodating volume from uterine autotransfusion after delivery. It also provides excellent pain control and minimizes the effect of sympathetic responses on the heart as a consequence of pain. Combined spinal–epidural anesthesia with very low dose infusion of bupivacaine (0.0625% to 0.04%) as a continuous epidural has also been used with success (170,128). Contraindications to regional anesthesia include the presence of an anticoagulated state. Cesarean delivery may be performed under general anesthesia or neuraxial anesthesia. The principles of anesthetic management in patients undergoing general anesthesia include maintenance of a low to normal heart rate and avoidance of large changes in blood pressure. An opioid-based technique for induction is helpful. This avoids the myocardial depression and vasodilation caused by large doses of agents such as thiopental and propofol. There should be adequate preparation for neonatal resuscitation following high dose narcotic induction in mothers undergoing general anesthesia. Use sufentanil and low dose thiopental for induction in a diabetic obese parturient with PPCM has been described (171).

In patients with severe cardiac dysfunction, inotropic support can be provided along with general anesthesia. A recent review by the National Heart, Lung, and Blood Institute suggests that patients with EF less than 35% benefit from anticoagulation therapy (172).

The administration of anticoagulation should be considered when placing neuraxial blocks in these patients. The ASRA (American Society of Regional Anesthesia) (173) guidelines should be followed. Monitoring usually includes an arterial line and a PAC. TEE is a very useful tool to assess ventricular function and wall motion when general anesthesia is used. Regional anesthesia for cesarean delivery has been performed with a combined spinal–epidural technique, but such a choice should be made on a case-by-case basis.

Postpartum Management

In the postpartum period, medical management is continued with close hemodynamic monitoring by a multidisciplinary team. ACE inhibitors or angiotensin receptor blockers can be used to reduce afterload and has shown some LV systolic improvement in heart failure patients (156,174). Warfarin as oral anticoagulant therapy can be started a few days after delivery and the interim period bridged with LMWH.

Annual echocardiographic assessment is recommended as follow-up (175). The overall prognostic value of ECG in PPCM has to be used with caution as only small numbers of patients have been studied (176,177). Presence of symptoms, side effects from treatment and medications, and LV systolic function should be monitored and patients with progressive deterioration as evidenced by ECG should be evaluated for cardiac transplantation. Younger patients, recent onset PPCM, and minimal end-organ damage signifies a better outcome after cardiac transplantation (174). In about 30% to 50% of patients normalization of left ventricle occurs over a period of 3 to 24 months (178). If LV function is less than

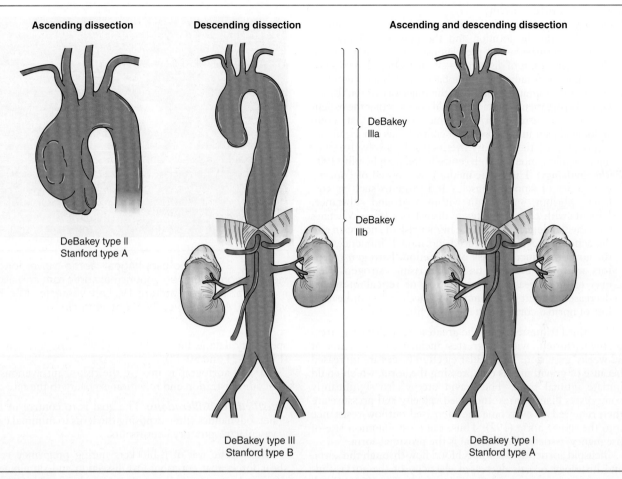

FIGURE 30-20 Classification schemes for aortic dissection based on which portions of the aorta are involved. Reproduced with permission from: Creager M, Dzau VS, Loscalzo J (eds): Vascular Medicine: A companion to Braunwald's heart disease. Philadelphia: WB Saunders, 2006.

25%, the chances of recovery are low. In subsequent pregnancies, patients with persistent LV dysfunction will progress to cardiac failure as compared with women whose LV function is restored. In addition, these patients have a higher incidence of premature deliveries and a mortality rate up to 19% during subsequent pregnancy (179–182).

Aneurysms and Dissection

Aortic aneurysm[1,2] is rare in young females, usually presenting in those with CHD, Marfan's syndrome or other connective tissue disorders, bicuspid aortic valve and coarctation, syphilis, or trauma (Fig. 30-20). Although aneurysms present rarely in pregnancy, they have high maternal morbidity due to dissections and other complications.

Immer and colleagues (183) reviewed the literature and assembled reports including 45 Type A dissections (40 prepartum and 5 postpartum), 12 Type B (7 prepartum and 5 postpartum), and four undefined aneurysms occurring during pregnancy. Maternal outcome was notably the poorest

in the prepartum Type A dissections, with 6/40 maternal deaths and 12/40 fetal deaths. Postpartum Type A dissection was associated with one maternal and one fetal death. In other reports, approximately one-half of aortic dissections in women younger than 40 years occurred during pregnancy, with an average age of 30 and average gestation of 32 weeks (184,185). A significant portion of these (43%) occurred in patients with Marfan's syndrome, Ehler–Danlos, Loeys–Dietz, or other genetic syndromes. Type B dissections occurring during pregnancy are very rare.

Awareness of the underlying syndrome is necessary for comprehensive management of the parturient with aortic disease. Marfan's syndrome occurs with an incidence of 1 in 5,000. Patients with Marfan's syndrome and aortic root diameter of more than 4 cm have 10% risk of dissection during pregnancy. Marfan's patients with normal aortic root diameters have a 1% risk of dissection (186,187). Ehler–Danlos that represents a group of syndromes affecting collagen, fibrillin, and other matrix proteins, has an incidence of one in 5,000 for all subtypes. EDs type IV, or vascular type, is associated with blood vessel rupture and visceral perforation and may carry severe life-threatening consequences. Aortic involvement is characteristic of type IV.

Loeys–Dietz syndrome is an autosomal dominant syndrome causing thoracic aneurysms which was recently recognized. Its defect is a mutation in the TGF-β gene. Most experts consider Loeys–Dietz syndrome to be an absolute contraindication to pregnancy because there is elevated risk of dissection even without prior aneurysmal dilation (188).

---

[1]Classification (DeBakey): Type I: Ascending and descending aorta involvement; Type II: Isolated-ascending aorta; Type III: Isolated-descending aorta (IIIA originates distal to the left subclavian artery and may extend to the diaphragm; IIIB involves the descending aorta below the diaphragm).

[2]Classification (Stanford): Type A: Involves the ascending aorta regardless of the entry site location; Type B: Involves the aorta distal to the origin of the left subclavian artery.

Clinical Manifestations

Signs and Symptoms: Aortic aneurysm can be asymptomatic depending on the location and the rate of development. Severe hypertension and preeclampsia may accompany the classical symptoms of dissection—sharp, tearing chest pain or abdominal pain radiating to the back (189). The presenting pain can be migratory, following the trajectory of the dissection. In a parturient, clinicians should note whether the patient is having concurrent uterine contractions, given that severe abdominal pain in the absence of contractions can mean dissection. Finally, the coronary arteries may be involved extending ischemic symptoms both centrally and peripherally (190).

Pathophysiology: The aortic media is composed of concentric circles of smooth muscles and proteins such as collagen, fibrillin, and elastin within a ground substance. Patients with connective tissue disorders such as Marfan's with medial deterioration have higher risk of aneurysm and dissection. Pregnancy-induced hormonal influences on the aorta may increase risk of dissection. Estrogen receptors are found in aortic tissue, and rising estrogen levels may cause increased fragmentation of reticulum fibers, decreases amount of acid mucopolysaccharides, and causes loss of normal corrugation of elastic fibers (191).

The third trimester poses the greatest hemodynamic stress on the parturient, with the greatest incidence of dissection at 32 weeks' gestation. Ventricular ejection forces are increased because of gravid uterus compressing the aorta, which could initiate intimal tears. The gravid uterus also significantly compresses iliac arteries. Increased velocity and pressure are then required to overcome the increased outflow resistance into the upper aorta (192). Thus, the most common site of pregnancy-associated dissection is the proximal aorta.

Bicuspid aortic valve disrupts blood flow through the aorta, and histology reveals decreased elasticity of the aorta, thus promoting aneurysm and dissection formation (193). Crack cocaine use promotes the development of aneurysm through its profound effects on the cardiovascular systems: Tachycardia, hypertension, increased myocardial contractility, and vasoconstriction. When compounded with the pregnancy-induced increased cardiac output, heart rate, etc., crack cocaine puts the parturient at higher risk of developing or worsening of an aortic aneurysm.

Management Considerations in Pregnancy: Aortic dissection during pregnancy carries a high mortality rate for both mother and fetus. The management principles should consider the type of dissection and gestational age. The Stanford type B dissections are usually managed medically. Type A dissections require emergency surgery. There are cases in the literature describing surgical repair during different stages of pregnancy and in the postpartum period. A review of acute aortic dissection complicating pregnancy suggests the following guidelines for management (194). If dissection occurs prior to 28 weeks' gestation, aortic repair with the fetus kept in utero is recommended. If the fetus is truly viable (i.e., after 32 weeks' gestation), primary cesarean delivery followed by aortic repair at the same operation is the treatment of choice. Between 28 and 32 weeks' gestation there is a dilemma, with the delivery strategy determined by the fetal condition. However, with the advances in neonatology these recommendations need to be reconsidered since improved outcomes have been shown in babies delivered as early as 24 weeks' gestation.

TTE is useful in the initial screening of patients with suspected aortic dissection. The sensitivity and specificity can be up to 75% and 90%, respectively. TEE overcomes many of the limitations associated with TTE and has sensitivity and

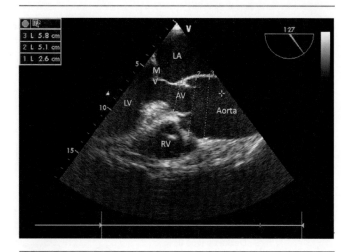

FIGURE 30-21 Mid-esophageal aortic valve long-axis view demonstrating an aneurismal aortic root and ascending aorta. LA, Left atrium; LV, Left ventricle; MV, Mitral valve; AV, Aortic valve; RV, Right ventricle.

specificity data as high as 99% and 98%, respectively (195) (Figs. 30-21 and 30-22).

CT and aortography involve the risk of intravenous contrast administration and radiation exposure to the fetus.

Anesthetic Considerations: The goal is to control maternal hemodynamics while exposing the fetus to minimal cardiovascular/respiratory depressants.

Prophylactic use of β-blockers during pregnancy reduces shear forces that contribute to dissection and simultaneously decrease heart rate. They are recommended for use if the aortic root is larger than 4 cm or progression of aortic root enlargement observed, but β-blockers should be used with caution because of side effects. These side effects may result in increased uterine tone, contractility, and decreased umbilical blood flow.

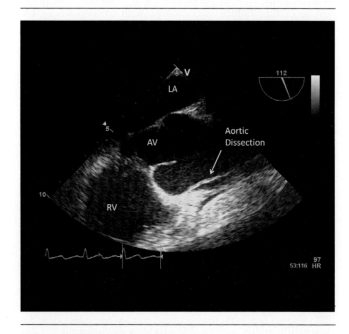

FIGURE 30-22 Mid-esophageal long axis view demonstrating an ascending aortic dissection. LA, Left atrium; RV, Right ventricle; AV, Aortic valve.

Acute ascending aortic dissections are surgical emergencies (DeBakey types I and II) while descending dissections can be managed medically. However, all of these require hemodynamic control; namely, decreasing ventricular ejection velocity and decreased systemic mean arterial pressure. Treatment agents used include nitroprusside, propranolol, metoprolol, esmolol, and nicardipine. However, nitroprusside causes fetal cyanide toxicity and β-blockers can cause fetal bradycardia and hypoglycemia through placental transfer (196).

Anesthesia for Acute Dissection
In the case of an acute aortic dissection, anesthesia should prepare standard ECG monitoring, two large-bore intravenous catheters, arterial catheter, central venous, PACs, and TEE (for dissections involving the ascending aorta). The site of invasive arterial monitoring is dependent on the type of dissection. Type 1 dissections should receive a left radial arterial line or femoral arterial line. Descending aortic dissections requiring surgical correction should have a right radial/brachial arterial line placed (cross-clamping of the aorta may include the left subclavian artery and loss of any left radial arterial pressure monitor). A modified rapid sequence induction can be used to rapidly secure an airway while maintaining hemodynamic stability (197).

Anesthesia for Vaginal Delivery
The anesthetic goal during labor and delivery in patients with risk for dissection is reduction of cardiovascular stress. Vaginal delivery in the setting of an aneurysm results in less blood loss than cesarean delivery and eliminates postoperative complications. However, vaginal delivery induces more hemodynamic instability. In particular, the second stage of delivery should be expedited. Women may labor on in a semi-upright position or on their left side to reduce stress on the aorta. Early epidural analgesia is recommended to promote hemodynamic stability and decreases shearing and tension forces on the aorta. However, Marfan's patients have an increased risk of dural ectasia with neuraxial analgesia, with subsequent dilution of anesthetic (198).

Anesthesia for Cesarean Delivery
A cesarean delivery is recommended if the aortic root dilation exceeds 40 mm or in the case of dissection. Cesarean delivery with concomitant aortic repair is recommended for type A dissection in parturients with viable fetuses.

As for vaginal delivery, regional anesthesia during cesarean confers the advantages of decreased vessel wall shearing forces and tension. Disadvantages in Marfan's patients arise from the increased rate of dural ectasia and technical difficulty of placement if the patient has scoliosis or has had scoliosis surgery in the past. In the event of dissection, resuscitation may prove difficult after neuraxial anesthesia because of sympathectomy (198).

Although no consensus has been established regarding anesthetic choice, general anesthesia may be advantageous in patients with acute dissection. Inhalational agents can decrease the force of cardiac ejection, and therefore, diminish the risk of aortic dissection. TEE is useful during cesarean delivery to monitor chronic dissection and risk factors such as aortic diameter greater than 40 mm (199). However, the hypertensive response to intubation, difficulty of the parturient airway, and the risk of uterine atony due to inhalational agents pose challenges that must be considered.

Complications: Patients should be monitored closely after delivery because dissection, both type A and B, can occur postpartum. Delivery relieves aortocaval compression and the autotransfusion of uteroplacental blood increases car-

TABLE 30-16 Cardioversion and Pregnancy

Theoretical Concerns
Amniotic fluid and hyperemic uterus are good conductors of electricity
Fetal V-fib
MAC vs. GETA—airway, full-stomach considerations
Careful FHR monitoring needed and LUD
Energy needed is unchanged (50–400 J)
Pad placement—anterior posterior vs. anterior apex

diac output (200). Gelpi et al. in 2008 (201) described two cases of aortic dissection in nonMarfan's, nonbicuspid aortic valve women after term cesarean delivery, suggesting that pregnancy itself is a risk factor for dissection.

Vascular changes do not normalize immediately after pregnancy (202), so predisposed patients continue to have increased risk. The hemodynamic stress of pregnancy accelerates the growth of the aortic root. In a follow-up study of Marfan's patients, growth of the aortic root in the pregnant patients averaged 0.28 mm/year after pregnancy versus 0.19 mm in the matched childless group (203). This effect was especially pronounced in patients with an aortic root diameter greater than 40 mm at baseline, with growth of 0.36 mm/year in Marfan patients who had been pregnant versus childless controls.

Primary Pulmonary Hypertension

Primary pulmonary hypertension (PPH) typically presents in women in the third decade of life (2:1 female to male prevalence) (204–206) (Table 30-16). Maternal outcome of pregnancy in patients with PPH are similar to that of pregnancy complicated by Eisenmenger's syndrome (160). Many of the physiologic changes in pregnancy contribute to the difficulties in managing pregnant patients with PPH (98).

Clinical Manifestations
Signs and Symptoms: The presenting symptom is typically dyspnea, though syncope, fatigue, chest pain, and palpitations may also be present. Symptoms usually appear late in the disease process and are due to a fixed cardiac output. Physical examination findings also present in late stages of the disease. A prominent pulmonic valve closure may be heard on auscultation as well as signs of tricuspid regurgitation (205). When right ventricular dysfunction becomes severe, prominent A waves can be noted on venous pressure tracings. Patients with late stages of the disease may be acyanotic, have poor peripheral pulses, and cool extremities.

Test Indicators: ECG typically reveals right ventricular hypertrophy, right atrial enlargement, and a right ventricular strain pattern. Chest x-ray shows enlarged pulmonary arteries, cardiomegaly, and usually clear lung fields. Pulmonary function testing is typically normal until late stages of the disease (205). Cardiac catheterization demonstrates isolated pulmonary hypertension with a normal wedge pressure. Vasodilator therapy effectiveness can be tested during right heart catheterization.

Pathophysiology: Pulmonary hypertension is present when mean pulmonary artery pressures are greater than 25 mm Hg at rest or greater than 30 mm Hg with exercise (207). With increasing pulmonary hypertension, right ventricular afterload and thus right ventricular pressure work increases. The right ventricle hypertrophies and eventually fails, causing an elevated right ventricular end-diastolic pressure and a decreased cardiac output. The elevation of end-diastolic pressure is reflected by an increase in CVP, resulting in passive congestion of the liver and peripheral edema. With progression of the disease, the right ventricle will become dilated, and tricuspid insufficiency will occur. Characteristically, throughout this course, neither PCWP nor left ventricular preload is elevated. The left ventricle usually functions well; however, left ventricular output declines because of the failing right ventricle.

Pregnancy-induced Changes: Pregnancy is accompanied by a broad spectrum of physiologic changes, including sympathetic, thrombogenic, mechanical (pulmonary capacity), and inflammatory changes, all of which can exacerbate substantial changes in pulmonary artery resistance and impedance. Both chronic and acute disturbances of these changes occur, especially during labor and delivery, which may readily exacerbate pulmonary hypertension and secondary right ventricular dysfunction.

Anesthetic Considerations: It is imperative that the degree of pulmonary hypertension and right ventricular failure be assessed before proceeding with an anesthetic plan. If possible, the reactivity of the pulmonary vasculature should be determined to assess responsiveness to pharmacologic vasodilation. In symptomatic patients, invasive monitoring with arterial line is needed. Pulmonary artery catheterization is critical to the management of patients with symptomatic pulmonary arterial hypertension (208,209).

Increases in PVR are not well tolerated. Hypercarbia, hypoxia, acidosis, lung hyperinflation, pharmacologic vasoconstrictors, and stress can markedly increase PVR and should be avoided. Ensuring adequate pain control or deep levels of anesthesia prior to stimulation will help avoid many of these pitfalls. Most vasopressors will affect the PVR as well as the SVR. If systemic hypotension is present, vasopressin (bolus or infusion) is the best option to increase the SVR with the least concomitant effect on the PVR.

Marked decreases in right ventricular volume and not well tolerated. Early correction of fluid and blood loss and avoidance of inferior vena caval obstruction are important to maintaining normal to slightly elevated CVP.

Marked decreases in SVR may not be well tolerated. Cardiac output is limited by a fixed right ventricular output, compromising the ability to compensate for decreases in SVR. Vasopressin is the vasopressor of choice in patients with severe pulmonary hypertension to correct decreases in SVR.

Right ventricular contractility may be compromised, and negative inotropes may result in marked depression of ventricular function.

Anesthesia for Vaginal and Cesarean Delivery

In parturients with primary pulmonary hypertension, pain, anxiety, and stress are especially detrimental because PVR may increase markedly. Adequate psychological support and analgesia are mandatory.

Vaginal Delivery: As noted in the anesthetic goals above, optimum pain control during labor and delivery is paramount in preventing increases in pulmonary artery pressures. Intravenous opioids may be adequate in some patients, though care is needed to prevent oversedation and hypercarbia. Augmentation with pudendal nerve blocks may be needed with this approach. Lumbar sympathetic anesthesia is the preferred approach for vaginal delivery in these patients (208–210). Epidural analgesia should be administered with low dose local anesthetic combined with an opioid. Dosing of the epidural should be done slowly

and cautiously. Intravenous fluids should be administered to maintain adequate preload to the heart. Small decreases in SVR should be allowed as aggressive corrective measures with vasoconstrictors may have deleterious effects on the PVR. Severe decreases in SVR require treatment with ephedrine, phenylephrine, or vasopressin.

Cesarean Delivery: Both general anesthesia (211,212) and regional anesthesia (208,213–218) have successfully been used during cesarean delivery in patients with pulmonary hypertension. Adequate anesthesia should be established prior to instrumentation of the airway as tracheal stimulation may precipitate marked increases in pulmonary hypertension. As with vaginal delivery, lumbar epidural anesthesia should be titrated slowly until surgical anesthesia is accomplished. Preoperative invasive arterial monitoring and central venous monitoring should be performed to monitor CVP and systemic blood pressure during epidural titration.

Complications: The most serious complication is right ventricular failure resulting from increases in pulmonary hypertension. Early signs may be subtle, progressive increases in CVP while other vital signs remain stable may indicate failure of the right ventricle. If right ventricular failure is suspected, hypercarbia, hypoxia, acidosis, and light anesthesia should be immediately ruled out. Once these common causes of pulmonary hypertension have been ruled out, treatments aimed at reducing right ventricular afterload should be started. Treatments aimed at reducing pulmonary hypertension are limited and experience with these in pregnancy is rare. Intravenous and inhaled prostaglandins (epoprostenol, iloprost) have been successfully used in a number of pregnant patients and are more readily available than inhaled nitric oxide (traditional agent in the treatment of pulmonary hypertension) (69,208,211–215,219). If signs of right ventricular failure develop, inotropes such as milrinone or isoproteronol should be started.

■ CARDIAC DYSRHYTHMIAS/ CARDIOVERSION

Most dysrhythmias occurring during pregnancy are benign and unlikely to be associated with underlying heart disease (Fig. 30-23). However, serious dysrhythmias, though infrequent, do occur in about 1/1,000 parturients (220,221).

Pregnancy can precipitate cardiac dysrhythmias not previously present in seemingly healthy individuals (221). More likely is occurrence of dysrhythmias during labor and delivery (221), when stresses associated with volume overload, increased heart rate, and hormonal changes increase myocardial excitation and precipitate dysrhythmia (222). More serious ventricular dysrhythmias, however, are likely associated with valvular or myocardial disease and increase maternal morbidity. It is important to consider the normal cardiovascular changes that occur during pregnancy and the medication or treatment effects on the fetus when evaluating and managing rhythm disturbances.

Of note are electrocardiographic changes. The increased heart rate that occurs during pregnancy can decrease the PR, QRS, and QT intervals, but usually there is no change in the amplitude of the P wave, QRS complex, and T wave in the electrocardiography (221). PACs commonly occur, and the electrical axis can shift, more commonly leftward, due to rotation of the heart secondary to the enlarged gravid uterus (221).

Pathogenesis: Cardiac rhythm disorders result from impaired impulse formation, impaired impulse conduction, or both (223). Tachydysrhythmias result from enhanced

Paddle Placement

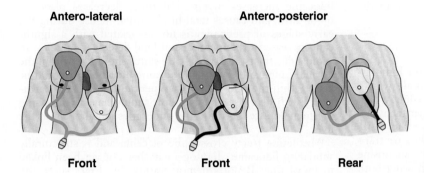

Antero-lateral

Front

Antero-posterior

Front   Rear

**Improved success 87% vs 76%
Lower energy required**

FIGURE 30-23 External cardioversion. Reprinted with permission from: Botto GL, Politi A, Bonini W, et al. External cardioversion of atrial fibrillation: Role of paddle position on technical efficacy and energy requirements. Heart 1999;82(6):726–730.

automaticity or unidirectional block with re-entry and bradydysrhythmias result from decreased automaticity or conduction block (223).

Effects of Pregnancy: Physiologic changes of pregnancy influence the pharmacology of antiarrhythmic drugs, given that a number of factors may affect drug levels (224):

1. Changes in gastric absorption, pH, and gastric motility, which affects the bioavailability of drugs
2. Reduced serum protein concentration and changes in protein binding affinity
3. Increased blood volume and concomitant increased volume of distribution, may decrease serum drug concentration and increase elimination half-life
4. Increased cardiac output can increase renal blood flow and glomerular filtration rate, and therefore, increase clearance of drugs by the kidneys
5. Increased progesterone levels may increase the metabolism of hepatically cleared medications
6. Placental transfer of antiarrhythmic drugs is better for low molecular weight and unionized, lipid-soluble drugs. Several undergo biotransformation in the placenta and fetal liver even as early as the eighth week of gestation.

Assessment of parturient with dysrhythmias should include careful history and examination, and comparative assessment of 12-lead ECG changes. Underlying causes and comorbidities must be considered including coronary artery disease, preeclampsia, alcohol abuse, illicit drug use, thyroid dysfunction, pulmonary disease, cardiomyopathy, and electrolyte imbalances. With any history of serious dysrhythmia, a comprehensive cardiology assessment during each stage of pregnancy is warranted.

Nonpharmacologic Treatment

Approaches are well established and include avoidance of caffeine, cigarettes, and strenuous exertion. Esophageal and endocardial pacing have been used in pregnancy with success for treatment of bradydysrhythmias, tachydysrhythmias, and refractory tachycardia (225).

Rarely, electrical cardioversion or catheter ablation is required during pregnancy (220). Direct current countershock up to 400 J has been used for termination of both supraventricular and ventricular dysrhythmias at all stages of pregnancy with no evidence of significant complication (222). Use of implantable cardioverter-defibrillator devices in

pregnant women at risk for malignant ventricular dysrhythmias appears to pose little risk (222), but clinical experience is limited.

When indicated, cardiopulmonary resuscitation (CPR) must be initiated without hesitation. Cesarean delivery should be considered after 25 weeks' gestation in an effort to save the fetus and improve CPR effectiveness for the mother (222). It is important to maintain left uterine displacement during resuscitation in pregnancy to alleviate aortocaval compression and improve effectiveness of CPR.

Pharmacologic Treatment

Medical treatment is typically reserved for patients that are experiencing debilitating symptoms or become hemodynamically compromised. With few exceptions, antiarrhythmic medications are safe. However, if medications are necessary, a conservative approach is advocated (fewer drugs, lower doses) using drugs that have been proven safe (225). The teratogenic risk is the greatest during the embryonic period, the first 8 weeks after fertilization (10 weeks after the last menstrual period); after that, organogenesis is essentially complete and the risk to the fetus is substantially reduced (222). Congenital malformations generally occur within the first trimester, whereas interference with fetal growth and development generally occurs within the second and third trimesters. Therefore, all medications should be avoided during the first trimester, if possible. These hazardous side effects depend on duration of exposure, drug type, genetic susceptibility, and exposure to the fetus.

Digoxin

Digoxin has been used safely and effectively in parturients for decades (226). Vagal effects of digoxin on the sinoatrial and atrioventricular nodes make this class of drugs an excellent choice for slowing heart rate, particularly in the presence of supraventricular tachycardia or atrial fibrillation (227). It is not associated with any fetal adverse outcomes or teratogenic effects when dosed appropriately. Observations of three women during their 11th and 12th weeks of pregnancy showed that less than 1% of the administered digoxin was detected in the fetus (228). On the other hand, digitalis toxicity during pregnancy has been associated with miscarriage and fetal death, likely due to maternal cardiac instability and subsequent uterine hypoperfusion (229). Enhanced renal function during pregnancy may decrease serum digoxin levels by 50% (220,229). Therefore, the digoxin serum level should be monitored regularly. The serum concentration in the third trimester may be difficult to assess as the result of a circulating digoxin-like substance that interferes with the radioimmune assay (222).

Adenosine

Adenosine is an endogenous purine nucleoside which modulates conduction through the atrioventricular node with a half-life of less than 2 seconds in a nonpregnant adult, which is effective in treating paroxysmal supraventricular tachycardias (220,222,226,229). Side effects such as hypotension, dizziness, flushing, and dyspnea are common, but they are transient and minor (220). The case reports describing adenosine use in pregnancy thus far have been positive, showing both efficacy and a lack of any direct adverse or teratogenic side effects on the fetus (226). In one report, an intravenous dose of 24 mg was administered without deleterious effects on the fetus (229).

Class IA Agents

Class IA agents are used in the treatment of ventricular and supraventricular dysrhythmias, including those associated with Wolff–Parkinson–White syndrome (226). In addition, quinidine can be used to treat atrial fibrillation and flutter. Teratogenicity has not been associated with quinidine, procainamide, or disopyramide (226,229). Of the IA agents, quinidine has the longest history of use during pregnancy (222,229). However, quinidine does have reported side effects (229) such as mild uterine contractions, premature labor, neonatal thrombocytopenia, depresses pseudocholinesterase activity by 60% to 70% (226), and spontaneous abortion or possible cranial nerve VIII injury at toxic doses.

Procainamide appears to be equally safe, is well tolerated over short-term therapy (months), and has the advantage of dosing intravenously; thus it is perhaps the best choice, especially for the acute treatment of undiagnosed wide-complex tachycardia (222). However, some practitioners do not consider procainamide a first-line treatment because a lupus-like syndrome can occur and rapid administration can precipitate hypotension and widening of the QRS complex.

Reported experience with disopyramide during pregnancy is limited. It is as effective as or better than procainamide or quinidine in suppressing premature ventricular contractions and can have fewer gastrointestinal side effects (226). In Europe, it has been found to be equal in potency to quinidine in the prevention and termination of supraventricular dysrhythmias (226). The most common side effects are dry mouth and urinary hesitancy, which reflect anticholinergic effects produced by this drug (227). This drug may increase the sensitivity of the neuromuscular junction to the effects of nondepolarizing muscle relaxants (227). There have been reported side effects (226) such as premature uterine contractions, low fetal weight, and placental abruption. Disopyramide should be used with caution in pregnancy, and likely reserved for refractory cases.

Class IB Agents

Lidocaine is not known to be teratogenic and has been used for the treatment of ectopic ventricular dysrhythmias and digitalis-induced ventricular irritability (220,227,229). When administered, the patient should be observed carefully for signs of toxicity (somnolence, tinnitus, dysgeusia,

and convulsions). Unexpectedly high fetal concentrations can occur due to ion trapping. High maternal blood levels of lidocaine (>5 μg/mL) are associated with neonatal depression (228). Although various studies have shown that lidocaine increases myometrial tone, decreases placental blood flow, and causes fetal bradycardia; its use during the early stages of pregnancy is not associated with a significant increase in the incidence of fetal defects (226,229). To avoid side effects, fetal acid–base status should be within the normal range and maternal lidocaine blood level should be kept within the mid to low therapeutic range (226). Parturients with decreased hepatic flow should have their dosing regimen adjusted as lidocaine undergoes metabolism in the liver.

Mexiletine freely crosses the placenta and is structurally similar to lidocaine. Teratogenicity has not yet been linked to mexiletine. Reports demonstrating the drug's successful use in pregnant women exist, but data in pregnant women are limited (229). Unlike lidocaine, mexiletine undergoes less than 10% first-pass hepatic metabolism, and bioavailability after oral administration is approximately 90% (226). There is little data regarding the safety of mexiletine in pregnancy. Isolated reports of fetal bradycardia, a small-for-gestational-age, low Apgar scores, and neonatal hypoglycemia have been associated with its use (226).

Tocainide is an orally effective amine analog of lidocaine that is used for suppression of symptomatic ventricular dysrhythmias (227). It commonly causes adverse effects such as nausea, vomiting, dizziness, tremor, paresthesia, confusion, and psychosis. Less common side effects include elevated liver enzymes, hepatitis, acute pulmonary edema, and lupus-like syndrome. Agranulocytosis, rash and fever, interstitial pneumonitis, and cardiodynamic effects such as pre-existing heart failure also have been reported (226). There is little information regarding the adverse effects of tocainide during pregnancy. Therefore, no recommendation regarding its use can be made until further investigation of the safety of the medication is performed.

Class IC Agents

Flecainide and propafenone appear to be relatively safe, although experience is limited (222). Flecainide has been used with clinical effectiveness and safety to treat several cases of maternal tachydysrhythmias (226). Neither of these drugs is known to be teratogenic. Both of these medications readily cross the placenta. Although the majority of reported cases have good outcomes, caution is still advised with flecainide use because of the reports of death of three fetuses. None of these deaths could be directly linked with this medication use. Use of these medications should be approached cautiously because the absence of information gathered from controlled studies does not allow clear recommendations regarding its application.

Class II Agents

β-blockers have been used extensively in pregnancy and are well tolerated. Propranolol, atenolol, and metoprolol have been widely used for a variety of indications, including hypertension, long QT syndrome, mitral stenosis, HOCM, and control of heart rate with both atrial and ventricular tachydysrhythmias (220,226). Propranolol is a useful drug for slowing ventricular responses during atrial fibrillation and for conversion of atrial flutter or paroxysmal atrial tachycardia to normal sinus rhythm (227). Esmolol has been increasingly used recently to control tachydysrhythmias because of its ease of treatability (228). There have been reports of IUGR, fetal bradycardia, polycythemia, apnea, hypoglycemia, prolonged labor, and hyperbilirubinemia, but these did not reach significance in randomized trials (220,222,225,226). Prospective clinical studies have shown the incidence of IUGR associated with propranolol to be approximately 4%, with normal-sized babies delivered in later pregnancies despite continued propranolol therapy (226). Other reports have linked propranolol use during pregnancy to the incidence of transient respiratory depression in infants at birth (229). While β-blockers have not been implicated in any fetal malformations, one small retrospective trial suggested an increase in fetal death with propranolol use during pregnancy (225,229). Atenolol is classified as a category D medication, because it has been associated with IUGR. Therefore, among pregnant patients, atenolol should be replaced with safer alternatives such as pindolol or acebutalol. However, the majority of cases had rare or minor side effects. It has been suggested that blockers with β_1 selectivity, intrinsic sympathetic activity, or α-adrenergic blocking activity might avoid β_2-mediated alterations in uterine relaxation or peripheral vasodilation and should be less likely to cause hypoglycemia (222,226,229). If necessary, glucagon may be administered during labor to counteract the bradycardic and hypoglycemic effects of β-blockade (229). Higher doses of β-blockers might need to be used to control heart rate during pregnancy despite adequate drug serum levels, suggesting a decreased sensitivity to the effects of β-blocker therapy (229).

Hurst and coworkers have made the following recommendations when using β-blocker therapy (229):

- When possible, avoid longer-duration therapy during the first trimester.
- Use the lowest dose possible.
- Discontinue therapy, if possible, at least 2 to 3 days before delivery to limit the drug's effect on uterine contractility and to prevent neonatal complications.

Class III Agents

The class III medications are characterized by delay of repolarization. Sotalol has recently received attention because of its superior efficacy in patients with ventricular dysrhythmias (222). However, sotalol should be used cautiously given the risk of developing torsade de pointes, and/or neonatal bradycardia (229).

Amiodarone has been used to treat refractory maternal atrial and ventricular dysrhythmias (220,227). Unlike other antiarrhythmics, amiodarone, and its metabolite, desethylamiodarone have a limited ability to cross the placenta, achieving fetal concentrations of only 9% and 14%, respectively, of the concentration in maternal serum (229). It has been shown to produce both coronary and peripheral vasodilation, likely by interfering with vascular smooth muscle excitation–contraction coupling (228). Initial reports suggested that this drug was safe, but subsequent reports have noted a high incidence of adverse fetal effects such as IUGR, preterm delivery, bradycardia, prolonged QT interval, spontaneous abortion, fetal goiter, and fetal hypothyroidism (220,222,228,229). The high iodine content in amiodarone, approximately 40% of its molecular weight, has been implicated in causing fetal hypothyroidism (220,226,229). Widerhorn et al. reported that the incidence of neonatal hypothyroidism associated with amiodarone was approximately 9% (229). Thus, treatment with amiodarone should be reserved for life-threatening conditions only (222).

Ibutilide is an intravenous antiarrhythmic approved for the acute conversion of atrial fibrillation and flutter of short duration (<30 days) (230). Studies with ibutilide have demonstrated that its ability to terminate atrial fibrillation falls off rapidly from the time of dysrhythmia onset (>50% efficacy on day 1) to an efficacy after 30 days of less than 10% (230). It has reasonable efficacy in terminating these rhythms with minimal associated hemodynamic effects and an acceptable safety profile. Unlike most other class III agents, ibutilide does not demonstrate significant reverse use dependence, greater effect at slower rates, which likely accounts for its effectiveness in terminating ongoing atrial fibrillation and flutter (230). The safety of ibutilide in early pregnancy is not established.

The effects of bretylium during pregnancy are unknown. Bretylium is effective in treating ventricular tachycardia and fibrillation that are unresponsive to other therapy, including lidocaine, procainamide, and repeated electrical shocks (227). Antiarrhythmic actions of bretylium are thought to be due to its actions on adrenergic receptors, which include stimulation of neurotransmitter release followed by prevention of the release of norepinephrine. There is only one case report in the literature regarding oral bretylium use during pregnancy, which resulted in no adverse reactions or complications (226,226). The known side effect of persistent hypotension could worsen hemodynamic instability, so it should be reserved for life-threatening situations where other options have failed (222).

Class IV Agents

The safety of the calcium channel blockers has not been thoroughly investigated in pregnant women. Verapamil has the most information regarding safety and clinical studies have not demonstrated adverse effects on either the patient or fetus (229). Verapamil gained wide acceptance in the treatment of paroxysmal supraventricular tachycardia and is also useful in slowing the ventricular response during atrial fibrillation or flutter (222,226). Subsequently, there were reports of maternal and fetal bradycardia, heart block, depression of contractility, and hypotension (222). Calcium entry blockers are relatively ineffective in suppressing ectopic pacemakers in the ventricles (227). Verapamil crosses the placenta to a limited degree. Murad et al. noted that fetal serum drug concentrations were 35% to 45% of maternal serum drug concentrations (220). These levels can decrease conduction at the atrioventricular node in the fetus.

Diltiazem has a similar electrophysiologic mechanism of action as verapamil. There are no reported adverse effects at this time. However, some animal studies have shown that large doses can cause skeletal abnormalities, decreased fetal weight, fetal death, and inhibition of uterine contractions (226,229). One retrospective analysis of 27 newborns exposed during the first trimester to diltiazem suggested a possible association with birth defects (229). Therefore, verapamil is the calcium channel blocker of choice during pregnancy. Adenosine and β-blockers are preferred over calcium antagonists to manage supraventricular tachycardia in pregnant women (222,229).

Anticoagulation

Protection against thromboembolism is recommended throughout pregnancy for all patients with atrial fibrillation, except those with lone atrial fibrillation or a low thromboembolic risk (225). When choosing the appropriate therapy, it is essential to consider the stage of the pregnancy. Heparin can be administered in the first trimester and in the terminal stages of pregnancy. Warfarin is contraindicated in the first trimester because it crosses the placenta and can cause spontaneous abortion, fetal hemorrhage, mental retardation, and birth malformations. All forms of anticoagulation can result in hemorrhage and pregnancy loss. Warfarin is relatively safe during the remainder of the pregnancy until just before delivery when it has to be discontinued (221). Unfractionated heparin does not cross the placenta, but the efficacy of high dose subcutaneous heparin for preventing thromboembolism in high-risk patients has not been established (225). LMWH has not been linked to teratogenic effects and does not cross the placenta. There are not any studies that evaluate the efficacy and safety of unfractionated or LMWH in preventing stroke in pregnant patients with atrial fibrillation. Lederer et al. reported that thrombolytic therapy during CPR may enhance the chance of successful electrical defibrillation after initially unsuccessful CPR due to sustained ventricular fibrillation in a nonpregnant patient (231).

Treatment of Specific Dysrhythmias

Atrial and Ventricular Premature Beats
Atrial and ventricular premature beats are usually benign unless the patient has cardiac structural abnormalities. In these cases the practitioner can provide reassurance with patient education. Chemical stimulants and other aggravating factors should be identified and discontinued. Medications are usually not needed unless the patient remains highly symptomatic, in which case β-blockers have been shown to alleviate anxiety and decrease the frequency of palpitations. β₁-selective β-blockers are a safer choice for asthmatic or bronchospastic patients. There is no indication for treatment with class III antiarrhythmic drugs because of their side effects and their risk for pro-dysrhythmia (224). Often, premature beats will decrease substantially in the postpartum period (225).

Atrioventricular Node-dependent Tachycardia
Atrioventricular node-dependent tachycardias require atrioventricular node conduction to sustain the tachycardia; atrioventricular node re-entry and atrioventricular re-entry are typical for this category (229). Paroxysmal atrial tachycardia is the most commonly encountered maternal dysrhythmia and is usually associated with too strenuous exercise (232).

In structurally normal hearts, the presence of paroxysmal atrial tachycardia does not increase maternal morbidity (228). When associated with mitral stenosis in parturients with RHD, paroxysmal atrial tachycardia is reportedly associated with a 14% incidence of heart failure and a 5.5% mortality rate (228). Moderate-to-severe mitral stenosis was present in 90% of patients and mitral regurgitation in 10% (228). Eighty-eight percent of the paroxysms lasting for more than 6 hours were associated with left ventricular failure, whereas paroxysms lasting less than 2 hours were not (228).

Recommendations include avoidance of aggravating factors and utilizing vagal maneuvers. Medications are needed if these recommendations fail to alleviate the symptoms, or if the symptoms are troublesome to the patient. Adenosine can be used for short-term management to alleviate the dysrhythmia. Verapamil and propranolol are acceptable alternatives. However, caution not to induce maternal hypotension and subsequent fetal hypoperfusion is advised when administering these drugs, especially verapamil (229). Another option is esophageal pacing. First-line prophylactic treatment used is digoxin or β-blocker. The class IC agents probably pose little risk and are efficacious.

If vagal maneuvers or drugs are ineffective at terminating VT, direct current cardioversion (10 to 50 J) is well tolerated and effective (224,229). In a very small number of pregnant patients with untreatable tachycardia refractory to both drugs and cardioversion, a "rescue" radiofrequency ablation is indicated with excellent results and no serious side effects for the pregnant women or the fetus (224).

Atrial Fibrillation/Atrial Flutter
Atrial flutter and atrial fibrillation are rare in pregnant patients in the absence of structural heart disease, underlying metabolic disturbances such as thyrotoxicosis, or electrolyte disturbances (221,224,225,229). Atrial flutter is rare and less common than atrial fibrillation. The presence of atrial fibrillation during pregnancy usually is associated with advanced rheumatic mitral valve disease, primarily dominant mitral stenosis (228,232). In one study, among 117 parturients in whom atrial fibrillation occurred, maternal mortality was 17%; fetal mortality, 50%; and heart failure developed in 52% of cases (228). If these dysrhythmias are not treated early with conversion to sinus rhythm or ventricular rate control, the risk of thromboembolism and detrimental fetal effects are increased. Class B or C β-blockers (avoid atenolol), digoxin, or calcium channel blockers (verapamil) are preferred for rate control. Nonspecific maintenance therapy for rhythm control is necessary. If these medications are effective, they should be continued for the entire pregnancy.

Early chemical cardioversion using quinidine, flecainide, propafenone, or ibutilide or direct current cardioversion within 48 hours of onset should be considered to avoid the need for anticoagulation (225). Rate-slowing drugs should be administered before starting quinidine because of its vagolytic effect on the AV node (224). Electrical cardioversion using the synchronized mode is usually successful with 50 to 100 J for atrial fibrillation and 25 to 50 J for atrial flutter (224,229). Amiodarone is effective against atrial fibrillation, but should be avoided during pregnancy if possible.

Wolff–Parkinson–White Syndrome
An increased incidence of dysrhythmias occurs during pregnancy in patients with Wolff–Parkinson–White syndrome (225). Atrial fibrillation has an increased incidence in patients with pre-excitation syndrome and may conduct rapidly over the bypass tract (229). β-blockers are the best choice for AV re-entrant tachycardia. Verapamil and digoxin should be avoided as they may enhance conduction of accessory pathways, particularly if a patient has atrial fibrillation (225). Class IA or IC medications should be administered with a β-blocker for long-term control. Electrical cardioversion is indicated for hemodynamically unstable patients.

Ventricular Tachycardia and Prolonged QT Syndrome
Ventricular tachycardia may be associated with drugs, electrolyte abnormalities, and eclampsia (220). Prolonged QT syndrome increases the risk of torsade de pointes and cardiac arrest during pregnancy (220). The increased heart rate that occurs in normal pregnancy may have a protective effect on the QT interval. Psychological and physical stresses are the major causes of ventricular tachycardia in parturients with no cardiac structural abnormalities. Ventricular tachycardia may be the presenting sign of PPCM, especially during the third trimester; ECG should be performed to assess left ventricular function (225). Most of these dysrhythmias respond well

to β-blockers. In fact, β-blocker therapy has been shown to decrease the risk of torsade de pointes related cardiac events (death, aborted cardiac arrest, or syncope) in patients with long QT syndrome, and, therefore, must be continued during pregnancy and postpartum period in women with this syndrome (221). Acute therapy for sustained ventricular tachycardia should start with lidocaine, and if ineffective, procainamide or sotalol is indicated (220,222). In addition, patients that have structurally normal hearts could benefit from flecainide. Episodes of syncopal ventricular tachycardia or ventricular fibrillation justify the placement of automatic implantable converter-defibrillator AICD (220). Electrical cardioversion is indicated for hemodynamically unstable patients.

BradyDysrhythmias

Symptomatic bradydysrhythmias are relatively uncommon in pregnant women. In a series of 92,000 pregnancies, complete AV block was observed in 0.02% (224). In some cases, sinus bradycardia or arrest has been attributed to the supine hypotensive syndrome of pregnancy, with uterine compression of inferior vena cava blood return causing a paradoxical sinus slowing (224,222). Prophylactic temporary pacing is recommended in patients with asymptomatic complete heart block before labor and delivery and if necessary permanent placement for symptomatic improvement (220–222,224). During labor, the use of epidural anesthesia is recommended to minimize maternal expulsive efforts, which might cause reflex bradycardia (220). (Fig. 30-24)

TABLE 30-17 Principles of Management During CPB in a Pregnant Patient

1. Monitor uterine tone and FHR (especially if fetus > 24 wk gestation)
2. Maintenance of a 15° left lateral tilt using a wedge under the right hip or a left lateral tilt of the table to prevent aortocaval compression
3. Maintenance of maternal hematocrit >28%
4. Maintenance of high maternal oxygen saturation
5. Normothermia
6. High flow rate (>2.5 L/min/m²)
7. Increased perfusion pressure (>70 mm Hg)
8. Minimize CPB time
9. Consider pulsatile perfusion
10. Stat pH management
11. Tocolytic therapy (e.g., magnesium sulfate, ritodrine, or terbutaline)
12. Perinatologist and obstetrician on standby if emergency delivery is required

Cardioversion During Pregnancy

Direct current (DC) cardioversion may be necessary during pregnancy. It is generally considered safe in all stages of pregnancy (Table 30-17 and Fig. 30-23). However, caution should be applied since the uterine muscle as well as the amniotic fluid are excellent conductors of electricity. Careful

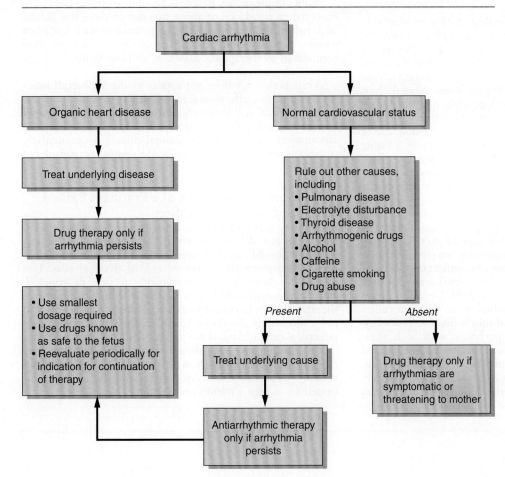

FIGURE 30-24 Management of cardiac dysrhythmias during pregnancy. Reproduced with permission from: Rotmensch HH, Rotmensch S, Elkayam U. Management of cardiac arrhythmias during pregnancy. Current concepts. Drugs. 1987 ;33(6):623–33.

fetal heart rate monitoring during the procedure is required and a multidisciplinary approach with the possibility for cesarean delivery and left uterine displacement to avoid aortocaval compression. Antacid prophylaxis and endotracheal intubation are advisable after the first trimester for anesthetic management of these procedures.

Successful external cardioversion (ECV) (50 to 400 J) after one or more attempts have been published in many case reports. Since 1965, 44 cases have been reported but there are limited data on perinatal outcome: 22 cases do not report pregnancy outcome and 13 cases report an uncomplicated continuation of pregnancy resulting in term vaginal deliveries (233). In two cases, fetal distress directly after the cardioversion was noted, necessitating an immediate cesarean delivery at 37 and 28 weeks of gestational age, respectively (234,235). Possible explanations are that the pads were placed extending beneath the apex on the ribs and the current could have reached the enlarged uterus.

The first case reported a notably hypertonic uterus, in the face of only a 50-J shock. The hypothesis was that it occurred as a result of cardioversion, the uterus became hypertonic and causing fetal bradycardia. Arguing against this is the fact that the current trajectory usually does not involve the uterus, with only a minimal current exposure to the fetal heart—small enough to have a high fibrillation threshold.

■ CARDIAC SURGERY

Cardiac Surgery During Pregnancy

Surgical morbidity and mortality are higher in the parturient than nonpregnant patients. Hence most parturients with cardiac disease should be managed medically, with cardiac surgery reserved for patients who fail intensive medical management.

Risk factors for maternal mortality during cardiac surgery include use of vasoactive drugs, age, type of surgery, reoperation, and maternal functional class. Risk factors for fetal mortality include maternal age greater than 35 years, functional class, repeat operation, emergency surgery, type of myocardial protection, and bypass time. Nonetheless, acceptable maternal and fetal perioperative mortality rates may be achieved through such measures as early preoperative detection of maternal cardiovascular decompensation, use of fetal monitoring, optimization of CPB, delivery of a viable fetus prior to the operation, and scheduling surgery on an elective basis during the second trimester. Physicians must have a firm understanding of the perioperative management of these complex, high-risk patients.

As reported in a number of studies, fetal and maternal mortality associated with intra-pregnancy cardiovascular surgery range between 20% to 30% and 2% to 6%, respectively. However, a recent retrospective, single-institution study reported on 21 pregnant patients undergoing cardiothoracic surgery, finding improved maternal and fetal outcomes as compared to older studies (236). Cesarean delivery prior to cardiac surgery resulted in no fetal mortality and minimal changes in maternal morbidity and mortality. If CPB is used, normothermic perfusion with high pressure is recommended. If surgery can be delayed to the third trimester, a cesarean delivery immediately before a cardiac operation should be considered (23,24,237). Finally, maternal and fetal outcome depend primarily on the underlying maternal status, gestational age, and the emergent nature of the operation, and not on the anesthetic agent used. See Table 30-8.

Cardiac Transplantation and Pregnancy

The first successful pregnancy after cardiac transplantation was reported by Lowenstein and colleagues (238). Potential risks to the prospective mother, and possible teratogenic effects from immunosuppressive drugs must be considered. Interestingly, the National Transplant Pregnancy Registry (established in 1991) has investigated pregnancy outcomes for transplant recipients, and long term implications. Comorbidities include chronic allograft dysfunction, development of diabetes, and onset of hypertension. Pregnancy-induced, increased cardiac workload is usually well tolerated by the transplanted heart. However, preconception counseling is critical, especially in circumstances in which PPCM or fetal cardiac defects are likely.

Consensus recommendations indicate that pregnancy is likely to be successful if there exists no evidence of rejection after 12 months, no evidence of infection, graft function remains stable, and immunosuppression therapy has been stabilized (239).

Maternal and Fetal Risks

Concerns include (1) hypertension and renal dysfunction secondary to use of immunosuppressant drugs; (2) inadequate absorption of drugs (due to hyperemesis gravidarum); (3) development of diabetes; (4) osteoporotic fractures; (5) autoimmune responses; (6) anemia; and (7) infection. The increased volume of distribution may mandate dose adjustment of medications during pregnancy (239–242).

Studies of pregnancy in recipients of heart transplants have reported an incidence of about two out of three live births, with half of those newborns being premature with low birth weight. Approximately one in ten of the pregnancies were terminated by therapeutic abortion, and one in five by spontaneous abortion (240).

While pregnancy does not appear to affect allograft function or rejection, effects on fetal well-being (low birth weight, pre-term birth, still birth) should be anticipated, with serial monitoring using fetal ultrasound and ECG. Screening for autoimmune disease and congenital infection—particularly toxoplasmosis, HBV, HCV, and CMV—must be considered (243,244).

Peripartum Management of a Pregnant Patient after Cardiac Transplantation

Stable pregnant patients can be delivered vaginally at term with cesarean delivery reserved for obstetric indications. Patients should receive continuous electrocardiographic monitoring given the increased risk of dysrhythmias. Use of invasive hemodynamic monitoring is case determined. Infection control is the key in the face of immunosuppressive therapy. Prophylactic antibiotics to prevent subacute bacterial endocarditis should be considered when valve or other structural cardiac defects are present (242).

Immunosuppressant medications should be continued during labor and after delivery, with serum levels of assayed for at least 1 month after delivery. Graft assessment must be continued for at least 1 month postpartum (245).

■ CARDIAC THERAPEUTICS

Cardiac Drugs and Their Effects on Pregnancy

Drug	Class	Indication	Commentary
Amiodarone	D	Ventricular dysrhythmia/ atrial fibrillation	Has been successfully used in pregnancy; however, high iodine content has been linked to transient fetal hypo/ hyperthyroidism (246,247).
Propranolol	C	Hypertension/ tachydysrhythmia	Reported increased incidence of IUGR. Newborns may suffer from bradycardia/hypoglycemia (248–250).
Labetalol	C	Hypertension	Rapid onset of action. Long history of safe use in pregnancy, though like other β-blockers, has been associated with IUGR (250–254).
Esmolol	C	Hypertension/ tachydysrhythmia	Short elimination half-life of 9 min may be beneficial in acute settings. Crosses placental membrane in pregnant ewes quickly (255). (May cause fetal β-blockade and contribute to neonatal distress if given concomitantly during a period of uteroplacental insufficiency (256,257).
Nicardipine	C	Stable angina/ hypertension	Used for tocolysis in pregnancy. Intravenous infusion effective and safe for treatment of hypertension in pregnancy (258–263). Pulmonary edema has been reported as a complication from nicardipine use (264,265).
Verapamil	C	Angina/atrial tachycardia/ hypertension	Has been successfully used in treatment of PSVT in pregnancy. (230,266–268). No known teratogenic effects, but may prolong fetal PR interval in pregnant ewes.
Hydralazine	C	Hypertension	Long history of use in pregnancy. Effects can last up to 6 h which make it difficult to titrate if hypotension develops. Associated with maternal hypotension and tachycardia. Fetal effects include fetal heart rate effects and a trend towards higher stillbirths with hydralazine use (269–271).
Nitroglycerine	C	Angina/hypertension	Commonly used as rapid-acting uterine relaxant. Minimal fetal side effects in pregnant ewes (31,272–274). Maternal hypotension and tachycardia may result from nitroglycerin use.
Adenosine	C	Supraventricular tachycardia	Multiple reports of safe use in the conversion of maternal SVT. Minimal fetal side effects reported in humans or animals (248,268,275,276).
Phenylephrine	C	Hypotension	Long history of use in perioperative period. Recent studies comparing phenylephrine to ephedrine report increased fetal pH, less nausea and vomiting, and better control of maternal blood pressure with phenylephrine use (277–281). May cause bradycardia and decrease in maternal cardiac output (279,282). May decrease rostral spread of spinal anesthetics (283).
Ephedrine	C	Hypotension	Has traditionally been the vasopressor of choice in treating hypotension associated with regional anesthesia in pregnancy. Recent evidence does not support ephedrine as superior to phenylephrine in treating hypotension in pregnancy. Recently found to be associated with decreased fetal pH, worse maternal blood pressure control, and increased nausea and vomiting (277–281,284).
Norepinephrine	D	Hypotension/shock	Used for severe hypotension when phenylephrine is not effective. Should be given through central venous access. May decrease uterine blood flow temporarily with no clear fetal side effects in pregnant sheep (285).
Epinephrine	C	Cardiac arrest/ hypotension/ low cardiac output states	Despite typically raising cardiac output, may decrease uterine blood flow in the animal model (286–288).
Isoproterenol	C	Low cardiac output states/ heart block	Invariably causes maternal tachycardia. Effect on uterine blood flow in the animal model is minimal with small doses of isoproterenol (287,289,290).

Drug	Class	Indication	Commentary
Dopamine	C	Hypotension/low cardiac output states/ decreased systemic vascular resistance	Effects vary depending on dose. Larger doses may decrease uterine blood flow despite raising maternal cardiac output in sheep (291–294). Human reports suggest possible lowering of fetal P_{O_2} in women treated with dopamine (295).
Milrinone	C	Low cardiac output states	An inodilator useful in patients with heart failure. Limited studies in pregnancy. Animal studies report either no change or an increase in uterine blood flow associated with milrinone use (296,297).
Heparin	C	Anticoagulation (cardiac surgery)/ risk for thrombotic events	Does not cross the placenta. Has been used in patients requiring anticoagulation in pregnancy but is associated with increased rates of thromboembolic complications (31,226,298,299). Pregnant patients may require higher doses of heparin (300).
Protamine	C	Reversal of heparin (cardiac surgery)	Associated with three common protamine reactions: Vasodilation, anaphylactoid, and pulmonary vasoconstriction. Limited published pregnancy-specific experience.
Warfarin	X	Risk for thrombotic events	Associated with teratogenicity. Facial anomalies associated with first trimester use (Between weeks 6 and 12). CNS abnormalities have been reported with use during second and third trimester use (31,226,298,299).
Lidocaine	B	Ventricular dysrhythmia	Long history of use in pregnancy. High maternal blood levels may be associated with fetal central nervous system depression (221,248). Supraclinical doses associated with transient decreases in uterine blood flow in pregnant ewes (241,301). Excreted in breast milk with no known side effects (302).

KEY POINTS

The anesthetic considerations for the pregnant patient with cardiac disease naturally vary according to the nature of the disease and its progression. However, several general guidelines can be offered.

- *Continue cardiac medications throughout pregnancy, labor, and delivery.*
- *Avoid marked changes in systemic or PVR.*
- *Prevent or treat factors that can increase a shunt.*
- *Avoid the use of myocardial depressants when ventricle is either compromised or at risk.*
- *Avoid any factors that can precipitate ventricular dysfunction or failure.*
- *Adapt anesthetic technique to the demands of the parturient's disease,* for example, regional techniques are applicable in the presence of many cardiac conditions, but not TOF, aortic or pulmonic stenosis, or pulmonary hypertension, when systemic and inhalational anesthesia are recommended.
- *Avoid any anesthetic agents or drugs that may contribute to marked changes in heart rate, blood volume, peripheral vasoconstriction, venous return, and ventricular filling volumes.*
- *Apply invasive hemodynamic monitoring where appropriate, but with the advent of ECG it has become the mainstay for noninvasive cardiovascular assessment of the pregnant woman with heart disease or suspected cardiac abnormality.* Pregnancy-related changes can be suitably assessed by the complementary use of quantitative pulsed and continuous Doppler and qualitative color Doppler technology. More recent and specific areas of clinical use including cardiac output estimation, contrast ECG minimizing fluoroscopy during cardiac catheterization, and TEE for selection of patients with mitral stenosis suitable for percutaneous catheter valvotomy.

REFERENCES

1. Mendelson CL. *Cardiac Disease in Pregnancy.* Medical Care, Cardiovascular Surgery, and Obstetric Management as Related to Maternal and Fetal Welfare. Philadelphia, PA: F.A. Davis Co; 1960.
2. Mendelson CL. Acute cor pulmonale and pregnancy. *Clin Obstet Gynecol* 1968; 11(4):992–1009.
3. Szekely P, Snaith L. Atrial fibrillation and pregnancy. *Br Med J* 1961;1(5237):1407–1410.
4. Ueland K. Cardiovascular diseases complicating pregnancy. *Clin Obstet Gynecol* 1978;21(2):429–442.
5. Burwell C, Metcalfe J. *Heart disease and pregnancy.* In: Boston: Little Brown; 1958:210.
6. Sugrue D, Blake S, MacDonald D. Pregnancy complicated by maternal heart disease at the National Maternity Hospital, Dublin, Ireland, 1969 to 1978. *Am J Obstet Gynecol* 1981;139(1):1–6.
7. Hess DB, Hess LW. Management of cardiovascular disease in pregnancy. *Obstet Gynecol Clin North Am* 1992;19(4):679–695.
8. International Journal of Gynecology & Obstetrics. Cardiac disease in pregnancy. ACOG technical bulletin number 168–June 1992. *Int J Gynaecol Obstet* 1993;41(3):298–306.
9. Niswander KR, Berendes H, Deutschberger J, et al. Fetal morbidity following potentially anoxigenic obstetric conditions. V. Organic heart disease. *Am J Obstet Gynecol* 1967;98(6):871–876.
10. Buehler JW, Kaunitz AM, Hogue CJ, et al. Maternal mortality in women aged 35 years or older: United states. *JAMA* 1986;255(1):53–57.
11. Steer PJ . Pregnancy and contraception. In: Gatzoulis MA, Swan L, Therrien J, Pantely GA, eds. *Adult Congenital Heart Disease: A Practical Guide.* London: Blackwell; 2005:16–35.
12. Avila WS, Rossi EG, Ramires JA, et al. Pregnancy in patients with heart disease: Experience with 1,000 cases. *Clin Cardiol* 2003;26(3):135–142.

13. Abdel-Hady ES, El-Shamy M, El-Rifai AA, et al. Maternal and perinatal outcome of pregnancies complicated by cardiac disease. *Int J Gynaecol Obstet* 2005;90(1):21–25.
14. Panchabhai TS, Patil PD, Shah DR, et al. An autopsy study of maternal mortality: A tertiary healthcare perspective. *J Postgrad Med* 2009;55(1):8–11.
15. Siu SC, Colman JM, Sorensen S, et al. Adverse neonatal and cardiac outcomes are more common in pregnant women with cardiac disease. *Circulation* 2002;105(18):2179–2184.
16. Oron G, Hirsch R, Ben-Haroush A, et al. Pregnancy outcome in women with heart disease undergoing induction of labour. *BJOG* 2004;111(7):669–675.
17. Balint OH, Siu SC, Mason J, et al. Cardiac outcomes after pregnancy in women with congenital heart disease. *Heart* 2010;96(20):1656–1661.
18. Khairy P, Ouyang DW, Fernandes SM, et al. Pregnancy outcomes in women with congenital heart disease. *Circulation* 2006;113(4):517–524.
19. Drenthen W, Pieper PG, Roos-Hesselink JW, et al. Outcome of pregnancy in women with congenital heart disease: A literature review. *J Am Coll Cardiol* 2007;49(24):2303–2311.
20. Ford AA, Wylie BJ, Waksmonski CA, et al. Maternal congenital cardiac disease: Outcomes of pregnancy in a single tertiary care center. *Obstet Gynecol* 2008;112(4):828–833.
21. Stangl V, Schad J, Gossing G, et al. Maternal heart disease and pregnancy outcome: A single-centre experience. *Eur J Heart Fail* 2008;10(9):855–860.
22. Klein LL, Galan HL. Cardiac disease in pregnancy. *Obstet Gynecol Clin North Am* 2004;31(2):429–459.
23. Martin SR, Foley MR. Intensive care in obstetrics: An evidence-based review. *Am J Obstet Gynecol* 2006;195(3):673–689.
24. Davies GA, Herbert WN. Congenital heart disease in pregnancy. *J Obstet Gynaecol Can* 2007;29(5):409–414.
25. Siu SC, Colman JM. Heart disease and pregnancy. *Heart* 2001;85(6):710–715.
26. Bevacqua BK. Supraventricular tachycardia associated with postpartum metoclopramide administration. *Anesthesiology* 1988;68(1):124–125.
27. Clarkson PM, Wilson NJ, Neutze JM, et al. Outcome of pregnancy after the mustard operation for transposition of the great arteries with intact ventricular septum. *J Am Coll Cardiol* 1994;24(1):190–193.
28. McCaffrey F, Sherman F. Pregnancy and congenital heart disease: The Magee Women's Hospital. *J Matern Fetal Med* 1995;4:152–159.
29. Shime J, Mocarski EJ, Hastings D, et al. Congenital heart disease in pregnancy: Short- and long-term implications. *Am J Obstet Gynecol* 1987;156(2):313–322.
30. Chatterjee K. The Swan-Ganz catheters: Past, present, and future. A viewpoint. *Circulation* 2009;119(1):147–152.
31. Chandrasekhar S, Cook CR, Collard CD. Cardiac surgery in the parturient. *Anesth Analg.* 2009;108(3):777–785.
32. American College of Obstetricians and Gynecologists. ACOG practice bulletin number 47, October 2003: Prophylactic antibiotics in labor and delivery. *Obstet Gynecol* 2003;102(4):875–882.
33. American Society of Anesthesiologists and Society of Cardiovascular Anesthesiologists Task Force on Transesophageal Echocardiography. Practice guidelines for perioperative transesophageal echocardiography. An updated report by the American Society of Anesthesiologists and the Society of Cardiovascular Anesthesiologists Task Force on Transesophageal Echocardiography. *Anesthesiology* 2010;112(5):1084–1096.
34. Armstrong S, Fernando R, Columb M. Minimally- and non-invasive assessment of maternal cardiac output: Go with the flow! *Int J Obstet Anesth* 2011;20(4):330–340.
35. Cleves A, Carolan-Rees G, Williams J, et al. *Cardio Q-ODM (Oesophageal Doppler Monitor) to Guide Intravenous Fluid Management in Patients Undergoing Surgery or in Critical Care.* External Assessment Centre Report. London: Cedar, Cardiff and Vale University Health Board; 2010.
36. Hoffman JI, Kaplan S, Liberthson RR. Prevalence of congenital heart disease. *Am Heart J* 2004;147(3):425–439.
37. Marelli AJ, Mackie AS, Ionescu-Ittu R, et al. Congenital heart disease in the general population: Changing prevalence and age distribution. *Circulation* 2007;115(2):163–172.
38. Warnes CA, Liberthson R, Danielson GK, et al. Task force 1: The changing profile of congenital heart disease in adult life. *J Am Coll Cardiol* 2001;37(5):1170–1175.
39. Cannesson M, Earing MG, Collange V, et al. Anesthesia for noncardiac surgery in adults with congenital heart disease. *Anesthesiology* 2009;111(2):432–440.
40. Engelfriet P, Boersma E, Oechslin E, et al. The spectrum of adult congenital heart disease in Europe: Morbidity and mortality in a 5 year follow-up period. The Euro Heart Survey on adult congenital heart disease. *Eur Heart J* 2005;26(21):2325–2333.
41. Yap SC, Drenthen W, Meijboom FJ, et al. Comparison of pregnancy outcomes in women with repaired versus unrepaired atrial septal defect. *BJOG* 2009;116(12):1593–1601.
42. Song YB, Park SW, Kim JH, et al. Outcomes of pregnancy in women with congenital heart disease: A single center experience in Korea. *J Korean Med Sci* 2008;23(5):808–813.
43. Fowler N. *Cardiac Diagnosis and Treatment.* 3rd ed. Hagerstown, MD: Harper and Row; 1976.
44. Zufelt K, Rosenberg HC, Li MD, et al. The electrocardiogram and the secundum atrial septal defect: A reexamination in the era of echocardiography. *Can J Cardiol* 1998;14(2):227–232.
45. Verheugt CL, Uiterwaal CS, van der Velde ET, et al. The emerging burden of hospital admissions of adults with congenital heart disease. *Heart* 2010;96(11):872–878.
46. Minette MS, Sahn DJ. Ventricular septal defects. *Circulation* 2006;114(20):2190–2197.
47. Yap SC, Drenthen W, Pieper PG, et al. Pregnancy outcome in women with repaired versus unrepaired isolated ventricular septal defect. *BJOG* 2010;117(6):683–689.
48. Fesslova' VM, Villa L, Chessa M, et al. Prospective evaluation from single centre of pregnancy in women with congenital heart disease. *Int J Cardiol* 2009;131(2):257–264.
49. Hoffman JI, Kaplan S. The incidence of congenital heart disease. *J Am Coll Cardiol* 2002;39(12):1890–1900.
50. Schneider DJ, Moore JW. Patent ductus arteriosus. *Circulation* 2006;114(17):1873–1882.
51. Campbell M. Natural history of persistent ductus arteriosus. *Br Heart J* 1968;30(1):4–13.
52. Green NJ, Rollason TP. Pulmonary artery rupture in pregnancy complicating patent ductus arteriosus. *Br Heart J* 1992;68(6):616–618.
53. Pollack KL, Chestnut DH, Wenstrom KD. Anesthetic management of a parturient with Eisenmenger's syndrome. *Anesth Analg* 1990;70(2):212–215.
54. Bailliard F, Anderson RH. Tetralogy of Fallot. *Orphanet J Rare Dis* 2009;4:2.
55. Gelson E, Gatzoulis M, Steer PJ, et al. Tetralogy of Fallot: Maternal and neonatal outcomes. *BJOG* 2008;115(3):398–402.
56. Reller MD, Strickland MJ, Riehle-Colarusso T, et al. Prevalence of congenital heart defects in metropolitan Atlanta, 1998–2005. *J Pediatr* 2008;153(6):807–813.
57. Nollert G, Fischlein T, Bouterwek S, et al. Long-term survival in patients with repair of tetralogy of Fallot: 36-year follow-up of 490 survivors of the first year after surgical repair. *J Am Coll Cardiol* 1997;30(5):1374–1383.
58. Alexiou C, Mahmoud H, Al-Khaddour A, et al. Outcome after repair of tetralogy of Fallot in the first year of life. *Ann Thorac Surg* 2001;71(2):494–500.
59. Bacha EA, Scheule AM, Zurakowski D, et al. Long-term results after early primary repair of tetralogy of Fallot. *J Thorac Cardiovasc Surg* 2001;122(1):154–161.
60. Veldtman GR, Connolly HM, Grogan M, et al. Outcomes of pregnancy in women with tetralogy of Fallot. *J Am Coll Cardiol* 2004;44(1):174–180.
61. Jones AM, Howitt G. Eisenmenger syndrome in pregnancy. *Br Med J* 1965;1(5451):1627–1631.
62. Meyer EC, Tulsky AS, Sigmann P, et al. Pregnancy in the presence of tetralogy of Fallot. Observations on two patients. *Am J Cardiol* 1964;14:874–879.
63. Jacoby WJ Jr. Pregnancy with tetralogy and pentalogy of Fallot. *Am J Cardiol* 1964;14:866–873.
64. Kirklin J, Karp R. *The Tetralogy of Fallot From a Surgical Viewpoint.* Philadelphia, PA: W.B. Saunders; 1970.
65. Meijer JM, Pieper PG, Drenthen W, et al. Pregnancy, fertility, and recurrence risk in corrected tetralogy of Fallot. *Heart* 2005;91(6):801–805.
66. Zuber M, Gautschi N, Oechslin E, et al. Outcome of pregnancy in women with congenital shunt lesions. *Heart* 1999;81(3):271–275.
67. Aggarwal N, Suri V, Kaur H, et al. Retrospective analysis of outcome of pregnancy in women with congenital heart disease: Single-centre experience from North India. *Aust N Z J Obstet Gynaecol* 2009;49(4):376–381.
68. Cannell DE, Vernon CP. Congenital heart disease and pregnancy. *Am J Obstet Gynecol* 1963;85:744–753.
69. Weiss BM, Hess OM. Pulmonary vascular disease and pregnancy: Current controversies, management strategies, and perspectives. *Eur Heart J* 2000;21(2):104–115.
70. Bloomfield DK. The natural history of ventricular septal defect in patients surviving infancy. *Circulation* 1964;29:914–955.
71. Copeland W, Wooley C, Ryan J, et al. Pregnancy and congenital heart disease. *Am J Obstet Gynecol* 1963;86:107–110.
72. Neilson G, Galea EG, Blunt A. Eisenmenger's syndrome and pregnancy. *Med J Aust* 1971;1(8):431–434.
73. Eisenberger V. Die angeborenen defecte der kammerscheidewand des herzens. *Z Klin Med* 1897;32:1.
74. Rudolph A. *Congenital Diseases of the Heart.* Chicago: Year Book Medical Publishers; 1974.
75. Ueland K. Cardiac surgery and pregnancy. *Am J Obstet Gynecol* 1965;92:148–162.
76. Avila WS, Grinberg M, Snitcowsky R, et al. Maternal and fetal outcome in pregnant women with Eisenmenger's syndrome. *Eur Heart J* 1995;16(4):460–464.
77. Baker JL, Russell CS, Grainger RG, et al. Closed pulmonary valvotomy in the management of Fallot's tetralogy complicated by pregnancy. *J Obstet Gynaecol Br Emp* 1963;70:154–157.

78. Cutforth R, Catchlove B, Knight LW, et al. The Eisenmenger syndrome and pregnancy. *Aust N Z J Obstet Gynaecol* 1968;8(4):202–210.

79. Martin JT, Tautz TJ, Antognini JF. Safety of regional anesthesia in Eisenmenger's syndrome. *Reg Anesth Pain Med* 2002;27(5):509–513.

80. Cole PJ, Cross MH, Dresner M. Incremental spinal anaesthesia for elective caesarean section in a patient with Eisenmenger's syndrome. *Br J Anaesth* 2001;86(5):723–726.

81. Lust KM, Boots RJ, Dooris M, et al. Management of labor in Eisenmenger syndrome with inhaled nitric oxide. *Am J Obstet Gynecol* 1999;181(2):419–423.

82. Goodwin TM, Gherman RB, Hameed A, et al. Favorable response of Eisenmenger syndrome to inhaled nitric oxide during pregnancy. *Am J Obstet Gynecol* 1999;180(1 Pt 1):64–67.

83. Geohas C, McLaughlin VV. Successful management of pregnancy in a patient with Eisenmenger syndrome with epoprostenol. *Chest* 2003;124(3):1170–1173.

84. Goodwin JF. Pregnancy and coarctation of the aorta. *Clin Obstet Gynecol* 1961;4:645–664.

85. Deal K, Wooley CF. Coarctation of the aorta and pregnancy. *Ann Intern Med* 1973;78(5):706–710.

86. Beauchesne LM, Connolly HM, Ammash NM, et al. Coarctation of the aorta: Outcome of pregnancy. *J Am Coll Cardiol* 2001;38(6):1728–1733.

87. Saidi AS, Bezold LI, Altman CA, et al. Outcome of pregnancy following intervention for coarctation of the aorta. *Am J Cardiol* 1998;82(6):786–788.

88. Szekely P, Snaith L. *Heart Disease and Pregnancy.* London: Churchill Livingstone; 1974.

89. Dizon-Townson D, Magee KP, Twickler DM, et al. Coarctation of the abdominal aorta in pregnancy: Diagnosis by magnetic resonance imaging. *Obstet Gynecol* 1995;85(5 Pt 2):817–819.

90. Dessole S, D'Antona D, Ambrosini G, et al. Pregnancy and delivery in young woman affected by isthmic coarctation of the aorta. *Arch Gynecol Obstet* 2000;263(3):145–147.

91. Lip GY, Singh SP, Beevers DG. Aortic coarctation diagnosed after hypertension in pregnancy. *Am J Obstet Gynecol* 1998;179(3 Pt 1):814–815.

92. Venning S, Freeman LJ, Stanley K. Two cases of pregnancy with coarctation of the aorta. *J R Soc Med* 2003;96(5):234–236.

93. Singh BM, Kriplani A, Bhatla N. Vaginal delivery in a woman with uncorrected coarctation of aorta. *J Obstet Gynaecol Res* 2004;30(1):24–26.

94. Manullang TR, Chun K, Egan TD. The use of remifentanil for cesarean section in a parturient with recurrent aortic coarctation. *Can J Anaesth* 2000;47(5):454–459.

95. Vriend JW, van Montfrans GA, van der Post JA, et al. An unusual cause of hypertension in pregnancy. *Hypertens Pregnancy* 2004;23(1):13–17.

96. Avanzas P, Garcia-Fernandez MA, Quiles J, et al. Pseudoaneurysm complicating aortic coarctation in a pregnant woman. *Int J Cardiol* 2004;97(1):157–158.

97. Walker E, Malins AF. Anaesthetic management of aortic coarctation in pregnancy. *Int J Obstet Anesth* 2004;13(4):266–270.

98. Cohen LS, Friedman WF, Braunwald E. Natural history of mild congenital aortic stenosis elucidated by serial hemodynamic studies. *Am J Cardiol* 1972;30(1):1–5.

99. Pansegrau DG, Kioshos JM, Durnin RE, et al. Supravalvular aortic stenosis in adults. *Am J Cardiol* 1973;31(5):635–641.

100. Parker BM. The course in idiopathic hypertrophic muscular subaortic stenosis. *Ann Intern Med* 1969;70(5):903–911.

101. Aboulhosn J, Child JS. Left ventricular outflow obstruction: Subaortic stenosis, bicuspid aortic valve, supravalvar aortic stenosis, and coarctation of the aorta. *Circulation* 2006;114(22):2412–2422.

102. Varghese PJ, Izukawa T, Rowe RD. Supravalvular aortic stenosis as part of rubella syndrome, with discussion of pathogenesis. *Br Heart J* 1969;31(1):59–62.

103. Roberts WC. The congenitally bicuspid aortic valve. A study of 85 autopsy cases. *Am J Cardiol* 1970;26(1):72–83.

104. Basso C, Boschello M, Perrone C, et al. An echocardiographic survey of primary school children for bicuspid aortic valve. *Am J Cardiol* 2004;93(5):661–663.

105. Siu SC, Silversides CK. Bicuspid aortic valve disease. *J Am Coll Cardiol* 2010;55(25):2789–2800.

106. Tzemos N, Silversides CK, Colman JM, et al. Late cardiac outcomes after pregnancy in women with congenital aortic stenosis. *Am Heart J* 2009;157(3):474–480.

107. Yap SC, Drenthen W, Pieper PG, et al. Risk of complications during pregnancy in women with congenital aortic stenosis. *Int J Cardiol* 2008;126(2):240–246.

108. Silversides CK, Colman JM, Sermer M, et al. Early and intermediate-term outcomes of pregnancy with congenital aortic stenosis. *Am J Cardiol* 2003;91(11):1386–1389.

109. Brickner ME, Hillis LD, Lange RA. Congenital heart disease in adults. First of two parts. *N Engl J Med* 2000;342(4):256–263.

110. Drenthen W, Pieper PG, Roos-Hesselink JW, et al. Non-cardiac complications during pregnancy in women with isolated congenital pulmonary valvar stenosis. *Heart* 2006;92(12):1838–1843.

111. Bentivoglio LG, Maranhao V, Downing DF. The electrocardiogram in pulmonary stenosis with intact septa. *Am Heart J* 1960;59:347–357.

112. Cayler GG, Ongley P, Nadas AS. Relation of systolic pressure in the right ventricle to the electrocardiogram; a study of patients with pulmonary stenosis and intact ventricular septum. *N Engl J Med* 1958;258(20):979–982.

113. Moller I, Wennevold A, Lyngborg KE. The natural history of pulmonary stenosis. Long-term follow-up with serial heart catheterizations. *Cardiology* 1973;58(4):193–202.

114. Campbell N, Rosaeg OP, Chan KL. Anaesthetic management of a parturient with pulmonary stenosis and aortic incompetence for caesarean section. *Br J Anaesth* 2003;90(2):241–243.

115. Autore C, Brauneis S, Apponi F, et al. Epidural anesthesia for cesarean section in patients with hypertrophic cardiomyopathy: A report of three cases. *Anesthesiology* 1999;90(4):1205–1207.

116. Tessler MJ, Hudson R, Naugler-Colville M, et al. Pulmonary oedema in two parturients with hypertrophic obstructive cardiomyopathy (HOCM). *Can J Anaesth* 1990;37(4 Pt 1):469–473.

117. Hurst J. *The Heart.* 4th ed. New York: McGraw-Hill; 1978.

118. Sonnenblick E, Lesch M. *Valvular Heart Disease.* New York: Grune & Stratton; 1974.

119. Spagnuolo M, Pasternack B, Taranta A. Risk of rheumatic-fever recurrences after streptococcal infections. Prospective study of clinical and social factors. *N Engl J Med* 1971;285(12):641–647.

120. Jones T. The diagnosis of rheumatic fever. *JAMA* 1944;126:481–484.

121. Seaworth BJ, Durack DT. Infective endocarditis in obstetric and gynecologic practice. *Am J Obstet Gynecol* 1986;154(1):180–188.

122. Cox SM, Leveno KJ. Pregnancy complicated by bacterial endocarditis. *Clin Obstet Gynecol* 1989;32(1):48–53.

123. al Kasab SM, Sabag T, al Zaibag M, et al. Beta-adrenergic receptor blockade in the management of pregnant women with mitral stenosis. *Am J Obstet Gynecol* 1990;163(1 Pt 1):37–40.

124. Ziskind Z, Etchin A, Frenkel Y, et al. Epidural anesthesia with the Trendelenburg position for cesarean section with or without a cardiac surgical procedure in patients with severe mitral stenosis: A hemodynamic study. *J Cardiothorac Anesth* 1990;4(3):354–359.

125. Baumgartner H, Hung J, Bermejo J, et al. Echocardiographic assessment of valve stenosis: EAE/ASE recommendations for clinical practice. *J Am Soc Echocardiogr* 2009;22(1):1–23; quiz 101–102.

126. Rahimtoola SH. The year in valvular heart disease. *J Am Coll Cardiol* 2006;47(2):427–439.

127. Clark SL, Phelan JP, Greenspoon J, et al. Labor and delivery in the presence of mitral stenosis: Central hemodynamic observations. *Am J Obstet Gynecol* 1985;152(8):984–988.

128. Hamlyn EL, Douglass CA, Plaat F, et al. Low-dose sequential combined spinal-epidural: An anaesthetic technique for caesarean section in patients with significant cardiac disease. *Int J Obstet Anesth* 2005;14(4):355–361.

129. Gomar C, Errando CL. Neuroaxial anaesthesia in obstetrical patients with cardiac disease. *Curr Opin Anaesthesiol* 2005;18(5):507–512.

130. Rapaport E. Natural history of aortic and mitral valve disease. *Am J Cardiol* 1975;35(2):221–227.

131. Zoghbi WA, Enriquez-Sarano M, Foster E, et al. Recommendations for evaluation of the severity of native valvular regurgitation with two-dimensional and Doppler echocardiography. *J Am Soc Echocardiogr* 2003;16(7):777–802.

132. Bonow RO, Carabello BA, Chatterjee K, et al. 2008 focused update incorporated into the ACC/AHA 2006 guidelines for the management of patients with valvular heart disease: A report of the American College of Cardiology/American Heart Association Task Force on Practice Guidelines (Writing Committee to Revise the 1998 Guidelines for the Management Of Patients With Valvular Heart Disease): Endorsed by the Society of Cardiovascular Anesthesiologists, Society for Cardiovascular Angiography and Interventions, and Society of Thoracic Surgeons. *Circulation* 2008;118(15):e523–e661.

133. Naidoo DP, Desai DK, Moodley J. Maternal deaths due to pre-existing cardiac disease. *Cardiovasc J S Afr* 2002;13(1):17–20.

134. Hustead ST, Quick A, Gibbs HR, et al. "Pseudo-critical" aortic stenosis during pregnancy: Role for Doppler assessment of aortic valve area. *Am Heart J* 1989;117(6):1383–1385.

135. Chuang ML, Parker RA, Riley MF, et al. Three-dimensional echocardiography improves accuracy and compensates for sonographer inexperience in assessment of left ventricular ejection fraction. *J Am Soc Echocardiogr* 1999;12(5):290–299.

136. Brian JE Jr, Seifen AB, Clark RB, et al. Aortic stenosis, cesarean delivery, and epidural anesthesia. *J Clin Anesth* 1993;5(2):154–157.

137. Colclough GW, Ackerman WE 3rd, Walmsley PN, et al. Epidural anesthesia for cesarean delivery in a parturient with aortic stenosis. *Reg Anesth* 1990;15(5):273–274.

138. Pittard A, Vucevic M. Regional anaesthesia with a subarachnoid microcatheter for caesarean section in a parturient with aortic stenosis. *Anaesthesia* 1998;53(2):169–173.

139. Ioscovich AM, Goldszmidt E, Fadeev AV, et al. Peripartum anesthetic management of patients with aortic valve stenosis: A retrospective study and literature review. *Int J Obstet Anesth* 2009;18(4):379–386.

140. Yentis SM, Dob DP. Caesarean section in the presence of aortic stenosis. *Anaesthesia* 1998;53(6):606–607.

141. Goertz AW, Lindner KH, Schutz W, et al. Influence of phenylephrine bolus administration on left ventricular filling dynamics in patients with coronary artery disease and patients with valvular aortic stenosis. *Anesthesiology* 1994;81(1):49–58.

142. Torsher LC, Shub C, Rettke SR, et al. Risk of patients with severe aortic stenosis undergoing noncardiac surgery. *Am J Cardiol* 1998;81(4):448–452.

143. Roth A, Elkayam U. Acute myocardial infarction associated with pregnancy. *Ann Intern Med* 1996;125(9):751–762.

144. James AH, Jamison MG, Biswas MS, et al. Acute myocardial infarction in pregnancy: A United States population-based study. *Circulation* 2006;113(12):1564–1571.

145. Roth A, Elkayam U. Acute myocardial infarction associated with pregnancy. *J Am Coll Cardiol* 2008;52(3):171–180.

146. Lewis CE, Funkhouser E, Raczynski JM, et al. Adverse effect of pregnancy on high density lipoprotein (HDL) cholesterol in young adult women. The CARDIA study. Coronary artery risk development in young adults. *Am J Epidemiol* 1996;144(3):247–254.

147. Elkayam U . Pregnancy and cardiovascular disease. In: Zipes DP, Libby P, Bonow RO, Braunwald E, eds. *Braunwald's Heart Disease: A textbook of Cardiovascular Medicine*. Philadelphia, PA: WB Saunders; 2005:1965–1983].

148. Shade GH Jr, Ross G, Bever FN, et al. Troponin I in the diagnosis of acute myocardial infarction in pregnancy, labor, and post partum. *Am J Obstet Gynecol* 2002;187(6):1719–1720.

149. Carpenter MW, Sady SP, Hoegsberg B, et al. Fetal heart rate response to maternal exertion. *JAMA* 1988;259(20):3006–3009.

150. Collins JS, Bossone E, Eagle KA, et al. Asymptomatic coronary artery disease in a pregnant patient. A case report and review of literature. *Herz* 2002;27(6):548–554.

151. Koul AK, Hollander G, Moskovits N, et al. Coronary artery dissection during pregnancy and the postpartum period: Two case reports and review of literature. *Catheter Cardiovasc Interv* 2001;52(1):88–94.

152. Heefner WA. Dissecting hematoma of the coronary artery. A possible complication of oral contraceptive therapy. *JAMA* 1973;223(5):550–551.

153. Lawal L, Lange R, Schulman S. Acute myocardial infarction in two young women without significant risk factors. *J Invasive Cardiol* 2009;21(1):E3–E5.

154. Skelding KA, Hubbard CR. Spontaneous coronary artery dissection related to menstruation. *J Invasive Cardiol* 2007;19(6):E174–E177.

155. Turrentine MA, Braems G, Ramirez MM. Use of thrombolytics for the treatment of thromboembolic disease during pregnancy. *Obstet Gynecol Surv* 1995;50(7):534–541.

156. Task Force on the Management of Cardiovascular Diseases During Pregnancy of the European Society of Cardiology. Expert consensus document on management of cardiovascular diseases during pregnancy. *Eur Heart J* 2003;24(8):761–781.

157. Chambers CE, Clark SL. Cardiac surgery during pregnancy. *Clin Obstet Gynecol* 1994;37(2):316–323.

158. Parry AJ, Westaby S. Cardiopulmonary bypass during pregnancy. *Ann Thorac Surg* 1996;61(6):1865–1869.

159. Pomini F, Mercogliano D, Cavalletti C, et al. Cardiopulmonary bypass in pregnancy. *Ann Thorac Surg* 1996;61(1):259–268.

160. Weiss BM, von Segesser LK, Alon E, et al. Outcome of cardiovascular surgery and pregnancy: A systematic review of the period 1984–1996. *Am J Obstet Gynecol* 1998;179(6 Pt 1):1643–1653.

161. Karahan N, Ozturk T, Yetkin U, et al. Managing severe heart failure in a pregnant patient undergoing cardiopulmonary bypass: Case report and review of the literature. *J Cardiothorac Vasc Anesth* 2004;18(3):339–343.

162. Iscan ZH, Mavioglu L, Vural KM, et al. Cardiac surgery during pregnancy. *J Heart Valve Dis* 2006;15(5):686–690.

163. Dufour P, Berard J, Vinatier D, et al. Pregnancy after myocardial infarction and a coronary artery bypass graft. *Arch Gynecol Obstet* 1997;259(4):209–213.

164. Cunningham FG, Pritchard JA, Hankins GD, et al. Peripartum heart failure: Idiopathic cardiomyopathy or compounding cardiovascular events? *Obstet Gynecol* 1986;67(2):157–168.

165. Melvin KR, Richardson PJ, Olsen EG, et al. Peripartum cardiomyopathy due to myocarditis. *N Engl J Med* 1982;307(12):731–734.

166. Hilfiker-Kleiner D, Sliwa K, Drexler H. Peripartum cardiomyopathy: Recent insights in its pathophysiology. *Trends Cardiovasc Med* 2008;18(5):173–179.

167. Lamparter S, Pankuweit S, Maisch B. Clinical and immunologic characteristics in peripartum cardiomyopathy. *Int J Cardiol* 2007;118(1):14–20.

168. Mastrobattista JM. Angiotensin converting enzyme inhibitors in pregnancy. *Semin Perinatol* 1997;21(2):124–134.

169. Bozkurt B, Villanueva FS, Holubkov R, et al. Intravenous immune globulin in the therapy of peripartum cardiomyopathy. *J Am Coll Cardiol* 1999;34(1):177–180.

170. VanHelder T, Smedstad KG. Combined spinal epidural anaesthesia in a primigravida with valvular heart disease. *Can J Anaesth* 1998;45(5 Pt 1):488–490.

171. Kaufman I, Bondy R, Benjamin A. Peripartum cardiomyopathy and thromboembolism; anesthetic management and clinical course of an obese, diabetic patient. *Can J Anaesth* 2003;50(2):161–165.

172. Pearson GD, Veille JC, Rahimtoola S, et al. Peripartum cardiomyopathy: National heart, Lung, and Blood Institute and Office of Rare Diseases (National Institutes of Health) workshop recommendations and review. *JAMA* 2000;283(9):1183–1188.

173. Horlocker TT, Wedel DJ, Rowlingson JC, et al. Regional anesthesia in the patient receiving antithrombotic or thrombolytic therapy: American Society of Regional Anesthesia and Pain Medicine Evidence-Based Guidelines (Third Edition). *Reg Anesth Pain Med* 2010;35(1):64–101.

174. Sliwa K, Fett J, Elkayam U. Peripartum cardiomyopathy. *Lancet* 2006;368(9536):687–693.

175. Goland S, Modi K, Bitar F, et al. Clinical profile and predictors of complications in peripartum cardiomyopathy. *J Card Fail* 2009;15(8):645–650.

176. Chapa JB, Heiberger HB, Weinert L, et al. Prognostic value of echocardiography in peripartum cardiomyopathy. *Obstet Gynecol* 2005;105(6):1303–1308.

177. Lampert MB, Weinert L, Hibbard J, et al. Contractile reserve in patients with peripartum cardiomyopathy and recovered left ventricular function. *Am J Obstet Gynecol* 1997;176(1 Pt 1):189–195.

178. Elkayam U, Akhter MW, Singh H, et al. Pregnancy-associated cardiomyopathy: Clinical characteristics and a comparison between early and late presentation. *Circulation* 2005;111(16):2050–2055.

179. Elkayam U, Tummala PP, Rao K, et al. Maternal and fetal outcomes of subsequent pregnancies in women with peripartum cardiomyopathy. *N Engl J Med* 2001;344(21):1567–1571.

180. Fett JD, Carraway RD, Dowell DL, et al. Peripartum cardiomyopathy in the Hospital Albert Schweitzer District of Haiti. *Am J Obstet Gynecol* 2002;186(5):1005–1010.

181. de Souza JL Jr, de Carvalho Frimm C, Nastari L, et al. Left ventricular function after a new pregnancy in patients with peripartum cardiomyopathy. *J Card Fail* 2001;7(1):30–35.

182. Fett JD, Fristoe KL, Welsh SN. Risk of heart failure relapse in subsequent pregnancy among peripartum cardiomyopathy mothers. *Int J Gynaecol Obstet* 2010;109(1):34–36.

183. Immer FF, Bansi AG, Immer-Bansi AS, et al. Aortic dissection in pregnancy: Analysis of risk factors and outcome. *Ann Thorac Surg* 2003;76(1):309–314.

184. Mandel W, Evans EW, Walford RL. Dissecting aortic aneurysm during pregnancy. *N Engl J Med* 1954;251(26):1059–1061.

185. Pedowitz P, Perell A. Aneurysms complicated by pregnancy. I. Aneurysms of the aorta and its major branches. *Am J Obstet Gynecol* 1957;73(4):720–735.

186. Lipscomb KJ, Smith JC, Clarke B, et al. Outcome of pregnancy in women with Marfan's syndrome. *Br J Obstet Gynaecol* 1997;104(2):201–206.

187. Rossiter JP, Repke JT, Morales AJ, et al. A prospective longitudinal evaluation of pregnancy in the Marfan syndrome. *Am J Obstet Gynecol* 1995;173(5):1599–1606.

188. Harris IS. Management of pregnancy in patients with congenital heart disease. *Prog Cardiovasc Dis* 2011;53(4):305–311.

189. Plunkett MD, Bond LM, Geiss DM. Staged repair of acute type I aortic dissection and coarctation in pregnancy. *Ann Thorac Surg* 2000;69(6):1945–1947.

190. Robinson R. Aortic aneurysm in pregnancy: A case study. *Dimens Crit Care Nurs* 2005;24(1):21–24.

191. Manalo-Estrella P, Barker AE. Histopathologic findings in human aortic media associated with pregnancy. *Arch Pathol* 1967;83(4):336–341.

192. Wheat MW. Intensive drug therapy. In: Dorghazi S, ed. *Aortic Dissection*. New York, NY: McGraw-Hill; 1983:55–60.

193. Nistri S, Sorbo MD, Basso C, et al. Bicuspid aortic valve: Abnormal aortic elastic properties. *J Heart Valve Dis* 2002;11(3):369–373; discussion 373–374.

194. Zeebregts CJ, Schepens MA, Hameeteman TM, et al. Acute aortic dissection complicating pregnancy. *Ann Thorac Surg* 1997;64(5):1345–1348.

195. Khan IA, Nair CK. Clinical, diagnostic, and management perspectives of aortic dissection. *Chest* 2002;122(1):311–328.

196. Briggs GG, Freeman RK, Yaffe SJ .Drugs in pregnancy and lactation. A Reference Guide to Fetal and Neonatal Risk. 4th edn. Baltimore, MD: Williams and Wilkins; 1994:808–813.

197. Skeehan TM, Cooper JR. Anesthetic management for thoracic aneurysms and dissections. In: Hensely FA, Martin DE, Graylee GP, eds. *A Practical Approach to Cardiac Anesthesia*.3rd edn. Philadelphia, PA: Lippincott Williams & Williams; 2003:624–625.

198. Lacassie HJ, Millar S, Leithe LG, et al. Dural ectasia: A likely cause of inadequate spinal anaesthesia in two parturients with Marfan's syndrome. *Br J Anaesth* 2005;94(4):500–504.

199. Ioscovich A, Elstein D. Images in anesthesia: Transesophageal echocardiography during cesarean section in a Marfan's patient with aortic dissection. *Can J Anaesth* 2005;52(7):737–738.

200. Singh SI, Brooks C, Dobkowski W. General anesthesia using remifentanil for cesarean delivery in a parturient with Marfan's syndrome. *Can J Anaesth* 2008;55(8):526–531.

201. Gelpi G, Pettinari M, Lemma M, et al. Should pregnancy be considered a risk factor for aortic dissection? Two cases of acute aortic dissection following cesarean section in non-Marfan nor bicuspid aortic valve patients. *J Cardiovasc Surg (Torino)* 2008;49(3):389–391.

202. Anderson RA, Fineron PW. Aortic dissection in pregnancy: Importance of pregnancy-induced changes in the vessel wall and bicuspid aortic valve in pathogenesis. *Br J Obstet Gynaecol* 1994;101(12):1085–1088.

203. Meijboom LJ, Vos FE, Timmermans J, et al. Pregnancy and aortic root growth in the Marfan syndrome: A prospective study. *Eur Heart J* 2005;26(9):914–920.

204. Ghamra ZW, Dweik RA. Primary pulmonary hypertension: An overview of epidemiology and pathogenesis. *Cleve Clin J Med* 2003;70(Suppl 1):S2–S8.

205. Runo JR, Loyd JE. Primary pulmonary hypertension. *Lancet* 2003;361(9368):1533–1544.

206. Galie N, Manes A, Uguccioni L, et al. Primary pulmonary hypertension: Insights into pathogenesis from epidemiology. *Chest* 1998;114(3 Suppl):184S–194S.

207. Rich S, Dantzker DR, Ayres SM, et al. Primary pulmonary hypertension. A national prospective study. *Ann Intern Med* 1987;107(2):216–223.

208. Bonnin M, Mercier FJ, Sitbon O, et al. Severe pulmonary hypertension during pregnancy: Mode of delivery and anesthetic management of 15 consecutive cases. *Anesthesiology* 2005;102(6):1133–1137; discussion 5A–6A.

209. Smedstad KG, Cramb R, Morison DH. Pulmonary hypertension and pregnancy: A series of eight cases. *Can J Anaesth* 1994;41(6):502–512.

210. Nootens M, Rich S. Successful management of labor and delivery in primary pulmonary hypertension. *Am J Cardiol* 1993;71(12):1124–1125.

211. O'Hare R, McLoughlin C, Milligan K, et al. Anaesthesia for caesarean section in the presence of severe primary pulmonary hypertension. *Br J Anaesth* 1998;81(5):790–792.

212. Monnery L, Nanson J, Charlton G. Primary pulmonary hypertension in pregnancy; a role for novel vasodilators. *Br J Anaesth* 2001;87(2):295–298.

213. Stewart R, Tuazon D, Olson G, et al. Pregnancy and primary pulmonary hypertension : Successful outcome with epoprostenol therapy. *Chest* 2001;119(3):973–975.

214. Weiss BM, Maggiorini M, Jenni R, et al. Pregnant patient with primary pulmonary hypertension: Inhaled pulmonary vasodilators and epidural anesthesia for cesarean delivery. *Anesthesiology* 2000;92(4):1191–1194.

215. Decoene C, Bourzoufi K, Moreau D, et al. Use of inhaled nitric oxide for emergency cesarean section in a woman with unexpected primary pulmonary hypertension. *Can J Anaesth* 2001;48(6):584–587.

216. Wong PS, Constantinides S, Kanellopoulos V, et al. Primary pulmonary hypertension in pregnancy. *J R Soc Med* 2001;94(10):523–525.

217. Kiss H, Egarter C, Asseryanis E, et al. Primary pulmonary hypertension in pregnancy: A case report. *Am J Obstet Gynecol* 1995;172(3):1052–1054.

218. Olofsson C, Bremme K, Forssell G, et al. Cesarean section under epidural ropivacaine 0.75% in a parturient with severe pulmonary hypertension. *Acta Anaesthesiol Scand* 2001;45(2):258–260.

219. Tacoy G, Ekim NN, Cengel A. Dramatic response of a patient with pregnancy induced idiopathic pulmonary arterial hypertension to sildenafil treatment. *J Obstet Gynaecol Res* 2010;36(2):414–417.

220. Tromp CH, Nanne AC, Pernet PJ, et al. Electrical cardioversion during pregnancy: Safe or not? *Neth Heart J* 2011;19(3):134–136.

221. Gowda RM, Khan IA, Mehta NJ, et al. Cardiac arrhythmias in pregnancy: Clinical and therapeutic considerations. *Int J Cardiol* 2003;88(2–3):129–133.

222. Page RL. Treatment of arrhythmias during pregnancy. *Am Heart J* 1995;130(4):871–876.

223. Yachimski P, Lilly LS. Valvular heart disease. In: Lilly L, ed. Pathophysiology of heart disease. Baltimore, MD: Lippincott Williams & Wilkins; 2003:195–202.

224. Trappe HJ. Acute therapy of maternal and fetal arrhythmias during pregnancy. *J Intensive Care Med* 2006;21(5):305–315.

225. Kron J, Conti JB. Arrhythmias in the pregnant patient: Current concepts in evaluation and management. *J Interv Card Electrophysiol* 2007;19(2):95–107.

226. Qasqas SA, McPherson C, Frishman WH, et al. Cardiovascular pharmacotherapeutic considerations during pregnancy and lactation. *Cardiol Rev* 2004;12(4):201–221.

227. Stoelting PK, Dierdorf SF, McCammon RL. Anesthesia and co-existing disease. 2nd edn. New York, NY: Churchill Livingstone; 1988.

228. Hughes SC, Levinson G, Rosen MA. Schnider and Levinson's anesthesia for obstetrics. Baltimore, MD: Lippincott Williams & Wilkins; 2001.

229. Chow T, Galvin J, McGovern B. Antiarrhythmic drug therapy in pregnancy and lactation. *Am J Cardiol* 1998;82(4A):58I–62I.

230. Burkart TA, Conti JB. Cardiac arrhythmias during pregnancy. *Curr Treat Options Cardiovasc Med* 2010;12(5):457–471.

231. Padosch SA, Milde AS, Martin E, et al. Thrombolytic therapy during cardiopulmonary resuscitation–is the initial cardiac rhythm a critical issue? *Acta Anaesthesiol Scand* 2002;46(5):620–621.

232. Beckmann CRB. *Obstetrics and Gynecology.* Baltimore, MD: Lippincott Williams & Wilkins; 2002.

233. Brown O. Direct current cardioversion during pregnancy. *BJOG* 2003;110(7):713–714.

234. Barnes EJ, Eben F, Patterson D. Direct current cardioversion during pregnancy should be performed with facilities available for fetal monitoring and emergency caesarean section. *BJOG* 2002;109(12):1406–1407.

235. Rotmensch HH, Rotmensch S, Elkayam U. Management of cardiac arrhythmias during pregnancy. Current concepts. *Drugs* 1987;33(6):623–633.

236. John AS, Gurley F, Schaff HV, et al. Cardiopulmonary bypass during pregnancy. *Ann Thorac Surg* 2011;91(4):1191–1196.

237. Barth WH Jr. Cardiac surgery in pregnancy. *Clin Obstet Gynecol* 2009;52(4):630–646.

238. Lowenstein BR, Vain NW, Perrone SV, et al. Successful pregnancy and vaginal delivery after heart transplantation. *Am J Obstet Gynecol* 1988;158(3 Pt 1):589–590.

239. McKay DB, Josephson MA, Armenti VT, et al. Reproduction and transplantation: Report on the AST consensus conference on reproductive issues and transplantation. *Am J Transplant* 2005;5(7):1592–1599.

240. Armenti VT, Radomski JS, Moritz MJ, et al. Report from the National Transplantation Pregnancy Registry (NTPR): Outcomes of pregnancy after transplantation. *Clin Transpl* 2004:103–114.

241. EBPG Expert Group on Renal Transplantation. European best practice guidelines for renal transplantation. Section IV: Long-term management of the transplant recipient. IV.10. Pregnancy in renal transplant recipients. *Nephrol Dial Transplant* 2002;17(Suppl 4):50–55.

242. Cardonick E, Moritz M, Armenti V. Pregnancy in patients with organ transplantation: A review. *Obstet Gynecol Surv* 2004;59(3):214–222.

243. Mastrobattista JM, Katz AR. Pregnancy after organ transplant. *Obstet Gynecol Clin North Am* 2004;31(2):415–428, vii.

244. Kostopanagiotou G, Smyrniotis V, Arkadopoulos N, et al. Anesthetic and perioperative management of adult transplant recipients in nontransplant surgery. *Anesth Analg* 1999;89(3):613–622.

245. Sivaraman P. Management of pregnancy in transplant recipients. *Transplant Proc* 2004;36(7):1999–2000.

246. Lomenick JP, Jackson WA, Backeljauw PF. Amiodarone-induced neonatal hypothyroidism: A unique form of transient early-onset hypothyroidism. *J Perinatol* 2004;24(6):397–399.

247. Magee LA, Downar E, Sermer M, et al. Pregnancy outcome after gestational exposure to amiodarone in Canada. *Am J Obstet Gynecol* 1995;172(4 Pt 1):1307–1311.

248. Fagih B, Sami M. Safety of antiarrhythmics during pregnancy: Case report and review of the literature. *Can J Cardiol* 1999;15(1):113–117.

249. Frishman WH, Chesner M. Beta-adrenergic blockers in pregnancy. *Am Heart J* 1988;115(1 Pt 1):147–152.

250. Magee LA, Elran E, Bull SB, et al. Risks and benefits of beta-receptor blockers for pregnancy hypertension: Overview of the randomized trials. *Eur J Obstet Gynecol Reprod Biol* 2000;88(1):15–26.

251. Pickles CJ, Symonds EM, Broughton Pipkin F. The fetal outcome in a randomized double-blind controlled trial of labetalol versus placebo in pregnancy-induced hypertension. *Br J Obstet Gynaecol* 1989;96(1):38–43.

252. el-Qarmalawi AM, Morsy AH, al-Fadly A, et al. Labetalol vs. methyldopa in the treatment of pregnancy-induced hypertension. *Int J Gynaecol Obstet* 1995;49(2):125–130.

253. Michael CA. Intravenous labetalol and intravenous diazoxide in severe hypertension complicating pregnancy. *Aust N Z J Obstet Gynaecol* 1986;26(1):26–29.

254. Macpherson M, Broughton Pipkin F, Rutter N. The effect of maternal labetalol on the newborn infant. *Br J Obstet Gynaecol* 1986;93(6):539–542.

255. Ostman PL, Chestnut DH, Robillard JE, et al. Transplacental passage and hemodynamic effects of esmolol in the gravid ewe. *Anesthesiology* 1988;69(5):738–741.

256. Eisenach JC, Castro MI. Maternally administered esmolol produces fetal beta-adrenergic blockade and hypoxemia in sheep. *Anesthesiology* 1989;71(5):718–722.

257. Ducey JP, Knape KG. Maternal esmolol administration resulting in fetal distress and cesarean section in a term pregnancy. *Anesthesiology* 1992;77(4):829–832.

258. Elatrous S, Nouira S, Ouanes Besbes L, et al. Short-term treatment of severe hypertension of pregnancy: Prospective comparison of nicardipine and labetalol. *Intensive Care Med* 2002;28(9):1281–1286.

259. Hanff LM, Vulto AG, Bartels PA, et al. Intravenous use of the calcium-channel blocker nicardipine as second-line treatment in severe, early-onset pre-eclamptic patients. *J Hypertens* 2005;23(12):2319–2326.

260. Magee LA, Schick B, Donnenfeld AE, et al. The safety of calcium channel blockers in human pregnancy: A prospective, multicenter cohort study. *Am J Obstet Gynecol* 1996;174(3):823–828.

261. Weber-Schoendorfer C, Hannemann D, Meister R, et al. The safety of calcium channel blockers during pregnancy: A prospective, multicenter, observational study. *Reprod Toxicol* 2008;26(1):24–30.

262. Aya AG, Mangin R, Hoffet M, et al. Intravenous nicardipine for severe hypertension in pre-eclampsia–effects of an acute treatment on mother and foetus. *Intensive Care Med* 1999;25(11):1277–1281.

263. Bartels PA, Hanff LM, Mathot RA, et al. Nicardipine in pre-eclamptic patients: Placental transfer and disposition in breast milk. *BJOG* 2007;114(2):230–233.

264. Vaast P, Dubreucq-Fossaert S, Houfflin-Debarge V, et al. Acute pulmonary oedema during nicardipine therapy for premature labour; report of five cases. *Eur J Obstet Gynecol Reprod Biol* 2004;113(1):98–99.

265. Oei SG. Calcium channel blockers for tocolysis: A review of their role and safety following reports of serious adverse events. *Eur J Obstet Gynecol Reprod Biol* 2006;126(2):137–145.

266. Klein V, Repke JT. Supraventricular tachycardia in pregnancy: Cardioversion with verapamil. *Obstet Gynecol* 1984;63(3 Suppl):16S–18S.

267. Byerly WG, Hartmann A, Foster DE, et al. Verapamil in the treatment of maternal paroxysmal supraventricular tachycardia. *Ann Emerg Med* 1991;20(5):552–554.

268. Joglar JA, Page RL. Antiarrhythmic drugs in pregnancy. *Curr Opin Cardiol* 2001;16(1):40–45.

269. Magee LA, Cham C, Waterman EJ, et al. Hydralazine for treatment of severe hypertension in pregnancy: Meta-analysis. *BMJ* 2003;327(7421):955–960.

270. Vigil-De Gracia P, Lasso M, Ruiz E, et al. Severe hypertension in pregnancy: Hydralazine or labetalol. A randomized clinical trial. *Eur J Obstet Gynecol Reprod Biol* 2006;128(1–2):157–162.

271. Vigil-De Gracia P, Ruiz E, Lopez JC, et al. Management of severe hypertension in the postpartum period with intravenous hydralazine or labetalol: A randomized clinical trial. *Hypertens Pregnancy* 2007;26(2):163–171.

272. Bootstaylor BS, Roman C, Parer JT, et al. Fetal and maternal hemodynamic and metabolic effects of maternal nitroglycerin infusions in sheep. *Am J Obstet Gynecol* 1997;176(3):644–650.

273. Mercier FJ, Dounas M, Bouaziz H, et al. Intravenous nitroglycerin to relieve intrapartum fetal distress related to uterine hyperactivity: A prospective observational study. *Anesth Analg* 1997;84(5):1117–1120.

274. Dayan SS, Schwalbe SS. The use of small-dose intravenous nitroglycerin in a case of uterine inversion. *Anesth Analg* 1996;82(5):1091–1093.

275. Elkayam U, Goodwin TM. Adenosine therapy for supraventricular tachycardia during pregnancy. *Am J Cardiol* 1995;75(7):521–523.

276. Mason BA, Ogunyemi D, Punla O, et al. Maternal and fetal cardiorespiratory responses to adenosine in sheep. *Am J Obstet Gynecol* 1993;168(5):1558–1561.

277. Ngan Kee WD, Khaw KS, Tan PE, et al. Placental transfer and fetal metabolic effects of phenylephrine and ephedrine during spinal anesthesia for cesarean delivery. *Anesthesiology* 2009;111(3):506–512.

278. Ngan Kee WD, Khaw KS. Vasopressors in obstetrics: What should we be using? *Curr Opin Anaesthesiol* 2006;19(3):238–243.

279. Lee A, Ngan Kee WD, Gin T. A quantitative, systematic review of randomized controlled trials of ephedrine versus phenylephrine for the management of hypotension during spinal anesthesia for cesarean delivery. *Anesth Analg* 2002;94(4):920–926, table of contents.

280. Ngan Kee WD, Lee A, Khaw KS, et al. A randomized double-blinded comparison of phenylephrine and ephedrine infusion combinations to maintain blood pressure during spinal anesthesia for cesarean delivery: The effects on fetal acid-base status and hemodynamic control. *Anesth Analg* 2008;107(4):1295–1302.

281. Ngan Kee WD, Khaw KS, Lau TK, et al. Randomised double-blinded comparison of phenylephrine vs ephedrine for maintaining blood pressure during spinal anaesthesia for non-elective caesarean section*. *Anaesthesia* 2008;63(12):1319–1326.

282. Dyer RA, Reed AR, van Dyk D, et al. Hemodynamic effects of ephedrine, phenylephrine, and the coadministration of phenylephrine with oxytocin during spinal anesthesia for elective cesarean delivery. *Anesthesiology* 2009;111(4):753–765.

283. Cooper DW, Jeyaraj L, Hynd R, et al. Evidence that intravenous vasopressors can affect rostral spread of spinal anesthesia in pregnancy. *Anesthesiology* 2004;101(1):28–33.

284. Ngan Kee WD, Lau TK, Khaw KS, et al. Comparison of metaraminol and ephedrine infusions for maintaining arterial pressure during spinal anesthesia for elective cesarean section. *Anesthesiology* 2001;95(2):307–313.

285. Hasaart TH, de Haan J. Effect of continuous infusion of norepinephrine on maternal pelvic and fetal umbilical blood flow in pregnant sheep. *J Perinat Med* 1986;14(4):211–218.

286. Marcus MA, Gogarten W, Vertommen JD, et al. Haemodynamic effects of repeated epidural test-doses of adrenaline in the chronic maternal-fetal sheep preparation. *Eur J Anaesthesiol* 1998;15(3):320–323.

287. Marcus MA, Vertommen JD, Van Aken H, et al. Hemodynamic effects of intravenous isoproterenol versus epinephrine in the chronic maternal-fetal sheep preparation. *Anesth Analg* 1996;82(5):1023–1026.

288. Hood DD, Dewan DM, James FM 3rd. Maternal and fetal effects of epinephrine in gravid ewes. *Anesthesiology* 1986;64(5):610–613.

289. Norris MC, Arkoosh VA, Knobler R. Maternal and fetal effects of isoproterenol in the gravid ewe. *Anesth Analg* 1997;85(2):389–394.

290. Marcus MA, Vertommen JD, Van Aken H, et al. Hemodynamic effects of intravenous isoproterenol versus saline in the parturient. *Anesth Analg* 1997;84(5):1113–1116.

291. Krasnow N, Rolett EL, Yurchak PM, et al. Isoproterenol and cardiovascular performance. *Am J Med* 1964;37:514–525.

292. Mahon WA, Reid DW, Day RA. The in vivo effects of beta adrenergic stimulation and blockade on the human uterus at term. *J Pharmacol Exp Ther* 1967;156(1):178–185.

293. Blanchard K, Dandavino A, Nuwayhid B, et al. Systemic and uterine hemodynamic responses to dopamine in pregnant and nonpregnant sheep. *Am J Obstet Gynecol* 1978;130(6):669–673.

294. Callender K, Levinson G, Shnider SM, et al. Dopamine administration in the normotensive pregnant ewe. *Obstet Gynecol* 1978;51(5):586–589.

295. Clark RB, Brunner JA 3rd. Dopamine for the treatment of spinal hypotension during cesarean section. *Anesthesiology* 1980;53(6):514–517.

296. Baumann AL, Santos AC, Wlody D, et al. Maternal and fetal effects of milrinone and dopamine (abstract). *Anesthesiology* 1989;71:A855.

297. Santos AC, Baumann AL, Wlody D, et al. The maternal and fetal effects of milrinone and dopamine in normotensive pregnant ewes. *Am J Obstet Gynecol* 1992;166(1 Pt 1):257–262.

298. Chan WS, Anand S, Ginsberg JS. Anticoagulation of pregnant women with mechanical heart valves: A systematic review of the literature. *Arch Intern Med* 2000;160(2):191–196.

299. Bates SM, Greer IA, Hirsh J, et al. Use of antithrombotic agents during pregnancy: The Seventh ACCP Conference on Antithrombotic and Thrombolytic Therapy. *Chest* 2004;126(3 Suppl):627S–644S.

300. Chunilal SD, Young E, Johnston MA, et al. The APTT response of pregnant plasma to unfractionated heparin. *Thromb Haemost* 2002;87(1):92–97.

301. McHenry MM, Smeloff EA, Davey TB, et al. Hemodynamic results with full-flow orifice prosthetic valves. *Circulation* 1967;35(4 Suppl):I24–I33.

302. Ortega D, Viviand X, Lorec AM, et al. Excretion of lidocaine and bupivacaine in breast milk following epidural anesthesia for cesarean delivery. *Acta Anaesthesiol Scand* 1999;43(4):394–397.

Asthma in Pregnancy

Uma Munnur • Venkata D. P. Bandi

■ INTRODUCTION

Asthma is one of the most common serious medical problems in pregnancy. Asthma is a risk factor for several maternal and fetal complications posing a special challenge for physicians treating asthmatic pregnant women (1). Evidence suggests a two-fold effect of asthma: It can impact adversely on the outcome of pregnancy, and pregnancy can alter the clinical status of the patient with the disease (2). Pregnant women with asthma are at increased risk of perinatal complications including preeclampsia, low birth weight, and premature delivery (3–5). Asthma exacerbations during pregnancy can have detrimental consequences for both mother and fetus. Active asthma management with a view to reduce the exacerbation rate will be clinically useful in reducing the perinatal complications, particularly preterm labor.

■ DEFINITION

Asthma is a chronic inflammatory disorder of the airways defined by the presence of the following three characteristic findings: Reversible airway obstruction (1), airway inflammation (2), and airway hyperresponsiveness (3). Airway obstruction produces the clinical manifestations of cough, dyspnea, and wheezing. Airway inflammation contributes to airway hyperresponsiveness, airflow limitation, respiratory symptoms, and chest tightness. Airway inflammation modulates the course of asthma by independently producing airway obstruction and enhancing airway responsiveness. Airway hyperresponsiveness is marked by exaggerated responses to a wide variety of bronchoconstrictor stimuli. The interaction of these features of asthma determines the clinical manifestations and severity of asthma and the response to treatment.

■ EPIDEMIOLOGY

Asthma is a common, potentially serious medical condition that complicates approximately 4% to 8% of pregnancies (6–8). In 2009, current asthma prevalence was 8.2% of the US population (24.6 million). It was higher among females, children, non-Hispanic Black and Puerto Rican ethnicity, and people below the poverty level. In 2007, there were 1.75 million asthma-related emergency department visits and 456,000 asthma hospitalizations (9). The prevalence of asthma attacks seems to be elevated among pregnant women who are younger, unmarried, or have a lower annual family income (8). In general, the prevalence and morbidity from asthma are increasing, although asthma mortality rates have decreased in recent years (10). Acute exacerbations that necessitate emergency care or hospitalization have been reported in 9% to 11% of pregnant women cared by asthma specialists (11). Fifty-five percent of women with asthma will experience at least one exacerbation during pregnancy (12).

■ PATHOPHYSIOLOGY AND PATHOGENESIS OF ASTHMA

Asthma is a chronic inflammatory disease characterized by a reversible airway obstruction and airway hyperreactiveness. In addition to increased sensitivity, there is airway narrowing and a deficient response of the airways and a lack of bronchodilatory response of the airways to deep inspiration. Asthmatics also have a progressive loss of airway distensibility due to loss of lung elastic recoil (13).

Airway obstruction may be caused by changes in smooth muscle. Even though the smooth muscle is hypertrophic, it does not show increased constriction when exposed to pharmacologic stimuli. However, the failure of the normal autonomic neural control mechanisms can result in impaired relaxation and subsequent obstruction. Narrowing of the airway lumen can also result from bronchial mucosal edema and inflammatory cell infiltrates. Reversible airway obstruction is defined as an obstruction on spirometry which is documented during acute asthmatic attacks with normal physiology between attacks. Reversibility can also be proven by either partial or complete resolution of obstruction following the administration of a short-acting bronchodilator.

Airway hyperresponsiveness is marked by exaggerated responses to a wide variety of bronchoconstrictor stimuli like methacholine, histamine, or specific antigens, and is the cornerstone feature of this disorder. Multiple factors lead to narrowing of the airway that in turn result in reduced airflow, such as smooth muscle contraction, thickening of the airway wall, and the presence of secretions within the airway lumen (14).

Airway inflammation primarily serves as a modulating influence in asthma. Inflammation is present in nearly all asthmatic patients. The process of inflammation involves the occurrence of airway wall edema and infiltration of the mucosa by a variety of inflammatory cells which include neutrophils, mast cells, helper T lymphocytes, macrophages, and eosinophils. These cells release mediators of inflammation, including histamine, leukotrienes, platelet activating factor, prostaglandins, thromboxanes, cytokines, and serotonin.

The major physiologic abnormality during an asthma attack is air trapping. The patient can inhale air into her lungs, but is not able to exhale it out. This increases the work of breathing as the patient tries to breathe with the hyperinflated lung. The overdistension of normal alveoli causes pressure on capillaries in the alveolar walls, causing decreased perfusion to overdistended alveoli and thus resulting in ventilation–perfusion mismatch. When asthma is severe, pulmonary hypertension results in a leftward shift of the interventricular septum, and there is a decrease in the stroke volume. On deep inspiration, systolic blood pressure decreases, resulting in pulsus paradoxus (13,15).

TABLE 31-1 Diagnosis of Asthma

Symptoms	Wheezing, Cough, Chest Tightness
Signs	Wheezing on auscultation (absent when limited airflow movement)
Diagnosis confirmation	Airway obstruction that is partially or completely reversible >12% increase in FEV_1 after administration of bronchodilator

DIAGNOSIS OF ASTHMA

Medical History

Diagnosis of asthma in pregnancy is no different than for a nonpregnant patient (Table 31-1). The classic symptoms of asthma include dyspnea, wheezing, cough, and chest tightness. The medical history should also include information about the pattern and severity of the symptoms, precipitating and aggravating factors, duration and course of the symptoms along with hospitalization, and mechanical ventilation. The diagnosis of asthma is usually straightforward since most patients have a history of asthma prior to conception. However, diagnostic testing is required in patients with clinical picture or response to therapy is atypical and also in patients who present with respiratory symptoms for the first time in pregnancy [16].

Current asthma control should be assessed according to the frequency, severity of symptoms, frequency of use of rescue therapy, history of exacerbations requiring the use of systemic corticosteroids, and the result of pulmonary function tests. Forced expiratory volume of air expired in one second (FEV_1) and peak flow rates do not change significantly during pregnancy and so can be used for assessing asthma control. Patients who have asthma that is well controlled and who are not receiving controller medications can be classified as having intermittent rather than persistent asthma [16].

Physical Examination

Important aspects of the examination are assessment of respiratory rate, speech (number of words between breaths), use of accessory muscles, ability to lie flat, and presence of pulsus paradoxus. Auscultation of the chest will reveal wheezing and a prolonged phase of expiration (which may be absent when there is limited airflow during an exacerbation).

Laboratory Studies

After obtaining a thorough history and examining the patient, pulmonary function tests are useful to document the severity and establish the reversibility of obstruction. Diagnostic testing is warranted in patients whose clinical picture or response to therapy is atypical or in patients who present with respiratory symptoms during pregnancy without history of asthma. Bronchoprovocation tests (with histamine) are used when the history and physical examination strongly suggest the presence of asthma but spirometry fails to reveal airway obstruction. FEV_1 is a standardized measure of airway obstruction and is used to reflect both asthma severity and degree of asthma control [16]. Methacholine, which is used to confirm hyperreactivity, is contraindicated during pregnancy because of the lack of data on the safety of such testing in pregnant patients. The demonstration of a reduced FEV_1 to forced vital capacity ratio along with a 12% or greater improvement in FEV_1 after the administration of inhaled albuterol confirms a diagnosis of asthma during pregnancy [16].

Patients with asthma, who have not been tested before for allergens, should undergo serologic testing for IgE antibodies to allergens such as dust mites, cockroaches, mold spores, and pets. Skin tests are generally not recommended during pregnancy because the potent antigens may be associated with significant systemic reactions [16]. Bronchial provocation tests are infrequently done in pregnancy. If the patient has a prior history of physician-diagnosed asthma, she usually is managed as an asthmatic [13].

EFFECTS OF ASTHMA ON PREGNANCY AND FETUS

Women with asthma have been reported to have higher risk for several complications of pregnancy which include preeclampsia, preterm birth, intrauterine growth retardation, congenital malformations, and perinatal mortality [17,18]. Other adverse outcomes that appear to be increased in asthmatics include postpartum hemorrhage, preterm labor, premature rupture of membranes, neonatal hypoxia, and transient tachypnea of the newborn. Data regarding the effect of maternal asthma on pregnancy have been conflicting, but the largest Swedish population based study on pregnant women with asthma found an association of preeclampsia, preterm birth, and lower birth weight [19]. The potential mechanisms proposed for this increased risk are: (1) Poor maternal asthma control leading to exacerbations and fetal hypoxia, (2) asthma medications like corticosteroids, and (3) common pathogenetic factors that cause both asthma and perinatal complications.

The need to induce labor and the rate of cesarean delivery also tend to be higher in asthmatic parturients [20]. Data suggests a strong association between poor asthma control with these increased risks. Better asthma control in pregnancy may improve pregnancy outcomes [16,17,21]. As a general rule, mild asthma is unchanged in pregnancy and severe asthma tends to worsen [22].

During acute exacerbations, potential mechanisms of increased perinatal morbidity and mortality include hypoxemia and hypocapnia [23]. Maternal hypocapnia can produce uterine vasoconstriction and hypoxemia can diminish fetal oxygen delivery, both of which are detrimental to the fetus.

EFFECT OF PREGNANCY ON ASTHMA

The effect of pregnancy on asthma is unpredictable. The course of asthma may improve, deteriorate, or remain unchanged during pregnancy. Asthma exacerbations can occur at any time during pregnancy, but are more common in the second and third trimesters. Asthma exacerbation is rare during labor and the peripartum period. Monitoring of asthma status during prenatal visits is encouraged. Monthly evaluation of asthma history and pulmonary function (spirometry or measurement with a peak flow meter) is recommended.

Some asthmatic pregnant women experience improvement in their symptoms during pregnancy. This is probably due to the increase in progesterone with advancing gestation which contributes to cyclic adenosine monophosphate (cAMP)-induced bronchodilation, thereby improving asthma and peak flow rates [24]. In the last 4 weeks of pregnancy, asthmatics have reduced wheezing, sleep interference, and interference with daily activities, most likely due to the hormonal changes.

The mechanism for asthma exacerbation during pregnancy is not very clear. Maternal cell-mediated immunosuppression may increase maternal susceptibility to viral infections, which seem to be the most common precipitators of severe asthma during pregnancy. Increase in progesterone during pregnancy has been associated with relaxation of smooth muscle of the lower esophageal sphincter tone which causes gastroesophageal reflux (GER). GER occurs in 45% to 89% of patients with asthma. In essence, some of the obvious factors responsible for the exacerbation include smoking, GER, and reducing asthma medications for fear of causing harm to the fetus.

■ MANAGEMENT OF ASTHMA

The general principles of asthma management during pregnancy do not significantly vary from the management of nonpregnant asthmatics. The ultimate goal for the asthmatic parturient is to have no limitation of activity, minimal symptoms, avoid exacerbations, maintain normal pulmonary function, minimal adverse effects of medications, and ultimately deliver a healthy neonate. The physician should be able to provide optimal therapy to maintain asthma control that improves maternal quality of life and allows for normal progression of pregnancy. Routinely, the anesthesiologist may not be responsible for the management of asthma, but having the knowledge of the currently available treatment options will improve the care during delivery. The anesthesiologist should be able to distinguish between asthma and other causes of wheezing and also should avoid drugs that could exacerbate asthma.

Good asthma control is defined as: (1) Minimal or no chronic symptoms day or night, (2) minimal or no exacerbations, (3) no limitation on activities, (4) maintenance of near normal pulmonary function, (5) minimal use of short-acting inhaled β-2 agonist, and (6) minimal or no adverse effects from medications (25).

Acute symptoms of asthma usually arise from bronchospasm and respond well to bronchodilator therapy. Acute and chronic inflammation can affect not only the airway caliber and airflow but also underlying bronchial hyperresponsiveness which enhances susceptibility to bronchospasm. Consultation with an asthma specialist is appropriate in moderate to severe asthmatic patients. The effective management of asthma during pregnancy relies on four basic components: (1) Objective measures for assessment and monitoring, (2) patient education, (3) avoidance of asthma triggers, and (4) pharmacologic therapy.

Objective Measures for Assessment and Monitoring

Monitoring of asthma status during prenatal visits is strongly recommended. Since the course of asthma is usually unpredictable, it improves for about one-third of women, unchanged in one-third, and worsens for one-third of women during pregnancy, monthly evaluations of asthma history and pulmonary function (spirometry is generally preferred but measurement with a peak flow meter is usually sufficient) are recommended. See Table 31-2 for assessment of control and severity classification. The peak expiratory flow rate (PEFR) correlates well with the FEV_1, and has the advantages that it can be measured reliably with inexpensive, disposable, portable peak flow meters. Self-monitoring of PEFR will provide valuable insight regarding the course of asthma throughout the day. In moderate to severe asthmatic patients, it would be important to use a peak flow meter twice daily to have an objective measure of the lung function. This evaluation will provide the treating physicians with objective evidence to either step down treatment, or to increase treatment as needed. Serial ultrasound examinations starting at 32 weeks' gestation may be considered for patients who have suboptimally controlled asthma (25).

Patient Education

Patient education regarding diagnosis and treatment of asthma is more important than ever during pregnancy. The patient must be able to understand the potential adverse effects of uncontrolled asthma on the well-being of the fetus, and that treating asthma with medications is safer than under treatment of asthma which may lead to both maternal and fetal hypoxia. Above all, the patient should be able to recognize symptoms of worsening asthma and be able to obtain appropriate treatment when need arises (Table 31-3). This requires an individualized management plan that is based on a joint agreement between the patient and the treating physician. Correct inhaler technique should be assured, and the patient also should understand how she can reduce her exposure and control the factors that exacerbate her asthma (26). Women who smoke must be informed regarding the adverse effects on the fetus along with fetal effects of uncontrolled asthma, and they should be strongly encouraged to quit smoking (17). They should also be advised to avoid exposure to second hand smoking if at all possible.

TABLE 31-2 Assessment of Asthma Control in Pregnant Women

Variable	Well-controlled Asthma Mild Intermittent	Asthma not Well Controlled Mild/ Moderate Persistent	Very Poorly Controlled Asthma Severe Persistent
Frequency of symptoms	≤2 days/wk	>2 days/wk	Throughout the day
Frequency of nighttime awakening	≤2 times/mo	1–3 times/wk	≥4 times/wk
Interference with normal activity	None	Some	Extreme
Use of short-acting β-agonist for symptom control	≤2 days/wk	>2 days/wk	Several times/day
FEV_1 or peak flow (% of the predicted or personal best value)	>80	60–80	<60
Exacerbations requiring use of systemic corticosteroid (no.)	0–1 in past 12 mos	≥2 in past 12 mos	

Data from: the National Asthma Education and Prevention Program: National Heart, Lung, and Blood Institute. National Asthma Education and Prevention Program Expert Panel Report 3: Guidelines for the Diagnosis and Management of Asthma. Bethesda, MD: National Institutes of Health; 2007. URL: http://www.nhlbi.nih.gov/guidelines/asthma/asthgdln.htm Last accessed Feb 19, 2012.

TABLE 31-3 Patient Education for Treatment of Asthma during Pregnancy

Topic	Recommendation
General information	Provide basic information about asthma and explain how asthma affects pregnancy and pregnancy affects asthma
Use of inhaler/technique	Demonstrate proper technique for specific device and ask patient to perform the technique
Adherence to treatment	Discuss self-reported adherence to treatment with controller medication and address barriers to optimal adherence like cost, convenience, concern about side effects of medications
Self-treatment plan	Provide schedule for maintenance medication and doses of rescue therapy for increased symptoms; explain how to recognize a severe exacerbation and when and how to seek urgent or emergency care

Adapted from: Schatz M, Dombrowski MP. Clinical practice: asthma in pregnancy. *N Engl J Med* 2009; 360(18):1862–1869.

Avoidance of Asthma Triggers

Limiting adverse environmental exposure during pregnancy is very important for controlling asthma. Avoiding or controlling triggers can reduce asthma symptoms, airway hyperresponsiveness, and the need for pharmacologic therapy. Approximately 75% to 85% of patients with asthma have positive skin tests to common allergens (17). The most common asthma triggers are animal dander, dust mites, cockroach antigens, pollens, and molds. Nonimmune triggers are tobacco smoke, air pollutants, drugs like aspirin and β-blockers. In patients with exercise-triggered asthma, use of a short-acting bronchodilator inhaler 5 to 60 minutes prior to exercise can significantly reduce the occurrence of exacerbations. All patients should be strongly encouraged to stop smoking (Table 31-4).

In 1993, the National Asthma Education and Prevention Program Expert Panel Report (NAEPP) published the *Report of the Working Group on Asthma and Pregnancy*, which reviewed the data from available studies, and presented recommendations for the pharmacologic management of asthma during pregnancy. Since then there have been new developments with introduction of new medications, availability of additional safety data, and treatment guidelines. All of these developments led to the update of the previous report and is published in *NAEPP Working Group Report on Managing Asthma During Pregnancy: Recommendations for Pharmacologic Treatment-Update 2004* (25).

TABLE 31-4 Asthma Triggers

Exercise
Viral infection
Animal with fur
Dust mites
Mold
Tobacco smoke
Pollen
Changes in weather
Strong emotional expression (laughing or crying hard)
Dust
Menstrual cycles

■ PHARMACOLOGIC THERAPY

Pharmacologic therapy of asthma during pregnancy is geared toward avoiding exacerbations and status asthmaticus. Management should begin prior to conception. Medications that are used to treat asthma fall into two main categories—bronchodilators and anti-inflammatory agents. The prophylactic use of antibiotics is not necessary. The goals of asthma therapy include: (1) Relieve bronchospasm; (2) protect the airways from irritant stimuli; (3) mitigate inflammatory response to an allergen exposure; and (4) resolve the inflammatory process in the airways reducing airway hyperresponsiveness (Table 31-5).

Bronchodilators

Inhaled β-2 agonists are powerful bronchodilators and are recommended for asthma treatment for all classes of severity. Albuterol is the first-line rescue inhaler for the rapid relief of acute bronchospasm. Short-acting β-adrenergic agonists (SABAs) are considered pregnancy category C and are generally safe during pregnancy. β-adrenergic agonists exert beneficial effects in patients with asthma by activating β-2 adrenergic receptors. SABAs represent the most effective therapy for acute exacerbations of asthma episodes. β-adrenergic agonists exert their beneficial effects by (1) direct smooth muscle relaxation in the airway; (2) enhanced mucociliary transport; (3) reduced airway edema; and (4) inhibition of cholinergic neurotransmission.

Routes of administration of β-adrenergic agonists include aerosol, oral, and parenteral. The aerosol route is generally preferred during pregnancy because high concentration of drugs can be delivered directly to the site of activity in the airways. This route minimizes maternal systemic effects and decreases fetal exposure. Albuterol is the preferred SABA because it has an excellent safety profile and has the most pregnancy-related safety data. Data are limited with regards to the effectiveness of long-acting β-adrenergic agonists (LABAs) during pregnancy, although there is justification for expecting LABAs to have a safety profile similar to that of albuterol.

There are a limited number of human studies that have investigated the fetal safety of chronic administration of β-adrenergic agonists. Schatz and colleagues prospectively conducted a study in 259 asthmatic parturients using β-adrenergic agonists. He found no association with congenital malformations, preterm delivery, intrauterine growth restriction, or perinatal mortality (27). These agents have been

TABLE 31-5 Pharmacologic Management of Asthma in Pregnancy

Medications	Adult Dose	Comments
Short-acting Inhaled β-2 Agonists		
Albuterol Nebulizer solution (5.0 mg/mL, 2.5 mg/3 mL, 1.25 mg/3 mL, 1.25 mg/3 mL, 0.63 mg/3 mL)	2.5–5 mg every 20 mins for 3 doses, then 2.5–10 mg every 1–4 h as needed, or 10–15 mg/hr continuously 4–8 puffs every 20 min up to 4 h, then every 1–4 h as needed	Only selective β-2 agonists are recommended. For optimal delivery, dilute aerosols to minimum of 3 mL and nebulize at gas flow of 6–8 L/min
System (injected) β-2 Agonists		
Epinephrine 1:1,000 (1 mg/mL)	0.3–0.5 mg every 20 min for 3 doses sq	No proven advantage of systemic therapy over aerosol
Terbutaline (1 mg/mL)	0.25 mg every 20 min for 3 doses sq	No proven advantage of systemic therapy over aerosol
Anticholinergics		
Ipratropium bromide Nebulizer solution (0.25 mg/mL)	0.5 mg every 30 min for 3 doses, then every 2–4 h as needed	May mix in same nebulizer with albuterol. Should not be used as first-line therapy: Should be added to β-2 agonist therapy
Ipratropium with albuterol Nebulizer solution (Each 3 mL vial contains 0.5 mg ipratropium bromide and 2.5 mg albuterol)	3 mL every 30 min for 3 doses, then every 2–4 h as needed	May mix in same nebulizer with albuterol. Should not be used as first-line therapy: Should be added to β-2 agonist therapy
Systemic Corticosteroids	(Dosages and comments apply to all three corticosteroids)	
Prednisone Methylprednisolone Prednisolone	120–180 mg/day in 3 or 4 divided doses for 48 h, then 60–80 mg/day until PEF reaches 70% of predicted or personal best	For outpatient "burst" use 40–60 mg in single or 2 divided doses for adults for 3–10 days

Adapted from: NAEPP Working Group Report on Managing Asthma During Pregnancy: Recommendations for Pharmacologic Treatment, 2004. *J Allergy Clin Immunol* 2005;115(1):34–46.

used for many years without any reports of teratogenicity and should not be restricted for fetal concerns. Optimal control of maternal symptoms of asthma seems to be more important than any detrimental effects of β-adrenergic agonists (23).

Inhaled Corticosteroids (ICSs)

Corticosteroids are the most effective treatment for the airway inflammation component of asthma and reduce the hyperresponsiveness of airways to allergens and triggers. ICSs are the preferred treatment for long-term control and have gained widespread popularity; they decrease the incidence of exacerbations by more than three-fold compared with patients not using ICS (10). In pregnancy, ICSs are preferred for the management of all levels of persistent asthma. The route of administration is effective and rinsing the mouth immediately after using the ICS will reduce local side effects as well as limit systemic absorption and therefore fetal exposure. Budesonide is the preferred ICS because more data are available on using budesonide in pregnant women than are available on other ICSs, and the data is reassuring. There seems to be no increased risk of adverse perinatal outcomes in pregnant women. Although budesonide is the preferred ICS, it is important to note that no data indicate that the other ICS preparations are unsafe during pregnancy. ICSs are considered category C except budesonide, which is category B as few or no studies are available on the use of other ICS formulations during pregnancy.

The NAEPP Working Group on Managing Asthma during Pregnancy conducted a systematic review of the evidence on the use of ICS during pregnancy and the conclusions are: (1) The risk of asthma exacerbations associated with pregnancy can be reduced and lung function (FEV$_1$) improved with the use of ICS therapy; (2) to date, no studies have related ICS use to any increased congenital malformations or other adverse perinatal outcomes; and (3) in studies using birth registries of newborns whose mothers were exposed to budesonide, information is reassuring regarding the safety of this medication during pregnancy (25).

Oral (Systemic) Corticosteroids

The findings from current review of the evidence on the safety of oral corticosteroids during pregnancy are conflicting. Oral corticosteroid use, especially during the first trimester, is associated with an increased risk for isolated cleft lip with or without cleft palate. Very few pregnant women who have oral steroid-dependent asthma were including in the studies, and length of exposure, dose, and timing of steroid administration were not well described in the studies. Oral corticosteroid use during pregnancy in women who have severe asthma is associated with an increased incidence of preeclampsia and delivery of both preterm and low birth weight infants. The available data makes it difficult to separate the effects of the corticosteroids on these outcomes from effects of severe asthma. As severe asthma has been associated with maternal/

fetal mortality, risk–benefit considerations favor the use of oral corticosteroid medication when indicated in the long-term management of severe asthma and exacerbations during pregnancy (25). Systemic corticosteroids are considered category C drugs.

Cromolyn Sodium

Cromolyn sodium belongs to a class of drugs that are thought to reduce inflammation and mediator release primarily by stabilizing mast cells and other cells. Cromolyn is used as an alternative treatment for mild asthma and adjunctive treatment for moderate and severe asthma. It blocks early and late bronchospasm and response to asthma triggers. It has anti-inflammatory properties and relaxes smooth muscle. It does appear to be safe during pregnancy, but experience with dosing is lacking (11). Cromolyn is considered a category B drug.

Theophylline

Theophylline is a methylxanthine that acts as a weak bronchodilator. It is useful for chronic therapy and is not helpful in acute exacerbations. It is associated with adverse effects such as insomnia, heartburn, palpitations, and nausea. Theophylline also has significant drug interactions as the rate of theophylline clearance is altered with use of certain medications, resulting in increased theophylline levels and toxicity. Some of the medications affecting the clearance are cimetidine, lorazepam, and erythromycin. Serum levels should be maintained between 5 and 12 μg/mL during pregnancy (11). The main advantage of theophylline is the long duration, up to 12 hours with the use of sustained release preparations.

Anticholinergics

Ipratropium bromide is a quaternary compound derivative of atropine and allows delivery of a higher concentration of anticholinergic agent to the lungs with less systemic absorption and decreased fetal concentrations. It leads to parasympathetic blockade that further accentuates the bronchodilating effect of β-agonists. It is labeled category B. Anticholinergics can be used in an acute exacerbation in the emergency room or hospital and are usually given in combination with β-agonists but they do not have any benefit in the long-term therapy of asthma.

Leukotriene Inhibitors

Leukotriene mediators have numerous biologic activities including augmentation of neutrophil and eosinophil migration, neutrophil and monocyte aggregation as well as increasing capillary permeability, and smooth muscle contraction. All of these effects contribute to the inflammation, edema, bronchoconstriction, and mucus secretion seen in asthmatic patients. Leukotriene inhibitors block the physiologic effects of these leukotrienes. Animal data regarding these drugs suggest that they are likely to be safe in pregnancy but human data is lacking (14). These drugs are labeled category B.

■ CONTROL OF FACTORS THAT AGGRAVATE ASTHMA

For patients with persistent asthma, the physician should evaluate the potential role of allergens. Skin testing or in vitro testing should be used to determine sensitivity to indoor inhalant allergens to which the patient is exposed and the significance of positive tests should be assessed. Patients with asthma should reduce the exposure to relevant allergens. Allergen immunotherapy should be considered when there

is clear evidence of a relationship between asthma symptoms and exposure to an allergen to which the patient is sensitive.

Exacerbations during pregnancy may require hospitalization. During pregnancy, approximately 5.8% of women are hospitalized with asthma exacerbation (28). Patients with asthma and pregnant women are two groups with significantly increased susceptibility to infection with influenza strains including seasonal and H_1N_1 influenza. In the early stages of the H_1N_1 pandemic in the United States, 7% of hospitalized patients were pregnant; and 22% of those women were asthmatics (29).

■ STEP THERAPY

Current pharmacologic therapy emphasizes treatment of airway inflammation to decrease airway hyperresponsiveness and prevent asthma symptoms. The step-care therapeutic approach uses the least amount of drug intervention necessary to control a patient's severity of asthma. Patients not optimally responding to treatment should be stepped up to more intensive medically therapy. Once control is achieved and sustained for several months, a step-down approach can be considered, but should be undertaken cautiously and gradually to avoid compromising the stability of the asthma control (30). See Figure 31-1 for a recommended stepwise approach for managing asthma during pregnancy.

■ MANAGEMENT OF ASTHMA EXACERBATION

Pregnant women with asthma exacerbation are considered high-risk patients and management should include a multidisciplinary approach between obstetricians, anesthesiologists, pulmonologists, and pediatricians (Fig. 31-2). Acute exacerbations cannot always be avoided. When a parturient comes to the hospital with an asthma exacerbation, peak flow should be compared with usual predictive values. An arterial blood gas should be taken keeping in mind that a pregnant woman usually has a baseline compensated respiratory alkalosis. Worsening of the alkalosis as a result of acute asthma exacerbation may lead to fetal hypoxia. Alkalosis lessens the placental blood flow and hypoxia may be more severe in the fetus than the mother (31). On the other hand, acute respiratory acidosis can manifest with patient exhaustion. Maternal acidosis can lead to inability of the fetus to unload CO_2 if the maternal venous and fetal umbilical artery CO_2 gradient is decreased (32).

Patients with acute exacerbation should be provided with oxygen supplementation to maintain oxygen saturation above 95%. Fluid status should be assessed, and intravenous fluids should be administered if necessary. The initial treatment should include the administration of inhaled albuterol every 20 minutes, to a maximum of 3 doses in the first hour. Ipratropium bromide (500 μg) can be given concomitantly in severe cases. Systemic corticosteroids, either orally or intravenously should be given to patients who show no improvement with the bronchodilator therapy. If the patient is taking theophylline at home, a stat theophylline level should be obtained.

Patients should be closely monitored and reassessed regarding the response to therapy. This should also include continuous fetal heart rate monitoring. The decision to hospitalize the patient or discharge home is based on the response in the first 4 hours. If there is any evidence of maternal fatigue, fetal distress, or signs of impending respiratory failure as evidenced by worsening $PaCO_2$, the patient should be appropriately transferred to the intensive care unit (ICU). A progressive increase in maternal $PaCO_2$, regardless of maintained oxygenation, is in itself an indication for intubation and ventilation to prevent hypercarbia, respiratory failure, and fetal acidosis. The basic goals of management of asthma exacerbation

Classify Severity: Clinical Feature Before Treatment or Adequate Control			Medications Required to Maintain Long-Term Control
	Symptoms /Day —— Symptoms/ Night	PEF or FEV$_1$ —— PEF Variability	Daily Medications
Step 4 Severe Persistent	Continual —— Frequent	≤ 60% —— > 30%	• Preferred treatment: - High-dose inhaled conticosteroid AND - Long-acting inhaled beta$_2$-agonist AND, if needed, - Conticoseroid tablets or syrup long term (2 mg/kg per day. Generally not to exceed 60mg per day). (Make repeat attempts to reduce systemic corticosteroid and maintain control with High-dose inhaled conticosteroid. *) • Alternative tpreatment: - High-dose inhaled conticosteroid* AND - Sustained released theophylline to serum concentration of 5-12 μg/ml.
Step 3 Moderate Persistent	Daily —— > 1 night/week	> 60% - < 80% —— > 30%	• Preferred treatment: EITHER - Low-dose inhaled conticosteroid* and long-acting inhaled beta$_2$-agonist OR - Medium-dose inhaled conticosteroid.* If needed (particularly in patients with recurring severe exacerbations): - Medium-dose inhaled conticosteroidl* and long-actiing inhaled beta$_2$-agonist. • Alternative treatment: - Low-dose inhaled corticosteroid* and either theophylline or leukotriene receptor antagonist.† If needed: - Medium-dose inhaled corticosteroid* and either theophylline or leukotriene receptor antagonist.†
Step 2 Mild Persistent	> 2 days/week but < daily —— > 2 nights/month	≥ 80% —— < 20%	• Preferred treatment: - Low-dose inhaled corticosteroid.* • Alternative treatment (listed alphabetically): cromolyn, leukotriene receptor antagonist † OR sustained-release theophylline to serum concentration of 5-12 μg/ml.
Step 1 Mild intermittent	≤ 2 days/week —— ≤ 2 nights/month	≥ 80% —— < 20%	• No daily medication needed. • Severe exacerbations may occur, separated by long periods of normal lung function and no symptoms. A course of systemic corticosteroid is recommended.
Quick Relief All Patients			• Short-acting bronchodilator: 2-4 puffs **short-acting inhaled beta$_2$-agonist‡** as needed for symptoms. • Intensity of treatment will depend on serverity of exacerbation: up 3 treatments at 20-minute intervals or a single nebulizer treatment as needed. Course of systemci corticosteroid may be needed. • Use of short-acting inhaled beta$_2$-agonist‡ > 2 times a week in intermittent asthma (daily, or increasing use in persistent asthma) may indicate the need to initiate long-term-control therapy.

Step down
Review treatment every 1-6 months; a gradual stepwise reduction in treatment may be possible.

Step up
If control is not maintained, consider step up. First, review patient medication technique, adherence, and environmental control.

Goals of Therapy: Asthma Control

• Minimal or no chronic symptoms day or night
• Minimal or not exacerbations
• No limitations on activities; no school/work missed

• Maintain (near) normal pulmonary function
• Minimal use of short-acting inhaled beta$_2$-agonist‡
• Minimal or no adverse effects from medications

Notes

• The stepwise approach is meant to assist, not replace, the clinical desionmaking required to meet individual patient needs.
• Classify severity: assign patient to most severe step in which any feature occurs (PEF is percent of personal best; FEV$_1$ is percent predicted).
• Gain control as quickly as possible (consider a short course of systemic corticosteroid), then step down to the least medication necessary to maintain control.
• Minimize use of short-acting inhaled beta$_2$-agonist‡ (e.g. use of approximately one canister a month even if not using it every day indicates inadequate control of asthma and the need to initiate or intensify long-term-control therapy).
• Provide education on self-management and controlling environmental factors that make asthma worse (e.g. allergens, irritants).
• Refer to an asthma specialist if there are difficulties controlling asthma or if Step 4 care is required. Referral may be considered if Step 3 care is required.

* There are more data on using budesonide during pregnancy than on using other inhaled corticosteroids.
† There are minimal data on using leukotriene receptor antagonists in humans during pregnancy, although there are reassuring animal data submitted to FDA.
‡ There are more data on using albuterol during pregnancy than on using other short-acting inhaled beta$_2$-agonists.

FIGURE 31-1 Stepwise approach to managing asthma in pregnancy and lactation: Treatment. From the NAEPP Working Group Report on Managing Asthma during pregnancy: Recommendations for Pharmacologic Treatment. Report can be accessed at: http://www.nhlbi.nih.gov/health/prof/lung/asthma/astpreg.htm. Last accessed Nov 4, 2011.

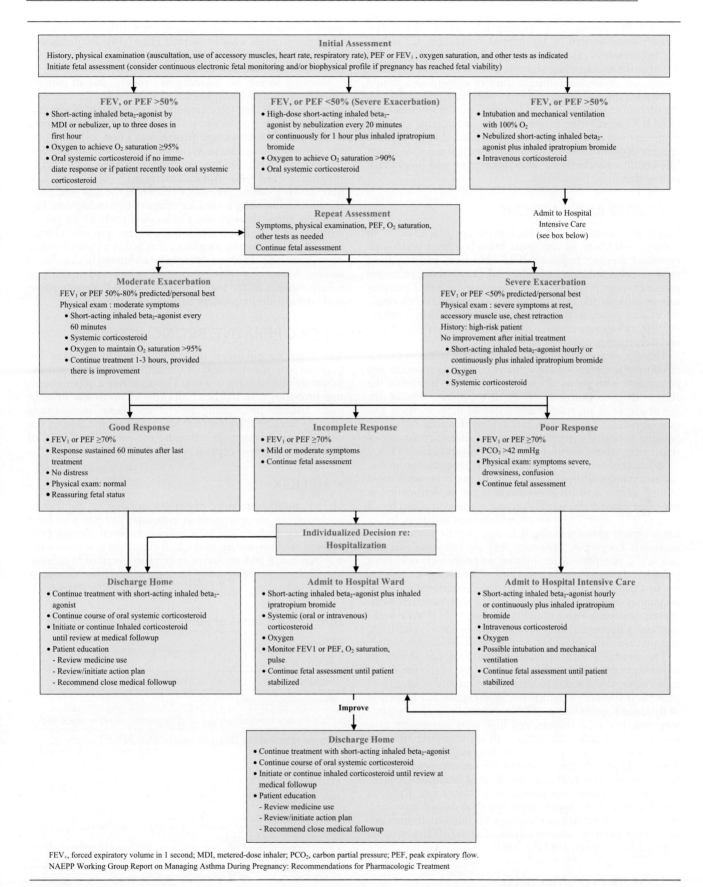

Initial Assessment
History, physical examination (auscultation, use of accessory muscles, heart rate, respiratory rate), PEF or FEV_1, oxygen saturation, and other tests as indicated
Initiate fetal assessment (consider continuous electronic fetal monitoring and/or biophysical profile if pregnancy has reached fetal viability)

FEV_1 or PEF >50%
- Short-acting inhaled beta$_2$-agonist by MDI or nebulizer, up to three doses in first hour
- Oxygen to achieve O_2 saturation ≥95%
- Oral systemic corticosteroid if no immediate response or if patient recently took oral systemic corticosteroid

FEV_1 or PEF <50% (Severe Exacerbation)
- High-dose short-acting inhaled beta$_2$-agonist by nebulization every 20 minutes or continuously for 1 hour plus inhaled ipratropium bromide
- Oxygen to achieve O_2 saturation >90%
- Oral systemic corticosteroid

FEV_1 or PEF >50%
- Intubation and mechanical ventilation with 100% O_2
- Nebulized short-acting inhaled beta$_2$-agonist plus inhaled ipratropium bromide
- Intravenous corticosteroid

Admit to Hospital Intensive Care
(see box below)

Repeat Assessment
Symptoms, physical examination, PEF, O_2 saturation, other tests as needed
Continue fetal assessment

Moderate Exacerbation
FEV_1 or PEF 50%-80% predicted/personal best
Physical exam : moderate symptoms
- Short-acting inhaled beta$_2$-agonist every 60 minutes
- Systemic corticosteroid
- Oxygen to maintain O_2 saturation >95%
- Continue treatment 1-3 hours, provided there is improvement

Severe Exacerbation
FEV_1 or PEF <50% predicted/personal best
Physical exam : severe symptoms at rest, accessory muscle use, chest retraction
History: high-risk patient
No improvement after initial treatment
- Short-acting inhaled beta$_2$-agonist hourly or continuously plus inhaled ipratropium bromide
- Oxygen
- Systemic corticosteroid

Good Response
- FEV_1 or PEF ≥70%
- Response sustained 60 minutes after last treatment
- No distress
- Physical exam: normal
- Reassuring fetal status

Incomplete Response
- FEV_1 or PEF ≥70%
- Mild or moderate symptoms
- Continue fetal assessment

Poor Response
- FEV_1 or PEF ≥70%
- PCO_2 >42 mmHg
- Physical exam: symptoms severe, drowsiness, confusion
- Continue fetal assessment

Individualized Decision re: Hospitalization

Discharge Home
- Continue treatment with short-acting inhaled beta$_2$-agonist
- Continue course of oral systemic corticosteroid
- Initiate or continue Inhaled corticosteroid until review at medical followup
- Patient education
  - Review medicine use
  - Review/initiate action plan
  - Recommend close medical followup

Admit to Hospital Ward
- Short-acting inhaled beta$_2$-agonist plus inhaled ipratropium bromide
- Systemic (oral or intravenous) corticosteroid
- Oxygen
- Monitor FEV1 or PEF, O_2 saturation, pulse
- Continue fetal assessment until patient stabilized

Admit to Hospital Intensive Care
- Short-acting inhaled beta$_2$-agonist hourly or continuously plus inhaled ipratropium bromide
- Intravenous corticosteroid
- Oxygen
- Possible intubation and mechanical ventilation
- Continue fetal assessment until patient stabilized

Improve

Discharge Home
- Continue treatment with short-acting inhaled beta$_2$-agonist
- Continue course of oral systemic corticosteroid
- Initiate or continue inhaled corticosteroid until review at medical followup
- Patient education
  - Review medicine use
  - Review/initiate action plan
  - Recommend close medical followup

FEV_1, forced expiratory volume in 1 second; MDI, metered-dose inhaler; PCO_2, carbon partial pressure; PEF, peak expiratory flow.
NAEPP Working Group Report on Managing Asthma During Pregnancy: Recommendations for Pharmacologic Treatment

FIGURE 31-2 Management of asthma exacerbations in pregnancy and lactation: Emergency and hospital-based care. From the NAEPP Working Group Report on Managing Asthma During Pregnancy: Recommendations for Pharmacologic Treatment. Report can be accessed at: http://www.nhlbi.nih.gov/health/prof/lung/asthma/astpreg.htm. Last accessed Nov 4, 2011.

are: (1) Preventing or correcting hypoxemia with either supplemental oxygen or mechanical ventilation, (2) reducing hypercarbia, (3) reversing bronchospasm with inhaled β-2 agonists and systemic steroids, and (4) avoiding maternal exhaustion. Systemic administration of epinephrine should be avoided if possible because of its vasoconstrictive effect on the uteroplacental circulation. If epinephrine is administered, close ICU monitoring is needed to avoid maternal and fetal complications (32). Assessment of the fetus during an acute episode depends on the stage of pregnancy. If the fetus is viable, continuous electronic fetal monitoring and biophysical profile should be considered.

■ STATUS ASTHMATICUS

Status asthmaticus is described as severe exacerbation of asthma, refractory to the usual bronchodilator and corticosteroid therapy, requiring ICU admission, and requiring mechanical ventilation; it can be fatal. Some of the asthmatic parturients can progress to status asthmaticus either antepartum or intrapartum despite adequate treatment. When respiratory compromise is severe enough and patient requires ventilatory support, maintenance of adequate fetal blood flow and oxygenation can be a challenge.

There is very limited literature regarding status asthmaticus during pregnancy. Elsayegh and colleagues reported five parturients with status asthmaticus who were treated in the ICU with good outcome. All the five patients were in different stages of pregnancy and required deep sedation and neuromuscular blockade to facilitate ventilation. All of the patients tolerated extreme hypercapnia during treatment of status asthmaticus without any evident adverse effects (33).

Sedation is necessary to achieve optimal ventilation in status asthmaticus. Propofol (category B) has been safely used as long as hypotension is avoided as it can be detrimental in pregnant patients due to the decrease in uteroplacental blood flow (33). Benzodiazepines are widely used sedatives in the nonpregnant patients in the ICU due to their amnestic and anxiolytic properties. However, they do cross the placenta and while not proven teratogenic in pregnancy, one must consider the risk–benefit ratio before initiating therapy in the first trimester. Benzodiazepine administration during late pregnancy and labor may be associated with neonatal withdrawal syndrome with irritability, tremor, and vigorous sucking, and a floppy infant syndrome with hypotonia, lethargy, and sucking difficulties (34).

The mortality rate of status asthmaticus has shown an improvement in the past few decades. One of the main reasons responsible for this reduction in mortality of ventilated patients is the use of permissive hypercapnia and reduction of dynamic hyperinflation (33,35). Normally, a slow respiratory rate, low tidal volume, and high peak inspiratory flow rate are set in asthmatic patients to allow greater time for exhalation. This also prevents air trapping (auto-PEEP or dynamic hyperinflation). Some of the known complications from dynamic hyperinflation are elevated intrathoracic pressure that can cause hypotension and barotrauma. Reduced ventilation leads to hypercapnia, which is usually tolerated, and resolves as the airflow obstruction is relieved. In humans, there have been no adverse effects of maternal hypercapnia induced for the period of labor (36).

■ CIGARETTE SMOKING

Cigarette smoking is one of the most significant preventable causes of perinatal morbidity and mortality. Approximately 80% of smoking women continue to do so during pregnancy (23). Multiple studies have shown that cigarette smoking is more common among pregnant women with asthma than in pregnant women without asthma (12,37,38). Roelands and colleagues have shown that pregnant smokers were 4 times more likely to have asthma (39).

Smoking should be discouraged strongly, and all patients should try to avoid environmental tobacco smoke exposure as much as possible. Smoking during pregnancy is a public health problem due to the many associated adverse effects. These include intrauterine growth restriction, placenta previa, abruptio placentae, preterm premature rupture of membranes, low birth weight, perinatal mortality, and ectopic pregnancy (14,39,40). Approximately 80% of women who quit smoking during pregnancy relapse in the first year postpartum, highlighting a need for effective continuing care that supports them through the challenging postpartum period when stress is high and motivations to stay quit may change (41). Morbidity during pregnancy that is due to smoking may be independent of asthma and may be additional to that due to asthma. Maternal smoking during pregnancy and exposure to tobacco smoke in the home deteriorate child's lung function and increase life-long risk of developing asthma (42).

■ PERIOPERATIVE BRONCHOSPASM

There are no published recommendations concerning the perioperative management of the asthmatic patient and the literature on this topic is scant. The occurrence of perioperative bronchospasm has been reported in up to 9% of asthmatic patients undergoing general anesthesia, immediately after endotracheal intubation. Smoking can also add to the risk of bronchospasm in asthmatic patients (43). Causes of perioperative bronchospasm are listed in Table 31-6.

■ HELIOX

Heliox, an 80:20 mixture of helium and oxygen, sometimes is considered for treatment in asthmatic patients who have respiratory acidosis and who fail conventional therapy (44). Helium is a low-density, biologically inert gas that lowers airway resistance and decreases respiratory work of breathing. Significant improvement may be noted within 10 to 20 minutes

TABLE 31-6 Causes of Perioperative Bronchospasm

Physiologic
Acute asthma
Exacerbation of chronic asthma
Pulmonary edema
Pulmonary embolism (air and amniotic fluid embolism)
Acute respiratory distress syndrome (ARDS)
Anatomic
Vocal cord dysfunction
Mucus plug in the airway
Mechanical
Obstruction of airway
Kinking of ETT
Endobronchial intubation
Anesthetic Complications
Aspiration
Drug reaction

of initiating therapy, but there is scant data on whether heliox can improve outcomes such as avert tracheal intubation, change intensive care and hospital admission rates and duration, or even affect mortality. One case report described the use of heliox in a pregnant, intubated asthmatic with status asthmaticus and respiratory failure but otherwise, the use of heliox has not been studied in pregnancy (45).

■ TERATOGENICITY

There is a lack of consensus in the literature about the effect of maternal asthma on the development of congenital malformations. A recent Canadian administrative database revealed that pregnant women with asthma have a 30% increased risk of any congenital malformation and a 34% increased risk of a major congenital malformation compared with nonasthmatic women. The authors concluded the disease itself, through fetal oxygen impairment, likely to play a role in this increased risk, but further research is needed to prove the effect of asthma and medications used to treat the disease (46,47).

In a recent study, women treated with bronchodilators during the periconceptional period had a risk of gastroschisis in their offspring approximately two times that of women not using these medications. No significant association was found between maternal use of asthma anti-inflammatory medications and gastroschisis. Since information on maternal asthma status/severity was not available, the effects of disease on the risk of gastroschisis cannot be ruled out. The authors recommend additional research in determining whether a real risk exists and for guiding asthma treatment (48,49).

Airway inflammation can cause maternal hypoxia and results in fetal oxygen impairment. There is evidence that oxygen levels in the fetus are tightly controlled in the first trimester of pregnancy and hypoxia in this crucial time can cause some malformations (2).

■ OBSTETRIC MANAGEMENT

When compared to a nonasthmatic parturient, the obstetric management in a pregnant asthmatic patient differs in the following aspects: (1) Induction of labor, (2) postpartum hemorrhage, and (3) treatment of hypertension.

Induction of Labor

Prostaglandins should be administered with caution in patients with asthma. Prostaglandin F_2-α constricts airways in vivo and in vitro. Airways of asthmatic subjects demonstrate an increased sensitivity to prostaglandin F_2-α, and when used for induction of labor, it can produce bronchospasm. Prostaglandin E_2 (PGE_2) dilates airways in vitro, but aerosols can provoke bronchospasm in asthmatic subjects in vivo, probably due to an irritant effect. Due to the possible risk of bronchospasm, alternate methods of induction of labor are preferred in known asthmatic parturients.

Towers and colleagues conducted a prospective study on 189 patients with a history of asthma or active asthma and exposed them to intravaginal PGE_2. None of the patients in the study experienced any evidence of clinical exacerbation of their disease. The authors recommend careful monitoring of asthmatic patients but support the use of PGE_2 in asthmatic parturients, if obstetrically indicated (50).

Postpartum Hemorrhage

Numerous outcome studies have shown that asthmatics have a higher incidence of postpartum hemorrhage than nonasthmatic patients. Probable reasons for this increased risk are:

(1) Abnormalities in smooth muscle and the neural regulation of contraction and (2) treatment with β-agonists (20).

Hemabate (15-methyl prostaglandin F_2-α) should be used with caution to treat postpartum hemorrhage in asthmatic patients. Recently, we had a morbidly obese parturient without history of asthma that developed bronchospasm after treatment with Hemabate for postpartum hemorrhage in our institution. Ergot alkaloids have also been associated with episodes of bronchospasm. Oxytocin is the preferred agent to treat postpartum hemorrhage in asthmatic patients as it does not affect airway tone and can be given in an increased concentration as long as hemodynamic stability is maintained. If hemorrhage is not controlled with oxytocin, risk–benefit ratio should be considered before using Hemabate or ergot alkaloids as hemorrhage can lead to a cardiovascular collapse. Medications to treat bronchospasm should be readily available when using Hemabate and ergot alkaloids.

Treatment of Hypertension

Blood pressure can be elevated during pregnancy due to preeclampsia or chronic hypertension. Schatz and colleagues found an increased incidence of preeclampsia in the asthmatic patients. Low dose aspirin is widely used for prevention of preeclampsia. However, conflicting results have been obtained from various studies (51,52). Aspirin should be used with caution in the asthmatic patient as it is a known trigger for bronchospasm in a certain subset of patients sensitive to aspirin (53).

β-adrenergic receptor antagonists are used as first-line treatment of hypertension in nonpregnant and nonasthmatic patients. Labetalol is commonly used to treat hypertension in the preeclamptic patients (54). All β-blockers, especially non–β-1 selective agents, may provoke bronchospasm and it would be preferable to avoid them. Vasodilators like hydralazine, calcium channel blockers, nitroglycerin, and nitroprusside can be safely used in the pregnant asthmatic patients with preeclampsia. These agents can cause or worsen hypoxemia as they affect ventilation–perfusion matching by interfering with hypoxic pulmonary vasoconstriction. Magnesium bolus and infusions are frequently (54) used in preeclamptic patients for seizure prophylaxis and it may have an added benefit in treatment of bronchospasm (55–57).

■ ANESTHETIC MANAGEMENT
Preoperative Assessment

During the preoperative evaluation, the anesthesiologist should obtain a thorough history and physical examination of the patient. The severity of the disease should be assessed and the patient should be examined for symptoms of wheezing, dyspnea, and cough. Information should also include frequency and severity of symptoms, course of asthma during pregnancy, date of most recent exacerbation, steroid dependency, and need for hospitalization or intubation. Patients with severe and frequent attacks are at increased risk for morbidity during the peripartum period.

Physical examination should focus on pulmonary system. Wheezing may be heard on chest auscultation. If air movement is markedly reduced, wheezing may not be audible. Additional signs of an acute exacerbation: Tachypnea, pulsus paradoxus, and use of accessory respiratory muscles.

In a mild asthmatic patient, there may be no need for any additional tests. If an exacerbation is suspected, chest x-ray, arterial blood gas, and pulmonary function tests can assist in diagnosis and management. Chest x-ray can help diagnose pneumonia. During an acute exacerbation of asthma, arterial blood gas measurement will often reveal hypoxemia and respiratory alkalosis. After a prolonged and severe asthmatic episode, arterial blood gas will show an increased carbon dioxide tension due to fatigue. PEFR can be measured at bedside with a peak flow meter and this is the most convenient indirect method to assess airway obstruction during labor.

Tocolysis

If preterm labor occurs during pregnancy, tocolytic therapy is often considered. Since most of the asthmatic patients are already receiving inhaled β-2 agonists, administration of systemic β-2 agonists can cause significant adverse effects. Magnesium sulfate can be safely used in this situation. Although the role of intravenous infusion of magnesium sulfate on the course of acute asthma has not been extensively studied, data from nonpregnant women suggest that it may have an added bronchodilator effect in patients with severe asthma (32,55). Indomethacin may induce bronchospasm, especially in aspirin-sensitive asthmatics, and therefore should be avoided. Calcium antagonists such as nifedipine are believed to be safe, but there is not enough data in the asthmatic patient to confirm this (32).

Labor and Delivery

All scheduled asthma medications should be continued during labor and delivery. Asthmatic patients should have optimized pulmonary status prior to induction of an anesthetic. A pulmonary physician should be consulted if there is any evidence of wheezing or chest tightness. If patients have received systemic corticosteroids in the past, "stress dose" of intravenous corticosteroids every 8 hours should be administered for 24 hours postpartum (16,32). During labor, epidural anesthesia is preferred and safe in the asthmatic patients. Drugs that can cause bronchospasm should be avoided if possible (Table 31-7).

Systemic Analgesics

The use of systemic opioids in asthmatic patients is controversial as it can lead to respiratory depression which may not be tolerated, and also some opioids like high-dose morphine can release histamine (58). Despite these concerns, the importance of analgesia in early labor takes a priority. Fentanyl and meperidine are commonly used opioids for analgesia during labor. Respiratory status should be carefully monitored when respiratory depressants are administered in the asthmatic patient.

Neuraxial Anesthesia for Vaginal Delivery and Cesarean Delivery

It is well known that neuraxial anesthesia results in decreased catecholamine levels and decreased oxygen consumption during labor. This offers great advantage especially in asthmatic

TABLE 31-7 Drugs Associated with Exacerbation of Asthma

Non–β-1 selective antagonists
Prostaglandin F_2-α
Ergot alkaloids
Sulfite agents
Aspirin
NSAIDs
Indomethacin

parturients and is strongly recommended. Anesthesia can be provided with spinal, epidural, or combined spinal–epidural (CSE) technique. There is a theoretical concern that patients on steroid therapy might have a greater risk for epidural or intrathecal infections (20).

Careful titration of local anesthetics should be used and a high block should be avoided as it can lead to a compromise of respiratory muscle function. Spinal anesthesia with a motor block of T_2 level or higher can significantly decrease the expiratory reserve volume. Spinal anesthesia for elective cesarean in healthy women has been shown to reduce forced vital capacity and PEFR (59). Epidural anesthesia may be preferable as it can be titrated to the desired level, recognizing that surgical anesthesia may not be as reliable and time pressures may not permit using a de novo epidural. In the stable asthmatic patient, neuraxial anesthesia is safe. In the woman with unstable asthma who may be dependent upon accessory muscles for effective respiration, neuraxial anesthesia may worsen the respiratory status. When epidural or intrathecal narcotics are used, the patient should be closely monitored for any respiratory depression.

General Anesthesia

General anesthesia is administered when neuraxial block is contraindicated. Exacerbation of bronchospasm is much more likely with placement of an endotracheal tube (60). Rapid sequence induction is commonly utilized in pregnant patients. Placement of endotracheal tube with lighter levels of anesthesia can further exacerbate bronchospasm as airway reflexes are not blunted completely.

The most commonly used induction agents are ketamine and propofol. Although there is not enough supporting evidence, ketamine is still the induction agent of choice because of the mild bronchodilatory properties secondary to the release of endogenous catecholamines. On the other hand, propofol is much more effective at blunting the airway reflexes and is thought to have a weak bronchodilating property. Intravenous lidocaine is useful as an adjuvant during induction as it can blunt the airway reflexes and also attenuate the hemodynamic response for intubation. The dose normally utilized is 1 mg/kg during induction. Aerosolized lidocaine should be avoided in the asthmatic patient as it has been shown to be an airway irritant (61).

Succinylcholine is normally used for rapid sequence induction for muscle relaxation. Rocuronium can safely be used as an alternative for intubation if contraindications to succinylcholine exist in the asthmatic patient. Atracurium can worsen bronchospasm due to histamine release and should be avoided. Vecuronium can be safely used during maintenance of muscle relaxation and if the cesarean delivery time is short, succinylcholine can be used as a drip and reversal agents can be avoided. Reversal of neuromuscular blockade with neostigmine can exacerbate airflow obstruction by increasing secretions and bronchospasm. However, glycopyrrolate or atropine can attenuate this response. Shibata and colleagues conducted a study on the rat tracheal models and suggested that edrophonium is less likely to cause bronchospasm than neostigmine (62).

Halogenated volatile anesthetics are also useful in asthmatics as they produce bronchodilation. Isoflurane and sevoflurane are commonly used for cesarean delivery. Caution should be used when using high alveolar concentrations of volatile anesthetics for control of bronchospasm after delivery as it can increase the risk of bleeding. Poorly controlled asthma is associated with perioperative pulmonary complications. Airway instrumentation may induce life-threatening bronchospasm, perioperative complications, and prolonged intensive care treatment. On the other hand, controlled asthma does not promote any added risk for complications (43). In nonpregnant patients with asthma, extubation can be done under deep anesthesia. As pregnant patients are at increased risk for aspiration, deep extubation is not possible. β-adrenergic agonists and steroids can be used during surgery and the patient should be extubated awake.

■ CYSTIC FIBROSIS

Cystic fibrosis (CF) involves the exocrine glands and epithelial tissues of the pancreas, sweat glands, and mucous glands in the respiratory, digestive, and reproductive tracts. CF is genetically transmitted with an autosomal recessive pattern of inheritance. In the United States, approximately 4% of Caucasian populations are heterozygous carriers of the CF gene. The disease occurs in 1 in 3,000 Caucasian live births (63). Survival of patients with CF has significantly improved over the past 3 decades and therefore more women with CF are able to reach reproductive age. Currently about 140 pregnancies in CF women are reported annually to the US Cystic Fibrosis Foundation Registry, with approximately 100 resulting in live births (14).

The physiologic changes associated with pregnancy are well tolerated by healthy parturients; but patients with CF may adapt poorly. During pregnancy, minute ventilation increases and upward displacement of the diaphragm leads to a decrease in residual volume. There is also a widening of the alveolar–arterial oxygen gradient that is most pronounced in the supine position. In CF patients, these changes may contribute to respiratory decompensation that can lead to increase in morbidity and mortality for both mother and fetus. In addition, women with CF and advanced lung disease may also suffer from pulmonary hypertension which adds to the increased morbidity and mortality during pregnancy.

Pregnancy in women with CF and mild disease is usually well tolerated. Parturients with severe disease have an associated increase in maternal and fetal morbidity and mortality. The potential risk to any individual with CF desirous of pregnancy should be assessed and counseling with the patient and her family in detail even before conception should be done. Management by a team, including the CF specialist, obstetrician, and maternal–fetal medicine specialist will help to optimize the outcome (64).

■ CONCLUSION

The National Asthma Education and Prevention Program (NAEPP) has found that "it is safer for pregnant women with asthma to be treated with medications than it is for them to have asthma symptoms and exacerbations" (65). The NAEPP emphasizes that maintaining adequate control of asthma during pregnancy is important for the health and well-being of both the mother and her fetus. Monitoring and making appropriate adjustments in therapy may be required to maintain lung function and improve blood oxygenation that ensures adequate oxygen supply to the fetus. The undertreatment of asthma in pregnant women may contribute to worsening of asthma symptoms in some pregnant women (66). If pregnant women with asthma discontinue medication, even mild asthma is likely to become significantly more severe (67).

Anesthetic considerations in a pregnant asthmatic should be proper evaluation of the parturient, and preventing or managing acute exacerbations of asthma. Neuraxial analgesia and anesthesia is safe to use in the stable asthmatic patient, but caution should be applied when considering high levels (above T_2) of neuraxial anesthesia in the unstable asthmatic woman.

Drugs that can cause bronchospasm should be avoided if at all possible, but when they are used, adequate measures to treat bronchospasm should be readily available.

KEY POINTS

- Pregnant women with asthma are at increased risk for perinatal complications such as preeclampsia, low birth weight, and premature delivery.
- Albuterol is the first-line rescue inhaler for the rapid relief of acute bronchospasm.
- ICSs are currently used for the management of persistent asthma because they are the most effective anti-inflammatory medication. Due to reassuring clinical experience, beclomethasone dipropionate is the preferred ICS during pregnancy.
- It is safer for pregnant women to be treated with medications than it is for them to have asthma symptoms and exacerbations.
- Smoking adds to the increased morbidity in the asthmatic patients.
- Neuraxial analgesia/anesthesia is safe in stable asthmatic patients; it eliminates the need for endotracheal intubation as long as a high block can be avoided.
- Drugs causing bronchospasm should be avoided if at all possible, but when used, adequate measures to treat bronchospasm should be readily available.

REFERENCES

1. Tamasi L, Horvath I, Bohacs A, et al. Asthma in pregnancy-immunological changes and clinical management. *Respir Med* 2011;105(2):159–164.
2. Rocklin RE. Asthma, asthma medications and their effects on maternal/fetal outcomes during pregnancy. *Reprod Toxicol* 2011;32(2):189–197.
3. Murphy V, Namazy J, Powell H, et al. A meta-analysis of adverse perinatal outcomes in women with asthma. *BJOG* 2011;118(11):1314–1323.
4. Aly H, Nada A, Ahmad T, et al. Maternal asthma, race and low birth weight deliveries. *Early Hum Dev* 2011;87(7):457–460.
5. Lim A, Stewart K, Konig K, et al. Systematic review of the safety of regular preventive asthma medications during pregnancy. *Ann Pharmacother* 2011;45:931–945.
6. From the Centers for Disease Control. Asthma–United States, 1980–1990. *JAMA* 1992;268(15):1995–1999.
7. Esplin MS, Clark SL. Outpatient management of asthma during pregnancy. *Clin Obstet Gynecol* 1998;41(3):555–563.
8. Kwon HL, Triche EW, Belanger K, et al. The epidemiology of asthma during pregnancy: Prevalence, diagnosis, and symptoms. *Immunol Allergy Clin North Am* 2006;26(1):29–62.
9. Akinbami LJ, Moorman JE, Liu X. Asthma prevalence, health care use, and mortality: United States, 2005–2009. *Natl Health Stat Report* 2011;32:1–14.
10. Dombrowski MP, Schatz M, ACOG Committee on Practice Bulletins-Obstetrics. ACOG practice bulletin: Clinical management guidelines for obstetrician-gynecologists number 90, February 2008: Asthma in pregnancy. *Obstet Gynecol* 2008;111(2 Pt 1):457–464.
11. Hardy-Fairbanks AJ, Baker ER. Asthma in pregnancy: Pathophysiology, diagnosis and management. *Obstet Gynecol Clin North Am* 2010;37(2):159–172.
12. Clifton V. Maternal asthma during pregnancy and fetal outcomes: Potential mechanisms and possible solutions. *Curr Opin Allergy Clin Immunol* 2006;6(5):307–311.
13. Mabie WC. Asthma in pregnancy. *Clin Obstet Gynecol* 1996;39(1):56–69.
14. Larson L, Mehta N, Paglia M, et al. Pulmonary disease in pregnancy. In: Powrie R, Greene M, Camann W, eds. *de Swiet's Medical Disorders in Obstetric Practice.* 5th ed. Hoboken, NJ: Wiley-Blackwell; 2010:1–46.
15. McFadden ER Jr, Gilbert IA. Asthma. *N Engl J Med* 1992;327(27):1928–1937.
16. Schatz M, Dombrowski MP. Clinical practice: asthma in pregnancy. *N Engl J Med* 2009;360(18):1862–1869.
17. Dombrowski MP, Schatz M. Asthma in pregnancy. *Clin Obstet Gynecol* 2010;53(2):301–310.
18. Siddiqui S, Goodman N, McKenna S, et al. Pre-eclampsia is associated with airway hyperresponsiveness. *BJOG* 2008;115(4):520–522.

19. Kallen B, Rydhstroem H, Aberg A. Asthma during pregnancy–a population based study. *Eur J Epidemiol* 2000;16(2):167–171.

20. Carlisle AS. Perioperative management of the pregnant patient with asthma. In: Hughes SC, ed. Shnider and Levison's Anesthesia for Obstetrics. Philadelphia, PA: Lippincott Williams & Wilkins; 2001:487.

21. Beckmann CA. The effects of asthma on pregnancy and perinatal outcomes. *J Asthma* 2003;40(2):171–180.

22. Gluck JC, Gluck PA. The effect of pregnancy on the course of asthma. *Immunol Allergy Clin North Am* 2006;26(1):63–80.

23. Lindeman KS. Respiratory disease in pregnancy. In: Chestnut DH, ed. *Chestnut's Obstetric Anesthesia Principles and Practice*. 4th ed. Philadelphia, PA: Mosby Elsevier; 2009:1109.

24. Murphy VE, Gibson PG. Asthma in pregnancy. *Clin Chest Med* 2011;32(1):93–110.

25. National Heart, Lung, and Blood Institute, National Asthma Education and Prevention Program Asthma and Pregnancy Working Group. NAEPP expert panel report - managing asthma during pregnancy: Recommendations for pharmacologic treatment-2004 update. *J Allergy Clin Immunol* 2005;115(1):34–46.

26. Namazy JA, Schatz M. Management of asthma during pregnancy. *Womens Health (Lond Engl)* 2006;2(3):405–413.

27. Schatz M, Zeiger RS, Harden KM, et al. The safety of inhaled beta-agonist bronchodilators during pregnancy. *J Allergy Clin Immunol* 1988;82(4):686–695.

28. Murphy VE, Gibson P, Talbot PI, et al. Severe asthma exacerbations during pregnancy. *Obstet Gynecol* 2005;106(5 pt 1):1046–1054.

29. Jain S, Kamimoto L, Bramley AM, et al. Hospitalized patients with 2009 H1N1 influenza in the United States, April–June 2009. *N Engl J Med* 2009;361(20):1935–1944.

30. Schatz M, Dombrowski MP, Wise R, et al. The relationship of asthma-specific quality of life during pregnancy to subsequent asthma and perinatal morbidity. *J Asthma* 2010;47(1):46–50.

31. Stenius-Aarniala BS, Hedman J, Teramo KA. Acute asthma during pregnancy. *Thorax* 1996;51:411–414.

32. Hanania NA, Belfort MA. Acute asthma in pregnancy. *Crit Care Med* 2005;33(10 Suppl):S319–S324.

33. Elsayegh D, Shapiro JM. Management of the obstetric patient with status asthmaticus. *J Intensive Care Med* 2008;23(6):396–402.

34. Wikner BN, Stiller CO, Bergman U, et al. Use of benzodiazepines and benzodiazepine receptor agonists during pregnancy: Neonatal outcome and congenital malformations. *Pharmacoepidemiol Drug Saf* 2007;16(11):1203–1210.

35. Shapiro JM. Management of respiratory failure in status asthmaticus. *Am J Respir Med* 2002;1(6):409–416.

36. Ivankovic AD, Elam JO, Huffman J. Effect of maternal hypercarbia on the newborn infant. *Am J Obstet Gynecol* 1970;107(6):939–946.

37. Murphy VE, Clifton VL, Gibson PG. The effect of cigarette smoking on asthma control during exacerbations in pregnant women. *Thorax* 2010;65(8):739–744.

38. Demissie K, Breckenridge MB, Rhoads GG. Infant and maternal outcomes in the pregnancies of asthmatic women. *Am J Respir Crit Care Med* 1998;158(4):1091–1095.

39. Roelands J, Jamison MG, Lyerly AD, et al. Consequences of smoking during pregnancy on maternal health. *J Womens Health (Larchmt)* 2009;18(6):867–872.

40. Committee opinion no. 471: Smoking cessation during pregnancy. *Obstet Gynecol* 2010;116(5):1241–1244.

41. Coleman-Cowger VH. Smoking cessation intervention for pregnant women: A call for extension to the postpartum period. *Matern Child Health J* 2012;16(5):937–940.

42. Leung DY, Szefler SJ. In utero smoke (IUS) exposure has been associated with increased prevalence of asthma and reduced lung function in healthy children. *J Allergy Clin Immunol* 2010;126(3):481–482.

43. Dewachter P, Mouton-Faivre C, Emala CW, et al. Case scenario: Bronchospasm during anesthetic induction. *Anesthesiology* 2011;114(5):1200–1210.

44. Cydulka RK. Acute asthma during pregnancy. *Immunol Allergy Clin North Am* 2006;26(1):103–117.

45. George R, Berkenbosch JW, Fraser RF, et al. Mechanical ventilation during pregnancy using a helium-oxygen mixture in a patient with respiratory failure due to status asthmaticus. *J Perinatol* 2001;21(6):395–398.

46. Blais L, Beauchesne MF, Lemiere C, et al. High doses of inhaled corticosteroids during the first trimester of pregnancy and congenital malformations. *J Allergy Clin Immunol.* 2009;124(6):1229–1234.e4.

47. Blais L, Forget A. Asthma exacerbations during the first trimester of pregnancy and the risk of congenital malformations among asthmatic women. *J Allergy Clin Immunol* 2008;121(6):1379–84, 1384.e1.

48. Lin S, Herdt-Losavio M, Gensburg L, et al. Maternal asthma, asthma medication use, and the risk of congenital heart defects. *Birth Defects Res A Clin Mol Teratol* 2009;85(2):161–168.

49. Lin S, Munsie JP, Herdt-Losavio ML, et al. Maternal asthma medication use and the risk of gastroschisis. *Am J Epidemiol* 2008;168(1):73–79.

50. Towers CV, Briggs GG, Rojas JA. The use of prostaglandin E2 in pregnant patients with asthma. *Am J Obstet Gynecol* 2004;190(6):1777–1780.

51. Trivedi NA. A meta-analysis of low-dose aspirin for prevention of preeclampsia. *J Postgrad Med* 2011;57(2):91–95.

52. Rossi AC, Mullin PM. Prevention of pre-eclampsia with low-dose aspirin or vitamins C and E in women at high or low risk: A systematic review with meta-analysis. *Eur J Obstet Gynecol Reprod Biol* 2011;158(1):9–16.

53. Stevenson DD, Szczeklik A. Clinical and pathologic perspectives on aspirin sensitivity and asthma. *J Allergy Clin Immunol* 2006;118(4):773–786.

54. Magee LA, Abalos E, von Dadelszen P, et al. How to manage hypertension in pregnancy effectively. *Br J Clin Pharmacol* 2011;72(3):394–401.

55. Silverman RA, Osborn H, Runge J, et al. IV magnesium sulfate in the treatment of acute severe asthma: A multicenter randomized controlled trial. *Chest* 2002;122(2):489–497.

56. Adams JY, Sutter ME, Albertson TE. The patient with asthma in the emergency department. *Clin Rev Allergy Immunol* 2011; May 20 (epub ahead of print).

57. Blake K. Review of guidelines and the literature in the treatment of acute bronchospasm in asthma. *Pharmacotherapy* 2006;26(9 pt 2):148S–155S.

58. Aviado DM. Regulation of bronchomotor tone during anesthesia. *Anesthesiology* 1975;42(1):68–80.

59. Lirk P, Kleber N, Mitterschiffthaler G, et al. Pulmonary effects of bupivacaine, ropivacaine, and levobupivacaine in parturients undergoing spinal anaesthesia for elective caesarean delivery: a randomized controlled study. *Int J Obstet Anesth* 2010;19(3):287–292.

60. Groeben H, Schlicht M, Stieglitz S, et al. Both local anesthetics and salbutamol pretreatment affect reflex bronchoconstriction in volunteers with asthma undergoing awake fiberoptic intubation. *Anesthesiology* 2002;97:1445–1450.

61. Fish JE, Peterman VI. Effects of inhaled lidocaine on airway function in asthmatic subjects. *Respiration* 1979;37(4):201–207.

62. Shibata O, Kanairo M, Zhang S, et al. Anticholinesterase drugs stimulate phosphatidylinositol response in rat tracheal slices. *Anesth Analg* 1996;82(6):1211–1214.

63. Ciavattini A, Ciattaglia F, Cecchi S, et al. Two successful pregnancies in a woman affected by cystic fibrosis: case report and review of the literature. *J Matern Fetal Neonatal Med* 2011;25(2):113–115.

64. Whitty JE. Cystic fibrosis in pregnancy. *Clin Obstet Gynecol* 2010;53(2):369–376.

65. National Asthma Education and Prevention Program. Expert Panel Report 3 (EPR-3): Guidelines for the Diagnosis and Management of Asthma-Summary Report 2007. *J Allergy Clin Immunol* 2007;120(5 Suppl):S94–138.

66. Louik C, Schatz M, Hernandez-Diaz S, et al. Asthma in pregnancy and its pharmacologic treatment. *Ann Allergy Asthma Immunol* 2010;105(2):110–117.

67. Belanger K, Hellenbrand ME, Holford TR, et al. Effect of pregnancy on maternal asthma symptoms and medication use. *Obstet Gynecol* 2010;115(3):559–567.

Neurologic and Neuromuscular Disorders

Stephanie R. Goodman • Suzanne Wattenmaker Mankowitz

There are a number of neuromuscular and neurologic diseases that can complicate pregnancy. Sometimes pregnancy affects the course of preexisting disease, either improving or worsening the severity. Conversely, the disease itself might affect the pregnancy, causing a number of obstetric and fetal complications. Lastly, some of these conditions have important anesthetic implications and need careful assessment and management in consultation with an obstetrician and neurologist. This chapter reviews many of the neuromuscular and neurologic diseases that can occur during the childbearing years.

■ NEUROMUSCULAR DISEASE IN PREGNANCY

Myasthenia Gravis

Myasthenia gravis (MG) is a chronic autoimmune disease of striated muscle that affects the neuromuscular junction. Most cases result from the production of autoantibodies toward postsynaptic acetylcholine receptors or, more rarely, through the production of antibodies against postsynaptic muscle-specific kinase (1). Other anti-muscle antibodies have also been identified (2). Immunoglobulin G has been the most abundant antibody detected at the neuromuscular junction. These antibodies result in impaired function and accelerated degradation of acetylcholine receptors as well as complement activation, which damages the postsynaptic surface. Thus, the end-plate potential may be disrupted, and synaptic transmission may be compromised (3).

MG affects twice as many women as men, with the peak incidence in women occurring in the third decade. MG affects approximately one in 20,000 pregnancies (4,5). The cardinal symptom of MG is weakness, worsening with activity and improving with rest. Patients frequently present with isolated ocular symptoms, commonly diplopia and ptosis. However, patients may also present with or ultimately develop bulbar symptoms. Bulbar involvement is characterized by dysarthria, dysphagia, and weakness of the neck and proximal muscles (1). The disease progresses in a craniocaudal fashion, and the majority of patients with bulbar symptoms develop generalized limb weakness. Weakness of the diaphragm and intercostal muscles may lead to dyspnea and myasthenic crisis. Respiratory failure occurs in few patients. The disease is characterized by relapses and remissions. The serum levels of antibodies do not always correlate with disease severity though decreased levels are usually associated with an improvement in the disease (2). Thymic abnormalities are common in patients with MG with most manifesting hyperplasia and 10% with thymomas. In addition, patients with MG often have other associated autoimmune diseases (6,7).

Myasthenia Gravis Treatment

Anticholinesterases are used to treat MG. These are taken daily and act by increasing the amount of acetylcholine available to bind to the postsynaptic receptors. Pyridostigmine is commonly used to inhibit the enzyme responsible for hydrolysis of acetylcholine. The drug peaks within 2 hours and its duration is 3–6 hours. Commonly, doses are less than 120 mg every 3 hours. It is very important to follow levels of cholinesterase inhibitors during pregnancy because altered pharmacokinetics can lead to cholinergic crisis. Overdose of anticholinesterases causes cholinergic crisis, which is characterized by paralysis, respiratory failure, hypersalivation, miosis, sweating, vomiting, diarrhea, lacrimation, bronchospasm, and bradycardia. Myasthenic crisis is another event that may occur but this is due to an exacerbation of MG. Myasthenic crisis results in respiratory compromise requiring mechanical ventilation. There are a number of factors that may precipitate a crisis including pregnancy, infection, surgery, stress, medications, hyperthermia, and thyroid dysfunction (8).

Symptomatic patients with MG should be treated with anticholinesterases, immunosuppressant drugs, corticosteroids, plasmapheresis, and immunoglobulin (2). These therapies are directed at decreasing the levels of antibodies and increasing acetylcholine availability. Thymectomy is usually recommended as the thymus may generate autoantigen and house cells that secrete acetylcholine receptor antibody. Although remission occurs in nearly 50% of patients with MG within 1 to 5 years after a thymectomy (5), the impact that thymectomy has on pregnant women with MG has not been determined. Many long-term immunosuppressants are contraindicated during pregnancy. Methotrexate is contraindicated; folic acid antagonists lead to fetal skeletal and craniofacial abnormalities. Azathioprine can also lead to congenital anomalies and has been assigned to pregnancy category D by the FDA, though many women have taken this medication throughout pregnancy without any adverse outcome. Cyclosporine does not seem to carry any major teratogenic risk. Plasmapheresis removes acetylcholine receptor antibodies and immunoglobulin down-regulates the immune system (2).

Pregnancy and Myasthenia Gravis

Pregnancy has a variable and unpredictable effect on MG. Our knowledge is limited by a paucity of literature on this subject. Approximately 30% to 40% of patients will have an exacerbation at some time during pregnancy, and 30% will enjoy a remission (2,9). Relapse seems to occur most commonly in the first trimester (8). However, one-third of all patients have exacerbations in the postpartum period (10). Neither the disease severity nor pregestational medication use before conception determines the relapse rate during pregnancy. Remissions may be due to increased α-fetoprotein in the second and third trimesters leading to decreased antibody binding to the acetylcholine receptor. Women who become pregnant within the first year of MG diagnosis may have a worse outcome compared to those that postpone pregnancy; disease duration is inversely related to disease severity (10). Thus, it is recommended that women delay pregnancy for at least 1 year after diagnosis. The overall maternal mortality is estimated at 3.4% to 4%. Mortality risk factors include myasthenic and cholinergic crises (5,9,10).

There is no convincing evidence that MG alone has adverse effects on pregnancy (2). However, should the patient with MG develop pregnancy-related or myasthenic-related complications, then significant maternal and fetal morbidity may occur. Complications such as acute respiratory distress, weakness, and iatrogenic myasthenic crisis can adversely affect both the mother and fetus. If the mother develops preeclampsia, the use of magnesium (to prevent eclampsia) can precipitate myasthenic crisis. Magnesium inhibits the release of acetylcholine at the neuromuscular junction and decreases the motor endplate sensitivity to acetylcholine (2,11). Some authors report an increased number of preterm births and premature rupture of membranes though further studies are needed to confirm these findings. There is a report of an increased perinatal death rate in babies born to mothers with MG, and there is a higher death rate due to fetal anomalies (2).

Fetal Effects of Myasthenia Gravis

The fetus of patients with MG may develop transient neonatal myasthenia and, rarely, arthrogryposis multiplex congenital, contractures caused by decreased movement secondary to acetylcholine receptor antibodies (2,8,12). Other neonatal complications include Potter's sequence, hyperbilirubinemia, and pulmonary hypoplasia. Ten to twenty percent of neonates born to mothers with MG will have neonatal MG. The infants usually display symptoms 12 to 48 hours after delivery which may last for up to 4 months. The infants may have poor sucking, hypotonia, and respiratory distress (2,5,8). Some infants will require anticholinesterases and respiratory support. The severity of disease in the mother does not predict the occurrence of neonatal MG. Maternal thymectomy may protect against neonatal MG (2,12,13).

Obstetric Anesthesia in Myasthenia Gravis

Parturients with MG should attempt to have a vaginal delivery (10). Surgical intervention presents several risks to parturients with MG (infection and crisis) and should be reserved for obstetrical reasons or for patients in crisis. These patients should be seen in consultation with an anesthesiologist prior to the onset of labor in order to rule out other associated diseases that could further complicate the patient's course. Diseases associated with MG include systemic lupus erythematosus, rheumatoid arthritis, ankylosing spondylitis, diabetes, multiple sclerosis, myocarditis, dysrhythmias, cardiomyopathy, and Crohn's disease (6,7). It is important to determine the duration, medication dose, and severity of the disease. Pulmonary function tests can help to determine which patients are at increased risk for needing respiratory support.

Labor and delivery may be a difficult time for the patient with MG. Cholinesterase inhibitors should be continued. Stress, pain, and exertion during the first stage of labor can exacerbate myasthenic symptoms and should be controlled with early epidural analgesia. Both epidural and combined spinal–epidural have been used successfully. Epidural analgesia curtails opioid-induced respiratory depression. Furthermore, titration of the analgesic level to T10 can help maintain good respiratory function during labor. In addition, the epidural can be extended should a cesarean delivery become necessary. This is especially important given that regional anesthesia is preferred to general anesthesia. Since the first stage of labor primarily involves smooth muscle, parturients tend to tolerate this stage well. However, neuraxial analgesia may exacerbate skeletal muscle weakness (4). A more dilute solution of local anesthetic may be used to reduce the extent of motor block (10). Some recommend a local anesthetic such as ropivacaine in order to reduce the extent of motor block (9,10). Amide local anesthetics should be used because ester local anesthetic duration can be prolonged by anticholinesterases (14,15). The second stage of labor may pose a problem for the patient as the expulsive effort required from the mother may lead to myasthenic crisis. This stage does require use of striated muscles. For this reason, assisted delivery with forceps or vacuum under epidural analgesia may be necessary. Several studies have shown an increase in assisted delivery in these parturients (15). All anesthetics that could cause respiratory depression or affect neuromuscular transmission should be avoided. Thus, most sedatives and opioids should not be given to these patients.

Cesarean delivery should be reserved for obstetric indications, as surgery itself is a trigger for myasthenic crisis (2,10,13). Cesarean delivery has been accomplished with both spinal and general anesthesia. Should a cesarean delivery become necessary in a patient with an epidural already in place, the regional anesthetic blockade can be extended with amide local anesthetics. Chloroprocaine should be avoided given the impaired hydrolysis of ester local anesthetics in the setting of anticholinesterase therapy (2,10). However, patients who have preexisting respiratory compromise may not be able to tolerate a high level of neuraxial anesthesia (10). Maternal hypoxemia may be caused by the decrease in forced vital capacity (FVC) and forced expiratory volume in 1 minute (FEV_1) from neuraxial anesthesia combined with the supine position, decreased functional residual capacity (FRC) of pregnancy, and myasthenia-induced intercostal muscle and diaphragm weakness. In order to maintain a level below T_4, many anesthesiologists prefer epidural to spinal anesthesia (10). Several authors have reported neuraxial anesthetic success with supplemental use of noninvasive ventilatory support such as bilevel positive airway pressure (BiPAP) (16,17).

General anesthesia should be avoided in MG patients, but if general anesthesia and neuromuscular blockade becomes necessary, there are several important considerations. Due to the reduction in functional acetylcholine receptors, patients with MG exhibit resistance to succinylcholine. A higher dose may overcome this resistance but can lead to a phase II block. In addition, chronic anticholinesterase therapy can decrease plasma cholinesterase levels which may lead to prolonged neuromuscular block with succinylcholine (11,18). For these reasons, routine use of depolarizing muscle relaxants in these patients is not recommended. However, some believe that the dose of succinylcholine commonly used is large enough that resistance should not pose a significant problem. Furthermore, the inhibition of plasma cholinesterase by anticholinergics may not have a clinical effect (19). Since parturients should undergo a rapid sequence induction given the risk of aspiration, rocuronium offers an alternative medication for neuromuscular blockade. However, the response to nondepolarizing neuromuscular relaxants is markedly exaggerated in MG patients, which can lead to a prolonged neuromuscular blockade. Even a defasciculating dose of a nondepolarizer can produce profound weakness. When these nondepolarizing muscle relaxants are used, the dose should be greatly reduced (10% to 25% of ED_{95} and monitored with a peripheral nerve stimulator) or avoided altogether if possible. Of

Regional Analgesia	Regional Anesthesia	General Anesthesia
• Institute early • May see increased weakness with local anesthetics • Usually well tolerated to T10 • Alleviates stress of labor though not much effort required as uterus is smooth muscle • Avoid magnesium • Use caution with opioids and benzodiazepines • Watch for myasthenic crisis during second stage	• Avoid esters in setting of anticholinesterases—potential for toxicity • May see prolonged block with lidocaine • Patients may not tolerate T4 level—may lead to respiratory compromise • Surgery may precipitate myasthenic crisis • Also watch for cholinergic crisis at all times while on pyridostigmine • Avoid aminoglycosides and other antibiotics	• Exhibit resistance to succinylcholine; larger doses may lead to prolonged paralysis • Extreme sensitivity to nondepolarizing muscle blockers. May have prolonged paralysis • Anticholinesterase therapy could precipitate cholinergic crisis • Magnesium combined with NDMR will lead to prolonged blockade • Post-op mechanical ventilation may be necessary

FIGURE 32-1 Anesthesia for myasthenia gravis.

note, in Europe, success has been reported with the use of rocuronium for a rapid sequence induction followed by sugammadex reversal (18). Volatile agents also contribute to neuromuscular relaxation, necessitating extreme caution on emergence (2,4,10,11). Given this property of volatile anesthetics, some have advocated induction and intubation with volatile agents alone (10). Reversal with cholinesterase inhibitors in MG can lead to a cholinergic crisis which mimics a myasthenic crisis, with paralysis and respiratory failure (10) (Fig. 32-1).

Due to the risk of prolonged weakness and respiratory depression, postoperative mechanical ventilation may be necessary. The duration of disease, presence of coexisting respiratory disease, and the peripartum pyridostigmine dose all influence the need for prolonged mechanical ventilation (4). Additional factors which are used to assess the need for postoperative ventilation in MG include: A forced expiratory flow 25% to 75% <3.3 L and <78% predicted, a FVC <2.6 L, and a maximum expiratory flow 50% <3.9 L/s and <80% predicted (16). All patients undergoing general anesthesia should be informed about the possibility of prolonged intubation. All patients with MG should be carefully observed in the postpartum period for an exacerbation of the disease.

Myotonic Syndromes

Myotonia refers to an abnormal delay in muscle relaxation after contraction, which is caused by skeletal muscle membrane hyperexcitability and inappropriate firing. This results in contracture states common to a number of muscle diseases that are collaboratively called myotonic disorders (20). Myotonia can be mild or severe; if severe, it interferes with activities of daily living such as walking and climbing stairs. Repeated contraction and relaxation may improve myotonia, which is called the "warming up" phenomenon. Medications used to treat myotonia include sodium channel antagonists such as procainamide, phenytoin, and mexiletine, tricyclic antidepressant drugs, benzodiazepines, calcium channel antagonists, and prednisone (21).

The most common disease within the myotonias is myotonic dystrophy. Myotonic dystrophy (DM) is currently divided into two types: Type 1 (DM1 or Steinert's disease) and type 2 (DM2 or proximal myotonic myopathy [PROMM]). Both are genetically inherited in an autosomal dominant manner and are trinucleotide repeat disorders. DM1 is caused by an abnormal repetition of CTG on chromosome 19 in the DM protein kinase gene, and DM2 is caused by a CCTG repeat on chromosome three in the ZNF9 gene (21). The severity of the disease generally depends on the amount of extra genetic material. DM1 severity seems to worsen in subsequent generations (22). Patients suffer from weakness, atrophy (face, neck, fingers, and limbs), cardiac conduction defects, cognitive dysfunction, cataracts, hypersomnia, insulin resistance, and muscle pain (20). DM2 is not as common as DM1, usually has less severe muscle weakness than DM1, and demonstrates less genetic anticipation (21).

Myotonia congenita (CM) is a less common myotonia and also has two main forms: The autosomal dominant form called Thomsen's disease and the autosomal recessive form called Becker's disease. These diseases are caused by a mutation in CLCN1, which is the skeletal muscle chloride channel that suppresses muscle membranes after potentials. In Thomsen's disease, the myotonia is more severe in the upper limbs and is often associated with muscular hypertrophy. Patients suffer from painless muscle stiffness. Becker's disease tends to be more severe and affects the lower limbs first (20).

DM is associated with an increased rate of obstetric complications. During pregnancy, some patients experience increased weakness while others remain undiagnosed until pregnancy when they become symptomatic. In pregnant patients with DM1, there is an increased incidence of fetal loss, premature delivery, and polyhydramnios (22). Some studies show that the incidence of preterm birth is as high as 50% in patients with DM1 who had clinical signs of the disease prior to pregnancy. These patients also have an increased risk of placenta previa (23). Since DM is an autosomal dominant disease, many fetuses are affected. One study has shown that the pregnancies with affected fetuses have a higher risk of preterm labor and polyhydramnios compared to those with unaffected fetuses (24). It is not known why the fetus influences preterm labor, but polyhydramnios is due to reduced swallowing of amniotic fluid by the affected fetus.

The disease may affect uterine smooth muscle, requiring forceps or other assisted delivery methods (22). The rate of cesarean delivery in these patients is twice as high as in unaffected patients (23). The risk of uterine atony is also increased. Tocolytic treatment with β-adrenergic agonists may precipitate myotonia and rhabdomyolysis, and magnesium may cause severe weakness and respiratory compromise. Women with DM2 do not seem to have a higher risk of fetal loss or polyhydramnios, but they may have worsening of symptoms during pregnancy and an increased risk of preterm labor (5). Pregnancy does not cause a worsening of the overall disease course in DM (22).

Patients with DM1 are also at increased risk of anesthetic and surgical complications. Triggers of myotonia, such as hypothermia and shivering, should be avoided; if laryngeal and respiratory muscles are involved, intubation can be challenging. Myotonic patients are at increased risk for aspiration due to laryngeal muscle weakness and poor esophageal motility (25). Myotonic contractions during surgical manipulation and electrocautery may interfere with surgical access (26). Laboring women may have decreased pulmonary reserve and are at increased risk for respiratory depression from intravenous opioids (5). Patients with DM1 have an increased sensitivity to induction agents and other sedatives (22). Due to the risk of cardiac arrhythmias, electrocardiographic monitoring should be used.

Local and regional anesthesia and analgesia are preferable to general anesthesia, but neither prevents myotonia from occurring (23). Epidural and spinal anesthesia have both been used successfully in DM, but a high thoracic block may not be tolerated for cesarean delivery in a patient with decreased cardiac or pulmonary reserve. Combined spinal–epidural has also been used successfully in DM for cesarean delivery (27,28). Patients with DM2 are not at risk from anesthesia to the same extent as patients with DM1 (29,30).

Succinylcholine should not be administered to patients with myotonia due to hyperkalemia and total body rigidity. The latter can cause difficulty with intubation and ventilation. Nondepolarizing neuromuscular relaxants should be used with caution because of their potentially long duration of action given the patient's preexisting weakness (25).

Although nondepolarizing neuromuscular relaxants usually do not cause a prolonged block, they do not counteract a succinylcholine-induced myotonia (20). Anticholinesterase medications may cause myotonia in patients with CM (21).

There are rare case reports of hyperthermia and acidosis in patients with CM undergoing general anesthesia. It is not certain that these were definitive cases of malignant hyperthermia (MH); one case was described without the administration of triggering agents. A recent review states: "It is highly unlikely that patients with any of the chloride channel myotonias have a risk of developing MH above that of the general population" (20) (Table 32-1). There are no case reports of MH in the setting of DM. It may be very difficult to make the diagnosis of MH when a patient has generalized skeletal muscle rigidity after receiving succinylcholine. Although quite unlikely, it is possible for a patient to have two genetic defects making them susceptible to both MH and myotonia (20).

Muscular Dystrophy

Muscular dystrophies (MDs) are a heterogeneous group of inherited neuromuscular disorders including Duchenne MD, Becker MD, limb-girdle MD, congenital MD, and facioscapulohumeral MD (FSHD). Some are X-linked and have a male preponderance, while others have an autosomal inheritance. These diseases all cause muscle weakness and are characterized pathologically by muscle fiber degeneration, necrosis, fibrosis, and sometimes inflammation. Traditionally, they have been classified based on pathologic, clinical, and inheritance patterns, but currently molecular diagnostic techniques are available to differentiate the many different forms of the disease (31).

TABLE 32-1 Tabular List of Myotonias, Genes Encoding Associated Channels, and Estimated Risk of Malignant Hyperthermia (MH) (in the Absence of a Family History of MH)

Disease	Gene	MH Risk

Chloride channelopathies
    Myotonia congenita, Becker, or Thomsen myotonia
    levior fluctuating *Myotonia congenita*
	CLCN1	Low

Sodium channelopathies
    HyperPP (adynamia episodica hereditaria)
    Paramyotonia congenita (Eulenburg's disease),
    PAM, HypoPP-2
	SCN4A	Low

Calcium channelopathies HypoPP-1	*CACNA1S*	Unclear
Expanded nucleotide repeats Myotonic dystrophy, type 1 (DM1, Steinert's disease)	Expanded trinucleotide repeat, CTG, 3' untranslated region of *DMPK* gene	Low

Myotonic dystrophy, type 2 (DM2, proximal
    myotonic dystrophy [PDM], proximal myotonic
    myopathy [PROMM])
	Tetranucleotide repeat, CCTC, of first
	intron, *ZNF9* gene
		Low

The table summarizes the known molecular genetics of the different myotonias and our estimation of associated risk of MH. Estimation of risk of MH emphasizes the underlying molecular pathology rather than phenotypic presentation. We have left the risk of MH for HypoPP-1 as "unclear," since the genetic change for this entity is in the same gene as one of the loci for MH though the mutations for the two diseases are in different parts of the same gene. Even in the absence of clinical reports of true MH in patients with HypoPP-1 we cannot exclude this possibility at our present state of knowledge.
PAM, potassium aggravated myotonias; HyperPP, hyperkalemic periodic paralysis; HypoPP, hypokalemic periodic paralysis; CLCN1, skeletal muscle chloride channel; SCN4A, sodium channel α-subunit; CACNA1S, α-I subunit of L-type, voltage-dependent calcium channel; MH, malignant hyperthermia.
Reprinted from: Parness J, Bandschapp O, Girard T. The myotonias and susceptibility to malignant hyperthermia. *Anesth Analg* 2009;109: 1054–1064.

TABLE 32-2 Pregnancy and Birth Complications in FSHD and National Data

	FSHD	National	*P*
Cesarean delivery, total	23.8	16.9	0.012
Cesarean delivery, primary	9.2	9.4	0.95
Forceps	19.0	7.1	0.0002
Vacuum	7.9	4.5	0.19
All operative vaginal deliveries	27.0	11.6	0.0001
Preterm birth (<37 weeks' gestation)	12.8	8.4	0.16
Low birth weight (<2,500 g)	16.4	5.6	0.0001
Miscarriage	16.2	15.6	0.87
Preterm labor	11.5	9	0.42
Premature rupture of membranes	11.5	10.7	0.81
Polyhydramnios	4.6	2	0.08
Preeclampsia	3.4	5	0.51
Gestational diabetes	4.6	5	0.86
Birth defects	1.3	5.5	0.71
Neonatal death	1.1	0.5	0.39
Early childhood death	1.1	0.8	0.71
Fetal distress, reported	11.5	3.6	0.0001
Fetal distress, confirmed	3.4	3.6	0.90
Infection, reported	5.7	1.5	0.0011
Infection, confirmed	3.4	1.5	0.11

FSHD, facioscapulohumeral muscular dystrophy.
Reprinted with permission from: Ciafaloni E, Pressman EK, Loi AM, et al. Pregnancy and birth outcomes in women with facioscapulohumeral muscular dystrophy. *Neurology* 2006;67:1887–1889.

FSHD is an autosomal dominant disease; women tend to be less severely affected than men. The disease is characterized by progressive weakness and wasting of the facial, shoulder girdle, and upper arm muscles (32). The progression of weakness is slow in this disease with only 20% of patients ever becoming wheelchair bound (22). This type of MD is not associated with a shortened life expectancy (33).

There is very little information regarding pregnancy and anesthesia for women with MD, especially since many women with these diseases decide against having children. Vaginal delivery may be attempted if there is no obstetric contraindication. One study involving a postal questionnaire of women with FSHD found an increased incidence of low birth weight babies (33) (Table 32-2). Cesarean delivery and forceps delivery were more common in patients with FSHD compared to national birth data (Fig. 32-2). This was thought to be due to abdominal and truncal weakness affecting the second stage of labor. Twenty-four percent of the women with FSHD reported worsening symptoms of weakness and falling that did not resolve postpartum (33).

Limb-girdle MD refers to a myopathy that involves progressive weakness of the limb-girdle musculature. There are many different forms described: Autosomal dominant, autosomal recessive, some with early onset in childhood, and others with a later onset. These patients have difficulty with walking, climbing stairs, and rising from a seated position. An older postal questionnaire that included nine women with limb-girdle MD suggests that these patients also have an increased incidence of operative deliveries but may suffer from a more marked progression of disease during pregnancy compared to those with FSHD (32).

Respiratory complications may be increased in patients with MD, especially if there is restrictive lung disease due to kyphoscoliosis (5). In severe forms of FSHD, patients may have weakness of accessory muscles of respiration and reduced vital capacity. Patients with limb-girdle MD may have weakness of the diaphragm (34). A recent case report describes a woman with limb-girdle MD who had severe restrictive lung

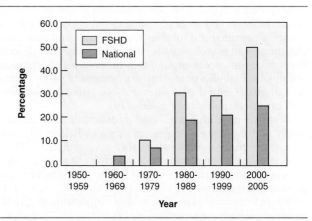

FIGURE 32-2 Cesarean delivery rates in FSHD (expressed in percentages). Reprinted with permission from: Ciafaloni E, Pressman EK, Loi AM et al. Pregnancy and birth outcomes in women with facioscapulohumeral muscular dystrophy. *Neurology* 2006;67:1887–1889.

TABLE 32-3 The Underlying Pathogenesis and the Response to Succinylcholine Versus Nondepolarizing Relaxants in Different Types of Myopathy

Disorder	Pathogenesis	Succinylcholine	Nondepolarizing Relaxants
Denervation	Upregulation of acetylcholine receptors	Hyperkalemia	Resistance
Myasthenia gravis	Autoimmune disease Anti-acetylcholine receptors' antibodies	Resistance	Sensitivity
Muscular dystrophy	X-linked recessive mutation resulting in abnormal dystrophin	Hyperkalemia, rhabdomyolysis	Sensitivity
Myotonic dystrophy	Autosomal dominant disorders Hyperexcitable muscles secondary to abnormal chloride or sodium channels	Myotonic contracture	Normal
Malignant hyperthermia	Dominant inheritance of abnormal ryanodine receptors	Hypermetabolism and muscular rigidity	Normal

Reprinted from: Baraka AS, Jalbout MI. Anesthesia and myopathy. *Curr Opin Anaesthesiol* 2002;15:371–376.

disease during pregnancy. She was treated with noninvasive positive pressure ventilation at 34 weeks' gestation and had a combined spinal–epidural placed for her emergency cesarean delivery without complications (35).

In pregnancy, patients with MD can be challenging to anesthetize. In addition to restrictive lung disease, they may also suffer from cardiomyopathies and pulmonary hypertension. Succinylcholine is contraindicated due to the expression of extrajunctional postsynaptic acetylcholine receptors, which can lead to hyperkalemic cardiac arrest and severe rhabdomyolysis (Table 32-3). It is also recommended that inhalation anesthetics be avoided in these patients due to reports of MH-like responses (36). Similar to the description of the myotonias, MH and MD are distinct genetic diseases, but the hyperkalemic arrest and rhabdomyolysis can mimic MH (37,38). Neuraxial anesthesia must be carefully titrated because significant cephalad spread can decrease inspiratory capacity and expiratory reserve volume, which may worsen already compromised ventilatory function (35).

Central Core Disease

Central core disease is a rare, inherited neuromuscular disease that is characterized by central cores on muscle biopsy and has the clinical features of a congenital myopathy. Affected patients are diagnosed in infancy with hypotonia and motor developmental delay. Common presenting symptoms include muscle stiffness and weakness. The distribution of weakness is usually proximal and involves the hip girdle and axial muscles though all muscles can be affected. Congenital dislocation of the hips, scoliosis, and foot deformities are frequent orthopedic complications that are associated with central core disease. Central core disease is not typically associated with cardiac or pulmonary disease (39).

Most patients with central core disease ambulate independently and the disease progresses very slowly if at all; however, some patients may suffer from severe disease. There is no cure, and management is supportive. Regular physical therapy helps to maintain muscle power and function and prevent contractures. Muscle atrophy can easily occur with prolonged immobilization; it is thus important to quickly mobilize patients postoperatively (39).

There is very little literature regarding central core disease and pregnancy. One study of women with MDs included five women with central core disease. During pregnancy, these women had difficulty climbing stairs, walking long distances, and carrying heavy weights. Many of these women had exacerbations of weakness and generalized fatigue during pregnancy and postpartum. There also seems to be an increased incidence of preterm births and assisted deliveries in central core disease patients (32).

Patients with central core disease are susceptible to MH. Central core disease and MH are both conditions that are caused by mutations in the skeletal muscle ryanodine receptor (RYR1) gene (40). A non-triggering anesthetic must be utilized for patients with central core disease; that is, succinylcholine and volatile anesthetics must be avoided. If clinical signs of MH do occur, dantrolene must be administered early in the course of the reaction (39).

Some central core disease patients may have facial abnormalities such as retrognathism and a high arched palate which can make airway management difficult (41). Due to severe scoliosis, Harrington rods, and scarring, one parturient with central core disease was administered total intravenous anesthesia with propofol and remifentanil for cesarean delivery and had no anesthetic complications (41). Postoperatively, these patients are at increased risk for pulmonary complications due to their inherent weakness and exaggerated response to sedatives and opioids. There are reports of safe neuraxial anesthetics used for vaginal delivery and cesarean delivery. However, intercostal muscle blockade from spinal or epidural anesthesia could place these patients at risk for respiratory impairment (42,43).

Charcot–Marie–Tooth Disease

Charcot–Marie–Tooth (CMT) disease is a group of genetically heterogeneous, inherited neuropathies, which are also called hereditary sensory and motor neuropathies. While rare, these are the most common hereditary neuromuscular disorders. CMT is caused by more than 40 gene mutations that are expressed in Schwann cells and neurons and produce axonal degeneration. Classically, patients with CMT manifest distal muscle weakness and atrophy, sensory loss, hyporeflexia, and skeletal abnormalities. Life span is normal, and patients usually remain ambulatory. Currently, there is no medical treatment for the disease (44).

While there is much in the literature regarding preimplantation and fetal diagnosis of CMT, there are few studies of how CMT affects pregnancy. One registry study, which included 49 parturients with CMT, found a higher rate of abnormal presentation, postpartum hemorrhage, operative and assisted delivery in CMT patients compared to non-CMT patients (45) (Table 32-4). Another study of CMT in

TABLE 32-4 Interventions during Birth and Obstetric Complications in Women with CMT (*n* = 108) and Reference Group (*n* = 2, 102, 971), Adjusted for Period of Birth

	CMT Group, *n* (%)	Reference Group, %	Odds Ratio	*p* Value[a]
Total interventions	36 (33.3)	22.5	1.4	0.09
Total operative delivery: Cesarean section and vacuum/forceps	32 (29.6)	15.3	1.9	0.002
Cesarean section				
Total	17 (15.7)	9.0	1.5	0.1
Elective[b]	3 (2.8)	2.0	1.4	0.6
Forceps	10 (9.3)	2.7	3.4	<0.001
Vacuum	6 (5.6)	3.9	1.3	0.6
Total complications	46 (42.6)	36.3	1.1	0.7
Presentation anomalies	10 (9.3)	4.5	2.0	0.04
Bleeding postpartum	13 (12.0)	5.8	2.0	0.02

[a]Pearson x^2, *p* value.
[b]Data from 1988 onward.
CMT, Charcot–Marie–Tooth.
Reprinted with permission from: Hoff JM, Gilhus NE, Daltveit AK. Pregnancies and deliveries in patients with Charcot-Marie-Tooth disease. *Neurology* 2005;64:459–462.

pregnancy found that 38% of parturients had worsening of their symptoms during pregnancy, but the authors did not find an effect of CMT on the pregnancy outcome (46).

These patients can have a wide spectrum of disability. Some patients have significant scoliosis, which can make neuraxial labor analgesia more challenging or impossible. CMT patients can develop a restrictive pattern of lung disease, which can worsen with pregnancy and require assisted ventilation. Both spinal and epidural anesthesia have been used successfully in CMT patients for vaginal and cesarean delivery (47). Combined spinal–epidural is a useful technique; a low dose spinal with incremental epidural boluses as needed minimizes the cardiovascular and respiratory effects of spinal anesthesia. Depending on the severity of disease, CMT patients could be sensitive to nondepolarizing neuromuscular relaxants and be at risk for succinylcholine-induced hyperkalemia. The literature suggests that succinylcholine is contraindicated in CMT, but a review of 86 nonpregnant surgical cases included many patients who received succinylcholine without complications (48). If general anesthesia is used, a period of postoperative ventilation may be necessary.

Motor Neuron Disorders

Amyotrophic Lateral Sclerosis

Amyotrophic lateral sclerosis (ALS) is a progressive neurologic disease that affects the upper and lower motor neurons and leads to irreversible muscle weakness and atrophy. Death usually occurs within 3 to 5 years of diagnosis and is due to respiratory paralysis. Riluzole, which blocks tetrodotoxin-sensitive sodium channels associated with damaged neurons, is the only treatment that slows the disease progression, but there is no cure. ALS affects men more than women and usually does not occur until after age 50, therefore, ALS during pregnancy is extremely rare. There are reported cases of uneventful pregnancies and deliveries, but there are also cases of respiratory failure during pregnancy (49).

Spinal Muscular Atrophy

Spinal muscular atrophy (SMA) is an autosomal recessive disease that causes degeneration of the anterior horn cells;

SMA is caused by a mutation or deletion of the Survival Motor Neuron-1 (SMN1) gene. There are four types, which are classified by the age of onset and the degree of motor impairment. SMA type 1 is the most severe form, also known as Werdnig–Hoffmann disease, with onset before 6 months of age, and patients are unable to sit. SMA type 2 has onset between 6 and 18 months of age, and patients are unable to stand. SMA type 3 has onset after 18 months of age, and patients are unable to walk. SMA type 4 has adult onset, and patients are able to walk. The treatment for SMA is supportive. Pulmonary complications are the main cause of morbidity and mortality from respiratory muscle weakness. SMA patients are also at risk for progressive scoliosis due to weak paraspinal muscles (50).

Severely affected women are discouraged from getting pregnant, but there are cases of women successfully delivering babies. One patient with SMA type 2 weighing 20 kg and with a vital capacity of 11% of predicted had two separate, uneventful cesarean deliveries at 28 weeks' gestation under general anesthesia after fiberoptic intubation. Her epidural attempts failed due to severe scoliosis (51). A review of pregnancy outcomes in 12 patients with SMA type 3 showed an increased risk of premature delivery, and 67% of patients had an exacerbation of muscle weakness during their second trimester (52). Most women with SMA are delivered by cesarean delivery, and some require mechanical ventilation to help reduce dyspnea and atelectasis (51). If magnesium is indicated for treatment of preeclampsia or preterm labor, great care must be given to its administration as these patients already have significant weakness.

Very little is written about the anesthetic management of labor and delivery in SMA patients. Due to severe scoliosis, SMA patients are at risk for difficult and possibly failed regional anesthesia, especially if they have had a surgical correction. It can be a challenge just to position wheelchair-dependent patients on an operating table for neuraxial anesthesia. Spinal anesthesia can lead to pulmonary decompensation if a severe restrictive deficit is already present (53). However, spinal anesthesia has been used successfully in SMA patients (54). General anesthesia is not without risk in SMA. Patients may have restricted mouth opening, which can make intubation difficult. They are also at risk for succinylcholine-induced hyperkalemia and sensitivity to nondepolarizing neuromuscular relaxants (51). Rocuronium can be used to facilitate intubation during rapid sequence induction of general anesthesia, but some authors recommend avoiding neuromuscular blockade entirely, especially if severe respiratory compromise is already present preoperatively. If nondepolarizing neuromuscular relaxants are administered, a prolonged duration of blockade should be anticipated as well as the possibility of postoperative mechanical ventilation (55).

■ NEUROLOGIC DISEASE IN PREGNANCY
Multiple Sclerosis

Multiple sclerosis (MS) is the most common disabling neurologic disease that affects young adults in the Western world. MS is an inflammatory and demyelinating disease that most commonly affects women, with a mean age of onset of 30 years. MS has both an autoimmune and genetic component, but the exact etiology is unknown. It is thought that patients with MS are exposed to a set of environmental agents, which trigger an autoimmune attack on the myelin sheath of central nervous system axons (56) and results in axonal loss and gliosis. A plaque is the hallmark pathologic lesion of MS and is due to focal loss of myelin. The most common areas to find macroscopic lesions are the spinal cord, optic nerves, brainstem/cerebellum, and the periventricular white matter. With ongoing axonal loss, the patient experiences irreversible disability and disease progression (56). MS is a clinical diagnosis, but detection of plaques on MRI is frequently used for confirmation (57).

Early symptoms of MS include tingling, numbness, and loss of balance, limb weakness, and blurred or double vision. Later symptoms of MS include worsening motor weakness, lack of coordination, intention tremor, spasticity, bladder dysfunction, fatigue, decreased respiratory function, and paroxysmal pain or paresthesias (58). The course of the disease is highly variable and is characterized by exacerbations and remissions. The majority of patients (80% to 90%) have a relapsing–remitting disease course that lasts about 20 years with relapses occurring an average of every 1 to 2 years. There is general agreement that a slower progression of MS is associated with a complete or near complete recovery from the first attack; many studies suggest that fewer relapses in the first 2 to 5 years are associated with slower disease progression (59). Other positive prognostic signs include female gender, younger age at onset, an initial presentation of either optic neuritis or sensory symptoms, and low baseline lesion load on MRI. It remains unclear how relapses affect the course of the disease and whether elimination of relapses early in the disease prevents secondary progression (56). MS is treated with a number of medications that are not recommended for use in pregnancy (60) (Table 32-5).

TABLE 32-5 Multiple Sclerosis Medications Not Recommended in Pregnancy

Azathioprine
Methotrexate
Mitoxantrone
Cyclophosphamide
Cyclosporin A
Interferon β-1-b and β-1-a
Glatiramer acetate

Pregnancy does not have a deleterious effect on the course of MS, and the majority of parturients report improvement during pregnancy. Several retrospective studies have shown a decrease in the relapse rate during pregnancy and an increase in the relapse rate postpartum (57). The Pregnancy in Multiple Sclerosis (PRIMS) study was a European multicenter, prospective, observational study involving 254 women with MS during 269 pregnancies (61). They found that the mean rate of relapse in the year prior to pregnancy was 0.7 ± 0.9 per woman per year, which decreased to 0.2 ± 1.0 in the third trimester and increased to 1.2 ± 2.0 during the first 3 months postpartum. Immunosuppression during pregnancy may explain the improvement seen in MS patients (57). The PRIMS study also found that while disability scores worsened during the study period, there was no postpartum acceleration of disability progression (61).

Two years later, a follow-up to the PRIMS study was published and found that while there was an increased risk of relapse in the first 3 months postpartum, the majority of women (72%) remained asymptomatic (62). The occurrence of a postpartum relapse was correlated with an increased relapse rate in the pre-pregnancy year, an increased relapse rate during the pregnancy, and a higher disability score at the onset of pregnancy. Postpartum relapse was not found to be correlated with breastfeeding, the use of epidural analgesia, the age of the patient at diagnosis of MS or at conception, the disease duration, the number of previous pregnancies, or the child's gender (62). Infection, stress, and hyperpyrexia may explain the increased frequency of MS relapses postpartum (58). Breastfeeding may be protective against MS relapses in the postpartum period (63).

Most studies do not find an increase in serious pregnancy-related complications or neonatal complications due to MS. Delivery itself is not more complicated in MS patients, and the delivery mode should be based solely on obstetrical criteria. However, there may be some bias in the literature due to the possibility that women with very disabling MS choose not to get pregnant (57). Some studies do find a higher rate of operative deliveries (forceps, vacuum, and cesarean delivery) and induced labors as well as a greater number of low birth weight or small for gestational age babies due to MS. It is postulated that perineal weakness, muscular spasticity, fatigue, and exhaustion may all play a role in these findings (64–66).

Patients with MS may have decreased maximal inspiratory and expiratory effort even if total lung volume and vital capacity are normal. Also, the central control of ventilation, and the response to an increase in $PaCO_2$ may be impaired. Women with MS should be monitored carefully for increased body temperature and treated aggressively with antipyretics; excessive surface warming should be avoided because there is some association of hyperthermia and worsening of MS symptoms (58). There is no evidence suggesting that any one particular intravenous or inhalational anesthetic is better for patients with MS. Succinylcholine may cause hyperkalemia if there is muscle wasting (58). In addition, MS patients may have a greater effect from residual neuromuscular blockade compared to normal patients, especially if they are taking baclofen for treatment of spasticity. Thus, ensuring the complete reversal of neuromuscular blocking agents is crucial (57).

Currently, there appears to be very little evidence to support the claim that neuraxial analgesia or anesthesia causes MS exacerbations. The concern has been that local anesthetics cause neurotoxicity when demyelinated areas of the spinal cord are exposed to them. In 1988, Bader et al. published a retrospective report of 20 women with MS that suggested an association between higher concentrations of epidural local anesthetic and MS relapse. Even then, the authors felt that there was no absolute contraindication to regional anesthesia for labor and delivery (67). The PRIMS study found no adverse effect on the rate of relapse or on the progression of disability from epidural analgesia (61). In 2006, a survey of UK anesthesiologists found that the majority were willing to perform regional anesthesia in parturients with MS provided that the patients understood the risk of relapse, full consent was given, and adequate follow-up provided (68). If there are lesions affecting the autonomic nervous system, the patient may suffer from hemodynamic instability during neuraxial analgesia and anesthesia; it is important to monitor these patients carefully (58). As with all autoimmune diseases, these patients may require supplemental steroids if they are chronically taking steroids in order to avoid an adrenal crisis, because they may not be able to increase their endogenous steroid production during the stress of labor and delivery.

When we offer patients with MS labor analgesia at Columbia University, we do a thorough assessment of the stage and severity of disease and document the patient's current neurologic status. We carefully explain that muscle weakness will occur due to the anesthetic, and that this is not due to an exacerbation of the disease. We also explain to the patient that it is not uncommon to experience a postpartum relapse, which occurs whether or not one has a neuraxial anesthetic.

Epilepsy

Epilepsy is a chronic seizure disorder that affects 0.3% to 0.6% of gestations (69). Most pregnant women with epilepsy enjoy uneventful pregnancies (70). Approximately 15% to 30% of women may experience an increase in seizure frequency during pregnancy. Seizures often occur in the peripartum period, and if they happen during labor, fetal heart rate deceleration may occur as a result. Seizure activity is likely related to both hormonal changes and the altered pharmacokinetics of antiepileptic drugs during pregnancy (69,71). Pregnant woman have a larger volume of distribution, increased renal clearance, decreased plasma protein binding, and decreased intestinal absorption. Thus, it is important to monitor drug levels during pregnancy. Folic acid administration to women being treated with antiepileptic drugs may decrease the incidence of fetal neural tube defects (70,72). There is evidence that remaining seizure-free for 9 to 12 months prior to pregnancy confers protection against seizures during pregnancy (73). It is therefore important to optimize medical treatment prior to conception.

There have been reports of maternal and neonatal complications in pregnant women with epilepsy. These include preeclampsia, spontaneous abortion, congenital malformations, placental abruption, small-for-gestational-age (SGA), stillbirth, intracranial hemorrhage, long-term fetal cognitive deficits, preterm delivery, and cesarean delivery (69,71,73). Congenital malformations have been associated with antiepileptic drugs; the incidence of congenital malformations in women taking antiepileptic drugs is estimated to be 2 to 3 times greater than average. Although all antiepileptic drugs are associated with congenital malformations, polytherapy and valproate seem to carry a higher risk (70). Given the lack of conclusive evidence about these complications, The American Academy of Neurology (AAN) has created guidelines for the treatment and counseling of pregnant women with epilepsy (72).

The AAN suggests that woman taking antiepileptic drugs probably do not have a substantially (that is, more than 2 times expected) increased rate of cesarean delivery nor do they have a significantly increased risk of preterm labor and delivery. Smokers with epilepsy, however, may have a substantially increased risk of preterm delivery. Furthermore, pregnant women with epilepsy do not have a substantially increased risk of late bleeding complications. The practice parameter update states that there is inadequate data to either support or refute the suggestion that epilepsy is associated with preeclampsia, pregnancy-related hypertension, spontaneous abortion, change in seizure frequency, or increased risk of status epilepticus (72). There is, however, probably an increased rate of SGA neonates in woman taking antiepileptic drugs though no substantially increased risk of perinatal death (72). The AAN concludes that valproate probably carries a higher risk of congenital malformations compared to other antiepileptic drugs, especially when taken as monotherapy in the first trimester. In addition, when used as part of polytherapy, valproate probably increases the risk of congenital malformations. It is thought that valproate is associated with fetal neural tube defects, facial clefts, and poor cognitive outcomes. Polytherapy in general is probably associated with both congenital malformations and reduced cognitive outcomes (72). Newer agents such as lamotrigine and levetiracetam are thought to be less teratogenic, although the data are derived from small and uncontrolled studies (70). Obviously, much larger, randomized, controlled trials are needed to confirm all of the above recommendations and findings.

Despite the concern about antiepileptic drugs, seizure control is critically important. Prolonged seizure activity has been associated with uterine contractions and fetal hypoxemia, bradycardia, intracranial hemorrhage, and acidosis (69,70). If a pregnant patient has a seizure, she should be given oxygen and airway support as needed and placed in the left lateral decubitus position. Benzodiazepines should be the first line of treatment to terminate the seizure. Other sedatives such as a barbiturate or propofol can also be effective. Dehydration, sleep deprivation, stress, treatment noncompliance, and some analgesics, such as meperidine and ketamine, can all precipitate seizures and should be avoided when possible.

Migraine Headaches

Migraine headache is described as moderate to severe unilateral pain that is pulsating in nature. It is frequently associated with nausea, vomiting, and photophobia and occurs three times more commonly in women than men. Most pregnant women with migraine headaches report remission or a significant improvement during pregnancy, particularly during the second and third trimesters. This is likely due, in part, to the hormonal changes associated with pregnancy, especially the increase in estrogen. A small percentage (4% to 8%) of pregnant women with migraine headaches experience a worsening of their headaches during pregnancy. Patients who continue to have migraine headaches at the end of the first trimester as well as those who have associated auras are less likely to improve during pregnancy (74,75). A small number of women experience their first migraine during pregnancy, often with aura. Many patients do have postpartum flares, although breastfeeding offers some protection against this (75,76).

It has generally been thought that pregnant women with migraine headaches do not have any adverse maternal or neonatal outcomes. However, while there are currently no known neonatal complications caused by migraine headaches, there is some evidence that pregnant women with migraine headaches may have an increased incidence of gestational hypertension and preeclampsia (74–77). Some authors suggest that pregnant women with migraine headaches share an association with vascular disorders such as stroke, deep vein thrombosis, myocardial infarction, and thrombophilias (74,76,78,79). However, larger prospective studies are needed to confirm whether pregnant women with migraine headaches carry any additional obstetric risk.

Many migraine medications are associated with congenital anomalies, intrauterine growth retardation, and other embryotoxic effects (Fig. 32-3). For this reason, medications

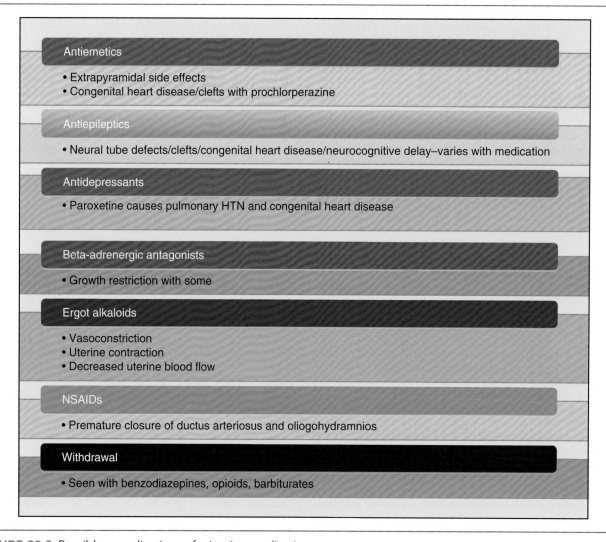

Antiemetics

- Extrapyramidal side effects
- Congenital heart disease/clefts with prochlorperazine

Antiepileptics

- Neural tube defects/clefts/congenital heart disease/neurocognitive delay–varies with medication

Antidepressants

- Paroxetine causes pulmonary HTN and congenital heart disease

Beta-adrenergic antagonists

- Growth restriction with some

Ergot alkaloids

- Vasoconstriction
- Uterine contraction
- Decreased uterine blood flow

NSAIDs

- Premature closure of ductus arteriosus and oliogohydramnios

Withdrawal

- Seen with benzodiazepines, opioids, barbiturates

FIGURE 32-3 Possible complications of migraine medications.

taken chronically to prevent attacks should, if possible, be discontinued during pregnancy. Some women will continue to have disability, pain, nausea, vomiting, and dehydration and may benefit from treatment when the headache occurs. Nonsteroidal anti-inflammatory drugs (NSAIDs), acetaminophen, triptans, antiemetics (ondansetron and metoclopramide), and opioids have been used to treat pregnant women with migraine headaches when they develop a migraine headache (76,80). Ergot alkaloids should not be used during pregnancy, and NSAIDs should not be used after 32 weeks gestation. Ergot alkaloids are associated with uterine contractions and decreased uterine blood flow while NSAIDs are linked to premature closure of the ductus arteriosus and persistent neonatal pulmonary hypertension (74,79). β-adrenergic antagonists, tricyclic antidepressants, selective serotonin reuptake inhibitors (except paroxetine which has been associated with cardiac anomalies), some antiepileptic drugs, as well as verapamil, may be used as preventative medications in patients with severe migraine (75,79,80). Pregnant women with migraine headaches should be advised to maintain good nutrition, exercise, and sleep patterns and to avoid nicotine and stress; relaxation and biofeedback may be helpful as well.

Neuropathies

Meralgia Paresthetica

Meralgia paresthetica is one of the most common pregnancy-related neuropathies. This sensory only palsy occurs when the lateral femoral cutaneous nerve is compressed as it passes around the anterior superior iliac spine, under or within the inguinal ligament. The nerve is easily subjected to compression and stretch, particularly as patients gain weight and become more lordotic. The deficit is usually unilateral although 8% to 12% of patients have bilateral involvement (81). The lateral femoral cutaneous nerve can also be injured in the lithotomy position or by retractors during cesarean delivery. Patients complain of tingling, burning, and numbness in the anterolateral thigh. The deficit usually recovers postpartum. Severe discomfort can be treated with medications such as local anesthetics, corticosteroid injections, anticonvulsants, and antidepressants. A nerve transposition is rarely indicated (5,81).

Carpal Tunnel Syndrome

Carpal tunnel syndrome is another common neuropathy that occurs during pregnancy, involving as many as 62% of parturients (5,82). Carpal tunnel syndrome occurs when the median nerve is compressed between the flexor retinaculum and the carpal bones. It may be either unilateral or bilateral. Patients present with paresthesias, pain, and numbness in the thumb, index finger, long finger, and radial side of the ring finger as well as thenar weakness with decreased grip strength. Pregnancy is a risk factor for the development of carpal tunnel syndrome. This may be due to edema, musculoskeletal changes, or relaxin-induced hypertrophy of the transverse carpal ligament. Carpal tunnel syndrome occurs more frequently in patients with preeclampsia, excessive weight gain, older primigravidas, smokers, and those who drink alcohol. Carpal tunnel syndrome most often occurs in the third trimester, and it may continue or begin with breastfeeding. In most women, carpal tunnel syndrome greatly improves within a few weeks postpartum or within 6 weeks after cessation of breastfeeding. However, some patients continue to have symptoms of carpal tunnel syndrome for many years (82). The earlier in pregnancy that carpal tunnel syndrome develops, the longer the symptoms may last. Treatment consists of splinting, steroids, diuretics, and physical therapy; surgery is rarely indicated (5,83–85).

Bell's Palsy

Bell's palsy is usually characterized by unilateral upper or lower facial paralysis, decreased taste on the anterior two-thirds of the tongue, hyperacusis, and inability to close the eyes with decreased lacrimation and absent corneal reflex. It arises from dysfunction of the facial nerve on the affected side and can be bilateral in 1% of cases (86). The incidence of Bell's palsy is thought to be slightly higher in pregnancy than in the general population with estimates of 45 per 100,000 cases, possibly due to the relative immunosuppression of pregnancy and viral reactivation (22,87). Bell's palsy almost always presents in the third trimester and, less commonly, in the postpartum period. Many authors have noted an association between Bell's palsy and preeclampsia as well as gestational hypertension (22,87,88).

The etiology of Bell's palsy remains controversial and is likely multifactorial (87,89). Nerve impingement from the increased edema seen in pregnancy has been implicated as the cause, as has the hypercoagulable, hormonal state of pregnancy, which may lead to thrombosis, vasospasm, or embolism of the vasa nervorum (22,87–89). Eighty percent of patients improve without treatment. If initiated early in the course of the illness, both prednisone and antiviral medications may be beneficial (22,87). Most patients enjoy a full recovery. However, there is some evidence that patients who have a full paralysis during pregnancy may have a worse outcome than the general population (87,88). The incidence, etiology, neonatal effects, and outcomes of Bell's palsy during pregnancy needs further study.

Guillain–Barré Syndrome

Guillain–Barré Syndrome (GBS) is an acute, inflammatory, demyelinating polyneuropathy that rarely occurs in woman of childbearing age. Thus, there is little information pertaining to parturients with GBS. Patients develop an acute, progressive, ascending, symmetric limb weakness or paralysis with variable sensory loss, areflexia, and possibly cranial nerve involvement. Two-thirds of GBS cases are preceded by a viral infection (often campylobacter jejuni and cytomegalovirus) within the previous month (5,83). Typically symptoms may worsen for up to a month followed by a period of stability prior to improvement (83). Complications include death in 3% to 8% of patients, although many authors report even higher rates (90,91), cardiac arrest, respiratory arrest, deep venous thrombosis and/or pulmonary embolism, aspiration pneumonia, and sepsis (83,92).

The incidence of GBS in pregnancy seems similar to the general population although some report an increased incidence of the disease postpartum (5,22,90,91). GBS does not appear to affect pregnancy, labor, or delivery. Given that the course of GBS is not altered by pregnancy, termination of pregnancy is not recommended (91). There are some authors who report an increased incidence of maternal and perinatal morbidity, namely respiratory failure and preterm delivery, although there are too few cases to make a definitive statement (5,90,93). Of note, there is one case report of neonatal GBS presumably from placental transfer of maternal antibodies (5). Early treatment may reduce both the need for mechanical ventilation as well as other complications (90,91,93,94). Plasmapheresis and immunoglobulin (IVIG) have not resulted in adverse neonatal outcomes and should be started within 2 weeks of disease onset. Anticoagulation is also indicated. Vaginal delivery is not contraindicated as uterine contractility is preserved; cesarean delivery should be reserved for obstetric indications.

Anesthetic management has been safely performed with either neuraxial or general anesthesia (90,91,95). It is important to be aware of the possibility of autonomic instability when administering anesthesia to these patients. Parasympathetic and sympathetic nervous system instability can lead to life-threatening arrhythmias as well as hypotension and hypertension. Vasoactive medications should therefore be administered with caution. If general anesthesia is used, it is important to note that there is a risk of hyperkalemia when using succinylcholine due to the proliferation of extrajunctional postsynaptic acetylcholine receptors as part of the disease pathophysiology. Patients may exhibit sensitivity to nondepolarizing neuromuscular relaxants and, if used, may require postoperative ventilation (5,90–92). Epidural analgesia has been performed safely, although there is one recent case report of worsening of symptoms (96). Epidural analgesia will blunt the hemodynamic response to labor although increased sensitivity to local anesthetics has been reported (91,92).

Posterior Reversible Encephalopathy Syndrome

Posterior reversible encephalopathy syndrome (PRES), although a rare entity, has been more frequently reported in the obstetric population in recent years. Patients usually present with a number of neurologic impairments such as seizures or status epilepticus, headache, altered mental status including coma, paresis, and visual loss or deficit (97–99). The identification of PRES and early treatment are critical in decreasing morbidity and mortality. The condition is usually transient and reversible.

Some predisposing risk factors for PRES include preeclampsia and eclampsia, autoimmune disease, cytotoxic or immunosuppressive medications, acute hypertension, immunocompromised states, and infection (97,99–102). The areas supplied by the posterior cerebral artery, the white matter of the posterior cerebral hemispheres, are most commonly involved. The posterior circulation may be more susceptible to disease because of decreased sympathetic innervation. Frontal lobes, basal ganglia, cerebellum, brainstem, and the spinal cord have also been affected, and the syndrome is usually bilateral (97,99–102).

The vasogenic edema of PRES can be appreciated with fluid attenuation inversion recovery (FLAIR) MRI (Fig. 32-4) (100,101). The pathophysiology of the vasogenic edema has not been fully elucidated. Theories include cerebral hypoperfusion resulting from vasospasm, ischemia, and endothelial dysfunction, leading to disruption of the blood–brain barrier. Alternatively, cerebral hyperperfusion may arise from increased cerebral perfusion pressure and altered

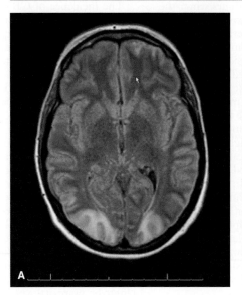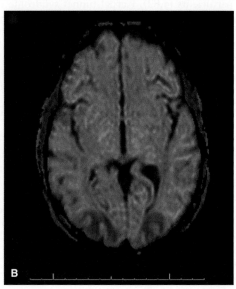

FIGURE 32-4 Typical MRI appearance of PRES: Bilateral posterior subcortical hyperintensities showing abnormal signal on FLAIR (**A**) without restricted diffusion (**B**) on diffusion weighted imaging. Reprinted with permission from: Pula JH, Eggenberger E. Posterior reversible encephalopathy syndrome. *Curr Opin Ophthalmol* 2008;19:479–484.

autoregulation in the cerebral vasculature. All of these triggers result in extravasation of fluid and vasogenic edema (97–102). Management is largely supportive and consists of controlling hypertension and seizure activity.

KEY POINTS

- Many neuromuscular diseases involve weakness of the respiratory muscles or restrictive lung disease so careful titration of neuraxial anesthesia is critical. Careful use of nondepolarizing neuromuscular relaxants is also advocated due to muscle weakness in many neuromuscular diseases.
- MG patients are resistant to succinylcholine and sensitive to non-depolarizing neuromuscular relaxants, and cesarean delivery can trigger a myasthenic crisis.
- There is no contraindication to neuraxial anesthesia in multiple sclerosis but there is a high rate of postpartum relapse.
- Seizures in pregnant women with epilepsy are common in the peripartum period, should be treated promptly, and are associated with fetal heart rate decelerations. Antiepileptic drugs are associated with congenital malformations, especially valproate.
- Pregnant women with migraines may have associated preeclampsia and vascular events.
- Myotonic dystrophy Type 1 is associated with preterm birth, placenta previa, cesarean delivery, and uterine atony. Avoid triggers of myotonia: Succinylcholine, hypothermia, shivering, and electrocautery in patients with myotonic disorders.
- Preeclampsia/eclampsia is a risk factor for PRES.
- Succinylcholine may cause massive hyperkalemia in many neuromuscular diseases including GBS, myotonia, MD, CMT disease, and SMA and can cause rhabdomyolysis in MD. Its use should be avoided in those patients.
- Patients with central core disease are susceptible to malignant hyperthermia.
- SMA is associated with severe scoliosis.

REFERENCES

1. Jani-Acsadi A, Lisak R. Myasthenia gravis. *Curr Treat Options Neurol* 2010;12:231–243.
2. Ferrero S, Esposito F, Biamonti M, et al. Myasthenia gravis during pregnancy. *Expert Rev Neurother* 2008;8:979–988.
3. Hughes BW, Moro De Casillas ML, Kaminski HJ. Pathophysiology of myasthenia gravis. *Semin Neurol* 2004;24:21–30.
4. Kuczkowski KM. Labor analgesia for the parturient with neurological disease: what does an obstetrician need to know? *Arch Gynecol Obstet* 2006;274:41–46.
5. Sax TW, Rosenbaum RB. Neuromuscular disorders in pregnancy. *Muscle Nerve* 2006;34:559–571.
6. Roh HS, Lee SY, Yoon JS. Comparison of clinical manifestations between patients with ocular myasthenia gravis and generalized myasthenia gravis. *Korean J Ophthalmol* 2011;25:1–7.
7. Venna N, Gonzalez RG, Zukerberg LR. Case records of the Massachusetts General Hospital. Case 39-2011. A woman in her 90s with unilateral ptosis. *N Engl J Med* 2011;365:2413–2422.
8. Kalidindi M, Ganpot S, Tahmesebi F, et al. Myasthenia gravis and pregnancy. *J Obstet Gynaecol* 2007;27:30–32.
9. D'Angelo R, Gerancher JC. Combined spinal and epidural analgesia in a parturient with severe myasthenia gravis. *Reg Anesth Pain Med* 1998;23:201–203.
10. Almeida C. Myasthenia gravis and pregnancy: anaesthetic management–a series of cases. *Eur J Anaesthesiol* 2010;27:985–990.
11. Mueksch JN, Stevens WA. Undiagnosed myasthenia gravis masquerading as eclampsia. *Int J Obstet Anesth* 2007;16:379–382.
12. Hoff JM, Daltveit AK, Gilhus NE. Myasthenia gravis in pregnancy and birth: identifying risk factors, optimising care. *Eur J Neurol* 2007;14:38–43.
13. Wen JC, Liu TC, Chen YH, et al. No increased risk of adverse pregnancy outcomes for women with myasthenia gravis: a nationwide population-based study. *Eur J Neurol* 2009;16:889–894.
14. Stafford IP, Dildy GA. Myasthenia gravis and pregnancy. *Clin Obstet Gynecol* 2005;48:48–56.
15. Djelmis J, Sostarko M, Mayer D, et al. Myasthenia gravis in pregnancy: report on 69 cases. *Eur J Obstet Gynecol Reprod Biol* 2002;104:21–25.
16. Terblanche N, Maxwell C, Keunen J, et al. Obstetric and anesthetic management of severe congenital myasthenia syndrome. *Anesth Analg* 2008;107:1313–1315.
17. Warren J, Sharma SK. Ventilatory support using bilevel positive airway pressure during neuraxial blockade in a patient with severe respiratory compromise. *Anesth Analg* 2006;102:910–911.
18. Unterbuchner C, Fink H, Blobner M. The use of sugammadex in a patient with myasthenia gravis. *Anaesthesia* 2010;65:302–305.
19. Baraka A, Tabboush Z. Neuromuscular response to succinylcholine-vecuronium sequence in three myasthenic patients undergoing thymectomy. *Anesth Analg* 1991;72:827–830.
20. Parness J, Bandschapp O, Girard T. The myotonias and susceptibility to malignant hyperthermia. *Anesth Analg* 2009;109:1054–1064.
21. Conravey A, Santana-Gould L. Myotonia congenita and myotonic dystrophy: surveillance and management. *Curr Treat Options Neurol* 2010;12:16–28.
22. Briemberg HR. Neuromuscular diseases in pregnancy. *Semin Neurol* 2007;27:460–466.
23. Rudnik-Schoneborn S, Zerres K. Outcome in pregnancies complicated by myotonic dystrophy: a study of 31 patients and review of the literature. *Eur J Obstet Gynecol Reprod Biol* 2004;114:44–53.

24. Rudnik-Schoneborn S, Nicholson GA, Morgan G, et al. Different patterns of obstetric complications in myotonic dystrophy in relation to the disease status of the fetus. *Am J Med Genet* 1998;80:314–321.

25. Bisinotto FM, Fabri DC, Calcado MS, et al. Anesthesia for videolaparoscopic cholecystectomy in a patient with Steinert disease. Case report and review of the literature. *Rev Bras Anestesiol* 2010;60:181–191.

26. Russell SH, Hirsch NP. Anaesthesia and myotonia. *Br J Anaesth* 1994;72:210–216.

27. O'Connor PJ, Caldicott LD, Braithwaite P. Urgent caesarean section in a patient with myotonic dystrophy: a case report and review. *Int J Obstet Anesth* 1996;5:272–274.

28. Campbell AM, Thompson N. Anaesthesia for caesarean section in a patient with myotonic dystrophy receiving warfarin therapy. *Can J Anaesth* 1995;42:409–414.

29. Weingarten TN, Hofer RE, Milone M, et al. Anesthesia and myotonic dystrophy type 2: a case series. *Can J Anaesth* 2010;57:248–255.

30. Kirzinger L, Schmidt A, Kornblum C, et al. Side effects of anesthesia in DM2 as compared to DM1: a comparative retrospective study. *Eur J Neurol* 2010;17:842–845.

31. Sewry CA. Muscular dystrophies: an update on pathology and diagnosis. *Acta Neuropathol* 2010;120:343–358.

32. Rudnik-Schoneborn S, Glauner B, Rohrig D, et al. Obstetric aspects in women with facioscapulohumeral muscular dystrophy, limb-girdle muscular dystrophy, and congenital myopathies. *Arch Neurol* 1997;54:888–894.

33. Ciafaloni E, Pressman EK, Loi AM, et al. Pregnancy and birth outcomes in women with facioscapulohumeral muscular dystrophy. *Neurology* 2006;67:1887–1889.

34. Klingler W, Lehmann-Horn F, Jurkat-Rott K. Complications of anaesthesia in neuromuscular disorders. *Neuromuscul Disord* 2005;15:195–206.

35. Allen T, Maguire S. Anaesthetic management of a woman with autosomal recessive limb-girdle muscular dystrophy for emergency caesarean section. *Int J Obstet Anesth* 2007;16:370–374.

36. Molyneux MK. Anaesthetic management during labour of a manifesting carrier of Duchenne muscular dystrophy. *Int J Obstet Anesth* 2005;14:58–61.

37. Birnkrant DJ, Panitch HB, Benditt JO, et al. American College of Chest Physicians consensus statement on the respiratory and related management of patients with Duchenne muscular dystrophy undergoing anesthesia or sedation. *Chest* 2007;132:1977–1986.

38. Yemen TA, McClain C. Muscular dystrophy, anesthesia and the safety of inhalational agents revisited; again. *Paediatr Anaesth* 2006;16:105–108.

39. Jungbluth H. Central core disease. *Orphanet J Rare Dis* 2007;2:25.

40. Klingler W, Rueffert H, Lehmann-Horn F, et al. Core myopathies and risk of malignant hyperthermia. *Anesth Analg* 2009;109:1167–1173.

41. Foster RN, Boothroyd KP. Caesarean section in a complicated case of central core disease. *Anaesthesia* 2008;63:544–547.

42. Waikar PV, Wadsworth R. A patient with severe central core disease. *Br J Anaesth* 2008;101:284.

43. Saito O, Yamamoto T, Mizuno Y. Epidural anesthetic management using ropivacaine in a parturient with multi-minicore disease and susceptibility to malignant hyperthermia. *J Anesth* 2007;21:113.

44. Patzko A, Shy ME. Update on Charcot-Marie-Tooth disease. *Curr Neurol Neurosci Rep* 2011;11:78–88.

45. Hoff JM, Gilhus NE, Daltveit AK. Pregnancies and deliveries in patients with Charcot-Marie-Tooth disease. *Neurology* 2005;64:459–462.

46. Rudnik-Schoneborn S, Rohrig D, Nicholson G, et al. Pregnancy and delivery in Charcot-Marie-Tooth disease type 1. *Neurology* 1993;43:2011–2016.

47. Greenwood JJ, Scott WE. Charcot-Marie-Tooth disease: peripartum management of two contrasting clinical cases. *Int J Obstet Anesth* 2007;16:149–154.

48. Antognini JF. Anaesthesia for Charcot-Marie-Tooth disease: a review of 86 cases. *Can J Anaesth* 1992;39:398–400.

49. Kawamichi Y, Makino Y, Matsuda Y, et al. Riluzole use during pregnancy in a patient with amyotrophic lateral sclerosis: a case report. *J Int Med Res* 2010;38:720–726.

50. Oskoui M, Kaufmann P. Spinal muscular atrophy. *Neurotherapeutics* 2008;5:499–506.

51. Flunt D, Andreadis N, Menadue C, et al. Clinical commentary: obstetric and respiratory management of pregnancy with severe spinal muscular atrophy. *Obstet Gynecol Int* 2009;2009:942301.

52. Rudnik-Schoneborn S, Zerres K, Ignatius J, et al. Pregnancy and spinal muscular atrophy. *J Neurol* 1992;239:26–30.

53. McLoughlin L, Bhagvat P. Anaesthesia for caesarean section in spinal muscular atrophy type III. *Int J Obstet Anesth* 2004;13:192–195.

54. Harris SJ, Moaz K. Caesarean section conducted under subarachnoid block in two sisters with spinal muscular atrophy. *Int J Obstet Anesth* 2002;11:125–127.

55. Habib AS, Helsley SE, Millar S, et al. Anesthesia for cesarean section in a patient with spinal muscular atrophy. *J Clin Anesth* 2004;16:217–219.

56. Rejdak K, Jackson S, Giovannoni G. Multiple sclerosis: a practical overview for clinicians. *Br Med Bull* 2010;95:79–104.

57. Ferrero S, Pretta S, Ragni N. Multiple sclerosis: management issues during pregnancy. *Eur J Obstet Gynecol Reprod Biol* 2004;115:3–9.

58. Dorotta IR, Schubert A. Multiple sclerosis and anesthetic implications. *Curr Opin Anaesthesiol* 2002;15:365–370.

59. Tremlett H, Zhao Y, Rieckmann P, et al. New perspectives in the natural history of multiple sclerosis. *Neurology* 2010;74:2004–2015.

60. Houtchens MK. Pregnancy and multiple sclerosis. *Semin Neurol* 2007;27:434–441.

61. Confavreux C, Hutchinson M, Hours MM, et al. Rate of pregnancy-related relapse in multiple sclerosis. Pregnancy in Multiple Sclerosis Group. *N Engl J Med* 1998;339:285–291.

62. Vukusic S, Hutchinson M, Hours M, et al. Pregnancy and multiple sclerosis (the PRIMS study): clinical predictors of post-partum relapse. *Brain* 2004;127:1353–1360.

63. Langer-Gould A, Huang SM, Gupta R, et al. Exclusive breastfeeding and the risk of postpartum relapses in women with multiple sclerosis. *Arch Neurol* 2009;66:958–963.

64. Dahl J, Myhr KM, Daltveit AK, et al. Pregnancy, delivery, and birth outcome in women with multiple sclerosis. *Neurology* 2005;65:1961–1963.

65. Kelly VM, Nelson LM, Chakravarty EF. Obstetric outcomes in women with multiple sclerosis and epilepsy. *Neurology* 2009;73:1831–1836.

66. Jalkanen A, Alanen A, Airas L. Pregnancy outcome in women with multiple sclerosis: results from a prospective nationwide study in Finland. *Mult Scler* 2010;16:950–955.

67. Bader AM, Hunt CO, Datta S, et al. Anesthesia for the obstetric patient with multiple sclerosis. *J Clin Anesth* 1988;1:21–24.

68. Drake E, Drake M, Bird J, et al. Obstetric regional blocks for women with multiple sclerosis: a survey of UK experience. *Int J Obstet Anesth* 2006;15:115–123.

69. Kaplan PW, Norwitz ER, Ben-Menachem E, et al. Obstetric risks for women with epilepsy during pregnancy. *Epilepsy Behav* 2007;11:283–291.

70. Hill DS, Wlodarczyk BJ, Palacios AM, et al. Teratogenic effects of antiepileptic drugs. *Expert Rev Neurother* 2010;10:943–959.

71. Walker SP, Permezel M, Berkovic SF. The management of epilepsy in pregnancy. *BJOG* 2009;116:758–767.

72. Harden CL, Hopp J, Ting TY, et al. Practice parameter update: management issues for women with epilepsy–focus on pregnancy (an evidence-based review): obstetrical complications and change in seizure frequency: report of the Quality Standards Subcommittee and Therapeutics and Technology Assessment Subcommittee of the American Academy of Neurology and American Epilepsy Society. *Neurology* 2009;73:126–132.

73. Harden CL, Sethi NK. Epileptic disorders in pregnancy: an overview. *Curr Opin Obstet Gynecol* 2008;20:557–562.

74. Contag SA, Mertz HL, Bushnell CD. Migraine during pregnancy: is it more than a headache? *Nat Rev Neurosci* 2009;5:449–456.

75. MacGregor EA. Migraine in pregnancy and lactation: a clinical review. *J Fam Plann Reprod Health Care* 2007;33:83–93.

76. Loder E. Migraine in pregnancy. *Semin Neurol* 2007;27:425–433.

77. Allais G, Gabellari IC, Borgogno P, et al. The risks of women with migraine during pregnancy. *Neurol Sci* 2010;31(Suppl 1):S59–S61.

78. Bushnell CD, Jamison M, James AH. Migraines during pregnancy linked to stroke and vascular diseases: US population based case-control study. *BMJ* 2009;338:b664.

79. Contag SA, Bushnell C. Contemporary management of migrainous disorders in pregnancy. *Curr Opin Obstet Gynecol* 2010;22:437–445.

80. Lucas S. Medication use in the treatment of migraine during pregnancy and lactation. *Curr Pain Headache Rep* 2009;13:392–398.

81. Paul F, Zipp F. Bilateral meralgia paresthetica after cesarian section with epidural analgesia. *J Peripher Nerv Syst* 2006;11:98–99.

82. Ablove RH, Ablove TS. Prevalence of carpal tunnel syndrome in pregnant women. *WMJ* 2009;108:194–196.

83. Mabie WC. Peripheral neuropathies during pregnancy. *Clin Obstet Gynecol* 2005;48:57–66.

84. Mondelli M, Rossi S, Monti E, et al. Long term follow-up of carpal tunnel syndrome during pregnancy: a cohort study and review of the literature. *Electromyogr Clin Neurophysiol* 2007;47:259–271.

85. Jurjevic A, Bralic M, Antoncic I, et al. Early onset of carpal tunnel syndrome during pregnancy: case report. *Acta Clin Croat* 2010;49:77–80.

86. Gilden DH. Clinical practice. Bell's Palsy. *N Engl J Med* 2004;351:1323–1331.

87. Vrabec JT, Isaacson B, Van Hook JW. Bell's palsy and pregnancy. *Otolaryngol Head Neck Surg* 2007;137:858–861.

88. Mylonas I, Kastner R, Sattler C, et al. Idiopathic facial paralysis (Bell's palsy) in the immediate puerperium in a patient with mild preeclampsia: a case report. *Arch Gynecol Obstet* 2005;272:241–243.

89. Shehata HA, Okosun H. Neurological disorders in pregnancy. *Curr Opin Obstet Gynecol* 2004;16:117–122.

90. Kocabas S, Karaman S, Firat V, et al. Anesthetic management of Guillain-Barré syndrome in pregnancy. *J Clin Anesth* 2007;19:299–302.

91. Chan LY, Tsui MH, Leung TN. Guillain-Barré syndrome in pregnancy. *Acta Obstet Gynecol Scand* 2004;83:319–325.

92. Alici HA, Cesur M, Erdem AF, et al. Repeated use of epidural anaesthesia for caesarean delivery in a patient with Guillain-Barré syndrome. *Int J Obstet Anesth* 2005;14:269–270.

93. Campos da Silva F, de Moraes Paula G, Dos Santos Esteves Automari CV, et al. Guillain-Barré syndrome in pregnancy: early diagnosis and treatment is essential for a favorable outcome. *Gynecol Obstet Invest* 2009;67:236–237.

94. Matsuzawa Y, Sakakibara R, Shoda T, et al. Good maternal and fetal outcomes of predominantly sensory Guillain-Barré syndrome in pregnancy after intravenous immunoglobulin. *Neurol Sci* 2010;31:201–203.

95. Hebl JR, Horlocker TT, Schroeder DR. Neuraxial anesthesia and analgesia in patients with preexisting central nervous system disorders. *Anesth Analg* 2006;103:223–228.

96. Wiertlewski S, Magot A, Drapier S, et al. Worsening of neurologic symptoms after epidural anesthesia for labor in a Guillain-Barré patient. *Anesth Analg* 2004; 98:825–827.

97. Gimovsky ML, Guzman GM, Koscica KL, et al. Posterior reversible encephalopathy with late postpartum eclampsia and short-term memory loss: a case report. *J Reprod Med* 2010;55:71–74.

98. Bartynski WS. Posterior reversible encephalopathy syndrome, part 2: controversies surrounding pathophysiology of vasogenic edema. *AJNR Am J Neuroradiol* 2008;29:1043–1049.

99. Torrillo TM, Bronster DJ, Beilin Y. Delayed diagnosis of posterior reversible encephalopathy syndrome (PRES) in a parturient with preeclampsia after inadvertent dural puncture. *Int J Obstet Anesth* 2007;16:171–174.

100. Bartynski WS. Posterior reversible encephalopathy syndrome, part 1: fundamental imaging and clinical features. *AJNR Am J Neuroradiol* 2008;29:1036–1042.

101. Pula JH, Eggenberger E. Posterior reversible encephalopathy syndrome. *Curr Opin Ophthalmol* 2008;19:479–484.

102. Thackeray EM, Tielborg MC. Posterior reversible encephalopathy syndrome in a patient with severe preeclampsia. *Anesth Analg* 2007;105:184–186.

CHAPTER

33

The Parturient with Intracranial and Spinal Pathology

Ellen M. Lockhart • Curtis L. Baysinger

INTRODUCTION

With the improvements in maternal care that have occurred over the last several decades, the relative percentage of maternal morbidity and mortality due to nonobstetric causes has risen. Trauma is the leading nonobstetric cause of maternal mortality and central nervous system trauma contributes significantly to the risk of both maternal and fetal death (1). Cerebrovascular events not associated with obstetric disease were responsible for 13.5% of nonobstetric maternal deaths in a recent survey of maternal death in the United States (2). Some diseases of the central nervous system and spinal cord found in the parturient most often predate pregnancy, such as tumors, idiopathic intracranial hypertension, hydrocephalus, and Arnold–Chiari malformation (ACM), while others have an increased incidence during pregnancy such as stroke due to either intracranial hemorrhage, and arterial or venous occlusive disease. Anesthesiologists may also be called upon to provide care for a parturient with brain death. Published data on pregnant women with these disorders is limited, so only case reports and small case series are available to guide neurosurgical, obstetric, and anesthetic management. A multidisciplinary approach to individual case management is most often required and should occur as early in pregnancy as practical. Neuraxial techniques for labor, and both vaginal and cesarean delivery, can be safely used in many cases.

INTRACRANIAL TUMORS DURING PREGNANCY

The incidence of new brain tumors during pregnancy is the same as for an age-matched nonpregnant population and occurs in approximately 90 pregnant women in the United States yearly (3). Malignant tumors comprise approximately 50% of brain tumors with a frequency of $3.6/10^6$ to $3.2/10^5$ live births (3). The distribution of primary tumor types also appears similar to that of the nonpregnant population (Table 33-1) (3). Pregnancy may aggravate the natural course of primary intracranial tumors by accelerating tumor growth, increasing peritumor edema due to the generalized fluid retention associated with pregnancy, blood vessel engorgement of the vessels feeding a tumor, and immunologic tolerance (4). In addition, the hormonal changes associated with pregnancy may influence the growth of some tumors as 90% of meningiomas and some gliomas exhibit progesterone receptor activity, and hormonal stimulation may accelerate the growth of preexisting pituitary tumors particularly prolactinomas (5). Choriocarcinoma is associated with a high percentage of brain metastases and is a tumor unique to pregnancy. Metastatic brain tumors would be expected to occur less frequently as systemic cancer is relatively rare in women of childbearing age (3).

TUMORS ENCOUNTERED DURING PREGNANCY

Gliomas are the most common intracranial tumor diagnosed during pregnancy and account for 38% of all tumors (Table 33-1) (3). Tumors less often arise from astrocytes or oligodendrocytes and are graded as to potential invasiveness: Low-grade (grade II), anaplastic (grade III), or glioblastoma multiforme/anaplastic astrocytoma (grade IV) (3). Tumor grading is important for gauging prognosis and guiding decisions as to surgical intervention during pregnancy (3). Urgent neurosurgical treatment of low-grade tumors is rarely necessary and resection can be delayed until later in pregnancy or after delivery (6) while high-grade lesions require prompt diagnosis and treatment regardless of gestational age (1).

Meningiomas are histologically benign, are usually slow growing, and arise from the membranous arachnoid layer. They eventually cause symptoms from compression of brain tissue. Pregnancy may accelerate the growth of preexisting meningiomas due to generalized fluid retention during pregnancy and resultant cerebral edema, and estrogen and progesterone effects may stimulate tumor growth, mediated through receptors for both hormones are commonly expressed in meningiomas (3). Surgical treatment, which is typically curative, can most often be delayed until after delivery.

Acoustic neuromas, which occur with greater frequency in patients with neurofibromatosis, arise from the vestibular portion of the vestibulocochlear nerve (8th cranial nerve) and present with progressive hearing loss, tinnitus, and dizziness (3). Like meningiomas, their size may increase dramatically during pregnancy, possibility linked to the high expression of estrogen receptors by these tumors, although these tumors are typically slow growing and surgical resection can be delayed (3,5).

Pituitary adenomas are diagnosed infrequently during pregnancy, although autopsy and MRI studies suggest that the incidence may be from 10% to 13% in adult women (3,5). They may present clinically as an endocrinopathy or with neurologic symptoms, often as visual field defects (5). Approximately, 23% of tumors produce no hormones, while 35% produce prolactin, with the rest more commonly producing growth hormone and ACTH, and rarely, TSH and FSH (5). Prolactin adenomas, may more likely than other pituitary tumors, enlarge during pregnancy due to the normal stimulatory effects of pregnancy on pituitary tissue to increase prolactin levels (3). Surgical resection is curative in 90% of microadenomas (5), but observation of pregnant women without significant imaging findings and or visual field defects is appropriate. Bromocriptine administration is effective in lowering prolactin levels and shrinking the size of prolactin secreting adenomas and is generally considered safe during pregnancy (6). Transsphenoidal surgical resection is necessary for large tumors and can be done safely during

TABLE 33-1 Distribution of Primary Intracranial Tumors in Pregnant and Nonpregnant Women (Excluding Pituitary Tumors)

Neoplasm	% of Brain Tumors	
	Pregnant	Nonpregnant
Glioma	38	36
Meningioma	28	29
Acoustic neuroma	14	15
Astrocytoma	7	5
Medulloblastoma	3	3

From: Stevenson CB, Thompson RC. The clinical management of intracranial neoplasms in pregnancy. *Clin Obstet Gynecol* 2005;48:24–37.

pregnancy in most large referral centers (3), while radiotherapy is reserved for recurrent disease and infrequently indicated during pregnancy (5).

Metastatic brain lesions do not occur more frequently in pregnancy than in nonpregnant women, except for choriocarcinoma which occurs in 1 in 50,000 term pregnancies and 1 in 30 molar pregnancies (7). Metastases to the brain occur in 4% to 17% of these women and an acute onset of neurologic symptoms may occur in association with hemorrhage into the tumor, which occurs often (7). Craniotomy is not often needed as radiation therapy and chemotherapy lead to a good overall prognosis (3).

The four most common presenting signs and symptoms of both primary and metastatic intracranial neoplasms during pregnancy are headache, nausea and vomiting (indicators of increased intracranial pressure), new onset of seizure activity, and progressive focal neurologic deficits (5,8,9). Unfortunately, headache occurs frequently during normal pregnancy and makes use of this symptom less helpful in pregnant women, but headache that has a gradual onset, an unremitting course, and is exacerbated by activities that increase intracranial pressure (cough, Valsalva maneuvers, etc.) should prompt investigation (3,8). Likewise, nausea and vomiting occur frequently during pregnancy, but persistence into the second and third trimesters suggests the need for further evaluation (10). The onset of new seizure activity

during the first and second trimesters requires prompt neuroradiologic evaluation as the likelihood of eclampsia is low (8). Focal seizures that occur in the third trimester, especially if not accompanied by hypertension and proteinuria, indicate the need for further investigation as eclamptic seizures usually exhibit generalized motor activity (3). The extent and type of focal neurologic deficit depends on the location of the tumor and the extent of its invasion of normal tissue. Brain edema and hemorrhage may also increase intracranial pressure and the significant intravascular volume expansion that accompanies pregnancy may cause rapid deterioration (5).

The diagnosis of brain tumors in pregnancy requires neuroimaging with MRI and CT which can be safely obtained throughout pregnancy (3,5,8–11). MRI is preferable to CT scanning for tumor diagnosis as it is more sensitive in detecting tumors, detects radiologic features that lead to a shorter differential diagnosis of tumor type and the grade of malignancy, and does not expose the mother or fetus to ionizing radiation (3,9). The increases in tissue temperature with scanners that use a magnetic field strength of 3 T is of little clinical consequence (11). Head CT scanning is very safe for the fetus as tight collimation and abdominal lead shielding reduces radiation exposure to approximately 1 mrem, equivalent to that of 2 weeks of background cosmic radiation, and no study has documented deleterious fetal effects (12). MRI and CT studies should involve the use of IV contrast material and the patient scanned before and after its use as the diagnostic information obtained far outweighs the risks it administer (3). The IV contrast material used for CT scanning is composed of iodinated compounds that are renally excreted with well-documented minimal risks for maternal allergic reaction and nephrotoxicity, and hypothyroidism in the fetus (11–13). Gadolinium has a much lower risk for allergic reaction (1:350,000) (12), and despite readily crossing the placenta, has not been associated with fetal adverse outcomes when administered during pregnancy (11–13).

Obstetric and neurosurgical management depend upon the size and location of the tumor, the potential for tumor growth during pregnancy, and the ability of the patient to accommodate increases in intracranial pressure (3,8). These considerations govern the progression of neurologic findings which guide clinical management (3,5,14). Ng and Kitchen have suggested an algorithm for the neurosurgical management of the pregnant patient with a brain neoplasm (Fig. 33-1) (14). Surgical removal of benign slower growing tumors

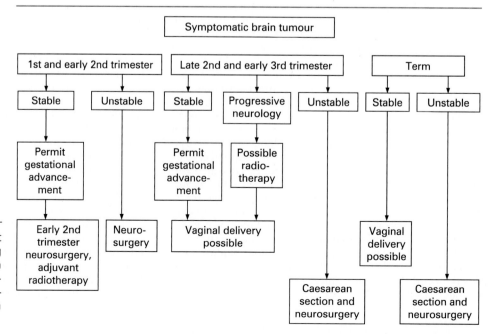

FIGURE 33-1 Management of intracranial tumors during pregnancy. From: Ng J, Kitchen N. Neurosurgery and pregnancy. *J Neurol Neurosurg Psychiatry* 2008;79:745–752, with permission.

can often be delayed until after delivery (5,6,14). Management of malignant tumors that create significant symptoms may require elective surgery during pregnancy as a delay can allow significant maternal deterioration and increase the risk for fetal wastage in association with emergency treatment (4). If surgery can be delayed until the chance of fetal survival is good, then cesarean delivery followed by craniotomy is a reasonable approach (3,5,14). Unfortunately, radiation therapy and maternal chemotherapy pose significant risks to the fetus, particularly if instituted during the first trimester, although the risk for teratogenicity is significantly reduced if these treatments can be delayed into the late second or early third trimester (3,5). Fetal exposure during radiation therapy can be minimized if appropriate shielding is employed (9,11,12). For many tumors, it may be reasonable to delay chemotherapy treatment until after delivery as it may offer only a small increase in maternal survival and delay may not reduce the benefits of its use (3).

The control of intracranial pressure is of great importance during labor and delivery. The classic work by Marx et al. documented a rise in CSF pressure of 53 cm H_2O during painful uterine contractions and rise of 70 cm H_2O during the second stage with maternal bearing down during contractions (15). These changes are well tolerated by women with normal intracranial compliance, but will likely lead to significant neurologic deterioration in women with impaired compliance. Patients with small pituitary tumors or small benign lesions should tolerate vaginal delivery well, but in patients with larger lesions labor analgesia is advised. Consideration may also be given to an instrumental vaginal delivery to minimize pushing during the second stage. Alternatively an elective cesarean delivery may be the best option for some patients, especially when regional anesthesia is contraindicated (3,5,6). A multidisciplinary approach as to the mode of delivery and other management that involves the obstetrician, neurosurgeon, neuroradiologist, anesthesiologist, midwife, and neonatologist is required (3,5,6,14).

Anesthetic management for labor and delivery or cesarean section is based upon the reports of individual case management or small case series (8). Successful epidural analgesia for labor and delivery has been reported (16,17) and would be expected to prevent the increase in intracranial pressure that would accompany painful labor (17) and the increases that would be expected during bearing down during the second stage of labor (4,16). One case report describes successful spinal anesthesia for cesarean section utilizing a 24 g pencil point needle in a patient with symptoms consistent with increased intracranial pressure (18) and another, successful cesarean delivery with spinal anesthesia (17); however, other case reports describe fatal brain stem herniation shortly after delivery in patients with unsuspected neoplasms who received an unintentional dural puncture during an epidural catheter placement (19,20). Other case reports of cerebral herniation in association with lumbar cerebrospinal fluid leak in other settings have been reported as well (21). However, cerebrospinal fluid drainage catheters are often employed during intracranial surgery to improve surgical exposure and reduce intracranial pressure most often without sequelae (22). Examination of these reports does not allow for the identification of those patients who would be at greatest risk for cerebral herniation in the setting of dural puncture during the performance of neuraxial anesthesia. In addition, injection of fluid into the epidural space is associated with increases in intracranial pressure (23). Studies in animal models of baseline elevated intracranial pressure show significant decreases in cerebral blood flow that accompany increases in intracranial pressure (24). The onset of new neurologic symptoms has been reported in one case report of epidural placement in a mother with an unsuspected cerebello-

pontine angle tumor and obstructive hydrocephalus (25). Such considerations lead many anesthesiologists to select cesarean delivery under general anesthesia in parturients with increased intracranial pressure (6,12) despite the loss of intraoperative monitoring of maternal neurologic status in an awake patient and the need to control rises in intracranial pressure that may accompany anesthetic induction and endotracheal intubation. However, general anesthesia may facilitate maternal blood pressure control and the management of maternal intracranial pressure through hyperventilation and drug administration (12). Several case reports support the safety of general anesthesia when used for emergent and urgent cesarean section due to fetal concerns (12,26).

■ ANESTHETIC MANAGEMENT OF THE PREGNANT PATIENT UNDERGOING NEUROSURGERY

A more detailed discussion of the anesthetic management of the parturient undergoing neurosurgery is described in Chapter 50. The management of general anesthesia for a procedure that combines delivery followed by tumor resection or cesarean delivery followed later by a neurosurgical procedure requires an understanding of the physiologic changes associated with pregnancy, and preparations to control maternal intracranial pressure and hemodynamics. The administration of medication to reduce the risk of aspiration, such as an oral or IV H2 receptor antagonist to reduce gastric acid secretion and oral sodium citrate to neutralize stomach acid should be given approximately 1 hour prior to induction (27). Preoperative placement of intra-arterial blood pressure monitoring is recommended to facilitate moment to moment blood pressure monitoring. Blood pressure should be maintained within narrow limits as hypertension can lead to increases in intracranial pressure (27) and hypotension to decreases in cerebral and uterine perfusion pressures (3). A rapid sequence induction should balance the need to protect the mother against the risk of aspiration and to control the intracranial pressure during endotracheal intubation. The administration of both thiopental and propofol reduces the hypertensive response associated with intubation and attenuates the intracranial pressure rises and cerebral metabolism (27), although propofol may be more effective in blunting maternal hypertension (28). Some anesthesiologists avoid the use of succinylcholine for fear that its administration will increase intracranial pressure, but others find this to be of little clinical significance (27). Other approaches to reduce the hypertensive response to tracheal intubation include the administration of a continuous sodium nitroprusside infusion, (29) small IV bolus dosing of nitroglycerin, (30) and moderate dosing of IV opioids (27). The short acting opioid remifentanil in doses of 1 µg/kg over 1 minute prior to intubation has been shown to be particularly effective and safe when used during cesarean delivery (31). IV magnesium sulfate in doses of 30 to 60 mg/kg may be effective as well as intravenous lidocaine in doses of 1 mg/kg (32). Aortocaval compression should be avoided by the use of left uterine displacement. Maternal ventilation during anesthesia should be set to keep maternal $PaCO_2$ values at 30 to 32 mm Hg, normal for the parturient at term. Although controlled hyperventilation can acutely reduce intracranial pressure, decreases in $PaCO_2$ of <25 mm Hg can lead to uterine artery vasoconstriction and a left shift of the maternal oxyhemoglobin dissociation curve and reduce fetal oxygen transfer (33). Prolonged severe hyperventilation is associated with poor patient outcomes in other populations of neurosurgical patients (30). Intravenous fluids that are administered intraoperatively should be isonatremic, isotonic, and glucose free to reduce the risk of cerebral edema associated with hypotonic, hyponatremic fluids and poor neurologic outcome associated with hyperglycemia (27). Diuretic administration may be indicated to control intracranial pressure. Although mannitol accumulates in the fetus and leads to fetal physiologic changes such as reduced urine production, hypernatremia, and dehydration (34), doses of 0.25 to 0.5 mg/kg appear to be safe (26,27). Furosemide causes a fetal diuresis in animal models but offers a safe alternative to osmotic diuretics (27). Patient positioning in a slight head-up posture can also be effective in reducing intracranial pressure as well as the use of low tidal volumes during positive pressure ventilation (27). Oxytocic drug administration has not been well studied in patients who have undergone neurosurgery, but 5 unit bolus dosing of oxytocin following delivery has been reported as safe in case reports (26). Hypotension can accompany its use and should be treated appropriately (35). The use of other oxytocics in this setting appears to not have been reported, but prostaglandin F2α administration may be associated with systemic and pulmonary hypertension (36). Ergometrine may create hypertension through its vasoconstrictor effect and thus increase intracranial pressure (37), while vaginal prostaglandin E1 administration is associated with little maternal hemodynamic effect (38).

▪ STROKE

As the direct obstetrical causes of maternal death have declined, cerebrovascular accidents have become a proportionally more important cause for maternal morbidity and mortality. Stroke during pregnancy is relatively rare, occurring at an estimated rate between 11 and 26 deliveries per 100,000, but is a cause of 12% of all maternal deaths (39). The death rates cited in older studies are widely variable, with rates as high as 210/100,000, but methodologic weaknesses and inclusion of data from underdeveloped countries may overestimate the rate in developed countries (40) which suggests a rate at the lower end of the range cited above (9 to 11 per 10,000 deliveries). However, one recent well-conducted review of data from approximately 1,000 United States hospitals identified a higher rate of 34.2/100,000 deliveries (40), which contrasts with a rate of 10.7/100,000 women-years reported among nonpregnant women of childbearing age (39). The stroke rate would be expected to be higher during pregnancy as the increases in hypercoagulability and venous stasis that accompany pregnancy, and the increased risk for endothelial trauma during delivery, would increase the risk for thrombotic stroke (8). The risk for stroke due to cerebral hemorrhage would also be increased due to the pregnancy-associated hypertensive disorders that affect up to 10% of all pregnancies (8).

Stroke can be broadly categorized into ischemic and hemorrhagic causes (8). Feske in a recent review of single and multiple hospital experiences with pregnancy-related stroke, noted that the causes were nearly evenly divided between both (41). Age greater than 35 years and black ethnicity convey increased risk (40). Significant risk factors associated with pregnancy and delivery are postpartum infection, pregnancy-related transfusion, increased parity, multiple gestation, and cesarean delivery (Table 33-2) (40). Cesarean delivery is more likely among women who have had a stroke prior to delivery and other pregnancy-related disorders associated with stroke such as preeclampsia (39). Maternal medical conditions that are most associated with pregnancy-related stroke include hypertension, heart disease, history of migraine headaches, lupus,

TABLE 33-2 Pregnancy and Postdelivery Complications and the Risk of Stroke

Complication	Odds Ratio	95% Confidence Interval
Hyperemesis	1.5	(0.8–2.8)
Preterm labor	0.8	(0.6–1.1)
Antepartum hemorrhage	1.5	(0.9–2.5)
Multiple gestation	0.2	(0.1–0.9)
Hypertensive disorders of pregnancy	4.4	(3.6–5.4)
Postpartum hemorrhage	1.8	(1.2–2.8)
Transfusion	10.3	(7.1–15.1)
Postpartum infection	25	(18.3–34)
Fluid and electrolyte imbalance	7.2	(5.1–10)

Data obtained from the Nationwide Inpatient from the Healthcare Cost and Utilization Project of the Agency for Healthcare research and Quality. Data from all records with pregnancy-related discharge codes (International Classification of Disease, Ninth Revision (ICD-9) for the years 2000–2001 were matched with ICD-9 codes for the complications of pregnancy associated with pregnancy-related stroke. Postpartum hemorrhage, hypertensive disorders of pregnancy, fluid and electrolyte imbalance, transfusion, and pregnancy related infection were associated with an increased risk of stroke by univariate analysis. Adapted from: James AH, Bushnell CD, Jamison MG, et al. Incidence and risk factors for stroke in pregnancy and the puerperium. *Obstet Gynecol* 2005;106:509–516, with permission.

sickle cell disease, smoking, alcohol and substance abuse, thrombophilias, and postpartum infection (Table 33-3) (40). Pregnancy-induced hypertension appears to convey the greatest risk as one large retrospective review found that 24% of cerebral infractions and 14% of intracerebral hemorrhages (ICHs) occurred in association with hypertensive disorders (42). Although one retrospective study found a risk for arterial strokes that increased during the third trimester and postpartum, that same study found that most strokes due to venous occlusion occurred in the puerperium (43). Virtually all studies note an increased risk of stroke regardless of cause during the third trimester and postpartum with the exception of those associated with hemorrhage due to intracranial arteriovenous malformations (AVMs) that occur throughout pregnancy (Fig. 33-2).

▪ INTRACRANIAL HEMORRHAGE

Intracranial hemorrhage occurs in 5 to 31 per 100,000 pregnancies (41) and is due to subarachnoid hemorrhage (SAH) and ICH. The reported percentage of pregnancy-related SAH due to cerebrovascular malformations ranges from 20% to 67% (45) with ruptured intracranial aneurysms affecting 77% of patients and arteriovenous malformation occurring in 23%, and other causes very rarely (46). ICH occurs during pregnancy at a rate of 7.1/100,000 at risk person years, which is higher than the rate of 5/10,000 at risk patient year for nonpregnant women (45). Both SAH and ICH convey substantial risk for maternal and fetal death. SAH accounts for 5% of all maternal deaths and is the third leading cause of nonobstetric maternal death (14). The in-hospital maternal

TABLE 33-3 **Medical Disease and Pregnancy-Related Stroke**

Medical Disease	Odds Ratio	95% Confidence Interval
Cardiovascular		
Hypertension	6.1	(4.5–8.1)
Heart disease	13.2	(10.2–17)
Hematologic		
Thrombophilia	16	(9.4–27.2)
Sickle cell disease	9.1	(3.7–22.2)
Anemia	1.9	(1.5–2.4)
Thrombocytopenia	6	(1.5–24.1)
Rheumatologic		
Lupus	15.2	(7.4–31.2)
Endocrinologic		
Diabetes	2.5	(1.3–4.6)
Obesity	1.4	(0.6–3.3)
Neurologic		
Migraine headaches	16.9	(9.7–29.5)
Lifestyle Factors		
Alcohol-substance abuse	2.3	(1.3–4.6)
Smoking	1.9	(1.2–2.8)

Data obtained from the Nationwide Inpatient from the Healthcare Cost and Utilization Project of the Agency for Healthcare research and Quality. Data from all records with pregnancy-related discharge codes (International Classification of Disease, Ninth Revision (ICD-9) for the years 2000–2001 were matched with ICD-9 codes for medical conditions associated with pregnancy-related stroke. All conditions were significantly associated with an increased risk of pregnancy-associated stroke except obesity by univariate analysis. Adapted from: James AH, Bushnell CD, Jamison MG, et al. Incidence and risk factors for stroke in pregnancy and the puerperium. *Obstet Gynecol* 2005;106:509–516, with permission.

mortality associated with maternal ICH was 20.3% in a recent survey of 10 years of data from 20% of United States non-Federal hospitals (45). Fetal mortality from maternal SAH was 25% in one survey (46).

■ SUBARACHNOID HEMORRHAGE

Most cases of SAH during pregnancy are caused by intracranial aneurysm bleeding, which occurs with an incidence of 3 to 20 per 100,000 deliveries, (42,47) with bleeding from AVMs less frequently a cause (14). The incidence of SAH due to aneurysmal bleeding is thought to increase with increasing gestational age due to the increases in maternal blood volume and changes in arterial wall strength that accompany pregnancy with an increased risk compared to nonpregnant women until 6 weeks postpartum (47). Most aneurysms are due to congenital or acquired defects in the muscularis or media of the arterial wall and 85% occur in the anterior cerebral circulation at the base of the brain at the bifurcations of arterial vessels (48). Maternal coagulopathy and uncontrolled hypertension are the risk factors for bleeding from both aneurysms and AVMs (49).

Aneurysms and AVMs that have not bled usually do not cause symptoms unless they are large enough to cause persistent headache or focal neurologic signs (49). The clinical presentation of SAH in pregnancy is the same as in nonpregnant women (14). A sudden onset of severe headache, usually with vomiting and photophobia, occurs in up to 97% of cases with periorbital pain, neck pain, nuchal rigidity, and frequently a positive Kernig's sign (14,50). Up to 60% of patients will report sentinel headaches that precede the SAH by several weeks (6,14). Loss of consciousness due to rapid increases in intracranial pressure that reduce cerebral perfusion can occur (51). Focal neurologic signs can occur due to acute vasospasm (51) and the electrocardiogram can show changes similar to those associated with myocardial ischemia as well as prolonged QRS complexes and tall and inverted T waves (8,14). The patient's presenting clinical condition is an important guide to prognosis and worsening grade on the World Federation of Neurological Surgeons scale (Table 33-4), a score that combines the Glasgow Coma Score (GCS) (Table 33-5) and assessment of best motor function, correlates with poorer outcome

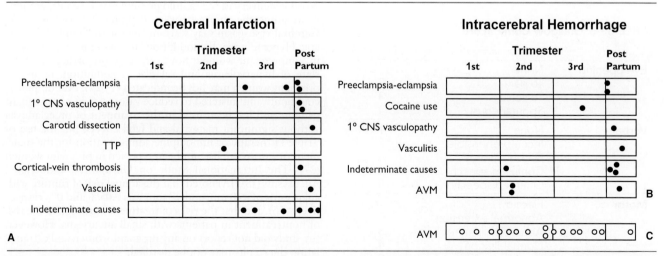

FIGURE 33-2 Timing of stroke during pregnancy and postdelivery. CNS, central nervous system; TTP, thrombotic thrombocytopenic purpura; AVM, arteriovenous malformation. The closed circles represent week of occurrence for cerebral infarcts (A) and ICH (B) as reported by Kittner SJ, Stern BJ, Feeser BR, et al. Pregnancy and the risk of stroke. *N Eng J Med* 1996;335:768–774. The open circles represent the week of occurrence for AVM-related hemorrhage (C) as reported by Horton JC, Chambers WA, Lyons SL, et al. Pregnancy and the risk of hemorrhage from cerebral AVMs. *Neurosurgery* 1990;27:867–871; discussion 871–872.

TABLE 33-4 World Federation of Neurological Surgeons (WFNS) Coma Grading Score

WFNS Grade	Glasgow Coma Score	Motor Deficit
I	15	Absent
II	14–15	Absent
III	14–13	Present
IV	12–7	Present or absent
V	6–3	Present or absent

From: Selo-Ojeme DO, Marshman LA, Ikomi A, et al. Aneurysmal subarachnoid haemorrhage in pregnancy. *Eur J Obstet Gynecol Reprod Biol* 2004;116:131–143, with permission.

(50). All patients with suspected SAH due to either aneurysm or AVM bleeding should undergo urgent neuroradiologic examinations with computed tomographic scanning and MRI studies, both with contrast, (6,11,14,39,47–51) and lumbar puncture looking for persistent blood staining and xanthochromia (14). Neurosurgical referral is mandatory to monitor for re-bleeding, and the management of vasospasm. Re-bleeds occur in 10% to 30% of patients within the next month following an aneurysmal rupture (14,52) and the chance of re-bleeding during pregnancy from an initial AVM bleed is 25% (52). Vasospasm occurs in 35% of patients with an aneurysmal rupture within 4 to 11 days, but less often following AVM bleeding (52) with significant morbidity and mortality in up to 75% of patients (51). Hydrocephalus occurs in 10% to 25% of patients with SAH, and a syndrome of inappropriate ADH secretion occurs infrequently (51).

Neurosurgical and medical management of the pregnant patient with SAH should be the same as in the nonpregnant patient (6,14,39,47–51,52) and a multidisciplinary approach involving the obstetrician, neurosurgeon, neuroradiologist, neonatologist, and anesthesiologist is required. In the patient with a ruptured aneurysm, the optimal time for surgical intervention is controversial (45,47–52); however, early operative

TABLE 33-5 Glasgow Coma Score

Category	Response	Score
Eye opening	None	1
	To pain	2
	To voice	3
	Spontaneously	4
Verbal	None	1
	Incomprehensible	2
	Garbled words	3
	Confused speech	4
	Oriented speech	5
Motor	Flaccid	1
	Abnormal extension	2
	Abnormal flexion	3
	Normal flexion	4
	Localizing pain	5
	Follow commands	6

From: Dodson BA, Rosen MA. Anesthesia for neurosurgery during pregnancy. In: Hughes SC, Levinson G, Rosen MA, eds. *Shnider and Levinson's Anesthesia for Obstetrics.* 4th ed. Philadelphia, PA: Lippincott Williams and Wilkins; 2002:509–527.

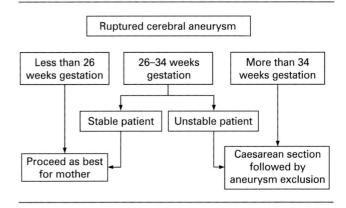

FIGURE 33-3 Management of ruptured cerebral aneurysm during pregnancy. From: Ng J, Kitchen N. Neurosurgery and pregnancy. *J Neurol Neurosurg Psychiatry* 2008;79:745–752, with permission.

intervention, either through endovascular embolization or through intracranial surgery to clip the aneurysm, is usually considered as early interventions reduce the incidence of vasospasm and re-bleeding (6,14,24,53). Ng and Kitchen have suggested an algorithm for the management of a ruptured aneurysm and the timing of a concurrent cesarean delivery based on patient stability and gestational age (Fig. 33-3) (14). Although case series of intracranial surgery for the clipping of aneurysms have uniformly reported good maternal and fetal outcomes (6,14,52), endovascular embolization has become the primary treatment modality for nonpregnant patients with SAH due to aneurysmal bleeding (54). These results may not be totally applicable to the pregnant patient as the International Subarachnoid Aneurysm Trial which reported on outcomes of surgical clipping versus endovascular coiling did not include any pregnant patients (54), although there have been several small case series reports of good outcomes (55). Practical problems include the need for systemic anticoagulation for up to 48 hours following endovascular coiling and the need to deliver general anesthesia in an area outside the conventional operating room environment (6,14). Preparations for possible delivery in the radiologic suite may be considerations in weighing the choice between clipping and coiling (6,14). Cerebral vasospasm may warrant the use of "Triple H" therapy: Hypervolemia, hemodilution, and systemic hypertension in nonpregnant women; however, since pregnancy creates a state of hypervolemia and relative hemodilution, its use in pregnant women may not be indicated (14,27). Nimodipine is commonly administered to reduce vasospasm in nonpregnant patients and has been used in the treatment of preeclampsia without significant maternal and fetal effects, but the use of Triple H therapy or nimodipine administration for the treatment of vasospasm has not been reported in pregnant women (27). The International Study on Unruptured Intracranial Aneurysms (ISUIA) noted that the annual risk of rupture with aneurysms of <10 mm and <7 mm was 0.05% and 0% respectively (56), and that the risks of treatment outweighed the risk of nontreatment in patients with small aneurysms. However, the study did not report on any pregnant women and extrapolating the results may not be justified.

In contrast with SAH due to aneurysm bleeding, surgical management of AVMs has not been shown to significantly lower maternal or fetal mortality and endovascular embolization is usually inadequate to completely treat many lesions (14). The management of known vascular malformations which have not bled in pregnant women has to be individualized recognizing that the risk of hemorrhage from an AVM during vaginal or cesarean delivery is low (14,45,56). If a neurovascular lesion has been successfully repaired, then no special care is required for labor and delivery (6,14,27,46–52). In a patient with an untreated aneurysm or AVM, maternal hemodynamic fluctuations should be minimized during delivery and current data does not suggest an advantage of cesarean over vaginal delivery (45,47,52,57). Most authors suggest an instrumental delivery under epidural analgesia to avoid bearing down during labor if labor and vaginal delivery are selected. There are fewer reports of anesthetic management for labor and delivery than for cesarean delivery in pregnant women who have untreated aneurysms, but most reports report successful outcomes when epidural analgesia is used for patients with both unrepaired aneurysms and AVMs who undergo either vaginal or cesarean delivery (8,58–62). Considerations for general anesthesia for cesarean delivery are the same as for other pregnant patients with neurosurgical disease and one case report attests to its safety (63). There are many case reports of anesthetic management of pregnant patients undergoing neurosurgical repair of intracranial vascular lesion, many in a combined procedure with cesarean delivery (64–67). In addition to the considerations outlined above and in Chapter 50, care must be taken to minimize the transmural pressure across the aneurysm wall, especially measures to minimize rises in mean arterial pressure during induction and intubation and drops in intracranial pressure until after the surgeon has opened the dura mater (64–67). The induction of controlled hypotension may be required and sodium nitroprusside use is safe when used for this purpose (64). Monitoring of the fetal heart rate response after 20 weeks of gestation is indicated to detect potential fetal compromise during the use of deliberate hypotension.

■ INTRACEREBRAL HEMORRHAGE

ICH occurs at a rate of 3.8 to 18.1 per 100,000 deliveries (40,42,43). A recent survey by Bateman et al. of discharge data from 20% of non-Federal United States hospital found a rate of 6.1/10,000 deliveries (45). Although older studies suggested that 20% to 67% of intracerebral bleeding was due to cerebrovascular malformations, (39,41–43,68) the more recent report by Bateman et al. reported a much lower associated incidence of 7.1% (45,69). The hypertensive disorders of pregnancy are a significant cause, as eclampsia or preeclampsia have been reported in 14% to 50% of patients with ICH (39,41–43,45) and it is the most common cause of death in eclamptic patients (8,40–42,44). Significant related risk factors in order of increasing strength of association are African-American race, advanced maternal age, alcohol and tobacco use, cocaine abuse, chronic hypertension with and without superimposed preeclampsia/eclampsia, and coagulopathy (40,45). Despite its rarity, ICH accounts for 7.1% of all maternal deaths (45). Most studies show the incidence to be higher postpartum with approximately 60% of ICH occurring after delivery (41,42,45).

Patients with ICH present with focal neurologic deficits and headache, nausea, vomiting, and other signs of increased intracranial pressure. Noncontrast CT scanning is the most sensitive test for diagnosis (8,11), but contrast CT and MRI scanning as well as angiography may be needed to plan indicated invasive interventions. Bleeding due to ICH should be differentiated from bleeding associated with SAH as the treatments are very different (47–51).

ICH does not often have a cause that can be corrected surgically, so care is supportive with treatment of associated hypertension and coagulopathy, if present, and control of intracranial pressure if indicated. Surgery may be indicated for an expanding hematoma or to prevent brain stem hernia-

tion (6,14). Obstetric management is focused on the timing of delivery as vaginal delivery may lead to increases in intracranial pressure due to pain during the first stage of labor and pushing during the second stage, but there is no evidence that a painless vaginal delivery with an assisted delivery during the second stage is more beneficial than cesarean delivery (42,43). If intracranial pressure has been controlled and a coagulopathy is not present, regional anesthesia would be preferred as it avoids the hypertensive response that accompanies airway management during general anesthesia (8,70). If a general anesthetic is required then the considerations for monitoring and maternal hemodynamic and intracranial pressure control as noted above apply.

■ SUBDURAL HEMATOMA

In the absence of brain trauma, subdural hematoma is an exceedingly rare cause of neurologic signs and symptoms in pregnant women, but should be part of the differential diagnosis in women with a coagulopathy, those who engaged in intense Valsalva maneuvers during labor, among those who have had a neuraxial block with dural puncture, or in women with preexisting intracranial hypotension (which may put tension on dural veins) (57). Most cases have been reported in postpartum women who have had an unintentional dural puncture (57,71), but some cases have been reported following spinal anesthesia using small bore needles (72) and some following uneventful epidural anesthesia without an obvious dural puncture (53,57). Zeidan et al. recently reviewed 25 cases of subdural hematoma following spinal anesthesia, most in nonobstetrical patients undergoing surgical procedures, and 21 cases following unintentional dural puncture, 19 of whom were obstetrical patients (73). Although parturients may be at greater risk for subdural hematoma formation after accidental dural puncture due to a greater CSF leak compared to nonpregnant patients (72), the incidence following either spinal anesthesia or epidural blockade is unknown (53,72), although Scott et al. estimated the incidence to be 1:500,000 following otherwise uncomplicated epidural anesthesia (53).

The patient can present with symptoms very soon after dural puncture, or many weeks thereafter (73). Some authors state that early blood patch placement may reduce the risk by relieving brain displacement (71,73), but others have noted subdural formation after successful epidural blood patch (74). Traction on the bridging vein due to brain displacement may lead to epidural bleeding as these veins have a nontortuous course from dural sinus through the epidural and subarachnoid space, are thinnest at the point they cross the epidural portion, and are thus more likely to rupture at their weakest point (72,75). Subdural hematomas can be managed either medically or surgically depending on severity of symptoms, size of the hematoma, presence of a midline shift on CT scan, and the initial response to medical therapy (76). Typically, hematomas less than 10 mm in size can be managed with therapies to reduce intracranial pressure, while those greater than 5 mm in size with midline shift or those greater than 10 mm will require surgical treatment (76). The anesthetic considerations outlined above concerning management of the pregnant/postpartum patient with increased intracranial pressure should guide the management of most cases.

■ MATERNAL BRAIN DEATH

Anesthesiologists may be called upon to help care for pregnant women who are receiving somatic support following brain death. Advanced life support techniques and advances in the care of the premature infant allow continuation of a

TABLE 33-6 Ischemic Stroke in Pregnancy (Including Central Venous Thrombosis)

Study	Embolism	Preeclampsia/ Eclampsia	CNS Angiopathy	Central Venous Thrombosis	Unknown	Other
Kittner et al. (44)	N/A	25	13	6	38	19[a]
Jaigobin et al. (45)	20[b]	20	N/A	40[b,c]	20	15[d]
Lanska et al. (46)	36	18	N/A	27	N/A	N/A

Data are % of the strokes recorded noted in the applicable study
[a]Carotid dissection, 1; thrombotic thrombocytopenic purpura, 1; postherpetic vasculitis, 1.
[b]Two patients had central venous thrombosis and preeclampsia.
[c]Seven of eight central venous thromboses occurred postpartum.
[d]Coagulopathy, 2; large artery disease, 1.
CNS, central nervous system; N/A, not applicable;
Adapted from: Feske SK. Stroke in pregnancy. *Semin Neurol* 2007;27:442–452, with permission.

pregnancy in the comatose parturient for the delivery of a potentially viable fetus. This creates medical, legal, and ethical challenges for the multidisciplinary team who is called upon to care for them (70,77–82). Brain death is defined as the irreversible cessation of brain stem function (83,84) in the patient in coma and should be differentiated from a persistent vegetative state defined as patients who have lost cerebral function and thus have no purposeful movement, but may have intact sleep–wake cycles, normal respiratory function, and some electroencephalographic activity (84). Somatic support of women with brain death to allow delivery of a viable neonate is made more difficult than in the patient in a persistent vegetative state by the loss of respiratory and thermoregulatory function, severe hemodynamic instability, and the greater likelihood of diabetes insipidus. However, both conditions require control of maternal seizures; identification and treatment of infection; mechanical ventilation; nutritional support; prevention of thromboembolism; frequent monitoring of fetal well-being; and monitoring of electrolytes, acid–base balance, and coagulation status (79,80). Although earlier reports of patients with brain death suggested that they had no more than a 14-day survival (77,83), a recent review by Powner and Bernstein (80) reported a survival range of 24 to 107 days in one series of pregnant women with delivery of infants from gestational age of 27 to 32 weeks, all of whom survived. They concluded that maintenance of placental perfusion was the most important priority for best fetal outcome, made more difficult in patients with severe hemodynamic instability as the uterine vasculature does not autoregulate to maintain appropriate perfusion in the face either maternal hyper- or hypotension. Bush et al.'s review of parturients with persistent vegetative states noted that deliveries occurred later in gestation compared to women with brain death and that fetal outcomes were good in centers with good neonatal support (79). All women with brain death and 10 of the 15 women who were in a persistent vegetative state underwent cesarean delivery (79,80).

■ ISCHEMIC STROKE

Ischemic stroke is rare and is due to occlusion of the arterial or venous cerebral circulation. Feske recently summarized seven retrospective reviews of ischemic stroke and found that cardioembolic events, arterial angiopathy, and preeclampsia were the most frequent causes of arterial occlusion (41). Rare causes included atherosclerosis, arterial dissection in association with trauma or arterial inflammation, preexisting maternal conditions associated with angiopathy (sickle cell disease, lupus, thrombotic thrombocytopenia

purpura, moyamoya disease, and migrainous headaches), or drug ingestion. Although cardiomyopathy is an established risk factor for cardioembolic stroke as the presence of left ventricular thrombosis is common (85), it was reported as a cause of only one stroke in Feske's recent review (41). Sinus and cortical vein thrombosis are the most frequent causes due to venous occlusion. A large portion of ischemic stroke is of unknown etiology (25%) and only a few cases are due to rare causes such as arterial dissection, disseminated intravascular coagulation, or in association with procoagulation syndromes (Table 33-6). Feske noted that reports of associated causes may differ due to differences in the populations studied, as studies involving Asian populations can be expected to have a higher proportion of cardioembolic causes, probably related to the higher incidence of rheumatic heart disease (41).

Stroke Due to Arterial Occlusion

Cerebral arterial occlusion as a cause of stroke is mostly related to preeclampsia–eclampsia (41). Although cerebral edema due to widespread endothelial injury or cerebral hemorrhage due to uncontrolled hypertension are more likely causes of cerebral dysfunction in hypertensive disorders of pregnancy (39–41,44,47), severe vasospasm and resultant thrombosis can cause infarction as well (86). Paradoxical embolism through a patent foramen ovale may be a frequent cause of cryptogenic stroke during pregnancy, but whether pregnancy increases its risk is unknown (47). Arterial occlusive stroke will present with focal neurologic findings related to the brain tissue affected. Arterial occlusion may more rarely occur in association with postpartum cerebral angiopathy, which is a group of reversible cerebral vasoconstrictive disorders affecting multiple vessels. More fully described below in the section on posterior reversible ischemic encephalopathy, it occurs in women with uncomplicated pregnancies, although it has also been reported to occur in women who have received vasoconstrictor drugs such as ergonovine and bromocriptine (47). It presents with headache, nausea, vomiting, changes in levels of consciousness, and focal neurologic deficits (47). The etiology is unknown, and its similarity to the clinical presentation of the neurologic complications of preeclampsia and subarachnoid-related vasospasm have lead some to suggest that the factors causing all these syndromes are similar (87). Multifocal segmental narrowing of cerebral arteries will be seen in radiologic studies, but sometimes an arterial biopsy is needed to differentiate it from arterial vasculitis (55). The treatment is supportive as the syndrome usually resolves over several weeks (47).

TABLE 33-7 Incidence of Pregnancy-Related Stroke in Published Series

Study	Ischemic	IC Hemorrhage	CVT	SAH	Study Type
	Pregnancy-Related Stroke Subtype and no. of Events per 100,000 Deliveries				
James et al. (42)	8.4	7.7	0.55	N/A	US Nationwide inpatient sample
Kittner et al. (44)	11	9	0.7	N/A	Retrospective, hospital based
Jaigobin et al. (45)	11.1	3.7	6.9	4.3	Retrospective, hospital based
Lanska et al. (46)	N/A	N/A	11.6	N/A	Retrospective, US Healthcare data

IC, intracerebral; CVT, central venous thrombosis; SAH, subarachnoid hemorrhage; N/A, not applicable.
Adapted from: Davie CA, O'Brien P. Stroke and pregnancy. *J Neurol Neurosurg Psychiatry* 2008;79:240–245, with permission.

Although a CT or MRI without contrast can in most cases distinguish hemorrhagic from ischemic stroke, if catheter-based angiographic therapies are contemplated, vascular imaging is required to define the vascular lesion (11,41). The most proven effective therapy for acute ischemic stroke is early thrombolysis with plasminogen activator or intra-arterial thrombolysis and mechanical clot removal (41,88,89). The major risk for thrombolysis is maternal cerebral hemorrhage, and subchorionic hematomas have been reported, but mostly good outcomes have been reported in studies of small groups of pregnant women (90). Treatment of associated underlying medical conditions is necessary to avoid stroke recurrence. While there are no systematic studies of anti-platelet or anti-coagulant drugs used to prevent stroke in women at risk or its recurrence following acute therapy, the use of low molecular weight heparins or aspirin in such women is widely advocated (39,41,47). Warfarin is associated with significant risk of fetal malformations if administered early in gestation and for fetal hemorrhage if administered later in pregnancy. The American Society of Regional Anesthesia guidelines for the use of regional anesthesia in anti-coagulated patients should be included in management decisions if neuraxial anesthesia is contemplated (91).

Stroke Due to Venous Occlusion

Cerebral vein thrombosis (CVT) is a common cause of stroke during and immediately following pregnancy, although the incidence reported varies widely in reported surveys (39,41) (Tables 33-6 and 33-7) and is reported with a higher incidence in developing countries (92). Data from the Healthcare Cost and Utilization Project estimates a risk of 11.6 cases per 100,000 births (44) and most cases occur during the second and third weeks postpartum (39,41,44,92). CVT presents with a wide variety of symptoms and signs as thrombosis of isolated cortical veins will present with focal sensory or motor deficit, while thrombosis of larger sinuses (cavernous, lateral, and sagittal) will often present with signs and symptoms of intracranial hypertension (41,44,92). Specific factors common to pregnancy thought to increase the risk compared to nonpregnant women are the hypercoagulability associated with pregnancy, dehydration, intracerebral blood flow stasis, and capillary damage that might occur during the second stage of labor (41,47,92). Additional risks during pregnancy are advanced maternal age, hyperemesis, cesarean delivery, a maternal inflammatory process, maternal hypertension, and thrombophilias (8,10,41,92). Although dural puncture is thought by some authors to increase the risk (44), others do not feel that needle trauma is sufficient injury to do so (92). The diagnostic dilemma of a positional headache in a patient who has received regional anesthesia may delay the diagnosis of CVT as many patients who ultimately were diagnosed with CVT were noted to present with a positional headache in one recent review (92). Most received epidural blood patching before changing signs and symptoms lead to

further evaluation for intracranial pathology without significant effect on neurologic outcome (92). One author has opined that epidural blood patch placement might protect against CVT in patients with low-pressure headache (93); however, a neurologic examination should be performed before epidural blood patch placement and an abnormality that cannot be attributed to deficits known to occur in association with low-pressure headache would warrant radiologic investigation (92).

The diagnosis is made by MRI venography, as the risk to the fetus of gadolinium administration is outweighed by the potential maternal benefit from early diagnosis (13,41). Acute anticoagulation appears to be the treatment of choice (41,92) and, although up to 50% of cases have an associated ICH (41,92), most retrospective series note a significantly lower mortality rate when full anticoagulation is instituted (39,41). The American Heart Association and American Stroke Association recommend that women at risk for stroke due to ischemia or thrombosis receive either unfractionated heparin therapy with partial thromboplastin therapy monitoring, low molecular weight heparin therapy with factor Xa monitoring, or warfarin therapy after 13 weeks of gestation with institution of low molecular weight heparin or unfractionated heparin therapy from the middle of the third trimester until delivery (94). Anesthetic management is guided by concerns over administering regional anesthesia to an anticoagulated patient and either regional or general anesthesia in a patient with possible increased intracranial pressure.

■ POSTERIOR REVERSIBLE ENCEPHALOPATHY SYNDROME

First described in 1996, Posterior Reversible Encephalopathy Syndrome (PRES) is a syndrome characterized by headache, seizures, altered mental status, and visual changes (blindness has been described, as posterior cerebral structures are most often involved with this syndrome), in association with a characteristic neuroradiologic picture (95). Although the syndrome occurs more often in nonpregnant patients with associated disease that can cause vascular damage such as uremia, hemolytic–uremic syndrome, and exposure to immunosuppressant drugs, 25% of cases have been reported in pregnant women (95–97). Most cases during pregnancy have been reported in association with preeclampsia (96–99), but a few others have occurred in healthy postpartum women (99,100). Some authors feel that the disorder is one of the group of postpartum cerebral angiopathy syndromes, mentioned above, as many times it is clinically indistinguishable from them (47). The pathophysiology is not well understood, but several authors feel that a breakdown in cerebral autoregulation occurs, similar to that which occurs in hypertensive encephalopathy in which loss of cerebral autoregulation, either due to or occurring with cerebral endothelial damage leads to vasogenic edema (39,95,101). Vasospasm is thus not thought to be a significant contributor and not routinely found on MRI imaging (101,102). Primary involvement of structures in the vertebrobasilar circulation is thought due to the reduced sympathetic innervation of the vessels in the posterior circulation which makes the characteristic lesions more commonly found in the occipital, posterioparietal, and temporal lobes (99). The brain MRI shows reversible parieto-occipital white matter edema on a fluid attenuated inversion recovery MRI, a normal diffusion-weighted imaging MRI which distinguishes vasogenic edema from that associated with cerebral infarction, and an increased apparent diffusion coefficient in posterior white matter indicating vasogenic edema in those areas where it is higher (101–103).

Treatment is supportive with aggressive treatment of the underlying condition (i.e., antihypertensive therapy), removal of medications associated with development of the syndrome, seizure prophylaxis, and control of intracranial hypertension if suspected (96–103). Although most case reports show resolution of the clinical syndrome and radiologic findings over a few months after presentation, irreversible damage can occur if the syndrome is not recognized early and appropriate therapy has begun (97,102). An early diagnosis may be difficult in the patient who has had regional anesthesia for delivery and initially presents with a complaint of headache without other symptoms and signs of neurologic deficit (104).

■ TRAUMATIC HEAD INJURY

Traumatic injury affects 6% to 8% of all pregnancies (105,106), and is the leading nonobstetric cause of maternal death in pregnancy, estimated to be 46% in some surveys (106). Fetal death exceeds that of maternal death by nearly threefold (107,108), placental abruption is the most frequent cause of fetal demise (109), and even seemingly minor trauma is associated with a significantly increased risk for placenta abruption (105,107–109). Although the GCS (Table 33-5) correlates poorly with fetal outcome (107), a GCS < 8 is one of the three most significant risk factors for fetal death (108). Neonatal outcomes at later delivery are significantly worse following intrapartum trauma when compared to other term neonates (107). Significant maternal head trauma occurs infrequently without other significant organ injury (106). Maternal head injuries are either open or penetrating and closed injuries can be either diffuse or focal in nature depending on the amount of brain tissue affected (8). Focal injuries are due to epidural, subdural, or intracerebral hematomas, or coup/countrecoup cerebral contusions (8).

Management of traumatic brain injury in the pregnant patient depends on the severity and type of brain injury. Since hypoxia and hypotension increase morbidity and mortality in all head-injured patients (110), the control of maternal blood pressure, oxygenation, ventilation, and cerebral perfusion and placental perfusion are top management priorities. Patients with a GCS < 9, who are unable to maintain their airway, or who are hypoxemic despite supplemental oxygen, should be endotracheally intubated and their ventilation controlled (110,111). Crystalloids should be used as opposed to colloids for resuscitation (112) and the patient should be positioned with the head of the bed elevated 30 degrees with the patient's head in a neutral position to facilitate venous drainage to lower ICP (110,111), and with left uterine displacement to avoid aortocaval compression. CT scanning should occur in all pregnant patients with known significant head injury shortly after presentation, just as in nonpregnant patients (11,105,110,111). Treatment of increased ICP should occur when pressures exceed 20 to 25 mm Hg, and hyperventilation, pharmacologic interventions (mannitol, furosemide, hypertonic saline, and steroids), hypothermia, and surgery are therapies that may be used (110,113). Hyperventilation may have detrimental effects on uterine blood flow as reductions of $PaCO_2$ to levels

required to have a significant effect in lowering intracranial pressure in the pregnant woman with already low $PaCO_2$ have been shown to cause uterine artery vasoconstriction (110,111). The beneficial effects of hyperventilation and diuretic therapy are usually short lived and are used to acutely reduce intracranial pressure until more definitive treatments can be instituted (110,111). Steroids can help accelerate fetal lung maturity, but their use is no longer recommended in head-injured patients due to an associated increase in mortality (113). The effects of hypertonic saline and hypothermia on the fetus are unknown and such therapies should be considered only as a last resort.

Surgical intervention should be considered for subdural and epidural hematoma evacuation, intracerebral hematoma with mass effect, in patients with GCS < 8 or in whom intracranial pressure is refractory to medical management, those patients with depressed skull fractures, or to place intracranial pressure monitors (8,105,110,113). There are no case series to help guide the time for optimal delivery after the initial presentation when delivery for acute fetal compromise due to placental abruption would be most likely. Interventions best for the mother may put the fetus in jeopardy, so the fetal risks due to preterm delivery need to be weighed against the fetal risk of prolonging the pregnancy. Cesarean delivery at the time of other acute or planned surgery should be considered (114). Anesthetic considerations are the same as in pregnant patients who have increased intracranial pressure undergoing craniotomy for the treatment of intracranial hemorrhage, outlined above. The treatment of each patient must be individualized as there are no case series that specifically review management of the head-injured parturient.

■ IDIOPATHIC INTRACRANIAL HYPERTENSION

Also labeled pseudotumor cerebri and benign intracranial hypertension, idiopathic intracranial hypertension is an increase in intracranial pressure without intracranial mass lesion or hydrocephalus and is a diagnosis of exclusion as many disorders can cause increases in intracranial pressure (Table 33-8) (115). Friedman and Jacobson recently proposed modifications to the modified Dandy criteria for diagnosis: CSF pressure greater than 25 mm H_2O measured in the lateral decubitus position without any other identifiable cause of elevated ICP seen; CSF of normal composition; and no mass, structural, or vascular lesion demonstrated on MRI or CT scanning (115). The most common presenting symptoms are headache and visual changes, with signs of papilledema. Abducens nerve and facial nerve palsies are less frequently observed (116). The cause is unknown, but decreased absorbance of CSF, increased intracranial venous pressure, and increased production of CSF have all been suggested as etiologies (115). The incidence in the general population is 1 to 2 cases per 100,000, with a female/male ratio of 3:1. Pregnancy does not appear to affect the outcome of the disorder, although symptoms worsen in 50% of women (116,117). Most cases during pregnancy present during the first 2 trimesters, and pregnancy itself does not appear to be a risk factor for the development of the disorder, although obesity seems to be an associated risk factor (117).

Since the disorder does not affect maternal or neonatal outcomes, therapy is directed toward the treatment of headache, maintenance of appropriate body weight, and monitoring for visual loss with quantitative visual field testing (116,117). If visual loss is significant, then treatment with repeated lumbar puncture or temporary spinal fluid drainage is indicated, but may not be effective long term (116–118). Steroid therapy is effective in a significant percentage of cases, but complications are increased when used for long periods of time in

TABLE 33-8 Conditions that may Increase Intracranial Pressure and Mimic Idiopathic Intracranial Hypertension

Medical disorders
Addison's disease
Hypoparathyroidism
Right heart failure with pulmonary hypertension
Sleep apnea
Renal failure
Severe anemia
Medications
Tetracycline
Vitamin A
Corticoisteroid withdrawal
Chordecone
Nalidixic acid
Lithium
Norplant® implant system
Obstruction to venous drainage
Central venous thrombosis

Adapted from: Friedman DI, Jacobson DM. Diagnostic criteria for idiopathic intracranial hypertension. *Neurology* 2002;59:1492–1495, with permission.

pregnant women (117). If visual loss is progressive, then lumboperitoneal (LP) shunting or optic nerve sheath decompression may be required (116–118).

Both single shot spinal and continuous spinal and epidural anesthesia have been used with success for vaginal and cesarean delivery (119–121). Since CSF pressures are typically uniform throughout the cranial vault, cerebellar herniation should not occur with lumbar puncture; however, inappropriately severe headache and signs of focal neurologic deficit would preclude the use of neuraxial anesthesia. These findings were present in the two reported cases of tonsillar herniation following lumbar puncture (122). Insertion of a spinal catheter may provide therapy and used for anesthesia for either vaginal (121) or cesarean delivery (123). While dosing of an epidural block might be expected to increase intracranial pressure in the parturient without an LP shunt, a shunt would allow safe epidural anesthesia. Some authors have expressed concern that safe neuraxial anesthesia requires radiologic studies to avoid trauma to an LP shunt, but others have performed successful intrathecal and epidural blockade without such studies citing minimal risk if the needle is placed above or below the surgical scar (124,125). Others advocate the use of general anesthesia over spinal anesthesia for fear that drug injected intrathecally may escape into the peritoneal space and make an adequate sensory block difficult to achieve (119); however, use of a combined spinal–epidural technique might avoid this theoretical concern.

■ MATERNAL HYDROCEPHALUS

Maternal hydrocephalus is most often due to conditions that predate pregnancy and many women will present with either ventriculoperitoneal or ventriculoatrial shunts in place. Improved care has allowed children with hydrocephalus following childhood acquired intracranial infection or intra-

cranial hemorrhage, congenital aqueductal stenosis, hydrocephalus in association with neural tube defects, the ACMs, and the Dandy–Walker syndrome to survive into childbearing years (126,127). The number of pregnant women with shunts has increased, although the percentage among pregnant women is unknown (8).

Although obstetric management is governed by obstetric and other medical factors in the presence of a well-functioning shunt (127), neurologic complications have been reported in older series to complicate 58% to 76% of pregnancies, a rate higher than that in the nonpregnant population of childbearing age (52). However, report of one newer case series showed that 84% of patients delivered without shunt malfunction during their pregnancy (127). If real, the reason for an increase in shunt malfunctions is unclear, with some authors hypothesizing mechanical problems due to changed anatomy and functional obstruction due to increased intraabdominal pressure (14). Detection of increased intracranial pressure may be difficult as headaches and visual changes occur frequently during pregnancy due to obstetric causes, but the threshold for neurosurgical consultation should be low and appropriate radiologic studies should be ordered as fetal risk from such testing is low (14,126,127). If CT and MRI studies are normal, then CSF cultures should be obtained (5). If shunt revision is required, then the principles of anesthetic care of the pregnant women with increased intracranial pressure as outlined above should be followed. One comprehensive series report noted that the incidence of vaginal delivery was 60.7% and the preferred mode of delivery. Indications for cesarean delivery are most often dictated by obstetric considerations (5,126,127), but simultaneous urgent delivery with a shunt revision in the parturient with rapid neurologic deterioration may be necessary (128). Prophylactic antibiotics are recommended during delivery (14,126,127), but evidence for their efficacy in preventing shunt infection during vaginal delivery is lacking (126). In the patient without increased intracranial pressure, regional anesthesia can be used safely, although concerns over an increase in shunt infection with spinal anesthesia probably limited its reported use in one series (127).

■ ARNOLD–CHIARI MALFORMATION

The ACM is a congenital anomaly that typically presents in the second to third decade of life with a posterior occipital headache made worse with a Valsalva maneuver and coughing, and signs and symptoms associated with lower cranial nerve, brain stem, cerebellar, and spinal cord dysfunction (129). The disorder is classified into types I–III depending on the degree of medullary, cerebellar tonsillar, and fourth ventricle herniation through the foramen magnum, with neuronal impairment of the medulla causing the most concern as respiratory failure can occur (130). An associated syringomyelia is found in up to 50% of women (8,130). Although increases in intracranial pressure have been thought to be a cause of a large part of the symptom complex, (130) cases of associated hydrocephalus are rare (130–132) and one recent review could not find reports of CSF pressure measurements in patients with ACM during pregnancy, labor, and delivery (130). Two recent reviews did not describe significant progression of symptoms during pregnancy, nor before or after delivery (130,133). The therapy for patients with progressive symptoms is a suboccipital craniotomy with decompression of the posterior fossa and placement of expansive dural grafts (133), although case reports of this surgery during pregnancy have not been described in the literature.

Most authors have expressed reservations in performing regional anesthesia for patients with an Arnold–Chiari I malformation, citing theoretical concerns that changes in the potential pressure CSF pressure gradient that might be present above and below the foramen magnum could cause further cerebellar tonsillar herniation (131,132). The safety of spinal anesthesia in particular has been questioned due to the temporal appearance of symptoms in previously undiagnosed patients following spinal anesthesia or accidental dural puncture (133,134). However, some case reports (131,132,135) suggest that epidural and spinal anesthesia for both vaginal and cesarean delivery in patients with corrected and uncorrected lesions can be used in selected patients. In addition, despite two small case series of patients with both previously diagnosed and unsuspected Arnold–Chiari I malformations which reported good neurologic outcomes when both epidural and spinal were used (129,133), regional anesthesia should be performed with caution in patients with ACM (133). If a regional anesthetic is chosen, slow careful dosing of an epidural block might be the best approach (136).

■ THE NEUROCUTANEOUS SYNDROMES

The neurocutaneous syndromes, or phakomatoses, are a heterogenous group of congenital disorders with diverse genetic, clinical, and pathologic features. Most are hereditary although some occur sporadically. The common features include involvement of organs of ectodermal origin (nervous system, eye, and skin), evolution of lesions in childhood and adolescence, and potential for malignant transformation of lesions. There are many syndromes in this category and this section will focus on those that are most common and thus more likely to affect the parturient.

The Neurofibromatoses

The neurofibromatoses are a group of autosomal dominant neurocutaneous syndromes which are associated with the formation of ectodermal and mesodermal tissue masses (137). Much of the potential morbidity is related to tumor location, and every major system can be affected. There are two clinically and genetically distinct types of neurofibromatoses, type I (NF1) and type II (NF2).

NF1 (formerly known as von Recklinghausen's disease) is more common, occurring in 1 in 2,500 to 3,000 live births (138). NF1 is associated with multiple cutaneous manifestations such as cafe au lait spots, axillary and inguinal freckling, multiple discrete dermal neurofibromas (benign peripheral nerve sheath tumors), and Lisch nodules in the iris. NF1 can have a remarkably variable clinical picture and learning disabilities are often present. Patients with NF1 have an approximately 10% lifetime risk of malignant transformation of preexisting tumors, or de novo malignancies (138). Epilepsy is diagnosed in about 6% of NF1 patients and is generally of a milder form (138).

The cardiovascular manifestations of NF1 deserve special mention as they are a frequent cause of premature death in these patients (139). Though severe complications from intracardiac and mediastinal neurofibromas have been reported during pregnancy (140), these are extremaly rare occurences. The three most common cardiovascular manifestations of NF1 are vasculopathy, hypertension, and congenital heart defects (139). There are several case reports of morbidity from arterial vasculopathy in pregnant patients with NF1, one with a ruptured pancreaticoduodenal artery (141) and another with brachial artery rupture (142). There is also an increased prevalence of the sympathetic nervous system tumors pheochromocytoma and ganglioneuroma in patients with NF1 (143). Pheochromocytomas are catecholamine secreting tumors with an incidence of approximately <0.2%/10,000 pregnancies (144). Although rare, pheochro-

mocytomas carry a high mortality rate if untreated, and prior to detection are often treated as gestational hypertension or preeclampsia (144). Most ganglioneuromas do not secrete catecholamine or steroid hormones (145).

There are several retrospective reviews of maternal outcomes in patients with NF1 (146,147) which seem to demonstrate trends toward high cesarean rates and intrauterine growth restriction (IUGR). The largest series by Dugoff and Sujansky (148) reported on 105 women with NF1 with a total of 247 pregnancies and 182 live births. The cesarean delivery rate was 36%. The authors noted increasing percentages of preeclampsia, preterm delivery, and IUGR reported in prior series (147). Of interest, 60% women reported growth of new neurofibromas during pregnancy and 52% noted enlargement of existing neurofibromas. Eighteen percent observed no changes in the size of their neurofibromas and no growth of new neurofibromas during pregnancy. This increase in size and number of cutaneous neurofibromas has previously been reported and can have implications for delivery of anesthesia (149).

NF2 is a much less common disorder, occurring in 1 in 33,000 to 40,000 live births. Cutaneous signs are either very limited or absent in NF2 and clinical manifestations are largely restricted to the nervous system and eye (138). The most common tumors associated with NF2 are vestibular schwannomas (acoustic neuromas). These usually appear during adolescence or in a person's early twenties; therefore NF2 can be diagnosed during pregnancy. In general these patients have a higher risk of central nervous system tumors, such as ependymomas, meningiomas, and rarely astrocytomas (146). These tumors can be on the dorsal root extending medially and laterally, within the vertebral canal, intradurally, or extramedullary masses (146). Since this disease is rare, there are no large outcome studies, and only case reports to help guide management. The concern for tumors that increase in size during pregnancy is also present in the case of NF2 (150). The obstetric management and mode of delivery in general should be based on the usual obstetric indications along with consideration of patient-specific details such as tumor type and location. These decisions are best made in consultation with obstetric anesthesiology, neurosurgery, neurology, and other required disciplines.

Anesthetic management of patients with NF1 and NF2 requires knowledge of underlying disease process and its implications (Table 33-9). There are clear differences between NF1 and NF2 yet much commonality with regard to anesthetic concerns. Knowledge of type and locations of tumor is important in the management of both disorders.

Many anesthetic concerns surround the provision of regional anesthesia. Placement of spinal or epidural anesthesia may be difficult in a patient with neurofibromatosis because of kyphoscoliosis and surface neurofibromas. Neurofibromas along the path of the needle may limit the safety of the procedure because of concerns of bleeding (151). Regional anesthesia may be even contraindicated in presence of tumors near the spinal cord or nerve roots. Given these concerns, imaging prior to placement of neuraxial anesthesia is potentially very important. In patients with NF1, spinal neurofibromas with clinical implications are reported in only about 5% of patients (152). However, MRI studies in randomly selected asymptomatic NF1 patients show that spinal neurofibromas are found in up to 38% of patients (152). There are many case reports of successful regional anesthesia after confirmation of absence of neuraxial tumor (69). As the clinical picture in NF1 is so variable and central tumors are not a hallmark of the disease, the requirement to image prior to central neuraxial anesthesia in an asymptomatic patient remains controversial, although most published reports recommend imaging prior to placement. The type of regional

TABLE 33-9 Systemic Considerations in Neurofibromatosis Type I

System	Potential Complications
Airway	• Neurofibromas of the oropharynx and trachea
Central nervous system	• Intracranial and spinal tumors • Vascular lesions • Learning disabilities, attention deficit hyperactivity disorder
Musculoskeletal	• Pseudoarthroses, sphenoid dysplasia • Osteoporosis • Scoliosis (typically cervical and upper thoracic) • Vertebral deformities
Cardiovascular	• Hypertension—essential and renovascular • Arterial vasculopathy • Cardiomyopathy
Gastrointestinal	• Gasrointestinal stromal tumors—typically of the proximal small bowel • Cardinoid tumors
Genitourinary	• Neurofibromas of bladder • Neurofibromas obstructing ureters and urethra • Neurofibromas of pelvis and perineum
Pulmonary	• Pulmonary fibrosis • Pulmonary hypertension • Intrapulmonary neurofibromas

Modified from: Hirsch NP, Murphy A, Radcliffe JJ. Neurofibromatosis: clinical presentations and anaesthetic implications. *Br J Anaesth* 2001;86(4):555–564.

anesthetic provided may factor into the decision as the risk of bleeding may be acceptable with a small bore spinal needle versus a larger bore epidural needle. As the presence of central nervous system tumors is much more likely to occur in NF2, most authors recommend intracranial and spine imaging prior to regional anesthesia in these patients (153).

Regardless of imaging, it is wise to perform a neurologic examination, and consider symptomology and history of prior central tumors prior to placement of regional anesthesia. It is also important to discuss risks and benefits of regional anesthesia with the patient and the care team, ideally in an antepartum setting. Monitoring of neurologic status during and after anesthesia is another important aspect of care. Anesthetic considerations are the same as in pregnant patients who have increased intracranial pressure as previously outlined. Deciding between general and regional anesthesia can pose a dilemma for the clinician and could lead to neurologic compromise if not managed appropriately.

Sturge–Weber Syndrome

Sturge–Weber syndrome (encephalotrigeminal angiomatosis) occurs approximately 1 in 20,000 to 50,000 live births (154). It occurs sporadically with a highly variable clinical course. Patients generally present with a large facial hemangioma of the trigeminal nerve distribution along with associated intracranial or intraocular vascular malformations (154) such as ipsilateral leptomeningeal angiomatosis and other venous anomalies (155). Vascular manifestations have also been noted on the spleen, pituitary, lungs, and other organs (156). This disorder is associated with seizures, hemiplegia, hemi-cerebral atrophy, glaucoma and other ocular manifestations, and developmental delay or mental retardation (157,156).

There are few case reports in pregnancy, therefore specific effects of pregnancy on the disorder or outcomes of pregnancy are unclear. Case reports include one patient who developed hemiplegia, hemianopia, and aphasia during the third trimester (158), and another with worsening intractable seizures who did not have a formal diagnosis until the early postpartum period (155).

Since the facial angiomas may involve the mouth, nose, palate, and larynx, careful evaluation of the airway is warranted prior to the initiation of any type of anesthesia. Stress and hypertension can cause marked expansion of this patient's hemangiomas and rupture of one of the hemangiomas covering the facial region has been reported (159). This can become an important issue for a laboring patient or one with preeclampsia. As patients with Sturge–Weber syndrome can have associated intracranial pathology, appropriate imaging and investigation should be done in order to aid management. It is also important to note that occasionally patients with large port-wine nevus may not have been evaluated for Sturge–Weber syndrome and appropriate consultation is warranted. Because of the potential for intracranial pathology, anesthetic management should be geared toward minimizing changes in intracranial and intraocular pressure.

Tuberous Sclerosis Complex

Tuberous sclerosis complex (TSC) is an autosomal dominant neurocutaneous syndrome which is characterized by the formation of multiple hamartomatous lesions (consisting of a disorganized local tissue mixture). These hamartomas are generally nonmalignant but can have significant morbidity and mortality, depending on their size and location. These lesions are most commonly found in the skin, brain, kidney, and lungs (160). Other common manifestations of the disease include epilepsy, developmental delay, mental retardation, autism, and psychiatric problems (161).

The presence of TSC seems to increase risks for maternal adverse outcome. King and Stamilio (162) reviewed 23 pregnancies in 17 mothers with TSC. There were four hemorrhages from ruptured renal masses, the preterm delivery rate was 35%, cesarean delivery rate was 33%, four developed preeclampsia, two experienced acute renal failure, and there were two perinatal demises. Of note, three cases of maternal TSC were diagnosed following recognition of affected offspring.

Anesthetic concerns are related to the specific tumor types and locations. Of particular concern are cardiac and renal tumors, spinal and intracranial tumors, pharyngeal tumors, and pulmonary involvement (lymphangiomyomatosis) (160). Careful airway evaluation and appropriate imaging prior to regional or general anesthesia is essential. Specific anesthetic management plans should be made using a multidisciplinary team approach and should include an assessment of the patient's ability to cooperate.

■ ACUTE SPINAL CORD INJURY

Acute spinal cord injury (ACSI) is usually the result of trauma and thus can be associated with significant morbidity. Fifteen percent of ACSIs involve young women of childbearing age (163). Initial management of ACSI involves neck stabilization, airway management, evaluation for other injuries, and hemodynamic stabilization. For the pregnant patient, especially one over 20 weeks of gestation, uterine displacement is an important aspect of maintaining hemodynamic stability Ensuring that the mother should receive all care, therapies, and imaging that is appropriate to her situation is of utmost importance.

Neurogenic (vasogenic) shock results from the disruption of autonomic nervous system control over vasoconstriction. This period of instability resulting from blockage of sympathetic tone can last from 1 to 3 weeks and can have significant implications for both the mother and fetus. It is characterized by profoundly decreased peripheral vascular resistance and cardiac output, leading to hypotension, profound or relative bradycardia, and hypothermia. It does not usually occur with spinal cord injury below the level of T6 and the higher the level of injury the more likely it is for the patient to exhibit severe symptoms. Shock associated with a spinal cord injury involving the lower thoracic cord must be considered hemorrhagic in nature until proven otherwise. Uteroplacental perfusion can be maintained with adequate fluid resuscitation and hemodynamic support (163).

Once neurogenic shock has resolved, 85% of patients with an injury above T6 will experience autonomic hyperreflexia (AH) (163). This occurs because of unopposed sympathetic activity above lesion and is triggered by sensory input below the level of the lesion. Stimuli such as bladder or bowel distension, muscle spasms, and uterine contractions can trigger this response. Milder reactions can be limited to flushing, piloerection, shivering, nausea, or headache. More severe consequences include severe to life-threatening hypertension with tachycardia or baroreceptor-induced bradycardia, and ventricular arrhythmias.

Much of the information on pregnant patients with ASCI comes from case reports. Individual outcomes can vary tremendously with associated injuries; however, several concerns arise from these case reports. Because of the risks or AH and neurogenic shock, patients with ASCI should be monitored and deliver at facility capable of invasive monitoring. It is important to distinguish preeclampsia and eclampsia from AH. It is unclear if patients with ASCI are at the risk of preterm delivery (164). Several potentially confounding factors exist, including the presence of associated injuries and the possible inability to feel contractions make it difficult to assess the true incidence of preterm labor.

The decision to deliver a fetus is a complicated one in the setting of ASCI. The fetal heart rate can be monitored as appropriate but the first priority must be the hemodynamic stability of the mother. In some situations a cesarean delivery is performed to promote stability of the mother, and in other instances there is a decision to maintain pregnancy with fetal and tocodynometric monitoring. These decisions are difficult ones and must be made in a multidisciplinary format.

Anesthetic management of the pregnant patient with ASCI is challenging as one must balance many concerns. General anesthesia is complicated by concerns for the mother and fetus, airway, and possibly head injury. Regional anesthesia in the setting of neurogenic shock, recent spinal surgery, an unstable spine, and associated injuries is often not an option.

■ CHRONIC SPINAL CORD INJURY

Once the acute phase concludes, and there is resolution of associated injuries, patients enter the phase of chronic spinal cord injury (CSCI). For some parturients, the spinal cord injury maybe very remote. Several small retrospective reviews (165,166) suggest that patients with CSCI have maternal and neonatal outcomes similar to normal pregnancy. It is unclear if patients with CSCI are truly at risk for preterm labor;

however, unattended delivery is a potential complication. Standard obstetric practice should generally dictate care in patients with CSCI (167).

There are several chronic medical issues associated with CSCI that can be aggravated during pregnancy. These include deep venous thrombosis, recurrent urinary tract infections, decubitus ulcers, anemia, and decreased pulmonary reserve requiring monitoring of respiratory status (167). These patients may be at greater risk for hypotension, and those with injuries above T6 are clearly at risk for autonomic hyperreflexia (168).

Assuming that they do not present with any of the standard contraindications to regional anesthesia, patients with CSCI should be given consideration for spinal or epidural anesthesia. Regional anesthesia in patients with CSCI can be difficult to perform for multiple reasons. Many patients have prior surgical stabilization, often with hardware in place. Thus, spinal and epidural techniques in patients with CSCI are associated with higher incidence of block failure, and incomplete analgesia. As patients are at risk for deep venous thrombosis, many will be on subcutaneous heparin which depending on dosing and formulation may delay or even contraindicate regional anesthesia.

Even in the face of the previously mentioned difficulties, reasonable attempts should be made to provide neuraxial anesthesia to patients with CSCI, especially those at risk for AH, even when the injury level would seem to preclude sensation of pain. This might even include attempts at placement under fluoroscopy. The potential for severe sudden hypertension is concerning as intracranial hemorrhage attributed to autonomic hyperreflexia has been reported in two laboring women (168). Neuraxial anesthesia is proven to prevent and treat autonomic hyperreflexia (168). Amniotomy, perineal stretching, and particularly labor are all triggers of autonomic hyperreflexia, even in patients with no prior history (168). Crosby et al. recommend that epidural analgesia with local anesthetic solution should be performed, tested, and activated if possible prior to the onset of labor (168). Because of the potential for hemodynamic instability, the authors recommend that invasive monitoring be available if needed. The use of epidural or spinal opioids alone has been met with mixed results. Epidural meperidine has been successful at controlling AH during labor (169) possibly due to its local anesthetic properties. Fentanyl alone in the epidural space is ineffective (170).

In the instance where regional anesthesia is impossible in a patient at risk for AH, general anesthesia has been reported to control blood pressure in patients with CSCI. In addition to all of the concerns of general anesthesia during pregnancy, the concentrations of volatile agent plus intravenous agents required to achieve this goal may lead to uterine atony and depression of the newborn, and thus is not an ideal anesthetic for obstetrics. For laboring patients who are unable to receive neuraxial analgesia, there are reports of the use of intravenous magnesium (171) with success. There are also various case reports of the use of vasoactive agents including hydralazine and anxiolytics (172) and sodium nitroprusside (173); however, blood pressure control tended to be poor with these methods.

■ SPINA BIFIDA

Spina bifida (SB), the most common permanently disabling birth defect in the United States, occurs when the neural tube fails to close during early embryonal development, resulting in a range of defects. SB can be divided into three anatomical variations. Myelomeningocele is the most severe form, in which the spinal cord and meninges protrude from a defect in the spine. The specific functional impairments depend on the level of the lesion, and the primary functional deficits include lower limb paralysis and sensory loss, bladder and bowel dysfunction, and cognitive dysfunction (174). The majority of these patients also have a history of hydrocephalus. With a meningocele, the spinal cord develops normally but the meninges protrude from the spinal opening. Symptoms of meningocele vary from those with few or no symptoms to incomplete paralysis with urinary and bowel dysfunction.

Spina bifida occulta (SBO) is the mildest form, yet deserves some discussion as there can be some confusion regarding its diagnosis and therefore the anesthetic management. SBO occurs when one or more vertebrae fail to fuse in the midline. Generally the spinal cord and meninges are normal and there are no skin defects. There may be no motor or sensory impairments evident at birth. It is thought to be present in up to 20% of the general population and may be discovered as an incidental finding. Subtle, progressive neurologic deterioration can become evident in later childhood or adulthood. In many instances, SBO is so mild that there is no disturbance in function at all.

Spinal dysraphism is often confused with or misdiagnosed as SBO. With spinal dysraphism the bony spinal defect is accompanied by spinal abnormalities such as intraspinous lipoma, dermal sinus tracts, dermoid cysts, fibrous bands, and diastematomyelia or split cord (175). In addition, spinal cord tethering is present in 35% to 87% of patients with spinal dysraphism (176,177). Approximately, 50% of patients with a tethered cord will have cutaneous manifestations such as tufts of hair, dimples, lipomas, hyperpigmentation, hemangiomas, or other skin abnormalities (176). SBO which was diagnosed incidentally in an asymptomatic patient with no neurologic complaints and a normal examination is unlikely to be associated with any further anomalies. In a patient with the aforementioned cutaneous manifestations, or with neurologic complaints or abnormalities on physical examination, the clinician should consider imaging in order to exclude intraspinal abnormalities (177).

Arata et al. (178) reported 17 women with SB who had a total of 29 pregnancies, with 23 pregnancies progressing to birth. Vaginal deliveries occurred in one of five pregnancies of women who were wheelchair dependent and in ten of eighteen pregnancies in independently mobile women, including seven of eight pregnancies of independently mobile women without ileal conduits. Cesarean deliveries were accompanied by postoperative complications in 10 women. The authors concluded that women with SB who become pregnant generally have a positive outcome, with relatively low complication rates.

Many of the anesthetic concerns with SB surround the provision of regional anesthesia. Regional anesthesia is not absolutely contraindicated although there are many potential problems. Because of scoliosis and prior operations, epidural or spinal placement may be difficult. There may also be VP shunts in place, infectious concerns, and unpredictable spread of local anesthesia depending on the specifics of the lesion. Tidmarsh and May (179) retrospectively reported on the labor analgesia of 16 patients with SB at their institution. Eight of the patients had SBO with no neural deficits, and eight had meningomyelocoele with deficits ranging from mild to moderate sensorimotor loss. All had normal sphincter function and none had indwelling VP shunts. Ten of the sixteen received epidural analgesia inserted above the level of the defect. Six of the ten had adequate analgesia. There was one asymmetric block which resolved with catheter manipulation, one dural puncture followed by subsequent successful epidural blockade, one excessively high block, and one block which failed to extend below the level of the lesion. Knowledge of the type of lesion, history of prior operations, assess-

ment of neurologic symptoms, and a neurologic examination are important aspects of anesthetic planning for the parturient with SB.

■ SYRINGOMYELIA

Syringomyelia involves the formation of a cyst or syrinx within the spinal cord. These cysts can enlarge over time, destroying part of the spinal cord. The most common cause of syringomyelia is Arnold–Chiari I malformation (ACMI) secondary to obstruction of the cerebrospinal fluid circulatory pathways. Other causes include neoplasm, meningitis, hemorrhage, arachnoiditis, and other postinflammatory states (129). Symptoms vary according to the size and location of the syrinx and can include pain and motor weakness, headaches, and decreased sensation. This condition is most commonly diagnosed in young adults at the age of 25 to 40 years (136); however, more widespread use of MRI is leading to earlier diagnosis. Progressive clinical symptoms usually begin years after the initiating event.

There are many forms of surgical intervention for syringomyelia, based on symptoms, etiology, and progression of disease. In general, drainage of a syrinx does not necessarily mean the elimination of the syrinx-related symptoms, but rather is aimed at stopping progression. Surgery results in stabilization or modest improvement in symptoms for most patients in the setting of motor neurologic deterioration as a consequence of posttraumatic syrinx/tethered cord (180). Lumboperitoneal shunts may lead to useful improvement in the symptoms of a patient with syringomyelia while avoiding the risk of neurologic deterioration inherent in myelotomies required for syrinx shunting procedures (181).

In terms of obstetric management, the optimal mode of delivery has not been established and an individualized decision is based on symptoms and in consideration of neurosurgical recommendations. Vaginal delivery does not seem to be contraindicated, especially in the presence of syringomyelia alone; however, there seems to be general concern about the effects of maternal expulsive efforts. Many authors of published reports chose to perform either elective cesarean delivery (136, 182,183) or operative vaginal delivery for this reason (183).

Most of the relevant reports describe patients with syringomyelia associated with Arnold–Chiari I malformations. Since there are few case reports of management of syringomyelia as a separate entity in pregnant patients, evidence is anecdotal. Most published cases report the use of general anesthesia, chosen over regional anesthesia mainly because of medicolegal concerns and fear of CSF pressure fluctuation (184). Most authors caution against the use of spinal anesthesia (136) especially in the presence of ACMI. There are reports of recurrent postdural puncture headache and neurologic symptoms up to several weeks after dural puncture (134,185). Nel et al. (136) recommend that when regional anesthesia is chosen, a slow establishment of an epidural block is best in order to avoid rapid compression of the subarachnoid space.

■ SPINAL VASCULAR MALFORMATIONS

Spinal vascular malformations are rare and present with a wide variety of clinical manifestations. These malformations can be responsible for severe morbidity if not treated appropriately. Symptoms can include sensorimotor deterioration, bowel and bladder dysfunction, radicular pain, and various localized complaints (186). The specific mechanisms of injury can be multifactorial and may include hemorrhage, arterial steal, mass effect, and venous hypertension (186). Clinical diagnosis is made on the basis of MRI and angiography (187). There are many types of classification systems which are beyond the scope of this chapter. We will discuss the most common lesions: AVMs, arteriovenous fistulas (AVFs), dural AVFs, and cavernous malformations.

Arteriovenous Malformations

AVMs are high-flow shunts of blood which are often thought to be the most clinically significant type of malformation as they are more likely than other lesions to hemorrhage (186). Some authors have concluded that there is a higher propensity for hemorrhage during pregnancy and the puerperium in AVM, and postulate a role for hormonal stimulation (188).

Arteriovenous Fistulas

AVFs represent a direct arteriovenous shunt located on the pial surface of the spinal cord (186). Most are located in the conus medullaris or the cauda equina (186). There seems to be no clear relationship between the size of the lesion and clinical symptoms. There is at least one reported case of an AVF in a pregnant patient who experienced an exacerbation of her neurologic symptoms and AVF growth which was thought to be triggered by pregnancy. She improved after delivery without interventional treatment. The authors concluded that careful follow up of neurologic findings is required to prevent unnecessary interventional procedures in pregnant women with spinal AVF (189).

Dural Arteriovenous Fistula

Dural AVFs are by far the most common vascular malformation to affect the spinal cord (186). However, they are more common in men and peak age of onset is in the fifth and sixth decades. Therefore the incidence in women of childbearing age is limited. These lesions are comprised of an arteriovenous shunt on the dura, usually arising from an intervertebral foramen (186).

Cavernous Malformations

Cavernous malformations (CM) are well-defined, grossly visible lesions that comprise 5% to 12% of spinal vascular tumors (190). They are more common in brain but also occur in the spinal cord and may reach a significant size. They are composed of a compact mass of sinusoidal-type vessels immediately in apposition to each other without any recognizable intervening neural parenchyma. There are several reports of cavernous malformations in pregnancy that either became symptomatic (188,191,192) or ruptured during pregnancy or the peripartum period (188,193). The evidence for increasing rates of hemorrhage and development of symptoms from CMs in female patients is inconsistent. Pregnancy and prior hemorrhage may be risk factors for repeated hemorrhages (193). Fortunately the need for emergent neurosurgery has been very rare (193). Most cases can be observed and treated after delivery. In the case of severe symptoms surgery has successfully preceded delivery (193).

It is recommended that the mode of delivery for patients with spinal vascular malformations should be based on the usual obstetric indications (188); however, the presentation and clinical course should clearly factor into this decision. Anesthetic management of the parturient with a spinal vascular malformation must take into account the anticipated mode of delivery. This decision should involve joint input from obstetric, neurosurgical, and obstetric anesthesia. The decision to pursue a vaginal delivery should include a plan for adequate pain management. The general consensus of published case reports seems to be that regional anesthesia

is relatively contraindicated. There are several case reports of neurologic decline in patients with undiagnosed AVM after spinal and epidural anesthesia in both pregnant and nonpregnant patients (194). Hirsch et al. (195) describe a patient who developed leg weakness 4 weeks after spontaneous vaginal delivery with epidural anesthesia. This weakness progressed to permanent paraplegia despite successful clipping of the newly diagnosed spinal AVM. Ong et al. (196) however report a case of successful spinal anesthesia for cesarean delivery in a symptomatic patient with cervical AVM. The authors chose spinal anesthesia over epidural anesthesia in order to avoid increases in transmitted pressure from the epidural space. Ong et al. (196) concluded that spinal cord AVM in the cervical region is not an absolute contraindication to spinal anesthesia. Despite the successful outcome of this case, regional anesthesia should be carefully weighed against the relative risks of general anesthesia and should be considered relatively contraindicated in patients with spinal vascular malformations. On the contrary, a patient with a small, incidentally discovered asymptomatic lesion which is distant from the site of needle placement may be appropriate for regional anesthesia. Knowledge of the size, location, and type of lesion; risk of hemorrhage; neurologic symptoms; and consultation with neurosurgical colleagues will help in assessing the patient specific risk of regional anesthesia.

■ SPINAL CORD TUMORS

Primary spinal cord tumors are rare compared to their intracranial counterparts and comprise 12% of central nervous system tumors during pregnancy (5). These intramedullary tumors infiltrate and destroy parenchyma, can extend over multiple cord segments, and can result in the formation of a syrinx. The most common signs and symptoms of spinal cord tumors include back pain, numbness and paresthesias, unilateral or bilateral weakness, ataxia, bowel or bladder dysfunction, mild spasticity, and gait difficulties. The most common types of tumors are astrocytoma, ependymoma, and hemangioblastoma, which represent over 70% of all spinal cord neoplasms. In adults, ependymomas are the most common tumor type, accounting for 40% to 60% of all intramedullary spinal tumors, with the mean age of presentation being 35 to 40 years (197).

There are multiple reports of parturients with undiagnosed ependymomas who experienced neurologic compromise and even paraplegia after spinal or epidural anesthesia (65,198). Compared with intracranial ependymomas, spinal ependymomas are less prevalent, occur in a younger population, and exhibit a better prognosis (199,200). Ependymomas are also encountered in patients with the neurofibromatoses.

Spinal metastatic disease most commonly spreads to the vertebrae from primary malignancies such as lung, breast, prostate, renal, and thyroid. Lymphomas may also spread to the spine (201). Neurologic compromise occurs when these metastases compress the spinal cord or nerve roots. There are several such examples reported in parturients, including paraplegia secondary to metastatic osteosarcoma (202), and paraspinal Wilms' tumor with metastatic to the spine (203).

Vertebral hemangiomas (VH) are benign and are present and asymptomatic in 10% of the population. They are more common in women, and tend to be located in the lumbar or thoracic regions (204). There are multiple reports of VH during pregnancy presenting as spinal cord syndromes with pain and neurologic deficits (204,205). They tend to present during the second and third trimesters and unlike their traditional distribution, tend to be reported in the upper thoracic spine during pregnancy (206). It is widely believed that these tumors tend to enlarge during pregnancy (206). The need for surgical intervention is variable, as many patients experience remission of symptoms after delivery (206). In patients who are symptomatic or experience rapid progression of deficits, surgical decompression should be considered.

Anesthetic and obstetric management of the parturient with primary and metastatic spinal tumors as well as those with vertebral hemangiomas is challenging. Mode of delivery is generally based on obstetric indications but must take into account stability of the spine, ability to adequately control pain, and other associated comorbidities. Regional anesthesia is not absolutely contraindicated, but appropriate spinal imaging and consultation with surgical and pain management colleagues are required in order to fully inform this decision.

■ SPINAL TUBERCULOSIS

Spinal tuberculosis (TB) or Pott's disease is much more common in developing nations, but can be encountered especially in patients who are immunocompromised or those who have immigrated from other countries. The incidence of neurologic complications is reported to be between 10% and 30%. Many patients may not display other manifestations of extraspinal TB, and some may have a reactivation of TB (207). Often only the anterior spinal wall is involved; however, cases of posterior involvement have been reported, one of which presented as an abscess 15 days after epidural labor analgesia (208).

The effect of pregnancy on the course of TB is controversial. Some experts feel that pregnancy does not seem to worsen tuberculosis (209). Others report that because of the high serum steroid levels and altered immune state associated with pregnancy, skeletal TB may have an aggressive behavior with rapid and profound vertebral destruction (207). This may result in earlier neurologic involvement.

Badve et al. (207) presented three cases of spinal TB during pregnancy complicated by neurologic deficits including back and neck pain, motor weakness, and bowel and bladder dysfunction. All progressed to paraparesis prior to treatment. All patients underwent surgical decompression and two experienced complete recovery. One patient had no recovery (207). The authors recommended that in cases of spinal TB during pregnancy not complicated by neurologic deficit or significant vertebral body destruction, conservative treatment is indicated. The authors further recommended that even though the surgical intervention was associated with significantly high blood loss in all the cases, pregnancy complicated by spinal TB with neurologic deficit should be treated with prompt surgical decompression and instrumented fusion after initiation of appropriate multidrug therapy.

There is little information in the literature to guide anesthetic management of patients with spinal TB. The location of the lesion, potential instability of the spine, neurologic symptoms, and history of recent spinal decompression will severely limit use of regional anesthesia in these patients.

KEY POINTS

■ Neuroimaging studies of the central nervous system should be undertaken in the parturient if needed for diagnosis as the maternal benefit exceeds the fetal risk in virtually all cases.

■ Neuraxial techniques for labor and delivery can be used for most intracranial lesions, but only case reports and small-case series are available to guide anesthetic care of the pregnant patient with intracranial pathology.

■ Regional anesthesia for labor and delivery of the pregnant patient with an intracranial tumor requires balancing the remote risk of cerebral herniation in most patients with possible increased intracranial pressure with the benefits of preventing increases in intracranial pressure offered by neuraxial anesthesia.

■ Anesthetic management of the pregnant patient with an aneurysm undergoing aneurysm repair should be tailored to avoid rises in arterial pressure and falls in intracranial pressure until the dura mater has been opened.

■ Following successful repair of a neurovascular lesion, no special care is required for the patient undergoing labor and delivery. In the patient with an unrepaired lesion, epidural analgesia and anesthesia is recommended.

■ Neuroimaging can in most cases distinguish between hemorrhagic and ischemic stroke.

■ A neurologic examination of the patient in whom an epidural blood patch is being contemplated should be performed and abnormality that cannot be attributed to intracranial hypotension should be investigated before the procedure is undertaken.

■ Continuous spinal analgesia for the laboring patient with idiopathic intracranial hypertension may offer therapy for increased intracranial pressure as well as be extended to provide anesthesia for cesarean delivery.

■ Several case reports show the safety of epidural and spinal anesthesia when used in the pregnant patient with Arnold–Chiari syndrome, but caution in performing regional anesthesia in the patient with suspected intracranial pressure seems prudent.

■ Autonomic hyperreflexia can be a potential source of significant morbidity and even mortality in the parturient as labor and delivery are potent stimuli. Regional anesthesia has been proven to be effective at prevention of autonomic hyperreflexia.

■ Regional anesthesia for the patient with a spinal lesion is not absolutely contraindicated but should be approached with caution.

REFERENCES

1. Oxford CM, Ludmir J. Trauma in pregnancy. *Clin Obstet Gynecol* 2009;52:611–629.
2. Berg CJ, Callaghan WM, Syverson C, et al. Pregnancy-related mortality in the United States, 1998 to 2005. *Obstet Gynecol* 2010;116:1302–1309.
3. Stevenson CB, Thompson RC. The clinical management of intracranial neoplasms in pregnancy. *Clin Obstet Gynecol* 2005;48:24–37.
4. Tewari KS, Cappuccini F, Asrat T, et al. Obstetric emergencies precipitated by malignant brain tumors. *Am J Obstet Gynecol* 2000;182:1215–1221.
5. Swensen R, Kirsch W. Brain neoplasms in women: a review. *Clin Obstet Gynecol* 2002;45:904–927.
6. Qaiser R, Black P. Neurosurgery in pregnancy. *Semin Neurol* 2007;27:476–481.
7. Seckl MJ, Sebire NJ, Berkowitz RS. Gestational trophoblastic disease. *Lancet* 2010;376:717–729.
8. Martinez-Tica J. Disorders of the central nervous system in pregnancy. In: Gampling DR DM, McKay RSF, eds. *Obstetric Anesthesia and Uncommon Disorders*. Cambridge: Cambridge University Press; 2008:167–189.
9. Zak IT, Dulai HS, Kish KK. Imaging of neurologic disorders associated with pregnancy and the postpartum period. *Radiographics* 2007;27:95–108.
10. Euliano T. A practical approach to obstetric anesthesia. In: Bucklin BA GDWD, ed. Philadelphia, PA: Lippincott Williams and Wilkins; 2009:435–455.
11. Baysinger CL. Imaging during pregnancy. *Anesth Analg* 2010;110:863–867.
12. Patel SJ, Reede DL, Katz DS, et al. Imaging the pregnant patient for nonobstetric conditions: algorithms and radiation dose considerations. *Radiographics* 2007;27:1705–1722.
13. Brass SD, Copen WA. Neurological disorders in pregnancy from a neuroimaging perspective. *Semin Neurol* 2007;27:411–424.
14. Ng J, Kitchen N. Neurosurgery and pregnancy. *J Neurol Neurosurg Psychiatry* 2008;79:745–752.

15. Marx GF, Zemaitis MT, Orkin LR. Cerebrospinal fluid pressures during labor and obstetrical anesthesia. *Anesthesiology* 1961;22:348–354.
16. Goroszeniuk T, Howard RS, Wright JT. The management of labour using continuous lumbar epidural analgesia in a patient with a malignant cerebral tumour. *Anaesthesia* 1986;41:1128–1129.
17. Finfer SR. Management of labour and delivery in patients with intracranial neoplasms. *Br J Anaesth* 1991;67:784–787.
18. Atanassoff PG, Alon E, Weiss BM, et al. Spinal anaesthesia for caesarean section in a patient with brain neoplasma. *Can J Anaesth* 1994;41:163–164.
19. Su TM, Lan CM, Yang LC, et al. Brain tumor presenting with fatal herniation following delivery under epidural anesthesia. *Anesthesiology* 2002;96:508–509.
20. Duffy GP. Lumbar puncture in the presence of raised intracranial pressure. *Br Med J* 1969;1:407–409.
21. Richards PG, Towu-Aghantse E. Dangers of lumbar puncture. *Br Med J (Clin Res Ed)* 1986;292:605–606.
22. Grady RE, Horlocker TT, Brown RD, et al. Neurologic complications after placement of cerebrospinal fluid drainage catheters and needles in anesthetized patients: implications for regional anesthesia. Mayo perioperative outcomes group. *Anesth Analg* 1999;88:388–392.
23. Hilt H, Gramm HJ, Link J. Changes in intracranial pressure associated with extradural anaesthesia. *Br J Anaesth* 1986;58:676–680.
24. Grocott HP, Mutch WA. Epidural anesthesia and acutely increased intracranial pressure. Lumbar epidural space hydrodynamics in a porcine model. *Anesthesiology* 1996;85:1086–1091.
25. Wakeling HG, Barry PC. Undiagnosed raised intracranial pressure complicating labour. *Int J Obstet Anesth* 1995;4:117–119.
26. Chang L, Looi-Lyons L, Bartosik L, et al. Anesthesia for cesarean section in two patients with brain tumours. *Can J Anaesth* 1999;46:61–65.
27. Wang LP, Paech MJ. Neuroanesthesia for the pregnant woman. *Anesth Analg* 2008;107:193–200.
28. Gin T, Gregory MA, Oh TE. The haemodynamic effects of propofol and thiopentone for induction of caesarean section. *Anaesth Intensive Care* 1990;18:175–179.
29. Rigg D, McDonogh A. Use of sodium nitroprusside for deliberate hypotension during pregnancy. *Br J Anaesth* 1981;53:985–987.
30. Muizelaar JP, Marmarou A, Ward JD, et al. Adverse effects of prolonged hyperventilation in patients with severe head injury: a randomized clinical trial. *J Neurosurg* 1991;75:731–739.
31. O'Hare R, McAtamney D, Mirakhur RK, et al. Bolus dose remifentanil for control of haemodynamic response to tracheal intubation during rapid sequence induction of anaesthesia. *Br J Anaesth* 1999;82:283–285.
32. El-Orbany M, Connolly LA. Rapid sequence induction and intubation: current controversy. *Anesth Analg* 2010;110:1318–1325.
33. Low JA, Boston RW, Cervenko FW. Effect of low maternal carbon dioxide tension on placental gas exchange. *Am J Obstet Gynecol* 1970;106:1032–1043.
34. Lumbers ER, Stevens AD. Changes in fetal renal function in response to infusions of a hyperosmotic solution of mannitol to the ewe. *J Physiol* 1983;343:439–446.
35. Dyer RA, van Dyk D, Dresner A. The use of uterotonic drugs during caesarean section. *Int J Obstet Anesth* 2010;19:313–319.
36. Granstrom L, Ekman G, Ulmsten U. Intravenous infusion of 15 methylprostaglandin F2 alpha (Prostinfenem) in women with heavy post-partum hemorrhage. *Acta Obstet Gynecol Scand* 1989;68:365–367.
37. Royal College of Obstetricians and Gynecologists. Prevention and treatment of post-partum Haemorrhage Royal College of Obstetricians and Gynecologists Greentop Guideline #52, 2009.
38. Ramsey PS, Hogg BB, Savage KG, et al. Cardiovascular effects of intravaginal misoprostol in the mid trimester of pregnancy. *Am J Obstet Gynecol* 2000;183:1100–1102.
39. Davie CA, O'Brien P. Stroke and pregnancy. *J Neurol Neurosurg Psychiatry* 2008;79:240–245.
40. James AH, Bushnell CD, Jamison MG, et al. Incidence and risk factors for stroke in pregnancy and the puerperium. *Obstet Gynecol* 2005;106:509–516.
41. Feske SK. Stroke in pregnancy. *Semin Neurol* 2007;27:442–452.
42. Kittner SJ, Stern BJ, Feeser BR, et al. Pregnancy and the risk of stroke. *N Engl J Med* 1996;335:768–774.
43. Jaigobin C, Silver FL. Stroke and pregnancy. *Stroke* 2000;31:2948–2951.
44. Lanska DJ, Kryscio RJ. Risk factors for peripartum and postpartum stroke and intracranial venous thrombosis. *Stroke* 2000;31:1274–1282.
45. Bateman BT, Schumacher HC, Bushnell CD, et al. Intracerebral hemorrhage in pregnancy: frequency, risk factors, and outcome. *Neurology* 2006;67:424–429.
46. Roman H, Descargues G, Lopes M, et al. Subarachnoid hemorrhage due to cerebral aneurysmal rupture during pregnancy. *Acta Obstet Gynecol Scand* 2004;83:330–334.
47. Treadwell SD, Thanvi B, Robinson TG. Stroke in pregnancy and the puerperium. *Postgrad Med J* 2008;84:238–245.
48. Rinkel GJ, Djibuti M, Algra A, et al. Prevalence and risk of rupture of intracranial aneurysms: a systematic review. *Stroke* 1998;29:251–256.
49. Dias MS, Sekhar LN. Intracranial hemorrhage from aneurysms and arteriovenous malformations during pregnancy and the puerperium. *Neurosurgery* 1990;27:855–865; discussion 65–66.
50. Selo-Ojeme DO, Marshman LA, Ikomi A, et al. Aneurysmal subarachnoid haemorrhage in pregnancy. *Eur J Obstet Gynecol Reprod Biol* 2004;116:131–143.
51. Barrow DL, Reisner A. Natural history of intracranial aneurysms and vascular malformations. *Clin Neurosurg* 1993;40:3–39.
52. Cohen-Gadol AA, Friedman JA, Friedman JD, et al. Neurosurgical management of intracranial lesions in the pregnant patient: a 36-year institutional experience and review of the literature. *J Neurosurg* 2009;111:1150–1157.
53. Scott DB, Hibbard BM. Serious non-fatal complications associated with extradural block in obstetric practice. *Br J Anaesth* 1990;64:537–541.
54. Ausman JI. ISAT study: is coiling better than clipping? *Surg Neurol* 2003;59:162–165; discussion 5–73; author reply 73–75.
55. Pumar JM, Pardo MI, Carreira JM, et al. Endovascular treatment of an acutely ruptured intracranial aneurysm in pregnancy: report of eight cases. *Emerg Radiol*;17:205–207.
56. Wiebers DO, Whisnant JP, Huston J, 3rd, et al. Unruptured intracranial aneurysms: natural history, clinical outcome, and risks of surgical and endovascular treatment. *Lancet* 2003;362:103–110.
57. Mashour GA, Schwamm LH, Leffert L. Intracranial subdural hematomas and cerebral herniation after labor epidural with no evidence of dural puncture. *Anesthesiology* 2006;104:610–612.
58. Stoodley MA, Macdonald RL, Weir BK. Pregnancy and intracranial aneurysms. *Neurosurg Clin N Am* 1998;9:549–556.
59. Yih PS, Cheong KF. Anaesthesia for caesarean section in a patient with an intracranial arteriovenous malformation. *Anaesth Intensive Care* 1999;27:66–68.
60. Hudspith MJ, Popham PA. The anaesthetic management of intracranial haemorrhage from arteriovenous malformations during pregnancy: three cases. *Int J Obstet Anesth* 1996;5:189–193.
61. Sharma SK, Herrera ER, Sidawi JE, et al. The pregnant patient with an intracranial arteriovenous malformation. Cesarean or vaginal delivery using regional or general anesthesia? *Reg Anesth* 1995;20:455–458.
62. Gupta A, Hesselvik F, Eriksson L, et al. Epidural anaesthesia for caesarean section in a patient with a cerebral artery aneurysm. *Int J Obstet Anesth* 1993;2:49–52.
63. Laidler JA, Jackson IJ, Redfern N. The management of caesarean section in a patient with an intracranial arteriovenous malformation. *Anaesthesia* 1989;44:490–491.
64. Newman B, Lam AM. Induced hypotension for clipping of a cerebral aneurysm during pregnancy: a case report and brief review. *Anesth Analg* 1986;65:675–678.
65. Jaeger K, Ruschulte H, Muhlhaus K, et al. Combined emergency caesarean section and intracerebral aneurysm clipping. *Anaesthesia* 2000;55:1138–1140.
66. Whitburn RH, Laishley RS, Jewkes DA. Anaesthesia for simultaneous caesarean section and clipping of intracerebral aneurysm. *Br J Anaesth* 1990;64:642–645.
67. Horton JC, Chambers WA, Lyons SL, et al. Pregnancy and the risk of hemorrhage from cerebral arteriovenous malformations. *Neurosurgery* 1990;27:867–871; discussion 871–872.
68. Bushnell CD, Hurn P, Colton C, et al. Advancing the study of stroke in women: summary and recommendations for future research from an NINDS-Sponsored Multidisciplinary Working Group. *Stroke* 2006;37:2387–2399.
69. Dounas M, Mercier FJ, Lhuissier C, et al. Epidural analgesia for labour in a parturient with neurofibromatosis. *Can J Anaesth* 1995;42:420–422; discussion 2–4.
70. Dodson BA, Rosen MA. Anesthesia for neurosurgery during pregnancy. In: Hughes SC LG, Rosen MA, eds. *Shnider and Levinson's Anesthesia for Obstetrics*. 4th ed. Philadelphia, PA: Lippincott Williams and Wilkins; 2002.
71. Kayacan N, Arici G, Karsli B, et al. Acute subdural haematoma after accidental dural puncture during epidural anaesthesia. *Int J Obstet Anesth* 2004;13:47–49.
72. Ramos-Aparici R, Segura-Pastor D, Edo-Cebollada L, et al. Acute subdural hematoma after spinal anesthesia in an obstetric patient. *J Clin Anesth* 2008;20:376–378.
73. Zeidan A, Farhat O, Maaliki H, et al. Does postdural puncture headache left untreated lead to subdural hematoma? Case report and review of the literature. *Middle East J Anesthesiol* 2010;20:483–492.
74. Davies JM, Murphy A, Smith M, et al. Subdural haematoma after dural puncture headache treated by epidural blood patch. *Br J Anaesth* 2001;86:720–723.
75. Yamashima T, Friede RL. Why do bridging veins rupture into the virtual subdural space? *J Neurol Neurosurg Psychiatry* 1984;47:121–127.
76. Bullock MR, Chesnut R, Ghajar J, et al. Surgical management of acute subdural hematomas. *Neurosurgery* 2006;58:S16–S24; discussion Si–Siv.
77. Hill LM, Parker D, O'Neill BP. Management of maternal vegetative state during pregnancy. *Mayo Clin Proc* 1985;60:469–472.

78. Field DR, Gates EA, Creasy RK, et al. Maternal brain death during pregnancy. Medical and ethical issues. *JAMA* 1988;260:816–822.

79. Bush MC, Nagy S, Berkowitz RL, et al. Pregnancy in a persistent vegetative state: case report, comparison to brain death, and review of the literature. *Obstet Gynecol Surv* 2003;58:738–748.

80. Powner DJ, Bernstein IM. Extended somatic support for pregnant women after brain death. *Crit Care Med* 2003;31:1241–1249.

81. Lane A, Westbrook A, Grady D, et al. Maternal brain death: medical, ethical and legal issues. *Intensive Care Med* 2004;30:1484–1486.

82. Farragher RA, Laffey JG. Maternal brain death and somatic support. *Neurocrit Care* 2005;3:99–106.

83. Black P. Brain death. *N Engl J Med* 1978;299:338–344.

84. Ashwal S, Cranford R. Medical aspects of the persistent vegetative state—a correction. The multi-society task force on PVS. *N Engl J Med* 1995; 333:130.

85. Crawford TC, Smith WTt, Velazquez EJ, et al. Prognostic usefulness of left ventricular thrombus by echocardiography in dilated cardiomyopathy in predicting stroke, transient ischemic attack, and death. *Am J Cardiol* 2004;93:500–503.

86. Zeeman GG, Fleckenstein JL, Twickler DM, et al. Cerebral infarction in eclampsia. *Am J Obstet Gynecol* 2004;190:714–720.

87. Dietrich HH, Dacey RG, Jr. Molecular keys to the problems of cerebral vasospasm. *Neurosurgery* 2000;46:517–530.

88. Group TNIoNDaSt-PSS. The national institute of neurological disorders and stroke. t-PA stroke study group. *N Engl J Med* 1995;333:1581–1587.

89. Smith WS, Sung G, Starkman S, et al. Safety and efficacy of mechanical embolectomy in acute ischemic stroke: results of the MERCI trial. *Stroke* 2005; 36:1432–1438.

90. Murugappan A, Coplin WM, Al-Sadat AN, et al. Thrombolytic therapy of acute ischemic stroke during pregnancy. *Neurology* 2006;66:768–770.

91. Horlocker TT, Wedel DJ, Rowlingson JC, et al. Regional anesthesia in the patient receiving antithrombotic or thrombolytic therapy: American Society of Regional Anesthesia and Pain Medicine Evidence-Based Guidelines (Third Edition). *Reg Anesth Pain Med* 2010;35:64–101.

92. Lockhart EM, Baysinger CL. Intracranial venous thrombosis in the parturient. *Anesthesiology* 2007;107:652–658; quiz 87–88.

93. Wilder-Smith E, Kothbauer-Margreiter I, Lammle B, et al. Dural puncture and activated protein C resistance: risk factors for cerebral venous sinus thrombosis. *J Neurol Neurosurg Psychiatry* 1997;63:351–356.

94. Sacco RL, Adams R, Albers G, et al. Guidelines for prevention of stroke in patients with ischemic stroke or transient ischemic attack: a statement for healthcare professionals from the American Heart Association/American Stroke Association Council on Stroke: co-sponsored by the Council on Cardiovascular Radiology and Intervention: the American Academy of Neurology affirms the value of this guideline. *Stroke* 2006;37:577–617.

95. Hinchey J, Chaves C, Appignani B, et al. A reversible posterior leukoencephalopathy syndrome. *N Engl J Med* 1996;334:494–500.

96. Krishnamoorthy U, Sarkar PK, Nakhuda Y, et al. Posterior reversible encephalopathy syndrome (PRES) in pregnancy: a diagnostic challenge to obstetricians. *J Obstet Gynaecol* 2009;29:192–194.

97. Macarthur A. Postpartum headache. In: Chestnut DH PL, Tsen LC, Wong CA, eds. *Obstetric Anesthesia*. 4th ed. Philadelphia, PA: Mosby-Elsevier; 2009:677–700.

98. Thackeray EM, Tielborg MC. Posterior reversible encephalopathy syndrome in a patient with severe preeclampsia. *Anesth Analg* 2007;105:184–186.

99. Prout RE, Tuckey JP, Giffen NJ. Reversible posterior leucoencephalopathy syndrome in a peripartum patient. *Int J Obstet Anesth* 2007;16:74–76.

100. Long TR, Hein BD, Brown MJ, et al. Posterior reversible encephalopathy syndrome during pregnancy: seizures in a previously healthy parturient. *J Clin Anesth* 2007;19:145–148.

101. McKinney AM, Short J, Truwit CL, et al. Posterior reversible encephalopathy syndrome: incidence of atypical regions of involvement and imaging findings. *AJR Am J Roentgenol* 2007;189:904–912.

102. Oehm E, Hetzel A, Els T, et al. Cerebral hemodynamics and autoregulation in reversible posterior leukoencephalopathy syndrome caused by pre-/eclampsia. *Cerebrovasc Dis* 2006;22:204–208.

103. Lamy C, Oppenheim C, Meder JF, et al. Neuroimaging in posterior reversible encephalopathy syndrome. *J Neuroimaging* 2004;14:89–96.

104. Torrillo TM, Bronster DJ, Beilin Y. Delayed diagnosis of posterior reversible encephalopathy syndrome (PRES) in a parturient with preeclampsia after inadvertent dural puncture. *Int J Obstet Anesth* 2007;16:171–174.

105. Chames MC, Pearlman MD. Trauma during pregnancy: outcomes and clinical management. *Clin Obstet Gynecol* 2008;51:398–408.

106. El-Kady D, Gilbert WM, Anderson J, et al. Trauma during pregnancy: an analysis of maternal and fetal outcomes in a large population. *Am J Obstet Gynecol* 2004;190:1661–1668.

107. El Kady D. Perinatal outcomes of traumatic injuries during pregnancy. *Clin Obstet Gynecol* 2007;50:582–591.

108. Ikossi DG, Lazar AA, Morabito D, et al. Profile of mothers at risk: an analysis of injury and pregnancy loss in 1,195 trauma patients. *J Am Coll Surg* 2005;200:49–56.

109. Rogers FB, Rozycki GS, Osler TM, et al. A multi-institutional study of factors associated with fetal death in injured pregnant patients. *Arch Surg* 1999;134:1274–1277.

110. Muench MV, Canterino JC. Trauma in pregnancy. *Obstet Gynecol Clin North Am* 2007;34:555–583, xiii.

111. Howell P. Trauma. In: Chestnut DH PL, Tsen LC, Wong CA, eds. *Obstetric Anesthesia*. Philadelphia, PA: Mosby-Elsevier; 2009:1149–1163.

112. Myburgh J, Cooper DJ, Finfer S, et al. Saline or albumin for fluid resuscitation in patients with traumatic brain injury. *N Engl J Med* 2007;357:874–884.

113. Bratton SL, Chestnut RM, Ghajar J, et al. Guidelines for the management of severe traumatic brain injury. VIII. Intracranial pressure thresholds. *J Neurotrauma* 2007;24 suppl 1:S55–S58.

114. Goldschlager T, Steyn M, Loh V, et al. Simultaneous craniotomy and caesarean section for trauma. *J Trauma* 2009;66:E50–E51.

115. Friedman DI, Jacobson DM. Diagnostic criteria for idiopathic intracranial hypertension. *Neurology* 2002;59:1492–1495.

116. Evans RW, Friedman DI. Expert opinion: the management of pseudotumor cerebri during pregnancy. *Headache* 2000;40:495–497.

117. Huna-Baron R, Kupersmith MJ. Idiopathic intracranial hypertension in pregnancy. *J Neurol* 2002;249:1078–1081.

118. Tang RA, Dorotheo EU, Schiffman JS, et al. Medical and surgical management of idiopathic intracranial hypertension in pregnancy. *Curr Neurol Neurosci Rep* 2004;4:398–409.

119. Abouleish E, Ali V, Tang RA. Benign intracranial hypertension and anesthesia for cesarean section. *Anesthesiology* 1985;63:705–707.

120. Kim K, Orbegozo M. Epidural anesthesia for cesarean section in a parturient with pseudotumor cerebri and lumboperitoneal shunt. *J Clin Anesth* 2000; 12:213–215.

121. Aly EE, Lawther BK. Anaesthetic management of uncontrolled idiopathic intracranial hypertension during labour and delivery using an intrathecal catheter. *Anaesthesia* 2007;62:178–181.

122. Paruchuri SR, Lawlor M, Kleinhomer K, et al. Risk of cerebellar tonsillar herniation after diagnostic lumbar puncture in pseudotumor cerebri. *Anesth Analg* 1993;77:403–404.

123. Heckathorn J, Cata JP, Barsoum S. Intrathecal anesthesia for cesarean delivery via a subarachnoid drain in a woman with benign intracranial hypertension. *Int J Obstet Anesth* 2010;19:109–111.

124. Kaul B, Vallejo MC, Ramanathan S, et al. Accidental spinal analgesia in the presence of a lumboperitoneal shunt in an obese parturient receiving enoxaparin therapy. *Anesth Analg* 2002;95:441–443, table of contents.

125. Bedard JM, Richardson MG, Wissler RN. Epidural anesthesia in a parturient with a lumboperitoneal shunt. *Anesthesiology* 1999;90:621–623.

126. Liakos AM, Bradley NK, Magram G, et al. Hydrocephalus and the reproductive health of women: the medical implications of maternal shunt dependency in 70 women and 138 pregnancies. *Neurol Res* 2000;22:69–88.

127. Bradley NK, Liakos AM, McAllister JP, 2nd, et al. Maternal shunt dependency: implications for obstetric care, neurosurgical management, and pregnancy outcomes and a review of selected literature. *Neurosurgery* 1998;43:448–460; discussion 60–61.

128. Freo U, Pitton M, Carron M, et al. Anesthesia for urgent sequential ventriculoperitoneal shunt revision and cesarean delivery. *Int J Obstet Anesth* 2009; 18:284–287.

129. Mueller DM, Oro J. Chiari I malformation with or without syringomyelia and pregnancy: case studies and review of the literature. *Am J Perinatol* 2005; 22:67–70.

130. Milhorat TH, Chou MW, Trinidad EM, et al. Chiari I malformation redefined: clinical and radiographic findings for 364 symptomatic patients. *Neurosurgery* 1999;44:1005–1017.

131. Agusti M, Adalia R, Fernandez C, et al. Anaesthesia for caesarean section in a patient with syringomyelia and Arnold-Chiari type I malformation. *Int J Obstet Anesth* 2004;13:114–116.

132. Semple DA, McClure JH. Arnold-chiari malformation in pregnancy. *Anaesthesia* 1996;51:580–582.

133. Chantigian RC, Koehn MA, Ramin KD, et al. Chiari I malformation in parturients. *J Clin Anesth* 2002;14:201–205.

134. Barton JJ, Sharpe JA. Oscillopsia and horizontal nystagmus with accelerating slow phases following lumbar puncture in the Arnold-Chiari malformation. *Ann Neurol* 1993;33:418–421.

135. Kuczkowski KM. Spinal anesthesia for cesarean delivery in a parturient with Arnold-Chiari type I malformation. *Can J Anaesth* 2004;51:639.

136. Nel MR, Robson V, Robinson PN. Extradural anaesthesia for caesarean section in a patient with syringomyelia and Chiari type I anomaly. *Br J Anaesth* 1998; 80:512–515.

137. Hirsch NP, Murphy A, Radcliffe JJ. Neurofibromatosis: clinical presentations and anaesthetic implications. *Br J Anaesth* 2001;86:555–564.

138. Ferner RE. The neurofibromatoses. *Pract Neurol* 2010;10:82–93.

139. Friedman JM, Arbiser J, Epstein JA, et al. Cardiovascular disease in neurofibromatosis 1: report of the NF1 Cardiovascular Task Force. *Genet Med* 2002; 4:105–111.

140. Nelson DB, Greer L, Wendel G. Neurofibromatosis and pregnancy: a report of maternal cardiopulmonary compromise. *Obstet Gynecol*; 116 suppl 2:507–509.

141. Serleth HJ, Cogbill TH, Gundersen SB, 3rd. Ruptured pancreaticoduodenal artery aneurysms and pheochromocytoma in a pregnant patient with neurofibromatosis. *Surgery* 1998;124:100–102.

142. Tidwell C, Copas P. Brachial artery rupture complicating a pregnancy with neurofibromatosis: a case report. *Am J Obstet Gynecol* 1998;179:832–834.

143. Mezitis SG, Geller M, Bocchieri E, et al. Association of pheochromocytoma and ganglioneuroma: unusual finding in neurofibromatosis type 1. *Endocr Pract* 2007;13:647–651.

144. Oliva R, Angelos P, Kaplan E, et al. Pheochromocytoma in pregnancy: a case series and review. *Hypertension* 2010;55:600–606.

145. Shi BB, Li HZ, Chen C, et al. Differential diagnosis and laparoscopic treatment of adrenal pheochromocytoma and ganglioneuroma. *Chin Med J (Engl)* 2009;122:1790–1793.

146. Segal D, Holcberg G, Sapir O, et al. Neurofibromatosis in pregnancy. Maternal and perinatal outcome. *Eur J Obstet Gynecol Reprod Biol* 1999;84:59–61.

147. Weissman A, Jakobi P, Zaidise I, et al. Neurofibromatosis and pregnancy. An update. *J Reprod Med* 1993;38:890–896.

148. Dugoff L, Sujansky E. Neurofibromatosis type 1 and pregnancy. *Am J Med Genet* 1996;66:7–10.

149. Ansari AH, Nagamani M. Pregnancy and neurofibromatosis (von Recklinghausen's disease). *Obstet Gynecol* 1976;47:25S–29S.

150. Sakai T, Vallejo MC, Shannon KT. A parturient with neurofibromatosis type 2: anesthetic and obstetric considerations for delivery. *Int J Obstet Anesth* 2005; 14:332–335.

151. Sahin A, Aypar U. Spinal anesthesia in a patient with neurofibromatosis. *Anesth Analg* 2003;97:1855–1856.

152. Wimmer K, Muhlbauer M, Eckart M, et al. A patient severely affected by spinal neurofibromas carries a recurrent splice site mutation in the NF1 gene. *Eur J Hum Genet* 2002;10:334–338.

153. Spiegel JE, Hapgood A, Hess PE. Epidural anesthesia in a parturient with neurofibromatosis type 2 undergoing cesarean section. *Int J Obstet Anesth* 2005;14:336–339.

154. Comi AM. Update on Sturge-Weber syndrome: diagnosis, treatment, quantitative measures, and controversies. *Lymphat Res Biol* 2007;5:257–264.

155. Dolkart LA, Bhat M. Sturge-Weber syndrome in pregnancy. *Am J Obstet Gynecol* 1995;173:969–971.

156. Batra RK, Gulaya V, Madan R, et al. Anaesthesia and the Sturge-Weber syndrome. *Can J Anaesth* 1994;41:133–136.

157. Thomas-Sohl KA, Vaslow DF, Maria BL. Sturge-Weber syndrome: a review. *Pediatr Neurol* 2004;30:303–310.

158. Chabriat H, Pappata S, Traykov L, et al. [Sturge-Weber angiomatosis responsible for hemiplegia without cerebral infarction in term pregnancy]. *Rev Neurol (Paris)* 1996;152:536–541.

159. Yamashiro M, Furuya H. Anesthetic management of a patient with Sturge-Weber syndrome undergoing oral surgery. *Anesth Prog* 2006;53:17–19.

160. Causse-Mariscal A, Palot M, Visseaux H, et al. Labor analgesia and cesarean section in women affected by tuberous sclerosis: report of two cases. *Int J Obstet Anesth* 2007;16:277–280.

161. Ess KC. Tuberous sclerosis complex: a brave new world? *Curr Opin Neurol* 2010;23:189–193.

162. King JA, Stamilio DM. Maternal and fetal tuberous sclerosis complicating pregnancy: a case report and overview of the literature. *Am J Perinatol* 2005;22:103–108.

163. Gilson GJ, Miller AC, Clevenger FW, et al. Acute spinal cord injury and neurogenic shock in pregnancy. *Obstet Gynecol Surv* 1995;50:556–560.

164. Catanzarite VA, Ferguson JE 2nd., Weinstein C, et al. Preterm labor in the quadriplegic parturient. *Am J Perinatol* 1986;3:115–118.

165. Baker ER, Cardenas DD, Benedetti TJ. Risks associated with pregnancy in spinal cord-injured women. *Obstet Gynecol* 1992;80:425–428.

166. Hughes SJ, Short DJ, Usherwood MM, et al. Management of the pregnant woman with spinal cord injuries. *Br J Obstet Gynaecol* 1991;98:513–518.

167. Baker ER, Cardenas DD. Pregnancy in spinal cord injured women. *Arch Phys Med Rehabil* 1996;77:501–507.

168. Crosby E, St-Jean B, Reid D, et al. Obstetrical anaesthesia and analgesia in chronic spinal cord-injured women. *Can J Anaesth* 1992;39:487–494.

169. Baraka A. Epidural meperidine for control of autonomic hyperreflexia in a paraplegic parturient. *Anesthesiology* 1985;62:688–690.

170. Abouleish EI, Hanley ES, Palmer SM. Can epidural fentanyl control autonomic hyperreflexia in a quadriplegic parturient? *Anesth Analg* 1989;68:523–526.

171. Maehama T, Izena H, Kanazawa K. Management of autonomic hyperreflexia with magnesium sulfate during labor in a woman with spinal cord injury. *Am J Obstet Gynecol* 2000;183:492–493.

172. Young BK, Katz M, Klein SA. Pregnancy after spinal cord injury: altered maternal and fetal response to labor. *Obstet Gynecol* 1983;62:59–63.

173. Ravindran RS, Cummins DF, Smith IE. Experience with the use of nitroprusside and subsequent epidural analgesia in a pregnant quadriplegic patient. *Anesth Analg* 1981;60:61–63.

174. Vinck A, Nijhuis-van der Sanden MW, Roeleveld NJ, et al. Motor profile and cognitive functioning in children with spina bifida. *Eur J Paediatr Neurol* 2010;14:86–92.

175. Ali L, Stocks GM. Spina bifida, tethered cord and regional anaesthesia. *Anaesthesia* 2005;60:1149–1150.

176. James HE, Walsh JW. Spinal dysraphism. *Curr Probl Pediatr* 1981;11:1–25.

177. Wood GG, Jacka MJ. Spinal hematoma following spinal anesthesia in a patient with spina bifida occulta. *Anesthesiology* 1997;87:983–984.

178. Arata M, Grover S, Dunne K, et al. Pregnancy outcome and complications in women with spina bifida. *J Reprod Med* 2000;45:743–748.

179. Tidmarsh MD, May AE. Epidural anaesthesia and neural tube defects. *Int J Obstet Anesth* 1998;7:111–114.

180. Bonfield CM, Levi AD, Arnold PM, et al. Surgical management of post-traumatic syringomyelia. *Spine* (Phila Pa 1976);35:S245–S258.

181. Oluigbo CO, Thacker K, Flint G. The role of lumboperitoneal shunts in the treatment of syringomyelia. *J Neurosurg Spine* 2010;13:133–138.

182. Murayama K, Mamiya K, Nozaki K, et al. Cesarean section in a patient with syringomyelia. *Can J Anaesth* 2001;48:474–477.

183. Parker JD, Broberg JC, Napolitano PG. Maternal Arnold-Chiari type I malformation and syringomyelia: a labor management dilemma. *Am J Perinatol* 2002;19:445–450.

184. Landau R, Giraud R, Delrue V, et al. Spinal anesthesia for cesarean delivery in a woman with a surgically corrected type I Arnold Chiari malformation. *Anesth Analg* 2003;97:253–255, table of contents.

185. Hullander RM, Bogard TD, Leivers D, et al. Chiari I malformation presenting as recurrent spinal headache. *Anesth Analg* 1992;75:1025–1026.

186. Jahan R, Vinuela F. Vascular anatomy, pathophysiology, and classification of vascular malformations of the spinal cord. *Seminars in Cerebrovascular Diseases and Stroke* 2002;2:186–200.

187. Krings T. Vascular malformations of the spine and spinal cord : Anatomy, classification, treatment. *Klin Neuroradiol* 2010.

188. Safavi-Abbasi S, Feiz-Erfan I, Spetzler RF, et al. Hemorrhage of cavernous malformations during pregnancy and in the peripartum period: causal or coincidence? Case report and review of the literature. *Neurosurg Focus* 2006;21:e12.

189. Kinoshita M, Asai A, Komeda S, et al. Spontaneous regression of a spinal extradural arteriovenous fistula after delivery by cesarean section. *Neurol Med Chir (Tokyo)* 2009;49:313–315.

190. Gross BA, Du R, Popp AJ, et al. Intramedullary spinal cord cavernous malformations. *Neurosurg Focus*; 29:E14.

191. Lopate G, Black JT, Grubb RL, Jr. Cavernous hemangioma of the spinal cord: report of 2 unusual cases. *Neurology* 1990;40:1791–1793.

192. Canavero S, Pagni CA, Duca S, et al. Spinal intramedullary cavernous angiomas: a literature meta-analysis. *Surg Neurol* 1994;41:381–388.

193. Flemming KD, Goodman BP, Meyer FB. Successful brainstem cavernous malformation resection after repeated hemorrhages during pregnancy. *Surg Neurol* 2003;60:545–547; discussion 7–8.

194. Eldridge AJ, Kipling M, Smith JW. Anaesthetic management of a woman who became paraplegic at 22 weeks' gestation after a spontaneous spinal cord haemorrhage secondary to a presumed arteriovenous malformation. *Br J Anaesth* 1998;81:976–978.

195. Hirsch NP, Child CS, Wijetilleka SA. Paraplegia caused by spinal angioma—possible association with epidural analgesia. *Anesth Analg* 1985;64:937–940.

196. Ong BY, Littleford J, Segstro R, et al. Spinal anaesthesia for caesarean section in a patient with a cervical arteriovenous malformation. *Can J Anaesth* 1996;43:1052–1058.

197. McCormick PC, Torres R, Post KD, et al. Intramedullary ependymoma of the spinal cord. *J Neurosurg* 1990;72:523–532.

198. Armstrong PA, Polley LS. Asymptomatic spinal cord neoplasm detected during induction of spinal anaesthesia. *Int J Obstet Anesth* 2010;19:91–93.

199. Henson JW. Spinal cord gliomas. *Curr Opin Neurol* 2001;14:679–682.

200. Leidinger W, Meierhofer JN, Ullrich V. [Unusual complication after combined spinal/epidural anaesthesia]. *Anaesthesist* 2003;52:703–706.

201. Klezl Z, Krbec M, Gregora E, et al. Rare presentation of non-Hodgkin lymphoma of the thoracolumbar spine in pregnancy with 7 years' survival. *Arch Orthop Trauma Surg* 2002;122:308–310.

202. Jones BP, Milliken BC, Penning DH. Anesthesia for cesarean section in a patient with paraplegia resulting from tumour metastases to spinal cord. *Can J Anaesth* 2000;47:1122–1128.

203. Corapcioglu F, Dillioglugil O, Sarper N, et al. Spinal cord compression and lung metastasis of Wilms' tumor in a pregnant adolescent. *Urology* 2004;64:807–810.

204. Vijay K, Shetty AP, Rajasekaran S. Symptomatic vertebral hemangioma in pregnancy treated antepartum. A case report with review of literature. *Eur Spine J* 2008;17 suppl 2:S299–S303.

205. Chi JH, Manley GT, Chou D. Pregnancy-related vertebral hemangioma. Case report, review of the literature, and management algorithm. *Neurosurg Focus* 2005;19:E7.

206. Lavi E, Jamieson DG, Granat M. Epidural haemangiomas during pregnancy. *J Neurol Neurosurg Psychiatry* 1986;49:709–712.

207. Badve SA, Ghate SD, Badve MS, et al. Tuberculosis of spine with neurological deficit in advanced pregnancy: a report of three cases. *Spine J*; 11:e9–e16.

208. Morau EL, Lotthe AA, Morau DY, et al. Bifocal tuberculosis highlighted by obstetric combined spinal-epidural analgesia. *Anesthesiology* 2005;103:445–446.

209. Tripathy SN. Tuberculosis and pregnancy. *Int J Gynaecol Obstet* 2003;80:247–253.

34

New Thoughts on Bleeding and Coagulation Disorders

Moeen K. Panni

■ INTRODUCTION

Pregnancy induces a protective hypercoagulable state (1) in preparation for the potential bleeding that may occur during delivery of the fetus (2). There are a number of clinical disorders occurring in pregnancy, however, that can predispose to bleeding, many of which are related to thrombocytopenic syndromes (3). Neuraxial anesthesia has been shown to be the optimal anesthetic technique for most parturients; however, it carries with it the risk of subsequent epidural hematoma formation, particularly in those with abnormalities in processes that prevent bleeding.

As newer and more potent anticoagulant medications have been introduced, many of which are used in parturients, additional risk of bleeding in the epidural space after neuraxial anesthesia now exists. While bleeding time studies are no longer routinely used clinically, due to their inaccuracy in predicting bleeding risks, the common standard laboratory coagulation tests such as prothrombin time (PT) and partial thromboplastin time (PTT) that are used, are limited in their application in the assessment of the risks of bleeding, especially in patients receiving these newer anticoagulant and antiplatelet medications. Point-of-care tests such as the thromboelastogram TEG® and TEG® Platelet Mapping™ assay (Haemoscope Corporation, Niles, IL, US), Sonoclot® Coagulation & Platelet Function Analyzer (Sienco Inc., Arvada, CO), Hemodyne™ Hemostasis Analyzer (Hemodyne, Richmond, VA), and platelet functional analyzers such as PFA-l00® (Dade-Behring, Dudingen, Switzerland) (4), the first three of which assay the entire coagulation system, are important tools in the anesthesiologist's repertoire to evaluate the risks of bleeding and benefits of using neuraxial techniques.

Anesthesia Options for the Obstetric Patient

There are a number of choices available to achieve analgesia during labor as well as anesthesia during operative delivery in obstetrics (5). Neuraxial techniques are safe and extremely effective in relieving labor pain; and they are the preferred methods of anesthesia in the obstetric operating room. While these are safe, as with all anesthetic techniques, there are definite risks associated with them that need to be balanced by the benefits of performing such procedures.

The choice of anesthetic technique selected in the obstetric operating room is based upon the clinical scenario that is presented and is influenced by several factors, including but not limited to the timing of cesarean delivery (elective, urgent, or emergent) as well as the indications for cesarean delivery (maternal, fetal, or both). If possible, instrumentation of the pregnant airway is avoided and neuraxial anesthesia is used whenever it is clinically feasible, weighing the risks and

benefits for each patient and clinical scenario. General anesthesia in the obstetric patient carries with it a markedly increased incidence of difficult airway compared to the non-obstetric patient (1:~300 vs.1:~2,000) (6), increased aspiration risk (7), chance of higher awareness under general anesthesia than in a non-obstetric patient (8), potentially detrimental anesthetic effects on the fetus, (9) and lack of maternal participation in the birth process (10). All of these reasons suggest that a regional technique should be chosen whenever possible.

The effects of anesthetic agents on obstetric patients have been debated since 1847 when James Simpson first described his use of inhalational labor analgesia in Scotland (11), shortly after the first public demonstration of ether anesthesia in Boston. While the increasing use of regional anesthesia has led to substantial reductions in maternal mortality (12), certain serious complications can result after the use of this technique, one of the most significant and serious being epidural hematoma (13). Epidural hematoma, characterized by symptomatic bleeding within the epidural space, may lead to compression, ischemia, nerve trauma, or paralysis.

Impact of Neuraxial Techniques on Bleeding

The epidural space has a rich venous plexus (14) which when injured can bleed, and if this bleeding continues, can potentially lead to peripheral and central neurologic compression. This can then lead to loss of neurologic function if prolonged, and if not relieved, to permanent damage and paralysis (15). The incidence of epidural hematoma is low (~1:150,000), but the frequency of it occurring increases with impairment of coagulation function along with the type of neuraxial technique that is employed.

Normal Mechanisms to Reduce Bleeding

After injury to any blood vessel, there are three main mechanisms that exist to prevent further bleeding: (i) Vessel wall contraction or spasm (16), (ii) Platelet activation and plugging (17) (Fig. 34-1), and (iii) Intravascular coagulation (18) (Fig. 34-2). Impairment in any of these components could potentially lead to spontaneous (15) or trauma-related epidural hematoma formation (i.e., due to neuraxial anesthesia needle or catheter damage to the epidural vessels) (19).

Blood Vessel Wall

Issues related to a defective blood vessel wall can lead to bleeding in any area of the body. In relation to regional anesthesia and the risk of epidural hematoma formation, the incidence is very low. Clinical conditions with a defective blood vessel wall structure include diseases such as scurvy (vitamin C deficiency) (20) and collagen vascular disease (Marfan's

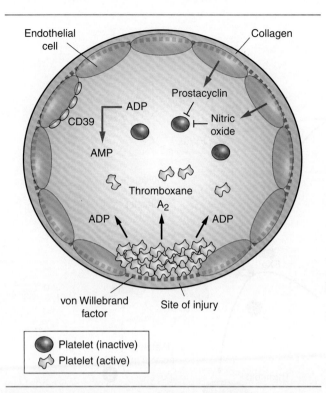

FIGURE 34-1 Formation of a platelet plug at sites of blood vessel damage. Reprinted with permission from: Brass S. Cardiovascular biology: Small cells, big issues. *Nature* 2001;409:145–147). Copyright © 2001, Rights Managed by Nature Publishing Group.

syndrome) (21), both of these having been reported as causes of epidural hematoma formation. Overall, defects in blood vessel walls are rare causes of epidural hematoma formation.

Platelet Function

Defects related to platelets are a more common cause of concern in obstetric patients, both in relation to quality and quantity of the platelets. Low platelet counts or thrombocytopenia can be defined as a platelet concentration <150,000/mm³ and is common (8%) in obstetric patients (3). Pregnancy-related gestational thrombocytopenia (GTP) is the most common subset of thrombocytopenic obstetric patients (75% of cases); in GTP, the platelet count is low but rarely drops <100,000/mm³ (3). Other common causes of thrombocytopenia in pregnancy result from patients with hypertensive disorders of pregnancy (PIH) (21% of cases), where the platelet counts can drop <100,000/mm³ but usually not <20,000/mm³. The decline in platelet counts may be more precipitous and is largely dependent upon the severity of the disease, e.g., in severe PIH or hemolysis elevated liver enzymes, low platelet counts (HELLP) syndrome (4% to 12% of cases). Less common causes of thrombocytopenia include idiopathic thrombocytopenia (ITP) (4% of cases), where the counts can routinely fall <20,000/mm³ (Table 34-1).

Spontaneous bleeding can result when platelet counts fall <20,000/mm³ and surgical bleeding (or bleeding after vaginal delivery) can occur when counts fall <50,000/mm³. The conventional wisdom was that it was relatively safe to perform neuraxial anesthesia in a patient with a platelet count >100,000/mm³. This data was interpolated from bleeding time studies (22), which have subsequently been shown to be subjective in their assessment, and in addition, may not correlate with the risk of epidural hematoma formation.

TABLE 34-1 Thrombocytopenia in Pregnancy (3)

Defined as any platelet concentration <150,000/mm³

1. Gestational thrombocytopenia (GTP) is the most common (75%)
   • Platelet count is low but rarely drops <100,000/mm³
2. Another common cause is pregnancy-induced hypertension (PIH) (21%)
   • Platelet counts can drop <100,000/mm³, but rarely <20,000/mm³
3. Less common cause is idiopathic thrombocytopenia (ITP) (4%)
   • Platelet counts can drop <20,000/mm³

Newer Dynamic Coagulation Test Use

While standard coagulation tests currently performed (i.e., PT and PTT) are used frequently to assess the coagulation status of patients, they do not provide information as to the risk assessment of platelet-related bleeding in thrombocytopenic patients. There are more specific tests for platelet function that have been developed such as the thromboelastogram TEG® (Haemoscope Corporation, Niles, IL) and the platelet functional analyzer PFA-l00® (Dade-Behring, Dudingen, Switzerland).

The thromboelastogram (TEG) is a viscoelastic test of the whole blood during the coagulation process, which can be used to evaluate the initialization, formation, and strength of clot formation (23). In the standard TEG, a small quantity of blood (0.36 mL) is rotated gently in a cuvette, which is set to mimic sluggish venous blood flow and so activates the coagulation system. This is concurrently followed by sensor rod placement into the blood sample. The strength and speed of clot formation is then measured with the results being quantified graphically. The typical trace can be seen in (Fig. 34-3).

Valuable information is then generated on the activity of the enzymatic coagulation system, platelet function, fibrinolysis, and other factors, which can be related to antithrombotic agents present. TEG has been used since the 1940s (23), but with technical development and improved standardization and reproducibility, it has been used recently in clinical settings at a much greater frequency. TEG is a dynamic test of coagulation, whose maximum amplitude (MA) value is a commonly used clinical variable that correlates to both platelet quantity and function. Sharma presented an elegant paper that showed that the TEG MA values start to become significantly abnormal at platelet counts <75,000/mm³ in patients with preeclampsia (24). This suggested that when a platelet count is seen above this value in preeclamptic patients, it may correlate to the patient having a normal coagulation profile.

While the absolute platelet count is important, its trend over time is equally important in the consideration in assessing the risk/benefit ratio of when to perform a neuraxial regional technique. As an example, if the patient's platelet count has been stable in the range 75,000 to 80,000/mm³, this would be a more reassuring value to the clinician than a platelet count of 85,000/mm³ if the prior count in that same patient a few hours earlier was substantially >100,000/mm³.

The quality of platelet function is another important clinical factor in determining the bleeding risk after neuraxial block placement. Platelet function in disease states varies. For example, ITP has relatively high functioning platelets ("survival of the fittest") (25), as compared with conditions such as preeclampsia and von Willebrand disease (26) where platelets may not be as effective.

Once the decision has been made to place a neuraxial block in a parturient with a low but clinically acceptable

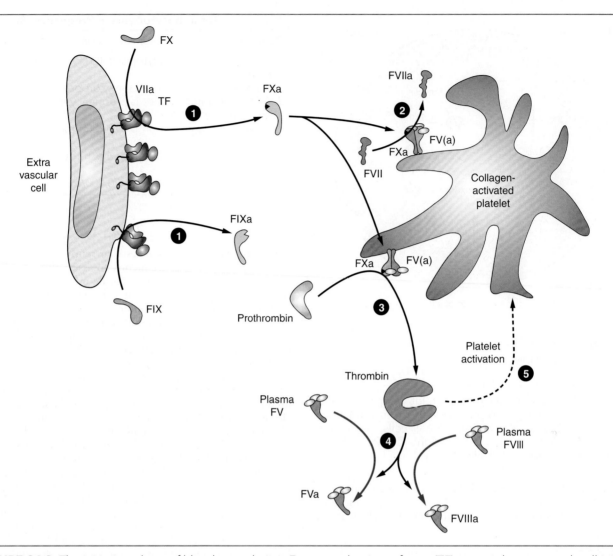

FIGURE 34-2 The initiation phase of blood coagulation. Extravascular tissue factor (TF) exposed upon vessel wall injury forms a complex with factor VII/activated factor VII (FVII/FVIIa). Reprinted with permission from: Eilertsen KE, Østerud B. Tissue factor: (patho)physiology and cellular biology. *Blood Coagul Fibrinolysis* 2004;15(7):521–538.

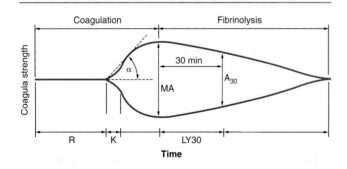

FIGURE 34-3 Major TEG parameters. R reflects coagulation factor activities, K and α show fibrinogen and coagula formation. MA indicates platelet function. LY30 reflects fibrinolysis. A30 is the amplitude 30 minutes after MA. Adapted with permission from: Reikvam H, Steien E, Hauge B, et al. Thrombelastography. *Transfus Apher Sci* 2009;40(2):119–123.

platelet count, additional safeguards need to be taken for these patients. These precautions would include utilization of the most atraumatic block needle available (e.g., small 27 gauge spinal needle would be more preferable than a large 17 gauge epidural Tuohy needle), placement by the most experienced provider on the team (not a good candidate for an anesthetic trainee), and extreme vigilance of that patient in the postanesthetic period (e.g., frequent neurologic checks and monitoring).

Intravascular Coagulation

In addition to thrombocytopenia, defective coagulation mechanisms, whether due to disease states or therapeutic agents, pose an increased risk of a neuraxial hematoma formation after a neuraxial anesthetic technique. With a normal coagulation mechanism in place, the risk of hematoma has been reported by Vandermeulen to be low after neuraxial anesthesia, ranging from 1:150,000 (epidural) to 220,000 (spinal) (27). The standard tests of coagulation (PT, PTT,

INR) are elevated in certain disease states (e.g., liver disease, severe preeclampsia) and by the actions of certain pharmacologic agents (e.g., warfarin, unfractionated heparin)—all of which increase the risk of hematoma formation. Using Vandermeulen's calculated background risk of 1:150,000 and actual reports of epidural hematoma in the literature, Schroeder performed a mathematical estimate and reported an increase in risk with defective coagulation mechanisms leading to a risk assessment of 1 in 40,800, 1 in 6,600, and 1 in 3,100 of hematoma formation in patients following spinal, single shot epidural, and epidural with epidural catheter placement, respectively (28).

Antithrombotic Medications

Pregnancy is a known hypercoagulable state, which may be a protective mechanism to reduce excessive bleeding during the labor and delivery process. The typical blood loss after a vaginal delivery ranges from 300 to 500 mL (29) while typical blood loss during a cesarean delivery may be up to 1,000 mL (30). Post-operative hemorrhage has been defined as a blood loss greater than 500 mL although the American College of Obstetricians and Gynecologists (ACOG) suggests an alternative definition for postpartum hemorrhage based on a decline in hematocrit level by 10 points after delivery (31). This hypercoagulable state of pregnancy is in part due to factors II, VII, VIII, IX, X, vWF, and fibrinogen being elevated during the course of gestation, and while protective against potential hemorrhage, these elevations can conversely lead to hypercoagulable complications such as thrombus formation, including deep vein thrombosis (DVT) and pulmonary embolism (PE). For these pathologic entities, the risk is 6 times higher in pregnant patients compared to non-pregnant patients, estimated at 1 per 1,000 deliveries (32).

Parturients with additional risk factors for thrombotic complications include those with factor V Leiden mutation, prothrombin G20210A mutation, antiphospholipid syndrome, antithrombin, protein C, and protein S deficiencies, and similar inherited or acquired thrombophilias. These patients often need anticoagulant medication to prevent thrombotic complications from occurring. Oral anticoagulants such as warfarin are effective in managing hypercoagulable disorders, but their use is contraindicated in pregnancy due to the risk of teratogenesis and other side effects (33). Some parturients are managed with daily subcutaneous unfractionated heparin injections, e.g., 5,000 units twice a day, which may have a less effective antithrombotic action than warfarin, but does still reduce the chance of thrombotic disease without significantly increasing the risk of hematoma formation under regional anesthesia (34).

More recently introduced low molecular weight heparins are also very effective antithrombotic agents that have a favorable pharmacologic profile; that is, they can be administered without routine follow-up laboratory monitoring and are given as weight-based medications. Their effectiveness in preventing thrombotic complications also leads to an equally effective increase in bleeding after neuraxial anesthesia (e.g., leading to possible epidural hematoma formation). Vandermeulen reviewed a total of 61 cases in the literature from 1904 to 1994, prior to widespread clinical use of low molecular weight heparins such as enoxaparin sodium (Lovenox®). Following the advent of low molecular weight heparin use, Wysowski summarized many more frequent reports of epidural hematoma (43 cases) from 1993 to 1998 (35), which led to the request by the FDA to manufacturers to include a black box warning of this potential complication in their product labeling. The black box warning on enoxaparin stated that epidural or spinal hematomas may occur in patients who receive

TABLE 34-2 FDA Black Box Warning for Patients Receiving Enoxaparin Sodium (Lovenox®) (36)

The risk of developing epidural or spinal hematomas is increased in patients with the following conditions:

- Use of indwelling (implanted) epidural catheters
- Use of other drugs that affect the coagulation system, including non-steroidal anti-inflammatory drugs (NSAIDs), platelet inhibitors, or other anticoagulants
- History of spinal deformity
- History of spinal surgery
- History of traumatic or repeated epidural or spinal punctures

enoxaparin injections while receiving neuraxial anesthesia or undergoing spinal puncture. Such hematomas can result in long-term or permanent paralysis. Additional risks outlined in the black box warning are highlighted in Table 34-2.

American Society of Regional Anesthesia and Pain Medicine Guidelines

In response to these more efficacious anticoagulant and antiplatelet agents being developed, the American Society of Regional Anesthesia and Pain Medicine (ASRA) convened three Consensus Conferences on Regional Anesthesia and Anticoagulation. The first conference took place in 1997 and subsequent conferences convened at 5-year intervals in 2002 and 2007. The most recently updated information regarding these recommendations is outlined in a 2010 issue of *Regional Anesthesia and Pain Medicine* (34). Some of these guidelines are highlighted in Tables 34-3–34-5, focusing on those recommendations that include relevant medications taken by obstetric patients. Other agents discussed in the guidelines include non-steroidal anti-inflammatory drugs (NSAIDs), which ASRA guidelines suggest do not have an added risk by themselves for epidural hematoma formation after neuraxial anesthesia, but recommends awareness that combinations of these agents with other more potent antiplatelet agents can be a concern, particularly the potent and long-lasting agents such as ticlopidine.

Recently introduced potent antithrombotic medications (e.g., enoxaparin, fondaparinux, ticlopidine) are being prescribed in greater frequency to pregnant patients and unfortunately may not reveal their bleeding risks as abnormal values on the

TABLE 34-3 ASRA Practice Advisory (Unfractionated Heparin) (34)

Recommendations for Patients Receiving Unfractionated Heparin:

1. There is *no contraindication* to the use of neuraxial techniques in patients receiving subcutaneous (mini-dose) heparin prophylaxis.
2. In debilitated patients receiving prolonged therapy (>4 days), check a platelet count to rule out heparin-induced thrombocytopenia.
3. *Intravenous unfractionated heparin* administration should be *delayed for 1 h* after needle placement.
4. Indwelling neuraxial *catheters* should be *removed 2–4 h after* the last heparin dose and the patient's coagulation status is evaluated.
5. Re-heparinization should occur *1 h after* catheter removal.

TABLE 34-4 ASRA Practice Advisory (LMWH Pre) (34)

Preoperative Considerations for Patients Receiving Low Molecular Weight Heparin (LMWH):

1. If heme ("bloody tap") occurs during placement, initiation of LMWH therapy should be *delayed for 24 h* postoperatively
2. Needle placement should occur at least *10–12 h* after LMWH administration (single daily dosing regimen)
3. Patients receiving *higher* (twice daily dosing regimen) doses of LMWH, such as enoxaparin 1 mg/kg every 12 h, will require delays of at least *24 h* to assure normal hemostasis at the time of insertion
4. Neuraxial techniques should be avoided in patients administered a dose of LMWH *2 h* preoperatively (general surgery patients), because needle placement would occur during peak anticoagulant activity

standard coagulation laboratory tests; however, patients taking them are susceptible to a higher risk of epidural hematoma formation with regional anesthesia.

TEG and other platelet function testing may be useful tools to help elucidate some of these effects on coagulation that are not captured in the standard laboratory assays. At this point, however, their use has not been incorporated in the ASRA guidelines as of yet, in the risk stratification of patients before proceeding with a neuraxial anesthetic block. This is based to some extent on the lack of published data validating the efficacy of these tests in assessing bleeding risk after neuraxial block and the lack of widespread availability of TEG in all clinical settings in which anesthesia is practiced. With the incidence of bleeding complications so low, it may be very difficult to perform an adequately powered prospective trial to ever validate these measures and quantify their use in risk assessment.

Point-of-care Testing and Assessment of Neuraxial Risk

ASRA guidelines are an excellent framework to work within, in the assessment of the coagulation status of the patient and

TABLE 34-5 ASRA Practice Advisory (LMWH Post) (34)

Postoperative Considerations for Patients Receiving Low Molecular Weight Heparin (LMWH):

1. When twice daily dosing is used, the first dose of LMWH should be administered *no earlier than 24 h postoperatively*
2. Indwelling *catheters* should be *removed prior* to initiation of LMWH
3. If a continuous technique is selected, the epidural catheter may be left indwelling overnight and removed the following day, with the first dose of LMWH administered at least *2 h* after catheter removal
4. When single daily dosing is used, the first dose should be administered 6–8 h postoperatively. The second dose should occur *no sooner than 24 h after the first dose.*
5. Indwelling neuraxial catheters may be safely maintained, but catheter should be removed a *minimum of 10–12 h* after the last dose of LMWH
6. *Subsequent LMWH* dosing should occur a *minimum of 2 h after* catheter removal

quantification of the risks and benefits in making the decision of whether to proceed with a neuraxial technique in a patient. It is important to use all clinical information available as even the current ASRA guidelines do not necessarily assure that all the anticoagulant medication is no longer present in the patient within the time frame that is suggested as being relatively safe to place a neuraxial technique. For example, with regard to low molecular weight heparin therapy, the case report described in the subsequent paragraph demonstrates the utilization of the TEG-heparinase assay to show anticoagulant medication activity still being present in a patient who was considered to be safe in the ASRA guidelines.

The TEG-heparinase assay (m-TEG®) is a modification to the standard TEG test, wherein clot formation is not dependent on thrombin-related effects on platelets. Reptilase (batroxobin) and factor XIII are added to heparinized samples to generate fibrin and crosslink fibrin, respectively. This produces a weak clot and platelet activation is then achieved by adding arachidonic acid (AA) or adenosine diphosphate (ADP), depending on the platelet pathway activation being assayed. This can allow for the assessment of any contribution of residual heparin activity in the lack of thrombin-related clot formation in standard TEG testing. Using a TEG-heparinase assay, the author and colleagues have reported a case in which there was still a significant presence of heparin activity at 24 hours following a dose of enoxaparin in a laboring parturient (37). At exactly 24 hours after the last dose of enoxaparin in this patient requesting epidural analgesia, a TEG assay performed showed a prolonged R time, which then normalized on a concurrent TEG-heparinase assay run at the same time (Fig. 34-4). This showed a significant residual presence of heparin activity, which was then taken into consideration in the decision to not perform the neuraxial block in this patient (37).

TEG testing, both standard as well as modified, has been used to guide target-directed transfusion therapy (38), guiding factor VII therapy after coronary artery bypass surgery (39) and to reduce bleeding risk (40), with many of the normal limitations of the standard coagulation tests overcome by TEG (41). TEG does not necessarily predict hypercoagulable thromboembolic events (42) nor has it been validated against a prospective study in assessing epidural hematoma formation. Suggestions have been made that TEG testing be used to confirm normal coagulation (43) before removing or inserting an epidural catheter. If, in addition to this, the use of platelet functional analyzer (PFA-100) is considered, it may add to the testing sensitivity in obstetric patients, to completely assess platelet function, but may not be likely necessarily in every clinical case setting (44).

While TEG (with or without heparinase modification) is very helpful in assessing low molecular weight heparin therapy, not all antiplatelet medication will lead to an abnormal MA value on the TEG trace. Aspirin and other NSAIDs inhibit platelets by inactivating cyclooxygenase, an enzyme that normally produces prostaglandin G2 and thromboxane A2 (TXA2). The effect of aspirin on cyclooxygenase-1 (COX-l) is irreversible so is maintained for the remaining life of the platelet (7 to 10 days), as platelets have no nuclei and so lack the ability to regenerate new COX-1. NSAIDs are weak antiplatelet drugs, because they affect only one of the several pathways that leads to platelet activation.

After damage to a vessel, platelets when exposed to disrupted collagen, will adhere via their surface glycoprotein (Gp) receptor complexes—a process facilitated by von Willebrand factor (vWF) bridges. This then leads to stimulation of phospholipase C (PLC) production and release of ADP alpha granules that then binds to $P_2Y_{1\&12}$ receptors on adjacent platelets resulting in substantial amplification of the whole

TEG® PATIENT HEMOSTASIS SUMMARY
3:58:32 PM

Patient name   Procedure name

Tracings

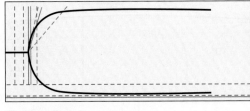 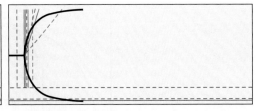

Ch 4 baseline
Kaolin 3/22/2007 11:10:22 AM

Ch 3 baseline
Kaolin with heparinase 3/22/2007 11:10:22 AM

FIGURE 34-4 TEG tracings. TEG values from venous blood sample taken 24 hours after the patient received a full dose of Lovenox. The first TEG shown indicates a regular kaolin TEG and the second TEG shown was run concurrently with the addition of heparinase. Adapted with permission from: Panni MK, Panni JK. Obstetric patient on lovenox therapy—evidence of heparin activity at 24 hours. *J Obstet Gyn* 2010;30(1):62–64.

pathway (4) (Fig. 34-5). More potent platelet inhibition is achieved with the newer thienopyridine derivatives (e.g., first generation ticlopidine, second generation clopidogrel, and third generation prasugrel) which inhibit ADP-induced platelet activation by binding covalently to the P_2Y_{12} receptor (4). These agents are not only more potent than NSAIDS but they can also act synergistically with them.

Regardless of the pathway of platelet activation or antagonism, the final step in the platelet aggregation pathway results from the binding of fibrinogen to newly exposed GpIIb/IIIa receptors on adjacent platelets. In the absence of this binding, platelet aggregation cannot occur. GpIIb/IIIa inhibitors block these receptors, thereby preventing platelet aggregation (4). GpIIb/IIIa inhibitors vary in their affinity for the GpIIb/IIIa receptor and their plasma half-life, but otherwise have a similar mechanism of action (e.g., Abciximab has high affinity and slow dissociation resulting in a biologic half-life of 12 to 24 hours). Eptifibatide and tirofiban have lower affinity and rapid dissociation resulting in a 2- to 4-hour half-life.

While standard TEG may be sensitive to many causes of impaired platelet function, it may be insensitive to some drug-induced causes of platelet dysfunction, due to the use of thrombin present in standard TEG cuvettes, which is normally produced through the intrinsic pathway of coagulation. Therefore, standard TEG testing is insensitive to the antiplatelet effects of COX-I inhibitors (aspirin and other NSAIDS) and P_2Y_{12} antagonists (ticlopidine and clopidogrel), which still allow for the clot formation using thrombin even if platelet function is impaired. However, standard TEG testing is sensitive to the effect of GpIIb/IIIa inhibitors, because their action is independent of thrombin. While most traditional point-of-care techniques cannot completely assess the effect of COX-I inhibitors and P_2Y_{12} antagonists, TEG® with Platelet Mapping™ has been shown to assess bleeding risk after cardiac surgery (45). Similar to modified TEG® testing, Platelet Mapping™ uses different activators for platelet activation and clot formation initiation, with up to four channels and comparisons between traces allowing for the measurement of percentage inhibition of antiplatelet drug (4). In addition to these newer antiplatelet agents, other applications of TEG could be applied to difficult-to-measure

agents (e.g., enoxaparin monitoring with and without heparinase) where the use of TEG is unmatched in this setting (46).

These specific alternative tests (e.g., TEG®, platelet function analyzers (PFA)) provide useful supplemental clinical information to the standard laboratory tests (PT and PTT) that may not always pick up the antithrombotic action of some of the newer pharmacologic agents, so as to assess enoxaparin activity (e.g., factor Xa levels) as well as the activity of other potent anticoagulant and antiplatelet agents. Neither TEG, PFA, or factor Xa levels, however, are recommended to be obtained by ASRA in their guidelines. This may be in part due to the lack of large studies to validate these tests against risk of hematoma formation after neuraxial anesthesia, given the low incidence of this complication and so necessitating recruitment of large numbers of patients in order to achieve an adequate study power. In addition, these new and sophisticated tests may not be available in every hospital setting and may place many institutions in a difficult position if these tests were required in the guidelines for routine assessments.

Clinical Decision-Making

It is recommended that the following elements be in place before the performance of regional anesthesia: A detailed history, firm assurance that the patient is not currently receiving anticoagulant medication, confirmation that the patient has not experienced any bleeding diathesis (e.g., easy bruising, frequent nose bleeds), and immediate laboratory evidence of a normal and stable platelet count (for those patients in whom there is a suspicion of thrombocytopenia, e.g., hypertensive parturients). As the risks of defective coagulation mechanisms increase, either through a disease process or pharmacologic effects on normal coagulation processes, a step-wise approach is required to assess the patient's clinical need and coagulation status in order to make an appropriate evidence-based decision of whether or not to proceed with regional anesthesia.

In patients who are only taking NSAIDs or subcutaneous unfractionated heparin, ASRA guidelines suggest there is no additional risk in performing neuraxial anesthesia. In patients who are taking regular intravenous heparin, following discontinuation of the heparin infusion, a normal PTT should be obtained before proceeding with a regional technique;

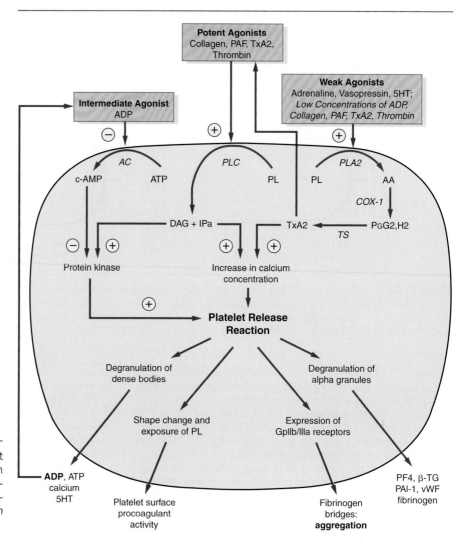

FIGURE 34-5 Pathways of platelet activation. Adapted with permission from: Gibbs NM. Point-of-care assessment of antiplatelet agents in the perioperative period: a review. *Anaesth Intensive Care* 2009;37(3):354–369.

similarly, a recent platelet count should be obtained if there were any suspicion of thrombocytopenia. If there is no time to obtain such a value (typically 1 hour in most hospital laboratories) and platelet function abnormalities are suspected, or if the patient is taking one of the newer potent anticoagulants which do not reveal themselves with abnormal PTT or platelet counts, then a point-of-care rapid test (e.g., TEG®) could be considered. While a standard TEG is not validated in studies of risk of hematoma formation, it is a very effective way to assess current coagulation status. If used with TEG® Platelet Mapping™ and heparinase modified TEG® testing, it can provide very useful clinical information of the patient's complete coagulation status and allow the provider to have an improved risk stratification of the patient. In addition, if newer anticoagulant medications are encountered in the patients, knowledge of the half-life of the medication could also guide the clinician to the time necessary to have the plasma levels and effectiveness of those medications decrease, in addition to the results of these laboratory investigations.

Having taken into consideration all the risks and benefits of neuraxial anesthesia, and if deciding to perform this procedure in a patient with a higher but acceptable risk/benefit ratio, the approach to neuraxial placement needs to be appropriately modified. The most experienced practitioner available should perform this with as minimal trauma as possible (minimal attempts with the smallest needle), and there needs to be increased patient vigilance including monitoring

of neurologic function at frequent, regular intervals. At the first signs of any potential issue such as severe back pain or prolonged motor block, the patient needs to have emergent imaging of their spinal cord. If an epidural hematoma is evident, urgent surgical decompression at the earliest opportunity is then indicated to preserve neurologic function (13).

■ SUMMARY

ASRA consensus statements give an excellent summary of practice guidelines and recommendations based on available evidence and the summative experience of experts in the field (34). The decision to perform a neuraxial anesthetic technique as well as optimal timing for removal of a catheter in a patient receiving antithrombotic or anticoagulant therapy is made by weighing the risks of neuraxial hematoma with the benefits of regional anesthesia for each patient (34). This risk versus benefit analysis may have a different emphasis in the obstetric population where there is a higher risk of complications from general anesthesia compared to the nonpregnant population who may require neuraxial anesthesia only for postoperative analgesia, when other analgesic techniques would be available for this. There is an expanding role here for the more frequent use of point-of-care whole blood coagulation testing (e.g., TEGs and platelet function analyzers) in obtaining the most complete information regarding the patient's coagulation status during this risk assessment.

More routine use of point-of-care whole blood coagulation testing such as the TEG assay will likely be employed in obtaining the most complete information of the patient's coagulation status, especially in high-risk parturients.

KEY POINTS

- Regional anesthesia is a safe and preferred method of anesthesia in parturients.
- Widespread use of regional anesthesia has led to dramatic reductions in maternal morbidity and mortality.
- Certain serious complications are associated with regional anesthesia, the most potentially devastating being epidural hematoma.
- The American Society of Regional Anesthesia and Pain Medicine (ASRA) consensus statements provide an excellent summary of practice guidelines or recommendations that are based on available evidence and the collective experience of experts in the field.
- The decision to perform a spinal or epidural anesthetic and the optimal timing of epidural catheter removal in a patient receiving antithrombotic or anticoagulant therapy should be made weighing the risks of neuraxial hematoma with the benefits of regional anesthesia for each patient.
- Consideration of the pharmacodynamics and pharmacokinetics of newer agents, along with the use of point-of-care testing of the whole blood coagulation process, would give much needed additional information in decision-making of whether or not to proceed with regional anesthesia.

REFERENCES

1. Cerneca F, Ricci G, Simeone R, et al. Coagulation and fibrinolysis changes in normal pregnancy. Increased levels of procoagulants and reduced levels of inhibitors during pregnancy induce a hypercoagulable state, combined with a reactive fibrinolysis. *Eur J Obstet Gynecol Reprod Biol* 1997;73(1):31–36.
2. Hellgren M. Hemostasis during normal pregnancy and puerperium. *Semin Thromb Hemost* 2003;29(2):125–130.
3. Levy JA, Murphy LD. Thrombocytopenia in pregnancy. *J Am Board Fam Pract* 2002;15(4):290–297.
4. Gibbs NM. Point-of-care assessment of antiplatelet agents in the perioperative period: a review. *Anaesth Intensive Care* 2009;37(3):354–369.
5. Wong CA. Advances in labor analgesia. *Int J Womens Health* 2010;1:139–154.
6. Munnur U, Suresh MS. Airway problems in pregnancy. *Crit Care Clin* 2004;20(4):617–642.
7. O'Sullivan G. Gastric emptying during pregnancy and the puerperium. *Int J Obstet Anesth* 1993;2(4):216–224.
8. Robins K, Lyons G. Intraoperative awareness during general anesthesia for cesarean delivery. *Anesth Analg* 2009;109(3):886–890.
9. Wang S, Peretich K, Zhao Y, et al. Anesthesia-induced neurodegeneration in fetal rat brains. *Pediatr Res* 2009;66(4):435–440.
10. Carlton T, Callister LC, Stoneman E. Decision making in laboring women: ethical issues for perinatal nurses. *J Perinat Neonatal Nurs* 2005;19(2):145–154.
11. Todman D. A history of caesarean section: from ancient world to the modern era. *Aust N Z J Obstet Gynaecol* 2007;47(5):357–361.
12. Hawkins JL, Koonin LM, Palmer SK, et al. Anesthesia-related deaths during obstetric delivery in the United States, 1979–1990. *Anesthesiology* 1997;86(2):277–284.
13. Al-Mutair A, Bednar DA. Spinal epidural hematoma. *J Am Acad Orthop Surg* 2010;18(8):494–502.
14. Bowen BC, DePrima S, Pattany PM, et al. MR angiography of normal intradural vessels of the thoracolumbar spine. *Am J Neuroradiol* 1996;17(3):483–494.
15. Chen CL, Lu CH, Chen NF. Spontaneous spinal epidural hematoma presenting with quadriplegia after sit-ups exercise. *Am J Emerg Med* 2009;27(9):1170.e3–1177.e3.
16. Sobey CG, Faraci FM. Subarachnoid haemorrhage: what happens to the cerebral arteries? *Clin Exp Pharmacol Physiol.* 1998;25(11):867–876.
17. Jennings LK. Mechanisms of platelet activation: need for new strategies to protect against platelet-mediated atherothrombosis. *Thromb Haemost* 2009;102(2):248–257.
18. Eilertsen KE, Østerud B. Tissue factor: (patho)physiology and cellular biology. *Blood Coagul Fibrinolysis* 2004;15(7):521–538.
19. Perrini P, Pieri F, Montemurro N, et al. Thoracic extradural haematoma after epidural anaesthesia. *Neurol Sci* 2010;31(1):87–88.
20. Verma S, Sivanandan S, Aneesh MK, et al. Unilateral proptosis and extradural hematoma in a child with scurvy. *Pediatr Radiol* 2007;37(9):937–939.
21. Subramaniam B, Panzica PJ, Pawlowski JB, et al. Epidural blood patch for acute subdural hematoma after spinal catheter drainage during hybrid thoracoabdominal aneurysm repair. *J Cardiothorac Vasc Anesth* 2007;21(5):704–708.
22. Ramanathan J, Sibai BM, Vu T, et al. Correlation between bleeding times and platelet counts in women with preeclampsia undergoing cesarean section. *Anesthesiology* 1989;71(2):188–191.
23. Reikvam H, Steien E, Hauge B, et al. Thromboelastography. *Transfus Apher Sci* 2009;40(2):119–123.
24. Sharma SK, Philip J, Whitten CW, et al. Assessment of changes in coagulation in parturients with preeclampsia using thromboelastography. *Anesthesiology* 1999;90(2):385–390.
25. Toltl LJ, Arnold DM. Pathophysiology and management of chronic immune thrombocytopenia: focusing on what matters. *Br J Haematol* 2011;152(1):52–60.
26. Torres R, Fedoriw Y. Laboratory testing for von Willebrand disease: toward a mechanism-based classification. *Clin Lab Med* 2009;29(2):193–228.
27. Vandermeulen EP, Van Aken H, Vermylen J. Anticoagulants and spinal–epidural anesthesia. *Anesth Analg* 1994;79(6):1165–1177.
28. Schroeder DR. Statistics: detecting a rare adverse drug reaction using spontaneous reports. *Reg Anesth Pain Med* 1998;23(6) (Suppl 2):183–189.
29. Pritchard JA, Wiggins KM, Dickey JC. Blood volume changes in pregnancy and the puerperium. I. Does sequestration of red blood cells accompany parturition? *Am J Obstet Gynecol* 1960;80:956–964.
30. Duthie SJ, Ghosh A, Ng A, et al. Intra-operative blood loss during elective lower segment caesarean section. *Br J Obstet Gynaecol* 1992;99(5):364–367.
31. American College of Obstetricians and Gynecologists. *Post-partum Hemorrhage.* ACOG Educational Bulletin Number 243:Washington, DC: ACOG. *Int J Gynaecol Obstet* 1998;61(1)79–86.
32. McColl MD, Ramsay JE, Tait RC, et al. Risk factors for pregnancy associated venous thromboembolism. *Thromb Haemost* 1997;78(4):1183–1188.
33. Hall JG, Pauli RM, Wilson KM. Maternal and fetal sequelae of anticoagulation during pregnancy. *Am J Med* 1980;68(1):122–140.
34. Horlocker TT, Wedel DJ, Rowlingson JC, et al. Regional anesthesia in the patient receiving antithrombotic or thrombolytic therapy: American Society of Regional Anesthesia and Pain Medicine Evidence-Based Guidelines (Third Edition). *Reg Anesth Pain Med* 2010;35(1):64–101.
35. Wysowski DK, Talarico L, Bacsanyi J, et al. Spinal and epidural hematoma and low molecular-weight heparin. *N Engl J Med* 1998;338(24):1774–1775.
36. http://www.accessdata.fda.gov/drugsatfda_docs/label/2009/020164s083lbl.pdf
37. Panni MK, Panni JK. Obstetric patient on lovenox therapy – evidence of heparin activity at 24 hours. *J Obstet Gyn* 2010;30(1):62–64.
38. Wang SC, Shieh JF, Chang KY, et al. Thromboelastography-guided transfusion decreases intraoperative blood transfusion during orthotopic liver transplantation: randomized clinical trial. *Transplant Proc* 2010;42(7):2590–2593.
39. Wasowicz M, Meineri M, McCluskey SM, et al. The utility of thromboelastography for guiding recombinant activated factor VII therapy for refractory hemorrhage after cardiac surgery. *J Cardiothorac Vasc Anesth* 2009;23(6):828–834.
40. Clements A, Jindal S, Morris C, et al. Expanding perfusion across disciplines: the use of thromboelastograph technology to reduce risk in an obstetrics patient with Gray Platelet Syndrome – A case study. *Perfusion* 2011;26(3):181–184.
41. Bischof D, Dalbert S, Zollinger A, et al. Thromboelastography in the surgical patient. *Minerva Anestesiol* 2010;76(2):131–137.
42. Dai Y, Lee A, Critchley LA, et al. Does thromboelastography predict postoperative thromboembolic events? A systematic review of the literature. *Anesth Analg* 2009;108(3):734–742.
43. Fazakas J, Tóth S, Füle B, et al. Epidural anesthesia? No of course. *Transplant Proc* 2008;40(4):1216–1217.
44. Beilin Y, Arnold I, Hossain S. Evaluation of the platelet function analyzer (PFA-100) vs. the thromboelastogram (TEG) in the parturient. *Int J Obstet Anesth* 2006;15(1):7–12.
45. Preisman S, Kogan A, Itzkovsky K, et al. Modified thromboelastography evaluation of platelet dysfunction in patients undergoing coronary artery surgery. *Eur J Cardiothorac Surg* 2010;37(6):1367–1374.
46. Carroll RC, Craft RM, Whitaker GL, et al. Thromboelastography monitoring of resistance to enoxaparin anticoagulation in thrombophilic pregnancy patients. *Thromb Res* 2007;120(3):367–370.

J. Sudharma Ranasinghe • Donald H. Penning

Obesity is a metabolic disease in which abnormal or excessive accumulation of adipose tissue represents greater than normal proportion of body mass. Obesity is increasing in prevalence amongst pregnant women across the United States (1). The prevalence of obesity is growing at an alarming rate worldwide, and by 2015 it is expected that approximately 700 million people will be obese (2). The World Health Organization also projects that by 2025, more than 50% of the United States population will have a BMI >30 kg/m² (Fig. 35-1).

In the United States obesity rates has reached epidemic proportions with extreme obesity (BMI >40 kg/m²) showing the greatest increase, particularly among women (3). According to the latest data from the National Health and Nutrition Examination Survey (NHANES) in 2007 to 2008, the prevalence of obesity was 32.2% among adult men and 35.5% among adult women in the United States (4) and certain ethnic groups are affected more than others (5). The dramatically increasing rate of obesity in the general population also extends to women of reproductive age. Obesity increases the risk for cesarean delivery significantly and thus also the need for anesthesia. Anesthesiologists are thus increasingly faced with the care for morbidly obese parturients.

Overweight and obesity are major risk factors for a number of chronic diseases, including diabetes, ischemic heart disease, stroke, hypertension, hypercoagulability, osteoarthritis, gall bladder disease, and several types of cancer. There is evidence that risk of chronic disease increases progressively from a BMI of 21 kg/m². Obesity caused by poor diet and physical inactivity is now the second leading cause of death in the United States (3). In pregnant women, obesity is associated with serious consequences on birth outcome (6).

■ DEFINITIONS

Body mass index (BMI) is a simple, clinically relevant measure of overweight and obesity in adult population. It can be easily computed and well correlated with the risk of mortality. It is defined as the total body weight (TBW) in kilograms divided by the square of the height in meters (kg/m²). The World Health Organization (WHO) defines "overweight" as a BMI ≥25, obesity as a BMI ≥30. Obesity is further categorized by BMI into Class I (30 to 34.9); Class II (35 to 39.9) and Class III obesity (>40). Morbid obesity is BMI ≥40 kg/m² and super obesity is classified as a BMI ≥50 kg/m² (7).

Although there are no pregnancy-specific definitions of obesity, the American College of Obstetricians and Gynecologists (ACOG) recommends using height and weight measured at the first prenatal visit to calculate the BMI. Pregnant women are considered obese when the BMI is ≥30 kg/m², and morbidly obese when the BMI is ≥40 kg/m². The maternal body weight is expected to increase during pregnancy due to increase in blood volume, fetus, placenta, amniotic fluid, and deposition of new fat and protein. The normal mean maternal weight increase during pregnancy is 17% of the pre-pregnancy weight or about 12 kg (8). However, it is important to recognize that the allowable weight gain during pregnancy varies by pre-pregnancy BMI (8) (Table 35-1). Obesity is an increasing problem in women of child-bearing age. According to the data from the NHANES survey, at least 60% of women of child-bearing age are overweight or obese (3).

There are several subgroups of obese individuals.

A. Simple obesity
B. Obesity hypoventilation syndrome (OHS) also referred to as "Pickwickian syndrome" comprises 5% to 10% of obese individuals. Fortunately, patients with OHS are usually not seen in labor and delivery due to two reasons: (1) This syndrome usually develops later in life and (2) patients with OHS are unlikely to get pregnant.
C. Obesity-related metabolic syndrome: Increasing incidence of obesity worldwide has led to the recognition of this obesity-related metabolic syndrome also referred to as syndrome X, which is characterized by "truncal" obesity, insulin resistance or glucose intolerance (hyperglycemia), altered lipid levels, low HDL cholesterol, and high LDL cholesterol—that foster plaque buildup in arteries prothrombotic state, high fibrinogen or plasminogen activator inhibitor-1 in the blood; proinflammatory state (e.g., elevated serum C-reactive protein), and hypertension (9). Obesity-related metabolic syndrome carries a different risk profile than obesity alone. These patients are at a greater risk for coronary artery disease (CAD), obstructive sleep apnea (OSA), hypercoagulability with predisposition to deep vein thrombosis (DVT), and pulmonary dysfunction.

■ PHYSIOLOGIC DISTURBANCES

Both obesity and pregnancy are associated with significant physiologic changes in multiple organ systems. Many of the physiologic effects of pregnancy and obesity are additive and can lead to considerable functional impairment and decreased physiologic reserves. Therefore, obstetric- and anesthetic-related complications are more frequent in obese parturients. A report of anesthesia-related maternal deaths in Michigan (1985 to 2003) confirms that obesity is an important risk factor for anesthesia-related maternal mortality (10). In the 2003–2005 Confidential Enquiries into Maternal and Child Health (CEMACH) report from the UK, there were six women who died from problems directly related to anesthesia, and obesity was a factor in four of them (11).

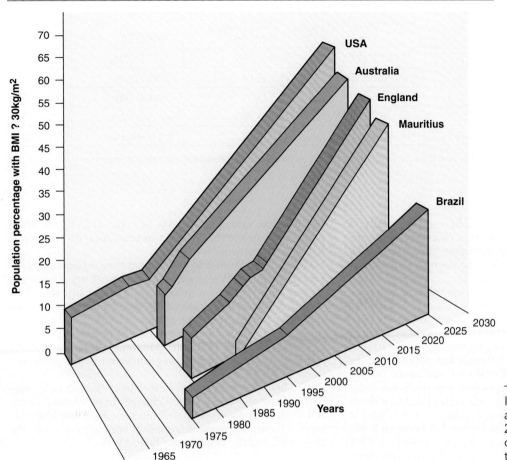

FIGURE 35-1 Projected prevalence of obesity in adults by 2025. The Global Challenge of Obesity and the International Obesity Task Force. http://www.iuns.org/

Respiratory Changes

Lung Volumes and Pulmonary Function Tests (PFTs)

Pregnancy is associated with significant anatomical and functional changes in the respiratory system. Similar to pregnancy, obesity reduces the expiratory reserve volume (ERV), residual volume (RV), and functional residual capacity (FRC). One would speculate that when an obese woman gets pregnant these changes in lung volumes will be markedly accentuated. However, according to a study by Eng et al. (12), such is not the case. They found that in obese women with reduced pre-pregnancy FRC, further reduction in pregnancy is limited.

TABLE 35-1 The National Institute of Medicine's Guidelines for Weight Gain in Pregnancy

Pre-pregnancy BMI	Recommended Weight Gain in kg/(lb)
<19.8 (low)	12.5–18 (28–40)
19.8–26.0 (normal)	11.5–16 (25–35)
26.1–29.0 (overweight)	7–11.5 (15–25)
>29 (obese)	≤6 (≤15)

Adapted with permission from: Stotland NE. Obesity and pregnancy. *BMJ* 2009;338:107–110.

The reason for this finding is not clear. In some respects, pregnancy may reduce some of the negative effects of obesity on respiratory system. Progesterone is a direct respiratory stimulant and increases the sensitivity of brainstem to carbon dioxide. The relaxing effect of progesterone on smooth muscle decreases airway resistance. Oxygenation and ventilation of obese pregnant women in the upright position seem to be intermediate between normal-weight–term pregnant women and obese, nonpregnant women (13) (Table 35-2).

During the third trimester of pregnancy, gravid uterus pushes the diaphragm in a cephalad direction.

It has been shown that the closing volume (CV) does begin to impinge on FRC as pregnancy advances. This is most likely from a reduction in RV and ERV (14). However, in contrast to obese parturients, this change does not worsen in normal-weight parturients upon taking the supine position (14). When the mass loading effect of obesity reduces FRC, it may fall at or below closing capacity leading to airway closure during tidal ventilation, especially in the dependent regions causing intrapulmonary shunting (15,16). Assumption of supine, lithotomy, or Trendelenburg position, use of abdominal straps to retract the panniculus cephalad, and induction of general anesthesia results in further reduction in FRC in the obese parturient (Fig. 35-2).

Shunt fractions of 10% to 25% of cardiac output have been reported in obesity (15). Therefore, unlike in normal-weight pregnancy, in obese parturients there is mismatching of ventilation–perfusion ratio with concomitant increase in

TABLE 35-2 Blood Gas Measurements by Pregnancy and Obesity Status

	PaO$_2$ (SD) mm Hg	PaCO$_2$ (SD) mm Hg	pH (SD)	Mean BMI (n)
Normal-weight–term pregnant	101.8 (1.0)	30.4 (0.06)	7.43 (0.006)	23.6 (20)
Obese term pregnant	85 (5.0)	29.7 (2.8)	7.44 (0.04)	43.5 (12)
Obese postpartum	86 (10)	35.5 (3)	7.44 (0.04)	41.4 (12)
Obese nonpregnant	76.7 (16.1)	41.3 (5.7)	Not available	39.5 (62)
Obese nonpregnant with sleep apnea	70.9 (11.7)	42.8 (5.0)	Not available	39.6 (40)

Reprinted with permission from: Mhyre JM. Anesthetic management for the morbidly obese pregnant woman. *Int Anesthesiol Clin* 2007;45: 51–70.

alveolar to arterial oxygen tension difference, especially in the supine position. Oxygen saturation measured in the sitting and supine position during normal ventilation may provide evidence of airway closure and the degree of pulmonary reserve.

Holley et al. (17) reported that in obese subjects with ERV less than 0.4 L (21% predicted), the distribution of a normal tidal breath was predominantly to the upper zones. This distribution pattern is similar to what is found in normal weight subjects at low lung volumes, i.e., upper lungs are predominantly ventilated at low lung volumes and opposite occurs at high lung volumes. Distribution of perfusion, on the other hand, remains gravity dependent and perfusion index increases approximately linearly with vertical distance down the lungs similar to normal-weight subjects (18). Thus, in obese subjects there is an abnormally low V/Q ratio in lower lung zones, which depends more on the amount of ERV reduction than to the degree of obesity. Even a very large increase in weight is not necessarily associated with severe decrease in ERV due to the fact that the increase in body mass may occur in lower half of the body, which would not interfere with the ERV (17). However, if the fat deposition occurs in the abdominal wall, this would cause an increase in abdominal pressure, and cause a considerable decrease

in ERV. The value of ERV may be taken as an approximate indicator as to whether a defect in ventilation distribution is likely in the parturient.

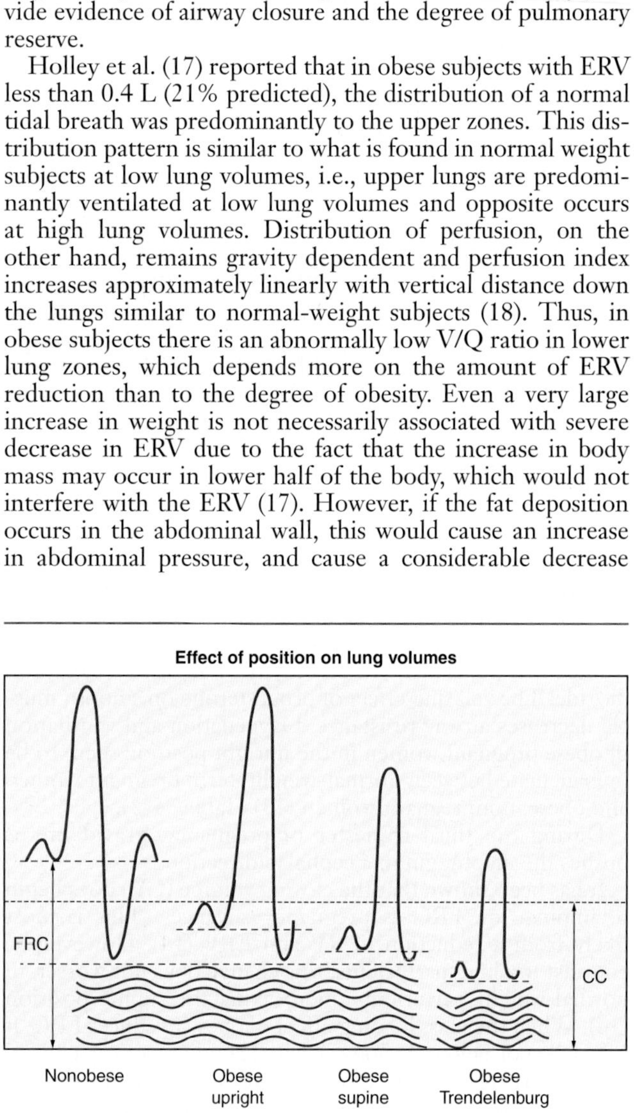

Classically, spirometric values other than maximum voluntary ventilation (MVV) are not affected in obesity. Therefore, an abnormal pulmonary function test (PFT) value should be considered as an indication of intrinsic lung disease and not caused by obesity, unless in extreme obesity where a significant reduction in vital capacity (VC) and total lung capacity (TLC) can be seen (19). The pulmonary diffusion capacity remains unchanged during pregnancy and is well preserved in obesity as well.

The lung parenchyma in obese subjects is essentially normal and the above-mentioned changes in pulmonary values reflect changes due to chest wall mechanics and low lung volumes. Obesity alters the relationship between the lungs, the chest wall, and the diaphragm (Table 35-3).

Work of Breathing

Early in pregnancy, the alveolar ventilation is increased, which is attributed to the respiratory stimulant effect of progesterone rather than a response to increased metabolism. In obesity, hyperventilation at rest occurs due to increased oxygen requirement and CO$_2$ production by the excess fat that is deposited in the body. Dempsey et al. (20) demonstrated that excess body weight increases oxygen consumption and CO$_2$ production in a linear fashion. Achieving this augmented ventilation imposes an additional physiologic burden, and work of breathing is increased tremendously in obesity. In patients with simple obesity, the total work of breathing may be increased up to twice normal. In patients with OHS, it is increased about 3 times above that of normal individual (21). The oxygen consumption in obesity is increased even more than the mechanical work of breathing, ranging 4 to 12 times normal thus reducing the efficiency of respiratory muscles in obesity (22).

Compared to normal pregnancy, the most significant pulmonary mechanics change in obesity, is that the chest compliance is reduced to a much greater extent. This change is due to the increased weight of the chest and abdominal wall from accumulation of fat in and around the ribs, the diaphragm, and the abdomen. It has been estimated that 33% of the increased work of breathing in obese subject is due to elastic work done on the chest wall (22). Sharp et al. (21) showed that in obesity the total respiratory compliance is reduced to one-third of normal. Naimark et al. (23) reported further significant reduction in respiratory compliance in obese subjects when assuming supine position as compared to normal-weight patients. Another factor that may contribute to increased work of breathing in obesity is due to an increase in total airway resistance, secondary to the lower lung volumes (24).

Effect of position on lung volumes

Nonobese   Obese upright   Obese supine   Obese Trendelenburg

FIGURE 35-2 Effect of position change on lung volumes in nonobese compared with markedly obese subjects. FRC, functional residual capacity; RV, residual volume; CC, closing capacity. Adapted with permission from: Vaughan RW. Pulmonary and cardiovascular derangements in the obese patient. In: Brown BR Jr, ed. *Anesthesia and the Obese Patient*. Philadelphia, PA: Davis. 1982:26.

TABLE 35-3 Resting Respiratory Changes in Pregnancy, Obesity, and Pregnancy and Obesity Combined

Parameter	Pregnancy	Obesity	Combined
Tidal volume	↑	↓	↑
Respiratory rate	↑	↑	↑
Minute volume	↑	↓ or ↔	↑
Inspiratory reserve volume	↑	↓	↑
Expiratory reserve volume	↓	↓↓	↓
Residual volume	↓	↓ or ↔	↓
Functional residual capacity	↓↓	↓↓↓	↓↓
Vital capacity	↔	↔ or ↓	↔ or ↓
FEV$_1$	↔	↓ or ↔	↔
FEV$_1$/VC	↔	↔	↔
Total lung capacity	↓	↓↓	↓
Compliance	↔	↓↓	↓
Work of breathing	↑	↑↑	↑
Airway resistance	↓	↑	↓
V/Q mismatch	↑	↑	↑↑
DLCO	↔	↔	↔
PaO$_2$	↑	↓↓	↓
PaCO$_2$	↓	↑	↓
A–a gradient	↔	↑	↑↑

↑, increase; ↓, decrease; ↔, no change (multiple arrows represent the degree of intensity). CO$_2$, carbon dioxide; FEV$_1$, forced expiratory volume in 1 s; V/Q, ratio of ventilation to perfusion; DLCO, diffusion capacity of lung for carbon monoxide; PaO$_2$, partial pressure of oxygen; PaCO$_2$, = partial pressure of carbon dioxide. Modified with permission from: Sarvanakumar et al. Obesity and obstetric anaesthesia. *Anesthesia* 2006;61: 36–48, from Blackwell Publishing.

During pregnancy, resting minute ventilation increases primarily due to increase in tidal volume. In contrast, obese individuals with increased chest wall mass show a tendency to rapid shallow breathing pattern. This particular breathing pattern optimizes the work of breathing thus avoiding diaphragmatic muscle fatigue (25). However, in obesity, with increasing ventilation when breathing frequency and dead space increases, rapid breathing may become uneconomical leading to ventilatory failure (26).

The adverse changes in the respiratory system illustrate that the obese parturient has minimal or absent pulmonary reserve and can develop hypoxemia rapidly.

Obstructive Sleep Apnea

Obesity is linked to many respiratory conditions which include asthma, OSA, OHS, pulmonary embolism, and aspiration pneumonia. With increased prevalence, obesity is now considered an emerging cause of chronic respiratory failure (27).

The prevalence of OSA in pregnancy is unknown and in many cases may be undiagnosed. It has been suggested that pregnancy may precipitate or exacerbate this condition (28). During normal pregnancy it is not uncommon to have upper airway congestion and edema; which in the obese parturient at risk can precipitate OSA. OSA is characterized by periodic apnea during sleep that produces hypoxia and sleep disruption. Obesity in pregnancy complicated by OSA can have adverse effects on the mother and the fetus. Repetitive significant

hypoxemia episodes concurrent with apneic episodes results in maternal hemodynamic consequences, such as elevation of maternal systemic and pulmonary artery pressures, right-sided heart failure and cardiac arrhythmias. Pulmonary vasoconstriction secondary to hypoxia and hypercapnia is believed to be the pathophysiology of this process. Pulmonary hypertension when superimposed by the physiologic changes of pregnancy and labor produces a lethal condition (29).

Maternal oxygen desaturation during apnea can result in fetal hypoxia as demonstrated by resultant fetal heart rate abnormalities. Episodic fetal hypoxia may result in intrauterine fetal growth retardation (30).

Careful history taking and prompt diagnosis by polysomnography would allow early treatment of OSA. Since daytime fatigue is very common in normal pregnancy, OSA is easily missed in this patient population. A recent systemic review and meta-analysis of clinical screening tests for OSA reported that the STOP questionnaire (S = **S**noring, T = **T**iredness, O = **O**bserved apnea, P = Elevated blood **p**ressure) is an excellent screening test for moderate-to-severe OSA (31) and must be ascertained preoperatively in the morbidly obese parturients. Patients who present with combination of high screening score, recurrent apneic episodes, and/or desaturations during immediate postoperative period were shown to be at increased risk of recurrent postoperative respiratory events (odds ratio = 21) (32). Therefore, these patients require close surveillance and postoperative monitoring to prevent adverse catastrophic respiratory events.

Nasal CPAP is the mainstay of therapy for OSA. Diagnosis of OSA early in the prenatal period allows initiation of CPAP therapy. CPAP has been used successfully with improved perinatal outcome, with no adverse effects during pregnancy (33).

Cardiovascular Changes

The blood volume and cardiac output increases during pregnancy beginning early first trimester. Obesity, on the other hand, independently increases blood volume and cardiac output to double that of pregnancy. The increased cardiac output is required to meet high metabolic demands related to increased fat and increased work of breathing. Cardiac output increases by 30 to 35 mL/min for every 100 g of fat tissue (34).

During normal pregnancy there is additional elevation of cardiac output during labor, and immediate postpartum period (125% increased from pre-pregnancy values). Obese parturients with reduced functional reserves may not be able to tolerate this dramatic increase in cardiac demand and is therefore at much higher risk during the peripartum period. In addition, obesity is a risk factor for peripartum cardiomyopathy, a potentially lethal disease (35).

The systemic vascular resistance decreases during normal pregnancy, and is about 20% below pre-pregnancy value at term (36). In an obese or morbidly obese parturient, due to generalized atherosclerosis, the arterial walls can be less compliant, thus the normal pregnancy–associated afterload reduction, may not occur to the same extent (37).

The combination of higher afterload and increased cardiac output contributes to the significant left ventricular hypertrophy that is found in obese parturients (37). In normal pregnancy, there is an increase in left ventricular diameter (38). However, this increase occurs without a corresponding enlargement in wall thickness. In contrast, cardiac adaptation to obesity results in left ventricular dilatation as well as ventricular hypertrophy (eccentric hypertrophy). Veille et al. (37) demonstrated significantly greater left ventricular posterior wall thickness and interventricular septal thickness with smaller radius-to-wall thickness in obese pregnant patients. This adaptation seems to be important to maintain normal systolic function in obese pregnant patients (Fig. 35-3).

In spite of hypertrophy, left ventricular size and function are shown to be normal in otherwise healthy obese pregnant women during the third trimester of pregnancy (37).

Up to about 15% of pregnant women at term experience a significant drop in blood pressure and bradycardia when they assume the supine position, the so-called supine hypotensive syndrome. This phenomenon is more pronounced in obese parturients since the fat pannus further contributes to pressure on the inferior vena cava in the supine position. Although left uterine decubitus (LUD) position is usually an effective measure to improve venous return, it may be very hard to achieve the LUD position in obese women due to the extra weight.

Tamoda et al. (39) studied the effects of obesity on maternal hemodynamic changes. They concluded that obesity during pregnancy is clearly a risk factor for hypertension, hemoconcentration, and poor cardiac function. Obese parturients secrete excess insulin from the pancreas since adipose tissue is resistant to insulin. This hyperinsulinemia is considered to be the main cause of hypertension (40). During pregnancy, hyperinsulinemia will be more severe due to the fat deposition and enhanced insulin secretion due to estrogen (41). The possible mechanism for hemoconcentration is also thought to be due to sympathetic nervous activity caused by

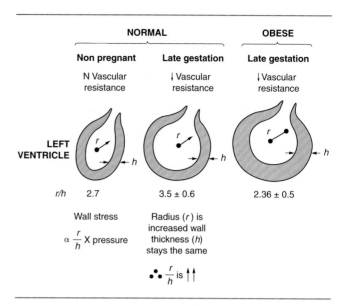

FIGURE 35-3 Cardiovascular effects of pregnancy. Illustration of radius-to-wall thickness ratio (r/h) in nonpregnant, pregnant, and obese pregnant patients. The ratio in obese pregnant patient was significantly smaller than in pregnant patients but similar to that of nonpregnant patients. Modified with permission from: Veille JC, Hanson R. Obesity, pregnancy, and left ventricular functioning during the third trimester. *Am J Obstet Gynecol* 1994;171:980–983.

hyperinsulinemia. Pre-pregnancy obesity is a significant risk factor for preeclampsia (42).

The hypertrophied myocardium that is found in morbidly obese population is vulnerable to serious arrhythmias. Drenick et al. (43) demonstrated that malignant arrhythmias can arise even with minor Q-Tc prolongations in morbidly obese patients undergoing stressful period (upper limit for a normal Q-T interval ranges from 0.425 to 0.44 seconds). Therefore, physiologic stresses should be minimized by appropriate measures in these patients. Screening and perioperative monitoring for Q-T interval prolongation, prophylactic beta-blockade during the stressful period, and avoidance of medications known to enhance sympathetic tone or to prolong the Q-T interval is recommended in this subset of morbidly obese patients (43).

There have been reports of sudden cardiac arrest with positional change in morbidly obese surgical patients (44). The mechanism of cardiovascular collapse was believed to be three-fold: (1) Further decrease in lung volume and vital capacity secondary to high intra-abdominal pressure in the supine position while there was an increase in the ventilation requirement; (2) inability to increase ventilation due to respiratory center dysfunction; (3) inability of the already failing hypoxic myocardium to handle the shift of blood to the central circulation on assuming the supine position.

Gastrointestinal Changes

Aspiration of gastric contents, although rare in the current obstetric practice, is a serious risk of general anesthesia. Obesity is associated with several risk factors that increase the risk for aspiration. These include increased incidence of emergent operative delivery (45–47), difficult mask ventilation (48), difficult intubation (47,49) gastro-esophageal reflux disease (50), and co-morbidities such as diabetes (41).

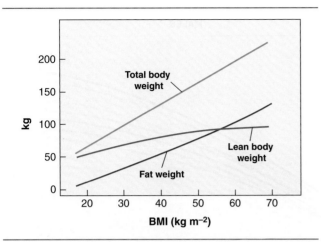

FIGURE 35-4 Relationship of TBW, fat weight, and LBW to BMI in a standard height male. LBW and fat weight were derived from the equations of Janmahasatian et al. Modified with permission from: Ingrande J, Lemmens HJM. Dose adjustment of anesthetics in the morbidly obese. *BJA* 2010;105:i16–i23.

Endocrine Changes

Gestational diabetes and type II diabetes are both more frequently associated with obesity (6,41). Optimum glucose control is of utmost importance in these patients for the best possible outcome in pregnancy. During labor, insulin therapy should be adjusted to achieve levels between 4 and 8 mmol/L to prevent neonatal hypoglycemia. Following delivery, further reduction in insulin dose is required to prevent maternal hypoglycemia (51).

Dose Adjustment of Anesthetic Drugs

In morbidly obese patients there are changes in the cardiac output, extra cellular fluid volume, and body composition, which alter the pharmacokinetic properties of most drugs (52,53).

Although fat mass accounts for most of the increase in TBW, it is poorly perfused and therefore its increase in obese patients will not show proportionate increase in the volume of distribution of lipophilic drugs as obesity increases (Fig. 35-4).

Lean body weight (LBW) is significantly correlated to cardiac output (54). Drug clearance also increases proportionately with LBW (53). These data suggests that the drug administration in morbidly obese patients should be based on LBW. Administration of drugs based on TBW may result in overdose.

Ideal body weight (IBW) is a term that describes the weight that people are expected to weigh based on age, sex, and height. There are numerous equations to calculate the IBW. Before the introduction of BMI, IBW was used to define obesity. A person weighing greater than 120% of IBW was considered obese, and greater than 200% as pathologic obese. Administration of drugs based on IBW may result in underdosing in the morbidly obese patient because it does not account for the associated changes in body composition in obesity (52). The LBW is estimated as 20% to 30% above the IBW (55).

Although LBW is the most appropriate for scaling drug doses, most equations to calculate LBW have limitations at extremes of obesity (52). Recently, Janmahasatian et al. (54) derived LBW equations for patients weighing between 40 and 220 kg. These data can be used to easily approximate LBW (Fig. 35-5).

There are alterations in pharmacodynamic properties of drugs also due to the effect of obesity on cardiac and respiratory functions. Morbidly obese patients show increased sensitivity to medications with respiratory and myocardial depressant effects.

Induction Agents

Thiopental and propofol are commonly used intravenous induction agents. Administration of these agents based on TBW may result in overdose and profound hemodynamic changes. When morbidly obese subjects were given propofol based on LBW, they required similar doses and had similar time to hypnosis as lean control subjects given propofol based on TBW (55).

Opioids

Morbidly obese patients show exaggerated respiratory depression with opioids and are more susceptible to obstruction of the upper airway and hypoxemia when administered in the perioperative period (56). Almost half of the adverse respiratory events secondary to opioids were reported in obese or morbidly obese patients. If opioids are required in this patient population, the dosing should be calculated according to LBW (53), titrate as needed. Serious consideration should be given to the need for continuous monitoring in a high dependency unit.

Inhalational Agents

Newer, less lipophilic, less soluble agents such as sevoflurane and desflurane show no difference in time to awakening in morbidly obese subjects when compared with lean subjects (57). Although isoflurane is more lipophilic than sevoflurane and desflurane, the effect of BMI on uptake is clinically insignificant for procedures lasting less than 2 to 4 hours.

Neuromuscular Blockers
Succinylcholine
The rapid onset and short duration of action makes succinylcholine the neuromuscular blocking agent of choice in morbidly obese patients. Two factors that determine the duration of action of succinylcholine, namely the pseudocholinesterase level and the amount of extracellular fluid, are increased in the morbidly obese patients (58). Therefore, a larger dose of succinylcholine based on TBW is recommended to achieve optimal intubating conditions (59). However, the longer time to 50% twitch recovery (which should allow adequate spontaneous ventilation) associated with the large dose based on TBW could be a disadvantage if problems were encountered during intubation and subsequent mask ventilation.

Nondepolarizing Muscle Relaxants
Intermediate acting drugs such as vecuronium, rocuronium, cisatracurium, or atracurium are commonly used in the current clinical practice. The dosing based on IBW is recommended to avoid prolonged recovery in obese (53) (Table 35-4).

■ PREGNANCY-RELATED PROBLEMS AND PERINATAL OUTCOME

Obesity complicates obstetric management because of the associated co-morbidities. Obesity increases the risk of emergency cesarean delivery in majority of the cohort studies (60,61). Obesity is shown to be a major predictor of maternal mortality and major complications (6). Maternal pregnancy–related complications such as gestational diabetes, gestational hypertension, preeclampsia, induction/augmentation of labor and cesarean section are significantly increased in

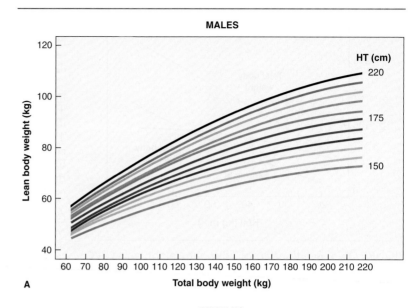

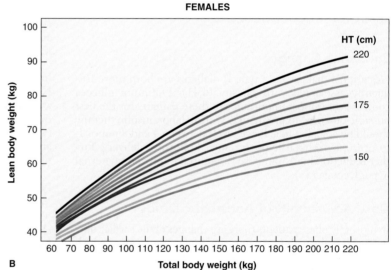

FIGURE 35-5 Estimated lean body weight for men and women with weights between 60 and 220 kg and heights between 150 and 200 cm. Estimates are derived from the equation of Janmahasatian et al. Modified with permission from: Lemmens JM. Perioperative pharmacology in morbid obesity. *Curr Opin Anesthesiol* 2010;23:85–91).

TABLE 35-4 Weight-Based Dosing Scalar Recommendation for Commonly Used IV Anesthetic Drugs

Drug	Dosing Scalar
Thiopental	Induction: LBW Maintenance: TBW
Propofol	Induction: LBW Maintenance: TBW
Fentanyl	LBW
Remifentanil	LBW
Succinylcholine	TBW
Vecuronium	IBW
Rocuronium	IBW
Atracurium	IBW
Cisatracurium	IBW

IBW, ideal body weight; LBW, lean body weight; TBW, total body weight. Adapted from: Ingrande J, Lemmens HJM. Dose adjustment of anesthetics in the morbidly obese. *BJA* 2010;105:i16–i23.

obese women (6). Barau et al. in a study involving more than 17,000 singleton live births demonstrated a significant linear association between maternal pre-pregnancy BMI and risk of caesarean section in term deliveries (45). Slow progress in labor has been observed before 7 cm of cervical dilation in overweight and obese parturients compared to normal-weight parturients (62). The monitoring of uterine contractions to ensure adequate labor also could be a challenging task in an obese parturient. Obesity seems to be an independent risk factor for fetal macrosomia. The morbidly obese patient, with or without diabetes, and with or without excessive weight gain during pregnancy is at increased risk of having a macrosomic fetus (45,62).

Fetal macrosomia (>4,000 g) may result in shoulder dystocia and birth trauma. Obesity, especially when combined with diabetes, may be associated with increase in birth defects such as neural tube defects and abdominal wall defects (63). In obese parturients, the *in utero* diagnosis of fetal defects are often delayed or missed because of difficult ultrasound imaging. The less than optimal imaging of anatomical structures of the fetal heart, spine, kidneys, diaphragm, and umbilical cord are associated with increasing BMI (64).

Obesity is the most prevalent risk factor for unexplained still birth (65). The mechanisms suggested include decreased ability to perceive changes in fetal movement, atherosclerosis affecting placental blood flow, and desaturation secondary to OSA (66). External fetal monitoring is difficult in the presence of maternal obesity; therefore, internal fetal monitoring may be more effective. Occasionally, the morbidly obese woman may be unaware of pregnancy until full term (67).

The perioperative complication rate is also increased (61,68) in obese women and include (1) increased intraoperative blood loss of >1,000 mL, (2) increased operative time, (3) increased postoperative wound infection and endometritis (even with elective cesarean delivery and antibiotic prophylaxis), and (4) need for vertical incision, which has a wound complication rate of 12%.

When planning for cesarean delivery, the care team should be aware of the longer time required to prepare and commence surgery in obese patients. Therefore, when an emergent or urgent cesarean delivery is required, the decision to delivery interval may be longer in obese parturients. Thomas et al. (69) demonstrated that prolonged decision to delivery intervals of more than 75 minutes may result in poor maternal and fetal outcomes, and therefore proper planning is required and all emergency caesarean deliveries should occur within this time. Currently, there are no studies that adequately address decision to delivery interval in obese patients.

Pregnancy Following Bariatric Surgery

Initial reports indicate that following bariatric surgery and adequate weight loss, many of the obesity-related detrimental effects on fertility and pregnancy are reversed (70). The American College of Obstetricians and Gynecology recommends that women should avoid pregnancy for 18 months after bariatric surgery, which is the rapid weight loss period (71). According to recent case reports, significant maternal and fetal problems can occur post-bariatric surgery (71–74) including mechanical obstructive problems or herniation due to the growing uterus. Vitamin B12, folate, and vitamin K deficiency may be present in up to 70% of post-bariatric surgery patients. These patients may present with peripheral neuropathy secondary to nutritional deficiency (72) or rapid weight loss (73). A thorough history and physical examination is mandatory before a neuraxial block is performed in these patients with neuropathy.

Adverse neonatal outcome due to vitamin K deficiency following pre-pregnancy bariatric surgery also has been reported (74). These include increased incidence of congenital abnormalities, small for gestational age, and intrauterine growth retardation.

■ ANESTHETIC MANAGEMENT

Transport and positioning: Standard operating room tables have a maximum weight limit of approximately 200 kg. Operating tables (Herculean tables) that will support up to 455 kg with extra width are available. Particular care should be taken to prevent pressure-related injuries. Patient should be properly secured on the operating table with strapping so as to achieve adequate LUD. Sufficient number of personnel should be available for safe transfer of patient to the operating room and table.

Vascular access: Peripheral venous access can be difficult and extravasations may not be immediately apparent. The use of ultrasound guided peripheral venous access, which is becoming increasingly popular, can be very helpful. Ultrasound guided central venous access may be necessary if the peripheral access is inadequate or unobtainable.

Monitoring: Noninvasive blood pressure measurement requires appropriately sized cuff; if the cuff is too small both systolic and diastolic readings will be overestimated. The forearm may be used if the upper arm is too large or conical shape. Invasive arterial pressure monitoring is necessary in some cases to accurately monitor the blood pressure.

Evaluation of the Airway

In obese patients, use of a single test such as Mallampati score alone, in predicting potential difficult airway in the obese parturient seems to have a lesser value when compared to lean patients. A study involving more than 100 morbidly obese patients, more than 50% of the difficult laryngoscopies were not detected by the Mallampati assessment alone. In contrast, the multivariate simplified airway risk (SAR) index, which combines several airway risk factors, resulted in a much greater ability to predict actual occurrence of grade 3–4 laryngeal views (49). Therefore, a complete airway evaluation including Mallampati score, mouth opening, evaluation of the dentition, ability to protrude the lower teeth beyond the upper teeth, thyromental distance, range of motion of the neck, and a measure of neck circumference should be performed just before any anesthetic procedure in obese parturients (see Chapter 22).

Aspiration Prophylaxis

Effective prophylactic measures increase gastric pH, reduce gastric volume, and therefore, decrease the risk of pneumonitis should aspiration occur.

Prophylactic measures include:

1. Antacid: All parturients should receive 30 mL of a nonparticulate acid, such as 0.3 molar sodium citrate, immediately before or within 20 minutes before induction of anesthesia.
2. For elective cesarean delivery, an H_2-receptor antagonist (ranitidine 150 mg or famotidine 20 mg) or a proton pump inhibitor (omeprazole 40 mg) should be administered orally the night before and again 60 to 90 minutes before the induction of anesthesia. Administration of metoclopramide 10 mg orally 60 minutes before or intravenously 30 minutes before induction of anesthesia increases the lower esophageal sphincter tone and accelerates gastric emptying (75), which is particularly beneficial in obese parturients.
3. For emergency cesarean delivery, metoclopramide 10 mg should be administered intravenously. In addition, ranitidine 50 mg or omeprazole 40 mg also should be given intravenously. Although ranitidine may not have an effect at the time of induction of anesthesia, there will be a decrease risk of aspiration pneumonitis at the time of extubation. Although H_2-receptor antagonists begin to work within 30 minutes of administration, the peak effect occurs in 60 to 90 minutes. The duration of action of the drug is long enough to cover emergence from anesthesia during cesarean delivery (76). Some obstetric units administer H_2-receptor antagonists orally every 6 hours to morbidly obese parturients in labor.

Antibiotic Prophylaxis

Because of the increased postoperative wound infection and endometritis in obese parturients (47,68), timely administration of antibiotic prophylaxis during cesarean delivery is important. According to the new ACOG guidelines (77) antibiotic prophylaxis should be administered within 60 minutes of the start of the cesarean delivery.

Thromboprophylaxis

The risk of thromboprophylaxis is increased in obese parturients. The incidence of thromboembolism was shown to be 2.5% in obese parturients and only 0.6% in the normal-weight parturient (6). Early ambulation and graduated compression stockings are recommended for obese parturients in the postpartum period (71). Thromboprophylaxis with postpartum low molecular weight heparin should be considered in obese parturients at high risk for venous thromboembolism (VTE), especially those on bed rest or having surgery (71).

Neuraxial Anesthesia and Analgesia Techniques for Labor and Delivery

Epidural for Labor Analgesia

Advantages
Neuraxial labor analgesia has been widely accepted as the most effective, safe and the least depressive form of intrapartum analgesia currently available. Effective pain control during labor can significantly improve maternal respiratory function, reduce oxygen consumption, and attenuate sympathetically mediated cardiovascular stress response (78,79). A functional epidural catheter *in situ* helps avoid the implementation and associated risks of general anesthesia and tracheal intubation should any urgent operative delivery be required. According to a prospective study by Hood et al. (47), 48% of laboring morbidly obese parturients required emergency cesarean section, compared with 9% of control laboring patients.

Potential Difficulties
Locating the epidural space and obtaining adequate neuraxial block may present unique challenges in this patient population: (1) Proper positioning of the patient and palpation of the midline may be difficult; (2) there is a high incidence of false loss of resistance when this technique is used to locate the epidural space due to the presence of fat pockets (47); (3) a high incidence of accidental dural puncture (47) and epidural venous puncture (80) also has been reported. Initial failure rate for epidural catheter placement in obese parturients can be as high as 42% and multiple attempts at catheter placement are common (47).

Early placement of epidural catheter should be encouraged to allow ample time for this potentially difficult procedure. Sitting position is preferable and landmarks may be easier to identify compared to the lateral position. In recent years, prior to placement of regional blocks, ultrasound has been used to identify the landmarks so as to facilitate proper epidural placement. Ultrasound (US) imaging in the transverse plane can reliably determine the skin puncture site, predict the depth to the epidural space, and thereby facilitate epidural catheter placement in obese parturients (81). A 5.0 MHz curved US array probe provides accurate measurements.

Clinkscales et al. (82) presented a mathematical formula that can be used to calculate the depth of skin to epidural space in centimeters relative to BMI and age:

$$\text{Depth} = 3.0 + (0.11 \times \text{BMI}) - (0.01 \times \text{age}) \text{ in centimeters}$$

One may use this formula to decide whether it is necessary to use an extra long epidural needle to locate the epidural space, in the absence of ultrasound equipment. Multiple studies (81,83), however, have reported that only a small percentage of obese patients have epidural space deeper than 8 cm. Therefore, in most cases a standard epidural needle is of adequate length and a longer needle should only be used when necessary. The long needles may bend more easily and are more difficult to steer in the intended direction and thus have greater potential for injury.

Frequent evaluation of the quality of the labor epidural block in these patients is vital because several investigators (47,84) have demonstrated high risk of epidural failure in obese patients. Any questionable catheters should be replaced promptly. One should be aware that opioid containing solutions can mask a malpositioned epidural catheter because of the pain relief caused by the absorption of opioids.

The epidural catheter may move as much as 2 cm out of the epidural space when an obese patient stretches her back with the catheter already secured to the skin (85). Therefore, it is recommended that the obese parturient should straighten the back in the upright sitting position or lateral position before securing the catheter (86).

Combined Spinal-epidural (CSE) for Labor Analgesia

The CSE technique offers the advantage of combining rapid onset of subarachnoid analgesia with the flexibility of continuous epidural analgesia. However, the function of the epidural catheter inserted under CSE technique is uncertain until after the duration of spinal analgesia wears off. Possible delayed recognition of nonfunctional catheter therefore is a concern in this high risk obese parturient with a possible difficult airway.

Continuous Spinal for Labor Analgesia

Continuous spinal technique is one of the most reliable regional techniques available for providing both analgesia and anesthesia in the morbidly obese parturient. However, its acceptance and usage is currently minimal due to limitations on the proper size needles and catheters. Currently, what are available for continuous spinal techniques in the United States include epidural kits with 17 or 18 G Tuohy-type epidural needle and 20 G epidural catheters or the Wiley Spinal continuous catheters. Because of the high incidence of post-dural puncture headache (PDPH) rate that accompany the use of the epidural needle and catheter, continuous spinal anesthesia is considered a less favorable routine option in obstetric patients. However, the incidence of PDPH appears to be lower in morbidly obese parturients compared to normal-weight parturients (87).

Morbid obesity increases the cesarean delivery rate. The need for emergent or urgent cesarean delivery during labor is also higher. The rate of epidural failure is shown to be higher in morbidly obese parturients (47). Therefore, a continuous spinal catheter can provide reliable rapid onset of surgical anesthesia with low dose local anesthetics.

It is important that the continuous spinal catheter is clearly labeled and strict sterility is maintained. Communication with all personnel involved in her care is crucial so as to avoid accidental administration of epidural doses of medications.

Anesthesia for Cesarean Delivery

Patient Positioning During Cesarean Delivery
Optimal positioning before the induction of anesthesia as shown in Figure 35-6B is critical prior to induction of general anesthesia in the morbidly obese parturient.

In this ramped position, the shoulders are elevated with blankets or the ramp/Troop elevation pillow under the patient's thorax and head allowing the breasts and soft tissues to fall away from the chin and to open up the neck area. Sniffing position is obtained by flexing the neck on the chest with blankets or pillows under the occiput and extending the head on the neck (atlanto-occipital extension) by tilting the head

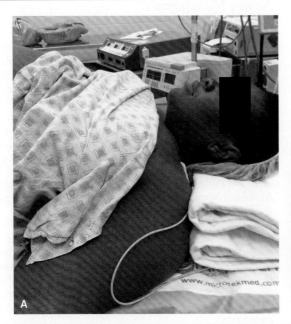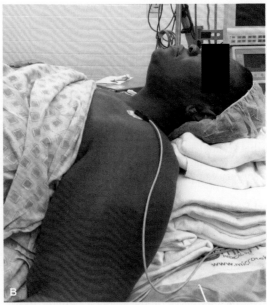

FIGURE 35-6 A: Morbidly obese parturient in the supine position. **B:** The same patient correctly positioned for laryngoscopy in the ramped position.

backwards. When morbidly obese patient is correctly positioned for laryngoscopy in the ramped position, an imaginary horizontal line can be drawn from the sternal notch to the external auditory meatus (88).

Even when counting on a neuraxial block for surgical anesthesia, patients should be positioned optimally on the operating room table in the ramped position, and devices to establish an airway should be immediately available.

In morbidly obese parturients the panniculus needs to be retracted to permit adequate surgical exposure. The panniculus can be retracted caudad, cephalad, or vertically depending on the surgical incision (Fig. 35-7). A panniculus may weigh over 70 kg in some patients. When a heavy panniculus is retracted cephalad, as commonly done to enable a Pfannenstiel incision, it can cause aortocaval compression, maternal hypotension, respiratory distress, nonreassuring fetal heart tones, and even fetal death (89).

Anesthetic Technique

The anesthetic options for cesarean delivery include neuraxial anesthesia and general anesthesia. Neuraxial techniques include epidural, single shot spinal, continuous spinal, and CSE.

Neuraxial Techniques

Epidural Anesthesia

Epidural anesthesia using a catheter technique offers the advantage of the ability to prolong the block and respiratory plus hemodynamic stability with titrated dosing. Epidural is the preferred technique if a functional catheter is already in place. The height of an epidural block for a given volume of local anesthetic is shown to be proportional to BMI and maternal weight, not height (83). Therefore, epidural local

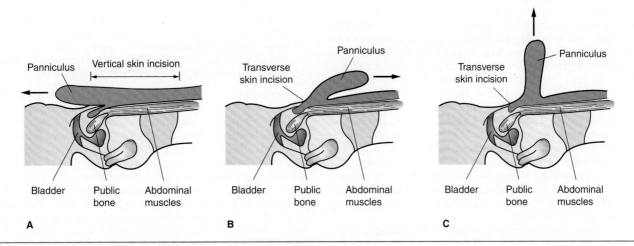

FIGURE 35-7 The panniculus is shown (**A**) retracted caudad to permit a vertical incision above; (**B**) retracted cephalad to permit a transverse Pfannenstiel incision; and (**C**) retracted vertically. Direction of retraction is shown by arrows. Modified with permission from: Hodgkins R, Husain FJ. Cesarean section associated with gross obesity. *Br J Anaesth* 1980;52:919–923.

anesthetics should be gradually titrated to avoid high block and its consequences.

Single Shot Spinal

Although spinal anesthesia provides quick onset, reliable, and dense surgical anesthesia for cesarean delivery, there are many concerns of using single shot spinal anesthesia in morbidly obese parturients. These include hemodynamic compromise due to sudden onset of high thoracic block and inability to prolong the block. In obese patients, the block can be often exaggerated. Large buttocks place the vertebral column in the Trendelenburg position; cerebral spinal fluid volume also shown to be decreased in obese patients (90). In most cases, surgery can exceed 2 hours (61).

Combined Spinal-epidural (CSE) Anesthesia

The CSE technique is the most common technique that is currently used in obese parturients undergoing cesarean delivery. The advantages with the CSE technique include: (1) It allows the spinal dose reduction; (2) reducing the dose helps to minimize hemodynamic effect of the block; (3) the quality of the sensory block and surgical anesthesia is superior to an epidural anesthesia; (4) the epidural catheter allows the option to extend the block with the indwelling epidural catheter.

Continuous Spinal Anesthesia

This technique offers the advantages of spinal anesthesia with the ability to prolong the block, and hemodynamic stability due to the possibility of incremental dosing.

General Anesthesia

General anesthesia is hazardous in the morbidly obese parturient. As reviewed earlier, there are a number of features of morbidly obese parturients that increase the risk of hypoxia during rapid sequence induction of anesthesia. However, general anesthesia may be required in emergency cesarean delivery or when regional anesthesia is contraindicated or technically difficult. Endotracheal intubation is an essential component of general anesthesia for cesarean delivery. Pregnancy alone increases the frequency of failed intubation rate by eight- to ten-fold when compared with nonpregnant population (91). Endotracheal intubation via direct laryngoscopy may be difficult or impossible in morbidly obese patients due to several reasons. These include increased amount of soft tissues of the upper airways, increased tongue size, large breasts, short neck with increased circumference, and difficult neck extension due to the presence of large posterior fat pad. One-third of the tracheal intubations are shown to be difficult in morbidly obese parturients, with a failure rate of 6% (47). Mask ventilation is also difficult or impossible in obese patients. BMI of 30 kg/m^2 or greater has been identified as one of the independent predictors for difficult mask ventilation grade 3, which is defined as inadequate mask ventilation or requiring two providers (48). Isono et al. demonstrated that in obese patients mandibular advancement (a helpful maneuver to relieve airway obstruction) does not improve retropalatal airway, as it may in nonobese persons (92). After induction of anesthesia there is reduced compliance and increased resistance of the lungs also due to a sharp decrease in lung volumes.

Therefore, pregnancy and obesity each independently increases the risk of failed or difficult intubation and ventilation. Both conditions also increase the oxygen consumption, reduce the FRC, and shorten the time before hypoxemia develops.

Airway Management

Prior to induction of general anesthesia of a morbidly obese parturient, anesthesiologist should ensure presence of additional experienced personnel and availability of difficult intubation equipment. The equipment should include videolaryngoscope, laryngeal mask airway (LMA size 3 and 4), Fastrach™ LMA, Combitube™ and percutaneous cricothyrotomy kit, connected to high pressure jet ventilator to maintain oxygenation and ventilation should attempts at intubation fail (93). The short-handled laryngoscope and small diameter endotracheal tube (6.5 or 7.0) should be prepared for intubation. An assortment of laryngoscope blades and various sizes of endotracheal tubes should be immediately available. Anesthesiologists should be familiar with the American Society of Anesthesiologists Practice Parameter on the Difficult Airway (93).

If difficulty with the airway is anticipated prior to induction of anesthesia, and it is not an emergency situation, the parturient should be prepared for awake fiberoptic intubation through oral route with adequate topicalization of the airway. If time permits, topicalization of the upper airway and "one quick look" with a laryngoscope to evaluate the upper airway in an awake patient can be performed before induction of anesthesia.

The videolaryngoscopy represents a recent addition to airway management. Videolaryngoscopy has been shown to provide a better view of the larynx and improvement in the intubation technique. It does not require alignment of oral–pharyngeal–tracheal axis which may be difficult to achieve in some cases. Its design makes it potentially useful for emergency situations. Marrel et al. (94) in a randomized study involving 80 morbidly obese patients found that the grade of laryngoscopy was significantly lower (at least one or two points on the Cormack–Lehane scale) with the videolaryngoscope compared with the direct vision laryngoscopy ($P <$ 0.001). It could possibly reduce the timing for intubation and the number of intubation attempts.

Refer to Chapter 22 for details on management of the difficult airway. However, a parturient requiring an emergent cesarean delivery may not be a candidate for awake fiberoptic intubation. In this situation, anesthesiologist should call for an experienced surgeon capable of performing emergency surgical airway in case intubation fails. Alternative methods of intubation should be readily available in case conventional laryngoscopy fails.

The alternative methods include:

1. Videolaryngoscope
2. Intubating LMA (Fastrach™ LMA). The Fastrach™ intubating LMA is shown to be associated with high success rate (96.3%) of tracheal intubation (95) in morbidly obese patients. It allows "blind" or fiberscope guided endotracheal tube placement through the LMA.

Fortunately, in recent years many airway devices/techniques have been introduced to facilitate intubation in difficult or failed airway situations. Various supraglottic devices are available to establish an artificial airway, if intubation fails. Currently, there are many other supraglottic and extraglottic devices to ensure airway control, The supraglottic devices are often effective and permit ventilation and oxygenation in "cannot intubate, cannot ventilate" situations. The LMA, first described by Archie Brain in 1983, can be considered as the device that paved the way for the supraglottic airway approach. The ProSeal LMA (PLMA) is especially helpful in parturients since it provides a separate channel opening into the upper esophagus for insertion of a standard gastric tube to prevent accidental gastric insufflation, and permits drainage of gastric fluid. Anesthesiologists should ensure that all these equipment are immediately available in the OB suite to be used in an emergency situation.

Anesthetic Induction, Maintenance, and Recovery

Preoxygenation

The aim of preoxygenation for 3 minutes with 100% oxygen with a tightly fitting mask utilizing tidal volume ventilation before induction of anesthesia is to optimize oxygen reserves and thereby increase the period of apnea without hypoxia. In urgent situations, 8 deep breaths of 100% oxygen over 60 seconds appear to be as effective as the 3-minute tidal volume method (96). However, it requires patient cooperation and high fresh gas flow at 10 L/min (See Figure 35.8).

McClelland et al. using a computational simulation found that labor and obesity both considerably accelerate preoxygenation and, more importantly, also decrease the time to arterial desaturation (97). They found that the safe period of apnea in obesity, particularly during labor, after induction of anesthesia and paralysis is as short as 40 seconds. This means after waiting for the onset of succinylcholine action there is probably time only for one attempt at tracheal intubation before a critical reduction in arterial oxygen saturation occurs with that in mind the first attempt should be the best attempt at intubation with adequate positioning, adequate maneuvers, and airway devices.

In an attempt to prolong safe apnea time, a number of preoxygenation methods have been studied. In morbidly obese patients, 30-degree reverse Trendelenburg position has been shown to prolong safe apnea time by at least 30% (98) as compared with the supine. However, head-up position has the risk of hypotension and increased difficulty with tracheal intubation. Gander et al. (99) demonstrated that application of positive end-expiratory pressure (PEEP) during induction of general anesthesia (100% oxygen through a CPAP device set at 10 cm H_2O for 5 minutes) increases

nonhypoxic apnea duration by 50% or 1 minute in morbidly obese patients. PEEP increases FRC, decreases atelectasis, and shunt.

However, the studies performed on nonpregnant women may not fully translate to pregnancy because of the effects of gravid uterus and physiologic changes of pregnancy; the effects on the uterine blood flow and the fetus are also not known.

Induction of Anesthesia

In hemodynamically stable patients with a favorable airway, rapid sequence induction may be performed with propofol. Etomidate is preferred for patients with cardiac dysfunction and ketamine may be the drug of choice for patients with significant blood loss. Succinylcholine is the drug of choice to achieve optimal laryngoscopic conditions in morbidly obese patient. Cricoid pressure should be applied concurrently by a skilled assistant. Proper placement of the endotracheal tube should be confirmed with capnography and bilateral auscultation prior to skin incision.

Exaggerated catecholamine response to laryngoscopy and intubation in hypertensive, obese parturients can be hazardous. A short acting vasodilator or antihypertensive agent should be prepared depending on the presence or absence of invasive monitoring such as an arterial line. Intravenous nicardipine or labetalol can be titrated in the absence of invasive monitoring. Additional muscle relaxation with intermediate duration nondepolarizing muscle relaxants may be required if surgery is technically difficult or prolonged in morbidly obese patients. Anesthesia can be maintained with 50% nitrous oxide/oxygen and 0.5 MAC isoflurane, sevoflurane, or desflurane. Some patients may require more than 50% oxygen to maintain satisfactory oxygen saturation. In those cases, additional hypnotic/amnestic agents should be considered.

In obese patients, intraoperative ventilation strategies to reduce atelectasis and improve oxygenation include recruitment maneuvers (35 to 55 cm H_2O for 6 seconds followed by the application of PEEP of 10 cm H_2O) and reverse Trendelenburg position. However, these maneuvers should be performed only when the patient is normovolemic and hemodynamic stabilization is reached after induction of anesthesia. The effect of these maneuvers on uterine blood flow and fetal well-being also should be taken into consideration.

Extubation

A recent report of pregnancy-associated deaths highlights the importance of continued vigilance during emergence from general anesthesia, especially in obese women. According to the report, anesthesia-related deaths occurred not during induction of general anesthesia but during emergence and recovery from airway obstruction or hypoventilation (10).

Spontaneous ventilation against an obstructed airway may also lead to rapid development of negative pressure pulmonary edema requiring reintubation. Therefore, an obese parturient with a difficult airway should be extubated fully awake. This means that the patient should be rational, oriented, and following commands in a clear manner. Full recovery of neuromuscular blockade should be proven by a monitor as well as by clinical criteria. Extubation in the semirecumbent position minimizes compression of the diaphragm by intra-abdominal contents, improves breathing, and reduces atelectasis. If the patient was on CPAP preoperatively, postoperative CPAP should be started immediately upon arrival in the PACU. If doubt exists about the adequacy of breathing, patient should remain intubated and should be transferred to an intensive care setting.

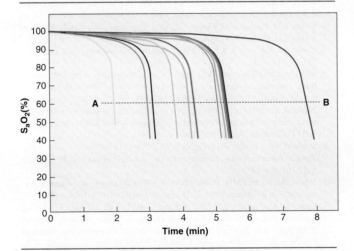

FIGURE 35-8 Time course of SaO_2 during apnea after 99% denitrogenation. The heavy dashed line represents the average pregnant subjects. Line AB transects subjects in the following order, left to right: BMI 50 and labor; BMI 35 and labor; labor; sepsis; BMI 35; twins; hypovolemia; average pregnant; anemia; preeclampsia. Modified with permission from: McClelland SH, Bogod DG, Hardman JG. Pre-oxygenation and apnoea in pregnancy: changes during labour and with obstetric morbidity in a computational simulation. *Anaesthesia* 2009;64:371–377.

Postoperative Care Following Cesarean Delivery

In the postoperative period, beach chair position, noninvasive respiratory support, aggressive physiotherapy, careful fluid management, adequate pain relief, and recovery in a high-dependency unit with O_2 saturation and end tidal CO_2 monitoring is essential to reduce pulmonary complications (9). Postoperative ambulation should be initiated early to reduce the risk of DVT, and formation of decubitus ulcers.

Because of the exaggerated respiratory depression with sedatives and opioids, postoperative pain management may be challenging in these patients. Neuraxial morphine is used commonly for postoperative pain relief following cesarean delivery. However, respiratory arrest has been reported after neuraxial morphine administration in high risk patients, such as patients with sleep apnea (100). Multimodal techniques that have been shown to improve postoperative analgesia and patient satisfaction while limiting opioid usage should be utilized more frequently in these patients. These techniques include neuraxial analgesia with low concentration local anesthetics, peripheral nerve blocks such as transverse abdominis plane (TAP) blocks (101), ilioinguinal block (102), or continuous incisional infusion of local anesthetic (103). Addition of acetaminophen and nonsteroidal anti-inflammatory drugs improve pain relief and helps to further reduce the opioid usage (101).

Effective respiratory monitoring is also critical to patient safety in clinical situations where hypoventilation, respiratory obstruction, and respiratory depression and arrest are not only a potential complication, but also a common theme in preventable deaths particularly in morbidly obese parturients. Although oximetry provides an excellent measure of oxygenation, it does not reflect adequacy in monitoring ventilation. During apnea, oxygen desaturation may not occur for several minutes, especially in patients receiving supplemental oxygen. The new technology Microstream® Capnography with Integrated Pulmonary Index technology may provide a better assessment of the patient's respiratory status which includes: (1) Accurate physiologic respiratory rate, (2) adequacy of ventilation represented by a numeric value for end tidal CO_2, (3) a breadth-to-breadth waveform that indicates any respiratory conditions such as hypoventilation, apnea, or airway obstruction whereas respiratory rate monitoring alone by itself does not provide complete factual information. As O_2 cannula is already part of patient care in the PACU, the Microstream® capnography integrates oxygen delivery and CO_2 sampling into a single line, and prevents the additional points of attachment to the patient. In the near future, capnography will become a standard of care for monitoring ventilation in high risk patients who are susceptible to hypoventilation and adverse respiratory events.

KEY POINTS

- Many of the effects of pregnancy and obesity on major organs are additive and can lead to decreased physiologic reserve and thus significant functional impairment. The obese parturient is at increased risk for diabetes, ischemic heart disease, stroke, hypertension, hypercoagulability, osteoarthritis, and gall bladder disease and pregnancy-associated complications. General anesthesia and anesthesia-related complications are much higher in the morbidly obese parturient. There are a number of features that increase the risk of hypoxia, morbidity and mortality during induction of anesthesia, intrapartum, emergence and postpartum period in these patients.

- Early placement of a neuraxial catheter during labor should be encouraged to allow ample time for this potentially difficult procedure. A functional epidural during labor avoids the risks of general anesthesia and tracheal intubation should any urgent operative intervention be required.
- Frequent evaluation of the quality of the labor epidural block in these patients is vital because of the high risk of epidural failure in obese patients. Any nonfunctioning catheters should be replaced promptly.
- A continuous spinal technique is a reliable regional technique available for providing both analgesia and anesthesia in the morbidly obese parturient. Strict sterility should be maintained to avoid infectious complications.
- When planning for cesarean delivery, the care team should be aware of the longer time required to prepare and commence surgery in obese patients.
- Even with a functioning neuraxial blockade for surgical anesthesia, the patient should be positioned optimally on the OR table in the ramped position, with immediate access to a difficult airway cart to establish an airway if necessary.
- Adequate preoperative assessment and preparation prior to induction of general anesthesia in a morbidly obese parturient is critical.
- A recent report of pregnancy-associated deaths highlights the importance of continued vigilance during emergence from general anesthesia, especially in obese women.
- Because of the exaggerated respiratory depression with sedatives, and opioids, implementation of multimodal analgesic techniques to improve postoperative analgesia and patient satisfaction, limiting opioid usage, and monitoring of oxygenation and ventilation is crucial to avoid postoperative adverse respiratory outcomes.

REFERENCES

1. Yeh J, Shelton JA. Increasing prepregnancy body mass index: analysis of trends and contributing variables. *Am J Obstet Gynecol* 2005;193:1994–1998.
2. World Health Organization. *Obesity and Overweight: Factsheet No 3011.* Geneva 2006.98.
3. McTigue K, Larson JC, Valoski A, et al. Mortality and cardiac and vascular outcomes in extremely obese women. *JAMA* 2006;296:79–86.
4. Flegal KM, Carroll MD, Ogden CL, et al. Prevalence and trends in obesity among US adults, 1999–2008. *JAMA* 2010;303:235–241.
5. Canoy D, Buchnan I. Challenges in obesity epidemiology. *Obes Rev* 2007;(8 Suppl 1):1–11.
6. Edwards LE, Hellerstedt WL, Alton IR, et al. Pregnancy complications and birth outcomes in obese and normal-weight women: effects of gestational weight change. *Obstet Gynecol* 1996;87:389–394.
7. National Institutes of Health. Clinical guidelines on the identification, evaluation, and treatment of overweight and obesity in adults-The evidence report. NIH Publication No. 98-4083 1998.
8. Stotland NE. Obesity and pregnancy. *BMJ* 2009;338:107–110.
9. Tung A. Anesthetic considerations with the metabolic syndrome. *Br J Anaesth* 2010;105:124–133.
10. Mhyre JM, Riesner MN, Polley LS, et al. A series of anesthesia-related maternal deaths in Michigan, 1985–2003. *Anesthesiology* 2007;106:1096–1104.
11. Lewis G. ed. Enquiry into Maternal and Child Health (CEMACH). Saving mothers' lives: Reviewing (Maternal) Deaths to Make Motherhood Safer 2003–2005. The Seventh Report on Confidential Enquiries into Maternal Deaths in the United Kingdom. London, CEMACH; 2007.
12. Eng M, Butler J, Bonica JJ. Respiratory function in pregnant obese women. *Am J Obstet Gynecol* 1975;123:241–245.
13. Mhyre JM. Anesthetic management for the morbidly obese pregnant woman. *Int Anesthesiol Clin* 2007;45:51–70.
14. Bevan DR, Holdcroft A, Loh L, et al. Closing volume and pregnancy. *Br Med J* 1974;1:13–15.
15. Craig DB, Wahba WM, Don HF, et al. "Closing volume" and its relationship to gas exchange in seated and supine positions. *J Appl Physiol* 1971;31:717–721.
16. Saravanakumar K, Rao SG, Cooper GM. Obesity and obstetric anaesthesia. *Anaesthesia* 2006;61:36–48.
17. Holley HS, Milic-Emili J, Becklake MR, et al. Regional distribution of pulmonary ventilation and perfusion in obesity. *J Clin Invest* 1967;46:475–481.

18. Anthonisen NR, Milic-Emili J. Distribution of pulmonary perfusion in erect man. *J Appl Physiol* 1966;21:760–766.

19. Ray CS, Sue DY, Bray G, et al. Effects of obesity on respiratory function. *Am Rev Respir Dis* 1983;128:501–506.

20. Dempsey JA, Reddan W, Rankin J, et al. Alveolar-arterial gas exchange during muscular work in obesity. *J Appl Physiol* 1966;21:1807–1814.

21. Sharp JT, Henry JP, Sweany SK, et al. The total work of breathing in normal and obese men. *J Clin Invest* 1964;43:728–739.

22. Unterborn J. Pulmonary function testing in obesity, pregnancy, and extremes of body habitus. *Clin Chest Med* 2001;22:759–767.

23. Naimark A, Cherniack RM. Compliance of the respiratory system and its components in health and obesity. *J Appl Physiol* 1960;15:377–382.

24. Douglas FG, Chong PY. Influence of obesity on peripheral airways patency. *J Appl Physiol* 1972;33:559–563.

25. Luce JM. Respiratory complications of obesity. *Chest* 1980;78:626–631.

26. Cournand A, Richards DW Jr, Bader RA, et al. The oxygen cost of breathing. *Trans Assoc Am Physicians* 1954;67:162–173.

27. Janssens JP, Derivaz S, Breitenstein E, et al. Changing patterns in long-term noninvasive ventilation: a 7-year prospective study in the Geneva Lake area. *Chest* 2003;123:67–79.

28. Kowall J, Clark G, Nono-Marcia G, et al. Precipitation of obstructive sleep apnea during pregnancy. *Obstet Gynecol* 1989;74:453–455.

29. Roberts NV, Keast PJ. Pulmonary hypertension and pregnancy–a lethal combination. *Anaesth Intensive Care* 1990;18:366–374.

30. Charbonneau M, Falcone T, Cosio MG, et al. Obstructive sleep apnea during pregnancy. Therapy and implications for fetal health. *Am Rev Respir Dis* 1991;144:461–463.

31. Ramachandran SK, Josephs LA. A meta-analysis of clinical screening tests for obstructive sleep apnea. *Anesthesiology* 2009;110:928–939.

32. Gali B, Whalen FX, Schroeder DR, et al. Identification of patients at risk for postoperative respiratory complications using a preoperative obstructive sleep apnea screening tool and postanesthesia care assessment. *Anesthesiology* 2009;110:869–877.

33. Edwards N, Blyton DM, Kirjavainen T, et al. Nasal continuous positive airway pressure reduces sleep-induced blood pressure increments in preeclampsia. *Am J Respir Crit Care Med* 2000;162:252–257.

34. Alexander JK, Dennis EW, Smith WG, et al. Blood volume, cardiac output, and distribution of systemic blood flow in extreme obesity. *Cardiovasc Res Cent Bull* 1962–1963;1:39–44.

35. Shnaider R, Ezri T, Szmuk P, et al. Combined spinal-epidural anesthesia for Cesarean section in a patient with peripartum dilated cardiomyopathy. *Can J Anaesth* 2001;48:681–683.

36. Clark SL, Cotton DB, Lee W, et al. Central hemodynamic assessment of normal term pregnancy. *Am J Obstet Gynecol* 1989;161:1439–1442.

37. Veille JC, Hanson R. Obesity, pregnancy, and left ventricular functioning during the third trimester. *Am J Obstet Gynecol* 1994;171:980–983.

38. Katz R, Karliner JS, Resnik R. Effects of a natural volume overload state (pregnancy) on left ventricular performance in normal human subjects. *Circulation* 1978;58:434–441.

39. Tomoda S, Tamura T, Sudo Y, et al. Effects of obesity on pregnant women: maternal hemodynamic change. *Am J Perinatol* 1996;13:73–78.

40. Kaplan NM. The deadly quartet. Upper-body obesity, glucose intolerance, hypertriglyceridemia, and hypertension. *Arch Intern Med* 1989;149:1514–1520.

41. Landon MB, Gabbe SG. Diabetes mellitus and pregnancy. *Obstet Gynecol Clin North Am* 1992;19:633–654.

42. Sibai BM, Gordon T, Thom E, et al. Risk factors for preeclampsia in healthy nulliparous women: a prospective multicenter study. The National Institute of Child Health and Human Development Network of Maternal-Fetal Medicine Units. *Am J Obstet Gynecol* 1995;172:642–648.

43. Drenick EJ, Fisler JS. Sudden cardiac arrest in morbidly obese surgical patients unexplained after autopsy. *Am J Surg* 1988;155:720–726.

44. Tsueda K, Debrand M, Zeok SS, et al. Obesity supine death syndrome: reports of two morbidly obese patients. *Anesth Analg* 1979;58:345–347.

45. Barau G, Robillard PY, Hulsey TC, et al. Linear association between maternal pre-pregnancy body mass index and risk of caesarean section in term deliveries. *BJOG* 2006;113:1173–1177.

46. Dempsey JC, Ashiny Z, Qiu CF, et al. Maternal pre-pregnancy overweight status and obesity as risk factor for cesarean delivery. *J Matern Fetal Neonatal Med* 2005;17:179–185.

47. Hood DD, Dewan DM. Anesthetic and obstetric outcome in morbidly obese parturients. *Anesthesiology* 1993;79:7210–7218.

48. Kheterpal S, Han R, Tremper KK, et al. Incidence and predictors of difficult and impossible mask ventilation. *Anesthesiology* 2006;105:885–891.

49. Voyagis GS, Kyriakis KP, Dimitriou V, et al. Value of oropharyngeal Mallampati classification in predicting difficult laryngoscopy among obese patients. *Eur J Anaesthesiol* 1998;15:330–334.

50. Nilsson M, Lundegårdh G, Carling L, et al. Body mass and reflux oesophagitis: an oestrogen-dependent association? *Scand J Gastroenterol* 2002;37:626–630.

51. de Valk HW, Visser GH. Insulin during pregnancy, labour and delivery. *Best Pract Res Clin Obstet Gynaecol* 2010. [Epub ahead of print].

52. Lemmens JM. Perioperative pharmacology in morbid obesity. *Curr Opin Anesthesiol* 2010;23:485–491.

53. Ingrande J, Lemmens HJM. Dose adjustment of anesthetics in the morbidly obese. *Br J Anaesth* 2010;105:i16–i23.

54. Janmahasatian S, Duffull SB, Ash S, et al. Quantification of lean bodyweight. *Clin Pharmacokinet* 2005;44:1051–1065.

55. Ingrande J, Brodsky JB, Lemmens HJ. Lean body weight scalar for the anesthetic induction dose of propofol in morbidly obese subjects. *Anesth Analg* 2010. [Epub ahead of print].

56. Benumof JL. Obesity, sleep apnea, the airway and anesthesia. *Curr Opin Anesthesiol* 2004;17:21–30.

57. Arain SR, Barth CD, Shankar H, et al. Choice of volatile anesthetic for the morbidly obese patient: sevoflurane or desflurane. *J Clin Anesth* 2005;17:13–19.

58. Bentley JB, Borel JD, Vaughan RW, et al. Weight, pseudocholinesterase activity, and succinylcholine requirement. *Anesthesiology* 1982;57:48–49.

59. Lemmens HJ, Brodsky JB. The dose of succinylcholine in morbid obesity. *Anesth Analg* 2006;102:438–442.

60. Vahratian A, Zhang J, Troendle JF, et al. Maternal prepregnancy overweight and obesity and the pattern of labor progression in term nulliparous women. *Obstet Gynecol* 2004;104:943–951.

61. Perlow JH, Morgan MA. Massive maternal obesity and perioperative cesarean morbidity. *Am J Obstet Gynecol* 1994;170:560–565.

62. Zhang J, Bricker L, Wray S, et al. Poor uterine contractility in obese women. *BJOG* 2007;114:343–348.

63. Rahaman J, Narayansingh GV, Roopnarinesingh S. Fetal outcome among obese parturients. *Int J Gynaecol Obstet* 1990;31:227–230.

64. Wolfe HM, Sokol RJ, Martier SM, et al. Maternal obesity: a potential source of error in sonographic prenatal diagnosis. *Obstet Gynecol* 1990;76:339–342.

65. Fretts RC. Etiology and prevention of stillbirth. *Am J Obstet Gynecol* 2005;193:1923–1935.

66. Davies GA, Maxwell C, McLeod L, et al. Obesity in pregnancy. *Int J Gynaecol Obstet* 2010;110:167–173.

67. Muppala H, Rafi J, Arthur I. Morbidly obese woman unaware of pregnancy until full-term and complicated by intraamniotic sepsis with pseudomonas. *Infect Dis Obstet Gynecol* 2007;2007:516–589.

68. Wall PD, Deucy EE, Glantz JC, et al. Vertical skin incisions and wound complications in the obese parturient. *Obstet Gynecol* 2003;102:952–956.

69. Thomas J, Paranjothy S, James D. National cross sectional survey to determine whether the decision to delivery interval is critical in emergency caesarean section. *BMJ* 2004;328:665.

70. Guelinekx I, Devlieger R, Vansant G, et al. Reproductive outcome after bariatric surgery: a critical review. *Hum Reprod Update* 2009;15:189–201.

71. ACOG committee opinion #315. Obesity in pregnancy. *Obstet Gynecol* 2005;106:671–675.

72. Kumar N. Nutritional neuropathies. *Neurol Clin* 2007;25:209–255.

73. Weyns FJ, Beckers F, Vanormelingen L, et al. Foot drop as a complication of weight loss after bariatric surgery: is it preventable? *Obes Surg* 2007;17:1209–1212.

74. Eerdekens A, Debeer A, Van Hoey G, et al. Maternal bariatric surgery: adverse outcomes in neonates. *Eur J Pediatr* 2010;169:191–196.

75. Brock-Utne JG, Dow TG, Welman S, et al. The effect of metoclopramide on the lower oesophageal sphincter in late pregnancy. *Anaesth Intensive Care* 1978;6:26–29.

76. Coombs DW, Hooper D, Colton T. Acid-aspiration prophylaxis by use of preoperative oral administration of cimetidine. *Anesthesiology* 1979;51:352–356.

77. ACOG Committee opinion no. 465: Antimicrobial prophylaxis for cesarean delivery: timing of administration. *Obstet Gynecol* 2010;116:791–792.

78. Von Ungern-Sternberg BS, Regli A, Bucher E, et al. The effect of epidural analgesia in labour on maternal respiratory function. *Anaesthesia* 2004;59:350–353.

79. Cascio M, Pygon B, Bernett C, et al. Labour analgesia with intrathecal fentanyl decreases maternal stress. *Can J Anaesth* 1997;44:605–609.

80. Chanimov M, Evron S, Haitov Z, et al. Accidental venous and dural puncture during epidural analgesia in obese parturients. *J Clin Anesth* 2010;22:614–618.

81. Balki M, Lee Y, Halpern S, et al. Ultrasound imaging of the lumbar spine in the transverse plane: the correlation between estimated and actual depth to the epidural space in obese parturients. *Anesth Analg* 2009;108:1876–1881.

82. Clinkscales CP, Greenfield ML, Vanarase M, et al. An observational study of the relationship between lumbar epidural space depth and body mass index in Michigan parturients. *Int J Obstet Anesth* 2007;16:323–327.

83. Watts RW. The influence of obesity on the relationship between body mass index and the distance to the epidural space from the skin. *Anaesth Intensive Care* 1993;21:309–310.

84. Dresner M, Brocklesby J, Bamber J. Audit of the influence of body mass index on the performance of epidural analgesia in labour and the subsequent mode of delivery. *BJOG* 2006;113:1178–1181.

85. Faheem M, Sarwar N. Sliding of the skin over subcutaneous tissue is another important factor in epidural catheter migration. *Can J Anaesth* 2002;49:634.

86. Hamilton CL, Riley ET, Cohen SE. Changes in the position of epidural catheters associated with patient movement. *Anesthesiology* 1997;86:778–784.

87. Faure E, Moreno R, Thisted R. Incidence of postdural puncture headache in morbidly obese parturients. *Reg Anesth* 1994;19:361–363.

88. Brodsky JB, Lemmens HJ, Brock-Utne JG, et al. Letter to the editor. Anesthetic considerations for bariatric surgery: proper positioning is important for laryngoscopy. *Anesth Analg* 2003;96:1841–1842.

89. Hodgkinson R, Husain FJ. Caesarean section associated with gross obesity. *Br J Anaesth* 1980;52:919–923.

90. Hogan QH, Prost R, Kulier A, et al. Magnetic resonance imaging of cerebrospinal fluid volume and the influence of body habitus and abdominal pressure. *Anesthesiology* 1996;84:1341–1349.

91. Vasdev GM, Harrison BA, Keegan MT, et al. Management of the difficult and failed airway in obstetric anesthesia. *J Anesthesia* 2008;22:38–48.

92. Isono S, Tanaka A, Tagaito Y, et al. Pharyngeal patency in response to advancement of the mandible in obese anesthetized persons. *Anesthesiology* 1997;87:1055–1062.

93. American Society of Anesthesiologists Task Force on Obstetric Anesthesia: Practice guidelines for obstetric anesthesia. *Anesthesiology* 2007;106:843–863.

94. Marrel J, Blanc C, Frascarolo P, et al. Videolaryngoscopy improves intubation condition in morbidly obese patients. *Eur J Anaesthesiol* 2007;24:1045–1049.

95. Frappier J, Guenoun T, Journois D, et al. Airway management using the intubating laryngeal mask airway for the morbidly obese patient. *Anesth Analg* 2003;96:1510–1515.

96. Chiron B, Laffon M, Ferrandiere M, et al. Standard preoxygenation technique versus two rapid techniques in pregnant patients. *Int J Obstet Anesth* 2004;13:11–14.

97. McClelland SH, Bogod DG, Hardman JG. Pre-oxygenation and apnoea in pregnancy: changes during labour and with obstetric morbidity in a computational simulation. *Anaesthesia* 2009;64:371–377.

98. Dixon BJ, Carden JR, Burn AJ, et al. Preoxygenation is more effective in the 25 degrees head-up position than in the supine position in severely obese patients: a randomized controlled study. *Anesthesiology* 2005;102:1110–1115.

99. Gander S, Frascarolo P, Suter M, et al. Positive end-expiratory pressure during induction of general anesthesia increases duration of nonhypoxic apnea in morbidly obese patients. *Anesth Analg* 2005;100:580–584.

100. Lamarche Y, Martin R, Reiher J, et al. The sleep apnoea syndrome and epidural morphine. *Can Anaesth Soc J* 1986;33:231–233.

101. Belavy D, Cowlishaw PJ, Howes M, et al. Ultrasound-guided transversus abdominis plane block for analgesia after Caesarean delivery. *Br J Anaesth* 2009;103:726–730.

102. Gucev G, Yasui GM, Chang TY, et al. Bilateral ultrasound-guided continuous ilioinguinal-iliohypogastric block for pain relief after cesarean delivery. *Anesth Analg* 2008;106:1220–1222.

103. Liu SS, Richman JM, Thirlby RC, et al. Efficacy of continuous wound catheters delivering local anesthetic for postoperative analgesia: a quantitative and qualitative systematic review of randomized controlled trials. *J Am Coll Surg* 2006;203:914–932.

Human Immunodeficiency Virus: Maternal and Fetal Considerations and Management

Roulhac D. Toledano • May C. M. Pian-Smith

The human immunodeficiency virus (HIV-1) was identified in 1983, and is now estimated to infect over 40 million people worldwide. Women of childbearing age comprise a growing proportion of those infected, with racial minorities in the United States affected disproportionately. An estimated 25% of infants born to these women, if untreated, will become infected with HIV. This chapter reviews the medical management of HIV-1-infected women, including early detection of infection in parturients, peripartum treatment options, and anesthetic considerations, with emphasis also on the pathogenesis of HIV and the multiorgan nature of the disease.

■ EPIDEMIOLOGY AND SCOPE OF THE DISEASE

While data most likely underestimate the true incidence of HIV-1 infection, roughly half of the 40 million individuals living with HIV worldwide are women (1). Of the industrialized countries, the United States is the most heavily affected, with an estimated 56,000 new cases annually (2). In 2006, more than 1.2 million individuals were living with HIV in the United States (3), and women comprised an estimated one-third of those infected. Of note, approximately one-quarter of these infected individuals are unaware of their HIV-positive status (4).

Both African American and Hispanic men, as well as women of ethnic and racial minority groups, are affected disproportionately in the U.S. epidemic. Indeed, the rate of new HIV and acquired immunodeficiency syndrome (AIDS) diagnoses in 2005 was 21 times higher among African American women than among white women (5). More recent statistics estimate that Blacks/African Americans account for 52% of all diagnoses of HIV infection in the United States and 44% of all persons living with an AIDS diagnosis (2). The rate of infection among Hispanics is roughly 3 times higher than that of the white population. From 2007 to 2010, males accounted for 79% of all diagnoses of infection among adults and adolescents, while the rate of HIV infection among women decreased slightly to 8/100,000 (6). Unprotected heterosexual intercourse and, secondarily, intravenous (IV) drug use with contaminated needles are the two main sources of HIV infection among female minority subgroups. Among all women, heterosexual intercourse is the primary source of infection.

In Western Europe, HIV infection is also becoming endemic, with both heterosexual transmission and cases imported from Africa accounting for a large proportion of new infections. In Eastern Europe and Asia the incidence of HIV infection is burgeoning, in large part due to IV drug use, the sex-trade industry, and subsequent secondary transmission to stable partners. In the Russian Federation and the Ukraine, women accounted for roughly 40% of the new infections in 2005, most likely acquired during heterosexual intercourse.

Sub-Saharan Africa, however, carries the greatest burden of HIV infection worldwide, with 70% of HIV-infected individuals; 68% of new infections; and more than 90% of the world's HIV-infected children and AIDS orphans (7). Statistics from the late 1990s indicate that more than 80% of the women infected with HIV worldwide were African. HIV infection rates among pregnant women in some urban centers in southern and eastern Africa reach an astounding 25% (8).

■ PATHOGENESIS OF HIV

HIV-1 is a single-stranded RNA virus that is related genetically, morphologically, and biologically to the lentivirus subfamily of retroviruses. Like other lentiviruses, HIV-1 has a complex viral genome and characteristically causes indolent infections with extensive central nervous system (CNS) involvement and long periods of clinical latency. HIV-1 infection begins when glycoproteins on the HIV lipid envelope interact with CD4 receptors and a variety of co-receptors, such as CCR5 and CXCR4, on host cells. The CD4 antigen complex was first detected on helper T cells, and was subsequently identified on B cells, macrophages, and monocytes. It is also located on placental cells, thereby providing a route for vertical transmission to the fetus in early pregnancy. Once the virus enters the cell it is copied by a reverse transcriptase enzyme into a double-stranded DNA, which can be inserted into the infected host's cells. Mutations during the process and the rapid rate of viral replication contribute to viral resistance and complicate drug therapy. The human immunodeficiency virus type 2 (HIV-2) is similar to HIV-1, but is more commonly encountered in West Africa and has a longer asymptomatic stage, lower transmission rate, and less pathogenic course than HIV-1 (9).

The most common mode of HIV-1 infection is via sexual transmission through the genital mucosa, although transmission also occurs by exposure to infected blood or blood products and by perinatal transfer from mother to child. In the United States, high-risk heterosexual transmission of HIV comprises the principal source of infection of women of all races and ethnicities, and accounts for at least 80% of new infections among women (10). Perinatal transmission can occur in utero, during labor and delivery, and postnatally from breastfeeding, although the majority occurs in the intrapartum period (11). Regardless of the mode of transmission, within 2 days the virus can be detected in peripheral lymphoid tissues and it can be cultured from the plasma within a week. Thereafter there is a rapid rise in plasma viremia, as the virus spreads to lymphoid organs and to the brain.

CD4+ T cells are infected early in the course of the disease, and play a key role in propagating the infection. The number of CD4+ cells declines sharply during initial infection and slowly rebounds as the immune system combats viral replication. An asymptomatic period marked by a balance between CD4+ cell production and destruction ensues, ending once viral replication outpaces the immune system's defenses. In general, the decline in CD4+ cells marks HIV progression from the initial infection and accounts for the profound immunodeficiency of advanced AIDS (12). Plasma viral load also serves as a marker for disease progression, and is extremely high during the acute infection and subsides during the latent stage. Patients tend to be highly infectious during the early stages of infection as a result of the high viral load. Acute infection manifests with transient flu-like symptoms of fever, fatigue, rash, headache, lymphadenopathy, pharyngitis, myalgia, arthralgia, and nausea, vomiting, and diarrhea.

■ SCREENING AND DIAGNOSTIC TESTS FOR HIV INFECTION DURING PREGNANCY

Since the mid-1990s, diagnosed cases of perinatally acquired HIV infection have declined by an estimated 90% in the United States (13). This sharp decline is attributed in part to routine HIV screening during pregnancy and the widespread availability of therapeutic drugs that prevent transmission. Preconceptual counseling for known carriers of HIV or early detection of HIV infection during pregnancy in patients whose HIV status is unknown, with subsequent counseling, are cornerstones of the prevention of mother-to-child transmission of HIV.

Currently, the Centers for Disease Control and Prevention (CDC), U.S. Public Health Service (USPHS), and the American College of Obstetricians and Gynecologists (ACOG) recommend HIV screening for all pregnant women. The so-called "opt-out" approach to prenatal HIV testing encourages health care providers to test routinely for HIV infection unless the woman specifically refuses. Under universal opt-out screening, all parturients are notified that they will receive an HIV test as part of the routine prenatal tests unless they decline. Additional written documentation of informed consent beyond that required for routine tests is not necessary. The HIV test should be performed early in pregnancy and should be repeated in the third trimester in particular "at-risk" populations, such as IV drug users, women whose partners are infected, women who themselves or whose partners have more than one sexual partner during pregnancy, women who exchange sex for money or drugs, or women who receive healthcare in areas with an elevated incidence of HIV/AIDS (14). A repeat test in the third trimester for all pregnant women, regardless of risk factors, is also considered cost-effective. If testing has not been performed prior to term gestation or if the HIV status remains unknown at the onset of labor, rapid HIV testing is recommended at the time of presentation to the labor and delivery unit, unless the patient declines. If maternal HIV status is still unknown postpartum, a rapid test is recommended. Newborns whose maternal HIV status is unknown should be tested as soon as possible after birth.

Several diagnostic tests, with varying degrees of sensitivity and specificity, are available to determine HIV status. The enzyme-linked immunosorbent assay (ELISA) detects antibodies to HIV in the patient's serum and is often the initial screening test for HIV. Rapid enzyme-linked immunoassay (EIA) blood and oral secretion tests are also available and are recommended during labor and delivery for women of unknown HIV status. Obstetrician–gynecologists may also choose to use rapid testing as their standard outpatient test (15). Currently, four rapid HIV antibody tests are available in the United States, two of which are approved for point-of-care. Results are interpreted visually; when HIV antibodies in

a positive specimen bind to HIV antigens affixed to the test strip, a color change occurs. Positive EIA tests are confirmed by a more specific test, such as a Western blot, immunofluorescence assay (IFA), or HIV RNA polymerase chain reaction (HIV RNA-PCR). In the event that a parturient of previous unknown HIV status presents in labor and has a positive rapid HIV test by the opt-out approach, delaying treatment for confirmatory tests is not feasible. The expectant mother should be counseled that her preliminary test is positive and that the newborn may be exposed to HIV. Immediate initiation of antiretroviral (ARV) prophylaxis should be recommended. Antiretroviral therapy (ART) for both the mother and child will be discontinued if the confirmatory test result is negative (16).

False-positive and false-negative results, as well as indeterminate confirmatory testing, occasionally occur. Both the EIA test and the Western blot test rely on the detection of antibodies to HIV antigens, yet there may be a period after initial infection during which adequate antibody levels have not yet formed or remain undetectable. During this "window period," a patient may be highly contagious despite negative test results. Immunosuppressive therapy may also account for false-negative results. False-positive EIA tests can be caused by autoimmune disease, hepatitis B immunization, and high parity, among other things. Indeterminate test results occur when a positive EIA test is followed by a Western blot result that is insufficient to make a definitive diagnosis. Causes of indeterminate results include partial seroconversion, organ transplantation, autoimmune disease, blood transfusions, and advanced AIDS. Repeat testing can be delayed if indeterminate test results occur early in pregnancy, as initiation of ARV prophylaxis in the absence of maternal indications is suggested after the first trimester (but no later than 28 weeks' gestation).

For patients with confirmed HIV disease, preconception counseling is highly advised. Counseling provides the opportunity to discuss modes of mother-to-child transmission, methods to avoid transmission, safe sex practices during pregnancy, means of optimizing maternal health and nutrition, when to initiate ART, and concerns about potential adverse effects of ARV therapy for both mother and fetus. Birth control options to prevent future pregnancies, smoking cessation initiatives, referrals for drug counseling, delivery options, and alternatives to breastfeeding might also be discussed. For women whose HIV-positive status is discovered during prenatal testing, similar subjects should be broached during that or subsequent prenatal visits.

■ HIV DISEASE: CLINICAL MANIFESTATIONS

It is estimated that up to 25% of HIV-1-infected people will require surgery at some stage during the course of their illness (17). Further, given the rising rate of infection among women of childbearing years, anesthesiologists will encounter infected patients in the labor and delivery suites with increasing frequency. HIV infection affects multiple organs, and the provision of care may be further complicated by opportunistic infections, substance abuse, social and domestic issues, therapeutic drugs, tumors, and the risk of viral transmission to the health care worker. The following sections review the multiple organ systems affected by HIV.

Neurologic Effects

Neurologic involvement occurs early in the course of HIV infection, but may manifest at any stage during the disease (Table 36-1). According to some sources, an estimated 80%

TABLE 36-1 Neurologic Manifestations of HIV Infection

Early (initial infection and latent phase)	Headache Retro-orbital pain Depression Irritability Peripheral neuropathies Visual disturbances
Late (AIDS)	Encephalopathy (AIDS dementia complex) Infectious/opportunistic meningitis Intracranial masses (TB, lymphoma, KS) Myopathy (including vacuolar myelopathy, chronic distal symmetric polyneuropathy) Autonomic dysfunction

of AIDS patients demonstrate neurologic abnormalities at autopsy, and roughly half suffer from overt signs and symptoms of CNS dysfunction (18). However, the frequency of HIV-1-related CNS disease has been reduced by a variety of highly effective ARV agents with improved brain penetration (19).

Like other lentiviruses, HIV-1 invades the CNS very soon after the initial systemic infection (20). During the earliest stage of primary infection, the HIV-1 virus can be isolated from the cerebrospinal fluid (CSF). Neurologic disturbances such as headache, retro-orbital pain, depression, irritability, peripheral neuropathies, and visual disturbances are not uncommon during this period of primary infection (21). An acute inflammatory demyelinating polyneuropathy similar to Guillain–Barre syndrome, cauda equina syndrome, and acute aseptic encephalitis have also been reported. In severe immunocompromised states or as the disease progresses to clinical AIDS, patients are more susceptible to diffuse encephalopathy (a.k.a., the AIDS dementia complex), infectious/opportunistic meningitis (e.g., cryptococcal or syphilitic), and focal intracranial masses, such as tuberculosis (TB), lymphomas, or, less commonly, Kaposi's sarcoma (KS).

Cerebrovascular complications, such as hemorrhage and vasculitis, may develop within cerebral tumors. In addition, CNS tumors can cause cerebral edema, elevated intracranial pressure, changes in cerebral hemodynamics, or overt cognitive dysfunction that renders the patient unable to consent to and cooperate for procedures. Myopathy and segmental or diffuse myelopathy also manifest in the late stages of infection. Vacuolar myelopathy, which affects the lateral and posterior columns of the thoracic cord, affects up to 20% of the AIDS population (22). While peripheral neuropathies may be seen during all stages of the HIV infection, patients with advanced HIV or AIDS frequently develop a chronic distal symmetric polyneuropathy, with clinical features of numbness, dysesthesias, paresthesias, weakness, and decreased deep tendon reflexes. Autonomic dysfunction, including diarrhea, syncope, and orthostatic hypotension, also can present in the later stages of HIV progression.

Pulmonary Manifestations

Pulmonary complications of HIV affect an estimated 70% of infected individuals at least once during the course of the disease (23). Causes include a variety of bacterial, viral, fungal, and parasitic opportunistic infections, as well as several noninfectious conditions. Upper respiratory tract infections, acute bronchitis, and acute sinusitis most often involve *Streptococcus pneumoniae*, *Haemophilus influenza*, and *Pseudomonas aeruginosa*. The clinical course of each of these conditions is similar in individuals with and without HIV, but HIV-infected individuals are prone to more frequent recurrences. Further, there is some evidence that bronchitis in HIV-positive patients progresses more frequently to bronchiectasis, and, in conjunction with cigarette smoking, can progress to emphysema earlier than in the non-HIV population. Bacterial pneumonia also occurs more frequently in HIV-infected individuals than in the general population. Common causative organisms include *S. pneumonia* and *H. influenza*, while *Staphylococcus aureus* and *P. aeruginosa*, as well as other gram-negative organisms, are implicated in patients with advanced disease. Abscesses, empyemas, and intrapulmonary cavitations are not uncommon complications of bacterial pneumonia in the HIV population. Viruses, too, can cause a clinical pneumonia and may play a critical role in producing other pulmonary and extrapulmonary complications of HIV, including neoplasms.

The outbreak of *Pneumocystis jiroveci* pneumonia (formerly *Pneumocystis carinii* pneumonia, PCP) among four homosexual men heralded the HIV/AIDS epidemic in the early 1980s. Despite the current widespread use of both highly active antiretroviral therapy (HAART) and prophylaxis against opportunistic infections, PCP still accounts for a large proportion of respiratory events in HIV-infected individuals. Patients susceptible to PCP generally have CD4+ counts of <200 cells/mm^3 and present with bilateral infiltrates and severe acute respiratory distress that can progress rapidly to respiratory failure. As a result, primary prophylactic therapy is often initiated when the CD4+ cell count begins to decline, when patients develop AIDS-defining diseases, or when constitutional features of HIV are present.

TB is another pulmonary complication that is strongly associated with systemic HIV and is particularly prevalent amongst IV drug users and, increasingly, among women of childbearing age. *Mycobacterium tuberculosis* infection can present at any stage during the HIV illness *de novo*, from primary infection, or as a result of reactivation of an earlier exposure. In the early stages of HIV infection, TB may present with lobe consolidation and cavitation, while in the more advanced stages patients can develop vague constitutional symptoms, extrapulmonary manifestations, and multidrug-resistant varieties that pose a significant mortality risk, as well as a public health threat (24). Other pulmonary infections that develop more often in the advanced stages of HIV/AIDS include *Mycobacterium avium* complex (MAC) and fungal infections, such as *Blastomyces dermatitidis*, *Coccidioides immitis*, *Cryptococcus neoformans*, *Aspergillus fumigatus*, and *Histoplasma capsulatum*.

Lymphomas, KS, and the immune reconstitution inflammatory syndrome (IRIS) are among the noninfectious conditions with potential pulmonary findings in HIV-positive individuals. KS can affect the trachea, bronchi, lung parenchyma, and mediastinal and hilar lymph nodes in patients with advanced disease, causing reduced lung volumes and airflow obstruction. Intrathoracic B-cell lymphoma tumors also present more commonly in later stages of HIV disease. Lymphoma has been implicated in creating pleural, pericardial, and peritoneal effusions, even in the absence of tumor masses. IRIS, a more recently recognized condition, appears to be associated with the proinflammatory effects that accompany the inhibition of viral replication with HAART and may have far-reaching effects on multiple organ systems (25).

Cardiac Manifestations

Cardiac complications of HIV infection appear on the rise due to both the increased incidence of HIV/AIDS worldwide and the improved longevity of HIV-infected patients since the advent of HAART. In addition, treatment for HIV infection itself may contribute to cardiac disease. Indeed, histopathologic evidence of myocarditis at autopsy has been reported in an estimated one-third of patients with AIDS (26). In another autopsy series, roughly 24% of patients with HIV/AIDS were found to have evidence of heart disease (27). Etiologies of heart disease in patients with HIV/AIDS have been reviewed recently and include direct effects of HIV on the myocardium, opportunistic infections, adverse effects of drug therapies, non-HIV cardiac risk factors such as hypercholesterolemia, insulin resistance, and hypertension that may be exacerbated by HAART, and lifestyle choices related to the mode of acquisition of HIV, such as IV drug abuse (27).

Patients with HIV/AIDS may present with pericardial disease, myocardial disease, including cardiomyopathy, myocarditis, secondary cardiac tumors, or drug-induced myocardial dysfunction, and endocardial disease secondary to bacterial or non-bacterial endocarditis. Offending agents range from TB, KS, lymphoma, candidiasis, histoplasmosis, cryptococcosis, aspergillosis, herpes simplex virus (HSV), cytomegalovirus (CMV), and toxoplasmosis to HIV itself. In addition, HAART is thought to contribute to myocardial dysfunction via an autoimmune response or by direct injury to the cardiac conduction system. Illicit drugs, such as cocaine and methamphetamines, and prescription drugs, including foscarnet, doxorubicin, pentamidine, amphotericin B, and interferon alpha, have also been implicated in cardiac toxicity in the HIV/AIDS population.

HIV-infected individuals are susceptible to other heart conditions, such as arrhythmias, coronary artery disease (CAD), pulmonary hypertension, vascular disease, aneurysms, and venous thrombosis. Drug toxicity from the prophylaxis and treatment of toxoplasmosis and PCP has been implicated in arrhythmias, although intrinsic myocardial disease and heart failure also contribute to conduction abnormalities in this patient population. CAD has been associated with an aging population infected with HIV/AIDS, with a hypercoagulable state, and with metabolic abnormalities, such as low high-density lipoprotein, hyperglycemia, and lipodystrophy, that have been linked to protease inhibitors (PIs) (28). In general, prolonged HAART therapy accelerates atherosclerosis and increases the risk of CAD and myocardial infarction. The etiology of pulmonary hypertension appears to be related to a hypercoagulable state, as well as to inflammatory and genetic factors (29). Roughly 0.5% of individuals with HIV develop pulmonary hypertension. More surprisingly, perhaps, the incidence of deep vein thrombosis is estimated to be 10 times higher in HIV-infected individuals than in the general population (27).

Hematologic Manifestations

Hematologic abnormalities of the HIV infection affect all cell lines and occur early in the course of disease. Indeed, a decline in the CD4+ T cell count (generally attributed to direct actions of HIV-1, to CD8+ T-lymphocyte activity, increased apoptosis, reduced production of T cells, and inhibitory cytokine activity) is the hallmark of the disease (30). In addition, anemia, thrombocytopenia, and coagulation disorders are common. Anemia is estimated to affect up to 90% of untreated patients infected with HIV, particularly at advanced stages of the infection (31). Women, infants and children, and patients in developing countries have a higher prevalence of anemia than other HIV-infected individuals. Iron deficiency, as well as vitamin and folic acid deficiencies, may contribute to this discrepancy. A shorter erythrocyte lifespan, impaired erythropoietin production,

inadequate bone marrow erythropoiesis, and opportunistic infections are other causes of anemia in the HIV-infected population. Bone marrow infiltration by infections or malignancies, immune-mediated effects, myelotoxicity of certain ARV drugs, and gastrointestinal (GI) blood loss must also be considered.

Thrombocytopenia in HIV-infected individuals is clinically similar to immune thrombocytopenic purpura (ITP) and is multifactorial in origin (32). Causes include a shortened platelet lifespan, increased splenic platelet sequestration, and ineffective platelet production. Underlying opportunistic infections, medications, malignancy, and comorbidities resulting in hypersplenism are among the secondary causes of thrombocytopenia. While HIV-associated thrombocytopenia can present at any time during the course of the HIV infection, its severity correlates with the disease progression. Both monotherapy with zidovudine (ZDV) and HAART have been demonstrated to improve HIV thrombocytopenia. However, thrombocytopenias, as well as other cytopenias, may be induced by ART (33). Corticosteroid treatment and intravenous immunoglobulin (IVIG), for the life-threatening thrombocytopenia, produce transient and variable results.

Other coagulation disorders associated with HIV infection, such as that seen in patients with the lupus anticoagulant, may contribute to a hypercoagulable state.

Gastrointestinal Manifestations

Gastrointestinal abnormalities associated with HIV commonly affect the oral cavity, esophagus, stomach, and the hepatobiliary system. While the widespread use of HAART has reduced the incidence of these complications, nausea, vomiting, diarrhea, and other gastrointestinal disturbances may be severe enough to cause electrolyte imbalances and cachexia. Oral manifestations of HIV can be categorized into infections (viral, bacterial, and fungal), neoplasms, salivary gland disease, and a series of miscellaneous lesions, some of which are associated with HAART (34). Oral candidiasis, HSV ulcers, and CMV outbreaks, among others, may cause painful, burning sores on the palate, tongue, and pharynx, as well as impair swallowing and pose an infectious or hemorrhagic risk during manipulation of the airway. Oral KS and intraoral non-Hodgkin's lymphoma (NHL) may cause ulcerations, bleeding, and pain in the tongue, tonsillar pillars, and palate.

Before the advent of HAART, roughly one-third of HIV-infected patients suffered from esophageal disease, most commonly associated with candidiasis (35). CMV and, less commonly, HSV are among the viral causes of esophageal disease, including ulceration or perforation of the GI tract. Idiopathic esophageal ulcer, a diagnosis of exclusion, may also present either alone or in combination with infectious sources of esophageal disease. Patients commonly present with odynophagia and dysphagia and tend to respond well to therapy once the causative agent is identified. Although the evidence suggests no increased incidence of gastroesophageal reflux (GERD) in HIV-infected individuals, reflux is not an uncommon complaint and should be treated as in non–HIV-infected patients. For patients presenting with dyspepsia, a less common clinical presentation of GERD, a work-up for other causes of upper abdominal pain affecting the HIV population, including gastroesophageal junction ulceration and gastric or duodenal mucosal disease, may be warranted. Other sources of gastric complaints include CMV and neoplasms, such as NHL and KS.

Hepatobiliary disease is also common among HIV-infected patients. Biliary tract disease can develop in the advanced stages of HIV infection. While several pathogens have been implicated, the precise etiology of AIDS cholangiopathy remains unclear. Hepatitis B virus (HBV), hepatitis C virus (HCV), CMV, KS, NHL, and mycobacterial infections are among the causes of parenchymal liver disease in this patient population. Importantly, approximately one-third of HIV-infected patients are co-infected with HCV infection; further, HIV/HCV co-infection accelerates the course of HCV-associated liver disease, although the mechanism of interaction between the two viruses is not completely understood (36). With the widespread use of HAART, end-stage liver disease (ESLD) resulting from HCV has emerged as an important cause of death among HIV-infected patients (37). HIV-infected individuals with ESLD are being considered with increasing frequency for orthotopic liver transplantation (OLT) (38).

Renal Manifestations

Renal complications of HIV are diverse and can be attributed directly to the HIV infection, to coincidental complications of the HIV infection, and to non–HIV-related comorbidities that predispose the aging HIV-infected population to chronic kidney disease (CKD). Glomerulonephropathies, including HIV-associated nephropathy (HIVAN), a variety of immune-complex–mediated conditions, and IgA nephropathy, are widely recognized complications of HIV and contribute to an increased incidence of hospitalizations for acute renal failure (ARF) among HIV-infected individuals compared to similarly matched controls without the virus (39). HIVAN, previously known as AIDS nephropathy, is characterized by profound proteinuria, hematuria, and azotemia and can present at any stage of the HIV disease. It disproportionately affects African American men and IV drug abusers, although HIVAN has been reported in all risk groups for HIV infection, including sexual partners of HIV-infected individuals and children born to HIV-infected mothers (40). The time course from onset of proteinuria to overt end-stage renal disease (ESRD) in patients with HIVAN is roughly 3 to 4 months. However, this ominous nephropathy may be prevented and treated with ART (41).

Many of the coincidental renal disorders in the HIV population reflect the severity of the underlying systemic disease process or its infectious, malignancy-related, or drug-associated complications. Bacteria, *Mycobacteria*, viruses (most commonly CMV), and fungi, such as *Candida*, *Aspergillus*, and *Cryptococcus*, have all been implicated in renal disorders in HIV-infected individuals. Lymphoma, amyloidosis, KS, and simple calcifications of the kidney are among the many infiltrative lesions affecting the HIV population. Fluid/electrolyte imbalances and a variety of respiratory and metabolic disorders associated with advanced HIV/AIDS in patients suffering from diarrhea, malnutrition, and malabsorption or CNS involvement are additional risk factors for ARF. ARF in the HIV population can also be attributed to prerenal causes such as hypovolemia and hypotension; interstitial disorders, including acute tubular nephrosis (ATN), rhabdomyolysis, hemolytic uremic syndrome (HUS), and thrombotic thrombocytopenic purpura (TTP); or postrenal tubular or ureteral obstruction. Drug therapies for both opportunistic infections and HIV have been implicated in several of these renal sequelae (42).

Chronic renal disease related to improved survival with HAART, the aging population with HIV infection, and comorbidities of hypertension and diabetes mellitus, among others, comprises an additional subgroup of renal disorders in HIV-infected individuals. African Americans, who make up a large and ever-growing percentage of newly infected individuals, may be at higher risk for developing CKD and ESRD due to their significantly higher risk for these comorbidities compared with Caucasians. Atherosclerotic renal artery stenosis, hepatitis C-related kidney disease, and non–HIV-related diseases that affect the general population, such as IgA nephropathy, also contribute to renal failure in the aging population, amongst injection drug users, and, disproportionately, in urban populations.

■ MODES OF TRANSMISSION: HIV INFECTION FROM MOTHER TO INFANT

Maternal-to-child transmission of HIV occurs in utero, intrapartum, and postpartum during breastfeeding, but most commonly occurs during labor and delivery. The mechanism of vertical transmission is not well understood, but it is speculated that transplacental transfusions of virus-contaminated blood during contractions or fetal exposure to virus-tainted cervicovaginal secretions and blood may be responsible (43). However, transplacental HIV transmission can also occur early in pregnancy, and the virus has been detected in specimens from elective abortions (44). Indeed, trophoblasts, which carry CD4+ receptors, demonstrate HIV viral sequences in pregnant HIV-infected individuals with no protective ARV therapy (45). Studies reporting that perinatal HIV transmission is reduced more effectively with ARV regimens that are initiated in the second trimester compared to regimens initiated later in pregnancy suggest that a significant proportion of in utero transmission occurs between 28 and 36 weeks' gestation (46).

During the postpartum period, mother-to-child transmission rates among breastfeeding infants may be as high as 40% (47). Although the mechanisms of HIV-1 transmission through breastfeeding are poorly understood, risk factors for transmission are linked to maternal, infant, and viral conditions, including CD4+ cell counts, viral loads in both breast milk and plasma, acuity of infection, duration of breastfeeding, breast health, infant prematurity, and presence or absence of oral thrush in the infant (48). Recent evidence suggests that HAART for lactating mothers reduces transmission via this route (49). Observational and clinical studies have also demonstrated a significant reduction of postnatal transmission with infant prophylaxis during breastfeeding, yet neither maternal nor infant therapy completely eliminates the risk of transmission associated with breastfeeding (50). Consequently, breastfeeding among HIV-infected women is not recommended in developed countries that have safe, affordable, and accessible alternative nutritional resources for infants.

Progress has been made toward quantifying the risk of mother-to-child transmission (Table 36-2), and recent data suggest that viral load correlates with the risk of vertical transmission. Specifically, studies report that at viral loads below 1,000 copies/mL, the rate of transmission is exceedingly low to nonexistent (51). Conversely, higher levels of HIV-1 RNA are associated with a greater risk of mother-to-child transmission. However, mother-to-child transmission has been observed in women with an undetectable viral load, and discordance between the plasma and genital tract viral loads, particularly in the presence of other genital tract infections, has been reported (52). Maternal use of ART during pregnancy is another independent determinant of mother-to-child transmission, suggesting a role for pre-exposure prophylaxis for the infant. Epidemiologic and clinical trials suggest that HIV-infected women receiving potent ARV combination drug therapy that reduces the viral load to low

TABLE 36-2 Risk Factors for Maternal-to-Child Transmission of HIV[a]

High Viral Load	Low CD4+ cell count
No Maternal ARV Therapy	Advanced HIV disease
Transplacental infection early in pregnancy	Poor nutritional status
	History of illicit drug or tobacco use
Transplacental transfusions during contractions	Presence of STDs
	Prolonged ROMs
Exposure to cervicovaginal secretions, blood	Chorioamnionitis
	Obstetrical interventions
Breastfeeding	Low birth weight
	Prematurity
	Genetic predisposition

[a]Current guidelines recommend antenatal and intrapartum maternal combination therapy and postnatal infant ARV.

or undetectable levels have very low rates of transmission (53). Other maternal factors associated with mother-to-child transmission include a low CD4+ cell count, advanced HIV disease, poor nutritional status, a history of illicit drug or tobacco use, and presence of sexually transmitted diseases (STDs). Obstetric factors include prolonged rupture of membranes (ROMs), chorioamnionitis, obstetrical interventions, such as amniocentesis or artificial ROM, and route of delivery. Low birth weight, prematurity, and genetic predisposition are among the fetal factors associated with mother-to-child transmission. Because of the multifactorial nature of perinatal transmission and the demonstrated efficacy of ART in reducing mother-to-child transmission, current guidelines recommend antenatal and intrapartum maternal combination therapy, as well as postnatal infant ARV, for prevention of perinatal transmission. Scheduled cesarean delivery in a parturient on ARV therapy and with an undetectable viral load does not appear to confer substantial benefit to the fetus. However, data remain insufficient to state unequivocally whether scheduled cesarean delivery confers any benefit in this setting (43). There appears to be little additional protective fetal benefit from elective cesarean delivery after the onset of labor or spontaneous ROM. Consequently, ACOG recommends scheduled cesarean delivery to decrease mother-to-child transmission at 38 weeks' gestation and prior to ROM and onset of labor in patients with HIV-1 RNA levels greater than 1,000 copies/mL or with an unknown HIV-1 RNA level.

■ ANTIRETROVIRAL THERAPY: AGENTS, INITIATION, AND ADVERSE EFFECTS

The morbidity and mortality associated with HIV/AIDS have decreased dramatically since the advent and widespread use of potent ART (54). In one of the biggest public health successes of the AIDS epidemic, the adherence to combined ART amongst HIV-seropositive parturients has reduced mother-to-child transmission to less than 2% in industrialized nations (55). The Department of Health and Human Services (DHHS) publishes and periodically updates current recommendations for ART online (56). Updated recommendations for ARV regimens for HIV-infected parturients are also available as a "living document" on the AIDS*info* website (52). In brief, combination drug regimens are considered the standard of care for HIV treatment and for the prevention of mother-to-child transmission. The major classes of pharmaceutical agents include nucleoside/nucleotide reverse transcriptase inhibitors (NRTIs), non-nucleoside reverse transcriptase inhibitors (NNRTIs),

protease inhibitors (PIs), fusion inhibitors, CCR5 antagonists, and integrase strand transfer inhibitors (INSTIs). In treatment-naïve patients, a triple therapy of two NRTIs with an NNRTI, a PI, or an INSTI is recommended for durable viral suppression.

While the benefit of ART must be weighed against the potential adverse effects to mother, fetus, and newborn, all HIV-infected parturients are encouraged to receive antepartum combination ARV therapy for fetal protection regardless of maternal indication. Intrapartum and postpartum infant ARV prophylaxis are also recommended, as ART reduces mother-to-child transmission both by reducing the maternal viral load and by providing pre- and post-exposure prophylaxis for the infant. In general, commonly used ARV drugs are considered safe during pregnancy and in early infancy, although the long-term toxicity to children with a history of exposure to ARV therapy remains unknown (55). Efavirenz (EFV), an NNRTI that has been associated with anencephaly, microphthalmia, and facial clefts in animal studies, as well as neural tube defects in humans, and tenofovir (TDF), an NRTI that has been associated with adverse fetal bone effects, are among the exceptions. Lactic acidosis and hepatic failure have been reported in parturients receiving stavudine (d4T) and didanosine (ddI), both NRTIs, throughout pregnancy. Although data are inconclusive and conflicting, these and other NRTIs have been linked also to mitochondrial toxicity in infants with a history of in utero exposure (57). Clinical manifestations of this rare, multisystem disorder include neuropathy, myopathy, cardiomyopathy, pancreatitis, and developmental delay. Fatal hepatotoxicity and hypersensitivity skin reactions have been reported in pregnant women receiving combination therapy with nevirapine (NVP), an NNRTI. Finally, there are conflicting data regarding risk of preterm labor in women receiving combination of ART with a protease inhibitor during pregnancy. However, PIs should not be withheld given the established benefits of this therapy for both maternal health and the prevention of mother-to-child transmission.

Combination ARV regimens for optimal prophylaxis in the pregnant population include two NRTIs and either an NNRTI or a PI. ZDV, an NRTI, should be included unless the parturient has documented resistance, has experienced toxicity, such as severe anemia, or is already on an effective suppressive regimen. Lamivudine (3TC), an NRTI often used in combination with ZDV, is another preferred agent based on extensive studies demonstrating its safety during pregnancy and efficacy in preventing mother-to-child transmission. Lopinavir/ritonavir (LPV/r), the only available coformulated boosted PI, is the preferred protease inhibitor during pregnancy, based also on efficacy studies. If maternal viral load is sufficiently low and in the absence of maternal indication, the triple regimen can be initiated after the first trimester. Patients who are already on a stable ART regimen when they become pregnant should not alter or disrupt therapy, with the exceptions of substituting another agent for EFV and possibly modifying PI dosage. Pharmacokinetics of NRTIs and NNRTIs are unchanged during pregnancy, but lower drug levels of PIs have been observed. As always, adherence to ART should be optimized during pregnancy in order to maximize viral suppression and prevent viral resistance; preconceptual and peripartum counseling may serve to promote adherence and help manage adverse side effects, such as nausea and vomiting.

ARV drugs have unique side effects, and may interact with other drugs or adversely affect a patient's anesthetic course. As a class, PIs have been associated with hyperlipidemia, glucose intolerance, hepatotoxicity, and GI disturbances. Since pregnant women may be prone to developing gestational diabetes, parturients who receive combination therapy with a PI should be monitored closely for signs and symptoms of hyperglycemia (58). If parturients experience severe nausea, vomiting, or abdominal pain that requires cessation of ART, they should be encouraged to stop, and later resume, all ARV agents simultaneously in order to minimize the emergence of drug resistance. Antiemetics may help reduce untoward GI side effects and simultaneously improve adherence to HAART. An additional concern associated with PIs is the inhibition of cytochrome P450, which is important in the metabolism of several drugs. In general, PIs may increase the effects of drugs metabolized by cytochrome P450. Ritonavir (RTV) has been shown to inhibit the metabolism of fentanyl, indicating a need to modify opioid dosing in patients receiving certain PIs (59). Caution with benzodiazepine administration with concomitant protease inhibitor therapy is advised on account of concerns for prolonged sedation. PIs also affect methadone metabolism, most likely resulting in significant reductions in methadone levels. Clinicians should be aware of the possibility of methadone withdrawal in patients on concomitant PI and methadone therapy. Clinicians should also bear in mind

that PIs have been associated with prolonged bleeding and an increased incidence of spontaneous bleeding in hemophiliac patients. Lastly, they have been associated with exaggerated vasoconstrictive responses. As a result, ergot alkaloids such as methergine should be avoided when uterine atony results in excessive postpartum bleeding in women receiving PIs. If alternative uterotonic agents are not available, methergine should be administered in low doses for a short duration in this setting.

Adverse effects of NNRTIs include several clinically significant drug interactions, hepatotoxicity, and skin rashes, including Stevens–Johnson syndrome (SJS). Rapid emergence of resistance to NNRTIs when administered as the sole ARV agent has also been reported. Certain NNRTIs induce cytochrome P450 and may decrease serum levels of anesthetic and sedative agents, including midazolam and fentanyl. Other drugs that may have significant interactions with NNRTIs, as well as PIs, as a result of the induction or inhibition of hepatic drug metabolism include lipid-lowering agents (e.g., statins), calcium channel blockers, azole antifungals, oral contraceptives, methadone, St. John's wort, immunosuppressants, anticonvulsants, antimycobacterials, macrolides, and other ARV agents. Both clinical hepatitis and asymptomatic elevation of liver function tests (LFTs), accompanied by nonspecific symptoms of anorexia, weight loss, or fatigue, are associated with NNRTIs as a class. A severe hypersensitivity reaction, marked by abrupt flu-like symptoms that may progress into fulminant hepatic failure, often accompanied by rhabdomyolysis, has been reported with NVP. NVP also has the strongest association with SJS and toxic epidermal necrosis, although other NNRTIs have been implicated. Complications of this severe skin reaction include fluid depletion, bacterial or fungal superinfection, and, ultimately, multiorgan failure.

Adverse effects of NRTIs include GI disturbances, headache, insomnia, hepatotoxicity, lipoatrophy, peripheral neuropathy, and skin reactions (Tables 36-3 through 36-5). ZDV may cause bone marrow suppression, as manifested by anemia and neutropenia. It is also associated with a higher incidence of nausea, vomiting, and abdominal pain compared with other

TABLE 36-3 Drugs for the Management of HIV Infection: NRTIs

Drug Class	Example Drugs	Class-wide Potential Side Effects	
NRTIs (nucleoside/ nucleotide reverse transcriptase inhibitors)	Abracavir (ABC), Didanosine (ddI), Emtricitabine (FTC), Lamivudine (3TC), Stavudine (d4T), Tenofovir (TDF), Zalcitabine (ddC), Zidovudine (ZDV)	• GI disturbances • headache • hepatotoxicity	• peripheral neuropathy • skin reactions
Specific Examples	**Potential Side Effects**		
Abracavir (ABC)	• Severe hypersensitivity reaction: nonspecific initial symptoms (myalgia, chills, fever, nausea, headache) can escalate (dyspnea, tachypnea, hypotension, overt respiratory distress, vascular collapse), especially upon rechallenge		
Didanosine (ddI)	• Hepatotoxicity associated with lactic acidosis and hepatic steatosis • Noncirrhotic portal hypertension	• Peripheral neuropathy	
Stavudine (d4T)	• Hepatic failure • Lactic acidosis • Mitochondrial toxicity • Peripheral neuropathy	• Rapidly progressive ascending demyelinating polyneuropathy, may evolve into frank respiratory paralysis and can present with lactic acidosis and increased creatine phosphokinase	
Zalcitabine (ddC)	• Peripheral neuropathy		
Zidovudine (ZDV)	• Nausea, vomiting, abdominal pain	• Hepatotoxicity associated with lactic acidosis and hepatic steatosis • Bone marrow suppression (anemia, neutropenia)	

TABLE 36-4 Drugs for the Management of HIV Infection: NNRTIs

Drug Class	Example Drugs	Class-wide Potential Side Effects	
NNRTIs (non-nucleoside reverse transcriptase inhibitors)	Efavirenz (EFV), Etravirine (ETR), Nevirapine (NVP)	• Hepatotoxicity • Clinical hepatitis • Asymptomatic elevation of LFTs • Induction of cytochrome P450, decreased serum levels of anesthetic and sedative agents (incl. midazolam, fentanyl) • Nonspecific symptoms of anorexia, weight loss, or fatigue	• Induction/inhibition of hepatic metabolism; Interactions with lipid-lowering agents, calcium channel blockers, methadone, St. John's wort, immunosuppressants, anticonvulsants, antimycobacterials, macrolides, other ARV agents • Skin rashes (incl. Stevens–Johnson syndrome)
Specific Example	**Potential Side Effects**		
Nevirapine (NVP)	• Hepatotoxicity • Hypersensitivity skin reactions (incl. Stevens–Johnson syndrome, toxic epidermal necrosis)		

NRTIs. Hepatotoxicity associated with lactic acidosis and hepatic steatosis has been reported with ZDV, d4T, and ddI; prolonged exposure to ddI has also been associated with non-cirrhotic portal hypertension. Patients with HBV co-infection may experience severe hepatic flare-ups when certain NRTIs are initiated or withdrawn. A severe hypersensitivity reaction marked initially by nonspecific symptoms such as myalgia, chills, fever, nausea, and headache has been reported with abacavir (ABC); the reaction can escalate to dyspnea, tachypnea, hypotension, overt respiratory distress, and vascular collapse. When patients susceptible to this hypersensitivity reaction are rechallenged with ABC, the reaction may be more intense, mimicking anaphylaxis. With regard to neurologic abnormalities associated with NRTIs, a rapidly progressive ascending demyelinating polyneuropathy that may evolve into frank respiratory paralysis has been reported, most frequently with d4T. This syndrome may mimic Guillain–Barré, and may present with concomitant lactic acidosis and markedly increased creatinine phosphokinase. Peripheral neuropathy is a common side effect of zalcitabine (ddC), d4T, and ddI, and appears to correlate with the severity of HIV infection. Lastly, severe skin reactions similar to those described with the use of NNRTIs have also been reported with NRTIs.

ANESTHESIA FOR LABOR AND DELIVERY

HIV-infected parturients may require anesthesia for nonobstetric surgery or obstetric procedures at any gestational age, for labor and delivery, for scheduled or emergent cesarean delivery, or for treatment of post-dural puncture headache (PDPH). When planning an anesthetic for any patient with a systemic disease, an understanding of the disease process, common comorbidities, the patient's current status, and the patient's therapeutic drug regimen is essential. Care of the HIV-infected parturient also entails a team approach involving multiple providers, including specialists in maternal–fetal medicine, infectious disease, pediatrics, and social services. While most HIV-infected parturients are otherwise healthy and present with a low viral load, others may present with opportunistic infections, malignancies, and other signs of advanced disease. Patients may be unaware of their disease state, may not have access to ART, or may choose not to take therapeutic agents. The anesthetic options for HIV-infected parturients must be considered carefully in advance given the complexity of HIV infection, the broad spectrum of clinical presentations of HIV disease, and fetal considerations. An understanding of strategies to prevent spread of HIV to the health care worker is also fundamental.

While regional anesthesia is the most common technique in obstetric anesthesia, general anesthesia is occasionally indicated for emergency cesarean deliveries. Specific clinical issues, such as severe coagulopathy or sepsis, and patient preference might also dictate the need for a general anesthetic. Despite early concerns linking immunologic changes to general anesthesia and cautionary recommendations against the use of inhalational agents in HIV-infected individuals, general anesthesia can be performed safely in parturients with

TABLE 36-5 Drugs for the Management of HIV Infection: PIs

Drug Class	Example Drugs	Class-wide Potential Side Effects	
PIs (protease inhibitors)	Atazanavir (ATV), Indinavir (IDV), Lopinavir/ritonavir (LPV/r), Nelfinavir (NFV), Ritonavir (RTV), Saquinavir (SQV)	• Glucose intolerance • Hepatotoxicity • GI disturbances • Exaggerated vasoconstrictive responses (with ergot alkaloids, e.g.) • Hyperglycemia (in cases of gestational diabetes) • Hyperlipidemia	• Inhibition of cytochrome P450, prolonged sedation (with benzodiazepines) • Reduced methadone levels, methadone withdrawal (concomitant PI/methadone therapy) • Prolonged bleeding, spontaneous bleeding (with coagulopathies or anticoagulants)
Specific Example	**Potential Side Effects**		
Ritonavir (RTV)	• Inhibition of fentanyl metabolism (opioid dosing modification needed)		

HIV (60). There is insufficient evidence to suggest that the transient depression of immune function that may accompany general anesthesia is clinically significant in the HIV-infected population; conclusive studies are lacking. Nonetheless, it may be prudent to consider all HIV patients and other potentially immunocompromised individuals as uniquely susceptible to infections (21). As always, universal sterile precautions are appropriate and must be implemented. Other factors that warrant consideration preoperatively include the patient's preexisting pulmonary, cardiovascular, hematologic, and neurologic status. Possible interactions of anesthetics with ARV agents, the possibility of space-occupying intracranial lesions that may alter cerebral hemodynamics, and dose adjustments in the settings of liver or kidney dysfunction or overt cachexia should also be taken into account. A chest x-ray is warranted if pulmonary manifestations are concerning, and a complete blood count (CBC), LFTs, and electrolytes should be reviewed before administering general anesthesia. In addition, HIV-infected parturients should receive periodic checks of HIV viral load, CD4+ cell counts, and fetal well being (e.g., ultrasound and nonstress test or biophysical profile), as indicated by the ARV regimen and/or obstetric standards.

With regard to regional anesthesia, epidural, combined spinal–epidural (CSE), and spinal techniques are considered safe in HIV-infected individuals (61). The CNS is infected early in the course of HIV infection, and there is no evidence that neuraxial instrumentation confers any additional risk of viral spread to the CNS. Nor do HIV-infected individuals appear to be at increased risk for infectious complications of neuraxial procedures, provided that strict aseptic techniques are maintained. Early concerns that the possible introduction of HIV-infected blood into the CSF might precipitate a CNS infection or that a preexisting infection, such as meningitis, in an HIV-positive patient might be exacerbated by a regional anesthetic have been addressed in several small studies (62). Hughes et al. prospectively followed 30 HIV-infected parturients who received regional anesthesia, IV opioids, or no analgesia during delivery and found no difference in neurologic, infectious, or immune function outcomes (63). A study by Gershon et al. comparing peripartum complications in 96 HIV-positive parturients who received general anesthesia, regional anesthesia, local anesthetics/IV sedation, or no anesthesia during delivery similarly found no difference in outcomes (61). In a more recent study, Avidan et al. found no increased incidence of perioperative complications, changes in immune function, or increases in viral load in 44 parturients undergoing cesarean delivery with spinal anesthesia compared with a control group of 45 HIV-negative parturients (64). Of note, all parturients in the latter study were receiving ART. Although the number of patients who received regional anesthesia in these studies is small, the evidence suggests that both epidurals and spinals can be performed without adverse sequelae in HIV-positive pregnant women.

All potential risks of regional anesthesia in HIV-infected individuals should be discussed with patients in advance. CNS manifestations of HIV may not be apparent until later in the course of the disease, and concern exists that future neurologic deficits may be ascribed to the neuraxial technique. Such concerns are unsubstantiated, as a temporal relationship between the epidural or spinal placement and the onset of neurologic deficits is unlikely (65). Nonetheless, given that peripheral neuropathy is the most frequent neurologic complication in HIV patients and that HIV-positive individuals are at high risk for other STDs that may affect the CNS (e.g., syphilis), thorough documentation of any preexisting deficit is recommended (66). It is also helpful to bear in mind that the hypotensive response to neuraxial blockade may be accentuated in patients with HIV-associated autonomic neuropathy. Special

caution to avoid infection, including wearing gowns and eye protection, when performing or assisting with invasive procedures in HIV-infected individuals, has also been recommended (67). Local infections at the anticipated site of neuraxial instrumentation must also be considered and may be a contraindication to regional anesthesia. HIV-induced thrombocytopenia is rarely severe enough to preclude regional anesthesia, yet a platelet count and a review of ART that may affect platelet function is prudent.

In the perioperative setting, anesthesiologists may face decisions related to the transfusion of blood products, including appropriate target hemoglobin levels, when to transfuse, and which specific products are needed. Patients with HIV infection not uncommonly have anemia, thrombocytopenia, and/or other coagulopathies associated with the disease, complications of HIV/AIDs, or ARV therapy. Treatment of such abnormalities should be determined on an individual basis, weighing relative risks and benefits. Historically, there is epidemiologic evidence that anemia is positively associated with increased mortality in HIV-infected patients (68). In a large observational cohort study by the CDC, treatment of anemia was strongly related to a decreased risk of death among HIV patients (69). However, a cohort study conducted by Moore and colleagues demonstrated that while gradual medical management of anemia with epoetin improved outcomes, blood transfusion was associated with shortened survival of HIV patients (70). Hypothesized mechanisms for this observation include increased susceptibility to blood-borne infectious contaminants in immunocompromised patients, transfusion-related immunosuppression (thought to be mediated by cytokines) (71), and transient activation of HIV expression and replication. Despite these concerns, there are circumstances in the perioperative setting, such as acute and ongoing blood loss, worsening coagulopathy, or severe anemia, in which transfusion of blood products may be appropriate. In these instances, relative risks and benefits need to be weighed carefully, with all patients, and there should be vigilant follow-up of patients for acute complications of transfusions (72).

Questions often arise regarding how to treat PDPH, a rare but potentially debilitating complication of neuraxial anesthesia. Historically, there were concerns that introducing HIV-infected blood into the epidural space or, in the case of an unintentional dural puncture, into the subarachnoid space might pose an unacceptable risk for introducing pathogens into the CNS. More recent research and clinical experience suggest that an epidural blood patch (EBP) is appropriate for treatment of PDPH in HIV-infected individuals. In one study, Tom et al. followed six HIV-seropositive males who received EBP therapy after PDPH from diagnostic lumbar punctures and found no adverse neurologic or infectious sequelae for 24 months afterward (73). It is generally accepted that CNS infection occurs early in the course of HIV, often before any symptoms appear, and therefore the EBP is unlikely to cause new CNS infection. Overall, the safety of regional anesthesia has been substantiated through both clinical studies and extensive clinical experience over the past quarter century. Just as in non–HIV-infected patients, regional anesthesia is indicated in the HIV-positive parturient in the absence of specific contraindications (74). Similarly, EBP remains the "gold standard" for treatment of PDPH if conservative measures fail for all patient populations, including HIV-positive individuals.

With regard to strategies to minimize transmission of HIV to the health care worker, preventing exposure to blood and body fluids remains the cornerstone of prevention (75). Gloves, masks, and eye shields are among the universal barrier precautions when contact with blood, CSF, amniotic fluid, and other infectious material is anticipated. Full-length gowns are indicated for situations in which gross contamination is likely. Avoiding percutaneous exposure to HIV-infected blood via needles or other sharp objects is another central aspect of health care provider safety. The risk for HIV transmission after percutaneous exposure is roughly 0.3% and correlates with exposure to a larger quantity of blood from the infected source, as might occur with a deep cut, injury with a hollow-bore needle, or injury with a needle that is visibly contaminated. If exposure to a potentially infected source occurs, immediate wound cleaning and risk assessment is advised. Post-exposure prophylactic therapy with ART is recommended.

▪ CONCLUSION

HIV infection has spread aggressively in the decades since the virus was first described, currently infecting over 40 million people worldwide. It is estimated that roughly half of those infected are women, giving rise to concerns for mother-to-child transmission among women of childbearing age. Without treatment, an estimated 25% of infants born to HIV-positive mothers will become infected in utero, during labor and vaginal delivery, or postpartum, during breastfeeding. Given that the number of HIV-infected females continues to rise, health care providers in obstetric suites will inevitably manage the HIV-positive patient with increasing frequency. HIV-infected parturients require early screening and counseling, careful evaluation for other comorbidities, timely administration of HAART, and anesthetic interventions, as indicated. Parturients may require anesthetic management at any stage during pregnancy for nonobstetric surgery, for emergent cesarean delivery, for labor analgesia, or for treatment of complications of neuraxial blockade, such as PDPH. While the HIV-seropositive parturient must be evaluated for the numerous potential complications of HIV disease, there are no unique contraindications to regional or general anesthesia or to the timely administration of an EBP. To be sure, universal precautions must be carefully observed to minimize the risk of occupational infection. Early screening for HIV, the increasing use of HAART, improved awareness of modes of mother-to-child transmission, and, ultimately, a vaccine for HIV will all contribute to improved maternal outcomes and a sharp decrease in vertical transmission.

KEY POINTS

- Women of childbearing age comprise a growing proportion of newly diagnosed HIV infections worldwide.
- Early detection of HIV infection in the parturient with subsequent counseling and prompt initiation of ART are integral components of the strategy to reduce mother-to-child transmission.
- HIV affects multiple organ systems and has numerous anesthetic implications.
- The anesthesia provider should be aware of the complexities of systemic HIV infection, as well as of the common drug interactions from ARTs.
- Neuraxial anesthesia techniques are considered safe in the HIV-infected parturient.
- EBP is the definitive procedure for treatment of PDPH in HIV-infected individuals unresponsive to conservative treatment.
- HCWs are encouraged to adhere to universal sterile precautions and avoid percutaneous needle stick injury in order to minimize risks of occupational exposure to HIV.

REFERENCES

1. Tuomala RE, Currier JS, Cu-Uvin S, et al. Human immunodeficiency virus infection in pregnancy. In: Powrie RO, Green MF, Camann W, eds. *de Swiet's Medical Disorders in Obstetric Practice*. 5th ed. West Sussex: Wiley-Blackwell; 2010: 464–476.
2. CDC. HIV Surveillance Report, 2009; vol.21. Available at: http://www.cdc.gov/hiv/topics/surveillance/resources/reports/
3. Hall HI, Song R, Rhodes P, et al. Estimation of HIV incidence in the United States. *JAMA* 2008;300:520–529.
4. Greenwald JL, Burstein GR, Pincus J. A rapid review of rapid HIV antibody tests. *Curr Infect Dis Rep* 2006;8:125–131.
5. www.unaids.org/pub/EpiReport/2006
6. CDC. HIV Surveillance Report 2010; vol. 22. Available at http://www.cdc.gov/hiv/topics/surveillance/resources/reports/
7. UNAIDS/WHO. *AIDS epidemic update, December 2001*. Geneva: Switzerland: UNAIDS/WHO; 2001.
8. De Cock KM, Fowler MG, Mercier E, et al. Prevention of mother-to-child HIV transmission in resource-poor countries. Translating research into policy and practice. *JAMA* 2000;282:1175–1182.
9. Levy JA. HIV pathogenesis: 25 years of progress and persistent challenges. *AIDS* 2009;23:147–169.
10. CDC. Subpopulation estimates for the HIV incidence surveillance system—United States, 2006. *MMWR Morb Mortal Wkly Rep* 2008;57:985–989.
11. Petropoulou H, Stratigos A, Katsambas AD. Human immunodeficiency virus infection and pregnancy. *Clin Dermatol* 2006;24:536–542.
12. Geleziunas R, Greene WC. Molecular insights into HIV-1 infection and pathogenesis. In: Sande MA, Volberding, eds. *The Medical Management of AIDS*. 6th ed. W.B. Saunders Co; 2000.
13. CDC. Racial/ethnic disparities among children with diagnoses of perinatal HIV infection—34 States, 2004–2007. *MMWR Morb Mortal Wkly Rep* 2010; 59:97–101.
14. CDC. Revised recommendations for HIV testing of adults, adolescents, and pregnant women in health-care settings. *MMWR Morb Mortal Wkly Rep* 2006;55:1–27.
15. ACOG Committee on Obstetric Practice. ACOG Committee Opinion No. 418. Prenatal and perinatal human immunodeficiency virus testing: expanded recommendations. *Obstet Gynecol* 2008;112:39–42.
16. www.cdc.gov/hiv/rapid_testing
17. Eichler A, Eiden U, Kessler P. AIDS and anesthesia. *Der Anaesthesist* 2000; 49:1006–1017.
18. Merrill JE, Chen IS. HIV-1, macrophages, glial cells, and cytokines in AIDS nervous system disease. *FASEB J* 1991;5:2391–2397.
19. Tardieu M. HIV-1-related central nervous system diseases. *Curr Opin Neurol* 1999;12:377–381.
20. Kramer-Hammerle S, Rothenaigner I, Wolff H, et al. Cells of the central nervous system as targets and reservoirs of the human immunodeficiency virus. *Virus Res* 2005;111:194–213.
21. Evron S, Glezerman M, Harow E, et al. Human immunodeficiency virus: anesthetic and obstetric considerations. *Anesth Analg* 2004;98:503–511.
22. Gabuzda DH, Hirsch MS. Neurologic manifestations of infection with human immunodeficiency virus. Clinical features and pathogenesis. *Ann Intern Med* 1987;107:383–391.
23. Miller R. HIV-associated respiratory diseases. *Lancet* 1996;348:307–312.
24. Beck JM, Rosen MJ, Peavy HH. Pulmonary complications of HIV infection. *Am J Respir Crit Care Med* 2001;164:2120–2126.
25. Dhasmana DJ, Dheda K, Raven P, et al. Immune reconstitution inflammatory syndrome in HIV-infected patients receiving antiretroviral therapy. Pathogenesis, clinical manifestations and management. *Drug* 2008;68:191–208.
26. Raj V, Joshi S, Pennell DJ. Images in cardiovascular medicine. Cardiac magnetic resonance of acute myocarditis in an human immunodeficiency virus patient presenting with acute chest pain syndrome. *Circulation* 2010;121: 2777–2779.
27. Gopal M, Bhaskaron A, Khalife WI, et al. Heart disease in patients with HIV/AIDS—an emerging clinical problem. *Curr Cardiol Rev* 2009;5:149–154.
28. Feigenbaum K, Longstaff L. Management of the metabolic syndrome in patients with human immunodeficiency virus. *Diabetes Educ* 2010;36:457–464.
29. Mesa RA, Edell ES, Dunn WF, et al. Human immunodeficiency virus infection and pulmonary hypertension. *Mayo Clin Proc* 1998;73:37–45.
30. Isgro A, Mezzaroma I, Aiuti A, et al. Recovery of hematopoietic activity in bone marrow from human immunodeficiency virus type-1-infected patients during highly active antiretroviral therapy. *AIDS Res Hum Retroviruses* 2000; 16:1471–1479.
31. Semba RD, Gray GE. Pathogenesis of anemia during human immunodeficiency infection. *J Invest Med* 2001;49:225–239.
32. Stasi R, Willis F, Shannon MS, et al. Infectious causes of chronic immune thrombocytopenia. *Hematol Oncol Clin North Am* 2009;23:1275–1297.

33. Koka PS, Reddy ST. Cytopenias in HIV infection: mechanisms and alleviation of hematopoietic inhibition. *Curr HIV Res* 2004;2:275–282.

34. Casiglia JW, Woo S. Oral manifestations of HIV infection. *Clin Dermatol* 2000;18:41–51.

35. Wilcox CM. Role of endoscopy in the investigation of upper gastrointestinal symptoms in HIV-infected patients. *Can J Gastroenterol* 1999;13:305–310.

36. Lo Re III V, Kostman JR, Amorosa VK. Management complexities of HIV/hepatitis C virus coinfection in the twenty-first century. *Clin Liver Dis* 2008;12:587–609.

37. Singal AK, Anand BS. Management of hepatitis C virus infection in HIV/HCV co-infected patients: clinical review. *World J Gastroenterol* 2009;15:3713–3724.

38. Miro JM, Aguero F, Laguno M, et al. Liver transplantation in HIV/hepatitis co-infection. *J HIV Ther* 2007;12:24–35.

39. Perazella MA. Acute renal failure in HIV-infected patients: a brief review of common causes. *Am J Med Sci* 2000;319:385–391.

40. Rao TKS. Renal complications in HIV disease. *Med Clin North Am* 1996;80:1437–1451.

41. Fine DM, Perazella MA, Lucas GM, et al. Renal disease in patients with HIV infection: epidemiology, pathogenesis, and management. *Drugs* 2008;68:963–980.

42. Izzedine H, Harris M, Perazella MA. The nephrotoxic effects of HAART. *Nephrology* 2009;5:563–573.

43. ACOG Committee on Obstetric Practice. ACOG Committee Opinion No. 234. Scheduled cesarean delivery and the prevention of vertical transmission of HIV infection. *Int J Gynaecol Obstet* 2001;73:279–281.

44. Lewis SH, Reynolds-Kohler C, Fox HE, et al. HIV-1 in trophoblastic and villous Hofbauer cells, and haematological precursors in eight-week fetuses. *Lancet* 1990;335:565–568.

45. Al-Husaini AM. Role of placenta in the vertical transmission of human immunodeficiency virus. *J Perinatol* 2009;29:331–336.

46. Lallemant M, Jourdain G, Le Couer S, et al. A trial of shortened zidovudine regimens to prevent mother-to-child transmission of human immunodeficiency virus type I. Perinatal HIV prevention trial (Thailand) investigators. *N Engl J Med* 2003;343:982–991.

47. Kourtis AP, Lee FK, Abrams EJ, et al. Mother-to-child transmission of HIV-1: timing and implications for prevention. *Lancet Infect Dis* 2006;6:726–732.

48. Coovadia H. Current issues in prevention of mother-to-child transmission of HIV-1. *Curr Opin HIV AIDS* 2009;4:319–324.

49. Chasela CS, Hudgens MG, Jamieson DJ, et al. Maternal or infant antiretroviral drugs to reduce HIV-1 transmission. *N Engl J Med* 2010;362:2271–2281.

50. Kumwenda N, Hoover DR, Mofenson LM, et al. Extended antiretroviral prophylaxis to reduce breast-milk HIV-1 transmission. *N Engl J Med* 2008;359:119–129.

51. Garcia PM, Kalish LA, Pitt J, et al. Maternal levels of plasma human immunodeficiency virus type I RNA and the risk of perinatal transmission. *NEJM* 1999;341:394–402.

52. Panel on Treatment of HIV-Infected Pregnant Women and Prevention of Perinatal Transmission. Recommendations for use of antiretroviral drugs in pregnant HIV-1-infected women for maternal health and interventions to reduce prenatal HIV transmission in the United States. May 24, 2010:1–117. Available at http://aidsinfo.nih.gov/Content Files/PerinatalGL.pdf

53. Cooper ER, Charurat M, Mofenson LM, et al. Combination antiretroviral strategies for the treatment of pregnant HIV-1 infected women and prevention of perinatal HIV-1 transmission. *J Acquir Immune Defic Syndr Hum Retrovirol* 2002;29:484–494.

54. Lopez-Jimenez F, Brito M, Aude YW, et al. Update in internal medicine. *Arch Med Res* 2000;31:329–352.

55. Rakhmanina NY, van den Anker JN, Soldin SJ. Safety and pharmacokinetics of antiretroviral therapy during pregnancy. *Ther Drug Monit* 2004;26:110–115.

56. Panel on Antiretroviral Guidelines for Adults and Adolescents. Guidelines for the use of antiretroviral agents in HIV-1-infected adults and adolescents. Department of Health and Human Services. December 1, 2009:1–161. Available at http://www.aidsinfo.nih.gov/ContentFiles/AdultandAdolescentGL.pdf

57. Blanche S, Tardieu M, Rustin P, et al. Persistent mitochondrial dysfunction and perinatal exposure to antiretroviral nucleosides analogues. *Lancet* 1999;354:1084–1089.

58. McGowan JP, Shah SS. Prevention of perinatal HIV transmission during pregnancy. *J Antimicrob Chemother* 2000;46:657–668.

59. Olkkola KT, Palkama VJ, Neuvonen PJ. Ritonavir's role in reducing fentanyl clearance and prolonging its half-life. *Anesthesiology* 1999;91:681–685.

60. Stevenson GW, Hall SC, Rudnick S, et al. The effect of anesthetic agents on the human immune response. *Anesthesiology* 1990;72:542–552.

61. Gershon RY, Manning-Williams D. Anesthesia and the HIV-infected parturient: a retrospective study. *Int J Obstet Anesth* 1997;6:76–81.

62. Grubert TA, Reindell D, Kashner, et al. Complications after cesarean section in HIV-1-infected women not taking antiretroviral treatment. *Lancet* 1999;354:1612–1613.

63. Hughes SC, Dailey PA, Landers D, et al. Parturients infected with human immunodeficiency virus and regional anesthesia: clinical and immunologic response. *Anesthesiology* 1995;82:32–37.

64. Avidan MS, Groves P, Blott M, et al. Low complication rate associated with cesarean section under spinal anesthesia for HIV-1 infected women on antiretroviral therapy. *Anesthesiology* 2002;97:320–324.

65. Wlody DJ. Human immunodeficiency virus. In: Chestnut DH, Polley LS, Tsen LC, Wong CA, eds. *Chestnut's Obstetric Anesthesia: Principles and Practice.* 4th ed. Philadelphia, PA: Mosby Elsevier; 2009:961–974.

66. Kuczkowski KM. Human immunodeficiency virus in the parturient. *J Clin Anesth* 2003;15:224–233.

67. American Society of Anesthesiologists Task Force on Infection Control. *Recommendations for infection control for the practice of anesthesiology.* Park Ridge, IL: American Society of Anesthesiologists; 1998.

68. Sullivan P. Associations of anemia, treatments for anemia, and survival in patients with human immunodeficiency virus infection. *J Infect Dis* 2002;185:S138–S142.

69. Sullivan PS, Hanson DL, Chu SY, et al. Epidemiology of anemia in human immunodeficiency virus (HIV)-infected persons: results from the multistate adult and adolescent spectrum of HIV disease surveillance project. *Blood* 1998;91:301–308.

70. Moore RD, Keruly JC, Chaisson RE, et al. Anemia and survival in HIV infection. *J Aquir Immune Defic Syndr Hum Retrovirol* 1998;19:29–33.

71. Kirkley SA. Proposed mechanisms of transfusion-induced immunomodulation. *Clin Diagn Lab Immunol* 1999;6:652–657.

72. Practice guidelines for perioperative blood transfusion and adjuvant therapies: an updated report by the American Society of Anesthesiologists Task Force on Perioperative Blood Transfusion and Adjuvant Therapies. *Anesthesiology* 2006;105:198–208.

73. Tom DJ, Gulevich SJ, Shapiro HM, et al. Epidural blood patch in the HIV-positive patient: review of clinical experience. *Anesthesiology* 1992;76:943–947.

74. Hughes SC, Dailey PA. Human immunodeficiency virus in the delivery suite. In: Hughes SC, Levinson G, Rosen MA, eds. *Shnider and Levinson's Anesthesia for Obstetrics.* 4th ed. Philadelphia, PA: Lippincott Williams & Wilkins; 2002:583–595.

75. CDC. Updated U.S. Public Health Service guidelines for the management of occupational exposures to HIV and recommendations for postexposure prophylaxis. *MMWR Morb Mortal Wkly Rep* 2005;54:1–17.

Renal and Hepatic Disorders in Pregnancy

Michael Paech

■ RENAL DISEASE

Introduction

Renal disease in pregnancy is uncommon, having an estimated incidence of 0.1% (1). It may be present as a consequence of renal disease prior to pregnancy (e.g., systemic lupus erythematosus [SLE], glomerulonephritis), occur antenatally or intrapartum as a result of an obstetric disorder that involves the kidney (e.g., preeclampsia, acute fatty liver of pregnancy [AFLP]), or develop shortly after pregnancy (e.g., acute renal failure [ARF] due to trauma, postpartum hemorrhage, or a thrombotic microangiopathy). The kidney is often involved in preexisting multisystem disorders (e.g., diabetic nephropathy, hypertensive nephropathy) because diabetes mellitus and hypertension account for more than 50% of cases of chronic renal failure in the general population. A few renal disorders are specific to the organ (e.g., urinary tract infection, some inherited diseases).

The obstetric outcomes of women with severe renal disease appear to have improved significantly in recent years, largely because of the use of erythropoietin for anemia, better management of hypertension, high-flux dialysis for end-stage or ARF, and progress in neonatal care (2). The anesthetic management of women with renal disease follows the principles that apply to the non-pregnant patient, with a variety of modifications because of the physiologic differences and pharmacologic considerations that pertain during pregnancy.

Changes in Renal Physiology During Pregnancy, and their Implications

There are a number of changes in renal anatomy and function, and in body fluids and electrolytes, during pregnancy (1,3–5) (Table 37-1). Kidney volume increases by 30% and size by 1 cm, mainly because of a 75% to 80% increase in renal blood flow that is a consequence of generalized vasodilation, mediated by increased progesterone, estrogen, nitric oxide, and the circulating ovarian hormone relaxin. The renal pelvis and calyces, and the ureters dilate, more markedly on the right side, mainly due to obstruction by the gravid uterus and congested right ovarian vein.

As well as renal blood flow, the glomerular filtration rate (GFR) increases very early in pregnancy—by 50% (from 100 to 150 mL/min) by the second trimester. The marked increase in creatinine clearance, in the presence of unchanged creatinine production, causes serum urea and creatinine to fall (normal range: 40 to 90 μmol/L; upper limit of range: 80 and 90 μmol/L [1.02 mg/dL] in the second and third trimesters, respectively). Proteinuria increases to a normal range maximum of 300 mg/24 h. Tubular reabsorption of glucose decreases, which contributes to the development of gestational diabetes. Women with severe renal disease may be unable to

mount an increase in GFR, such that any further insult, such as hemorrhage or the administration of nephrotoxic drugs (e.g., a non-steroidal anti-inflammatory drug [NSAID]), can cause a serious decline in renal function. Tubular reabsorption of bicarbonate decreases, producing a 4 to 5 μmol/L (4 to 5 mEq/L) decrease in serum bicarbonate, which compensates for the respiratory alkalosis of pregnancy. The healthy kidney increases production of vitamin D, renin, and erythropoietin. Total body water increases by 6 to 8 L and plasma osmolality falls. Those who are unable to increase production adequately may develop normochromic normocytic anemia, vitamin D deficiency, and a reduced plasma volume.

Of note, a normal or slightly raised serum urea and/or creatinine during pregnancy may indicate significant renal impairment. A serum creatinine greater than 70 μmol/L (0.8 mg/dL) during the first trimester warrants further assessment of renal function. The physiologic fall in serum albumin and edema of late pregnancy can mimic nephrotic syndrome. Women presenting with early onset preeclampsia, including proteinuria, may have unrecognized chronic renal disease so should be reviewed by a nephrologist. Any proteinuric preeclampsia is associated with an increased risk of postpartum microalbuminemia, although estimated GFRs are similar to healthy women.

The physiologic changes of pregnancy take up to 3 months to disappear, so postpartum monitoring and review of women with renal dysfunction or preeclamptic proteinuria is required.

Chronic Renal Disease: Maternal and Fetal Implications

Chronic renal disease is found in 1 in 750 to 3,000 pregnancies (6). It may be clinically and biochemically silent, but even in early stages impact on pregnancy outcomes. In addition, although the impact may be clinically undetectable, pregnancy adversely affects abnormal renal function, by means of exacerbation of endothelial dysfunction, and alteration in immune function and inflammatory processes.

Most women have mild renal dysfunction (serum creatinine <124 μmol/L or 1.4 mg/dL) (Table 37-2) and well-controlled hypertension prior to pregnancy, and suffer little or no apparent adverse effect on long-term renal function. There is some evidence to suggest they have more obstetric complications such as preterm and cesarean delivery, and need for neonatal intensive care (7), but most women have good outcomes if antenatal care is adequate.

The severity of renal impairment and of hypertension correlate with pregnancy outcome (1,6), so for women in stages 3 to 5 (which represents moderate to severe disease with serum creatinine 124 to 220 μmol/L or 1.4 to 2.5 mg/dL) (Table 37-2); or who have heavy proteinuria, poorly controlled hypertension or recurrent urinary tract infection

TABLE 37-1 Changes in Renal Anatomy and Physiology in Pregnancy

Parameter	Direction of Change	Approximate Magnitude
Kidney volume	Increases	30% increase
Urinary tract	Dilates	
Renal blood flow	Increases	50%
GFR	Increases	50%
Creatinine clearance	Increases	40–65%
Protein excretion	Increases	Max. normal 300 mg/day
Glucose excretion	Increases	
Calcium and amino acid excretion	Increases	
Plasma volume	Increases	50%
Total body water	Increases	6–8 L
Plasma osmolality	Decreases	5–10 mOsmol/kg
Anion gap	Decreases	To 5–11
Serum bicarbonate	Decreases	4–5 μmol/L
Serum sodium	Decreases	
Serum potassium	No change	

GFR, glomerular filtration rate.

adapt poorly to the pregnancy-induced increases in renal blood flow. They are more likely to suffer not only poor obstetric outcomes (infertility, miscarriage, perinatal death) but also a subsequent decline in renal function (6,8).

About 20% of women with early onset preeclampsia, with proteinuria, have undetected chronic renal disease and of those with established moderate or severe chronic renal disease, 40% to 80% develop preeclampsia (1,4). After preeclampsia, the absolute risk of end-stage renal disease remains very low but preeclampsia is a marker for chronic kidney disease, increasing the relative risk significantly (9).

Most aspects of prognosis and management during pregnancy relate to clinical features and the severity of renal dysfunction, rather than to the specific type of disease. Early antenatal assessment by specialists, monitoring of renal function, blood pressure, and proteinuria (Table 37-3); and when appropriate midstream urine for infection and kidney ultrasound for urologic obstruction, is used to detect problems and guide intervention (4). Ultrasonography is an important imaging tool of the renal tract that is complimented by magnetic resonance imaging, especially for renal masses.

Acute Renal Failure During Pregnancy

ARF in pregnancy has multiple causes (Table 37-4) but is a rare event (incidence 1% to 3%; dialysis required in 1 in 10 to 15,000 pregnancies). Maternal mortality from ARF is 5% to 30%, the higher rate associated with sepsis. ARF is usually a complication of common obstetric complications, such as severe preeclampsia, postpartum hemorrhage or puerperal sepsis but also occurs with very uncommon disorders, for example, AFLP or hemolytic uremic syndrome (HUS). Bilateral renal cortical necrosis in addition to acute tubular necrosis is more likely, especially in older women (8). Patients who show delayed recovery may need renal biopsy, but the vast majority of patients return to normal renal function (10).

Pseudo-renal failure results from systemic reabsorption of urea and creatinine from the peritoneal cavity after bladder rupture, in association with uterine rupture or prolonged vaginal delivery when the bladder has not been catheterized. It presents with ascites, ileus, and laboratory parameters of ARF or is an incidental finding at explorative surgery (11).

Renal Replacement Therapy (Dialysis) During Pregnancy

Acute renal replacement therapy is based on experience in non-pregnant patients and may prove inadequate unless the physiologic changes of pregnancy are taken into account. The anesthesiologist should liaise with the patient's nephrologist, obstetrician and dialysis nurse to determine the patient's

TABLE 37-2 Severity of Chronic Renal Disease

Stage	GFR	Estimated GFR (mL/min/1.73 m^2)	Serum Creatinine (μmol/L:mg/dL)
1	Normal	>90	to 90:1.02
2	Mild disease	60–89	106–124:1.2–1.4
3	Moderate disease	30–59	124–220:1.4–2.5
4	Severe disease	15–29	Above 220:2.5
5	Renal failure	<15	

GFR, glomerular filtration rate.

TABLE 37-3 Monitoring of Renal Disease During Pregnancy

Parameter	Details
Urine	4–6 weekly checks for infection, proteinuria, hematuria
Blood pressure	Regular review aiming for 120–140 systolic and 70–90 diastolic blood pressure, with treatment
Renal function	Check serum urea and creatinine, more frequently in grade 3–5 disease and later pregnancy. Protein:creatinine ratio estimation is convenient (>30 mg/μmol abnormal).
Blood count/picture	Check hemoglobin aiming for 100–110 g/L with iron and erythropoietin
Renal tract	Ultrasound at 12 wks gestation and repeat if suggestion of obstruction

TABLE 37-4 Causes of Acute Renal Failure During Pregnancy

Severe preeclampsia
Acute fatty liver of pregnancy
Acute deterioration of chronic renal disease
Renal insults, especially sepsis and obstetric hemorrhage, but also drug toxicity and hyperemesis gravidarum
Urinary tract obstruction
Hemolytic uremic syndrome and thrombotic thrombocytopenic purpura
Multiple myeloma and other myeloproliferative disorders

current hemoglobin, blood pressure, fluid and electrolyte status, use of anticoagulants and dialysis requirement.

Among women already on dialysis, pregnancy rates are low (incidence 1.5%) (8) but improvements in dialysis regimens (12) and the widespread use of erythropoietin (in higher doses) has reduced anovulation and improved fertility rates and pregnancy outcomes (2,13). Protein restriction can be decreased, which improves maternal and fetal nutrition.

Dialysis may also be required in women with renal impairment who become pregnant and then reach end-stage renal failure—this population produces babies of higher birth weight (14). Indications for dialysis include refractory volume overload, hyperkalemia, maternal blood pH <7.2, serum creatinine of 350 to 400 μmol/L (4 to 4.5 mg/dL) or a GFR below 20 mL/min (1). Maternal hypertension occurs in 30% to 50% of dialyzed women, 10% develop preeclampsia and hypertension worsens in 20%. Anemia is common, because red blood cell production is outstripped by the increase in plasma volume, such that up to a 2-fold increase in erythropoietin dose may be required to maintain an adequate concentration of hemoglobin (5,15).

Successful pregnancy outcomes are increasing in these women, with better outcomes generally among those who have been on dialysis for shorter periods before becoming pregnant and those who reach later gestations before requiring dialysis. Preterm delivery (spontaneous or iatrogenic), polyhydramnios, and growth retardation are very common and combined fetal and neonatal death rate continues to be approximately 30% (2,13,14). Attention has been directed to improving fetal outcome by increasing the time spent on dialysis, usually by increasing its frequency (often daily to achieve >20 hours per week) and a predialysis serum urea of 5 to 8 μmol/L (30 to 50 mg/dL) (5,12). Heparinization should target the lowest therapeutic level to reduce the risk of obstetric hemorrhage and low-dose aspirin may be warranted to prevent preeclampsia in women at risk (5). The success of pregnancy among women receiving continuous ambulatory peritoneal dialysis, and the associated perinatal mortality, appears similar to that among women receiving hemodialysis (15). Peritonitis develops in a small percentage, is likely to cause miscarriage or premature labor (2,14), and, in addition to hemoperitoneum, may indicate surgery.

Renal Transplantation

Although they remain lower, pregnancy rates improve dramatically among women of reproductive age who have been transplanted, especially if they are stable, with no or minimal proteinuria, well-controlled blood pressure, no pelvicalyceal distension, serum creatinine <133 μmol/L (1.5 mg/dL) and on low doses of prednisolone, azathioprine, and cyclosporine (5). Successful pregnancy is also possible after simultaneous pancreas–kidney transplant (16).

Short-term graft function is maintained during pregnancy too, provided renal function is good and immunosuppression regimens are stable (4,17). Long-term graft function is rarely adversely affected (17). Triple immunosuppressive therapy should be continued throughout pregnancy, although mycophenolate mofetil is contraindicated based on recent evidence of adverse fetal and neonatal outcomes (4,18).

The most common maternal problems are preexisting and steroid-induced hypertension, urinary tract infection, preeclampsia and steroid-induced impaired glucose tolerance (5). Birth defects are not increased but fetal loss can be high as a result of preterm birth, small for gestational age infants and neonatal mortality. Long-term childhood development of children of transplanted mothers appears normal. Acute rejection during pregnancy is rare, but should be treated with steroids and immunoglobulin, with the safety of anti-lymphocyte globulins and rituximab unknown (5,19).

Kidney donors have similar obstetric outcomes to the general population but compared to predonation pregnancies have a higher fetal loss (approximately 20% vs. 10%), gestational diabetes, gestational hypertension, and preeclampsia (20).

Anesthetic Considerations for Pregnant Women with Renal Disorders

Preoperative Assessment

Severe renal impairment affects most body systems, mandating a systematic preoperative assessment. In the cardiovascular system, symptoms and signs of hypertension and accelerated atherosclerosis are common. Hyperkalemia, hypermagnesemia and chronic metabolic acidosis are common biochemical features. Intestinal absorption of calcium is decreased and phosphate excretion impaired, so hyperphosphatemia develops, calcium is deposited in soft tissues, and in chronic renal failure, osteomalacia occurs. The electrocardiogram should be reviewed for signs of hyperkalemia, which may cause ventricular dysfunction and acute arrhythmias; and for Q–T prolongation, reflecting hypocalcemia.

TABLE 37-5 Safety of Drugs Used in Pregnancy-related Renal and Liver Disease

Drug	FDA Category	Comments
Antiemetics		
Metoclopramide	B	Appears safe in pregnancy
Ondansetron	B	More first trimester information required, appears safe thereafter
Prochlorperazine	C	Reports of anomalies but causation uncertain. Extrapyramidal effects possible in neonates.
Promethazine	C	Possible neonatal respiratory depression
Anticoagulants		
Aspirin	C/D	Low dose may be safe. Potential growth retardation, bleeding, and acidosis. Near delivery use and premature closure of ductus arteriosus.
Enoxaparin	B	Inadequate evidence but widely used.
Heparin	C	Does not cross placenta
Anti-hypertensives		
ACE inhibitors, ARBs	C/D	Avoid. Major anomalies in first trimester and later oligohydramnios, renal failure, skull hyperplasia, death
β-blockers	C/D	Growth retardation, bradycardia, hypotension
Calcium channel blockers	C	Animal embryopathy but inadequate human data
Other		
Ursodeoxycholic acid	B	Low risk
Prednisolone	C	Low risk. Possible increase cleft palate, adrenal insufficiency
Azathioprine	D	Low risk
Cyclosporine	C	Low risk
Tacrolimus	C	Probably safe
Lamivudine	C	Low risk
Interferon	C	Not recommended
Mycophenolate mofetil	C	Limited data but not recommended

C/D, C in first trimester and D in second and third trimesters; ACE, angiogenesis-converting enzyme; ARB, angiogenesis receptor blocker.

In chronic renal failure, hypoalbuminemia and low plasma oncotic pressure predispose to the development of pulmonary edema in the presence of fluid overload. A decrease in surfactant production increases the risk of postoperative atelectasis and impaired response to infection increases the risk of pneumonia.

Glucose intolerance and gestational diabetes mellitus are common, as is normochromic normocytic anemia, although widespread use of recombinant erythropoietin has decreased the incidence of chronic anemia. There is an increased risk of gastric irritation and gastrointestinal hemorrhage. Nausea and vomiting are common in the uremic patient, but more likely to have other etiologies in the pregnant woman with renal disease. Central nervous system manifestations of renal dysfunction, such as confusion or convulsions, are rarely encountered during pregnancy, and are sinister signs of end-stage disease.

Drug Therapy

Knowledge about drug safety during pregnancy is important (Table 37-5). Of particular clinical relevance is the fact that angiotensin-converting enzyme (ACE) inhibitors and angiotensin II receptor blockers (ARBs) cause a 3-fold increase in teratogenic effects and up to 25% fetal and neonatal loss, not only in early pregnancy but with administration in the second and third trimesters, so are contraindicated. Any drug with

activity at the fetal renin–angiotensin–aldosterone axis should be discontinued or avoided during pregnancy. NSAIDs are nephrotoxic and must also be avoided. Diuretics are usually avoided except for women with diabetic nephropathy and volume-dependent hypertension. Nifedipine is probably preferable to a β-agonist for tocolysis, because the latter drugs cause hypokalemia and are dangerous in salt-losing interstitial renal diseases. Magnesium sulfate undergoes renal excretion, so infusion rates in preeclampsia and eclampsia need to be reduced and serum concentrations monitored (1).

Immunosuppressive drugs such as cyclophosphamide and mycophenolate mofetil are fetotoxic, but cyclosporin, azathioprine, tacrolimus, and steroids are non-teratogenic and considered safe, with sirolimus unknown (4,5,16,21,22).

Renal dysfunction alters the pharmacokinetics of many drugs. Low serum albumin and metabolic acidosis may increase the free-drug concentration of some drugs, volumes of distribution are often increased, renal replacement therapy may alter drug concentrations and the activity of drugs eliminated in part or largely by the kidneys is prolonged. This may mandate monitoring of drug levels and dose adjustment (Table 37-6), including during general anesthesia.

Breast-feeding is recommended despite chronic renal failure. Most drugs of relevance, for example, prednisolone (prednisone), ACE inhibitors, and azathioprine, have negligible breast milk transfer and are considered safe. Others such as the

TABLE 37-6 **Drug Dosing in Renal Failure**

Analgesics	
Fentanyl, alfentanil, remifentanil	No change
Morphine, diamorphine	Not cleared by dialysis. Avoid because of accumulation of active metabolites morphine-3-glucuronide and morphine-6-glucuronide
Codeine, dihydrocodeine	Accumulation of morphine metabolites may prolong effect
Oxycodone	Decrease dose by approximately 50%
Buprenorphine	No change
Acetaminophen (paracetamol)	No change
Non-steroidal anti-inflammatory drugs	Contraindicated due to further reduction in GFR
Tramadol	Reduce dose or increase dose interval because active metabolites accumulate
Anesthetics	
Propofol, thiopental, ketamine	No change
Isoflurane, desflurane	No change
Sevoflurane	Avoid due to potential fluoride accumulation and toxicity
Succinlycholine (suxamethonium), atracurium, cisatracurium	No change
Vecuronium, rocuronium, pancuronium	No change but avoid repeat dosing due accumulation
Drugs with Sedative Effects	
Midazolam	Reduce dose
Clonidine	No change
Phenothiazines, butyrophenones	No change
Antibiotics	
Penicillins, cephalosporins	Reduce dose by approximately 50%
Gentamicin	Reduce dose, increase dose interval and monitor levels
Cardiovascular Drugs	
α-adrenergic blockers, calcium channel blockers, nitroglycerin (glyceryl trinitrate)	No change
β-adrenergic blockers	Reduce dose
Anti-arrhythmic drugs	No change
Digoxin	Reduce dose and monitor levels
Methyldopa	Prolonged duration due renal excretion
Diuretics	Usually avoid
Other Drugs	
Metoclopramide	No change
Ranitidine	Reduce dose by approximately 50%
Low molecular weight heparins	Reduce dose
Oxytocin	No change but caution with fluid overload
Ergonovine, ergometrine	No change
Magnesium	Reduce dose and monitor levels
Cyclosporin, tacrolimus	Avoid if possible but increase dose if required
Azathioprine	Avoid if possible and use minimum effective dose if required

immunosuppressive drugs cyclosporin and tacrolimus transfer into breast milk but are also considered acceptable to use during lactation.

Anesthetic Assessment and General Anesthesia

Patients with mild renal disease but normal renal function and blood pressure present no particular concerns. In contrast, there are many factors to consider when anesthetizing women with moderate to severe renal impairment, end-stage renal failure, or on dialysis. Such patients should be identified as high risk early in pregnancy and appropriate monitoring and management plans established, in liaison with obstetric, nephrology and anesthetic colleagues. For obstetric anesthesia, general recommendations in non-pregnant patients apply (23), but specific issues need consideration (24).

The maternal intravascular volume should be assessed with a view to maintaining blood pressure, renal and placental perfusion. Large fluid or blood volume loss may be poorly tolerated and central venous pressure monitoring can be considered. Arterial blood pressure monitoring is useful if there is severe hypertension or large blood loss is anticipated or occurs. Electrolyte disorders may need correction, with hyperkalemia (>6.0 mEq/L or 6.0 μmol/L) treated using intravenous glucose, insulin, β-adrenergic agonists or dialysis.

Treatment of diabetes is likely to require insulin and dextrose infusions and anemia should be sought and corrected, taking care to avoid blood transfusion of patients who have adapted to low hemoglobin levels. Erythropoietin, initially at a dose increase of 50%, is indicated if hemoglobin concentration is <8 g/dL (80 g/L), aiming to achieve a target of 10 to 11 g/dL (100 to 110 g/L) or a transferrin saturation >30% (1,5). Intravenous iron infusion may be indicated but smaller doses should be given to minimize the risk of fetal iron toxicity. Renal patients are prone to delayed gastric emptying and full precautions against gastric aspiration are advisable. Drugs that are primarily excreted by the kidneys should be avoided or the dosage altered (Table 37-6).

Patients on steroids are at increased infection risk and if taking doses above 7.5 to 10 mg/day, additional steroid cover is required (1). Infection control is particularly important in transplanted or other immunosuppressed women, who have higher rates of urinary tract and cytomegalovirus infection (1).

Prolonged responses to succinylcholine (suxamethonium) have been reported due to pseudo-cholinesterase deficiency despite normal genotype. During ventilation, hypercarbia leads to extracellular acidosis, causing intracellular potassium to move into the extracellular compartment and exacerbate hyperkalemia. In the presence of hypermagnesemia, non-depolarizing muscle relaxants are potentiated. Potassium release following the use of succinylcholine is not increased, but normal potassium release may evoke arrhythmias. Uremia disrupts the blood–brain barrier, resulting in exaggerated responses to induction agents. Neuromuscular blocking drugs with renal excretion should be avoided, making atracurium and cisatracurium preferable to vecuronium or rocuronium. Smaller doses of epidural morphine are advised because of impaired excretion of morphine 3- and 6-glucoronide, so fentanyl is the preferred systemic opioid because it has no active metabolites. NSAIDs are renotoxic and should not be used.

Patients with renal impairment are prone to thrombosis, so anti-thrombotic therapy is frequently indicated. They are also at increased risk of infection, so strict asepsis is required when undertaking invasive procedures. Great care must be taken of arteriovenous fistulae, which should be protected and padded during childbirth or anesthesia. Intravenous cannula must be sited well away from fistulae, using the opposite limb whenever possible.

Patients with osteomalacia are prone to fractures, especially under regional block, so careful attention to positioning and movement is needed. Postoperative sodium and water retention is exaggerated if the concentrating ability of the kidney is impaired, yet hypovolemia may result from fluid loss as a result of pyrexia, vomiting, surgery or hemorrhage.

Consideration must be given to the most appropriate care setting after delivery. High-dependency care, where close monitoring of fluid and electrolyte balance can continue, is often required.

Neuraxial Techniques

Peripheral neuropathies should be documented preoperatively prior to a regional technique, and the possibility of co-existing autonomic neuropathy with delayed gastric emptying remembered.

There is no evidence supporting additional benefits from regional versus general anesthesia in pregnant women with renal impairment. The safety of neuraxial block is not proven but appears acceptable in the absence of platelet or coagulation abnormalities. Before regional block, fluid loading is best avoided, because small increases in end-diastolic volume may result in pulmonary edema. Epidural insertion is generally considered safe in renal patients and has also been used for patients undergoing renal transplantation (25), but a number of potential hazards exist, including epidural hematoma (26). The activity of concomitant low molecular weight heparin therapy must be considered and the platelet count may be normal or low, especially when superimposed preeclampsia exists. Although standard coagulation tests tend to be normal, patients with moderate to severe renal disease can have reduced von Willebrand factor activity (27), so ideally specific hematologic tests will have been performed during early pregnancy.

At acute presentation for labor or delivery, thromboelastography has been suggested but is of unproven utility (28). Abnormal bleeding can be treated with D-desmethyl-arginine vasopressin (DDAVP) and the role of recombinant factor VIIa should be considered.

The disposition of epidural bupivacaine is unaltered, even among those having renal transplantation (25). As a result of a hyperdynamic circulation and acidosis on the binding and pharmacokinetics of local anesthetics, the onset of subarachnoid block may be faster, the dermatomal spread increased by one or two segments, but the duration of the block reduced (29).

Diseases with Renal Involvement in Pregnancy

Diabetic Nephropathy

This develops after 10 to 15 years in type 1 diabetics, and complicates approximately 5% of insulin-dependent diabetic pregnancies. Preconception assessment and monitoring are recommended. Although diabetic nephropathy increases the perinatal risk, the babies of women with microalbuminuria and well-preserved renal function have a very good prognosis (5). ACE inhibitors need to be stopped and anti-hypertensive therapy switched to safer drugs such as methyldopa, labetalol, or nifedipine. Pregnancy is more likely to be complicated by preeclampsia (especially if overt nephropathy is present) and urinary infection, but does not appear to affect disease progression. Given that few diabetic women of reproductive age have significant renal impairment, maternal outcomes are also usually excellent (30).

Glomerulonephritis

This term is a non-specific descriptor of a range of conditions in which the glomerulus is inflamed, whether as a primary renal disease or part of a systemic illness. Diagnosis and division into pathologic sub-categories is based on clinical findings and renal biopsy, which has a low complication rate in pregnancy but may not be indicated unless it alters therapy. Patients present with acute symptomatic disease (hematuria, edema, rising creatinine) or chronic asymptomatic disease (microhematuria, proteinuria, slow rising creatinine). Nephrotic syndrome is associated with diuretic-resistant edema and hypertension may require treatment with ACE inhibitors and ARBs, though these increase the risk of acute kidney injury and hyperkalemia. Thromboembolism can occur due to increased loss of anticoagulants.

Post-infectious glomerulonephritis is unusual in pregnancy, but occurs particularly after streptococcal throat infection (31). Pregnancy outcome is determined by the severity of renal impairment and the presence of lupus nephritis (32).

Systemic Lupus Erythematosus

SLE is a multisystem autoimmune disease, principally of women of reproductive age. Hypertension is due to lupus nephritis, which is present in 60% of patients within 3 years of initial presentation. Some patients are anti-cardiolipin IgG and IgM antibody positive and others have lupus anticoagulant, which is associated with poorer pregnancy outcomes. Pregnancy increases the risk of a flare in renal or hematologic disease (32). Women with lupus nephritis who conceive are usually in a quiescent phase and adequately controlled, so experience good outcomes. The absence of uterine artery Doppler abnormalities and lupus flares are good prognostic indicators (33). If the nephritis is active, perinatal outcome is poorer and these women show increased organ damage after pregnancy (5). Overall, compared with women without lupus nephritis, those with nephritis are more likely to have fetal abnormalities, pregnancy-induced hypertension and low birth weight infants, but pregnancy outcomes are otherwise similar (34).

Management is based on low-dose steroid therapy (<20 mg/day reduces the risk of inducing hypertension or gestational diabetes), acceptable drugs such as hydroxychloroquine and azathioprine, and in those with lupus anticoagulant, aspirin and low molecular weight heparin (given twice daily to account for increased excretion during pregnancy) (35).

Approximately 2% of the children of mothers with SLE will develop the disease, which is polygenic with environmental precipitants.

Anti-phospholipid Syndrome

Anti-phospholipid syndrome, which occurs in isolation or is associated with other autoimmune diseases, is characterized by significant pregnancy morbidity, especially recurrent pregnancy loss and recurrent arterial and venous thromboses. The kidney is a major target, with pathology including nephropathy, renal artery stenosis and thrombosis, renal infarction and widespread renal vasculature changes (36). During early pregnancy, aspirin is recommended, as is low molecular weight heparin, especially if there have been previous complications. Women with SLE who are also anti-phospholipid antibody positive have higher rates of nephritis and hypertension (37).

Urinary Tract Infection

Dilatation of the renal tract and urinary stasis predispose to this infection, which is the most common cause of abdominal pain in pregnancy and which may trigger preterm labor (3,38).

Bacteriuria is present in 3% to 7% of pregnant women, urinary tract infection in 2% to 30% and acute pyelonephritis in 1%, usually presenting during the second trimester (3,39). Women experiencing recurrent infection should be

monitored closely for deterioration of renal function, using renal ultrasound and laboratory testing. Prophylactic antibiotic therapy may reduce further infections and preserve renal function. Pyelonephritis is most often caused by *Escherichia coli* and group B *Streptococcus*, so ceftriaxone is a good initial choice of antibiotic. Urinary tract infection is associated with preterm delivery and growth retardation but not increased perinatal mortality (40).

Some women present with septic shock, hemolysis, thrombocytopenia, pulmonary edema and adult respiratory distress syndrome, mandating intensive care (41). It is postulated that low colloid osmotic pressure and plasma fibronectin concentrations during pregnancy explain the apparent increase in vulnerability to pulmonary complications (42).

A rare complication of obstruction and urinary tract infection is non-traumatic rupture of the renal tract. In one series, five patients required nephrectomy; one died before surgery and there were two fetal intrauterine deaths (43).

Reflux Nephropathy and Urinary Stone Disease

Hydronephrosis is a normal physiologic change that commences in the first trimester of pregnancy. It promotes urinary stasis and predisposes to urolithiasis, urinary tract infection and pyelonephritis. These complications are associated with abortion, hypertension, preterm delivery, and fetal growth retardation (40).

Reflux nephropathy is common in women of child-bearing age and renal scarring is an important cause of urinary tract infection and later renal impairment. Some women with severe reflux may benefit from ureteric re-implantation prior to pregnancy or from early dialysis to improve fetal outcome. Scarring occurs in 50% of women who experience bacteriuria in pregnancy, so if bacteriuria is detected, rotating courses of antibiotics are appropriate to prevent symptomatic infection (38).

Urinary tract obstruction may also arise from pelvo-ureteric junction obstruction, ureterocele or most commonly, calculi. Symptomatic calculi are not more common in pregnancy (incidence 1 in 1,500 to 2,500), because excretion of both stone-forming substances and inhibitors (magnesium, citrate, glycosaminoglycans, acute glycoproteins) is increased (3,44). Ureteric stones are twice as common as renal and are mostly calcium phosphate (hydroxyapatite), followed by calcium oxalate (44). The diagnosis of renal colic is difficult because flank pain and other symptoms mimic several other conditions in pregnancy, but overt or microscopic hematuria is almost always present (44,45). Enhanced spiral CT has replaced intravenous urography as the imaging modality of choice in non-pregnant patients but despite the sensitivity and specificity being far less, routine ultrasound evaluation is performed first in pregnancy, to avoid issues of radiation exposure (46). Up to 40% of patients with symptomatic urolithiasis go into preterm labor (45,46).

A third of patients with stones require intervention and those with sepsis and obstruction may need drainage and stone retrieval in addition to intravenous fluids, antibiotics, and analgesics. Seventy to 90% of these patients recover after conservative treatment, such as epidural analgesia or β-adrenergic blockade to stimulate ureteric contractility (44). Even non-calculus hydronephrosis may require ureteric stents or percutaneous nephrostomy, which can be performed with ultrasound or fluoroscopic guidance (with pelvic shielding), under regional or general anesthesia. Extracorporeal lithotripsy may induce labor or harm fetal hearing, so is best avoided, but flexible ureteroscopy with stone baskets or pneumatic or laser lithotripsy is safe and has high rates of success (44,47).

Autosomal Dominant Polycystic Kidney Disease

Autosomal dominant polycystic kidney disease (ADPKD) is an inherited disorder of membrane proteins with incomplete penetrance and a 5% new mutation rate, resulting in a prevalence of 1 in 400 to 1,000 live births (48). Fifty percent of patients ultimately require renal replacement therapy as a consequence of renal cyst enlargement, making the disease the most common genetic cause of renal failure. Cysts are also commonly found in the liver and pancreas but are usually asymptomatic. Intracranial aneurysms are found in 1 in 20 patients but hypertensive or ischemic stroke is more common than hemorrhage. Mitral valve prolapse can occur. New pharmacotherapies are being developed based on animal models of the disease and include tolvaptan, a vasopressin type 2 receptor antagonist, octreotide, rapamycin, sirolimus, and everolimus (48).

The clinical presentation is typically later in life, so pregnant women are usually asymptomatic, declining renal function being associated with increasing multiparity and moderate to severe disease at conception. The aims of preconception counseling and specialist referral are control of hypertension and treatment of complications, because 25% of affected women develop hypertension and 11% develop preeclampsia. Normotensive women with normal renal function generally have uncomplicated pregnancies (49).

Systemic Sclerosis (Scleroderma)

Pregnancy, in women with systemic sclerosis (scleroderma) that is stable, is usually uneventful, although risks include hypertension, renal crises and fetal intrauterine growth retardation. Symptoms other than gastro-esophageal reflux may improve, but monitoring for renal and cardiovascular complications is warranted (50,51). Therapy with oral hydroxychloroquine and intravenous immunoglobulin, but not cyclophosphamide, is appropriate and appears safe.

Tuberous Sclerosis

Tuberous sclerosis is a multisystem autosomal dominant disorder characterized by benign growths in the skin, brain, kidney, and lungs. These hamartomas may cause seizures or renal hemorrhage if angiomyolipomas, which are present in 50% of patients and often multiple and bilateral (52). Few pregnancies in women with tuberous sclerosis have been reported, although anesthesia is usually not a concern and both epidural analgesia and general anesthesia for cesarean delivery are described (52). The management of a pregnant woman with chronic non-malignant pain from the disease is also reported (53).

Vasculopathic Diseases

Wegener's granulomatosis and *Churg–Strauss syndrome* are small vessel vasculitides associated with anti-neutrophil cytoplasmic antibodies (ANCAs). Blood vessel walls become inflamed and necrotic, causing fever, night sweats, and weight loss. Those with Churg–Strauss syndrome develop eosinophilic and granulomatous lesions and asthma worsens, but as the disease mostly affects males, pregnancy is rare (54). In Wegener's granulomatosis, upper respiratory tract disease, epistaxis, nasal bridge collapse, and ARF are features (55).

Treatment in non-pregnancy is with high-dose steroids and cyclophosphamide, but the latter is contraindicated during pregnancy. Plasma exchange may be required and maternal mortality is high. Patients who enter remission within 4 to 6 weeks become ANCA negative and pregnancy should be avoided until in remission. The placenta appears unaffected by the vasculitic pathology, so fetal mortality and morbidity is low. *Moyamoya disease* is a vascular stenotic or occlusive disease, predominantly among those of Asian ethnicity. It typically involves the cerebrovascular circulation but renal artery stenosis may be present (56).

Takayasu's arteritis is a rare chronic inflammatory disease, predominantly of women of child-bearing age, affecting the aorta and its main branches, including the renal arteries. Successful pregnancy while on prednisolone, adalimumab, and initially leflunomide has been described, but generally pregnancy should only be contemplated during remission, because the higher intravascular volume exacerbates aortic regurgitation, hypertension, and cardiac failure (57). If anesthesia is required, organ ischemia should be evaluated and intravascular volume optimized. Monitoring may be difficult in a pulseless patient. Titrated regional techniques providing stable hemodynamics and allowing monitoring of the cerebral circulation are recommended (57).

Thrombotic Microangiopathy

Thrombotic thrombocytopenic purpura (TTP) and *HUS* are rare, potentially fatal diseases that share features with severe preeclampsia and AFLP, such as thrombocytopenia and microangiopathic hemolytic anemia, making them difficult to diagnose. Pregnancy may precipitate an acute episode, and TTP is now thought to be due to a deficiency of von Willebrand factor-cleaving metalloprotease (ADAMTS13). They are managed using fresh frozen plasma, plasmapheresis, blood products, and in some cases steroids pre- and post-delivery, to improve the platelet count (58–60).

HUS (when not associated with *E. coli* toxin in children especially) is a sporadic or familial disease characterized by non-immune hemolytic anemia, thrombocytopenia and in two-thirds of cases, renal failure (from platelet thrombi formation in the renal microcirculation, possibly in association with retained placental fragments of generalized endothelial disorders) (9,58–60). Predisposing conditions are systemic disease, malignant hypertension, malignancy, and TTP. The incidence of HUS during pregnancy is estimated as 1 in 25,000 and presentation may be antepartum (associated with preeclampsia) or postpartum (presenting as ARF).

The maternal mortality rate from these diseases is 5% to 25%, largely due to extrarenal complications such as left ventricular failure, but the severity and duration of renal failure predicts long-term outcome. Patients needing dialysis for more than 28 days are very unlikely to recover normal renal function. Perinatal mortality is high (30% to 80%) (58). There is no clear benefit from delivery of the baby, but intrauterine death and iatrogenic preterm delivery are common.

The anesthesiologist is most likely to encounter a pregnant woman with one of these disorders when critical care or delivery is necessary. Full blood count and renal function should be reviewed. Plasmapheresis is required if there are signs of ongoing disease 8 to 72 hours post-delivery.

Goodpasture's Syndrome, Alport's Syndrome, Bartter's Syndrome, and Gitelman's Syndrome

Goodpasture's syndrome is an autoimmune disease characterized by anti-glomerular basement membrane antibodies directed against collagen IV in renal and alveolar basement membranes. Patients develop severe progressive glomerulonephritis and hemoptysis from pulmonary hemorrhage. Management includes steroids, immunosuppression with cytotoxic drugs (to prevent further renal damage) and intermittent plasmapheresis (to clear circulating anti-basement membrane antibodies from the circulation). There are very few case reports of successful pregnancy, with superimposed preeclampsia, declining renal function and progression to end-stage renal disease postpartum likely (61,62). *Alport's syndrome* is a rare inherited disease associated with various mutations (most often X-linked) in the gene for basement membrane type IV collagen. The diagnosis is based on clinical findings, renal biopsy and molecular genetic testing, with features including variable progression of glomerulonephritis and sometimes cochlear or ocular involvement, particularly sensorineural deafness (62). Little is known about the impact of pregnancy on this vasculopathic disease, with both no change in a woman with mild disease, and severe rapid deterioration to renal failure in another with well-controlled disease, reported (63). *Bartter's syndrome* is a rare autosomal recessive disorder of chloride transport in the ascending loop of Henle, characterized by severe hypokalemia, metabolic alkalosis, hyperaldosteronism, and normotension (64). Clinical manifestations include growth restriction, muscle weakness, cramps, polyuria, and polydipsia. Obstetric and anesthetic management is directed toward restoration of normal serum potassium levels, but hypokalemia may persist irrespective of aggressive replacement therapy using intravenous and oral supplements. Hyperventilation-induced hypocapnia can exacerbate the reduction in serum potassium and effective regional analgesia for laboring patients is recommended. Potassium-sparing diuretics (amiloride and spironolactone) are used, as ACE inhibitors are contraindicated. Regional-induced hypotension is a potential issue due to vasopressor resistance (65) but pregnancy appears to be associated with good outcomes (48,64). *Gitelman's syndrome* is a rare (incidence 1 in 40,000) autosomal recessive defect of a co-transporter in the renal tubules, that leads to urinary wasting of magnesium, sodium, potassium, and calcium but rarely progresses to end-stage renal disease. As well as replacing magnesium and potassium (full correction may not be possible) and organizing electrocardiograms and serial monitoring, 50% of patients have a prolonged Q–T interval, so drugs causing further prolongation must be avoided (65).

Renal Tubular Acidosis

Renal tubular acidosis is characterized by inadequate renal hydrogen ion excretion, despite normal glomerular filtration. Type 1 renal tubular acidosis is inherited in an autosomal dominant manner and affects the distal tubules, while Type 2 affects the proximal tubules. Both result in hyperchloremic metabolic acidosis, with a normal anion gap. There are few reports of pregnancy, one describing two pregnancies, both complicated by hypertension but free of adverse maternal or fetal events (66).

Renal Tumors

The management of cancers such as nephroblastoma (Wilm's tumor) or clear cell carcinoma in young adults who fall pregnant and are then diagnosed with a malignant renal mass is unchanged during pregnancy, although early delivery may be required (67). Magnetic resonance imaging is the best method of diagnosis, following antenatal ultrasound, and avoids fetal irradiation. Wilm's tumor has an excellent prognosis after surgery, chemotherapy, and radiotherapy and laparoscopic nephrectomy can be safely performed during pregnancy (68).

■ LIVER AND BILIARY DISEASE

Introduction

Abnormalities of liver function tests (LFTs) and jaundice are uncommon (0.3% to 3%) in pregnancy, and approximately 1 in 500 women develop serious hepatic disease (69,70). Derangements of LFTs are mainly associated with acute liver disease from preeclampsia, acute fatty liver, and acute viral hepatitis (71,72). Diagnosis may be difficult because serologic testing takes time, and liver biopsy is usually contraindicated by coagulopathy or is not appropriate as a primary investigation.

Expert multidisciplinary input is often of benefit in preventing disease progression and determining the optimum timing of delivery. The safest imaging is ultrasonography, but MRI without contrast (gadolinium has unknown fetal effects) is also safe (70). If hepatobiliary surgery is required, the optimal timing is usually during the second trimester (73). With severe liver disease, maternal and perinatal mortality are potentially very high (74).

Various congenital and acquired liver diseases present during pregnancy (Table 37-7). The most common disease is viral hepatitis (especially chronic hepatitis B), but a number of uncommon diseases unique to pregnancy (e.g., hyperemesis gravidarum, intrahepatic cholestasis of pregnancy [IHCP], AFLP) are frequent causes of fetal mortality and occasionally, maternal mortality. Women with cirrhosis, portal hypertension, acute liver failure, or hepatic rupture pose major anesthetic challenges.

A number of hepatic disorders worsen during pregnancy, for example, choledocal cysts that rupture, hepatic adenomas that grow, acute intermittent porphyria (AIP) that is triggered, esophageal varices associated with portal hypertension that hemorrhage, and acute hepatitis that progresses to hepatic failure. In contrast, several uncommon liver disorders confer minimal or no risk of adverse maternal and fetal outcome. Examples are the hyperbilirubinemias, which are relatively benign disorders characterized by elevations of unconjugated bilirubin (Gilbert's disease) or conjugated bilirubin (Dubin–Johnson and Rotor syndromes). Bilirubin concentrations rise during pregnancy in about 50% of women affected by these disorders, but fetal outcomes are very good.

Several multisystem diseases involve the liver (e.g., SLE, hemochromatosis, hepatic porphyrias, hydatid disease) but the most common and potentially serious of these is preeclampsia. This disease is considered in detail elsewhere.

Changes in Hepatic Physiology and their Implications

The size of the liver does not change significantly during pregnancy and hepatic blood flow remains unchanged despite the other major cardiovascular changes, thus reducing significantly the proportion of cardiac output delivered. The portal and esophageal venous pressure rises in late pregnancy and in response to estrogen some women develop stigmata of liver disease, for example, spider nevi or palmar erythema. The normal range of laboratory tests changes, with serum alkaline phosphatase (ALP) rising steadily to a 300% increase, largely because of production by a placental isoenzyme. Other enzymes alter marginally—those indicative of liver damage, such as serum aspartate aminotransferase (AST) and alanine aminotransferase (ALT), remain unchanged (75) (Table 37-8).

Pharmacokinetic changes altering drug disposition include a larger volume of distribution, reduced clearance of drugs dependent on hepatic blood flow, and dilutional reduction in serum albumin (often to 30 g/L) and plasma protein concentrations. Serum globulins change slightly (Table 37-8).

Synthesis of coagulation factors increases, with production of fibrinogen, factors VII, VIII, IX, X, and von Willebrand factor. Coagulation tests remain in the normal range. Ceruloplasmin levels may reach normal in some patients with Wilson's disease and transferrin and several specific binding proteins (e.g., those for thyroxine, vitamin D, and corticosteroids) increase. There are minor changes in porphyrin metabolism and serum bilirubin remains unchanged. Serum triglyceride and cholesterol concentrations increase progressively to term (Table 37-8).

TABLE 37-7 Classification of Liver Disease in Pregnancy

Category	Specific Disease	Most Common Trimester of Presentation
Pregnancy-related	Hyperemesis gravidarum	1
	Intrahepatic cholestasis of pregnancy (IHCP)	2–3
	Preeclampsia (HELLP syndrome) with or without liver hematoma/rupture	Late 2, 3
	Acute fatty liver of pregnancy (AFLP)	3, postpartum
Chronic	Autoimmune hepatitis	1–3
	Chronic viral hepatitis (B and C)	1–3
	Cirrhosis and portal hypertension	1–3
	Wilson's disease	1–3
	Primary sclerosing cholangitis and primary biliary cirrhosis	1–3
Coincidental	Acute viral hepatitis (A and E)	1–3
	Other acute hepatitis	1–3
	Budd–Chiari syndrome	1–3, postpartum
	Drug-induced hepatotoxicity	1–3
	Acute cholelithiasis	1–3
	Other biliary and pancreatic disease	1–3
	Liver hematoma/rupture	3, postpartum
	Sepsis	3, postpartum
	Hydatid disease	1–3

HELLP, hemolysis, elevated liver enzymes, low platelets.

TABLE 37-8 Relevant Hepatic and Biochemical Changes in Normal Pregnancy

Parameter	Alteration from Non-pregnancy	Trimester of Maximum Change
Hemoglobin	Decreased	2
White cell count	Increased	2
Platelet count	Nil or slight decrease	
Bilirubin	Nil	
Alanine aminotransferase (ALT)	Nil	
Aspartate aminotransferase (AST)	Nil	
Alkaline phosphatase (ALP)	Increase 100–300%	3
Gamma-glutamyltransferase (GGT)	Nil or slight decrease	
Lactate dehydrogenase (LDH)	Nil or slight increase	3
Prothrombin time	Nil	
Serum albumin	Decreased 20–60%	2
α-globulin	Slight increase	3
β-globulin	Slight increase	3
γ-globulin	Nil or slight decrease	3
Serum fibrinogen	Increases 50%	2
Ceruloplasmin	Increase	3
Transferrin	Increase	3
Von Willebrand factor	Increase	2
α-fetoprotein	Moderate increase	3
Triglyceride	100–300% increase	3
Cholesterol	50–100% increase	3

Acute Liver Failure

Acute liver failure during pregnancy results from loss of hepatocellular function as a result of acute disease—fulminant viral hepatitis, AFLP, severe preeclampsia, hepatotoxin poisoning (e.g., α-methyldopa or acetaminophen [paracetamol] overdose), and rarely flares or deterioration of sickle cell disease, hereditary hemorrhagic telangiectasia (Osler–Weber–Rendu syndrome), Wilson's disease or cirrhosis (precipitated by variceal bleeding or infection). Cardiovascular changes include low systemic vascular resistance and increased cardiac output, a picture similar to septic shock. Hypoxemia results from respiratory pathologies such as pulmonary edema or infection, pleural effusion or adult respiratory distress syndrome, or from hypoventilation associated with cerebral edema. The hepatorenal syndrome is characterized by oliguria, renal failure, and transient diabetes insipidus. Hypoglycemia is a consequence of defective gluconeogenesis and inadequate insulin uptake. Disseminated intravascular coagulation and fluid and electrolyte abnormalities are frequently present and supportive care, plasmapheresis, extracorporeal perfusion, and steroids have potential treatment roles. The maternal and fetal mortality of liver failure is high, in one series of 26 patients being 40% and 60%, respectively (74).

Hepatic Rupture

Hepatic rupture is a rare, potentially catastrophic event, most commonly due to trauma (76). Spontaneous rupture also occurs because of tumors, subcapsular hematoma associated with severe preeclampsia (incidence 1%), abscesses (pyogenic, amoebic, parasitic), or cocaine abuse. Rupture complicating preeclampsia usually occurs in late pregnancy or peripartum, producing intraparenchymal hematoma in the superior and anterior sections of the right lobe and rupturing along the inferior edge of the right lobe (77).

Diagnostic features of rupture are acute right upper quadrant pain, peritonism, and hypovolemia. The preferred imaging is contrast CT scan, but unstable patients must be diagnosed using abdominal ultrasound, diagnostic peritoneal lavage or at explorative laparotomy. Both fetal and maternal mortality approach 30% to 50% (70). In stable patients and those with contained hematomas, a non-operative approach based on observation and transfusion is preferred. Unstable patients require hepatic angiography, early arterial embolization, or explorative surgery, followed by surgical packing, oversewing, ligation, or partial resection.

Liver Transplantation

Approximately 75% of women receiving a liver transplant are of reproductive age and transplantation restores fertility, so that successful pregnancy becomes common. Up to 70% of these women deliver a healthy baby, despite higher rates of cholestasis, anemia, intrauterine infection, and preterm delivery (78). It is recommended that pregnancy is deferred for 1 year post-transplant but pregnancy does not appear to accelerate graft rejection or impair liver function, provided immunosuppressive therapy is continued (70). Mycophenolate mofetil is associated with first trimester pregnancy loss and an increased risk of congenital malformation, so should be ceased (22). Tacrolimus and cyclosporin can be continued but breast-feeding is not advised (70).

Anesthesia for the post-transplant patient requires attention to the physiologic effects on the transplanted liver, preservation of liver function, and problems associated with immunosuppression (79).

Anesthetic Considerations for Pregnant Women with Liver Disease

General aims of general anesthesia are to maintain liver and renal blood flow and avoid hepatotoxicity; various diseases have specific aims (Table 37-9). Propofol is a suitable intravenous anesthetic for induction because it has normal pharmacokinetics in cirrhosis and does not alter hepatic blood flow, although it may be associated with higher hepatic oxygen consumption than desflurane (80–82). Desflurane appears to be the volatile anesthetic of choice because it has negligible hepatic metabolism (83), but hepatic blood flow is not as well maintained as with propofol anesthesia (82). Prolonged administration of isoflurane causes mild derangement of hepatocellular function in healthy individuals

TABLE 37-9 Key Anesthetic Implications of Certain Liver Diseases

Hyperemesis Gravidarum	Prescribe appropriate antiemetic therapy. Correct fluid and electrolyte imbalances
Intrahepatic Cholestasis of Pregnancy (IHCP)	Check liver function and coagulation status. Prepare for cesarean delivery. Prepare for postpartum hemorrhage
Acute fatty liver of pregnancy (AFLP)	Optimize medical condition in a critical care environment. Correct coagulopathy, hypoglycemia and other abnormalities. Plan for anesthesia for cesarean delivery (regional anesthesia unless contraindicated due to coagulopathy or patient encephalopathic). For general anesthesia, use anesthetic and analgesic drugs appropriate in severe hepatic dysfunction. Prepare for peripartum or postpartum hemorrhage. Organize postoperative critical care and monitoring
Wilson's disease	Check and monitor liver function; coagulation status. Consider implications of esophageal varices or bulbar involvement. Use anesthetic techniques and drugs appropriate to patients with severe liver dysfunction. Prepare for postpartum hemorrhage
Budd–Chiari syndrome	Monitor liver function, coagulation status, hematology. Consider implications of anticoagulant therapy. Use anesthetic drugs appropriate for patients with severe liver dysfunction.

(83) and nitrous oxide should be avoided. Succinylcholine (suxamethonium) is not contraindicated but may cause prolonged neuromuscular block in the presence of a low plasma cholinesterase (84). Atracurium and cisatracurium are the preferred non-depolarizing neuromuscular blocking drugs, because others have hepatic metabolism and rocuronium shows great individual variability among patients with hepatic impairment (85).

The anesthesiologist should be aware of drugs used in liver (and renal) disease and their classifications in pregnancy (Table 37-5). Health care workers are at risk of contracting hepatitis through blood contact, mandating special care and the application of universal precautions. Patients with liver disease may have an increased risk of thromboembolism or postpartum hemorrhage, important considerations when planning anesthetic and postoperative care.

In the presence of fulminant hepatic failure, exaggerated responses to anesthetics and opioid analgesics occur, because of poor metabolism and central depression associated with encephalopathy. Hepatic blood flow is altered by changes in carbon dioxide levels, positive pressure ventilation, volume shifts and particularly blood pressure, which shows no autoregulation (81).

The anesthesiologist may be required to manage an elective or emergency cesarean delivery (86,87) or an urgent liver transplantation. The two most serious issues to address are coagulopathy and encephalopathy (manifesting as restlessness, confusion, asterixis, seizures, psychosis, or coma). There are a number of anesthetic options (88), with regional anesthesia often contraindicated by coagulopathy, obtundation, or surgical needs. General anesthesia may reduce hepatic blood flow because of controlled ventilation and anesthetic drug effects, but propofol induction can be followed by either volatile anesthetic or an infusion (87). Prolonged drug responses are likely, making close monitoring and titration essential. Most patients will require continued postoperative ventilation and intensive care, and some hemodialysis or plasmapheresis. Acetaminophen (paracetamol) dosing should be greatly reduced because hepatic glutathione depletion may allow centrizonal necrosis after normal doses (89).

Diseases with Hepatic Involvement in Pregnancy

Hyperemesis Gravidarum
Most women experience nausea and vomiting in early pregnancy. For some this persists well into the second trimester, but intractable and protracted nausea and vomiting leading to inadequate hydration and nutrition, 5% loss of body weight, and fluid and electrolyte abnormalities, is known as hyperemesis gravidarum. The reported incidence varies widely, from 0.3% to 2% (70,90) and the severe vomiting usually resolves by 20 weeks' gestation, but may continue. The etiology probably involves interplay of hormonal, gastric motility and autonomic nervous system effects, with risk factors obesity, multiple pregnancy, younger age, diabetes, hydatidiform mole (70), and porphyria (91). Only in the most severe cases is fetal outcome poor, despite low birth weight.

Vomiting results in maternal dehydration, ketosis, weight loss, reflux esophagitis, and electrolyte disturbances, especially severe hyponatremia, hypokalemia, and hypochloremic alkalosis. Biochemical hyperthyroidism, due to elevated human chorionic gonadotropin levels, is present in 60% (70) and 15% to 50% of patients have reversible LFT abnormalities because of malnutrition in the presence of high estrogen levels (69,90). Serum unconjugated bilirubin and ALP concentrations increase slightly and transaminases such as ALT may increase 20-fold (to 1,000 U/L) (70,90). Rare complications are esophageal rupture, pneumomediastinum, renal failure, aspiration, and Wernicke's encephalopathy from thiamine deficiency.

Hospitalization for a few days (sometimes multiple admissions) is required for symptomatic treatment and monitoring. Most antiemetic drugs are safe in pregnancy, including metoclopramide, droperidol, antihistamines, and 5-hydroxytryptamine$_3$ receptor antagonists. The anesthesiologist may be consulted about antiemetic therapy and needs to be aware of current treatment, which might include histamine$_2$ receptor blockers or proton pump inhibitors for esophagitis, rehydration with intravenous fluids (sodium-containing crystalloid, with potassium as needed), parenteral or enteral nutrition with correction of vitamin deficiencies using pyridoxine, folate and thiamine, and psychological support.

Intrahepatic Cholestasis of Pregnancy
IHCP is the most common liver disease unique to pregnancy. It is the second most frequent cause of cholestasis during pregnancy, after viral hepatitis, with other causes, drug-induced cholestasis and primary biliary cirrhosis (92). Cardinal features are pruritus, abnormal liver function in the absence of other liver disease, and resolution after delivery. In most countries the prevalence of IHCP lies between 0.1% and 1%, but in Sweden and Chile it reaches 5% to 15% in certain populations (69,70,72,75,90), with the highest rates among multiple pregnancies and after assisted reproductive technology (93,94).

IHCP is a heterogeneous genetic disorder of complex etiology, involving mutations in genes encoding bile salt transporters within the hepatocytes and the biliary system. There are environmental and hormonal triggers, with risk factors a family history or cholestasis secondary to oral contraceptives (70,93,94). There is genetically determined dysfunction of the canalicular bile salt export pump and multidrug resistance protein 3, which encodes the pump protein that transports phospholipids. One severe form is due to ABCB4 gene mutations associated with loss of canalicular translocators (69,70,71).

Approximately 80% of cases present after 30 weeks' gestation, as estrogen and progestagens peak, with symptoms progressing in severity as pregnancy advances. Pruritus follows reduction in bile flow and reduced bile and bile acid excretion, typically starting in the extremities (palms and soles) before extending to the trunk and face. It is often severe, disrupting sleep at night and responding poorly to treatment with topical therapy. Mild conjugated hyperbilirubinemia and jaundice are uncommon, occurring in 10% to 25% of those affected, so cholelithiasis and other liver diseases should be excluded. Malaise, nausea, abdominal discomfort and subclinical steatorrhea from vitamin K deficiency are also possible, although pain warrants investigation for viral hepatitis or cholelithiasis. There are often 2- to 20-fold elevations of serum aminotransferases (concentrations usually <250 U/L), ALT more so than AST. The diagnosis of IHCP is clinical, since although there is a 10- to 100-fold increase in serum bile acids, some patients have normal levels. Total bile acid concentrations >10 μmol/L are diagnostic and >40 μmol/L indicates severe disease with poorer prognosis (70,95). Resolution begins within 24 hours of delivery and is usually complete in 2 to 6 weeks (93), although recurrence in subsequent pregnancy is likely (94) and in rare familial forms, fibrosis may occur (70).

The fetus is not at risk from very mild disease but risks rise in proportion to maternal bile salt concentration (in contrast, bilirubin does not cross the placenta significantly). Preterm labor is common (30% to 40%), neonatal respiratory distress may be a consequence of the disease as well as preterm birth, and there are higher rates of meconium aspiration and late stillbirth clustered around 38 weeks' gestation, with perinatal mortality approximately 3% (93,95). Induction of labor at 37 weeks is controversial but commonplace, because complications of prematurity and cesarean rates are high (95). Fetal distress in labor is also common, mandating close intrapartum monitoring. The neonate should receive vitamin K therapy to prevent intracranial bleeding.

Despite inadequate levels of evidence, pruritus and abnormal liver function appears to be improved by use of ursodeoxycholic acid 15 mg/kg/day in 2 divided doses. This hydrophilic bile acid stimulates biliary secretion of bile salt export pump, reduces bile salt and sulfated progesterone metabolite concentrations (70), and displaces toxic bile acids (cholic acid and chenodeoxycholic acid, products of cholesterol metabolism) from hepatic membranes (92–95). Pruritus is relieved and the drug well tolerated. The anesthesiologist should assess the severity of liver dysfunction and check for rare cases of coagulation disturbance. Prophylactic oral vitamin K is sometimes given empirically against fat-soluble vitamin deficiency and consequent maternal postpartum hemorrhage.

Acute Fatty Liver of Pregnancy

AFLP is a rare, potentially fatal metabolic disorder with an estimated population incidence of 1 in 20,000 (96) and referral hospital based incidence of 1 in 1 to 15,000 pregnancies (69,70,72,75,90) (Table 37-10). It usually presents in the third trimester, often close to term, and infrequently after delivery, with prodromal malaise and vomiting for several days to 2 weeks, then more severe abdominal pain, polydipsia, headache, or infrequently encephalopathy. Jaundice is mild and complications include renal failure, acute respiratory distress, diabetes insipidus, and pancreatitis (96,97) (Table 37-10). More severe jaundice suggests preeclampsia, viral hepatitis, cholestasis, or bile duct obstruction. Pruritus is uncommon (incidence 5% to 30%) and the liver size is normal.

The diagnosis of AFLP is clinical, supported by early laboratory coagulation abnormalities (although elevated fibrin degradation products and low fibrinogen are less common), later liver dysfunction (aminotransferases moderately elevated between 100 and 1,000 U/L), low blood glucose, and renal dysfunction (early elevation of serum creatinine and ammonia and metabolic acidosis from high serum lactate levels) (Table 37-10). Profound hypoglycemia is common, due to depression of glucose-6-phosphatase activity, and indicative of more severe disease. Cholesterol, triglycerides and antithrombin are low. Marked neutrophil leukocytosis to 30,000/mm³ with left shift, microangiopathic hemolytic anemia and thrombocytopenia, are very common. Some patients also have preeclampsia with hemolysis, elevated liver enzymes, low platelets (HELLP), the main distinguishing features of AFLP being hypoglycemia, hyperammonemia, more severe coagulopathy, less severe thrombocytopenia, and less right upper quadrant pain or hypertension (98) (Table 37-11). Abdominal ultrasound may show ascites or a bright liver (96) and excludes gallstones, while diagnostic liver biopsy is almost always precluded by the bleeding risk.

This disease affects women of all ages, races, and ethnicities and may appear after several normal pregnancies, but is more common in nulliparous women, multiple pregnancy, and preeclampsia (69,96). Metabolic, synthetic and excretory functions of the liver are abnormal due to fat infiltration and inflammation (72). AFLP occurs in 30% to 80% of women heterozygous for long-chain 3-hydroxyacyl-CoA dehydrogenase (LCHAD) deficiency, one of four enzymes that are part of a mitochondrial trifunctional protein complex responsible for long-chain fatty acid oxidation in the liver. If the fetus is homozygous (even heterozygous) and unable to oxidize 3-hydroxy fatty acids sufficiently it may present in infancy or after extended fasting with a hypoglycemic, Reye-like syndrome. Preceding this, excess fetal fatty acids transfer to the mother where they impair mitochondrial function and accumulate as microvesicles in hepatocytes. AFLP is also associated with deficiencies in carnitine palmitoyltransferase I and medium- and short-chain acyl-CoA dehydrogenase.

Supportive therapy in an intensive care unit is required. Invasive monitoring and dextrose infusions to correct hypoglycemia, hemodialysis for renal failure, desmopressin for diabetes insipidus, and blood products for correction of coagulopathy, are often needed. About 50% of cases have coagulopathic bleeding, requiring blood product transfusion. Coagulopathy may worsen postpartum, when antithrombin levels fall further. Mortality is due to gastrointestinal hemorrhage and sepsis. In women with preeclampsia, adjustment of magnesium doses is necessary if renal impairment is present. Patients who develop encephalopathy need lactulose and may require intubation and ventilation, mandating general anesthesia for cesarean delivery.

TABLE 37-10 Diagnostic Features of Acute Fatty Liver of Pregnancy

Feature	Frequency Outside Normal Range	Typical Range of Values
Low blood glucose	Very common	1–8 μmol/L
High bilirubin	Almost always	15–650 μmol/L
Coagulopathy	Extremely common	APTT 20–100 s
High serum urate	Extremely common	50–850 μmol
High serum creatinine	Common	60–400 μmol/L
High transaminases	Almost always	AST 40–3,000 IU/L ALT 20–1,100 IU/L
Low platelet count	Very common	15–450 × 10⁹/L
High ammonia	Common	15–70 μmol

Six or more of: Vomiting, abdominal pain, polyuria/polydipsia, encephalopathy, elevated bilirubin, urate, transaminases or ammonia, hypoglycemia, leukocytosis, ascites, renal impairment, coagulopathy, microvesicular steatosis on liver biopsy.
APTT, activated partial thromboplastin time; AST, aspartate aminotransferase; ALT, alanine aminotransferase.

TABLE 37-11 Differences Between Severe Preeclampsia with HELLP Syndrome and Acute Fatty Liver of Pregnancy

Symptom or Feature	Severe Preeclampsia (HELLP)	AFLP
Incidence	0.2–0.6%	0.005%
Parity	Nulliparous, multiple pregnancy	Multiparous, older age
Vomiting	Possible	Common
Epigastric pain	Common	Possible
Hypertension	Common	Possible
Proteinuria	Common	Possible
Hyperuricemia	Common	Very common
Elevated creatinine	Possible	Common
Transaminases	Mild to 20-fold elevation	Variable but to 500-fold elevation
APTT	Normal	Prolonged
Glucose	Normal	Low
Ammonia	Normal	High
Platelet count	Low or very low	Low–normal
Fibrinogen	Normal or high	Low
Encephalopathy	No	Sometimes
Maternal mortality	1–10%	5–20%

HELLP, hemolysis, elevated liver enzymes, low platelets.

After resuscitation and stabilization, usually within 24 hours of presentation, expedited delivery is mandated. Most women who enter spontaneous labor show evidence of fetal compromise, so about 75% of women with AFLP undergo cesarean delivery (96). Common neonatal problems arise due to prematurity, growth retardation, intrapartum hypoxia, and hypoglycemia. Although intensive care is needed for several days because of the risk of maternal hypoglycemia and hemorrhage, recovery is rapid over a few days, with resolution of disseminated intravascular coagulopathy and restoration of normal liver function within 4 weeks. Recurrence is unusual but genetic counseling should be offered. Greater awareness of the disease, intensive therapy and prompt delivery of the fetus have resulted in a significant fall in maternal mortality over the past 25 years, such that reported maternal case fatality rates of 7% to 18% probably exceed current rates (96). Unfortunately, perinatal mortality (usually stillbirth) is 10-fold normal (96), at 10% or more. Neonates with LCHAD deficiency can experience failure to thrive, hepatic failure, cardiomyopathy, and hypoglycemia.

The anesthesiologist should assist with multidisciplinary optimization of medical care, and initiate intensive monitoring of maternal physiology and neurologic status. Blood pressure, blood glucose, fluid and electrolytes, coagulation, and acid–base status need regular assessment. Arterial cannulation is invaluable and good venous access via a central venous or peripherally inserted central catheter assists with infusion of dextrose-containing fluids, maintenance of adequate urinary output, treatment of hypertension, and replacement of electrolytes. Prophylactic H_2-receptor antagonists are prescribed and coagulation defects corrected using IV vitamin K and blood products if clinical bleeding occurs. Successful urgent liver transplant has been used in cases with raised intracranial pressure or deteriorating neurologic function.

Anesthesia is tailored to the situation (88,96), with regional anesthesia more likely to preserve hepatic blood flow provided blood pressure is maintained (99), but contraindicated in at least half the cases by fetal compromise or coagulation abnormalities and hematoma risk (96). General anesthesia may worsen encephalopathy but is often the method of choice for cesarean delivery (84,100,101). Strategies to reduce rises in intracranial pressure (obtunding the responses to intubation and extubation, avoiding coughing or venous obstruction in the head and neck, avoiding hypercarbia) are warranted if encephalopathy is present. Care with laryngoscopy to minimize airway trauma and avoidance of intramuscular injections, acetylsalicylic acid and NSAIDs are also recommended.

Hepatitis

Autoimmune hepatitis is a chronic disease of uncertain origin affecting women of child-bearing age. It reduces fertility because of associated hypothalamic–pituitary dysfunction, making it rare in pregnancy. Severity varies and concurrent autoimmune diseases may confound the diagnosis. Immunotolerance in pregnancy usually has a positive effect on disease progression, but disease flares occur in 20% to 35% and in 10% to 50% postpartum (102). Fetal outcomes are highly variable. Treatment with immunosuppressive therapy is usually continued, but the cytokine shift from a T-helper type 1 cytotoxic profile to a T-helper type 2 anti-inflammatory profile, mediated by high estrogen levels, allows a reduction in drug dose or even temporary elimination (103). Both prednisolone and azathioprine are safe to continue and if ceased, should be resumed post-delivery. The major fetal risk is premature delivery, leading to fetal mortality of 20% and perinatal or maternal mortality of 3% to 4% (102).

Peliosis hepatitis is a rare infective disease, sometimes noted in immunodeficient patients, caused by the gram-negative bacteria genus Bartonella, which also causes "cat scratch disease." Opportunistic infections present with angiomatosis, liver and spleen vasculitis, and endocarditis. Patients may be asymptomatic or develop portal hypertension, liver failure, or intraperitoneal hemorrhage. Therapies include antibiotics and hepatic artery embolization (103). *Drug-induced hepatitis*, from amoxicillin–clavulanic acid or methyldopa, for example, is usually transient.

Viral hepatitis is the most common cause of hepatitis, hepatic dysfunction, and jaundice during pregnancy. Acute hepatitis can usually be distinguished from other causes of acute liver disease by the high liver transaminase concentrations (often 10-fold normal). A number of other viruses cause acute hepatitis during the systemic infection phase, especially among immunosuppressed patients. In addition to hepatitis A and E, these include the herpes simplex virus (HSV), which is more likely to cause fulminant hepatitis than in non-pregnancy, cytomegalovirus, Epstein–Barr virus and, in Africa, Crimean-Congo hemorrhagic fever. In HSV there may be fever, oropharyngeal or genital lesions, coagulopathy and very high serum AST and ALT, but near normal bilirubin levels. Treatment with antiviral drugs is indicated but prognosis is poor and maternal mortality 40% to 75% (70,104).

Hepatitis A, B, C, D and E virus may present as acute or chronic disease, with hepatitis B (HBV) and C (HCV) the most important for chronic liver disease. Only hepatitis E (HEV) appears to be more severe in pregnancy, but an impact on maternal obstetric and fetal outcomes is likely if disease is fulminant. The risk of vertical intrapartum transmission varies with each virus, being greatest with HBV and HEV.

Hepatitis A virus (HAV) varies in prevalence geographically, but is endemic in Africa, Asia, and Central America. It shows fecal–oral transmission and affects approximately 1 in 1,000 pregnant women in the United States, with most infections asymptomatic or subclinical. Symptoms are similar to non-pregnancy, although pruritus is more common because of high estrogen levels and disease more severe with advancing age (70). Serum AST and ALT levels are significantly elevated and IgM anti-HAV is present in acute infection, followed by development of acquired immunity (anti-HAV IgG-positive serostatus) over a few weeks. Both inactivated vaccine for high-risk women and post-exposure immunoglobulin prophylaxis are safe during pregnancy. Although vertical transmission to the fetus or neonate is very rare, perinatal transmission may occur, so immunoglobulin can be given to the neonate and close household contacts. Breastfeeding should be encouraged.

Hepatitis B virus (HBV) is a highly infectious double-stranded enveloped virus transmitted by cutaneous (especially needle sharing) or mucosal (especially sexual) exposure, and vertically from mother to fetus. It is one of the most common infections in the world, with over 350 million chronic carriers worldwide and prevalence of 1% to 3%. Most acute infections (incidence 1 in 500 to 1,000 pregnancies in the United States) present 6 weeks to 6 months after exposure and are sub-clinical, although nausea, vomiting, abdominal pain, and jaundice occur with similar severity to non-pregnancy. The diagnosis is made by detection of HBV surface antigen in the serum or other secretions, and is confirmed by detection of IgM antibodies to HBV core antigen. After the acute phase hepatitis e (envelope) antigen antibody develops (anti-HBe) and patient infectivity decreases, but remains if HBsAg is present. About 5% of immunocompetent adult patients become carriers (105).

Chronic infection in pregnancy has a prevalence of 0.1% to 6% depending on ethnicity, and these women usually do well (106), although poorer perinatal outcome may result from preterm labor and low birth weight. All pregnant women should be tested for HBsAg toward the end of the first trimester and vaccination during pregnancy is considered safe. Post-delivery flares, with or without HBeAg seroconversion, may be triggered by rapidly falling cortisol levels.

Since most women have mild disease and the antiviral drugs have limited safety data in pregnancy, antiviral treatment is usually deferred until after delivery and those on treatment have it ceased, unless they are at high risk of a flare. Transplacental transmission of HBV occasionally occurs in early pregnancy (rate: 10%), but is common in later pregnancy, rising to 90% in the third trimester for HBeAg-positive women. The neonates of women with high viral loads may benefit from third trimester maternal treatment. The best safety data are for lamivudine, with tenofovir or telbivudine alternatives (70,105), although no antiviral drug has confirmed safety during lactation (105,106). Passive immunization with HBIg (immune globulin) within 12 hours of birth, and active immunization starting within 7 days of birth and continuing over the first 6 months of neonatal life, is highly effective in preventing neonatal disease, but 5% to 10% of children of HBeAg-positive women still become chronically infected.

Hepatitis C virus (HCV) is a blood borne virus endemic in Asia, the eastern Mediterranean region and Africa in particular, but also prevalent now (2% to 3% worldwide) among patients with a history of intravenous drug use, blood transfusion prior to the introduction of screening, tattooing, body piercing, and organ transplantation. HCV causes up to 20% of acute viral hepatitis, although the 6 to 9 week illness is often subclinical or mild. Approximately 70% of those infected progress to chronic asymptomatic infection, and later cirrhosis (incidence 20% by 40 years post-viral acquisition), liver failure or hepatocellular carcinoma (1.5% to 4% of those with cirrhosis) can ensue (107).

LFTs are usually normal among carriers of HCV but a number of obstetric complications (maternal cholestasis, congenital malformation, preterm delivery, low birth weight, and higher perinatal mortality) (108) are increased. Treatment with interferon and ribavirin often fails to clear the infection and should only be instituted after pregnancy due to teratogenicity and serious adverse effects.

The risk of sexual transmission is very low, but vertical transmission from mother to fetus occurs in approximately 6% of women who are HCV polymerase chain reaction (PCR) positive. Quantitative HCV-RNA testing is a marker of the risk of vertical transmission, and is more likely to be positive in the presence of co-infection with human immunodeficiency virus (HIV) and certain HCV genotypes (70). Transmission is most likely at the time of delivery through contact with contaminated vaginal secretions, but the role of elective cesarean delivery in reducing transmission has not been determined. Both HBV and HCV are detectable in human milk but breast-feeding is considered safe (70). Neonatal surveillance is with HCV antibody screening at about 12 months (maternal antibody is detectable for up to 18 months) or HCV-RNA by PCR within the first few months of life.

Hepatitis D virus (HDV) is a single-stranded RNA virus that requires the presence of HBV to replicate. HDV causes more severe disease and higher rates of chronicity and cirrhosis than hepatitis B. Infection appears rare in pregnant women and children, suggesting that vertical transmission is uncommon.

Hepatitis E virus (HEV) is a single-stranded RNA virus endemic to developing countries that commonly causes acute hepatitis via fecal–oral spread. Disease during pregnancy, especially in the late second or third trimesters, is more severe and may be fulminant, leading to very high mortality (up to 50%) (109). Depending on the viral load, vertical intrapartum transmission to the newborn occurs in 33% to 50%, with neonatal hepatic failure (107) and chronic infection both reported (110).

Hepatitis G virus is detected by reverse-transcriptase PCR. It has similar epidemiology to HIV and transmission similar to HCV, but significant liver disease is unlikely. Vertical transmission appears very common but free of adverse effect on the infant.

Cirrhosis, Portal Hypertension and Budd–Chiari Syndrome

Cirrhosis is caused by a number of conditions, especially chronic hepatitis B, C, D, and E or alcoholism, but due to hormonal derangements that cause anovulation, is rare in women of child-bearing age (rate 1 in 2,500) and even rarer in pregnancy (1 in 6,000) (111). Improvements in care have resulted in higher conception rates and better obstetric outcomes among women with well-compensated cirrhosis (111), although 25% experience deterioration in liver function and maternal mortality is 10% (70).

Elevation of portal venous pressure predisposes to esophageal varices, which bleed in 15% to 25% of pregnant women with cirrhosis and 50% of those with known portal hypertension. Screening is advised in the second trimester and β-blockers can be commenced if indicated (70,90). Diversion of blood through the azygous venous system and reflux esophagitis further predispose to variceal bleeding, ascites and portal hypertensive encephalopathy. Hematemesis, especially during later pregnancy, is associated with mortality of 20% to 50% (112). Screening for splenic artery aneurysms is also warranted, and these considered for surgical or interventional radiologic therapy, because the incidence of rupture is up to 2.5% (69).

Portal hypertension may also be present without cirrhosis, secondary to portal vein thrombosis or congenital hepatic fibrosis. Non-cirrhotic portal hypertension is much more common in Asian countries, but is associated with better outcomes (113). Essential thrombocythemia may cause recurrent abortion, placental infarction, or intra-abdominal mesenteric, portal, and hepatic venous thromboses, leading to portal hypertension.

Therapy includes albumin, diuretics, ultrasound-guided paracentesis for ascites, and non-selective β-blockers such as propranolol to lower portal pressure, despite their association with fetal growth restriction, neonatal hypoglycemia or bradycardia. Endoscopic band ligation is used in preference to chemical sclerotherapy for acute variceal hemorrhage (111). Octreotide is not of established safety but has been used for acute bleeding, as has transjugular intrahepatic portosystemic shunt (TIPS) placement. Surgical splenorenal or portocaval shunts or liver transplantation are a last resort after life-threatening hemorrhage (114), but those patients with existing shunts are at lower risk of hematemesis and the outcome of pregnancy is usually good (111). Fifty percent of patients with cirrhosis and significant portal hypertension develop either acute variceal bleeding, severe anemia (as a result of chronic illness or bleeding varices), thrombocytopenia (as a result of hypersplenism), or rupture of a splenic artery aneurysm (incidence approximately 2% and associated with very high maternal and fetal mortality). Hepatic function may deteriorate because of bleeding, sepsis, hypotension, or drugs. Drugs with anti-platelet activity potentiate the bleeding risk; impaired acetaminophen (paracetamol) and morphine-3- and -6-glucuronide metabolism result in hepatotoxicity or central nervous system depression respectively, making opioids without active metabolites (e.g., fentanyl) preferable. Intra-abdominal surgery on patients with advanced cirrhosis is associated with very high 30-day mortality (60% or more), especially if urgent or associated with concurrent coagulopathy (115).

Spontaneous abortion and preterm birth rates are doubled and neonatal mortality is increased. When vaginal delivery is planned, provided both coagulation tests and the platelet count are adequate, regional analgesia is useful in preventing straining during delivery (116). If general anesthesia is required, the principles of anesthesia that pertain to severe liver disease are applicable.

Budd–Chiari syndrome occurs in women of child-bearing age and is characterized by thrombotic obstruction of hepatic veins or the inferior vena cava, leading to liver ischemia and portal hypertension. Presentation during pregnancy is exceptionally rare, although some cases present postpartum, usually between the fourth day and third week after delivery (117). The etiology is uncertain, but anti-cardiolipin antibodies may be present and the condition is associated with several pro-thrombotic conditions, such as polycythemia rubra vera, paroxysmal nocturnal hemoglobinuria, inherited thrombophilias (e.g., antithrombin, protein C or S deficiency, factor V Leiden) and malignancy.

The hypercoagulable state of pregnancy is a concern for those women with the condition who contemplate falling pregnant. Liver biopsy shows congestion and centrilobular liver necrosis (118) and the clinical presentation with hepatomegaly, ascites, and liver failure may be insidious over months or acute. The diagnosis is made with ultrasound Doppler flow studies, venography, or magnetic resonance imaging. Initial presentation during pregnancy carries high maternal mortality (119). Known cases that are well treated before pregnancy have very high rates of early fetal loss, especially in those with factor II gene mutation (120), but show good maternal and fetal outcome after 20 weeks' gestation. Vaginal delivery is encouraged because of the risks of difficult surgery (large pelvic collateral veins), bleeding, and thrombosis associated with cesarean delivery. Management is antenatal anticoagulation with heparin and postpartum warfarin, but the obstruction may prove resistant to anticoagulation, thrombolytic therapy, and other attempts at revascularization (118). The TIPS procedure is technically more difficult in late pregnancy, so surgical shunts or liver transplantation may be necessary.

Liver Tumors

Pregnancy complicated by hepatocellular carcinoma, cholangiocarcinoma, hepatic adenoma, hemangioma, or focal nodular hyperplasia (a vascular benign tumor) is very rare and many such tumors are found incidentally. Hepatocellular carcinoma is either a very rare primary malignancy or more often, secondary to chronic HBV or HCV infection. Maternal mortality is high, possibly influenced by estrogen-stimulated acceleration. Benign hepatic adenomas are almost exclusive to women and stimulation of tumor growth during pregnancy results in a 25% incidence of hemorrhagic rupture into the abdominal cavity (69). Hemangioma is the most common benign tumor of the liver and spontaneous rupture is rare, but potentially fatal.

Termination of pregnancy may be recommended and surgical resection of symptomatic or >5 cm hepatic tumors is recommended. Successful surgical options are partial hepatectomy in the second trimester or preoperative arterial embolization prior to surgery for acute rupture. Cirrhosis and metastatic disease need consideration during assessment and planning for anesthesia. Intraoperative fetal monitoring is warranted if the fetus is viable. If resection is attempted, massive hemorrhage should be expected and full preparations are mandatory, including consideration of cell salvage.

Hepatolenticular Degeneration (Wilson Disease)

Hepatolenticular degeneration (Wilson disease) is a rare (prevalence 1 in 20 to 30,000) (121) autosomal recessive disorder involving multiple gene mutations of ATP7B which codes for a copper-transporting ATPase. This reduces copper excretion into bile and inhibits the plasma copper binding transport protein ceruloplasmin, leading to copper damage to the liver, brain, and other organs, although renal function is usually maintained.

As well as liver disease, up to 50% of patients have movement abnormalities similar to Parkinson's disease, recurrent miscarriage or golden deposits of copper in Descemet's membrane of the cornea (Kayser–Fleischer rings). Treatment is with chelators such as penicillamine or trientine, but in pregnancy the safest chelating agent is zinc (122). Copper chelation restores fertility and in asymptomatic patients without significant liver disease or portal hypertension, the fetus is unlikely to suffer liver toxicity and outcomes are good. Estrogen induces a rise in plasma ceruloplasmin, so clinical improvement or remission may occur.

Pregnancy is rarely reported and descriptions of obstetric anesthesia are also rare (123). Anesthetic assessment should be that of hepatic dysfunction, thrombocytopenia, coagulopathy, and bulbar neurologic involvement. Skin problems may warrant care with pressure from face masks or at intravascular sites. For patients on penicillamine, neuromuscular blocking drugs should be monitored because of an associated myasthenic syndrome (123). Regional techniques are valuable if not contraindicated, although cranial nerve involvement may mandate general anesthesia.

Hemochromatosis

Hemochromatosis is one of the most common genetic diseases, with estimated prevalence 1 in 300, autosomal recessive inheritance and over-representation in men. Women with juvenile idiopathic hemochromatosis and iron overload may have multiple endocrine dysfunction, heart failure, and hypopituitarism. There is little information about pregnancy, other than a successful case after regular phlebotomy to restore serum ferritin and iron levels and conception through assisted reproductive technology (124).

Hepatic Porphyrias

There are a number of acute and non-acute hepatic porphyrias, arising from defects in the heme biosynthesis pathways, with AIP the most severe. The prevalence of AIP, an autosomal dominant disease with incomplete penetrance, is 1 to 10 per 100,000. Although up to one-third of women present for the first time in pregnancy or the postpartum period (69), case series involving pregnancy are rare. In AIP, porphobilinogen deaminase activity is markedly reduced and disease is triggered by drugs and hormones that stimulate aminolevulinic acid synthetase in the liver. Pregnancy is associated with increased excretion of porphobilinogens and coproporphyrins but not to the extent of porphyric attacks, which cause abdominal pain, gastrointestinal symptoms, autonomic disturbance, neuropathies, and mental changes (125).

Attacks are prevented by administration of oral or parenteral glucose and hematin. The effect of pregnancy on the disease is unpredictable, but fasting, vomiting, or hormonal changes are triggers that make flares more common. Pregnancy outcomes are variable but generally satisfactory, with fetal loss 10% or more. Crises are most frequently triggered by drugs and maternal mortality in hospitalized patients is less than 10% (69,91).

The anesthesiologist should assess mental status, peripheral neuropathy, and bulbar dysfunction. Regional anesthesia may be suitable in the absence of an acute crisis (126). General anesthesia should be induced with propofol (127), while volatile anesthetics, opioids, and neuromuscular blocking drugs are safe (128,129).

Hydatid Disease

Hydatid disease (cystic echinococcosis) is a parasitic disease found worldwide, but is most prevalent in the Mediterranean, Middle and Far East, Australasia, Africa, and South America, where the incidence reaches 200 per 100,000. In the United States and Europe the incidence is much lower (approximately 0.5 per 100,000), but probably increasing because of immigration. Primarily a disease of sheep and cattle, humans are accidental hosts, with the adult worm containing eggs transmitted in canine feces. Larvae develop in the intestine, penetrate into the portal circulation and invade the liver, spleen, mesentery, and pelvis, although not placenta, so the neonate is not exposed (130). Cysts are often asymptomatic, being diagnosed on ultrasound, with infection confirmed by an indirect hemagglutination test. Larger cysts (>5 cm) may rupture, causing life-threatening anaphylaxis and peritoneal infection (131).

Although reduced cellular immunity favors echinococcosis growth, the disease is rare during pregnancy, with a rate of less than 1 in 20 to 30,000 in endemic areas (132) and few published reports. Drug treatment is with anti-helmintics, such as praziquantel, albendazole, and mebendazole, which do not reduce cyst size but inhibit the polymerization of tubulin to microtubules, blocking glucose absorption, causing glycogen depletion and cellular autolysis. Albendazole shows teratogenicity and embryotoxicity in rat but not sheep models and appears safe after the first trimester (131,132). Drug therapy is usually reserved for recurrent disease or when surgery is impossible, although the World Health Organization does not recommend surgery during pregnancy because of the risk of intra-abdominal dissemination or anaphylaxis from spill of cyst content. Nevertheless, urgent surgery including partial hepatectomy, may be mandated by cyst torsion, rupture, or obstruction to labor (130).

Acute Cholecystitis

Cholelithiasis during pregnancy occurs most commonly during the second and third trimesters and early postpartum period as serum lipid concentrations peak, bile acid excretion is reduced, and intestinal motility slows. Increased biliary cholesterol forms monohydrate crystals that agglomerate to produce gallstones, detectable in 10% of the pregnant population and associated with higher parity (133,134). Despite gallstones, acute cholecystitis is uncommon, having a prevalence of 0.01% to 0.1% and associations with maternal obesity and elevated serum leptin (134). The clinical presentation is similar to non-pregnancy, features being right upper quadrant pain, tenderness, fever, and leukocytosis.

The course of cholecystitis is unchanged by pregnancy and ultrasound imaging is indicated to identify gallstones or biliary sludge, followed by magnetic resonance cholangiopancreatography (75). Endoscopic retrograde cholangiopancreatography (ERCP) to detect common bile duct stones is also safe provided the uterus is shielded with lead to minimize fetal exposure to radiation.

Most women respond to conservative management with analgesia, antibiotics, intravenous fluid, and fasting, but the relapse rate is over a third, so surgery is often required. Cholecystectomy (rate: 1 to 8 per 10,000 pregnancies) is the second most common non-gynecologic operation performed during pregnancy and is best deferred until the second trimester. Laparoscopic and even open cholecystectomy is associated with good maternal and fetal outcomes, even if disease is severe (135). Treatment delays may lead to pancreatitis, which confers a poorer fetal prognosis, and surgery in the third trimester is less safe (134).

Anesthetic management follows the usual principles of anesthesia during pregnancy (136,137).

Primary Biliary Cirrhosis

Primary biliary cirrhosis is a rare disease, primarily of women aged 30 to 60 years, with an estimated prevalence 1 in 13,000 (138,139) and an association with other autoimmune disorders. The diagnosis is made by detection of IgG auto-antibodies to mitochondrial pyruvate dehydrogenase or by liver biopsy, demonstrating slowly progressive destruction of intrahepatic bile ducts, portal inflammation, and scarring. The clinical spectrum and natural history varies, with most patients asymptomatic but some having pruritus, jaundice, and fatigue. The serum ALP and GGT are raised, as may be aminotransferases and bilirubin. Infertility is common and pregnancy rare, with maternal health and fetal outcomes unclear but probably poor (75,111,138).

Management is with ursodeoxycholic acid before pregnancy and again after the first trimester (140). Methotrexate is teratogenic, so must be avoided, and liver transplantation is the only definitive therapy for advanced disease.

Primary Sclerosing Cholangitis
Primary sclerosing cholangitis is a rare chronic inflammatory, fibrotic disease of bile ducts that leads to cirrhosis and the need for liver transplantation. The etiology is unclear and no medical therapy is effective, although ursodeoxycholic acid may improve liver biochemistry. Complications include metabolic bone disease, cholangitis, and cholangiocarcinoma (141).

Most cases occur in men with inflammatory bowel disease, so few pregnancies have been reported. Pruritus is prominent, the course of the disease appears unaltered, and neonatal outcome appears good (142).

Choledochal Cysts
Choledochal cysts are very rare, having a prevalence of 1 in 100,000. They present with abdominal pain, jaundice and a mass, although the latter can be obscured by the uterus during pregnancy, delaying the diagnosis (made using ultrasound, magnetic resonance imaging, or if need be cholangiography) until complications arise (143). Cyst growth, obstruction and compression during labor increase the risk of rupture (144), so elective cesarean delivery is often recommended. Definitive surgery is delayed until after delivery if possible (69,143,145).

The anesthesiologist is likely to encounter these patients at emergency explorative laparotomy for bile drainage or at elective excision, with reconstructive hepaticoenterostomy (145).

Pancreatitis
Acute pancreatitis is rare in pregnancy (prevalence up to 1 in 1,000) and mostly associated with gallstones or less frequently excess alcohol intake or viral illness. Patients present most commonly in the third trimester, possibly due to the lithogenic effect of estrogen, and complications occur in less than 5% (146). With early recognition (the diagnosis being made on the basis of abnormal serum amylase and lipase tests, although LFTs may be normal) and better care, including the safe performance of ERCP, mortality is very much lower than in the past (146).

KEY POINTS

- Renal disease in pregnancy is uncommon (approximate incidence 1 in 1,000) and results from renal disease prior to pregnancy, multisystem or organ-specific diseases, obstetric disorders involving the kidney, or complications of pregnancy or childbirth.
- The obstetric outcomes of women with severe renal disease appear to have improved significantly in recent years, largely because of the use of erythropoietin for anemia, better management of hypertension, high-flux dialysis for end-stage or acute renal failure, and progress in neonatal care.
- The anesthetic management of women with renal disease follows the principles that apply to the non-pregnant patient, with a variety of modifications because of the physiologic differences and pharmacologic considerations that pertain during pregnancy. Neuraxial techniques are frequently appropriate.
- Abnormalities of LFTs and jaundice are uncommon, but approximately 1 in 500 women develop serious hepatic disease.
- Various congenital and acquired liver diseases present during pregnancy, the most common being viral hepatitis, but diseases unique to pregnancy (e.g., IHCP and AFLP) are frequent causes of fetal mortality and rarely, maternal mortality. Women with cirrhosis, portal hypertension, acute liver failure, or hepatic rupture pose major anesthetic challenges.
- The anesthesiologist may be required to manage critically ill women with acute hepatic failure; or those requiring cesarean delivery or urgent liver transplantation. Serious issues to address include coagulopathy and encephalopathy and general aims are maintenance of liver and renal blood flow, avoidance of hepatotoxicity and cross-infection, and management of risks such as thromboembolism and postpartum hemorrhage.
- There are a number of anesthetic options for women with liver disease, with neuraxial anesthesia sometimes contraindicated by coagulopathy, obtundation, or surgical needs.

REFERENCES

1. Vidaeff AC, Yeomans ER, Ramin SM. Pregnancy in women with renal disease. Part 1: General principles. *Am J Perinatol* 2008;25:385–398.
2. Yang LY, Thia EWH, Tan LK. Obstetric outcomes in women with end-stage renal disease on chronic dialysis: a review. *Obstet Med* 2010;3:48–53.
3. Williams DJ. Renal disease in pregnancy. *Curr Obstet Gynaecol* 2004;14:166–174.
4. Maynard SE, Thadhani R. Pregnancy and the kidney. *J Am Soc Nephrol* 2009;20:14–22.
5. Podymow T, August P, Akbari A. Management of renal disease in pregnancy. *Obstet Gynecol Clin North Am* 2010;37:195–210.
6. Williams D, Davison J. Chronic kidney disease in pregnancy. *BMJ* 2008;336:211–215.
7. Piccoli GB, Attini R, Vasario E, et al. Pregnancy and chronic kidney disease: a challenge in all CKD stages. *Clin J Am Soc Nephrol* 2010;5:844–855.
8. Krane NK, Hamrahian M. Pregnancy: kidney diseases and hypertension. *Am J Kidney Dis* 2007;49:336–345.
9. Vikse BE, Irgens LM, Leivestad T, et al. Preeclampsia and the risk of end-stage renal disease. *N Engl J Med* 2008;359:800–809.
10. Hassan I, Junejo AM, Dawani ML. Etiology and outcome of acute renal failure in pregnancy. *J Coll Physicians Surg Pak* 2009;19:714–717.
11. Png KS, Chong YL, Ng CK. Two cases of intraperitoneal bladder rupture following vaginal delivery. *Singapore Med J* 2008;49:e327–e329.
12. Haase M, Morgera S, Bamberg C, et al. A systematic approach to managing pregnant dialysis patients—the importance of an intensified haemodiafiltration protocol. *Nephrol Dial Transplant* 2005;20:2537–2542.
13. Holley L, Reddy SS. Pregnancy in dialysis patients: A review of outcomes, complications, and management. *Semin Dial* 2003;16:384–387.
14. Chou CY, Ting IW, Lin TH, et al. Pregnancy in patients on chronic dialysis: a single center experience and combined analysis of reported results. *Eur J Obstet Gynecol Reprod Biol* 2008;136:165–170.
15. Jakobi P, Ohel G, Szylman P, et al. Continuous ambulatory peritoneal dialysis as the primary approach in the management of severe renal insufficiency in pregnancy. *Obstet Gynecol* 1992;79:808–809.
16. Bramham K, Lightstone L, Taylor J, et al. Pregnancy in pancreas-kidney transplant recipients: report of three cases and review of the literature. *Obstet Med* 2010;3:73–77.
17. Kashanizadeh N, Nemati E, Sharifi-Bonab M, et al. Impact of pregnancy on the outcome of kidney transplantation. *Transplant Proc* 2007;39:1136–1138.
18. Zachariah MS, Tomatore KM, Venuto RC. Kidney transplantation and pregnancy. *Curr Opin Organ Transplant* 2009;14:386–391.

19. Areia A, Galvao A, Pais MS, et al. Outcome of pregnancy in renal allograft recipients. *Arch Gynecol Obstet* 2009;279:273–277.

20. Ibrahim HN, Akkina SK, Leister E, et al. Pregnancy outcomes after kidney donation. *Am J Transplant* 2009;9:825–834.

21. Petri M. The Hopkins Lupus Pregnancy Center: ten key issues in management. *Rheum Dis Clin North Am* 2007;33:227–235.

22. Sifontis NM, Coscia LA, Constantinescu S, et al. Pregnancy outcomes in solid organ transplant recipients with exposure to mycophenolate mofetil or sirolimus. *Transplantation* 2006;82:1698–1702.

23. Stoelting RK, Dierdorf SF. Renal diseases. In: Tracy TM, ed. *Anaesthesia and Co-existing disease*. 3rd ed. Churchill Livingstone; 1993.

24. Dhir S, Fuller J. Case report: pregnancy in hemodialysis-dependent end-stage renal disease: anesthetic considerations. *Can J Anaesth* 2007;54:556–560.

25. Hammouda GE, Yahya R, Atallah MM. Plasma bupivacaine concentrations following epidural administration in kidney transplant recipients. *Reg Anesth* 1996;21:308–311.

26. Basta M, Sloan P. Epidural haematoma following epidural catheter placement in a patient with chronic renal failure. *Can J Anaesth* 1999;46:271–273.

27. Winearls CG. Chronic renal failure. Ch 20.5.1. In: Warrell DA, Cox TM, Firth JD, Benz EJ Jr, eds. *Oxford Textbook of Medicine*. 4th ed. Oxford University Press; 2003.

28. Steer PL. Anaesthetic management of a parturient with thrombocytopenia using thromboelastography and sonoclot analysis. *Can J Anaesth* 1993;40:84–85.

29. Orko R, Pitkanen M, Rosenberg PH. Subarachnoid anaesthesia with 0.75% bupivacaine in patients with chronic renal failure. *Br J Anaesth* 1986;58:605–609.

30. Landon MB. Diabetic nephropathy and pregnancy. *Clin Obstet Gynecol* 2007; 50:998–1006.

31. Fervenza F, Green A, Lafayette RA. Acute renal failure due to post-infectious glomerulonephritis during pregnancy. *Am J Kidney Dis* 1997;29:273–276.

32. Alexopoulos E, Bili H, Tampakoudis P, et al. Outcome of pregnancy in women with glomerular disease. *Ren Fail* 1996;18:121–129.

33. Madazli R, Bulut B, Erenel H, et al. Systemic lupus erythematosus and pregnancy. *J Obstet Gynaecol* 2010;30:17–20.

34. Gladman DD, Tandon A, Ibanez D, et al. The effect of lupus nephritis on pregnancy outcome and fetal and maternal complications. *J Rheumatol* 2010; 37:754–758.

35. Ruiz-Irastorza G, Khamashta MA. Managing lupus patients during pregnancy. *Best Pract Res Clin Rheumatol* 2009;23:575–582.

36. D'Cruz D. Renal manifestations of the antiphospholipid syndrome. *Curr Rheumatol Rep* 2009;11:52–60.

37. Mecacci F, Bianchi B, Pieralli A, et al. Pregnancy outcome in systemic lupus erythematosus complicated by anti-phospholipid antibodies. *Rheumatology (Oxford)* 2009;48:246–249.

38. Vidaeff AC, Yeomans ER, Ramin SM. Pregnancy in women with renal disease. Part II: Specific underlying conditions. *Am J Perinatol* 2008;25:399–405.

39. Sharma P, Thapa L. Acute pyelonephritis in pregnancy: a retrospective study. *Aust N Z J Obstet Gynaecol* 2007;47:313–315.

40. Cunningham FG, Leveno KJ, Hankins GD, et al. Respiratory insufficiency associated with pyelonephritis during pregnancy. *Obstet Gynecol* 1984;63:121–123.

41. Ridgway LE, Martin RW, Hess LW, et al. Acute gestational pyelonephritis. The impact on colloid osmotic pressure, plasma fibronectin, and arterial oxygen saturation. *Am J Perinatol* 1991;8:222–226.

42. Meyers SJ, Lee RV, Munschauer RW. Dilatation and non-traumatic rupture of the urinary tract during pregnancy: A review. *Obstet Gynecol* 1985;66:809–815.

43. Mazor-Dray E, Levy A, Schlaeffer F, et al. Maternal urinary tract infection: is it independently associated with adverse pregnancy outcome? *J Matern Fetal Neonatal Med* 2009;22:124–128.

44. Charalambous S, Fotas A, Rizk DE. Urolithiasis in pregnancy. *Int Urogynecol J Pelvic Floor Dysfunct* 2009;20:1133–1136.

45. Cheriachan D, Arianayagam M, Rashid P. Symptomatic urinary stone disease in pregnancy. *Aust N Z J Obstet Gynaecol* 2008;48:34–39.

46. McAleer SJ, Loughlkin KR. Nephrolithiasis and pregnancy. *Curr Opin Urol* 2004;14:123–127.

47. Andreoiu M, MacMahon R. Renal colic in pregnancy: Lithiasis or physiological hydronephrosis? *Urology* 2009;74:757–761.

48. Chow CL, Ong AC. Autosomal dominant polycystic kidney disease. *Clin Med* 2009;9:278–283.

49. Rizk D, Chapman AB. Cystic and inherited kidney diseases. *Am J Kidney Dis* 2003;42:1305–1317.

50. Steen VD. Scleroderma and pregnancy. *Rheum Dis Clin North Am* 1997;23: 133–147.

51. Miniati I, Guiducci S, Mecacci F, et al. Pregnancy in systemic sclerosis. *Rheumatology (Oxford)* 2008;47(Suppl 3):iii16–iii18.

52. Causse-Mariscal A, Palot M, Visseaux H, et al. Labor analgesia and caesarean section in women affected by tuberous sclerosis: report of two cases. *Int J Obstet Anesth* 2007;16:277–280.

53. Byrd LM, Jadoon B, Lieberman I, et al. Chronic pain and obstetric management of a patient with tuberous sclerosis. *Pain Med* 2007;8:199–203.

54. Cormio G, Cramarossa D, Di Vagno G, et al. Successful pregnancy in a patient with Churg-Strauss syndrome. *Eur J Obstet Gynecol Reprod Biol* 1995;60:81–83.

55. Parnham AP, Thatcher GN. Pregnancy and active Wegener's granulomatosis. *Aust N Z J Obstet Gynaecol* 1996;36:361–363.

56. Matsumoto Y, Asada M, Mukubou M. Postpartum subarachnoid hemorrhage due to Moyamoya disease associated with renal artery stenosis. *J Obstet Gynaecol Res* 2009;35:787–789.

57. Ioscovich A, Gislason R, Fadeev A, et al. Peripartum anesthetic management of patients with Takayasu's arteritis: case series and review. *Int J Obstet Anesth* 2008;17:358–364.

58. D'Angelo A, Fattorini A, Crippa L. Thrombotic microangiopathy in pregnancy. *Thromb Res* 2009;123(Suppl 2):S56–S62.

59. Dashe JS, Ramin SM, Cunningham FG. The long-term consequences of thrombotic microangiopathy (thrombotic thrombocytopenic purpura and hemolytic uremic syndrome) in pregnancy. *Obstet Gynecol* 1998;91:662–668.

60. Gammill HS, Jeyabalan A. Acute renal failure in pregnancy. *Crit Care Med* 2005;33(Suppl):S372–S384.

61. Hatfield T, Steiger R, Wing DA. Goodpasture's disease in pregnancy: case report and review of the literature. *Am J Perinatol* 2007;24:619–621.

62. Hudson BG, Tryggvason K, Sundaramoorthy M, et al. Alport's syndrome, Goodpasture's syndrome, and type IV collagen. *New Engl J Med* 2003;348:2543–2556.

63. Matsuo K, Tudor EL, Baschat AA. Alport syndrome and pregnancy. *Obstet Gynecol* 2007;109:531–532.

64. Luqman A, Kazmi A, Wall BM. Barrter's syndrome in pregnancy: a review of potassium homeostasis in gestation. *Am J Med Sci* 2009;338:500–504.

65. Roelofse JA, Van der Westhuijzen AJ. Anaesthetic management of a patient with Bartter's syndrome undergoing orthognathic surgery. *Anesth Prog* 1997; 44:71–75.

66. Shanbhag S, Neil J, Howell C. Anaesthesia for caesarean section in a patient with Gitelman's syndrome. *Int J Obstet Anesth* 2010;19:451–453.

67. Fowe TF, Magee K, Cunningham FG. Pregnancy and renal tubular acidosis. *Am J Perinatol* 1999;16:189–191.

68. Lee D, Abraham N. Laparoscopic radical nephrectomy during pregnancy: case report and review of the literature. *J Endourol* 2008;22:517–518.

69. Cappell MS. Hepatic disorders severely affected by pregnancy: medical and obstetric management. *Med Clin North Am* 2008;92:739–760.

70. Joshi D, James A, Quaglia A, et al. Liver disease in pregnancy. *Lancet* 2010; 375:594–605.

71. Devarbhavi H, Kremers WK, Dierkhising R, et al. Pregnancy-associated acute liver disease and acute viral hepatitis: differentiation, course and outcome. *J Hepatol* 2008;49:930–935.

72. Kondrackiene J, Kupcinskas L. Liver diseases unique to pregnancy. *Medicina (Kaunas)* 2008;44:337–345.

73. Jabbour N, Brenner M, Gagandeep S, et al. Major hepatobiliary surgery during pregnancy: safety and timing. *Am Surg* 2005;71:354–358.

74. Tank PD, Nadanwar YS, Mayedeo NM. Outcome of pregnancy with severe liver disease. *Int J Obstet Gynaecol Obstet* 2002;76:27–31.

75. Mackillop L, Williamson C. Liver disease in pregnancy. *Postgrad Med J* 2010; 86:160–164.

76. Icely S, Chez RA. Traumatic liver rupture in pregnancy. *Am J Obstet Gynecol* 1999;180:1030–1031.

77. Coelho T, Braga J, Sequeira M. Hepatic hematomas in pregnancy. *Acta Obstet Gynecol Scand* 2000;79:884–886.

78. Armenti VT, Constantinescu S, Moritz MJ, et al. Pregnancy after transplantation. *Transplant Rev (Orlando)* 2008;22:223–240.

79. Avraamides EJ, Craen RA, Gelb AW. Anaesthetic management of a pregnant, post liver transplant patient for dental surgery. *Anaesth Intensive Care* 1997;25:68–70.

80. Servin F, Cockshott ID, Farinotti R, et al. Pharmacokinetics of propofol infusions in patients with cirrhosis. *Br J Anaesth* 1990;65:177–183.

81. Gelman S. General anaesthesia and hepatic circulation. *Can J Physiol Pharmacol* 1987;65:1762–1779.

82. Meierhenrich R, Gauss A, Muhling B, et al. The effect of propofol and desflurane anaesthesia on human hepatic blood flow: a pilot study. *Anaesthesia* 2010;65:1085–1093.

83. Schmidt CC, Suttner SW, Piper SN, et al. Comparison of the effects of desflurane and isoflurane anaesthesia on hepatocellular function assessed by alpha glutathione S-transferase. *Anaesthesia* 1999;54:1204–1209.

84. Thomas SD, Boyd AH. Prolonged neuromuscular block associated with acute fatty liver of pregnancy and reduced plasma cholinesterase. *Eur J Anaesthesiol* 1994;11:245–249.

85. Servin FS, Lavaut E, Kleef U, et al. Repeated doses of rocuronium bromide administered to cirrhotic and control patients receiving isoflurane. *Anesthesiology* 1996;84:1092–1100.

86. Sato T, Hashiguchi A, Mitsuse T. Anesthesia for caesarean delivery in a pregnant woman with acute hepatic failure. *Anesth Analg* 2000;91:1441–1442.

87. Chan WH, Lee TS, Lin CS, et al. Anesthetic management for cesarean section in a pregnant woman with impending liver failure—a case report. *Acta Anaesthesiol Sin* 1999;37:141–146.

88. Gregory TL, Hughes S, Coleman MA, et al. Acute fatty liver of pregnancy: three cases and discussion of analgesia and anesthesia. *Int J Obstet Anesth* 2007;16:175–179.

89. Larson AM, Polson J, Fontana RJ, et al. Acetaminophen-induced acute liver failure: results of a United States multicenter, prospective study. *Hepatology* 2005;42:1364–1372.

90. Lee NM, Brady CW. Liver disease in pregnancy. *World J Gastroenterol* 2009;15:897–906.

91. Wolff C, Armas Merino R. Porphyria and pregnancy. Review of 17 women. *Rev Med Chil* 2008;136:151–156.

92. Arrese M. Cholestasis during pregnancy: rare hepatic diseases unmasked by pregnancy. *Ann Hepatol* 2006;5:216–218.

93. Geenes G, Williamson C. Intrahepatic homeostasis of pregnancy. *World J Gastroenterol* 2009;15:2049–2066.

94. Pathak B, Sheibani L, Lee RH. Cholestasis of pregnancy. *Obstet Gynecol Clin North Am* 2010;37:269–282.

95. Mays JK. The active management of intrahepatic cholestasis of pregnancy. *Curr Opin Obstet Gynecol* 2010;22:100–103.

96. Knight M, Nelson-Piercy C, Kurinczuk JJ, et al. A prospective national study of acute fatty liver of pregnancy in the UK. *Gut* 2008;57:951–956.

97. Moldenhauer JS, O'Brien JM, Barton JR, et al. Acute fatty liver of pregnancy associated with pancreatitis: a life threatening complication. *Am J Obstet Gynecol* 2004;190:502–505.

98. Brown MA, Passaris G, Carlton MA. Pregnancy-induced hypertension and acute fatty liver of pregnancy: atypical presentations. *Am J Obstet Gynecol* 1990;163:1154–1156.

99. Antognini JF, Andrews S. Anaesthesia for caesarean section in a patient with acute fatty liver of pregnancy. *Can J Anaesth* 1991;38:904–907.

100. Corke PJ. Anaesthesia for caesarean section in a patient with acute fatty liver of pregnancy. *Anaesth Intensive Care* 1995;23:215–218.

101. Holzman RS, Riley LE, Aron E, et al. Perioperative care of a patient with acute fatty liver of pregnancy. *Anesth Analg* 2001;92:1268–1270.

102. Czaja AJ. Special clinical challenges in autoimmune hepatitis: The elderly, males, pregnancy, mild disease, fulminant onset, and nonwhite patients. *Semin Liver Dis* 2009;29:315–330.

103. Omori H, Asahi H, Takahashi M, et al. Peliosis hepatitis during postpartum period: successful embolization of hepatic artery. *J Gastroenterol* 2004;39:168–171.

104. Norvell J, Blei A, Jovanovic BD, et al. Herpes simplex virus hepatitis: an analysis of the published literature and institutional cases. *Liver Transpl* 2007;13:1428–1434.

105. Tran TT. Management of hepatitis B in pregnancy: weighing the options. *Cleve Clin J Med* 2009;76(Suppl 3):S25–S29.

106. Jonas MM. Hepatitis B and pregnancy: an underestimated issue. *Liver Int* 2009;29:133–139.

107. Giles M, Hellard M, Sasadeusz J. Hepatitis C and pregnancy: An update. *Aust N Z J Obstet Gynaecol* 2003;43:290–293.

108. Safir A, Levy A, Sikuler E, et al. Maternal hepatitis B or hepatitis C carrier status as an independent risk factor for adverse perinatal outcome. *Liver Int* 2010;30:765–770.

109. Kumar A, Beniwal M, Kar P, et al. Hepatitis E in pregnancy. *Int J Gynaecol Obstet* 2004;85:240–244.

110. Aggarwal R, Naik S. Epidemiology of hepatitis E: current status. *J Gastroenterol Hepatol* 2009;24:1484–1493.

111. Tan J, Surti B, Saab S. Pregnancy and cirrhosis. *Liver Transpl* 2008;14:1081–1091.

112. Harnett MJ, Miller AD, Hurley RJ, et al. Pregnancy, labour and delivery in a Jehovah's Witness with esophageal varices and thrombocytopenia. *Can J Anesth* 2000;47:1253–1255.

113. Sumana G, Dadhwal V, Deka D, et al. Non-cirrhotic portal hypertension and pregnancy outcome. *J Obstet Gynaecol Res* 2008;34:801–804.

114. Duke J. Pregnancy and cirrhosis: management of hematemesis by Warren shunt during third trimester gestation. *Int J Obstet Anesth* 1994;3:97–102.

115. Aranha GV, Greenlee HB. Intraabdominal surgery in patients with advanced cirrhosis. *Arch Surg* 1986;121:275–277.

116. Heriot JA, Steven CM, Sattin RS. Elective forceps delivery and extradural anaesthesia in a primigravida with portal hypertension and oesophageal varices. *Br J Anaesth* 1996;76:325–327.

117. Khuroo MS, Datta DV. Budd-Chiari syndrome following pregnancy. Report of 16 cases with roentgenologic, hemodynamic and histologic studies of the hepatic outflow tract. *Am J Med* 1980;8:113–121.

118. Lee WM. Pregnancy in patients with chronic liver disease. *Gastroenterol Clin North Am* 1992;21:889–903.

119. Dilawari JB, Bambery P, Chawla Y, et al. Hepatic outflow obstruction (Budd-Chiari syndrome). Experience with 177 patients and a review of the literature. *Medicine (Baltimore)* 1994;73:21–36.

120. Rautou PE, Angermayr B, Garcia-Pagan JC, et al. Pregnancy in women with known and treated Budd-Chiari syndrome: maternal and fetal outcomes. *J Hepatol* 2009;51:47–54.

121. Bihl J. The effect of pregnancy on hepatolenticular degeneration. *Am J Obstet Gynecol* 1973;78:1182–1183.

122. Brewer GJ. Novel therapeutic approaches to the treatment of Wilson's disease. *Expert Opin Pharmacother* 2006;7:317–324.

123. El Dawlatly AA, Bakhamees H, Seraj MA. Anesthetic management for cesarean section in a patient with Wilson's disease. *Middle East J Anesthesiol* 1992;11:391–397.

124. Farina G, Pedrotti C, Cerani P, et al. Successful pregnancy following gonadotropin therapy in a young female with juvenile idiopathic hemochromatosis and secondary hypogonadotrophic hypogonadism. *Haematologica* 1995;80:335–337.

125. Kanaan C, Veille JC, Lakin M. Pregnancy and acute intermittent porphyria. *Obstet Gynecol Surv* 1989;44:244–249.

126. McNeill MJ, Bennet A. Use of regional anaesthesia in a patient with acute porphyria. *Br J Anaesth* 1990;64:371–373.

127. Kantor G, Rolbin SH. Acute intermittent porphyria and caesarean delivery. *Can J Anaesth* 1992;39:282–285.

128. Jensen NF, Fiddler DS, Striepe V. Anesthetic considerations in porphyrias. *Anesth Analg* 1995;80:591–599.

129. Harrison GG, Meissner PN, Hift RJ. Anaesthesia for the porphyric patient. *Anaesthesia* 1993;48:417–421.

130. Manterola C, Espinoza R, Munoz S, et al. Abdominal echinococcosis during pregnancy: clinical aspects and management of a series of cases in Chile. *Trop Doct* 2004;34:171–173.

131. van Vliet W, Scheele F, Sibinga-Mulder L, et al. Echinococcosis of the liver during pregnancy. *Int J Gynecol Obstet* 1995;49:323–324.

132. Montes H, Soetkino R, Carr-Locke DL. Hydatid disease in pregnancy. *Am J Gastroenterol* 2002;97:1553–1555.

133. Ko CW, Beresford SA, Schulte SJ, et al. Incidence, natural history, and risk factors for biliary sludge and stones during pregnancy. *Hepatology* 2005;41:359–365.

134. Mendez-Sanchez N, Chavez-Tapia NC, Uribe M. Pregnancy and gall bladder disease. *Ann Hepatol* 2006;5:227–230.

135. Lu EJ, Curet MJ, El-Sayed MD, et al. Medical versus surgical management of biliary tract disease in pregnancy. *Am J Surg* 2004;188:755–759.

136. Graham G, Baxi L, Tharakan T. Laparoscopic cholecystectomy during pregnancy: a case series and review of the literature. *Obstet Gynecol Surv* 1998;53:566–574.

137. Steinbrook RA, Bhavani-Shankar K. Hemodynamics during laparoscopic surgery in pregnancy. *Anesth Analg* 2003;93:1570–1571.

138. Goh SK, Gull SE, Alexander GJ. Pregnancy in primary biliary cirrhosis complicated by portal hypertension: report of a case and review of the literature. *BJOG* 2001;108:760–762.

139. Rinella ME. Primary biliary cirrhosis. *Ann Hepatol* 2006;5:198–200.

140. Poupon R, Chretien Y, Chazouilleres O, et al. Pregnancy in women with ursodeoxycholic acid-treated primary biliary cirrhosis. *J Hepatol* 2005;42:418–419.

141. Silveira MG, Lindor KD. Clinical features and management of primary sclerosing cholangitis. *World J Gastroenterol* 2008;14:3338–3349.

142. Janczewska I, Olsson R, Hultcrantz R, et al. Pregnancy in patients with primary sclerosing cholangitis. *Liver* 1996;16:326–330.

143. Hewitt PM, Krige JE, Bornman PC, et al. Choledochal cyst in pregnancy: a therapeutic dilemma. *J Am Coll Surg* 1995;181:237–240.

144. Benchellal ZA, Simon E, d'Alteroche L, et al. Choledochal cyst rupture during pregnancy. *Gastroenterol Clin Biol* 2009;33:390–391.

145. Singham J, Yoshida EM, Scudamore CH. Choledochal cysts. Part 3 of 3: Management. *Can J Surg* 2010;53:51–56.

146. Tang SJ, Rodriguez-Frias E, Singh S, et al. Acute pancreatitis during pregnancy. *Clin Gastroenterol Hepatol* 2010;8:85–90.

Anesthesia for the Pregnant Patient with Immunologic Disorders

Stephen H. Halpern • Margaret Srebrnjak

■ INTRODUCTION

The role of the immune system is to rid the body of foreign material such as bacteria, viruses, and other foreign matter. However, in predisposed individuals, an overreaction to foreign antigens can occur, resulting in a wide variety of pathologic states and syndromes. Some immunologically mediated disorders are acute and life-threatening, such as anaphylaxis, while others are chronic, such as rheumatoid disease and allograft rejection. None of these preclude pregnancy.

Immunologic responses are divided into two major divisions, the innate immune response and the adaptive immune response. The innate immune system is a non-specific and immediate reaction to a foreign allergen and does not change regardless of how many times an infectious agent is encountered. It includes physical barriers, such as the epidermis and mucous, as well as elements of the immune system such as natural killer cells, phagocytes, cytokines, and complement. Complement factors are a group of serum and cell surface proteins, which cause an amplifying series of enzymatic reactions when activated; they can cause direct cell lysis, facilitate phagocytosis of the foreign cell, or cause the release of mediators (1).

Higher organisms have also developed an antigen-specific immunologic reaction called adaptive immunity that works in concert with innate immunity. Specifically, an individual will respond, more rapidly and robustly, to specific antigens on subsequent exposure, using T and B cells. It is a reaction with "memory," since it relies on an initial exposure (2).

When an antigen is presented and recognized by antigen-specific T cells and B cells, priming, activation, and differentiation occur. B cells proliferate and differentiate into antigen-specific memory cells and plasma cells. Plasma cells secrete antibodies, such as immunoglobulin (Ig) A, G, or E, whose role is to neutralize toxins, activate complement, and facilitate phagocytosis of foreign cells. Only IgG crosses the placenta (1). T cells also proliferate and differentiate into memory cells as well as effector T cells.

There are four classic hypersensitivity reactions that lead to tissue injury. Similar mechanisms also cause autoimmune diseases. For the purpose of this chapter, the classification works well for both (Table 38-1). Recently, several subcategories under Type IV hypersensitivity have been included as our understanding of immune reactions has expanded (2).

Type I Hypersensitivity (IgE-mediated Reactions)

Immediate hypersensitivity or anaphylaxis is a reaction that requires the recognition of antigens by membrane-bound IgE on mast cells in the tissues and basophils in blood. A single cell may be armed with specific IgE molecules for many different antigens. When an allergen is re-encountered, a change in the shape of the cell membrane occurs resulting in degranulation and the release of vasoactive peptides and chemotactic factors. The immediate reaction is mostly carried out by mast cells with basophils being activated and recruited a few hours later (2).

Inhalation of antigens and subsequent mediator release leads to bronchoconstriction and mucous secretion; ingestion of antigens causes diarrhea and vomiting; and subcutaneous antigens produce urticaria and angioedema. With intravascular antigen exposure, systemic activation occurs, causing increased capillary permeability, hypotension, tissue swelling, and smooth muscle contraction (Fig. 38-1) (2).

Anaphylaxis Terminology

Defining anaphylaxis is a challenge. Some interpret it as a broad term describing a severe, life-threatening, generalized hypersensitivity reaction, while others define it as a specific IgE-mediated reaction (3,4). Recently, National Institute of Allergy and Infectious Disease/Food Allergy and Anaphylaxis Network proposed clinical criteria for the diagnosis (Table 38-2).

Anaphylactoid reactions appear similar to IgE-mediated hypersensitivity, but do not involve antibodies or a previous exposure. Mechanisms include, non-specific complement activation and direct histamine release. For example, most muscle relaxants and opioids release histamine directly from mast cells. Unlike anaphylaxis, many anaphylactoid reactions can be attenuated with antihistamines, corticosteroids, and the slow administration of drugs. Most drugs can cause both types of reactions (5).

Type II Hypersensitivity (Antibody-mediated Cytotoxic Reactions)

The antibody-mediated cytotoxic immune response is initiated by the binding of circulating IgM or IgG antibodies with cell surface or tissue-matrix antigens, which have been modified to make the antigen foreign. The antigens may be normal red blood cell antigens like those in autoimmune hemolytic anemia or they may be altered such as when penicillin attaches to red blood cells and initiates a drug-induced hemolytic anemia (1,2).

Once antibodies bind to the cells, the complement cascade is initiated. Activated complements C3 and C5, also known as anaphylatoxins, work directly to cause mast cell degranulation. Some complement factors enhance phagocytosis of the targeted cell by macrophages, neutrophils, and eosinophils; others form a membrane-attack complex that perforates the cell membrane causing cell lysis and death. This mechanism is responsible for disorders such as erythroblastosis fetalis, immune thrombocytopenia, and myasthenia gravis (1,2).

TABLE 38-1 Major Types of Immune-mediated Hypersensitivity Reactions

Mechanism	Antigen	Effector Mechanism	Examples
Type I Hypersensitivity (Immediate)	Soluble allergen	Mast cell–bound IgE • Histamine, tryptase, carboxy-peptidase, serotonin, PAF	Anaphylactic shock Allergic rhinitis Angioedema Urticaria
Type II Hypersensitivity (Cytotoxic)	Cell-surface Ag Tissue-matrix Ag	IgG or IgM • Phagocytes, NK cells • Complement	Hemolytic transfusion reactions Erythroblastosis fetalis ITP Graves' disease
Type III Immune complex mediated	Soluble Ag	IgG • Phagocytes, NK cells • Complement	SLE SBE
Type IV Delayed-type hypersensitivity	Soluble Ag Soluble Ag Cell-associated Ag	T_H 1 cell • Release cytokines to attract macrophages T_H 2 cell • Release cytokines to attract eosinophils and stimulate B cells T_C cell	Tuberculin test Contact dermatitis RA (in part) Multiple sclerosis Chronic rhinitis Chronic asthma Allograft rejection (in part)

Ag, antigen; IgE, immunoglobulin E; IgG, immunoglobulin G; IgM, immunoglobulin M; PAF, platelet activating factor; ITP, immune thrombocytopenic purpura; SLE, systemic lupus erythromatosus; SBE subacute bacterial endocarditis; T_H 1, Type I helper T cell; T_H 2, Type II helper T cell; T_C, cytotoxic T cell; RA, rheumatoid arthritis

Adapted from: Salmon JE. Mechanisms of immune-mediated tissue injury. In: Goldman L, Ausiello D, eds. *Cecil Medicine*. 23rd ed. Philadelphia, PA: Saunders Elsevier; 2008:266–270.

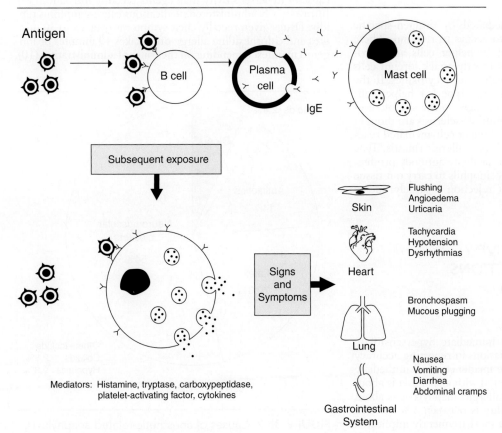

FIGURE 38-1 Mechanisms of IgE-mediated reactions.

TABLE 38-2 Clinical Criteria for Diagnosing Anaphylaxis

Anaphylaxis is highly likely when any *one of the following three criteria* are fulfilled:

1. Acute onset of an illness *(minutes to several hours)* with involvement of the skin, mucosal tissue, or both *(e.g., generalized hives, pruritus or flushing, swollen lips–tongue–uvula)*
   AND AT LEAST ONE OF THE FOLLOWING
   a. Respiratory compromise *(e.g., dyspnea, wheeze-bronchospasm, stridor, reduced PEF, hypoxemia)*
   b. ↓BP or associated symptoms of end-organ dysfunction *(e.g., hypotonia [collapse], syncope, incontinence)*
2. TWO OR MORE OF THE FOLLOWING that occur rapidly after exposure *to a likely allergen for that patient* (minutes to several hours):
   a. Involvement of the skin–mucosal tissue *(e.g., generalized hives, itch-flush, swollen lips–tongue–uvula)*
   b. Respiratory compromise *(e.g., dyspnea, wheeze-bronchospasm, stridor, reduced PEF, hypoxemia)*
   c. ↓ BP or associated symptoms *(e.g., hypotonia [collapse], syncope, incontinence)*
   d. Persistent gastrointestinal symptoms *(e.g., crampy abdominal pain, vomiting)*
3. ↓ BP after exposure to *known allergen for that patient* (minutes to several hours)
   • Systolic BP of less than 90 mm Hg or greater than 30% decrease from that person's baseline

PEF, Peak expiratory flow; BP, blood pressure
Data from: Sampson HA, Munoz-Furlong A, Campbell RL, et al. Second symposium on the definition and management of anaphylaxis: summary report-Second National Institute of Allergy and Infectious Disease/Food Allergy and Anaphylaxis Network symposium. *J Allergy Clin Immunol* 2006;117:391–397.

Type III Hypersensitivity (Immune Complex Diseases)

Immune complex diseases occur when small, soluble antigen–antibody complexes deposit in vascular beds, glomerular and pulmonary basement membranes, and serous cavities. Complement is activated and inflammation occurs. The prototypical Type III autoimmune disease is systemic lupus erythematosus (SLE). Patients with SLE develop circulating IgG against native cellular elements such as DNA (2).

Type IV Hypersensitivity (Delayed-type Reactions)

Delayed hypersensitivity is mediated by antigen-specific effector T cells that require 1 to 3 days to respond. These T cells include antigen-specific T helper cells and cytotoxic T cells. Cytotoxic T cells directly attack foreign cells while antigen-specific T helper cells release cytokines. In the tuberculin test or contact dermatitis, Type I T helper cells release cytokines to signal macrophages to the site of reaction. Rheumatoid arthritis and multiple sclerosis are thought to be caused in part by a Type I T helper cell–mediated reaction. With chronic asthma and chronic allergic rhinitis, Type II T helper cells use cytokines to facilitate antibody production from B cells and to attract eosinophils to carry out tissue inflammation. Chronic allograft rejection is largely due to cytotoxic T cell function (2).

■ TYPE I HYPERSENSITIVITY (IgE-MEDIATED REACTIONS)

Allergy to Anesthetic and Non-anesthetic Agents

Epidemiology

The incidence of perioperative immediate hypersensitivity is poorly defined because of variations in reporting accuracy and completeness. However, the incidence of all immediate hypersensitivity reactions associated with anesthesia is about 1:5,000, while the incidence of allergic anaphylaxis is about 1:10,000. The associated mortality is between 3% and 9% (6). Neuromuscular blockers are most frequently implicated

as a cause of perioperative anaphylaxis, followed by latex, and antibiotics (Fig. 38-2).

There are no specific risk factors for allergy to medications. However, patients who have had a previous, uninvestigated severe reaction during anesthesia are at increased risk of recurrence (7). It is unrelated to atopy, a history of multiple allergies, genetics, allergy to non-anesthetic drugs, or a history of multiple chemical sensitivities (8). Although asthma does not increase the incidence of anaphylaxis during anesthesia, it *is* a risk factor for severe respiratory symptoms (7).

Presentation

In general, agents that have been used for long, continuous periods before the onset of an acute reaction are less likely a cause of hypersensitivity than agents recently introduced (9). Intravenously administered medications cause symptoms rapidly. Drugs given rectally elicit symptoms over 15 to 30 minutes and chlorhexidine allergy often takes 10 minutes or longer to manifest depending on the route of administration (10).

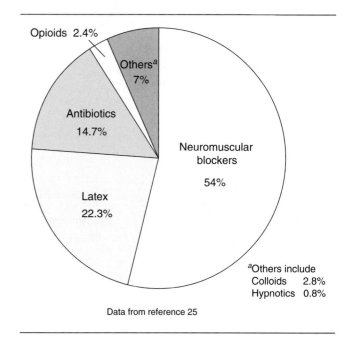

Data from reference 25

FIGURE 38-2 Causes of anesthetic-related anaphylaxis.

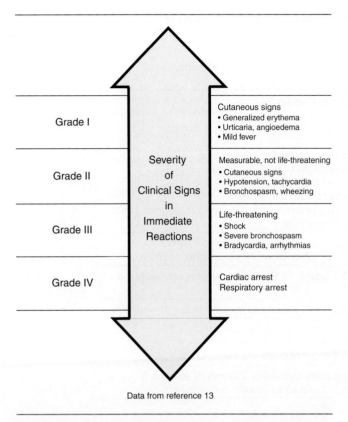

Grade I		Cutaneous signs • Generalized erythema • Urticaria, angioedema • Mild fever
Grade II	Severity of Clinical Signs in Immediate Reactions	Measurable, not life-threatening • Cutaneous signs • Hypotension, tachycardia • Bronchospasm, wheezing
Grade III		Life-threatening • Shock • Severe bronchospasm • Bradycardia, arrhythmias
Grade IV		Cardiac arrest Respiratory arrest

Data from reference 13

FIGURE 38-3 Grading of the severity of the clinical signs of immediate hypersensitivity.

Presentation of anaphylaxis is variable but if symptoms occur rapidly, it is more likely the reaction will be severe and life-threatening (11). In addition, anaphylaxis produces more severe symptoms than anaphylactoid reactions (12). A four-point grading scale may be useful to describe the severity of the reaction (Fig. 38-3) (13).

The awake patient may complain of pruritus around the lips, tongue, ear canal, eyes, palms, and genitalia. They also complain of a metallic taste in the mouth, headache, and a feeling of impending doom. Gastrointestinal symptoms include nausea, vomiting, and abdominal cramps. With progressive angioedema, they may have hoarseness, dysphonia, shortness of breath, chest pain, and eventual cardiovascular collapse. Female patients may also complain of uterine cramps (11).

During general anesthesia, common initial features include pulselessness, desaturation, and difficulty with ventilation (7). Low oxygen saturation can occur as a result of mucus plugging, bronchospasm, or impaired circulation. Skin manifestations are less helpful since draping can obscure urticaria and angioedema, and in severe cases, cardiovascular collapse may occur before skin signs appear. Overall, cutaneous symptoms can be absent in 33% of patients (14) but some of these appear after blood pressure is restored. Cardiovascular symptoms typically include tachycardia and hypotension but in 10% of cases, bradycardia is a prominent feature due to profound hypovolemia (4,7). In very severe cases, the patient may also develop disseminated intravascular coagulation (DIC) (11).

Management
Management of the parturient should include: (1) Remove or discontinue the offending agent, (2) administer 100% oxygen and maintain an open airway, (3) call for help and administer epinephrine for Grade III and IV reactions, and (4) maintain venous return by displacing the uterus to the left or positioning the patient in the full left lateral position. Pharmacologic treatment is discussed in Table 38-3.

It is important to administer intravenous epinephrine and maintain intravascular volume. While epinephrine is not used for Grade I reactions, it is indicated for Grade III or IV reactions. Electrocardiographic monitoring is needed since epinephrine can provoke ventricular arrhythmias. Patients on β blockers can have a blunted response to epinephrine, often requiring large volumes of fluid, high doses of epinephrine, and glucagon. Other resuscitative drugs should be considered in epinephrine-resistant anaphylaxis, such as dopamine, norepinephrine, or vasopressin. In Grade IV cases, as much as 35% to 50% of the intravascular fluid can transfer to the extravascular space within 10 minutes; large volumes of colloid or crystalloid may be required and therapy should be initiated early (7).

Histamine receptor blocking drugs and corticosteroids may be useful adjuncts. Antihistamines are particularly effective for angioedema and urticaria but the value of corticosteroids for reducing the risk of a recurrence has not been proven. Corticosteroids decrease late swelling of the pharynx and larynx. Salbutamol or albuterol are indicated for bronchoconstriction, but should not replace epinephrine in instances of severe bronchospasm and cardiovascular collapse (7). Patients have also been given tranexamic acid when anaphylaxis has been associated with DIC (11).

Anaphylaxis usually resolves in 2 to 8 hours in the absence of secondary pathology (4), but continued vigilance is mandatory since reactions may recur 1 to 72 hours after onset, in up to 23% of patients (11).

Specific Considerations in the Pregnant Patient
During anaphylaxis, the fetus is not exposed to maternal toxic inflammatory mediators such as histamine, as they are metabolized by the placenta. Since maternal IgE does not cross the placenta, an immune reaction should not occur in the fetus. However, the fetus is vulnerable to inadequate placental perfusion secondary to maternal hypotension. While epinephrine may cause uterine artery vasoconstriction, it should be used in effective doses to terminate the anaphylactic reaction. The use of ephedrine is controversial (15), as it may not effectively correct maternal hypotension.

Left uterine displacement should be used after 20 weeks' gestation to avoid aortocaval compression. The American Heart Association advocates that critically ill parturients who are at risk for cardiac arrest should be placed in the full lateral position to maintain venous return, blood pressure, cardiac output, and fetal oxygenation (16).

For an urgent or emergency cesarean delivery, regional anesthesia can be considered if the patient is hemodynamically stable and the fetus is not in distress. If the patient experienced oropharyngeal or laryngeal edema, immediate airway management may be indicated. Observation for airway obstruction should continue for several hours in case relapse occurs (11).

Specific Allergies
Local Anesthetic Agents
Many patients experience adverse reactions to local anesthetics (LAs) but only less than 1% are due to immune hypersensitivity reactions (17). When patients are referred for LA allergy testing, other allergens such as chlorhexidine or latex are found much more frequently to be responsible for the reaction (18). Both Type I and Type IV hypersensitivity reactions occur, with delayed-type hypersensitivity being more common (17).

Immediate hypersensitivity caused by LAs, presents with the typical symptoms of anaphylaxis within minutes of injection. Delayed-type hypersensitivity manifests as contact

TABLE 38-3 Pharmacologic Management of Anaphylaxis in the Parturient

Ephedrine	Grade II reactions (moderate): • BOLUS: 10 mg IV every 1–2 min Switch to epinephrine if there is no response or severity increases
Epinephrine	Grade II reactions (moderate): • BOLUS: 10–20 μg IV • Sc/im 200–500 μg (lateral thigh) every 5 min until IV obtained Grade III reactions (severe): • BOLUS: 100–200 μg IV every 1–2 min • INFUSION: 1–4 μg/min Grade IV reactions/Cardiac Arrest: • BOLUS: 1–3 mg IV over 3 min (3–5 mg over next 3 min) INFUSION: 4–10 μg/min
Fluid	IV crystalloid 5–10 mL/kg over 5 min • 1,000–2,000 mL, after 30 mL/kg switch to colloids
Diphenhydramine	25–50 mg IV (Grade II–IV reactions require epinephrine first)
Ranitidine	50 mg IV (Grade II–IV reactions require epinephrine first)
Salbutamol or Albuterol	Inhalation: 2.5–5 mg in 3 mL saline nebulized BOLUS: Salbutamol 100–200 μg INFUSION: Salbutamol 5–25 μg/min
Glucocorticoids	Hydrocortisone hemisuccinate 200 mg IV every 6 h (Grade II–IV reactions require epinephrine first)
Other vasopressors: 1. Dopamine: 2–20 μg/kg/min 2. Glucagon: 1–5 mg IV over 5 min, then 5–15 μg/min • Consider early with patient on β blockers 3. Norepinephrine: 5–10 μg/kg/min 4. Vasopressin: Bolus: 2–10 IU IV until response	

IV, intravenous; μg, micrograms; sc, subcutaneous; im, intramuscular.

dermatitis from topical preparations or localized edema from dental injections. Type IV reactions appear within 1 to 3 days but some occur as soon as 2 hours, causing difficulty in differentiating them from a Type I immediate reaction (17).

Local anesthetics are divided into two groups, based on their chemical structure. The benzoic acid or ester LAs (Group I) includes drugs such as benzocaine, chloroprocaine, and tetracaine. Allergy in Group I is much more common due to the metabolite, para-aminobenzoic acid, or preservatives such as methylparaben or metabisulfites (19). The amide group (Group II) includes bupivacaine, lidocaine, and ropivacaine, and reports of true hypersensitivity allergy are rare. Cross-reactivity among ester LAs is common, but not with amides. There is little evidence that ester LAs cross-react with amide LAs (7).

Ideally, the pregnant patient who has experienced an adverse response to LAs should be seen prior to pregnancy for testing. However, pregnant patients can undergo skin testing for LAs, after informed consent if clinically indicated. After a comprehensive history, a common protocol for diagnosing LA allergy includes the administration of skin tests followed by a provocative challenge (12); a summary appears in Table 38-4. If the offending agent *is unknown*, the challenge should consist of LAs likely to be used in labor and delivery such as preservative-free bupivacaine and lidocaine.

If the offending LA *is known*, it is best to use an LA with the other chemical structure. However, since substantial cross-reactivity among amides has not been well documented, another amide can also be considered if the suspicion of LA allergy is low (20).

TABLE 38-4 Approach to the Parturient with a History of Adverse Reactions to Local Anesthetics

1. History
   a. Determine nature of reaction and LA implicated
   b. If the history is suggestive of immediate LA allergy
      • Consultation from allergist if possible
      • Identify if LA is ester or amide
      • Weigh risks and benefits of skin and challenge testing
      • Obtain informed consent if testing is considered
   c. Perform test near term or when patient presents for delivery
2. Which LA agent?
   If LA is *known*: Test with LA with other structure, or another amide
   If LA is *unknown*: Test with LA to be used for labor and delivery
3. Perform challenge tests
   a. Perform test in area with resuscitative facilities and monitoring
   b. Intravenous catheter should be placed and the patient fasted
   c. Notify obstetrical and neonatal team

General Anesthetic Agents

Induction Agents

Propofol is currently mixed with a solution vehicle including soy and egg lecithins (extracted from egg yolks). There had been concern that patients allergic to soy or eggs may have reactions to propofol administered intravenously. However, in a small study of 25 egg-allergic patients, all propofol skin tests were negative (19). More commonly, propofol causes direct mast cell activation especially with higher doses (11,21). The estimated incidence of anaphylaxis with propofol is 1 in 60,000 (19). The incidence of thiopental allergy is estimated at 1 in 30,000 administrations. Etomidate, ketamine, and benzodiazepines are exceedingly rare causes for IgE-mediated anaphylaxis (19). There are no reported cases of anaphylaxis to inhalational anesthetics (4).

Neuromuscular Blockers

Neuromuscular blocking agents are among the most common agents to cause perioperative anaphylaxis and may cause a reaction on first exposure. This may be due to the structural similarity between neuromuscular blocking agents and certain chemicals found in toothpastes, detergents, cough medicines, and shampoos. Succinylcholine is the most common neuromuscular blocker implicated (4). The incidence of cross-reactivity among muscle relaxants lies between 60% and 70% (7).

Opioids

Most reactions to opioids such as morphine, codeine, and meperidine are secondary to direct mast cell mediator release from skin mast cells rather than IgE mechanisms. As a result, skin tests are invariably positive, even in normal control subjects. However, fentanyl, sufentanil, and remifentanil do not directly stimulate skin mast cells, so skin tests may be helpful. The incidence of cross-reactivity is unknown, although cases have been described in which meperidine, and methadone have cross-reacted with morphine antibodies, despite having different chemical structures (21).

Non-anesthetic Drugs

Oxytocin

Synthetic oxytocin has rarely been implicated in severe anaphylactic reactions (22). The test itself must be interpreted cautiously, since oxytocin can be irritating to the skin (23). Latex allergy should always be considered when symptoms of anaphylaxis occur soon after the administration of oxytocin since oxytocin may facilitate the development of symptoms in latex-allergic patients (24).

Antibiotics

Penicillins and cephalosporins elicit approximately 70% of the allergic reactions to antibiotics (7). With the recent Group B streptococcus infection prevention guidelines, it has become a more pressing issue in the parturient. Early cephalosporins were known to contain trace amounts of penicillin and cross-reactivity was often demonstrated. However, current drug preparations have a low level of cross-reactivity (11). A cross-sensitivity rate of 8% to 10% is often quoted; however, many of these reactions are related to skin rashes that are not immunologic in origin (19). First generation cephalosporins are more likely to cross-react with penicillin than third generation agents (7).

Non-steroidal Anti-inflammatory Drugs (NSAIDs)

NSAIDs are increasingly recognized as a cause of anaphylactoid reactions due to the inhibition of cyclooxygenase and the generation of excessive leukotrienes. The onset is usually 10 minutes after intravenous administration, 30 minutes after rectal dosing and up to 1 hour after oral administration (10). Since aspirin and NSAIDs do not initiate specific IgE antibodies, allergy can only be established by an oral challenge (21). Cross-reactions occur between aspirin and most of the NSAIDs (5).

Chlorhexidine

Chlorhexidine is increasingly recognized as a cause for both Type I and Type IV hypersensitivity reactions. It is often overlooked as a cause of anaphylaxis, since reactions are delayed up to 10 minutes. Reactions can be triggered by cutaneous, mucosal, or parenteral application (21).

Synthetic Colloids

Synthetic colloids, such as hydroxyethyl starch, gelatins, and dextran-containing colloids cause 3% of all perioperative hypersensitivity reactions (25). The vast majority of reactions occur after 30 minutes and are non-allergic in nature (10). Gelatins and dextrans cause more reactions than hetastarch (25) with estimates of IgE-mediated anaphylaxis, ranging from 0.06% to 0.35% (7).

Allergy to Latex

Epidemiology

The introduction of universal precautions in the 1980s increased the use of latex-containing gloves and medical equipment, with a subsequent increase in the incidence of latex allergy and sensitivity to 1.4% and 7%, respectively (25). More recently, latex avoidance in the workplace and the restriction of powdered latex gloves may be reducing the incidence of allergy (26,27).

Latex sensitivity is defined as the presence of positive skin tests or positive in vitro tests to latex; patients are frequently asymptomatic until a threshold of exposure triggers an *allergic* reaction. Latex allergy is defined as the presence of allergic symptoms when there is contact with latex in a latex-sensitive person (9). The most dramatic presentation for latex allergy is the IgE-mediated reaction, although Type IV allergic contact dermatitis is four times more common (28).

Three high-risk groups for latex allergy have been identified—health care workers, workers with occupational exposure, and children with spina bifida and genitourinary abnormalities (11). Among health care workers, the prevalence of latex sensitivity ranges from 12.5% to 15.8% with the majority being asymptomatic (29). Exposure is most often from latex-contaminated aerosolized cornstarch powder that is added to latex gloves to make them easier to put on. Latex proteins from the gloves attach to the cornstarch during processing and storage, and eventually disperse with manipulation (30).

Latex allergy and sensitivity may affect over half of the patients with spina bifida. Interestingly, studies show they are allergic to different latex proteins than hospital workers probably as a result of parenteral and mucous membranes exposure rather than through inhalation (30).

There are other risk factors for latex allergy including specific food allergies and atopy. Fruits such as chestnuts, bananas, kiwis, and avocados may have peptides that cross-react with latex (25,30). Atopic patients are also at high risk for latex sensitivity if they have occupational exposure (27).

Presentation

The clinical manifestations of latex anaphylaxis can differ depending on whether exposure is outside or inside the hospital setting. Typical histories outside the surgical suite include oral itching, facial redness, or swelling to latex toy balloons or during dental examinations (30). Vaginal symptoms occur with the use of condoms. Contact urticaria on the hands is commonly described when wearing latex gloves, and bronchospasm and rhinoconjunctivitis typically occurs with exposure to latex glove powder (9). Severe reactions may result in cardiovascular collapse (11).

In the hospital, symptoms of vaginal pruritus and swelling have been described at the time of examination, delivery, or immediately peripartum. Airborne exposure can lead to rhinitis, conjunctivitis, and bronchospasm, rarely leading to cardiovascular collapse and fetal distress (31). The signs and symptoms of anaphylaxis due to latex may occur from 20 minutes to an hour after exposure, making it difficult to differentiate from intravenously administered agents (11).

Pregnancy itself may be associated with higher rates of latex sensitivity (24). During cesarean delivery, symptoms of latex anaphylaxis may follow the intravenous injection of oxytocin, leading to misdiagnosis. It is possible that latex proteins released from surgical gloves during the skin and uterine incision enter the circulation after the administration of oxytocin. The contracting placental site provides the portal of entry causing symptoms. Alternatively, the reaction may occur because oxytocin has structural similarity to latex, or oxytocin may form part of the epitope of the latex antigen.

Management

Many hospitals have formulated policies and procedures for detection and management of patients with latex allergy or sensitivity. They have also taken the initiative to decrease the risk of latex sensitivity among their staff. Suggestions regarding the management of latex allergy patients appear in Table 38-5.

Testing for latex allergy can be difficult because numerous different latex proteins have been implicated in IgE-mediated immunologic reactions. In addition, skin test extracts are not commercially available. "Home-made" preparations have been produced, however due to the wide variability of glove protein content; latex skin tests have a limited sensitivity and

specificity. Serologic tests that identify latex IgE are available but not sufficiently sensitive for screening purposes (11).

Elective procedures on known latex-sensitive individuals should be carried out in a "latex-free" environment and should be performed at the start of the day (9). Airborne latex may persist in significant quantities, particularly on scrub suits (32). Synthetic gloves should be used when preparing equipment for the medical procedure in a latex-sensitive patient (4). Ideally, all latex products should be avoided but in reality, certain latex devices are more apt to cause a reaction than others, depending on the method of manufacture. Dry natural rubber, such as that used for syringe plungers and vial stoppers contain much less protein than surgical gloves made from latex concentrate and are less likely to cause reactions (30). Since it is not mandatory to identify the latex content of vial stoppers, guidelines advocate removal of the stopper or restrict use to a single puncture (33).

Hand Dermatitis

Hand dermatitis, both allergic contact dermatitis and common irritant dermatitis, are known risk factors for IgE-mediated latex reactions. The abraded skin may provide a portal of entry into the bloodstream for a variety of latex allergens (27).

Allergic contact dermatitis (Type IV hypersensitivity) is caused by a hypersensitivity to the various chemicals added to the latex mixture during manufacture, rather than the latex proteins themselves. The reactions appear 24 to 48 hours after a repeated exposure. Signs and symptoms include erythematous or scaling patches with blistering (30).

Irritant dermatitis is caused by moisture under the gloves, other workplace chemicals, and repeated hand washing. It is a non–immune-mediated reaction, characterized by pruritus, irritation, scaling, and cracking at the site of contact. It appears minutes to hours after exposure (9).

TABLE 38-5 Recommendations for the Management of Latex-sensitive and Latex-allergic Patients

Identify and Prioritize	• Identify the latex sensitive patient • Arrange in vivo and in vitro testing if possible • Notify the entire health care team • Arrange list so patient is first of the day • Place sign on operating/labor room door "Latex Allergy"
Patient Preparation	• Antihistamines and corticosteroids not recommended • Prepare all medication and equipment with non-latex gloves • A latex-free cart with supplies should be available • Cotton wrappings to protect skin from latex based blood pressure cuffs or tubing • Avoid latex esmarchs, tapes, tourniquets, drains, and urinary catheters
Gloves	• NO low protein latex gloves • Use alternatives: Styrene, styrene-butadiene, neoprene, and polyvinylchloride
Syringes	• Glass or non-natural latex syringes are preferred • Regular syringes are acceptable providing that drugs are freshly drawn and administered (within 6 h)
Medications	• Glass ampoules • Remove rubber stopper from vial *or* one puncture through fresh vial
Intravenous sets	• Tape over injection ports and use stopcocks. • Avoid buretrols • Regular intravenous bags or minibags may be used • Add medications through port to be spiked

Investigation of Anaphylaxis

Acute Assessment

If anaphylaxis is suspected, patients should be referred to an allergist to confirm that anaphylaxis has occurred and to identify the offending agent. Blood for serum tryptase levels should be drawn immediately and within 2 hours of symptoms, and again at 24 hours.

Histamine can be tested in the blood and urine. Since elevations in plasma histamine return to baseline within 60 minutes, samples must be drawn quickly (34). Similar to tryptase, it is elevated in both allergic and non-allergic mechanisms and its absence does not preclude an anaphylactic reaction (7). In addition, false negative values have been identified in pregnancy (12).

Allergy Testing

When allergy tests are performed after a reaction, many centers advocate waiting 4 to 6 weeks from the event before skin and in vitro tests are administered. It allows the levels of immunoglobulins and mediators to return to prereaction levels (7).

Skin Testing

Skin prick tests and intradermal testing involve exposing mast cells in the skin to specific antigens (in drugs or products). Both are performed on the upper back or the volar surface of the forearm. If specific IgE on the mast cells encounters the corresponding antigen, a skin reaction occurs, confirming a Type I reaction (5). It is more sensitive than in vitro testing and is the diagnostic procedure of choice for detecting IgE-mediated allergies (11). Appropriate positive (histamine or codeine) and negative (saline) controls should be used.

There is difficulty in studying some anesthetic agents, such as opioids and neuromuscular blockers, since standard solutions cause direct histamine release. Guidelines have been developed for the appropriate dilution of drugs for skin tests (12).

Skin prick tests are performed using a hypodermic needle which is passed through a drop of testing reagent at a 45-degree angle to the skin. The skin is gently lifted, causing a small break in the epidermis and a minute amount of allergen penetrates and interacts with the mast cells. The site is compared to positive and negative controls after 15 minutes. The mean diameter of the wheal (calculated by adding the longest diameter to the diameter at 90 degrees divided by 2) should be at least 3 mm more than the negative control (35).

Intradermal tests consist of injecting larger amounts of diluted allergen into the dermis at various volumes. Criteria for positive reactions are similar to those of skin prick tests (35). Experience in the interpretation of intradermal skin tests is necessary due to a relatively high incidence of reactions caused by direct histamine release. A true positive is more likely if a patient reacts to very dilute solutions (10).

Skin prick tests are less likely to cause systemic reactions than intradermal skin tests (4). Case reports of true anaphylaxis during testing are rare, with rates of 0.1% and 0.3% for antibiotics and neuromuscular blockers, respectively (36). Fatalities are extremely uncommon.

Local Anesthetic Skin Testing and Provocative Challenge in Pregnancy

Pregnancy is not a contraindication to allergy testing (12). Anesthesiologists may need to perform allergy testing for local anesthetics in pregnant patients during labor and delivery in order to perform a regional block. This should be done at a time when the risks and benefits of the procedure can be explained to the patient. If the history suggests an immediate reaction, then skin tests and the performance of a provocative challenge by the anesthesiologist before epidural placement would follow. Fetal monitoring and appropriate resuscitative equipment should be available.

Intradermal skin tests alone may give a high false positive rate because of injection trauma, skin distension, and localized histamine release. Provocative challenge testing is considered the gold standard for the diagnosis of LA allergy. It involves injecting a series of small aliquots of testing reagent into the subcutaneous tissue and observing for local or systemic reactions. Several large series testing hundreds of patients with a history suggestive of "local anesthetic allergy" have shown that provocative challenge testing is not only safe but clearly the test of choice (35). A suggested protocol appears in Table 38-6.

In Vitro Testing

Ideal tests in pregnancy include in vitro tests because they only require patient sera. Specific IgE antibody levels in the serum sample can be measured using radioimmunoassay. Significant levels are not proof that a particular drug is responsible, only that the patient is sensitized (7). The assays are limited by their low sensitivity. Tests such as the leukocyte histamine release test and the basophil activation test represent emerging tools for diagnosis. However, their role in confirming specific allergy has not yet been validated (25).

TABLE 38-6 Suggested Protocol for Skin Prick Tests and Progressive Challenge for Local Anesthetics

Initial Test	Skin Prick Test: Undiluted LA[a]		
Step	Route	Volume (mL)	Dilution
1	Subcutaneous	0.1	Undiluted LA[a]
2	Subcutaneous	0.5	Undiluted LA
3	Subcutaneous	1.0	Undiluted LA
4	Subcutaneous	2.0	Undiluted LA

[a]15 min interval in between
Positive challenge test: Presence of local wheal and erythema or systemic anaphylactic symptoms

[a]Consider dilutions of 1:100 or 1:1,000 with a history of severe reactions (Thyssen JP, Menne T, Elberling J, et al. Hypersensitivity to local anaesthetics-update and proposal of evaluation algorithm. *Contact Derm* 2008;59:69–78.)

LA, local anesthetic.

Preventing an Allergic Reaction

Skin testing is not recommended for preoperative screening if there is no prior history of an anesthetic reaction because many subjects screened for allergy to, for example, neuromuscular blockers have a positive test despite no previous exposure (19). When the offending agent is known, avoidance is the best management since no treatment can reliably prevent anaphylactic reactions. The use of corticosteroids and histamine receptor blocking drugs preoperatively is not recommended and may mask the early signs and symptoms of anaphylaxis (19). However, there is a role for these drugs in reducing the incidence of side-effects from contrast media and medications that cause direct histamine release (10). When the offending agent is unknown, regional anesthesia is prudent and products with latex or chlorhexidine should be avoided. When general anesthesia is chosen, inhalational agents are preferred and both neuromuscular blockers and histamine-releasing drugs should not be given.

Differential Diagnosis of Anaphylaxis

Urticaria and Angioedema

There is a broad differential diagnosis to anaphylaxis because of the numerous conditions that may present with urticaria and angioedema (see Fig. 38-4). They can occur together or in isolation.

Urticaria is defined as superficial skin wheals of various sizes, with or without erythema. It is caused by histamine and other mediators released from mast cells and basophils. Patients may complain of pruritus or, occasionally, burning sensations. Acute urticaria typically lasts 1 to 24 hours, and can be associated with infection, medications, or certain foods (37). If urticaria occurs, continuously or intermittently for 6 weeks, it is considered chronic urticaria, of which 80% to 90% are idiopathic (38). Common triggers include pressure, heat cold, and exercise.

Angioedema is a condition that involves swelling of the deep dermal and subcutaneous/submucosal tissues due to the mediator bradykinin (39). It is non-pruritic and non-pitting, lasting up to 72 hours. It can be associated with pain instead of pruritus, and often involves the mucous membranes (37). The chronic forms of angioedema are not associated with urticaria and are not responsive to antihistamines (39).

Mastocytosis

Mastocytosis is a heterogeneous group of diseases characterized by an increase in mast cells in the skin, lymph nodes, liver, spleen, gastrointestinal tract, and bone marrow. There are several different variants including: Cutaneous mastocytosis, indolent systemic mastocytosis, aggressive systemic mastocytosis, and mast cell leukemia. Treatment depends on the type of mastocytosis, with the benign forms being managed with antihistamines and supportive therapy (40).

Patients with cutaneous mastocytosis have fixed, pigmented, reddish brown macules, or papules over their body known as urticaria pigmentosa. It is estimated to occur with an incidence between 1 in 1,000 and 1 in 8,000 of individuals. Systemic mastocytosis is much less frequent occurring in 10% of those with urticaria pigmentosa (41).

The clinical manifestations of mastocytosis are the symptoms of overwhelming mast cell degranulation resulting in elevated serum levels of tryptase, histamine, and other mediators. Skin features include hives, flushing, and pruritus. Systematic symptoms often include abdominal pain, nausea and vomiting, diarrhea, and gastroesophageal reflux. Profound hypotension and vascular collapse can be life-threatening; however, bronchospasm is not a prominent finding (42). Episodes can be triggered by trauma, extremes of temperature, spicy foods, alcohol, NSAIDs, and histamine-releasing drugs (41,42).

In benign cutaneous or systemic mastocytosis, treatment includes antihistamines and occasionally corticosteroids, in both non-pregnant and pregnant patients (40,43). Life-threatening hypotension is treated with epinephrine that also helps to stabilize the mast cell membrane (41).

Prior to surgical procedures, pretreatment with antihistamines and corticosteroids has been advocated to prevent attacks but is not always effective (41).

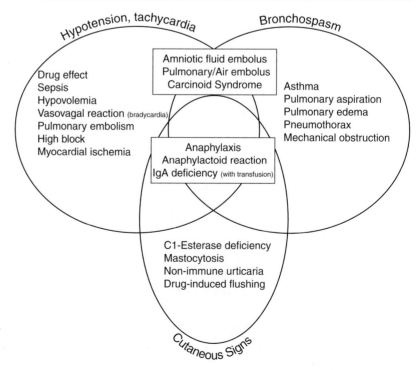

FIGURE 38-4 Differential diagnosis of anaphylaxis.

During pregnancy, particularly the first and second trimesters, and postpartum, half of the parturients may have a worsening of urticaria pigmentosa lesions, pruritus, flushing, and abdominal pain. Labor itself does not seem to exacerbate symptoms and labor pain can be treated with neuraxial analgesia, provided there are no local broken pustules that may be secondarily infected. Some clinicians use premedication with antihistamines during labor and delivery. Epinephrine is given if indicated (43). Medications for general anesthesia should include non–histamine-releasing drugs and active patient warming (42). Neonatal outcomes appear unaffected by maternal mastocytosis (43).

C1-esterase Inhibitor Deficiency

C1-esterase inhibitor (C1-INH) deficiency is a group of disorders characterized by deficient or dysfunctional levels of C1-INH. CI-INH is necessary to prevent unchecked activation of the complement cascade and parts of the fibrinolytic system. In hereditary angioedema, attacks usually occur in late childhood, while acquired forms of C1-INH deficiency have been associated with lymphoproliferative disorders and autoimmune diseases in adults.

Clinically, C1-INH features intermittent subcutaneous or submucosal edema in any part of the skin, respiratory tract, and gastrointestinal tract. Symptoms include recurrent, nonpruritic edema and abdominal pain. The presence of urticaria should lead to a search for another diagnosis. Fifty to seventy-five percent of patients have life-threatening airway obstruction at some point due to angioedema of the pharyngeal and laryngeal structures; symptoms include voice change and dysphagia, and the mortality rate is 15% to 33% (44). Abdominal edema can lead to nausea, vomiting, diarrhea, or the symptoms of an acute abdomen (45). With severe angioedema, the patient is at risk for hypotension and shock, due to diarrhea and the re-distribution of intravascular fluid into swollen intestinal tissue (46).

Typically, symptoms develop over several hours and subside over 2 to 5 days. However, abdominal pain may occur suddenly and airway obstruction can occur over 20 minutes (44). Common triggers include infection, dental work, minor trauma, snoring, anxiety, and emotional upset (45).

Acute attacks are treated with appropriate doses of C1-INH concentrate, which can start alleviating symptoms within 30 minutes and reduce the duration of attacks to a mean of 15 hours. The effects of C1-INH concentrate can last up to 2 days. Hereditary angioedema is not treated with antihistamines, corticosteroids, or epinephrine (44,45).

Long-term treatment includes anti-fibrinolytics and androgens to reduce the frequency and severity of attacks. Anti-fibrinolytics inhibit plasminogen activation and "spare" endogenous C1-INH. Tranexamic acid is not teratogenic and has been used during pregnancy in patients not at risk for thrombosis. Androgens are relatively contraindicated in parturients due to potential virilizing effects in female fetuses (44).

Information from reported cases indicates that attacks decrease in the second and third trimester and most patients have an uncomplicated peripartum period (46). However, abdominal pain may be attributed to hereditary angioedema and obscure serious obstetric disorders. Perineal edema may cause urethral obstruction (44) or appear as the first sign of angioedema leading to irreversible shock (47).

Regional analgesia is advised to lessen pain, anxiety, and the risk associated with airway manipulation (44). If general anesthesia is required, appropriate prophylaxis with C1-INH is required and common induction agents, muscle relaxants, and inhalational agents can be used (45).

Prophylaxis during pregnancy may include tranexamic acid or regular doses of C1-INH replacement. C1-INH concentrate can be given prophylactically, for both vaginal and operative deliveries or on reserve in the event that the patient develops symptoms. If C1-INH concentrate is not available, two units fresh frozen plasma can be used (44). A comparison of systemic mastocytosis and hereditary angioedema appears in Table 38-7.

IgA Deficiency

IgA deficiency is a disorder characterized by low levels of immunoglobulin A in serum and mucous secretions. It occurs with a prevalence of 1 in 500 individuals. A significant proportion of affected individuals produce IgG antibodies to IgA. If the patient has high antibody titers, a severe transfusion reaction can occur with the administration of blood products. Overall, the risk of a severe hypersensitivity reaction is low. Under normal circumstances, patients may be asymptomatic or suffer from recurrent sinus, respiratory, or gastrointestinal infections. Systemic lupus erythematosus (SLE) and rheumatoid arthritis have been associated with the deficiency (48).

■ TYPE II HYPERSENSITIVITY (ANTIBODY-MEDIATED CYTOTOXIC REACTION)

Erythroblastosis Fetalis

Erythroblastosis fetalis or, hemolytic disease of the newborn (HDN), is a condition in which specific maternal IgG antibodies (which freely cross the placenta) attach to antigens on fetal red blood cells, leading to fetal anemia and extramedullary hematopoiesis. The red blood cell antigen commonly involved includes the rhesus D (RhD) antigen, although other blood groups such as the ABO and Kell systems can be

TABLE 38-7 Comparison of Systemic Mastocytosis and Hereditary Angioedema

	Systemic Mastocytosis	Hereditary Angioedema
Treatment	Antihistamines Corticosteroids Epinephrine	C1-INH Anti-fibrinolytics
Anesthetic Implications		
Pretreatment	Antihistamines Corticosteroids	C1-INH Fresh frozen plasma
Airway	Usual	Manipulations cause pharyngeal and laryngeal angioedema
Medications	Avoid histamine-releasing drugs	Common agents acceptable
Regional	Acceptable	Encouraged

responsible (49). With the routine use of anti-D (antibodies against RhD antigens) prophylaxis for RhD negative mothers, the incidence and severity of HDN has fallen dramatically (50).

Pathophysiologically, an RhD negative mother produces antibodies when exposed to blood cells from a fetus that is RhD (paternally inherited) positive. The first pregnancy does not usually prompt maternal antibody production until delivery; therefore, it is the subsequent pregnancies which are affected (51).

Prior to the detection and treatment of HDN, most fetuses were either miscarried, stillborn, or developed hydrops fetalis. The syndrome of hydrops fetalis is initiated by profound fetal anemia and extramedullary hematopoiesis. Anemia impairs oxygen delivery leading to endothelial damage and leaky capillary membranes. Extramedullary hematopoiesis results in impaired hepatic protein synthesis, hepatosplenomegaly, and elevated portal and umbilical venous pressures. Eventually, extravasation of fluid occurs, producing ascites, pleural effusions, pericardial effusions, scalp edema, subcutaneous edema, and polyhydramnios (50).

During pregnancy, antibody titers are measured in the RhD antigen negative mother and the presence of the RhD antigens in the fetus are assayed (51). Until recently, the main investigation for fetal genotype-testing was amniocentesis. However, new and sophisticated tests have taken advantage of the normal presence of cell-free fetal DNA in maternal serum. From this, the fetal Rh genotype can be determined. An RhD antigen negative fetus does not require follow-up but an RhD antigen positive fetus requires close monitoring during the entire pregnancy (50).

Follow-up includes serial maternal antibody titers and tests to estimate the degree of fetal anemia. When maternal antibody titers against RhD reach a critical level, the risk of fetal hydrops rises significantly and prompts further investigation. Fetal anemia can be estimated by sampling amniotic fluid for hyperbilirubinemia or by measuring the peak velocity of blood flow in the middle cerebral artery by Doppler ultrasound. Studies show Doppler ultrasound is superior in accuracy and safety, and may supplant amniocentesis (50).

Many affected fetuses can be managed after delivery with phototherapy. However, when serial tests during pregnancy indicate progressive anemia, invasive fetal hemoglobin testing is performed. If anemia is significant, intraperitoneal or umbilical vein blood transfusions can temporarily reverse the complications until the fetus can be delivered. Fetal immobilization is required for both procedures, which can be accomplished indirectly with maternal sedation or, more commonly by injecting a neuromuscular blocking agent, directly into the umbilical vein. Vecuronium is commonly used (51).

With proper prenatal monitoring, most parturients and newborns have a relatively uncomplicated course. However, if a fetus at risk is not treated, fetal organomegaly and ascites can lead to dystocia necessitating cesarean delivery.

■ TYPE III HYPERSENSITIVITY REACTIONS (IMMUNE COMPLEX MEDIATED)

Systemic Lupus Erythematosus

SLE is a multisystem chronic inflammatory disease caused primarily by autoantibodies and immune complexes. The diagnostic criteria for the disease include a characteristic malar rash, non-erosive arthritis of peripheral joints, serositis, renal dysfunction, neurologic manifestations, hematologic disorders, and abnormal circulating antibodies including antinuclear antibody. The disease is nine times more common in women than in men and has an increased incidence

in African Americans compared to Caucasians (52). While maternal mortality has greatly improved, patients with SLE continue to have a mortality rate 20 times higher than the pregnant woman without SLE (53).

Patient Considerations

The signs and symptoms associated with SLE may be mild and confined to one organ system or fulminating, leading rapidly to death. Fever, weight loss, and fatigue may be the first signs of the disease. The skin may be affected, causing the classic malar "butterfly rash." Involvement of mucous membranes with painful ulcerations in the pharynx, mouth, or vagina may also occur (52).

The heart may be affected in a number of ways. Pericarditis with chest pain occurs in over 50% of patients with SLE but progression to cardiac tamponade is uncommon. It may be caused by coronary arteritis, myocarditis, or focal necrosis and atrophy of the myocardium. Some patients develop cardiac valvular lesions (Libman–Sacks endocarditis) that are usually asymptomatic. The cardiovascular system is best evaluated by physical examination. An electrocardiogram (ECG) may be useful to assess rhythm abnormalities and ischemic changes.

Polyserositis is relatively common, with pleurisy occurring in 50% of cases. If the patient is dyspneic, the respiratory system should be assessed to rule out pulmonary vasculitis, infarction, hemorrhage, pleural effusions, and pulmonary hypertension.

Lupus nephritis is common and accounts for the majority of fatalities due to SLE. A urinalysis, blood urea nitrogen, serum creatinine, serum electrolytes, and blood sugar should be measured. Hypokalemia and glucose intolerance are common in patients receiving corticosteroids. Casts in the urine sediment indicate active nephritis.

There may be several coagulation defects in patients with SLE. Patients may have thrombophilia, or thrombocytopenia due to antiplatelet antibodies and splenomegaly. In addition, specific circulating anticoagulants may be present with factor VIII inhibitors being the most common (54). Their presence contraindicates the use of regional block.

The presence of high anti-phospholipid antibody titers and a history of recurrent venous or arterial clotting and fetal loss characterize the anti-phospholipid antibody syndrome. This antibody is often reported as the "lupus anticoagulant" because in the laboratory it causes an elevated activated thromboplastin time, although clinically, it causes thrombosis. While this syndrome is often treated with immunosuppressants such as corticosteroids, other therapy such as low molecular weight heparin and/or aspirin may also be used in an attempt to reduce the incidence of thrombosis. These therapies may contraindicate use of regional anesthesia (55).

Many of the neurologic complications of SLE are due to vasculitis or complications related to steroid treatment. Patients can develop psychosis, transverse myelopathy, cranial nerve palsies, and peripheral neuropathy. Intracerebral bleeding or status epilepticus may lead to death. Findings of polyarthralgia or arthritis follow the same distribution as rheumatoid arthritis but are usually milder and not deforming. Avascular necrosis of the head of the femur may result from either chronic steroid therapy or vasculitis.

Obstetrical Considerations

Pregnancy increases the incidence of lupus flares in 30% to 60% of patients (56). Lupus flares can occur at any time and are more common in parturients with renal involvement, active urine sediment (casts and red cells), or falling complement levels. They consist of arthralgias, anemia, thrombocytopenia, worsening hypertension, proteinuria, renal dysfunction, encephalopathy, abdominal pain, and hepatic failure. As pregnancy advances, a lupus flare becomes very difficult to differentiate from preeclampsia, which is also more common in lupus patients (53). Treatment of a lupus flare includes high doses of corticosteroids and antihypertensive agents while preeclampsia is treated by delivery of the fetus.

Approximately 10% of infants have neonatal lupus erythematosus as a result of transplacental passage of anti-SSA/Ro or anti-SSB/La. Of these, approximately half have skin manifestations that resemble those seen in the adult. Cardiac manifestations include complete heart block, cardiomyopathy, and valvular lesions (57). Neonates are often premature and growth restricted (53).

Analgesia and Anesthesia for Labor and Delivery

Analgesia for vaginal delivery can include opioids, inhalational analgesia, and epidural analgesia. Before any neuraxial technique, there should be a detailed examination of the neurologic system and complete review of the coagulation status. Intrathecal or epidural opioids, with or without local anesthetic may be useful. Although a fixed neurologic deficit is not an absolute contraindication to regional block, it should be documented. If raised intracranial pressure is suspected, options other than regional blockade should be considered.

Cesarean delivery is more common in patients with lupus. Provided the coagulation and neurologic status is normal, it can be performed safely under regional or general anesthesia. Cross-matching of blood products may be a problem due to irregular circulating antibodies, therefore blood should be available in advance. Hourly urine output using a Foley catheter should be measured. An arterial line may be placed to monitor blood pressure if hypertension is difficult to control. If severe renal disease is present, a central venous or pulmonary artery catheter may be required to assess and optimize fluid status and cardiac output.

When general anesthesia is indicated, a rapid sequence induction may need to be modified for extremely ill patients. If myocardial function is poor, a reduced dose of induction agent combined with an opioid such as fentanyl may be required. Succinylcholine is still used as a muscle relaxant to facilitate endotracheal intubation. If there is a history of a recent stroke with paralysis, a non-depolarizing muscle relaxant such as rocuronium should be used, since succinylcholine can trigger massive hyperkalemia. Agents that require renal excretion to terminate their action should be avoided if renal failure is present. Finally, the delivery should take place in a facility that is prepared to take care of the infant should it be affected with neonatal SLE.

Progressive Systemic Sclerosis (Scleroderma)

Scleroderma or progressive systemic sclerosis (PSS) is a generalized disorder, characterized by excessive deposits of connective tissue in the skin and viscera and is associated with microvascular and immunologic changes (58). The disease is five times more common in women than men with an average age of onset of 40 years. Fifty percent of patients with scleroderma may become pregnant, in part as a result of the trend toward delayed pregnancy (59). It is classified as an autoimmune disorder because autoimmune hemolytic anemia, hypergammaglobulinemia, rheumatoid factor, and numerous autoantibodies have been found in patients with this disease. However, the immunopathologic mechanism is still unknown.

Patient Considerations

The most striking findings of scleroderma are the cutaneous changes. The skin becomes sclerosed and thickened from the dermis to the subcutaneous tissue, starting with the digits and extending proximally to include the trunk. The fetus may be difficult to assess clinically if the tissue over the abdomen is severely affected. The skin of the face may become tightly adherent to underlying structures, limiting the patient's ability to open her mouth, creating difficulties with intubation.

Raynaud's phenomenon is a hallmark feature of PSS. Its presence is associated with a decrease in renal blood flow in some patients. In addition, coronary vascular spasm may occur, causing arrhythmias and angina in patients with anatomically normal coronary arteries. The myocardium may show focal or generalized fibrosis leading to congestive heart failure (60). During pregnancy, aspirin and antihypertensive agents are prescribed to treat some of these complications.

Pulmonary function is often impaired. Interstitial fibrosis may lead to pulmonary hypertension, a restrictive lung defect, and a decrease in diffusing capacity. In pregnancy, the gravid uterus and an increased metabolic rate may further aggravate hypoxemia. Hypoxia may increase pulmonary artery pressures further, leading to cor pulmonale. Arterial blood gasses and chest x-rays may be required.

Almost 50% of patients with scleroderma have proteinuria, hypertension, and azotemia. Patients with diffuse, rapidly progressing skin thickening are more likely to suffer a renal crisis, which is characterized by progressive renal failure and malignant hypertension. These patients may present with severe headaches, hypertensive encephalopathy, retinopathy, seizures, and left ventricular failure. Renal crisis is a leading cause of mortality. While the condition may respond to a number of antihypertensive agents, angiotensin converting enzyme inhibitors appear to be most effective. This class of drugs is not generally recommended in pregnancy because of potential risks to the neonate such as refractory hypotension and oliguria, but it may be life saving for the mother.

The entire gastrointestinal tract can be involved with PSS. Swallowing may be difficult due to tongue and palate pathology. Abnormalities of esophageal motility, lower esophageal sphincter competence, and peptic strictures increase the risk of aspiration. Malabsorption can result in malnutrition and an elevated prothrombin time due to lack of vitamin K.

The small joints of the hands and feet are often arthritic exhibiting severe deformities, and positioning can be problematic.

Obstetric Considerations

Parturients with scleroderma are high-risk pregnancies. A recent American study compared 149 pregnant scleroderma patients to a cohort of unaffected parturients. Patients with PSS were more likely to have hypertensive disorders (odds ratio 4.0, 95% confidence interval 2.4 to 6.6) and intrauterine growth restriction (odds ratio 3.7, 95% confidence interval 1.5 to 9.0), presumably as a result of scleroderma-associated microvascular abnormalities associated with the disease (61).

Analgesia and Anesthesia for Labor and Delivery

The pregnant patient with severe PSS poses several difficult anesthetic management problems. Often there is a lack of suitable peripheral veins for intravenous therapy. Large veins in the forearm or a central vein should be cannulated, since Raynaud's phenomena can lead to digit necrosis and gangrene if cool fluids are infused. Patients should be kept warm to limit vascular spasm. Blood pressure may be difficult to measure due to skin changes, but indwelling arterial catheters should be avoided if possible because these may provoke distal vasospasm and gangrene.

Epidural analgesia is appropriate for the relief of labor pain or operative delivery, provided coagulation parameters are normal. Performance of the epidural block may be technically difficult due to skin changes or arthritis in the lumbar spine. Early case reports suggested that the action of local anesthetics were enhanced in patients with scleroderma, but the difference may not be clinically significant.

Cesarean delivery has been performed successfully under spinal anesthesia (62). Vasopressors should be given judiciously to avoid severe hypertension and vasospasm. For the same reasons, ergot preparations should be used with caution. If general anesthesia is required, several precautions should be noted. In patients with impaired esophageal motility, an attempt should be made to empty the lower esophagus of secretions with an orogastric tube. A non-particulate antacid can be given but if there is esophageal pathology, oral antacids may not be adequate. An H$_2$ antihistamine, such as ranitidine may be useful to reduce gastric acid secretion and metoclopramide may accelerate gastric emptying. Facial deformities may make tight placement of an anesthetic mask and preoxygenation problematic. If a difficult intubation is suspected because of restricted mouth opening, awake fiberoptic oral intubation under local anesthesia may be the safest way to secure the airway. If oral intubation fails, a tracheostomy may be required. Intraoperative monitoring is often difficult in patients with PSS, and the benefits of using each monitoring device must be weighed against the risks. Ideally non-invasive methods are preferred in stable patients. However, skin and subcutaneous tissue changes may make non-invasive blood pressure and oxygen saturation monitoring inaccurate (60).

■ TYPE IV HYPERSENSITIVITY (CELL-MEDIATED REACTIONS)

Rheumatoid Arthritis

Rheumatoid arthritis (RA) is a chronic inflammatory disease of diarthrodial joints that is frequently combined with the dysfunction of other organ systems. It is more common in females and can occur in any age group. The etiologic factors of the disease, point in part, to a Type IV cell-mediated immune mechanism. Juvenile rheumatoid arthritis is a similar disease with an onset before age 16 years. This condition can result in crippling sequelae by childbearing age.

Patient Considerations

The patient with RA suffers from multisystem complications. The musculoskeletal changes of the airway are often the most challenging for the anesthesiologist.

The severity of joint involvement ranges from mild inflammation and thickened synovium to articular cartilage destruction and ankylosis. The ankylosis can result in a significant restriction of joint movement. Tendons and ligaments may also be weakened, leading to instability and subluxation.

The cervical spine is involved in up to 85% of patients with RA but most are asymptomatic. Atlanto-axial subluxation with cord or nerve root compression, presents with symptoms of headache, subjective upper extremity pain, or objective long track signs (63). X-rays of the cervical spine including anteroposterior, open mouth, and flexion/extension views may show odontoid erosions, subaxial subluxations, apophyseal joint erosions, and disk space narrowing. If these are not available, one should assume that the neck is unstable.

Ankylosis of the temporomandibular joint, particularly in patients with juvenile rheumatoid arthritis, may make mouth opening so restricted that oral endotracheal intubation is difficult. Observing for at least a 4 cm opening when the parturient opens her mouth can test the temporomandibular joint. The patient should also be viewed from the side to note micrognathia.

Cricoarytenoid arthritis is present in about 59% of patients with RA. Approximately 14% have constriction of the glottic opening leading to stridor and obstructive sleep apnea (64). Complaints of hoarseness, wheezing, sore throat, and dysphagia, suggest cricoarytenoiditis and recurrent aspiration pneumonitis from vocal cord dysfunction and gastroesophageal reflux disease. A full otolaryngologic examination using indirect or direct fiberoptic laryngoscopy can diagnose these problems.

Visceral involvement may occur in patients with long-standing disease. Cardiac and respiratory reserve may be reduced with the progression of pregnancy as well as with labor and delivery.

Cardiac function may be compromised due to pericardial effusions, conduction defects, valvular heart disease, and cardiomyopathies. Lung manifestations include restrictive lung disease secondary to pleural effusions, kyphosis, and (to a lesser extent) fixation of the ribs by arthritis (64). As the gravid uterus becomes larger, this restriction may become more severe because of impaired diaphragmatic excursion.

Other skeletal abnormalities include deformities of the hips that limit flexion and abduction, a concern for positioning with vaginal delivery. Bony pelvic abnormalities increase the risk of cephalopelvic disproportion and cesarean delivery. Restricted movement of the lumbar vertebral column or deformities may complicate the performance of a neuraxial block. An ultrasound assessment may be helpful in demonstrating calcification in the midline ligaments.

Medications are often continued during pregnancy. Corticosteroids and NSAIDs such as salicylates, indomethacin, naproxen, and diclofenac are not known to be teratogenic. Other, agents such as methotrexate, leflunomide, and other biologic therapies are contraindicated (65). Large doses of aspirin near the time of delivery predispose patients to delayed and prolonged labor and an increased risk of blood loss during delivery (66). Physiologic maternal anemia can be aggravated by iron deficiency secondary to gastrointestinal loss. NSAIDs may cause reversible premature closure of the ductus arteriosus in the third trimester. This effect is less prominent with COX-2 inhibitors (65). In addition, newborns exposed to high doses of aspirin in utero may have an increased incidence of central nervous system bleeding after delivery. Platelet function may be impaired for days after discontinuing the drug.

The use of NSAIDs does not increase the risk of epidural hematoma after neuraxial blockade in these patients (55).

Analgesia and Anesthesia for Labor and Delivery

History, physical examination, and laboratory investigations should reflect the patient's medical condition. For patients with mild disease, that is, those with no joint deformities and limited drug therapy, the methods for administering pain relief during labor and delivery are the same as those in normal pregnancy. All patients on NSAIDs should have large intravenous access and blood available for delivery because of the potential risk of postpartum hemorrhage (66).

Anesthesia for vaginal delivery can be managed in the usual fashion with the following in mind. If the patient has severe airway abnormalities, early epidural should be encouraged if coagulation is normal. The use of opioids in these patients should be used with caution, as sedation may lead to the loss of muscle tone resulting in upper airway obstruction. Severe contractures and osteoporosis, secondary to steroid treatment or immobility, may be present. The range of motion (ROM) of each of the large joints should be determined before any neuraxial blockade so that over extension and dislocation do not occur under anesthesia. It is particularly important to test the hip joints by maximally abducting and flexing them before placing the patient in stirrups. The ROM and positioning should be done carefully to avoid pathologic fractures. Peripheral neuropathies should be assessed and documented, although it is not an absolute contraindication to regional anesthesia.

Patients with long-standing, crippling RA are likely to require a cesarean delivery because of hip joint or pelvic bony involvement. For elective cesarean delivery, lumbar epidural, spinal, or general anesthesia can be used. If there are upper airway deformities or cervical spine abnormalities, conduction anesthesia is preferred if technically possible.

If general anesthesia is used in patients with severe airway deformities, the airway must be secured while the patient is awake using fiberoptic intubation. This technique limits cervical spine manipulation before permanent neurologic damage occurs. Topical anesthesia of the upper airway is required and small doses of an opioid or benzodiazepine for anxiolysis may be useful. Glycopyrrolate, which has limited transplacental passage, will decrease airway secretions. A tracheostomy under local anesthesia may be necessary if other options fail. Several pillows can support the head if there is a preexisting severe flexion deformity of the neck. Otherwise the neutral position is ideal. The arms may have to be placed at the sides if there is restriction of shoulder movement. Patients with hip contractures may require pillows under the knees.

If an emergency cesarean delivery is required in a patient with a severely deformed upper airway, the experience of the anesthesiologist and the operating team determines the conduct of anesthesia. Extension of an epidural, rapid spinal anesthesia, or awake intubation prior to general anesthesia are options. If the operating team has had experience using local anesthesia, an abdominal wall field block using chloroprocaine and supplemental sedation may be necessary. While chloroprocaine has a short duration of action, there is no need to worry about local anesthetic toxicity because of its rapid metabolism. Therefore sufficient volume can be used to ensure patient comfort. After the procedure, the patient must be fully awake with a return in full muscle function before extubation. If glottic narrowing is severe, she should be observed for several hours following extubation in an area where re-intubation or emergency tracheostomy can be performed.

Transplanted Organs and Pregnancy

Overview

Transplantation allows women whose health and fertility have been restored by an organ transplant to conceive. Manipulation of the cell-mediated immune system allows successful organ transplantation. Although most parturients with a transplanted organ have healthy newborns and an intact functioning graft, they continue to be at high risk for complications (67). The anesthetic considerations for the parturient with an allograft are summarized in Figure 38-5.

Pregnancy is usually considered after the first year, provided that allograft function is stable and there have been no episodes of rejection within that year. At that point immunosuppressant doses are low and viral prophylaxis has been completed (67). When formulating an anesthetic plan, the history, physical examination, and laboratory investigations should reflect the extent of the parturient's systemic disease and obstetrical history. In some patients, the primary disease that led to the transplant may continue to require attention. In lung recipients, cystic fibrosis is associated with failure of the exocrine pancreas and obstructive biliary disease. In liver recipients, Wilson's disease causes significant neurologic, renal, and cardiac complications. Similarly, long-standing diabetic changes may not improve following pancreatic allografts or continue to progress in renal transplant patients.

Parturients on chronic immunosuppression have an increased the risk of opportunistic and reactivated infections. The risk of cytomegalovirus (CMV), in the mother and fetus, is particularly high immediately after transplantation due to higher levels of immunosuppression. Extra time may be needed to find CMV-free blood (68). The risk of urinary tract infections, regardless of the transplant allograft approaches 40% (69). Since infection is a major cause of morbidity and mortality, invasive procedures should only be used if the benefits outweigh the risks.

Transplant patients have 100 times the risk of malignant disease. The mechanism may include chronic immunosuppression, loss of immune surveillance, and chronic antigenic stimulation (70). For example, 5 years after cardiac transplantation, 22% of recipients die from malignancy with skin cancers, the most common diagnosis (71).

Hypertension, renal dysfunction, and diabetes are significant co-morbidities in all solid organ recipients, particularly with regimens that include cyclosporine and corticosteroids. Hypertension is most frequent among kidney and kidney-pancreas transplant patients and least frequent among liver recipients. Hyperglycemia is often a reflection of corticosteroid dosing, as seen in lung recipients who suffer a 27% incidence of diabetes (72).

All transplant patients have a higher incidence of preeclampsia and hypertension. Unlike non-transplant patients, where serum uric acid levels help in diagnosis, transplant patients often have elevated uric acid levels secondary to immunosuppressant therapy (67).

Neonatal support is imperative. Maternal complications such as preeclampsia and premature rupture of amniotic membranes (PROM) contribute to the 50% incidence of prematurity and low birth weight, especially in pancreas and lung recipients (72). This compares to rates in the general population of 5% to 15% (73).

Pregnancy does not increase the risk of allograft rejection in any solid organ transplant (67). Good graft function is associated with successful maternal and fetal outcomes and poor graft function should alert the anesthesia care team of the potential for increased morbidity and mortality (72). In renal recipients, fever, graft tenderness, and graft swelling suggests rejection which may require higher doses of immunosuppression or additional monitoring (73). In addition, previous transplant surgery may make cesarean delivery more difficult (69,73).

Most centers recommend stress-doses of corticosteroids for both vaginal and cesarean delivery. A discussion of the appropriate doses for corticosteroids and other immunosuppressants appear in the subsequent delivery on immunosuppressants.

The Parturient with a Cardiac Allograft

Common indications for cardiac transplantation include: Valvular and congenital heart disease, as well as, ischemic, viral, infiltrative, and idiopathic dilated cardiomyopathy. The 5-year patient and graft survival is 69% and 67%, respectively (69). Cardiac recipients with previous peripartum cardiomyopathy are not at risk of recurrence in subsequent pregnancies (74). One cause of the high morbidity and mortality is attributed to premature multi-vessel coronary artery stenosis, known as cardiac allograft vasculopathy (CAV). The incidence ranges between 30% and 60% after 5 years (69).

In non-transplant patients, pregnancy increases blood volume by 40% and cardiac output (CO) by 30% (74). Labor increases CO 30% further, but it is the immediate postpartum period in which the most significant changes occur. Following the autotransfusion of 500 mL of blood, the CO

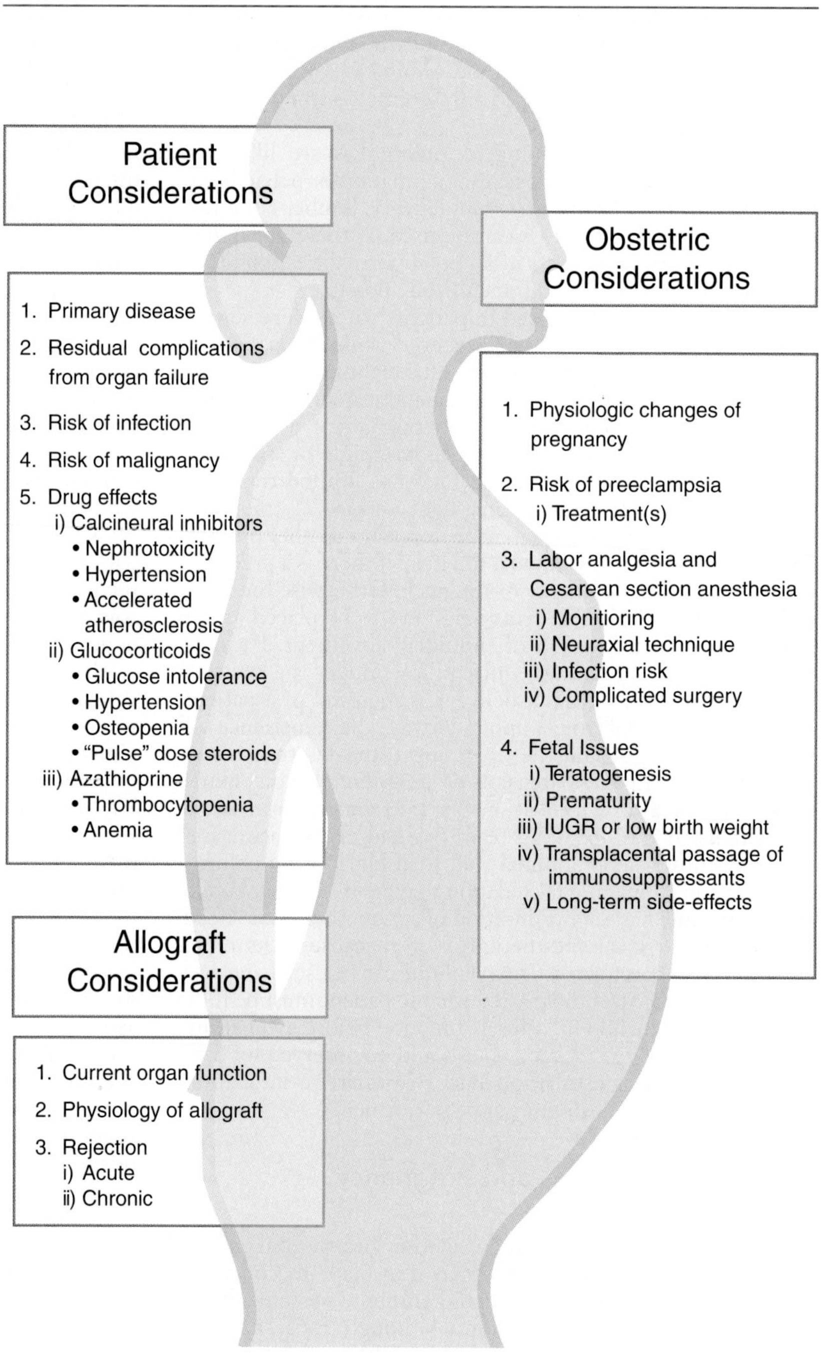

Patient Considerations

1. Primary disease
2. Residual complications from organ failure
3. Risk of infection
4. Risk of malignancy
5. Drug effects
   i) Calcineural inhibitors
      • Nephrotoxicity
      • Hypertension
      • Accelerated atherosclerosis
   ii) Glucocorticoids
      • Glucose intolerance
      • Hypertension
      • Osteopenia
      • "Pulse" dose steroids
   iii) Azathioprine
      • Thrombocytopenia
      • Anemia

Obstetric Considerations

1. Physiologic changes of pregnancy
2. Risk of preeclampsia
   i) Treatment(s)
3. Labor analgesia and Cesarean section anesthesia
   i) Monitioring
   ii) Neuraxial technique
   iii) Infection risk
   iv) Complicated surgery
4. Fetal Issues
   i) Teratogenesis
   ii) Prematurity
   iii) IUGR or low birth weight
   iv) Transplacental passage of immunosuppressants
   v) Long-term side-effects

Allograft Considerations

1. Current organ function
2. Physiology of allograft
3. Rejection
   i) Acute
   ii) Chronic

FIGURE 38-5 Anesthetic considerations in the parturient with an allograft.

reaches a peak of 60% above normal (75). Although the cardiac recipient can only reach a CO of 60% to 70% of normal due to chronotropic limitations and higher required filling pressures (76), they seem to compensate well with no evidence of adverse sequelae (69).

The Denervated Heart

After transplantation, when the heart is fully denervated, it beats at an intrinsic rate of 90 to 110 beats per minute (77). It has an impaired sympathetic response to exercise, hypovolemia, intubation, and the pain associated with labor and delivery (78). It also fails to produce a bradycardic parasympathetic response with carotid sinus massage and valsalva maneuvers. Heart rate and contractility increase as a result of circulating catecholamines in response to a particular stress. Catecholamines or cardiac pacing can be used to treat bradycardia; β blockers can decrease the heart rate and block the effects of circulating catecholamines (77). Drugs such as pancuronium and phenylephrine may not cause tachycardia or bradycardia respectively in the absence of an intact autonomic nervous system. Reversal of paralysis with neostigmine may cause bradycardia in some patients due to direct muscarinic receptor action (79). A muscarinic antagonist such as atropine or glycopyrrolate can be administered but direct chronotropic agents should be available to treat significant bradycardia (80).

The transplanted heart is considered preload-dependent and sensitive to hypovolemia. It relies on fluid volume to increase cardiac output since autonomic input is required to produce reflex tachycardia (77). Hypotension should be treated with fluids and direct acting vasoconstrictors, such as phenylephrine. Ephedrine has both direct and indirect actions and may only result in a small increase in heart rate and blood pressure (80).

Coronary autoregulation is intact and flow remains dependent on pH and arterial carbon dioxide tension (80). Over several years, re-innervation of the heart occurs with sympathetic nerve re-growth much more common than parasympathetic (81). This phenomenon explains how some cardiac recipients develop angina and rarely vasovagal responses.

Patient Assessment
Patients with a cardiac allograft must have a detailed assessment of exercise capabilities as well as the usual anesthetic history and physical examination performed. A thorough review of the laboratory investigations, ECG, echocardiogram, previous cardiac biopsies, and angiogram can help formulate anesthetic management. Some findings are typical and inconsequential while others necessitate further investigation.

In cardiac recipients without evidence of re-innervation, myocardial ischemia is silent (80). Symptoms of paroxysmal dyspnea and a poor exercise tolerance may indicate ischemia. The ECG is distinctive, with two P waves and incomplete or complete right bundle branch block (77). Non-lethal ectopic ventricular beats that occur in all patients immediately after transplantation usually decrease over the subsequent months (80). Pacemakers are necessary in 5% of cardiac recipients and should be evaluated for functionality during pregnancy (68). If late bradyarrhythmias occur, ischemia of the allograft sinoatrial node and allograft rejection should be considered (82).

Valvular lesions can include mitral regurgitation and moderate to severe tricuspid regurgitation. Left ventricular function is usually normal, although, diastolic dysfunction is common immediately after transplantation. Graft rejection can occur at any time and presents as fever, fatigue, atrial and ventricular dysrhythmias, silent myocardial ischemia, and congestive heart failure (80).

Analgesia and Anesthesia for Labor and Delivery
The mode of delivery is dependent on obstetrical indications. Cesarean delivery offers no specific advantage and does not prevent cardiac overload postpartum. With adequate prehydration, an epidural or a combined spinal–epidural can help minimize the hyperdynamic cardiovascular responses of labor and postoperative pain. Treatment of bradycardia and hypotension should be consistent with management of the denervated heart. Continuous electrocardiographic monitoring is recommended as a result of the high incidence of dysrhythmias and ischemia (83).

Cesarean delivery can be safely managed with non-invasive monitoring if the parturient has a normal exercise tolerance. If invasive monitoring is indicated, strict asepsis is required. Cautious extension of a labor epidural is safe for cesarean delivery. The precipitous drop in preload associated with spinal anesthesia may not be tolerated (68). When general anesthesia is indicated, anesthetic requirements are similar to those in the non-transplant patient (77), although, judicious use of all agents is prudent (79).

The American College of Obstetricians and Gynecologists guidelines for antibiotic prophylaxis for infective endocarditis do not recommend prophylaxis for vaginal or cesarean delivery regardless of the cardiac lesion. However, if there is an established infection such as chorioamnionitis or pyelonephritis, the underlying infection should be treated including treatment for endocarditis prophylaxis in high-risk patients (84). The American Heart Association guidelines consider patients with a cardiac transplant *and* cardiac valvulopathy as high risk for infective endocarditis and recommend prophylactic antibiotics (85).

The Parturient with a Lung Allograft
Lung transplantation is performed for a number of end-stage conditions such as chronic obstructive pulmonary disease, emphysema, cystic fibrosis, pulmonary fibrosis, and primary pulmonary hypertension. The reported 5-year patient and graft survival for all lung transplants is 47% and 46%, respectively (69). Declining lung function, fever, fatigue, and dyspnea is often attributed to obliterative bronchiolitis, a form of chronic graft rejection (78). The incidence is 60% to 70% after 5 years (79). The number of lung transplant recipients who become pregnant is extremely small and the incidences of rejection and poor obstetric outcome are much less favorable than patients with other solid organ transplants (86).

During pregnancy there are many physiologic changes to the respiratory system decreasing the reserve. In the absence of rejection, lung recipients adapt well to the changes of pregnancy (83).

Donor Lung
Lung transplantation causes a number of changes to lung physiology. Lymphatic disruption requires meticulous fluid management particularly early after transplantation in order to avoid pulmonary edema (79). Evidence in the canine model indicates that lymphatic drainage can re-establish within 2 to 4 weeks (87). Double lung transplants can be performed en bloc with denervation of the carina, or sequentially without resection of the carina, which allows for the preservation of the cough reflex (79). However, any degree of decline in the cough reflex with impaired mucociliary transport and silent aspiration, leaves the recipient more prone to infection. Preliminary studies indicate that the transplanted lung may re-innervate over the site of the anastomosis with recovery of the cough reflex after the first year (88).

Peak lung function occurs 6 months following transplantation with virtually normal lung function in those with double lung transplants. Pulmonary artery pressures, pulmonary vascular resistance, and pulmonary vasoconstriction in response to hypoxia, function immediately. Arterial blood gasses return to normal within a few weeks, but persistent hypercapnia can indicate diaphragmatic or allograft dysfunction. Bronchial hyper-responsiveness causing bronchoconstriction can occur and is responsive to β agonists. In patients with single lung transplants, 60% to 80% of pulmonary perfusion and ventilation is toward the transplanted lung (79).

Patient Assessment
Patients with a lung or heart–lung allograft must have a detailed assessment of exercise capabilities as well as the usual anesthetic history and physical examination performed. Particular attention should be given for signs and symptoms of infection or chronic rejection (obliterative bronchiolitis). Regular pulmonary function tests should be performed during pregnancy, and chest radiographs and invasive procedures should be performed if clinically indicated (83). Hypercapnia and a wide alveolar–arterial oxygen gradient on arterial blood gasses should trigger further investigation (79).

Lung recipients have an incidence of diabetes of 27%, likely due to the higher levels of corticosteroids required for the control of rejection (72).

Analgesia and Anesthesia for Labor and Delivery
The mode of delivery is dependent on obstetrical indications (72). Regional analgesia for labor is acceptable but fluid boluses should be given judiciously (78). In the supine position, the vast majority of pulmonary blood flow travels to the transplanted lung (in single lung transplants). When placing

the epidural in the lateral position, the transplanted lung should be non-dependent to prevent hypoxemia (79).

Standard monitors for cesarean delivery are appropriate in stable patients (79). The incidence of gastroesophageal reflux is high in lung recipients and there is evidence linking it to chronic allograft rejection (89). Therefore aspiration prophylaxis should be considered. Continuous epidural anesthesia reduces the risk of airway manipulation and allows the patient to continue lung physiotherapy in pain-controlled circumstances postoperatively (79). Special care should be taken to prevent paralysis of the intercostal muscles that may lead to respiratory insufficiency. When general anesthesia is indicated, assessment of the airway should note the possibility of subglottic stenosis from a previous tracheostomy or prolonged ventilation (79). Strictures may also occur at the site of tracheal or bronchial anastomoses (79,89). Mechanical ventilation should incorporate low volume protective ventilation with airway pressures less than 35 mm Hg and PEEP at or below 5 mm Hg (89).

The Parturient with a Liver Allograft

Liver transplantation dramatically improves fertility in patients with chronic liver disease. Most women of reproductive age resume normal menses within 8 weeks of transplantation. If pregnancy occurs within a year of transplantation there is a high risk of complications, possibly because of high circulating cytokinin levels. Registry data suggests that pregnancy results in about an overall 70% live birth rate but the incidence of hypertension, preeclampsia, and infection occurs in more than one-third of patients. Pregnancy does not seem to alter the incidence of graft failure (90).

In non-transplant pregnancies alkaline phosphatase levels (ALP) rise due to placental ALP after the second trimester. Liver transaminases and other serum proteins remain normal (91). Any elevations in liver enzymes remote from the transplant surgery can indicate rejection and the need for additional immunosuppressants (69).

Patient Assessment

The cardiorespiratory changes associated with end-stage liver disease improve steadily in the months following transplantation (78). The liver's ability to metabolize drugs or produce proteins is considered adequate if the INR or prothrombin time is normal (92). When biochemical abnormalities occur, preeclampsia and HELLP syndrome should be differentiated from acute rejection. Liver biopsies may be necessary for a clear diagnosis (90).

Analgesia and Anesthesia for Labor and Delivery

The mode of delivery is dependent on obstetrical indications and additional monitoring will depend on concurrent medical conditions. Regional analgesia and anesthesia has been used effectively in liver transplant patients when there is normal liver and coagulation function. If general anesthesia is employed for cesarean delivery, standard medications are acceptable in the absence of renal impairment. Isoflurane may be the vapor of choice, since it causes vasodilation of the hepatic circulation (92), although sevoflurane and desflurane are good alternatives.

Liver transplantation during pregnancy may be required acutely if there is hepatic rupture secondary to HELLP syndrome or hepatic failure due to fulminant viral hepatic failure. Management of the fetus has included delivery, if the fetus is viable, or continuation of the pregnancy with successful neonatal outcomes (93).

The Parturient with a Renal Allograft

Long-standing insulin-dependent diabetes mellitus, hypertension, and collagen vascular disorders are common primary conditions that can lead to chronic renal failure. Despite transplantation these disorders continue to have a significant impact on anesthetic management. Patient survival after kidney transplantation at 5 years is 86%, with graft survival of 72% (69).

In pregnant patients, the glomerular filtration rate (GFR) reaches a peak of 60% above normal at the end of the second trimester (94). Well-functioning renal allografts mirror these changes (70). However, with moderate or severe renal impairment the increase in GFR will be blunted or may not occur. Physiologic hydronephrosis occurs in all pregnancies and is caused by compression of the ureter by the enlarging uterus. It can lead to urinary reflux and an increased risk of pyelonephritis (94).

Patient Assessment

The assessment of a patient with a renal transplant involves a meticulous evaluation of the renal, cardiorespiratory, and neurologic systems.

Patients with prepregnancy graft dysfunction have a greater risk of preeclampsia, graft rejection, and preterm delivery (72). Hypertension occurs in 60% to 80% of patients (94) while transient proteinuria occurs in 40% in the third trimester (73). These findings make the diagnosis of preeclampsia problematic, necessitating the need for a renal biopsy. Ultimately, 33% of patients are diagnosed with preeclampsia (67), which is four times higher than the general pregnant population (72). Common anti-hypertensive agents used in parturients include methyldopa, labetalol, nifedipine, and thiazide diuretics.

The prevalence of coronary artery disease (CAD) can approach 92% in renal recipients who had renal failure from childhood. Although CAD does not improve following transplant surgery, uremic cardiomyopathy can resolve to a variable degree (95).

Kidney transplantation can also improve uremic peripheral neuropathies but has little effect on autonomic neuropathic dysfunction (96). Signs and symptoms of autonomic neuropathy include: Silent myocardial ischemia, postural hypotension, diarrhea, delayed gastric emptying, and the loss of heart rate variability with deep breathing and Valsalva maneuvers.

Analgesia and Anesthesia for Labor and Delivery

Vaginal delivery is tolerated well in renal recipients. In rare instances, the allograft can cause labor dystocia or can be damaged with high vaginal or cervical lacerations (69). Regional techniques are good options for analgesia or anesthesia in the renal transplant patient providing that there is no evidence of coagulopathy. When there is underlying kidney dysfunction, fluid loading should be done cautiously.

Cesarean delivery can be indicated for typical obstetrical reasons or for dystocia from pelvic osteodystrophy from the effects of chronic renal failure, dialysis, and prolonged steroid use (70). If gastroparesis is present, antacid prophylaxis should be considered. Positioning and intravenous access should take into account any preexisting arteriovenous fistulas. Surgery may be prolonged and difficult, secondary to the previous abdominal surgery. Reports of injury to the transplanted kidney and ureter have been reported. The transplanted ureter is often found superior to the uterine artery as it runs from the retroperitoneal pelvic kidney coursing over the lower uterine segment to the bladder (69).

When general anesthesia is required, a rapid sequence induction is indicated. Precautions for a difficult intubation are needed in recipients with long-standing diabetes mellitus and stiffness at the atlanto-occipital joint (97). In the presence of myocardial dysfunction, reduced doses of induction agents, meticulous fluid management, and additional monitoring may be necessary. The choice of general anesthetic agents should be based on current renal function. Sevoflurane is metabolized in the liver to inorganic fluoride, which is nephrotoxic. Isoflurane and desflurane are not metabolized and therefore are better choices (95).

The pharmacokinetics and pharmacodynamics of fentanyl, alfentanil, sufentanil, and remifentanil are not altered by kidney disease and can be used without modifying the dose. In the setting of renal dysfunction, active metabolites of meperidine and morphine can accumulate. High levels of normeperidine may cause seizures and metabolites of morphine may have a prolonged effect (95). NSAIDs are known to be nephrotoxic and are not recommended (79).

The Parturient with a Pancreas Allograft

Pancreatic transplantation has allowed many insulin-dependent diabetics the freedom from insulin injections with improved glycemic control. Patient survival after isolated pancreas transplantation at 5 years is 80%, with graft survival of 49% (69). Almost 80% of those who receive a pancreatic transplant, simultaneously receive a kidney allograft (97). Morbidities are similar to those with kidney transplants except for a higher risk of infection, premature delivery, and lower mean newborn birth weights (94). Parturients with functioning pancreatic grafts produce adequate amounts of endogenous insulin to deal with the common problem of insulin resistance in the second and third trimesters (72).

Patient Considerations

Pancreatic allografts may not reverse the effects of diabetic complications but they may prevent further deterioration of nerve structure and function. Unfortunately, macrovascular complications such as CAD continue to progress (97). When euglycemia is not maintained during pregnancy, graft rejection should be suspected (72).

Analgesia and Anesthesia for Labor and Delivery

Management of analgesia and anesthesia is similar to those with kidney transplants. The location of the pelvic pancreatic allograft leaves it at risk for injury; therefore special care should be used during cesarean delivery. Postoperatively, extra emphasis on respiratory monitoring is required due to a diabetic-related impaired response to hypoxia (97).

Medications used in Autoimmune Diseases and Transplantation

Immunosuppressants can be prescribed for a number of conditions including autoimmune diseases and transplantation. Reports of newer agents for the treatment of autoimmune disorders are limited with respect to pregnancy. However, agents used in transplant patients have a significantly longer history in the literature. See Table 38-8 for the FDA classification of drug safety in pregnancy.

Tumor necrosis factor inhibitors such as infliximab, etanercept, and adalimumab have been introduced for the treatment of rheumatoid arthritis. They show no increase in miscarriage, prematurity or congenital structural malformations. Other drugs such as leflunomide, abatacept, and rituximab are not typically recommended during pregnancy because the teratogenic potential is unknown (98).

Many patients with autoimmune diseases are also prescribed NSAIDs. Platelet function may be impaired for days after NSAIDs are discontinued, depending on the drugs. NSAIDs

TABLE 38-8 FDA Classification of Drug Safety in Pregnancy

- Category A—tested and safe
- Category B—extensive experience in pregnancy and appear
- Category C—insufficient safety data and may cause problems for mother and fetus
- Category D—clear health risk to the fetus
- Category X—shown to cause birth defects and should not be given in pregnancy

Drug	Category
Corticosteroids	
Prednisone	C
Betamethasone	C
Dexamethasone	C (D in the first trimester)
Non-steroidal Anti-inflammatory drugs	
Aspirin	B
Naproxen	C (prescribe with caution in the last trimester)
Diclofenac	C (D after 30 wks)
Indomethasone	C (D after 30 wks)
Antimetabolites	
Methotrexate	X
Cyclo-oxygenase inhibitors	
Celecoxib	C
Tumor necrosis factor inhibitors	
infliximab	B
etanercept	B
adalimumab	B
leflunomide	X
abatacept	C
rituximab	C
Immunosuppressants	
azathioprine	D
calcineurin inhibitors	C
tacrolimus	C
cyclosporine	
Others	
mycophenalate mofetil	D

and aspirin do not pose enough of a risk that would interfere in the performance of neuraxial blocks (55). After 20 weeks' gestation, all NSAIDs can cause constriction of the ductus arteriosus and impair fetal renal function. NSAIDs should be withdrawn at week 32 gestation. High dose aspirin and indomethacin given close to delivery can cause bleeding tendencies and hemorrhage in the central nervous system in the newborn. COX-2 inhibitors can be used throughout gestation (99).

Transplant patients are often on multiple medications, such as glucocorticoids, azathioprine, or calcineurin inhibitors such as tacrolimus or cyclosporine. It may be a single drug or the combination of medications that predispose to maternal hypertension, preeclampsia, prematurity, and IUGR. All of these immunosuppressants cross the placenta and with the exception of mycophenolate mofetil, none are proven teratogenic at therapeutic doses in humans (67). Common side-effects are described in Table 38-9.

There is significant experience in pregnant patients with the calcineurin inhibitors, cyclosporine, and tacrolimus. Cyclosporine can cause gingival hyperplasia which can be

TABLE 38-9 Side-effects of Common Immunosuppressants

	Corticosteroids	Azathioprine	Tacrolimus	Cyclosporine
Cardiovascular	Hypertension		Dyspnea Palpitations	Hypertension
Neurologic	Psychosis **Mood changes**		Tremor Parasthesias Seizures Focal neurologic deficits	Tremor Palmer and plantar parasthesias **Seizure** Confusion
Gastrointestinal	Peptic ulcer disease	**Hepatotoxicity** Pancreatic dysfunction Nausea and vomiting	Nausea and vomiting	Nausea and vomiting Mild hepatic dysfunction
Hematologic Renal and metabolism	Glucose intolerance Salt and water retention Adrenal suppression	**Myelosuppression** Thrombocytopenia	Nephrotoxicity Hyperkalemia **Glucose intolerance**	Nephrotoxicity Hyperkalemia **Hypomagnesemia** Hyperuricemia Inhibition of insulin secretion
Musculoskeletal	**Myopathy** Osteoporosis Osteonecrosis	Arthralgias		
Others	**Weight gain** **Increased risk of** **infection** Cataracts	Increased risk of neoplasia and infection	Increased risk of neoplasia	Increased risk of neo- plasia and infection Gingival hyperplasia
Fetus/Newborn	IUGR **Adrenal insufficiency**	IUGR Neonatal bone marrow sup- pression (correlates with maternal suppression)	Mild reversible renal dysfunc- tion	IUGR

problematic during airway manipulation (68). In addition, it is more likely than tacrolimus to produce renal artery vasoconstriction and nephrotoxicity (73) and in some cases can lead to renal failure (68). Cyclosporine and tacrolimus also lower the seizure threshold, so hyperventilation should be avoided under general anesthesia (68,80). In addition, they may prolong the effect of muscle relaxants due to drug-induced changes in liver metabolism (80).

Azathioprine is dose-limited due to myelosuppression and thrombocytopenia. In the pregnant patient, neonatal myelo-suppression can also occur. It crosses the placenta readily but the fetus cannot convert it to its teratogenic metabolite. While sporadic cases of congenital malformations have occurred, azathioprine is commonly used (100).

Corticosteroids have many complications that can affect pregnancy, including hypertension and hyperglycemia (99). They also increase the risk of PROM, prematurity, and IUGR. The mechanism for PROM could be due to abnormalities in the membrane itself or from alterations in maternal corticotrophin-releasing hormone (released centrally) making spontaneous labor more likely (100).

Vaginal or cesarean delivery may be complicated by poor wound healing and limited options for patient positioning. Accelerated bone loss and osteonecrosis increases the risk of damage to joints, tendons, and ligaments with positioning for delivery. Neuraxial analgesia can increase the risk further since the patient is unable to determine her limits of flexion and extension.

Maternal adrenal suppression is a concern at prednisone doses greater than 5 mg per day (94). However, doses less than this can cause suppression in some patients leading many centers to give stress dose steroids to all transplant recipients (94). Stress doses should consist of hydrocortisone 50 to

100 mg intravenously at delivery and every 8 hours thereafter until oral steroids are tolerated (73).

Fetal exposure to prednisone, cortisol, and methylprednisolone is minimal since the placenta metabolizes all but 10% of the active drug (99). However, both betamethasone and dexamethasone cross the placenta and reach high concentrations in the fetal circulation.

■ SUMMARY

Immunologic disorders in the parturient may be manifest as acute, life-threatening events or chronic illnesses. Anaphylaxis to drugs or physical agents may occur unexpectedly and must be treated considering the special conditions associated with pregnancy. Parturients with conditions such as collagen vascular diseases or other chronic disorders may conceive, but their pregnancies are complicated by the primary disease process, end organ damage, and drug side-effects. Many of these considerations, along with organ rejection, also apply to parturients with organ transplants. A team approach to planning and care of these patients is needed.

KEY POINTS

■ Acute hypersensitivity reactions to drugs and environmental agents can occur unexpectedly in the parturient. Treatment of reactions should take both mother and fetus into account. Physical maneuvers such as uterine tilt or rapid surgical removal of the fetus may be necessary to optimize the outcome.

- Chronic diseases with an immunologic basis do not preclude pregnancy. Management will depend on the severity of the disease, ongoing pharmacologic management, and interactions with obstetrical considerations.
- Parturients with transplanted organs require special care. Organ dysfunction and rejection may occur and may mimic obstetrical conditions such as preeclampsia. Management will depend on maternal underlying disease, the state of the transplant, ongoing drug therapy, and obstetrical requirements.

REFERENCES

1. Eales L. Cells and tissues of the immune system. In: Eales L, ed. *Immunology for Life Scientists.* 2nd ed. Chichester: Wiley; 2003:1–26.
2. Salmon JE. Mechanisms of immune-mediated tissue injury. In: Goldman L, Ausiello D, eds. *Cecil Medicine.* 23rd ed. Philadelphia, PA: Saunders Elsevier; 2008:266–270.
3. Sampson HA, Munoz-Furlong A, Campbell RL, et al. Second symposium on the definition and management of anaphylaxis: summary report-Second National Institute of Allergy and Infectious Disease/Food Allergy and Anaphylaxis Network symposium. *J Allergy Clin Immunol* 2006;117:391–397.
4. Harper NJ, Dixon T, Dugue P, et al. Suspected anaphylactic reactions associated with anaesthesia. *Anaesthesia* 2009;64:199–211.
5. Kroigaard M, Garvey LH, Gillberg L, et al. Scandinavian clinical practice guidelines on the diagnosis, management and follow-up of anaphylaxis during anaesthesia. *Acta Anaesthesiol Scand* 2007;51:655–670.
6. Mertes PM, Tajima K, Regnier-Kimmoun MA, et al. Perioperative anaphylaxis. *Med Clin North Am* 2010;94:761–789.
7. Dewachter P, Mouton-Faivre C, Emala CW. Anaphylaxis and anesthesia: controversies and new insights. *Anesthesiology* 2009;111:1141–1150.
8. Fisher MM, Doig GS. Prevention of anaphylactic reactions to anaesthetic drugs. *Drug Safety* 2004;27:393–410.
9. Hepner DL, Castells MC. Latex allergy: an update. *Anesth Analg* 2003;96:1219–1229.
10. Ewan PW, Dugue P, Mirakian R, et al. BSACI guidelines for the investigation of suspected anaphylaxis during general anaesthesia. *Clin Exp Allergy* 2010;40:15–31.
11. Lieberman P, Nicklas RA, Oppenheimer J, et al. The diagnosis and management of anaphylaxis practice parameter: 2010 update. *J Allergy Clin Immunol* 2010;126:477–480.
12. Mertes PM, Laxenaire MC, Lienhart A, et al. Reducing the risk of anaphylaxis during anaesthesia: guidelines for clinical practice. *J Invest Allergol Clin Immunol* 2005;15:91–101.
13. Ring J, Messmer K. Incidence and severity of anaphylactoid reactions to colloid volume substitutes. *Lancet* 1977;1:466–469.
14. Malinovsky JM, Decagny S, Wessel F, et al. Systematic follow-up increases incidence of anaphylaxis during adverse reactions in anesthetized patients. *Acta Anaesthesiol Scand* 2008;52:175–181.
15. Chaudhuri K, Gonzales J, Jesurun CA, et al. Anaphylactic shock in pregnancy: a case study and review of the literature. *Int J Obstet Anesth* 2008;17:350–357.
16. Vanden Hoek TL, Morrison LJ, Shuster M, et al. Part 12: cardiac arrest in special situations: 2010 American heart association guidelines for cardiopulmonary resuscitation and emergency cardiovascular care. *Circulation* 2010;122(18 Suppl 3):S829–S861.
17. Thyssen JP, Menne T, Elberling J, et al. Hypersensitivity to local anaesthetics-update and proposal of evaluation algorithm. *Contact Derm* 2008;59:69–78.
18. Harboe T, Guttormsen AB, Aarebrot S, et al. Suspected allergy to local anaesthetics: follow-up in 135 cases. *Acta Anaesthesiol Scand* 2010;54:536–542.
19. Hepner DL, Castells MC. Anaphylaxis during the perioperative period. *Anesth Analg* 2003;97:1381–1395.
20. Nicklas RA, Bernstein IL, Li JT, et al. XVIII. Local Anesthetics. *J Allergy Clin Immunol* 1998;101(6 Pt 2):S510–S511.
21. Ebo DG, Fisher MM, Hagendorens MM, et al. Anaphylaxis during anaesthesia: diagnostic approach. *Allergy* 2007;62:471–487.
22. Pant D, Vohra VK, Pandey SS, et al. Pulseless electrical activity during caesarean delivery under spinal anaesthesia: a case report of severe anaphylactic reaction to Syntocinon. *Int J Obstet Anesth* 2009;18:85–88.
23. Maycock EJ, Russell WC. Anaphylactoid reaction to Syntocinon. *Anaesth Intens Care* 1993;21:211–212.
24. Draisci G, Zanfini BA, Nucera E, et al. Latex sensitization: a special risk for the obstetric population? *Anesthesiology* 2011;114:565–569.
25. Mertes PM, Lambert M, Gueant-Rodriguez RM, et al. Perioperative anaphylaxis. *Immunol Allergy Clin N Am* 2009;29:429–451.
26. Allmers H, Schmengler J, John SM. Decreasing incidence of occupational contact urticaria caused by natural rubber latex allergy in German health care workers. *J Allergy Clin Immunol* 2004;114:347–351.
27. American Society of Anesthesiologists Committee on occupational health of operating room personnel, task force on latex sensitivity. Natural rubber latex allergy: considerations for anesthesiologists. Illinois: American Society of Anesthesiologists; 2005. http://ecommerce.asahq.org/publicationsAndServices/latexallergy.pdf. Last accessed July 21, 2011.
28. Hamann CP. Natural rubber latex protein sensitivity in review. *Am J Cont Derm* 1993;4:4–21.
29. Brown RH, Schauble JF, Hamilton RG. Prevalence of latex allergy among anesthesiologists: identification of sensitized but asymptomatic individuals. *Anesthesiology* 1998;89:292–299.
30. Cullinan P, Brown R, Field A, et al. Latex allergy. A position paper of the British Society of Allergy and Clinical Immunology. *Clin Exper Allergy* 2003;33:1484–1499.
31. Eckhout GV, Ayan S. Anaphylaxis due to airborne exposure to latex in a primigravida. *Anesthesiology* 2001;95:1034–1035.
32. Swanson MC, Bubak ME, Hunt LW, et al. Quantification of occupational latex aeroallergens in a medical center. *J Allergy Clin Immunol* 1994;94(3 Pt 1):445–451.
33. Heitz JW, Bader SO. An evidence-based approach to medication preparation for the surgical patient at risk for latex allergy: is it time to stop being stopper poppers? *J Clin Anesth* 2010;22:477–483.
34. Lieberman P. Definition and criteria for the diagnoses of anaphylaxis. In: Castells MC, ed. *Anaphylaxis and Hypersensitivity Reactions.* Totowa, NJ: Humana Press; 2011:1–12.
35. Bernstein IL, Li JT, Bernstein DI, et al. Allergy diagnostic testing: an updated practice parameter. *Ann Allergy Asthma Immunol* 2008;100(3 Suppl 3):S1–S148.
36. Dewachter P, Mouton-Faivre C. What investigation after an anaphylactic reaction during anaesthesia? *Cur Opinion Anaesthesiol* 2008;21:363–368.
37. Frigas E, Park MA. Acute urticaria and angioedema: diagnostic and treatment considerations. *Am J Clin Derm* 2009;10:239–250.
38. Najib U, Sheikh J. The spectrum of chronic urticaria. *Allergy Asthma Proc* 2009;30:1–10.
39. Banerji A, Sheffer AL. The spectrum of chronic angioedema. *Allergy Asthma Proc* 2009;30:11–16.
40. Arock M, Valent P. Pathogenesis, classification and treatment of mastocytosis: state of the art in 2010 and future perspectives. *Exp Rev Hematol* 2010;3:497–516.
41. Vaughan ST, Jones GN. Systemic mastocytosis presenting as profound cardiovascular collapse during anaesthesia. *Anaesthesia* 1998;53:804–807.
42. Villeneuve V, Kaufman I, Weeks S, et al. Anesthetic management of a labouring parturient with urticaria pigmentosa. *Can J Anesth* 2006;53:380–384.
43. Worobec AS, Akin C, Scott LM, et al. Mastocytosis complicating pregnancy. *Obst Gynecol* 2000;95:391–395.
44. Gompels MM, Lock RJ, Abinun M, et al. C1 inhibitor deficiency: consensus document. *Clin Exp Immunol* 2005;139:379–394.
45. Levy JH, Freiberger DJ, Roback J. Hereditary angioedema: current and emerging treatment options. *Anesth Analg* 2010;110:1271–1280.
46. Duvvur S, Khan F, Powell K. Hereditary angioedema and pregnancy. *J Mat Fetal Neonatal Med* 2007;20:563–565.
47. Chinniah N, Katelaris CH. Hereditary angioedema and pregnancy. *Aust N Z J Obstet Gynaecol* 2009;49:2–5.
48. Latiff AH, Kerr MA. The clinical significance of immunoglobulin A deficiency. *Ann Clin Biochem* 2007;44(Pt 2):131–139.
49. Roberts IA. The changing face of haemolytic disease of the newborn. *Early Hum Dev* 2008;84:515–523.
50. Illanes S, Soothill P. Management of red cell alloimmunisation in pregnancy: the non-invasive monitoring of the disease. *Prenat Diagn* 2010;30:668–673.
51. Moise KJ Jr. Management of rhesus alloimmunization in pregnancy. *Obst Gynecol* 2008;112:164–176.
52. Hahn BH, Tsao BP. Systemic lupus erythematosis and related syndromes. In: Firestein GS, Budd RC, Harris ED Jr, McInnes IB, Ruddy S, Sergent JS, eds. *Kelly's Textbook of Rheumatology.* 8th ed. Philadelphia, PA: Saunders Elsevier; 2009:1233–1310.
53. Clowse ME, Jamison M, Myers E, et al. A national study of the complications of lupus in pregnancy. *Am J Obstet Gynecol* 2008;199:127.e1–127.e6.
54. Reece EA, Romero R, Hobbins J. Coagulopathy associated with factor VIII inhibitor. A literature review. *J Reprod Med* 1984;29:53–58.
55. Horlocker TT, Wedel DJ, Rowlingson JC, et al. Executive summary: regional anesthesia in the patient receiving antithrombotic or thrombolytic therapy: American Society of Regional Anesthesia and Pain Medicine Evidence-Based Guidelines (Third Edition). *Reg Anesth Pain Med* 2010;35:102–105.
56. D'Cruz DP, Khamashta MA, Hughes GR. Systemic lupus erythematosus. *Lancet* 2007;369:587–596.
57. Hornberger LK, Al Rajaa N. Spectrum of cardiac involvement in neonatal lupus. *Scand J Immunol* 2010;72:189–197.

58. Ebert EC. Gastric and enteric involvement in progressive systemic sclerosis. *J Clin Gastroenterol* 2008;42:5–12.

59. Steen VD. Pregnancy in scleroderma. *Rheum Dis Clin North Am* 2007;33:345–358,vii.

60. Roberts JG, Sabar R, Gianoli JA, et al. Progressive systemic sclerosis: clinical manifestations and anesthetic considerations. *J Clin Anesth* 2002;14:474–477.

61. Chakravarty EF, Khanna D, Chung L. Pregnancy outcomes in systemic sclerosis, primary pulmonary hypertension, and sickle cell disease. *Obstet Gynecol* 2008;111:927–934.

62. Bailey AR, Wolmarans M, Rhodes S. Spinal anaesthesia for caesarean section in a patient with systemic sclerosis. *Anaesthesia* 1999;54:355–358.

63. Dreyer SJ, Boden SD. Natural history of rheumatoid arthritis of the cervical spine. *Clin Orthop Relat Res* 1999;366:98–106.

64. Matti MV, Sharrock NE. Anesthesia on the rheumatoid patient. *Rheum Dis Clin North Am* 1998;24:19–34.

65. Ostensen M. Management of early aggressive rheumatoid arthritis during pregnancy and lactation. *Expert Opin Pharmacother* 2009;10:1469–1479.

66. James AH, Brancazio LR, Price T. Aspirin and reproductive outcomes. *Obstet Gynecol Surv* 2008;63:49–57.

67. McKay DB, Josephson MA. Pregnancy in recipients of solid organs—effects on mother and child. *N Engl J Med* 2006;354:1281–1293.

68. Blasco LM, Parameshwar J, Vuylsteke A. Anaesthesia for noncardiac surgery in the heart transplant recipient. *Cur Opin Anaesthesiol* 2009;22:109–113.

69. Mastrobattista JM, Gomez-Lobo V. Society for Maternal-Fetal M. Pregnancy after solid organ transplantation. *Obstet Gynecol* 2008;112:919–932.

70. Davison JM, Bailey DJ. Pregnancy following renal transplantation. *J Obstet Gynaecol Res* 2003;29:227–233.

71. Taylor DO, Edwards LB, Boucek MM, et al. Registry of the International Society for Heart and Lung Transplantation: twenty-fourth official adult heart transplant report-2007. *J Heart Lung Transplant* 2007;26:769–781.

72. Armenti VT, Constantinescu S, Moritz MJ, et al. Pregnancy after transplantation. *Transplant Rev* 2008;22:223–240.

73. Alston PK, Kuller JA, McMahon MJ. Pregnancy in transplant recipients. *Obstet Gynecol Surv* 2001;56:289–295.

74. Wasywich CA, Ruygrok PN, Wilkinson L, et al. Planned pregnancy in a heart transplant recipient. *Intern Med J* 2004;34:206–209.

75. Carlin A, Alfirevic Z. Physiological changes of pregnancy and monitoring. *Best Pract Res Clin Obstet Gynaecol* 2008;22:801–823.

76. Mettauer B, Levy F, Richard R, et al. Exercising with a denervated heart after cardiac transplantation. *Ann Transplant* 2005;10:35–42.

77. Cheng DC, Ong DD. Anaesthesia for non-cardiac surgery in heart-transplanted patients. *Can J Anesth* 1993;40:981–986.

78. Kostopanagiotou G, Smyrniotis V, Arkadopoulos N, et al. Anesthetic and perioperative management of adult transplant recipients in nontransplant surgery. *Anesth Analg* 1999;89:613–622.

79. Keegan MT, Plevak DJ. The transplant recipient for nontransplant surgery. *Anesthesiol Clin North America* 2004;22:827–861.

80. Ashary N, Kaye AD, Hegazi AR, et al. Anesthetic considerations in the patient with a heart transplant. *Heart Disease* 2002;4:191–198.

81. Uberfuhr P, Frey AW, Reichart B. Vagal reinnervation in the long term after orthotopic heart transplantation. *J Heart Lung Transplant* 2000;19:946–950.

82. Allard R, Hatzakorzian R, Deschamps A, et al. Decreased heart rate and blood pressure in a recent cardiac transplant patient after spinal anesthesia. *Can J Anesth* 2004;51:829–833.

83. Wu DW, Wilt J, Restaino S. Pregnancy after thoracic organ transplantation. *Semin Perinatol* 2007;31:354–362.

84. American College of Obstetricians and Gynecologists Committee on Obstetric Practice. ACOG Committee Opinion No. 421, November 2008: antibiotic prophylaxis for infective endocarditis. *Obstet Gynecol* 2008;112:1193–1194.

85. Wilson W, Taubert KA. Gewitz M, et al. Prevention of infective endocarditis: guidelines from the American Heart Association: a guideline from the American Heart Association Rheumatic Fever, Endocarditis, and Kawasaki Disease Committee, Council on Cardiovascular Disease in the Young, and the Council on Clinical Cardiology, Council on Cardiovascular Surgery and Anesthesia, and the Quality of Care and Outcomes Research Interdisciplinary Working Group. *Circulation* 2007;116:1736–1754.

86. McKay DB, Josephson MA. Pregnancy after kidney transplantation. *Clin J Am Soc Neph* 2008;3(Suppl 2):S117–S125.

87. Ruggiero R, Muz J, Fietsam R Jr, et al. Reestablishment of lymphatic drainage after canine lung transplantation. *J Thorac Cardiovasc Surg* 1993;106:167–171.

88. Duarte AG, Terminella L, Smith JT, et al. Restoration of cough reflex in lung transplant recipients. *Chest* 2008;134:310–316.

89. Rosenberg AL, Rao M, Benedict PF. Anesthetic implications for lung transplantation. *Anesthesiol Clin North America* 2004;22:767–788.

90. Bonanno C, Dove L. Pregnancy after liver transplantation. *Semin Perinatol* 2007;31:348–353.

91. Degli Esposti S, Reinus J. Gastrointestinal and hepatic disorders in the pregnant patient. In: Feldman M, Friedman L, Brandt L, eds. *Sleisenger and Fordtran's Gastrointestinal and Liver disease*. 9th ed. Philadelphia, PA: Saunders Elsevier; 2010:626.

92. Steadman RH. Anesthesia for liver transplant surgery. *Anesthesiol Clin North America* 2004;22:687–711.

93. Zarrinpar A, Farmer DG, Ghobrial RM, et al. Liver transplantation for HELLP syndrome. *Am Surg* 2007;73:1013–1016.

94. Fuchs KM, Wu D, Ebcioglu Z. Pregnancy in renal transplant recipients. *Semin Perinatol* 2007;31:339–347.

95. Lemmens HJ. Kidney transplantation: recent developments and recommendations for anesthetic management. *Anesthesiol Clin North America* 2004;22:651–662.

96. Solders G, Persson A, Wilczek H. Autonomic system dysfunction and polyneuropathy in nondiabetic uremia. A one-year follow-up study after renal transplantation. *Transplantation* 1986;41:616–619.

97. Larson-Wadd K, Belani KG. Pancreas and islet cell transplantation. *Anesthesiol Clin North America* 2004;22:663–674.

98. Ostensen M, Lockshin M, Doria A, et al. Update on safety during pregnancy of biological agents and some immunosuppressive anti-rheumatic drugs. *Rheumatology* 2008;47(Suppl 3):28–31.

99. Ostensen M, Khamashta M, Lockshin M, et al. Anti-inflammatory and immunosuppressive drugs and reproduction. *Arthritis Res Ther* 2006;8:209.

100. Fuchs KM, Coustan DR. Immunosuppressant therapy in pregnant organ transplant recipients. *Semin Perinatol* 2007;31:363–371.

Julio B. Delgado • Michael Frölich

◼ INTRODUCTION

Diagnosis and treatment of psychiatric disorders during pregnancy and the postpartum period is a topic of significant relevance due to the high prevalence of these conditions and the multiple barriers to provide an appropriate diagnosis as well as effective and safe treatment. It is now more commonly acknowledged that new onset and exacerbation of psychiatric disorders during pregnancy and the postpartum period are frequent problems that may require a multidisciplinary approach to provide effective and timely diagnosis and treatment thereby minimizing the inherent risks secondary to treatment or lack of an early and effective intervention. Physicians who treat women during the childbearing years should be able to appropriately screen and provide guidance to effectively diagnose, refer, and treat patients who have a history of primary psychiatric disorders or exhibit symptoms which require a psychiatric evaluation. Empirical approaches to treatment are not ideal and consultation with psychiatry should be considered to provide safe and effective treatment minimizing morbidity to the mother and potential serious implications to the child. Pharmacologic treatment during pregnancy implies unique risks including neonatal exposure but untreated psychiatric illness can be more risky. The decision to treat includes many factors. A detailed history that addresses psychiatric issues and a careful assessment of the potential scenarios that affect the course of the specific condition during pregnancy and the postpartum period need to be carefully evaluated. In addition, consultation with psychiatry should be considered. In the absence of a thorough evaluation and planning, the consequences may be significant. The rationale to screen patients for psychiatric symptoms even before conception allows for better planning and better access to effective care.

Epidemiology

In general, psychiatric diseases affect both genders and all socioeconomic and ethnic groups. It is interesting to note that mental disease often affects highly functional and creative individuals. The association between mental illness and art is reflected in the painting *Broken Lines* by the German artist G. Schetelig (Fig. 39-1). The specific incidence and prevalence of most psychiatric disorders during pregnancy and the postpartum period has been described by Bijl (1,2). Therefore, there now exists a good understanding of the potential implications of having a primary psychiatric disorder prior to conception, the potential risks of developing a new condition, and the changes in the course of these illnesses during pregnancy and the postpartum period. According to Bijl's findings, roughly 40% of the adult population under 65 years of age has experienced at least one **Diagnostic & Statistical Manual of Mental Disorders, Third Edition, Revised** (DSM-III-R) disorder in their

lifetime. Among them, 23% have experienced a disorder within the preceding year. No gender differences were found in overall morbidity, but there was certainly a gender difference in the disease incidence as shown in Table 39-1. Depression, anxiety, and alcohol abuse and dependence were most prevalent; there was a high degree of comorbidity between them.

Diagnosis and Initial Evaluation during Pregnancy

Psychiatric disorders are some of the most prevalent conditions in mankind and produce significant morbidity in the general population and in women during the reproductive years. Regardless of their high prevalence, they are frequently undiagnosed, untreated, or misdiagnosed. An appropriate evaluation and accurate diagnosis are critical components in the process of providing successful treatment. Many nonpsychiatric physicians feel uncomfortable approaching, diagnosing, and treating psychiatric disorders. The reasons are many including negative attitudes toward patients with psychiatric disease. Frequently, there is a basic lack of knowledge and understanding of the nature and relevance of diagnosing and treating primary disorders or psychiatric manifestations of other conditions. A systematic approach in the evaluation, diagnosis, and treatment is based on reliable evidence that allows a clear specific diagnosis and more effective treatments. The diagnostic criteria are based on the DSM-IV produced by the American Psychiatric Association (APA). This manual of mental disorders provides the basic parameters for diagnosing specific psychiatric syndromes and entities based on reliable evidence that allows a methodic approach to classifying and diagnosing specific conditions, which correlates well with specific therapeutic approaches. The DSM-IV should be consulted for the diagnostic parameters and classification of psychiatric disorders. This chapter will emphasize a diagnostic approach based on basic signs and symptoms to facilitate an efficient and practical way to assessing, diagnosing, and planning appropriate and timely interventions initiated and provided by the anesthesiologist. An accurate diagnosis is the main initial goal to provide effective treatment.

The initial approach should facilitate the patient's description of her symptoms and concerns after the physician formulates open-ended questions to elicit general information to evaluate the presence of a primary psychiatric syndrome, to explore personality features, or to recognize the presence of a personality disorder. Such information may not be easily obtained if a structured set of concrete questions is the initial interaction. It is important to keep an open-minded approach exploring groups of signs and symptoms before diagnosing specific entities. Regardless of this initial flexibility, the anesthesiologist remains in control of the interviewing process by providing the necessary structure to the evaluation and

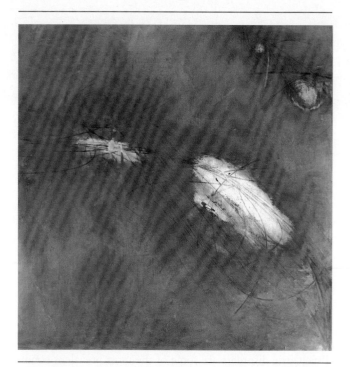

FIGURE 39-1 Creativity and Madness: Many psychiatrists have been intrigued by the definite link between creativity and madness. This female painter illustrates this concept by using broken (disconnected) lines that embody the madness of a painting that is in perfect harmony with color and shape. (*Broken Lines* by Gesine Schetelig, reprinted with permission.)

subsequently inquiring about the presence of specific symptoms but at the same time facilitating the description of the patient's perceived problems to orient the diagnostic process and to make a preliminary impression. The rationale to consider obtaining a formal psychiatric consultation will depend on the patient's history, severity of symptoms, and the patient's and the physician's preference. For patients who are actively suicidal, psychotic, manic, or where the diagnosis is completely unclear, a psychiatric consultation should be requested.

When the emotions, behavior, or thought processes of a patient appear unconventional or generate concern, a formal assessment should be initiated to rule out the possibility of a psychiatric disorder, a medical condition with psychiatric manifestations, or the consequences of substance abuse.

Specific Syndromes with Anesthetic Implications

Mood Disorders
Mood is the perception of the world through the patient's eyes; it can be pathologically lowered, elevated, or it may excessively cycle between the two. True mood disorders are not the typical reactions to life stressors but prolonged and abnormal affective stages that require an appropriate evaluation.

Major Depression
As indicated above, the presence of depression during the childbearing years is 2 to 3 times more common in women (3,4) with the highest incidence in the age group from 25 to 44 and a lifetime risk of up to 25%. Depression is a recurrent disorder with a high risk of suicide and a progressively worsening course if it is not appropriately treated.

The problems of mental illness (in general) and depression (in particular) have long been misjudged. One in six persons in the United States will, at some point, deal with major depression. Depression is also a leading cause of medical disability in women in the United States (5). Recent studies suggest that 10% of gravid women meet criteria for major depression (6,7) and up to 18% show depressive symptoms during gestation (8). Variable prevalence rates noted within the scientific literature reflect the variety of methods for screening subjects, whether subjects report symptoms themselves or whether trained researchers collected the data.

Gender differences in the expression of affective disorders have been attributed to the impact of hormonal influence, socialization, and genetics. The negative influence of maternal depression on maternal and child health, psychological well-being and other possible outcomes are significant (9). Because women are more likely to experience first time depression beginning at puberty and because reproductive life transitions are associated with relapse and recurrent episodes, the urgency to treat depression as fully and as early as possible is of critical importance.

The main clinical manifestations consistent with the presence of clinically significant depression are feelings of sadness, guilt, inadequacy, hopelessness or helplessness, irritability, difficulty concentrating, low energy level, insomnia or hypersomnia, anorexia, decreased libido, social isolation, anhedonia, decreased psychomotor activity, and suicidal thoughts.

Patients who have five or more of the above symptoms for a time period greater than 2 weeks fulfill criteria for the diagnosis of major depression and require treatment. The precipitating causes are diverse and include genetic factors, environmental factors, or other medical conditions. It is important not to assume that the clinical syndrome is just a consequence of the specific stressors but instead it is a clinical condition that requires specific treatment. Appropriate treatment will allow the patient a much faster recovery and will improve her ability to deal effectively with the ongoing stressors that may have precipitated the episode. The magnitude of the symptoms and the presence of feelings of hopelessness, guilt, or suicidal ideation are significant parameters that clearly suggest the presence of major depression. The clinical course can be acute or chronic, but a major depressive episode without treatment can produce significant morbidity for several months or may precipitate suicide. Depression can be effectively treated with psychotherapy, electroconvulsive therapy (ECT), or pharmacologic interventions. Specific therapeutic approaches will be discussed later.

One of the most significant components of the assessment in the patient with depression is evaluating the potential for suicide. Women attempt suicide more frequently than men. A detailed approach to evaluating the potential risk factors includes:

- The presence of a clinical syndrome consistent with major depression
- History of previous suicide attempts, impulsive behavior, substance abuse
- History of physical or sexual abuse or significant recent losses
- Family history of suicide
- A plan to commit suicide and access to the means to implement the plan
- History of a severe personality disorder

A suicide risk assessment is an inherent component of every mental status examination and should be evaluated in more detail in patients with a history of previous suicide attempts, severe character pathology with impulsivity, and acts of self-destructive behavior. Passive suicidal thoughts should be differentiated from the true intentions of self-inflicting lethal harm. If the above assessment is consistent with a high risk of suicide,

TABLE 39-1 Incidence Rate of Psychiatric Diseases by Gender and Incidence Rate Ratio

	Women	95% CI	Men	95% CI	IRR (f/m)	95% CI	Wald χ^2	p-value
Mood disorders	3.25	(2.48–4.02)	1.34	(0.89–1.79)	**2.39**	(1.55–3.68)	28	<0.000
Major depression	3.9	(3.06–4.69)	1.72	(1.23–2.24)	**2.23**	(1.53–3.26)	27.6	<0.000
Dysthymia	0.39	(0.14–0.60)	0.39	(0.17–0.63)	0.93	(0.39–2.22)	1309.6	0.869
Bipolar disorder	0.43	(0.19–0.68)	0.17	(0.02–0.33)	2.37	(0.75–7.54)	2805.7	0.143
Anxiety disorders	4.56	(3.62–5.46)	1.62	(1.13–2.13)	**2.58**	(1.73–3.86)	25.2	<0.000
Panic disorder	1.3	(0.88–1.75)	0.28	(0.09–0.49)	**4.17**	(1.98–8.77)	26.8	<0.000
Agoraphobia (without panic)	1.14	(0.75–1.56)	0.41	(0.18–0.65)	**2.57**	(1.23–5.35)	13.1	0.012
Simple phobia	3.17	(2.46–3.87)	1.34	(0.91–1.77)	**2.41**	(1.57–3.69)	23.3	<0.000
Social phobia	1.12	(0.72–1.54)	0.75	(0.43–1.07)	1.42	(0.77–2.60)	4.8	0.258
Generalized anxiety disorder	0.98	(0.61–1.37)	0.45	(0.22–0.72)	1.86	(0.95–3.66)	11.6	0.07
Obsessive-compulsive disorder	0.39	(0.15–0.60)	0.17	(0.03–0.33)	1.76	(0.52–5.99)	2708.2	0.366
Substance use disorders	0.99	(0.61–1.36)	2.96	(2.22–3.71)	**0.27**	(0.15–0.50)	53.7	<0.000
Alcohol abuse	0.91	(0.55–1.27)	4.09	(3.28–4.92)	**0.2**	(0.12–0.35)	57.5	<0.000
Alcohol dependence	0.18	(0.02–0.34)	0.82	(0.48–1.16)	**0.2**	(0.06–0.70)	12.7	0.012
Drug abuse	0.07	(−0.03–0.18)	0.48	(0.23–0.73)	**0.05**	(0.01–0.43)	2186.9	0.006
Drug dependence	0.32	(0.12–0.54)	0.21	(0.05–0.38)	1.42	(0.40–5.07)	2740.3	0.586
Schizophrenia	0.1	(−0.02–0.21)	—	—	—	—	—	—
Eating disorders	0.14	(0.00–0.28)	0.07	(−0.02–0.17)	1.91	(0.34–10.74)	1335.5	0.463
One or more DSM-III-R diagnoses	6.94	(5.65–8.19)	4.45	(3.44–5.47)	1.54	(1.12–2.14)	22.5	0.009

Adapted from: Bijl RV, De Graaf R, Ravelli A, et al.; Gender and age-specific first incidence of DSM-III-R psychiatric disorders in the general population. Results from the Netherlands Mental Health Survey and Incidence Study (NEMESIS). *Soc Psychiatry Psychiatr Epidemiol* 2002;37:372–379. IR, new cases per 100 person-years at risk; IRR, incidence rate ratio, the ratio between the IRs for women and for men (controlled for age). Rows with a light gray background represent psychiatric diagnoses with a higher female incidence; rows with a dark gray background represent psychiatric diagnoses with a higher male incidence.

psychiatry should always be consulted and the patient should be under constant supervision until the evaluation is complete.

Postpartum depression should be differentiated from the transitory and limited symptoms induced by changes in hormone levels ("baby blues"); such symptoms are more consistent with emotional lability rather than true depression. For patients with moderate to severe cases of depression, treatment with antidepressants or ECT may be necessary. ECT provides a very rapid and effective treatment that appears to be safe during or after pregnancy.

Numerous tools including the Edinburgh Postpartum Depression Scale can be used to screen for depression during pregnancy and postpartum. Common symptoms of depression (sleep, energy, and appetite change) may be misinterpreted as normative experiences of pregnancy. Other classical symptoms are continuous depressed mood, loss of interest in activities, irritability and restlessness, having unwarranted guilt feelings, excessive sleep, appetite disturbances, and concentration or memory difficulties. However, only a small number (18%) of women meet most criteria for major depressive disorder. Women typically do not seek treatment during pregnancy and postpartum but patients report that when providers speak to them about their depression, they are more

likely to seek treatment (10). Some depressive disorders may be secondary to medical conditions or medications; the diagnosis will rest on physical signs and symptoms, medical history, and medication history. Laboratory testing (e.g., thyroid function tests, B_{12}, and folate levels) may aid in reaching an accurate diagnosis and uncovering medical problems partially or fully responsible for the psychiatric presentation.

Mania or Hypomania
Mania or hypomania are specific clinical syndromes which are most of the times the manifestation of manic depressive disorder but can also be induced by other medical conditions or substance abuse. Hypomania is characterized by increased energy and self-confidence but does not impair contact with reality unless it evolves into a true manic episode. The main clinical manifestations consistent with a manic syndrome are:

- An expansive affect, a persistently elevated mood with frequent feelings of grandiosity with or without irritability
- Increased physical activity, increased energy, decreased need for sleep and reckless behavior

Treatment is important as untreated depression during pregnancy may have unfavorable outcomes for both women and children. Complications of pregnancy associated with depression include inadequate weight gain, underutilization of prenatal care, increased substance use, and premature birth. Human studies demonstrate that perceived life-event stress as well as depression and anxiety predicted lower birth weight, decreased Apgar scores, smaller head circumference, and small-for-gestational-age-babies. Because management of depressed pregnant women also includes care of a growing fetus, treatment may be complicated and primary care providers should consider a multidisciplinary approach including an obstetrician, psychiatrist, and pediatrician to provide optimal care (11).

Several antidepressants have been studied in the treatment of severe depression. Although onset of antidepressant efficacy may differ for individual patients, the onset may require 4 to 6 weeks of treatment with most agents, whereas full efficacy may require 8 to 12 weeks (12,13). Selective serotonin reuptake inhibitors (SSRIs) are often used as a first-line treatment of depressive disorders because of their specificity, therapeutic safety margin, and a favorable side-effect profile (14). They also effectively treat anxiety disorders and other psychiatric comorbidities frequently associated with depression (15,16). Serotonin–norepinephrine reuptake inhibitors (SNRIs) are also effective in treating depression and anxiety. They may be particularly helpful when other drugs show little effect and in specific chronic pain conditions (17). However, they tend to be more expensive. Tricyclic antidepressants (TCAs) are older, less expensive agents that act primarily by inhibiting serotonin and norepinephrine reuptake. They are effective as antidepressants and are also used to treat chronic pain (18). They interact with many other receptors and thereby produce side effects that may limit tolerability and compliance (19).

The major concern with drug therapy during pregnancy has been the question about teratologic drug effects. However, there appears to be no association of exposure to SSRIs during pregnancy and lactation and major fetal malformations. However, some minor perinatal complications have been reported. Prenatal antidepressant use was associated with lower gestational age at birth and an increased risk of preterm birth. Presence of depressive symptoms was not associated with this risk. These results suggest that medication status, rather than depression, is a predictor of gestational age at birth (20). With linked population health data and propensity score matching, prenatal SSRI exposure was associated with an increased risk of low birth weight and respiratory distress, even when maternal illness severity was accounted for (21). As for most drugs, data on the long-term developmental outcomes of children exposed to SSRIs in utero and during breastfeeding are limited (22).

Women with histories of depression who are euthymic in the context of ongoing antidepressant therapy should be aware of the association of depressive relapse during pregnancy with antidepressant discontinuation (23).

Anesthesia and Electroconvulsive Therapy in Pregnancy

In severe psychotic depression, severe melancholic depression, resistant depression, and in patients intolerant of antidepressant medications and those with medical illnesses which contraindicate the use of antidepressants (e.g., renal, cardiac, or hepatic disease), electroconvulsive therapy (ECT) may be indicated (24).

Maternal effects of ECT are caused by the cardiovascular responses consisting of generalized autonomic nervous system stimulation with initial parasympathetic outflow, followed immediately by a sympathetic response. The cerebrovascular system responds with a marked increase in cerebral blood flow in response to increased cerebral oxygen

consumption that results in dramatic elevation of intracranial pressure. Methohexital (0.75 to 1.0 mg/kg intravenously) is the most frequently used agent for induction of anesthesia for ECT. Alternatively, propofol (1.5 to 2 mg/kg IV) can be used safely. Muscle relaxation is usually accomplished with succinylcholine (0.5 to 1.0 mg/kg IV) (25,26). The risk associated with ECT during pregnancy is that of inducing premature contractions that may be refractory to tocolytic therapy. Ishikawa et al., recommend the use of an inhalational technique to reduce uterine activity associated with ECT (27).

Anesthetic Considerations

There are few studies of perioperative outcomes in patients with serious mental illness. The available literature suggests that patients with schizophrenia, compared with those without mental illness, may have higher pain thresholds, higher rates of death and postoperative complications, and differential outcomes (e.g., confusion, ileus) by anesthetic technique (28). A small dose of ketamine improves postoperative depressive state and relieves postoperative pain in depressed patients and is a suitable anesthetic for depressed patients. NMDA receptor antagonists are reported to be effective for improving depression. It remains unclear whether ketamine, which is an NMDA receptor antagonist, postoperatively affects the psychological state in depressed patients (29). The incidence of postoperative confusion in depressed patients with fentanyl was significantly lower than that of depressed patients without fentanyl (30). As the anesthetic management of depressed patients is becoming increasingly more complex, anesthesiologists should be familiar with medical illness and abnormal response (31). Patients receiving serotonergic antidepressants show significantly higher, but clinically unimportant, intraoperative blood loss, without an increase in perioperative transfusion requirements (32). Recent evidence suggests that preoperative executive dysfunction and depression may predict postoperative delirium; however, the combined effect of these risk factors remains unknown. Preoperative executive dysfunction and depressive symptoms are predictive of postoperative delirium among noncardiac surgical patients. Executive tasks with greater complexity are more strongly associated with postoperative delirium relative to tests of basic sequencing (33). Research has established that antidepressants administered to depressed patients should be continued before anesthesia. Discontinuation of antidepressants did not increase the incidence of hypotension and arrhythmias during anesthesia but increased symptoms of depression and delirium or confusion (30).

Anesthetic Concerns (Major Depression)

Early detection of depression during pregnancy is critical because depression can adversely affect birth outcomes and neonatal health and, if left untreated, can persist after the birth.
Untreated postpartum depression can impair mother–infant attachments and have cognitive, emotional, and behavioral consequences for children (Ryan et al., 2005).
Patients treated by antidepressants may have high postoperative pain scores.
Patients treated by antidepressants may have a mildly increased bleeding risk.
Patients treated by antidepressants may be at higher risk for temporary postoperative cognitive dysfunction.
Antidepressant therapy should be continued; the risk of intraoperative arrhythmias does not appear to be increased.

Bipolar Disorders

The spectrum and diagnosis of bipolar disorder (BPD) is based on the predominance of manic (euphoric) and depressive episodes, including BPD I, BPD II, and BPD not otherwise specified (NOS). BPDs with predominantly depressive symptoms are thought to have a combined lifetime prevalence of 3.5% compared to a prevalence rate of 1.0% for BPD I, which consists of one or more manic episodes (34). Surprisingly little is known about the course and treatment of these disorders during pregnancy and the postpartum period. Brief hypomanic symptoms occur in the early puerperium in as many as 15% of women, and there is preliminary evidence that postpartum depression in some patients may be related to BPD II or BPD NOS, which have predominantly depressive episodes.

Unfortunately, there are no psychopharmacological studies on the acute or maintenance treatment of bipolar postpartum depression to guide clinical decision-making. Also, there is a lack of screening instruments designed specifically for use before or after delivery in women with suspected bipolar disorder. A prospective study of 89 pregnant women with BPD including 28 women with BPD II reported that the overall recurrence rate was two-fold greater (35) among women who discontinued versus continued mood stabilizers during pregnancy. Data on the effectiveness and safety of antidepressants are lacking since patients with BPD are routinely excluded from studies on the use of antidepressants during pregnancy or after delivery. Women who are on antidepressants should be carefully watched for cycle acceleration or a mood switch to hypomania or mania. There is increasing usage of neuroleptics for the depressive and maintenance phase of BPD but there are limited data on their use in pregnancy. In one study, placental passage, defined as the ratio of umbilical cord to maternal plasma concentrations, was highest for olanzapine followed by haloperidol, risperidone, and quetiapine (36). Due to reports of gestational diabetes, women on atypical neuroleptics need to be monitored closely (37–39). Exposure to atypical neuroleptics during pregnancy is also associated with increased infant birth weight and large for gestational age births (40). In general, patients suffering from BPD should be on antidepressants in combination with mood stabilizers. They need to be monitored closely for impending signs of mood instability.

Treatment of Bipolar Disorder during Pregnancy and the Postpartum Period

The priorities regarding the approach to treat BPD during pregnancy are: (1) The severity of the illness, (2) the clinical course with and without medications in the past, (3) the history of discontinuation attempts, and (4) the response to specific medication. Each phase during pregnancy and postpartum represents variable risk; the best therapeutic approach depends on the severity of the illness. Abrupt discontinuation of treatment is not the standard any longer due to the very high rates of relapse (41) mainly when cessation is done suddenly. This risk is significantly reduced by continued mood stabilizer treatment. Treatment planning for pregnant women with BPD should consider the significant morbidity associated with discontinuation of maintenance treatment. Patients with a history of multiple relapses represent the greater challenge and ideally should remain on a mood stabilizer before and during pregnancy. The teratogenic risk of using lithium during the first trimester is small comparing it with the potential implications of relapse during pregnancy. Relapse of BPD during pregnancy is particularly dangerous and requires aggressive medical treatment with exposure to multiple psychotropics at high dosages.

Treatment during the postpartum period is critical due to the very high risk of relapse; the ideal approach has been extensively documented and consists of prophylaxis with mood stabilizers or neuroleptics mainly for the patients who were not undergoing treatment during pregnancy (42). Treatment with lithium can be reintroduced within the first 48 hours postdelivery or can be initiated in the last 3 weeks prior to delivery. The rationale to decrease lithium dose before delivery is particularly risky because it is taking place at the time of greatest risk of relapse. A more reasonable option is to follow the patient closely by monitoring lithium levels during labor and delivery as well as during the first postpartum days to adjust the dose as necessary and to minimize the risk of relapse. Therapeutic drug monitoring plays an important role in psychiatric pharmacotherapy during pregnancy to ensure that an adequate dose is given to achieve a therapeutic effect while avoiding excessive fetal exposure (43). The use of anticonvulsants and antipsychotics during the postpartum period is an option when lithium treatment has not been effective or well tolerated.

Lithium has a low teratogenic risk of Ebstein's anomaly following first trimester exposure (0.05 % to 0.1%). Additional risks of lithium exposure later in pregnancy include neonatal hypotonia and cyanosis; there are also sporadic cases of neonatal hypothyroidism.

Anticonvulsants including valproic acid have a much higher teratogenic risk including neural tube defects, cardiovascular malformations, craniofacial abnormalities, and other CNS structural abnormalities. Due to the inherent risks, therapeutic options should be discussed with the patient, her family, and other physicians involved in her care to facilitate the implementation of a safe and effective strategy.

Anesthetic Considerations

Some pregnant patients with a bipolar disorder may receive one or several mood stabilizers. It is important to realize that the therapeutic levels of these drugs may fluctuate, and the anesthesiologist should be aware of potential drug toxicity and drug interactions. Lithium may increase the effects of certain antiemetic agents (such as promethazine and prochlorperazine) and the neuroleptic drug haloperidol. Side effects of the latter are tremor and tardive dyskinesia. Lithium itself has a narrow therapeutic to toxic ratio. Plasma lithium concentrations should be maintained as 0.4 to 1.0 mmol/L. Levels greater than 2 mmol/L may result in toxic effects such as polyuria, polydipsia, cardiac rhythm disturbances, nausea, and vomiting. Severe toxic effects are renal failure, disorientation, convulsions, coma, and death. (44,45).

Anxiety Disorders

Anxiety is a sense of fear without a specific cause, which is usually associated to physical manifestations. It is a common human experience that becomes a pathologic condition when it induces disabling symptoms and interferes with the patient's capacity to function and with her quality of life. As stated above, anxiety disorders are very prevalent conditions in mankind and some of them are more common in women. The primary anxiety disorders include panic disorder (PD) with or without agoraphobia, specific phobias, generalized anxiety disorder, post-traumatic stress disorder (PTSD), and obsessive-compulsive disorder (OCD). The diagnostic approach should include a standard evaluation to rule out medical or toxic etiologies.

PD is a condition characterized by relapsing episodes of panic attacks, which can develop with or without specific precipitating factors; the onset of symptoms is more frequent in young adults and in the context of a recent traumatic event.

The presence of this condition without treatment significantly affects quality of life-inducing maladaptive behavioral changes. Panic attacks are frequently confused with symptoms of pulmonary, neurologic, or cardiac disease that generate additional anxiety and multiple unnecessary medical workups. A detailed history is frequently the best diagnostic instrument. Panic attacks consist of acute exacerbations of anxiety with sensation of impending doom with duration of up to 20 minutes. The main symptoms consist of shortness of breath, fear of dying or going crazy, chest pain, tremors, perspiration, feelings of detachment, lightheadedness, and paresthesias. The presence of agoraphobia, which can also be diagnosed independently of panic attacks, induces more avoidant behavior and increases the potential for disability. Agoraphobia is the fear and avoidance of situations where the patient may not be able to escape, and exposure to such conditions will typically generate great anxiety or will trigger a panic attack. PD with agoraphobia is 3 times more common in women and without agoraphobia is twice as common.

Specific phobias are characterized by the severe irrational fear of specific objects or situations that the patient most of the times knows represent no real threat. These conditions can generate disability because they induce avoidance and impair the patient's ability to interact with others, to perform at work, or to carry out other activities of daily living. Specific phobias are probably more common in women and have a lifetime prevalence of up to 10%.

Generalized Anxiety Disorder

Generalized anxiety disorder (GAD) is defined as excessive and uncontrollable worry and anxiety about everyday life situations. It is a chronic disorder, and is associated with substantial somatization, high rates of comorbid depression and other anxiety disorders, and significant disability (46).

There is now growing realization that many women suffer from new onset or worsening of anxiety disorders during pregnancy. Uguz et al. noted that the rate of any mood or anxiety disorder was 19.4% in the pregnant women. Major depression (5.5%) and obsessive-compulsive disorder (5.2%) were the most common diagnoses in the pregnant women. The results suggest that pregnancy is not a risk factor for the development of mood and anxiety disorders (47).

Generalized anxiety disorder is a condition characterized by an inherent inability to relax and an excessive tendency to worry in such a way that anxiety is consistently present in most aspects of the patient's life. The main symptoms include excessive worrying, difficulty relaxing, concentration and working memory deficits, insomnia, irritability, and low energy level.

Anxiety disorders are common problems facing obstetricians and gynecologists. Women are at least twice as likely to present with most anxiety disorders. The anxiety disorders are PD (with and without agoraphobia), OCD, PTSD, social phobia, and generalized anxiety disorder (GAD). Approximately 30% of women experience some type of anxiety disorder during their lifetime. Women with these disorders may experience profound changes in their symptoms during pregnancy and the postpartum period.

Anxiety disorders are common during the perinatal period, with reported rates of obsessive-compulsive disorder and generalized anxiety disorder being higher in postpartum women than in the general population (48). In addition, some evidence exists that anxiety disorders can affect pregnancy outcomes (49). It appears that anxiety disorders are associated with increased preeclampsia risk (50).

The SSRIs are the first-line treatment for most anxiety disorders because of data supporting their efficacy, the minimal need for dosage titration, the overall favorable side-effect profile, and the length of available clinical experience (51).

Anxiety symptoms in pregnancy have been associated with adverse fetal and infant outcomes. Furthermore, having an anxiety disorder during pregnancy is one of the strongest risk factors for postnatal depression. Optimal control of the psychiatric disorder should be maintained during pregnancy, the postpartum period, and thereafter. All pregnancies wherein a mother has a serious psychiatric disorder should be considered high risk and the mother and the fetus must be carefully monitored (52).

Antianxiety medications such as benzodiazepines (BZDs) are frequently and appropriately used to ameliorate the anxiety symptoms of depression, dysthymic disorder, PD, agoraphobia, obsessive-compulsive disorder, generalized anxiety disorder, eating disorder, and many personality disorders. Pregnancy may be accompanied by anxiety necessitating therapeutic intervention by anxiolytic drugs like BZD (53). Anxiety and depression during pregnancy increase the risk for an adverse pregnancy outcome and neurodevelopmental problems in the child (54). The risk of teratogenicity with pharmacotherapy must be considered, but judicious tapering and cessation of medication during high-risk periods can minimize it (55). For these reasons, it has been recommended that nonpharmacologic treatment, such as cognitive-behavioral therapy, should be first-line treatment in pregnant women with GAD or PD (56).

Panic Disorder

Little is known about the effect of pregnancy and the puerperium on the risk for and course of anxiety disorders (57,58). In a meta-analysis, 41% (88 out of 215) of the pregnancies that were described in these studies were associated with improvement of PD symptoms during the pregnancy, while 38% of the described pregnancies exhibited onset or exacerbation of PD in the postpartum period (59). Panic manifestations were fewer during pregnancy and more frequent in the postpartum period when compared with the control period. Women who had never been pregnant had significantly more panic manifestations than women with prior pregnancies. Breastfeeding and miscarriages appear not to have a significant effect. Women with postpartum panic reported more psychosocial stress events during this period. Possible reasons for postpartum panic and the protective effects of pregnancy include psychosocial or hormonal factors and other neurobiologic changes. Current study findings support the need to examine PD and trait anxiety as potential risk factors for alcohol use among pregnant and nonpregnant women in the community (60). Postpartum panic coincides with a sudden drop of hormones after delivery (61).

Obsessive-compulsive Disorder

People with OCD have persistent, upsetting thoughts (obsessions) and use rituals (compulsions) to control the anxiety these thoughts produce. The rituals end up controlling them most of the time. One-third of the adults with OCD develop symptoms as children. Women who are unmarried or abusing drugs are more likely to present with OCD, which is thought to be a familial and genetic disorder, particularly when one considers symptom dimensions instead of categorical diagnosis and when the disorder begins at an early age (62).

Treatment of Anxiety Disorders

OCD usually responds well to treatment with certain medications and/or exposure-based psychotherapy, in which people face situations that cause fear or anxiety and become less sensitive (desensitized) to them. Antidepressants were developed to treat depression but are also effective for anxiety disorders. Many antidepressants may be classified as selective serotonin reuptake inhibitors, or SSRIs. Fluoxetine

(Prozac®), sertraline (Zoloft®), escitalopram (Lexapro®), paroxetine (Paxil®), and citalopram (Celexa®) are some of the SSRIs commonly prescribed for PD and OCD. Other commonly used antidepressants are the TCAs, imipramine (Tofranil®) and clomipramine (Anafranil®), and monoamine oxidase inhibitors (MAOIs). The MAOIs most commonly prescribed for anxiety disorders are phenelzine (Nardil®), followed by tranylcypromine (Parnate®), and isocarboxazid (Marplan®) which are useful in treating PD and social phobia.

Clonazepam (Klonopin®) is used for social phobia and GAD, lorazepam (Ativan®) is helpful for PD, and alprazolam (Xanax®) is useful for both PD and GAD. When used to treat PD during pregnancy, clonazepam did not appear to be directly related to any obstetric complications during pregnancy, labor, or delivery. There was no evidence of neonatal toxicity or withdrawal syndromes in infants born to mothers who took clonazepam during pregnancy. Absence of serious maternal or neonatal compromise following clonazepam use during pregnancy in these mothers and infants is somewhat reassuring (63). Other forms of treatment include β-blockers, psychotherapy, and cognitive-behavioral therapy.

Anesthetic Considerations in Anxiety Disorders

Anesthetic concerns in patients with anxiety disorders deal with preoxygenation and several potential drug side effects and interactions described in the literature. Two syndromes, the serotonin syndrome and the neuroleptic malignant syndrome (NMS), deserve to be mentioned.

Preoxygenation with a facemask may not be tolerated in many patients with anxiety disorder. An alternative approach has been described whereby patients breathe through the elbow piece of the circle system and preferably have a nose clamp in place to avoid co-inhalation of room air (64). Although drug interaction probably remains the most potentially serious problem, current evidence suggests that psychiatric medication need not be discontinued prior to anesthesia and surgery. Discontinuation of medication may constitute its own hazards. Most interactions can be predicted and appropriate precautions taken. The use of meperidine is contraindicated for patients receiving MAOIs (65).

Anesthetic Considerations (Anxiety Disorders)

Preoxygenation with a face mask may not be tolerated. As an alternative, patients may breathe through the elbow piece of the circle system and preferably have a nose clamp in place.
Psychiatric medication need not be discontinued prior to anesthesia and surgery.
Meperidine is contraindicated for patients receiving MAOIs.
SSRIs fall into Category C of the United States Food and Drug Administration classification regarding safety of use during pregnancy.
Adjustment of local anesthetic dose may be necessary as SSRIs inhibit the cytochrome P450 system and affect local anesthetic metabolism.
TCAs' side effects may be related to the antimuscarinic properties of the TCAs. Such side effects are relatively common and may include dry mouth, dry nose, blurry vision, lowered gastrointestinal motility or constipation, urinary retention, cognitive and/or memory impairment, and increased body temperature.

MAOIs can interact with SSRIs to result in the "serotonin syndrome", characterized by confusion, hallucinations, increased sweating, muscle stiffness, seizures, blood pressure and cardiac rhythm changes.
NMS develops during the use of neuroleptics. The four main manifestations are high fever, altered consciousness, a variety of autonomic symptoms, and severe extrapyramidal symptoms, which are observed in typical cases of NMS.

Like most drugs used for anesthesia, antianxiety medications are neurotropic drugs. It is therefore important to consider these effects when devising the anesthetic plan. Some of the newest antidepressants are selective serotonin reuptake inhibitors, or SSRIs. Examples are Fluoxetine (Prozac®), sertraline (Zoloft®), escitalopram (Lexapro®), paroxetine (Paxil®), and citalopram (Celexa®). SSRIs fall in the Category C of the United States Food and Drug Administration classification regarding safety of use during pregnancy (66). Animal reproduction studies have shown an adverse effect on the fetus, and there are no adequate and well-controlled studies in humans. SSRIs are usually compatible with breastfeeding, but individual variations in infant exposure may occur. There is no conclusive evidence that SSRIs increase the risk for malformations, but paroxetine and possibly fluoxetine use in early pregnancy may be associated with a small increased risk for cardiovascular malformations (67). Adjustment of local anesthetic dose may be necessary as SSRIs inhibit the cytochrome P450 system and affect local anesthetic metabolism. Because there are no specific interactions between SSRIs and anesthetic agents, SSRIs are generally considered safe to use during the perioperative period. However, discontinuation of SSRIs during the perioperative period may lead to the development of withdrawal symptoms (66). Moreover, reinstituting the drugs at patients' previous dosage, which may be the maximum dosage for some patients, may lead to the development of serotonin syndrome. Confusion, hallucinations, increased sweating, muscle stiffness, seizures, blood pressure, and cardiac rhythm changes characterize this syndrome.

TCAs' side effects may be related to their antimuscarinic properties. Such side effects are relatively common and may include dry mouth, dry nose, blurry vision, lowered gastrointestinal motility or constipation, urinary retention, cognitive and/or memory impairment, and increased body temperature (68). Other side effects may include drowsiness, anxiety, emotional blunting (apathy/anhedonia), confusion, restlessness, dizziness, akathisia, hypersensitivity, changes in appetite and weight, sweating, sexual dysfunction, muscle twitches, weakness, nausea and vomiting, hypotension, tachycardia, and arrhythmias.

MAOIs are the oldest class of antidepressant medications. Patients treated with MAOIs cannot eat a variety of foods (including cheese and red wine) that contain tyramine or take certain medications, including some contraceptives and analgesics (such as ibuprofen). These combinations may result in severe hypertensive episodes. MAOIs can interact with SSRIs to result in the "serotonin syndrome" (69).

NMS develops during the use of neuroleptics (70). The four main manifestations are high fever, altered consciousness, a variety of autonomic symptoms, and severe extrapyramidal symptoms, which are observed in typical cases of NMS. However, many cases have not exhibited sufficient clinical manifestations because of better awareness and early diagnosis in recent years. NMS shares common features with malignant hyperthermia. While a caffeine-halothane contracture test is positive in the skeletal muscle of malignant hyperthermia patients, the results of the tests are inconclusive in NMS cases. Studies on the pathophysiology suggest that the occurrence of peripheral sympathetic nervous system hyperactivity plays a central role in the pathophysiology of NMS. When NMS is suspected, all neuroleptics must be discontinued immediately. Dehydration occurs in many cases, and fluid replacement may result in improvement in mild cases. Antipyretic drugs are generally ineffective against the fever, and complications such as respiratory failure, rhabdomyolysis, renal failure, and disseminated intravascular coagulation (DIC) may adversely affect the outcome.

Substance Abuse-related Disorders

Substance abuse complicates between 10% and 25% of pregnancies and has been associated with increased perinatal morbidity and mortality. The mechanisms of action of certain drugs predispose to specific types of complications, but the explanations for obstetrical effects of other drugs are more obscure. The impact of maternal substance abuse is reflected in the 2002–2003 National Survey on Drug Use and Health. Among pregnant women in the 15 to 44 age group, 4.3%, 18%, and 9.8% used illicit drugs, tobacco, and alcohol, respectively. Maternal pregnancy complications following substance use include increases in sexually transmitted disorders, placental abruption, and HIV-positive status (71). The effects of drugs on the infants of pregnant drug abusers include an increased risk of low birth weight, preterm delivery, possible teratogenic effects, fetal dependence and withdrawal, and possible neurobehavioral effects (72,73). Short-term and long-term neurobehavioral problems have been documented also in infants born to substance-abusing mothers (71).

Tobacco and alcohol are the substances most abused during pregnancy. Ethanol is the human teratogen that produces the most serious neurobehavioral effects on the fetus. Cocaine is associated with spontaneous abortions, premature labor, precipitous labor, stillbirths, meconium staining, and abruptio placentae. Heroin use during pregnancy has been associated with low birth weight, miscarriage, prematurity, microcephaly, and intrauterine growth retardation. Marijuana is not scientifically linked to significant teratogenic effects. Since most substance abusers use multiple drugs, a positive screen for marijuana may indicate a high-risk patient. Cigarette smoking has been associated with spontaneous abortions, premature rupture of membranes, preterm delivery, perinatal death, low birth weight infants, and deficits in learning and behavior (74,75). Pregnant substance-abusing women should be identified and targeted for HIV counseling and testing. In addition, drug rehabilitation should be strongly advocated (76).

Alcohol-related Disorders

The use of alcohol and drugs during pregnancy is a major public health problem in the United States. Detailed surveys estimate that 14% of pregnant women report alcohol use during the previous month, and 1.3% of women report binge drinking (77). Alcohol abuse during pregnancy can inhibit brain growth, resulting in reduced brain size and reduced reserve capacity (and therefore less ability to compensate for loss of function later in life) (78). Fetal alcohol syndrome (FAS) is a specific polydystrophic pattern of malformations with the following diagnostic criteria: Maternal alcohol dependence or alcohol abuse during pregnancy, pre- and postnatal deficiency of growth in weight, height and head circumference, typical facial features, and structural injuries of the central nervous system with complex brain dysfunction. Fetal alcohol effects or the so-called

"alcohol-related neurodevelopmental disorders" with predominant neurotoxic effects and a large spectrum of cerebral dysfunctions are more frequently encountered than FAS. These remain mostly unrecognized and overlooked. They are difficult to diagnose with the symptoms being unspecific. Alcohol in pregnancy is nowadays the most important and the most frequent toxic substance for the embryo and the fetus; it is one of the most frequent causes of mental retardation. The diagnosis is based on the careful maternal history and on the clinical findings; there are no biochemical parameters of assessment. The risk of addiction development in these children is assumed to be more than 20% (79).

Anesthetic Considerations of Alcohol
Use in Pregnancy

The consequences of long-term alcohol abuse include a three- to five-fold increased risk of postoperative infection, prolonged intensive care unit stays, and longer hospital stays (80). The cause of the higher infection rates is an altered immune response in long-term alcoholic patients (81). Alcohol use increases perioperative morbidity and mortality. The most ominous effects of chronic alcoholism are related to withdrawal, a serious and potentially life-threatening complication. Prophylaxis for withdrawal should be started preoperatively with BZDs or in combination with clonidine. Haloperidol is the drug of choice for emerging symptoms of alcohol withdrawal with productive psychosis. The most obvious implication for anesthesia is the choice of a rapid sequence induction to reduce the risk of aspiration (82).

Cocaine-related Disorders

Cocaine use prevalence rates have risen in recent years, with 722,000 teens and adults reporting first time cocaine use in 2009. This is equivalent to about 2,000 new cocaine initiates per day (83). Most cocaine users also abuse other drugs—mostly alcohol and marijuana (84,85).

Maternal sequelae of cocaine use appear to be related to the drug's detrimental effect on the cardiovascular system. Plasma catecholamine levels increase after acute cocaine exposure (2). The cardiovascular effect may be augmented by the sensitization of α-adrenergic receptors by progesterone (86). Pregnant cocaine users are at increased risk for migraines, cocaine-induced hypertension, stroke, and myocardial infarction (87). These effects may be accentuated by the administration of indirect acting vasopressors such as ephedrine (88).

Untoward fetal effects of maternal cocaine use include premature rupture of membranes, preterm labor, placental abruption, small-for-gestational-age-infants, and low (<2,500 g) and very low (750–1,500 g) birth weight newborns (89). A number of birth defects have been associated with cocaine use including genitourinary, cardiac, and limb anomalies. The reproductive toxic and putative teratogenic effects of cocaine are probably associated with its well-known pharmacologic action causing vasoconstriction. From preliminary studies, it would appear that methamphetamine also produces reproductive toxic effects similar to those of cocaine (90).

Opioid-related Disorders

Pregnant women dependent on opioids require careful treatment to minimize harm to the fetus and neonate and improve maternal health. Opioid maintenance therapy is the recommended treatment approach during pregnancy. Treatment decisions must include psychiatric comorbidities and the concomitant consumption of other drugs (91).

Anesthetic Implications of Drug Use during Pregnancy

The rate of cocaine use has increased more rapidly in women than men, placing such women at increased risk of adverse consequences such as HIV infection and physical abuse (92). Because illicit substance use is so prevalent, if untoward reactions occur during an otherwise uneventful anesthetic, the possibility of drug abuse should be considered (93).

Regardless of the drug(s) ingested and clinical manifestations, it is always difficult to predict the exact anesthetic implications in chemically dependent patients (94,95). Cocaine and amphetamine-abusing patients are at risk for hypertension, cardiac arrhythmias, and myocardial ischemia (96), and it should be recognized that propranolol may exaggerate hypertension by blocking β-receptors and enhancing the α-adrenergic effects of cocaine (97). Hydralazine, labetalol, and nitroglycerin are appropriate antihypertensive drugs in cocaine-addicted parturients (98). All volatile anesthetics may enhance the proarrhythmogenic effects of cocaine and amphetamines (99,100).

Anesthetic considerations for the opioid-addicted parturient are the maintenance of narcotic therapy to avoid acute withdrawal. For the same reason, opioid antagonists should be avoided. The symptoms of withdrawal, if they occur, can be treated with clonidine or doxepine (96). Acute withdrawal and delirium tremens are major concerns in the alcohol-abusing parturient. In this situation, the intravenous administration of ethanol may also be considered.

The effects of general anesthesia in the substance-abusing parturient are somewhat unpredictable and depend on the degree and combination of drug exposure. While stimulants may exaggerate the hypertensive effects of laryngoscopy, marijuana and ethanol may enhance the myocardial depressant effects of volatile anesthetics. The neurologically impaired drug user should be considered at risk for aspiration. Regional anesthesia is not contraindicated; however, increased risks for infection and coagulopathy should be considered (95).

Schizophrenia and Other Psychotic Disorders

Psychotic disorders are a heterogeneous group of disorders that are characterized during the active phase by the presence of a thought disorder which significantly impairs the patient's capacity to process information, to think logically and as a consequence significantly impairs the perception of reality. The main primary psychiatric disorders include schizophrenia, schizoaffective disorder, brief psychotic disorders, and delusional disorder. The differential diagnosis and classification of these disorders is based on the specific symptoms, duration, severity, the presence of an affective component, and the degree of compromise of intellectual domains. The presence of perceptual disturbances, true hallucinations, or unusual delusions is more consistent with schizophrenia; if such symptoms are associated with a significant affective component, they are more suggestive of schizoaffective disorder. Delusional disorder is typically restricted to a specific fixed delusional belief and brief psychotic disorders have a limited duration and a complete resolution without residual deficits after the acute episode. Negative symptoms (lack of social interactions with others, apathy) are more consistent with schizophrenia.

The possibility of a nonprimary psychiatric origin including other medical conditions or a toxic etiology should be a consideration mainly in patients who do not have a history of psychosis. The onset of schizophrenia in women typically takes place in the mid-20s to mid-30s, a decade later than in men and has a better prognosis.

The implications of having a psychosis are variable; for the patients who are compliant with treatment, the possibility of living a more independent life is a reasonable expectation but they have significant limitations in their capacity to care for children. Medical treatment is now a lot more effective and many patients go into remission with a long-term improvement in their prognosis. Regardless of the many improvements in the diagnosis and treatment of psychotic disorders, the possibility of not diagnosing or overlooking the manifestations of a psychosis in a pregnant patient will have severe consequences, which will develop at a particularly challenging time—during labor or in the operating room.

The incidence of *schizophrenia* in the general population ranges from approximately 1% to 2%, and the peak age of onset in women are 25 to 35 years, which are also the peak childbearing years. Schizophrenia has been associated with a number of adverse obstetric complications and pregnancy outcomes (e.g., low birth weight) as well as poor neonatal conditions (e.g., hypotonia, lethargy, tremors, extrapyramidal symptoms). All of these conditions resolved spontaneously within 2 to 3 weeks after birth, and there were no apparent long-term adverse effects (101).

Bipolar Disorder

Bipolar disorder has a lifetime prevalence of 1% to 5% and a substantial risk of long-term morbidity, comorbidity, and disability (102). Bipolar disorder is also associated with high rates of premature mortality, which is largely due to suicide but is also related to the effects of accidents, substance abuse, and general medical disorders (103). The clinical presentation of bipolar patients may include mania and/or depression in addition to more minor mood fluctuations that accompany the emotional and physical changes of pregnancy. The key issue in the differential diagnosis is to rule out medical, surgical, medication, and substance etiologies of mania that are potentially reversible (104). Maintenance of euthymia during pregnancy is critical because relapse during this period strongly predicts a difficult postpartum course.

Drugs used to treat schizophrenia and psychotic disorders are first-generation (conventional) antipsychotics (e.g., promethazine, chlorpromazine, prochlorperazine, haloperidol, perphenazine, trifluoperazine, loxapine, thioridazine, flupenthixol, fluphenazine) and second-generation antipsychotics (e.g., clozapine, risperidone, olanzapine, quetiapine, ziprasidone, aripiprazole, paliperidone) (105). To date, no definitive association has been found between use of antipsychotics during pregnancy and an increased risk of birth defects or other adverse outcomes. The side-effect profile of these drugs is listed in Table 39-2 (102).

Women suffering from schizophrenia and bipolar disorders are suitable candidates for regional anesthesia if their symptoms are well controlled with appropriate antipsychotic therapy. Kudoh et al. showed that intravenous general anesthesia with ketamine, propofol, and fentanyl is associated with a lower incidence of postoperative psychotic symptoms when compared to sevoflurane-based anesthesia (111).

Personality Disorders

Personality disorders are a group of psychiatric conditions in which a person's long-term (chronic) behaviors, emotions, and thoughts are very different from their culture's expectations and cause serious problems with relationships and work. These disorders include antisocial, avoidant, borderline, dependent, histrionic, narcissistic, OCD, paranoid, schizoid, and schizotypal personality disorder. They often affect women in the childbearing age. Thus, the anesthesia care provider should at a minimum be aware of

TABLE 39-2 Pregnancy Outcomes of Women with Psychiatric Disorders Treated with Antipsychotic Medications during Pregnancy

Study	Medications and Numbers of Subjects	Findings
Slone et al., 1977 (106)	FGAs (N = 1,309)	No differences in rates of birth defects, perinatal mortality, birth weight, or IQ compared with the general population.
Diav-Citrin et al., 2005 (107)	Haloperidol (N = 215)	No increased risk for birth defects
McKenna et al., 2005 (108)	Olanzapine (N = 60) Risperidone (N = 49) Quetiapine (N = 36) Clozapine (N = 6)	Prospective comparative study of 151 women exposed to SGAs: No increased risk for birth defects, small increased risk for low birth weight.
Manufacturers' registries (data as reported in 2007)	Clozapine (N = 523) Risperidone (N = 250) Olanzapine (N = 242) Quetiapine (N = 446)	Prospective and retrospective data; no pattern of birth defects identified.
Coppola et al., 2007 (109)	Risperidone (N = 713 women exposed during pregnancy; N = 68 prospectively reported with known outcome).	No increased risk for birth defects or other adverse outcomes in the 68 cases with known outcome.
Newham et al., 2008 (40)	SGAs (N = 25), FGAs (N = 45), Reference group (N = 38)	SGA exposure: Significantly higher incidence of infants being large for gestational age than in both comparison groups; mean birth weight significantly higher than those exposed to FGAs. FGAs: Significantly lower mean birth weight and higher incidence of being small for gestational age than reference group.
Reis et al., 2008 (110)	Exposed to anti-psychotics during pregnancy (N = 570), FGAs (N = 460), SGAs (N = 101)	Small (OR, 1.52) increased risk of defects with no pattern

SGA, second-generation (atypical) antipsychotic; FGA, first-generation (conventional or typical) antipsychotic.
Einarson A. Risks/safety of psychotropic medication use during pregnancy—motherisk update 2008. *Can J Clin Pharmacol* 2009;16(1), e58–e65.

these conditions (112). Epidemiologic studies have shown that the majority of substance-abusing women have one or more types of comorbid mental disorders with antisocial personality being extremely high compared with samples of non–substance-abusing women (113). It is also important to understand that childbearing women with avoidant, dependent, and obsessive-compulsive personality disorders have increased risk of new-onset major depression during the postpartum period (114).

Post-traumatic Stress Disorder (PTSD)

PTSD is an anxiety disorder which develops as a consequence of exposure to a traumatic event that induces horror or a sense of helplessness; the patient may or may not recall the event in detail but will experience chronic recurrent anxiety, avoidance or feelings of guilt, nightmares, flashbacks, or symptoms of hyperarousal when exposed to situations that remind her of the event. The lifetime prevalence of PTSD is variable and can be as high as 15% according to the exposure to different types of violence or abuse including child abuse, spousal abuse, and rape. Inquiring about a history of abuse and the impact in the patient's life should be part of the initial evaluation of the pregnant patient.

Obsessive-compulsive Disorder (OCD)

OCD is somewhat different from other personality disorders. It is a familial and genetic disorder and individuals with OCD from the community may present with other psychiatric conditions such as mood and anxiety disorders. The prevalence rate of OCD is 3.5% among the women in the third trimester of pregnancy. The most common obsessions are contamination (80.0%) and symmetry/exactness (60.0%), whereas the most common compulsions are cleaning/washing (86.7%) and checking (60.0%) (115). Pregnancy and childbirth are frequently associated with the onset of OCD or worsening of symptoms in those with preexisting disorder. In addition, there appears to be continuity between OCD onset and/or exacerbation across the reproductive life cycle, at least with menstruation and pregnancy (116).

Therapy typically is not based on behavioral intervention but, in some cases, medication may be useful. Antianxiety medications such as BZDs are frequently and appropriately used to ameliorate the anxiety symptoms of depression, paranoia, schizoid personality disorder, PD, agoraphobia, and obsessive-compulsive disorder. Pregnancy may be accompanied by anxiety necessitating therapeutic intervention by anxiolytic drugs like BZDs. Keeping in view the potential risks of teratogenicity and direct neonatal toxicity, BZDs with established safety records should be used, while avoiding exposure in the first trimester, especially with multidrug regimens, and prescribing the lowest dose for the shortest duration (53).

Eating Disorders

The most common eating disorders are anorexia nervosa and bulimia nervosa. Eating disorder behaviors during pregnancy are associated with complications such as preterm delivery, low birth weight, intrauterine growth restriction, cesarean delivery, and low Apgar scores (117). The anesthesia provider should recognize that patients with eating disorders may present with electrolyte, cardiovascular, and thermo-regulatory alterations thereby modifying the anesthetic plan accordingly.

While eating disorders typically lead to poor nutrition and, in extreme cases cachexia, it should be recognized that obesity is an important risk factor for anesthesia-related maternal mortality (118). Epidemiologic evidence clearly shows that being overweight contributes to menstrual disorders, infertility, miscarriage, poor pregnancy outcome, impaired fetal well-being, and diabetes mellitus (119). Anesthesia-related complications are more frequent in obese parturients. Most authors agree that regional anesthesia is the preferred technique for cesarean delivery in obese patients. Efforts to establish early labor epidural analgesia should be optimized in order to be able to avoid general anesthesia when unplanned cesarean delivery is required (120).

Antipsychotic Therapy during Pregnancy

There are several preliminary considerations in the process of choosing a psychiatric medication during pregnancy (121,122). Essentially all drugs taken by a pregnant woman reach her fetus. Multiple factors determine the degree of fetal exposure include dose, maternal absorption, distribution and elimination, bidirectional placental transfer, and fetal distribution and elimination. Factors that influence the degree of exposure include favorable pH gradients across the placenta, lipophilicity, and protein-binding characteristics. All psychoactive drugs appear to be easily distributed to the fetus with differences in their rate and extent of transfer. There is increasing recognition of the role of drug transporters in the disposition of psychoactive drugs that regulate access to the brain (122). At this point, it is not clear how transporters modify the exposure of the fetus but eventually they may become the tools to minimize fetal drug exposure. The main clinical goals are reproductive safety and efficacy to minimize the risk of miscarriage, the risk of teratogenesis, or neonatal toxicity including withdrawal syndromes (121). The risk of long-term neuropsychiatric sequelae is harder to evaluate, but it appears to be a more relevant factor with the use of antiepileptic drugs and in particular with valproic acid (123).

The FDA has developed a risk classification system that is not always consistent with the available data and is not always based on human studies. This system classifies medications into five different risk categories: A, B, C, D, and X. Category A includes medications that are considered safe to be used during pregnancy, Category D includes drugs with positive evidence of risk, and Category X includes medications that are clearly contraindicated during pregnancy. Category B includes medications with an intermediary risk between A and C. Category C includes most psychotropic medications; this category includes medications where human studies have not been done or the information is limited so the potential risk cannot be ruled out. No psychotropic medications are classified as Category A. This classification system is partially reliable and not always helpful; other sources of information need to be consulted to provide more specific recommendations.

Risk of Teratogenesis

Teratogenesis is a consequence of using an agent that produces organ malformation. The major organ systems develop during the first 12 weeks of intrauterine life. For each system, there are critical periods of development where specific teratogenic effects can take place. Neural tube defects occur during the first 4 weeks after conception, and cardiovascular defects develop during the first 4 to 9 weeks.

Prenatal exposure to most antidepressants has not revealed a statistically increased risk of congenital malformations. The information regarding low reproductive risk for fluoxetine and citalopram has been relatively well established; the information regarding other SSRIs and SNRIs is more limited with most of these medications classified as Category C except for paroxetine, which has been classified as D due to possible increase of cardiovascular malformations and perinatal complications. TCAs have been classified as Category D mainly due to risks of fetal anticholinergic effects, but there is no significant association between fetal exposure to TCAs and significant risks of major congenital anomalies. Among the TCAs, desipramine and nortryptyline are in principle the best options due to their lower anticholinergic effects. MAOIs may produce a hypertensive crisis and have been associated with possible congenital malformations; ideally, they should not be used during pregnancy. The information regarding bupropion is controversial with possible increased risk of cardiovascular malformations, but its use in pregnancy is not absolutely contraindicated. A list of possible teratogenic effects of antidepressant drugs is provided in Table 39-3.

Risks of Miscarriage

Antidepressants do not increase the risk of miscarriage. Some reports have suggested an increase in rates of spontaneous abortion in patients treated with SSRIs during the first trimester; such increases were not of statistical significance and a possible explanation is the inherent risk of complications secondary to the mood disorder per se.

Risk of Neonatal Toxicity or Perinatal Syndromes

This category represents a wide range of physical and behavioral symptoms in the acute neonatal period that have been attributed to the in utero exposure to antidepressants. The incidence of these events appears to be low and transitory. A withdrawal syndrome induced by TCAs has been described; the symptoms predominantly consist of irritability, urinary retention, and nonmechanical bowel obstruction. Such symptoms are mild and of short duration. Withdrawal seizures have been reported only with clomipramine (124). Several studies have implicated SSRI exposure to respiratory distress, shorter gestational age, jitteriness, feeding problems, and lower Apgar scores. The relevance of these reports is controversial and the magnitude of changes in the Apgar scores is minimal. Most of these reports do not consider the impact of the mood disorder on the perinatal outcome. The most significant cases of neonatal withdrawal with SSRIs are present in neonates exposed to paroxetine proximate to delivery, which has been associated with respiratory distress and hypoglycemia. The specific nature of these syndromes remains controversial, and the clinical course of most neonates is benign with no clear evidence of long-term problems.

The rationale to consider lowering the dose of antidepressants in women with severe depression before delivery in an effort to reduce the risk of neonatal toxicity is questionable and significantly increases the risk of relapse at a critical time. Regardless of the FDA labeling warnings about the potential complications of these syndromes, there is no clear evidence of significant clinical relevance including no long-term neurobehavioral sequelae including cognition and language development (125) or increased adverse obstetrical or neonatal outcomes following prenatal exposure to antidepressants including SSRIs and TCAs (126). On the other hand, there is documentation of evidence of developmental delay in the children of women who experienced clinical depression during pregnancy (43).

TABLE 39-3 Potential Teratogenic Effects of Anti-depressant Drugs (127–155)

Selective Serotonin Reuptake Inhibitors (SSRIs)		
Medication	**Potential Risk(s)**	**Recommendation**
Citalopram (Celexa)	Persistent pulmonary hypertension of the newborn (PPHN) (when taken during the last half of pregnancy) Septal heart defects Craniosynostosis Omphalocele	May be considered as an option during pregnancy
Fluoxetine (Prozac, Sarafem)	PPHN (when taken during the last half of pregnancy)	May be considered as an option during pregnancy
Paroxetine (Paxil)	Fetal heart defects (when taken during the first 3 months of pregnancy) PPHN (when taken during the last half of pregnancy) Anencephaly Craniosynostosis Omphalocele	Should be avoided during pregnancy
Sertraline (Zoloft)	PPHN (when taken during the last half of pregnancy) Septal heart defects Omphalocele	May be considered as an option during pregnancy
Tricyclic Antidepressants (TCAs)		
Amitriptyline	Limb malformation (suggested in early studies, but not confirmed by newer studies)	May be considered as an option during pregnancy
Nortriptyline (Pamelor)	Limb malformation (suggested in early studies, but not confirmed by newer studies)	May be considered as an option during pregnancy
Monoamine Oxidase Inhibitors (MAOIs)		
Phenelzine (Nardil)	Severe increase in blood pressure	Should be avoided during pregnancy
Tranylcypromine (Parnate)	Severe increase in blood pressure	Should be avoided during pregnancy
Other Antidepressants		
Bupropion (Wellbutrin)	No established risks during pregnancy	May be considered as an option during pregnancy

KEY POINTS

- Diagnosis and treatment of *psychiatric disorders during pregnancy* and the postpartum period is a topic of significant relevance due to the high prevalence of these conditions and the multiple barriers to provide an appropriate diagnosis and an effective and safe treatment. Approximately 40% of the adult population under 65 years of age has experienced at least one DSM-III-R disorder in their lifetime. Among them, 23% have experienced a disorder within the preceding year.
- The presence of *depression* during the childbearing years is 2 to 3 times more common in women. Antidepressants administered to depressed patients should be continued before anesthesia.
- Some pregnant patients with a *bipolar disorder* may receive one or several mood stabilizers (e.g., lithium). It is important to realize that the therapeutic levels of these drugs may fluctuate, and the anesthesiologist should be aware of potential drug toxicity and drug interactions.
- Preoxygenation with a facemask may not be tolerated in many patients with *anxiety disorder*. An alternative approach has been described whereby patients breathe through the elbow piece of the circle system and preferably have a nose clamp in place to avoid co-inhalation of room air.
- The consequences of long-term *alcohol abuse* include a three- to five-fold increased risk of postoperative infection, prolonged intensive care unit stays, and longer hospital stays.
- Pregnant cocaine users are at increased risk for migraines, cocaine-induced hypertension, stroke, and myocardial infarction. These effects may be accentuated by the administration of indirect acting vasopressors such as ephedrine. Untoward fetal effects of *maternal cocaine use* include premature rupture of membranes, preterm labor, placental abruption, small-for-gestational-age-infants, and low birth weight newborns.

REFERENCES

1. Bijl RV, Ravelli A, van Zessen G. Prevalence of psychiatric disorder in the general population: results of The Netherlands Mental Health Survey and Incidence Study (NEMESIS). *Soc Psychiatry Psychiatr Epidemiol* 1998;33(12): 587–595.
2. Birnbach D. Substance abuse. In: Chestnut D, ed. *Obstetric Anesthesia: Principles and Practice*. St. Louis, MO: Mosby; 1999:1027–1040.
3. Sloan DM, Kornstein SG. Gender differences in depression and response to antidepressant treatment. *Psychiatr Clin North Am* 2003;26(3):581–594.

4. Sloan DM, Sandt AR. Gender differences in depression. *Womens Health (Lond Engl)* 2006;2(3):425–434.

5. Meltzer-Brody S, Hartmann K, Miller WC, et al. A brief screening instrument to detect posttraumatic stress disorder in outpatient gynecology. *Obstet Gynecol* 2004;104(4):770–776.

6. Altshuler LL, Cohen LS, Moline ML, et al. Treatment of depression in women: a summary of the expert consensus guidelines. *J Psychiatr Pract* 2001;7(3):185–208.

7. Miller IW, Keitner GI, Schatzberg AF, et al. The treatment of chronic depression, part 3: psychosocial functioning before and after treatment with sertraline or imipramine. *J Clin Psychiatry* 1998;59(11):608–619.

8. Marcus SM, Flynn HA, Blow FC, et al. Depressive symptoms among pregnant women screened in obstetrics settings. *J Womens Health (Larchmt)* 2003;12(4):373–380.

9. Burt VK, Quezada V. Mood disorders in women: focus on reproductive psychiatry in the 21st century–Motherisk update 2008. *Can J Clin Pharmacol* 2009;16(1):e6–e14.

10. Marcus SM. Depression during pregnancy: rates, risks and consequences–Motherisk Update 2008. *Can J Clin Pharmacol* 2009;16(1):e15–e22.

11. Marcus SM, Heringhausen JE. Depression in childbearing women: when depression complicates pregnancy. *Prim Care* 2009;36(1):151–165, ix.

12. Watanabe N, Omori IM, Nakagawa A, et al. Mirtazapine versus other antidepressants in the acute-phase treatment of adults with major depression: systematic review and meta-analysis. *J Clin Psychiatry* 2008;69(9):1404–1415.

13. Trivedi MH, Rush AJ, Wisniewski SR, et al. Evaluation of outcomes with citalopram for depression using measurement-based care in STAR*D: implications for clinical practice. *Am J Psychiatry* 2006;163(1):28–40.

14. Papakostas GI. The efficacy, tolerability, and safety of contemporary antidepressants. *J Clin Psychiatry* 2010;71(Suppl E1):e03.

15. Fava M, Alpert JE, Carmin CN, et al. Clinical correlates and symptom patterns of anxious depression among patients with major depressive disorder in STAR*D. *Psychol Med* 2004;34(7):1299–1308.

16. Ravindran LN, Stein MB. The pharmacologic treatment of anxiety disorders: a review of progress. *J Clin Psychiatry* 2010;71(7):839–854.

17. Stahl SM, Grady MM, Moret C, et al. SNRIs: their pharmacology, clinical efficacy, and tolerability in comparison with other classes of antidepressants. *CNS Spectr* 2005;10(9):732–747.

18. Atkinson JH, Slater MA, Williams RA, et al. A placebo-controlled randomized clinical trial of nortriptyline for chronic low back pain. *Pain* 1998;76(3):287–296.

19. Snyder SH, Yamamura HI. Antidepressants and the muscarinic acetylcholine receptor. *Arch Gen Psychiatry* 1977;34(2):236–239.

20. Suri R, Altshuler L, Hellemann G, et al. Effects of antenatal depression and antidepressant treatment on gestational age at birth and risk of preterm birth. *Am J Psychiatry* 2007;164(8):1206–1213.

21. Oberlander TF, Warburton W, Misri S, et al. Neonatal outcomes after prenatal exposure to selective serotonin reuptake inhibitor antidepressants and maternal depression using population-based linked health data. *Arch Gen Psychiatry* 2006;63(8):898–906.

22. Misri S, Burgmann A, Kostaras D. Are SSRIs safe for pregnant and breastfeeding women? *Can Fam Physician* 2000;46:626–628, 631–623.

23. Cohen LS, Altshuler LL, Harlow BL, et al. Relapse of major depression during pregnancy in women who maintain or discontinue antidepressant treatment. *JAMA* 2006;295(5):499–507.

24. Sonawalla SB, Fava M. Severe depression: is there a best approach? *CNS Drugs* 2001;15(10):765–776.

25. Gaines GY 3rd, Rees DI. Anesthetic considerations for electroconvulsive therapy. *South Med J* 1992;85(5):469–482.

26. Prieto Martin RM, Palomero Rodriguez MA, de Miguel Fernandez P, et al. [Electroconvulsive therapy in the third trimester of pregnancy: a case report]. *Rev Esp Anestesiol Reanim* 2006;53(10):653–656.

27. Ishikawa T, Kawahara S, Saito T, et al. [Anesthesia for electroconvulsive therapy during pregnancy–a case report]. *Masui* 2001;50(6):991–997.

28. Copeland LA, Zeber JE, Pugh MJ, et al. Postoperative complications in the seriously mentally ill: a systematic review of the literature. *Ann Surg* 2008; 248(1):31–38.

29. Kudoh A, Katagai H, Takazawa T. Increased postoperative pain scores in chronic depression patients who take antidepressants. *J Clin Anesth* 2002; 14(6):421–425.

30. Kudoh A, Katagai H, Takazawa T. Antidepressant treatment for chronic depressed patients should not be discontinued prior to anesthesia. *Can J Anaesth* 2002;49(2):132–136.

31. Kudoh A. [Preoperative evaluation, preparation and prognosis in depressed patients]. *Masui* 2010;59(9):1116–1127.

32. van Haelst IM, Egberts TC, Doodeman HJ, et al. Use of serotonergic antidepressants and bleeding risk in orthopedic patients. *Anesthesiology* 2010; 112(3):631–636.

33. Smith PJ, Attix DK, Weldon BC, et al. Executive function and depression as independent risk factors for postoperative delirium. *Anesthesiology* 2009;110(4):781–787.

34. Sharma V. Management of bipolar II disorder during pregnancy and the postpartum period–Motherisk Update. 2008. *Can J Clin Pharmacol* 2009;16(1):e33–e41.

35. Viguera AC, Whitfield T, Baldessarini RJ, et al. Risk of recurrence in women with bipolar disorder during pregnancy: prospective study of mood stabilizer discontinuation. *Am J Psychiatry* 2007;164(12):1817–1824; quiz 1923.

36. Newport DJ, Calamaras MR, DeVane CL, et al. Atypical antipsychotic administration during late pregnancy: placental passage and obstetrical outcomes. *Am J Psychiatry* 2007;164(8):1214–1220.

37. Dickson RA, Hogg L. Pregnancy of a patient treated with clozapine. *Psychiatr Serv* 1998;49(8):1081–1083.

38. Gentile S. Clinical utilization of atypical antipsychotics in pregnancy and lactation. *Ann Pharmacother* 2004;38(7-8):1265–1271.

39. Nguyen HN, Lalonde P. [Clozapine and pregnancy]. *Encephale* 2003;29(2):119–124.

40. Newham JJ, Thomas SH, MacRitchie K, et al. Birth weight of infants after maternal exposure to typical and atypical antipsychotics: prospective comparison study. *Br J Psychiatry* 2008;192(5):333–337.

41. Viguera AC, Koukopoulos A, Muzina DJ, et al. Teratogenicity and anticonvulsants: lessons from neurology to psychiatry. *J Clin Psychiatry* 2007;68(Suppl 9):29–33.

42. Viguera AC, Nonacs R, Cohen LS, et al. Risk of recurrence of bipolar disorder in pregnant and nonpregnant women after discontinuing lithium maintenance. *Am J Psychiatry* 2000;157(2):179–184.

43. Deave T, Heron J, Evans J, Emond A. The impact of maternal depression in pregnancy on early child development. *BJOG* 2008;115(8):1043–1051.

44. Dunne FJ. Lithium toxicity: the importance of clinical signs. *Br J Hosp Med (Lond)* 2010;71(4):206–210.

45. Blake LD, Lucas DN, Aziz K, et al. Lithium toxicity and the parturient: case report and literature review. *Int J Obstet Anesth* 2008;17(2):164–169.

46. Davidson JR, Zhang W, Connor KM, et al. A psychopharmacological treatment algorithm for generalised anxiety disorder (GAD). *J Psychopharmacol* 2010;24(1):3–26.

47. Uguz F, Gezginc K, Kayhan F, et al. Is pregnancy associated with mood and anxiety disorders? A cross-sectional study. *Gen Hosp Psychiatry* 2010;32(2):213–215.

48. Ross LE, McLean LM. Anxiety disorders during pregnancy and the postpartum period: A systematic review. *J Clin Psychiatry* 2006;67(8):1285–1298.

49. Levine RE, Oandasan AP, Primeau LA, et al. Anxiety disorders during pregnancy and postpartum. *Am J Perinatol* 2003;20(5):239–248.

50. Qiu C, Williams MA, Calderon-Margalit R, et al. Preeclampsia risk in relation to maternal mood and anxiety disorders diagnosed before or during early pregnancy. *Am J Hypertens* 2009;22(4):397–402.

51. Brown CS. Depression and anxiety disorders. *Obstet Gynecol Clin North Am* 2001;28(2):241–268.

52. Einarson A. Risks/safety of psychotropic medication use during pregnancy–Motherisk Update 2008. *Can J Clin Pharmacol* 2009;16(1):e58–e65.

53. Iqbal MM, Sobhan T, Aftab SR, et al. Diazepam use during pregnancy: a review of the literature. *Del Med J* 2002;74(3):127–135.

54. King NM, Chambers J, O'Donnell K, et al. Anxiety, depression and saliva cortisol in women with a medical disorder during pregnancy. *Arch Womens Ment Health* 2010;13(4):339–345.

55. Vythilingum B. Anxiety disorders in pregnancy. *Curr Psychiatry Rep* 2008; 10(4):331–335.

56. Rubinchik SM, Kablinger AS, Gardner JS. Medications for panic disorder and generalized anxiety disorder during pregnancy. *Prim Care Companion J Clin Psychiatry* 2005;7(3):100–105.

57. Northcott CJ, Stein MB. Panic disorder in pregnancy. *J Clin Psychiatry* 1994;55(12):539–542.

58. Marchesi C. Pharmacological management of panic disorder. *Neuropsychiatr Dis Treat* 2008;4(1):93–106.

59. Hertzberg T, Wahlbeck K. The impact of pregnancy and puerperium on panic disorder: a review. *J Psychosom Obstet Gynaecol* 1999;20(2):59–64.

60. Meshberg-Cohen S, Svikis D. Panic disorder, trait anxiety, and alcohol use in pregnant and nonpregnant women. *Compr Psychiatry* 2007;48(6):504–510.

61. Bandelow B, Sojka F, Broocks A, et al. Panic disorder during pregnancy and postpartum period. *Eur Psychiatry* 2006;21(7):495–500.

62. Fontenelle LF, Hasler G. The analytical epidemiology of obsessive-compulsive disorder: risk factors and correlates. *Prog Neuropsychopharmacol Biol Psychiatry* 2008;32(1):1–15.

63. Weinstock L, Cohen LS, Bailey JW, et al. Obstetrical and neonatal outcome following clonazepam use during pregnancy: a case series. *Psychother Psychosom* 2001;70(3):158–162.

64. Keifer RB, Stirt JA. Preoxygenation. *Anesthesiology* 1995;83(2):429.

65. Sedgwick JV, Lewis IH, Linter SP. Anesthesia and mental illness. *Int J Psychiatry Med* 1990;20(3):209–225.
66. Udechuku A, Nguyen T, Hill R, et al. Antidepressants in pregnancy: a systematic review. *Aust N Z J Psychiatry* 2010;44(11):978–996.
67. Ellfolk M, Malm H. Risks associated with in utero and lactation exposure to selective serotonin reuptake inhibitors (SSRIs). *Reprod Toxicol* 2010;30(2):249–260.
68. Furukawa TA, McGuire H, Barbui C. Meta-analysis of effects and side effects of low dosage tricyclic antidepressants in depression: systematic review. *BMJ* 2002;325(7371):991.
69. Ables AZ, Nagubilli R. Prevention, recognition, and management of serotonin syndrome. *Am Fam Physician* 2010;81(9):1139–1142.
70. Nisijima K, Shioda K, Iwamura T. Neuroleptic malignant syndrome and serotonin syndrome. *Prog Brain Res* 2007;162:81–104.
71. Bell GL, Lau K. Perinatal and neonatal issues of substance abuse. *Pediatr Clin North Am* 1995;42(2):261–281.
72. Glantz JC, Woods JR Jr. Obstetrical issues in substance abuse. *Pediatr Ann* 1991;20(10):531–539.
73. Shankaran S, Lester BM, Das A, et al. Impact of maternal substance use during pregnancy on childhood outcome. *Semin Fetal Neonatal Med* 2007;12(2):143–150.
74. Bennett AD. Perinatal substance abuse and the drug-exposed neonate. *Adv Nurse Pract* 1999;7(5):32–36; quiz 37–38.
75. Bolnick JM, Rayburn WF. Substance use disorders in women: special considerations during pregnancy. *Obstet Gynecol Clin North Am* 2003;30(3):545–558, vii.
76. Sprauve ME. Substance abuse and HIV pregnancy. *Clin Obstet Gynecol* 1996;39(2):316–332.
77. CDC. Population-Based Prevalence of Perinatal Exposure to Cocaine. *MMWR—Morbidity and Mortality Weekly Report* 1995;45(41):887–891.
78. Fein G, Di Sclafani V. Cerebral reserve capacity: implications for alcohol and drug abuse. *Alcohol* 2004;32(1):63–67.
79. Loser H. [Alcohol and pregnancy–embryopathy and alcohol effects]. *Ther Umsch* 2000;57(4):246–252.
80. Spies C, Tonnesen H, Andreasson S, et al. Perioperative morbidity and mortality in chronic alcoholic patients. *Alcohol Clin Exp Res* 2001;25(5 Suppl ISBRA):164S–170S.
81. Lau A, von Dossow V, Sander M, et al. Alcohol use disorder and perioperative immune dysfunction. *Anesth Analg* 2009;108(3):916–920.
82. Vagts DA, Iber T, Noldge-Schomburg GF. [Alcohol–a perioperative problem of anaesthesia and intensive care medicine]. *Anasthesiol Intensivmed Notfallmed Schmerzther* 2003;38(12):747–761.
83. SAaMHSA NIoDA. Results From the 2008 National Survey on Drug Use and Health: National Findings. U.S. Department of Health and Human Services. Rockville, MD; 2009.
84. Bandstra ES, Vogel AL, Morrow CE, et al. Severity of prenatal cocaine exposure and child language functioning through age seven years: a longitudinal latent growth curve analysis. *Subst Use Misuse* 2004;39(1):25–59.
85. Beeghly M, Martin B, Rose-Jacobs R, et al. Prenatal cocaine exposure and children's language functioning at 6 and 9.5 years: moderating effects of child age, birthweight, and gender. *J Pediatr Psychol* 2006;31(1):98–115.
86. Woods JR Jr, Plessinger MA. Pregnancy increases cardiovascular toxicity to cocaine. *Am J Obstet Gynecol* 1990;162(2):529–533.
87. Gingras JL, Weese-Mayer DE, Hume RF Jr, et al. Cocaine and development: mechanisms of fetal toxicity and neonatal consequences of prenatal cocaine exposure. *Early Hum Dev* 1992;31(1):1–24.
88. Kuczkowski KM. The cocaine abusing parturient: a review of anesthetic considerations. *Can J Anaesth* 2004;51(2):145–154.
89. MacGregor SN, Keith LG, Chasnoff IJ, et al. Cocaine use during pregnancy: adverse perinatal outcome. *Am J Obstet Gynecol* 1987;157(3):686–690.
90. Zimmerman EF. Substance abuse in pregnancy: teratogenesis. *Pediatr Ann* 1991;20(10):541–544, 546–547.
91. Winklbaur B, Kopf N, Ebner N, et al. Treating pregnant women dependent on opioids is not the same as treating pregnancy and opioid dependence: a knowledge synthesis for better treatment for women and neonates. *Addiction* 2008;103(9):1429–1440.
92. OoAS S. The DASIS Report: Cocaine Route of Administration Trends: 1995–2005. Drug and Alcohol Services Information System (DASIS) Rockville, MD; 2007.
93. Ludlow J, Christmas T, Paech MJ, et al. Drug abuse and dependency during pregnancy: anaesthetic issues. *Anaesth Intensive Care* 2007;35(6):881–893.
94. Kuczkowski KM. Anesthetic implications of drug abuse in pregnancy. *J Clin Anesth* 2003;15(5):382–394.
95. Kuczkowski KM. The effects of drug abuse on pregnancy. *Curr Opin Obstet Gynecol* 2007;19(6):578–585.
96. Kuczkowski KM. Labor analgesia for the drug abusing parturient: is there cause for concern? *Obstet Gynecol Surv* 2003;58(9):599–608.
97. Kuczkowski KM, Birnbach D, van Zundert A. Drug abuse in the parturient. *Sem Anesthesiol Periop Med Pain* 2000;19:216–224.
98. Hollander JE. The management of cocaine-associated myocardial ischemia. *N Engl J Med* 1995;333(19):1267–1272.
99. Boylan JF, Cheng DC, Sandler AN, et al. Cocaine toxicity and isoflurane anesthesia: hemodynamic, myocardial metabolic, and regional blood flow effects in swine. *J Cardiothorac Vasc Anesth* 1996;10(6):772–777.
100. Murphy JL Jr. Hypertension and pulmonary oedema associated with ketamine administration in a patient with a history of substance abuse. *Can J Anaesth* 1993;40(2):160–164.
101. Sacker A, Done DJ, Crow TJ. Obstetric complications in children born to parents with schizophrenia: a meta-analysis of case-control studies. *Psychol Med* 1996;26(2):279–287.
102. Hirschfeld RM, Lewis L, Vornik LA. Perceptions and impact of bipolar disorder: how far have we really come? Results of the national depressive and manic-depressive association 2000 survey of individuals with bipolar disorder. *J Clin Psychiatry* 2003;64(2):161–174.
103. Tondo L, Isacsson G, Baldessarini R. Suicidal behaviour in bipolar disorder: risk and prevention. *CNS Drugs* 2003;17(7):491–511.
104. Hilty DM, Kelly RH, Hales RE. Diagnosis and treatment of bipolar disorder in pregnant women. *Prim Care Update Ob Gyns* 2000;7(3):105–112.
105. Einarson A, Boskovic R. Use and safety of antipsychotic drugs during pregnancy. *J Psychiatr Pract* 2009;15(3):183–192.
106. Kudoh A, Katagai H, Takazawa T. Anesthesia with ketamine, propofol, and fentanyl decreases the frequency of postoperative psychosis emergence and confusion in schizophrenic patients. *J Clin Anesth* 2002;14(2):107–110.
107. Chaudron LH, Nirodi N. The obsessive-compulsive spectrum in the perinatal period: a prospective pilot study. *Arch Womens Ment Health* 2010;13(5):403–410.
108. Hans SL. Demographic and psychosocial characteristics of substance-abusing pregnant women. *Clin Perinatol* 1999;26(1):55–74.
109. Akman C, Uguz F, Kaya N. Postpartum-onset major depression is associated with personality disorders. *Compr Psychiatry* 2007;48(4):343–347.
110. Uguz F, Gezginc K, Zeytinci IE, et al. Obsessive-compulsive disorder in pregnant women during the third trimester of pregnancy. *Compr Psychiatry* 2007;48(5):441–445.
111. Forray A, Focseneanu M, Pittman B, et al. Onset and exacerbation of obsessive-compulsive disorder in pregnancy and the postpartum period. *J Clin Psychiatry* 2010;71(8):1061–1068.
112. James DC. Eating disorders, fertility, and pregnancy: relationships and complications. *J Perinat Neonatal Nurs* 2001;15(2):36–48; quiz 32 p following 82.
113. Mhyre JM, Riesner MN, Polley LS, Naughton NN. A series of anesthesia-related maternal deaths in Michigan, 1985–2003. *Anesthesiology* 2007;106(6):1096–1104.
114. Norman RJ, Clark AM. Obesity and reproductive disorders: a review. *Reprod Fertil Dev* 1998;10(1):55–63.
115. Roofthooft E. Anesthesia for the morbidly obese parturient. *Curr Opin Anaesthesiol* 2009;22(3):341–346.
116. Cohen LS, Wang B, Nonacs R, et al. Treatment of mood disorders during pregnancy and postpartum. *Psychiatr Clin North Am* 2010;33(2):273–293.
117. DeVane CL, Stowe ZN, Donovan JL, et al. Therapeutic drug monitoring of psychoactive drugs during pregnancy in the genomic era: challenges and opportunities. *J Psychopharmacol* 2006;20(4 Suppl):54–59.
118. Meador KJ, Baker GA, Browning N, et al. Cognitive function at 3 years of age after fetal exposure to antiepileptic drugs. *N Engl J Med* 2009;360(16):1597–1605.
119. Bromiker R, Kaplan M. Apparent intrauterine fetal withdrawal from clomipramine hydrochloride. *JAMA* 1994;272(22):1722–1723.
120. Nulman I, Rovet J, Stewart DE, et al. Child development following exposure to tricyclic antidepressants or fluoxetine throughout fetal life: a prospective, controlled study. *Am J Psychiatry* 2002;159(11):1889–1895.
121. Pearson KH, Nonacs RM, Viguera AC, et al. Birth outcomes following prenatal exposure to antidepressants. *J Clin Psychiatry* 2007;68(8):1284–1289.
122. Slone D, Siskind V, Heinonen OP, et al. Antenatal exposure to the phenothiazines in relation to congenital malformations, perinatal mortality rate, birth weight, and intelligence quotient score. *Am J Obstet Gynecol* 1977;128(5):486–488.
123. Diav-Citrin O, Shechtman S, Ornoy S, et al. Safety of haloperidol and penfluridol in pregnancy: a multicenter, prospective, controlled study. *J Clin Psychiatry* 2005;66(3):317–322.
124. McKenna K, Koren G, Tetelbaum M, et al. Pregnancy outcome of women using atypical antipsychotic drugs: a prospective comparative study. *J Clin Psychiatry* 2005;66(4):444–449; quiz 546.
125. Coppola D, Russo LJ, Kwarta RF Jr, et al. Evaluating the postmarketing experience of risperidone use during pregnancy: pregnancy and neonatal outcomes. *Drug Saf* 2007;30(3):247–264.
126. Reis M, Kallen B. Maternal use of antipsychotics in early pregnancy and delivery outcome. *J Clin Psychopharmacol* 2008;28(3):279–288.

127. Stopping antidepressant use while pregnant may pose risks. National Institute of Mental Health. http://www.nimh.nih.gov/science-news/2006/stopping-anti-depressant-use-while-pregnant-may-pose-risks.shtml. Accessed Aug. 20, 2009.

128. How is depression treated and diagnosed? National Institute of Mental Health. http://www.nimh.nih.gov/health/publications/women-and-depression-discovering-hope/how-is-depression-diagnosed-and-treated.shtml. Accessed Aug. 20, 2009.

129. Misri S, Lusskin SI. Management of depression in pregnant women. http://www.uptodate.com/contents/depression-in-pregnant-women-management. Accessed Oct. 02, 2012.

130. Louik C, Lin AE, Werler MM, et al. First-trimester use of selective serotonin reuptake inhibitors and the risk of birth defects. N Engl J Med 2007;356:2675.

131. Wisner KL, Sit DK, Hanusa BH, et al. Major depression and antidepressant treatment: impact on pregnancy and neonatal outcomes. Am J Psychiatry 2009;166:557.

132. Chambers CD, Hernandez-Diaz S, Van Marter LJ, et al. Selective serotonin-reuptake inhibitors and risk of persistent pulmonary hypertension of the newborn. N Engl J Med 2006;354:579.

133. Freeman MP. Antenatal depression: Navigating the treatment dilemmas. Am J Psychiatry 2007;164:1162.

134. Parry BL. Assessing risk and benefit: to treat or not to treat major depression during pregnancy with antidepressant medication. Am J Psychiatry 2009; 166:512.

135. Hendrick V, Altshuler L. Management of major depression during pregnancy. Am J Psychiatry 2002;159:1667.

136. Yonkers KA, Wisner KL, Stewart DE, et al. The management of depression during pregnancy: a report from the American Psychiatric Association and the American College of Obstetricians and Gynecologists. Obstet Gynecol 2009;114:703.

137. Depression during pregnancy: treatment recommendations. American College of Obstetricians and Gynecologists. http://www.acog.org/from_home/publications/press_releases/nr08-21-09-1.cfm. Accessed Aug. 21, 2009.

138. Drugs: treatment challenges of depression in pregnancy and the possibility of persistent pulmonary hypertension in newborns. U.S. Food and Drug Administration. http://www.fda.gov/Drugs/DrugSafety/PublicHealthAdvisories/ucm124348.htm. Accessed Sept. 2, 2009.

139. Sackett JC, Weller RA, Weller EB. Selective serotonin reuptake inhibitor use during pregnancy and possible neonatal complications. Curr Psychiatry Rep 2009;11:253.

140. Maschi S, Clavenna A, Campi R, et al. Neonatal outcome following pregnancy exposure to antidepressants: a prospective controlled cohort study. BJOG 2008; 115:283.

141. Dell D. Mood and Anxiety Disorders. Clinical Update on Women's Health Care. Seattle, WA, 2008;7:1 http://www.clinicalupdates.org/.

142. The American College of Obstetricians and Gynecologists Committee on Practice Bulletins—Obstetrics. Use of psychiatric medications during pregnancy and lactation. ACOG Practice Bulletin 2008;92:1.

143. Paxil (prescribing information). Research Triangle Park, NC.: GlaxoSmithKline; 2009. http://us.gsk.com/products/assets/us_paxil.pdf. Accessed Sept. 2, 2009.

144. Prozac (prescribing information). Indianapolis, Ind.: Eli Lilly and Company; 2009. http://pi.lilly.com/us/prozac.pdf?reqNavId=undefined. Accessed Sept. 2, 2009.

145. Zoloft (prescribing information). New York, NY.: Pfizer; 2009. http://media.pfizer.com/files/products/uspi_zoloft.pdf. Accessed Sept. 2, 2009.

146. Wellbutrin (prescribing information). Research Triangle Park, NC.: GlaxoSmithKline; 2009. http://us.gsk.com/products/assets/us_wellbutrin_tablets.pdf. Accessed Sept. 2, 2009.

147. Celexa (prescribing information). St. Louis, Mo.: Forest Pharmaceuticals; 2009. http://www.frx.com/pi/celexa_pi.pdf. Accessed Sept. 2, 2009.

148. Health care guideline: Major depression in adults in primary care. Bloomington, Minn.: Institute for Clinical Systems Improvement. http://www.icsi.org/depression_5/depression_major_in_adults_in_primary_care_3.html. Accessed Sept. 3, 2009.

149. Cohen LS, Altshuler LL, Harlow BL, et al. Relapse of major depression during pregnancy in women who maintain or discontinue antidepressant treatment. JAMA 2006;295:499.

150. Alwan S, Reefhuis J, Rasmussen SA, et al. The use of selective serotonin-reuptake inhibitors in pregnancy and the risk of birth defects. N Engl J Med 2007;356:2684.

151. Passov V (expert opinion). Mayo Clinic, Rochester, Minn. Sept. 18, 2009.

152. Pedersen LH, Henriksen TB, Vestergaard M, et al. Selective serotonin reuptake inhibitors in pregnancy and congenital malformations: Population based cohort study. Br Med J 2009;339:b3569.

153. Moore KM (expert opinion). Mayo Clinic, Rochester, Minn. Sept. 25, 2009.

154. Cunningham FG, et al. Williams Obstetrics. 22nd ed. New York, N.Y.: McGraw Hill Companies Inc.:2005. http://www.accessmedicine.com/resourceTOC.aspx?resourceID=46. Accessed Sept. 27, 2009.

155. Berger MS. Neurosurgery and surgery of the pituitary. In: Doherty GM, ed. Current Surgical Diagnosis and Treatment. 12th ed. New York, N.Y.: McGraw Hill Companies Inc.: 2006. http://www.accessmedicine.com/content.aspx?aID=2068298. Accessed Sept. 27, 2009.

CHAPTER

40

Parturient with Pre-existing Congenital Anomalies

David G. Mann

■ GENERAL APPROACH TO PATIENT WITH A PRE-EXISTING CONGENITAL ANOMALY

A pre-existing congenital anomaly is frequently the result of some genetic syndrome, which is composed of several recognizable phenotypic traits that occur together in a specific association. It is believed that this association of phenotypic traits is the result of a specific genetic defect. Currently a geneticist (or dysmorphologist) identifies the syndrome or association using the patient's phenotype; however, in the future, more of these diagnoses will be made using molecular genetics to identify the patient's chromosomal defect(s) which resulted in the particular phenotype and inheritance pattern. Some of the more common genetic disorders (syndromes) are diagnosed using conventional karyotyping, chromosomal microarray (CMA), or fluorescence in situ hybridization (FISH), performed on peripheral blood lymphocytes. Presumably the genetic basis for many syndromes and associations which do not currently have a known cause will be determined. The term association is used when a constellation of several recognizable phenotypic traits occur together, either without a known genetic cause, or with a variety of genetic causes. Unfortunately, the distinction between a syndrome and an association frequently is not clear, and these terms are routinely used interchangeably. Historically patients with genetic syndromes and associations received care from our colleagues in pediatric anesthesia. However, given the advances in pediatric anesthesiology and surgery over the last 50 years, these children with syndromes have grown up to become the parturient with a pre-existing congenital anomaly. As such, many of these women will require analgesia for labor and delivery, anesthesia for surgical deliveries, and/or non-obstetric therapeutic procedures performed during pregnancy. The implication is that obstetric anesthesiologists should expect to encounter patients with a syndrome more frequently. This chapter will first review the general approach to the pregnant patient with a genetic syndrome, and then review in more detail some syndromes associated with challenges in providing anesthetic care. Finally, a listing of selected syndromes associated with anesthetic management issues will be presented.

■ AIRWAY CONSIDERATIONS

Airway management is always a central consideration for the obstetric anesthesiologist and many genetic syndromes are associated with an abnormal airway even before the pregnancy-induced changes to the airway occur. Some of the most common are syndromes associated with mandibular hypoplasia, including Crouzon syndrome (craniofacial dysostosis), Pierre Robin sequence (PRS), Treacher Collins syndrome (TCS) (mandibulofacial dysostosis), and Goldenhar syndrome (hemifacial microsomia). Other conditions include cleft lip and palate, high-arched palate with small mouth opening, cervical vertebral fusion limiting neck movement, and soft tissue obstruction from macroglossia or other causes. Eliciting a thorough preoperative history of airway issues, including snoring, airway obstruction while sleeping, and acute life-threatening events, is extremely important. Speaking with the parturient in order to identify and review any previous anesthetics and tracheal intubations is crucial, and whenever possible examining the previous anesthetic records or speaking to the previous anesthesiologist and/or otolaryngologist is also important. An examination of the airway for mouth opening, visualization of the pharynx, and soft palate, and neck range of motion, should only be performed by an experienced anesthesiologist. Finally, existing imaging studies such as chest, neck, and facial radiographs, CT scans, or MRI scans should be reviewed. It may be prudent to obtain airway imaging studies given that the radiation exposure risks to a properly shielded third-trimester fetus are minimal when compared to the risks to the parturient and her fetus in a "can't intubate, can't ventilate" scenario. A management plan, specific for this parturient's difficult airway should be developed. Details of difficult airway management are presented in Chapter 24.

■ CARDIAC MANIFESTATIONS

Many genetic syndromes include a cardiac component, and the importance of a thorough cardiac history and physical examination cannot be overemphasized. In the presence of an abnormal cardiac examination consisting most often of murmurs, the cardiac anatomy and pathophysiology must be understood, and any recent diagnostic studies such as echocardiography must be reviewed. Many of these women will be followed by a pediatric cardiologist who should be contacted in order to discuss specific issues related to this patient's cardiopulmonary physiology. Echocardiographic studies should be interpreted by a cardiologist who is comfortable with congenital cardiac lesions, both repaired and unrepaired, and the pregnancy-induced changes in cardiopulmonary physiology. Some congenital anomalies are associated with cardiac conduction abnormalities mandating that an electrocardiogram be performed and reviewed. The pathophysiology and anesthetic management of common cardiac diseases (Ebstein's anomaly, Eisenmenger's syndrome, Long QT syndrome, and Wolff–Parkinson–White syndrome) are discussed in Chapter 30.

NEURODEVELOPMENTAL ABNORMALITIES

Some genetic syndromes include central or peripheral nervous systems anomalies, such as the neuromuscular disorders and neurocutaneous syndromes. For these types of anomalies, assessing the location of the lesion (e.g., lumbar epidural space, intracardiac, etc.), changes in intracranial pressure (ICP), and pre-existing peripheral neuromuscular deficits or paresthesias is extremely important. Other syndromes are associated with neurodevelopmental delay without obvious anatomic malformations. These neurodevelopmental changes may include a generalized lag in intellectual development, difficulties with gross or fine motor skills, abnormal speech and language development, and/or behavioral issues. It is important to assess the neurodevelopmental status of any parturient with a genetic syndrome as the chronologic age may differ significantly from the developmental age. This may make the induction of either neuraxial or general anesthesia challenging and require changes in the approach to preoperative preparation, communication, premedication, and/or the presence of the parturient's support personnel. Many of these women will have experienced multiple medical encounters and interventions, and therefore may be very anxious in the pre-anesthetic period.

VASCULAR ACCESS

Some genetic syndromes are associated with limb abnormalities that make conventional intravenous (IV) access challenging. For these women, IV access should be obtained by an experienced anesthesiologist recognizing that the available options are limited and alternate sites may need to be utilized. These alternate sites may include scalp or anterior chest wall veins, external or internal jugular veins, or subclavian veins if the limbs are unavailable. As noted above, women with genetic syndromes have frequently had multiple hospitalizations and procedures making peripheral venous access potentially difficult or impossible, and further, the central veins may be thrombosed or stenotic from previous catheterizations. Noting the absence of typical superficial veins and the presence of cutaneous collaterals should increase the suspicion of difficult IV access. Consider additional studies, that is, ultrasound or MRI to plan for vascular access. In some cases, obtaining the assistance of an interventional radiologist may be warranted.

ORTHOPEDIC CONSIDERATIONS

Deformities of the spine (scoliosis, kyphosis, etc.), large joints (hip dysplasia), and limbs (contractures) occur commonly in patients with genetic syndromes. Severe scoliosis or kyphosis should prompt an evaluation of the woman's respiratory and cardiac status as this may initiate planning for postoperative ventilation and intensive care monitoring. Neuraxial anesthesia/analgesia may be technically challenging to administer and achieving an adequate block may be difficult when spread of the drug is impaired or unpredictable. Positioning of anesthetized patients with these problems must be done very carefully to avoid injury.

OTHER CONSIDERATIONS

Devising a rational and safe anesthetic plan for parturients with rare disorders, or disorders with which the anesthesiologist is not familiar, may be challenging. Consulting a reference source (typically found in the pediatric anesthesia literature) will be necessary in order to become familiar with the issues involved in the specific syndrome. An excellent general source

is the U.S. National Institutes of Health website which can be found at health.nih.gov/category/GeneticsBirthDefects (1). Other published resources are available; including both general review articles (2,3) and textbooks (4). It is becoming more prudent for the obstetric anesthesiologist to have these resources at hand since parturients with pre-existing congenital anomalies will be presenting more frequently. If the first presentation coincides with her time of delivery, a thorough literature search may not be possible. Recall that the patient, her family, and other caregivers may be extremely knowledgeable of the condition, and may be able to offer valuable information about how the parturient has previously responded to specific interventions.

MANAGEMENT OF COMMON IMPORTANT SYNDROMES

Trisomy 21 (Down Syndrome)

Down syndrome (DS), or Trisomy 21, is the most commonly identified genetic form of mental retardation, and the leading genetic cause of specific birth defects and medical conditions (5). Defying the notion that women with Trisomy 21 are infertile, Lin et al. reported 31 pregnancies in 27 women (6), so DS is discussed here to establish a template for approaching the parturient with a pre-existing genetic disorder.

DS patients have a number of characteristic facial features that vary by ethnicity, which include microbrachycephaly, midface hypoplasia with small nose, eyes, ears, upslanting palpebral fissures, and relatively large tongue. Also common are single transverse palmar creases, atlantoaxial instability, and pelvic hypoplasticity with joint laxity. Issues with neurodevelopment include mental retardation, developmental delay, and hypotonia. Congenital heart disease (CHD) occurs in about 50% of DS patients, typically consisting of complete atrioventricular canal defects, but may be ventricular septal defects (VSDs), tetralogy of Fallot (ToF), or others. Lesions with hemodynamically significant shunts will most likely have been surgically repaired; introducing possible iatrogenic (in addition to congenital) conduction system dysfunction. In addition, DS patients tend to develop pulmonary hypertension, earlier and to greater severity, than non-DS patients with the same congenital cardiac lesion. DS patients with unrepaired CHD should be evaluated for Eisenmenger syndrome. Particularly in patients with cyanosis, pulmonary hypertension, subacute bacterial endocarditis, and/or stroke, the pulmonary artery pressures should be evaluated; echocardiography is usually sufficient for this purpose. It has been reported that most DS adults have no clinically significant cardiac disease; although mitral valve prolapsed (MVP) may be a late development.

Airway obstruction occurs in patients with DS. In children this is caused by a relatively flat midface with a constricted oropharyngeal space, small nasal passages, and the relatively large tongue, tonsils, and adenoids. The resulting obstructive sleep apnea may further exacerbate any pulmonary hypertension. Despite the propensity for upper airway obstruction, most DS patients are easy to mask ventilate and intubate using direct laryngoscopy.

Atlantooccipital instability occurs in up to 15% of DS patients. This is defined as excessive movement on cervical flexion–extension radiographs. However, only 2% of these patients are symptomatic and no radiographic study conclusively predicts the risk of spinal cord compromise. Therefore, cervical spine (C-spine) imaging is not indicated in asymptomatic DS patients before receiving an anesthetic (7). Eliciting a history of neck pain or neurologic symptoms with neck movement is important for every DS parturient. Anesthetics involving C-spine manipulation must be approached very cautiously during both airway management and surgical positioning. Careful handling includes avoiding extreme C-spine flexion, extension, and rotation, as well as maintaining the C-spine in the neutral position whenever possible.

Gastrointestinal issues include duodenal atresia or an annular pancreas, and esophageal atresia/tracheoesophageal fistula (EA/TEF). The DS parturient may present with residual tracheal stenosis or malesia if she underwent a TEF repair in infancy. Celiac disease is reported to occur in 5% to 15% of DS children and no data exists on the prevalence in DS adults (7).

Between 3% and 54% of DS patients have thyroid disorders and the frequency of occurrence increases with age (7). This is particularly important during periods of physiologic stress, as during parturition or the perioperative period, where a subclinical state may be unmasked. The hypothyroid state may affect cardiac function by desensitizing the myocardium to both endogenous and exogenous catecholamines. This makes thyroid function testing in the DS parturient seem prudent.

Finally, vascular access may be challenging in DS parturients. Peripheral IV access may be difficult with increased adipose tissue; internal jugular access may be difficult with a short-webbed neck and increased adipose tissue; and radial arterial access may be difficult given the small caliber of this artery (8).

DIFFICULT AIRWAY SYNDROMES: CROUZON SYNDROME (CRANIOFACIAL DYSOSTOSIS), GOLDENHAR SYNDROME (HEMIFACIAL MICROSOMIA), PIERRE ROBIN SEQUENCE, TREACHER COLLINS SYNDROME

For the obstetric anesthesiologist, a difficult airway to perform tracheal intubation is expected to result from pregnancy-induced changes to the normal airway; whereas our pediatric anesthesiologists expect syndromes which manifest mandibular anomalies, hemifacial microsomia, and/or micrognathia to be the cause; so they (and now we) must evaluate every patient in order to identify these abnormal airways. A number of craniofacial syndromes lead to mandibular anomalies (e.g., Apert syndrome), craniofacial dysostosis (e.g., Crouzon syndrome), hemifacial microsomia (e.g., Goldenhar syndrome), and micrognathia, including the Pierre Robin sequence and TCS. To date, only a few case reports exist addressing the anesthetic management of parturients with difficult airway syndromes, such as Crouzon syndrome (9) and TCS (10).

Apert syndrome is characterized by midfacial malformations such as hypoplasia or underdevelopment of the midface complex, craniosynostosis, and symmetric syndactyly of both hands and feet. Reportedly it occurs in approximately 1:60,000 births (11), approximately 20% to 30% of Apert patients are developmentally delayed, and many will need staged surgery in order to ameliorate their turribrachycephaly (cone-shaped skull) and midface hypoplasia. The craniofacial surgeries are intended to create a cranial vault that will accommodate the growing brain to ameliorate increases in ICP. However, in Apert's patients, raised ICP also results from abnormal intracranial venous drainage, hydrocephalus, and airway obstruction; and is known to recur despite successful treatment (12). A number of factors contribute to their difficult airway. The midface grows more slowly and the forward development stops before 10 years of age; therefore, the deepest part of the face occurs just above the nose. Frequently the maxilla is hypoplastic causing a V-shaped maxillary arch. The soft

palate tends to be long and thick, and the hard palate tends to be short resulting in a constricted, highly arched palate. Excess soft tissue occurs on the hard palate and its size increases with age. In addition, the midface hypoplasia causes a reduction in the caliber of the nasopharyngeal passages leading to difficult, noisy breathing (13). Up to 20% of children with craniofacial deformities will require tracheostomy for airway management, 48% of these are in craniosynostosis (e.g., Apert syndrome) patients. Nearly all of these children will be decannulated following staged surgical interventions (14). As would be expected following tracheostomy decannulation, there is an increased incidence of laryngomalacia, cartilaginous tracheal sleeves, and bronchomalacia in patients with Apert syndrome (15) and the upper airway obstruction and sleep apnea may lead to increasing airway compromise with age, unlike other anomalies such as Pierre Robin syndrome (16). An additional airway complication stems from the C-spine fusion which occurs in >60% of these patients, occurring most commonly at C3–C4 and C5–C6 (17). In a review of craniofacial airway abnormalities, Nargozian C notes that a small midface and proptosis may make mask ventilation challenging because of difficulties in obtaining a good mask fit, the tongue may occlude the oral airway by filling the relatively smaller oral cavity, and small nasopharyngeal passages increase the airflow resistance. Tracheal intubation becomes increasingly difficult as neck mobility decreases and smaller than expected endotracheal tubes (ETTs) may be necessary because of tracheal abnormalities (18). Issues for the anesthesiologist to address include both alterations in ICP, and airway management with abnormalities of the oropharynx, possibly the C-spine, and possibly distal airway changes following tracheostomy reversal.

Crouzon syndrome is characterized by maxillary hypoplasia, craniosynostosis, midface underdevelopment and ocular proptosis. It is estimated to occur in approximately 1:60,000 live births (19). All Crouzon syndrome patients have ocular proptosis. Their craniosynostosis, premature cranial suture fusion, leads to a variety of cranial malformations including brachycephaly (broad, short head), scaphocephaly (long, narrow head), trigonocephaly (triangular-shaped head when viewed from above), and cloverleaf skull (actually shaped like a cloverleaf). Many will need staged surgery in order to ameliorate their craniosynostosis and midface hypoplasia. A number of factors contribute to a difficult airway. As with Apert's, the midface grows more slowly and forward development arrests. Both the length and width of the maxilla is reduced, and is pushed back farther than normal causing an arched appearance. In addition, the midface hypoplasia causes a reduction in the caliber of the nasopharyngeal passages leading to difficult, noisy breathing (13). Progressive C-spine fusion occurs in approximately 18% of these patients, most commonly at C2–C3 and C5–C6 and "butterfly" vertebrae are particularly prevalent (20). Sculerati et al. reported that 20% of children with craniofacial deformities will require tracheostomy for airway management, 48% of these are in craniosynostosis (e.g., Crouzon syndrome) patients. Nearly all of these children will be decannulated following staged surgical interventions (14). This would give rise to an increased incidence of cartilaginous tracheal sleeve, challenging mask ventilation, and decreasing neck mobility with increasing difficulties in tracheal intubation in patients with Crouzon syndrome. The overriding issue for the anesthesiologist to address is airway management with abnormalities of the oropharynx, possibly the C-spine, and possibly distal airway changes following tracheotomy reversal. In caring for a Crouzon's parturient with preeclampsia and morbid obesity, Martin et al. reported successful use of an epidural catheter for labor analgesia. A cesarean delivery became necessary for obstetric indications. The patient experienced progressive respiratory failure unresponsive to non-invasive ventilation. A general endotracheal anesthetic was indicated for respiratory failure; an awake fiberoptic intubation was only successful on the third attempt, with the use of an intubating laryngeal mask airway (AMA). Following delivery, an elective tracheostomy was performed for postoperative management of the patient's respiratory failure (9).

Goldenhar syndrome, a hemifacial microsomia variant, arises from (typically unilateral) disordered developmental of the first and second branchial arches. It affects approximately 1 in 5,600 live births and is characterized by malformations of the external/middle ear with sensorineural hearing loss, the mandible (hypoplasia), the eye such as microphthalmus and epibulbar dermoids, and the vertebrae such as C-spine malformations, cervicothoracic scoliosis, and spina bifida occulta. The phenotypic spectrum of Goldenhar syndrome ranges from the very mild hemifacial asymmetry with preauricular ear tags or pits to severe facial deformity and mandibular hypoplasia (21). Goldenhar syndrome patients have a high incidence of congenital C-spine malformations, such as odontoid hypoplasia with C1–C2 instability significant enough to require surgical fusion (22). Difficulties with airway management and tracheal intubation occur commonly due to the mandibular hypoplasia, restricted mouth opening following jaw/temporomandibular joint reconstruction, C-spine instability or limited flexion following spinal fusion, and tracheal deviation with significant cervicothoracic scoliosis (18). Techniques such as fiberoptic or video-assisted laryngoscopy are frequently required for airway management (23,24). Congenital heart defects are reported in approximately 32% of these patients, frequently involving defects of the conotruncus (39%) and septum (32%) (25). Issues for the anesthesiologist to address include both airway management with abnormalities of the oropharynx, possibly the C-spine, and possibly distal airway changes following tracheotomy reversal as well as cardiac function with repaired or unrepaired congenital heart defects.

PRS is composed of retrognathia, glossoptosis, airway obstruction, and high-arched midline soft palate cleft in 50% (26). The defining criteria for PRS are variable; some do not require a cleft palate and others require respiratory compromise as part of the definition. This results in a wide range when estimating the incidence; but approximately 1 per 8,500 live births, with childhood mortality occurring in approximately 25%. Deformational (isolated) PRS, accounting for approximately 40%, results from physical forces in utero inhibiting normal mandible/palatal development. Isolated PRS has a good prognosis since post-natal mandibular catch-up growth is expected. Malformational PRS (part of another syndrome) has a less favorable prognosis and is most associated with Stickler syndrome and velocardiofacial syndrome. In the neonatal period, minimal intervention may be required for mildly affected patients whereas prone positioning, continuous positive airway pressure, endotracheal intubation, or tracheostomy may be required for patients with significant upper airway obstruction. Early in their life, a gastrostomy may be required as feeding difficulties are common and surgical repair of the cleft palate and mandible may significantly improve the outcome. Numerous airway management techniques for patients with PRS are reported in the literature. In the parturient with isolated PRS, an experienced anesthesiologist should perform the airway assessment, review prior anesthetic records, and contact prior anesthesiologists for information regarding this woman's airway and intubation history, then develop a plan for managing her airway in the event that this becomes necessary.

TCS is a disorder of bilateral facial development, which affects approximately 1 in 50,000 live births. Characteristics of TCS include maxilla/zygoma/mandible hypoplasia, lateral downward palpebral fissure sloping, lower eyelid coloboma, external and middle ears malformation, and macrostomia, high palate, and a blind fistula between the angles of the mouth and ears. These patients require extensive bony facial reconstruction which spans decades, including the eyelid coloboma to protect the cornea, orbital and zygomatic reconstruction, external ear reconstruction, and mandibular advancement when bony growth is complete (26). Sculerati et al. reported that 20% of children with craniofacial deformities will require tracheostomy for airway management, 41% of these are in mandibulofacial dysostoses (e.g., TCS) patients. Nearly all of these children will be decannulated following staged surgical interventions (14). In children, the mask ventilation and tracheal intubation difficulties result from the mandibular hypoplasia and high-arched palate and these difficulties may become impossibilities when TMJ abnormalities are present as well (18). It should be presumed that tracheal intubation will become more difficult as the patient grows (27). Both successes and failures for numerous airway management techniques in TCS patients have been reported. In the TCS parturient, an experienced anesthesiologist should perform the airway assessment, review prior anesthetic records and contact prior anesthesiologists for information regarding this woman's airway and intubation history (recalling that the level of difficulty is expected to increase from the prior intubation), and then develop the plan for managing her airway in the event that this becomes necessary. Morillas et al. reported successfully inserting a LMA-Fastrach® for an emergent cesarean section under general anesthesia; however, blind endotracheal intubation was unsuccessful and the surgery was completed using the LMA (10).

■ CARDIAC SYNDROMES: EBSTEIN'S ANOMALY, LONG QT SYNDROME, NOONAN SYNDROME, AND UHL ANOMALY

Although obstetric anesthesiologists care for parturient's with each of these syndromes, only Noonan syndrome and the Uhl anomaly are discussed, since numerous reports addressing the anesthetic management for labor and delivery in these patients exist. Other cardiac syndrome, such as Ebstein's anomaly and Long QT syndrome, are covered in Chapter 30 of this text.

Noonan syndrome, occurring in approximately 1:2,500 live births, is characterized by cardiac defects and distinctive facial features including hypertelorism with downslanting palpebral fissures, ptosis, and low-set posteriorly rotated ears. Cardiovascular manifestations of this syndrome include pulmonary valve stenosis (60%), hypertrophic cardiomyopathy (20%), atrial septal defects (10%), VSDs (5%), and patent ductus arteriosus (3%) (28). Airway abnormalities may include a high-arched palate and micrognathia, which combined with a prominent trapezius muscle leading to neck webbing, may result in a challenging airway to manage (6). Other defects include a "shield chest" and abnormal lymphatic drainage resulting in lymphedema (28). Scoliosis, usually thoracic, is present in approximately 30% of these patients; (29) which combined with a "shield chest" and the changes in functional residual capacity during pregnancy may significantly compromise pulmonary function. Spinal deformities may contribute to difficulty placing an epidural catheter or controlling the block level in those patients with a lumbar spinal curvature may be technically challenging (30). Although these patients may have coagulation or platelet defects including factor XI deficiency, von Willebrand's disease, or thrombocytopenia, (31) which should be considered before placing a neuraxial block, there are numerous reports of successful delivery under spinal anesthesia, (30,32,33) epidural anesthesia/analgesia, (34) combined spinal–epidural anesthesia, (35) and general anesthesia, where the difficult airway was managed by performing an awake fiberoptic intubation (36,37). Dadabhoy et al. reported a failed lumbar epidural placement due to technical difficulty locating the epidural space although a spinal was placed without difficulty; (30) and Grange et al. reported the successful use of 1-deamino-8-D arginine vasopressin (DDAVP) to treat post-partum bleeding attributed to coagulopathy (37). Previously there was concern of MH susceptibility based on a single case report of a possible association; however, there are no other reports or genetic studies establishing a link and many reports of successful anesthetics using both halothane and succinylcholine (38).

Uhl anomaly (arrhythmogenic right ventricular cardiomyopathy [ARVC]) is a familial disease characterized by right ventricular structural and functional abnormalities that result from the replacement of myocardial tissue by fat and fibrous tissue which seems to progress (including possible involvement of the left ventricle) following an inflammatory reaction. Its estimated prevalence is 1:5,000, and it occurs 3 times more frequently in men. The clinical presentation involves phases. No symptoms occur during the "concealed phase"; however, these patients are at risk for sudden cardiac death during exertion. During the "electrical phase," symptomatic arrhythmias occur and morphologic abnormalities are discernable with conventional imaging. Disease progression may result in biventricular heart failure ultimately resembling dilated cardiomyopathy (39). This anomaly was identified post-mortem in 35% of patients during a retrospective analysis of unexpected sudden cardiac death in healthy patients related to surgery and/or anesthesia and included women undergoing cesarean delivery (40). Treatment for the arrhythmias in ARVC include anti-arrhythmic drugs and/or implantable cardioverter-defibrillator (ICD); however, for preventing sudden death, the ICD is superior to anti-arrhythmic drugs (41). In order to avoid labor pain-induced tachycardia and to facilitate an instrumented delivery, the successful use of epidural analgesia has been reported (42,43). In the case reported by Doyle et al, an implantable cardiac defibrillator was placed at 21 weeks' gestation (42). Successful use of general anesthesia for cesarean delivery has also been reported (44).

▪ EPIDERMOLYSIS BULLOSA

Epidermolysis bullosa (EB), a group of bullous skin disorders, is characterized by blister formation resulting from mechanical trauma. EB is generally divided into three major types: EB simplex, involving only the epidermis; junctional EB, involving the basement membrane; and dystrophic EB, involving primarily the dermis (45). Severity of the clinical manifestations is variable, with dystrophic EB (DEB) being the most severe form. Most DEB patients will have blisters and wounds presenting at birth or shortly thereafter. The blister size is variable and the healing process leads to atrophic scarring with contracture development, occurring most commonly on the hands, feet, elbows, and knees (46). Friction, from scratching or other mechanical forces, is very damaging in EB. Oral, pharyngeal, and esophageal blistering is common in EB, leading to mouth and tongue contractures. Extremity contractures can cause scarring that is severe enough to create pseudosyndactyly. Corneal scarring may also occur. Treatment for EB involves avoiding friction and shearing forces by using special clothing and feeding techniques, blister drainage and treatment with silver sulfadiazine for large infected lesions, special dressings made of hydrofiber foam and coated with silicone, and topical corticosteroids.

For parturients with EB, the most important anesthetic concept is that friction and shearing forces, not direct pressure, cause new bullae formation. Neck contractures and pharyngeal bullae present distinct challenges to airway management; therefore, assessment of the airway should be performed by an experienced anesthesiologist. Fortunately, the veins are typically easy to visualize and cannulate. Minimizing the number of transfers for these patients is prudent since sliding would cause shearing forces between the patient and both the stretcher and operating room bed which would contribute to bullae formation. Assiduously avoiding adhesives when attaching monitors, IV cannulae, or airway devices are also recommended. Peripheral IV cannulae may be secured using a single suture. Other suggested maneuvers include use of a clip on pulse oximetry probe, cutting away the adhesive portion of the ECG electrode and securing the gel portion to the skin with paraffin gauze or a gelpad, padding the skin with Webril® soft gauze before applying a non-invasive blood pressure cuff, avoiding both nasopharyngeal and rectal temperature probes, thoroughly lubricating the facemask with petroleum jelly or protecting it with paraffin gauze, and taking care to avoid shearing forces on the skin between the facemask and the patient's face and neck. Generally, orotracheal intubation is preferred, using an ETT that is one-half size smaller than normal; with gentle laryngoscopy the incidence of new laryngeal or pharyngeal bullae is low (46). Anticipated difficult airway management, with contractures or severe intraoral bullae, requires careful planning and may include the availability of videolaryngoscopy, fiberoptic bronchoscopy, and LMAs. A well-lubricated LMA can be used for airway maintenance, with little risk of new severe intraoral bullae formation, but airway maintenance using a facemask for long time periods should be avoided. Non-depolarizing muscle relaxants may be used, but succinylcholine should be avoided. Standard IV induction agents, maintenance agents, and both opioid and regional anesthesia (epidural catheters should be secured using a soft silicone-type tape) have been safely used in EB patients. Emergence from anesthesia and tracheal extubation must be carefully done, taking care to avoid shearing forces on the face; intraoral suctioning must also be gently done. Avoiding the use of a conventional facemask for supplemental oxygen administration in postanesthesia recovery is important; the oxygen concentration may be increased by blowing humidified oxygen over the face with 22 mm corrugated oxygen tubing. The patient should be evaluated for the formation of new bullae postoperatively and the anesthesia team should communicate with the patient's dermatologist regarding any changes in treatment plan after the anesthetic. There are published reports of successful vaginal deliveries without anesthesia, (47) and cesarean deliveries performed under general endotracheal anesthesia, (48) lumbar epidural anesthesia, (49,50) and spinal anesthesia (47,49,51).

▪ NEUROCUTANEOUS SYNDROMES (PHAKOMATOSES): NEUROFIBROMATOSIS (VON RECKLINGHAUSEN DISEASE), STURGE–WEBER SYNDROME, TUBEROUS SCLEROSIS, VON HIPPEL–LINDAU SYNDROME

Phakomatoses (neuroectodermal diseases) are characterized by ipsilateral or midline skin lesions, central nervous system (CNS) (often neuraxial) neoplasm's or arteriovenous malformations (AVMs), and ocular anomalies. Craniofacial asymmetry, seizures, intracranial hypertension are also characteristics of most phakomatoses and some (Tuberous Sclerosis, Sturge–Weber) are associated with congenital heart defects while others (von Hippel–Lindau [VHL], Neurofibromatosis) are uniquely associated with pheochromocytomas (52).

Neurofibromatosis (NF) or von Recklinghausen disease occurs in both peripheral nervous system and CNS form. NF Type 1, the most common phacomatosis with an estimated prevalence of 1:5,000, is characterized by café au lait macules, schwannomas or neurofibromas involving cranial and peripheral nerves, axillary/inguinal freckling, optic gliomas, Lisch nodules (hamartomas of the iris), and a distinctive osseous lesion. In NF-1, the neurofibromas are generally benign tumors that most commonly affect the cranial nerves (most commonly the trigeminal nerve, CN-5) with symptoms resulting from compression. Nearly all adults have Lisch nodules (hamartomas of the iris), and optic nerve gliomas, which lead to visual defects, occur in 15% to 20% of NF-1 patients. Other CNS findings include aqueductal stenosis, Chiari malformations, as well as cervical and occipital AVMs. Skin manifestations include café au lait spots, freckles, and cutaneous neurofibromas while visceral lesions include pheochromocytomas and intestinal, hepatic, or bladder neurofibromas. NF Type 2 has an estimated prevalence of 1:50,000 with the most prominent manifestation being acoustic (usually bilateral) neuromas leading to progressive hearing loss followed by tinnitus and imbalance. Visual changes occur with compression of cranial nerve 6 (CN-6), while facial numbness or weakness can occur with compression of CN-5 and cranial nerve 7 (CN-7), respectively. CNS tumors, such as gliomas, ependymomas, and meningiomas occur. Skin manifestations, such as café au lait spots and cutaneous neurofibromas, are less common than in NF-1 (53). Some of the issues followed by the obstetrician during the pregnancy include changes in tumor character (54–56), number and/or size (57), and/or obstructing delivery (58,59); tumor hemorrhage (60–62); hypertensive disorders both with (63) and without (64) pheochromocytoma, which span gestational hypertension, pre-eclampsia (65), HELLP syndrome (66), eclampsia (67), and renovascular hypertension (66). Issues for the experienced anesthesiologist to consider when selecting either regional or general anesthesia for these women start with the pregnancy-associated increase in both number and size of the neurofibromas attributed to NF-1 tumor expression of the progesterone receptor (68). The basis for choosing general over regional anesthesia would include symptoms and/or imaging studies suggesting neuraxial tumor growth, significant coagulopathy, or pheochromocytoma. Although successful general endotracheal anesthetics have been administered (61,69,70), a number of issues should be considered. First, airway management may be difficult; oral neurofibromas occur, commonly causing macroglossia, which are generally sessile and may bleed following trauma; tumors occurring in the neck or larynx, causing dysphagia, hoarseness, and/or stridor, may compromise the airway (71); and C-spine abnormalities, many asymptomatic, may be present in nearly 44% of patients (72). Tracheostomy has been required following complete airway obstruction following induction of anesthesia (73) and failed fiberoptic intubation (74). Second, cardiopulmonary compromise may occur with spontaneous hemothorax (62), mediastinal masses (55,56,75), and elevated blood pressures from renal artery stenosis (66,76), or pheochromocytoma (63). Abnormal responses to both depolarizing and nondepolarizing neuromuscular blockade have been reported (77,78). However, Richardson et al. demonstrated minimal risk of abnormal response to either drug class in patients with

NF-1 with appropriate dosing (79). Tumor growth occurs in both NF-1 and NF-2 in response to hormonal changes, making neuraxial imaging before performing a regional anesthetic strongly recommended (80). Following negative imaging studies, epidural analgesia/anesthesia has been used successfully in both NF-1 (81) and NF-2 (80) parturients; however, epidural hematoma has been reported as a complication (82). Rasko et al. demonstrated in vitro that normal platelet aggregation in NF-1 patients requires higher collagen concentrations (83), although it is unclear that this finding changes the risk of placing a neuraxial block. Further, Lighthall et al. reported the successful use of DDAVP to correct an intraoperative coagulopathy in a woman with NF-1, although the authors express their uncertainty that DDAVP alone resolved the bleeding (84).

Sturge–Weber syndrome is characterized by hemifacial cutaneous hemangiomas (port-wine stain) associated with brain and meningeal angiomata. Optic nerve damage from increased intraocular pressure is present in up to 60% of patients with choroidal hemangiomas. Meningeal angiomas, commonly in the occipitoparietal region, are vascular anomalies leading to abnormal cerebral venous drainage and elevated ICP. Other neurologic manifestations include seizure disorder and migraine headaches (53). Anesthetic issues to consider would include intracranial bleeding from changes in ICP or arterial blood pressure; ocular manifestations resulting from changes in intraocular pressure or intraocular hemorrhage; changes in drug metabolism with chronic anticonvulsant medication; and difficulty airway management, both mask ventilation with facial hemangiomas and tracheal intubation with intraoral or tracheolaryngeal hemangiomas, which may obstruct the view under direct laryngoscopy or hemorrhage following trauma (85). Successful cesarean delivery is reported; however, the anesthetic administered for the surgery is not discussed (86,87).

Tuberous sclerosis is a heterogeneous disorder, estimated prevalence between 1:10,000 and 1:26,500, with diagnostic criteria divided into primary, secondary, and tertiary features. The primary features include facial angiofibromas, ungula fibromas, cortical tubers, a subependymal nodule or giant-cell astrocytoma, multiple subependymal nodules protruding into the ventricle, and multiple retinal astrocytomas. The secondary features include a cardiac rhabdomyoma, retinal hamartoma or achromatic patch, cerebral tubers, noncalcified subependymal nodules, a shagreen patch, forehead plaques, pulmonary lymphangiomyomatosis, a renal angiomyolipoma, and renal cysts. The tertiary features include random enamel pits, hamartomatous rectal polyps, bone cysts, infantile spasms, gingival fibromas, nonrenal angiomyolipomas, and cerebral white matter migration tracts of heterotopias. Although the diagnosis is made using a combination of these features, the most common (70% to 90% of patients) presenting feature is seizures and most (50% to 60% of patients) display mental retardation. Cortical tubers and subependymal nodules are characteristic CNS findings; when the subependymal nodules coalesce to form a tumor, they are referred to as a "subependymal giant-cell astrocytoma" and may obstruct cerebrospinal fluid (CSF) flow to produce hydrocephalus. The skin manifestations include facial adenoma sebaceum, ash leaf patches, and subungual fibromas. Renal tumors include angiomyolipoma and renal cell carcinoma while 30% of patients have a cardiac rhabdomyoma (53). Pulmonary lymphangioleiomyomatosis occurs in approximately 26% of patients with tuberous sclerosis, has a high incidence of pneumothorax, causing impaired gas transfer associated with either obstructive or restrictive pulmonary physiology. Despite the pulmonary lymphangioleiomyomatosis, pneumothoraces during pregnancy are rare although reports of their occurrence exist and the recurrence rate is high (88). Pregnancy has been associated with renal complications including increased arterial pressures, renal failure requiring hemodialysis, and renal tumor rupture (89–92) as well as with no renal complications (93,94). Pulmonary complications include pneumothoraces and worsening function (95) as well as no pulmonary complications (93,96) or in one report associated with improved pulmonary function (97). The question regarding the exacerbating effects of pregnancy on either pulmonary or renal complications is still debated; however, Mitchell et al. demonstrated that pregnancy does not increase this risk (98). The anesthesiologist, as directed by symptoms, should assess and possibly image the CNS lesions and characterize their impact on both ICP and neuraxial anesthesia; perform an airway examination to identify potentially obstructive lesions; perform a cardiac work-up to assess both function and any intracardiac tumors, perform a pulmonary work-up to assess both function and any intrapulmonary or mediastinal lesions; and perform a renal work-up to assess function and any hamartomas. There are reports of successful lumber epidural analgesia (88,99) provided for labor and delivery, and both spinal (94) and general anesthesia (99,100) for cesarean delivery. An additional issue in these patients, described by Byrd et al., is chronic pain. They report the management of a woman with chronic flank pain, adequately controlled with an indwelling intrathecal morphine pump, for the delivery of her fourth child. During labor the intrathecal infusion was continued unchanged and analgesia was supplemented with a gaseous mixture of $50\%O_2/50\%N_2O$. This provided adequate analgesia until the late second stage of labor. However, she delivered before additional pain relief could be administered. The authors noted that in the primarily visceral pain of early labor, the intrathecal morphine and N_2O provided reasonably complete analgesia; however, the somatic pain occurring later required local anesthetics, which could be delivered into the epidural space via an epidural catheter or the intrathecal space via the in situ pump/catheter. They also discussed potential complications with both of these alternatives (101). Lee et al. reported a woman who developed retinal changes, parafoveal exudates and serous retinal detachment, during pregnancy but did not state a definite causal relationship in their occurrence (102).

VHL syndrome is rare, with an incidence of 1:36,000, is diagnosed using three criteria; CNS hemangioblastomas, visceral lesions (renal, pancreatic), and a family history; and is estimated to cause maternal morbidity at a rate of 5.4% (103). VHL is characterized by hemangiomas occurring as bilateral retinal angiomata leading to exudative retinal detachment in 40% of patients and intracranial (usually cerebellar) hemangioblastoma which are prone to hypertensive hemorrhage in 60% of patients. In approximately 10% of these patients, the hypertension is likely due to a pheochromocytoma and in 25% from a renal tumor (53). Pregnancy is associated with the enlargement of existing and the development of new hemangioblastomas, which may result in spinal cord compression from the increased spinal venous pressure and/or hemangioma size (103). Spinal cord hemangiomas, usually cervicothoracic but also thoracolumbar or lumbosacral, may occur in 5% to 28% of patients. Typical symptoms of cerebellar hemangioblastomas, including headache, dizziness, vomiting, ataxia, behavioral changes, and seizures, result from pressure to surrounding structures. These symptoms, headaches and visual disturbances (from intracranial hemangiomas) in the setting of elevated blood pressures (from a pheochromocytoma) would mimic other obstetric complications such as pregnancy-induced hypertension (104). Malignant hypertension in pregnancy from pheochromocytoma

is rare, and frequently unrelated to VHL, with only several hundred unilateral cases and a full order of magnitude fewer bilateral cases reported (105,106). Typical presenting symptoms are hypertension and the triad of episodic headaches, palpitations, and diaphoresis. Other symptoms include dizziness, chest pain, dyspnea, visual changes, arrhythmias, seizures, congestive heart failure, postural hypotension, anxiety attacks, flushing/pallor, abdominal pain, or symptoms from hemorrhage into the tumor. These symptoms resemble those of preeclampsia, thyrotoxicosis, cocaine intoxication, cerebral hemorrhage, and malignant hyperthermia. The diagnosis begins with detecting abnormal levels of catecholamines and their metabolites in the urine and imaging studies to localize the tumor (107). Maternal and fetal mortality are both increased, although early detection, proper medical management, and surgical excision improve the outcome. Timing the surgery during pregnancy is problematic: Surgical exposure is better with a smaller gravid uterus, but there is increased risk of fetal demise in early gestation (106). Medical management of pheochromocytoma in pregnancy includes some combination of alpha-adrenergic antagonists with adjuvant calcium-channel antagonists followed by beta-adrenergic antagonists. Although the optimal mode of delivery for women with unresected tumor(s) is unknown, an elective cesarean section followed by surgical tumor resection has been suggested (107). General endotracheal anesthesia for these procedures has been successfully administered (108). Severe hypotension from sympathectomy-induced vasodilation would theoretically relatively contraindicate neuraxial anesthesia; however, epidural anesthesia has been used for pheochromocytoma resection in a non-pregnant patient (109). Invasive monitoring would be utilized such as an intra-arterial blood pressure monitor for beat-to-beat analysis of labile blood pressures from acute changes in serum catecholamine levels and/or vasoactive drugs; a central venous pressure catheter (and possibly a pulmonary artery pressure catheter) for monitoring post-partum fluid shifts and for delivering vasoactive drugs or volume-expanding fluids. Post-partum these women continue to be at risk for ventricular failure and pulmonary edema, which would necessitate intensive care level monitoring. Numerous additional complications of VHL during pregnancy have been reported including eclampsia (110), increased intracranial hypertension (104,110,111), abdominal pain from a pancreatic cyst (110), paraplegia from a thoracic intramedullary hemorrhage (112), quadriplegia from a hemorrhagic cervical lesion (113), and lumbosacral pain from filum terminale hemangioblastomas (114). The anesthesiologist should assess/image the CNS to identify lesions that would alter ICP and/or impact the performance of neuraxial anesthesia. For a vaginal delivery, these women are at risk of hemorrhage from an intracranial hemangioma during labor and delivery. Both the arterial and CSF pressures increase with contractions and the CSF pressure increases again with a valsalva maneuver during the second stage of labor; leading to an increase in ICP if cerebral compliance is reduced by an intracranial tumor. Adequate epidural analgesia during labor would mitigate these changes by reducing the arterial pressure associated with contractions and abolishing the patients "bearing-down" reflex in response to painful contractions (104). For elective cesarean delivery, there are reports of successful general (115,116), epidural (104,112,117–119), and spinal anesthetics (120). Some issues to consider when selecting between these include potential cerebellar herniation from dural puncture, rupture of a spinal hemangioblastoma with a needle, bleeding from hemangioblastomas with increased blood pressures associated with endotracheal intubation and extubation, and cardiovascular instability from anesthetic medications.

■ NEUROMUSCULAR DISORDERS: MUSCULAR DYSTROPHIES INCLUDING DUCHENNE MUSCULAR DYSTROPHY, AND LIMB-GIRDLE MUSCULAR DYSTROPHY; CORE MYOPATHIES INCLUDING CENTRAL CORE DISEASE, MULTIMINICORE DISEASE, AND NEMALINE ROD MYOPATHY; KING-DENBOROUGH SYNDROME, MITOCHONDRIAL MYOPATHY

The neuromuscular disorders are particularly challenging given that both cardiomyopathy and arrhythmias are common manifestations. The cardiomyopathy appears to arise from the significant overlap between the genetic mutation affecting skeletal muscle and the myocardium. Formally assessing myocardial function with echocardiography is warranted but complicated in patients with respiratory compromise or who are wheelchair bound as the imaging windows are poor. In these cases, cardiac MRI can assess ventricular dysfunction and hypertrophy as well as provide information on impairment of myocardial contractility and relaxation from fibrosis. Cardiac biomarkers are used for patients in respiratory distress in order to distinguish primary respiratory disease from heart failure; however, these markers have not yet been extensively studied in patients with neuromuscular disease. Unfortunately, the pathophysiology leading to arrhythmias is less-well defined, but may involve diffuse myocardial fibrosis affecting the conduction system (121). Women with neuromuscular disease may have baseline respiratory dysfunction from muscle weakness and/or scoliosis. It should be assumed that these women will be particularly sensitive to respiratory depression from opioids, especially when receiving magnesium for obstetric indications as occurred in a parturient with congenital fiber-type disproportion myopathy (122). Neuromuscular disorders present another significant concern to the anesthesiologist, namely their potential association with susceptibility to malignant hyperthermia (MH). A definitive link between the individual neuromuscular disorders and MH susceptibility has been particularly elusive. In a 2009 editorial, Litman eloquently outlined the problems associated with establishing this definitive relationship. First, establishing a definitive causal relationship in clinical medicine is difficult without prospective randomized controlled trials or cohort studies, which are impossible to perform for rare events, leaving generalizations derived from case control studies, case reports, and case series. An additional confounding factor is that these historical reports were not associated with a genetic linkage and pedigree analysis which are important in modern analyses. Second, even internationally recognized authoritative experts in the field are unable to delineate which disorders are closely linked to MH susceptibility (except for central core myopathy, multiminicore myopathy, King-Denborough syndrome, and Brody myopathy which are closely linked). For these entities, there is strong clinical and genetic (for central core and multiminicore disease) evidence of such a link. Third, MH-triggering agents may produce life-threatening hyperkalemia and rhabdomyolysis when administered to patients with disorders such as Duchenne and Becker muscular dystrophy, although not with mitochondrial myopathies, glycogen storage myopathies, and Noonan syndrome. Succinylcholine will likely produce muscle rigidity, unrelated to MH, in patients with myotonia (123).

Muscular dystrophies are characterized by muscle wasting and weakness, where the muscle fibers vary in size, undergo degeneration/regeneration, and are replaced by connective tissue and fat; whereas congenital myopathies, although similar, lack the necrotic/degenerative changes (124).

Duchenne muscular dystrophy (DMD) is an X-linked recessive disorder that occurs in 1:3,500 live *male* births; but is presented here since the "manifesting carrier" female may undergo labor and cesarean delivery (125). The classic symptoms in boys include an abnormal gait with calf hypertrophy and difficulty rising from the floor (Gowers sign) by 5 years of age, leading to wheelchair dependence followed by scoliosis, respiratory insufficiency, cardiomyopathy, then death. The serum creatine kinase (CK) is elevated by 10 to 100 times from birth. DMD arises from a mutation of the dystrophin gene causing a severe reduction or absence of the dystrophin protein in myocytes. Becker muscular dystrophy (BMD) results from a separate mutation of the same gene leading to a truncated, partially functional dystrophin protein which manifests milder symptoms. Progressive weakness of respiratory muscles leads to pulmonary compromise with hypercapnia, and up to 90% have dilated cardiomyopathy by 18 years of age. Wheelchair dependence promotes progression of scoliosis that may require spinal fusion. Oropharyngeal muscle involvement may cause chewing/swallowing difficulties leading to choking, although frank aspiration is rare. Manifesting carriers occur in 1:100,000 live female births and approximately 2% to 5% manifest symptoms. These symptoms are less severe, ranging from muscle pain/cramps on exertion to proximal girdle weakness that rarely leads to wheelchair dependence. DMD carriers have a 10% life-time risk for developing cardiomyopathy (126).

It appears that neither patients with DMD nor BMD are at increased risk of malignant hyperthermia; although life-threatening rhabdomyolysis and hyperkalemia are associated with exposure to volatile anesthetics and succinylcholine, respectively (127). Anesthetic considerations include aspiration risk with oropharyngeal muscle weakness, assessment of respiratory function with thoracic deformities and muscle weakness, cardiac function with coincident cardiomyopathies, and the risk of rhabdomyolysis and hyperkalemia with exposure to volatile anesthetics and succinylcholine, respectively. Cesarean delivery has been performed under combined spinal–epidural anesthesia (125) in a DMD manifesting carrier.

Limb-girdle muscular dystrophy (LGMD) is a group of muscular dystrophies related by the common clinical feature of limb-girdle muscle weakness, with an overall frequency estimated as 1:15,000. The subgroups are named based on the deficient protein and molecular genetic defect, making a muscle biopsy the key diagnostic step. The phenotypic subtypes vary by their onset age, weakness pattern (proximal vs. distal), and the presence/distribution of muscle hypertrophy, as well as the presence/absence of elevated serum CK, contractures, respiratory or cardiac involvement (126). Anesthetic considerations include assessment of respiratory function with thoracic deformities and muscle weakness, cardiac function with coincident cardiomyopathies, and the risk of rhabdomyolysis and hyperkalemia with exposure to volatile anesthetics and succinylcholine respectively associated with any muscle wasting condition. Cesarean delivery has been performed under epidural anesthesia (128) on a patient with LGMD and severe lumbar lordosis; under combined spinal–epidural (129) on a patient with LGMD and severe restrictive lung disease requiring non-invasive positive pressure ventilation; and under combined epidural and general anesthesia (130) in a patient whose pulmonary insufficiency acutely deteriorated intraoperatively.

Core myopathies are congenital myopathies which share the common clinical feature of muscle weakness, possibly respiratory and/or bulbar muscles, but differ in their underlying molecular mechanism; unlike the muscular dystrophies, they do not usually involve the myocardium (131). Core myopathies have histopathologic derangements in their cellular core, identified following a muscle biopsy, which helps differentiate them from one another. This core derangement is increasingly being attributed to mutations in the skeletal muscle ryanodine receptor (RYR1) gene, which encodes the principle sarcoplasmic reticulum calcium release channel involved in excitation–contraction coupling (132). Mutations to this RYR1 gene are identified in up to 70% of families with MH susceptibility; although to date, this association has no proven diagnostic utility (131).

Central core disease (CCD) is a congenital myopathy, of unknown prevalence, characterized by hypotonia, muscle weakness, and skeletal abnormalities but not cardiac defects. These patients are susceptible to malignant hyperthermia (133). Although a definitive genotype–phenotype correlation defining the risk of MH in these patients is lacking, the clinical and genetic evidence for a relation is strong enough to recommend that non-triggering anesthetics be used (131). Cardiac and respiratory involvement is unusual and serum CK is typically normal. The hip girdle and axial muscles are typically involved given the proximal distribution of the muscle weakness, although bulbar weakness is unusual. Scoliosis is common as is ligamentous laxity (134). Anesthetic considerations include assessment of respiratory function with thoracic deformities and muscle weakness, cardiac function based on patient symptoms, and the risk of malignant hyperthermia with exposure to volatile anesthetics and/or succinylcholine. Cesarean delivery has been performed under general endotracheal total IV anesthesia (135) for a parturient with CCD.

Multiminicore disease (MmD) is a rare congenital myopathy, with an estimated incidence of 0.06:1,000 live births, where the classical phenotype is characterized by spinal rigidity, scoliosis, and respiratory impairment. Axial muscle weakness, proximal more than distal, affecting the flexors of the neck/trunk, shoulder girdle, and inner thighs is common. Progressive scoliosis with respiratory impairment, disproportionately affected compared to other muscle weakness, may lead to secondary cardiac failure. Another form has external ophthalmoplegia and less respiratory impairment; while still another has a predominant hip-girdle weakness and hand involvement, little scoliosis, and sparing of the respiratory and bulbar muscles (136). Given that the moderate form, with hand involvement, is associated with RYR1 mutations and that MmD shows significant overlap with CCD, it would seem prudent to treat these patients as MH susceptible (131). Anesthetic considerations include an assessment of respiratory function with thoracic deformities and the disproportionately affected respiratory muscle weakness, cardiac function with significant respiratory impairment, and the presumed risk of malignant hyperthermia with exposure to volatile anesthetics and succinylcholine. Epidural analgesia (137,138) has been used in a parturient with MmD for two vaginal deliveries.

Nemaline myopathy (CNM) is characterized by marked scoliosis, spinal rigidity, and respiratory impairment (139). Although rare, with an estimated incidence of 2:100,000 live births (131), it is usually fatal when presenting in infancy; a nonprogressive course occurs with presentation during childhood; and a variable course occurs with presentation during adulthood, from mild weakness to fatal hypertrophic cardiomyopathy. Features of childhood presentation include a narrow face, high-arched palate, kyphoscoliosis, finger abnormalities and clubbed feet; the weakness is more proximal than distal; and the extra-ocular muscles are spared despite palatal and pharyngeal muscle involvement (140). Heard et al. reported the successful use of both succinylcholine, with an abnormal response, and pancuronium, with a normal response (141); however, it would seem prudent to avoid neuromuscular blocking agents whenever possible. An association with MH susceptibility seems unlikely (131). Anesthetic concerns include aspiration risk with pharyngeal muscle involvement, assessment of the potentially difficult airway, assessment of cardiac function with potential hypertrophic cardiomyopathy, and the risk of rhabdomyolysis and hyperkalemia with exposure to volatile anesthetics and succinylcholine respectively associated with any muscle wasting condition. Cesarean delivery has been performed under general (142,143) and epidural (144) anesthesia in patients with CNM. However, these anesthetics were not without complications. The GETA reported by Stackhouse et al. was for the patient's fifth cesarean delivery and required multiple intubation attempts. The authors noted the patient's prior anesthetic management for her deliveries included one regional and three general anesthetics (one following a failed regional technique) (142). Use of a lumbar epidural reported by Wallgren-Pettersson et al. was complicated by an uneven block height during the surgery (144).

King-Denborough syndrome is characterized by facial anomalies such as malar hypoplasia, downslanting palpebral fissures, ptosis/blepharophimosis, micrognathia, malocclusion, a high-arched palate, and low-set ears; congenital myopathy with proximal muscle weakness and elevated serum CK levels, kyphoscoliosis and/or lumbar lordosis; and susceptibility to malignant hyperthermia (MH) (145). Anesthetic concerns include assessment of the potentially difficult airway, assessment of respiratory function, cardiac function with significant respiratory impairment, and the risk of malignant hyperthermia with exposure to volatile anesthetics and succinylcholine. Although predominately seen in males, there are reports of parturients requiring nightly ventilator support via permanent tracheostomy for chronic respiratory failure, undergoing successful labor and assisted vaginal delivery under lumbar epidural analgesia (146,147).

Mitochondrial myopathy is a group of disorders characterized by derangements in metabolic homeostasis, specifically, mitochondrial dysfunction resulting in defects of oxidative phosphorylation. This mitochondrial dysfunction disrupts the production of adenosine triphosphate (ATP) resulting in lactic acidosis and the inability to utilize glucose. As such, tissues (organs) with very high oxidative metabolism rates are affected primarily where CNS manifestation may include visual/hearing impairment, seizures, and ataxia; renal tubular acidosis may result from renal involvement; dystonia and weakness are skeletal muscle manifestations; dysphagia, pseudo-obstruction, and constipation would suggest gastrointestinal involvement; and diabetes mellitus, hypoparathyroidism, and hypothyroidism are symptoms of endocrine organ involvement. Some of these disorders manifest during infancy and are differentiated in part by their confusing blend of characteristics. Examples would include encephalopathy as the cardinal feature of Leigh syndrome, seizures/ataxia for MERRF (myoclonic epilepsy with ragged-red fibers) syndrome, dementia and stroke-like symptoms for MELAS (mitochondrial encephalomyopathy with lactic acidosis and stroke-like episodes) which may also involve hypertrophic cardiomyopathy. Adult onset of mitochondrial myopathies may involve insidious neurologic dysfunction or persistent muscle pain/weakness or fatigue; hepatic insufficiency may be subclinical; and renal involvement usually presents as Toni–Debre–Fanconi syndrome (148). The mitochondrial disorders pose an interesting challenge to the anesthesiologist given that anesthetic drugs affect mitochondrial function, although the *in vivo* extent of the alteration is not yet known. IV anesthetic drugs depress CNS carbohydrate metabolism, oxygen consumption, and energy production. For example, clinical doses of opioids inhibit glucose, lactate, and pyruvate oxidation in neural tissues. Propofol decreases oxygen consumption and ATP production in neural synaptosomes, reduces cardiac mitochondrial electron flow, and uncouples electron transport from ATP production. Barbiturates inhibit oxidative phosphorylation in the brain, heart, and liver, and seem to "uncouple" ATP production from metabolic activity. Volatile agents depress some mitochondrial function in vitro at high concentrations, exacerbated by adding nitrous oxide (N_2O), even though N_2O alone does not. Finally, local anesthetics disrupt oxidative phosphorylation similar to the IV agents (149). In this setting, anesthetic concerns for these patients would include decreased anesthetic requirements with neuronal impairment, intrinsic skeletal muscle hypotonia possibly compromising postoperative respiratory function, cardiomyopathy and/or conduction abnormalities, glucose dysregulation with prolonged fasting, and abnormal drug effect/metabolism with depressed hepatorenal function/reserve (148,149). Successful cesarean deliveries for various mitochondrial myopathies, using epidural anesthesia both with (150) and without (151) the use of non-invasive ventilator support are reported. The use of epidural anesthesia for the MELAS syndrome has also been reported (152). In addition, Diaz-Lobato et al. report two successful cesarean deliveries in a patient requiring non-invasive ventilator support without addressing the anesthesia (153).

KEY POINTS

- Pre-existing congenital anomalies are frequently the result of a genetic syndrome which is a constellation of recognizable traits, often involving multiple organ systems. Developing a plan to care for these women requires an organized approach, giving consideration to the organ systems both individually and collectively.
- Airway management, spanning the initial assessment, endotracheal intubation (if indicated) and extubation should be performed by the most experienced anesthesiologist. An assessment of atlantoaxial stability should be routinely performed. Recall that for some "difficult airway" syndromes the intubation may become easier (PRS) or harder (TCS) with age.
- Cardiac structural/functional anomalies require the anesthesiologist to understand the specific anatomy and pathophysiology. Studies that evaluate cardiovascular function should be interpreted by a cardiologist, both familiar and comfortable with the woman's specific pathophysiology, which would ideally be the pediatric cardiologist who has followed her from childhood into adulthood. Cardiac conduction anomalies require the anesthesiologist to understand both an existing defect and the defects most likely to arise during the peripartum period. Consultation with an electrophysiologist, to identify effective pharmacotherapies, would be prudent.
- Neurodevelopmental anomalies span behavioral issues, deficits in fine or gross motor skills, peripheral neuromuscular deficits/lesions or paresthesias, and central neuromuscular deficits/lesions or altered ICP. Behavioral issues may be challenging during the induction of neuraxial or general anesthesia. Identifying the lesion type and anatomic location starts the work-up, which would include an assessment of how such a lesion would impact the induction of neuraxial and/or general anesthesia.
- Vascular malformations found in some neurocutaneous syndromes may lead to hemodynamically significant shunts, impact the ICP by restricting venous drainage, or be associated with coagulopathies. These effects as well as the actual anatomic location may contraindicate placing a neuraxial block.
- Neuromuscular disorders are associated with cardiomyopathies and arrhythmias, and both should be assessed. Central core myopathy, multiminicore myopathy, King-Denborough syndrome, and Brody myopathy are closely linked to MH susceptibility. And succinylcholine may cause life-threatening hyperkalemia and rhabdomyolysis when administered to patients with some of these disorders, such as Duchenne and Becker muscular dystrophies.
- Vascular access may be challenging as a result of limb abnormalities or a history of multiple procedures/hospitalizations. Recall that central veins may be thrombosed or stenotic from previous catheterizations.
- These women present a host of challenges and a multidisciplinary approach to every patient seems warranted.

REFERENCES

1. U.S. National Institutes of Health, Health Information: Genetics/Birth Defects, available: health.nih.gov/category/GeneticsBirthDefects.
2. OMIM-Online Mendelian Inheritance in Man. Hamosh A, ed. 2011.
3. OJRD-Orphanet Journal of Rare Diseases. Ayme S, Dallapiccola B, Donnai D, eds. 2011.
4. Baum VC, O'Flaherty JE, eds. *Anesthesia for Genetic, Metabolic, and Dysmorphic Syndromes of Childhood*, 2nd ed. Lippincott Williams & Wilkins; 2006.
5. Butler MG, Hayes BG, Hathaway MM, et al. Specific genetic diseases at risk for sedation/anesthesia complications. *Anesth Analg* 2000;91:837–855.
6. Lin AE, Basson CT, Goldmuntz E, et al. Adults with genetic syndromes and cardiovascular abnormalities: clinical history and management. *Genet Med* 2008; 10:469–494.
7. Cohen WI. Current dilemmas in Down syndrome clinical care: celiac disease, thyroid disorders, and atlanto-axial instability. *Am J Med Genet C Semin Med Genet* 2006;142C:141–148.
8. Sulemanji DS, Donmez A, Akpek EA, et al. Vascular catheterization is difficult in infants with down syndrome. *Acta Anaesthesiol Scand* 2009;53:98–100.
9. Martin TJ, Hartnett JM, Jacobson DJ, et al. Care of a parturient with pre-eclampsia, morbid obesity, and Crouzon's syndrome. *Int J Obstet Anesth* 2008; 17:177–181.
10. Morillas P, Fornet I, de Miguel I, et al. Airway management in a patient with Treacher Collins syndrome requiring emergent cesarean section. *Anesth Analg* 2007;105:294.
11. Cohen MM Jr, Kreiborg S, Lammer EJ, et al. Birth prevalence study of the Apert syndrome. *Am J Med Genet* 1992;42:655–659.
12. Marucci DD, Dunaway DJ, Jones BM, et al. Raised intracranial pressure in Apert syndrome. *Plast Reconstr Surg* 2008;122:1162–1168.
13. Horbelt CV. Physical and oral characteristics of Crouzon syndrome, Apert syndrome and Pierre Robin sequence. *Gen Dent* 2008;56:132–134.
14. Sculerati N, Gottlieb MC, Zimbler MS, et al. Airway management in children with major craniofacial anomalies. *Laryngoscope* 1998;108:1806–1812.
15. Papay FA, McCarthy VP Eliachar I, et al. Laryngotracheal anomalies in children with craniofacial syndromes. *J Craniofac Surg* 2002;13:351–364.
16. McGill T. Otolaryngologic aspects of Apert syndrome. *Clin Plast Surg* 1991; 18:309–313.
17. Thompson DNP, Staney SF, Hall CM, et al. Congenital cervical spinal fusion: a study in Apert syndrome. *Pediatr Neurosurg* 1996;25:20–27.
18. Nargozian C. Airway in patients with craniofacial abnormalities. *Paediatr Anaesth* 2004;14:53–59.
19. Cohen MM Jr, Kreiborg S. Birth prevalence studies of the Crouzon syndrome: comparison of direct and indirect methods. *Clin Genet* 1992;41:12–15.
20. Anderson PJ, Hall C, Evans RD, et al. Cervical spine in Crouzon syndrome. *Spine* 1997;22:402–405.
21. Rollnick BR, Kaye CI, Nagatoshi K, et al. Oculoauriculovertebral dysplasia and variants: phenotypic characteristics of 294 patients. *Am J Med Genet* 1987; 26:361–375.
22. Healey D, Letts M, Jarvis JG. Cervical spine instability in children with Goldenhar's syndrome. *Can J Surg* 2002;45:341–344.
23. Ozlu O, Simsek S, Alacakir H, et al. Goldenhar syndrome and intubation with the fiberoptic bronchoscope. *Paediatr Anaesth* 2008;18:793–794.
24. Khalil S, Vinh B. Successful intubation of a child with Goldenhar syndrome, who previously failed intubation, using an Airtraq. *Paediatr Anaesth* 2010;20: 204–205.

25. Digilio MC, Calzolari F, Capolino R, et al. Congenital heart defects in the oculo-auriculo-vertebral spectrum (Goldenhar syndrome). *Am J Med Genet A* 2008; 146A:1815–1819.

26. Hunt JA, Hobar PG. Common craniofacial anomalies: the facial dysostoses. *Plast Reconstr Surg* 2002;110:1714–1725.

27. Inagawa G, Miwa T, Hiroki K. Change in difficult intubation with growth in a patient with Treacher Collins syndrome. *Anesth Analg* 2004;99:1874.

28. Van der Burgt I. Noonan syndrome. *Orphanet J Rare Dis* 2007;2:4.

29. Lee CK, Chang BS, Hong YM, et al. Spinal deformities in Noonan syndrome: a clinical review of 60 cases. *J Bone Joint Surg Am* 2001;83:1495–1502.

30. Dadabhoy ZP, Winnie AP. Regional anesthesia for cesarean section in a parturient with Noonan's syndrome. *Anesthesiology* 1988;68:636–638.

31. Sharland M, Patton MA, Talbot S, et al. Coagulation-factor deficiencies and abnormal bleeding in Noonan's syndrome. *Lancet* 1992;339:19–21.

32. Magboul MM. Anaesthetic management of emergency caesarean section in a patient with Noonan's syndrome—case report and literature review. *Middle East J Anesthesiol* 2000;15:611–617.

33. Engemise S, Croucher C. Pregnancy following oocyte donation in a woman with Noonan's syndrome and a balanced robertsonian translocation a case report. *Arch Gynecol Obstet* 2007;276:185–187.

34. McBain J, Lemire EG, Campbell DC. Epidural labour analgesia in a parturient with Noonan syndrome: a case report. *Can J Anaesth* 2006;53:274–278.

35. Cullimore AJ, Smedstad KG, Brennan BG. Pregnancy in women with Noonan syndrome: report of 2 cases. *Obstet Gynecol* 1999;93:813–816.

36. McLure HA, Yentis SM. General anaesthesia for caesarean section in a parturient with Noonan's syndrome. *Br J Anaesth* 1996;77:665–668.

37. Grange CS, Heid R, Lucas SB, et al. Anaesthesia in a parturient with Noonan's syndrome. *Can J Anaesth* 1998;45:332–336.

38. Benca J, Hogan K. Malignant hyperthermia, coexisting disorders and enzymopathies: risks and management options. *Anesth Analg* 2009;109:1049–1053.

39. Marcus FI, McKenna WJ, Sherrill D, et al. Diagnosis of arrhythmogenic right ventricular cardiomyopathy/dysplasia proposed modification of the task force criteria. *Circulation* 2010;121:1533–1541.

40. Tabib A, Loire R, Miras A, et al. Unsuspected cardiac lesions associated with sudden unexpected perioperative death. *Eur J Anaesthesiol* 2000;17:230–235.

41. Corrado D, Leoni L, Link MS, et al. Implantable cardioverter-defibrillator therapy for prevention of sudden death in patients with arrhythmogenic right ventricular cardiomyopathy/dysplasia. *Circulation* 2003;23:3084–3091.

42. Doyle NM, Monga M, Montgomery B, et al. Arrhythmogenic right ventricular cardiomyopathy with implantable cardioverter defibrillator placement in pregnancy. *J Matern Fetal Neonatal Med* 2005;18:141–144.

43. Lee LC, Bathgate SL, Macri CJ. Arrhythmogenic right ventricular dysplasia in pregnancy: a case report. *J Reprod Med* 2006;51:725–728.

44. Koenig C, Katz M, Gertsch M, et al. Pregnancy and delivery in a patient with Uhl anomaly. *Obstet Gynecol* 1991;78:932–934.

45. Bello YM, Falabella AF, Schachner LA. Management of epidermolysis bullosa in infants and children. *Clin Dermatol* 2003;21:278–282.

46. Herod J, Denyer J, Goldman A, et al. Epidermolysis bullosa in children: pathophysiology, anaesthesia and pain management. *Paediatr Anaesth* 2002;12:388–397.

47. Baloch MS, Fitzwilliams B, Mellerio J, et al. Anaesthetic management of two different modes of delivery in patients with dystrophic epidermolysis bullosa. *Int J Obstet Anesth* 2008;17:153–158.

48. Berryhill RE, Benumof JL, Saidman LJ, et al. Anesthetic management of emergency cesarean section in a patient with epidermolysis bullosa dystrophica polydysplastica. *Anesth Analg* 1978;57:281–283.

49. Broster T, Placek R, Eggers GW Jr. Epidermolysis bullosa: anesthetic management for cesarean section. *Anesth Analg* 1987;66:341–343.

50. Price T, Katz VL. Obstetrical concerns of epidermolysis bullosa. *Obstet Gynecol Surv* 1988;43:445–449.

51. Garcia I, Munoz C, Lopez-Gil MV, et al. Tratamiento anestesico para cesarea en una paciente con epidermolisis bullosa distrofica recesiva. *Rev Esp Anestesiol Reanim* 2009;56:569–571.

52. Diaz JH. Perioperative management of children with congenital phakomatoses. *Paediatr Anaesth* 2000;10:121–128.

53. Kerrison JB, Newman NJ. Phacomatoses. *Neurosurg Clin N Am* 1999;10:775–787.

54. Ginsburg DS, Hernandez E, Johnson JW. Sarcoma complicating von Recklinhausen disease in pregnancy. *Obstet Gynecol* 1981;58:385–387.

55. Posma E, Aalbers R, Kurniawan YS, et al. Neurofibromatosis type 1 and pregnancy: a fatal attraction? Development of malignant schwannoma during pregnancy in a patient with neurofibromatosis type 1. *BJOG* 2003;110:530–532.

56. Kellogg A, Watson WJ. Malignant schwannoma in pregnancy: a case report and literature review. *Am J Perinatol* 2010;27:201–204.

57. Bolten J, Jansen ENH, de Graaff R. Von Recklinghausen neurofibromatosis (VRNF) and pregnancy. A single case study. *Clin Neurol Neurosurg* 1987;89:181–184.

58. Griffiths ML, Theron EJ. Obstructed labour from pelvic neurofibroma. *S Afr Med J* 1978;53:781.

59. Baker VV, Hatch KD, Shingleton HM. Neurofibrosarcoma complicating pregnancy. *Gynecol Oncol* 1989;34:237–239.

60. Ansari AH, Nagamani M. Pregnancy and neurofibromatosis (von Recklinhausen's disease). *Obstet Gynecol* 1976;47:25S–29S.

61. Sangupta BS, Wynter HH. Pregnancy in a Jamaican with von Recklinghausen's disease. *West Indian Med J* 1978;27:81–85.

62. Brady DB, Bolan JC. Neurofibromatosis and spontantous hemothorax in pregnancy: two case reports. *Obstet Gynecol* 1984;63:35S–38S.

63. Humble RM. Pheochromocytoma, neurofibromatosis, and pregnancy. *Anaesthesia* 1967;22:296–303.

64. Edwards JN, Fooks M, Davey DA. Neurofibromatosis and severe hypertension in pregnancy. *Br J Obstet Gynaecol* 1983;90:528–531.

65. Sharma JB, Gulati N, Malik S. Maternal and perinatal complications in neurofibromatosis during pregnancy. *Int J Gynecol Obstet* 1991;34:221–227.

66. Hagymasy L, Toth M, Szucs N, et al. Neurofibromatosis type 1 with pregnancy-associated renovascular hypertension and the syndrome of hemolysis, elevated liver enzymes, and low platelets. *Am J Obstet Gynecol* 1998;179:272–274.

67. Sherman SJ, Schwartz DB. Eclampsia complicating a pregnancy with neurofibromatosis. A case report. *J Reprod Med* 1992;37:469–472.

68. McLauglin ME, Jacks T. Progesterone receptor expression in neurofibromas. *Cancer Res* 2003;63:752–755.

69. Sakai T, Vallejo MC, Shannon KT. Parturient with neurofibromatosis type 2: anesthetic and obstetric considerations for delivery. *Int J Obstet Anesth* 2008;17:170–173.

70. Kapur S, Kumar S, Eagland K. Anesthetic management of a parturient with neurofibromatosis 1 and Charcot-Marie-Tooth disease. *J Clin Anesth* 2007;19:405–406.

71. Holt GR. ENT manifestations of von Recklinghausen's disease. *Laryngoscope* 1978;88:1617–1632.

72. Yong-Hing K, Kalamchi A, MacEwen D. Cervical spine abnormalities in neurofibromatosis. *J Bone Joint Surg Am* 1979;61:695–699.

73. Crozier WC. Upper airway obstruction in neurofibromatosis. *Anaesthesia* 1987;42:1209–1211.

74. Wulf H, Brinkmann G, Rautenberg M. Management of the difficult airway. A case of failed fiberoptic intubation. *Acta Anaesthesiol Scand* 1997;41:1080–1082.

75. Nelson DB, Greer L, Wendel G. Neurofibromatosis and pregnancy: a report of maternal cardiopulmonary compromise. *Obstet Gynecol* 2010;116(Suppl 2):507–509.

76. Krishna G. Neurofibromatosis, renal hypertension, and cardiac dysrhythmias. *Anesth Analg* 1975;54:542–545.

77. Yamashita M, Matsuki A, Oyama T. Anaesthetic considerations on von Recklinghausen's disease (multiple neurofibromatosis). Abnormal response to muscle relaxants. *Anaesthetist* 1977;26:317–318.

78. Naguib M, Al-Rajeh SM, Abdulatif M, et al. Response of a patient with von Recklinghausen's disease to succinylcholine and atracurium. *Middle East J Anesthesiol* 1988;9:429–434.

79. Richardson MG, Setty GK, Rawoof SA. Responses to nondepolarizing neuromuscular blockers and succinylcholine in von Recklinghausen neurofibromatosis. *Anesth Analg* 1996;82:382–385.

80. Spiegel JE, Hapgood A, Hess PE. Epidural anesthesia in a parturient with neurofibromatosis type 2 undergoing cesarean section. *Int J Obstet Anesth* 2005;14:336–339.

81. Duounas M, Mercier FJ, Lhuissier C, et al. Epidural analgesia for labour in a parturient with neurofibromatosis. *Can J Anaesth* 1995;42:420–424.

82. Esler MD, Durbridge J, Kirby S. Epidural haematoma after dural puncture in a parturient with neurofibromatosis. *Br J Anaesth* 2001;87:932–934.

83. Rasko JE, North KN, Favaloro EJ, et al. Attenuated platelet sensitivity to collagen in patients with neurofibromatosis type 1. *Br J Haematol* 1995;89:582–588.

84. Lighthall GK, Morgan C, Cohen SE. Correction of intraoperative coagulopathy in a patient with neurofibromatosis type 1 with intravenous desmopression (DDAVP). *Int J Obstet Anesth* 2004;13:174–177.

85. Batra RK, Gulaya V, Madan R, et al. Anaesthesia and the Sturge-Weber syndrome. *Can J Anaesth* 1994;41:133–136.

86. Dolkart LA, Bhat M. Sturge-Weber syndrome in pregnancy. *Am J Obstet Gynecol* 1995;173:969–971.

87. Zanconato G, Papadopoulos N, Lampugnani F, et al. Uncomplicated pregnancy associated with Sturge-Weber angiomatosis. *Eur J Obstet Gynecol Reprod Biol* 2008;137:125–126.

88. McLoughlin L, Thomas G, Hasan K. Pregnancy and lymphangioleiomyomatosis: anaesthetic management. *Int J Obstet Anesth* 2003;12:40–44.

89. Rattan PK, Knuppel RA, Scerbo JC, et al. Tuberous sclerosis in pregnancy. *Obstet Gynecol* 1983;62:21s–22s.

90. Lewis EL, Palmer JM. Renal angiomyolipoma and massive retroperitoneal hemorrhage during pregnancy. *West J Med* 1985;143:675–676.

91. Petrikovsky BM, Vintzileos AM, Cassidy SB, et al. Tuberous sclerosis in pregnancy. *Am J Perinatol* 1990;7:133–135.

92. Forsnes EV, Eggleston MK, Burtman M. Placental abruption and spontaneous rupture of renal angiomyolipoma in a pregnant woman with tuberous sclerosis. *Obstet Gynecol* 1996;88:725.

93. Carter SM, Chazotte C, Caride D. Pregnancy courses in a patient with tuberous sclerosis. *Obstet Gynecol* 1996;88:724.

94. Cleary-Goldman J, Sanghvi AV, Nakhuda GS, et al. Conservative management of pulmonary lymphangioleomyomatosis and tuberous sclerosis complicated by renal angiomyolipomas in pregnancy. *J Matern Fetal Neonatal Med* 2004; 15:132–134.

95. Wilson AM, Slack HL, Soosay SA, et al. Lymphangioleiomyomatosis. A series of three case reports illustrating the link with high oestrogen states. *Scott Med J* 2001;46:150–152.

96. Yigla M, Bentur L, Benizhak O, et al. Pulmonary lymphangioleiomyomatosis: prolonged survival espite multiple pregnancies and no hormonal intervention. *Respirology* 1996;3:213–215.

97. Borro JM, Morales P, Baamonde A. Tuberous sclerosis and pregnancy; report of a case with renal and pulmonary involvement. *Eur J Obstet Gynecol Reprod Biol* 1987;26:169–173.

98. Mitchell AL, Parisi MA, Sybert VP. Effects of pregnancy on the renal and pulmonary manifestations in women with tuberous sclerosis complex. *Genet Med* 2003;5:154–160.

99. Causse-Mariscal A, Palot M, Visseaux H, et al. Labor analgesia and cesarean section in women affected by tuberous sclerosis: report of two cases. *Int J Obstet Anesth* 2007;16:277–280.

100. Cho SY, Kim KH, Jeon WJ. Caesarean delivery under general anaesthesia for a woman with undiagnosed tuberous sclerosis complex and lymphangioleiomyomatosis. *Anaesth Intensive Care* 2009;37:142–143.

101. Byrd LM, Jadoon B, Lieberman I, et al. Chronic pain and obstetric management of a patient with tuberous sclerosis. *Pain Med* 2007;8:199–203.

102. Lee SJ, Kim YH, Lee JH, et al. Development of parafoveal exudates and serous retinal detachment in a pregnant woman with tuberous sclerosis. *Gynecol Obstet Invest* 2002;53:188–190.

103. Hayden MG, Gephart R, Kalanithi P, et al. Von Hippel-Lindau disease in pregnancy: a brief review. *J Clin Neurosci* 2009;16:611–613.

104. Delisle MF, Valimohamed F, Money D, et al. Central nervous system complications of von Hippel-Lindau disease and pregnancy; perinatal considerations: case report and literature review. *J Matern Fetal Med* 2000;9:242–247.

105. Kothari A, Bethune M, Manwaring J, et al. Massive bilateral phaeochromocytomas in association with von Hippel-Lindau syndrome in pregnancy. *Aust N Z J Obstet Gynaecol* 1999;39:381–384.

106. Phupong V, Witoonpanich P, Snabboon T, et al. Bilateral pheochromocytoma during pregnancy. *Arch Gynecol Obstet* 2005;271:276–279.

107. Kolomeyevskaya N, Blazo M, Van den Vayver I, et al. Pheochromocytoma and von Hippel-Lindau in pregnancy. *Am J Perinatol* 2010;27:257–263.

108. Joffe D, Robbins R, Benjamin A. Caesarean section and phaeochromocytoma resection in a patient with von Hippel-Lindau disease. *Can J Anaesth* 1993; 40:870–874.

109. Cousins MJ, Rubin RB. Intraoperative management of phaeochromocytoma with total epidural sympathetic blockade. *Br J Anaesth* 1974;46:78–81.

110. Gimbert P, Chauveau D, Richard S, et al. Pregnancy in von Hippel-Lindau disease. *Am J Obstet Gynecol* 1999;180:110–111.

111. Naidoo K, Bhigjee AI. Multiple cerebellar haemangioblastomas symptomatic during pregnancy. *Br J Neurosurg* 1998;12:281–284.

112. Ogasawara KK, Ogasawara EM, Hirata G. Pregnancy complicated by von Hippel-Lindau disease. *Obstet Gynecol* 1995;85:829–831.

113. Kurne A, Bakar B, Arsava EM, et al. Pregnancy associated quadriparesis in a patient with von Hippel-Lindau disease. *J Neurol* 2003;250:234–235.

114. Ortega-Martinez M, Cabezudo JM, Fernandez-Portales I, et al. Multiple filum terminale hemangioblastomas symptomatic during pregnancy. *J Neurosurg Spine* 2007;7:254–258.

115. Boker A, Ong BY. Anesthesia for cesarean section and posterior fossa craniotomy in a patient with von Hippel-Lindau disease. *Can J Anaesth* 2001;48:387–390.

116. Razvi SAH, Stefak Y, Bird J. Caesarean section for a woman with von Hippel-Lindau disease. *Int J Obstet Anesth* 2009;18:294–295.

117. Mattews AJ, Halshaw J. Epidural anaesthesia in von Hippel-Lindau disease. Management of childbirth and anaesthesia for caesarean section. *Anaesthesia* 1986;41:853–855.

118. Wang A, Sinatra RS. Epidural anesthesia for cesarean section in a patient with von Hippel-Lindau disease and multiple sclerosis. *Anesth Analg* 1999;88:1083–1084.

119. Demiraran Y, Ozgon M, Utku T, et al. Epidural anaesthesia for caesarean section in a patient with von Hippel-Lindau disease. *Eur J Anaesthesiol* 2001; 18:330–332.

120. McCarthy T, Leighton R, Mushambi M. Spinal anaesthesia for caesarean section for a woman with von Hippel-Lindau disease. *Int J Obstet Anaesth* 2010; 19:461–462.

121. Hsu DT. Cardiac manifestations of neuromuscular disorders in children. *Paediatr Respir Rev* 2010;11:35–38.

122. Robins K, Lyons G. Opioid-Related narcosis in a woman with myopathy receiving magnesium. *Int J Obstet Anesth* 2007;16:367–369.

123. Litman RS, Rosenberg H. Malignant hyperthermia-associated diseases: state of the art uncertainty. *Anesth Analg* 2009;109:1004–1005.

124. Turbidy N, Fontaine B, Eymard B. Congenital myopathies and congenital muscular dystrophies. *Curr Opin Neurol* 2001;14:575–582.

125. Molyneux MK. Anaesthetic management during labour of a manifesting carrier of Duchenne muscular dystrophy. *Int J Obstet Anesth* 2005;14:58–61.

126. Manzur AY, Muntoni F. Diagnosis and new treatments in muscular dystrophies. *Postgrad Med J* 2009;85:622–630.

127. Gurnaney H, Brown A, Litman RS. Malignant hyperthermia and muscular dystrophies. *Anesth Analg* 2009;109:1043–1048.

128. Pash MP, Balaton J, Eagle C. Anaesthetic management of a parturient with severe muscular dystrophy, lumbar lordosis, and a difficult airway. *Can J Anaesth* 1996;43:959–963.

129. Allen T, Maguire S. Anaesthetic management of a woman with autosomal recessive Limb-Girdle muscular dystrophy for emergency caesarean section. *Int J Obstet Anesth* 2007;16:370–374.

130. Ekblad U, Kanto J. Pregnancy outcome in an extremely small woman with muscular dystrophy and respiratory insufficiency. *Acta Anaesthesiol Scand* 1993; 37:228–230.

131. Klingler W, Rueffert H, Lehmann-Horn F, et al. Core myopathies and risk of malignant hyperthermia. *Anesth Analg* 2009;109:1167–1173.

132. Jungbluth H, Muntoni F, Ferreiro A. ENMC International Workshop: Core Myopathies, 9–11th March 2007, Naarden, The Netherlands. *Neuromuscul Disord* 2008;18:989–996.

133. Sewry CA, Muller C, Davis M, et al. Spectrum of pathology in central core disease. *Neuromuscul Disord* 2002;12:930–938.

134. Jungbluth H. Central core disease. *Orphanet J Rare Dis* 2007;2:25.

135. Foster RN, Boothroyd KP. Caesarean section in a complicated case of central core disease. *Anaesthesia* 2008;63:544–547.

136. Jungbluth H. Multi-minicore disease. *Orphanet J Rare Dis* 2007;2:31.

137. Osada H, Masuda K, Seki K, et al. Multi-minicore disease with susceptibility to malignant hyperthermia in pregnancy. *Gynecol Obstet Invest* 2004;58:32–35.

138. Saito O, Yamamoto T, Mizuno Y. Epidural anesthetic management using ropivacaine in a parturient with multi-minicore disease and susceptibility to malignant hyperthermia. *J Anesth* 2007;21:113.

139. Jungbluth H, Sewry CA, Counsell S, et al. Magnetic resonance imaging of muscle in nemaline myopathy. *Neuromuscul Disord* 2004;14:779–784.

140. Riggs JE, Bodensteiner JB, Schochet SS Jr. Congenital myopathies/dystrophies. *Neurol Clin N Am* 2003;21:779–794.

141. Heard SO, Kaplan RF. Neuromuscular blockade in a patient with nemaline myopathy. *Anesthesiology* 1983;59:588–590.

142. Stackhouse R, Chelmow D, Dattel BJ. Anesthetic complications in a pregnant patient with nemaline myopathy. *Anesth Analg* 1994;79:1195–1197.

143. Eskandar OS, Eckford SD. Pregnancy in a patient with nemaline myopathy. *Obstet Gynecol* 2007;109:501–504.

144. Wallgren-Pettersson C, Hulesmaa VK, Paatero H. Pregnancy and delivery in congenital nemaline myopathy. *Acta Obstet Gynecol Scand* 1995;74:659–661.

145. Chitayat D, Hodgkinson KA, Ginsburg O, et al. King syndrome: a genetically heterogenous phenotype due to congenital myopathies. *Am J Med Genet* 1992; 43:954–956.

146. Habib AS, Millar S, Deballi P, et al. Anesthetic management of a ventilator-dependent parturient with the King-Denborough syndrome. *Can J Anaesth* 2003; 50:589–592.

147. Abel DE, Grotegut CA. King syndrome in pregnancy. *Obstet Gynecol* 2003; 101:1146–1149.

148. Muravchick S. Clinical implications of mitochondrial disease. *Adv Drug Deliv Rev* 2008;60:1553–1560.

149. Muravchick S, Levy RJ. Clinical implications of mitochondrial dysfunction. *Anesthesiology* 2006;105:819–837.

150. Yuan N, El-Sayed YY, Ruoss SJ, et al. Successful pregnancy and cesarean delivery via non-invasive ventilation in mitochondrial myopathy. *J Perinatol* 2009;29:166–169.

151. Rosaeg OP, MacLeod JP. Anaesthetic management for labour and delivery in the parturient with mitochondrial myopathy. *Can J Anaesth* 1996;43:403–407.

152. Mautua M, Torres A, Ibarra V, et al. Anesthetic management of an obstetric patient with melas syndrome: case report and literature review. *Int J Obstet Anesth* 2009;17:370–373.

153. Diaz-Lobato S, Gomez Mendieta MA, Moreno Garcia MS, et al. Two full-term pregnancies in a patient with mitochondrial myopathy and chronic ventilatory insufficiency. *Respiration* 2005;72:654–656.

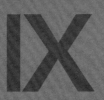

ETHICAL, MEDICAL, AND SOCIAL CHALLENGES AND ISSUES

CHAPTER

41

Informed Consent and Other Ethical and Legal Issues in Obstetric Anesthesia

William J. Sullivan • M. Joanne Douglas

■ INTRODUCTION

Ethical dilemmas exist in medicine when there is more than one possible solution to a problem and those solutions are incompatible with each other. Where there are ethical dilemmas "moral obligations demand . . . that a person adopt each of two (or more) alternative but incompatible actions" (1). One method for solving these ethical dilemmas, and the one adopted commonly by the western medical community, is to use the framework of the four prima facie principles of principle-based ethics: Autonomy (patient choice), beneficence (do good, prevent harm, remove harm), non-maleficence (do no harm), and justice (treat like cases alike) (1) and weigh their relative merits in each situation (2).

Obstetric anesthesiologists will encounter ethical and legal challenges in their anesthetic practice. In obstetrics there may be several competing interests: The obstetric caregivers, the woman herself, and the fetus. Ethical challenges may result from a conflict between the woman and anesthesiologist, who may have opposing views as to what is best for the woman and her fetus. This results in a conflict between the ethical principle of beneficence and possibly non-maleficence (by the physician) and the ethical principle of autonomy (the woman's right to choose).

■ INFORMED CONSENT

The most common legal and ethical challenge the obstetrical anesthesiologist will face in day-to-day practice will be informed consent. Informed consent is the legal method by which society enforces respect for the ethical principle of patient autonomy. The principle of patient autonomy is relatively new and has replaced the centuries old paternalistic approach of the physician who decided what was best for the patient (2–5). Informed consent involves recognition that the patient has a choice as to whether or not to accept the recommended treatment.

Honoring patient autonomy demonstrates respect for the patient and her beliefs and this process involves more than following a list of informed consent requirements (Table 41-1). Although these elements are essential there may be other factors involved. For example, a woman may come from a different cultural background where the husband or other family members may be the decision maker(s) (6). The physician must be certain that the woman wants someone else to make her decision (7) and this is best done by talking with the woman in the absence of the family and, if there is a language

barrier, using an impartial interpreter (6). If the physician is satisfied that the woman agrees to an alternate decision maker then the physician should respect and work with that decision maker. The act of appointing someone else to make a decision is in itself the exercise of autonomy (1). Autonomous choice is a right—not a duty of patients (1). As not all women from a particular culture follow the same rules, the physician has to recognize that belonging to a particular culture does not mean that everyone from that culture follows all or any particular rule.

To understand informed consent is first to understand that the requirements and the legal remedies for the "informed" part of informed consent differ from the "consent" part of informed consent. To avoid confusion some authors advocate the use of two separate terms such as "consent" and "informed choice" (or "informed decision") instead of the phrase "informed consent" (8). However, "informed consent" is fully embedded in western society and the terminology is unlikely to change (9).

■ CONSENT PART OF INFORMED CONSENT

The requirement for consent has long been part of the common law. Touching another (other than in an emergency or in normal societal living) without consent is a battery (in some jurisdictions called an assault or trespass to the person) for which damages can be awarded even if there has been no injury. As Justice Cardozo put it almost a 100 years ago, "every human being of adult years has a right to determine what shall be done with his own body; and a surgeon who performs an operation without his patient's consent commits an assault for which he is liable in damages" (10).

Consent can be implied when the patient cooperates with a procedure, for example, putting up one's arm for a vaccination implies consent to be vaccinated (11,12). Consent can be given with restrictions. Conversely, a battery can be committed even where an initial consent for the procedure was obtained. Examples of this are:

1. If consent is for a specific physician to administer an anesthetic and another physician does so, then there is no consent for that second physician. The second physician, in administering the anesthetic without consent, commits a battery (13) (unless it is an emergency and the first physician is not available).

TABLE 41-1 Basic Elements of Informed Consent (1,5)

1. The patient must have capacity.
2. Consent must be given voluntarily.
3. The patient must be informed (disclosure).
4. The patient must be able to understand the information supplied and the physician must believe the information was understood.
5. The patient must consent.

TABLE 41-2 Standards of Care used to Determine Disclosure

1. Physician (or professional) standard of care: What would a reasonable physician disclose?
2. Objective patient standard of care: What would a reasonable person in the patient's circumstances want to know?
3. Subjective patient standard of care: What would this particular patient want to know?

2. If consent is given for an epidural and without further consent, a general anesthetic is given instead, that is a battery (again, unless it is an emergency).
3. If a woman says, "please, don't touch my left arm" and the anesthesiologist inserts an intravenous in her left arm, the physician commits a battery (14).
4. If consent is withdrawn by a capable patient, and the physician continues with the medical procedure (unless not to continue would seriously endanger the life or health of the woman), that is a battery.

The patient must have capacity in order to give consent. If consent is not given voluntarily then there is no consent and any resultant procedure is a battery. The voluntariness of the consent can be affected by undue influence (usually when consent is sought by a person in a position of authority). Coercion is a form of undue influence that carries with it a threat (overt or implied). Other influences, such as opinions or recommendations from their physician, family, and/or friends, can impact on the patient's decision-making process in giving consent. Provided these influences do not control her decision (and seldom will they), the patient's consent is considered voluntary. There can be no intentional misrepresentation or fraud in obtaining consent. If there is and the procedure goes ahead it is a battery.

Consent does not make a morally wrong act ethically acceptable nor does it make a legally prohibited act lawful. Female circumcision is legally prohibited in most nations as well as considered a morally wrong act. Where female circumcision is legally prohibited consent does not change that legal prohibition nor make it morally right.

■ INFORMED PART OF INFORMED CONSENT

The requirement for the informed part of informed consent is a relatively recent development in the law. The American judges in the Nuremberg trials of Nazi doctors in 1948 developed the Nuremberg Code to govern human participation in research. Section 1 of the Code in part says: The subject should be advised of the "nature, duration and purpose of the experiment; the method and means by which it is to be conducted; all inconveniences and hazards reasonably to be expected; and the effects upon his health or person which may possibly come from his participation . . ." (15).

The words "informed consent" were not used, but in essence Section 1 of the Nuremberg Code recognized the importance of the "informed" requirement for consent (15). In the 1950s the courts began to recognize this principle for health care (16). However, it was only in the last 40 years that the informed part of informed consent, as we know it today, became firmly embedded in the law in the United States and Canada (17,18). The practical reason for the informed part of informed consent was succinctly put by Justice Robinson in Canterbury v. Spence in 1972.

"True consent to what happens to one's self is the informed exercise of a choice, and that entails an opportunity to evalu-

ate knowledgeably the options available and the risks attendant upon each. The average patient has little or no understanding of the medical arts, and ordinarily has only his physician to whom he can look for enlightenment with which to reach an intelligent decision" (17).

Where there has not been consistency is in determining what standard of care is required for disclosure of information. The main standards are the physician standard where the required disclosure is what a reasonable physician in the same field would tell a patient (19) and the objective patient standard where the test is what a reasonable patient in the patient's circumstances would want to know (17) (Table 41-2).

Approximately half of the states in the United States (20) as well as Canada (18) have adopted the "objective patient" standard with the other half of the states choosing the physician standard (20). A few states have the "subjective patient standard" defined as what information would that particular patient want (20) but almost all of the states and Canada were concerned that setting a subjective standard for disclosure would be unfair to a physician (17,18).

The basis for the objective patient standard rather than the physician standard is the argument that physicians should not set the standard of disclosure, as it is the patient's need for information that is the governing principle (17,18). The objective patient standard requires that "The scope of the physician's communications to the patient then must be measured by the patient's need, and that need is the information material to the decision" (17). However, in some jurisdictions a physician's personal knowledge of the patient may indicate additional information is required.

The determination of what in any circumstance is a risk that must be disclosed has been an ongoing challenge for both courts and physicians, whatever the standard, but particularly when using the objective patient standard. The governing principle is that the patient should have the necessary information to make an informed decision (Table 41-3). That information includes risks material to the decision and are those risks which a reasonable person in the patient's circumstances would want to know. If the patient has personal knowledge of risks that the physician fails to disclose (whatever standard) the patient cannot later successfully sue on the basis that the physician failed to disclose those risks.

TABLE 41-3 Disclosure Requirements in Obtaining Informed Consent

1. The condition for which the procedure is proposed;
2. The nature and technique of doing the procedure (what will be done);
3. The risks associated with the procedure;
4. The risks of not having the procedure;
5. The benefits of the procedure;
6. Any reasonable alternative procedure;
7. The answers to questions posed by the patient relevant to the procedure.

Whatever method is used to impart the information about the procedure and whomever may be tasked to impart this information, the ultimate responsibility for informed consent lies with the person performing the procedure. The anesthesiologist may delegate the consenting process to a nurse or resident but the anesthesiologist caring for the patient still remains responsible (21,22).

■ CAPACITY AND COMPREHENSION

In order to give consent the patient must have capacity. If the pregnant woman has capacity no one else's consent is required, including that of the husband. Some jurisdictions may require that a third party consent for underage (minor) patients (23). If the patient lacks capacity to give consent, and there is no consent from a substitute decision maker, it is a battery if the physician performs the procedure (unless it is an emergency). Capacity only goes to the proposed medical treatment. A patient may have no knowledge of world events but if she can understand "the nature and purpose of the treatment and the reasonably foreseeable consequences of giving or refusing consent then she is capable" (5). In most jurisdictions there is a legal presumption of capacity for the purposes of consenting or refusing consent to health care (24). A modern proviso to this is the requirement that the patient understands that the proposed treatment applies to her situation. Refusal of a recommended treatment by a patient is not proof of incapacity (25). The use of the words competence, capacity, and capability can sometimes be confusing. Often competency is considered a legal term as in "now that she is 18 years old she is legally competent to make her own decisions." The American Society of Anesthesiologists (ASA) in their Manual on Professional Liability define competence as "a patient's legal authority to make decisions" and capacity as "a determination (made by medical professionals) that patient has the ability to make a specific decision at a specific time" (26). The Oxford Dictionary of Current English defines "capacity" as "legal competence" and defines "capability" as "ability, power" (27). The important consideration is that whatever label is used in obtaining consent, it applies solely to the patient's mental ability at that time to give or refuse consent to that particular procedure. Pain or pain medication does not affect necessarily the woman's ability to fulfill the legal requirements for consent (28,29).

Part of the requirement to successfully obtain informed consent is to take reasonable steps to ensure that the patient understands the information provided (30). This is particularly so when the patient has apparent comprehension problems, such as those that may arise from language difficulties (30). Providing the information by way of a booklet or a video does not resolve the physician's obligation to be reasonably satisfied that the information is understood nor does asking the patient if she has any questions on the booklet or video (31). One way to test for comprehension is to ask the patient to repeat back in her own words what has been said to her.

An appreciation of the ethical principle of respect for autonomy is helpful in meeting the legal requirement of obtaining informed consent. When the physician wants to be reasonably certain (whatever standard) that the patient knows and understands the risks, benefits, and alternatives to a proposed procedure and understands that the patient cannot exercise her autonomy without that knowledge, the requirements for informed consent become clear.

If the patient lacks capacity (and depending on state law this can include being a minor) to give consent then the physician cannot act, except in an emergency, and must obtain consent from a legally authorized third party or substitute decision maker (32). Who can be a substitute decision maker will depend on the law of the jurisdiction in which the procedure is to be done. Ways in which it can be done include by state statute authorizing a person (generally on the basis of relationship) to be the decision maker, through proxy advance directives and by medical or durable powers of attorney. The substitute decision maker is not free to apply his or her values to health care decision making for the incapable patient. Any decision is first based on the patient's known preferences (substitute judgment) and if they're not known then on the patient's best interests (what a reasonable person in that patient's circumstances would decide) (3). Proxy advance directives and powers of attorney for substitute medical decision making are valid only if the legal requirements for their creation are met. If there is no statutory or other legal provision for a substitute decision maker then a court order is usually necessary to either authorize the procedure or to appoint a substitute decision maker.

■ INFORMED CONSENT AND NEGLIGENCE

Informed consent has nothing to do with whether or not the physician carrying out the medical procedure has met the required standard of care. An action for negligence in carrying out a medical procedure is separate and apart from an action for failure to obtain informed consent. The physician can carry out the procedure without negligence but could be found liable for damages if informed consent was not obtained.

Courts in the United States and Canada have been consistent in holding as a policy decision that the failure to obtain the informed part of informed consent is negligence, but not a battery. The same requirements that a patient must show in an action alleging negligence against a physician in carrying out a medical procedure are also required in an action alleging a physician failed to properly "inform" a patient (17,18) (Table 41-4).

Two of the four requirements (Table 41-4) in a negligence action are relatively straightforward and are usually easily met. If the physician treats the patient then a duty of care is established. It is unlikely that there would be a lawsuit if the patient were not injured. Whether the physician has adequately disclosed sufficient information is more difficult to determine. Most actions against physicians alleging failure to obtain informed consent are unsuccessful (11). In addition to the patient failing to show the standard of care was not met (disclosure), the lawsuit is often unsuccessful because causation was not established (the fourth requirement for negligence) (33) (Table 41-4). In almost all jurisdictions the test for causation is whether the reasonable person in the patient's circumstances would have refused consent if that information had been available (17). Courts often find that consent would still have been given, even if the missed information had been provided.

During the development of the informed consent concept the courts were concerned that if a patient was injured and a

TABLE 41-4 To Establish Negligence

1. The physician must owe a duty of care to the patient.
2. The physician must have breached the standard of care owing to the patient.
3. The patient must have suffered an injury resulting in damages.
4. The breach of the standard of care must have caused the injury.

subjective test of causation were applied (would that particular patient have refused consent if the missing information had been available at the time) then the physician "would be in jeopardy of the patient's hindsight and bitterness" (17).

■ EXCEPTIONS TO OBTAINING INFORMED CONSENT

There are several circumstances under which it is permissible to proceed with care without obtaining informed consent:

1. Waiver: The patient has a right to be informed and therefore can waive that right (34). The physician, however, must be certain as to the patient's decision and should explore, if possible, the reasons behind that decision.
2. Emergency: When the patient is incapable of consenting and there is serious risk to the patient's life or health requiring an immediate medical procedure and when there is no one readily available with the legal authority to give consent, the physician can, in law, proceed without consent (17,35). However, the physician must be careful in determining that the patient does need immediate medical attention to preserve life or health. It may be prudent for the physician to obtain a second opinion confirming the immediate necessity for the procedure and the degree of risk. Proceeding because it is convenient to do so does not constitute an emergency and to do so is a battery.
3. Therapeutic privilege: Information can be withheld if disclosure makes it impossible for the patient to make a rational decision or disclosure would cause psychological damage to the patient. For example, the physician fears that a severely depressed patient might become suicidal upon hearing his diagnosis (17,35). Such withholding is known as "therapeutic privilege." Unless therapeutic privilege is confined in its scope, it not only undermines the principle of informed consent, but it could also seriously erode the patient's right to information (17). Courts have become increasingly circumspect of claims of therapeutic privilege. One approach to the exception of therapeutic privilege is that it can be used only if the physician reasonably believes "the disclosure in itself, would physically or mentally harm the patient to some significant degree" (36). The fact that disclosure may cause the patient to reject the treatment because of fear or any other reason is irrelevant (37,38).

■ DOCUMENTATION OF CONSENT

It is vital to document the informed consent procedure. A written informed consent document signed by the patient is not in itself documentation of that procedure. It is not sufficient that a patient sign a form saying that they have been informed about the procedure and that they consent to it (38). There has to be a full discussion about the procedure, the potential risks and benefits, any alternatives to the proposed procedure (and their risks and benefits), and any questions that the patient might have must be answered and explored. If an interpreter was used for obtaining the consent that should be documented, as well as the name of the interpreter. It is the woman herself who must give the consent, unless she specifically assigns that responsibility to someone else. The anesthesiologist also should document whether the woman was provided with written material and any additional information about what took place (e.g., the woman who says "I don't want to know anything. Just get on with it"). It is the woman's autonomous right to waive the right to information as well as to give informed consent.

In the past a separate written consent for any anesthetic (obstetric or non-obstetric) usually was not required as anesthesia consent was considered part of the surgical consent. A written informed consent document, however, can serve to remind anesthesiologists that a full discussion of the proposed anesthetic (technique, risks, benefits, and alternatives) is essential and in most cases provides some documentation that this discussion did occur.

On admission to hospital, the patient may be requested to sign a generalized consent form which agrees to her receiving care from a wide variety of health care professionals (surgeons, anesthesiologists, trainees) and for them to perform whatever tests or treatment they deem appropriate. This type of consent may be of little value as it is vague with respect to the specific procedures that might be done and it does not inform the patient of any risks associated with those procedures or of not having the procedures. Patients often believe that they are required to sign the document, as presented, in order to receive health care which may mean that consent is not being given voluntarily (39). Relying solely on this type of consent and giving an anesthetic may be a battery and certainly would not satisfy the requirement to inform the patient.

■ OBTAINING INFORMED CONSENT FROM A LABORING PARTURIENT

The question often arises about whether it is possible to obtain informed consent for an epidural from a parturient who is experiencing pain or who has received opioid analgesia. Studies on laboring parturients that examined postpartum recall of information provided during the informed consent process (such as complications of an epidural) or at antenatal classes found that women were unable to recall much of the information that was provided (40,41). While these studies suggest that women were incapable at the time of the consent, the degree of recall was similar to that found in non-obstetric surgical populations, where presumably the patients were not encumbered by pain or opioids at the time of the consent (42). A postpartum patient may not recall the information provided before her labor epidural but this does not mean that she did not understand the information at the time of informed consent (43).

Studies suggest that neither pain (41) nor opioid analgesia (28) interferes with the consent process for most women requesting labor analgesia. Although there are limitations to these studies they indicate that women want to be informed of all of the risks and that pain and opioid medication do not appear to affect their ability to give consent (43).

■ COMMUNICATION

In one study, women indicated that they would prefer to receive information about epidural analgesia prior to labor (44). Ideally, anesthesiologists would have the opportunity to meet each pregnant woman prior to labor. This would establish a physician–patient relationship and allow an early and full discussion of the available anesthetic care and its benefits, side effects, and risks. The woman would have the opportunity to ask questions about analgesia and anesthesia and subsequently be better informed if anesthetic services were required. Unfortunately, most anesthesiologists rarely meet a woman prior to a request for an anesthetic with the exception of those referred to an anesthesia clinic. As a result there is limited time in which to establish a relationship. An obstetrical anesthesiologist may meet the woman for the first time during a period of high stress (e.g., during the pain of labor or on the way to the operating room for an emergency cesarean delivery) making effective communication difficult. The informed consent process is a way to establish a relationship (albeit a brief one) and to involve the woman in her own care. Even during an emergency the anesthesiologist should provide expeditiously as much information as possible about the woman's anesthetic care (technique, benefits, risks, alternatives), based on her particular circumstances (43).

Repeated visits by the anesthesiologist, while the woman is in the labor suite (or postpartum) to ensure that she has adequate analgesia will strengthen the relationship between the woman and her anesthesiologist. This is particularly important in the event of a maternal or neonatal complication, whether or not it is anesthetic-related. Poor communication and failure to establish a patient–physician relationship may lead to questions about what was done and why it was done. Failure to communicate may increase the chances of legal action by the woman (26).

▪ WAYS TO PROVIDE INFORMATION ABOUT ANESTHESIA

Organizations such as the Society for Obstetric Anesthesia and Perinatology in the United States, the Obstetric Anaesthetists' Association in the United Kingdom and the ASA have developed pamphlets or websites that provide information about epidural analgesia for labor and anesthesia for cesarean delivery. (The ASA publication is titled, planning your childbirth: Pain relief during labor and delivery.) Ideally this material would be available through prenatal classes and in antenatal clinics in order to allow pregnant women to consider their choices for analgesia/anesthesia for labor and delivery (45).

Most would agree that providing written information about anesthetic care is a good idea but does written information help the woman to understand the risks and benefits of epidural analgesia? Studies by White et al. (46) and Gerancher et al. (47) found that the addition of written information to a verbal discussion about epidural labor analgesia improved women's knowledge. However, providing written information does not eliminate the need for the anesthesiologist to have a full discussion with the woman requesting labor analgesia. A pamphlet or other means of providing the information such as a video is an aid and can serve as a catalyst for a full discussion with the anesthesiologist.

How does one communicate with the parturient that says "I don't care about the complications, just give me the epidural"? Although some anesthesiologists consider this sufficient reason to not have a full discussion explaining the procedure and alternatives one should not automatically decide to forego the explanation. Many women say this as they are concerned that a discussion may delay the provision of pain relief. The belief of the authors is that one should attempt to communicate at least the major risks of the epidural to the woman while preparing to initiate it. The woman still may refuse to have the discussion and, if this happens, it should be documented in her chart. The woman not only has the right to receive full information before giving informed consent she also has the right to refuse to receive information. Attempting to establish communication with the woman and providing the information will help avoid a later complaint about lack of information (particularly if there is an adverse reaction, such as a postdural puncture headache).

▪ INFORMATION TO DISCLOSE

The intent of informed consent is that the patient has the necessary information to make a decision about the proposed procedure so the benefits and risks of the procedure (and of having it or not having it) must be discussed, as well as the

procedure itself. If there are alternative procedures these too should be discussed with their risks and benefits, and if those alternatives are only available at another hospital that too should be disclosed. The extent of the disclosure will depend on the facts, and, even in jurisdictions where the physician standard of disclosure applies, the physician should also consider what a reasonable person in the patient's circumstances would want to know. Informed consent exists so the patient can make a reasoned decision, and providing sufficient information is the ethical duty of the physician, whatever the legal standard of disclosure.

Most obstetric patients want to know all the risks and complications of an anesthetic, whether it is for labor analgesia or operative delivery, and it is essential that these be disclosed as part of informed consent (29). In the past some anesthesiologists limited discussion about risks of anesthesia, for fear that a patient would refuse to have the procedure. This concern is not a legal or ethical reason to limit disclosure (48).

The recommendation for disclosure of risks is that one should disclose risks that are common, even if the injury may be minimal, and risks where the injury may be serious, whether rare or not (26). The patient also should be told about the consequences if the injury should occur (e.g., paralysis with an epidural hematoma). Courts have held that all risks need not be disclosed, only those that are material, but any risks that may be raised by patients require full disclosure. This underlines the importance of asking the woman at the end of the discussion if she has any questions and then fully answering them.

It is important to discuss the chance of a particular risk occurring. Putting the risk in the context of risks that the woman will understand may allay anxiety (49,50). It also affirms respect for the woman's autonomy, as she will be able to judge the magnitude of the risk relative to her own experience.

▪ REFUSAL BY THE ANESTHESIOLOGIST TO ADMINISTER A NON-RECOMMENDED ANESTHETIC

This ethical dilemma places the woman's autonomy against the anesthesiologist who does not want to cause harm (beneficence or non-maleficence). This situation may arise when a woman states that she wants or does not want a specific anesthetic, for example, refusing a general anesthetic when there are contraindications to a neuraxial technique. Anesthesiologists may argue that the woman's decision interferes with the anesthesiologist's autonomy. Unfortunately, there is no easy answer to this dilemma, particularly if the situation is an emergency. If the anesthesiologist proceeds with an anesthetic without consent, that is a battery, but if the requested anesthetic is administered and there is a complication (which can be predicted because of the woman's particular circumstances) then a claim of negligence could be made.

There often are reasons for the woman's choice of or refusal for a particular anesthetic. For example, Simon et al. reported two cases of emergency cesarean delivery where the women did not want a neuraxial anesthetic, because of a needle phobia (51). While this eliminated the possibility of neuraxial anesthesia it also severely altered the generally accepted method of an intravenous induction of general anesthesia. (One of the women refused an intravenous while the other refused an intravenous induction due to fears that it might cause pain, even though she already had intravenous access.) Both women agreed to an inhalation induction and the one who did not have an intravenous agreed to its insertion once consciousness was lost (51). Both cases resulted in positive outcomes for the mothers and their neonates. If alternatives had not been explored in these two cases following the women's refusal, the outcome could have been different as cesarean delivery was deemed necessary by the obstetrician.

In the situation where the woman refuses the recommended anesthetic, the anesthesiologist should explore, as quickly as possible, the reasons for the woman's wishes and determine if any alternatives would be acceptable. If there are none, the anesthesiologist can refuse to provide the non-recommended treatment (43). If the anesthesiologist is prepared to administer the non-recommended treatment then the informed consent process must be extensive, including reasons as to why her choice is not recommended. This discussion should preferably take place in the presence of another anesthesiologist, and should be fully documented, including who was present at the time. Generally, however, courts have said that consent under these circumstances does not change the physician's requirement to meet the standard of care (25).

■ REFUSAL OF CONSENT

The capable patient can always refuse consent for any reason and the reason does not have to be disclosed (52,53). The principle of autonomy allows the patient to refuse without giving reasons. It is, however, important that the anesthesiologist explore, if possible, the reasons for refusal and the risks involved with such refusal. This discussion should be fully documented. This patient right also allows the woman to refuse to be informed (54), but again the anesthesiologist must try to determine the reasons for refusal and ensure that there is full documentation.

■ WITHDRAWAL OF CONSENT

Respect for patient autonomy means that the patient has the right to withdraw consent to a medical procedure, subject to two provisos. First, the patient must have the mental capacity to do so, and second, stopping the procedure at the time of consent withdrawal must not seriously endanger her life or health. Withdrawal of consent can be verbal, even if the consent was in writing, and no reasons are necessary for the withdrawal. If the woman says "stop" or any other expression that could be interpreted as withdrawal of consent, the challenge for the physician is to determine whether she is, in fact, withdrawing consent or whether the words are an expression of fear or concern. If there is doubt the procedure should be stopped, unless to do so would result in death or serious harm. If the woman has withdrawn consent and then changes her mind and decides to continue the procedure, it is necessary to obtain consent again. The physician does not have to repeat all of the information but only provide that which is pertinent to the situation from the time that consent was withdrawn. If the physician continues the procedure after the woman has withdrawn consent that is a battery.

■ BIRTH PLANS

In principle, birth plans are helpful in expressing what the woman wants and does not want pertaining to her care. In practice they can be difficult when the woman does not (and often cannot) know the degree of pain or potential risks that may occur because of her choices expressed in the birth plan (55). It always is open to the capable woman to override her birth plan, for example, to give consent to an epidural when her birth plan says she does not want that procedure. As noted earlier, providing information to the woman prior to labor about the risks and benefits of labor analgesia may help her to make an informed choice. Providing this information is advisable even when the birth plan rejects it. That way if

the woman changes her mind and asks for an epidural she already has the needed information.

The challenge arises when the woman's birth plan states "no epidural" and goes on to say that even if she changes her mind and asks for one, it is not to be given to her. This is the classic Ulysses Directive whereby the woman is afraid that the pain of labor will be so great that she will ask for an epidural and therefore states in her a birth plan that no matter what she says she is not to be given an epidural (4). There is disagreement as to what is ethically right under these circumstances. One position is that it is unethical "to withhold pain relief from a greatly distressed woman actually begging for an epidural solely because of a statement written in her birth plan" (55). The opposite position is "acceding to her apparent immediate request does not respect her long-term preferences" (56). There is uncertainty in the law on this issue. The capable person can revoke previous withholding of consent (including in an advance directive), but given that the purpose of a Ulysses Directive is to act on her written instructions, even when she states she has changed her mind, administering an epidural under these circumstances runs some risk of committing a battery.

■ MATERNAL AUTONOMY VERSUS DOING GOOD TO THE FETUS (FETAL BENEFICENCE)

Rarely, obstetricians and anesthesiologists are caught in the dilemma of a woman who refuses consent to an intervention, even though she or her fetus may be at risk of morbidity or death. The ethical principles in this situation are the woman's autonomy (right to choose) as opposed to the physician's wish to do good or prevent harm to the woman and her fetus (beneficence and non-maleficence). This conflict can occur when the woman refuses the obstetrician's recommendation that an urgent or emergent cesarean delivery be performed, for example, for a placenta previa (woman and fetus at risk) or a non-reassuring fetal heart rate tracing (fetus at risk). Because of the unique relationship between the woman and her fetus, any situation in which the woman's life is at risk will potentially affect the fetus. If the woman dies before delivery, the fetus will die unless a perimortem cesarean delivery is performed. Even with that intervention the fetus may suffer harm.

The law on forced intervention (performing a procedure without consent in a capable patient by order of the court) depends on the country and state jurisdiction. In Canada and the United Kingdom as of this writing the law is clear, the fetus does not have rights until it is born and so the courts will not intervene with respect to the capable woman's choice (57,58). The Angela Carder case in the United States confirmed that autonomy of the capable woman is paramount in almost all circumstances (59). The court noted, "indeed some may doubt that there could ever be a situation extraordinary or compelling enough to justify a massive intrusion into a person's body such as a cesarean section, against that person's will" (59). However, other state courts have ordered forced obstetrical intervention (60).

Refusal of consent to an intervention can have serious implications for a woman in certain states. For example, in Utah in 2004 Melissa Rowland was charged with the homicide of her stillborn fetus from a delay in performing a cesarean delivery due to an initial refusal of consent (61). To avoid the murder charge Ms. Rowland subsequently pleaded guilty to a charge of child endangerment.

A court ruling in favor of forced obstetric intervention has profound implications for the obstetric anesthesiologist, who may be asked to administer an anesthetic to an unwilling woman who may be uncooperative and combative. When faced with an ethical dilemma such as this the anesthesiologist should ascertain the facts (medical and other reasons for refusal), consult with others as appropriate, consider all of the alternatives and their risks, and try to find a solution that will allow the woman to give consent.

Simon et al. reported on two women who refused consent for cesarean delivery based on their fear of needles (51). With a full understanding of their reason for refusal the anesthesiologist collaborated with the women to arrive at a solution—inhalation induction—that allowed them to consent to the cesarean delivery. Although the solution posed additional risks to the women they accepted these risks after full disclosure. Although these cases resulted in consent being given for cesarean delivery, an anesthesiologist could be asked to administer anesthesia for a court-ordered obstetric intervention in a woman who is incapable or one who is capable but continues to refuse consent. In this situation the anesthesiologist must ensure that the court order includes provision for anesthesia, not just the cesarean delivery.

■ LITIGATION AND THE OBSTETRIC ANESTHESIOLOGIST

Obstetrics is considered a high-risk specialty with respect to litigation. Sixty percent to seventy percent of all medical malpractice claims in the United Kingdom are obstetric claims (62). Sixty percent of obstetrical negligence claims in the United States are for neonatal death or brain injury and have arisen out of events during labor and delivery (63). As labor and delivery is the period of time when an anesthesiologist is most likely to be involved in a case it is not surprising that obstetrical litigation claims often include the anesthesiologist, even if they provided exemplary care. In the majority (78%) of obstetric anesthesia claims for neonatal death/brain damage anesthetic care was not a contributing factor (64).

The ASA Closed Claims Project compared obstetric cases pre- and post-1990 with respect to obstetric anesthesia litigation (64). This type of comparison not only shows trends in litigation, but also points out areas where improvement in obstetric anesthesia care can be focused. Comparing post-1990 experience to earlier data, the number of claims related to cesarean delivery decreased as did the proportion associated with general anesthesia (64). The use of capnography, pulse oximetry, and implementation of the Difficult Airway Algorithm (65) likely contributed to these improvements.

The use of general anesthesia decreased during the period of review, with a corresponding increase in the use of neuraxial anesthesia, and the proportion of claims due to complications of neuraxial anesthesia (e.g., maternal nerve injury, back pain, high neuraxial block) increased (64).

Other important changes included decreases in the proportion of claims due to maternal mortality, and neonatal mortality or brain damage and claims with substandard care (64).

Where anesthetic care contributed to neonatal death/brain injury the major contributing factors were anesthesia delay (due to lack of in-house anesthesia coverage), repeated efforts to administer neuraxial anesthesia rather than general anesthesia, communication failure between obstetrician and anesthesiologist regarding urgency of cesarean delivery, and substandard anesthetic care (failure to detect and appropriately treat high block).

The report from Davies et al. highlighted several areas where anesthetic care could be improved to possibly prevent litigation (64). These include improving communication (not only with respect to urgency of cesarean delivery but also alerting the anesthesiologist to potential high-risk cases), improving the response to difficult intubation and improved

diagnosis, and resuscitation of a high neuraxial block (64). Other areas which need to be addressed by obstetric anesthesiologists are prevention, early detection and appropriate followup of intraoperative awareness (66), and improvement in postoperative monitoring and detection of postoperative respiratory events (67). Changing demographics with respect to the increasing rate of obesity (68) and older maternal age (69) will lead to increasing complexity in obstetric anesthesiology care and potentially a greater risk of complications and possible litigation.

Even when exemplary care is provided for obstetric anesthesia, an obstetric anesthesiologist may still be sued. To decrease the likelihood of this event, it is important to establish a physician–patient relationship through good communication, obtain informed consent for all procedures, adhere to the required standard of anesthetic care including adequate preoperative evaluation, ensure that protocols and equipment are in place to manage anesthetic-related complications (such as unexpected high block), and contemporaneously document informed consent, anesthetic management and any unexpected events (26) (Table 41-5).

In the event of an adverse outcome it is now recognized that a frank discussion with the patient (and sometimes the patient's family) reduces the chances of legal action against the physician (26,70). Some jurisdictions in the United States and most of Canada have an apology act or similar legislation that protects the physician from the apology being used in a lawsuit against the physician (71). However, it is prudent for the anesthesiologist to contact his or her insurer or hospital-risk manager before making an apology or disclosing any details of the event.

When an anesthesiologist is notified of a threat of litigation the medical malpractice insurer and risk manager should be contacted immediately. They will then advise the anesthesiologist as to how to proceed. Generally they will require the anesthesiologist to make detailed notes on the case and date and sign them, obtain a copy of the pertinent records (and, of course, not alter the medical record in any way), and to not discuss the case with anyone outside of protected peer review settings (26).

There are times when the obstetric anesthesiologist will be asked to be an expert witness in a lawsuit. The ASA Manual

TABLE 41-5 Questions to Ask Yourself to Avoid or Lessen the Impact of Litigation

1. Have I fully informed the patient?
2. Have I adequately documented that discussion and my subsequent anesthetic management?
3. Am I prepared to check the patient frequently during her labor anesthetic or have I designated an adequately trained individual to detect early signs of complications while I am looking after other parturients?
4. In the event of an adverse event related to my anesthetic care am I prepared and able to intervene promptly? If not, have I designated another anesthesiologist to take my place?
5. Do I have the appropriate equipment to provide the necessary intervention, e.g., airway equipment in the event of a high block in the labor room?
6. When an adverse event has occurred have I completely documented the event, the management of that event and have I (subject to my insurer's requirement) talked to the woman and her family to explain what happened and documented that?
7. Are there sufficient safeguards in place to ensure safe postanesthetic care on the postpartum unit?

on Professional Liability describes the role of expert witnesses and their importance in a lawsuit (26). An expert witness is asked to provide an honest evaluation of the anesthetic care provided. The testimony of an expert witness is to assist the court, not the parties to the lawsuit.

KEY POINTS

- Informed consent shows respect for the woman's autonomy.
- The capable woman can accept, refuse, or withdraw consent for treatment.
- To obtain informed consent one has to present all of the information needed to allow the woman to make an informed decision.
- One should not rely on a written consent as satisfying the legal requirements for informed consent.
- The anesthesiologist should document that informed consent took place and what was discussed.
- Claims against obstetric anesthesiologists related to general anesthesia have decreased while those related to neuraxial anesthesia have increased.
- If there is threat of litigation the anesthesiologist's insurer and risk manager should be immediately advised.

REFERENCES

1. Beauchamp TL, Childress JF. *Principles of Biomedical Ethics*. 6th ed. New York, NY: Oxford University Press; 2009.
2. Mason JK, Laurie GT. *Mason & McCall Smith's Law and Medical Ethics*. 7th ed. Oxford: Oxford University Press; 2006.
3. Jonsen AR, Siegler M, Winslade WJ. *Clinical Ethics*. 6th ed. New York, NY: McGraw-Hill; 2006.
4. Brooks H, Sullivan WJ. The importance of patient autonomy at birth. *Int J Obstet Anesth* 2002;11:196–203.
5. Pickard EI, Robertson GB. *Legal Liability of Doctors and Hospitals in Canada*. 4th ed. Toronto, ON: Thomson Canada; 2007.
6. Blackhall LJ, Murphy ST, Frank G, et al. Ethnicity and attitudes toward patient autonomy. *JAMA* 1995;274:820–825.
7. Dworkin G. Autonomy and behavior control. *Hastings Cent Rep* 1976;6:23–28.
8. Appelbaum PS, Lidz CW, Meisel A. *Informed Consent: Legal Theory and Clinical Practice*. New York, NY: Oxford University Press; 1987.
9. Healy J. *Medical Negligence: Common Law Perspectives*. London: Sweet & Maxwell; 1999.
10. Schloendorff v. Society of New York Hospital 105 N.E. 92 (N.Y. 1914).
11. Knapp RM. Legal view of informed consent for anesthesia during labor. *Anesthesiology* 1990;72:211.
12. O'Brien v. Cunard Steam Ship Co. 28 N.E. 266 (Mass. 1891).
13. Perna v. Pirozzi 457 A. 2d 431 (N. J. 1983).
14. Allan v. New Mount Sinai Hospital (1980), 11C.C.L.T. 299.
15. Annas GJ, Grodin MA, eds. *The Nazi Doctors and the Nuremberg Code. Human Rights in Human Experimentation*. New York, NY: Oxford University Press; 1992.
16. Salgo v. Leland Stanford Jr University Board of Trustees 317 P.2d 179 (Cal. Ct. App. 1957).
17. Canterbury v. Spence, 464 F.2d 772 (D.C. Cir. 1972).
18. Reibl v. Hughes (1980), 114 D.L.R. (3d) 1@108 (2 S.C.R 880).
19. Natanson v. Klein, 186 Kan. 393.350 P. 2d 1093 (1960).
20. King JS, Moulton BW. Rethinking informed consent: the case for shared medical decision-making. *Am J Law Med* 2006;32:429–501.
21. Schanczl v. Singh [1988] 2W.W.R. 465 (Alta. Q.B.).
22. Auler v. Van Natta, 686 N.E. 2d 172, 175–176.
23. Guttmacher Institute Report: www.guttmacher.org/sections/adolescents.php
24. Lane v. Candura 376 N.E. 2d 1232 (1978).
25. Miller RD. *Problems in Health Care Law*. 9th ed. Sudbury, MA: Jones & Bartlett Publishers; 2006.
26. ASA Committee on Professional Liability. Manual on Professional Liability. American Society of Anesthesiologists; 2010.
27. Thompson D. ed. *The Oxford Dictionary of Current English*. 2nd ed. Oxford: Oxford University Press; 1992.
28. Pattee C, Ballantyne M, Milne B. Epidural analgesia for labour and delivery: informed consent issues. *Can J Anaesth* 1997;44:918–923.
29. Jackson A, Henry R, Avery N, et al. Informed consent for labour epidurals: what labouring women want to know. *Can J Anaesth* 2000;47:1068–1073.
30. Cirlariello v. Schacter (1993) 100 D.L.R. (4th) 609 (S.C.C.).
31. Byciuk v. Hollingsworth (2004) A.J. NO. 620.
32. Albala v. N.Y. 429 N.E. 2d 786 (1981).
33. Hastings v. Baton Rouge Hospital 498 So. 2d 713 (La. Ct. App. 1986).
34. Stoer v. Association of Thoracic & Cardiovascular Surgeons, 635 A.2d 1047, 1055–56 (Pa. Super. Ct. 1993).
35. Hall MA, Bobinski MA, Orentlicher D. *Health Care Law and Ethics*. 7th ed. Austin, TX: Wolters Kluwer; 2007.
36. Somerville M. Structuring the issues in informed consent. *McGill Law J* 1981: 26:740–808.
37. Pittman Estate v. Bain (1994) 112 D.L.R. (4th) 257.
38. Meisel A, Kuczewski M. Legal and ethical myths about informed consent. *Arch Intern Med* 1996;156:2521–2526.
39. Rizzo v. Schiller 445 S.E.2d 153 (Va. 1994).
40. Swan HD, Borshoff DC. Informed consent–recall of risk information following epidural analgesia in labour. *Anaesth Intensive Care* 1994;22:139–141.
41. Affleck PJ, Waisel DB, Cusick JM, et al. Recall of risks following labor epidural analgesia. *J Clin Anesth* 1998;10:141–144.
42. Garden AL, Merry AF, Holland RL, et al. Anaesthesia information–what patients want to know. *Anaesth Intensive Care* 1996;24:594–598.
43. Hoehner PJ. Ethical aspects of informed consent in obstetric anesthesia–new challenges and solutions. *J Clin Anesth* 2003;15:587–600.
44. Beilin Y, Rosenblatt MA, Bodian CA, et al. Information and concerns about obstetric anesthesia: a survey of 320 obstetric patients. *Int J Obstet Anesth* 1996;5: 145–151.
45. Smedstad KG. Informed consent for epidural analgesia in labour. *Can J Anaesth* 2000;47:1055–1059.
46. White LA, Gorton P, Wee MYK, et al. Written information about epidural analgesia for women in labour: did it improve knowledge? *Int J Obstet Anesth* 2003;12:93–97.
47. Gerancher JC, Brice SC, Dewan DM, et al. An evaluation of informed consent prior to epidural analgesia for labor and delivery. *Int J Obstet Anesth* 2000;9: 168–173.
48. Plaat F, McGlennan A. Women in the 21st century deserve more information: disclosure of material risk in obstetric anaesthesia. *Int J Obstet Anesth* 2004;13:69–70.
49. Kelly GD, Blunt C, Moore PAS, et al. Consent for regional anaesthesia in the United Kingdom: what is material risk? *Int J Obstet Anesth* 2004;13:71–74.
50. Jenkins K, Baker AB. Consent and anaesthetic risk. *Anaesthesia* 2003;58:962–984.
51. Simon GR, Wilkins CJ, Smith L. Sevoflurane induction for emergency caesarean section: two case reports in women with needle phobia. *Int J Obstet Anesth* 2002;11:296–300.
52. In re Fetus Brown, 689 N.E. 2d 397 (Ill. App. Ct. 1997).
53. Cruzan v. Director, Missouri Department of Health 497 U.S. 261 (1990).
54. Liang BA. What needs to be said? Informed consent in the context of spinal anesthesia. *J Clin Anesth* 1996;8:525–527.
55. Scott WE. Ethics in obstetric anaesthesia. *Anaesthesia* 1996;51:717–718.
56. Thornton J, Moore M. Controversies in obstetric anaesthesia. *Int J Obstet Anesth* 1995;4:41–42.
57. Winnipeg Child and Family Services v. D.F.G. 1997 3 S.C.R. 925.
58. Re MB [1997] 2 FCR 541.
59. Re A.C. 573 A.2d 1235 (DC App. 1990).
60. In Re Baby Doe 632 NE 2d, 326.
61. Minkoff H, Paltrow L. Melissa Rowland and the rights of pregnant woman. *Obstet Gynecol* 2004;10:1234–1236.
62. Chandraharan E, Arulkumaran S. Medico-legal problems in obstetrics. *Curr Obstet Gynaecol* 2006;16:206–210.
63. Cohen WR, Schifrin BS. Medical negligence lawsuits relating to labor and delivery. *Clin Perinatol* 2007;34:345–360.
64. Davies JM, Posner KL, Lee LA, et al. Liability associated with obstetric anesthesia. A closed claims analysis. *Anesthesiology* 2009;110:131–139.
65. American Society of Anesthesiologists Task Force on Management of the Difficult Airway. Practice guidelines for management of the difficult airway: an updated report. *Anesthesiology* 2003;98:1269–1277.
66. Robins K, Lyons G. Intraoperative awareness during general anesthesia for cesarean delivery. *Anesth Analg* 2009;109:886–890.
67. Mhyre JM, Riesner MN, Polley LS, et al. A series of anesthesia-related maternal deaths in Michigan, 1985–2003. *Anesthesiology* 2007;106:1096–104.
68. Gunatilake RP, Perlow JH. Obesity and pregnancy: clinical management of the obese gravida. *Am J Obstet Gynecol* 2011;204:106–119.
69. Yogev Y, Melamed N, Bardin R, et al. Pregnancy outcome at extremely advanced maternal age. *Am J Obstet Gynecol* 2010;203:558.e1–e7.
70. Pelt JL, Faldmo LP. Physician error and disclosure. *Clin Obstet Gynecol* 2008;51: 700–708.
71. www.perfectapology.com/medical-errors.html

Substance Abuse and the Drug-addicted Mother

John T. Sullivan

INTRODUCTION

The primary concerns for obstetric anesthesiologists in managing parturients with a history of substance abuse include understanding and managing the acute intoxication, chronic use and its associated comorbidities, acute withdrawal, and recognizing the impact of substance abuse on obstetric and neonatal outcomes. This chapter will discuss exposure to illicit substances, as well as alcohol, tobacco, and caffeine, as they also affect obstetric outcomes and anesthetic management. Making the diagnosis of substance abuse requires a combination of obtaining a thorough history, communication with obstetric colleagues, laboratory analysis, but frequently it depends simply on good clinical judgment. It is noteworthy that many pregnant women abuse multiple substances and that it is often difficult to ascertain the impact of the individual substances from the impact of other associated comorbidities. There is also a strong association between substance abuse and coexisting psychiatric illness, domestic violence, and poor prenatal care.

PREVALENCE

It is difficult to establish the exact prevalence of substance abuse during pregnancy due to the primary reliance on self-reporting. However, comprehensive epidemiologic statistics are maintained by several government agencies in the United States to monitor trends in the use of illicit drugs, alcohol, and tobacco. The most valuable of these include the Substance Abuse and Mental Health Service Administration (SAMHSA) (1) which is a part of the US Department of Health and Human Services (HHS) and the National Institute on Drug Abuse (NIDA) (2) which is a division of the National Institute of Health. In 2009, approximately 8.7% of all individuals in the United States greater than age 12 reported using illicit substances in the month prior to the survey (1). Unfortunately, the peak incidence of use by age generally corresponds with childbearing years for women and abuse of many substances is also associated with risky sexual behaviors that may lead to pregnancy. The rate for illicit drug use in the prior month among pregnant women has been reported to be approximately 4.5% in the United States as compared with 10.6% of nonpregnant respondents (3). There is a range of reported rates from different populations around the world but the variance appears to be more attributable to what has been measured rather than different use prevalence. For example, in the United Kingdom, the incidence of known drug abuse amongst 15 and 39 year olds is 11% (4). In Sao Paolo, Brazil, pregnant teenagers reported to have positive drug testing (hair analyses) in the third trimester 6% (used cocaine, 4% used marijuana, 1.7% used cocaine, and 3% used both drugs) is 6% (5). In South Australia, 3%

of pregnant women were identified as substance abusers in a 2-year retrospective review at a single institution including 1.1% with opioid dependence (6). The prevalence of substance abuse can also be estimated using psychiatric diagnostic criteria for substance abuse, which is generally defined as "the self-administration of various drugs or substances that deviate from medically or socially accepted use" (7). Using specific DSM IV criteria, 9% of the US population, or 27 million people, met these criteria in the last year with nearly 70% using alcohol alone. It is not clear how many also were pregnant from this methodology (1). Extrapolating from survey data, it can be conservatively estimated that approximately 225,000 infants could be exposed to illicit substances either in utero or in the immediate postpartum period (8).

The rate of illicit substance abuse among surveyed subjects in recent years in the United States has been relatively stable (Fig. 42-1). Individual substances and how they are administered or mixed with other agents fluctuate with social trends and it is important for anesthesiologists in many centers to keep abreast of these developments in evaluating and treating pregnant women who are using illicit drugs. The most widely used illicit substance in the general population of the United States is marijuana (Fig. 42-2). Of course, it is important to note that legal substances (caffeine, alcohol, and tobacco) are the most commonly used by pregnant women.

A greater prevalence of substance abuse has been weakly associated with younger age, ethnic minority status, urban location, unemployment and less education (3). However, these associations may track more closely with individual substances, particularly illicit substances, whereas an underlying rate of use of some form of substance use is found in nearly all demographics. Susceptibility to substance abuse is multifactorial but there is likely a strong genetic component. Substance abuse, including but not limited to alcohol and opioid abuse, is more prevalent in people with some genetic subtypes (9). The work has implications for both the screening and treatment of pregnant patients.

GENERAL CONSIDERATIONS

Substance abuse, in general, is associated with increased risk of obstetric and neonatal complications. These include an increase in preterm birth ([RR] 2.5, 95% confidence interval [CI] 1.6 to 3.8), low birth weight (RR 3.6, CI 2.4 to 5.4), intrauterine growth restriction (RR 3.82, CI 2.4 to 6.1), and placental abruption (RR 2.74, CI 1.1 to 7) (10,11). There may be a lower incidence of preeclampsia of which tobacco use may be a cofounder as it has been independently shown to reduce that complication (12). Patients who are abusing substances or are at risk for abusing substances should ideally receive early antenatal assessment and intervention to eliminate or minimize the exposure.

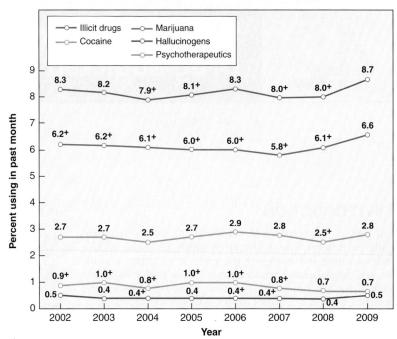

FIGURE 42-1 Past month use of selected illicit drugs among persons aged 12 or older, 2002 to 2009. From: Substance Abuse and Mental Health Services Administration (2010). Results from the 2009 National Survey on Drug Use and Health: Volume I. Summary of National Findings (Office of Applied Studies, NSDUH Series H-38A, HHS Publication No. SMA 10-4586 Findings). Rockville, MD.

†Difference between this estimate and the 2009 estimate is statistically significant at the .05 level.

Substance abuse is also associated with an increased incidence of other medical comorbidities. These include psychiatric disorders (AOR 8.8, 95% CI 6.5 to 11.9), viral (AOR 23.5, 95% CI 8.8 to 62.7) and bacterial (AOR 6.1, 95% CI 3.5 to 10.4) infections, skin diseases (AOR 3.9, 95% CI 2 to 7.8), and trauma and poisoning (AOR 4.2, 95% CI 3.1 to 5.6) (13,14) (Table 42-1). There is also an alarmingly high rate of mortality among those with a history of substance abuse (7.9% of a cohort of 524 pregnant, substance-abusing women in Finland died within 9 years compared with 0.2% of controls) (13).

Patients who are acutely intoxicated may be uncooperative at admission and this has several practical and ethical implications. Important information exchange and establishing trust between patient and health care providers can be compromised, and the validity of obtaining informed consent may be questioned (15).

For anesthesiologists, cooperation, including maintaining relative immobility during neuraxial procedures, is a serious limitation in performing these techniques safely and efficiently.

Some commonly abused substances may create symptoms that mimic other medical conditions or complications of pregnancy. The use of stimulants, including cocaine and amphetamines, has been associated with hypertension and proteinuria which may mimic preeclampsia. Seizure activity and mental status changes are associated with the acute intoxication or withdrawal from many substances which may be confused with eclampsia.

Parturients with a history of substance abuse utilize parenteral labor analgesia at a greater rate than nonsubstance-using controls (11), require more frequent analgesic interventions during cesarean delivery with regional anesthesia (6), and

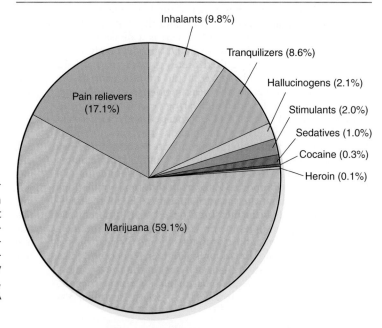

FIGURE 42-2 First specific drug associated with initiation of illicit drug use among past year illicit drug initiates aged 12 or older, 2009. From: Substance Abuse and Mental Health Services Administration (2010). Results from the 2009 National Survey on Drug Use and Health: Volume I. Summary of National Findings (Office of Applied Studies, NSDUH Series H-38A, HHS Publication No. SMA 10-4586 Findings). Rockville, MD.

TABLE 42-1 **Prevalence and Odds Ratios (adjusted for clinical site) of Selected Maternal Medical Conditions and Pregnancy/Labor and Delivery Characteristics, by Exposure Group**

	Exposure Status				OR (99% CI)		
	Exposed (n = 1,185)	Cocaine Only (n = 717)	Opiates Only (n = 100)	None-exposed (n = 7,442) (%)	Exposed	Cocaine Only	Opiates Only
Hepatitis	2.9	2.2	4	0.6	4.8 (2.6–8.9)	3.7 (1.7–8.1)	7.2 (1.8–29)
HIV tested	31.4	29.6	27.1	27.7	1.1 (1–1.4)	1 (0.8–1.3)	0.9 (0.5–1.6)
Positive result	12	12.2	4.2	1.9	8.2 (4.3–15.4)	8.2 (3.9–17.3)	4.3 (0.3–65.3)
AIDS	0.9	0.8	1	0.1	19.5 (4.1–91.6)	17.7 (3.2–98)	71.7 (2.1–2,431.4)
Syphilis	11.3	12.1	0	1.5	6.7 (4.8–9.6)	7.2 (4.8–10.6)	
Gonorrhea	4.5	4.2	1	1.8	1.9 (1.3–3)	1.7 (1–2.9)	0.5 (0–6.5)
Treated urinary tract infection	11.7	11.7	12	11.2	1.2 (0.9–1.5)	1.1 (0.8–1.6)	1.3 (0.6–2.9)
Chronic hypertension	3.9	3.4	7	2.6	1.3 (0.9–2.1)	1.1 (0.6–2)	3 (1.1–8.4)
Psychiatric/nervous/ emotional illness	2.4	2.1	2	1	4 (2.2–7.4)	4 (1.8–8.9)	1.7 (0.3–11.1)
Hospitalizations (total)	11.5	10.3	14	10.8	1.1 (0.8–1.4)	0.9 (0.7–1.3)	1.1 (0.5–2.4)
Violence	0.7	0.7	0	0	18.9 (3–120.3)	19.6 (2.7–144.7)	
Detoxification	1.2	1.3	0	0	46.9 (8.4–263.3)	54.4 (8.6–344.2)	
Drugs administered during pregnancy (total)	71	67.7	90	83.4	0.6 (0.5–0.7)	0.5 (0.4–0.7)	1.8 (0.7–4.4)
Anesthetics	44.4	39.6	72	59.9	0.6 (0.5–0.7)	0.5 (0.4–0.7)	1.6 (0.9–2.9)
Psychoactive drugs	0.9	0.8	1	0.5	2.8 (1.1–7.1)	2.7 (0.8–9.1)	1.8 (0.1–25.2)
Pain/sedation medications	35.3	31.4	65	44.7	0.9 (0.7–1.1)	0.8 (0.6–1)	2.6 (1.5–4.8)
Drugs administered during hospitalization	14.1	13.2	21	17.6	0.9 (0.7–1.2)	0.8 (0.6–1.1)	1.8 (0.9–3.5)
Preeclampsia	4.4	3.5	10	6	0.6 (0.4–0.9)	0.5 (0.3–0.9)	2 (0.8–4.8)
Bleeding							
Placenta previa	1.5	1.4	2	0.8	1.9 (1–3.9)	1.7 (0.7–4.2)	2.4 (0.4–16)
Abruptio placentae	3	2.8	1	1.2	2.3 (1.4–3.9)	2.1 (1.1–4)	0.7 (0.1–10.1)
Prolonged rupture of membranes	8.9	8.8	7	5	1.8 (1.3–2.4)	1.7 (1.2–2.5)	1.3 (0.5–3.6)
Evidence of fetal distress	8.8	7.8	15	7.8	1 (0.7–1.3)	0.8 (0.6–1.2)	1.7 (0.8–3.6)
If yes, emergency cesarean delivery	66.3	67.9	60	65	1 (0.5–1.8)	1.1 (0.5–2.4)	0.9 (0.2–3.4)
Prenatal care by physician	77.3	75.6	94	97.1	0.1 (0.1–0.2)	0.1 (0.1–0.2)	0.5 (0.1–1.4)
Median visits (n)	7	6	12	11	P < 0.001	P < 0.001	P < 0.032

Data are expressed as percentages.
AIDS, Acquired immunodeficiency syndrome; *HIV,* human immunodeficiency virus; *OR,* odds ratio. n = 8,627.
Reprinted with permission from: Bauer CR, Shankaran S, Bada HS, et al. The Maternal Lifestyle Study: Drug exposure during pregnancy and short-term maternal outcomes. *Am J Obstet Gynecol* 2002;186:487–495.

have a higher incidence of inadequate postcesarean analgesia (6). This observed difference is likely multifactorial including both physical and psychological etiologies. Nonpregnant patients with current opioid and cocaine abuse have been reported to have lower pain thresholds compared with historical controls in ice water immersion, which is a commonly used test to delineate population difference in pain experience (16). Because of this difference as well as the complexities in coordinating care, and greater degree of obstetric and neonatal comorbidity, parturients with a history of substance abuse can be expected to consume a disproportional amount of medical resources when admitted for delivery (17).

■ DIAGNOSIS

Confirming a history of substance abuse in a pregnant patient is typically made by a combination of clinical intuition, interview methodology, and laboratory analysis. Depending on the specific substance used, it is not uncommon to deny use when directly questioned; for example, 66% of parturients with subsequent urinalyses positive for cocaine denied using it at admission (18) and almost 60% denied use in a study examining a broader toxicologic screening (19).

In the absence of universal laboratory screening in admitted parturients, it is important to identify historical elements

TABLE 42-2 Federal Workplace Cutoff Values[a]

Substance	Initial Drug Test Level (Immunoassay) (ng/mL)	Confirmatory Drug Test Level (GC–MS) (ng/mL)
Marijuana metabolites[b]	50	15
Cocaine metabolites[c]	300	150
Opiate metabolites	2,000	2,000
Phencyclidine	25	25
Amphetamines	1,000	500
Methamphetamine[d]	Incomplete data	500

[a]GC – MS = gas chromatography – mass spectrometry.
[b]Delta-9-tetrahydrocannabinol-9-carboxylic acid.
[c]Benzoylecgonine.
[d]Specimen must also contain amphetamine at a concentration greater than or equal to 200 ng/mL.
From: Moeller KE, Lee KC, Kissack JC. Urine drug screening: Practical guide for clinicians. *Mayo Clin Proc* 2008;83:66–76.

and behaviors associated with general substance abuse. These include a history of physical or sexual abuse, tobacco use, and lack of prenatal care (20). General clinical signs such as altered mental status, uncooperativeness or combativeness, as well as signs associated with specific substances such as miosis with opioid use or hypertension with stimulants may be the first hints leading to a diagnosis of substance abuse.

There are a variety of published screening methods for detecting substance abuse (21). Short, direct questioning of patients using these instruments can be effective and efficient. The T-ACE (Tolerance, Annoyance, Cut Down, and Eye Opener) (22) and TWEAK (Tolerance, Worried, Eye-openers, Amnesia, and K [C] Cut Down) (23) instruments have been designed to identify alcohol abuse. The 4 P's (24) and 4 P's Plus (25) are appropriate questionnaires to use in screening for a wider number of substances and can detect lower levels of use in pregnant women with moderate to excellent sensitivity (81% to 95%) for detection of alcohol or illicit substance use in pregnancy (26). Longer, written questionnaires such as the Substance Abuse Subtle Screening Inventory (SASSI) have been shown to be very sensitive and specific as screening methods but are time consuming and require patient cooperation (27). They may be more valuable in an outpatient setting and have been shown to be particularly valuable in detecting chronic alcohol abuse. It should be noted that the short, direct screening tools, when used alone with their limited sensitivity and specificity, will ultimately fail in detecting a large number of patients who are currently using illicit substances. Ultimately, they need to be paired with physician judgment and laboratory analysis to detect substance use more effectively. How widely laboratory screening is used is institutionally variable and represents independent clinical practices and resource utilization decisions more than established standards.

■ LABORATORY SCREENING METHODOLOGY

Substance abuse can be diagnosed by analyzing urine, saliva, sweat, hair, meconium, and other biologic samples, although for the obstetric anesthesiologist, urinalysis is currently the most practical method for making a time-sensitive decision, in an acute care environment (28). The process of screening analysis may involve enzyme, fluorescence polarization, or radioimmunoassay techniques. These techniques are rapid, less expensive than alternatives, and considered to have sufficient sensitivity for clinically relevant substance abuse.

Liquid or gas chromatography or mass spectrometry are rarely used for screening but may be used by laboratories to confirm positive results obtained from the screening technique. Individual cutoff values and confirmatory values have been adopted by the Federal Government for workplace screening to minimize false positives (29) (Table 42-2). Urinalysis drug screening batteries vary but a typical panel may include amphetamines, cocaine metabolites, marijuana metabolites, methadone, PCP, propoxyphene, opiates, benzodiazepines, fentanyl, meperidine, and tramadol. It is of clinical importance to recognize the windows of detection for individual substances (29) (Table 42-3).

The cost of urinalysis is nominal; however, it is not common to routinely screen all obstetric patients. The cost effectiveness of screening all obstetric patients, however, could be justified depending on the prevalence of substance abuse in any given patient population. Alternatives to testing urine include testing samples of hair, saliva, sweat, meconium, and the placenta. Most of these alternatives are currently not practical to use in acute decision making in obstetric patients.

■ MANAGEMENT FOR SPECIFIC SUBSTANCES

Ethyl Alcohol

Epidemiology

Alcohol is one of the most commonly abused substances by pregnant women worldwide. Perhaps, since it is legal and commonly accepted in most cultures, its moderate use in pregnancy remains prevalent. In the United States, among pregnant women aged 15 to 44, 10% reported current alcohol use, 4.4% reported binge drinking (defined as having more than five drinks on at least one occasion), and 0.8% reported heavy drinking (defined as consuming at least five drinks on at least five of the last 30 days). These rates are substantially lower for nonpregnant women of the same age (3). Binge drinking during the first trimester was reported by 11.9%, which has implications for teratogenesis. It is estimated that at least 80,000 infants are born annually in the United States to a mother who drank five or more drinks on one or more occasions during pregnancy (30).

Systemic Effects

Ethyl alcohol is a central nervous system depressant. It has transient stimulant properties at low doses followed by a progressive depressant effect on the central nervous system ranging from hypnosis to death. It is absorbed in the

TABLE 42-3 Length of Time Drugs of Abuse can be Detected in Urine

Drug	Time
Alcohol	7–12 h
Amphetamine	48 h
Methamphetamine	48 h
Barbiturate	
Short-acting (e.g., pentobarbital)	24 h
Long-acting (e.g., phenobarbital)	3 wk
Benzodiazepine	
Short-acting (e.g., lorazepam)	3 d
Long-acting (e.g., diazepam)	30 d
Cocaine metabolites	2–4 d
Marijuana	
Single use	3 d
Moderate use (4 times/wk)	5–7 d
Daily use	10–15 d
Long-term heavy smoker	30 d
Opioids	
Codeine	48 h
Heroin (morphine)	48 h
Hydromorphone	2–4 d
Methadone	3 d
Morphine	48–72 h
Oxycodone	2–4 d
Propoxyphene	6–48 h
Phencyclidine	8 d

Data from: American Psychiatric Association. Diagnostic and Statistical Manual of Mental Disorders, 4th edition (DSM-IV), American Psychiatric Association, 4th ed. (Text revision) 2000. Washington, DC; Keegan J, Parva M, Finnegan M, et al. Addiction in pregnancy. *J Addict Dis* 2010;29:175–191; Landau R, Cahana A, Smiley RM, et al. Genetic variability of mu-opioid receptor in an obstetric population. *Anesthesiology* 2004;100:1030–1033; Pinto SM, Dodd S, Walkinshaw SA, et al. Substance abuse during pregnancy: Effect on pregnancy outcomes. *Eur J Obstet Gynecol Reprod Biol* 2010;150:137–141; Ludlow JP, Evans SF, Hulse G. Obstetric and perinatal outcomes in pregnancies associated with illicit substance abuse. *Aust N Z J Obstet Gynaecol* 2004;44:302–306; Castles A, Adams EK, Melvin CL, et al. Effects of smoking during pregnancy. Five meta-analyses. *Am J Prev Med* 1999;16:208–215; Moeller KE, Lee KC, Kissack JC. Urine drug screening: Practical guide for clinicians. *Mayo Clin Proc* 2008;83:66–76.

gastrointestinal tract and metabolized by hepatic microsomal oxidative pathways which are inducible with chronic exposure.

Acute alcohol intoxication is associated with progressive impairment of cognitive function and neuromuscular coordination, intravascular volume depletion resulting from reduced free water absorption in the distal convoluting tubules of the kidneys, and metabolic abnormalities (31). In addition, alcohol intoxication may reduce normal hemodynamic compensatory mechanisms in response to hypotension or hemorrhage (32).

Chronic alcohol abuse is associated with abnormalities in the effects of administered drugs as well as a wide range of potential systemic comorbidities including cardiac, pulmonary and liver disease, and neuropathy. Drug effects in the setting of chronic alcoholism are unpredictable due to alterations in hepatic metabolism, volumes of distribution, and plasma protein binding. Hemodynamic instability may result from intravascular volume depletion, autonomic instability, cardiomyopathy, and an increased shunt fraction with the presence of varices. Alcoholic cardiomyopathy typically presents after 10 years of alcohol abuse but its onset may be unpredictable. The most common manifestation is dilated cardiomyopathy with global depression of ventricular function and a resultant decrease in cardiac output. There is also an association of drinking alcohol and hypertension (33).

Alcoholism has been associated with pneumonia and pulmonary tuberculosis, presumably due to suppressed immune function (34). It has also been associated with an increase in developing acute respiratory distress syndrome (ARDS) in critically ill patients although the mechanism is not clearly defined (35). Chronic alcohol ingestion has been associated with hepatitis, decreased synthetic function of the liver resulting in hypoalbuminemia and coagulopathy, and ultimately end-stage hepatic failure.

Chronic alcohol ingestion leads to cognitive dysfunction including Wernike–Korsakoff syndrome, autonomic dysfunction, and peripheral neuropathy. Autonomic neuropathy may also result in hemodynamic instability and delayed gastric emptying. Peripheral neuropathy is present in 70% of nonpregnant ethanol abusers (34).

Patients with chronic alcohol abuse have been reported to have increased gastric volumes, acidity, and delayed gastric emptying as compared with nonalcohol-abusing patients (36). This phenomenon has not been confirmed in the obstetric population and, it is not clear if this does actually translate to a higher incidence or morbidity from aspiration. Esophageal varices associated with cirrhosis can present a risk for bleeding spontaneously or in association with any instrumentation of the esophagus. Chronic pancreatitis is a rare but problematic complication of alcoholism. Because the condition is very painful, it is common that patients may already be exposed to opioids, which may alter requirements for labor analgesia.

Alcohol withdrawal should be anticipated after hospital admission and presumed alcohol abstinence. It typically presents following 24 to 48 hours of abstinence and manifests with tremor, agitation, seizures, and hallucination. The most concerning effect of acute alcohol withdrawal is the development of delirium tremens that can be life threatening.

Effects on Pregnancy and the Fetus

Although the effects of heavy alcohol use in pregnancy have been well defined, the evidence defining the effects of lower levels of alcohol consumption are somewhat less clear. Low-to-moderate alcohol consumption may be associated with miscarriage, stillbirth, intrauterine growth restriction, prematurity, low birth weight, and being small for gestational age a birth. (37–39). In addition, a higher rate of neonatal mortality has been reported in association with as little as four drinks per week or three binge episodes during pregnancy in the Danish National Birth Cohort (40). Identification of mothers who are at risk (relative risk for neonatal mortality of 1.98 for those consuming one or two drinks per day, and 3.53 for those consuming three or more drinks per day, in comparison with nondrinkers) can result in facilitating appropriate treatment and may likely improve pregnancy outcomes.

With regards to teratology, unfortunately, maternal alcohol consumption remains the source of one of the most preventable birth defects and childhood disabilities in the United States (41). **Fetal alcohol syndrome** is defined as the presence of particular neonatal facial features (small palpebral fissures, flat midface with short upturned nose, thin upper lip) and significant impairment in neurodevelopment and physical growth. **Fetal alcohol spectrum disorders** (FASD) encompass a range of anatomic and behavioral defects related to in utero exposure to alcohol. The combined rate of FASD and alcohol-related neurodevelopment disorders has been reported at 9.1 per 1,000 live births in the United States (34). This translates into approximately 40,000 infants in the United States being born with FASD each year. The combined cost of managing this illness is estimated to be $6 billion annually (42). Amidst the gravity of this problem, controversies exist as to whether there are thresholds of consumption below which it is safe for fetal development, since moderate alcohol consumption is prevalent and FASD has been primarily associated with heavy, chronic, or binge alcohol consumption.

Anesthetic Considerations and Management

In the setting of acute alcohol intoxication, particularly with the aspiration prone physiology of pregnancy, the first priority in anesthetic management should be an assessment of the patient's ability to protect her airway. There should be careful consideration of the influence of intoxication on subsequently administered medications, particularly systemically administered analgesics known to be synergistic with alcohol, on mental status and respiratory depression. In the setting of acute intoxication, additive effects should be expected between alcohol and opioids, benzodiazepines, hypnotics, and volatile anesthetics. With regard to anesthetic choices for the intoxicated parturient, neuraxial analgesia or anesthesia may be superior to either parenteral analgesia for labor or general anesthesia for cesarean delivery to avoid these drug interactions. However, in the setting of chronic alcohol abuse, coagulopathy and systemic infection may present as contraindications to neuraxial anesthesia and should be ruled out.

Other anesthetic considerations in the acutely intoxicated parturient include assessing hemodynamic stability as well as intravascular volume and metabolic status. Intravascular depletion and resulting metabolic acidosis are frequently present in patients acutely intoxicated with alcohol which may require intravenous volume replacement, more intensive monitoring and caution with analgesic and anesthetic interventions known to induce hypotension.

In the setting of chronic alcohol abuse, anesthetic considerations include those related to decreased synthetic function of the liver (coagulopathy, altered drug responses), hemodynamic management (cardiomyopathy, autonomic dysfunction), neurologic dysfunction (gastroparesis, peripheral neuropathy), and the prevention of withdrawal. Coagulopathy may increase the risk of epidural hematoma and contraindicate neuraxial anesthesia as well as complicate the management of any hemorrhage management. Coagulation status should be evaluated before initiating neuraxial anesthesia if hepatic dysfunction is suspected. Compromised hepatic synthetic function can be associated with decreased plasma cholinesterase activity. The implication may be primarily prolonged activity of succinylcholine. The degree to which the activity may be prolonged is unknown in the pregnant patient and, given succinylcholine's generally short plasma half-life, it should not be considered as an absolute contraindication. Another manifestation of decreased synthetic function of the liver, as well as malnutrition that often accompanies chronic alcoholism, is hypoalbuminemia. This may increase the effects of many anesthetic plasma protein-bound drugs including sodium thiopental. Hypoalbuminemic patients may also be more prone to developing pulmonary edema due to decreased intravascular oncotic pressure.

Autonomic neuropathy that may accompany chronic alcohol abuse may affect heart rate and blood pressure stability, which could result in exaggerated hemodynamic responses to dosing neuraxial anesthetics, as well as from the effects of general anesthetic induction and maintenance. In addition, dilated cardiomyopathy may decrease cardiac output and electrocardiography alone is not sensitive in identifying this disorder (33). Echocardiography should be conducted with any clinical suspicion for this condition. With regards to induction agents for general anesthesia, sodium thiopental has been described to have predictable effects in the setting of chronic alcoholism (42), although this phenomenon has not been independently tested in the setting of pregnancy.

With a very high prevalence of peripheral neuropathy in chronic alcohol abuse, it would be helpful to conduct a thorough neurologic examination on admission. At the very least, this condition may confound the evaluation of any postpartum peripheral neuropathy and it may actually be implicated as a risk factor for it. Autonomic dysfunction contributes to delayed gastric emptying in alcoholics, which may influence practitioners to adopt more restrictive fasting policies when applicable and this pathophysiology should be incorporated into any risk–benefit decision making regarding the use of neuraxial versus general anesthesia (43). With esophageal varices often present in chronic alcohol abusers, judgment should be exercised about the relative merits of passing an oro- or nasogastric tube to decompress the stomach during a general anesthetic to reduce the risk of vomiting and aspiration.

Finally, a plan should be established for prophylaxis against acute withdrawal during labor. Benzodiazepines form the cornerstone of management for both the prophylaxis and treatment of acute alcohol withdrawal (44). In addition, any electrolyte abnormalities should be addressed and thiamine replenished beginning early in admission.

Nicotine

Epidemiology

Tobacco smoking has been firmly established as a risk for increasing the incidence of several complications of pregnancy. Although the primary active ingredient of tobacco is nicotine, there are numerous other potentially toxic substances identified in tobacco smoke. The rate of smoking among women of childbearing age indicate both a lower rate of smoking among women who are pregnant compared with nonpregnant women, and a slight reduction in the prevalence of both groups over time (3) (Fig. 42-3). In contradistinction, among teenagers aged 15 to 17, there is a higher rate of smoking among pregnant (20.6%) versus nonpregnant (13.9%) women. With an overall prevalence of 15.3%, smoking represents one of the most commonly abused legal substances (3).

Systemic Effects

Although there are many active substances inhaled in tobacco smoke, the principal one is nicotine. Nicotine increases maternal heart rate, blood pressure, and systemic vascular resistance (45). Uterine artery blood flow is decreased, which is believed to be secondary to increased uterine artery vascular resistance (46). Carboxyhemoglobin levels, which impair oxygen transport, can be expected to be in the 3% to 8% range in mothers who smoke as compared with 1% in nonsmokers. Carboxyhemoglobin is even more concentrated in the fetus (47) (Table 42-4).

Effects on Pregnancy and the Fetus

Tobacco smoking has been strongly associated with low birth weight, placental abruption, respiratory impairment in neonates, and sudden infant death syndrome (SIDS) (12).

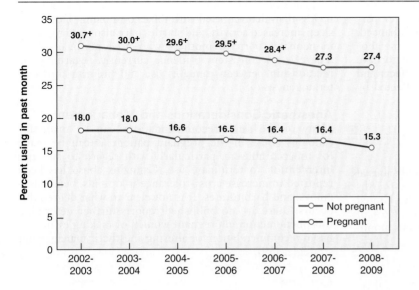

+Difference between this estimate and the 2008-2009 estimate is statistically significant at the .05 level.

FIGURE 42-3 Past month cigarette use among women aged 15 to 44, by pregnancy status: Combined years 2002 to 2003 to 2008 to 2009. From: Substance Abuse and Mental Health Services Administration (2010). Results from the 2009 National Survey on Drug Use and Health: Volume I. Summary of National Findings (Office of Applied Studies, NSDUH Series H-38A, HHS Publication No. SMA 10-4586 Findings). Rockville, MD.

Smoking has also been implicated in a higher rate of PPROM, ectopic pregnancy, spontaneous abortion, and preterm delivery (Table 42-5). There is also a greater incidence of fetal heart rate abnormalities including decreased beat to beat variability in smokers (48). Of the many other potentially toxic substances present in tobacco smoke, cyanide is one of the more noteworthy ones. Cyanide has been reported to reduce vitamin B12, which has been implicated in the fetal growth retardation associated with maternal smoking (49). There is, however, an interesting and incompletely explained beneficial effect of tobacco smoking in reducing the incidence of preeclampsia (45).

The increase risk of SIDS in the children of smokers has been well documented including an apparent dose–response effect: unadjusted odds ratios ranging from 1.6 to 2.5 in individual racial groups for mothers who smoked one to nine cigarettes per day and 2.3 to 3.8 for women who smoked greater than ten cigarettes per day (50).

TABLE 42-4 Data for 134 Women Who Smoked During Pregnancy and Labor[a]

	Mean ± SE (Range)
Age (yr)	25.2 ± 4.28 (16–40)
No. of cigarettes/day during pregnancy	18.6 ± 7.18 (1–35)
No. of cigarettes during labor	4 ± 5.44 (1–20)
Time of last cigarette before delivery (h)	3.2 ± 2.55 (0.25–12)
Maternal HbCO level	
On arrival at hospital (%)	5.6 ± 2.55 (1.2–14.3)
At delivery (%)	3.6 ± 1.97 (0.1–12.5)
Fetal HbCO level in cord blood (%)	9.2 ± 2.66 (2.1 ± 18.5)

[a]HbCO, carboxyhemoglobin.
From: Goodman JD, Visser FG, Dawes GS. Effects of maternal cigarette smoking on fetal trunk movements, fetal breathing movements and the fetal heart rate. *Br J Obstet Gynaecol* 1984;91:657–661.

Anesthetic Considerations and Management

Perhaps the most important intervention to be made with pregnant smokers, although it is more an obstetrician's responsibility, is to engage them in an aggressive smoking cessation program early in pregnancy to minimize obstetric and anesthetic complications. Nicotine replacement strategies have been used in pregnancy (pregnancy category C and D) and are likely to be safer than continuing to smoke, because at a minimum, they reduce the nonnicotine agents present in smoke (51). Smoking cessation success rates, which have been improved in recent years, are due in part to the multimodal therapy and nicotine tapering programs. Many antidepressants commonly used in multimodal therapy have fetal considerations. The risks of using any of these agents must be weighed against continued fetal nicotine exposure. Nonetheless, more intensive smoking cessation programs report higher success rates even though there is a high rate of recidivism following delivery (30). It is not clear if cessation of smoking immediately before delivery is advantageous. Abstinence from tobacco for 48 hours improves available oxygen in the blood but may not reduce peripartum respiratory complications (52).

TABLE 42-5 Pooled Odds Ratios and Confidence Intervals for the Relationship of Smoking to Five Pregnancy Complications

Condition	Pooled OR	Lower 95% CL	Upper 95% CL
Placenta previa	1.58	1.04	2.12
Abruptio placenta	1.62	1.46	1.77
Ectopic pregnancy	1.77	1.31	2.22
Preterm PROM	1.7	1.18	2.25
Preeclampsia	0.51	0.38	0.64

From: Benowitz NL, Jacob P 3rd, Jones RT, et al. Interindividual variability in the metabolism and cardiovascular effects of nicotine in man. *J Pharmacol Exp Ther* 1982;221:368–372.

In the setting of continued tobacco abuse, the existing advantages of neuraxial analgesia and anesthesia over parenteral opioids or general anesthesia are further enhanced. Nicotine exposure has been reported to alter the metabolism of many drugs. Benzodiazepines are reported to have increased effects; many opioids have decreased effects and sodium thiopental has been reported to be not affected by nicotine exposure (53).

Cannabis

Epidemiology

Cannabis, or marijuana, is one of the most commonly abused substances by pregnant women accounting for three-fourths of illicit substance abuse (54). Marijuana use in the United States has been relatively stable over the last decade; 6.6% of individuals (12 and older) reported use in the previous month in the 2009 survey (3).

Systemic Effects

Cannabis contains the active ingredient delta-9-tetrahyrdocannibinol (THC) that is a hallucinogen. It is most commonly inhaled by smoking but can also be ingested. It causes euphoria, mild tachycardia, and elevated blood pressure. The time of onset is approximately 10 to 15 minutes and the duration of effect lasts for up to 3 to 5 hours. As with tobacco smoking, smoking cannabis is associated with pulmonary diseases and elevated levels of carboxyhemoglobin in the maternal blood. Cannabis smoking has been reported to transiently increase maternal heart rate and blood pressure, and causes myocardial depression, but it is not clear if these are serious clinical considerations (55). An acute effect of cannabis is to increase anxiety, which frequently manifests as paranoia and has implications for communication and the development of a trusting relationship between obstetric patients and their health care providers. There have been isolated case reports describing an unexpected degree of airway edema immediately following cannabis smoking (56). It is not clear how prevalent this is with cannabis, or if this should alter management in the pregnant patient presuming a thorough airway examination is already being performed.

Effects on Pregnancy and the Fetus

There is conflicting evidence regarding the impact of cannabis on obstetric outcomes. THC accumulates in fat-rich tissues and crosses the placenta readily, which may lead to more chronic exposure for the fetus than that which may be estimated by the duration of the physiologic effects in the mother (55). Decreased birth weights have been reported in infants of marijuana users but the relationship appears to be less than that reported with tobacco smoking. Decreased sleep, increased activity, and startles have also been reported in neonates born to mothers who used marijuana (57). There is no consistent evidence currently, regarding the relationship between cannabis use and preterm births or teratogenesis (58).

Anesthetic Considerations and Management

Many of the same recommendations can be made for cannabis abuse in the pregnant patient as can be made for tobacco abusers, particularly with regard to an early intervention to terminate use. Cannabis abuse has been reported to increase cross-tolerance to opioids, benzodiazepines, and barbiturates. It is not clear to what degree this occurs; there are no published reports further describing this phenomenon in pregnant women or making evidence-based recommendation for altering anesthetic management strategies (59).

Cocaine

Epidemiology

Cocaine is a commonly abused drug in pregnancy although its use may be declining in the United States relative to other stimulants. In 1998, it accounted for approximately 10% of overall illicit drug use in the United States (2). When surveyed in 2009, 0.7% of adults reported use of cocaine in the previous month (3).

Systemic Effects

Cocaine, an ester local anesthetic, causes decreased reuptake of dopamine, serotonin, and tryptophan at presynaptic nerve terminals in the central nervous system, which results in euphoria and increased alertness (60). It also activates the sympathetic nervous system by inhibition of presynaptic catecholamine uptake, which results in substantial increases in heart rate, blood pressure, vasoconstriction, and dysrhythmia; and these relationships may not necessarily be dose dependent (61). In addition, cocaine-induced coronary vasospasm and increased sensitivity to circulating catecholamines, in combination with the tachycardia and hypertension, all contribute to an increased risk of developing myocardial ischemia and infarction. The severe hypertension resulting from cocaine has also been implicated in maternal subarachnoid hemorrhage, seizures, and aortic dissection (62). Animal experiments confirm that the onset and resolution of cocaine's hemodynamic effects are rapid (Table 42-6); however, it is difficult to extrapolate the relationship between dose and degree of heart rate, and blood

TABLE 42-6 Effect of Cocaine on UBF and Maternal and Fetal Heart Rate (HR) and MAP

Parameter (± SD)	Experimental Time After Bolus Maternal Cocaine Administration					
	Baseline	7 min	30 min	60 min	90 min	120 min
Maternal (n = 5)						
HR (bpm)	98 (17)	97 (11)	101 (12)	100 (14)	101 (15)	100 (15)
MAP (mm Hg)	108 (10)	129 (11)	111 (8)	107 (8)	105 (6)	106 (6)
UBF (% baseline)	100 (10)	62 (19)	78 (13)	98 (8)	100 (10)	100 (7)
Fetal (n = 5)						
HR (bpm)	164 (15)	14S (11)	182 (20)	175 (12)	176 (22)	178 (17)
MAP (mm Hg)	49 (7)	57 (5)	47 (9)	46 (11)	48 (5)	47 (6)

From: Oriol NE, Bennett FM, Rigney DR, et al. Cocaine effects on neonatal heart rate dynamics: Preliminary findings and methodological problems. *Yale J Biol Med* 1993;66:75–84.

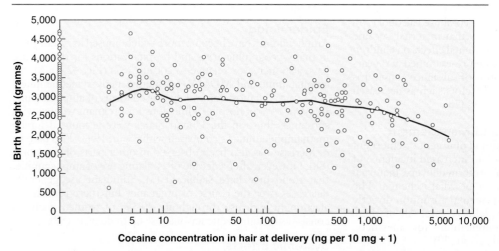

FIGURE 42-4 Smoothed scatter plot of birth weights (g) by cocaine concentration (ng/10 mg) in the mother's hair at delivery among 339 women, New York City, 1990 to 1992. Reprinted with permission from: Kain ZN, Mayes LC, Pakes J, et al. Thrombocytopenia in pregnant women who use cocaine. *Am J Obstet Gynecol* 1995;173:885–890.

pressure changes in these experiments in humans. It is noteworthy that the cocaine-induced mild increases in heart rate and blood pressure has profound effects in reducing uterine perfusion presumably due to selective uterine artery vasoconstriction (63). In addition to inhaling the powder form, the free base of cocaine can be inhaled or smoked. Smoking cocaine has been reported to be associated with exacerbation of asthma, thermal airway injury, pneumothorax, pulmonary hemorrhage, noncardiogenic pulmonary edema, and pulmonary infarction (64).

There is conflicting evidence with regard to the association of chronic cocaine abuse and thrombocytopenia. One retrospective cohort study of 1,907 pregnant women reported an incidence of thrombocytopenia of 6.7% (7/104) in cocaine-using women as compared with 1.5% (5/331) of pregnant women who did not use any drugs (65). In another retrospective review of 7,547 obstetric admissions, there was actually a lower incidence of thrombocytopenia (2.5%) in patients with urine tests positive for cocaine as compared with those who had negative urine cocaine results (4.7%) (66). Cocaine and other stimulants are unique among illicit drugs in that it is associated with hyperthermia. The mechanism for this appears to be increased heat production from the induced hypermetabolic state and also diminished heat dissipation, specifically reduced sweating and cutaneous vasodilation, via altered central thermoregulatory processes (67). This can be particularly deleterious for the heat-sensitive fetus although there is no evidence of specific negative outcomes associated with cocaine hyperthermia.

Effects on Pregnancy and the Fetus

Cocaine abuse has been associated with a wide range of adverse obstetric outcomes including placental abruption, intrauterine growth retardation (IUGR), preterm labor, and fetal heart rate abnormalities (68). There is a substantial increased risk for placental abruption with cocaine abuse (OR 3.9, 95% CI 2.8 to 5.5) presumably due to the associated hypertension and uterine artery vasoconstriction (69). IUGR is higher with maternal cocaine abuse (70) (OR 2.15, 95% CI 1.75 to 2.64) which may be as a direct result of the drug, or a higher rate of concurrent smoking (71), or other substance abuse-related comorbidities such as malnutrition. A more specific analysis has been reported in an investigation using hair sampling analysis which showed that the relationship between cocaine and IUGR was specifically associated with the heavier use of cocaine (Fig. 42-4), and exposure late in pregnancy was necessary for the association (72).

Cocaine use has been associated with earlier presentation in labor. It is not clear to what degree these earlier admissions represent preterm labor as opposed to admissions for an evaluation of fetal status (64), placental abruption, or the management of other comorbidities (Table 42-7). Cocaine abuse may masquerade as preeclampsia. In a case series of 11 patients who had recently abused cocaine and presented with clinical symptoms presumed to be preeclampsia, 2 out of 11 also had measurable proteinuria (73). Seizure activity, which has been reported in 3% of cocaine-related emergency admissions in nonpregnant adults (74), could be presumed to be eclampsia particularly when associated with other clinical features of cocaine abuse. Unlike preeclampsia, cocaine abuse, if terminated while hospitalized, should be associated with transient and not progressive hypertension, and it should not be associated with elevated liver transaminases or creatinine levels.

Cocaine use has been associated with decreased FHR variability (75). Cocaine readily crosses the placenta, and neonates born to cocaine-abusing mothers have been reported to demonstrate low birth weight, transient irritability, and perhaps, some congenital malformations including craniofacial abnormalities.

TABLE 42-7 Comparison of Patients with Negative and Positive Urine Toxicology Screens

	Cocaine (+) (n = 102)	Cocaine (−) (n = 48)	p
Maternal age (yr)	28.8 ± 4.8	28 ± 5.2	NS
Gestational age (wk)	34.9 ± 4.2	37 ± 5	<0.01
"Presumed fetal jeopardy"	39 (38.2%)	10 (20.8%)	<0.05
Cigarette smoking	80 (78.4%)	22 (45.8%)	<0.001
Denied cocaine use	68 (66%)	48 (100%)	

Values presented as mean ± sd or n (%).
From: Haim DY, Lippmann ML, Goldberg SK, et al. The pulmonary complications of crack cocaine. A comprehensive review. *Chest* 1995;107:233–40.

However, it is not clear if this is a direct effect of cocaine abuse per se or related to a high prevalence of co-abused alcohol (76). Also, there is no convincing evidence that maternal cocaine abuse itself has long-standing developmental effects on children born to cocaine-abusing mothers when re-examined at 6 years of age (77). As with most other forms of substance abuse, it is difficult to separate other associated factors such as decreased maternal care with behavioral outcomes (78).

Anesthetic Considerations and Management

Cocaine abuse increases the likelihood of urgent or emergent anesthetic management because of an increased incidence of fetal distress, placental abruption, preterm delivery, maternal seizure, severe hypertension, and myocardial ischemia. The higher rates of fetal distress and placental abruption directly contribute to a higher cesarean delivery rate. All of these complications have profound implications for anesthetic decision making and resource utilization (79).

There is no single optimal strategy for managing severe hypertension associated with cocaine abuse. Beta blockers administered alone are relatively contraindicated due to concerns about unopposed alpha agonist activity in a setting of existing vasoconstriction (80). Hydralazine was initially considered the drug of choice in this setting although its tendency to further worsen tachycardia must be considered. Animal experiments evaluating the use of hydralazine in the setting of cocaine toxicity demonstrate a reduction in mean arterial pressure (MAP) but also a commensurate equivalent reduction in uterine blood flow (UBF) (81). Nitroglycerine is an excellent antihypertensive choice in this setting because it has beneficial coronary dilating properties and it may preserve UBF better than hydralazine but it also exacerbates tachycardia. Multimodal therapy or agents that have mixed receptor activity such as labetalol perhaps represent a better approach in this setting because of effective control of blood pressure and heart rate, but there is limited published evidence regarding the effect of multimodal therapy on UBF in the setting of cocaine intoxication. In addition, caution should be exercised when administering other anesthetic agents such as ketamine which may compound the tachycardia and hypertension. Managing hypotension in the setting of cocaine intoxication is more effective with a direct-acting vasopressor such as phenylephrine, and indirect-actiing ephedrine may be less effective due to neurotransmitter's depletion (82). Given the possibility of cocaine-induced coronary ischemia, obtaining an ECG should be considered if cocaine abuse is confirmed or highly likely.

Cocaine-abusing patients have been reported to have altered pain perception. This may be explained by changes in mu and kappa opioid receptor densities (83). The duration of intrathecal opioid (sufentanil) analgesia has been shown to be reduced in patients that abuse cocaine (84), which may require compensation with a greater volume or concentration of epidural local anesthetic.

With regards to general anesthesia, laryngoscopy following induction is a period of particular concern for exacerbating severe hypertension in the cocaine-abusing parturient. A strategy of using rapid-onset, short-acting agents, timed to correspond to this stimulation, should be employed. Both acute (85) and chronic (86) cocaine intoxication increase the minimum alveolar concentration of volatile anesthetics. Prolonged blockade from succinylcholine has been reported presumably due to an effect of chronic cocaine on plasma cholinesterase levels (72). Neither the prevalence nor the degree of this interaction is well described. This phenomenon may not necessarily contraindicate the use of succinylcholine given its relatively short duration of action, but this observation should be incorporated into any decision to use a neuromuscular blocking which is always a balance of aspiration risk, onset time, duration, and other factors.

Amphetamines

Epidemiology

Amphetamines have become more widely abused in recent years in many geographic areas and hospitalizations for their abuse have also increased relative to cocaine (87) (Fig. 42-5). Methamphetamine and MDMA (3,4-methylenedioxymethamphetamine) are the most commonly abused forms of amphetamine. In 2006, 24% of hospital admissions for pregnant women with substance abuse in the United States were accounted for by methamphetamine as compared with 8% in 1994. This pattern of increase has also been observed in other parts of the world (88). However, after a decade of escalating use of amphetamine, that trend may have stabilized (3). Stimulant use generally decreases over the course of pregnancy but there remains an alarmingly high use throughout; 29.3% of women maintain consistently high frequency of abuse up to delivery (89).

Systemic Effects

Amphetamines are sympathomimetic amines that exert their effects by increasing the levels of dopamine and norepinephrine in the central nervous system. Increased alertness and euphoria are associated with their use. Other common clinical findings are tachycardia, elevated blood pressure, dysrhythmias, hyperreflexia, and proteinuria (59). Amphetamine abuse is also associated with maternal fever, seizures, myocardial ischemia, cerebrovascular accidents, and there is also an

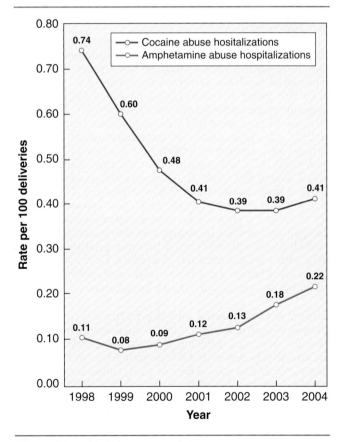

FIGURE 42-5 Hospitalization ratios for amphetamine or cocaine abuse among pregnant women. The statistical test for the linear trends is significant for both diagnosis groups ($P < 0.001$). Reprinted with permission from: Cox S, Posner SF, Kourtis AP, et al. Hospitalizations with amphetamine abuse among pregnant women. *Obstet Gynecol* 2008;111:341–347.

TABLE 42-8 Perinatal Outcomes

Perinatal Characteristics	Methamphetamine Users (n = 273)	Control Patients (n = 34,055)	p^a
Preterm delivery	139 (52)	5,627 (17)	<0.001
1-min Apgar score less than 4	16 (6)	665 (2)	<0.001
5-min Apgar score less than 7	16 (6)	328 (1)	<0.001
Cesarean delivery	79 (29)	7,730 (23)	<0.02
Neonatal mortality	11 (4)	325 (1)	<0.001
Maternal obstetric + intensive care unit admissions	6 (2)	95 (0.3)	<0.001

Data are n (%) unless otherwise specified.
^{a}p from x test.
From: Good MM, Solt I, Acuna JG, et al. Methamphetamine use during pregnancy: Maternal and neonatal implications. *Obstet Gynecol* 2010;116:330–334.

increased risk of death often related to hypertensive events such as cerebrovascular accidents (90). Amphetamines have been associated with an increase in maternal temperature believed to be related to adrenergic receptor stimulation in the hypothalamus (91). This elevated temperature has been implicated as a contributing factor in the deaths of several nonpregnant patients who have abused amphetamines (92). It is not clear if elevated maternal temperature from stimulant abuse carries the same association of greater neonatal morbidity and mortality that has been reported with infection-related fever (93).

Effects on Pregnancy and the Fetus
Amphetamine abuse is associated with an increase in several obstetric and neonatal complications (94) (Table 42-8). More intensive management of amphetamine-abusing parturients can be expected due to an increase in these complications as well as for increased incidences of placental abruption (87), fetal heart rate abnormalities (95), and interventions for hemodynamic manipulations.

Amphetamine use has been confused with preeclampsia due to a similar presentation with hypertension and possible proteinuria (96). It may be difficult to distinguish these diagnoses but elevations in creatinine and liver transaminases would be more suggestive of preeclampsia. Stimulant use has generally not been reported to be associated with teratogenesis but a case cluster of gastroschisis has been reported in the western United States with methamphetamine abuse (97).

Anesthetic Considerations and Management
Women who have used stimulants, specifically amphetamines, have been reported to require more pharmacologic analgesia, both parenteral opioids and regional analgesia, for labor. This effect was not as strong as that for women with a history of opioid use but it may impact clinical decision making and resource utilization (11). It can also be expected that neuraxial analgesia placement may be more challenging or potentially contraindicated in a combative, amphetamine-abusing parturient. In addition to the logistic consideration in managing an uncooperative patient, there may be ethical dilemmas in providing such care in the first place without a robust informed consent process. Chronic amphetamine use has been associated in nonpregnant patients with catecholamine depletion which may result in diminished effectiveness of indirect-acting vasopressors such as ephedrine (98). An alternative, direct-acting

agent may be a wiser choice to treat hypotension. As with managing patients with cocaine intoxication, caution should be exercised in using agents that would further increase heart rate or blood pressure. In managing general anesthetics, acute amphetamine intoxication has been reported to decrease MAC whereas chronic use has been reported to increase MAC (99).

Opioids

Epidemiology
The prevalence of illicit opioid abuse in pregnant women in one large retrospective review was reported to be 1.1% (6). But it has also been estimated that up to 4.4% of pregnant women used some form of opioid analgesics during pregnancy "without appropriate medical oversight" (3). Despite a modest decline in the abuse of many illicit substances, there has been a recent increase in the rate of nonmedical use of prescription pain relievers between 2002 and 2009. In this survey, only 4.8% obtained pain relievers from a drug dealer or stranger while 55.3% of those surveyed obtained these drugs from a friend or relative for free (3).

Systemic Effects
Opioids may be administered by intravenous, oral, nasal, and transdermal routes, all of which may be accompanied by life-threatening respiratory depression. Less commonly observed by anesthesiologists are the wide range of systemic symptoms associated with maternal opioid withdrawal of which the most common include dysphoric mood, nausea, vomiting, muscle aches, lacrimation, rhinorrhea, pupillary dilation, sweating, diarrhea, yawning, fever, and insomnia (7). Predictable time courses for acute opioid withdrawal (Table 42-9) demonstrate that even patients addicted to opioids with the longest durations can manifest during normal obstetric admissions without drug replacement. There has been substantial experience with using methadone as a replacement agent but there is emerging evidence that buprenorphine may be associated with less neonatal abstinence syndrome (NAS) (100). Methadone (30 to 100 mg/d oral) is a synthetic opioid with a long half-life of 12 to 100 hours (usually 25 to 30 in long-term users), which blocks opioid cravings for 24 to 36 hours (59). Buprenorphine (2 to 32 mg/d sublingual, 35 to 75 µg/h transdermal patch) is a partial opioid with a half-life of 3 to 44 hours (101) and has the advantages of a low level of physical

TABLE 42-9 Time Course of Opioid Withdrawal

Opioid	Onset	Peak Intensity	Duration
Meperidine Fentanyl	2–6 h	6–12 h	4–5 d
Morphine Heroin	6–18 h	36–72 h	7–10 d
Methadone	24–48 h	3–21 d	6–7 wk

From: Wang JK, Nauss LA, Thomas JE. Pain relief by intrathecally applied morphine in man. *Anesthesiology* 1979;50:149–151.

dependence, easy medical withdrawal, and low overdose potential as compared with methadone (102). Both agents are categorized as pregnancy category C (103). Opioid replacement therapy and refraining from other substance abuse have also been associated with many beneficial obstetric outcomes including reduced fetal mortality; increased birth weights; and decreased HIV infection, preeclampsia, and NAS (104). Additional treatment options for opioid withdrawal include alpha adrenergic blockade such as clonidine, as well as generally supportive management of hemodynamics and suppression of autonomic hyperactivity (105).

Effects on Pregnancy and the Fetus

Opioid abuse during pregnancy has been associated with an increased rate of spontaneous abortion, IUGR, preterm labor, preterm, premature rupture of membranes (PPROM), placental insufficiency, placental abruption, preeclampsia, chorioamnionitis, low Apgar scores, postpartum hemorrhage, and thrombophlebitis (106). Opioids parenterally administered for acute labor pain have been reported to reduce fetal heart rate variability and reduce 1-minute APGAR scores (107). It is likely that chronically administered opioids have less effect on fetal monitoring. There is no evidence that opioids are teratogenic.

Anesthetic Considerations and Management

Unlike most other abused substances, opioids are used universally in the analgesic and anesthetic management of obstetric patients. This carries, in addition to all the management issues related to the comorbidities of substance abuse, specific management issues related to concurrent opioid use and dosing.

Analgesic requirements are higher in opioid-abusing patients due to upregulation of opioid receptors and likely other complex and incompletely described neural mechanisms including a decrease in endogenous opioids as well as other behavioral phenomenon (16). In the setting of acute pain, analgesic administration is typically guided by simple patient request. With a history of chronic opioid administration, it may be more predictable to incorporate objective physiologic criteria, such as respiratory rate, into an analgesic titration strategy. Extreme caution should be exercised with the use of opioid antagonists including partial or mixed agonist/antagonists. A seemingly benign intervention such as the administration of a small dose of naloxone or buprenorphine for pruritus has been reported to precipitate withdrawal (108).

Expert opinion suggests that a greater reliance on regional anesthesia techniques in the opioid-dependent patient is beneficial (109). Analgesic responses to neuraxial local anesthetic techniques should be predictable but there is evidence, at least in nonpregnant patients with chronic opioid use, that standard intrathecal opioid doses may be less effective. For example, patients with terminal cancer require higher intrathecal opioid doses for effective analgesia (110). However, strategies for appropriate dose escalation in the setting of labor analgesia for

a patient with chronic opioid use have not been established. In addition to standard contraindications to regional anesthesia in opioid-abusing parturients, serious consideration should be given to the appropriateness of patient consent and cooperation. There may be a higher rate of neuraxial infection in the substance-abusing population but the absolute rate is likely still very low and must be weighed against the benefits of neuraxial analgesia and anesthesia (111). In managing general anesthetics in parturients, it can be assumed that acute opioid use would decrease the anesthetic requirement whereas chronic opioid exposure would increase requirements (97).

A common dilemma, not necessarily restricted to opioid abuse, resolves around managing parturients with a history of successfully rehabilitated substance abuse. Peripartum pain management is a legitimate concern for many of these patients and it may include a fear of being undertreated for pain or recidivism if they have been successfully rehabilitated and are re-exposed to opioids. It is likely that some of the anxiety associated with being undertreated for pain itself, in addition to the receptor upregulation, may be responsible for the higher reported utilization of both parenteral opioids and neuraxial analgesia in labor (11).

Ease in obtaining intravenous access may be challenging in a patient who has chronically used peripheral veins for injections. This has been reported in 16.5% of intravenous drug users (6). This often necessitates seeking central venous access. Given the risk of endocarditis in patients with a history of intravenous opioid abuse, it is unclear if routine echocardiographic evaluation would improve clinical outcomes. In a series of 23 patients with substance abuse, 2D echocardiography identified two previously undiagnosed valvular vegetations which were treated with antibiotics during labor (112).

Caffeine

Epidemiology

Caffeine is the most widely ingested pharmacologically active substance worldwide and its effects during pregnancy remain controversial. Because caffeine is a legal substance and is ingested orally, it is possible to more accurately quantify dosages compared with illicit substances. That being said, caffeine dosages vary widely in consumed products, depending on portion and type of foods and beverages (19). There is also "wide interindividual variation in caffeine metabolism" reported to be attributable to differential CYP1A2 activity (113).

Systemic Effects

Caffeine is a moderate stimulant which exerts its effects via the metabolite methylxanthine on several central nervous system pathways including dopamine, serotonin, and norepinephrine receptors (114). Patients consuming caffeine may experience increased alertness as well as tachycardia, hypertension, and arrhythmias.

Effects on Pregnancy and the Fetus

It is controversial whether moderate amounts of caffeine (<200 mg/d) consumed during pregnancy have any measurable effects on fetal development or obstetric outcomes. There have been several epidemiologic studies, primarily retrospective in study design, evaluating this relationship. Evidence is conflicting regarding the effect of moderate caffeine ingestion on preterm labor (115), although meta-analysis of these studies shows no important relationship (115). An association with spontaneous abortion, intrauterine growth restriction, and low birth weight has also been reported in some studies with moderate caffeine consumption during pregnancy (116,117). It is not clear whether higher caffeine consumption (>200 mg/d) is associated with greater obstetric outcome risks (118). It is unlikely that caffeine confers any significant teratogenic effect given its prevalent use, but, of reported observations, one study described an increase in orofacial defects (119) and another reported an increase in cryptorchidism in the offspring of mothers who consumed approximately three cups of coffee per day (120).

Anesthetic Considerations

Some of the same physiologic considerations apply to caffeine-consuming pregnant patients as those who have ingested mild stimulants although the concerns about arrhythmia, tachycardia, and hypertension are likely much lower on a dosing continuum. Perhaps, the most impactful effect of caffeine use on anesthetic management is the impact of its withdrawal both during the labor and in the postpartum period. The effects of caffeine withdrawal include headache, poor mood, decreased energy, and flu-like symptoms, which may manifest during prolonged labors or in hospitalized women (121). Caffeine withdrawal headache may be confused with postdural puncture headache, although the latter has a more prominent postural component.

Inhalants and Solvents

Epidemiology

Toluene-based solvents that are commonly found in household cleaners and paints are inhaled recreationally for their hallucinogenic effects. It is not clear what the prevalence of this abuse is in pregnant women but it is likely less common than other agents previously described in this chapter.

Systemic Effect

Chronic inhalation is associated with the development of permanent damage to the central nervous system (diffuse cerebral atrophy and cerebellar degeneration) (122) and renal tubular acidosis with associated maternal electrolyte disturbances and neonatal acidemia (123). Acute respiratory distress, increased airway resistance, pulmonary hypertension, ARDS, and liver toxicity have also been reported in pregnant women exposed to solvents (124).

Effects on Pregnancy and the Fetus

Regarding obstetric outcomes, solvent abuse has been associated with intrauterine growth restriction, preterm delivery, and higher prenatal mortality (125). Exposure in the first trimester is very likely teratogenic with a similar presentation to fetal alcohol syndrome with growth retardation, microcephaly, and dysmorphic facies (123).

Anesthetic Considerations and Management

There is very little published evidence that may be helpful to guide management for abuse of inhaled solvents in pregnancy. Correcting the metabolic (rental tubular acidosis) and electrolyte abnormalities (hyperchloremia, hypokalemia, hypomagnesemia, and hypophosphatemia) with intravenous fluid and electrolyte supplementation should be of primary importance for both maternal and fetal well-being. Sodium bicarbonate should be considered to reverse severe metabolic acidosis.

Hallucinogens

Epidemiology and Effects on Pregnancy and the Fetus

Hallucinogenic agents are infrequently abused by pregnant patients and have been reported to be associated with fetal growth restriction, premature labor, meconium, and neonatal withdrawal syndrome (97). Commonly abused hallucinogens include ketamine, lysergic acid diethylamide (LSD), and phencyclidine 1-(1-phenylcyclohexyl) piperidine more commonly referred to as PCP.

Anesthetic Considerations and Management

There is a limited amount of evidence in the medical literature to help guide care in this clinical setting but the following general considerations may be warranted. The abuse of ketamine has been associated with tachycardia and hypertension, and may require caution with subsequently administered sympathomimetics (126). Ketamine abuse may be confused with preeclampsia. There is no evidence that ketamine abuse is associated with hyperthermia. Ketamine, although generally not associated with substantial respiratory depression, can be synergistic with opioids to that effect. A prolongation of succinylcholine has been reported presumably due to decreased plasma cholinesterase and its value as a rapid-onset agent should be weighed against this possible unpredictability (127).

■ NEONATAL WITHDRAWAL

The management of infants born to mothers with a history of substance abuse is outside the scope of this chapter; however, there are important considerations for the obstetric anesthesiologist even if not directly involved in neonatal resuscitation. The majority of infants born to mothers with a broad range of substance-abuse problems are observed to have some withdrawal symptoms (128). These symptoms of NAS are systemic (129) (Table 42-10) and require a comprehensive management plan (100). It is important for anesthesiologists to recognize the potential need for increased resuscitative support for these infants and communicate the substance abuse history to the neonatologists.

■ MATERNAL COMORBIDITIES

Coexisting Psychiatric Illness

There is a substantially higher prevalence of coexisting psychiatric disorders among substance-abusing pregnant women (10.3%) compared with nonsubstance-abusing pregnant women (1.4%) (130). The most common diagnoses among opioid-dependent women were reported to be hypomania, generalized anxiety disorder, major depressive disorder, and dysthymia. Pharmacologic treatment for these diagnoses involves most commonly anxiolytics (35.4%), SSRIs (24%), as well as mixed neurotransmitter uptake inhibitors, tricyclic antidepressants, antipsychotics, and mood stabilizers (106). The impact of these medications on anesthetic care must be considered in addition to substances being abused (131). (See Chapter on Co-existing Psychiatric Disease).

Infectious Complications

Coexisting infectious disease is a serious concern in the pregnant, substance-abusing patients. Although the principal concern is in patients injecting substances intravenously under poor sterile conditions (e.g., endocarditis, systemic abscesses, cellulitis) or sharing needles (e.g., hepatitis, HIV), there are also infectious risks (e.g., tuberculosis) associated with malnutrition, immunosuppression, engaging in higher risk sexual practices, homelessness, poor access to health care, and noncompliance with medical treatment regimens (132). HIV infection is not believed to be a contraindication to neuraxial labor analgesia as the virus penetrates the central nervous system early in the illness and worsened outcomes have not been observed in this patient population (133). There are, however, numerous important drug interactions to consider in the substance-abusing parturient, particularly those concurrently taking antiviral therapy for HIV (131).

TABLE 42-10 Clinical Signs of Opioid Withdrawal

Neurological system
  High-pitched crying
  Irritability
  Increased wakefulness
  Hyperactive deep tendon reflexes
  Increased muscle tone
  Tremors
  Exaggerated moro reflex
  Seizures, generalized
  Intraventricular hemorrhage

Gastrointestinal
  Poor feeding
  Uncoordinated and constant sucking
  Vomiting
  Diarrhea
  Dehydration

Autonomic signs
  Increased sweating
  Nasal stuffiness
  Fever
  Mottling

Other signs
  Poor weight gain
  Increased rapid eye movement sleep
  Poor organization of sleep states
  Skin excoriation

From: Suresh S, Anand KJ. Opioid tolerance in neonates: Mechanisms, diagnosis, assessment, and management. *Semin Perinatol* 1998; 22:425–433.

■ CONCLUSION

Substance abuse complicates the management of obstetric anesthesia because it is associated with an increase in comorbid medical conditions, as well as obstetric and neonatal complications, and it alters the predictability of administered medications including many anesthetics. It is important to identify which substances have been used as many of the management decisions are specific to the class of drug used. Ultimately, establishing a system that effectively screens for substance abuse among parturients and a practice that ensures safe and effective obstetric anesthetic care is advised.

KEY POINTS

■ The rate for illicit drug use in the previous month among pregnant women has been reported to be approximately 4.5% in the United States.

■ Substance abuse is associated with increased risk of obstetric and neonatal complications including an increase in preterm birth, low birth weight, intrauterine growth restriction, and placental abruption.

■ Substance abuse is associated with an increased incidence of medical comorbidities including psychiatric disorders, viral and bacterial infections, skin diseases, trauma, and poisoning.

■ Screening questionnaires have limited sensitivity and specificity in detecting substance abuse and should be paired with physician judgment and laboratory analysis to be more effective.

■ Parturients with a history of substance abuse utilize parenteral labor analgesia at a greater rate, require more

frequent analgesic interventions during cesarean delivery with regional anesthesia, and have a higher incidence of inadequate postcesarean analgesia.

■ The use of cocaine and amphetamines has been associated with hypertension and proteinuria that may mimic preeclampsia.

■ Acute alcohol intoxication is associated with additive effects with opioids, benzodiazepines, hypnotics, and volatile anesthetics, and it is associated with intravascular volume depletion and metabolic acidosis. Chronic alcohol use is associated with a wide range of comorbidities including coagulopathy and systemic infection that may contraindicate regional anesthesia, and plans should be established to prevent withdrawal during the course of labor.

■ Cocaine abuse increases the likelihood of urgent or emergent anesthetic management due to a higher rate of fetal distress, placental abruption, preterm delivery, maternal seizure, severe hypertension, myocardial ischemia, and cesarean delivery. It is associated with increased maternal heart rate, blood pressure, and dysrhythmia, which may be best managed by multimodal therapy or mixed receptor antihypertensive agents. Hypotension may be best treated with direct-acting vasopressor such as phenylephrine. There is conflicting evidence whether cocaine abuse is associated with thrombocytopenia.

■ Chronic opioid abuse is associated with higher analgesic requirements; however, there is little evidence to support dosing modifications for neuraxial opioids. Acute withdrawal can be precipitated in the mother and neonate with very small doses of opioid antagonist or mixed agonist/antagonist.

REFERENCES

1. http://oas.samhsa.gov/
2. http://www.nida.nih.gov/nidahome.html
3. Substance Abuse and Mental Health Services Administration. (2010). Results from the 2009 National Survey on Drug Use and Health: Volume I. Summary of National Findings (Office of Applied Studies, NSDUH Series H-38A, HHS Publication No. SMA 10-4586 Findings). Rockville, MD.
4. Morrison C, Siney C. Maternity services for drug misusers in England and Wales: A national survey. *Health Trends* 1995;27:15–17.
5. Mitsuhiro SS, Chalem E, Barros MC, et al. Prevalence of cocaine and marijuana use in the last trimester of adolescent pregnancy: Socio-demographic, psychosocial and behavioral characteristics. *Addict Behav* 2007; 32:392–397.
6. Cassidy B, Cyna AM. Challenges that opioid-dependent women present to the obstetric anaesthetist. *Anaesth Intensive Care* 2004;32:494–501.
7. American Psychiatric Association. Diagnostic and Statistical Manual of Mental Disorders, 4th edition (DSM-IV), American Psychiatric Association, 4th ed. (Text revision) 2000. Washington, DC.
8. Keegan J, Parva M, Finnegan M, et al. Addiction in pregnancy. *J Addict Dis* 2010;29:175–191.
9. Landau R, Cahana A, Smiley RM, et al. Genetic variability of mu-opioid receptor in an obstetric population. *Anesthesiology* 2004;100:1030–1033.
10. Pinto SM, Dodd S, Walkinshaw SA, et al. Substance abuse during pregnancy: Effect on pregnancy outcomes. *Eur J Obstet Gynecol Reprod Biol* 2010;150:137–141.
11. Ludlow JP, Evans SF, Hulse G. Obstetric and perinatal outcomes in pregnancies associated with illicit substance abuse. *Aust N Z J Obstet Gynaecol* 2004; 44:302–306.
12. Castles A, Adams EK, Melvin CL, et al. Effects of smoking during pregnancy. Five meta-analyses. *Am J Prev Med* 1999;16:208–215.
13. Kahila H, Gissler M, Sarkola T, et al. Maternal welfare, morbidity and mortality 6-15 years after a pregnancy complicated by alcohol and substance abuse: A register-based case-control follow-up study of 524 women. *Drug Alcohol Depend* 2010;111:215–221.
14. Bauer CR, Shankaran S, Bada HS, et al. The Maternal Lifestyle Study: Drug exposure during pregnancy and short-term maternal outcomes. *Am J Obstet Gynecol* 2002;186:487–495.
15. Byrne MW, Lerner HM. Communicating with addicted women in labor. *MCN Am J Matern Child Nurs* 1992;17:22–26.

16. Compton MA. Cold-pressor pain tolerance in opiate and cocaine abusers: Correlates of drug type and use status. *J Pain Symptom Manage* 1994;9:462–473.

17. Kelly JJ, Davis PG, Henschke PN. The drug epidemic: Effects on newborn infants and health resource consumption at a tertiary perinatal centre. *J Paediatr Child Health* 2000;36:262–264.

18. Birnbach DJ, Browne IM, Kim A, et al. Identification of polysubstance abuse in the parturient. *Br J Anaesth* 2001;87:488–490.

19. Christmas JT, Knisely JS, Dawson KS, et al. Comparison of questionnaire screening and urine toxicology for detection of pregnancy complicated by substance use. *Obstet Gynecol* 1992;80:750–754.

20. Howell EM, Heiser N, Harrington M. A review of recent findings on substance abuse treatment for pregnant women. *J Subst Abuse Treat* 1999;16:195–219.

21. Shields AL, Howell RT, Potter JS, et al. The Michigan Alcoholism Screening Test and its shortened forms: A meta-analytic inquiry into score reliability. *Subst Use Misuse* 2007;42:1783–1800.

22. Sokol RJ, Martier SS, Ager JW. The T-ACE questions: Practical prenatal detection of risk-drinking. *Am J Obstet Gynecol* 1989;160:863–868.

23. Russell M, Martier SS, Sokol RJ, et al. Detecting risk drinking during pregnancy: A comparison of four screening questionnaires. *Am J Public Health* 1996;86:1435–1439.

24. Chasnoff IJ, Neuman K, Thornton C, et al. Screening for substance use in pregnancy: A practical approach for the primary care physician. *Am J Obstet Gynecol* 2001;184:752–758.

25. Chasnoff IJ, McGourty RF, Bailey GW, et al. The 4P's Plus screen for substance use in pregnancy: clinical application and outcomes. *J Perinatol* 2005;25:368–374.

26. Yonkers KA, Gotman N, Kershaw T, et al. Screening for prenatal substance use: Development of the Substance Use Risk Profile-Pregnancy scale. *Obstet Gynecol* 2010;116:827–833.

27. Horrigan TJ, Piazza NJ, Weinstein L. The substance abuse subtle screening inventory is more cost effective and has better selectivity than urine toxicology for the detection of substance abuse in pregnancy. *J Perinatol* 1996;16:326–330.

28. Kintz P. Drug testing in addicts: A comparison between urine, sweat, and hair. *Ther Drug Monit* 1996;18:450–455.

29. Moeller KE, Lee KC, Kissack JC. Urine drug screening: Practical guide for clinicians. *Mayo Clin Proc* 2008;83:66–76.

30. Bobo JK. Tobacco use, problem drinking, and alcoholism. *Clin Obstet Gynecol* 2002;45:1169–1180.

31. Cicero TJ. Neuroendocrinological effects of alcohol. *Annu Rev Med* 1981;32:123–142.

32. Mathis KW, Zambell K, Olubadewo JO, et al. Altered hemodynamic counter-regulation to hemorrhage by acute moderate alcohol intoxication. *Shock* 2006;26:55–61.

33. Eckardt MJ, Harford TC, Kaelber CT, et al. Health hazards associated with alcohol consumption. *JAMA* 1981;246:648–666.

34. Sampson PD, Streissguth AP, Bookstein FL, et al. Incidence of fetal alcohol syndrome and prevalence of alcohol-related neurodevelopmental disorder. *Teratology* 1997;56:317–326.

35. Moss M, Steinberg KP, Guidot DM, et al. The effect of chronic alcohol abuse on the incidence of ARDS and the severity of the multiple organ dysfunction syndrome in adults with septic shock: An interim and multivariate analysis. *Chest* 1999;116:97S–98S.

36. Nimmo WS. Effect of anaesthesia on gastric motility and emptying. *Br J Anaesth* 1984;56:29–36.

37. Henderson J, Gray R, Brocklehurst P. Systematic review of effects of low-moderate prenatal alcohol exposure on pregnancy outcome. *BJOG* 2007;114:243–252.

38. Makarechian N, Agro K, Devlin J, et al. Association between moderate alcohol consumption during pregnancy and spontaneous abortion, stillbirth and premature birth: A meta-analysis. *Can J Clin Pharmacol* 1998;5:169–176.

39. Jaddoe VW, Bakker R, Hofman A, et al. Moderate alcohol consumption during pregnancy and the risk of low birth weight and preterm birth. The generation R study. *Ann Epidemiol* 2007;17:834–840.

40. Strandberg-Larsen K, Gronboek M, Andersen AM, et al. Alcohol drinking pattern during pregnancy and risk of infant mortality. *Epidemiology* 2009;20:884–891.

41. Centers for Disease Control and Prevention (CDC). Update: Trends in fetal alcohol syndrome—United States, 1979–1993. *MMWR Morb Mortal Wkly Rep* 1995;44:249–251.

42. http://www.fasdcenter.samhsa.gov/

43. May JA, White HC, Leonard-White A, et al. The patient recovering from alcohol or drug addiction: Special issues for the anesthesiologist. *Anesth Analg* 2001;92:1601–1608.

44. McKeon A, Frye MA, Delanty N. The alcohol withdrawal syndrome. *J Neurol Neurosurg Psychiatry* 2008;79:854–862.

45. Benowitz NL, Jacob P 3rd, Jones RT, et al. Interindividual variability in the metabolism and cardiovascular effects of nicotine in man. *J Pharmacol Exp Ther* 1982;221:368–372.

46. Albuquerque CA, Smith KR, Johnson C, et al. Influence of maternal tobacco smoking during pregnancy on uterine, umbilical and fetal cerebral artery blood flows. *Early Hum Dev* 2004;80:31–42.

47. Bureau MA, Monette J, Shapcott D, et al. Carboxyhemoglobin concentration in fetal cord blood and in blood of mothers who smoked during labor. *Pediatrics* 1982;69:371–373.

48. Goodman JD, Visser FG, Dawes GS. Effects of maternal cigarette smoking on fetal trunk movements, fetal breathing movements and the fetal heart rate. *Br J Obstet Gynaecol* 1984;91:657–661.

49. Walsh RA. Effects of maternal smoking on adverse pregnancy outcomes: Examination of the criteria of causation. *Hum Biol* 1994;66:1059–1092.

50. MacDorman MF, Cnattingius S, Hoffman HJ, et al. Sudden infant death syndrome and smoking in the United States and Sweden. *Am J Epidemiol* 1997;146:249–257.

51. Wisborg K, Henriksen TB, Jespersen LB, et al. Nicotine patches for pregnant smokers: A randomized controlled study. *Obstet Gynecol* 2000;96:967–971.

52. Davies JM, Latto IP, Jones JG, et al. Effects of stopping smoking for 48 hours on oxygen availability from the blood: A study on pregnant women. *Br Med J* 1979;2:355–356.

53. Pearce AC, Jones RM. Smoking and anesthesia: Preoperative abstinence and perioperative morbidity. *Anesthesiology* 1984;61:576–584.

54. Ebrahim SH, Gfroerer J. Pregnancy-related substance use in the United States during 1996–1998. *Obstet Gynecol* 2003;101:374–379.

55. Zuckerman B, Frank DA, Hingson R, et al. Effects of maternal marijuana and cocaine use on fetal growth. *N Engl J Med* 1989;320:762–768.

56. Mallat A, Roberson J, Brock-Utne JG. Preoperative marijuana inhalation—an airway concern. *Can J Anaesth* 1996;43:691–693.

57. Curet LB, Hsi AC. Drug abuse during pregnancy. *Clin Obstet Gynecol* 2002;45:73–88.

58. van Gelder MM, Reefhuis J, Caton AR, et al. Characteristics of pregnant illicit drug users and associations between cannabis use and perinatal outcome in a population-based study. *Drug Alcohol Depend* 2010;109:243–247.

59. Ludlow J, Christmas T, Paech MJ, et al. Drug abuse and dependency during pregnancy: Anaesthetic issues. *Anaesth Intensive Care* 2007;35:881–893.

60. Fleming JA, Byck R, Barash PG. Pharmacology and therapeutic applications of cocaine. *Anesthesiology* 1990;73:518–531.

61. Kuczkowski KM. Cocaine abuse in pregnancy—anesthetic implications. *Int J Obstet Anesth* 2002;11:204–210.

62. Plessinger MA, Woods JR Jr. Maternal, placental, and fetal pathophysiology of cocaine exposure during pregnancy. *Clin Obstet Gynecol* 1993;36:267–278.

63. Penning DH, Dexter F, Henderson JL, et al. Bolus maternal cocaine administration does not produce a large increase in fetal sheep cerebral cortical glutamate concentration. *Neurotoxicol Teratol* 1999;21:177–180.

64. Haim DY, Lippmann ML, Goldberg SK, et al. The pulmonary complications of crack cocaine. A comprehensive review. *Chest* 1995;107:233–240.

65. Kain ZN, Mayes LC, Pakes J, et al. Thrombocytopenia in pregnant women who use cocaine. *Am J Obstet Gynecol* 1995;173:885–890.

66. Gershon RY, Fisher AJ, Graves WL. The cocaine-abusing parturient is not at an increased risk for thrombocytopenia. *Anesth Analg* 1996;82:865–866.

67. Crandall CG, Vongpatanasin W, Victor RG. Mechanism of cocaine-induced hyperthermia in humans. *Ann Intern Med* 2002;136:785–791.

68. Kain ZN, Rimar S, Barash PG. Cocaine abuse in the parturient and effects on the fetus and neonate. *Anesth Analg* 1993;77:835–845.

69. Hulse GK, Milne E, English DR, et al. Assessing the relationship between maternal cocaine use and abruptio placentae. *Addiction* 1997;92:1547–1551.

70. Hulse GK, English DR, Milne E, et al. Maternal cocaine use and low birth weight newborns: A meta-analysis. *Addiction* 1997;92:1561–1570.

71. Birnbach DJ, Stein DJ, Grunebaum A, et al. Cocaine screening of parturients without prenatal care: An evaluation of a rapid screening assay. *Anesth Analg* 1997;84:76–79.

72. Kuhn L, Kline J, Ng S, et al. Cocaine use during pregnancy and intrauterine growth retardation: New insights based on maternal hair tests. *Am J Epidemiol* 2000;152:112–119.

73. Towers CV, Pircon RA, Nageotte MP, et al. Cocaine intoxication presenting as preeclampsia and eclampsia. *Obstet Gynecol* 1993;81:545–547.

74. Koppel BS, Samkoff L, Daras M. Relation of cocaine use to seizures and epilepsy. *Epilepsia* 1996;37:875–878.

75. Oriol NE, Bennett FM, Rigney DR, et al. Cocaine effects on neonatal heart rate dynamics: Preliminary findings and methodological problems. *Yale J Biol Med* 1993;66:75–84.

76. Snodgrass SR. Cocaine babies: A result of multiple teratogenic influences. *J Child Neurol* 1994;9:227–233.

77. Frank DA, Augustyn M, Knight WG, et al. Growth, development, and behavior in early childhood following prenatal cocaine exposure: A systematic review. *JAMA* 2001;285:1613–1625.

78. Strathearn L, Mayes LC. Cocaine addiction in mothers: Potential effects on maternal care and infant development. *Ann N Y Acad Sci* 2010;1187:172–183.

79. Kain ZN, Mayes LC, Ferris CA, et al. Cocaine-abusing parturients undergoing cesarean section. A cohort study. *Anesthesiology* 1996;85:1028–1035.

80. Ramoska E, Sacchetti AD. Propranolol-induced hypertension in treatment of cocaine intoxication. *Ann Emerg Med* 1985;14:1112–1113.

81. Vertommen JD, Hughes SC, Rosen MA, et al. Hydralazine does not restore uterine blood flow during cocaine-induced hypertension in the pregnant ewe. *Anesthesiology* 1992;76:580–587.

82. Schindler CW, Tella SR, Erzouki HK, et al. Pharmacological mechanisms in cocaine's cardiovascular effects. *Drug Alcohol Depend* 1995;37:183–191.

83. Kreek MJ. Cocaine, dopamine and the endogenous opioid system. *J Addict Dis* 1996;15:73–96.

84. Ross VH, Moore CH, Pan PH, et al. Reduced duration of intrathecal sufentanil analgesia in laboring cocaine users. *Anesth Analg* 2003;97:1504–1508.

85. Stoelting RK, Creasser CW, Martz RC. Effect of cocaine administration on halothane MAC in dogs. *Anesth Analg* 1975;54:422–424.

86. Bernards CM, Kern C, Cullen BF. Chronic cocaine administration reversibly increases isoflurane minimum alveolar concentration in sheep. *Anesthesiology* 1996;85:91–95.

87. Cox S, Posner SF, Kourtis AP, et al. Hospitalizations with amphetamine abuse among pregnant women. *Obstet Gynecol* 2008;111:341–347.

88. Wouldes T, LaGasse L, Sheridan J, et al. Maternal methamphetamine use during pregnancy and child outcome: What do we know? *N Z Med J* 2004; 117:U1180.

89. Della Grotta S, LaGasse LL, Arria AM, et al. Patterns of methamphetamine use during pregnancy: Results from the Infant Development, Environment, and Lifestyle (IDEAL) Study. *Matern Child Health J* 2010;14:519–527.

90. Perez JA Jr, Arsura EL, Strategos S. Methamphetamine-related stroke: Four cases. *J Emerg Med* 1999;17:469–471.

91. Chi ML, Lin MT. Involvement of adrenergic receptor mechanisms within hypothalamus in the fever induced by amphetamine and thyrotropin-releasing hormone in the rat. *J Neural Transm* 1983;58:213–222.

92. Henry JA, Jeffreys KJ, Dawling S. Toxicity and deaths from 3,4-methylenedioxymethamphetamine ("ecstasy"). *Lancet* 1992;340:384–387.

93. Petrova A, Demissie K, Rhoads GG, et al. Association of maternal fever during labor with neonatal and infant morbidity and mortality. *Obstet Gynecol* 2001;98:20–27.

94. Good MM, Solt I, Acuna JG, et al. Methamphetamine use during pregnancy: Maternal and neonatal implications. *Obstet Gynecol* 2010;116:330–334.

95. Little BB, Snell LM, Gilstrap LC 3rd. Methamphetamine abuse during pregnancy: Outcome and fetal effects. *Obstet Gynecol* 1988;72:541–544.

96. Elliott RH, Rees GB. Amphetamine ingestion presenting as eclampsia. *Can J Anaesth* 1990;37:130–133.

97. Elliott L, Loomis D, Lottritz L, et al. Case-control study of a gastroschisis cluster in Nevada. *Arch Pediatr Adolesc Med* 2009;163:1000–1006.

98. Johnston RR, Way WL, Miller RD. Alteration of anesthetic requirement by amphetamine. *Anesthesiology* 1972;36:357–363.

99. Fischer SP, Healzer JM, Brook MW, et al. General anesthesia in a patient on long-term amphetamine therapy: Is there cause for concern? *Anesth Analg* 2000;91:758–759.

100. Ebner N, Rohrmeister K, Winklbaur B, et al. Management of neonatal abstinence syndrome in neonates born to opioid maintained women. *Drug Alcohol Depend* 2007;87:131–138.

101. Elkader A, Sproule B. Buprenorphine: Clinical pharmacokinetics in the treatment of opioid dependence. *Clin Pharmacokinet* 2005;44:661–680.

102. Kakko J, Heilig M, Sarman I. Buprenorphine and methadone treatment of opiate dependence during pregnancy: Comparison of fetal growth and neonatal outcomes in two consecutive case series. *Drug Alcohol Depend* 2008;96:69–78.

103. Jones HE, Johnson RE, Jasinski DR, et al. Randomized controlled study transitioning opioid-dependent pregnant women from short-acting morphine to buprenorphine or methadone. *Drug Alcohol Depend* 2005;78:33–38.

104. Martin PR, Arria AM, Fischer G, et al. Psychopharmacologic management of opioid-dependent women during pregnancy. *Am J Addict* 2009;18:148–156.

105. Gowing L, Farrell M, Ali R, et al. Alpha2-adrenergic agonists for the management of opioid withdrawal. *Cochrane Database Syst Rev* 2009:CD002024.

106. Kaltenbach K, Berghella V, Finnegan L. Opioid dependence during pregnancy. Effects and management. *Obstet Gynecol Clin North Am* 1998;25:139–151.

107. Wong CA, Scavone BM, Peaceman AM, et al. The risk of cesarean delivery with neuraxial analgesia given early versus late in labor. *N Engl J Med* 2005; 352:655–665.

108. Sun HL. Naloxone-precipitated acute opioid withdrawal syndrome after epidural morphine. *Anesth Analg* 1998;86:544–545.

109. Mitra S, Sinatra RS. Perioperative management of acute pain in the opioid-dependent patient. *Anesthesiology* 2004;101:212–227.

110. Wang JK, Nauss LA, Thomas JE. Pain relief by intrathecally applied morphine in man. *Anesthesiology* 1979;50:149–151.

111. Koppel BS, Tuchman AJ, Mangiardi JR, et al. Epidural spinal infection in intravenous drug abusers. *Arch Neurol* 1988;45:1331–1337.

112. Henderson CE, Terribile S, Keefe D, et al. Cardiac screening for pregnant intravenous drug abusers. *Am J Perinatol* 1989;6:397–399.

113. Grosso LM, Bracken MB. Caffeine metabolism, genetics, and perinatal outcomes: A review of exposure assessment considerations during pregnancy. *Ann Epidemiol* 2005;15:460–466.

114. Nehlig A, Daval JL, Debry G. Caffeine and the central nervous system: Mechanisms of action, biochemical, metabolic and psychostimulant effects. *Brain Res Brain Res Rev* 1992;17:139–170.

115. Maslova E, Bhattacharya S, Lin SW, et al. Caffeine consumption during pregnancy and risk of preterm birth: A meta-analysis. *Am J Clin Nutr* 2010; 92:1120–1132.

116. CARE Study Group. Maternal caffeine intake during pregnancy and risk of fetal growth restriction: A large prospective observational study. *BMJ* 2008; 337:a2332.

117. Weng X, Odouli R, Li DK. Maternal caffeine consumption during pregnancy and the risk of miscarriage: A prospective cohort study. *Am J Obstet Gynecol* 2008; 198:279.e1–279.e8.

118. American College of Obstetricians and Gynecologists. ACOG Committee Opinion No. 462: Moderate caffeine consumption during pregnancy. *Obstet Gynecol* 2010;116:467–468.

119. Collier SA, Browne ML, Rasmussen SA, et al. Maternal caffeine intake during pregnancy and orofacial clefts. *Birth Defects Res A Clin Mol Teratol* 2009; 85:842–849.

120. Mongraw-Chaffin ML, Cohn BA, Cohen RD, et al. Maternal smoking, alcohol consumption, and caffeine consumption during pregnancy in relation to a son's risk of persistent cryptorchidism: A prospective study in the Child Health and Development Studies cohort, 1959–1967. *Am J Epidemiol* 2008;167:257–261.

121. Silverman K, Evans SM, Strain EC, et al. Withdrawal syndrome after the double-blind cessation of caffeine consumption. *N Engl J Med* 1992;327:1109–1114.

122. Kuczkowski KM. Solvents in pregnancy: An emerging problem in obstetrics and obstetric anaesthesia. *Anaesthesia* 2003;58:1036–1037.

123. Wilkins-Haug L, Gabow PA. Toluene abuse during pregnancy: Obstetric complications and perinatal outcomes. *Obstet Gynecol* 1991;77:504–509.

124. Reyes de la Rocha S, Brown MA, Fortenberry JD. Pulmonary function abnormalities in intentional spray paint inhalation. *Chest* 1987;92:100–104.

125. Jones HE, Balster RL. Inhalant abuse in pregnancy. *Obstet Gynecol Clin North Am* 1998;25:153–167.

126. Weiner AL, Vieira L, McKay CA, et al. Ketamine abusers presenting to the emergency department: A case series. *J Emerg Med* 2000;18:447–451.

127. White PF, Way WL, Trevor AJ. Ketamine—its pharmacology and therapeutic uses. *Anesthesiology* 1982;56:119–136.

128. Dawkins JL, Tylden E, Colley N, et al. Drug abuse in pregnancy: Obstetric and neonatal problems. Ten years' experience. *Drug Alcohol Rev* 1997;16:25–31.

129. Suresh S, Anand KJ. Opioid tolerance in neonates: Mechanisms, diagnosis, assessment, and management. *Semin Perinatol* 1998;22:425–433.

130. Kennare R, Heard A, Chan A. Substance use during pregnancy: Risk factors and obstetric and perinatal outcomes in South Australia. *Aust N Z J Obstet Gynaecol* 2005;45:220–225.

131. McCance-Katz EF. Drug interactions associated with methadone, buprenorphine, cocaine, and HIV medications: Implications for pregnant women. *Life Sci* 2011;88:953–958.

132. Sprauve ME. Substance abuse and HIV pregnancy. *Clin Obstet Gynecol* 1996; 39:316–332.

133. Hughes SC, Dailey PA, Landers D, et al. Parturients infected with human immunodeficiency virus and regional anesthesia. Clinical and immunologic response. *Anesthesiology* 1995;82:32–37.

Jehovah's Witness: Ethical and Anesthetic-related Issues

Connie Khanh Vu Lan Tran

■ INTRODUCTION

The care of a Jehovah's Witness parturient can pose an ethical dilemma for the anesthesia care team since we are usually the ones who are responsible for transfusion during the perioperative period. On the one hand, we would like to respect the patient's autonomy but on the other hand as medical doctors we have taken an oath to do no harm. In order to provide the best care to these challenging patients, the healthcare providers should understand the religious background of the Jehovah's Witnesses, the ethical principles and medicolegal ramifications and the treatments which Jehovah's Witnesses may be amenable to accept.

■ HISTORICAL BACKGROUND

Jehovah's Witnesses is a Christian denomination founded by Charles Taze Russell in Pennsylvania in the 1870s (1). Initially started out as a bible study group, it is now one of the most rapidly growing religious groups in the world with more than 7 million members worldwide and 1.15 million members in the United States, according to its 2009 census (2). The group is officially known as the Watchtower Bible and Tract Society and since 1931 its members are called Jehovah's Witnesses based on biblical passages (*Isaiah 43:10 to 12 and Hebrews 12:1, 2*) (3). Jehovah's Witnesses have a close knitted community and usually meet three times a week in the Kingdom Hall for religious discussion based upon topics from its official publications, The Watchtower and Awake! Jehovah's Witnesses believe in the literal interpretation of the bible and salvation is dependent on being faithful to the word of Jehovah. Life on earth is a temporary period and death is a period of no conscious existence. All will be judged on Judgment Day and only the faithful and sin-free witnesses will be granted eternal life on paradise earth and the wicked will suffer eternal damnation (2). Jehovah's Witnesses are known for their house to house ministry, refusal to recognize secular authority and salute flags, pledge allegiance, join service organizations, enlist in the military, vote in public elections, or take any interest in civil government and within the medical community for the refusal for blood transfusion (2–4).

In 1945 the Watchtower, the official journal of the Jehovah's Witnesses, published the first stance against blood transfusion. The article warned its members against taking blood directly into the human body and to respect the sanctity of blood; however, no punitive measure for accepting blood transfusion was mentioned. The source of this belief is based on literal translation of the several passages from the Bible (*Genesis 3, 4, Leviticus 17:10 to 16*, and *Acts 15:28 to 29*).

Jehovah's Witnesses consider receiving blood products intravenously to be the same as "eating blood," similar to an intravenous feeding of a sugar solution to feed the patient (4,5). The official position of the Watch Tower Bible and Tract Society is that blood is sacred and once blood leaves the body, it must be disposed; therefore, preoperative donated autologous blood and allogeneic whole blood are prohibited. Jehovah's Witnesses who accepted blood transfusion are at risk for eternal damnation and eternal salvation is forfeited. Since 1961, individuals who "partake" blood can be "disfellowshipped" or excommunicated from the church and other members are required to refrain from spiritually socializing with the disfellowshipped member. This shunning from the community can cause great anguish to the disfellowshipped member (6–8). Administration of blood to a Jehovah's Witness against her wish has been likened by Witnesses to rape (9). If a Jehovah's Witness received blood against her will, she will not be disfellowshipped but she may have deep and lasting psychological effects (9). In June 2000, The Watchtower magazine published an article which clarified its position on blood transfusion. Blood is divided into four major components: Red blood cells, white blood cells, plasma, and platelets. A Jehovah's Witness is prohibited from receiving these major components; however, the utilization of minor components of each major component such as hemoglobin-based blood substitute, interferons, interleukins, albumin, globulins, clotting factors, and wound healing factors is left to each member's conscientious decision (Fig. 43-1) (10,7). This position was reaffirmed in the section "Questions from Readers" in the June 2004 Watchtower.

Jehovah's Witnesses carry an Advance Medical Directive/Release pocket-sized card which stated that no blood be administered under any circumstances (11,2). This card is renewed every year. The patient can also write in the blood factions and alternative treatments that are personally acceptable.

The Watch Tower and Tract Society established a network Hospital Liaison Committee worldwide to provide physicians information on the religious views of a Jehovah's Witness patient. There are more than 1,600 committees worldwide with some 120 in the United States (11). One can contact the Hospital Liaison Committee at anytime by phone (718-560-4300) or email (his@jw.org) for support (11). Jehovah's Witnesses have also championed bloodless medicine and surgery programs where blood is avoided and alternative techniques such as optimizing preoperative red blood cell production, oxygenation, and prophylactic angiographic embolization are offered (12). In the United States, many hospitals have developed these bloodless programs not only to treat Jehovah's Witnesses but also for blood conservation (13–15). The Society for the Advancement of Blood Management was founded in 2001 to improve patient outcomes through optimal blood management. Its website (www.sabm.org) provides a list of hospitals with bloodless medicine and surgery programs.

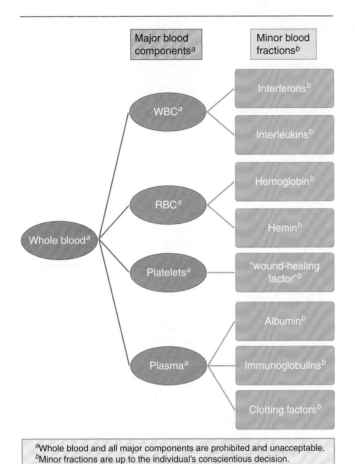

[a]Whole blood and all major components are prohibited and unacceptable.
[b]Minor fractions are up to the individual's conscientious decision.
Adapted from: Watchtower magazine; June 15, 2004:29–31.

FIGURE 43-1 Jehovah's Witnesses official position on blood

Within the Jehovah's Witnesses' community, there is a group who disagree with the Watch Tower Bible and Tract Society's blood ban policy. The Associated Jehovah's Witnesses for Reform on Blood seek to change the blood policy which they viewed as misguided policy and biblical misinterpretation of blood by a high-control religious group (6,16). Muramoto noted that "the significance of the reform movement for physicians is awareness of a growing diversity of values and beliefs among individual Jehovah's Witnesses. Such diversity requires physicians to scrutinize the patient's premolded medical directive more closely and take a more individualized approach" (16).

■ ETHICAL PRINCIPLES

In caring for patients, a physician subscribes to the four principles of medical ethics. Each of the principles is equally important and efforts must be made to avoid violation of any one of them (17). *Autonomy* or "self-rule" is the right to choose or refuse recommended treatment. *Beneficence* or "doing good" compels the physician to act in a manner that is beneficial to the patient. *Non-maleficence* is the obligation not to harm or cause injury and *Justice* is the fair distribution of benefits, risks, and cost. Traditionally, beneficence and non-maleficence played a central role in medical ethics but within the past 30 years, autonomy and justice have become more prominent (18). The principle of autonomy is the foundation of informed consent and a person's right for self-determination. A person must be competent and have the capacity to give consent. An informed

consent must occur prior to any treatment or intervention. The consent is considered informed if it has the following elements (9,18):

1. The nature or purpose of the decision or procedure
2. Reasonable alternatives to the proposed intervention
3. The relevant risks, benefits, and uncertainties related to each alternative
4. Assessment of the patient understanding
5. Decision to accept or refuse an intervention is voluntarily and free from pressure

Muramoto and Elder have argued that Jehovah's Witnesses do not have autonomy since there is organized intimidation from the church and members are given insufficient information about blood transfusion (6,19). Malyon and Ridley responded that in caring for Jehovah's Witnesses, the physician must respect the patient's autonomy and beliefs and that faith transcends rationality (8,20).

The principle of justice has also come into question when caring for Jehovah's Witnesses. Savulescu pointed out that in demanding for alternative treatments other than blood transfusion; Jehovah's Witnesses are receiving more expensive alternative treatments (21). By providing care for a patient, the physician enters into a patient–doctor relationship in which the physician has a moral obligation to always act in the patient's best interest. The physician's desire for non-maleficence and beneficence may come into conflict with the patient's autonomy and society's justice (22–25).

When the four principles come into conflict in a difficult clinical situation, the physician may use different perspectives and frameworks to solve the problem. The *virtue-based* approach relies on qualities of character that dispose health professionals to make choices and decisions that achieve the well-being of patients (26). There is no comprehensive list of virtues but five are applicable to medical practitioner: Trustworthiness, integrity, discernment, compassion, and conscientiousness (27). By using virtue ethics as a framework to a medical dilemma, the physician takes into account the emotions and motivations of the involved parties and arrive at a creative solution. Virtue ethicists recognize that tragic dilemmas can rarely be resolved to the complete satisfaction of all parties and that any conclusion is likely to leave some remainder of pain and regret (27).

The *care-based ethics* or the ethic of care emphasizes the commitment, empathy, compassion, caring, and love instead of the impartial principles. Good ethical decisions result from personal caring in relationships and the impact of different possible actions on those relationships (26). The *communitarian ethics* assumes that human beings are social animals and whose lives are lived out within social, political, and cultural institutions and practices (28). The need of the community may supersede personal autonomy. An example of communitarian ethics is the need to balance a patient's claims of privacy and confidentiality against risks to others (26). The *case-based* approach to an ethical decision uses previous similar cases as precedent for the current one. Past decisions about moral rights and wrongs in cases serve as a form of authority for decisions in new cases (29). The difficulty in the case-based approach is in determining the similarities and differences among the cases (26).

According to the American Medical Association Code of Medical Ethics, Opinion 8.115, if it is not an emergency situation, the physician may terminate the doctor–patient relationship by transferring the care to another physician who is willing to treat the patient without using blood (30). However, physicians have resorted to the legal system when patients rejected the medical recommendation for blood transfusion.

■ LEGAL CONSIDERATIONS

The First Amendment of the United States Constitution, as extended to the individual States by the Fourteenth Amendment, guarantees the absolute right of every individual to freedom in his religious belief (31). A religious belief is a constitutional guaranteed freedom but religious practice is not an absolute guaranteed legal protection. Courts have upheld a variety of laws on the theory that society has an overriding interest in protecting the lives of its citizens (31). There are no statue laws regarding religious freedom since this is covered by the Constitution; however, there are multiple case laws regarding religious practice. Case laws are the resulting court rulings from individual cases and may be inconsistent due to different jurisdictions and individual states laws. Case laws tend to change over time due to the changing values of society (32).

The case of *Schloendorff v New York Hospital* (1914) is often cited as the landmark case for patient's autonomy or the right of a competent adult to accept or refuse care and need of consent for medical procedures. Mary Schloendorff had agreed to have an examination under ether but did not want any surgery done. However, during the examination, the surgeon decided to perform a hysterectomy in order to remove the fibroids. She developed severe postoperative complications with loss of fingers and injuries to her legs. She sued the hospital for surgery performed without her consent and as a result, she was maimed for life (33). Judge Benjamin Cardozo wrote in the court's opinion that "every human being of adult years and sound mind has a right to determine what shall be done with his own body, and a surgeon who performs an operation without his patient's consent commits an assault for which he is liable in damages. This is true except in cases of emergency where the patient is unconscious and where it is necessary to operate before consent can be obtained" (34). Unfortunately, Ms. Schloendorff's claim was rejected because a non-profit hospital could not be held liable for the actions of the doctor who is considered an independent contractor.

The law is clear on a competent adult who knows the nature and consequences of his actions. The competent adult may make a decision about her healthcare that may be contrary to the physician's recommendations. This right is reiterated in The Patient Self-Determination Act of 1990, which became effective in 1991. The act requires facilities which received Medicare or Medicaid funding to provide in writing to each adult patient describing the person's legal rights according to the laws of the state in which he or she resides. The patient can accept or refuse medical treatment and has the right to an advance directive (35,36).

Minors have no legal rights and remain under parental jurisdiction until they reach the age of majority but the state has a duty and interest in preserving the health of minors (37). This principle is known as "Parens Patriae" which the state acts as "the father of the people" in order to preserve the basic right of a minor to grow up and become an adult (38). Courts usually intervene in cases involving minors with imminent threat to life or limb by failure to receive blood because of the parent's religious belief. In 1944, the milestone cases of *Prince v Massachusetts* which concerned a child distributing Jehovah's Witness magazine accompanied by an aunt, Justice Rutledge wrote "Parents may be free to become martyrs themselves. But it does not follow they are free, in identical circumstances, to make martyrs of their children before they have reached the age of full and legal discretion when they can make that choice for themselves" (39).

When it comes to a pregnant woman's rights, the courts have been asked to assert the rights of the woman and that of her unborn child. The *Roe v Wade*'s decision in 1973 allows the state to prohibit abortion when the fetus attains the point of viability. However, the state's interest in protecting the life of the fetus is limited by the mother's own interests in the preservation of her life and health (40). With the improvement of fetal monitoring, more cesarean deliveries are done to safely deliver the baby. In the 1980s, physicians and hospitals would resort to the court system to compel a pregnant woman to undergo a cesarean delivery when the woman refused the recommended surgery (41). The Supreme Court of Georgia in 1981 ordered a pregnant woman at 39 weeks' gestation with a diagnosis of placenta previa to undergo a cesarean delivery in *Jefferson v. Griffin Spalding County Hospital*. Mrs. Jessie Jefferson has refused to consent for a cesarean delivery based upon religious belief and faith in God. This is the first case in which the court ordered a pregnant woman to undergo surgery in order to save a viable fetus and establishes a pregnant woman's duty to protect the health of a viable fetus and fetal right to such protection and the first time a court asserts jurisdiction over a fetus in order to transfer custody of the fetus to the state (42). The court's decision in *Jefferson* was based upon the physician's opinion that there was a 99% chance that the baby would not survive and a 50% chance that the mother would not survive a vaginal birth and that the *Roe* analysis allowed the state to protect a viable fetus which derived from the statutes that prohibit abortion (40,42). The court's conclusion is that the state interest in protecting the potential life of a viable fetus outweighed the mother's right to refuse medical treatment, to practice her religion, and right to parental autonomy.

There is a lack of U.S. Supreme Court opinion on maternal rights versus fetal rights. However, there are inconsistent state case laws regarding the right of a pregnant woman to refuse medical treatments. Because of the different state laws, maternal–fetal rights remain a highly emotional charged issue.

The state of Illinois is a strong maternal right state (43). In 1988, the Illinois Supreme Court determined in the case of *Stallman v. Youngquist* that the mother is not liable to her child for accidental prenatal injury. The father sued the mother on behalf of his child who had suffered injury due to an automobile accident which occurred when the mother was driving when she was 5 months pregnant. The court held that the child does not have the right to recover against its mother and that "judicial scrutiny into the day-to-day lives of pregnant women would involve an unprecedented intrusion into the privacy and autonomy of the citizens of this State" (43). The landmark decision of the Stallman case is that the Illinois Supreme Court determined that fetal rights are not superior to maternal rights.

In 1994, the Illinois Court of Appeals upheld with the lower court's decision to refuse to order a cesarean delivery *In re Baby Boy Doe*. The case involved a pregnant woman at 37 weeks' gestation who had refused to undergo a cesarean delivery upon the recommendation of her doctor because of placenta insufficiency, citing religious reasons. The court's opinion was based upon the previous Illinois cases including *Stallman* and stated that "a woman's right to refuse invasive medical treatment, derived from her rights to privacy, bodily integrity, and religious liberty, is not diminished during pregnancy. The woman retains the same right to refuse invasive treatment, even of lifesaving or other beneficial nature that she can exercise when she is not pregnant. The potential impact upon the fetus is not legally relevant; to the contrary, the *Stallman* court explicitly rejected the view that the woman's rights can be subordinated to fetal rights" (40,43). The patient delivered vaginally a healthy baby boy 3 weeks after the court's petition.

In *re Fetus Brown*, a court order was obtained to forcefully transfuse Darlene Brown after a surgery to remove a urethral mass at 34 and 3/7 weeks pregnant. She had refused blood transfusion during surgery because of her Jehovah's Witness' belief and no blood was given; but after surgery her hemoglobin level was 4.4 g/dL and continued to drop to 3.4 g/dL on postoperative day 2. Her doctor, who feared that without a blood transfusion Darlene Brown and her fetus would not survive, asked the hospital to request a court intervention so that a blood transfusion can be given to save the patient's and her viable fetus' lives since blood transfusion was considered minimally invasive to Mrs. Brown. The Illinois circuit court citing the state's interest in a viable fetus appointed the hospital administrator as a temporary custodian for Fetus Brown who then consented to blood transfusion based on the physician's recommendation. Darlene Brown had to be sedated and restrained during the transfusion. She delivered a healthy infant a few days later. Brown appealed to the Illinois Court of Appeals contending that as a competent adult under federal and Illinois law, she has an absolute right to refuse medical advice and treatment and to overturn the trial court's order appointing a temporary custodian to blood transfusion for the benefit of her fetus (44). The Illinois Court of Appeal agreed to hear the case even though the issues had become moot since Brown had delivered and the hospital custody was terminated. The court considered the case since the issue may come up again in the future and the issue is "a public one requiring authoritative determination for the future guidance of public officials, especially given the emergency and expedited nature of such proceedings" (44). In examining the case, the court had to determine the right of a competent adult to refuse medical treatment to the state's four interests in refusal of treatment cases:

1. Preservation of life
2. Prevention of suicide
3. Protection of third parties
4. Maintaining the ethical integrity of the medical profession

In the first interest, the court found that the state had an interest in preserving the life of both mother and fetus. However, the court held that "the State may not override a pregnant woman's competent treatment decision, including refusal of recommended invasive medical procedures, to potentially save the life of the viable fetus" (43,44). The court also found that "blood transfusion is an invasive procedure that interrupts a competent adult's bodily integrity."

The second State's interest in prevention of suicide was not an issue since Darlene Brown was willing to accept all possible treatments except blood transfusion. The third State's interest in protection of third parties was also determined to be not an issue since the husband and extended family were willing to take care of Darlene Brown's two other minor children. The court looked at the State's interest in protecting the viable fetus. The court noted that this was not an abortion case so *Roe v. Wade* was not applicable. The court also noted that the fetus was not considered a minor for the purpose of the Illinois Juvenile Court Act, therefore, "cannot separate the mother's valid treatment refusal form the potential adverse consequences to the viable fetus" (44). The court observed that the fourth State's interest in maintaining the ethical integrity of the medical profession did not "provide a definitive solution" but cited the American Medical Association board of Trustees' recommendation that "judicial intervention is inappropriate when a woman has made an informed refusal of a medical treatment designed to benefit her fetus" (43,44). Based on the above reasons, the Illinois Court of Appeals ruled that the circuit court erred in appointing a guardian for Fetus Brown in order to consent for blood transfusion for Darlene Brown.

■ MEDICAL COMMUNITIES POSITION ON MATERNAL–FETAL RIGHTS

The American Medical Association's Code of Medical Ethics recognizes the patient's right to make medical decisions based on informed consent. There are certain conditions which the American Medical Association Board of Trustees has proposed which may be reasonably to obtain legal intervention. The medical treatment must pose insignificant or no health risks for the woman, involve minimal invasion of the woman's body integrity, and clearly prevent substantial and irreversible fetal harm (45). These three conditions are difficult to obtain and have limited practical usefulness in clinical situations.

The American College of Obstetricians and Gynecologists has ethical guidelines for its members concerning the care of a pregnant patient. The Committee on Ethics publishes and updates its opinions on issues such as informed consent, informed refusal, ethical decision making, and maternal decision making. The ACOG Committee Opinion number 321, states that it "strongly opposes the criminal prosecution of pregnant women whose activities may appear to cause harm to their fetuses. Efforts to use legal system specifically to protect the fetus by constraining women's decision making or punishing them for their behavior erode a woman's basic rights to privacy and bodily integrity and are neither legally nor morally justified" (46). In fact, ACOG Committee on Ethics maintains that "judicial authority should not be used to implement treatment regimens aimed at protecting the fetus, for such actions violate the pregnant woman's autonomy."

The American Society of Anesthesiologists (ASA) also has Guidelines for the Ethical Practice of Anesthesiology and last amended in 2008 which affirms the AMA principles of medical ethics. The ASA introduced the Syllabus on Ethics which was published in 1999 to help provide an ethic curriculum in the anesthesiologist's training. In the section of Informed Consent for Jehovah's Witnesses, the Syllabus emphasizes that "by entering into a covenant with a Jehovah's Witness patient, the anesthesiologist accepts the patient's belief that receiving a transfusion will prevent him or her from eternal salvation.... If the anesthesiologist cannot agree to a patient's desires, the anesthesiologist has both the right and obligation to withdraw from that patient's care" and transfer care to another provider.

■ ANESTHETIC CARE OF A JEHOVAH'S WITNESS PARTURIENT

Communication is one of the core competencies mandated by the Accreditation Council for Graduate Medical Education that all residents must demonstrate. Open communication between the obstetric team and the anesthesia team is a must in the care of a parturient. All healthcare providers who are willing and able to offer medical care to a Jehovah's Witness parturient should be identified in the obstetric and anesthesia team. Ideally, a multidiscipline meeting should be done in the early prenatal period since women who are Jehovah's Witnesses have an increased risk of maternal mortality and morbidity due to obstetric hemorrhage (47–49). Because of this risk, Gyamfi suggested that the Jehovah's Witness parturient should be evaluated by a maternal–fetal medicine specialist prior to the third trimester and deliver at a tertiary center (50).

Maternal hemorrhage is the second leading cause of maternal death and permanent brain damage from 1990 or later according to the ASA Closed Claims Project (51). This trend is also reflected in Berg's report of pregnancy-related death in the United States from 1998 to 2005 (52). Blood transfusion can minimize the risk of maternal death due to hemorrhage but not if the patient refuses blood transfusion. Singla examined the data at Mount Sinai Medical Center over a 10-year period and reported that Jehovah's Witness parturients are at a 44-fold increased risk of maternal death (49). Massiah reported a 65-fold increased risk of maternal death due to hemorrhage in the Jehovah's Witness parturients in the United Kingdom over a 14-year period (48). Another large study from the Netherlands also showed that Jehovah's Witnesses are at a six times increased risk for maternal death and 130 times increased risk for maternal death due to obstetric hemorrhage and at 3.1 times increased risk for serious maternal morbidity because of obstetric hemorrhage (47).

In order to provide optimal care for the Jehovah's Witness parturients, a plan of care must be developed at each institution to guide healthcare providers.

■ PRENATAL CARE

Once a parturient notified her obstetrician of her refusal to accept blood transfusion during her prenatal care, her doctor should formulate a plan of care specifically for her needs. Routine prenatal laboratory studies should be done and the patient's hematocrit should be maintained at 40% or greater. Anemia should be worked up, and iron supplement and vitamin C which boosts the absorption of iron in the gastrointestinal tract should be given (50). Erythropoietin, which is a glycoprotein produced mainly by the kidneys and stimulates the production of red blood cells, has been used and proposed if patient remains anemic despite iron supplement. Commercially available recombinant human erythropoietin may contain albumin but the newest formula of darbepoetin alfa does not contain any blood fraction. Erythropoiesis-stimulating agents are usually given with folate and iron sulfate. However, the Food and Drug Administration issued a black box warning in 2008 due to findings that erythropoietin-stimulating agents shortened overall survival and/or increased the risk of tumor progression or recurrence in clinical studies of patients with breast, non-small cell lung, head and neck, lymphoid, and cervical cancers (53).

Healthcare providers should not assume that all Jehovah's Witnesses refuse blood products since a review by Gyamfi showed that about 50% of the Jehovah's Witness parturients agreed to accept blood or blood products (54). The parturient's decision should be her own and not influenced by others; therefore, an in-depth discussion of her risks for hemorrhage and what type of blood products the patient is willing to accept should be obtained individually. Jehovah's Witnesses may carry the Medical Power of Attorney form which differs depending on her state of residency. The example form is a legal document in the state of Texas. This form allows the parturient to direct her care regarding blood transfusion of minor components and refusal of whole blood and major components. Jehovah's Witnesses renew this form yearly and usually carry this form (Fig. 43-2). There is also a worksheet that is available to Jehovah's Witnesses which explains what medical treatments are unacceptable and what can be accepted based upon the patient's conscientious decisions (Fig. 43-3). Informed consent should be obtained and outlined what the Jehovah's Witness patient would accept or refuse. At Ben Taub General Hospital, a part of Harris County Hospital District, patients who refuse blood transfusion are asked to sign the refusal to authorize administration of blood or blood products and release from liability and the form is co-signed by two other family members (Fig. 43-4).

Multidisciplinary meeting should be held prior to the patient's due date if she has additional co-morbidities and should include the obstetricians, maternal–fetal medicine specialists, anesthesiologists, interventional radiologists for possible placement of embolization catheter or vascular balloons, hematologists, other surgical services, neonatologists, and nursing staff (55). Ideally, a departmental guideline or protocol should have been developed for the care of a Jehovah's Witness parturient such as described by Gyamfi at Mount Sinai Medical Hospital (50). A plan of care should be understood by all parties.

■ BLOODLESS SURGERY

Many hospitals have developed bloodless medicine and surgery program to minimize allogeneic blood transfusion. The proponents of bloodless surgery program cited the decreased risk of blood-borne infections, transfusion reactions, and medical errors during the banking of autologous blood and the decreased supply of donated blood (56,57). The principles of bloodless surgery involve steps taken preoperatively, intraoperatively, and postoperatively to reduce blood loss and increase available oxygen supply (see Table 43-1).

■ INTRAOPERATIVE MANAGEMENT

When the parturient arrives in the Labor and Delivery Unit, the anesthesia team should perform a complete history and physical, with emphasis on airway examination and intravenous access, review laboratory data, verify the informed consent, and document what the Jehovah's Witness parturient is willing to accept. Anesthetic plans including risks and benefits of regional or general anesthesia, acute normovolemic hemodilution, cell salvage, postoperative pain management, and possible intensive care unit admission should be discussed with the patient (58,59). If the parturient has known risks of hemorrhage such as previous abdominal surgery or cesarean delivery and placenta accreta or placenta previa, then a planned cesarean delivery with possible hysterectomy should be scheduled preferably as the first case of the day. Once the anesthesia team has evaluated the patient, two large-bore peripheral intravenous catheters should be placed. Consideration should be given to insertion of central and arterial lines. There is a plan for placement of pelvic arterial embolization to control intraoperative bleeding; the patient is then seen by the interventional radiology team for temporary balloon occlusion placement with fluoroscopic guidance and angiographic confirmation. This involves the placement of an angioplasty balloon in each of the proximal internal arteries which can be inflated intraoperatively to decrease pelvic blood flow. The balloons are usually deflated at the end of the surgical procedure to inspect for bleeding and removed under fluoroscopic guidance (55). Prophylactic balloon occlusions of internal iliac arteries have been shown to decrease blood loss and transfusion requirement in patients with placenta accreta undergoing cesarean delivery and hysterectomy (60–62).

■ ACUTE NORMOVOLEMIC HEMODILUTION

Jehovah's Witnesses may accept acute normovolemic hemodilution as part of blood conservation techniques especially if a closed circuit is used. This will satisfy the requirement that blood is continuous with the body (63). Introduced in the 1970s as a means to reduce intraoperative loss of red blood cells and allogeneic blood transfusion during surgery, Estella et al. reported its first usage in an obstetrical case in a Jehovah's Witness parturient in 1997 (64). Candidates for acute normovolemic hemodilution must have a hemoglobin

Medical Power of Attorney

DISCLOSURE STATEMENT

INFORMATION CONCERNING THE MEDICAL POWER OF ATTORNEY

THIS IS AN IMPORTANT LEGAL DOCUMENT. BEFORE SIGNING THIS DOCUMENT, YOU SHOULD KNOW THESE IMPORTANT FACTS:

Except to the extent you state otherwise, this document gives the person you name as your agent the authority to make any and all health-care decisions for you in accordance with your wishes, including your religious and moral beliefs, when you are no longer capable of making them yourself. Because "health care" means any treatment, service, or procedure to maintain, diagnose, or treat your physical or mental condition, your agent has the power to make a broad range of health-care decisions for you. Your agent may consent, refuse to consent, or withdraw consent to medical treatment and may make decisions about withdrawing or withholding life-sustaining treatment. Your agent may not consent to voluntary inpatient mental health services, convulsive treatment, psychosurgery, or abortion. A physician must comply with your agent's instructions or allow you to be transferred to another physician.

Your agent's authority begins when your doctor certifies that you lack the competence to make health-care decisions.

Your agent is obligated to follow your instructions when making decisions on your behalf. Unless you state otherwise, your agent has the same authority to make decisions about your health care as you would have had.

It is important that you discuss this document with your physician or other health-care provider before you sign it to make sure that you understand the nature and range of decisions that may be made on your behalf. If you do not have a physician, you should talk with someone else who is knowledgeable about these issues and can answer your questions. You do not need a lawyer's assistance to complete this document, but if there is anything in this document that you do not understand, you should ask a lawyer to explain it to you.

The person you appoint as agent should be someone you know and trust. The person must be 18 years of age or older or a person under 18 years of age who has had the disabilities of minority removed. If you appoint your health- or residential-care provider (e.g., your physician or an employee of a home health agency, hospital, nursing home, or residential-care home, other than a relative), that person has to choose between acting as your agent or as your health- or residential-care provider; the law does not permit a person to do both at the same time.

Page 1 of 4

You should inform the person you appoint that you want the person to be your health-care agent. You should discuss this document with your agent and your physician and give each a signed copy. You should indicate on the document itself the people and institutions who have signed copies. Your agent is not liable for health-care decisions made in good faith on your behalf.

Even after you have signed this document, you have the right to make health-care decisions for yourself as long as you are able to do so and treatment cannot be given to you or stopped over your objection. You have the right to revoke the authority granted your agent by informing your agent or your health- or residential-care provider orally or in writing, or by your execution of a subsequent medical power of attorney. Unless you state otherwise, your appointment of a spouse dissolves on divorce.

This document may not be changed or modified. If you want to make changes in the document, you must make an entirely new one.

You may wish to appoint an alternate agent in the event that your agent is unwilling, unable, or ineligible to act as your agent. Any alternate agent you appoint has the same authority to make health-care decisions for you.

THIS POWER OF ATTORNEY IS NOT VALID UNLESS IT IS SIGNED IN THE PRESENCE OF TWO COMPETENT ADULT WITNESSES. AT LEAST ONE OF YOUR TWO WITNESSES MUST BE A PERSON WHO IS NOT:

(1) **the person you have appointed as your agent or alternate agent;**
(2) a person related to you by blood or marriage;
(3) a person entitled to any part of your estate after your death under a will or codicil executed by you or by operation of law;
(4) your attending physician;
(5) an employee of your attending physician;
(6) an employee of a health-care facility in which you are a patient if the employee is providing direct patient care to you or is an officer, director, partner, or business office employee of the health-care facility or of any parent organization of the health-care facility; or
(7) a person who at the time this power of attorney is executed, has a claim against any part of your estate after your death.

Page 2 of 4

Medical Power of Attorney

1. I, ______________________ (print or type full name), fill out this document to set forth my treatment instructions and to appoint a health-care agent in case of my incapacity.
2. I am one of Jehovah's Witnesses, and I direct that **NO TRANSFUSIONS of whole blood, red cells, white cells, platelets, or plasma** be given me under any circumstances, even if health-care providers believe that such are necessary to preserve my life. I refuse to predonate and store my blood for later infusion.
3. **Regarding minor fractions of blood:** [initial those that apply]
(a) ____ I REFUSE ALL (b) ____ I REFUSE ALL EXCEPT: ______
(c) ____ I may be willing to accept some minor blood fractions, but the details will have to be discussed with me if I am conscious or with my health-care agent in case of my incapacity.
4. **Regarding medical procedures involving the use of my own blood,** except diagnostic procedures, such as blood samples for testing: [initial those that apply]
(a) ____ I REFUSE ALL (b) ____ I REFUSE ALL EXCEPT: ______
(c) ____ I may be willing to accept certain medical procedures involving my blood, but the details will have to be discussed with me if I am conscious or with my health-care agent in case of my incapacity.
5. **Regarding end-of-life matters:** [initial one of the two choices]
(a) ____ I do not want my life to be prolonged if, to a reasonable degree of medical certainty, my situation is hopeless.
(b) ____ I want my life to be prolonged as long as possible within the limits of generally accepted medical standards, even if this means that I might be kept alive on machines for years.
6. **Regarding other health-care instructions** (such as current medications, allergies, and medical problems):
7. I give no one (including my agent) any authority to disregard or override my instructions set forth herein. Family members, relatives, or friends may disagree with me, but any such disagreement does not diminish the strength or substance of my refusal of blood or other instructions.
8. Apart from the matters covered above, I appoint the person named below as my agent to make health-care decisions for me. I give my agent full power and authority to consent to or to refuse treatment (including artificial nutrition and hydration) on my behalf, to consult with my doctors and receive copies of my medical records, and to take legal action to ensure that my wishes are honored. If my first appointed agent is unavailable, unable, or unwilling to serve, I appoint an alternate agent below to serve with the same power and authority.

Page 3 of 4

9. I have been provided with a disclosure statement (pages 1 and 2) explaining the effect of this document. I have read and understand the information contained in the disclosure statement.

Signature Date

Address

10. TWO WITNESSES MUST SIGN BELOW; HOWEVER, ONLY THE FIRST WITNESS MUST COMPLY WITH THE FOLLOWING STATEMENT:

STATEMENT OF FIRST WITNESS

I am not the person appointed as agent or alternate agent by this document. I am not related to the principal (the person who signed this document above) by blood or marriage. I would not be entitled to any portion of the principal's estate on the principal's death. I am not the principal's attending physician or an employee of the attending physician. I have no claim against any portion of the principal's estate on the principal's death. Furthermore, if I am an employee of a health-care facility in which the principal is a patient, I am not involved in providing direct patient care to the principal and am not an officer, director, partner, or business office employee of the health-care facility or of any parent organization of the health-care facility.

Signature of first witness / Date Signature of second witness / Date

Address Address

HEALTH-CARE AGENT*

Name:
Address:
Telephone(s):

* Note: The person you appoint as agent should be someone you know and trust. The person must be 18 years of age or older or a person under 18 years of age who has had the disabilities of minority removed. If you appoint your health- or residential-care provider (e.g., your physician or an employee of a home health agency, hospital, nursing home, or residential-care home, other than a relative), that person has to choose between acting as your agent or as your health- or residential-care provider; the law does not permit a person to do both at the same time.

ALTERNATE HEALTH-CARE AGENT*

Name:
Address:
Telephone(s):

Medical Power of Attorney

NO BLOOD

Page 4 of 4

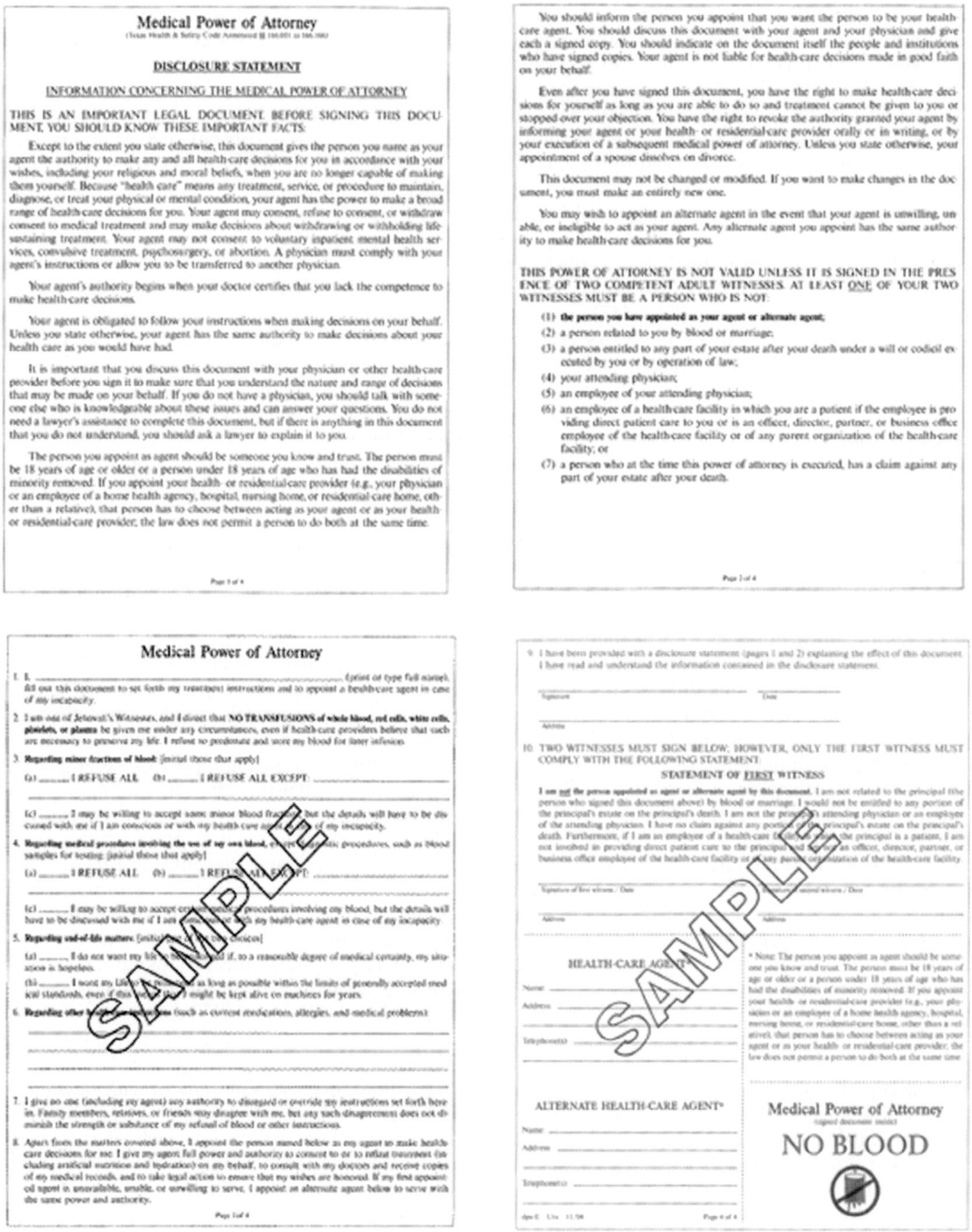

FIGURE 43-2

level at least in the upper limit of the norm or above 12 g/dL, no history of cardiovascular or clotting deficiencies, and the predicted blood loss during the surgery must be more than 50% of the circulating volume or not less than 1,500 mL (32,64–66). The basis of acute normovolemic hemodilution is that by removing the blood prior to surgical incision and replacing it with a crystalloid or colloid, the blood loss during surgery will contain fewer red cells per volume and reinfusion of blood after the control of surgical blood loss will be that of whole blood containing not only red blood cells but also platelets and clotting factors. Hemodilution decreases blood viscosity resulting in an increase in microcirculatory flow and cardiac output (32,57). The volume of blood to be removed can be determined by using the formula (32,65):

$$\text{Blood volume to remove} = \text{EBV} \times \frac{\text{Hct}_i - \text{Hct}_f}{\text{Hct}_m}$$

EBV = estimated blood volume (L) (kg of body weight × 0.8)
Hct_i = initial hematocrit
Hct_f = final desired hematocrit
Hct_m = mean value of initial and final desired hematocrit

The procedure is done intraoperatively and prior to surgical incision (Fig. 43-5A and B). Blood is removed from a central or peripheral vein into a citrated blood bag from blood bank which is connected to another intravenous line

WORK SHEET 1

Unacceptable to Christians	Your Personal Decision		
Whole Blood	Fractions		Choices You Need to Make
PLASMA	**ALBUMIN—UP TO 4% OF PLASMA** A protein extracted from plasma. Types of albumin are found also in plants, in foods such as milk and eggs, and in the milk of a nursing mother. Albumin from blood is sometimes used in volume expanders to treat shock and severe burns. These preparations may contain up to 25% albumin. Minute amounts are used in the formulation of many other medicines, including some formulations of erythropoietin (EPO). **IMMUNOGLOBULINS—UP TO 3% OF PLASMA** Protein fractions that may be used in some medicines that fight viruses and diseases, such as diphtheria, tetanus, viral hepatitis, and rabies. They may also be used to guard against some medical conditions that threaten the life of a developing baby and to counteract the effects of snake or spider venom. **CLOTTING FACTORS—LESS THAN 1% OF PLASMA** There are various proteins that help blood to clot in order to stop bleeding. Some are given to patients who tend to bleed easily. They are also used in medical glues to seal wounds and to stop bleeding after surgery. One combination of clotting factors is known as cryoprecipitate. **Note:** Some clotting factors are now made from nonblood sources.		__I accept albumin or __I refuse albumin __I accept immunoglobulins or __I refuse immunoglobulins __I accept blood-derived clotting factors or __I refuse blood-derived clotting factors
RED CELLS	**HEMOGLOBIN—33% OF RED CELLS** A protein that transports oxygen throughout the body and carbon dioxide to the lungs. Products being developed from human or animal hemoglobin could be used to treat patients with acute anemia or massive blood loss. **HEMIN—LESS THAN 2% OF RED CELLS** An enzyme inhibitor derived from hemoglobin that is used to treat a group of rare genetic blood disorders (known as porphyria) that affect the digestive, nervous, and circulatory systems.		__I accept hemoglobin or __I refuse hemoglobin __I accept hemin or __I refuse hemin
WHITE CELLS	**INTERFERONS—A TINY FRACTION OF WHITE CELLS** Proteins that fight certain viral infections and cancers. Most interferons are not derived from blood. Some are made from fractions of human white blood cells.		__I accept blood-derived interferons or __I refuse blood-derived interferons
PLATELETS	At present, no fractions from platelets are being isolated for direct use in medical treatment.		

WORK SHEET 2

	Your Personal Decision	
PROCEDURES INVOLVING THE MEDICAL USE OF YOUR OWN BLOOD		
*Note: The methods of applying each of these medical procedures vary from physician to physician. You should have your physician explain exactly what is involved in any proposed procedure to ensure that it is in harmony with Bible principles and with your own conscientious decisions.		
Name of Treatment	What it Accomplishes	Choices You Need to Make (You might want to speak to your physician before accepting or refusing any of these procedures)
CELL SALVAGE	**Reduces blood loss.** Blood is recovered during surgery from a wound or body cavity. It is washed or filtered and then, perhaps in a continuous process, returned to the patient.	_I accept _I might accept* _I refuse
HEMODILUTION	**Reduces blood loss.** During surgery, blood is diverted to bags and replaced with nonblood volume expander. Thus the blood remaining in the patient surgery is diluted, containing fewer red blood cells. During or at the end of the surgery, the diverted blood is returned to the patient.	_I accept _I might accept* _I refuse
HEART–LUNG MACHINE	**Maintains circulation.** Blood is diverted to an artificial heart–lung machine where it is oxygenated and directed back into the patient.	_I accept _I might accept* _I refuse
DIALYSIS	**Functions as an organ.** In hemodialysis, blood circulates through a machine that filters and cleans it before returning it to the patient.	_I accept _I might accept* _I refuse
EPIDURAL BLOOD PATCH	**Stops spinal fluid leakage.** A small amount of the patient's own blood is injected into the membrane surrounding the spinal cord. It is used to seal a puncture site that is leaking spinal fluid.	_I accept _I might accept* _I refuse
PLASMAPHERESIS	**Treats illness.** Blood is withdrawn and filtered to remove plasma. A plasma substitute is added, and the blood is returned to the patient. Some physicians may want to use plasma from another person to replace that from the patient's blood. If so, this option would be unacceptable to a Christian.	_I accept _I might accept* _I refuse
LABELING OR TAGGING	**Diagnoses or treats illness.** Some blood is withdrawn, mixed with medicine, and returned to the patient. The length of time one's blood is outside the body may vary.	_I accept _I might accept* _I refuse
PLATELET GEL; AUTOLOGOUS (MEANING "MADE FROM YOUR OWN BLOOD")	**Seals wounds, reduces bleeding.** Some blood is withdrawn and concentrated into a solution rich in platelets and white cells. This solution is applied on surgical sites or wounds. **Note:** In some formulations, a clotting factor taken from cow's blood is used.	_I accept _I might accept* _I refuse

FIGURE 43-3 Jehovah's Witnesses' worksheets

**HARRIS COUNTY
HOSPITAL DISTRICT**

1. I._____ ("Patient"), and the undersigned members of the Patient's family, having been informed of the Patient's need for blood and the risks to the Patient's health if the Patient does not receive blood or blood products, refuse to authorize or consent to the administration of any blood or blood products to the Patient and specifically direct that such not be administered to the Patient by anyone.

   (CIRCLE WHICHEVER of a) or b) applies:)

   a) The Patient's refusal is based upon membership in the religious organization known as Jehovah's Witnesses, which limits the acceptance of blood by its members, and the Patient's desire to adhere to those religious tenets and beliefs.

   b) My reason for refusal is_____

   _____

2. I (We) understand the Patient has a condition_____
   which causes or results in blood loss. I (We) understand that when the amount of blood loss reaches a certain point, there can be serious impairment of the Patient's health or even death, and the administration of blood or blood products is medically indicated and necessary. Although the physicians cannot guarantee that administration of blood or blood products would prevent the Patient's death or serious impairment, the use of blood or blood products does lessen the potential for such injuries by attempting to correct or replace the blood loss.

3. I (We) understand that refusal to authorize the use of blood or blood products can and will in all likelihood result in Patient's death, or at a minimum serious impairment of the Patient's health, such as brain damage. I (We) understand there is no effective substitute for blood or blood products.

4. I (We) understand that a decision by the Patient at a later time to authorize the use of blood, after the need for blood has arisen, may be too late and administration of blood or blood products at that time may not correct the blood loss or prevent serious impairment or death.

5. In consideration for honoring the Patient's request, the Patient's and the undersigned family members, individually and on behalf of the Patient RELEASE AND AGREE TO HOLD HARMLESS Harris County Hospital District and any of its employees who participate in Patient's health care;
   _____; _____; and Baylor College of Medicine
   (Physician)   (Physician):
   or The University of Texas and any of its employees who participate in Patient's health care from any and all liability for honoring this refusal to authorize the administration of blood or blood products or for failing to administer blood or blood products when such would be medically indicated and appropriate. I (We) fully accept all responsibility for injuries to the Patient, including death, which may result from the failure to administer blood or blood products by the above parties.

6. I (We) certify that this form has been fully explained to me (us), that I (we) have read it or have had it read to me (us), * and that I (we) understand its contents. I (We) believe I (we) have sufficient information to make this decision to refuse the use of blood or blood products in any treatment of the Patient and to release the health care providers from liability in this regard.

READ TO PATIENT BY	PRINTED NAME		DATE	TIME

PATIENT'S SIGNATURE	PRINTED NAME		DATE	TIME
WITNESS'S SIGNATURE	PRINTED NAME		DATE	TIME
FAMILY MEMBER'S SIGNATURE	PRINTED NAME	RELATIONSHIP	DATE	TIME
WITNESS'S SIGNATURE	PRINTED NAME		DATE	TIME
FAMILY MEMBER'S SIGNATURE	PRINTED NAME	RELATIONSHIP	DATE	TIME
WITNESS'S SIGNATURE	PRINTED NAME		DATE	TIME

* Translated Into _____

REFUSAL TO AUTHORIZE ADMINISTRATION OF
BLOOD OR BLOOD PRODUCTS
AND
RELEASE FROM LIABILTY

CHART

FIGURE 43-4 Example of consent for refusal to authorize administration of blood or blood products and release from liability

connected to the patient. At the same time, either a crystalloid 3 mL for every 1 mL of blood or a colloid 1 mL for every 1 mL of blood is given to replace the blood drawn. However, keep in mind that hydroxyethyl starch can cause coagulopathy when given in large amounts (32). Blood collected can be kept at room temperature up to 6 hours. The last unit collected should be given back to the patient first and the first unit given last since the first collected unit has the highest concentration of hemoglobin and clotting factors (65,66). Despite touting the benefits of acute normovolemic hemodilution, the published data show minimal evidence to recommend the use of this technique alone to reduce the need for allogeneic blood and may not be adequate in massive obstetric hemorrhage (65,67). Yet it should be taken into

TABLE 43-1 Goals of Bloodless Surgery

Preoperative	Intraoperative	Postoperative
• Iron, folate, vitamin B$_{12}$ supplement • Erythropoietin	• Meticulous hemostasis and hemostasis agents • Microsampling laboratory testing • Hemodilution • Cell salvage • Volume expanders	• Increased hemopoiesis • Microsampling • Cell salvage • Hyperbaric oxygen therapy • Nutritional support

Adapted from: "Medical Alternatives to Blood Transfusion" brochure. Watchtower Bible and Tract Society of New York, Inc. 2001; and Gohel MS, Bulbulia RA, Slim FJ, et al. How to approach major surgery where patients refuse blood transfusion (including Jehovah's Witnesses). *Ann R Coll Surg Engl* 2005;87(1):3–14.

consideration in the management of the Jehovah's Witnesses who refused blood transfusion and are at high risk for peripartum bleeding.

■ CELL SALVAGE

The use of intraoperative cell salvage when massive obstetrical bleeding is expected has been recommended by many worldwide medical societies including the American College of Obstetrics and Gynecology, the Royal College of Obstetricians and Gynaecologists, the ASA, the Association of Anaesthetists of Great Britain and Ireland, and the United Kingdom National Institute for Health and Clinical Excellence (68–70) (Fig. 43-6). Many Jehovah's Witnesses will accept cell salvage especially if it is a closed circuit since cell salvage is not prohibited but left to the member's personal decision (63). To reduce the amount of amniotic fluid collected by the cell salvage system, two suction devices are used on the field. One suction device is used initially up until the delivery of the fetus, placenta, and amniotic fluid. At that point, a second suction device which is connected to the cell salvage system is used. However, Sullivan recently demonstrated that the use of one suction device has no significant difference in the amount of amniotic fluid, heparin, and fetal red cells from that of using two suction devices (71). The

blood is collected from the operative site through a dual lumen suction tubing in which an anticoagulant, either heparin or citrate, is fed to the suction tip and immediately mixed with the shed blood. It is then passed through a filter and collected in a reservoir before episodic or non-continuous hemoconcentration and washing in a differential centrifugation bowl. Less dense elements such as plasma, platelets, activated clotting factors, and complements are all removed with the centrifugation and washing process. The blood then is returned to the patient at a concentration of hematocrit of 50% to 80% and a leucocyte depletion filter may be used to reduce further unwanted particulates prior to reinfusion in the patient (65,66,72–74).

The use of intraoperative cell salvage has been delayed in obstetric patients due to the theoretical risks of amniotic fluid embolism and maternal–fetal anti-D alloimmunization (73,75). However, there have been over 800 intraoperative cell salvage procedures in obstetric surgeries and more than 400 obstetric patients transfused with salvaged blood reported in the literature (73). There has been only one fatal obstetric case which the authors attributed to the use of cell salvage reported in the literature. The patient was a Jehovah's Witness with severe pre-eclampsia and HELLP syndrome whose preoperative hemoglobin was 7.1 g/dL and had received up to 200 mL of cell-salvaged blood. Due to the lack of infor-

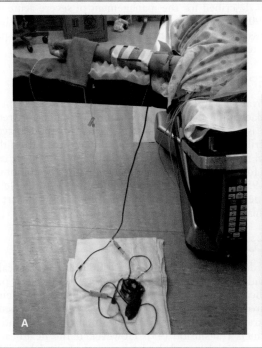
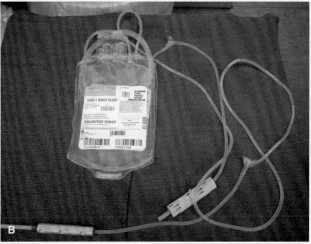

FIGURE 43-5 (**A** and **B**) Acute normovolemic hemodilution

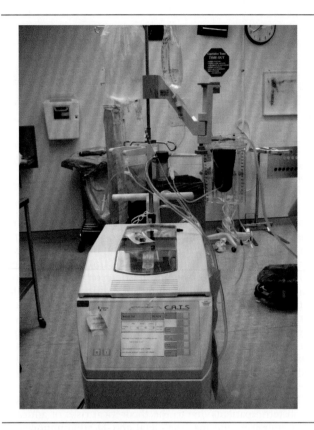

FIGURE 43-6 Cell salvage

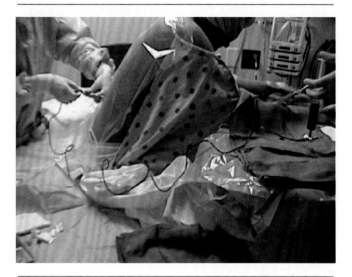

FIGURE 43-7 Continuous epidural blood patch

mation from this case report, it is generally not accepted by most authorities that the fatality was caused by amniotic fluid embolism from cell-salvaged blood (72,75,76). Amniotic fluid embolism occurs in 1 in 8,000 to 80,000 parturients so that a randomized controlled trial to establish the safety of cell salvage in cesarean delivery would require 25,000 to 250,000 cases in order to obtain a study with the power of 80% to detect a 5-fold increase in incidence (77,78). This large number of cases makes it difficult to perform a randomized controlled trial. Waters, Catling, and Sullivan showed that the use of leucocyte depletion filters with washed blood reduce amniotic components (71,79,80). However, cell salvage systems cannot differentiate between maternal and fetal red blood cells Hence the presence of fetal red blood cells in the salvaged blood may increase the risk of maternal alloimmunization in case of incompatibility between mother and fetal antigens (72,74,81,82). Anti-D immunoglobulin should therefore be given to prevent Rhesus immunization of Rhesus negative mothers who received cell-salvaged blood (72–74,81).

There is growing evidence that cell salvage can be safely use in obstetric hemorrhage especially when in combination with leucocyte depletion filter (73,82–85). It can be cost effective when compared to allogeneic blood transfusion when massive blood loss is expected (86). Intraoperative cell salvage can be life saving for obstetric patients with massive hemorrhage and in particular Jehovah's Witnesses who refuse allogeneic transfusion but will accept closed circuit cell salvage.

■ OTHER INTRAOPERATIVE CONSIDERATIONS

The management of massive blood loss in obstetrics is the same for all patients with the exception of refusal to accept blood transfusion in Jehovah's Witnesses. Meticulous surgical techniques to minimize blood loss, the use of crystalloids

and colloids for volume expanders, and pharmacologic agents such as topical hemostatic agents and recombinant products such as Factor VIIa have been advocated by Jehovah's Witnesses to manage anemia without blood transfusion (4,14,48,87). Anesthetic techniques such as controlled hypotensive anesthesia to reduce mean arterial blood pressure to 50 mm Hg and muscle paralysis will decrease oxygen consumption thereby off-setting the low oxygen delivery from anemia (88). As a last resort, surgeons may need to perform Cesarean hysterectomy to control bleeding (60).

■ POSTPARTUM MANAGEMENT

Jehovah's Witnesses who are anemic in the postpartum period should be given iron, vitamin B_{12}, and folic acid. Recombinant human erythropoietin may be used to increase red blood cell production (14,57,48). ICU care may be needed in the postoperative period and the use of hyperbaric oxygen has been described for the management of severe acute anemia (89,90,48). Blood samplings should be limited to the most necessary tests and using small volume sampling or point of care testing will help conserve blood (14,87,91).

■ EPIDURAL BLOOD PATCH

Jehovah's Witnesses who experience postdural puncture headache may accept an epidural blood patch for treatment if it is a closed circuit system. A few methods have been described but all involved a continuous circuit from the epidural needle to the intravenous line with a stopcock connection for blood aspiration and injection into the epidural space (92–95) (Fig. 43-7). This is in alignment with the Jehovah's Witnesses' belief that the diverted blood is still part of the circulatory system (63,95).

■ CONCLUSION

In order to provide optimal care to any patient, the healthcare provider must have understanding not only of the patient's medical history and current conditions but also of their social environment and beliefs. Jehovah's Witnesses patients can frustrate physicians with their refusal of blood and blood products transfusion (43). However, if the healthcare provider can understand the background of the Jehovah's Witnesses' belief, the four principles of medical ethics and legal precedents involving parturients' refusal of medical care and the medical community's position on women's rights, then optimal care is ensured for the patient. Physicians and healthcare providers also have rights and can refuse care of a patient and transfer the care over to a colleague providing it is not a clinical emergency (50). Just like any beliefs, there is a wide range of practices; therefore, it behooves the physician to find out what the patient will or will not accept. The physician should conduct the interview with the patient alone so that there will be no outside influences. Once the patient's wishes are known, the healthcare team should honor them. Patient's confidentiality is a must in medical practice. Informed consent should be obtained and most hospital will have an additional blood refusal form which requires completion.

Jehovah's Witnesses provide a hospital liaison committee network in response to the medical community's concerns in caring for its members. Physicians and other healthcare providers can access the hospital liaison committee by calling 718-560-4300 24 hours a day. A local committee member will contact and provide support services to physicians and patients if needed.

When caring for the Jehovah's Witness parturient, the anesthesiologist should be a part of the medical team in the prenatal period. The anesthesia team should have a plan for preoperative, intraoperative, and postoperative care of any patient who may be at risk for hemorrhage. Acute normovolemic hemodilution and cell salvage take time to set up. Recombinant Factor VIIa may not be readily available. By having a plan of care or protocol for patients who refuse blood or blood product transfusion, the healthcare team will be prepared and equipped to take care of these patients. The physician must also be willing to accept the patient's decision and realize that even in the best of care the patient may still die when no blood is given (50,88).

KEY POINTS

- Jehovah's Witnesses is a Christian religious community whose teachings forbid its members to partake blood or risk eternal damnation.
- According to Jehovah's Witnesses, blood is divided into four major components which are further divided into minor fractions. Jehovah's Witnesses believe that accepting whole blood or its four major components violates God's laws, as does preoperative autologous blood donation. However, accepting the minor fractions is permissible based upon the individual's conscientious decision. Healthcare providers can obtain support services from the Hospital Liaison Committee provided by Jehovah's Witnesses.
- There is wide variation of beliefs regarding acceptance of blood among Jehovah's Witnesses; therefore, the healthcare provider must discuss with each individual patient what she would or would not accept and be willing to abide to the patient's informed decision.
- Jehovah's Witnesses usually carry a Medical Power of Attorney form which can delineate their transfusion preferences.
- The four principles of medical ethics are autonomy, beneficence, non-maleficence, and justice. Each principle has an equal weight to each other.
- When the four ethical principles come into conflict, healthcare providers have used different ethical frameworks and legal system in attempts to resolve the conflict.
- The law and all medical societies support the woman's autonomy.
- Jehovah's Witnesses parturients have a higher risk of maternal morbidities and mortalities.

- Multidisciplinary medical care team should be involved early in the care of a high-risk parturient and a care plan should be made. Each hospital should have a protocol on the management of patients who refuse blood or blood products transfusion and healthcare providers who are willing to care for these patients.
- Cell salvage and acute normovolemic hemodilution have been safely used in obstetric patients despite the concerns of amniotic fluid embolism and fetal red cell contamination. Jehovah's Witnesses may accept these therapies.
- Epidural blood patch with a closed circuit has been acceptable for Jehovah's Witnesses.
- Even with the best alternative management in patients refusing blood or blood products transfusion, patients may not survive massive hemorrhage.

REFERENCES

1. "Russell, charles taze 1852–1916." American decades. 2001. *encyclopedia.com.* (January 17, 2011). [Internet]. Available from: http://www.encyclopedia.com/doc/1G2-3468300259.html.
2. [Internet]. Available from: http://www.watchtower.org.
3. Rothenberg DM. The approach to the Jehovah's witness patient. *Anesthesiol Clin North America* 1990;8(3):589–607.
4. Hughes DB, Ullery BW, Barie PS. The contemporary approach to the care of Jehovah's witnesses. *J Trauma* 2008;65(1):237–247.
5. Questions From Readers. The Watchtower, July 1, 1951, 414–416.
6. Elder L. Why some Jehovah's witnesses accept blood and conscientiously reject official watchtower society blood policy. *J Med Ethics* 2000;26(5):375–380.
7. Muramoto O. Bioethical aspects of the recent changes in the policy of refusal of blood by Jehovah's witnesses. *BMJ* 2001;322(7277):37–39.
8. Ridley DT. Jehovah's witnesses' refusal of blood: Obedience to scripture and religious conscience. *J Med Ethics* 1999;25(6):469–472.
9. Hivey S, Pace N, Garside JP, et al. Religious practice, blood transfusion, and major medical procedures. *Paediatr Anaesth* 2009;19(10):934–946.
10. Questions from Readers. The Watchtower, June 15, 2000, 29–31.
11. Hospital Liaison Committee Network for Jehovah's Witnesses. Watch Tower Bible and Tract Society of Pennsylvania. 2001.
12. Clinical Strategies for Avoiding and Controlling Hemorrhage and Anemia Without Blood Transfusion in Surgical Patients. Watch Tower and Bible Tract Society of Pennsylvania. 2001, 1–14.
13. Doyle DJ. Blood transfusions and the Jehovah's witness patient. *Am J Ther* 2002;9(5):417–424.
14. Rogers DM, Crookston KP. The approach to the patient who refuses blood transfusion. *Transfusion* 2006;46(9):1471–1477.
15. Sarteschi LM. Jehovah's witnesses, blood transfusions and transplantations. *Transplant Proc* 2004;36(3):499–501.
16. Muramoto O. Recent developments in medical care of Jehovah's witnesses. *West J Med* 1999;170(5):297–301.
17. Finnerty JJ, Chisholm CA. Patient refusal of treatment in obstetrics. *Semin Perinatol* 2003;27(6):435–445.
18. Rajput V, Bekes CE. Ethical issues in hospital medicine. *Med Clin North Am* 2002;86(4):869–886.
19. Muramoto O. Bioethics of the refusal of blood by Jehovah's witnesses: Part 1. Should bioethical deliberation consider dissidents' views? *J Med Ethics* 1998;24(4):223–230.
20. Malyon D. Transfusion-free treatment of Jehovah's witnesses: Respecting the autonomous patient's motives. *J Med Ethics* 1998;24(6):376–381.
21. Savulescu J. The cost of refusing treatment and equality of outcome. *J Med Ethics* 1998;24(4):231–236.
22. Gillon R. Ethics needs principles – four can encompass the rest – and respect for autonomy should be "first among equals". *J Med Ethics* 2003;29(5):307–312.
23. Gillon R. Four scenarios. *J Med Ethics* 2003;29(5):267–268.
24. Macklin R. Applying the four principles. *J Med Ethics* 2003;29(5):275–280.
25. Campbell AV. The virtues (and vices) of the four principles. *J Med Ethics* 2003;29(5):292–296.
26. American College of Obstetrics and Gynecology. ACOG committee opinion no. 390, December 2007. Ethical decision making in obstetrics and gynecology. *Obstet Gynecol* 2007;110(6):1479–1487.
27. Gardiner P. A virtue ethics approach to moral dilemmas in medicine. *J Med Ethics* 2003;29(5):297–302.
28. Callahan D. Principlism and communitarianism. *J Med Ethics* 2003;29(5):287–291.
29. Beauchamp TL. Methods and principles in biomedical ethics. *J Med Ethics* 2003;29(5):269–274.

30. Smith ML. Ethical perspectives on Jehovah's witnesses' refusal of blood. *Cleve Clin J Med* 1997;64(9):475–481.

31. Layon AJ, D'Amico R, Caton D, et al. And the patient chose: Medical ethics and the case of the Jehovah's witness. *Anesthesiology* 1990;73(6):1258–1262.

32. Benson KT. The Jehovah's witness patient: Considerations for the anesthesiologist. *Anesth Analg* 1989;69(5):647–656.

33. Lombardo PA. Phantom tumors and hysterical women: Revising our view of the Schloendorff case. *J Law Med Ethics* 2005;33(4):791–801.

34. Schloendorff v. Society of New York Hospital, 211 N.Y. 125, 105 N.E. 92 (1914).

35. Kring DL. The patient self-determination act: Has it reached the end of its life? *JONAS Healthc Law Ethics Regul* 2007;9(4):125–131, quiz 132–133.

36. Wolf SM, Boyle P, Callahan D, et al. Sources of concern about the patient self-determination act. *N Engl J Med* 1991;325(23):1666–1671.

37. Woolley S. Children of Jehovah's witnesses and adolescent Jehovah's witnesses: What are their rights? *Arch Dis Child.* 2005;90(7):715–719.

38. Goldman EB, Oberman HA. Legal aspects of transfusion of Jehovah's witnesses. *Transfus Med Rev* 1991;5(4):263–270.

39. Prince v. massachusetts, 321 US 158 (1944).

40. Arch RR. The maternal-fetal rights dilemma: Honoring a woman's choice of medical care during pregnancy. *J Contemp Health Law Policy* 1996;12(2):637–673.

41. "Fetal rights." [Internet];2005.

42. Finamore EP. Jefferson v. Griffin spalding county hospital authority: Court-ordered surgery to protect the life of an unborn child. *Am J Law Med* 1983;9(1):83–101.

43. Levy JK. Jehovah's witnesses, pregnancy, and blood transfusions: A paradigm for the autonomy rights of all pregnant women. *J Law Med Ethics* 1999; 27(2):171–189.

44. Illinois. Appellate Court, First District, Fifth Division. In re brown. *North East Rep Second Ser* 1997;689:397–406.

45. Pinkerton JV, Finnerty JJ. Resolving the clinical and ethical dilemma involved in fetal-maternal conflicts. *Am J Obstet Gynecol* 1996;175(2):289–295.

46. ACOG Committee on Ethics. ACOG committee opinion #321: Maternal decision making, ethics, and the law. *Obstet Gynecol* 2005;106(5 Pt 1):1127–1137.

47. Van Wolfswinkel ME, Zwart JJ, Schutte JM, et al. Maternal mortality and serious maternal morbidity in Jehovah's witnesses in the Netherlands. *BJOG* 2009;116(8):1103–1108; discussion 1108–1110.

48. Massiah N, Athimulam S, Loo C, et al. Obstetric care of Jehovah's witnesses: A 14-year observational study. *Arch Gynecol Obstet* 2007;276(4):339–343.

49. Singla AK, Lapinski RH, Berkowitz RL, et al. Are women who are Jehovah's witnesses at risk of maternal death? *Am J Obstet Gynecol* 2001;185(4):893–895.

50. Gyamfi C, Gyamfi MM, Berkowitz RL. Ethical and medicolegal considerations in the obstetric care of a Jehovah's witness. *Obstet Gynecol* 2003;102(1):173–180.

51. Davies JM, Posner KL, Lee LA, et al. Liability associated with obstetric anesthesia: A closed claims analysis. *Anesthesiology* 2009;110(1):131–139.

52. Berg CJ, Callaghan WM, Syverson C, et al. Pregnancy-related mortality in the United States, 1998 to 2005. *Obstet Gynecol* 2010;116(6):1302–1309.

53. Crouch Z, DeSantis ER. Use of erythropoietin-stimulating agents in breast cancer patients: A risk review. *Am J Health Syst Pharm* 2009;66(13):1180–1185.

54. Gyamfi C, Berkowitz RL. Responses by pregnant Jehovah's witnesses on health care proxies. *Obstet Gynecol* 2004;104(3):541–544.

55. Barth WH Jr, Kwolek CJ, Abrams JL, et al. Case records of the Massachusetts general hospital. Case 23-2011. A 40-year-old pregnant woman with placenta accreta who declined blood products. *N Engl J Med* 2011;365(4):359–366.

56. Cogliano J, Kisner D. Bloodless medicine and surgery in the OR and beyond. *AORN J* 2002;76(5):830–837, 839, 841.

57. Gohel MS, Bulbulia RA, Slim FJ, et al. How to approach major surgery where patients refuse blood transfusion (including Jehovah's witnesses). *Ann R Coll Surg Engl* 2005;87(1):3–14.

58. Fuller AJ, Carvalho B, Brummel C, et al. Epidural anesthesia for elective cesarean delivery with intraoperative arterial occlusion balloon catheter placement. *Anesth Analg* 2006;102(2):585–587.

59. Harnett MJ, Carabuena JM, Tsen LC, et al. Anesthesia for interventional radiology in parturients at risk of major hemorrhage at cesarean section delivery. *Anesth Analg* 2006;103(5):1329–1330; author reply 1330.

60. Gonsalves M, Belli A. The role of interventional radiology in obstetric hemorrhage. *Cardiovasc Intervent Radiol* 2010;33(5):887–895.

61. Carnevale FC, Kondo MM, de Oliveira Sousa W Jr, et al. Perioperative temporary occlusion of the internal iliac arteries as prophylaxis in cesarean section at risk of hemorrhage in placenta accreta. *Cardiovasc Intervent Radiol* 2011;34(4):758–764.

62. Tan CH, Tay KH, Sheah K, et al. Perioperative endovascular internal iliac artery occlusion balloon placement in management of placenta accreta. *AJR Am J Roentgenol* 2007;189(5):1158–1163.

63. Questions from Readers. The Watchtower, October 15, 2000, 30–31.

64. Estella NM, Berry DL, Baker BW, et al. Normovolemic hemodilution before cesarean hysterectomy for placenta percreta. *Obstet Gynecol* 1997;90(4 Pt 2):669–670.

65. Liumbruno GM, Bennardello F, Lattanzio A, et al. Recommendations for the transfusion management of patients in the peri-operative period. II. The intra-operative period. *Blood Transfus* 2011;9(2):189–217.

66. Pacheco LD, Saade GR, Gei AF, et al. Cutting-edge advances in the medical management of obstetrical hemorrhage. *Am J Obstet Gynecol* 2011;205(6):526–532.

67. Yoong W, Ridout A, Madgwick K. Reducing blood transfusion in obstetrics. *J Obstet Gynaecol* 2010;30(4):337–338.

68. Committee on Obstetric Practice. ACOG committee opinion. Placenta accreta. Number 266, January 2002. American college of obstetricians and gynecologists. *Int J Gynaecol Obstet* 2002;77(1):77–78.

69. American College of Obstetricians and Gynecologists. ACOG practice bulletin: Clinical management guidelines for obstetrician-gynecologists Number 76, October 2006: Postpartum hemorrhage. *Obstet Gynecol* 2006;108(4):1039–1047.

70. American Society of Anesthesiologists Task Force on Obstetric Anesthesia. Practice guidelines for obstetric anesthesia: An updated report by the American society of anesthesiologists task force on obstetric anesthesia. *Anesthesiology* 2007;106(4):843–863.

71. Sullivan I, Faulds J, Ralph C. Contamination of salvaged maternal blood by amniotic fluid and fetal red cells during elective caesarean section. *Br J Anaesth* 2008;101(2):225–229.

72. Liumbruno GM, Meschini A, Liumbruno C, et al. The introduction of intra-operative cell salvage in obstetric clinical practice: A review of the available evidence. *Eur J Obstet Gynecol Reprod Biol* 2011;159(1):19–25.

73. Liumbruno GM, Liumbruno C, Rafanelli D. Intraoperative cell salvage in obstetrics: Is it a real therapeutic option? *Transfusion* 2011;51(10):2244–2256.

74. Esper SA, Waters JH. Intra-operative cell salvage: A fresh look at the indications and contraindications. *Blood Transfus* 2011;9(2):139–147.

75. Catling S, Joels L. Cell salvage in obstetrics: The time has come. *BJOG* 2005;112(2):131–132.

76. Catling S, Haynes SL. Coagulopathy during intraoperative cell salvage in a patient with major obstetric haemorrhage. *Br J Anaesth* 2011;106(5):749; author reply 750.

77. Geoghegan J, Daniels JP, Moore PA, et al. Cell salvage at caesarean section: The need for an evidence-based approach. *BJOG* 2009;116(6):743–747.

78. Catling S, Wrench I. Cell salvage at caesarean section: The need for an evidence-based approach. *BJOG* 2010;117(1):122–123; author reply 123–124.

79. Waters JH, Biscotti C, Potter PS, et al. Amniotic fluid removal during cell salvage in the cesarean section patient. *Anesthesiology* 2000;92(6):1531–1536.

80. Catling SJ, Williams S, Fielding AM. Cell salvage in obstetrics: An evaluation of the ability of cell salvage combined with leucocyte depletion filtration to remove amniotic fluid from operative blood loss at caesarean section. *Int J Obstet Anesth* 1999;8(2):79–84.

81. Ashworth A, Klein AA. Cell salvage as part of a blood conservation strategy in anaesthesia. *Br J Anaesth* 2010;105(4):401–416.

82. Tanqueray T, Allam J, Norman B, et al. Leucocyte depletion filter and a second suction circuit during intra-operative cell salvage in obstetrics. *Anaesthesia* 2010;65(2):207; discussion 207–208.

83. Allam J, Cox M, Yentis SM. Cell salvage in obstetrics. *Int J Obstet Anesth* 2008;17(1):37–45.

84. Ralph C, Faulds J, Sullivan I. Cell salvage and leucocyte depletion filters. *Anaesthesia.* 2010;65(12):1228–1229.

85. Ralph CJ, Sullivan I, Faulds J. Intraoperative cell salvaged blood as part of a blood conservation strategy in caesarean section: Is fetal red cell contamination important? *Br J Anaesth* 2011;107(3):404–408.

86. Waters JR, Meier HH, Waters JH. An economic analysis of costs associated with development of a cell salvage program. *Anesth Analg* 2007;104(4):869–875.

87. Heard JS, Quinn AC. Jehovah's witnesses—surgical and anaesthetic management options. *Anaesth Intens Care.* 2010;11(2):62–64.

88. Gyamfi C, Berkowitz RL. Management of pregnancy in a Jehovah's witness. *Obstet Gynecol Clin North Am* 2007;34(3):357–365, ix.

89. Greensmith JE. Hyperbaric oxygen reverses organ dysfunction in severe anemia. *Anesthesiology* 2000;93(4):1149–1152.

90. McLoughlin PL, Cope TM, Harrison JC. Hyperbaric oxygen therapy in the management of severe acute anaemia in a Jehovah's witness. *Anaesthesia* 1999;54(9):891–895.

91. Berend K, Levi M. Management of adult Jehovah's witness patients with acute bleeding. *Am J Med* 2009;122(12):1071–1076.

92. Bearb ME, Pennant JH. Epidural blood patch in a Jehovah's witness. *Anesth Analg* 1987;66(10):1052.

93. Kanumilli V, Kaza R, Johnson C, et al. Epidural blood patch for Jehovah's witness patient. *Anesth Analg* 1993;77(4):872–873.

94. Brimacombe J, Clarke G, Craig L. Epidural blood patch in the Jehovah's witness. *Anaesth Intensive Care* 1994;22(3):319.

95. Jagannathan N, Tetzlaff JE. Epidural blood patch in a Jehovah's witness patient with post-dural puncture cephalgia. *Can J Anaesth* 2005;52(1):113.

Trauma During Pregnancy: Maternal Resuscitation, Rapid Response Team, and Protocols

Sally Radelat Raty • Kenneth L. Mattox • Uma Munnur • Andrew D. Miller • Mihaela Podovei

▪ INTRODUCTION

Trauma during pregnancy is a significant contributor to both maternal and fetal morbidity and mortality in the United States. Motor vehicle accidents are the leading cause of injury-related maternal death, followed by violence and assault. Trauma is associated with first trimester pregnancy loss, premature labor, placental abruption, uterine rupture, and stillbirth (1). The ultimate goal is to provide the most advantageous care to both the mother and fetus, ordering diagnostic testing, and making therapeutic decisions with both patients in mind. As a rule, providing optimal care to the mother enhances fetal well-being and survival; however, when there is conflict between care that favors the mother's survival and care that favors the survival of the fetus, the interests of the mother take priority.

▪ EPIDEMIOLOGY

In the United States, an estimated 5% to 8% of women experience trauma during pregnancy. Trauma is the leading cause of non-obstetric death in the pregnant patient, and 20% of affected women require emergency surgery. The World Health Organization reports statistics on the top ten causes of death for women during their reproductive years according to country income (2). In low-income countries, HIV/AIDS (cause #1) and maternal conditions (cause #2) account for 41.8% of deaths within this age group. Trauma-related injuries including fires (#5), self-inflicted injuries (#6), and road traffic accidents (#8) are in the top ten causes of death for women during their reproductive years and in aggregate, account for 9.4% of deaths in this group. In middle-income countries, trauma-related injuries including road traffic accidents (#3), self-inflicted injuries (#4), and violence (#9) together account for 15.3% of deaths in this age group. In high-income countries, trauma-related injuries including road traffic accidents (#1), self-inflicted injuries (#2), and violence (#7) together account for 22.9% of deaths in this age group. Pregnancy itself does not worsen maternal survival; rather, maternal survival after trauma is related to the overall injury severity (3). The rate of trauma admissions rises with each trimester of pregnancy; 8% occur in the first trimester, 40% in second trimester, and 52% in the third trimester (4). Trauma is responsible for 0.3% to 0.4% of maternal hospital admissions (5). Although most pregnant trauma victims are eventually able to continue their pregnancies at home, as many as 38% remain hospitalized until delivery (4).

The major risk factors for maternal trauma include age less than 25 years, African American or Hispanic, use of alcohol or illicit drugs, domestic violence, improper seat belt use, and low socioeconomic status. Drugs and alcohol are factors in about 20% of maternal trauma (5). Education about the use of illicit drugs and alcohol during pregnancy in high-risk women may play a preventive role in maternal trauma. Proper seat belt use should also play a major role in preventing injuries. The American College of Obstetricians and Gynecologists (ACOG) and the National Highway Traffic Safety Administration recommend that women use a three point restraint system while in a motor vehicle, with the lap portion of the belt beneath the protuberant abdomen, snuggly across the highest portion of the thighs, and the shoulder strap worn to the side of the uterus, between the breasts and mid-clavicle (never directly across the protuberant abdomen) (6,7).

▪ MATERNAL INJURIES

Connolly and colleagues found that motor vehicle accidents are the most common injury in pregnant patients comprising 55%, followed by falls 22%, assaults 22%, and burns 1% (8) (Table 44-1). Younger pregnant patients are at a higher risk for trauma than older patients (9). Head injury and hemorrhagic shock are the major causes of maternal death following trauma.

▪ FETAL INJURIES

Motor vehicle accidents are the leading cause of fetal deaths related to maternal trauma comprising 82%, followed by firearm injuries 6%, and falls 3% (9). Maternal death accounted for 11% of fetal deaths (9). Fetal loss in the first trimester is not secondary to any direct uterine trauma but usually is due to maternal hypotension and hypoperfusion of the uterus (10). Providing optimal maternal care is the best strategy to optimize fetal survival. In early pregnancy, the only way to save the fetus is to save the mother (5).

▪ PRE-HOSPITAL CARE

Pregnancy should be a consideration in any female trauma patient of reproductive age. If possible, a brief obstetric history should be obtained as part of the initial evaluation.

If the history reveals a gestational age above 18 to 20 weeks, left uterine displacement should be maintained in patients placed in the supine position. If no obstetric history can be elicited, but the patient has obvious signs of pregnancy, the gestational age is advanced enough to deserve pregnant patient considerations. The following table shows a correlation between the size of the uterus and the gestational age (Table 44-2).

If a trauma patient is pregnant, the guidelines for Advanced Trauma Life Support (ATLS) and pre-hospital care should be similar to those of the non-pregnant patient. Stabilizing the mother takes priority. In taking care of the mother, there are a few considerations specifically related to pregnancy:

1. Institute lateral decubitus or maintain left uterine displacement in supine position. If injury to the spine is

TABLE 44-1 Causes of Maternal Trauma

Motor vehicle accidents
Violence and assault
Gunshots
Stab wounds
Strangulation
Falls
Suicide
Burns

suspected, the patient can be placed on a rigid board and the entire board tilted 30 degrees (11).
  - Rationale: Beginning at 18 to 20 weeks, the uterus causes aortocaval compression in supine position, decreasing the preload to the heart and potentially decreasing the cardiac output.
2. Start supplemental oxygen. Consider securing the airway early. In securing the airway, consider the need for early intubation against the higher probability of difficult airway.
  - Rationale: Oxygen consumption during pregnancy increases by 40% above non-pregnant levels. In addition, pregnant patients have decreased oxygen reserve (functional residual capacity [FRC] declines, tidal volume and minute ventilation increase, and closing capacity can be higher than the FRC). Weight gain, edema, engorgement of the airway mucosa, and increased mucosal friability, make airway instrumentation more likely to be difficult (12). Maternal hypoxia can cause fetal hypoxia and acidosis.
3. Secure intravenous access above the diaphragm with two large bore catheters.
  - Rationale: Aortocaval compression is responsible for a 30% decrease in cardiac output in the supine position during the third trimester. Caval compression decreases the venous return to the heart and increases the venous pressure in the lower extremities, with higher blood loss from pelvic or lower extremity trauma. Fluid resuscitation below the diaphragm may not be as effective as fluid administration above the diaphragm in improving cardiac output and supporting maternal hemodynamic stability.

TABLE 44-2 Gestational Age and Uterine Location

Gestational Age (wks)	Location of the Top of the Uterus
8	Just above pubis
12	Halfway between pubis and umbilicus
16	Two-thirds between pubis and umbilicus
20	At umbilicus
26	Just above umbilicus
32	Halfway between umbilicus and xyphoid
36	Three-fourths of the way between umbilicus and xyphoid
40	Near xyphoid

Adapted from: Mattox KL, Goetzl L. Trauma in pregnancy. *Crit Care Med* 2005;33:S385–S389.

4. Assess and treat hypotension. If transfusion is required and cross-matched or type-specific blood is not yet available, O-negative packed red blood cells (PRBCs) are a rational choice.
  - Rationale: During pregnancy, heart rate increases by only 10 to 15 beats/min and blood pressure drops by only 5 to 10 mm Hg. Any marked tachycardia or hypotension should not be considered to be normal physiologic changes of pregnancy. Lacking autoregulation, the uterus is very sensitive to changes in maternal blood pressure, and fetal well-being depends on adequate uterine blood flow.
5. If a chest tube is required, the insertion point should be one or two intercostal spaces higher than in the non-pregnant trauma patient (13).
  - Rationale: Beginning in the second trimester, the uterus becomes an abdominal organ, with upward displacement of the intra-abdominal contents and the diaphragm. The elevated position of the diaphragm requires adjustment of the chest tube insertion point to avoid abdominal injury during placement.
6. Consider the use of Military Anti-Shock Trousers (MAST)/pneumatic anti-shock garments for lower extremity trauma, but inflation of the abdominal portion is contraindicated (10).
7. Transport an injured third trimester patient to a trauma center as soon as possible even if the injuries lack apparent severity.
  - Rationale: Absence of abdominal tenderness or other "classic" abdominal signs in pregnancy does not exclude abdominal trauma. In a retrospective study of 203 trauma patients (victims of interpersonal violence), five out of eight fetal death cases occurred without apparent maternal injury (14). Fetal death with minor maternal injury was also documented in other series (15). Third trimester pregnancy at the time of traumatic injury is an independent risk factor for the need for specialized care in a trauma center (3,7,16).

■ CARE IN THE EMERGENCY DEPARTMENT (ED)

Primary Survey

The emergency room primary survey for a trauma pregnant patient should be similar to the survey of a non-pregnant patient (17). While continuing the measures instituted for the pre-hospital care (left lateral displacement of the uterus, administration of supplemental O$_2$, establishment of intravenous access), the primary survey should take 30 to 60 seconds and include assessment of the airway, breathing, circulation, and neurologic examination including a Glasgow coma score (7). If the cervical spine has been immobilized, inline stabilization should be maintained throughout the primary and secondary surveys. In addition to the differential diagnoses common to trauma patients, the pregnant trauma patient may have preeclampsia, eclampsia, placental abruption, or uterine rupture.

Secondary Survey

The secondary survey should include a comprehensive, head-to-toe inspection, palpation, and auscultation, with focus on the mechanism of injury, weapons used (if any), alcohol or drug involvement, and seat belt use. Obtaining a detailed past medical, surgical, and obstetric history is a priority with special attention paid to determination of the gestational age of the fetus. See Figure 44-1 flow diagram for clinical assessment of a pregnant trauma patient more than 20 weeks of gestation.

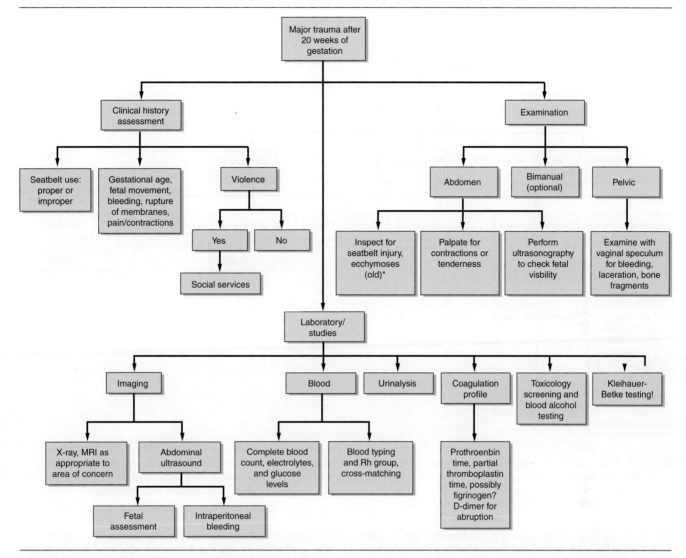

FIGURE 44-1 Clinical assessment of the pregnant trauma patient more than 20 weeks of gestation. [a]Old ecchymoses—suggestive of domestic abuse. [b]Detects maternal–fetal hemorrhage and allows calculation of immune globulin (RhoGAM, Ortho-Clinical Diagnostics, Inc., Rochester, NY) dosing in Rh-negative women (immune globulin 300 μg covers up to 15 mL of red cells bleed). Reprinted with permission from: Brown H. Trauma in pregnancy. *Obstet Gynecol* 2009;114(1):147–160.

As soon as the patient arrives in the ED, an obstetric consultation should be requested and fetal monitoring should be initiated. In addition to standard monitoring and resuscitation protocols, a vaginal examination, fetal heart rate monitoring and obstetric ultrasound are essential; vaginal bleeding is strongly associated with placental abruption and fetal loss (3). Placement of a urinary catheter provides a valuable monitor of both urine output and fluid resuscitative efforts and establishes the presence or absence of hematuria (18). Fetal heart tracing may give an earlier warning of impending maternal cardiovascular collapse than will maternal pulse and blood pressure alone. Thus, fetal monitoring is an important monitor of well-being for both mother and fetus. A normal fetal heart rate is 120 to 160 beats/min. Signs of fetal compromise include tachycardia, bradycardia, loss of variability, and recurrent decelerations.

In most series of blunt abdominal trauma during pregnancy, more than 70% of fetal losses result from abruptio placentae. The other less common causes of fetal loss are fetal–maternal hemorrhage and direct fetal injury (19). Considerable work has been done to establish screening tools and develop algorithms aimed at early detection of abruptio placentae. The

presence of frequent uterine activity has been the most sensitive predictor of abruption. In one study, all patients that developed abruption had at least eight uterine contractions per hour during the initial 4-hour monitoring (20,21).

Continuous electronic fetal monitoring is the current standard of care following maternal trauma. Fetal monitoring should be initiated as soon as possible after maternal injury if the gestational age is >24 weeks (viable pregnancy). The duration of monitoring depends on the case scenario and institutional practice but in general, is maintained for at least 4 to 6 hours, and up to 24 hours for non-catastrophic trauma (22,23). Four-hour monitoring was advocated by Pearlman et al. who successfully identified all of the patients who developed abruption based on the uterine activity pattern recorded during the initial 4 hours of continuous monitoring. Pearlman advises continuing fetal monitoring past 4 hours in patients who have continued contractions (four or more per hour), rupture of amniotic membranes, vaginal bleeding, serious maternal injury, or fetal tachycardia, late decelerations, or non-reactive non-stress test (19,24). If fetal tachycardia or a non-stress test is non-reactive, monitoring is continued

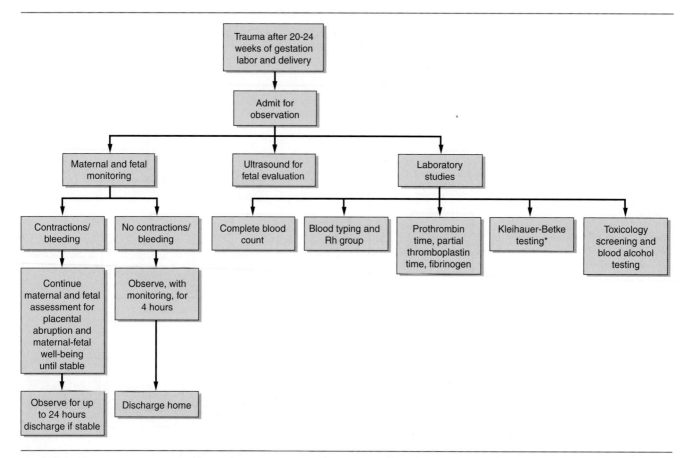

FIGURE 44-2 Labor and delivery observation after maternal trauma. [a]Detects maternal–fetal hemorrhage and allows calculation of immune globulin (RhoGAM, Ortho-Clinical Diagnostics, Inc., Rochester, NY) dosing in Rh-negative women (immune globulin 300 μg covers up to 15 mL of red cells bleed). Reprinted with permission from: Brown H. Trauma in pregnancy. *Obstet Gynecol* 2009;114(1):147–160.

for 24 hours (22). Some experts recommend 24-hour fetal monitoring for high-risk mechanisms of injury (i.e., ejections, lack of restraints, pedestrian collisions, assaults, Injury Severity Score (ISS) >9) (23). See Figure 44-2 for flow diagram of recommended observation protocol after maternal trauma.

The ISS is an anatomical scoring system that provides an overall score for patients with multiple injuries. Six body regions (head, face, chest, abdomen, extremities, including pelvis, and external) are scored separately. Each injury is allocated to one of the six body regions and is assigned an Abbreviated Injury Score (AIS). The AIS can take a value of 0 (no injury) to 6 (non-survivable single organ injury) and is scored in terms of "threat to life." Only the highest AIS score in each body region is used. The three most severely injured body regions have their score squared and added together to produce the ISS score (23).

The ISS score takes values from 0 to 75. If an injury is assigned an AIS of 6 (non-survivable injury), the ISS score is automatically assigned to 75. The ISS score is virtually the only anatomical scoring system in use and correlates linearly with mortality, morbidity, hospital stay, and other measures

of severity (Table 44-3). Its weaknesses are that any error in AIS scoring increases the ISS error. Many different injury patterns can yield the same ISS score and injuries to different body regions are not weighted. Also, as a full description of patient injuries is not known prior to full investigation and operation, the ISS (along with other anatomical scoring systems) is not useful as a triage tool (25).

Initial laboratory studies should include complete blood count (CBC), coagulation studies (prothrombin time [PT], activated partial thromboplastin time [PTT], International Normalization Ratio [INR], fibrinogen), electrolytes, and urinalysis. Arterial blood gasses (ABGs) including the measurement of serum bicarbonate or serum lactate may be indicated following significant trauma. The strong correlation between maternal trauma and substance misuse favor toxicology testing. Sending a sample of blood to the blood bank for type and cross-match with request for rapid determination of type, Rh status and antibody status is critically important. The Kleihauer–Betke (KB) test measures the amount of fetal hemoglobin transferred into the maternal circulation (fetal–maternal hemorrhage) and should be obtained on every injured pregnant patient (17,26). The KB test has particular utility in Rh-negative mothers but may be relevant in any pregnant patient. The test can be used to determine the need for Rh immune globulin and to identify the few patients for whom the quantity of immune globulin given is insufficient. A positive KB test may predict higher risk of preterm labor independent of the Rh status, and may indicate the need for longer fetal monitoring. One study showed an increased incidence of abruption in those with a positive test (26,27).

TABLE 44-3 ISS and Degree of Injury

ISS Score	Injury Grade
1–9	Minor injury
10–15	Moderate injury
16–24	Moderate/severe injury
≥25	Severe injury

The Focused Abdominal Ultrasonography for Trauma (FAST) has an 80% to 85% sensitivity and a 98% to 100% specificity for free peritoneal fluid in pregnant patients. It is safe and rapid to perform and should be the first line diagnostic examination in abdominal trauma (7,17,26,28). In most cases, a computerized tomography (CT) scan will be used to further evaluate the pregnant patient following blunt trauma. Even so, a rapid fetal survey to assess the fetal heart rate, placental position, and abnormalities should be performed in any pregnant trauma patient (29). With the advent of bedside ultrasound and rapid CT scans, routine use of diagnostic peritoneal lavage (DPL) in the evaluation of traumatically injured patients has fallen out of favor. If performed during pregnancy, DPL should be performed using the supraumbilical approach in an open technique (26).

Other diagnostic studies including cervical spine, chest, abdomen, and pelvis images should be obtained for indications similar to those in the non-pregnant trauma patient. Radiation exposure to the fetus can be minimized by shielding the uterus whenever possible during imaging procedures (7). In 2010, the Eastern Association for the Surgery of Trauma (EAST) published their practice guidelines for the diagnosis and management of injury in the pregnant patient (30). Their recommendations are evidence-based, using a classification based upon level of evidence: Level I—randomized controlled trials (there were none); Level II—data collected prospectively and analyzed retrospectively i.e., cohort, observational, and case control studies; Level III—retrospective data collection and analysis, i.e., clinical series and reviews, and expert opinion. These are the guidelines (30):

Level I

There are no level I standards.

Level II

a. All pregnant women >20 weeks of gestation who suffer trauma should have cardiotocographic monitoring for a minimum of 6 hours. Monitoring should be continued and further evaluation should be carried out if uterine contractions, a non-reassuring fetal heart rate pattern, vaginal bleeding, significant uterine tenderness or irritability, serious maternal injury, or rupture of amniotic membranes is present.

b. KB analysis should be performed in all pregnant patients >12 weeks of gestation.

Level III

a. The best initial treatment for the fetus is the provision of optimum resuscitation of the mother and the early assessment of the fetus.

b. All the female patients of childbearing age with significant trauma should have a β-HCG performed and be shielded for x-rays whenever possible.

c. Concern about possible effects of high-dose ionizing radiation exposure should not prevent medically indicated maternal diagnostic x-ray procedures from being performed. During pregnancy, other imaging procedures not associated with ionizing radiation should be considered instead of x-rays when possible.

d. Exposure to <5 radiation absorbed dose (rad) has not been associated with an increase in fetal anomalies or pregnancy loss and is herein deemed to be safe at any point during the entirety of gestation.

e. Ultrasonography and magnetic resonance imaging are not associated with known adverse fetal effects. However, until more information is available, magnetic resonance imaging is not recommended for use in the first trimester.

f. Consultation with a radiologist should be considered for purposes of calculating estimated fetal dose when multiple diagnostic x-rays are performed.

g. Perimortem cesarean delivery should be considered in any moribund pregnant woman above 24 weeks of gestation.

h. Delivery in perimortem cesareans must occur within 20 minutes of maternal death but should ideally start within 4 minutes of the maternal arrest. Fetal neurologic outcome is related to delivery time after maternal death.

i. Consider keeping the patient tilted left side down 15 degrees to keep the pregnant uterus off the vena cava and prevent supine hypotension syndrome.

j. Obstetric consult should be considered in all cases of injury in pregnant patients.

■ PREGNANCY EFFECTS ON DIAGNOSTIC STUDIES

Imaging

The indications for imaging studies of the injured patient are similar for both pregnant and non-pregnant patients. Physiologic changes of pregnancy have implications on the results, and should be considered when interpreting imaging.

Ionizing Radiation Exposure During Pregnancy

During radiologic imaging, the fetus receives approximately 30% of the total radiation dose and should be shielded from exposure whenever possible (3,7). Regarding radiation exposure to the embryo and fetus, ACOG published a committee opinion on diagnostic imaging during pregnancy stating that "Undergoing a single diagnostic x-ray procedure does not result in radiation exposure adequate to threaten the well-being of the developing pre-embryo, embryo, or fetus and is not an indication for therapeutic abortion. When multiple diagnostic x-rays are anticipated during pregnancy, imaging procedures not associated with ionizing radiation, such as ultrasonography and magnetic resonance imaging, should be considered" (31).

The fetus is most susceptible to ionizing radiation exposure during organogenesis (2 to 7 weeks after conception) and the fetal period (8 to 15 weeks after conception) (32). Non-cancer health effects have not been detected at any stage of gestation after exposure to less than 5 rad. Spontaneous abortion, growth restriction, and mental retardation may occur at higher exposure levels. For example, a 15 rad exposure results in 6% incidence of mental retardation, 3% incidence of childhood cancer, and 15% incidence of microcephaly (3,7). Table 44-4 presents a more comprehensive list of dose-related non-cancer radiation effects.

Exposure to ionizing radiation increases the risk of childhood cancer regardless of the dose (32). One to two rad fetal exposures increase the risk of leukemia by a factor of 1.5 to 2 over natural incidence, with 1 in 2,000 children exposed to ionizing radiation developing leukemia as compared to the 1 in 3,000 background rate (31,33). ACOG states that risk of radiation-induced carcinogenesis is not likely to exceed 1 in 1,000 children per rad, and therapeutic abortion should not be recommended solely on the basis of exposure to diagnostic radiation (31). For a better understanding of the amount of radiation exposure, one would have to consider that 1 rad is the equivalent of a mother undergoing 100 chest x-rays or just a single abdominal CT scan. Table 44-5 provides a more comprehensive list of exposure doses that the fetus receives during common radiologic procedures (32).

When interpreting imaging of a pregnant patient, the gestational age is relevant, and certain findings are normal with pregnancy. For example, a normal chest x-ray in a pregnant patient will include mild cardiomegaly, widened mediasti-

TABLE 44-4 **Radiation Dose and Effects on Developing Fetus**

Acute Radiation Dose	Up to 2 wks Post-conception	2–7 wks Post-conception	8–15 wks Post-conception	16–25 wks Post-conception	26–38 wks Post-conception
<5 rad	Non-cancer health effects not detectable				
5–50 rad	Incidence of failure to implant may increase slightly, but surviving embryos probably will not have substantial non-cancer health effects	Incidence of major malformations may increase slightly; growth restriction possible	Growth restriction possible; IQ reduction possible (≤15 points); incidence of severe mental retardation ≤20%	Non-cancer health effects unlikely	
>50 rad	Incidence of failure to implant is likely large, but surviving embryos probably will not have substantial non-cancer health effects	Incidence of miscarriage may increase, substantial risk of major malformations (neurologic and motor deficiencies); growth restriction likely	Incidence of miscarriage probably will increase; growth restriction likely; IQ reduction (>15 points); incidence of severe mental retardation >20%; incidence of major malformations probably will increase	Incidence of miscarriage may increase; growth restriction, IQ reduction and severe mental retardation possible; incidence of major malformations may increase	Incidence of miscarriage and neonatal death may increase

Adapted from: Williams PM, Fletcher S. Health effects of prenatal radiation exposure. *Am Fam Physician* 2010;82(5):488–493. URL: www.aafp.org/afp. Last accessed January 2011.

num, increased antero-posterior diameter, and prominence of pulmonary vasculature. A normal pelvic x-ray may show widening of the sacroiliac joints and symphysis pubis (7,17).

Ultrasound

In the 40 years of clinical use, the ultrasound has demonstrated no significant health risks to either the fetus or the

TABLE 44-5 **Fetal Radiation Exposure During Common Radiologic Procedures**

Procedure	Fetal Exposure
Radiography	
Chest (2 views)	<0.01 rad
Abdomen	0.1–0.3 rad
Intravenous pyelography	0.358–1.398 rad
Hip and femur	0.051–0.37 rad
Barium enema	0.7–3.986 rad
Lumbar spine	0.346–0.62 rad
Pelvis	0.04–0.238
Computer Tomography	
CT scan of chest	0.1–0.45 rad
CT scan of head	<0.05 rad
CT scan of abdomen (10 slices)	0.24–2.6 rad
CT scan of lumbar spine	3.5 rad
CT scan of pelvis	0.73–4.6 rad

Adapted from: Williams PM, Fletcher S. Health effects of prenatal radiation exposure. *Am Fam Physician* 2010;82(5):488–493. URL: www.aafp.org/afp. Last accessed January 2011.

mother. Tissue temperature increases are not expected to exceed 0.5°C for even prolonged examinations with modern scanners and are unlikely to have significant fetal side effects (29). Ultrasonography should be the first imaging test used in the evaluation of suspected maternal intra-abdominal pathology because it does not expose the mother or the fetus to ionizing radiation (29).

Laboratory

Pregnancy induces profound physiologic adaptations in most if not all organ systems, and laboratory tests will reflect these adaptations (34). Normal laboratory values in a pregnant patient may be quite different from what is considered normal in the non-pregnant patient. The injured pregnant patient whose laboratory values fall within the normal ranges for the non-pregnant patient may in fact be quite ill. For example, the non-pregnant normal values of a $PaCO_2$ of 40 mm Hg or a creatinine of 1.1 mg/dL are abnormal values in pregnancy (34). Table 44-6 lists normal ranges in pregnant women for common laboratory tests.

■ CHANGES OF PREGNANCY AS THEY APPLY TO TRAUMA

In the traumatically injured pregnant patient, both physiologic and anatomic changes of pregnancy can affect both evaluation and management strategies. Throughout evaluation and treatment of the injured pregnant patient, every effort must be made to avoid aortocaval compression by the gravid uterus. Placing a 30-degree wedge beneath the patient's right hip or if the patient is secured to a backboard, tilting the entire board laterally to the left by 30 degrees effectively relieves the compression and can restore preload back to the heart.

TABLE 44-6 Normal Range for Laboratory Values in Pregnancy

	Non-pregnant Adult	First Trimester	Second Trimester	Third Trimester
Hematology				
Hemoglobin (g/dL)	12–15.8	11.6–13.9	9.7–14.8	9.5–15.0
Hematocrit (%)	35.4–44.4	31.0–41.0	30.0–39.0	28.0–40
Platelets ($\times 10^9$/L)	165–415	174–391	155–409	146–429
WBC ($\times 10^3$/mm^3	3.5–9.1	5.7–13.6	5.6–14.8	5.9–16.9
Coagulation				
Fibrinogen (mg/dL)	233–496	244–510	291–538	373–619
Partial thromboplastin time, activated (s)	26.3–39.4	24.3–38.9	24.2–38.1	24.7–35.0
Prothrombin time (s)	12.7–15.4	9.7–13.5	9.5–13.4	9.6–12.9
Chemistry				
Albumin (g/dL)	4.1–5.3	3.1–5.1	2.6–4.5	2.3–4.2
Anion gap (mmol/L)	7–16	13–17	12–16	12–16
Bicarbonate (mmol/L)	22–30	20–24	20–24	20–24
Urea Nitrogen (mg/dL)	7–20	7–12	3–13	3–11
Creatinine (mg/dL)	0.5–0.9 (females)	0.4–0.7	0.4–0.8	0.4–0.9
Blood Gas				
pH	7.38–7.42 (arterial)	7.36–7.52 (venous)	7.40–7.52 (venous)	7.41–7.53 (venous)
PaO$_2$ (mm Hg)	90–100	93–100	90–98	92–107
PaCO$_2$ (mm Hg)	38–42	Not reported	Not reported	25–33
Bicarbonate (HCO$_3^-$) (mEq/L)	22–26	Not reported	Not reported	16–22

Data from: Abbassi-Ghanavati M, Greer LG, Cunningham FG. Pregnancy and laboratory studies: a reference table for clinicians. *Obstet Gynecol* 2009;114(6):1326–1331.

Airway and Pulmonary Changes

Compared to the non-pregnant patient, the airway of the pregnant patient is normally more engorged and edematous and is associated with an up to ten-fold higher incidence of difficult intubation (12). The addition of a cervical spine collar (c-collar), commonly placed after blunt trauma and falls, compounds the challenge of managing the airway particularly if the patient requires emergent surgical intervention. If the cervical spine can be "cleared" prior to intubation, the c-collar should be removed to facilitate intubation. Often, this is not possible, and intubation must be performed while the head and cervical spine are held with inline stabilization. Regardless of the presence or absence of a c-collar, the anesthesiologist must prepare for the likelihood of a difficult intubation in any pregnant patient. Airway rescue devices including video-assisted equipment and intubating laryngeal mask airways should be within arm's reach before attempting any airway interventions. Securing the airway via the oral route is much preferred over the nasal route because of the risk of bleeding and epistaxis common with even minor trauma to the engorged nasal mucosa. The increase in tidal volume in pregnant patients is largely responsible for the 50% increase in minute ventilation. At the same time, the enlarging pregnant abdomen causes a 20% decrease in FRC. These two physiologic pulmonary changes make the pregnant patient particularly susceptible to hypoxemia. A decrease in minute ventilation from any cause can lead to profound hypoxemia in the pregnant patient (12). Given the common presence of airway edema, the higher frequency of difficult intubations, and the limited respiratory reserve in pregnant patients, early

rather than delayed intubation is prudent (13,17). Even short periods of maternal hypoxemia can lead to fetal acidosis and hypoxemia causing direct fetal distress. Hyperventilation and alkalosis can cause uterine vasoconstriction and a leftward shift of the oxyhemoglobin dissociation curve with a decrease in oxygen delivery to the fetus. If the injured pregnant patient is hemodynamically stable and has a non-reassuring airway examination, video-assisted or fiberoptic awake oral intubation provides the safest route. Elevated progesterone levels of pregnancy lower the sphincter tone at the gastroesophageal junction and predispose the patient to aspiration upon induction of anesthesia. Early administration of antacids and motility stimulants even before any decision regarding the need for surgery, is reasonable given the morbidity associated with aspiration and the relative safety of the prophylactic regimen (most commonly ranitidine and metoclopramide). Post-intubation, PaO$_2$ and PaCO$_2$ should be maintained at values normal for pregnancy (see Table 44-6). Frequent blood gasses may be required to adjust ventilation, so early placement of an arterial line should be considered.

Hematologic and Cardiovascular Changes

Plasma volume and total blood volume increase dramatically during pregnancy by 25% to 40% and 40% to 50%, respectively. While red cell mass also increases, it does so to a much smaller extent, and dilutional anemia in pregnancy is common. Since mild tachycardia, hypotension relative to the non-pregnant patient, and a decreased central venous pressure can be present in the normal, uninjured pregnant patient; these classic signs of hemorrhage cannot be automatically extrapolated to the pregnant patient (17,35). Normal electrocardiographic changes of pregnancy can include sinus tachycardia, ectopic beats, left axis deviation, inverted or flattened T-waves and Q-waves in II, II and AVF (7). Pregnant patients can lose up to 2 to 3 L of blood before showing the classic signs of hypovolemia, making a normal blood pressure after trauma essentially meaningless (36). Tachypnea may be one of the earliest clinical signs of hypovolemia (36). Other signs of hypoperfusion must be sought by measuring serum bicarbonate or serum lactate levels (35). The metabolic alkalosis of normal pregnancy translates into a decreased ability to buffer an acid load from any cause (endogenous or exogenous). The increase in oxygen consumption in the pregnant patient places both the mother and the fetus at increased risk for hypoperfusion when the hemoglobin concentration declines by even a small percentage. Even mild levels of hypoperfusion leading to anaerobic metabolism can result in acidemia in the pregnant patient. The physiologic response to fluid challenges can be very helpful in determining the volume status of the injured pregnant patient. A decrease in heart rate, an elevation of blood pressure, or increased urine output after a fluid challenge may be interpreted as signs of hypovolemia and/or blood loss (36). So called "hypotensive resuscitation" commonly employed in trauma centers is not a reasonable option for the pregnant patient because blood flow to the uterus is not autoregulated and is dependent on the mother's blood pressure. However, uteroplacental perfusion can decline 20% even when maternal blood pressure is unchanged. Fetal monitoring may be one of the best ways to monitor both fetal and maternal well-being with a decline in fetal heart rate or a lack of beat to beat variability signaling that both patients may be compromised.

Throughout pregnancy, leukocyte, fibrinogen, and factors VIII, IX, and X increase while circulating levels of a plasminogen activator (involved in the breakdown of blood clots) decline. These changes in the coagulation factors predispose the pregnant patient to not only thromboembolic events, made more likely if immobilization after trauma is prolonged, but also disseminated intravascular coagulation following placental abruption (37). Uninjured, healthy pregnant women have venous stasis from vena caval compression by the gravid uterus and are hypercoagulable secondary to increased production of coagulation factors by the liver, and thus satisfy two elements of Virchow's triad that describe the risk factors for thrombotic events. The third element of the triad is vascular injury. Use of low-dose heparin, compression stockings or sequential compression devices, and early ambulation or physical therapy during bed confinement can be used to decrease the risk of thrombotic events.

Gastrointestinal and Abdominal Changes

Pregnant patients appear to have decreased peritoneal sensitivity and may not exhibit any of the classic peritoneal signs (tenderness, rebound, guarding) despite significant abdominal injury. Other diagnostic tests including ultrasonography and CT scan can provide more reliable information about intra-abdominal injuries. Prior to 12 weeks of gestation, the uterus is a pelvic organ and is somewhat protected from trauma by the bony pelvis. By 12 weeks of gestation, the enlarging uterus "escapes" the protection of the bony pelvic structures, becomes an abdominal organ and as such, has an increased risk of injury from both blunt and penetrating trauma (17). The gradual upward displacement of the abdominal organs throughout the progression of pregnancy by the enlarging uterus changes the dissipation of energy in blunt trauma and confers relative "protection" to the abdominal organs in penetrating trauma. Injury to the bowel is less common in pregnant patients than in the non-pregnant patient (38).

However, gunshot wounds to the pregnant abdomen cause fetal injury in 70% and fetal death in 4% to 70% of cases (7).

Should abdominal exploration of the patient be necessary, the surgical team should not allow the gravid uterus to impede a thorough examination of all abdominal organs and structures. Nonetheless, an exploratory laparotomy is not an automatic indication for delivery by cesarean, either during laparotomy or subsequently (1). A sterilely draped ultrasound probe on the surgical field should be used periodically to monitor the well-being of the fetus. Ultrasound results, including estimated fetal heart rate, should be recorded in the anesthesia record. For pregnancies beyond 24 weeks of gestation, an obstetric team should be immediately available for cesarean if the maternal or fetal condition becomes significantly compromised (1).

Renal and Pelvic Changes

As the uterus enlarges, the bladder is pushed forward and slightly cephalad making it more susceptible to injury. In addition, the increased glomerular filtration rate of pregnancy tends to keep the bladder somewhat distended, making it more susceptible to injury, including rupture. The normal pregnancy-induced increase in progesterone can cause laxity at both the symphysis pubis and the sacroiliac (SI) joints. By 7 months of gestation, the normal widening at the symphysis pubis and the SI joints on imaging can be confused with pelvic fractures and/or pelvic diastasis with suspected retroperitoneal hematoma (17). In the non-pregnant patient, pelvic fractures with retroperitoneal hemorrhage are frequently treated in the interventional radiology suite with embolization. However, the extensive radiation exposure that attends an embolization procedure makes this an ill-advised choice for the pregnant patient except in the direst circumstances.

Fetal skull and brain trauma resulting from maternal pelvic fractures are most common when the fetal head is engaged in the pelvis and confer a nearly 25% fetal mortality rate (7). Uterine rupture is relatively rare after trauma and accounts for less than 1% of all injures during pregnancy. However, uterine rupture secondary to trauma carries a 10% maternal mortality and a nearly 100% fetal mortality. Trauma-related uterine rupture should be suspected after rapid deceleration or direct compression injuries. Cessation of uterine contractions, severe abdominal or rebound tenderness, an asymmetric uterus, vaginal bleeding, and/or the ability to palpate fetal parts through the abdominal wall should raise the clinician's suspicion for uterine rupture.

Central Nervous System and Intracranial Changes

Preeclampsia can lead to debilitating headaches, blurred vision, dizziness, and seizures. Blurred vision, dizziness and seizures may predispose the afflicted patient to trauma especially as the driver of a motor vehicle. Further, seizures and loss of consciousness associated with preeclampsia can mimic the signs and symptoms of head injury. Preeclampsia can lead to intracerebral hemorrhage and a true neurosurgical emergency. Pregnancy leads to an increase in the pituitary gland size by 35% (39). Hypotension can lead to ischemic injury of the enlarged pituitary with subsequent development of pituitary insufficiency or Sheehan's syndrome.

■ RESUSCITATION

The goals of resuscitation are to control bleeding, replace volume deficits in order to restore adequate perfusion pressure and oxygen delivery to vital organs and the uterus, and to prevent and/or treat coagulopathy. All trauma patients should have two large bore intravenous lines placed as soon as possible. Given the risk of aortocaval compression by the gravid uterus and the associated decrease in venous return from the lower extremities, the upper extremities are usually the best location for intravenous access. However, injury to the chest, particularly penetrating injuries, may cause disruption of the vasculature leading from the arms to the heart and necessitate the placement of intravenous lines below the diaphragm as well. MAST can be used to provide compression of the lower extremities to promote confinement of the blood volume to the central compartment. However, inflation of the abdominal portion of the trousers is contraindicated in pregnant patients because of the risk of extreme compression of the uterus causing compromise of the placental blood supply (10). The use of pre-warmed fluids, active fluid warmers, forced air body warmers, a warm room, the lowest acceptable fresh gas flows, and blankets over all exposed areas exclusive of the surgical field are crucial to preventing hypothermia. The detrimental effects of hypothermia include coagulopathy, shivering with increased oxygen consumption, a leftward shift in the oxyhemoglobin curve impairing oxygen delivery, and delayed metabolism of some medications. Given the edema formation commonly present in pregnant patients, choosing colloid rather than crystalloids may be the more prudent choice for intravascular volume replacement. However, if total body water is depleted, resuscitation must include appropriate amounts of crystalloid. The use of normal saline as a resuscitative fluid is not recommended due to the risk of developing hyperchloremic metabolic acidosis following massive infusion (6).

The use of vasopressors is common during care of the critically injured non-pregnant patient. However, in the pregnant patient, volume repletion rather than vasopressor use is preferable as a strategy to maintain blood pressure and improve cardiac output (17). While epinephrine and norepinephrine will often be effective in restoring maternal blood pressure, both medications compromise uterine blood flow and should be avoided if at all possible. Ephedrine and dopamine (5 mcg/kg/min) can improve maternal hemodynamic condition while maintaining blood flow to the uterus.

Massive transfusion is often defined as transfusion of >10 units PRBCs in a 24-hour period, though some variation in the definition exists. In the non-pregnant patient, initiation of a massive transfusion protocol implies a systematic approach to the transfusion of PRBCs, fresh frozen plasma (FFP), platelets, and fibrinogen. Current recommendations in massive transfusion situations include maintaining a transfusion ratio of FFP:PRBCs of 1:1.5, the platelet count >100×10^9/L and the fibrinogen level >1.5 g/L (40). Scheduled blood draws throughout resuscitation during massive transfusion should include hemoglobin, PT, aPTT, INR, fibrinogen, D-dimer, and CBC. Use of recombinant activated factor VII (rFVIIa) is not currently recommended for use in trauma unless other, more conventional methods of managing coagulopathy have failed. Arterial thrombotic events following the use of rFVIIa are estimated to be between 1:10 and 1:100 (40). Given the risk of thrombotic events in pregnant patients, use of rFVIIa is best avoided in the case of managing trauma.

■ BURNS

Contact Burns

Burns in the pregnant patient are relatively rare and mortality is directly related to the burned surface area, depth, type, and location of the burn. Early intubation of the pregnant patient presenting with evidence of burns of the airway (soot in the nares or mouth, singed nasal hair, hoarseness, stridor) is prudent given their propensity for pre-existing airway edema. Fluid requirements should be calculated using the Parkland formula (i.e., percent of body surface area burned multiplied by the patient's weight in kilograms multiplied by 4 mls). The resultant product is the amount of crystalloid that should be administered in the first 24 hours following the burn with one-half of the fluid given in the first 8 hours, and the remaining half given over the next 16 hours. Burns cause an increase in the release of prostaglandins that can stimulate preterm uterine contractions. In the hemodynamically stable burned patient, a course of tocolytics may be effective to mitigating the effects of the increased prostaglandin release (35). Carboxyhemoglobin levels should be serially measured to determine the efficacy of oxygen therapy. Carboxyhemoglobin does cross the placenta creating fetal carboxyhemoglobinemia. Hyperbaric oxygen (HBO) therapy is a reasonable choice in patients with extensive burn injury and/or evidence of significantly elevated carboxyhemoglobin levels. There is a paucity of studies addressing the safety and/or hazards of HBO therapy in pregnant patients. However, Elkharrat et al. enrolled 44 pregnant women who had sustained carbon monoxide intoxication in a prospective study in order to assess HBO tolerance (41). Their patients received HBO for 2 hours at 2 atmospheres of pressure, and the authors concluded that with their HBO doses and duration, HBO is safe for pregnant women and their fetuses and should be initiated for carbon monoxide intoxication.

Electrical Burns

Electrical burns can cause electrothermal injury of skin and underlying tissue, flame burns secondary to ignition of clothing or surrounding structures, cardiac injury, cardiac dysrhythmias including cardiac arrest, and respiratory arrest. Electrical current passing from hand to hand rarely passes through the uterus. However, electrical current passing between hand and foot often includes the uterus in its path and is nearly always fatal to the fetus (7).

■ MANAGEMENT OF MATERNAL CARDIAC ARREST

Maternal resuscitation is the most effective method of fetal resuscitation. If the pregnant patient is in a healthcare facility, a rapid response by the health care team is required to minimize the interval between the cardiac arrest and the subsequent delivery so as to allow for the best maternal and fetal outcome even in trauma. Should a pregnant patient suffer cardiac arrest, immediate resuscitation efforts should include chest compressions, calling for assistance, and establishing oxygenation, ventilation, and vascular access in order to optimize circulation. Lastly, an important factor to consider prior to an emergent cesarean delivery is the gestational age of the fetus.

The principles of cardiopulmonary resuscitation (CPR) for the late-term pregnant woman are based on the American Heart Association (AHA) advanced cardiac life support (ACLS) recommendations (Fig. 44-3). During CPR in pregnancy, the team needs to follow the revised 2010 AHA guidelines with modifications to compensate for the altered anatomy and physiology of pregnancy as delineated above (11). The major modifications include: (1) Prompt airway management, (2) meticulous attention to lateral displacement of uterus and avoidance of aortocaval compression, (3) optimal performance of chest compressions in the lateral tilt position, (4) caution in the use of sodium bicarbonate, (5) search for reversible causes such as magnesium toxicity, and (6) early consideration of perimortem cesarean delivery so as to optimize CPR and survival of mother and baby.

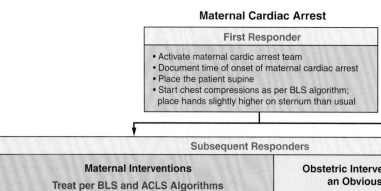

Maternal Cardiac Arrest

First Responder

- Activate maternal cardic arrest team
- Document time of onset of maternal cardiac arrest
- Place the patient supine
- Start chest compressions as per BLS algorithm; place hands slightly higher on sternum than usual

Subsequent Responders

Maternal Interventions

Treat per BLS and ACLS Algorithms

- Do not delay defibrillation
- Give typical ACLS drugs and doses
- Ventilate with 100% oxygen
- Monitor waveform capnography and CPR quality
- Provide post-cardiac arrest care as appropriate

Maternal Modifications

- Start IV above the diaphragm
- Assess for hypovolemia and give fluid bolus when required
- Anticipate difficult airway; experienced provider preferred for advanced airway placement
- If patient receiving IV/IO magnesium prearrest, stop magnesium and give IV/IO calcium chloride 10 mL in 10% solution, or calcium gluconate 30 mL in 10% solution
- Continue all maternal resuscitative interventions (CPR, positioning, defibrillation, drugs, and fluids) during and after cesarean section

Obstetric Interventions for Patient with an Obviously Gravid Uterus*

- Perform manual left uterine displacement (LUD) – displace uterus to the patient's left to relieve aortocaval compression
- Remove both internal and external fetal monitors if present

Obstetric and neonatal teams should immediately prepare for possible emergency cesarean section

- If no ROSC by 4 minutes of resuscitative efforts, consider performing immediate emergency cesarean section
- Aim for delivery within 5 minutes of onset of resuscitative efforts

*An obviously gravid uterus is a uterus that is deemed clinically to be sufficiently large to cause aortocaval compression

Search for and Treat Possible Contributing Factors (BEAU-CHOPS)

Bleeding/DIC
Embolism: coronary/pulmonary/amniotic fluid embolism
Anesthetic complications
Uterine atony
Cardiac disease (MI/ischemia/aortic dissection/cardiomyopathy)
Hypertension/preeclampsia/eclampsia
Other: differential diagnosis of standard ACLS guidelines
Placenta abruptio/previa
Sepsis

FIGURE 44-3 Maternal cardiac arrest algorithm. From: 2010 American Heart Association. Reprinted with permission from: Vanden Hoek TL, Morrison LJ, Shuster M, et al. Part 12: Cardiac arrest in special situations: 2010 American Heart Association guidelines for cardiopulmonary resuscitation and emergency cardiovascular care. *Circulation* 2010;122(18):S829–S861.

Patient positioning has emerged as an important strategy to improve the quality of CPR and resultant compression force. The gravid uterus can compress the inferior vena cava, impeding venous return and thereby reducing stroke volume and cardiac output. Therefore, to relieve aortocaval compression during chest compressions and optimize the quality of CPR, it is reasonable to perform manual left uterine displacement in the supine position initially. If this technique is unsuccessful, a few solutions are recommended, including use of (1) sand bag under the right hip, (2) a human wedge (i.e., tilting the patient on the bent knees of a kneeling rescuer), and (3) the Cardiff wedge, a large wedge-shaped board on which resuscitation takes place (3). Caution should be used in cases of potential neck injury, with particular attention taken to stabilize the head and neck when patient is turned to the side. Chest compressions should be performed slightly higher on the sternum than normally recommended to adjust for the elevation of the diaphragm and abdominal contents caused by the gravid uterus.

There should be no delay in delivering usual ACLS drugs during the management of cardiac arrest during pregnancy.

The AHA guidelines state that the first rescuer on the scene should deliver one shock by automated external defibrillator (AED) before initiating CPR. There is a paucity of evidence-based data to show whether the defibrillation requirements change during pregnancy. Nanson and colleagues measured the transthoracic impedance (TTI) registered by a defibrillator in 45 women at term pregnancy. They repeated the measurements at 6 to 8 weeks postpartum in 42 out of the 45 women after the physiologic changes of pregnancy had resolved. The TTI at term was 91.3 and post-delivery the TTI was 91.6. There was no statistical difference (42). Defibrillation should follow the standard recommended defibrillation energies. There is no documented evidence of adverse effects on the fetus. Fetal monitors should be removed before delivering shocks. Medications should be administered based on traditional ACLS guidelines. Although vasopressors may decrease uterine blood flow, they should be given at recommended doses in order to maximize the chances of a return of spontaneous circulation.

Perimortem Cesarean Delivery

Perimortem cesarean delivery is defined as a cesarean initiated after CPR has been initiated. The recommendation to perform a perimortem cesarean within 4 minutes of maternal cardiac arrest was introduced in 1986 by Katz and colleagues (43). They recommended a "4-minute rule" from the maternal arrest to the initiation of the cesarean delivery, with the fetus being delivered within 5 minutes. This approach was based on the assumptions that CPR is ineffective in the third trimester because of aortocaval compression, and that fetal and perhaps maternal outcomes would be optimized by timely delivery. Emptying the uterus results in a 60% to 80% increase in cardiac output and an increase in maternal survival rates. Since the initial description, numerous case reports have described often dramatic reversal of the maternal hemodynamic collapse, even in refractory situations (44). The original report advocating prompt cesarean delivery as an important tool of maternal resuscitation was based on theory and one case report (45). The "5-minute rule" from arrest to delivery is now recommended by the AHA when the intrauterine gestation is greater than 24 weeks. If initial resuscitation is not effective during cardiac arrest in pregnancy, delivering the fetus within 5 minutes may facilitate maternal and fetal survival.

The performance of a perimortem cesarean delivery is a challenging aspect of maternal resuscitation. Adherence to the AHA's "5-minute rule" means that the rapid response team must rapidly assess the patient, institute appropriate resuscitation, and prepare for imminent delivery. The rapid response multidisciplinary team must be knowledgeable and skilled in appropriate CPR techniques for the pregnant patient. In addition, the resuscitation team leader should also consider the need for an emergency hysterotomy (cesarean delivery) protocol as soon as a pregnant woman develops a cardiac arrest. Speed is of the essence once the decision is made to deliver the baby. The procedure should be performed by the most skilled provider proficient in cesarean delivery. The best survival for infants greater than 24 to 25 weeks of gestation results when delivery occurs no more than 5 minutes after the maternal cardiac arrest. Katz conducted a Medline search and concluded that published reports from 20 years support, but fall far from proving, that perimortem cesarean delivery within 5 minutes of maternal cardiac arrest improves maternal and neonatal outcomes (45).

The decision to perform a perimortem cesarean delivery is based on the viability of the fetus. Survival of the fetus after a perimortem cesarean delivery is: (1) 70% when delivered in less than 5 minutes, (2) 13% within 6 to 10 minutes, and (3) 12% within 11 and 15 minutes (43). Perimortem cesarean is recommended even in a pregnant trauma patient as it may result in fetal salvage. Fetal survival after 45 minutes of CPR is reported in a 27-year parturient with multiple penetrating injuries with perimortem cesarean delivery performed in the emergency department (46). In severe trauma cases, CPR can be difficult due to massive blood loss. Even in cases of massive trauma, immediate delivery should be considered if the prognosis for the mother is very poor, and the fetus is beyond 24 weeks of gestation.

Post-resuscitation Management

Very few randomized controlled clinical trials deal specifically with supportive care following cardiopulmonary–cerebral resuscitation (CPCR) from cardiac arrest. Initial objectives of post-resuscitation care are to (1) optimize cardiopulmonary function and systemic perfusion, especially to the brain, (2) identify precipitating cause of the arrest, (3) institute measures to prevent recurrence, and (4) institute measures that may improve long-term, neurologically intact survival (47).

Therapeutic hypothermia after cardiac arrest has been demonstrated to abate the neurologic injury and increase the likelihood of a neurologically intact survival (48). Unfortunately, pregnant patients have been excluded from therapeutic hypothermia protocols for cerebral protection. Rittenberger and colleagues describe the first case of therapeutic hypothermia applied to the post-arrest care of a pregnant woman followed by a successful delivery and favorable outcome. The authors recommend that therapeutic hypothermia should be considered in pregnant women status post-cardiac arrest and return of spontaneous circulation (49).

■ SUMMARY

In order to have the best outcome for mother and baby, rapid response multidisciplinary team training in resuscitation of the pregnant patient is mandatory. Developed in the United Kingdom, the Managing Obstetric Emergencies and Trauma (MOET) course offers a structured curriculum during which obstetricians, anesthesia providers, and emergency personnel learn how to provide appropriate and timely care to the traumatically injured pregnant patient. The newly modified ACLS protocols and drug therapies similar to that implemented in non-pregnant patients must be followed. Hospitals must develop multidisciplinary rapid response teams comprised of experts in obstetrics, anesthesiology, internal medicine, surgery, and nursing who are skilled in the care of pregnant patients under the most demanding clinical circumstances. Incorporation of team training through simulation and "mock" drills provides the needed practice in a safe environment and prepares the team for optimum performance when treating atraumatically injured pregnant patient.

KEY POINTS

- Motor vehicle accidents are the leading cause of injury-related maternal death, followed by violence and assault.
- Providing optimal care to the mother enhances fetal well-being and survival.
- Pregnancy itself does not worsen maternal survival; rather, maternal survival after trauma is related to the overall injury severity.
- Pregnancy should be a consideration in any female trauma patient of reproductive age. If possible, a brief obstetric history should be obtained as part of the initial evaluation.
- If a trauma patient is pregnant, the guidelines for ATLS and pre-hospital care should be similar to those of the non-pregnant patient with the addition of left uterine displacement during transport to minimize aortocaval compression.
- The emergency room primary survey for a trauma pregnant patient should be similar to the survey of a non-pregnant patient.
- The secondary survey should include a comprehensive, head-to-toe inspection, palpation, and auscultation, with focus on the mechanism of injury, weapons used (if any), alcohol or drug involvement, and seat belt use.
- As soon as the patient arrives in the ED, an obstetric consultation should be requested and fetal monitoring should be initiated.
- Fetal heart tracing may give an earlier warning of impending maternal cardiovascular collapse than will maternal pulse and blood pressure alone.
- The presence of frequent uterine activity has been the most sensitive predictor of abruption.
- The indications for imaging studies of the injured patient are similar for both pregnant and non-pregnant patients. Ultrasonography should be the first imaging test used

in the evaluation of suspected maternal intra-abdominal pathology because it does not expose the mother or the fetus to ionizing radiation. The FAST has an 80% to 85% sensitivity and a 98% to 100% specificity for free peritoneal fluid in pregnant patients. It is a safe and rapid to perform and should be the first line diagnostic examination in abdominal trauma.

- Pregnancy induces profound physiologic adaptations in most if not all organ systems, and laboratory tests will reflect these adaptations.

- In the traumatically injured pregnant patient, both physiologic and anatomic changes of pregnancy can affect both evaluation and management strategies.

- The goals of resuscitation are to control bleeding, replace volume deficits in order to restore adequate perfusion pressure and oxygen delivery to vital organs and the uterus, and to prevent and/or treat coagulopathy. Maternal resuscitation is the most effective method of fetal resuscitation. If the pregnant patient is in a healthcare facility, a rapid response by the health care team is required to minimize the interval between the cardiac arrest and the subsequent delivery so as to allow for the best maternal and fetal outcome even in trauma.

- The major modifications in CPR recommendations for pregnant women include: (1) Prompt airway management, (2) meticulous attention to lateral displacement of uterus and avoidance of aortocaval compression, (3) optimal performance of chest compressions in the lateral decubitus position, (4) caution in the use of sodium bicarbonate, and (5) early consideration of perimortem cesarean delivery so as to optimize CPR and survival of mother and baby.

- For perimortem cesarean deliveries, experts recommended a "4-minute rule" from the maternal arrest to the initiation of the cesarean delivery, with the fetus being delivered within 5 minutes.

- Hospitals must develop multidisciplinary rapid response teams comprised of experts in obstetrics, anesthesiology, internal medicine, surgery, and nursing who are skilled in the care of pregnant patients under the most demanding clinical circumstances.

REFERENCES

1. Brown H. Trauma in pregnancy. *Obstet Gynecol* 2009;114(1):147–160.
2. World Health Organization. Ten leading causes of death in females by age and country income group, 2004. Available at: http://gamapserver.who.int/gho/interactive_charts/women_and_health/causes_death/chart.html. Accessed May 1, 2012.
3. Shah A, Kilcline BA. Trauma in pregnancy. *Emerg Med Clin North Am* 2003; 21:615–629.
4. Howell P. In: Chestnut DH, ed. *Chestnut's Obstetric Anesthesia Principles and Practice.* 4th ed. Philadelphia, PA: Mosby Inc; 2009:1149–1163.
5. Fisgus JR, Tyagaraj K, Mahboobi SK. In: Smith CE, ed. *Trauma Anesthesia.* 1st ed. New York, NY: Cambridge University Press; 2008:402–416.
6. Oxford CM, Ludmir J. Trauma in pregnancy. *Clin Obstet Gynecol* 2009;52(4): 611–629.
7. Hill CC, Pickpaugh J. Trauma and surgical emergencies in the obstetric patient. *Surg Clin North Am* 2008;88(2):421–440.
8. Connolly AM, Katz VL, Bash KL, et al. Trauma in pregnancy. *Am J Perinatol* 1997;14(6):331–336.
9. Weiss HB, Songer TJ, Fabio A. Fetal deaths related to maternal injury. *JAMA* 2001; 286(15):1863–1868.
10. Mattox KL, Goetzl L. Trauma in pregnancy. *Crit Care Med* 2005;33: S385–S389.
11. Vanden Hoek TL, Morrison LJ, Shuster M, et al. Part 12: Cardiac arrest in special situations: 2010 American Heart Association guidelines for cardiopulmonary resuscitation and emergency cardiovascular care. *Circulation* 2010;122(18):S829–S861.
12. Munnur U, Suresh MS. Airway problems in pregnancy. *Crit Care Clin* 2004; 20:617–642.
13. Meroz Y, Elchalal U, Ginosar Y. Initial trauma management in advanced pregnancy. *Anesthesiol Clin* 2007;25:117–129.
14. Poole GV, Martin JN Jr, Perry KG, et al. Trauma in pregnancy: the role of interpersonal violence. *Am J Obstet Gynecol* 1996;174:1873–1877.
15. Agran PF, Dunkle DE, Winn DG, et al. Fetal death in motor vehicle accidents. *Ann Emerg Med* 1987;16:1355–1358.
16. Goodwin TM, Breen MT. Pregnancy outcome and fetomaternal hemorrhage after noncatastrophic trauma. *Am J Obstet Gynecol* 1990;162:665–671.
17. Clark A, Bloch R, Gibbs M. Trauma in pregnancy. *Trauma Reports* 2011; 12(3):1–11.
18. Coleman MT, Trianfo VA, Rund DA. Nonobstetric emergencies in pregnancy: trauma and surgical conditions. *Am J Obstet Gynecol* 1997;177(3):497–502.
19. Pearlman MD. Motor vehicle crashes, pregnancy loss and preterm labor. *Int J Gynaecol Obstet* 1997;57(2):127–132.
20. Pearlman MD, Tintinallli JE, Lorenz RP. A prospective controlled study of outcome after trauma during pregnancy. *Am J Obstet Gynecol* 1990;162:1502–1507.
21. Williams JK, McClain L, Rosemurgy AS, et al. Evaluation of blunt abdominal trauma in the third trimester of pregnancy: maternal and fetal considerations. *Obstet Gynecol* 1990;75(1):33–37.
22. Grossman NB. Blunt trauma in pregnancy. *Am Fam Physician* 2004;70(7):1303–1310.
23. Curet MJ, Schermer CR, Demarest GB, et al. Predictors of outcome in trauma during pregnancy: identification of patients who can be monitored for less than 6 hours. *J Trauma* 2000;49(1):18–24.
24. Pearlman MD, Tintinalli JE, Lorenz RP. Blunt trauma during pregnancy. *N Engl J Med* 1990;323(23):1609–1613.
25. Baker SP, O'Neill B, Haddon W Jr, et al. The injury severity score: a method for describing patients with multiple injuries and evaluating emergency care. *J Trauma* 1974;14(3):187–196.
26. Cusick SS, Tibbles CD. Trauma in pregnancy. *Emerg Med Clin North Am* 2007;25(3):861–872.
27. Muench MV, Baschat AA, Reddy UM, et al. Kleihauer-Betke testing is important in all cases of maternal trauma. *J Trauma* 2004;57(5):1094–1098.
28. Goodwin H, Holmes JF, Wisner DH. Abdominal ultrasound examination in pregnant blunt trauma patients. *J Trauma* 2001;50(4):689–693.
29. Baysinger CL. Imaging during pregnancy. *Anesth Analg* 2010;110(3):863–867.
30. Barraco RD, Chiu WC, Clancy TV, et al. Practice management guidelines for the diagnosis and management of injury in the pregnant patient: the EAST Practice Management Guidelines Work Group. *J Trauma* 2010;69(1):211–214.
31. ACOG Committee Opinion. Number 299, Guidelines for diagnostic imaging during pregnancy. *Obstet Gynecol* 2004:104;647–651.
32. Williams PM, Fletcher S. Health effects of prenatal radiation exposure. *Am Fam Physician* 2010;82(5):488–493.
33. Brent RL. The effect of embryonic and fetal exposure to x-ray, microwaves, and ultrasound: counseling the pregnant and nonpregnant patient about these risks. *Semin Oncol* 1989;16(5):347–368.
34. Abbassi-Ghanavati M, Greer LG, Cunningham FG. Pregnancy and laboratory studies: a reference table for clinicians. *Obstet Gynecol* 2009;114(6):1326–1331.
35. Hull SB, Bennett S. The pregnant trauma patient: assessment and anesthetic management. *Int Anesthesiol Clin* 2007;45(3):1–18.
36. Plaat F. Anaesthetic issues related to postpartum haemorrhage (excluding antishock garments). *Best Pract Res Clin Obstet Gynaecol* 2008;22(6):1043–1056.
37. Todd ME, Thompson JH Jr, Bowie EJ, et al. Changes in blood coagulation during pregnancy. *Mayo Clin Proc* 1965;40:370–383.
38. Ruffolo DC. Trauma care and managing the injured pregnant patient. *J Obstet Gynecol Neonatal Nurs* 2009;38(6):704–714.
39. Petrone P, Asensio JA. Trauma in pregnancy: assessment and treatment. *Scand J Surg* 2006;95:4–10.
40. Lier H, Bottiger BW, Hinkelbein J, et al. Coagulation management in multiple trauma: a systematic review. *Intensive Care Med* 2011;37(4):572–582.
41. Elkharrat D, Raphael JC, Korach JM, et al. Acute carbon monoxide intoxication and hyperbaric oxygen in pregnancy. *Intensive Care Med* 1991;17(5):289–292.
42. Nanson J, Elcock D, Williams M, et al. Do physiologic changes in pregnancy change defibrillation energy requirements? *Br J Anaesth* 2001;87(2):237–239.
43. Katz VL, Dotters DJ, Droegemueller W. Perimortem caesarean delivery. *Obstet Gynecol* 1986;68(4):571–576.
44. DePace NL, Betesh JS, Kotler MN. Postmortem cesarean delivery with recovery of both mother and offspring. *JAMA* 1982;248(8):971–973.
45. Katz V, Balderston K, DeFreest M. Perimortem cesarean delivery: were our assumptions correct. *Am J Obstet Gynecol* 2005;192(6):1916–1920.
46. Yildirim C, Goksu S, Kocoglu H, et al. Perimortem cesarean delivery following severe maternal penetrating injury. *Yonsei Med J* 2004;45(3):561–563.
47. Suresh MS, LaToya Mason C, Munnur U. Cardiopulmonary resuscitation and the parturient. *Best Pract Res Clin Obstet Gynaecol* 2010;24(3):383–400.
48. Bernard SA, Gray TW, Buist MD, et al. Treatment of comatose survivors of out-of-hospital cardiac arrest with induced hypothermia. *N Engl J Med* 2002;346(8):557–563.
49. Rittenberger JC, Kelly E, Jang D, et al. Successful outcome utilizing hypothermia after cardiac arrest in pregnancy: a case report. *Crit Care Med* 2008; 36(4):1354–1356.

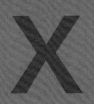

CHAPTER

45

Utilization of Crisis Resource Management and Simulation in Maternal and Neonatal Safety

Stephen D. Pratt

◼ INTRODUCTION

The twentieth century saw dramatic improvements in the quality of health care. Medical advances like the discovery of antibiotics and vaccines improved the treatment and prevention of infectious diseases. Chemotherapy and advances in surgical techniques made cancer a survivable disease. Public health initiative dramatically decreased death from modifiable causes like smoking and motor vehicle accidents. Maternal death rates from both obstetric and anesthesia causes were dramatically reduced. With these advances, however, came a significant increase in the complexity of delivering health care. By the end of the twentieth century and into the beginning of the twenty-first century, concerns about the safety of the healthcare system began to be raised. The system itself became a leading cause of patient harm and death. Hospital acquired infections caused by bacteria made more virulent by widespread use of antibiotics became major causes of patient harm. Clinician error became a leading cause of hospital death. This brought an emphasis on patient safety alongside the established focus on quality of care. The practices of obstetrics and obstetric anesthesia have led the way in this patient safety movement.

Most clinicians have now heard that tens of thousands of patients die each year in the United States due to medical error (1–3), that hundreds of thousands more are injured (4), and that the economic cost of these errors runs into the tens of billions of dollars. The recommendations that medical institutions adopt the teamwork concepts of Crew Resource Management (CRM) and use simulation to improve patient safety have been widely made (3,5–7). Sadly, these recommendations have not been well implemented, and now more than a decade after the Institute of Medicine (IOM) recommended these changes (8,9), adverse events due to medical error remain common (2,10). Many factors may influence the difficulty in adopting teamwork and simulation into medical practice. Leape suggested that the very culture of medicine, often associated with a "finger-pointing environment," (11) is not conducive to a teamwork approach (8). A lack of understanding of what CRM is or what is needed to make it succeed almost certainly plays a role (12,13). (A thorough discussion of CRM and its utility in the clinical setting is provided later in this chapter.) Inherent differences between the aviation and medical industries are also likely to inhibit the proliferation of CRM. For instance, cockpit crews frequently are assigned to fly only one type of aircraft and may only fly a small number of flight paths. In contrast, medical staff—especially those in acute care areas like obstetrics—must care for whatever patients arrive on the unit. Machines (airplanes) respond much more consistently to a given set of parameters than do people (patients), who are likely to have their own, idiosyncratic reaction to nearly every treatment. The culture of aviation is very different from that in medicine. Most pilots support a relatively flat hierarchy, which then facilitates open communication and teamwork. Physicians are less supportive of a flat hierarchy (14). Cockpit crews are also more likely than medical staff to understand the negative impact that emotional stress, production pressure, and fatigue can have on performance (15). Finally, while the emotional impact of an adverse event or medical error can be devastating to medical staff (16,17), the caregiver does not directly suffer the impact of the error. The fact that a pilot may die due to his or her mistake adds a compelling reason to take any step necessary to prevent accidents.

◼ SCOPE OF THE PROBLEM IN OBSTETRICS

The practice of obstetrics poses particular challenges to both the need for and implementation of teamwork and other patient safety practices. Most importantly, it is the only medical environment that can have a 200% mortality rate. Every action that a health care team takes to care for the mother may also impact the safe care of the unborn child. The birth of a baby is an inherently private and personal experience. Families may anticipate the birth experience in the same way they look forward to a wedding, graduation, or other significant life transition. Superimposing a team of previously unknown care providers may not fit these plans. Parturition frequently takes place literally behind closed doors in the privacy of a labor room. This is part of the private nature of the process, but it makes it difficult for team members to monitor the safe conduct of the birth. This is in stark contrast to the cockpit crew who sit within feet of each other and have ready access to outside experts (air traffic control) monitoring their performance. Finally, the physician leaders of the labor and delivery process are very different from pilots. They are frequently not on the unit. An obstetrician may be in his/her office throughout most of a parturient's labor. The obstetric anesthesiologist may have duties in the main operating room and may come to the labor floor for only a few minutes to place a labor epidural. Teamwork is clearly difficult when much of the team is not physically present.

While estimates of the number of women and babies that die or are harmed due to medical error during obstetric care do not currently exist to the same extent that they do for the general medical population, available evidence does suggest that the patient safety crisis is as problematic in obstetrics and obstetric anesthesia as it is in the rest of the medical community. Labor and delivery is the most common cause for hospitalization in the United States, and cesarean delivery is the most common operation in the United States. Thus, the exposure to medical error is high for the parturient and her fetus. Perhaps 9% of deliveries are associated with a maternal or fetal complication (18). It has been estimated that up to 87% of perinatal adverse events are preventable, with poor teamwork protocol violations and unavailable staff being the common problems (19). Substandard care contributes to approximately 50% of maternal deaths, with poor communication and teamwork being primary factors in the substandard care (20–22). Up to 72% of neonatal adverse events can similarly be attributed to poor communication (23). Among obstetric cases that go to litigation, poor communication and teamwork is identifiable in 43% (24). Anesthesia, specifically failed or esophageal intubation, remains a leading cause of maternal death, and anesthesia care often indirectly contributes to poor maternal outcomes.

Even when no complication occurs, the care provided during parturition is often substandard. Up to 85% of women with preeclampsia receive substandard treatment for their blood pressure (25), a statistic that would likely improve with better teamwork and more involvement by an obstetric anesthesiologist. Communication on the labor ward is often inadequate. Simpson found that obstetric nurses and obstetricians may communicate for only several minutes over the entire course of labor (26). Obstetric anesthesia handoffs are frequently short, interrupted by clinical care, and poorly structured (27). Poor communication and coordination of care has been identified in 43% of closed malpractice claims in obstetrics (28). Using in situ simulated eclampsia drills, Thompson et al. found that timely communication with senior obstetric staff was a recurrent problem (29). Similarly, Daniels et al. demonstrated that obstetric residents communicated poorly with their pediatric team members during a simulated emergent delivery. While 63% called for pediatric help during the simulated maternal cardio-pulmonary arrest, only 10% gave helpful information to the pediatricians when they arrived (30). Obstetric care providers often do not value patient safety initiatives (31). Finally, and perhaps most telling, many obstetric care providers do not grade their own institutions highly with regard to safety, and 30% would not want to be delivered in their own institution.

The final reasons to encourage both teamwork and simulation is to help identify areas of clinical weakness and to maintain skills in infrequently encountered clinical scenarios. Obstetricians are prone to making the same errors repeatedly when practicing uncommon events in the simulated environment (32). Up to half of the cases of failed tracheal intubation, the leading cause of anesthesia-related maternal death, are improperly managed (33). This is likely related to the decreased frequency of general anesthesia use in the obstetric

population and thus a decreased exposure to the maternal airway (34–36). Better teamwork during these crisis events and the ability to practice them using simulation are likely to improve care and decrease adverse outcomes.

Despite all the challenges described above, and hopefully because of the great need, some of the greatest successes in both teamwork and simulation have occurred in obstetrics. The first literature demonstrating improvements in outcomes associated with both team training and simulation were published in obstetrics.

■ WHAT IS CREW RESOURCE MANAGEMENT: AN OVERVIEW

While CRM is not universally defined and no standard CRM training program exists, Salas et al. define CRM as a "family of *instructional strategies* that seek to improve *teamwork in the cockpit* by applying well-tested training *tools* (e.g., simulators, lectures, videos) targeted at specific *content* (i.e., teamwork knowledge, skills, and attitudes [KSAs])" (37). It has also been referred to as "Airmanship," "Captaincy," and "Crew Cooperation" (38). The roots of CRM date back to a NASA workshop in 1979 entitled *Resource Management on the Flight deck* (39). This conference was designed to help spread research indicating that poor interpersonal communication, decision making, and leadership were leading causes of air traffic accidents. The term Cockpit Resource Management was used at this conference to describe training processes designed to improve these interpersonal aspects of cockpit management. The first versions of this CRM focused largely on the psychological aspects of the captain's managerial style (12,39). Since then, CRM has evolved through several generations to include a greater focus on the management of the cockpit crew, training of all crew members (flight attendants, dispatchers, maintenance staff, etc.), and a greater emphasis on the impact of human factors on error. The current (fifth) iteration of CRM, however, is the first to focus specifically on error management (12,39). Current CRM training teaches that error is inevitable ("normalizing error" (39), and that human performance is limited (40). Strategies have been developed to prevent error whenever possible, to trap error when it occurs, and finally to mitigate the impact of error when the first two fail (12,39). Specific tools and behaviors are included in CRM training to help accomplish each of these goals.

■ CRM BEHAVIORS AND SKILLS

While CRM does not represent a specific training program, a defined set of KSAs at both the team and individual level are commonly included in most CRM education. The most important attitude is that participants must believe that error, including their own error, is inevitable and that working as a team is likely to reduce these errors. They must be willing to advocate for safety whenever risk is identified and to listen to risk concerns, irrespective of hierarchy. Some of the early concepts are identified in Table 45-1. While these concepts exist to some degree in most CRM training, they may be

TABLE 45-1 Early Crew Resource Management Concepts

Situation awareness	Effective communication	Mission planning
Group dynamics	Risk management	Human factors
Workload management	Stress awareness	Decision making

Adapted from: Department of the Air Force, Air Traffic Control Training Series. Crew Resource Management (CRM). Basic Concepts. December, 1998. http://www.af.mil/shared/media/epubs/AT-M-06A.pdf. Accessed Jan 25, 2011.

difficult to define or measure, and not intuitive to the learner. More recently, Salas (41) suggests that there is a set of "big five" team behaviors necessary for successful teamwork:

- **Leadership:** "The ability to direct and coordinate the activities of other team members, assess team performance, develop team knowledge skills and abilities, motivate team members, plan and organize, and establish a positive atmosphere."
- **Mutual performance monitoring:** "The ability to apply appropriate task strategies to develop common understanding of the team environment. This includes an understanding of team mate workload, fatigue, stress, skills, and the environment external to the team itself."
- **Back-up behaviors:** "A person's ability to anticipate other team members' needs through knowledge about their responsibilities."
- **Adaptability:** "The ability to adjust team strategies and alter the course of action based on information gathered from the environment through the use of back-up behavior and reallocation of intrateam resources."
- **Team orientation:** "An attitude characterized by a propensity to take other's behavior and input into account during group interaction and the belief in the importance of team goals over individual members' goals."

These behaviors are supported by shared mental models (the development and articulation of a shared vision regarding plans), closed loop communication (the use of specific communication techniques outlined in Table 45-2), and mutual trust. Other important concepts in CRM training include: **Situation Awareness** (the state of knowing the conditions of the team and environment that could influence the team's performance), **Conflict Resolution** (the ability to rapidly and professionally resolve differences of opinion about appropriate actions when making or modifying plans), **Team Structure** (clearly identifying the members and the leader of the team so all members know their role and the role of the other members) (42). Finally, several team behaviors help

to ensure that the teamwork KSAs occur. Team briefings before scheduled activities allow for planning, development of shared mental models, and defining of roles. Team meetings allow the entire team to come together at predetermined time or ad hoc to discuss general plans, concerns (current or anticipated), staffing problems (current or anticipated), and other issues that might impact team functioning. Team meetings help the team to maintain normal operation and prevent crisis. Debriefing after all activities, especially crisis intervention, allows the team to learn from both successes and failures, and thus to improve future performance.

■ TEACHING CRM

The best way to teach teamwork has not been established and is controversial (43,44). Within aviation, CRM concepts are generally embedded into simulation scenarios that pilots must perform twice a year. However, options range from a high-fidelity simulation center, to didactic lectures, to the development of clinical protocols that help standardize the team behaviors. In reality, any teaching method will likely use a combination of techniques; those who endorse high-fidelity simulators generally include some didactic teaching, and classroom-based models often allow participants to practice teamwork behaviors in simulated scenarios. Some have advocated that a combination of methods may be best and may even act synergistically to teach teamwork and to bring the behaviors to the clinical environment (13,45). Irrespective of the teaching method, it is clear that CRM education should not be a single experience but must be part of an ongoing educational process (13,39).

■ CRM IN MEDICINE

Aviation and healthcare share much in common. They are both complicated, highly technical fields that depend on the well-coordinated interactions of multiple team members. Staff must often make decision with incomplete information,

TABLE 45-2 Specific Communication Techniques

SBAR	Defined technique for communication of relevant patient information. Stands for: **S**ituation **B**ackground **A**ssessment **R**ecommendation
2-challenge rule	A patient safety concern must be articulated at least twice if it is not addressed to ensure that the leader has heard and understood the concern. The second time might include additional information or a question about why the leader believes the current plan is safe.
DESC Script	Structured language to describe and defuse conflict or concern. It stands for: **D**escribe the problem **E**xplain consequences of the problem **S**uggest alternative(s) Reach **C**onsensus
Check back	Closed-loop communication between the sender and receiver to ensure that the receiver has heard and understands the message correctly. The receiver must repeat sender's message and the sender confirm its accuracy.
Call out	Calling aloud important decision or action during evolving events. It helps staff know what is happening and enables them to anticipate next steps.

and both must be able to quickly adapt to changes in the plans. Most importantly, both have historically worked with steep hierarchies, and poor performance can lead to fatal consequences. Despite this, there has been relatively little adoption of formal CRM-based training in medicine, although many of the concepts have been shown to be important to patient safety. Aviation-based team training has been shown to improve attitude toward patient safety among operating room staff (46–49). Surrogate measures have been shown to improve with teamwork processes, including operating room dosing of antibiotics and deep vein thrombosis (DVT) prophylactic medications (50), staff knowledge of planned surgical procedures (51), and efficacy of communication among operating room staff (48). Improvements in patient outcomes have been seen in the operating room (52,53) and emergency room (49) environment with formal team training.

A much larger body of literature demonstrates that even without full team training, the use of specific CRM-based team behaviors may improve outcomes in the general medical literature. Use of pre-procedure briefings has been shown to decrease perioperative mortality (54) and wrong side surgery (55). Use of structured, multidisciplinary rounds may decrease post-operative intensive care unit (ICU) admissions (56) and hospital (57) length of stay. Improved leadership is associated with better teamwork during resuscitation efforts (58).

■ CRM IN OBSTETRICS

Fortunately, obstetrics is one of the areas in which formal CRM-based team training has been implemented and assessed. Obstetric teamwork training itself, whether through simulation or classroom-based courses, has consistently been associated with improvements in staff attitudes toward patient safety and teamwork when assessed at the time of the training (20,28,59–62). The training is generally well received (20,59,62). These attitudes toward patient safety and teamwork can be translated to the clinical environment (24,60,61,63). Using the Safety Attitudes Questionnaire (SAQ) (64), Pratt et al. found that clinician attitudes toward patient safety were significantly higher among labor and delivery staff who had been through classroom-based team training than among those working on other units who had not been trained (60). The SAQ is a single page (double sided) questionnaire with 60 items and

demographics information (age, sex, experience, and nationality). It assesses staff perceptions of safety in six categories (see Table 45-3). Gardner developed a 6-hour, multidisciplinary simulation course involving obstetricians, anesthesiologists, obstetric nurses, and midwives. Self-assessment of teamwork and communication more than 1 year after course completion demonstrated improvements in both areas. In addition, most clinicians felt that their clinical practice had changed because of the course (28). Finally, Haller et al. trained 239 obstetric nurses, physicians, midwives, and other labor and delivery staff in a 2-day, classroom-based, CRM-style course. Initial reactions to the course and evidence that participants learned the CRM concepts were both very positive. Surveys of the staff over the next year demonstrated improvements in attitudes toward patient safety, stress recognition, work conditions, and job satisfaction. Participants also reported improved availability of clinical information and "feeling part of a bigger family" (61).

The impact of team training on clinician teamwork behaviors has been poorly evaluated in obstetrics. While improvements in various teamwork behaviors have been demonstrated after training in other clinical environments (48,49), this has not been formally evaluated on labor and delivery units. This may be in part because measuring teamwork is an imprecise science and not easily done in obstetrics (65). Robertson et al. did evaluate the impact of simulation-based team training on teamwork behaviors among obstetric nurses, midwives, and attending and resident obstetricians within the simulator (66). The authors found that teamwork task completion improved from 24% to 40% in the first simulated scenario to 80% to 100% in the fourth. However, it is unclear whether the behaviors learned in the simulators were transferred to the clinical setting.

Improvements in patient outcomes are the ultimate measure of the impact of team training. A large, prospective randomized trial evaluating the impact of a classroom-based CRM course based on the MedTeams curriculum previously developed for the emergency room failed to demonstrate improvements in patient outcomes in obstetrics. The authors did find a 10-minute (~33%) improvement in the time from decision to incision in emergent cesarean deliveries. Inadequate power, high staff turnover, and a short implementation time for the teamwork behaviors may have contributed to the negative results (18).

TABLE 45-3 Safety Attitudes Questionnaire Categories of Patient Safety

Category Definition	Examples
Teamwork climate: Perceived quality of collaboration between personnel	1. Disagreements are appropriately resolved (i.e., what is best for the patient) 2. Our doctors and nurses work together as a well-coordinated team
Job satisfaction: Positivity about the work experience	1. I like my job 2. This is a good place to work
Perceptions of management: Approval of managerial action	1. Management supports my daily efforts 2. Management is doing a good job
Safety climate: Perceptions of a strong and proactive organizational commitment to safety	1. I would feel perfectly safe being treated here 2. Personnel frequently disregard rules or guidelines
Working conditions: Perceived quality of the work environment and logistical support (staffing, equipment, etc.)	1. Our levels of staffing are sufficient to handle the number of patients 2. The equipment is adequate
Stress recognition: Acknowledgement of how performance is influenced by stressors	1. I am less effective at work when fatigued 2. When my workload becomes excessive, my performance is impaired

Adapted from: Sexton J.B, Helmreich RL, Neilands TB, et al. The Safety Attitudes Questionnaire: psychometric properties, benchmarking data, and emerging research. *BMC Health Serv Res* 2006;6:44.

TABLE 45-4 Adverse Outcome Index with Weights

Outcome	Points
Maternal death	750
Intrapartum death in infant >2,500 g and >37 wks' gestation	400
Intrapartum uterine rupture	100
Unplanned maternal admission to ICU	65
Birth trauma	65
Return to OR/labor and delivery	40
Admission to NICU for >24 h in infant >2,500 g and >37 wks' gestation	35
APGAR <7 at 5 min	25
Maternal blood transfusion	20
Third or fourth degree perineal tear	5

ICU, intensive care unit; OR, operating room; NICU, neonatal ICU.
Data Adapted from: Mann S, Pratt S, Gluck P, et al. Assessing quality in obstetrical care: Development of standardized measures. *Jt Comm J Qual Patient Saf* 2006;32(9):497–505.

However, others have demonstrated improvements in patient outcomes associated with both classroom and simulation-based team training. Pratt et al. trained more than 220 labor and delivery staff in a classroom-based CRM teamwork course. In addition, the authors described a structured implementation process involving the use of templates, structured language, coaches, and three types of formal teams that helped to translate the behaviors to the clinical environment. The authors used a measure of adverse events called the Adverse Outcomes Index (AOI) (Table 45-4) (67). AOI, a weighted composite measure of ten adverse events, was used to measure the impact of CRM training on their labor and delivery unit. They found that obstetric complication rates and overall severity decreased by 23% and 13.2% respectively among more than 19,000 women who delivered after the implementation of teamwork. The severity of the outcomes among those who had an adverse event also decreased, suggesting improved team response to evolving events. They did not measure teamwork behaviors on the unit, and thus could not draw a direct causal relationship between the training and the improved outcomes (60). Similarly, Pettker described a multi-step process designed to improve safety on their labor and delivery unit. This included the development of clinical protocols, fetal monitoring certification, a safety nursing committee, and team training. The entire process required nearly 2 years to implement. The adverse event rate, as measured by the AOI, decreased by nearly 28% in the second half of the study period (see Fig. 45-1) (68). In addition, the percentage of nurses and physicians that reported a "good teamwork climate" increased from 16.4% and 39.5% respectively to 72.2% and 88.7%. Using a similar multi-step model that mandated CRM-based team training, Grunebaum et al. described a dramatic drop in the number of sentinel events on their obstetrics unit (69). Team training was the first of 19 individual safety steps implemented over a 6-year period. The unit experienced three to five sentinel events per year at the start of the program. This number dropped to three total events over the last five years (0.6/year). Shea-Lewis described a 43% reduction in the rate of adverse obstetric events after the implementation of a CRM-based team training curriculum in an intermediate-sized community hospital (70). Finally, in a landmark paper, Draycott et al. developed a 1-day course that combined didactic and simulation training in both teamwork behaviors and obstetric crisis management. All obstetric care providers at a large, urban

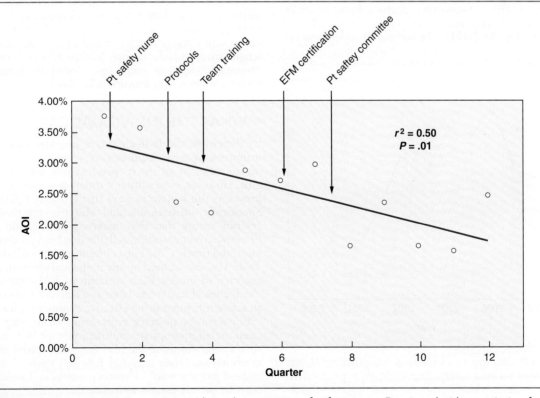

FIGURE 45-1 Adverse event rate over time with implementation of safety steps. Reprinted with permission from: Pettker CM, Thung SF, Norwitz ER, et al. Impact of a comprehensive patient safety strategy on obstetric adverse events. *Am J Obstet Gynecol* 2009;200(5):492.e1–492.e8.

TABLE 45-5 Change in Hypoxic Ischemic Encephalopathy (HIE) Rates after Team Training

Apgar score and HIE before (1998–1999) and after (2001–2003) introduction of training in obstetric emergencies

	1998–1999 ($n = 8,430$)	2001–2003 ($n = 11,030$)	Relative Risk
5-min Apgar ≤6, n (rate per 10,000)	73 (86.6)	49 (44.4)	0.51 (0.35–0.74)
HIE, n (rate per 10,000)	23 (27.3)	15 (13.6)	0.50 (0.26–0.95)
Moderate/severe HIE, n (rate per 10,000)	16 (19.0)	11 (10.0)	0.53 (0.24–1.13)

Reprinted with permission from: Draycott T, Sibanda T, Owen L, et al. Does training in obstetric emergencies improve neonatal outcome? *BJOG* 2006;113(2):177–182.

center were required to attend the course in multidisciplinary sessions. Evaluation of more than 19,000 deliveries during the 2 years prior to and 3 years after training demonstrated a 50% risk reduction in the rate of neonatal hypoxic ischemic encephalopathy (HIE) after the training (Table 45-5) (71). While it was unclear whether the improvement was related to better individual clinical care or better teamwork, the decrease in the rate of hypoxic brain injury is impressive.

As with the general medical literature, the use of elements of CRM-type teamwork behaviors without full team training has also been shown to improve provider care and patient outcomes in obstetrics. The implementation of an obstetric-specific rapid response team has been associated with improved outcomes (72). This effort used protocols to ensure role clarity, structured language, and simulation to allow the teams to practice. Similarly, Skupski et al. developed an obstetric rapid response team specifically for maternal hemorrhage. Guidelines helped define roles of the team members and improved communication processes were created. These efforts were associated with a decrease in maternal mortality due to hemorrhage (73). Clark described a system-wide approach to improving outcomes in obstetrics. This included many CRM concepts without formal training in teamwork. The authors described improved outcomes, fewer cesarean deliveries, and a drop in malpractice claims associated with these changes (Fig. 45-2) (21). The use of a shoulder dystocia

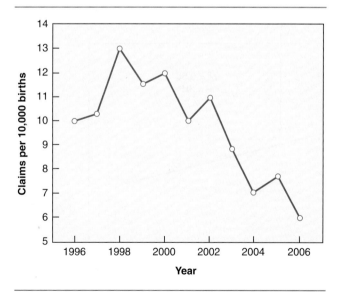

FIGURE 45-2 Change in obstetrical malpractice claims with improved patient safety. Reprinted with permission from: Clark S, Belfort MA, Byrum SL, et al. Improved outcomes, fewer cesarean deliveries, and reduced litigation: results of a new paradigm in patient safety. *Am J Obstet Gynecol* 2008;199(2):105.e1–105.e7.

protocol has been used to improve role clarity, situation awareness, shared mental models, and communication—all CRM concepts (74).

■ IMPORTANCE OF IMPLEMENTATION

The successful transition of the skills learned during teamwork education, whether using classroom or simulation-based training, to the clinical environment requires significant implementation efforts, feedback, and sustaining behaviors (42). Pratt et al. described a year-long process to train and fully implement the teamwork behaviors (60). Pettker et al. required nearly 3 years to train their staff, develop appropriate clinical protocols, and effectively implement the teamwork skills on the labor and delivery units (68). Implementation is slow even in smaller private practice units (70). Coaching of the teamwork behaviors may help the successful transition from the classroom to the clinical unit (42,60,63). In a follow-up study to the prospective randomized trial of team training by Nielsen et al., the RAND (**R**esearch and **D**evelopment) Corporation found significant variation in the degree to which team behaviors had actually taken root in the clinical environment. Early emphasis on effective communication, pre-procedure briefings, and team meetings appears to be predictive of successful teamwork. Failure to train the entire staff (largely due to budgetary constraints) and challenges from outside factors (staff shortages, constructions projects, competing initiatives) tended to undermine the implementation of teamwork behaviors (63).

■ WHAT THE INDIVIDUAL CAN DO

By definition, the individual care provider cannot perform teamwork. A team requires two or more individuals working together in an interdependent way toward a common goal. However, even without formal team training, individual providers can behave in ways that facilitate CRM concepts. Specifically, obstetricians and obstetric anesthesia providers can ensure that they meet communication standards. Effective communication is defined as being complete, clear, brief, and timely (75). The communication tools described in Table 45-2 can be used by any individual clinician and can be expected of others. Even without a CRM-trained environment, clinical leaders on labor and delivery units should take an active role in ensuring effective communication.

Physicians on obstetric units should ensure that they communicate all appropriate information with their team members. Communicating the plan may seem trivial and obvious in obstetrics, "*Have a healthy baby and mother*," or "*place an epidural for pain relief.*" However, nurses and resident physicians frequently cannot articulate the specific goals for their patients, largely because the goals have never been communicated (56). An example of a specific plan for one anesthesia provider might be: *Place a labor epidural in patient "Smith," perform a pre-operative assessment for the scheduled cesarean delivery, and then administer an epidural bolus to patient "Jones."* As seen in this example, the plans made for one patient may dramatically impact the safety of the rest of the unit and vice versa. By clearly articulating the plan, the anesthesiologist facilitates feedback and potential change to the plan. Clinicians should communicate their location, how they can be reached, and who will cover their patients during an emergency if they are off the unit. Anesthesia providers frequently must cover surgical cases in the operating room while also being responsible for the labor and delivery floor. Finally, physicians should develop structured processes for handing off or transferring the responsibility of patient care. One of the specific recommendations of the IOM report was decreased reliance on individual vigilance and an increased attention to handoffs (3). However, there is still no large-scale structured process for handoffs. Obstetric anesthesia handoffs are frequently inadequate (27). Obstetric anesthesia providers should develop formalized systems for handing off responsibility of their patients, ideally face-to-face. Structured communication techniques such as *S*ituation, *B*ackground, *A*ssessment, *R*ecommendations (SBAR) should be used whenever possible.

Perhaps the most important communication behavior that obstetric care providers can perform is to actively work to foster an atmosphere conducive to patient safety. Patient safety is predicated on trust, open communication, and effective interdisciplinary teamwork. Some physicians undermine the atmosphere of trust with disruptive or abusive behavior. A Joint Commission Sentinel Event Alert indicated that *"intimidating and disruptive behaviors can foster medical errors, contribute to poor patient satisfaction and to preventable adverse outcomes, increase the cost of care, and cause qualified clinicians, administrators and managers to seek new positions in more professional environments"* (76). It has been estimated that 3% to 5% of physicians present a problem with disruptive behavior. Rosenstein et al. have demonstrated the negative effects that aggressive and disruptive behaviors have on patient safety and staff retention in the perioperative setting (77). Similar behaviors have been described in obstetrics. Veltman found that 60.7% of labor and delivery units noted disruptive behavior, generally occurring at least monthly. 41.9% of the units indicated that adverse patient outcomes had occurred as a direct result of these behaviors, and 39.3% stated that nurses had left the unit due to the intimidation (78). In another survey, 34% of nurses stated that they had been concerned about a physician's performance, but only 1% actually shared these concerns (79). Obstetric nurses have described explicit episodes of aggressive behavior (26).

Physicians can help create an open and trusting communication atmosphere by asking other team members to raise safety concerns, by expressly giving them permission to question unclear orders, or by encouraging them to challenge apparently dangerous actions. Openly communicating in this way during a briefing prior to surgery (e.g., cesarean delivery) can set the tone for better communication throughout the procedure (48). Physicians should thank staff who question their behavior, even if the questioner is wrong, because the act of questioning done for patient safety should be encouraged.

■ ADDITIONAL VALUE OF TEAMWORK

Team training may lead to improvements not related to patient care or even directly due to the team training. For instance, improved staff satisfaction has been linked to the implementation of CRM-based behaviors (60,61,68). This benefit can be especially important in units with nursing shortages, high turnover rates, or absenteeism.

The ability to identify unsafe conditions (latent errors) on a labor and delivery unit may also improve with better teamwork (60). Flattening of the hierarchy may encourage staff to speak up when they identify potentially unsafe systems. Physicians frequently fail to follow well-established guidelines and protocols. Team members advocating for safety may also be better able to enforce guidelines. The implementation of a patient safety culture has been associated with the successful implementation of practice guidelines and protocols (68).

Finally, CRM-based team training has the potential to decrease medical malpractice litigation in three distinct but clearly interrelated ways. First, and most important, the improved communication, coordination of care, plan development, shared mental models, and subsequent reduced error rate lead to improved outcomes and thus fewer suits (21,80,81). Clinicians simply cannot be sued if there is no injury. Clark et al. demonstrated a 50% decrease in obstetric-related ligation over an 8-year period with the implementation of a systemic change in practice that included CRM principles (21). Grunebaum found that a comprehensive obstetric safety program was associated with a nearly 90% average decrease in malpractice costs and an absolute savings of more than $75,000,000 (69). This program included the development of guidelines, physician and nurse clinical education programs, new staff positions, medication safety initiatives, and other safety projects. The individual impact of team training could not be determined.

Improved patient satisfaction with the clinical care provided, even in the face of an adverse event, is the second way that improved teamwork could decrease medical malpractice claims. Patients or their families are more likely to sue their healthcare providers when they feel angry toward them (82) or when they want to know what happened to cause the adverse event (83). Physicians who score lowest on the patient satisfaction surveys are more likely to be sued (84). Recent data suggest that disclosing errors to patients and helping them to understand how an adverse event occurred actually decreases the likelihood of being sued (85,86). Improved teamwork has the potential to improve patient satisfaction, both by improving the care provided as outlined above and by improving communication with the patient and their family.

Although working in teams clearly improves staff satisfaction, little data exist on the impact of team training on patient satisfaction. Morey et al. measured patient and staff satisfaction before and after the implementation of team training in the emergency department. They found that although staff satisfaction improved with improved teamwork, patient satisfaction did not. High baseline patient satisfaction may have limited their ability to influence this outcome (49). Meterko et al. demonstrated that patient satisfaction was independently associated with a higher teamwork culture score on the basis of patient and staff surveys (87). However, they could not demonstrate a direct causal relationship. Although dissatisfied patients are more likely to file a malpractice suit and it seems that improved teamwork does have the ability to improve patient satisfaction even when an adverse event occurs, a direct link between improved teamwork and fewer law suits has not yet been established.

The final way that team training could work to limit malpractice liability is to actually make cases more defensible when the clinician does get sued. This might occur in several ways. Clearly, if team-based obstetric care becomes the community standard, then failure to meet this standard would place the clinicians and hospital at increased risk should a suit be brought against them. However, even without this standard, teamwork might add defenses in a medical malpractice case. If the plan of care for a patient is reviewed by the entire team, and all agree with that plan, it may become very difficult to make a plaintiff case that the plan was negligent. Further, as one of the goals of teamwork is for team members to help each other carry out their plans and to identify errors and high-risk situations, clinicians working in teams may be more able to demonstrate that the plans were carried out or appropriately changed as the clinical situation changed. Finally, nurses are taught that accurate documentation is their best defense against medicolegal action (88). However, if nursing documentation contradicts that of other clinicians, this clearly increases the medicolegal risk for parts or all of the team. Pronovost et al. demonstrated that only 10% of house officers and ICU nurses could articulate the goals for each patient in the ICU (56). After the implementation of a multidisciplinary team meeting each morning, they were able to improve this number to 95%. Clearly, it is easier to both deliver a clear and concise message to patients or their families and to document similar plans when the entire team knows the plan. By reviewing, agreeing upon, and communicating patient care plans, effective teams may be able to minimize these "chart wars" that can undermine effective defense of a malpractice case. All of this is only speculative at this point as the impact of teamwork on the legal defense of malpractice cases has not been tested in the courts.

■ SIMULATION

Medical simulation is the second major patient safety recommendation designed to decrease error, lessen the likelihood of harm to patients when error does occur, and improve individual and team performance in both routine and emergent situations. As noted above, simulation is often used as an educational tool for CRM-based team training. However, simulation can also be a powerful tool to teach clinical skills, assess the safety of the work environment, and evaluate the abilities of clinical staff. Each of these uses has been described in the labor and delivery environment and each contributes to improved safety of the parturient and her baby.

History of Medical Simulation

At its most fundamental, simulation is defined as "an imitation of some real thing, state of affairs, or process. The act of simulating something generally entails representing certain key characteristics or behaviors of a selected physical or abstract system" (89). It has been described as an old art but a young science. Simulation in obstetrics may predate recorded history but certainly dates to the ninth century when the use of wax or wooden figures helped teach the processes of childbirth (24,90). Mannequin torsos, known as "phantoms," were developed in the 1600s to teach midwives the stages and processes of normal or abnormal births. Made of wicker, wood, or glass, these birth "simulators" evolved over the ensuing 300 years. Some models were full size with articulating limbs and simulated placentas. Some were transparent to allow the learner to see the internal processes of the pelvis. Some even used a stillborn fetus. The descendants of the phantoms, plastic pelvises, and cardboard cervical dilation trainers, can be seen on nearly every academic obstetric unit. Modern medical simulation began in the 1960s with the advent of Resusci® Anne (designed to teach CPR) and the Sim One simulator (designed to teach manual and decision-making tasks to anesthesiologists) (91). In the 1990s, Eggert et al. developed a life-sized obstetric mannequin called "Noelle." Noelle was designed with an indwelling audible heart tone simulator and a motor designed to "push" the fetus out (24). Currently, approximately 20 maternal or fetal/neonatal simulators or task trainers exist in obstetrics. These simulators have all largely been designed to help teach specific tasks related to the birthing process, and it was not until recently that simulation began to be used to assess and teach teamwork, crisis management, and the concepts of CRM.

The field of anesthesia has produced some of the most prolific researchers in the modern use of simulation, with much of this attention focused specifically on *obstetric* anesthesia. Gaba is credited with the introduction of CRM concepts into medical simulation with the development of Anesthesia Crisis Resource Management training (ACRM) (92). ACRM sought to teach anesthesia staff to better communicate and coordinate care as well as to practice rare clinical events. Only over the past decade have these concepts been applied to obstetric care. Task simulators in obstetric anesthesia and research into the ability to assess clinician performance have also grown over the past decade.

While it is clear that a non-threatening culture of safety is essential to the overall success of any patient safety initiative, the specific components associated with effective simulation training have not been fully elucidated (93). In order to be effective, a simulator must provide a high degree of physical, emotional, and conceptual realism (or fidelity) (24). High-fidelity is not necessarily the same as high-technology simulation. The simulation should be able to realistically mimic the emotional, physical, and physiologic environment irrespective of the degree of technology (93). Simulation appears to be better than didactic teaching of obstetric emergencies (30,94). Both local (in situ) and off-site simulation center methods have been effective (95,96). The use of live actors may improve the realism of the experience and educational response (97). The addition of specific team training education does not appear to add to the simulation training of specific clinical skills (20). However, for some skills training, advanced technology with realistic feedback may help improve simulation training (95). Finally, multidisciplinary training should be used whenever possible (93).

Simulation to Teach Skills

In Obstetrics

For most of its history, obstetric simulation has been used to teach or improve clinical skills. This remains largely true today. Reviews on the impact of obstetric skills simulation on obstetric and neonatal outcomes have been published (98,99). In a recent systematic review of simulation in obstetrics, Merien described the use of simulation to teach a wide variety of clinical skills including the management of eclampsia, maternal hemorrhage, fetal shoulder dystocia, breech extraction, and adult and neonatal resuscitation (99). Simulation sessions were generally 1 to 2 days in length; they were conducted either on site within the local hospital or at formal simulation centers. Clinical skills or knowledge base consistently increased after simulation training. Of the eight studies reviewed, only one demonstrated improvements in clinical outcomes associated with the use of simulation. The authors delineated the advantages and disadvantages of using high-fidelity simulation as an educational tool in obstetrics (see Fig. 45-3).

Both hospital-based simulation and center-based simulation training have been shown to increase the knowledge of obstetricians and midwives in the management of obstetrics emergencies (20,96). Simulation improves the performance of basic tasks in the management of eclampsia (94,96). Training in shoulder dystocia improves skills and knowledge (95). These skills are retained for up to 12 months (100). Obstetricians have even been trained to manage an unexpected high spinal in a simulated laboring patient (101). The use of simulation has been shown to greatly improve obstetricians' estimates of maternal blood loss during post-partum hemorrhage (102,103).

Advantages
- Provision of a safe environment for both patient and trainees in risky procedures
- The opportunity for multidisciplinary team training and specific behavioral skills
- Unlimited exposure to uncommon, complicated, and important clinical events
- The ability to plan simulator-based clinical training rather than waiting for a specific available situation
- The possibility to stop an intervention to allow discussion and give immediate feedback
- The opportunity to repeat an intervention or practice alternative techniques
- The ability to test new technology and learn how these can be used without exposing patient to risk

Disadvantages
- High costs
- Lack of capable trainers
- Lack of good educational training programs
- Lack of studies investigating cost-effectiveness

FIGURE 45-3 Advantages and disadvantages of educational use of high-fidelity simulators. Reprinted with permission from: Merien A.E, van de Ven J, Mol BW, et al. Multidisciplinary team training in a simulation setting for acute obstetric emergencies: a systematic review. *Obstet Gynecol* 2010;115(5):1021–1031.

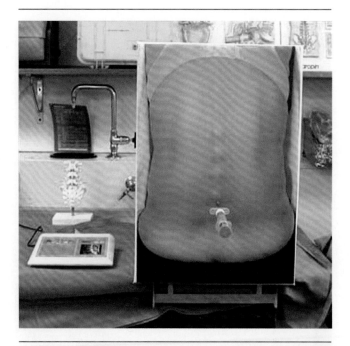

FIGURE 45-4 High-tech epidural simulator. Reprinted with permission from: Friedman Z, Siddiqui N, Katznelson R, et al. Clinical impact of epidural anesthesia simulation on short- and long-term learning curve: High- versus low-fidelity model training. *Reg Anesth Pain Med* 2009; 34(3):229–232.

The assessment of the impact of simulation training on knowledge and performance is nearly always done in the simulation center. The learners are assessed before the training, taken through a set of simulated events, and then assessed again at the simulator. Little data exist on the impact of obstetric simulation on task performance in the clinical environment. Sorensen et al. implemented a mandatory in situ obstetric skills training program (104). They found that clinicians liked the training and believed that it improved their ability to manage a series of obstetric emergencies. More importantly, the simulation experience led to a series of changes in clinical guidelines and protocols on the clinical unit. It is not clear whether the clinicians' performance in the clinical environment actually improved. Draycott published the only study to date to evaluate the impact of simulation on obstetric outcomes (71). The authors compared the rates of neonatal HIE before and after the implementation of a simulation program in obstetric emergencies. All obstetric staff at the authors' institution were required to attend a 1-day training session. The curriculum consisted of didactic courses on obstetric emergencies and teamwork in the morning. In the afternoon, participants attended six simulated obstetric emergencies. In analyzing more than 27,000 births, the author found that the overall rate of HIE and the rate of severe HIE had dropped by approximately 50%. This improvement was associated with a nearly 23% increase in the emergency cesarean section rate. The authors' assumption was that clinical skills improved, but this was not directly measured.

In Anesthesia
Simulators have also been used to teach obstetric anesthesia skills, although it has been argued that they are a waste of time and money (105,106). Several epidural simulators have been described. More than 20 years ago, Leighton described how to make an epidural simulator from a banana, a slice of bread,

a balloon, and an intubating pillow (107). This "green grocer" simulator appears to be as effective as a very high-technology simulator (Fig. 45-4) in teaching residents to place an epidural (although it is not clear that either simulator is better than nothing) (108). Glassenberg designed a virtual epidural simulator in which the user interacts with a virtual spine on a computer screen using a pen designed to provide haptic feedback (109). Magill et al. described the development of a hands-on epidural needle insertion simulator that used a series of cables and computer-driven actuators to simulate the movement of the needle through tissues (110). Both the Glassenberg and Magill models accurately recreated the forces required to penetrate the various tissue layers between the skin and the epidural space, but neither has been demonstrated to improve clinician performance or resident education.

The accuracy of maternal blood loss among obstetric anesthesia personnel has also been improved using both live (111) and web-based simulated training (112). Toledo et al. found that during massive maternal hemorrhage, clinicians underestimated maternal blood loss by 38% (range 20% to 59%) (112). The error grew worse as actual blood loss increased. Study participants attended didactic lectures on blood loss and then interacted in three low-volume and two high-volume blood loss stations using mannequins and equipment usually found in a delivery room (Fig. 45-5). This decreased the average underestimation to only 4%.

Finally, with the high rate of failed intubation in obstetrics (33,34), the high frequency with which the maternal airway is mismanaged (33), and the decreasing experience with general anesthesia in the parturient, practicing airway drills have been argued as the most compelling reason for simulated skills training in obstetric anesthesia (35,36,113). Goodwin et al. demonstrated that task completion by anesthesia trainees was generally poor during a simulated failed intubation in a

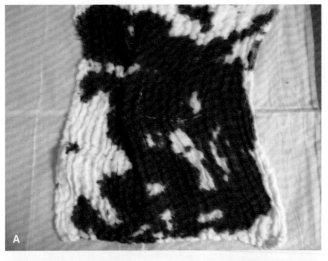

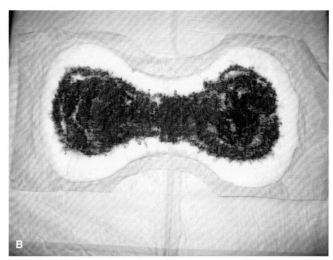

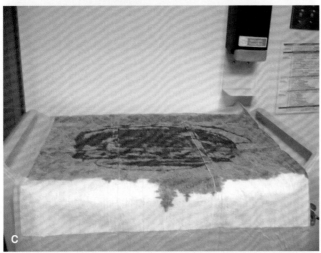

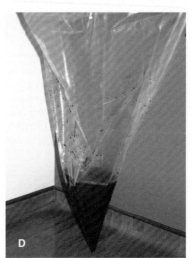

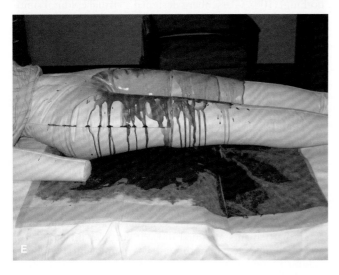

FIGURE 45-5 Web-based maternal blood loss simulator. (**A**) Laparotomy sponge; (**B**) perineal pad; (**C**) large blue under-the-buttocks pad; (**D**) vaginal delivery drape; (**E**) blood spill on a mannequin on a labor and delivery bed. Reprinted with permission from: Toledo P, McCarthy RJ, Burke CA, et al. The effect of live and web-based education on the accuracy of blood-loss estimation in simulated obstetric scenarios. *Am J Obstet Gynecol* 2010; 202(4):400.e1–400.e5.

parturient. However, they found significant improvement in task performance after education and participation in simulated failed intubations in a pregnant mannequin (114). Similar findings have been demonstrated in the performance of cardio-pulmonary resuscitation during pregnancy (115).

As with obstetrics, the use of simulators to teach skills in obstetric anesthesia holds promise and appears to be effective when assessed in the simulated environment. Much more research is

required to determine if the skills obtained in the simulator can be effectively transferred to the clinical environment.

Simulation to Assess Clinician Performance

The simulated environment can be used to assess individual clinician performance. By definition, the skills training scenarios described above all assess individual and group performance before and after training in the simulator. However, others have used a single simulator session to help identify clinical weaknesses and areas for improvement. This has been used to assess basic anesthesia technical performance in the general operating room among novice anesthesia residents (116) and to measure the response to anesthesia emergencies among residents and attending anesthesia staff (117–119). Scavone et al. developed and validated an objective scoring system to assess resident performance during simulated general anesthesia in a parturient. They found that senior residents scored higher on the assessment (120). Maslovitz found that obstetricians made recurrent mistakes when dealing with simulated eclampsia, post-partum hemorrhage, shoulder dystocia, and vaginal breech extraction (32). For example, more than 80% of the time, teams provided improper ventilation techniques and treated magnesium toxicity incorrectly in the eclampsia drill. The authors suggested that simulation can help to both train clinicians in the management of unusual events and identify specific weaknesses that can be highlighted during this training.

To date, no one has described the use of simulation as part of a formal peer review process. The American Board of Anesthesiology Maintenance of Certification in Anesthesiology (ABA MOCA) Program currently requires clinicians to spend time in a simulated environment but does not require an assessment of their performance during the simulation. Based on current understanding of the science, any attempt to use simulation to determine the fitness of a clinician to perform his or her clinical duties should be undertaken with great caution. No data exist demonstrating that performance in the simulated environment predicts performance in the clinical arena. Performance anxiety, lack of understanding of the simulated environment, even boredom, and a whole host of other factors might cause a very competent clinician to perform poorly in a simulator or vice versa.

Simulation to Assess the Work Environment

Recently, there has been a growing emphasis on the use of simulation within the clinical environment (in situ). With in situ simulation, a simulator mannequin or actor portrays a patient on the actual unit where clinicians practice. Usually a single specific event (or drill) is rehearsed, but multiple events can be practiced at once. Common drill scenarios in obstetrics include maternal hemorrhage, eclampsia, failed intubation, cardiac arrest, and shoulder dystocia (5,29,121). The advantages of in situ simulation include the ability to train the entire staff on the unit at once, the ability to identify weaknesses within the system of care that are potential barriers to safe care, the ability to include other areas within the hospital in the drill (e.g., laboratories, blood bank, code teams), and the ability to train without leaving one's clinical environment. Disadvantages include distracting caregivers from their clinical responsibilities, the need for significant organization, and potential significant cost (122). More than half of the obstetrics units in England and Wales conduct in situ drills, and nearly half of these perform them at least monthly (123). No data exist on the prevalence of in situ simulation in the United States, but the dearth of published reports would suggest that it is not nearly as common as in England.

Thompson et al. employed eclampsia drills on their unit and found recurrent communication and coordination failures, inefficiencies, and deficiencies in clinical skills (29). The deficiencies identified led to immediate and concrete changes on the unit (Fig. 45-6). Similarly, Riley studied teamwork behaviors during simulated, in situ crises in six hospitals ranging from 700 to 3,300 deliveries per year (121). They found generally fair scores in teamwork behaviors (leadership, situation awareness, closed-loop communication, and shared

- Difficulty summoning senior staff urgently
  Rapid activation of team through one call from switchboard
- Multiple protocols for managing eclampsia in different clinical areas, many out of date
  Development and dissemination of an evidence based protocol for eclampsia
- Deficiencies in the skills and knowledge of individuals in the management of eclampsia: Positioning of the fitting patient; choice of first line anticonvulsant; safe administration of magnesium Immediate individual feedback and education; didactic instruction on magnesium administration in eclampsia protocol
- Time wasted fetching individual items for management of seizures
  Creation of strategically placed "eclampsia boxes" containing all necessary equipment and protocol for eclampsia
- Variable presentation of magnesium in drug cupboards
  Liaison with pharmacy to ensure consistency of magnesium ampoules supplied
- Confusion about staff roles, resulting in inefficient activity
- Clear division of tasks in management protocol

FIGURE 45-6 Problems identified during drills, and solutions. Reprinted with permission from: Thompson S, S. Neal, V. Clark. Clinical risk management in obstetrics: eclampsia drills. *BMJ* 2004;328(7434):269–271.

mental model). These scores tended to decrease as the acuity of the simulated scenario increased. The authors made several important observations about how the team performed. First, the mother was the only member of the team who was present throughout all stages of the crisis. This demonstrated the importance of including her as an active member of the team whenever possible. Second, they identified that with 208 clinicians on their unit, there are *381 million* possible combinations of staff that could make up the teams on any given shift. Thus, while the staff may know each other well as individuals and believe that they communicate and perform well together, these assumptions can and did lead to miscommunications and errors. Osman et al. conducted eclampsia and maternal hemorrhage drills in three hospitals (124). They found that general medical care was within accepted standards. However, they also identified multiple systems problems within each unit that hindered the quality of the care provided. These included: Lack of a fetal Doppler monitor in the emergency ward, delays in fetal heart tone assessment; inadequate/absence of antihypertensive medications; and delays in reaching both resident and attending physicians. In each instance, the problems identified were quickly corrected by changes in protocols. The simulation allowed these latent errors to be identified without placing patients at risk.

Finally, several authors have described in situ simulation techniques that are mobile in order to bring standard simulation education to many labor and delivery units. Deering et al. created the Mobile Obstetric Emergencies Simulator (MOES) (125). This course was designed to: (1) Be mobile; (2) provide a standardized curriculum; (3) evaluate teamwork and clinical competency; (4) incorporate debriefing; (5) track performance over time; and (6) be cost effective. The course includes a 6-hour training course in teamwork (75), followed by two simulated scenarios in each of seven obstetric emergencies.

These are followed by structured debriefing based on objective performance measures. This system is attractive, but results on its efficacy have not yet been published.

Similarly, Johanson describes the Management of Obstetric Emergencies and Trauma (MOET) course (126). This mobile 2-day course uses classroom and low-fidelity simulation to teach skills and teamwork in a series of obstetric emergencies. MOET has been effectively implemented in the United Kingdom (127), Armenia (128), Bangladesh (129), and Iraq (130). It appears to improve both clinician knowledge and technical skills.

Jha et al. developed the Simulated Delivery Suite (SiDeS) management course (62). This course is divided into six sessions: (1) Teamwork, (2) prioritizing the delivery suite board, (3) patient management, (4) clinical algorithms, (5) an interactive session based on case reports from the **Confidential Enquiries into Maternal Deaths**, and (6) a simulated 8-hour shift on a busy labor and delivery unit. This course is different from others because it uses simulation and didactic lectures not only to manage emergent or rare events but also to teach techniques to keep the labor suite running "normally" and thus avoid emergent events. The authors describe the implementation of three SiDeS courses with generally positive evaluations from clinicians. It is unclear if this training will improve clinician performance or obstetric outcomes.

Simulation to Teach Teamwork

Teaching teamwork, the last major use of simulation discussed in this context, is the one that has received the most attention. Fundamentally, teamwork training is a subset of skills training with an emphasis on non-technical skills. However, because these non-technical skills are frequently not well taught and are under appreciated in the clinical arena, team training is presented as a separate use of simulation. The simulated environment offers the perfect opportunity to practice the skills needed to function as a team (communication behaviors, leadership skills, cross-monitoring, etc.). Since these skills are best practiced in a clinical environment, the teamwork training is generally embedded into the simulation of an emergent clinical event, thus allowing the learners to practice both the clinical and teamwork skills. Teamwork training simulation can occur in either a formal simulation center or in situ.

Simulation can be used to define and measure the quality and effectiveness of teamwork behaviors. Using very low-level simulated scenarios and structured interviews of clinicians deemed to have superior clinical skill, Bahl defined the non-clinical skills required to perform an operative vaginal delivery (131). In this study, seven non-technical skills were identified in high-performing clinicians; all were very similar to CRM training (Table 45-6). In addition, being calm, confident, but knowing his/her limitations were cited as important attributes to "maintaining professional behavior." In a similar study, Siassakos and colleagues analyzed the communication patterns during a simulated maternal hemorrhage (132). They found that commands and enquiries were the most common types of communications, accounting for more than 59% of all events. Interestingly, skills training in the management of maternal hemorrhage led to a decrease in required communication events of 35% to 47%, without evidence of a decline in the quality of care. Teamwork training improved communication further by increasing the percentage of commands that were directed to an individual (versus being spoken "in the air") from 26% to 71%. This led directly to an improvement in task performance.

TABLE 45-6 Non-technical Skills Identified in High-performing Clinicians

Teamwork Category during Operative Vaginal Delivery	How Measured
Situation awareness	Gather information Analyze information Anticipate events
Decision making	Consider all options Implement and review plans Informed consent
Task management	Gather team Identify resources Re-evaluate each step Document events Debrief
Professional relationship with mother	Gain her confidence Ensure her cooperation Tailor care to her expectations Communicate with mother Maintain mother's dignity Allow partner participation
Maintaining professional behavior with staff	Calm Confident/assertive Able
Teamwork and communication	Clear communication Aware of team members' capabilities Respectful of team members
Cross monitoring	Ability to question practice

Adapted from: Bahl R., D.J. Murphy, B. Strachan. Non-technical skills for obstetricians conducting forceps and vacuum deliveries: qualitative analysis by interviews and video recordings. *Eur J Obstet Gynecol Reprod Biol* 2010;150(2):147–151.

Others have used simulation specifically to teach teamwork in the obstetric environment. Miller et al. were able to take more than 700 clinicians through 35 in situ simulations in six different obstetric units (133). The study was designed to measure teamwork and communication—not clinical effectiveness or technical abilities. They observed consistent teamwork failures related to communication, situation awareness, and shared mental models. An example of teamwork failure to develop a shared mental model is explicitly described as follows: "*The nurse notes that the laboring patient suddenly has severe unrelenting uterine pain and ruptures membranes with bloody fluid; the fetal heart rate changes to bradycardia. She calls the physician. Upon entering the room, the physician sees the patient in pain, notes the bleeding, and asks the patient questions. Instead of stating a clear sense of urgency directly, the nurse "hints and hopes" by calling out that the fetal heart rate is "90," or "now 60," and, "I have the Operating Room team on standby.*"

Multiple authors have found that teamwork training in the simulated environment is well liked (59,62,66), associated with improved teamwork skills (at least as measured in the simulated environment) (59,66), and improves the clinical performance of the team (also in the simulator). Robertson et al. demonstrated that clearly identifying roles was an important teamwork skill, and that as team went through a series of simulated obstetric crises, the task completion rate improved as role clarity improved (66). Daniels demonstrated that obstetric residents frequently failed to adequately distribute workloads or communicate effectively as a leader in simulated obstetric emergencies. These teamwork failures led to delays in care and could have a significant negative impact on actual clinical outcomes (30). Gum designed an interdisciplinary simulation in team training that helped to improve teamwork skills, including leadership and collaboration, and a sense of trust and mutual respect among the staff (134).

Despite the apparent benefits of teaching teamwork in the simulated environment, it has not been well established that this teamwork alters clinical behaviors or patient outcomes. It has been argued that when simulation is used to teach clinical skills in obstetrics, the addition of specific teamwork training is not needed or helpful (20,135). Further, it is unlikely that any single teamwork training course can alter attitudes; changes in work culture can only be achieved through repetitive training (134). Contrary to this view, Gardner surveyed obstetric providers after simulation training in crisis management and teamwork (28). A total of 176 participants from obstetrics, labor and delivery nursing, and anesthesiology participated in a 6-hour course. Each clinician participated in three separate simulated scenarios followed by a formal debriefing session. Initial assessment of the course was favorable. One year later, the majority indicated that since the course they communicate more effectively (87%), debrief more thoroughly (45%), and respond better to crisis (90%). These findings were based on self-assessment, so their validity is unclear; nonetheless, they do suggest that the use of simulation to teach teamwork may improve team behaviors in the clinical environment. As stated above, Draycott et al. found that neonatal outcomes improved after all obstetric care providers completed a 1-day course at a simulation center (71). This is the only study to demonstrate an improvement in patient outcomes associated with simulation. However, the authors taught both technical and teamwork skills in the didactic and simulation portions of the course, and so it is unclear which component—if any—was associated with the improved outcomes. More research is clearly needed to determine the role of simulation in the effective implementation of CRM-based teamwork concepts into clinical medicine.

Debriefing

Debriefing is an important part of both CRM training and effective teamwork in the clinical environment. Effective feedback is a critical part of the educational simulation experience (136). Verbal, computerized, and video-assisted methods have been used to allow participants to review and learn from their experiences in the simulator (137,138). The use of simulation in obstetrics (whether to teach skills and team behaviors or to assess the in situ environment) has generally included active feedback and debriefing as an important component of the educational process (24,30,32,124,125). Gardner dedicated twice as much time to debriefing of the simulation scenarios as to the running of the simulations. The debriefing was used to teach CRM principles using educational videos and provided in-depth analysis of the team's performance to learn how well they adhered to these principles. The debriefing occurred after each of the three simulation sessions. This allowed lessons learned from one scenario to be incorporated into the next (28).

Debriefing is also critical to the success of a well-functioning team. The ability to reflect upon and learn from one's practice allows clinicians and teams to improve future performance. Debriefing in the clinical environment can occur either on a routine basis (e.g., at the end of each shift or after every surgical procedure), or it can occur after critical incidents. Care should be taken to ensure that debriefings are considered part of the peer review process. Salas et al. described 12 evidence-based best practices for medical team debriefing (139). These practices are summarized below:

- Debriefs must be diagnostic. Whether performed at regular intervals or only after critical incidents, debriefs should be aimed at identifying and improving team weaknesses.
- They should occur in a supportive environment. Time, adequate space, and a positive attitude about the importance of debriefing is essential.
- Encourage team members to attend to the teamwork processes during the debriefing. This helps the team members to improve their knowledge of teamwork behaviors. It also helps to de-emphasize the medical care, for which other environments (e.g., Morbidity and Mortality Conferences) may be better suited.
- Leaders must be educated on leading a debriefing: This includes creation of an agenda, reviewing conclusions, encouraging participation, and focusing on teamwork processes. The creation of a non-judgmental atmosphere is also important (140).
- Ensure that team members feel comfortable: This includes both emotional comfort (a non-judgmental atmosphere) and physical comfort (all participants should be able to interact).
- Focus on a few critical issues. This allows time to be effectively used to solve specific problems.
- Describe the specific teamwork interactions that were involved in the incident. Was leadership established? Did supporting behavior occur? Was a shared mental model created?
- Support feedback with objective indicators. Explicitly describing specific examples of teamwork failure allows team members to better accept the feedback.
- Provide outcome feedback later and less frequently than process feedback. Outcome feedback is less useful as the team has less direct control over outcomes. Process or behavioral feedback allows team members to improve specific behaviors in the future.
- Provide both individual and team-oriented feedback. Team failures might include failure to establish a mental model. Individual feedback might include when an individual did not perform a specific task.
- Shorten the time between task performance and feedback as much as possible. Whenever possible, debriefs should occur soon after the event so team members are better able to link behaviors to the feedback and improve future events.
- Record conclusions and goals. This allows future debriefs to learn from past events and the team to look for trends over time.

The creation of a non-judgmental atmosphere is critical to effective feedback whether after a simulated or real clinical event. Avoiding judgmental questions (whether positive or negative) when leading a debriefing creates a more supportive atmosphere and may also help better identify teamwork strengths upon which the team can build as well as concerns that need to be addressed. Rudolph et al. described "debriefing with good judgment" (140). This technique focuses on the advocacy and inquiry feedback technique. Rather than asking, "Why didn't you give pressors when the mother's blood pressure dropped after the spinal?", the leader might advocate, "The blood pressure dropped after the spinal and this can negatively affect uterine perfusion" and then ask, "What were your thoughts about what was happening at that time?" This avoids judgment and assumptions; furthermore, it allows the team member to express his/her frame of reference. Education can then occur about the frame of reference ("I thought that a systolic blood pressure of 80 mm Hg was fine") and not simply with regard to behavior ("You should have given a pressor for that blood pressure").

■ CONCLUSION

Modern medical practice is highly complex. This complexity may lead to errors, and these errors may lead to patient harm. The ability to prevent errors from occurring, trap errors when they do occur, and mitigate the impact of errors on patients is essential to safe medical practice. The use of simulation and teamwork based on CRM has proven effective at improving safety in other highly complex and dangerous industries. In obstetrics and obstetric anesthesia, CRM-based teamwork has been shown to improve clinician attitudes toward safety and patient outcomes. Simulation can improve technical and non-technical skills and can be used to assess clinical performance. It is an effective and safe way to identify latent errors within the labor and delivery environment.

KEY POINTS

- Maternal and neonatal morbidity and mortality are frequently caused by medical error and/or substandard care. Poor communication and teamwork are frequently cited as causes for substandard care.
- CRM offers a defined set of team and individual behaviors that help to improve communication, better utilize resources and coordination of care, resolve conflicts, and identify and mitigate errors. CRM-based team training has been demonstrated to improve clinician attitudes toward patient safety and decrease adverse events in obstetrics.
- Simulation is an effective way to teach CRM concepts.
- Simulation is effective in teaching both obstetric and obstetric anesthesia skills.
- Simulation is effective in assessing the performance of these skills by individual providers.
- In situ (within one's clinical environment) simulation is an effective and safe way to identify hidden problems (latent errors) that could pose a threat to patients. Once identified, improvements can be made to enhance the safety of the environment.
- The transfer of CRM concepts to the clinical environment requires a significant coaching and sustainment effort that may take years to successfully implement.
- Improved teamwork can lead to a culture of safety that may improve patient safety and the malpractice environment in ways not directly related to the teamwork training.

REFERENCES

1. Leape L. Scope of problem and history of patient safety. *Obstet Gynecol Clin North Am* 2008;35(1):1–10.
2. Adverse events in hospitals: national incidence among medicare beneficiaries. 2010 [cited 2010 12/14]; Available from: http://oig.hhs.gov/oei/reports/oei-06-07-00471.pdf.
3. Kohn LT, Corrigan J, Donaldson MS. *To Err is Human: Building a Safer Health System*. Washington, DC: National Academy Press; 2000;xxi:287.
4. Preventing Medication Errors: Quality Chasm Series. 2006 2/7/2011]; Available from: http://www.iom.edu/Reports/2006/Preventing-Medication-Errors-Quality-Chasm-Series.aspx.
5. Birnbach D. Can medical simulation and team training reduce errors in labor and delivery? *Anesthesiol Clin* 2008;26(1):159–168.
6. Salas E, DiazGranados D, Weaver SJ, et al. Does team training work? Principles for health care. *Acad Emerg Med* 2008;15(11):1002–1009.
7. Main EK, Bingham D. Quality improvement in maternity care: promising approaches from the medical and public health perspectives. *Curr Opin Obstet Gynecol* 2008;20(6):574–580.
8. Leape LL, Berwick DM. Five years after To Err Is Human: what have we learned? *JAMA* 2005;293(19):2384–2390.
9. Wachter RM. Patient safety at ten: unmistakable progress, troubling gaps. *Health Aff (Millwood)* 2010;29(1):165–173.
10. Landrigan CP, Parry GJ, Bones CB, et al. Temporal trends in rates of patient harm resulting from medical care. *N Engl J Med* 2010;363(22):2124–2134.
11. Liang BA. The adverse event of unaddressed medical error: identifying and filling the holes in the health-care and legal systems. *J Law Med Ethics* 2001;29(3–4):346–368.
12. Salas E, Wilson KA, Burke CS, et al. Myths about Crew Resource Management Training. *Ergonomics in Design* 2002(Fall):5.
13. Salas E, Wilson KA, Murphy CE, et al. What Crew Resource Management Training will not do for Patient Safety: Unless. *J Patient Saf* 2007;3(2):3.
14. Sexton JB. Error, stress, and teamwork in medicine and aviation: cross sectional surveys. *BMJ* 2000;320(7237):745–749.
15. Manser T. Teamwork and patient safety in dynamic domains of healthcare: a review of the literature. *Acta Anaesthesiol Scand* 2009;53(2):143–151.
16. Wu AW. Medical error: the second victim. The doctor who makes the mistake needs help too. *BMJ* 2000;320(7237):726–727.
17. Scott SD, Hirschinger LE, Cox KR, et al. The natural history of recovery for the healthcare provider "second victim" after adverse patient events. *Qual Saf Health Care* 2009;18(5):325–330.
18. Nielsen PE, Goldman MB, Mann S, et al. Effects of teamwork training on adverse outcomes and process of care in labor and delivery: a randomized controlled trial. *Obstet Gynecol* 2007;109(1):48–55.
19. Forster AJ, Fung I, Caughey S, et al. Adverse events detected by clinical surveillance on an obstetric service. *Obstet Gynecol* 2006;108(5):1073–1083.
20. Crofts JF, Ellis D, Draycott TJ, et al. Change in knowledge of midwives and obstetricians following obstetric emergency training: a randomised controlled trial of local hospital, simulation centre and teamwork training. *BJOG* 2007;114(12):1534–1541.
21. Clark S. Improved outcomes, fewer cesarean deliveries, and reduced litigation: results of a new paradigm in patient safety. *Am J Obstet Gynecol* 2008;199(2): 105.e1–105.e7.
22. Berg CJ, Chang J, Callaghan WM, et al. Pregnancy-related mortality in the United States, 1991–1997. *Obstet Gynecol* 2003;101(2):289–296.
23. Preventing infant death and injury during delivery. Joint Commission Sentinel Event Alert 2004 July 21 [cited 30; Available from: http://www.jointcommission.org/Sentinel_Event_Alert__Issue_30_Preventing_infant_death_and_injury_during_delivery_Additional_Resources/.
24. Gardner R, Raemer DB. Simulation in obstetrics and gynecology. *Obstet Gynecol Clin North Am* 2008;35(1):97–127, ix.
25. Schutte JM, Schuitemaker NW, van Roosmalen J, et al. Substandard care in maternal mortality due to hypertensive disease in pregnancy in the Netherlands. *BJOG* 2008;115(6):732–736.
26. Simpson KR, James DC, Knox GE. Nurse-physician communication during labor and birth: implications for patient safety. *J Obstet Gynecol Neonatal Nurs* 2006;35(4):547–556.
27. Sabir N, Yentis SM, Holdcroft A. A national survey of obstetric anaesthetic handovers. *Anaesthesia* 2006;61(4):376–380.
28. Gardner R, Walzer TB, Simon R, et al. Obstetric simulation as a risk control strategy: course design and evaluation. *Simul Healthc* 2008;3(2):119–127.
29. Thompson S, Neal S, Clark V. Clinical risk management in obstetrics: eclampsia drills. *BMJ* 2004;328(7434):269–271.
30. Daniels K, Lipman S, Harney K, et al. Use of simulation based team training for obstetric crises in resident education. *Simul Healthc* 2008;3(3):154–160.
31. Stumpf PG, Anderson B, Lawrence H, et al. Obstetrician-gynecologists' opinions about patient safety: costs and liability remain problems; are mandated reports a solution? *Womens Health Issues* 2009;19(1):8–13.
32. Maslovitz S, Barkai G, Lessing JB, et al. Recurrent obstetric management mistakes identified by simulation. *Obstet Gynecol* 2007;109(6):1295–300.
33. Rahman K, Jenkins JG. Failed tracheal intubation in obstetrics: no more frequent but still managed badly. *Anaesthesia* 2005;60(2):168–171.
34. Hawthorne L, Wilson R, Lyons G, et al. Failed intubation revisited: 17-yr experience in a teaching maternity unit. *Br J Anaesth* 1996;76(5):680–684.
35. Lipman S, Carvalho B, Brock-Utne J. The demise of general anesthesia in obstetrics revisited: prescription for a cure. *Int J Obstet Anesth* 2005;14(1):2–4.
36. Tsen LC, Pitner R, Camann WR. General anesthesia for cesarean section at a tertiary care hospital 1990–1995: indications and implications. *Int J Obstet Anesth* 1998;7(3):147–152.
37. Salas E, Fowlkes JE, Stout RJ, Milanovich DM, Prince C. Does CRM training improve teamwork skills in the cockpit? Two evaluation studies. *Human Factors* 1999;41(2):18.
38. Crew Resource Management (CRM) Training. 2006; Available from: http://www.caa.co.uk/docs/33/CAP737.PDF.
39. Helmreich RL, Merritt AC, Wilhelm JA. The evolution of Crew Resource Management training in commercial aviation. *Int J Aviat Psychol* 1999;9(1):19–32.
40. Pizzi LT, Goldfarb N, Nash DB. Crew resource management and its applications in medicine. In: D.B. Shojania KG, McDonald KM, Wachter RM, eds. *Making Health Care Safer: A Critical Analysis of Patient Safety Practices*. Agency for Healthcare Research and Quality; 2001.

41. Salas E, Sims D, Burke CCS. Is there a "Big Five" in Teamwork? *Small Group Research* 2005;36(5):5.

42. Mann S, Pratt SD. Team approach to care in labor and delivery. *Clin Obstet Gynecol* 2008;51(4):666–679.

43. Gaba. What Does Simulation Add to Teamwork Training?. WebM&M 2006; Available from: http://www.webmm.ahrq.gov/perspective.aspx?perspectiveID=20.

44. Pratt SD, S.B. Team training: classroom training vs. high-fidelity simulation Web M+M 2006; Available from: http://www.webmm.ahrq.gov/perspective.aspx?perspectiveID=21.

45. Cooper JB. Are simulation and didactic crisis resource management (CRM) training synergistic? *Qual Saf Health Care* 2004;13(6):413–414.

46. Grogan EL, Stiles RA, France DJ, et al. The impact of aviation-based teamwork training on the attitudes of health-care professionals. *J Am Coll Surg* 2004;199(6):843–848.

47. Gore DC, Powell JM, Baer JG, et al. Crew resource management improved perception of patient safety in the operating room. *Am J Med Qual* 2010; 25(1):60–63.

48. Lingard L, Regehr G, Orser B, et al. Evaluation of a preoperative checklist and team briefing among surgeons, nurses, and anesthesiologists to reduce failures in communication. *Arch Surg* 2008;143(1):12–17.

49. Morey JC, Simon R, Jay GD, et al. Error reduction and performance improvement in the emergency department through formal teamwork training: evaluation results of the MedTeams project. *Health Serv Res* 2002;37(6):1553–1581.

50. Awad SS, Fagan SP, Bellows C, et al. Bridging the communication gap in the operating room with medical team training. *Am J Surg* 2005;190(5):770–774.

51. Makary MA, Mukherjee A, Sexton JB, et al. Operating room briefings and wrong-site surgery. *J Am Coll Surg* 2007;204(2):236–243.

52. Uhlig PN, Brown J, Nason AK, et al. John M. Eisenberg Patient Safety Awards. System innovation: Concord Hospital. *Jt Comm J Qual Improv* 2002; 28(12):666–672.

53. Neily J, Mills PD, Young-Xu Y, et al. Association between implementation of a medical team training program and surgical mortality. *JAMA* 2010; 304(15):1693–1700.

54. Haynes AB, Weiser TG, Berry WR, et al. A surgical safety checklist to reduce morbidity and mortality in a global population. *N Engl J Med* 2009;360(5):491–499.

55. Defontes J, Surbida S. Preoperative safety briefing project. *Perm J* 2004;8(3):7.

56. Pronovost P, Berenholtz S, Dorman T, et al. Improving communication in the ICU using daily goals. *J Crit Care* 2003;18(2):71–75.

57. Friedman DM, Berger DL. Improving team structure and communication: a key to hospital efficiency. *Arch Surg* 2004;139(11):1194–1198.

58. Cooper S, Wakelam A. Leadership of resuscitation teams: "Lighthouse Leadership'. *Resuscitation* 1999;42(1):27–45.

59. Freeth D, Ayida G, Berridge EJ, et al. Multidisciplinary obstetric simulated emergency scenarios (MOSES): promoting patient safety in obstetrics with teamwork-focused interprofessional simulations. *J Contin Educ Health Prof* 2009; 29(2):98–104.

60. Pratt SD, Mann S, Salisbury M, et al. John M. Eisenberg Patient Safety and Quality Awards. Impact of CRM-based training on obstetric outcomes and clinicians' patient safety attitudes. *Jt Comm J Qual Patient Saf* 2007;33(12):720–725.

61. Haller G, Garnerin P, Morales MA, et al. Effect of crew resource management training in a multidisciplinary obstetrical setting. *Int J Qual Health Care* 2008;20(4):254–263.

62. Jha V, Kaufmann S, Duffy S. Simulated delivery suite (SiDeS) management course: An innovative methods for future training in obstetrics. *Innov Educ Teach International* 2003:40:6.

63. Farley DO, Sorbero ME, Lovejoy S, Salisbury M. Achieving Strong Teamwork Practices in Hospital Labor and Delivery Units. 2010 12/14/2010; Available from: http://www.rand.org/pubs/technical_reports/TR842.html.

64. Sexton JB, Helmreich RL, Neilands TB, et al. The Safety Attitudes Questionnaire: psychometric properties, benchmarking data, and emerging research. *BMC Health Serv Res* 2006;6:44.

65. Morgan PJ, Pittini R, Regehr G, et al. Evaluating teamwork in a simulated obstetric environment. *Anesthesiology* 2007;106(5):907–915.

66. Robertson B, Schumacher L, Gosman G, et al. Simulation-based crisis team training for multidisciplinary obstetric providers. *Simul Healthc* 2009;4(2):77–83.

67. Mann S, Pratt S, Gluck P, et al. Assessing quality obstetrical care: development of standardized measures. *Jt Comm J Qual Patient Saf* 2006;32(9):497–505.

68. Pettker CM, Thung SF, Norwitz ER, et al. Impact of a comprehensive patient safety strategy on obstetric adverse events. *Am J Obstet Gynecol* 2009; 200(5):492.e1–492.e8.

69. Grunebaum A, Chervenak F, Skupski D. Effect of a comprehensive obstetric patient safety program on compensation payments and sentinel events. *Am J Obstet Gynecol* 2011;204(2):97–105.

70. Shea-Lewis A. Teamwork: crew resource management in a community hospital. *J Healthc Qual* 2009;31(5):14–18.

71. Draycott T, Sibanda T, Owen L, et al. Does training in obstetric emergencies improve neonatal outcome? *BJOG* 2006;113(2):177–182.

72. Gosman G, Baldisseri MR, Stein KL, et al. Introduction of an obstetric-specific medical emergency team for obstetric crises: implementation and experience. *Am J Obstet Gynecol* 2008;198(4):367.e1–367.e7.

73. Skupski DW, Lowenwirt IP, Weinbaum FI, et al. Improving hospital systems for the care of women with major obstetric hemorrhage. *Obstet Gynecol* 2006; 107(5):977–983.

74. Grobman. Development and implementation of a team-centered shoulder dystocia protocol. *Simul Healthc* 2010;5(4):5.

75. TeamSTEPPS; Available from: http://team.ahrq.gov/abouttoolsmaterials.htm#online.

76. Behaviors that undermine a culture of safety. *Sentinel Event Alert* 2008;(40):1–3. Available from: http://www.jointcommission.org/SentinelEvents/SentinelEvent Alert/sea_40.htm.

77. Rosenstein AH, O'Daniel M. Impact and implications of disruptive behavior in the perioperative arena. *J Am Coll Surg* 2006;203(1):96–105.

78. Veltman LL. Disruptive behavior in obstetrics: a hidden threat to patient safety. *Am J Obstet Gynecol* 2007;196(6):587.e1–587.e4; discussion 587.e4–587.e5.

79. Maxfield D, Grenny J, McMillan R, et al. SilenceKills; The Seven Crucial Conversations for Healthcare. Available from: http://www.silencekills.com/PDL/SilenceKills.pdf.

80. Hanscom R. Medical Simulation from an insurer's perspective. *Acad Emerg Med* 2008;15(11):984–987.

81. Collins DE. Multidisciplinary teamwork approach in labor and delivery and electronic fetal monitoring education: a medical-legal perspective. *J Perinat Neonatal Nurs* 2008;22(2):125–132.

82. Nisselle P. Angered patients and the medical profession. *Med J Aust* 1999; 170(12):576–577.

83. Hampshire M. Why patients sue. *Nurs Stand* 2000;14(48):14–15.

84. Stelfox HT, Gandhi TK, Orav EJ, et al. The relation of patient satisfaction with complaints against physicians and malpractice lawsuits. *Am J Med* 2005;118(10):1126–1133.

85. Studdert DM, Mello MM, Gawande AA, et al. Disclosure of medical injury to patients: an improbable risk management strategy. *Health Aff (Millwood)* 2007;26(1):215–226.

86. Landis NT. Disclosure of errors may have financial benefit. *Am J Health Syst Pharm* 2000;57(4):312.

87. Meterko M, Mohr DC, Young GJ. Teamwork culture and patient satisfaction in hospitals. *Med Care* 2004;42(5):492–498.

88. Kilmer DM. Documentation—the nurses' defense. *Pa Nurse* 2007;62(1):19, 29.

89. Fanning R, Gaba D. Simulation-based learning as an educational tool. In: Stonemetz J, Ruskin K, eds. *Anesthesia Informatics*. New York, NY: Springer; 2008:459–479.

90. Macedonia CR, Gherman RB, Satin AJ. Simulation laboratories for training in obstetrics and gynecology. *Obstet Gynecol* 2003;102(2):388–392.

91. Denson JS, Abrahamson S. A computer-controlled patient simulator. *JAMA* 1969;208(3):504–508.

92. Howard SK, Gaba DM, Fish KJ, et al. Anesthesia crisis resource management training: teaching anesthesiologists to handle critical incidents. *Aviat Space Environ Med* 1992;63(9):763–770.

93. Siassakos D, Crofts JF, Winter C, et al. The active components of effective training in obstetric emergencies. *BJOG* 2009;116(8):1028–1032.

94. Fisher N, Bernstein PS, Satin A, et al. Resident training for eclampsia and magnesium toxicity management: simulation or traditional lecture? *Am J Obstet Gynecol* 2010;203(4):379.e1–379.e5.

95. Crofts JF, Bartlett C, Ellis D, et al. Training for shoulder dystocia: a trial of simulation using low-fidelity and high-fidelity mannequins. *Obstet Gynecol* 2006;108(6):1477–1485.

96. Ellis D, Crofts JF, Hunt LP, et al. Hospital, simulation center, and teamwork training for eclampsia management: a randomized controlled trial. *Obstet Gynecol* 2008;111(3):723–731.

97. Crofts JF, Bartlett C, Ellis D, et al. Patient-actor perception of care: a comparison of obstetric emergency training using manikins and patient-actors. *Qual Saf Health Care* 2008;17(1):20–24.

98. Black RS, Brocklehurst P. A systematic review of training in acute obstetric emergencies. *BJOG* 2003;110(9):837–841.

99. Merien AE, van de Ven J, Mol BW, et al. Multidisciplinary team training in a simulation setting for acute obstetric emergencies: a systematic review. *Obstet Gynecol* 2010;115(5):1021–1031.

100. Crofts JF, Bartlett C, Ellis D, et al. Management of shoulder dystocia: skill retention 6 and 12 months after training. *Obstet Gynecol* 2007;110(5):1069–1074.

101. Eason M, Olsen ME. High spinal in an obstetric patient: a simulated emergency. *Simul Healthc* 2009;4(3):179–183.

102. Maslovitz S, Barkai G, Lessing JB, et al. Improved accuracy of postpartum blood loss estimation as assessed by simulation. *Acta Obstet Gynecol Scand* 2008; 87(9):929–934.

103. Dildy GA 3rd, Paine AR, George NC, et al. Estimating blood loss: can teaching significantly improve visual estimation? *Obstet Gynecol* 2004;104(3):601–606.

104. Sorensen JL, Løkkegaard E, Johansen M, et al. The implementation and evaluation of a mandatory multi-professional obstetric skills training program. *Acta Obstet Gynecol Scand* 2009;88(10):1107–1117.

105. Gardiner J. Simulators in obstetric anaesthesia are a waste of time. *Int J Obstet Anesth* 2006;15(1):44–46.

106. Donald F. Simulators in obstetric anaesthesia are a waste of time. *Int J Obstet Anesth* 2006;15(1):46–49.

107. Leighton BL. A greengrocer's model of the epidural space. *Anesthesiology* 1989;70(2):368–369.

108. Friedman Z, Siddiqui N, Katznelson R, et al. Clinical impact of epidural anesthesia simulation on short- and long-term learning curve: High- versus low-fidelity model training. *Reg Anesth Pain Med* 2009;34(3):229–232.

109. Glassenberg R, Glassenberg S. Development of a tactile feedback simulator for placement of an epidural or spinal needle. *Anesthesiology* 2004;101:A-1358.

110. Magill JC, Byl MF, Hinds MF, et al. A novel actuator for simulation of epidural anesthesia and other needle insertion procedures. *Simul Healthc* 2010;5(3):179–184.

111. Toledo P, McCarthy RJ, Hewlett BJ, et al. The accuracy of blood loss estimation after simulated vaginal delivery. *Anesth Analg* 2007;105(6):1736–1740.

112. Toledo P, McCarthy RJ, Burke CA, et al. The effect of live and web-based education on the accuracy of blood-loss estimation in simulated obstetric scenarios. *Am J Obstet Gynecol* 2010;202(4):400.e1–400.e5.

113. Nair A, Alderson JD. Failed intubation drill in obstetrics. *Int J Obstet Anesth* 2006;15(2):172–174.

114. Goodwin M. Simulation as a training and assessment tool in the management of failed intubation in obstetrics. *Int J Obstet Anesth*. 2001;10(4):273–277.

115. Einav S, Matot I, Berkenstadt H, et al. A survey of labour ward clinicians' knowledge of maternal cardiac arrest and resuscitation. *Int J Obstet Anesth* 2008;17(3):238–242.

116. Forrest FC, Taylor MA, Postlethwaite K, et al. Use of a high-fidelity simulator to develop testing of the technical performance of novice anaesthetists. *Br J Anaesth* 2002;88(3):338–344.

117. Byrne AJ, Jones JG. Responses to simulated anaesthetic emergencies by anaesthetists with different durations of clinical experience. *Br J Anaesth* 1997;78(5):553–556.

118. Schwid HA, Rooke GA, Carline J, et al. Evaluation of anesthesia residents using mannequin-based simulation: a multiinstitutional study. *Anesthesiology* 2002;97(6):1434–1444.

119. Murray DJ, Boulet JR, Avidan M, et al. Performance of residents and anesthesiologists in a simulation-based skill assessment. *Anesthesiology* 2007;107(5):705–713.

120. Scavone BM, Sproviero MT, McCarthy RJ, et al. Development of an objective scoring system for measurement of resident performance on the human patient simulator. *Anesthesiology* 2006;105(2):260–266.

121. Riley W, Hansen H, Gürses AP, et al. The Nature, Characteristics and Patterns of Perinatal Critical Events Teams. Available from: http://www.ahrq.gov/downloads/pub/advances2/vol3/Advances-Riley_58.pdf.

122. Gaba DM. The future vision of simulation in healthcare. *Simul Healthc* 2007;2(2):126–135.

123. Anderson ER, Black R, Brocklehurst P. Acute obstetric emergency drill in England and Wales: a survey of practice. *BJOG* 2005;112(3):372–375.

124. Osman H, Campbell OM, Nassar AH. Using emergency obstetric drills in maternity units as a performance improvement tool. *Birth* 2009;36(1):43–50.

125. Deering S, Rosen MA, Salas E, et al. Building team and technical competency for obstetric emergencies: the mobile obstetric emergencies simulator (MOES) system. *Simul Healthc* 2009;4(3):166–173.

126. Johanson RB, Cox C, O'Donnell E, et al. Managing Obstetric Emergencies and Trauma (MOET). Structured skills training using models and reality-based scenarios. *Obstetrician and Gynaecologist* 1999;1:7.

127. Jyothi NK, Cox C, Johanson R. Management of obstetric emergencies and trauma (MOET): regional questionnaire survey of obstetric practice among career obstetricians in the United Kingdom. *J Obstet Gynaecol* 2001;21(2):107–111.

128. Johanson RB, Menon V, Burns E, et al. Managing Obstetric Emergencies and Trauma (MOET) structured skills training in Armenia, utilising models and reality based scenarios. *BMC Med Educ* 2002;2:5.

129. Johanson R, Akhtar S, Edwards C, et al. MOET: Bangladesh—an initial experience. *J Obstet Gynaecol Res* 2002;28(4):217–223.

130. Ryan JM, Macnad C, Mathieson A, et al. MOET in Iraq: enabling Iraqi doctors to develop a teaching model for obstetric emergencies and trauma. *The Obstetrician & Gynaecologist* 2004;6:5.

131. Bahl R, Murphy DJ, Strachan B. Non-technical skills for obstetricians conducting forceps and vacuum deliveries: qualitative analysis by interviews and video recordings. *Eur J Obstet Gynecol Reprod Biol* 2010;150(2):147–151.

132. Siassakos D, Draycott T, Montague I, et al. Content analysis of team communication in an obstetric emergency scenario. *J Obstet Gynaecol* 2009;29(6):499–503.

133. Miller KK, Riley W, Davis S, et al. In situ simulation: a method of experiential learning to promote safety and team behavior. *J Perinat Neonatal Nurs* 2008;22(2):105–113.

134. Gum L, Greenhill J, Dix K. Clinical simulation in maternity (CSiM): interprofessional learning through simulation team training. *Qual Saf Health Care* 2010;19(5):e19.

135. Draycott T, Crofts J. Structured team training in obstetrics and its impact on outcome. *Fetal Matern Med Rev* 2006;17(3):9.

136. Salas E, Wilson KA, Burke CS, et al. Using simulation-based training to improve patient safety: what does it take? *Jt Comm J Qual Patient Saf* 2005;31(7):363–371.

137. Savoldelli GL, Naik VN, Park J, et al. Value of debriefing during simulated crisis management: oral versus video-assisted oral feedback. *Anesthesiology* 2006;105(2):279–285.

138. Welke TM, LeBlanc VR, Savoldelli GL, et al. Personalized oral debriefing versus standardized multimedia instruction after patient crisis simulation. *Anesth Analg* 2009;109(1):183–189.

139. Salas E, Klein C, King H, et al. Debriefing medical teams: 12 evidence-based best practices and tips. *Jt Comm J Qual Patient Saf* 2008;34(9):518–527.

140. Rudolph JW, Simon R, Rivard P, et al. Debriefing with good judgment: combining rigorous feedback with genuine inquiry. *Anesthesiol Clin* 2007;25(2):361–376.

Near Misses and Maternal Mortality

Joy L. Hawkins

■ INTRODUCTION

The subspecialty of obstetric anesthesia has made tremendous efforts in the area of patient safety. Obstetric anesthesiologists have documented their practices and followed up on efforts to improve them. For example, three workforce surveys have documented how care is provided and hospitals are staffed in low and high volume delivery services (1). Obstetric anesthesiologists have updated the American Society of Anesthesiologists (ASA) practice guidelines, with evidence-based recommendations for care (2). There are published reviews of anesthesia-related maternal mortality from international (3), national (4), and state (5) sources that document how adverse outcomes occur so anesthesiologists can address and prevent them. The ASA Closed Claims Project database has extracted the obstetric anesthesia liability cases for review, reflection, and improvement of care (6). Team training and simulation have been used to improve performance in emergency situations on labor and delivery (7). Patient safety has clearly been at the forefront of obstetric anesthesia care. This chapter will review our understanding of maternal morbidity and mortality, both current status and areas where efforts can be focused to achieve further improvement.

The Centers for Disease Control and Prevention (CDC) published their U.S. maternal mortality data from 1991 to 1997 in 2003 (8). They noted that although death from complications of pregnancy has decreased by 99% since 1900, there have been no further decreases in the last two decades. In the 2003 report there were 4,200 pregnancy-related deaths with an overall mortality ratio of 11.8 deaths per 100,000 live births, a substantial increase from the 7 to 8/100,000 reported since 1982. In 1999 the national maternal mortality rate was 13.2 deaths per 100,000 live births. The appearance of an increase may be due to better methods of ascertainment, but it is certainly not decreasing and is still far from the Healthy People 2010 objective for maternal mortality of 3.3/100,000 live births. Those at greatest risk in their report were women of black race, women >34 years of age, and women who received no prenatal care. Among women who died after a live birth, the leading causes of death were embolism and hypertensive disorders of pregnancy.

A maternal death is devastating to all involved; after all, only in the obstetric patient can mortality be 200%. The most recent CDC report that reviewed US maternal mortality from 1998 to 2005 showed that although infant mortality has declined steadily due to increased survival of preterm infants and prevention of Sudden Infant Death Syndrome (SIDS), maternal mortality has not declined reaching 14.5/100,000 live births (9). This is the highest aggregate pregnancy-related mortality ratio of any period in the previous 20 years. Reasons for the lack of improvement are unclear but may include an actual increase, changes in coding from ICD-9 to ICD-10 and improved ascertainment from linkage of death certificates to live birth and fetal death certificates. Mortality remains 3 to 4 times higher for African-American women than white women. The causes of pregnancy-related deaths are shown in Figure 46-1. Non-cardiovascular medical conditions are now the most common cause of death (13% of deaths), followed by hemorrhage (12%), hypertensive disorders of pregnancy (12%), cardiovascular conditions (12%), cardiomyopathy (11%), infection (11%), and thrombotic pulmonary embolism (10%). Since their last report (8), deaths due to hemorrhage and hypertension continue to decrease, while those due to medical conditions, especially cardiac, continue to increase. Among deaths after a live birth, hypertensive disorders of pregnancy, cardiomyopathy, non-cardiovascular medical conditions and cardiovascular conditions were most common. Anesthetic deaths account for 1.2% of maternal deaths, and have fallen to tenth among the most common causes of maternal mortality in the United States (Table 46-1).

■ ALL-CAUSE MATERNAL MORTALITY IN THE UNITED STATES

Since 1991, the United States' CDC has defined maternal deaths as those that occur within 1 year of delivery (rather than the 42 days used previously) and that are related to the pregnancy (10). By extending the definition to 1 year after delivery, the percentage of deaths due to cardiomyopathy increased because those deaths often occur after a lengthy illness, but are still related to the pregnancy. Many maternal deaths (perhaps over 30%) are missed because the cause of death on the death certificate does not include the fact that she was pregnant. For example, if a woman dies of a pulmonary embolism but the death certificate does not record that she was pregnant, it would not be classified as a maternal death. The CDC asks states to link maternal death certificates with live birth or fetal death certificates, thus increasing identification of maternal deaths. This increased ascertainment may be the reason for an apparent increase in pregnancy-related deaths.

In the United States mothers are having their children at older ages. How does the change in demographics affect outcomes? Using the CDC database, investigators looked at maternal mortality in women having children after age 35 (11) and after age 50 (12). Although the actual risk of mortality was low, the risk ratio for deaths in all categories (hemorrhage, embolism, hypertension, cardiomyopathy, etc.) was increased after age 35. The authors note ". . . it is clear that for both the woman and her fetus, achieving pregnancy before age 35 is the safest course to follow." There were only 539 births among women aged 50 and older, but the risk of

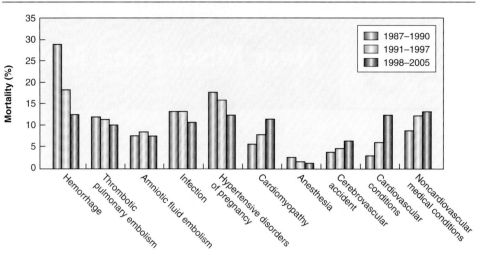

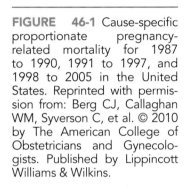

FIGURE 46-1 Cause-specific proportionate pregnancy-related mortality for 1987 to 1990, 1991 to 1997, and 1998 to 2005 in the United States. Reprinted with permission from: Berg CJ, Callaghan WM, Syverson C, et al. © 2010 by The American College of Obstetricians and Gynecologists. Published by Lippincott Williams & Wilkins.

preterm labor and low birth weight was higher, leading to increased fetal morbidity and mortality. Physicians have little or no control over the age when women choose to become pregnant, but they can certainly have more awareness of the increased risk to the mother when they are over age 35.

Ascertainment may also be improved when access to medical records is improved. A very large retrospective review of maternal deaths in a large US health care delivery system (HCA, the Hospital Corporation of America) examined the details of 95 maternal deaths in 1.5 million deliveries (6.5 deaths per 100,000 pregnancies) between 2000 and 2006 (13). Leading causes of death were preeclampsia, pulmonary thromboembolism, amniotic fluid embolism, hemorrhage, and cardiac disease. The most common preventable causes were failure to adequately control blood pressure in hypertensive women, failure to adequately diagnose and treat pulmonary edema in women with preeclampsia, failure to pay attention to vital signs following cesarean delivery, and hemorrhage following cesarean delivery. Rate by mode of delivery was strikingly different: 0.2/100,000 for vaginal and 2.2/100,000 for cesarean deliveries, or 11 times higher during cesarean delivery. That is a sobering statistic as cesarean delivery rates continue to rise and operative deliveries may be done solely for maternal request. Anesthesia is not listed as a cause of death in their series, but a personal communication with the author indicated there were two deaths attributed

to anesthetic management. One involved an unrecognized intravascular injection of local anesthetic through an epidural catheter and the second involved an anaphylactic reaction to antibiotics given by the anesthesiologist at the time of cesarean delivery. The conclusions from their study were that most maternal deaths in the United States are not preventable and occur in low risk pregnancies. Segregating delivery services into high and low risks will never be completely successful. The authors also state that universal thromboembolism prophylaxis for cesarean deliveries is the best way to decrease maternal mortality, but add that since neuraxial anesthesia is the most common anesthetic technique for cesarean delivery, pneumatic compression devices should be used in preference to anticoagulation.

A perinatal network of physicians was also able to do a detailed evaluation of their cases of maternal mortality, "near miss" morbidity, and severe morbidity (14). *The data showed that 41% of the deaths, 46% of the "near misses," and 17% of the severe morbidities should have been preventable.* Cardiac causes, stroke, and embolic diagnoses were higher among the deaths. Hemorrhage and infection were highest in the near-miss group, and preeclampsia was highest in the severe morbidity group. Patient factors were involved in 13% to 20%, systems issues in 33% to 47%, and provider issues in 90%. *In all groups, incomplete or inappropriate management was cited as the major factor.*

Other perinatal networks are also attempting to gather more complete data on maternal mortalities. A review of maternal deaths from 1992 to 1998 in a 10-hospital urban perinatal network in the United States found a strikingly higher maternal mortality ratio than that reported nationally; 22.8 maternal deaths per 100,000 live births rather than the reported national rate at the time of 7.5/100,000 (15). The group was able to identify all maternal deaths in their perinatal network, and because they formed a peer-review committee, they were able to review each case in detail. The deaths were deemed potentially preventable in 37%, and there was a provider factor identified in >80%. Pulmonary embolus and cardiac disease together accounted for 40% of the pregnancy-related deaths. There was only one anesthesia-related death, and it was attributed to central nervous system depression in a patient who was receiving multiple narcotics, as well as other potentially depressive medications during labor.

Using similar methodology, a state-maintained database was used to determine the incidence and causes of maternal mortality (16). They reported a high overall delivery mortality rate of 16.4/100,000 live births, which they also attributed to improved detection. Anesthesia-related mortality

TABLE 46-1 **Causes of Pregnancy Related Death during Live Birth in the United States, 1998–2005**

Hypertensive disorders	15.0%
Cardiomyopathy	13.3%
Cardiovascular conditions	12.5%
Non-cardiovascular conditions	11.3%
Hemorrhage	9.7%
Thrombotic pulmonary embolism	9.7%
Infection	9.2%
Amniotic fluid embolism	9.0%
Cerebrovascular accident	7.0%
Anesthesia complications	1.2%

Adapted from: Berg CJ, Callaghan WM, Syverson C, et al. Pregnancy-related mortality in the United States from 1998–2005. *Obstet Gynecol* 2010;116:1302–1309.

accounted for 5.2% of the deaths. Unfortunately, since it was an anonymous database, no further information could be obtained about the specifics of each case. Perinatal networks and state maternal mortality committees are able to more accurately identify all maternal deaths in their area and may provide more in-depth information to use in prevention programs.

A state maternal mortality committee in North Carolina identified all pregnancy-related deaths between 1995 and 1999, and determined the incidence of preventable deaths (17). Overall, 40% of deaths were preventable, but almost all deaths due to hemorrhage or exacerbation of a chronic disease were considered preventable. In contrast, almost none of the deaths due to amniotic fluid embolism or stroke were preventable. The most frequent cause of death was comorbidity associated with cardiomyopathy. Race was another factor that also influenced outcome. Among African-American women, 46% of deaths were potentially preventable compared to 33% of deaths among white women. The mortality ratio was 42/100,000 live births among African Americans, as compared to 12.3/100,000 among whites.

To summarize the common themes in all-cause maternal mortality studies:

- Approximately 40% of deaths are preventable.
- Provider issues contribute to most maternal deaths.
- The most common causes of maternal death are cardiac and non-cardiac medical conditions, thromboembolism, hemorrhage, hypertensive disorders, and cardiomyopathy. Coexisting medical conditions in pregnancy are now the most common cause of maternal death.
- Race plays a role with the deaths being more common amongst the African-American population.
- Older mothers are at higher risk.
- Deaths occur in low-risk as well as high-risk pregnancies.

Even when anesthesia is not the direct cause of death, anesthetic care contributes to the quality of the outcomes. The 2003–2005 Confidential Enquiry into Maternal and Child Health reviewed maternal deaths and found 31 cases due to other causes in which anesthesia contributed (3). These contributions included failure of the anesthesiologist to recognize serious illness or comorbidities, less than optimal anesthetic management of hemorrhage including delayed diagnosis, poor resuscitation in sepsis, inadequate control of hypertension in preeclampsia, and issues related to maternal obesity. Obstetric anesthesiologists must be prepared to handle disastrous complications associated with hemorrhage, thrombotic or amniotic fluid embolism, hypertension and sepsis as well as maternal coexisting diseases. Peripartum hemorrhage requires participation from everyone on the labor and delivery team.

A study of the epidemiology of postpartum hemorrhage in the United States from 1995 to 2004 found that postpartum hemorrhage complicated 2.9% of all deliveries and was associated with 19% of all in-hospital deaths after delivery (18). Although hemorrhage due to placental abnormalities can be severe, atony accounts for 79% of cases. Risk factors for uterine atony include age <20 or >40, cesarean delivery, hypertensive disorders, polyhydramnios, chorioamnionitis, multiple gestation, retained placenta, and antepartum hemorrhage, but other than extremes of age and cesarean delivery, risk factors were present in only 39% of cases. In other words, postpartum hemorrhage caused by uterine atony resulting in transfusion often occurs in the absence of recognized risk factors. Another cause of peripartum hemorrhage is uterine rupture. A review of 41 cases of uterine rupture found that only half occurred in women with a prior cesarean delivery, and of the remaining cases, only one-third had had uterine

surgery of other types (19). Nine uterine ruptures occurred before labor and the rest during labor. Results of studies such as these point out that parturients at risk of serious hemorrhage may be difficult to identify. Hospitals must adopt protocols for management of postpartum hemorrhage that include medications, operative and non-operative maneuvers, and massive transfusion protocols to guide care and prevent treatment delays.

Two studies reviewed obstetric morbidity in the United States. The first examined severe obstetric morbidity from 1998 to 2005 from the Nationwide Inpatient Sample of the Healthcare Cost and Utilization Project (20). They found that complications increased from 0.64% to 0.81% of delivery hospitalizations, with significant increases in renal failure, pulmonary embolism, adult respiratory distress syndrome, shock, blood transfusion, and ventilation. Increases paralleled the rising cesarean delivery rate during this time. Maternal age, parity, multiple births, and most comorbidities did not contribute to these outcomes. Only the increases in pulmonary embolism and blood transfusion were not accounted for by the rise in cesarean delivery rates from 21% to 30%. The second study used the National Hospital Discharge Survey data to estimate rates of intrapartum morbidity during 2001 to 2005 and compared them with rates during 1993 to 1997 (21). They did not find an increase in intrapartum obstetric complications even though the cesarean delivery rate increased from 21.8% to 28.3%. Rates of pregnancies complicated by preexisting medical conditions such as chronic hypertension, preeclampsia, gestational and preexisting diabetes, asthma and postpartum hemorrhage did increase by 20%, while rates of third- and fourth-degree lacerations and some infections decreased.

ANESTHESIA-RELATED MATERNAL MORTALITY

The epidemiology of maternal morbidity and mortality due to a direct anesthetic cause has been reviewed in several ways. The Healthcare Cost and Utilization Project State Inpatient Database was used to identify women in the New York state who experienced an anesthesia-related complication during labor and delivery from 2002 to 2005 (22). Significant risk factors for an anesthetic complication were cesarean delivery, rural area, preexisting medical condition, Caucasian race, and scheduled admission. Anesthetic complications occurred in 0.46% of women, but when complications occurred, mortality increased 22-fold. Spinal headache accounted for a third of the complications. Anesthesia-related causes of maternal mortality have become so uncommon, they are rarely mentioned in studies of all-cause maternal mortality. Data from the CDC shows that anesthesia-related maternal mortality in the United States has fallen by 59% since 1979 and stabilized at about 1 death per million live births (4). Results from the triennial reports in the United Kingdom are similar (Table 46-2).

In 1987 the CDC established an ongoing National Pregnancy Mortality Surveillance System to monitor maternal deaths at the national level and conduct epidemiologic studies of the deaths of pregnant women (23). Health departments in all 50 states, the District of Columbia, and New York City provide the CDC with copies of maternal death certificates with patient and provider identification removed. When available, linked birth certificates or fetal death records are also provided. These records are available since 1979 (4). The CDC has no legal ability to obtain medical records, autopsy reports, or other information that could provide detailed data, but some conclusions can be made. Using national statistics on cesarean delivery rates, the number of

TABLE 46-2 Pregnancy-related Mortality due to Anesthesia in the United States versus the United Kingdom

Triennium	United States[a]	United Kingdom[b]
1979–1981	4.3	8.7
1982–1984	3.3	7.2
1985–1987	2.3	1.9
1988–1990	1.7	1.7
1991–1993	1.4	3.5
1994–1996	1.1	0.5
1997–1999	1.2	1.4
2000–2002	1.0	3.0

[a]Pregnancy-related deaths due to anesthesia per million live births (limited to deaths associated with delivery of live births/stillbirths).
[b]Rate per million maternities.
Adapted from: Hawkins JL, Chang J, Palmer SK, et al. Anesthesia-related maternal mortality in the United States: 1979–2002. *Obstet Gynecol* 2011;117:69–74.

deaths reported to the CDC in each year, and estimates of the proportion of cesarean deliveries done under regional or general anesthesia each year (1), case fatality rates and risk ratios by type of anesthesia can be calculated (Table 46-3). In the 1980s, general anesthesia for cesarean delivery appeared to be much riskier than regional anesthesia. Since then, deaths associated with general anesthetics appear to be declining, while deaths associated with regional anesthesia may be increasing.

General versus Regional Anesthesia for Cesarean Delivery

Between 1979 and 1990, the number of deaths from general anesthesia remained relatively stable, but the number of deaths associated with regional anesthesia declined markedly, leading to a large risk ratio between the two techniques. This occurred despite the fact that regional anesthesia was being used more often for cesarean delivery in virtually every hospital (1,24). The decline in regional anesthetic deaths occurred in the mid-1980s, coincident with the withdrawal of 0.75% bupivacaine, increasing awareness of local anesthetic toxicity and inadvertent intrathecal injections, and increased use of test dosing.

From 1991 to 1996, the case fatality rate for general anesthesia fell. The improvement in mortality due to general anesthesia may be related to the development of improved monitoring techniques during general anesthesia. Standards for the use of pulse oximetry were published by the ASA in 1989 and required its use during every anesthetic, capnography became a requirement in 1995, and the ASA introduced the Difficult Airway Algorithm in 1993.

From 1997 to 2002, the case fatality rate for general anesthesia continued to fall as anesthesiologists became facile using the laryngeal mask airway and similar rescue devices to maintain ventilation in the difficult airway scenario. Two reviews from UK looked at failed intubations between 1993–1998 and 1999–2003 (25,26). The failed intubation rate was stable at 1:249 and 1:238 respectively, but there were no maternal deaths. Common themes in both surveys were that most failed intubations were emergencies after hours performed by trainees, and in over half of the cases the hospital's failed intubation protocol was not followed, that is, providers were giving a second dose of succinylcholine, giving repeated doses of hypnotic, and making over 3 attempts at laryngoscopy.

The relative risk of general anesthesia versus regional anesthesia has fallen to 1.7 in the most recent data from the CDC, with a 95% confidence interval 0.6 to 4.6, $p = 0.2$ (Table 46-3). There may be no real difference in fatality rates between the two techniques in modern practice. However, in contrast to the continued decline in case fatality rates for general anesthesia over the last 18 years (32.3 to 6.5 deaths per million general anesthetics), there is a continuing rise in case fatality rates for regional anesthesia (from 1.9 to 3.8 deaths per million regional anesthetics).

Despite recent improvements, the results in Table 46-3 show that general anesthesia has been riskier than regional anesthesia in the obstetric patient. Some of the factors that increase the risk of maternal morbidity or mortality during general anesthesia may include:

- General anesthesia requires that the airway be secured, and airway management with intubation has been shown to be more difficult in the obstetric patient than the surgical patient (25–27).
- General anesthesia is often chosen in emergencies when our preparation and preoperative examination of the patient is not optimal.
- General anesthesia is used in our highest risk patients who have contraindications to the use of regional anesthesia (e.g., hemorrhage, HELLP, cardiac lesions) or when attempts at regional have failed (e.g., morbid obesity). These patients often have increased risk factors for a difficult airway.
- Residency training programs may not provide trainees with adequate exposure to general anesthesia on their obstetric rotations because anesthesiologists, patients, and obstetricians prefer regional anesthesia (28).

TABLE 46-3 Case Fatality Rates and Risk Ratios by Type of Anesthesia in the United States, 1979–2002

Year of Death	Case Fatality Rates General Anesthetics[a]	Case Fatality Rates Regional Anesthetics[a]	Risk Ratios
1979–1984	20.0	8.6	2.3
1985–1990	32.3	1.9	16.7
1991–1996	16.8	2.5	6.7
1997–2002	6.5	3.8	1.7 (p = NS)

[a]Per million general or regional anesthetics.
Adapted from: Hawkins JL, Chang J, Palmer SK, et al. Anesthesia-related maternal mortality in the United States: 1979–2002. *Obstet Gynecol* 2011;117:69–74.

A review performed at a large tertiary care obstetric facility found general anesthesia was used in only about 5% of cesarean deliveries between 1990 and 1995 (29). The indications for cesarean delivery in patients receiving general anesthesia were non-reassuring fetal heart tracing, placenta previa or abruption, maternal disease (primarily HELLP, preeclampsia, or ITP), abnormal presentation, and cord prolapse. These can be the most emergent situations and highest risk patients. Their incidence of difficult intubation was about 1.3% with a single maternal mortality due to an unrecognized difficult airway. The same group updated their data to include the years 2000 to 2005 (30). They found the rate of general anesthesia for cesarean had declined, and ranged from 0.4% to 1.0% per year. The most common indications for general anesthesia were lack of time for regional anesthesia in an emergency situation followed by maternal contraindication to regional anesthesia, primarily severe preeclampsia and HELLP syndrome. Only one case of difficult intubation occurred and there was no adverse maternal outcome.

A nationwide study by the Maternal-Fetal Medicine Units Network quantified anesthesia-related complications associated with cesarean delivery in 37,142 cesarean procedures for singleton gestations (31). They found that 93% of mothers received a regional anesthetic with a 3% failure rate and rare maternal morbidity. General anesthesia was used when the decision-to-incision interval was less than 15 minutes (38% of the general anesthetics) or when ASA status was ≥ 4, (odds ratio 6.9). There was one maternal death in which the anesthetic was directly implicated. It occurred during an attempted awake fiberoptic intubation when the patient became hypoxic and had a cardiac arrest.

How will anesthesiologists maintain their skills in airway management for cesarean delivery when it is used so infrequently? Consider an anesthesiologist in practice at a hospital with 1,500 deliveries per year. If the cesarean delivery rate is 30%, there will be 450 cases each year, and if 5% are done using general anesthesia there will be roughly 22 cases per year. With multiple anesthesiologists in the group, some members will do no general anesthetics for cesarean delivery. It would appear that providing organized airway management programs for residents and practitioners will be necessary so they are prepared for obstetric airway emergencies. Regional anesthetic complications may also involve airway management. Several cases in the ASA Closed Claims database occurred during regional anesthetics when the block became too high for adequate ventilation and the airway could not be secured, leading to hypoxia and/or aspiration (6). There will be times when general anesthesia is the most appropriate choice for the patient, for example hemorrhage with hemodynamic instability or umbilical cord prolapse. In these cases it should not be avoided. The mortality rate was only 6.5 per million general anesthetics in the most recent data from the CDC, a remarkable safety record.

Sources of Detailed Information About Cases of Anesthetic Maternal Mortality

Acquiring detailed information about adverse outcomes related to anesthesia is crucial. The Confidential Enquiries into Maternal Deaths (CEMD) in the United Kingdom 2000 to 2002 marked 50 years of this medical audit (32). The leading cause of death in this report was again thromboembolism, as it was in the United States. There were seven deaths due to anesthesia, all involving general anesthesia. Unrecognized esophageal intubation occurred in three cases, all performed by trainees without senior backup. Another two patients had hypoventilation inadequately managed leading to cardiac arrest. One obese woman died from aspiration after a difficult

intubation scenario. One woman developed anaphylaxis during cesarean delivery, probably due to succinylcholine. There were another 20 deaths in which anesthetic management contributed to adverse outcomes, either because of lack of multidisciplinary cooperation, lack of appreciation of the severity of illness, poor perioperative care, or inadequate response during major hemorrhage.

The triennial report on maternal deaths that occurred between 2003 and 2005 was published in 2007 (33). The leading overall causes of maternal death were cardiac pathology and thromboembolism. Over half the women who died were obese, leading one of the authors to say "Obesity represents one of the greatest and growing threats to the childbearing population." Anesthesia deaths were eighth in frequency, but all were associated with substandard care and deemed avoidable as judged by the reviewers. An accompanying editorial notes: "As in the last report, among anesthetic deaths, 100% are classed as avoidable; elsewhere criticism of anesthetists is widespread . . . The overall impression is that obstetric anesthesia has not resolved its recurrent problems and is adding to the list" (34). Provider issues continued to be a common theme. The six deaths due to anesthesia included two obese women in early pregnancy, anesthetized by trainees, who suffered postoperative respiratory failure. Another obese woman with asthma had postoperative respiratory failure following cesarean delivery under spinal anesthesia. One woman had her bupivacaine epidural infusion connected in error to her intravenous line, and one died of complications of central venous access. The cause of death is unclear in the final case. In another 31 cases anesthesia care contributed. These were related to unrecognized or under-managed comorbidities or peripartum hemorrhage. Recommendations focus on protocols for management of morbidly obese women including antepartum anesthetic consultation, experienced practitioners supervising trainees during care of morbidly obese women, better blood pressure control in severe preeclampsia, and better recognition and aggressive management of obstetric hemorrhage. Although practice differs to some degree between the United States and the United Kingdom, the ability of the CEMD to review cases in detail is far superior than what is available in the United States.

The Centre for Maternal and Child Enquiries (CMACE) published the Eighth Report on Confidential Enquiries into Maternal Deaths in the United Kingdom in 2011 (35). There were 7 women (3%) who died from problems directly associated with their anesthetic; a rate of 0.31/100,000 maternities. Six of the seven, or 86%, were considered to have had substandard anesthetic or perioperative care. Four deaths related to loss of the airway: One at induction for an emergency cesarean, another postoperatively when a tracheotomy tube came out in the ICU and could not be replaced, a third who aspirated on emergence from general anesthesia for an emergency cesarean delivery, and a fourth from respiratory depression while receiving intravenous patient-controlled analgesia postoperatively. A fifth died following general anesthesia for abortion from a cardiac arrest that may have been related to her substance abuse history that was unknown to the anesthesiologist. A sixth death was caused by circulatory collapse from a blood transfusion reaction. An autopsy in the final case found an abscess in the lumbar and lower thoracic spinal canal after an uneventful spinal anesthetic, and she died of acute hemorrhagic disseminated leukoencephalitis. There were a further 18 deaths to which anesthetic care contributed, primarily failure to recognize acute severe illness such as sepsis, preeclampsia, anaphylaxis, and hemorrhage (35). CMACE also looks at intensive care issues for the obstetric patient (36). A common theme is late recognition of the severity of the parturient's illness, leading to delay in referral and transfer for specialist clinical care. For the first time in this report, sepsis is the leading cause of direct maternal death. Uncontrolled hemorrhage caused by uterine atony or amniotic fluid embolism is also an important issue in the intensive care unit.

In the United States, a state review of maternal deaths in Michigan found that 8 of 855 deaths were anesthesia-related, and in another 7 anesthesia contributed (5). All of the anesthesia-related deaths occurred during emergence or recovery from general anesthesia (not induction) and involved hypoventilation or airway obstruction. Obesity and African-American race were common factors associated with these deaths. In three cases inadequate supervision was an associated factor; two in which the nurse anesthetist was supervised by the operating obstetrician and one in which the anesthesiologist was absent for emergence from general anesthesia. All these cases raise the question of appropriate Post Anesthesia Care Unit (PACU) management after general anesthesia and additional monitoring for obese patients at risk for sleep-obstructed breathing. An accompanying editorial notes that each anesthesia practice must establish protocols that reduce risks associated with emergence from general anesthesia and during recovery (i.e., which PACU should we use after general anesthesia for cesarean delivery, main O.R. or Labor and Delivery (L&D)?) and address risks associated with obesity and obstructive sleep apnea (37). A survey of obstetric anesthesia directors found that 45% of their hospitals had no postanesthesia recovery training for L&D nursing staff and that 43% of obstetric anesthesia directors described L&D PACU care as inferior to the main operating room (38). These were fairly large delivery services with a median of 2,550 deliveries per year and a 30% cesarean delivery rate with 5% done under general anesthesia. The authors note that both the ASA and the American Society of Peri-Anesthesia Nurses (ASPAN) have guidelines that apply to all postoperative patients including cesarean deliveries, regardless of their recovery locations.

With obesity now so prevalent and obstructive sleep apnea a common comorbidity in the obese parturient, the L&D nursing and anesthesia teams should be well aware of the ASA "Practice Guidelines for the Perioperative Management of Patients with Obstructive Sleep Apnea" (39). Their recommendations on postoperative management include use of regional techniques for postoperative pain control where possible, multimodal analgesia to minimize use of systemic opioids, resumption of Continuous Positive Airway Pressure (CPAP) if used preoperatively, keeping the patient in a non-supine position, and continuous pulse oximetry on a monitored unit for patients at increased risk of obstruction or hypoxemia. The ASA "Practice Guidelines for the Prevention, Detection, and Management of Respiratory Depression Associated with Neuraxial Opioid Administration" suggest that patients receiving neuraxial morphine are at no increased risk of respiratory depression over those receiving parenteral opioids, and recommend respiratory and sedation monitoring every hour for the first 12 hours and every two hours for 24 hours when neuraxial morphine is used (40).

The Doctors Insurance Company reported on 22 anesthesiology malpractice claims filed after maternal cardiac arrests on labor and delivery wards between 1998 and 2006 (41). Outcomes were poor: 10/22 died, 11 had anoxic brain damage, and only 1 woman left the hospital neurologically intact. Thirteen cases were respiratory arrests following epidurals or spinals. Eight followed labor epidural placement with unintentional subarachnoid blocks (all occurring within 30 minutes of placement) and five occurred during spinal anesthetics for cesarean delivery. None of the cases that occurred in the operating room had audible alarms on the monitors at the time of arrest, making delay in response likely. In seven cases resuscitation of the mother was delayed because a decision was made to move her to the operating room, either to facilitate delivery or because airway equipment was not available in the labor room. The one woman who survived neurologically intact had ventilation with an Ambu bag begun immediately, and the obstetrician delivered the baby within minutes of the arrest. These outcomes indicate that any delay in ventilation or blood pressure support of the mother is devastating. Seven additional cases involved postpartum hemorrhage with delay in diagnosis and treatment with blood products. There were often systems issues involving communication, but the anesthesia care contributed to the arrest. Two cases involved preeclampsia, with arrest occurring at induction of anesthesia—one spinal anesthetic and one general anesthetic. Hypovolemia might have been involved. Only one case involved general anesthesia with a difficult airway.

Two surveys questioned physicians about their knowledge of cardiac arrest on L&D (42,43). Both concluded there was inadequate and limited knowledge among obstetric, anesthesia and emergency medicine personnel about basic concepts of resuscitation of the parturient. Test questions evaluated whether they knew the following management points:

- Maintain uterine displacement at all times.
- Maintain cricoid pressure during mask ventilation.
- Intubate immediately if possible.
- Use a higher sternal location for chest compressions.
- Do not change paddle placement during shock.
- Defibrillate even if the baby is not yet delivered.
- Use normal doses of medications per Advanced Cardiac Life Support (ACLS) protocols, including pressors.
- Perform cesarean delivery within 4 to 5 minutes of unsuccessful resuscitation with no cardiac rhythm.

This is an ideal area for simulation and team training to assess knowledge and improve outcomes for a rare event on L&D. Simulated obstetric crises leading to cardiac arrest found the teams made multiple errors in performance of both physical and cognitive tasks (44). Given that these simulations occurred in tertiary care high-risk obstetric centers where the teams knew the purpose of the simulation, one can only assume the performance at low volume emergency rooms or small hospitals would be worse.

Anesthesia personnel may be involved in the management of intrapartum cardiac arrest due to embolism, a leading cause of pregnancy-related death. In one case report, an amniotic fluid embolism occurred shortly after artificial rupture of membranes during labor, and successful resuscitation of the mother occurred only after cesarean delivery of the fetus in the labor room by the obstetrician while Cardiopulmonary Resuscitation (CPR) was ongoing (45). In another case, an air embolism occurred during cesarean delivery for placenta previa (46). Three anesthesia providers were unable to place a central line to aspirate air, and she could not be resuscitated. Although embolism is not an anesthesia-related cause of maternal mortality, anesthesia providers are always involved in treatment and resuscitation.

The 2009 ASA Closed Claims Project update of their obstetric anesthesia claims contrasted those claims occurring before 1990 with those claims occurring after 1990 through 2003, and there are some significant differences (6). Causes of maternal death or permanent brain damage due to general or regional anesthesia in the two time periods are shown in Table 46-4. The most common causes during general anesthesia were difficult intubation and maternal hemorrhage. In four of the cases, general anesthesia was induced despite the fact that preoperative assessment indicated tracheal intubation would be difficult. The most common cause of injury

TABLE 46-4 Causes of Maternal Death or Permanent Brain Damage in the American Society of Anesthesiologists Closed Claims Project, 1990 and Later

Type of Injury	Overall n = 69 (%)	General Anesthesia n = 28 (%)	Regional Anesthesia n = 41 (%)
High neuraxial block	15 (22)	0 (0)	15 (37)
Maternal hemorrhage	11 (16)	8 (29)	3 (7)
Embolic events	8 (12)	2 (7)	6 (15)
Difficult intubation	7 (10)	7 (25)	0 (0)
Preeclampsia/HELLP	5 (7)	3 (11)	2 (5)
Medication	5 (7)	0 (0)	5 (12)
Inadequate oxygenation/ ventilation	3 (4)	1 (4)	2 (5)
Aspiration of gastric contents	2 (3)	1 (4)	1 (2)
Neuraxial cardiac arrest	2 (3)	0 (0)	2 (5)
Hypertensive intracranial hemorrhage	2 (3)	1 (4)	1 (2)
Central venous catheter cx	1 (1)	1 (4)	0 (0)
Chorioamnionitis/ARDS	1 (1)	1 (4)	0 (0)
Airway obstruction	1 (1)	1 (4)	0 (0)
Others/unknown	6 (9)	2 (7)	4 (10)

Percentages do not sum to 100% due to rounding error.
ARDS, adult respiratory distress syndrome; HELLP, Hemolysis, elevated liver enzymes, low platelet count.
Adapted from: Davies JM, Posner KL, Lee LA, et al. Liability associated with obstetric anesthesia: A closed claims analysis. *Anesthesiology* 2009;110:131–139.

in regional anesthesia claims was high neuraxial block—12 during epidural and 3 during spinal anesthetics. Although most claims are related to cesarean deliveries (58%), those related to vaginal delivery are increasing. Compared to claims prior to 1990, claims for maternal death and brain damage are decreasing, but nerve injury claims are increasing and are now the most common cause of a lawsuit. Claims with substandard care decreased from 39% to 22%, payment was made less frequently (42% vs. 58% previously), and the median payment made also decreased from $455K to $222K; all positive findings. However, there were negative findings as well. Cases related to undetected intrathecal catheters increased, and providers were not always prepared to treat hypotension or airway emergencies when placing labor epidurals. Four cases describe patients requiring transfer to an operating room for resuscitation because there was no airway equipment in the labor room. These mistakes may be contributing to the increase in case fatality rates from regional anesthesia.

■ ANESTHETIC CAUSES OF NEAR MISSES AND MATERNAL MORBIDITY

Management of the Difficult Airway in Obstetrics

The incidence of failed intubation with standard direct laryngoscopy in obstetric patients was first reported to be 1:280 in 1985 (47). This compares to an incidence of failed intubation in the general operating room of 1:2230; seven times the chance of dealing with a failed intubation while you are providing general anesthesia on labor and delivery. Multiple reports in the years since have found the incidence to be remarkably similar even while maternal mortality during general anesthesia has declined (4). Two prospective audits in the United Kingdom from 1993 to 1998 (25) and 1999 to 2003

(26) found the incidence of failed intubation to be 1:249 and 1:238, respectively. However, there were no maternal mortalities or adverse outcomes in either report. An Australian prospective observational study reviewed 1,095 general anesthetics for cesarean delivery during 2005 to 2006 and found a failed intubation rate of 1:274, but the laryngeal mask airway was successfully used in all cases with no maternal mortalities (48). The most common indication for general anesthesia was the need for immediate delivery, obstetrician or patient request, and failed regional anesthesia. A large tertiary care hospital in the UnitedStates reviewed their general anesthetics during 2000 to 2005 (29). They found the incidence of general anesthesia was only 0.6% with most being done because of urgency or maternal medical conditions. There was only one difficult intubation with no maternal mortalities. They note that anesthesiologists retain their skills with difficult airway equipment in non-obstetric patients. The ASA Closed Claims Project also found that although claims for difficult intubation did not change since 1990 compared to before, there were no claims for esophageal intubation (Table 46-4). Claims for aspiration fell to less than 1% and those for inadequate oxygenation or ventilation fell from 5% pre-1990 to 1% from 1990 to 2003. Closed Claims data may also indicate that anesthesiologists' skill with difficult airway equipment and adherence to difficult airway algorithms have improved maternal outcomes (49). Difficult airways in obstetric patients may be just as common, but adverse outcomes seem increasingly rare.

All personnel on L&D should be familiar with the ASA' Difficult Airway Algorithm (50). Anesthesiologists should educate the nursing and obstetric teams about their roles in the failed intubation scenario. In addition, there should be airway supplies on L&D with a variety of airway adjuncts for managing the difficult airway. General operating rooms have a difficult airway cart, and L&D should have the same access to its own emergency equipment. The ASA Practice Guidelines for Obstetric Anesthesia (2) state that "Labor and delivery units should have equipment and personnel readily available to manage airway emergencies. Basic airway equipment should be immediately available during the provision of regional anesthesia. In addition, portable equipment for difficult airway management should be readily available in the operative area of labor and delivery units."

A "prophylactic regional anesthetic" should be considered when the anesthesiologist anticipates a difficult airway (2). If the anesthesia team recognizes a patient has a difficult airway, the obstetrician and anesthesiologist should discuss placement of a continuous epidural or spinal catheter as soon as she is committed to delivery. In "*Guidelines for Perinatal Care, 6th ed.*" risk factors that should initiate an anesthetic consultation are listed, including those that might indicate a difficult airway (51). It goes on to say "Strategies thereby can be developed to minimize the need for emergency induction of general anesthesia in women for whom this would be especially hazardous. For those patients at risk, consideration should be given to the planned placement in early labor of an intravenous line and an epidural or spinal catheter with confirmation that the catheter is functional." In the event there is fetal distress or other need to proceed emergently to the operating room, regional anesthesia can be provided expediently. In addition, the obstetric team should understand that starting a case emergently will take extra time to place a regional anesthetic or to secure the airway. Administer aspiration prophylaxis to any patient with a potentially difficult airway as soon as operative delivery is anticipated. Medications such as H_2-receptor blocking agents may take an hour for maximum effectiveness. Have extra, experienced hands available at induction of general anesthesia. Other anesthesiology providers should be made aware when there is a patient with a difficult airway on L&D so they can be prepared to assist if airway management becomes necessary.

Despite best efforts, occasionally anesthesiologists have an unsuspected difficult airway and intubation is unsuccessful (52). If mask ventilation is difficult or impossible, move immediately to a laryngeal mask airway or other method of ventilation. Because of the parturient's higher metabolic rate and lower functional residual capacity, she will become hypoxic and suffer neurologic injury faster than the nonpregnant patient. If the situation deteriorates and cardiopulmonary resuscitation is necessary, ". . . standard resuscitative measures and procedures, including left uterine displacement should be taken. In cases of cardiac arrest, the American Heart Association has stated the following: "Several authors now recommend that the decision to perform a perimortem cesarean delivery should be made rapidly, with delivery accomplished within 4 to 5 minutes of the arrest." (2,53).

Reports from the United States (5) and Great Britain (3) indicate that extubation and recovery are now at-risk times for loss of the airway. Anesthesiologists and L&D nursing staff must be alert to the increased risk in the postoperative period posed by parturients who are obese or have obstructive sleep apnea and are receiving magnesium for preeclampsia or require neuraxial or systemic opioids for pain control. They may require additional monitoring or recovery in a step-down unit elsewhere in the hospital (39,40).

Aspiration of Gastric Contents

Through increased awareness of the difficult airway, consistent use of rapid sequence induction and cuffed endotracheal tubes, fasting guidelines, use of antacids, H_2-receptor antagonists and metoclopramide, and predominant use of regional anesthesia, cases of aspiration have become extremely rare.

Although rare, aspiration has been reported as a cause of death in both the ASA Closed Claims analysis (6) and in the Confidential Enquiries in Great Britain (33). Aspiration is frequently associated with a difficult or failed intubation. Encouraging use of regional anesthesia seems to be an obvious solution, but aspiration can also occur during a high spinal or epidural block when the patient cannot cough or clear her airway effectively. In addition to NPO policies, decreasing the volume and acidity of gastric contents pharmacologically should be considered before any cesarean delivery (2), but there are no outcome studies to prove use of these medications is beneficial (54). Opiates are known to delay gastric emptying, so regional analgesia for labor should be favored in patients with a suspected difficult airway. Both the ASA Practice Guidelines for Obstetric Anesthesia (2) and several American College of Obstetricians and Gynecologists' statements (51) support modest amounts of clear liquids in labor but oppose any intake of solid foods. The ASA Guidelines go on to say ". . . patients with additional risk factors of aspiration (e.g., morbid obesity, diabetes, difficult airway), or patients at increased risk for operative delivery (e.g., non-reassuring fetal heart rate pattern) may have further restrictions of oral intake, determined on a case-by-case basis." Anesthesiologists should teach their nursing colleagues on L&D the correct method of providing cricoid pressure, and provide training for them on the steps in the difficult airway algorithm. This is an ideal use of simulation and team training.

Local Anesthetic Systemic Toxicity (LAST)

Local anesthetic toxicity was the leading cause of death during regional anesthesia in the 1980s (55); however, its occurrence has decreased markedly and the Closed Claims project had no cases after 1990 (49). Newer local anesthetics such as ropivacaine and levobupivacaine may have a better safety profile than bupivacaine, but lidocaine still has the best safety profile of the amide drugs. Prevention of local anesthetic toxicity centers on aspiration of the epidural catheter, incremental dosing, and use of a test dose. The incidence of undetected intravascular placement of a multiorifice epidural catheter after negative aspiration is estimated to be only 0.6% (56).

The ideal test dose for the parturient has been controversial. A test dose is administered through the epidural catheter with two markers; one which would show whether the catheter is in a blood vessel to prevent local anesthetic systemic toxicity, and another which would show whether the catheter is in the cerebrospinal fluid (CSF) to prevent an extremely high block or "total spinal." A number of different drugs and techniques have been used with varying degrees of success. Epinephrine is the most commonly used agent to test for intravascular placement of an epidural catheter, but dose–response curves in parturients are different from that in nonpregnant patients, epinephrine can adversely affect uterine blood flow, the specificity is poor in a laboring patient whose heart rate varies with contractions, and there are adverse maternal consequences if the patient has preeclampsia or chronic hypertension. Other test dose regimens advocated for the parturient include 2-chloroprocaine, air, fentanyl or sufentanil, aspiration and fractionation only without a marker, and isoproterenol (only theoretical pending neurotoxicity studies). A systematic review of studies for detection of intravascular epidural catheter placements found 100 μg fentanyl reliably produced sedation, drowsiness or dizziness within 5 minutes after injection in pregnant patients with a sensitivity of 92 to 100 (57). Accidental intravenous injection of fentanyl would certainly have less adverse consequences for the fetus and mother than accidental intravenous injection of 15 μg epinephrine.

The American Society of Regional Anesthesia (ASRA) published a practice advisory on local anesthetic systemic toxicity (LAST) that provides recommendations for prevention and treatment. Methods of prevention include using the smallest total dose (volume × concentration) that will be clinically effective, dosing in small increments, frequent aspiration, intravascular markers such as fentanyl or epinephrine, and for peripheral nerve blocks, consideration of ultrasound guidance (58). Treatment of LAST will include stopping any seizures with benzodiazepines or induction agents. ACLS algorithms should be modified with smaller initial doses of epinephrine, use of amiodarone, consideration of lipid emulsion therapy with 1.5 mL/kg 20% solution, and avoiding vasopressin, calcium channel blockers, beta blockers, and lidocaine (59). The mechanism of action of lipid therapy is probably reduced binding of local anesthetic to cardiac tissue due to their solubility in the lipid phase (a "lipid sink") and a positive metabolic effect on cardiac myocytes. Animal studies have shown that epinephrine in doses higher than 10 μg/kg worsens recovery from bupivacaine systemic toxicity by increasing lactate levels and impairing lipid resuscitation (60).

High Spinal or Epidural Block

Preventing a high spinal or epidural block also involves test dosing to detect inadvertent injection of local anesthetic into the CSF. The incidence of subarachnoid injection after negative aspiration of an epidural catheter is quite rare, with an incidence of 0.06% to 0.0008% (61). The extent of spinal block depends on the number of milligrams of local anesthetic given, baricity of the solution, the volume used, and the position of the patient. The best indicator of an inadvertent subarachnoid injection in the laboring parturient is onset; if she is comfortable within one contraction, the catheter is subarachnoid until proven otherwise. Most cases of high neuraxial block in the ASA Closed Claims report were related to epidural catheters that had migrated subarachnoid (80%) rather than spinal anesthetics (20%) (6).

If a "total" spinal occurs, there are two problems to be addressed: (1) Lack of preload and an empty heart causing hypotension and decreased cardiac output, and (2) paralysis of the respiratory muscles leading to hypoventilation and aspiration. Treatment involves airway management with ventilation and intubation, fluids, pressors, left uterine displacement and elevation of the legs to promote venous return and improve cardiac output. Airway equipment and vasopressors must be immediately available to prevent adverse maternal outcome (6,41). The best maternal outcome results from rapid airway management and pressors with delivery of the fetus within 5 minutes if cardiac arrest occurs.

Obstetric Hemorrhage

Although hemorrhage is not a direct anesthetic cause of death, massive hemorrhage in the parturient will always require participation of the anesthesiologist. The anesthesiologist can strongly influence patient outcome in a negative or positive way. The ASA Closed Claims analysis contained 10 maternal deaths due to an inability of the anesthesiologist to keep up with blood loss (6). The causes of hemorrhage were subcapsular hepatic bleeding in a preeclamptic patient, placenta previa, placenta accreta or percreta, and uterine rupture. The Confidential Enquiry from 2003 to 2005 also describes 17 maternal deaths from hemorrhage with suboptimal anesthetic management contributing to adverse outcomes (35). Many failures were due to delayed recognition because of failure to interpret the vital signs correctly, administration of cold fluids and blood products, failure to appropriately use invasive monitoring, and poor perioperative management of women with placenta accreta. Having adequate help from additional anesthesia providers is key.

Recent literature from war trauma and from major vascular surgery indicates that survival may be improved by transfusing packed red blood cells (PRBCs) and plasma (FFP) in a 1:1 ratio (62). Fibrinogen levels can be used to predict the severity of postpartum hemorrhage (63). If the fibrinogen level is less than 200 at the time of initial diagnosis of hemorrhage, there is a 100% positive predictive value that they will require at least 4 units PRBC. The mechanism appears to be consumption of fibrinogen related to exposure of tissue factor on the endometrial surface. Another new therapy for intractable hemorrhage is recombinant activated factor VII (rFVIIa). The Australian and New Zealand Haemostasis Registry reported on 110 cases of administration of rFVIIa to obstetric patients (64). They reported a high success rate of 76%, with 64% responding to the first dose. There were two thromboembolic events but no related mortality. rFVIIa is expensive, and lack of randomized controlled trials reserves its use for intractable obstetric hemorrhage when other therapies have failed. Dosing should begin with 40 μg/kg.

■ CONCLUSIONS

In summary, there is room for both optimism and improvement (65). Anesthesia-related maternal mortality rates are improving (Table 46-2). In the early 1980s test dosing and incremental dosing of epidural catheters was accepted, and spinal bupivacaine became the standard spinal local anesthetic. In the 1990s anesthesiologists began requiring better monitoring with pulse oximetry and capnography, the laryngeal mask airway and other rescue devices became widely available, and the ASA difficult airway algorithm became standard teaching. In 2000 lipid emulsion was adopted as standard therapy for local anesthetic systemic toxicity and the ASA revised their practice guidelines to emphasize that L&D units should have the same staffing and equipment as the general operating rooms and PACUs. Obstetric anesthesiologists have focused their efforts and attention on areas of concern and accomplished notable improvements in outcomes. However, anesthesiologists are likely to be challenged in the future by parturients who are older, have more comorbidities such as congenital heart disease, are increasingly obese, and are more likely to require a cesarean delivery. Continuing development of new strategies will be needed to prevent and treat morbidity and mortality in obstetric patients (66).

In contrast to the success in obstetric anesthesia, the United States' overall maternal mortality ratio is worse than that of 40 other countries, leading Amnesty International to condemn the US record for maternal health as a public health emergency and a human rights crisis (65,67). Care of the parturient is a team effort that will involve the anesthesiologist as a perioperative physician. A Joint Commission Sentinel Alert (68) suggested actions that can help hospitals and providers prevent maternal death:

1. Educate physicians and other clinicians who care for women with underlying medical conditions about the additional risks that could be imposed if pregnancy were added. Communicate identified pregnancy risks to all members of the health care delivery team.
2. Identify specific triggers for responding to changes in the mother's vital signs and clinical condition, and develop and use protocols and drills for responding to changes, such as hemorrhage and preeclampsia.

3. Educate emergency room personnel about the possibility that a woman, whatever her presenting symptoms, may be pregnant or may have recently been pregnant. Many maternal deaths occur before the woman is hospitalized or after she delivers and is discharged. Knowledge of pregnancy may affect the diagnosis or appropriate treatment.
4. Refer high-risk patients to the care of experienced prenatal care providers with access to a broad range of specialized services.
5. Make pneumatic compression devices available for patients undergoing cesarean delivery who are at high risk for pulmonary embolism.
6. Evaluate patients who are at high risk for thromboembolism for low molecular weight heparin for postpartum care (68).

More information should be available to review individual cases when a bad outcome or a "near miss" occurs. Access to all information about maternal mortalities should be required in an environment free of concerns about legal liability. In that environment anesthesiologists can analyze why mishaps occurred and research ways to prevent them in the future. Valuable information can be gained from studying "near misses" and the ways in which mortalities or adverse outcomes were avoided in those instances. Anesthesiologists should be able to learn from each other's mistakes so as not to repeat them.

KEY POINTS

- Anesthesia complications are a rare cause of maternal mortality in the United States, accounting for less than 1.2% of maternal deaths. The most common causes of death are coexisting conditions, both non-cardiovascular and cardiac, hypertensive disorders, hemorrhage, cardiomyopathy, infection, and thromboembolism.
- Studies of maternal mortality from all causes show that about 40% are preventable, provider issues contribute to most deaths, there are racial differences, older mothers are more at risk, and deaths occur in both low- and high-risk pregnancies.
- Inadequate anesthesia care can contribute to maternal death from other causes such as hemorrhage and coexisting disease. Anesthesia providers can influence outcomes in a negative or positive way.
- The incidence of difficult intubation in the parturient has been reported to be 1 in 240 to 280 patients in several reports, but rarely results in maternal death since the advent of difficult airway algorithms and difficult airway devices such as supraglottic airways.
- Deaths during general anesthesia are declining in the United States while deaths during regional anesthesia may be increasing, with high blocks the most common cause of death. In current obstetric anesthesia practice, there appears to be no difference in case fatality rates between general or regional anesthesia for cesarean delivery.
- General anesthesia is currently used in less than 5% of cesarean deliveries, so exposure of anesthesiologists to obstetric airway management is very limited. Most general anesthetics are done during emergency (STAT) cesareans or in patients with significant comorbidities, i.e., the sickest patients and most hurried cases.
- Recent reports indicate that respiratory compromise at extubation and emergence are an increasing source of maternal morbidity and mortality. Although the ASA Practice Guidelines for Obstetric Anesthesia state that recovery

room (PACU) care on L&D must be equivalent to that provided in the main operating room, 45% of obstetric anesthesia directors report that their hospitals have no PACU training for L&D nurses, and 43% of directors describe their L&D PACU as inferior to the main operating room.
- When a maternal cardiac arrest occurs antepartum, delivery of the fetus should be accomplished within 4 to 5 minutes if an effective cardiac rhythm has not been reestablished, to improve resuscitation of the mother.
- In addition to low dose epinephrine and ACLS protocols, 20% lipid emulsion should be immediately available on L&D and administered in a dose of 1.5 mL/kg if a parturient has sustained LAST resulting in cardiac arrest.
- Based on results from war trauma and major vascular surgeries, survival of massive hemorrhage may be improved by transfusion of PRBCs and FFP in a 1:1 ratio with early administration of platelets. rFVIIa may also be considered for intractable hemorrhage.

REFERENCES

1. Bucklin BA, Hawkins JL, Anderson JR, et al. Obstetric anesthesia workforce survey. *Anesthesiology* 2005;103:645–653.
2. ASA Task Force on Obstetric Anesthesia. Practice guidelines for obstetric anesthesia. An updated report. *Anesthesiology* 2007;106:843–863.
3. Cooper GM, McClure JH. Anaesthesia chapter from saving mothers' lives; reviewing maternal deaths to make pregnancy safer. *Br J Anaesth* 2008;100:17–22.
4. Hawkins JL, Chang J, Palmer SK, et al. Anesthesia-related maternal mortality in the United States: 1979–2002. *Obstet Gynecol* 2011;117:69–74.
5. Mhyre JM, Riesner MN, Polley LS, et al. A series of anesthesia-related maternal deaths in Michigan, 1985–2003. *Anesthesiology* 2007;106:1096–1104.
6. Davies JM, Posner KL, Lee LA, et al. Liability associated with obstetric anesthesia: A closed claims analysis. *Anesthesiology* 2009;110:131–139.
7. Pettker CM, Thung SF, Norwitz ER, et al. Impact of a comprehensive patient safety strategy on obstetric adverse events. *Am J Obstet Gynecol* 2009;200:492.e1–e8.
8. Berg CJ, Chang J, Callaghan WM, et al. Pregnancy-related mortality in the United States, 1991–1997. *Obstet Gynecol* 2003;101:289–296.
9. Berg CJ, Callaghan WM, Syverson C, et al. Pregnancy-related mortality in the United States from 1998–2005. *Obstet Gynecol* 2010;116:1302–1309.
10. Berg CJ, Atrash HK, Koonin LM, et al. Pregnancy-related mortality in the United States, 1987–1990. *Obstet Gynecol* 1996;88:161–167.
11. Callaghan WM, Berg CJ. Pregnancy-related mortality among women aged 35 years and older, United States, 1991–1997. *Obstet Gynecol* 2003;102:1015–1021.
12. Salihu HM, Shumpert MN, Slay M, et al. Childbearing beyond maternal age 50 and fetal outcomes in the United States. *Obstet Gynecol* 2003;102:1006–1014.
13. Clark SL, Belfort MA, Dildy GA, et al. Maternal death in the 21st century: Causes, prevention, and relationship to cesarean delivery. *Am J Obstet Gynecol* 2008;199:36.e1–e5.
14. Geller SE, Rosenberg D, Cox SM, et al. The continuum of maternal morbidity and mortality: factors associated with severity. *Am J Obstet Gynecol* 2004;191:939–944.
15. Panting-Kemp A, Geller SE, Nguyen T, et al. Maternal deaths in an urban perinatal network, 1992–1998. *Am J Obstet Gynecol* 2000;183:1207–1212.
16. Panchal S, Arria AM, Labhsetwar SA. Maternal mortality during hospital admission for delivery: a retrospective analysis using a state-maintained database. *Anesth Analg* 2001;93:134–141.
17. Berg CJ, Harper MA, Atkinson SM, et al. Preventability of pregnancy-related deaths. Results of a state-wide review. *Obstet Gynecol* 2005;106:1228–1234.
18. Bateman BT, Berman MF, Riley LE, et al. The epidemiology of postpartum hemorrhage in a large, nationwide sample of deliveries. *Anesth Analg* 2010;110:1368–1373.
19. Porreco RP, Clark SL, Belfort MA, et al. The changing specter of uterine rupture. *Am J Obstet Gynecol* 2009;200:269.e1–e4.
20. Kuklina EV, Meikle SF, Jamieson DJ, et al. Severe obstetric morbidity in the United States: 1998–2005. *Obstet Gynecol* 2009;113:293–299.
21. Berg CJ, MacKay AP, Qin C, et al. Overview of maternal morbidity during hospitalizations for labor and delivery in the United States: 1993–1997 and 2001–2005. *Obstet Gynecol* 2009;113:1075–1081.
22. Cheesman K, Brady JE, Flood P, et al. Epidemiology of anesthesia-related complications in labor and delivery, New York State, 2002–2005. *Anesth Analg* 2009;109:1174–1181.

23. Koonin LM, Atrash HK, Rochat RW, et al. Maternal mortality surveillance, United States, 1980–1985. *MMWR* 1988;37:19–29.

24. Hawkins JL, Gibbs CP, Orleans M, et al. Obstetric anesthesia work force survey, 1981 versus 1992. *Anesthesiology* 1997;87:135–143.

25. Barnardo PD, Jenkins JG. Failed tracheal intubation in obstetrics: A 6-year review in a UK region. *Anaesthesia* 2000;55:685–694.

26. Rahman K, Jenkins JG. Failed tracheal intubation in obstetrics: No more frequent but still managed badly. *Anaesthesia* 2005;60:168–171.

27. Samsoon GL, Young JR. Difficult intubation: A retrospective study. *Anaesthesia* 1987;42:487–490.

28. Searle RD, Lyons G. Vanishing experience in training for obstetric general anaesthesia: An observational study. *Int J Obstet Anesth* 2008;17:233–237.

29. Tsen LC, Pitner R, Camann WR. General anesthesia for cesarean section at a tertiary care hospital 1990-1995: Indications and implications. *Int J Obstet Anesth* 1998;7:147–152.

30. Palanisamy A, Mitani AA, Tsen LC. General anesthesia for cesarean delivery at a tertiary care hospital from 2000–2005: A retrospective analysis and 10-year update. *Int J Obstet Anesth* 2011;20:10–16.

31. Bloom SL, Spong CY, Weiner SJ, et al. Complications of anesthesia for cesarean delivery. *Obstet Gynecol* 2005;106:281–287.

32. Cooper GM, McClure JH. Maternal deaths from anaesthesia. An extract from why mothers die 2000–2002, the confidential enquiries into maternal deaths in the United Kingdom. Chapter 9: Anaesthesia. *Br J Anaesth* 2005;94:417–423.

33. Lewis G, ed. *The confidential enquiry into maternal and child health (CEMACH). Saving mother's lives: Reviewing maternal deaths to make motherhood safer – 2003–2005. The Seventh Report on Confidential Enquiries into Maternal Deaths in the United Kingdom.* London: CEMACH; 2007.

34. Lyons G. Saving mother's lives: Confidential enquiry into maternal and child health 2003–5. *Int J Obstet Anesth* 2008;17:103–105.

35. McClure J, Cooper G. (on behalf of the Centre for Maternal and Child Enquiries). Chapter 8: Anaesthesia. *BJOG* 2011;118(suppl 1):102–108.

36. Clutton-Brock T. (on behalf of the Centre for Maternal and Child Enquiries). Chapter 16: Critical care. *BJOG* 2011;118(suppl 1):173–180.

37. D'Angelo R. Anesthesia-related maternal mortality; a pat on the back or a call to arms? *Anesthesiology* 2007;106:1082–1084.

38. Wilkins KK, Greenfield MLVH, Polley LS, et al. A survey of obstetric perianesthesia care unit standards. *Anesth Analg* 2009;108:1869–1875.

39. ASA Task Force on Obstructive Sleep Apnea. Practice guidelines for the perioperative management of patients with obstructive sleep apnea. *Anesthesiology* 2006;104:1081–1093.

40. ASA Task Force on Neuraxial Opioids. Practice guidelines for the prevention, detection, and management of respiratory depression associated with neuraxial opioid administration. *Anesthesiology* 2009;110:218–230.

41. Lofsky AS. Doctors Company reviews maternal arrest cases. APSF Newsletter Summer 2007; 28–30.

42. Cohen SE, Andes LC, Carvalho B. Assessment of knowledge regarding cardiopulmonary resuscitation of pregnant women. *Int J Obstet Anesth* 2008;17:20–25.

43. Einav S, Matot I, Berkenstadt H, et al. A survey of labour ward clinicians' knowledge of maternal cardiac arrest and resuscitation. *Int J Obstet Anesth* 2008;17:238–242.

44. Lipman SS, Daniels KI, Carvalho B, et al. Deficits in the provision of cardiopulmonary resuscitation during simulated obstetric crises. *Am J Obstet Gynecol* 2010;203:179.e1–e5.

45. Finegold H, Alaedin D, Ryan R, et al. Successful resuscitation after maternal cardiac arrest by immediate cesarean section in the labor room. *Anesthesiology* 2002;96:1278.

46. Kostash MA, Mensink F. Lethal air embolism during cesarean delivery for placenta previa. *Anesthesiology* 2002;96:753–754.

47. Lyons G. Failed intubation. *Anaesthesia* 1985;40:759–762.

48. McDonnell NJ, Paech MJ, Clavisi OM, et al. Difficult and failed intubation in obstetric anaesthesia: An observational study of airway management and complications associated with general anaesthesia for caesarean section. *Int J Obstet Anesth* 2008;17:292–297.

49. Leighton BL. Why obstetric anesthesiologists get sued. *Anesthesiology* 2009;110:8–9.

50. ASA Task Force on Management of the Difficult Airway. Practice guidelines for management of the difficult airway. *Anesthesiology* 2003;98:1269–1277.

51. The American Academy of Pediatrics and The American College of Obstetricians and Gynecologists. *Guidelines for Perinatal Care*, 6th ed. Washington, D.C.; 2007:154–155.

52. Mhyre JM, Healy D. The unanticipated difficult intubation in obstetrics. *Anesth Analg* 2011;112:648–652.

53. Vanden Hoek TL, Morrison LJ, Shuster M, et al. Part 12: Cardiac arrest in special situations: 2010 American Heart Association guidelines for cardiopulmonary resuscitation and emergency cardiovascular care. *Circulation* 2010;122:S829–S861.

54. ASA Committee on Standards and Practice Parameters. Practice guidelines for preoperative fasting and the use of pharmacologic agents to reduce the risk of pulmonary aspiration: application to healthy patients undergoing elective procedures. *Anesthesiology* 2011;114:495–511.

55. Hawkins JL, Koonin LM, Palmer SK, et al. Anesthesia-related deaths during obstetric delivery in the United States, 1979–1990. *Anesthesiology* 1997;86:277–284.

56. Pan PH, Bogard TD, Owen MD. Incidence and characteristics of failure in obstetric neuraxial analgesia and anesthesia: a retrospective analysis of 19,259 deliveries. *Int J Obstet Anesth* 2004;13:227–233.

57. Guay J. The epidural test dose: A review. *Anesth Analg* 2006;102:921–929.

58. Neal JM, Bernards CM, Butterworth JF, et al. ASRA practice advisory on local anesthetic systemic toxicity. *Reg Anesth Pain Med* 2010;35:152–161.

59. Weinberg GL. Treatment of local anesthetic systemic toxicity (LAST). *Reg Anesth Pain Med* 2010;35:188–193.

60. Hiller DB, DiGregorio G, Ripper R, et al. Epinephrine impairs lipid resuscitation from bupivacaine overdose. *Anesthesiology* 2009;111:498–505.

61. Leighton BL, Topkis WG, Gross JB, et al. Multiport epidural catheters: Does the air test work? *Anesthesiology* 2000;92:1617–1620.

62. Johansson PI, Stensballe J, Rosenberg I, et al. Proactive administration of platelets and plasma for patients with a ruptured abdominal aortic aneurysm: evaluating a change in transfusion practice. *Transfusion* 2007;47:593–598.

63. Charbit B, Mandelbrot L, Samain E, et al. The decrease of fibrinogen is an early predictor of the severity of postpartum hemorrhage. *J Thromb Haemost* 2007;5:266–273.

64. Phillips LE, McLintock C, Pollock W, et al. Recombinant activated factor VII in obstetric hemorrhage: Experiences from the Australian and New Zealand haemostasis registry. *Anesth Analg* 2009;109:1908–1915.

65. Mhyre JM. What's new in obstetric anesthesia in 2009? An update on maternal patient safety. *Anesth Analg* 2010;111:1480–1487.

66. Arendt KW, Segal S. Present and emerging strategies for reducing anesthesia-related maternal morbidity and mortality. *Curr Opin Anaesthesiol* 2009;22:330–335.

67. Hogan MC, Foreman KJ, Naghavi M, et al. Maternal mortality for 181 countries, 1980–2008: A systematic analysis of progress towards Millennium Development goal 5. *Lancet* 2010;375:1609–1623.

68. The Joint Commission Sentinel Alert, Issue 44, Preventing Maternal Death, January 26, 2010. http://www.jointcommission.org/sentinel_event_alert_issue_44_preventing_maternal_death/

Global Perspective on Obstetric Anesthesia

Holly A. Muir • Medge D. Owen

■ MATERNAL MORTALITY—A GLOBAL CRISIS

Nearly every minute, a woman dies somewhere in the world from complications arising during pregnancy and childbirth. This accounts for 350,000 to 500,000 maternal deaths each year, many of which are preventable (1,2). More women's lives are lost every year during childbirth than deaths that resulted from the 2004 Asian tsunami and the 2010 Haitian earthquake combined. Yet unlike natural disasters, maternal mortality receives relatively little media attention. Maternal mortality remains a silent disaster of wide-scale proportion. This chapter seeks to call attention to this silent crisis by offering a discussion of maternal death, the roles and challenges of anesthesia provision, and the impact of current anesthesia outreach projects and educational missions. In an effort to promote greater understanding throughout this discussion, the following key terms are defined, as they are pertinent to this offering of global perspectives on obstetric anesthesia.

- *Maternal death* is defined as the death of a woman while pregnant or within 42 days of termination of pregnancy, regardless of the site or duration of pregnancy, from any cause related to or aggravated by the pregnancy or its management.
- The *maternal mortality ratio (MMR)* is the number of maternal deaths per 100,000 live births. It is commonly used to describe and compare maternal death rates between countries.
- The *lifetime risk of maternal death* estimates the probability of maternal death during a woman's reproductive life.

Maternal mortality is considered a basic health indicator that reflects the overall adequacy of a country's healthcare system. While maternal mortality has dramatically decreased in industrialized nations over the past 80 years, this has not occurred in many low- and middle-income countries (LMICs). The disparity between countries is extreme (Fig. 47-1) (1,2). The MMR is <25/100,000 in the United States, Canada, and UK; 280/100,000 in South Central Asia; 640/100,000 in sub-Saharan Africa; and an overwhelming 1,400/100,000 in Afghanistan resulting in a range of lifetime risk of maternal death of 1 in 7,600 compared to 1 in 11 (Table 47-1) (2).

In 2008, eleven countries including Afghanistan, Bangladesh, the Democratic Republic of Congo, Ethiopia, India, Indonesia, Kenya, Nigeria, Pakistan, Sudan, and Tanzania comprised 65% of all maternal deaths (2). Over the past decade, the worldwide distribution pattern of maternal mortality has remained relatively consistent, although the absolute numbers have declined since 1990 (Fig. 47-2) (1,2). This is somewhat unclear, however, because gross underestimates

of maternal death are likely in countries where death rates are the highest due to poorly developed data collection and death registration systems (3).

For every maternal death, it is estimated that 30 women suffer morbidity such as chronic anemia, stress incontinence, infertility, vaginal fistulae, chronic pelvic pain, emotional depression, and/or physical exhaustion. Maternal death is also frequently associated with fetal and neonatal death, with conservative worldwide estimates predicting approximately 3.7 million neonatal deaths and 3.3 million stillbirths each year (4). The persistence of high maternal mortality and morbidity in developing countries represents a pervasive neglect of women's most fundamental human rights. Such neglect primarily affects poor, disadvantaged, and powerless women in a continuum of pain and suffering.

Maternal mortality is not just a woman's problem. In many circumstances, women financially support and maintain the cultural traditions of their families. The premature death of a mother deeply penetrates into a community's social and cultural fiber, placing burden not only on the individual family but also on society as a whole. Maternal death in dependent societies often negatively impacts other vulnerable family members such as infants, young children, and the elderly.

■ A CALL FOR ACTION

In September 2000, a declaration was adopted by 189 nations during the United Nations Millennium Summit to heighten awareness of global economic and health disparity. Eight Millennium Development Goals (MDGs) were created to be achieved by 2015 (Fig. 47-3). MDG 5 calls for a 75% reduction of maternal death by 2015—which would require an annual 5.5% decline. Globally, this decline has only been 2.5% since 1990 (5). Among countries with the highest MMR, 30 have made poor progress; 23 of these are in sub-Saharan Africa. One challenge has been in obtaining accurate data. A number of agencies, including the World Health Organization (WHO), the United Nations International Children's Fund (UNICEF), the United Nations Fund for Population Activities (UNFPA), and the World Bank are collaborating to provide accurate statistics.

The UN Millennium Project identified four broad categories to explain why countries are failing to meet MDGs. These include poor governance, poverty traps, poverty pockets, and policy neglect (6). With poor governance, low-income countries fail to provide citizens equal protection under the law. Corruption, mismanagement, and economic instability are rampant. Even many well-intentioned governments have insufficient human resources and infrastructure to maintain effective public services that include healthcare.

Second, poverty traps prevent society from carrying out initiatives to overcome hunger, disease, and infrastructure frailty

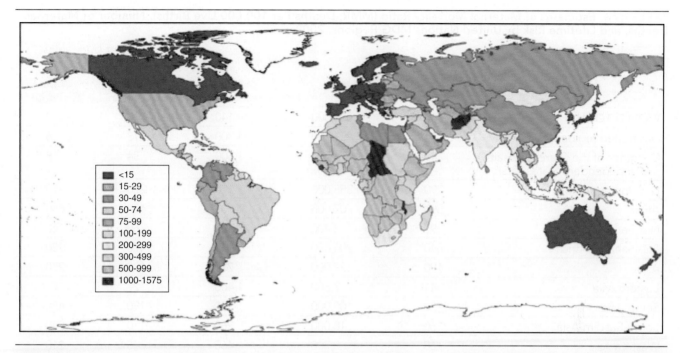

FIGURE 47-1 World map of maternal mortality WHO, UNICEF, UNFPA, The World Bank. Trends in maternal mortality 1990–2008; estimates developed by WHO, UNICEF, UNFPA, and the World Bank. Geneva: World Health Organization 2010. Reprinted from: Hogan MC, Foreman KJ, Naghavi M, et al. Maternal mortality for 181 countries, 1980–2008: a systematic analysis of progress towards Millennium Development Goal 5. *Lancet* 2010;375:1609–1623, with permission from Elsevier, Inc.

in order to achieve economic stability. A vicious cycle ensues whereby poverty results in low rates of savings, tax revenues, and foreign investment and simultaneously high rates of violence, brain drain, population growth, and environmental degradation. Poverty traps are common where geographical conditions are unfavorable. In sub-Saharan Africa, for example, poor road infrastructure, through difficult terrain, produces high transportation cost that limits commerce. Tropical diseases (such as malaria) and agricultural compromise, due to rain dependence in arid regions, are also problematic. One

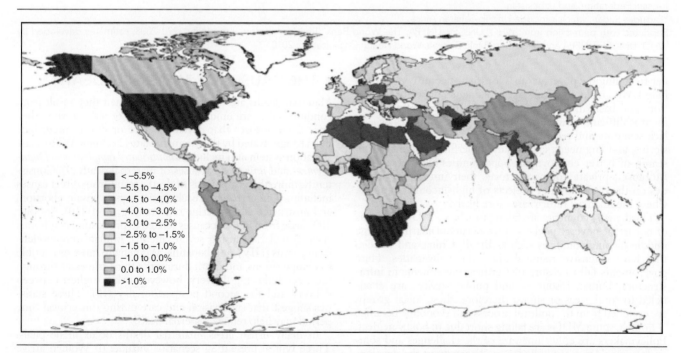

FIGURE 47-2 Global map demonstrating percent decline in MMR since 1990—WHO, UNICEF, UNFPA, The World Bank. Trends in maternal mortality 1990–2008: estimates developed by WHO, UNICEF, UNFPA, and The World Bank. Geneva: World Health Organization 2010. Reprinted from: Hogan MC, Foreman KJ, Naghavi M, et al. Maternal mortality for 181 countries, 1980–2008: a systematic analysis of progress towards Millennium Development Goal 5. *Lancet* 2010;375:1609–1623, with permission from Elsevier, Inc.

TABLE 47-1 Estimates of Maternal Mortality Ratio (MMR, Deaths Per 100,000 Live Births), Number of Maternal Deaths, and Lifetime Risk by United Nations MDG Regions, 2008

Region	Estimated MMR[a]	Number of Maternal Deaths[a]	Lifetime Risk of Maternal Death[a]; 1 in	Range of Uncertainty on MMR Estimates	
				Lower Estimate	Upper Estimate
WORLD TOTAL	260	358,000	140	200	370
Developed regions[b]	14	1,700	4,300	13	16
Countries of the Commonwealth of Independent States (CIS)[c]	40	1,500	1,500	34	48
Developing regions	290	355,000	120	220	410
Africa	590	207,000	36	430	850
Northern Africa[d]	92	3,400	390	60	140
Sub-Saharan Africa	640	204,000	31	470	930
Asia	190	139,000	220	130	270
Eastern Asia	41	7,800	1,400	27	66
South Asia	280	109,000	120	190	420
South-Eastern Asia	160	18,000	260	110	240
Western Asia	68	3,300	460	45	110
Latin America and the Caribbean	85	9,200	490	72	100
Oceania	230	550	110	100	500

[a]The MMR and lifetime risk have been rounded according to the following scheme: <100, no rounding; 100–999, rounded to nearest 10; and >1,000, rounded to nearest 100. The numbers of maternal deaths have been rounded as follows: <1,000, rounded to nearest 10; 1,000–9,999, rounded to nearest 100; and >10,000, rounded to nearest 1,000.

[b]Includes Albania, Australia, Austria, Belgium, Bosnia and Herzegovina, Bulgaria, Canada, Croatia, Czech Republic, Denmark, Estonia, Finland, France, Germany, Greece, Hungary, Iceland, Ireland, Italy, Japan, Latvia, Lithuania, Luxembourg, Malta, Montenegro, Netherlands, New Zealand, Norway, Poland, Portugal, Romania, Serbia, Slovakia, Slovenia, Spain, Sweden, Switzerland, the former Yugoslav Republic of Macedonia, the United Kingdom, and the United States of America.

[c]The CIS countries are Armenia, Azerbaijan, Belarus, Georgia, Kazakhstan, Kyrgyzstan, Tajikistan, Turkmenistan, the Republic of Moldova, the Russian Federation, and Uzbekistan.

[d]Excludes Sudan, which is included in sub-Saharan Africa.

Reprinted with permission from: WHO, UNICEF, UNFPA, The World Bank. Trends in maternal mortality 1990–2008: estimates developed by WHO, UNICEF, UNFPA and The World Bank. Geneva: World Health Organization; 2010.

key to ending the poverty trap is for high-income countries to help LMIC make the necessary investments in health, education, and basic infrastructure (6). Sustainability of advancement is difficult, however, since developing countries usually lack scientific and technologic communities. Scientists, physicians, and engineers, chronically underfunded, emigrate in search of better employment opportunities elsewhere (7,8). Moreover, private companies focus their innovation activities on the problems and projects of high-income countries, where the financial returns are more likely.

Third, many countries are failing to achieve MDGs because of persistent poverty pockets. This occurs primarily in large middle-income countries such as Brazil, China, and Mexico that have extensive regional and ethnic diversities. Here governments fail to ensure that critical investments in infrastructure, human resources, and public services are channeled to rural areas or slums; therefore, these social groups are excluded from the political process and economic benefits.

Fourth, some MDGs are falling short due to policy neglect. Policymakers are either unaware of the challenges and solutions or neglect core public issues. Throughout the developing world, neglect is especially common with girls and women in regards to education, healthcare, and legal protection against violence. Reaching the MDGs would bring tremendous benefits worldwide (6).

■ THE CAUSES OF MATERNAL DEATH

Maternal deaths are described as *direct* when they result from conditions that are unique to pregnancy, or *indirect* when they arise from diseases that develop before or during pregnancy that are aggravated by the pregnant state (2). A new WHO classification system also includes *unanticipated complications of management* and *unknown* as causes of maternal death (9). Consistently, more than two-thirds of deaths result from direct causes including hemorrhage, preeclampsia, sepsis, unsafe abortion, and obstructed labor/uterine rupture (Fig. 47-4) (10). Another 20% arise from indirect causes related to preexisting conditions such as malaria causing severe anemia, human immunodeficiency virus (HIV), and hepatitis. Women are most susceptible to complications and death during the third trimester through the week following delivery; however, risk is highest between delivery and the second postpartum day (10). These statistics suggest that supervision and care during this critical time period may help reduce maternal death.

In many urban areas, maternal deaths occur in hospitals. Three typical presenting scenarios include: (i) Women arrive moribund, too late to benefit from any emergency care; (ii) women arrive with complications that could have been prevented had they received timely and effective interventions; and (iii) women arrive for normal delivery that subsequently develop

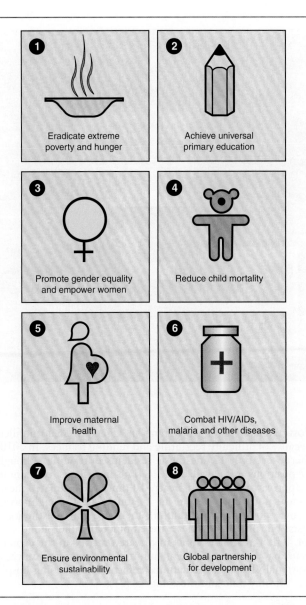

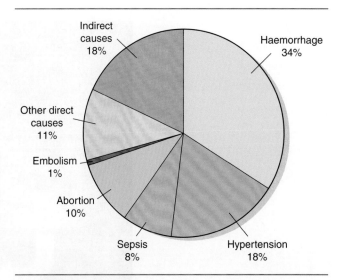

FIGURE 47-4 Causes of maternal mortality (WHO, UNICEF, UNFPA, and the World Bank. Geneva: World Health Organization 2010). Reproduced with permission from: UNICEF "A global overview of maternal mortality" available at: http://www.childinfo.org/maternal_mortality.html. Original data source from WHO, Systematic Review of Causes of Maternal Death from Preliminary Data, 2010.

FIGURE 47-3 The millennium development goals: Eight interlinked development and health goals set in 2000 (baseline 1990, target 2015). Reprinted from: Joy Lawn. Are the millennium development goals on target? *BMJ* 2010;341:c5045, with permission from BMJ Publishing Group Ltd.

serious complications, either naturally or through iatrogenic factors, and die with or without having received emergency care (10). The latter two scenarios raise concerns regarding the quality of hospital care. Numerous studies have shown that delays in recognition and treatment of life-threatening complications, as well as substandard practices, contribute directly to maternal deaths (11,12). In cases where women arrive in a moribund state, it is likely that problems exist with referrals between facilities, or there are community barriers—which might be physical, cultural, or financial—to accessing care (10,13).

Community barriers include late recognition, by women and families of the need to seek care that is either intentional or unintentional, and transportation difficulties in reaching hospitals (13). Most women labor in their houses for several days and go to hospital only as a last resort because delivery is considered "natural," not as an "illness" requiring hospitalization.

Unfortunately, death during labor or delivery may also be accepted as normal and inevitable (13). In addition, a lack of health education and/or poor reputation of health care facilities leave many patients unconvinced or frankly afraid of the value of modern obstetric management (13,14). A woman may deliberately stay in the house hoping to achieve normal vaginal delivery. A random questionnaire administered to a group of rural women in the Akosombo district of Ghana revealed that about 70% of women associated hospital confinement with severe discomfort, especially related to cesarean delivery (14). Others have a natural disinclination toward cesarean delivery because their peer groups insult them openly if they have been unable to deliver vaginally, considered the "natural" way (14). A lack of support and privacy in the hospital is a factor keeping some away and women may associate surgery with mortality (13). Furthermore, it is a status symbol to have large families and women believe that cesarean delivery will limit the number of children that they may bear (14). In some cultures, a pregnant woman with complications or a woman in labor cannot be taken to the hospital without the husband's consent, further delaying care (13,14). These social issues, along with the physical impediments of travel to referral centers, put lives of the mother and the fetus in peril.

The poorest and most remote communities illustrate the highest magnitude of delay (Fig. 47-5). Elements we take for granted, such as a passable road or gas to power a vehicle, are frequently absent and represent insurmountable barriers that result in untimely deaths. Some maternal deaths are so remote that the women are not even given the justice of becoming a statistic to be analyzed. In Egypt, the MMR was more than twice as high in the nomadic Frontier region than in the Metropolitan area (120 vs. 48 deaths per 100,000) (15). In Afghanistan, the differences are most striking, with mortality being 418/100,000 in the capital city of Kabul compared with 6,507/100,000 in the remote district of Ragh (16).

The enormity of this global crisis can be overwhelming to the point of creating inactivity. When one dissects the layers of problems, however, it boils down to few common needs: Access to a suitable facility to receive care, a sufficient number of competently trained medical staff, and a sustainable source of supplies and equipment.

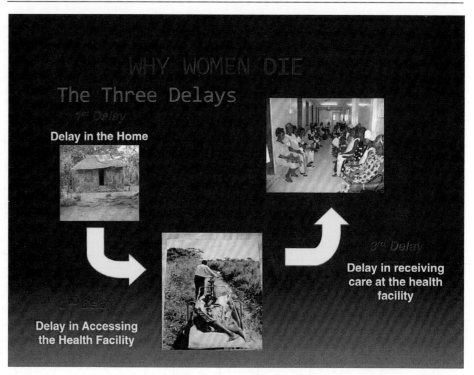

FIGURE 47-5 The cycle of delay. Reprinted with permission from Kybele, Inc.

■ THE ROLE AND CHALLENGES OF ANESTHESIA PROVISION

The importance of trained anesthesia providers for achieving MDG 5 becomes apparent when one recognizes the necessity of surgery in managing obstetric emergencies. Obstetric anesthesia as a subspecialty does not exist in most developing countries, yet hospitals within most countries treat obstetric complications that require surgery, including obstructed labor, ruptured uterus, eclampsia, and hemorrhage (17). The WHO recommends a cesarean delivery rate of 5% to 10%; however, in sub-Saharan Africa, the rate is frequently less than 1%, due in part to poor availability of anesthesia personnel (18,19). In many parts of Asia and Africa, anesthesia is administered by the surgeon or inadequately trained nonphysician providers working alone (14,18). The most dire example is described in Afghanistan where maternal mortality rates are among the highest in the world (1,400 maternal deaths per 100,000 live births). In an article by Hill, an obstetrician practicing in Afghanistan, a single photo of her operating theater paints a big picture (Fig. 47-6) (20). Strikingly absent is the complete lack of anesthesia equipment. Anesthesia for cesarean delivery may simply consist of local infiltration by the surgeon with some physical and chemical (ketamine ± benzodiazepine) restrain provided by midwives or nurses (14,20).

As a medical specialty, anesthesia does not command much clout worldwide (17,19). Anesthesia providers are in extreme shortage throughout much of Africa and Asia (Fig. 47-7), and even within rural areas of developed countries (19,21–24). Physician anesthesiologists in developing countries often leave in search of more lucrative opportunities abroad (19,21) creating a situation known as "brain drain." Currently in Uganda, for example, there are 14 physician anesthesiologists in a population of 30 million—approximately one anesthesiologist per every 2 million people (19). By comparison, in the United States, the ratio is 1:4,000 and in UK, 1:5,000. Most Ugandan anesthesia providers work in cities, in conditions that would still be considered austere by Western standards.

Postgraduate training programs in Uganda remain unfilled because of difficulty recruiting and funding trainees. In 2010, there were only 12 anesthesia residents in training although 47 positions were available (21). The annual cost of training is approximately $3,500, nearly 10 times the estimated mean annual household income in Uganda (21). In neighboring Kenya (population 32 million), there are 120 anesthesiologists, but only 13 of these are employed in the public sector. The remainder works in private practice in the capital, Nairobi. There are several hundred surgeons at Kenyatta National Hospital, the national referral and teaching hospital, but only nine anesthesiologists (21).

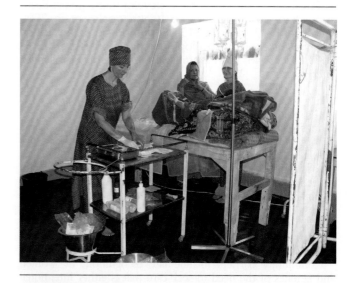

FIGURE 47-6 OR set up in Afghanistan. Reprinted from: Hill JC. Dying to give birth: obstructed labour in the Hindu Kush. *Obstet Gynaecol* 2005;7:267–270, with permission from John Wiley & Sons, Inc.

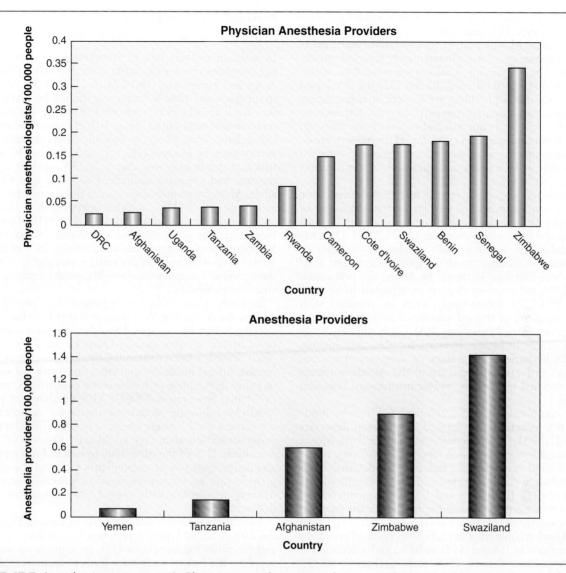

FIGURE 47-7 Anesthesia manpower. **A:** Physician anesthesia providers per 100,000 people in low- and middle-income countries (LMICs). **B:** Physician and nonphysician anesthesia providers per 100,000 people in LMICs. Reprinted from: Dubowitz G, Detlefs S, McQueen KA. Global anesthesia workforce crisis: a preliminary survey revealing shortages contributing to undesirable outcomes and unsafe practices. *World J Surg* 2010;34:438–444. Copyright © 2009, with permission from Springer.

In LMIC, the response to the critical shortage of anesthesia providers has varied. In general, it is common to reduce the required training period for medical practitioners or to create opportunities for nonmedical personnel to conduct anesthesia. As a result, the backgrounds of anesthesia providers across the world vary dramatically. In Africa, anesthesia is predominantly provided by nonphysicians, usually as nurse anesthetists or clinical officers, some with up to 2 years of clinical training and others with no formal training—just on the job experience (14,19,22,24). China has a large portion of its care given by nurse anesthetists (50% to 90%). In some areas of central Asia (e.g., Mongolia), physician anesthesiologists are the norm and paramedical providers virtually unheard of (24). India is unique because subspecialty trained anesthesiologists can provide services for liver transplant a few miles away from a sparsely staffed community health center where anesthesia is given by the surgeon either in the form of local infiltration or a spinal, then monitored by an untrained nurse (25). India has not allowed training of nurse anesthetists or medical officers, despite a critical shortage of anesthesia providers in rural areas. India has an MMR of 540/100,000 live births. Given the enormous Indian population, this country alone may represent more than 20% of all maternal deaths (25).

■ ANESTHESIA AS A CAUSE OF MATERNAL DEATH

Many global initiatives are striving to improve emergency obstetrical services, and these, by necessity, should also include a model of safe anesthesia care (18,23,26–28). Anesthesia significantly contributes to maternal mortality and is associated with as many as 3% to 9% of hospital-based maternal deaths each year in developing countries (12,22,23,26,29–31). Considering the high number of maternal deaths in many countries, the impact of anesthesia is real.

Emergency cesarean delivery remains one of the most common surgical procedures conducted worldwide, although capabilities to perform it are insufficient in many areas, as previously stated. For this reason, it is not surprising that perioperative mortality rates are estimated to be as high as 1% to 2% (14,18). A publication from Togo revealed a 3.8% incidence of perioperative maternal mortality. In this report, 96% of cesarean deliveries were conducted under general anesthesia (GA) resulting in 3 cases of aspiration, 1 esophageal intubation, 1 pulmonary aspiration, and 1 post-operative hypoxic event from inadequately reversed muscle relaxation. The remaining deaths were related to issues involving blood and fluid resuscitation (32). In developed countries, anesthesia providers are leaders in resuscitation and intensive care for patients in peril. In many low-income nations, this skill set is not integral to anesthetic training, which undoubtedly increases mortality. Hypertensive crisis, hemorrhagic shock, and sepsis are common preoperative problems that make surgery and anesthesia administration hazardous (24).

Most reported anesthesia-related maternal deaths occur during the administration of GA for cesarean delivery in both healthy and medically compromised patients in both developed and developing countries (23,24,29–31,33). Difficult intubation, unrecognized esophageal intubation, or premature extubation result in gastric aspiration and/or hypoxemia that lead to death. In Africa, the prevalence of use of GA for cesarean delivery is reported to be over 85% (23,29,31,32). Interestingly, even in countries with sufficient numbers of trained anesthesia providers and the availability of regional anesthesia (RA), GA is still frequently preferred (27,29,30,34,35). Reasons for this may include fear of RA by patients, reluctance of surgeons to operate on "awake" patients, unfamiliarity of the anesthesiologists with the regional techniques, and/or institutional tradition (19,34,35).

Airway complications that accompany GA can be minimized if RA techniques are utilized for cesarean deliveries (18,23,26,27,29,31,33). Indeed, the use of spinal anesthesia for cesarean delivery in both developed and developing countries has been associated with a reduction of maternal death (27,33), although death reported with spinal anesthesia has increased (26,33). In the US and UK, the contribution of anesthesia to maternal mortality has fallen over the past two decades as anesthesia practices have become safer (33). In the study by Hawkins, maternal mortality was reduced over time with an increase in RA use (55% to 84%) and a decrease in GA use for cesarean delivery (41% to 16%) (Fig. 47-8) (33). Fortunately, the adoption of spinal anesthesia for cesarean delivery does appear to be on the rise in many low resource centers (36,37); however, safety for all types of anesthesia provision is paramount.

■ ANESTHESIA DRUG AND EQUIPMENT LIMITATIONS

In addition to their lack of anesthesia providers, developing countries chronically suffer from the lack of anesthesia drugs and equipment (18,19,24,26,27,29,31,34). Operating room space and time is frequently limited by availability of functional anesthesia equipment. Frequently, broken equipment cannot be repaired due to lack of biomedical engineering support, even when the needed repairs are simple. In a survey done by Hodges (19), respondents from 97 anesthetists in Uganda indicated that only 23% of their operating theaters had adequate equipment to safely give GA to an adult. Most frequently absent were pulse oximeters (74%), an oxygen source (22%), a tilting operating table (23%), and appropriate-sized endotracheal tubes (21%) (19). In addition, succinylcholine was only reliably available 54% of the time. Vasopressors of any type were not available 28% of the time. Tables 47-2–47-4 indicate the relative availability of many of the agents and supplies most would consider essential to provide safe anesthesia.

Similarly, many lacked the equipment to provide spinal anesthesia. A striking 59% indicated that they had no local anesthetic suitable for spinal anesthesia at least some of the time. Spinal needles, usually Quincke tip (22 gauge), are often reused, whether intended by the manufacturer to be or not. Spinal headache and infection rates are unknown in many developing or low-income countries. One report in Ghana, however, did find a 33% incidence of postural headache following spinal anesthesia for cesarean delivery using a no. 22 gauge Quincke needle (36). Overall, the respondents felt that they could only provide safe spinal anesthesia 21% of the time. Due to lack of both equipment and drugs, only 6% of respondents reported the ability to provide safe anesthesia (regional or general) for cesarean delivery in centers with over 32,000 cumulative annual deliveries (19).

Even fairly sophisticated countries in Eastern Europe and the former Soviet Union report lack of necessary equipment and monitors for anesthesia (38). In addition to anesthesia supplies, the lack of antibiotics leads to an increased risk of infection, and the lack of water and electricity leads to the inability to clean instruments or administer care (14). Sterilization techniques vary from country to country with some methods having questionable efficacy (Fig. 47-9).

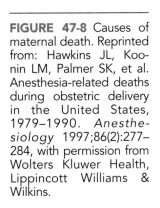

FIGURE 47-8 Causes of maternal death. Reprinted from: Hawkins JL, Koonin LM, Palmer SK, et al. Anesthesia-related deaths during obstetric delivery in the United States, 1979–1990. *Anesthesiology* 1997;86(2):277–284, with permission from Wolters Kluwer Health, Lippincott Williams & Wilkins.

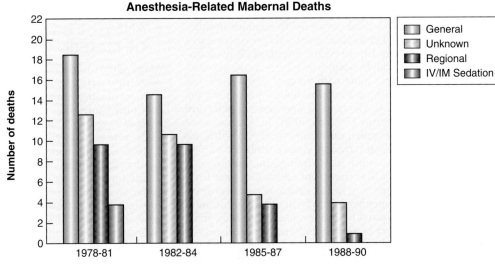

TABLE 47-2 **Availability of Critical Anesthesia Agents in Uganda**

n = 91	Always Available	Sometimes Available	Never Available	Do Not Know
Ketamine	84 (92%)	3 (3%)	4 (4%)	0
Thiopental	54 (59%)	22 (24%)	14 (15%)	1
Suxamethonium	50 (54%)	21 (23%)	18 (19%)	2
Non-depolarizing relaxant	14 (15%)	11 (12%)	63 (69%)	3
Neostigmine	15 (16%)	6 (6%)	63 (69%)	7
Halothane	35 (38%)	15 (16%)	36 (39%)	5
Ether	62 (68%)	19 (20%)	9 (9%)	1
Pethidine/morphine	41 (45%)	28 (30%)	20 (21%)	2
Naloxone	9 (9%)	15 (16%)	55 (60%)	12
Atropine	77 (84%)	6 (6%)	6 (6%)	2

Reprinted from: Hodges SC, Mijumbi C, Okella M, et al. Anaesthesia services in developing countries: defining the problems. *Anaesthesia* 2007;62:4–11, with permission from John Wiley & Sons, Inc.

TABLE 47-3 **Availability of Anesthesia Agents in Uganda**

n = 91	Always	Sometimes	Never	Do Not Know
Adrenaline	68 (74%)	17 (18%)	3 (3%)	3
Ephedrine/metaraminol/ phenylephrine	41 (45%)	20 (21%)	26 (28%)	4
Spinal local anesthetic	36 (39%)	26 (28%)	28 (30%)	1
Local anesthetics for blocks	64 (70%)	17 (18%)	7 (7%)	3
Magnesium	18 (19%)	35 (38%)	36 (39%)	2
Hydralazine	28 (30%)	31 (34%)	28 (30%)	4
Diazepam	74 (81 %)	16 (17%)	0 (0%)	1
Labetalol	27 (29%)	27 (29%)	28 (30%)	9
Oxytocin	52 (57%)	29 (31%)	7 (7%)	3
Ergometrine	74 (81 %)	13 (14%)	1 (1%)	3
Oxygen	58 (63%)	23 (25%)	10 (10%)	0
Intravenous fluid	62 (68%)	25 (27%)	2 (2%)	0
Nitrous oxide	0 (0%)	3 (3%)	84 (92%)	4
Blood for transfusion	21 (23%)	54 (59%)	15 (16%)	1

Reprinted from: Hodges SC, Mijumbi C, Okella M, et al. Anaesthesia services in developing countries: defining the problems. *Anaesthesia* 2007;62:4–11, with permission from John Wiley & Sons, Inc.

TABLE 47-4 **Availability of Essential Supplies and Equipment**

n = 91	Always Available	Sometimes Available	Never Available	Do Not Know
Electricity	18 (19%)	60 (65%)	13 (14%)	0
Generator	45 (49%)	34 (37%)	9 (9%)	3
Running water	51 (56%)	32 (35%)	8 (8%)	0
Disinfectant	63 (69%)	21 (23%)	6 (6%)	1
Sterile gloves	73 (80%)	18 (19%)	0 (0%)	0
Non-sterile gloves	66 (72%)	25 (27%)	0 (0%)	0
Bleach	49 (53%)	30 (32%)	9 (9%)	3
Brush for cleaning tracheal tube	21 (23%)	13 (14%)	51 (56%)	6
Hemoglobin measurement	52 (57%)	20 (21%)	17 (18%)	2
Glucose measurement	30 (32%)	27 (29%)	27 (29%)	7

Reprinted from: Hodges SC, Mijumbi C, Okella M, et al. Anaesthesia services in developing countries: defining the problems. *Anaesthesia* 2007;62:4–11, with permission from John Wiley & Sons, Inc.

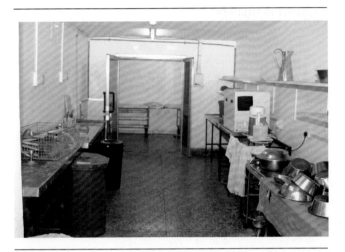

FIGURE 47-9 Sterilization room in a major referral hospital in Africa. Photograph reprinted with permission from Kybele, Inc.

Well-intentioned donors frequently send vast amounts of supplies and equipment abroad to help alleviate the vast need. Unfortunately, the drugs and equipment often remain unused because of expiration, installation difficulty, missing parts, or electrical incompatibility. In any given hospital in a low-income country, one does not have to look far to find storage rooms filled with donated equipment that cannot be used.

■ OTHER LIMITING FACTORS— BLOOD AVAILABILITY

Obstetric patients frequently consume blood products, and inefficient blood supplies put the patient at risk, even for routine cesarean delivery. For example, 60% of the 10,000 to 13,000 blood-unit consumption at Korle Bu Teaching Hospital in Accra, Ghana, is used for obstetrics (annual delivery rate of 10,000 to 11,000) (14).

This is in the face of a very poorly developed national blood bank service. Statistics from the national blood bank show that only 25% to 30% of the donated blood comes from the general public (14). More commonly, directed donation from relatives is used to obtain blood. In some situations, this may be given in advance of surgery, but frequently, it is given in the throngs of an acute hemorrhage when adding extra time for maternal and donor crossmatch can be deadly. Lab facilities are often limited or unavailable in many areas. Crossmatching is a relatively simple procedure that can be easily done using reagents with some basic training. It may be a useful technique to master if working in a very remote region.

■ DEFINING MINIMUM STANDARDS FOR SAFE ANESTHESIA

The World Federation of Societies of Anaesthesiologists (WFSA) has defined the minimum required equipment standards for the provision of safe anesthesia (Fig. 47-10) (39). The WFSA maintains an ongoing educational campaign to improve anesthesia safety worldwide. One such endeavor, the Lifebox project (www.lifebox.org), promotes the availability of pulse oximetry worldwide. This project is in partnership with the WHO Safe Surgery Saves Lives project (www.who.int/patientsafety/safesurgery) and represents a giant step forward in attempts to improve the global environment in which surgery is performed.

■ ANESTHESIA OUTREACH AND EDUCATIONAL MISSIONS

On a smaller scale, many organizations send teams to work in underserved areas to help provide surgery and anesthesia. Many anesthesia teams initially go with a broad focus of providing general surgical care but soon find that they are providing anesthesia for maternal and trauma care. Once in an underserviced area, one can quickly see the benefits that well-trained anesthesia personnel offer to safety and delivery outcomes. Also apparent are the lack of resources for providing care (35).

In addition to service provision, medical education is also being provided from the international community (17,26–28,40). Several charitable organizations exist primarily to support obstetric anesthesia education in developing countries (Fig. 47-11). Mothers of Africa (www.mothersofafrica.org) links anesthesia departments in Togo, Benin, and Liberia to the University Hospital of Wales (40). Kybele (www.kybeleworldwide.org) is a US-based non-governmental organization (NGO) that recruits medical volunteers from a multinational and multidisciplinary base to create country-specific programs that promote childbirth and anesthesia safety (28,35). Both organizations provide theoretical and practical teaching and conduct 1- to 2-week training programs at regular intervals (28,35,40). This builds relationships and trust with local hosts, encouraging long-term sustainability. It is vitally important to observe medical practices within host hospitals as care is actually provided. Only there can gaps between theoretical knowledge and practical application be observed. For example, while working in Togo and Benin, Morris found that despite knowledge of aortocaval compression, there is reluctance to tilt the table or place a wedge under the patient's hip (40). Gaps were also noted in applying extubation criteria and in assessing the level of spinal anesthesia prior to surgery start (40).

Numerous other organizations and societies have had long-standing interests in improving anesthesia care in the developing world through teaching and training, which impact obstetric anesthesia both directly and indirectly. Most notable are the WFSA (www.anaesthesiologists.org), the American Society of Anesthesiologists (ASA) Committee on Overseas Training Program, recently renamed the ASA Committee on Global Humanitarian Outreach (www.asahq.org/GHO), Canadian Anesthesiologists' Society International Education Foundation (www.cas.ca/casief/), Obstetric Anaesthetists' Organization (www.oaa-anaes.ac.uk), Health Volunteers Overseas (www.hvousa.org), and more recently, the Alliance for Surgery and Anesthesia Presence (www.asaptoday.org) and the Society for Obstetric Anesthesia and Perinatology International Outreach Committee (www.soap.org).

In addition, a multitude of global health programs are emerging within academic anesthesia departments. It is hoped that research efforts associated with these partnerships can better define and quantitate the global anesthesia crisis (21). Currently, anesthesia global health electives exist for anesthesia faculty, fellows, and residents at Duke, Wake Forest Baptist, Medical University of South Carolina, Vanderbilt, University of California-San Francisco, Emory, University of Utah, University of Virginia, Dalhousie University, McGill University, and Stanford, although there are undoubtedly more. Individuals involved both teach and learn in global health settings through the provision of clinical care, education, equipment distribution, and research. It is imperative that these endeavors primarily benefit the needs of the host community, as voiced by the host community, and not the needs and egos of the donors. To be most effective, teaching must be tailored to the environment, teachers must be flexible and adaptable to unfamiliar and austere settings, local champions must be found to be the ultimate change agents, and ongoing support

Level 1-Small hospital	Level 2-District hospital-100-300 beds with OR	Level 3-Referral hospital-300-1000 beds with intensive care
• Performs normal delivery/ D & C but no CS • Staffed by paramedical personnel, nurse, midwives, anesthetic officers (non MD) • Drugs-ketamine, lidocaine, benzodiazapine, narcotic, epinephrine, atropine, volatile agent • Equipment-bag and mask, foot powered suction, stethescope, BP cuff, thermometer, pulse Ox, O_2 supply, laryngoscope, bougie' gloves, IV infusion supplies, suction catheters, airways and ET tubes	• Can perform CS and other routine minor surgeries • Staffed by-medical officers (MD), trained anesthesia personnel, midwives, nurses and visiting specialists • Drugs-as above plus thiopental or propofol, suamethonium, nondepolarizer relaxant, neostigmine, spinal lidocaine and or bupivacaine, hydralazie, furosemide, dextrose 50%, aminiphylline, ephedrine, hydrocortisone • Equipment-complete adult and pediatric anesthesia, resuscitation and airway management systems, monitors to include capnography, ECG, pulse Ox, NIBP, nerve stimulator and temp, defibrillator, spinal anesthesia supplies, ECG electrodes, nasogastric tubes, suction catheters, adults and pediatric IV infusion sets, airway management supplies sized from 3.0-8.5 with accompanying oral and nasal airways, bougies	• Complex surger including cardiac and neurosurgery, major trauma and prolonged life support, has ventilators in OR and ICU and hemodialysis • Staffed by clinical officers with specialist in anesthesia and surgery • Drugs as above with addition of propofol, selection of neuromuscular blocking agents and volatile agents, inotropes, antiarrhythmics, nitroglcerine infusion, CaCl 10%, KCl 20% • Equipment-as for level 2 plus-anesthetic ventilator, electric or pneumonic suction, O_2 analyzer, warming blankets and overbed heaters, infant incubator, laryngeal masks, anesthetic agent analyzer, pressure bags, disposable anesthesia for airway management and ventilation

FIGURE 47-10 Required anesthesia equipment—2008. Adapted in part from: World Federation of Societies of Anaesthesiologists®. 2008 International Standards for a Safe Practice of Anaesthesia. Available at: http://www.operationgivingback.facs.org/stuff/contentmgr/files/a384bb3c7b77e154ad25c6136d7be344/miscdocs/wfsa___2008_international_standards_for_a_safe_practice_of_anesthesia.pdf

and continuity are needed (28). This ultimately requires personal commitment of participants beyond the excitement of the initial interaction and a willingness to repeat the journey, sacrificing vacation and personal time away from family.

Despite the interest in improving the global burden of healthcare, there is little coordination or communication between nonprofit organizations, academic programs, and the host facilities they serve. There is no central registry of what is being attempted by whom (17), although some attempts have been recently made to do so through websites associated with the American College of Surgeons' Operation Giving Back (www.operationgivingback.facs.org), the Society for

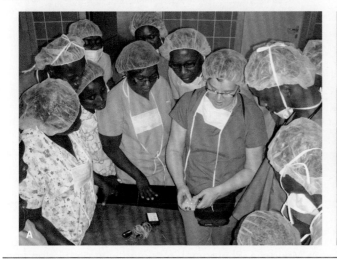
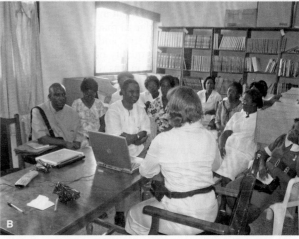

FIGURE 47-11 Eager students in a major referral center in Africa. Photograph reprinted with permission from Kybele, Inc.

Pediatric Anesthesia (www.pedsanesthesia.org), The Journal of the American Medical Association (www.jamacareercenter.com/volunteer_opportunities.cfm), and The International Health Volunteers Organization (www.internationalhealthvolunteers.org). Best practices and outcome data are lacking despite the outpouring of good will. There is often overlap and inefficiency, to the point that some groups do not know of others working within the same foreign hospital. The questions every organization operating outreach programs have to ask are: Is there any lasting good? Has progress been sustained or do practices revert back to the old status quo when the visitors have gone (17)?

Lasting change is more likely to result from education and training than from donations of equipment and drugs (40). As with all external interventions, measurement of outcomes and the impact of the programs are essential for evaluation and improvement for the future.

■ LABOR ANALGESIA

Efforts are underway by individuals and nongovernmental organizations to train anesthesia providers in RA techniques for cesarean delivery and labor analgesia (17,26,35,40). Labor analgesia may seem unnecessary in countries with limited resources but represents an index of healthcare quality and compassion (41). The provision of pain relief is now considered a basic human right although cultural and financial barriers impede treatment in many developing countries (28,35). Providing analgesia during labor could encourage patients to seek earlier hospital admission in urban settings and would promote multidisciplinary patient care with anesthesiologists outside the operating room (28). Earlier intervention by anesthesia providers could potentially improve patient outcomes in cases of hemorrhage or hypertensive crisis (14,18,27,28,41). One confounding issue existing in middle-income countries is poor remuneration of academic faculty. Resultantly, senior consultants often pursue private practice simultaneously with their teaching commitments, which limit trainees' exposure to supervision and learning opportunities for RA techniques (17).

A recent survey in Nigeria suggests that despite agreement regarding the benefit of regional anesthesia techniques, unfamiliarity with the techniques limited their use. Among the respondents, 93% indicated that they regularly used spinal anesthesia whenever a surgical procedure is amenable to a regional technique. Only 15% reported regular use of epidural techniques and 26% indicated that they never performed an epidural block. The majority of anesthesiologists in Nigeria (59%) reported only occasional use of epidural techniques (42).

Additional research needs to be conducted surrounding the provision of low-dose spinal labor analgesia in resource poor settings. One small study was carried out in Indonesia that utilized single-dose spinal labor analgesia that consisted of bupivacaine (2.5 mg), morphine (250 μg), and clonidine (45 μg) (43). It was difficult to assess the quality or duration of analgesia; however, maternal satisfaction was reported to be high. In areas where the epidural technique is sparely utilized, there is greater potential risk of inadvertent dural puncture, total spinal, intravenous local anesthetic toxicity, and infection. Advantages of a single shot spinal include more familiarity with the spinal technique and lower local anesthetic consumption, good from a resource-sparing standpoint. Disadvantages include limited duration of analgesia from single shot spinal, postdural puncture headache if two or more spinals are performed or large-gauge and/or cutting-tip needles are used, and sterility concerns. Surveys from Togo and Nigeria found that women would accept neuraxial analgesia if given the opportunity to receive it (44,45). In a separate Nigerian survey, parturients thought to most benefit from labor analgesia included those who were nulliparous, young, preterm, and those with induced labor or instrumental delivery (46). Education on RA across the whole spectrum of anesthesia care is needed and should be a focus of western visitors.

■ TEACHING ANESTHESIA IN LOW RESOURCE SETTINGS—WHAT TO EXPECT

In many countries, the most commonly used agents for the induction of GA are thiopental or ketamine followed by succinylcholine to facilitate tracheal intubation. For anesthesia maintenance, however, ketamine, halothane, or ether are most commonly used with or without muscle relaxants (14,19,24,27,34). In healthcare settings where spinal anesthesia is conducted, 0.5% hyperbaric bupivacaine is the usual preparation for cesarean delivery and other lower abdominal or extremity surgical procedures. Fentanyl and morphine may be available; however, morphine preparations often contain preservatives and should not be given by the intrathecal route.

Standard anesthetic drugs can be hard to secure (Fig. 47-12). In very remote rural settings, anesthesia for cesarean delivery may be conducted with intravenous ketamine or face-mask open drop ether as the sole anesthetic with spontaneous ventilation (14,19,20,24,47). Practitioners of this method claim that it is safer for untrained, unequipped anesthesia providers who should not attempt intubation or spinal anesthesia (24,47).

When planning a trip, it is useful to take the time to try to determine the resources available to you prior to your arrival. In some sparsely resourced areas, many things considered essentials for basic anesthesia practice may be absent. This may be something as basic as an oxygen source! Once resources are determined, it may be important for you to bring what you consider critical for your comfort. It is equally as important for one to think about how to best use available resources.

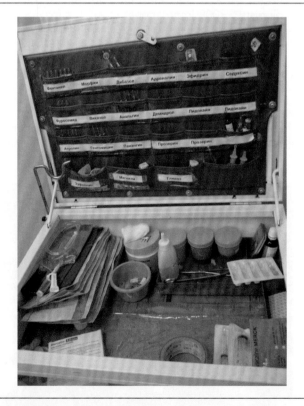

FIGURE 47-12 Complete anesthesia medication supply in Mongolia. Photograph reprinted with permission from Kybele, Inc.

■ ANESTHESIA MACHINES

Anesthesia equipment can be very basic (Fig. 47-13). An anesthesia machine, if available, may be an older model possibly lacking basic safety features such as an oxygen fail-safe device and disconnect alarms (Fig. 47-14). The anesthesia machine may have a drawover vaporizer, the most common of which are the EMO (Epstein, Macintosh, Oxford), OMV (Oxford Miniature Vaporizer), and the Tec series (previously known as the PAC [Portable Anesthesia Complete] series). A drawover system is designed to provide anesthesia without a consistent supply of compressed gasses. Atmospheric air is used as the main carrier gas and is drawn by the patient's inspiratory effort through the vaporizer, where the volatile agent, normally ether or halothane, is added (48,49).

The mixture is inhaled by the patient via a nonrebreathing valve (Fig 47-15). During drawover anesthesia, the patient draws air through the vaporizer, which must have a very low resistance to the intermittent gas flow which is generated. The volume of air passing through the vaporizer is determined by the patient's tidal volume and respiration rate. Considerable variations in flow through the vaporizer occur, depending on the type and depth of anesthesia, the patient's age, and the mode of ventilation—spontaneous or assisted. As air flows through the vaporizer, vapor from the agent being used is picked up. This mixes with air bypassing the vaporizing chamber to create an admixture that determines the final concentration. These devices often work in parallel with a self-inflating bag or bellows for controlled ventilation (48,49).

The drawover device has several desirable qualities. It is robust, compact, and portable; in addition, it has low purchase and operational costs, requires straightforward maintenance, and does not dependent on compressed gasses (48). It is often the preferred delivery system even when modern equipment is available (Fig. 47-16).

■ VOLATILE INHALATIONAL AGENTS AND COMPRESSED GASSES

Ether is a common volatile agent used in these devices that most western trained providers have little or no experience with. It has a pungent smell and high blood solubility which prolongs anesthetic induction and delays emergence. In addition, it produces with postoperative nausea and vomit-

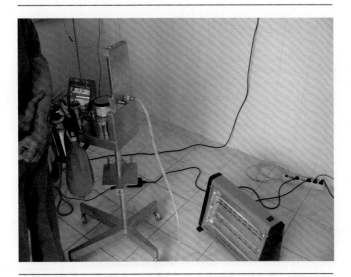

FIGURE 47-13 Basic anesthesia set-up and space heater for warmth. Photograph reprinted with permission from Kybele, Inc.

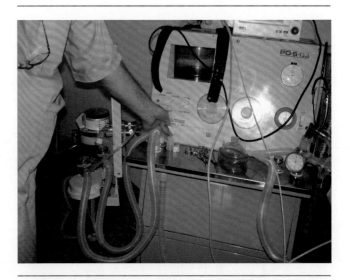

FIGURE 47-14 An unfamiliar anesthesia machine in the Republic of Georgia. Photograph reprinted with permission from Kybele, Inc.

ing. Ether is highly flammable posing explosion risks in the operating room. Explosion can be encountered if oxygen is added and a source of ignition, such as cautery, is present. This risk may be minimized by limiting the use of oxygen and keeping the cautery unit away from the anesthesia circuitry (49).

Ether nevertheless has some advantages that actually enhance its safety; it increases cardiac output and is a respiratory stimulant. It has a better safety margin than other volatile agents during spontaneous ventilation when oxygen is unavailable (49). The utility and safety of ether is further enhanced by performing an intravenous induction and administration after tracheal intubation. This technique is recommended for obstetric delivery because airway protection is required.

Halothane is widely used in low resource settings. It offers the advantages of nonflammability, a pleasant smell, and quicker induction of anesthesia than ether. It poses disadvantages, principally cardiovascular and respiratory depression, which can cause disastrous hypotension and hypoxia if monitors cannot be utilized (49). Sometimes, newer inhalational agents may be available including both isoflurane and sevoflurane.

Often, nitrous oxide is unavailable, as can be oxygen. Oxygen concentrators are, therefore, used to compress room air to a pressure of 4 bar, which passes through a zeolite column to absorb nitrogen, producing up to 96% oxygen. If excessive flows are demanded, the delivered concentration is reduced. Small concentrators, which meet WHO's standards can deliver 4 L/min of oxygen (>90%) consuming approximately 350 W (thus electricity or an AC generator are required). Concentrators are usually the cheapest source of oxygen at roughly 30% to 50% the cost of cylinders (50).

■ ALTERNATIVE ANESTHETIC TECHNIQUES

Ketamine may be the only anesthetic agent available in some areas. Ketamine is very versatile, however, in that it is inexpensive, has a good safety profile, is easy to store (does not require refrigeration), and has a wide range of applications.

Ketamine is a phencyclidine derivative and acts through an antagonist action at N-methyl-D-aspartate (NMDA) receptors throughout the central nervous system. Ketamine is metabolized in the liver to an active metabolite, norket-

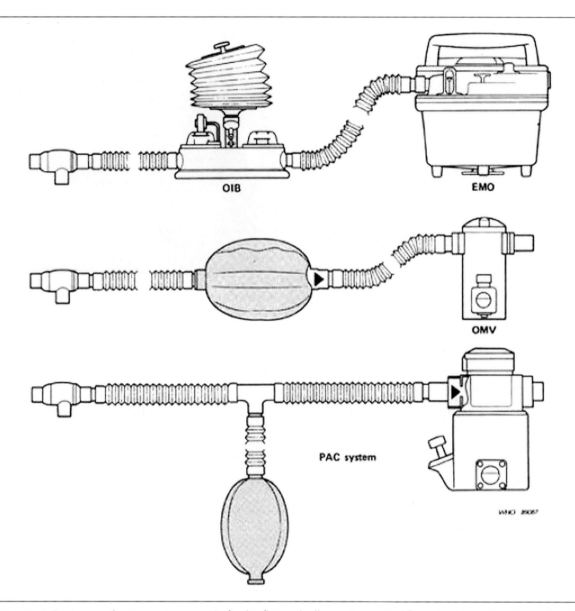

FIGURE 47-15 Basic anesthesia equipment, Oxford inflating bellows. Reprinted from: Dobson MB. Anaesthesia at the district hospital, 2nd ed., with permission from World Health Organization, Geneva, 2000;57–72.

amine, which is renally excreted. The elimination half-life is 2 to 3 hours in adults. Ketamine can be administered by many routes as it is both water and lipid soluble. Intravenous, intramuscular, oral, rectal, subcutaneous, epidural, and transnasal routes have all been described. Following intravenous administration, bioavailability is 90%; with oral or rectal routes, bioavailability is only 16% (51).

During ketamine anesthesia, the airway is usually well maintained with some preservation of pharyngeal and laryngeal reflexes. Despite this, in situations when patients have a "full stomach" (as with obstetric patients), airway protection is usually warranted. There is a small risk of laryngospasm during spontaneous ventilation with ketamine anesthesia. A slow intravenous infusion is recommended to prevent apnea; however, if apnea occurs, it usually resolves quickly with airway support. Ketamine has bronchodilator properties and can improve acute bronchospasm. Bronchodilation occurs by two mechanisms: One induces catecholamine release stimulating β-2 adrenergic receptors and the other inhibits vagal pathways by acting directly on bronchial smooth muscle to produce an anticholinergic effect (52).

Ketamine increases blood pressure, stroke volume, and heart rate. It has minimal effect on systemic vascular resistance; thus, it is an ideal agent for the patient with hemodynamic compromise (51).

Ketamine produces dissociative anesthesia often characterized by a patient whose eyes are open but without response to surgical stimuli. Patients may become restless, however, which can be problematic. This is overcome by increasing the dose or adding a benzodiazepine. In the recovery period, a patient who has received ketamine anesthesia can become agitated and complain of vivid and frightening hallucinations. This can be prevented and/or treated with small doses of benzodiazepine (51).

Ketamine is a potent anesthetic and may be used as the sole anesthetic intraoperatively. Coadministration of opiates reduces the amount of ketamine required for anesthetic maintenance, also shortening recovery time, and reducing ketamine-related side effects. Of note, the addition of opiates increases the risk of intraoperative respiratory depression.

The intravenous induction ketamine dose is 1 to 2 mg/kg. Doses should be reduced in hemodynamically unstable

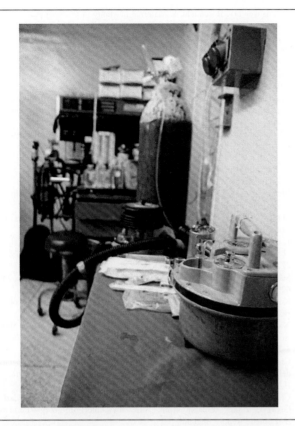

FIGURE 47-16 This picture demonstrates a recurrent situation. In the foreground we see an EMO anesthesia system, apparently in current use with the likely dysfunctional modern anesthesia machine pushed into the background. The drawover systems have a simpler maintenance and higher reliability.

patients. Ketamine can increase salivation so atropine or glycopyrrolate pretreatment can be beneficial.

Anesthesia maintenance can be achieved using intermittent boluses of intravenous ketamine (0.5 mg/kg) titrated to the patient's heart rate, blood pressure, and movement. Alternatively, a ketamine infusion can be used for maintenance. Mixing 500 mg of ketamine in a 500 mL bag of saline or dextrose will yield a 1 mg/mL solution. In the absence of an infusion pump, the drip rate can be manually adjusted according to the patient's response. In patients with spontaneous ventilation, a dose of 2 drops/kg/min with a non-micro drip intravenous chamber (15 drops/mL volume ratio) can provide effective maintenance (51). Paralyzed, ventilated patients will require less. Generally, a ketamine infusion should be discontinued 10 to 20 minutes before the end of surgery to avoid prolonged emergence. This technique for laparotomy yields optimal surgical conditions when administered with a muscle relaxant.

Intramuscular (IM) ketamine induction is possible when IV access is unavailable. Ketamine (5 to 10 mg/kg) is coadministered with atropine (20 mg/kg) IM in the same syringe with an approximately 5-minute onset time. This approach is commonly used in children, but it also works for adults who are fearful of healthcare providers. Similarly, sedation can be provided with IM ketamine (2 mg/kg) and atropine (20 mg/kg) with a 5- to 10-minute onset yielding a docile patient who can cooperate with either IV insertion or inhalational induction (51). The IV ketamine preparation can also be given orally (adult dose: 500 mg of ketamine with diazepam 5 mg; pediatric dose: 15 mg/kg) (51).

Ketamine is useful in acute and chronic pain states (53–55). Studies have demonstrated that intraoperative ketamine use reduces postoperative morphine consumption likely related to NMDA receptor antagonism. Low-dose ketamine can provide effective postoperative analgesia with tolerable side effects in most patients and can treat severe pain when morphine is unavailable. Both IV and oral administration routes are effective; however, patients experience fewer side effects with oral ketamine. Oral ketamine is not palatable and should be mixed with a sweet liquid like fruit juice for administration to children (51). Side effects are minimized by using the lowest possible doses. For adult patients in severe pain, a 0.5 to 1 μg/kg IM loading dose is used, followed by an infusion of 60 to 180 μg/kg/h, or 4 to 12 mg/h for a 70 kg adult (51). When used in a situation where anesthesia supervision is not immediately available, 50 mg of ketamine is added to 500 mL saline or dextrose yields a 0.1 mg/mL solution. Infusing 40 to 120 mL/h over 4 to 12 hours in a typical 70 kg adult is effective and safe as an analgesic regimen. Even if the entire volume is inadvertently administered, the patient should remain hemodynamically stable with intact airway reflexes (51).

■ SUMMARY

Maternal mortality remains an unrelenting challenge in developing nations in large part because emergency obstetric services are inadequate to treat life-threatening complications that accompany many pregnancies. Maternal deaths result from not reaching a hospital or reaching a hospital too late. Even within hospitals, there are a myriad of delays and inadequacies in the availability of medication, equipment, blood products, and access to prompt cesarean delivery and multidisciplinary care. In particular, the provision of anesthesia in low resource settings is woefully insufficient. All these factors place pregnant patients and their fetuses at risk. Maternal deaths that result from hospital inefficiencies fuel mistrust of the health system creating a vicious cycle whereby patients wait too long to seek care. It is imperative to strengthen health systems worldwide to improve maternal and newborn outcomes. Trained anesthesia providers, working individually or collectively through organizations, can and should play a vital role.

KEY POINTS

- There are at least 350,000 maternal deaths each year, many of which occur in sub-Saharan Africa and south Asia.
- Maternal deaths are most likely during labor, delivery, and the immediate postpartum period; a substantial number occur within hospitals.
- For every maternal death, it is estimated that 30 women suffer morbidity such as chronic anemia, stress incontinence, infertility, vaginal fistulae, chronic pelvic pain, emotional depression, and/or physical exhaustion.
- In 2000, the WHO recognized maternal mortality as one of the eight millennium development goals—Goal no. 5 is to reduce the MMR by three-quarters, between 1990 and 2015.
- Emergency cesarean delivery remains one of the most common surgical procedures conducted worldwide, although capabilities to perform it are insufficient in many areas.
- Many global initiatives are striving to improve emergency obstetrical services; these, by necessity, should include a model of safe anesthesia care because 3% to 9% of hospital-based maternal deaths result from anesthesia difficulties.
- Most anesthesia-related maternal deaths in low-income countries occur during the administration of general

anesthesia whereby failed intubation or premature extubation lead to aspiration and hypoxia.

■ The availability of drugs and equipment to provide safe anesthesia is one of the biggest barriers to care in low-income countries. Ketamine remains one of the most common agents available, offering flexibility in administration.

■ The provision of pain relief is more than a luxury—it is now considered a basic human right. Labor analgesia encourages woman to seek hospital care and engages anesthesia personnel in care.

■ Improving communication and coordination between non-profit organizations, academic programs, and the host facilities they serve is critical for success in improving the global burden of healthcare.

REFERENCES

1. Hogan MC, Foreman KJ, Naghavi M, et al. Maternal mortality for 181 countries, 1980–2008: a systematic analysis of progress towards Millennium Development Goal 5. *Lancet* 2010;375:1609–1623.
2. WHO, UNICEF, UNFPA, The World Bank. Trends in maternal mortality 1990–2008: estimates developed by WHO, UNICEF, UNFPA and The World Bank. Geneva: World Health Organization; 2010. Available from: http://www.who.int/reproductivehealth/publications/monitoring/9789241500265/en/index.html
3. Graham W, Hussein J. The right to count. *Lancet* 2004;363:67–68.
4. Neonatal and perinatal mortality: country, regional and global estimates 2006. Geneva: World Health Organization. 2006; Available from: http://www.who.int/reproductivehealth/docs/neonatal_perinatal_mortality/text.pdf
5. Hill K, Thomas K, AbouZahr C, et al. Estimates of maternal mortality worldwide between 1990 and 2005: an assessment of available data. *Lancet* 2007;370:1311–1319.
6. Sachs JD, McArthur JW. The Millennium Project: a plan for meeting the Millennium Development Goals. *Lancet* 2005;365:347–353.
7. Hooper CR. Adding insult to injury: the healthcare brain drain. *J Med Ethics* 2008;34:684–687.
8. Ahmad OB. Brain drain: the flight of human capital. *Bull World Health Organ* 2004;82(10):797–798.
9. Say L, Chou D. Better understanding of maternal deaths-the new WHO cause classification system. *BJOG* 2011;118(suppl 2):15–17.
10. Ronsmans C, Graham WJ, Lancet Maternal Survival Series steering group. Maternal mortality: who, when, where and why. *Lancet* 2006;368:1189–1200.
11. van den Broek N, Graham W. Quality of care for maternal and newborn health: the neglected agenda. *BJOG* 2009;116(suppl 1):18–21.
12. Wagaarachchi PT, Fernando L. Trends in maternal mortality and assessment of substandard care in a tertiary care hospital. *Eur J Obstet Gynecol Repord Biol* 2002;101:36–40.
13. Thaddeus S, Maine D. Too far to walk: maternal mortality in context. *Soc Sci Med* 199438(8):1091–1110.
14. Kwawukume EY. Caesarean section in developing countries. *Best Pract Res Clin Obstet Gynaecol* 2001;15:165–178.
15. Gipson R, El Mohandes A, Campbell O, et al. The trends of maternal mortality in Egypt from 1992–2000: an emphasis on regional differences. *Matern Child Health J* 2005;9:71–82.
16. Bartlett LA, Mawji S, Whitehead S, et al. The Afghan Maternal Mortality Study Team. Where giving birth is a forecast of death: maternal mortality in four districts of Afghanistan, 1999–2002. *Lancet* 2005;365:864–870.
17. Howell P. Supporting the evolution of obstetric anaesthesia through outreach programs. *IJOA* 2009;18:1–3.
18. Clyburn P, Morris S, Hall J. Anaesthesia and safe motherhood. *Anaesthesia* 2007;62:21–25.
19. Hodges SC, Mijumbi C, Okello M, et al. Anaesthesia services in developing countries: defining the problems. *Anaesthesia* 2007;62:4–11.
20. Hill JC. Dying to give birth: obstructed labour in the Hindu Kush. *Obstet Gynaecol* 2005;7:267–270.
21. Dubowitz G. Global health and global anesthesia. *Int Anesthesiol Clin* 2010;48:39–46.
22. Walker IA, Wilson IH. Anaesthesia in developing countries-a risk for patients. *Lancet* 2008;371:968–969.
23. Rout C. Maternal mortality and anaesthesia in Africa: a South African perspective. *IJOA* 2002;11:77–80.
24. Fenton PM. Obstetric anesthesia in the developing world. In: Palmer CM, D'Angelo R, Paech MJ, eds. *Handbook of Obstetric Anesthesia*. Oxford: BIOS Scientific Publishers; 2002:244–255.
25. Mavalankar DV, Rosenfield A. Maternal mortality in resource-poor settings: policy barriers to care. *Am J Public Health* 2005;95:200–203.
26. Dyer RA, Reed AR, James JF. Obstetric anaesthesia in low-resource settings. *Best Pract Res Clin Obstet Gynaecol* 2010;24:401–412.
27. Fenton PM, Whitty CJM, Reynolds F. Caesarean section in Malawi: prospective study of early maternal and perinatal mortality. *BMJ* 2003;327:587–591.
28. Engmann C, Olufolabi A, Srofenyoh E, et al. Multidisciplinary team partnerships to improve maternal and neonatal outcomes: The Kybele experience. *Int Anesthesiol Clin* 2010;48:109–122.
29. Enohumah KO, Imarengiaye CO. Factors associated with anesthesia-related maternal mortality in a tertiary hospital in Nigeria. *Acta Anaesthesiol Scand* 2006;50:206–210.
30. Cetin M, Sumer H, Timuroglu T, et al. Maternal mortality in the last decade at a university hospital in Turkey. *Int J Gynecol Obstet* 2003;83:301–302.
31. McKenzie AG. Operative obstetric mortality at Harare Central Hospital 1992–1994: an anaesthetic view. *IJOA* 1998;7:237–241.
32. Tomta K, Maman FO, Agbetra N, et al. Maternal deaths and anesthetics in the Lomé (Togo) University Hospital. *Sante* 2003;13:77–80.
33. Hawkins JL, Koonin LM, Palmer SK, et al. Anesthesia-related deaths during obstetric delivery in the United States, 1979–1990. *Anesthesiology* 1997;86(2):277–284.
34. Schnittger T. Regional anaesthesia in developing countries. *Anaesthesia* 2007;62:44–47.
35. Kopic D, Sedensky M, Owen M. The impact of a teaching program on obstetric anesthesia practices in Croatia. *IJOA* 2009;18:4–9.
36. Nafiu OO, Salam RA, Elegbe EO. Post dural puncture headache in obstetric patients: experience from a West African teaching hospital. *IJOA* 2007;16:4–7.
37. Crawford-Sykes A, Scarlett M, Hambleton IR, et al. Anaesthesia for operative deliveries at the University Hospital of the West Indies: a change of practice. *West Indian Med J* 2005;54(3):187–191.
38. Chkhatarashvili K, Chikovani I, Asatiani T. Assessment of Perinatal Care in Georgia. 2006; Available from: http://www.unicef.org/georgia/Perinatal_Assessment_Report_final.pdf
39. International Standards for a Safe Practice of Anaesthesia 2008; Available from: http://www.anaesthesiologists.org/guidelines/practice/2008-international-standards-for-a-safe-practice-of-anaesthesia
40. Morris S, Clyburn P, Harries S, et al. Mothers of Africa–an anaesthesia charity. *Anaesthesia* 2007;62:108–112.
41. Grady K. Building capacity for anaesthesia in low resource settings. *BJOG* 2009;116:15–17.
42. Okafor UV, Ezegwui HU, Ekwazi K. Trends of different forms of anaesthesia for caesarean section in South-eastern Nigeria. *J Obstet Gynaecol* 2009;29(5):392–395.
43. Kuczkowski KM, Chandra S. Maternal satisfaction with single-dose spinal analgesia for labor pain in Indonesia: a landmark study. *J Anesth* 2008;22:55–58.
44. Ouro-Bang'Na Maman AF, Agbetra N, Djibril A, et al. Knowledge and acceptance of obstetric peridural analgesia: survery of pregnant women in Togo. *Med Trop* 2007;67(2):159–162.
45. Oladokun A, Eyelade O, Morhason-Bello I, et al. Awareness and desirability of labor epidural analgesia: a survey of Nigerian women. *IJOA* 2009;18:38–42.
46. Olayemi O, Adeniji RA, Udoh ES, et al. Determinants of pain perception in labour among parturients at the University College Hospital, Ibadan. *J Obstet Gynaecol* 2005;25(2):128–130.
47. Maltby J, Malla DS, Dangol H. Open drop ether anaesthesia for caesarean section: a review of 420 cases in Nepal. *Can Anaesth Soc J* 1986;33:651–656.
48. Simpson S. Drawover anaesthesia review. Update in *Anaesthesia* 2002;15:13–18; Available from: http://www.nda.ox.ac.uk/wfsa/html/acrobat/update15.pdf
49. Dobson MB. Draw-over *Anaesthesia*. 1993; Available from: http://update.anaesthesiologists.org
50. Dobson MB. Oxygen concentrators for district hospitals. Update in *Anaesthesia* 1999;10;1–4; Available from: http://www.nda.ox.ac.uk/wfsa/html/u10/u1011_01.htm
51. Craven R. Ketamine. *Anaesthesia* 2007;62:48–53.
52. Lau TT, Zed PJ. Does ketamine have a role in managing severe exacerbation of asthma in adults? *Pharmacotherapy* 2001;21:1100–1106.
53. Subramaniam K, Subramanium B, Steinbrook RA. Ketamine as adjuvant analgesic to opioids: a quantitative and qualitative systematic review. *Anesth Analg* 2004;99:482–495.
54. Schmid RL, Sandler AN, Katz J. Use and efficacy of low-dose ketamine in the management of acute postoperative pain: a review of current techniques and outcomes. *Pain* 1999;82:111–125.
55. Correll GE, Maleki J, Gracely EJ, et al. Subanaesthetic ketamine infusion therapy: a retrospective analysis of a novel therapeutic approach to complex regional pain syndrome. *Pain Med* 2004;5:263–275.

ANESTHETIC CONSIDERATIONS FOR REPRODUCTIVE, IN-UTERO AND NON-OBSTETRIC PROCEDURES

CHAPTER

48

In vitro Fertilization and Reproductive Technologies

Roanne L. Preston • Katherine L. Cheesman

■ INTRODUCTION

In 2010, Robert Edwards received the Nobel Prize for Physiology or Medicine, 32 years after the first "test tube baby" was delivered in the United Kingdom in 1978 by his obstetrical colleague Patrick Steptoe (1). Since this time the number of babies born as a result of artificial reproductive techniques has been exponential; the US Centers for Disease Control (CDC) estimates that assisted reproductive technology (ART) now accounts for slightly more than 1% of total US births (2) and 12% of women of childbearing age in the United States have used an infertility clinic.

There are many definitions for assisted reproductive techniques or technologies. The CDC was required to define ART by the Fertility Clinic Success Rate and Certification Act of 1992 and defined ART to include "all fertility treatments in which both the egg and sperm are handled." In general, it involves surgically removing eggs from a woman's ovaries, combining them with sperm in a laboratory and returning them to the woman's body or donating them to another woman (2). It does not include techniques where only the sperm is handled, that is, intrauterine or artificial insemination, or when the woman only uses drugs to stimulate egg production without intending to have the eggs removed, or techniques such as timed intercourse. The term in vitro fertilization (IVF) is commonly used but actually refers to only one technique of ART—the various techniques are described later in the chapter. ART is further categorized by whether the procedure uses the woman's own eggs (non-donor) or eggs from another woman (donor) and whether the embryos used were newly fertilized (fresh) or, previously fertilized, frozen, and then thawed (frozen).

In the year 2007, there were 142,435 ART cycles performed at 430 clinics in the United States, resulting in 43,412 live births and 57,569 infants (56% singleton and 26% multiple infant births). Sixteen percent of these cycles used frozen embryos, the percentage of live births from frozen embryos is usually smaller than from fresh embryos (29.9% vs. 35.9%) because some embryos do not survive the freezing process; however, it is important to understand that transfer of frozen embryos are less expensive and invasive than fresh embryo transfers as the woman does not need to undergo ovarian stimulation therapy and oocyte retrieval (2) (Figs. 48-1, 48-2).

Reasons for using ART are varied. In 2007, infertility diagnoses for woman using fresh oocytes or embryos included male factors such as low sperm count or function representing 18.5% of cases, followed by diminished ovarian reserve in 10.3%, tubal factors in 9%, ovulatory dysfunction in 6.6%, and endometriosis in 4.7% of cases (2) (Fig. 48-3). Ethnic background does not seem to affect pregnancy outcomes or the type of ART, except that African Americans are more likely to have a tubal factor causing infertility than Caucasian women (3).

Delayed childbearing is occurring with increasing frequency and maternal age is the most important factor determining ART outcome (2). Advancing maternal age is associated with a decreased response to ovarian stimulation, lower retrieved oocyte numbers, and lower rates of fertilization and embryo cleavage (4). Increasing numbers of older women are presenting to ART clinics with infertility primarily due to reduced ovarian reserve; in 2007, 61% of women using ART were over the age of 35 years, and 20% were over the age of 41 years, making the average age for all women using ART being 36 years (Fig. 48-4). The vast majority of women younger than 35 years of age used their own eggs (96%), whereas 75% of women older than 44 years of age used donor eggs. Forty percent of cycles amongst women younger than 35 years of age resulted in live births compared to 5% in women aged 43 to 44 years, and 2% among women older than 44 years (2) (Fig. 48-5). In addition to these fertility considerations, the aging mother with potential comorbidities may present greater challenges for care by the anesthesiologist.

■ THE ART CYCLE

The human ovary normally produces one dominant follicle on every menstrual cycle, which has one mature egg inside it. Most forms of ART involve producing multiple eggs by artificially stimulating the ovary to produce multiple follicles (5). The ART cycle begins with downregulation of the pituitary gland and ovaries using a gonadotrophin-releasing hormone (GnRH) agonist or antagonist given subcutaneously for approximately 2 weeks, the intent of which is to shut down the ovaries and prevent the development of the single dominant follicle. After 2 weeks, the ovaries are then stimulated, by either a mixture of follicle-stimulating hormone (FSH) and luteinizing hormone (LH), or FSH alone; these drugs are given subcutaneously or intramuscularly for about 10 days. Follicular maturation is monitored every 2 to 3 days by ultrasound and blood tests. When there are approximately four to eight follicles human chorionic gonadotrophin (hCG) is given.

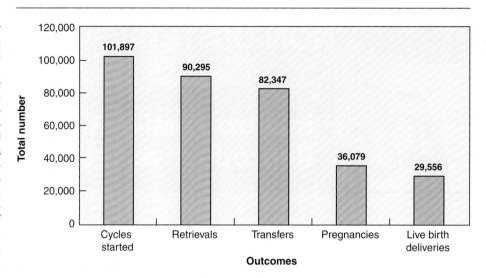

FIGURE 48-1 2007 US data on outcomes of ART cycles using fresh non-donor oocytes or embryos. Adapted from: Centers for Disease Control and Prevention, American Society for Reproductive Medicine, Society for Assisted Reproduction Technology. 2007 Assisted Reproductive Technology Success Rates: National Summary and Fertility Clinic Reports, Atlanta. In: US Department of Health and Human Services, Centers for Disease Control and Prevention; 2009. http://www.cdc.gov/art/ART2007/index.htm. Last accessed January 16, 2011.

hCG acts as a surrogate for the normal mid-cycle surge of LH that causes resumption of meiosis within the oocytes and preparation for fertilization. Ovulation predictably occurs 36 to 40 hours after hCG administration and retrieval is timed within this period (typically 32 to 34 hours following hCG). Delayed retrieval is inadvisable as spontaneous ovulation may occur leading to reduced numbers of mature oocytes or, more seriously, can lead to ovarian hyperstimulation syndrome (OHSS). The oocytes can be retrieved laparoscopically, but presently are more commonly retrieved by transvaginal oocyte retrieval (TVOR), which involves insertion of a specialized transvaginal ultrasound probe with an attached needle into the vagina (Fig. 48-6). The needle is then inserted through the fornix of the vagina into a follicle under ultrasound guidance, and the follicular contents are aspirated. The contents are then washed and examined under a microscope by an embryologist to look for oocytes; typically five to fifteen oocytes are collected during a single procedure. The next steps depend on the particular technique of ART.

■ ART TECHNIQUES

In vitro Fertilization (IVF)

This is the most commonly used assisted reproductive technique. Under controlled conditions in a laboratory, the retrieved oocytes are combined with sperm in a culture medium. After 8 to 12 hours, samples are examined for signs of fertilization, and any successfully created embryos are then observed. Three to six days following retrieval, one or two embryos are then drawn into a catheter and transferred through the cervix into the uterus. This procedure is similar to a pap smear—generally not painful, and analgesia or sedation is not normally required (5).

Gamete Intrafallopian Transfer (GIFT)

Retrieved oocytes are examined for quality and maturation, and then combined with sperm in a transfer catheter and immediately placed, with laparoscopic guidance, through the fimbriated end of one or both of the fallopian tubes;

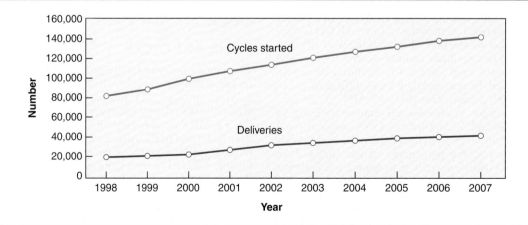

FIGURE 48-2 US data on number of ART cycles performed versus live birth deliveries using ART 1998 to 2007. Adapted from: Centers for Disease Control and Prevention, American Society for Reproductive Medicine, Society for Assisted Reproduction Technology. 2007 Assisted Reproductive Technology Success Rates: National Summary and Fertility Clinic Reports, Atlanta. In: US Department of Health and Human Services, Centers for Disease Control and Prevention; 2009. http://www.cdc.gov/art/ART2007/index.htm. Last accessed January 16, 2011.

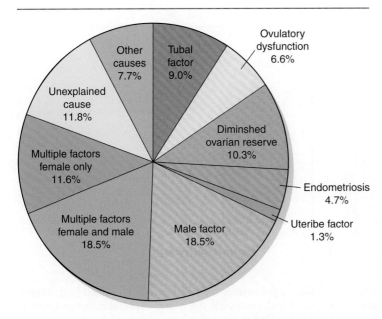

FIGURE 48-3 Diagnoses among couples who had ART cycles using fresh non-donor oocytes or embryos. Adapted from: Centers for Disease Control and Prevention, American Society for Reproductive Medicine, Society for Assisted Reproduction Technology. 2007 Assisted Reproductive Technology Success Rates: National Summary and Fertility Clinic Reports, Atlanta. In: US Department of Health and Human Services, Centers for Disease Control and Prevention; 2009. http://www.cdc.gov/art/ART2007/index.htm. Last accessed January 16, 2011.

fertilization therefore occurs in vivo. Oocyte retrieval can be performed laparoscopically at the same time as the gamete transfer in a single procedure under general anesthesia, or oocytes may have been previously retrieved transvaginally; there is no evidence that the collection technique alters clinical pregnancy or live birth rates. GIFT has the disadvantage that fertilization cannot be confirmed prior to transfer and it also requires patent fallopian tubes (6).

Zygote Intrafallopian Transfer (ZIFT)

ZIFT is procedurally similar to GIFT, but fertilization is first confirmed and the embryo or zygote is then implanted directly into the fallopian tube, via laparoscopy, usually under general anesthesia. This avoids the need for laparoscopic surgery if fertilization does not occur. But, it may require two operations if the oocytes are initially retrieved laparoscopically. ZIFT has a higher success rate than IVF or GIFT (2) (Fig. 48-7).

Intracytoplasmic Sperm Injection (ICSI)

This technique is often used for male infertility when there is little or no sperm in the semen or in the fertilization of cryopreserved oocytes. Individual sperm are injected directly into the cytoplasm of the egg. It has higher pregnancy success rate, but the risks of genetic anomalies appears to be increased, this may be due to the fact that the technique bypasses several phases of normal fertilization which act as a natural screening for genetic problems (7).

■ ANESTHETIC CONSIDERATIONS

Population

The population demographics of women seeking ART are changing. While the majority of women are healthy and infertility problems are related to male factors or gynecologic factors such as endometriosis, tubal dysfunction, or polycystic ovarian syndrome (see Fig. 48-3), many women are now presenting with coexisting illnesses such as thyroid dysfunction or tuberculosis, which are often the cause for their infertility (5). Thorough review of their underlying disease and regular medications should be undertaken to prevent adverse outcomes due to potential drug interactions or precipitation of underlying disease. With advances in cryopreservation of oocytes it is likely that more women will be undergoing oocyte retrieval who have cancer and are already on, or about to start, cytotoxic treatment (8). In addition, the aging nulliparous woman may present with systemic diseases such as type 2 diabetes and essential hypertension. Obesity is a major problem in North America and a leading cause of infertility (9). ART procedures are technically harder in the obese woman for a number of reasons including poorer ultrasound

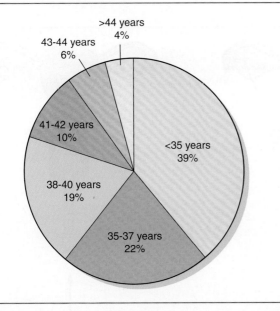

FIGURE 48-4 ART use by maternal age group as percentage of total cycles in US 2007. Adapted from: Centers for Disease Control and Prevention, American Society for Reproductive Medicine, Society for Assisted Reproduction Technology. 2007 Assisted Reproductive Technology Success Rates: National Summary and Fertility Clinic Reports, Atlanta. In: US Department of Health and Human Services, Centers for Disease Control and Prevention; 2009. http://www.cdc.gov/art/ART2007/index.htm. Last accessed January 16, 2011.

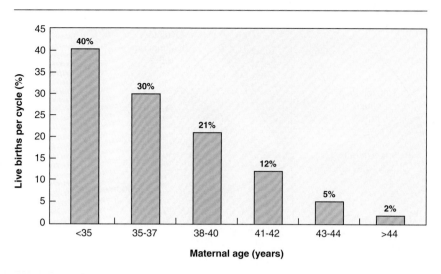

FIGURE 48-5 Percentage of cycles started that resulted in live births by age group in 2007. Adapted from: Centers for Disease Control and Prevention, American Society for Reproductive Medicine, Society for Assisted Reproduction Technology. 2007 Assisted Reproductive Technology Success Rates: National Summary and Fertility Clinic Reports, Atlanta. In: US Department of Health and Human Services, Centers for Disease Control and Prevention; 2009. http://www.cdc.gov/art/ART2007/index.htm. Last accessed January 16, 2011.

visualization, necessity for longer probes, and challenges in patient positioning for the procedure. Obese patients also have more comorbidities including type 2 diabetes and hypertension. Anesthesia problems typically include desaturation and airway management difficulties during sedation; for these reasons spinal anesthesia may be more appropriate (9).

ART has provided the means for women in whom pregnancy and childbirth may be life-threatening to conceive, such as the woman with ongoing organ dysfunction despite organ transplantation, or with primary pulmonary hypertension. She now has the opportunity to produce genetic offspring by undergoing oocyte retrieval, ART, and surrogacy. These women are a challenge to care for from preconception through to delivery and require an ongoing interdisciplinary team approach, including anesthesiologists (10,11).

Women presenting for ART are often under a high degree of social and emotional stress and depression is not uncommon (12). This is often further aggravated by the hormonal manipulation that occurs during ovarian stimulation. Anxiety about the medical procedures is often compounded by stress from financial issues and concerns about missing work. Management of this anxiety is important, and may require an increased dose of anxiolytics and/or propofol for moderate ("conscious") sedation compared to women with more typical procedural anxiety (13).

Anesthesia and Reproductive Success

The success rate of live births from ART is still only 30% and the underlying factors are still not well understood. In

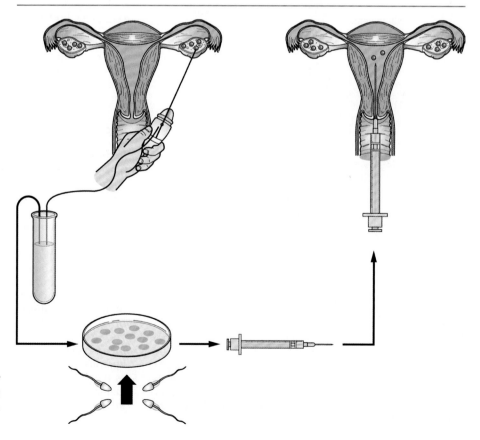

FIGURE 48-6 Transvaginal oocyte retrieval and transfer procedure. Courtesy of Dr. Caroline Dean.

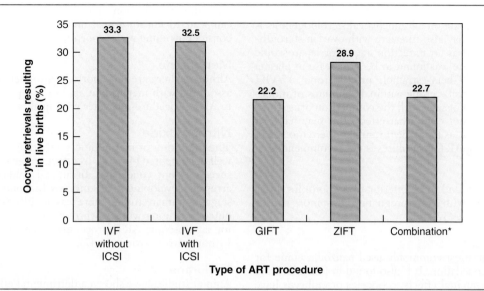

FIGURE 48-7 Percentages of oocyte retrievals that resulted in live births by type of ART procedure 2007. Adapted from: Centers for Disease Control and Prevention, American Society for Reproductive Medicine, Society for Assisted Reproduction Technology. 2007 Assisted Reproductive Technology Success Rates: National Summary and Fertility Clinic Reports, Atlanta. In: US Department of Health and Human Services, Centers for Disease Control and Prevention; 2009. http://www.cdc.gov/art/ART2007/index.htm. Last accessed January 16, 2011. *Combination of IVF with or without ICSI and either GIFT or ZIFT.

the early days of ART, oocyte retrieval was performed laparoscopically under general anesthesia. In 1987, Boyers et al. (14) and Hayes et al. (15) reported that the first oocytes collected laparoscopically under general anesthesia fertilized more often than the last oocytes collected, suggesting that general anesthesia may have a detrimental effect on fertilization of oocytes. It was unknown if the main contributory factor was the pneumoperitoneum or the anesthetic agents themselves. This led to interest in exploring the effects of anesthetic agents on oocyte fertilization and embryo implantation, and research into which anesthetic technique provides the best outcome—a successful live birth. Unfortunately, much of the evidence to date is marred by lack of specific details about the anesthetic agents used, limited data set from small studies or case reports/case series, and failure to control confounding factors such as procedure duration and maternal age.

The carbon dioxide (CO_2) pneumoperitoneum may be one of the causes of the lower fertilization rate seen in oocytes retrieved laparoscopically under general anesthesia. One hundred percent CO_2 is the ideal insufflation gas as its high blood solubility facilitates rapid absorption from the peritoneal cavity post surgery, it is noncombustible, and it minimizes the chance of life-threatening gas embolism. However, there is evidence to suggest that it may have direct adverse effects on fertilization, most likely due to the decrease in follicular pH that occurs subsequent to CO_2 diffusing into the follicle during the procedure (16).

Improvements in transvaginal ultrasonography enabling the operator to directly visualize the follicles, then puncture and aspirate a follicle has bypassed the need for general anesthesia and the potential harmful effects of the pneumoperitoneum. It also means that the procedures do not have to necessarily be done in a hospital, nor require the presence of an anesthesiologist. In addition to being less invasive than laparoscopic procedures, TVOR is associated with higher pregnancy rates (17).

Anesthetic Drugs
Propofol
The pharmacokinetic profile of propofol makes it ideal for procedures such as oocyte retrieval, providing a rapid onset and short duration of action as well as analgesic and antiemetic effects; however, its use in TVOR is controversial. Due to its high lipid solubility and large volume of distribution, propofol is of course present in follicular fluid (18), and concentrations are related to dose and duration of administration (19). The controversy is over whether it has a significant effect on fertilization, embryo implantation, and live birth rate. Some animal studies have shown a detrimental effect of propofol on oocyte cleavage, fertilization, and term pregnancy in mice (20,21) but others have shown no significant effect (22). The majority of current evidence from human studies suggests that it has no detrimental effect on embryo fertilization, cleavage, or pregnancy rates (23–26). Only Vincent et al. who compared propofol–nitrous oxide anesthesia to an isoflurane–nitrous oxide combination, found a significantly lower pregnancy rate (29% vs. 54%) (27). This conflicting evidence of detrimental effect on ART outcomes suggests it would be sensible to limit the duration of exposure to propofol during ART procedures in order to limit accumulation of drug in the follicular fluid.

Thiopentone
Thiopentone too has been found in follicular fluid when used as an induction agent (28) but there is no difference in the rate of clinical pregnancy in women who receive thiopentone (5 mg/kg) compared to propofol (2.7 mg/kg) for induction of general anesthesia during GIFT procedures (29) or differences in fertilization rate, cleavage rate, implantation rate, or pregnancy rate when it was used as an induction agent for oocyte retrieval (30).

Etomidate

The effect of etomidate on adrenocortical steroidogenesis is well known, but it may also interfere with ovarian steroidogenesis. When used as an induction agent for laparoscopic oocyte retrieval, there was found to be a decrease in plasma concentration of 17-beta-estradiol, progesterone, 17-OH progesterone, and testosterone within 10 minutes of induction; this trend was not seen with the comparison drug, thiopentone (31). It is not clear what effects this may have on pregnancy outcomes, as the patient numbers were too small, but its usage during ART procedures is not recommended.

Methohexital

Methohexital was found to be inferior to propofol for sedation during TVOR with lower pregnancy rates, more nausea and a longer recovery (32).

Benzodiazepines

Midazolam is the most commonly used benzodiazepine for procedures under sedation. It is also found in follicular fluid (33), but no detrimental effects to oocytes or embryos have been detected (34,35). Animal studies with doses as high as 35.0 mg/kg did not prevent or impair in vivo fertilization (36). Midazolam is often used in conjunction with other anesthetic drugs including propofol, fentanyl, alfentanil, and remifentanil. It has been shown to be as effective and safe as a fentanyl–propofol combination in patients undergoing TVOR (37–39).

Ketamine

Sedation with ketamine and midazolam has been proposed as a safe alternative to general anesthesia with fentanyl–propofol–isoflurane for TVOR with no differences in outcome of embryos transplanted (34).

Alfentanil

The rapid onset and short duration of alfentanil makes it an attractive opioid for ART procedures. While levels are detectable in the follicular fluid (33), they are ten-fold less than serum concentrations (39). When compared with fentanyl for sedation there was no difference in pregnancy outcome, yet induction was quicker and patients were less drowsy at the end of the procedure (40).

Fentanyl

Transfer into follicular fluid occurs but no adverse effects on reproduction have been reported. Animal studies show no effect on the fertilization or cleavage of sea urchin eggs exposed to fentanyl, even at large doses (41).

Remifentanil

The pharmacokinetic properties of remifentanil make it an attractive option for sedation for TVOR or for total intravenous anesthesia. When used during general anesthesia for TVOR compared to sedation with midazolam and propofol, there were no differences in cleavage or pregnancy rates (38). When used for monitored anesthetic care (MAC) compared to general anesthesia with propofol–nitrous oxide–alfentanil, patients who underwent MAC with remifentanil had higher pregnancy rates (30.6% vs. 17.9%) (42). In comparison with local anesthesia alone, a remifentanil infusion for sedation provided superior procedural conditions and there was no difference found in oocyte quality or embryo score in a retrospective analysis of over 500 cases (43).

Morphine

In an animal study using doses equivalent to 50 mg of morphine in humans, 26% to 33% of oocytes showed polyspermy (abnormal fertilization of an egg by multiple sperm), which can lead to chromosomal abnormalities (44). One should consider avoiding use of morphine for ART procedures.

Meperidine

Although there are no reported reproductive adverse effects associated with meperidine, its use as a premedication prior to ART procedures provides poor quality sedation (45).

Nitrous Oxide

The inhibition of methionine synthetase by nitrous oxide is well documented (46), but its effect on fertilization and ART success is not conclusive. In animal studies, nitrous oxide arrested development of embryos but only at the two-cell stage. In human studies, there was no difference in pregnancy outcome among women who underwent general anesthesia for laparoscopic ART procedures using isoflurane with or without nitrous oxide (26,47).

Isoflurane

Animal studies have shown a detrimental effect of isoflurane on mice embryo development (48). This was further seen when human sera, collected from women undergoing laparoscopic gynecologic surgery with nitrous oxide–isoflurane or nitrous oxide–morphine–fentanyl, was used to incubate mouse embryos and showed a decrease in embryo fertilization rates (49). Human studies have shown that exposure time may have an effect; there were significantly lower fertilization rates in the last oocytes retrieved compared to the first oocytes during laparoscopic oocyte collection (14). However, Beilin et al. found no difference in pregnancy rates following general anesthesia for GIFT procedure using isoflurane compared to propofol, nitrous oxide, or midazolam (26).

Enflurane

When compared with halothane, implantation and pregnancy rates were higher using enflurane (50,51).

Halothane

Animal studies have shown delayed oocyte maturation in mice exposed to halothane but there was no increase in lethal mutations or implantations (52). In human studies halothane was found to have higher first and second trimesters miscarriage rates compared to enflurane (50) and a lower implantation rate (51). It is one of the few anesthetic drugs in which there appears to be agreement it should be avoided for ART procedures (53).

Sevoflurane

While there is no evidence that sevoflurane is genotoxic, the potential degradation product compound A has been associated with the induction of sister chromatid exchange (an indicator of DNA mutation) in Chinese hamster ovary cells in vitro (54).

Desflurane

There is no published information on the use of desflurane in anesthesia for ART procedures.

Antiemetics

ART is associated with higher estradiol levels, which increases the incidence of emesis (55). Regular use of dopamine antagonists such as droperidol and metoclopramide during the ART cycle should be avoided as these drugs induce hyperprolactinemia, which impairs ovarian follicle maturation (56). However, the risks of transient hyperprolactinemia from drugs given perioperatively to prevent nausea and reduce aspiration risk is unclear; some studies have indicated that low levels of prolactin were associated with higher pregnancy rates (57) whereas others have shown that transient hyperprolactinemia was associated with a better oocyte quality and higher fertilization rate (58,59).

The 5-HT$_3$ receptor antagonists are very effective antiemetic agents in the perioperative period, and therefore are naturally used during ART procedures. This is despite the lack of safety data on use of serotonin antagonists in early pregnancy, or understanding of potential reproductive effects. 5-HT$_3$ receptors are found diffusely in the body, with a diverse array of functions. The 5-HT$_3$ antagonist GR38032F, which became ondansetron, was found to be highly toxic to DBA/2 mice in phase II trials, inducing abnormal neurobehavior prior to death (60). Both Sweden and Australia have attempted to collect outcome data on the effects of antiemetics used in early pregnancy to treat nausea and vomiting of pregnancy (NVP) through their national databases, but the data set size remains small (61,62). The Swedish data collected from 1995 to 2002 showed no differences in pregnancy outcomes amongst the different antiemetics used to treat NVP; however, 68% of women were prescribed meclozine with minimal data on ondansetron (61). The Australian data cover only 176 pregnancy outcomes, of which the majority received ondansetron, and shows no differences in miscarriage or major malformation rates amongst the different antiemetics used (62). North American opinion as of 2002 did not support use of the newer drugs as first-line agents for NVP and recommends that phenothiazines, antihistamine H$_1$ receptor antagonists, and doxylamine–pyridoxine be used as they are efficacious with no known association with adverse fetal outcomes (63). Only one study has been published on the placental transfer of ondansetron (64). The study involved 41 women undergoing first trimester terminations; each received three doses of 8 mg of ondansetron pre-procedure. Tissue concentrations of ondansetron were determined, showing a fetal–maternal ratio of 0.41 (0.31 to 0.52), with higher concentrations in fetal tissue than amniotic fluid.

In summary, there is insufficient evidence to recommend serotonin antagonists as first-line treatment for nausea/vomiting associated with anesthesia for ART procedures.

Non-steroidal Anti-inflammatory Drugs (NSAIDs)

The safety of NSAIDs in ART is not clear, although they are widely used as an analgesic periprocedurally (53). NSAIDs inhibit prostaglandin synthesis, which has been shown to lead to abnormal implantation and higher miscarriage rates in both animals and humans (65). In animal studies, both non-selective and selective COX-2 inhibitors cause a significant increase in postimplantation loss in rats (66). The selective COX-2 inhibitor meloxicam has been shown to inhibit rabbit ovulation, with potential for use as a nonhormonal contraceptive, hence its use in women undergoing ART should be avoided (67). There is also evidence in the general population that the use of NSAIDs is associated with an increased miscarriage rate (68). The use of aspirin to improve ART outcomes remains unproven though used in some centers; meta-analysis of numerous randomized trials found no benefit or risk of miscarriage (69).

Local Anesthetics

Comparing the effects of local anesthetics used in ART is difficult as their pharmacokinetic profile is dependent on their site of administration, that is, paracervically, intrathecally, or epidurally. Mouse oocytes incubated in lidocaine, chloroprocaine, and bupivacaine all showed abnormal fertilization and embryo development; however, detrimental effects from bupivacaine were only seen at high concentrations (70).

Procaine and tetracaine both delayed the natural response of the oocytes to extrude cortical granules preventing polyspermy, thereby increasing the likelihood of multiple sperms fertilizing the oocyte leading to chromosomal abnormalities (71). Lidocaine has been found to cause teratogenic effects in rat embryos; however, concentrations were much higher than clinically relevant (72). These animal studies may not be relevant to humans as oocytes are washed prior to fertilization; therefore, concentrations clinically are much lower. Moreover, the concentration reaching follicular fluid during spinal anesthesia is likely very low.

Anesthetizing Locations

Oocyte retrieval can be performed safely under ultrasound guidance with sedation, and can therefore be performed in a procedure room, negating the need for expensive operating rooms and personnel. Many ART procedures are performed in satellite sites such as freestanding surgical centers and office-based environments not necessarily attached to a hospital. The benefit of using a separate facility includes having a specialized team and environment, to not only provide an efficient dedicated service, but also to promote a relaxed personal environment to accommodate the psychosocial needs of the couple.

The practice of delivering sedation by non-anesthesia personnel in non-hospital facilities is well established and there are published guidelines by the American Society of Anesthesiologists (ASA) to guide the facility when setting up their protocols (73) (Table 48-1). The disadvantages of using a

TABLE 48-1 Minimum Requirements in a Procedure Room

- Reliable source of oxygen adequate for the length of the procedure. Back-up supply available.
- Reliable source of suction. Suction apparatus that meets operating room standards is strongly encouraged.
- Airway equipment available:
  - Self-inflating hand resuscitator bag capable of administering at least 90% oxygen as a means to deliver positive pressure ventilation.
  - Airway devices, such as laryngeal mask airway, laryngoscope blades, and endotracheal tubes.
- Adequate monitoring equipment to allow adherence to the ASA's "Standards for Basic Anesthetic Monitoring."
  - Blood pressure
  - Oxygen saturation
  - Electrocardiographic monitoring (EKG)
  - Availability of capnography
- Immediate availability of an emergency cart with a defibrillator, emergency drugs, and other equipment adequate to provide cardiopulmonary resuscitation.
- Appropriate post sedation management protocol.
- Written protocols for cardiopulmonary emergencies including anaphylaxis and local anesthetic toxicity as well as other internal and external disasters such as fire. All facility personnel should be trained in the facility's written emergency protocols

ASA, American Society of Anesthesiologists.
Adapted from: American Society of Anesthesiologists. Standards Guidelines and Statements: Basic Anesthetic Monitoring, Standards for (Effective July 1, 2011); Nonoperating Room Anesthetizing Locations, Statement on (2008). http://www.asahq.org/For-Healthcare-Professionals/Standards-Guidelines-and-Statements.aspx. Last accessed January 16, 2011.

non–hospital-based surgical/procedural facility include the lack of immediate facilities and anesthesiology staff in the event of a complication. It is therefore vital that the facility has a written protocol in place for the safe and timely transfer of patients to a prespecified alternate care facility when extended or emergency services are needed to protect the health or well-being of the woman. Patients should be screened by medical history and physical examination to assess risks and comorbidities, including airway assessment and aspiration risks, and consultation with an anesthesiologist made when appropriate.

■ ANESTHESIA FOR SPECIFIC ART PROCEDURES

Transvaginal Ultrasound-guided Oocyte Retrieval (TVOR)

Retrieving oocytes using guidance with transvaginal ultrasound is less invasive than the laparoscopic approach but is still one of the most stressful and painful procedures performed during ART (74). Although there are small studies of transvaginal single follicle aspiration being performed without the use of anesthesia (75), most centers offer some form of anesthesia—either neuraxial anesthesia, moderate sedation, local anesthetic to the vaginal wall and/or paracervical block or a combination of these approaches. Bokhari et al. in the United Kingdom reported the use of sedation in 46% of centers, general anesthesia in 28% and regional anesthesia in 14% (53). In the United States, Ditkoff et al. reported that in 1997 the commonest form of anesthesia was sedation, used in 95% of cases (76).

The procedure generally takes about 20 to 30 minutes and can be done as a day case. It therefore requires an anesthetic technique that is quick, easily reversible, and provides good pain relief. In addition, the chosen technique must minimize patient movement that can potentially make insertion of the probe and aspiration of follicles difficult, as well as increase the risk of trauma to surrounding tissues and organs. Options include local anesthesia, sedation, regional anesthesia, and electroacupuncture.

Local Anesthesia

Paracervical block provides adequate analgesia for puncturing of the vaginal wall but does not prevent the discomfort or pain experienced upon follicular aspiration. It is generally performed in conjunction with small amounts of intravenous sedation (77). This technique may offer the advantage of negating the need for anesthetic personnel and thus can be performed outside the hospital environment.

Sedation

Moderate sedation/analgesia (conscious sedation) has been defined by the ASA as "a drug-induced depression of consciousness during which patients respond purposefully to verbal commands, either alone or accompanied by light tactile stimulation. No interventions are required to maintain a patent airway, and spontaneous ventilation is adequate. Cardiovascular function is usually maintained (78)." While it does not require the presence of an anesthesiologist, it does requires a specially trained "sedation practitioner" who should be skilled in sedation techniques and airway management, and be able to recognize patients who are at risk for complications and whose sedation should be provided by an anesthesiologist. The type and method of providing sedative drugs is highly variable and facility/practitioner dependent. Close communication with the surgeon is important

to pre-empt the pain of needle insertion with a small dose of opioid, as well as knowing when to cease drug administration to allow for a fast emergence. Many ART programs offer monitored anesthesia care that is anesthesiologist led and allows for conversion from moderate sedation to general anesthesia, thus preventing the need to cancel oocyte collection mid-procedure should the patient not tolerate moderate sedation. In many US centers, deep sedation (perhaps better characterized as general anesthesia with a natural airway), utilizing propofol as the principal agent, has become popular.

Regional Anesthesia

Neuraxial blockade, by either epidural or spinal anesthesia, provides excellent pain relief with minimal sedation of the woman. In addition, there is lower absorption of agent into the systemic circulation and subsequently lower accumulation within the follicular fluid. It is associated with a lower incidence of nausea and oversedation when compared with general anesthesia or sedation (79,80). It has the added benefit that the partner may be in the room adding to the couple's experience, alleviating anxiety and improving satisfaction. Botta et al. showed no difference in fertilization, cleavage, or pregnancy rates between patients with epidural anesthesia compared with propofol sedation (79), and Lewin et al. showed improved outcomes in fertilization, cleavage, and pregnancy rates with neuraxial techniques as compared to general anesthesia (6).

The nerve supply to the ovaries is from the ovarian plexus, formed by the renal ganglion and superior mesenteric ganglion, from the lesser and least splanchnic nerves (T10 to T12). Ideally, one aims for a sensory block that allows the woman to be pain free but with minimal motor block so that she is able to move herself onto the bed and be able to position her legs into the lithotomy position. With short surgical times the dose of local anesthetic can be reduced. Using 1.5% lidocaine as opposed to 5% can significantly shorten recovery times, and the addition of fentanyl 10 μg can further reduce the dose of lidocaine, with improved comfort levels and no increase in side effects such as urinary retention, ambulation readiness, or discharge home (81,82). Concern over the association of lidocaine with post spinal pain syndrome led Tsen et al. to investigate the use of bupivacaine as an alternative (83); they compared 3.75 mg of 0.75% hyperbaric bupivacaine with 25 μg fentanyl to 30 mg of 1.5% lidocaine with 25 μg fentanyl, and found no differences in onset time, maximum block height, intraoperative and postoperative analgesia, full sensory and motor recovery or side effects, but did find that the bupivacaine group took significantly longer time to void and subsequently time to discharge was increased (159.05 +/− 37.80 minutes vs. 125.53 +/− 37.54 minutes). While the study was not powered to investigate post spinal pain syndrome, one patient in the lidocaine group did develop typical symptoms. Tidmarsh and May used 2.5 mg of bupivacaine with 25 μg fentanyl intrathecally and showed preservation of motor power but did not report on time to void (80). Bupivacaine is clinically an acceptable alternative to lidocaine, but in a busy ambulatory care centre, delayed discharge of patients has financial and staffing implications making it potentially unpopular.

Other considerations for use of neuraxial blockade include the occurrence of significant side effects, such as postdural puncture headache, prolonged motor blockade, urinary retention, nerve damage, epidural or spinal hematoma, and infection. In addition, it can be time-consuming to perform, requires specialized anesthesia personnel and should be performed in a hospital environment.

Electroacupuncture

This is an emerging practice, originally more time-consuming than conventional anesthesia but recent improved techniques have increased its accessibility. It may have benefits relating to its actions as an anxiolytic, as well as improving uterine blood flow (84). When used in combination with a paracervical block and compared with alfentanil plus paracervical block, electroacupuncture showed improved patient satisfaction and preference, despite higher procedural visual analog scores (85). Whether it improves ART success remains unknown (84).

At the present time there is insufficient data to recommend the optimal drugs or technique for providing anesthesia for a woman undergoing TVOR, and patient preference will always be a confounding factor. Kim et al., in a meta-analysis, reviewed 115 studies published between the years 1966 and 1999 for prospective trials examining the outcomes of local or regional anesthesia and general anesthesia on ART success (86). Only four trials met inclusion criteria so they could not definitively recommend any particular anesthetic type. A 2009 Cochrane review by Kwan et al. reviewed 390 reports with 12 papers meeting inclusion criteria, and failed to find sufficient evidence to support any one method of moderate sedation or analgesia as superior in terms of pregnancy outcomes, pain relief, or patient satisfaction (87).

Finally, while there is no definite link between anesthetic technique and decreased fertilization rates, we must continue to examine our practices to ensure that anesthesia drugs and/or our techniques help optimize ART outcomes.

ART-requiring Laparoscopy

Both GIFT and ZIFT procedures are performed laparoscopically. Most are performed under general anesthesia; however, neuraxial blockade is also an option thereby avoiding the need for potentially harmful drugs. The major disadvantages of laparoscopy are the pneumoperitoneum, the effect of CO_2 and other physiologic consequences; and the Trendelenburg position, which itself may have a detrimental effect on perfusion of the reproductive organs and therefore affect procedure success. The extent of the cardiovascular changes depends on the intra-abdominal pressure (IAP) used; at levels below 15 mm Hg, venous return is increased as blood is "squeezed" out of the splanchnic venous bed, causing an increase in cardiac output. At levels of 15 to 25 mm Hg, venous return decreases as the inferior vena cava is compressed along with the surrounding collateral vessels leading to decreased cardiac output and hypotension. It is advisable to limit the IAP to below 15 mm Hg during laparoscopic ART procedures, especially if the procedure is being performed under neuraxial blockade. The induction of pneumoperitoneum with the patient in the horizontal position rather than in the head-down position can decrease the severity of these hemodynamic changes (88), and finally, while the majority of women undergoing these techniques are healthy, the population demographic is changing and we are likely to

have to anesthetize women in the future in whom the physiologic changes associated with laparoscopic surgery could present significant challenges to maintaining homeostasis.

■ COMPLICATIONS OF ART

Although complications are rare, the most serious are obstetrical—preterm delivery, multiple pregnancy, and OHSS. In addition, there are procedural complications.

Procedural

Aragona et al. reviewed the clinical problems in a series of 7,098 TVORs and reported a total of six cases of severe clinical complications (0.08%, 95% confidence interval 0.03 to 0.18): Four patients with severe peritoneal bleeding requiring surgical treatment and two patients with pelvic abscesses (89). The incidence of pelvic abscess in this study was low compared to a previous review of 2,495 cases in the Netherlands showing a higher frequency at 0.24% (90) and which found it was associated with a history of pelvic adhesions.

Obstetrical

Preterm Delivery

The risk of preterm birth is higher amongst infants conceived by ART than the general population: 13% versus 11% (2). The risk of preterm delivery is increased for multiple births: 62% of twins and 96% of triplets deliver prematurely, as well as the risks conferred by low birth weight, other complications of preterm delivery include cerebral palsy, retinopathy of prematurity, and bronchodysplasia with associated significant ongoing care costs (91).

Multiple Births

Thirty-one percent of live births from ART cycles in 2007, using fresh non-donor eggs or embryos, resulted in multiple infant births (29.4% twins and 1.8% triplets or more), as opposed to 11% in the general population (2). From 1980 to 1997, the number of twin pregnancies rose by 50% and the number of higher order pregnancy rose by 404% (91). The risks for both the mother and infant(s) are greatly increased and open the discussion about the appropriate number of embryos to transfer. Maternal risks from carrying multiple fetuses include increased incidence of gestational diabetes, preeclampsia, abruption, placenta previa, vasa previa, and a higher cesarean delivery rate (Table 48-2). Neonatal risks include early pregnancy loss, preterm delivery, and low birth weight (<2,500 g). Polyhydramnios, oligohydramnios, and twin-to-twin transfusion syndrome are all significant morbidities associated with multiple gestations, and in addition, monozygote twinning is more common with ART (91).

Many countries, because of the increased health-care requirements of women carrying multiple gestations, are

TABLE 48-2 Rates of Major Maternal Complications Resulting from Multiple Order Pregnancies

Number of Fetuses	Preterm Labor	Preterm Delivery[a]	Gestational Diabetes Mellitus	Preeclampsia
1	15%	10%	3%	6%
2	40%	50%	5%–8%	10%–12%
3	75%	92%	7%	25%–60%
4	>95%	>95%	>10%	>60%

[a]Delivery at <37 weeks of gestation.

Redrawn from: ASRM Practice Committee. Multiple pregnancy associated with infertility therapy. *Fertil Steril* 2006;86:S106–S110, with permission.

scrutinizing the issue of transferring more than one embryo. In the United States, the number of embryos transferred is at the discretion of the doctor and patient but the American Society for Reproductive Medicine currently recommends no more than two embryos be transferred in women under the age of 35, two or three in those 35 to 37 years, three or four embryos or two blastocysts in those 38 to 40 years, and in those 41 to 42 years, no more than five embryos or three blastocysts (92). The Society of Obstetricians and Gynecologists of Canada recommend a maximum of two embryos be transferred if the woman is under the age of 35 years, and no more than four embryos should be transferred in the over-39 age group, recognizing that these women have decreased implantation rates with their own eggs. In women with good health and high likelihood of success, consideration should be made to transfer only one embryo (93). Many patients and physicians are reluctant to reduce the number of embryos transferred for fear of a reduction in the probability of pregnancy; this is particularly relevant when patients finance the treatments themselves and may not be able to afford multiple attempts. Many couples remain unaware of the higher maternal and neonatal risks associated with multiple births.

Selective reduction of pregnancy decreases preterm delivery but is associated with profound ethical dilemmas. The procedure normally takes place around 12 weeks of gestation and involves either injection of potassium chloride into the gestational sac of the selected fetus or by radiofrequency ablation of the umbilical cord; both are done under ultrasound guidance with local anesthesia, similar to an amniocentesis procedure. There is an approximately 3% to 5% miscarriage rate of the remaining fetus associated with this procedure (94).

Ectopic and Heterotopic Pregnancies

The incidence of ectopic pregnancy after ART varies from less than 5% to as high as 11% in those patients with a tubal factor for their infertility, compared to an incidence of approximately 2% after natural conception (95). The risk for a heterotopic pregnancy, where there is a normal intrauterine pregnancy coexisting with an ectopic pregnancy, is about 1% as compared to 0.015% in the general population (96). These women may require general anesthesia for salpingectomy and removal of the ectopic gestation; the risk of spontaneous abortion of the remaining fetus is high, but successful outcomes have been reported (96). Surprisingly, the rate of ectopic pregnancy is not increased in procedures such as GIFT and ZIFT where the embryo is placed directly into the fallopian tube. Anesthesia technique should take into account the remaining fetus—a hemodynamically stable technique to maximize placental perfusion, and use of drugs that have minimal effects on the remaining fetus.

Ovarian Hyperstimulation Syndrome

Diagnosis

OHSS is a rare and potentially life-threatening iatrogenic complication of ovarian hyperstimulation that complicates 1% to 10% of IVF cycles (97). It is characterized by ovarian enlargement due to multiple, large ovarian follicles or cysts and results in acute fluid shifts into the extravascular space causing profound intravascular volume depletion, ascites, oliguria, electrolyte imbalance, pleural effusion, hemoconcentration, hypercoagulability, and thromboembolism (97). OHSS is classified as mild, moderate, or severe. Severe OHSS has a prevalence of only 0.5% to 2%, but the estimated mortality rate is 1:400,000 to 1:500,000 per stimulated cycle with death usually secondary to a thromboembolic event (97,98). Overall, OHSS results in hospitalization in 1.9% of patients

undergoing ART procedures; however, with increasing numbers of women undergoing ART the number of women presenting with OHSS is likely to increase (98).

There are two forms of OHSS: Early onset occurs pre-retrieval within 3 to 7 days after hCG administration, and late onset, which occurs when the treatment is successful and is thought to be the consequence of endogenous hCG released by the trophoblast. If the treatment does not lead to pregnancy, early onset OHSS usually resolves on its own within a few days, whereas late onset OHSS can persist for weeks and is clinically more difficult to treat (98). The exact pathogenesis of OHSS remains unknown, but is thought to be related to ovarian release of vasoactive, angiogenic substances that increase vascular permeability leading to extravasation of protein-rich fluid; vascular endothelial growth factor (VEGF) is currently thought to be the main factor (99). Administration of hCG for final follicle maturation and triggering of ovulation seems to be the pivotal stimulus of OHSS in a susceptible patient. Risk factors for developing OHSS include previous OHSS, younger age, and women with ovulation disorders such as polycystic ovarian syndrome (98).

Prevention

Completely eliminating the risk of OHSS is achieved only by cancelling the cycle with the potential to cryopreserve the embryos, but many couples decide to accept the risk and continue with embryo transfer. Withholding the hCG for a few days ("coasting") or using a lower dose of hCG may help; future work lies in the use of dopamine agonists to inhibit VEGF (98,100).

Treatment

OHSS is a self-limiting disease and women with mild or moderate hyperstimulation can be treated on an ambulatory basis with bed rest and careful observation. Severe OHSS may include renal failure, hepatic damage, thromboembolic phenomena, acute respiratory distress syndrome, disseminated intravascular coagulation, and multiorgan failure, and is therefore best managed by an experienced team in a critical care unit; it is advisable to transfer any patient to such a unit if development of severe OHSS is imminent (100). Treatment is directed at maintaining intravascular blood volume with intravenous fluid infusions, often titrated using invasive cardiac monitoring. Assisted ventilation is sometimes required. Prevention of thromboembolism is important; thromboembolic stockings should be used as well as subcutaneous heparin 5,000 to 7,500 units daily or low-molecular-weight heparin and, in the immobile patient, compression boots should also be used.

Abdominal paracentesis in patients with significant ascites is often required to reduce abdominal pressure and is performed by ultrasonographic-guided transvaginal paracentesis (100). Surgical management is reserved for only the extreme cases of a ruptured cyst, ovarian torsion, or internal hemorrhage and may be lifesaving, but can further aggravate electrolyte imbalances and increase morbidity (100). The underlying pregnancy may perpetuate and exacerbate life-threatening OHSS, and therapeutic abortion may need to be considered.

Anesthesia may be required for transvaginal drainage of ascites, emergency laparotomy, or for termination of pregnancy. Anesthetic management should be as for any hypovolemic patient, with selection and titration of anesthetic agents to prevent further hypotension. Due to the raised abdominal pressure and frequent nausea and vomiting seen in OHSS patient, a rapid sequence induction would be appropriate, but it is important to check potassium levels which may be high due to renal failure or electrolyte imbalance. Transvaginal paracentesis can be performed under sedation in a similar set up as used for TVOR. Positioning the patient in slight reverse Trendelenburg during the procedure appears to cause less pulmonary compromise than does the supine position, and possibly allows for better fluid drainage (100).

OTHER TOPICS

Oocyte and Ovarian Tissue Cryopreservation

The technologic advances in the area of oocyte cryopreservation are continually expanding and will likely result in the procedure becoming common practice in the next 20 years. It has a number of advantages including allowing for flexibility in timing if the initial treatment cycles had to be halted for reasons such as development of ovarian hyperstimulation or inability of the partner to produce an adequate sperm sample, and reducing the cost of ART by removing the need for repeated doses of hormone treatment and follicle assessment. It also provides an option for women who choose or require to postpone childbirth until advanced age, and can provide a means to circumvent the ethical and legal issues of embryo cryopreservation (8). One of the most beneficial uses of the technology is the preservation of fertility in women requiring cytotoxic therapies to treat malignancy; for many cancer survivors, fertility is recognized as a critical component of quality of life. However, oocyte cryopreservation is not an option for some cancer sufferers who do not have enough time to undergo ovarian stimulation or in whom hormone therapy may accelerate tumor growth. For such women, there is the option of ovarian tissue cryopreservation; tissue can be harvested laparoscopically as a day procedure and cryopreserved without needing to delay the start of cancer therapy. Caution is necessary in certain malignancies, most significantly hematologic, due to the potential risk that transplanted tissue may harbor cancer cells that could induce recurrence of malignancy once reimplanted (8).

With respect to outcomes from use of cryopreserved oocytes, Noyes et al. reported in 2010 on 900 live births via oocyte cryopreservation techniques, reporting that there were no differences in the rate of congenital anomalies compared with naturally conceived infants (101).

FUTURE DIRECTIONS

Over the past 30 years the area of ART has expanded exponentially, and over the next 20 years it will continue to grow. With improvements in drug therapy, surgical skills, and technology, ART is becoming accessible to a wider patient population—the older woman with age-related systemic disease, the obese woman, and the post-chemotherapy woman. These women are likely to present a challenge not only during the assisted pregnancy but also throughout their entire pregnancy and delivery. With individual countries introducing guidelines restricting the number of embryos transferred there is hope that the number of high-order pregnancies and the associated maternal and neonatal risks will be eliminated. Reduction in multiple pregnancies will hopefully also reduce the number of preterm and low–birth-weight infants born following ART. Despite the many positive advances, ART will continue to provoke ongoing moral, ethical, and religious debates as it becomes more accessible worldwide. Long-term outcome data still needs to be collected and thoroughly examined to ensure the safe practice of varying new techniques and drugs so that these medical advances not only produce a higher successful live birth rate, but also more importantly healthy infants and healthy mothers. As anesthesiologists, we should continually examine our practice and techniques to ensure our choices have minimal impact on ART success.

KEY POINTS

- There is an ever increasing diversity of women undergoing ART: Older women, obese women, and women who have undergone cancer treatment. These women may have significant comorbidities
- There are no conclusive human studies to suggest significant effects of most anesthetic drugs on live births; however, there are animal studies that indicate some detrimental effects on early reproductive function
- Anesthetic drugs/adjuncts to avoid are halothane, etomidate, methohexital, morphine, and NSAIDs
- Anesthetic drugs/adjuncts to be cautious about are propofol (high dose or long duration of use), 5-HT_3 receptor antagonists, and sevoflurane
- Prolonged general anesthesia for laparoscopic procedures (GIFT, ZIFT) may affect fertilization rates as the absorbed CO_2 diffuses into the follicles lowering pH
- Most common ART procedure is TVOR, which can be performed under moderate or deep sedation, or light general anesthesia as a day case procedure in a non-hospital location without the need for an anesthesiologist. Appropriate protocols must be in place to manage complications of the procedure or anesthetic
- Complications of ART are rare, the most serious are multiple pregnancy and OHSS

REFERENCES

1. Steptoe PC, Edwards RG. Birth after the reimplantation of a human embryo. *Lancet* 1978;2(8085):366.
2. Centers for Disease Control and Prevention, American Society for Reproductive Medicine, Society for Assisted Reproduction Technology. 2007 Assisted Reproductive Technology Success Rates: National Summary and Fertility Clinic Reports, Atlanta. In US Department of Health and Human Services, Centers for Disease Control and Prevention 2009. http://www.cdc.gov/art/ART2007/index.htm. Last accessed January 16, 2011.
3. Bendikson K, Cramer DW, Vitonis A, et al. Ethnic background and in vitro fertilization outcomes. *Int J Gynaecol Obstet* 2005;88:342–346.
4. Spandorfer SD, Bendikson K, Dragisic K, et al. Outcome of in vitro fertilization in women 45 years and older who use autologous oocytes. *Fertil Steril* 2007;87:74–76.
5. Balen AH. *Infertility in Practice*. 3rd ed. London: Informa Healthcare; 2008.
6. Lewin A, Margalioth EJ, Rabinowitz R, et al. Comparative study of ultrasonically guided percutaneous aspiration with local anesthesia and laparoscopic aspiration of follicles in an in vitro fertilization program. *Am J Obstet Gynecol* 1985;151:621–625.
7. Bonduelle M, Wennerholm UB, Loft A, et al. A multi-centre cohort study of the physical health of 5-year-old children conceived after intracytoplasmic sperm injection, in vitro fertilization and natural conception. *Hum Reprod* 2005;20:413–419.
8. The Practice Committee of the American Society for Reproductive Medicine. Ovarian tissue and oocyte cryopreservation. *Fertil Steril* 2006;86:S142–S147.
9. Egan B, Racowsky C, Hornstein MD, et al. Anesthetic impact of body mass index in patients undergoing assisted reproductive technologies. *J Clin Anesth* 2008;20:356–363.
10. Douglas NC, Shah M, Sauer MV. Fertility and reproductive disorders in female solid organ transplant recipients. *Semin Perinatol* 2007;31:332–338.
11. Metzler E, Ginsburg E, Tsen LC. Use of assisted reproductive technologies and anesthesia in a patient with primary pulmonary hypertension. *Fertil Steril* 2004;81:1684–1687.
12. Gelbaya TA. Short and long-term risks to women who conceive through in vitro fertilization. *Hum Fertil (Camb)* 2010;13:19–27.
13. Hong JY, Jee YS, Luthardt FW. Comparison of conscious sedation for oocyte retrieval between low-anxiety and high-anxiety patients. *J Clin Anesth* 2005; 17:549–553.
14. Boyers SP, Lavy G, Russell JB, et al. A paired analysis of in vitro fertilization and cleavage rates of first- versus last-recovered preovulatory human oocytes exposed to varying intervals of 100% CO_2 pneumoperitoneum and general anesthesia. *Fertil Steril* 1987;48:969–974.

15. Hayes MF, Sacco AG, Savoy-Moore RT, et al. Effect of general anesthesia on fertilization and cleavage of human oocytes in vitro. *Fertil Steril* 1987;48:975–981.

16. Daya S, Wikland M, Nilsson L, et al. Effect on fertilization of intra-peritoneal exposure of oocytes to carbon dioxide. *Hum Reprod* 1987;2:603–606.

17. Tanbo T, Henriksen T, Magnus O, et al. Oocyte retrieval in an IVF program. A comparison of laparoscopic and transvaginal ultrasound-guided follicular puncture. *Acta Obstet Gynecol Scand* 1988;67:243–246.

18. Coetsier T, Dhont M, De Sutter P, et al. Propofol anaesthesia for ultrasound guided oocyte retrieval: Accumulation of the anaesthetic agent in follicular fluid. *Hum Reprod* 1992;7:1422–1424.

19. Christiaens F, Janssenswillen C, Verborgh C, et al. Propofol concentrations in follicular fluid during general anaesthesia for transvaginal oocyte retrieval. *Hum Reprod* 1999;14:345–348.

20. Janssenswillen C, Christiaens F, Camu F, et al. The effect of propofol on parthenogenetic activation, in vitro fertilization and early development of mouse oocytes. *Fertil Steril* 1997;67:769–774.

21. Tatone C, Francione A, Marinangeli F, et al. An evaluation of propofol toxicity on mouse oocytes and preimplantation embryos. *Hum Reprod* 1998;13:430–435.

22. Alsalili M, Thornton S, Fleming S. The effect of the anaesthetic, propofol, on in-vitro oocyte maturation, fertilization and cleavage in mice. *Hum Reprod* 1997;12:1271–1274.

23. Rosenblatt MA, Bradford CN, Bodian CA, et al. The effect of a propofol-based sedation technique on cumulative embryo scores, clinical pregnancy rates, and implantation rates in patients undergoing embryo transfers with donor oocytes. *J Clin Anesth* 1997;9:614–617.

24. Ben-Shlomo I, Moskovich R, Golan J, et al. The effect of propofol anaesthesia on oocyte fertilization and early embryo quality. *Hum Reprod* 2000;15:2197–2199.

25. Christiaens F, Janssenswillen C, Van Steirteghem AC, et al. Comparison of assisted reproductive technology performance after oocyte retrieval under general anaesthesia (propofol) versus paracervical local anaesthetic block: A case-controlled study. *Hum Reprod* 1998;13:2456–2460.

26. Beilin Y, Bodian CA, Mukherjee T, et al. The use of propofol, nitrous oxide, or isoflurane does not affect the reproductive success rate following gamete intra-fallopian transfer (GIFT): A multicenter pilot trial/survey. *Anesthesiology* 1999;90:36–41.

27. Vincent RDJ, Syrop CH, Van Voorhis BJ, et al. An evaluation of the effect of anesthetic technique on reproductive success after laparoscopic pronuclear stage transfer: Propofol/nitrous oxide versus isoflurane/nitrous oxide. *Anesthesiology* 1995;82:352–358.

28. Endler GC, Stout M, Magyar DM, et al. Follicular fluid concentrations of thiopental and thiamylal during laparoscopy for oocyte retrieval. *Fertil Steril* 1987;48:828–833.

29. Pierce ET, Smalky M, Alper MM, et al. Comparison of pregnancy rates following gamete intrafallopian transfer (GIFT) under general anesthesia with thiopental sodium or propofol. *J Clin Anesth* 1992;4:394–398.

30. Huang HW, Huang FJ, Kung FT, et al. Effects of induction anesthetic agents on outcome of assisted reproductive technology: A comparison of propofol and thiopental sodium. *Chang Gung Med J* 2000;23:513–519.

31. Heytens L, Devroey P, Camu F, et al. Effects of etomidate on ovarian steroidogenesis. *Hum Reprod* 1987;2:85–90.

32. Hein THA, Suit TC, Douning LK, et al. Effect of intravenous sedation on the outcome of transvaginal oocyte retrieval: A comparative study of propofol and methohexital-based techniques. *J Clin Anesth* 1997;9:617.

33. Soussis I, Boyd O, Paraschos T, et al. Follicular fluid levels of midazolam, fentanyl, and alfentanil during transvaginal oocyte retrieval. *Fertil Steril* 1995;64:1003–1007.

34. Ben-Shlomo I, Moskovich R, Katz Y, et al. Midazolam/ketamine sedative combination compared with fentanyl/propofol/isoflurane anaesthesia for oocyte retrieval. *Hum Reprod* 1999;14:1757–1759.

35. Ben-Shlomo I, Amodai I, Levran D, et al. Midazolam–fentanyl sedation in conjunction with local anesthesia during oocyte retrieval for in vitro fertilization. *J Assist Reprod Genet* 1992;9:83–85.

36. Swanson RJ, Leavitt MG. Fertilization and mouse embryo development in the presence of midazolam. *Anesth Analg* 1992;75:549–554.

37. Casati A, Valentini G, Zangrillo A, et al. Anaesthesia for ultrasound guided oocyte retrieval: Midazolam/remifentanil versus propofol/fentanyl regimens. *Eur J Anaesthesiol* 1999;16:773–778.

38. Hammadeh ME, Wilhelm W, Huppert A, et al. Effects of general anaesthesia vs. sedation on fertilization, cleavage and pregnancy rates in an IVF program. *Arch Gynecol Obstet* 1999;263:56–59.

39. Shapira SC, Chrubasik S, Hoffmann A, et al. Use of alfentanil for in vitro fertilization oocyte retrieval. *J Clin Anesth* 1996;8:282–285.

40. Shapira SC, Magora F, Katzenelson R, et al. Fentanyl vs alfentanil anesthesia for in vitro fertilization. *Harefuah* 1991;121:17–18.

41. Bruce DL, Hinkley R, Norman PF. Fentanyl does not inhibit fertilization or early development of sea urchin eggs. *Anesth Analg* 1985;64:498–500.

42. Wilhelm W, Hammadeh ME, White PF, et al. General anesthesia versus monitored anesthesia care with remifentanil for assisted reproductive technologies: Effect on pregnancy rate. *J Clin Anesth* 2002;14:1–5.

43. Milanini MN, D'Onofrio P, Melani Novelli AM, et al. Local anesthesia versus intravenous infusion of remifentanil for assisted reproductive technologies. A retrospective study. *Minerva Ginecol* 2008;60:203–207.

44. Cardasis C, Schuel H. The sea urchin egg as a model system to study effects of narcotics on secretion. In: Ford DH, ed. *Tissue Responses to Addictive Drugs.* New York, NY: Spectrum; 1976:631–640.

45. Sephton VC, Shaw A, Cowan CM, et al. Sedation and analgesia for transvaginal oocyte retrieval: An audit resulting in a change of clinical practice. *Hum Fertil (Camb)* 2001;4:94–98.

46. Baden JM, Serra M, Mazze RI. Inhibition of fetal methionine synthase by nitrous oxide. *Br J Anaesth* 1984;56:523–526.

47. Rosen MA, Roizen MF, Eger II EI, et al. The effect of nitrous oxide on in vitro fertilization success rate. *Anesthesiology* 1987;67:42–44.

48. Chetkowski RJ, Nass TE. Isofluorane inhibits early mouse embryo development in vitro. *Fertil Steril* 1988;49:171–173.

49. Matt DW, Steingold KA, Dastvan CM, et al. Effects of sera from patients given various anesthetics on preimplantation mouse embryo development in vitro. *J In Vitro Fert Embryo Transf* 1991;8:191–197.

50. Critchlow BM, Ibrahim Z, Pollard BJ. General anaesthesia for gamete intra-fallopian transfer. *Eur J Anaesthesiol* 1991;8:381–384.

51. Fishel S, Webster J, Faratian B, et al. General anesthesia for intrauterine placement of human conceptuses after in vitro fertilization. *J In Vitro Fert Embryo Transf* 1987;4:260–264.

52. Basler A, Rohrborn G. Lack of mutagenic effects of halothane in mammals in vivo. *Anesthesiology* 1981;55:143–147.

53. Bokhari A, Pollard BJ. Anaesthesia for assisted conception: A survey of UK practice. *Eur J Anaesthesiol* 1999;16:225–230.

54. Eger II EI, Laster MJ, Winegar R, et al. Compound A induces sister chromatid exchanges in Chinese hamster ovary cells. *Anesthesiology* 1997;86:918–922.

55. Coburn R, Lane J, Harrison K, et al. Postoperative vomiting factors in IVF patients. *Aust N Z J Obstet Gynaecol* 1993;33:57–60.

56. Kauppila A, Leinonen P, Vihko R, et al. Metoclopramide-induced hyperprolactinemia impairs ovarian follicle maturation and corpus luteum function in women. *J Clin Endocrinol Metab* 1982;54:955–960.

57. Forman R, Fishel SB, Edwards RG, et al. The influence of transient hyperprolactinemia on in vitro fertilization in humans. *J Clin Endocrinol Metab* 1985;60:517–522.

58. Mendes MC, Ferriani RA, Sala MM, et al. Effect of transitory hyperprolactinemia on in vitro fertilization of human oocytes. *J Reprod Med* 2001;46:444–450.

59. Doldi N, Papaleo E, De Santis L, et al. Treatment versus no treatment of transient hyperprolactinemia in patients undergoing intracytoplasmic sperm injection programs. *Gynecol Endocrinol* 2000;14:437–441.

60. Hendrie C. The 5HT3 antagonist GR38032F is highly toxic in DBA/2 mice. *Psychopharmacology* 1990;101:429–430.

61. Asker C, Norstedt Wikner B, Kallen B. Use of antiemetic drugs during pregnancy in Sweden. *Eur J Clin Pharmacol* 2005;61:899–906.

62. Einarson A, Maltepe C, Navioz Y, et al. The safety of ondansetron for nausea and vomiting of pregnancy: A prospective comparative study. *BJOG* 2004;111:940–943.

63. Magee LA, Mazzotta P, Koren G. Evidence-based view of safety and effectiveness of pharmacologic therapy for nausea and vomiting of pregnancy (NVP). *Am J Obstet Gynecol* 2002;186:S256–S261.

64. Siu SS, Chan MT, Lau TK. Placental transfer of ondansetron during early human pregnancy. *Clin Pharmacokinet* 2006;45:419–423.

65. van der Weiden RM, Helmerhorst FM, Keirse MJ. Influence of prostaglandins and platelet activating factor on implantation. *Hum Reprod* 1991;6:436–442.

66. Shafiq N, Malhotra S, Pandhi P. Comparison of nonselective cyclo-oxygenase (COX) inhibitor and selective COX-2 inhibitors on preimplantation loss, postimplantation loss and duration of gestation: an experimental study. *Contraception* 2004;69:71–75.

67. Salhab AS, Gharaibeh MN, Shomaf MS, et al. Meloxicam inhibits rabbit ovulation. *Contraception* 2001;63:329–333.

68. Li DK, Liu L, Odouli R. Exposure to non-steroidal anti-inflammatory drugs during pregnancy and risk of miscarriage: Population based cohort study. *BMJ* 2003;327:368.

69. Siristatidis CS, Dodd SR, Drakeley AJ. Aspirin for in vitro fertilisation. *Cochrane Database Syst Rev* 2011;(8):CD004832.

70. Schnell VL, Sacco AG, Savoy-Moore RT, et al. Effects of oocyte exposure to local anesthetics on in vitro fertilization and embryo development in the mouse. *Reprod Toxicol* 1992;6:323–327.

71. Ahuja KK. In-vitro inhibition of the block to polyspermy of hamster eggs by tertiary amine local anaesthetics. *J Reprod Fertil* 1982;65:15–22.

72. Fujinaga M. Assessment of teratogenic effects of lidocaine in rat embryos cultured in vitro. *Anesthesiology* 1998;89:1553–1558.

73. American Society of Anesthesiologists. Standards Guidelines and Statements: Basic Anesthetic Monitoring, Standards for (Effective July 1, 2011); Nonoperating Room Anesthetizing Locations, Statement on (2008). http://www.asahq.org/For-Healthcare-Professionals/Standards-Guidelines-and-Statements.aspx. Last accessed January 16, 2011.

74. Ng EH, Miao B, Ho PC. A randomized double-blind study to compare the effectiveness of three different doses of lignocaine used in paracervical block during oocyte retrieval. *J Assist Reprod Genet* 2003;20:8–12.

75. Ramsewak SS, Kumar A, Welsby R, et al. Is analgesia required for transvaginal single-follicle aspiration in in vitro fertilization? A double-blind study. *J Assist Reprod Genet* 1990;7:103–106.

76. Ditkoff EC, Plumb J, Selick A, et al. Anesthesia practices in the United States common to in vitro fertilization (IVF) centers. *J Assist Reprod Genet* 1997;14:145–147.

77. Hammarberg K, Wikland M, Nilsson L, et al. Patients' experience of transvaginal follicle aspiration under local anesthesia. *Ann N Y Acad Sci* 1988;541:134–137.

78. American Society of Anesthesiologists. Practice guidelines for sedation and analgesia by non-anesthesiologists. *Anesthesiology* 2002;96:1004–1017.

79. Botta G, D'Angelo A, D'Ari G, et al. Epidural anesthesia in an in vitro fertilization and embryo transfer program. *J Assist Reprod Genet* 1995;12:187–190.

80. Tidmarsh MD, May AE. Spinal analgesia for transvaginal oocyte retrieval. *Int J Obstet Anesth* 1998;7:157–160.

81. Manica VS, Bader AM, Fragneto R, et al. Anesthesia for in vitro fertilization: a comparison of 1.5% and 5% spinal lidocaine for ultrasonically guided oocyte retrieval. *Anesth Analg* 1993;77:453–456.

82. Martin R, Tsen LC, Tzeng G, et al. Anesthesia for in vitro fertilization: The addition of fentanyl to 1.5% lidocaine. *Anesth Analg* 1999;88:523–526.

83. Tsen LC, Schultz R, Martin R, et al. Intrathecal low-dose bupivacaine versus lidocaine for in vitro fertilization procedures. *Reg Anesth Pain Med* 2001;26:52–56.

84. Andersen D, Løssl K, Andersen AN, et al. Acupuncture on the day of embryo transfer: A randomized controlled trial of 635 patients. *Reprod Biomed Online* 2010;21:366–372.

85. Stener-Victorin E, Waldenstrom U, Nilsson L, et al. A prospective randomized study of electro-acupuncture versus alfentanil as anaesthesia during oocyte aspiration in in-vitro fertilization. *Hum Reprod* 1999;14:2480–2484.

86. Kim WO, Kil HK, Koh SO, et al. Effects of general and locoregional anesthesia on reproductive outcome for in vitro fertilization: a meta-analysis. *J Korean Med Sci* 2000;15:68–72.

87. Kwan I, Bhattacharya S, Knox F, et al. Conscious sedation and analgesia for oocyte retrieval during IVF procedures: A Cochrane review. *Hum Reprod* 2006;21:1672–1679.

88. Odeberg S, Ljungqvist O, Svenberg T, et al. Haemodynamic effects of pneumoperitoneum and the influence of posture during anaesthesia for laparoscopic surgery. *Acta Anaesthesiol Scand* 1994;38:276–283.

89. Aragona C, Mohamed MA, Espinola MSB, et al. Clinical complications after transvaginal oocyte retrieval in 7,098 IVF cycles. *Fertil Steril* 2011;95:293–294.

90. Roest J, Mous HV, Zeilmaker GH, et al. The incidence of major clinical complications in a Dutch transport IVF programme. *Hum Reprod Update* 1996;2:345–353.

91. The Practice Committee of the American Society for Reproductive Medicine. Multiple pregnancy associated with infertility therapy. *Fertil Steril* 2006;86:S106–S110.

92. The Practice Committee of the American Society for Reproductive Medicine and the Practice Committee of the Society for Assisted Reproductive Technology. Guidelines on the number of embryos transferred. *Fertil Steril* 2009;92:1518–1519.

93. Society of Obstetricians and Gynecologists of Canada. Guidelines for the number of embryos to transfer following in vitro fertilization No. 182, September 2006. *Int J Gynaecol Obstet* 2008;102:203–216.

94. Wimalasundera RC. Selective reduction and termination of multiple pregnancies. *Semin Fetal Neonatal Med* 2010;15:327–335.

95. Strandell A, Thorburn J, Hamberger L. Risk factors for ectopic pregnancy in assisted reproduction. *Fertil Steril* 1999;71:282–286.

96. Chin HY, Chen FP, Wang CJ, et al. Heterotopic pregnancy after in vitro fertilization-embryo transfer. *Int J Gynaecol Obstet* 2004;86:411–416.

97. Brinsden PR, Wada I, Tan SL, et al. Diagnosis, prevention and management of ovarian hyperstimulation syndrome. *Br J Obstet Gynaecol* 1995;102:767–772.

98. Humaidan P, Quartarolo J, Papanikolaou EG. Preventing ovarian hyperstimulation syndrome: guidance for the clinician. *Fertil Steril* 2010;94:389–400.

99. Rizk B, Aboulghar M, Smitz J, et al. The role of vascular endothelial growth factor and interleukins in the pathogenesis of severe ovarian hyperstimulation syndrome. *Hum Reprod Update* 1997;3:255–266.

100. Whelan JG, Vlahos NF. The ovarian hyperstimulation syndrome. *Fertil Steril* 2000;73:883–896.

101. Noyes N, Porcu E, Borini A. Over 900 oocyte cryopreservation babies born with no apparent increase in congenital anomalies. *Reprod Biomed Online* 2009;18:769–776.

In Utero Fetal Surgery and Ex Utero Intrapartum Therapy (EXIT)

David G. Mann • Olutoyin A. Olutoye

■ INTRODUCTION

The majority of prenatally diagnosed fetal conditions are amenable to medical or surgical intervention following delivery. However, there are a few that benefit from interventions during pregnancy. For conditions that may benefit from fetal intervention, the basic framework of understanding includes (a) the natural history of the untreated disease "in utero" must be documented before clinical application of the fetal procedure, (b) there must be sound pathophysiologic rationale to develop a prenatal treatment strategy, (c) there is a demonstration of safety and efficacy of the fetal procedure in an appropriate animal model, and (d) inclusion and exclusion selection criteria have been developed for treatment (1).

In utero fetal surgery can be performed via a percutaneous approach or through a uterine incision (hysterotomy). Percutaneous procedures are usually ultrasound guided and include intrauterine transfusions and shunt placements. In addition, fetoscopic procedures for laser photocoagulation of abnormal placental anastomoses, or placement of tracheal plugs for tracheal occlusion in congenital diaphragmatic hernia (CDH), can also be performed percutaneously.

Procedures performed via a hysterotomy or uterine incision are of two types: Open fetal surgery in which surgery is performed during pregnancy on mid-gestation fetuses and the pregnancy is allowed to continue to near term, and ex utero intrapartum therapy (EXIT) in which a procedure or surgery is performed on fetuses just prior to delivery.

This chapter will describe the indications for fetal intervention via the percutaneous and open approach as well as the anesthetic management for these different procedures.

■ PERCUTANEOUS FETAL INTERVENTIONS

A variety of procedures are performed percutaneously. Some require fetal analgesia while other procedures, which do not involve the fetus directly, may not warrant direct administration of medication to the fetus. Specific discussion of fetal medications will be addressed where indicated. Maternal anesthesia and/or analgesia required for percutaneous interventions will be discussed at the end of the description of the various procedures.

Intrauterine Transfusions

Hemolytic disease of the newborn, mostly the result of Rhesus alloimmunization, was previously a significant cause of perinatal mortality. However, elucidation of the pathophysiology, development of diagnostic tools, and effective prophylaxis has reduced its occurrence to a rarity (2). Red-cell alloimmunization may occur when a blood-type incompatibility (Rh-D or Kell) exists between mother and fetus. Fetal red blood cells that cross the placenta may stimulate the production of maternal antibodies resulting in red blood cell hemolysis in the fetus, and fetal anemia. While Rh-D alloimmunization is the most common etiology of fetal anemia, Kell alloimmunization, severe fetomaternal hemorrhage, placental chorioangiomas, homozygous α-thalassemia, and parvovirus B19 can also cause fetal anemia that may require fetal blood transfusion (2).

The incidence of rhesus D (Rh-D) alloimmunization is approximately 6/1,000 live births. As this is a rare entity, experts suggest that affected patients should be referred to a maternal–fetal medicine specialist experienced in treating red-cell alloimmunization in pregnancy, as some patients will require treatment with an intrauterine fetal transfusion (3). Intrauterine transfusion involves insertion of a needle through the maternal abdominal wall, uterus, and into a fetal vein (umbilical or intrahepatic approach) under ultrasound guidance. Transfusion may also be via the intraperitoneal or intracardiac approach although the intracardiac approach is usually utilized as a last resort.

For these procedures, drugs are administered to the fetus following maternal sedation or local anesthetic infiltration into the maternal abdomen. Fetal immobility is important for this procedure as fetal movement may result in laceration of the vessel at the puncture site with hemorrhage into the amniotic cavity particularly when transfusion is via a fetal intravascular approach (2). In order to prevent fetal movement, a neuromuscular blocking drug is administered directly to the fetus. Fetal analgesia is also provided with direct administration of opioids to the fetus particularly with the intrahepatic, intraperitoneal, or intracardiac approach. Further details of fetal analgesia and immobility and maternal sedative/anesthetic requirements for percutaneous procedures are discussed later in the chapter.

Intrauterine transfusion procedures are safe, with an overall survival rate of approximately 90% and a complication rate of approximately 3% (4). Possible complications that may occur during transfusion include inadvertent uterine artery puncture leading to arterial spasm and fetal bradycardia; tamponade, hemopericardium, or arrhythmias following cardiac puncture; cord accidents causing fetal distress; volume overload, preterm rupture of membranes, or preterm labor (2). Complications that have been reported following the procedure include rupture of membranes (0.1%), intrauterine infection (0.3%), fetal and neonatal death (0.7% and 0.9%, respectively), as well as emergency cesarean section (2.0%) (5).

Shunts

Lesions characterized by fluid-filled spaces amenable to decompression via shunt placement or aspiration, may be identified by ultrasound during pregnancy. These lesions include lower urinary tract obstruction (LUTO) which may cause an obstructive uropathy (6); congenital cystic adenomatoid malformations (CCAMs) or idiopathic pleural effusions (IPEs), both of which may cause pulmonary hypoplasia and cardiac failure from compression of mediastinal structures (6). Fetuses with any of these fluid-filled lesions may benefit from placement of shunts such as a vesicoamniotic or thoracoamniotic shunt to divert fluid from the enclosed space into the amniotic sac. These shunts are intended to halt or reverse the pathophysiologic changes resulting from obstruction of the normal fluid egress.

Lower Urinary Tract Obstruction (LUTO)

An enlarging fluid-filled fetal bladder may result from LUTO. This occurs most commonly in male fetuses with urethral abnormalities such as posterior urethral valves or urethral atresia. However, anterior urethral valves, meatal stenosis, and a hypoplastic mid-urethra may also lead to LUTO. LUTO is less common in female fetuses in which it may occur as a result of abnormal cloacal development. This type of obstruction can also be associated with congenital syndromes such as megacystis-microcolon syndrome, megacystis-megaureter syndrome, Trisomy 21, and Trisomy 18 (6). Complete urethral obstruction can lead to bladder distention and hydroureteronephrosis, possibly causing renal fibrocystic dysplasia in the fetus. Oligohydramnios occurs as a result of decreased urine entering the amniotic space and pulmonary hypoplasia may also occur due to decreased amniotic fluid entering the fetal lungs. Secondary deformities of the face and extremities have also been noted to occur in these patients (Potter's syndrome) (7). Postnatal morbidity and mortality depends on pulmonary development and renal function. Oligohydramnios with urethral obstruction occurring in early mid-gestation is associated with an estimated 95% mortality rate (8).

Determining prenatal renal injury in obstructive uropathy has been challenging. The prognosis for postnatal renal and pulmonary function have been separated into "good" and "poor" based on fetal urine characteristics as well as other findings such as the ultrasound appearance of fetal kidneys (9). Favorable and poor prognostic indicators based on urine values are shown in Table 49-1.

Technically, the fetal bladder must be drained at least three times with 24- to 48-hour intervals between each drain and within a 5- to 7-day period in order to establish the pattern (increasing or decreasing) of hypertonicity. The first drainage would collect urine that has been collecting in the fetal bladder for an unknown period of time and would not reflect current function. The second drainage would collect urine present in the upper renal system that drained into the

bladder following the first "decompressing" drainage and still would not reflect the current function. Finally, the third drainage will collect recently formed urine that adequately represents the current underlying renal function. Increasing urinary hypertonicity is reflective of progressive or advanced renal dysfunction, depicts a "poor prognosis" for the fetus, and renders the fetus ineligible for in utero therapy. Decreasing hypertonicity is believed to reflect the potential for renal salvage, and in this situation, in utero intervention may be beneficial (10).

For eligible cases of LUTO, in utero therapy involves insertion of a vesicoamniotic shunt that diverts urine from the obstructed fetal bladder into the amniotic sac. This temporizing therapy is intended to "decompress" the developing kidneys in order to halt and possibly reverse renal damage; hence, a neonatal procedure will likely still be necessary following delivery. Under ultrasound visualization, a shunt trocar is inserted percutaneously through the maternal abdominal wall, uterus, and into the amniotic sac near the lower fetal abdomen. The trocar tip is positioned inferolateral to the abdominal cord insertion site. Color Doppler confirms preservation of the umbilical arteries as the trocar is passed through the fetal abdominal wall and into the bladder. A shunt is deployed through the trocar with one "coiled" end positioned in the fetal bladder, a straight channel spanning the fetal abdominal wall, and the other "coiled" end placed in the amniotic sac. Shunt position and the initiation of bladder drainage are confirmed by ultrasound at the end of the procedure.

Possible complications of this procedure include chorioamnionitis, premature rupture of the fetal membranes, preterm labor, intraplacental bleeding, and iatrogenic gastroschisis. Shunts may also become dislodged with an occurrence rate of approximately 40% (6). Subsequent delivery of treated fetuses is managed by routine obstetrical indications, with vaginal delivery occurring typically at a gestational age of 34 to 35 weeks. Biard et al. (11) reported on long-term outcomes of fetuses with LUTO: The final postnatal diagnoses are most commonly posterior urethral valves (39%) and prune belly syndrome (39%). The overall 1-year survival rate is 91%, with mortality attributable to pulmonary hypoplasia. In the same review, at a median of 5.8 years, spontaneous voiding was possible in 61% of cases; renal function was "acceptable" in 44%, "mildly insufficient" in 22%; and 34% of affected fetuses' required renal transplant. In addition, 44% had persistent respiratory problems, 66.5% experienced poor growth, and 50% had frequent urinary tract infections.

Congenital Cystic Adenomatoid Malformation (CCAM)

An enlarging fluid-filled chest mass may result from a congenital cystic adenomatoid malformation or CCAM. The pathophysiology of CCAM is discussed in more detail later in this chapter. Thoracoamniotic shunt placement may be indicated for CCAMs with a dominant large cyst causing fetal cardiac failure (hydrops) or resulting in a mass effect severe enough to cause pulmonary hypoplasia or hemodynamic instability from significant mediastinal shift. Placement of a thoracoamniotic shunt diverts cystic fluid from within the CCAM into the amniotic sac and has been shown to reduce CCAM volumes by approximately 70% (12). It can also potentially reverse the hydrops (13).

Under ultrasound visualization, a shunt trocar is percutaneously passed through the maternal abdominal wall and uterus into the amniotic sac near the fetal thorax. The trocar tip is positioned at the superolateral left aspect of a left thoracic macrocyst to encourage superolateral involution of the cyst. The midclavicular line is avoided in order to decrease potential interference with restoration of the normal position

TABLE 49-1 Prognostic Urinalysis Values for Postnatal Renal and Pulmonary Function in Obstructive Uropathy

	Good Prognosis	Poor Prognosis
Sodium	<90 mmol/L	>100 mmol/L
Chloride	<80 mmol/L	>90 mmol/L
Osmolality	<180 mOsm/L	>200 mOsm/L
Calcium	<7 mg/dL	>8 mg/dL
Total protein	<20 mg/dL	>40 mg/dL
β2-microglobulin	<6 mg/L	>10 mg/L

Urine specimens between 18 and 22 weeks' gestation, are collected after 3 to 4 bladder draining episodes, with 1 to 2 days interval in-between sampling.

With permission from: Mann S, Johnson MP, Wilson RD. Fetal thoracic and bladder shunts. *Semin Fetal Neonatal Med* 2010;15(1):28–33.

of mediastinal structures (6). The shunt is deployed through the trocar as described for urinary tract obstruction and its position is confirmed by ultrasound.

This procedure can be complicated by catheter dislodgement, thrombus material occlusion of the catheter, premature rupture of the fetal membranes, preterm labor, fetal hemorrhage, and postnatal rib deformities at placement site (6). Subsequent delivery is managed by routine obstetrical indications and survival rates up to 74% have been reported (14).

Idiopathic Pleural Effusion (IPE)

IPE is another space-occupying lesion of the thorax that produces pathophysiologic effects similar to lung lesions. The resultant mass effect may lead to pulmonary hypoplasia or mediastinal shift with resulting hydrops. Thoracocentesis is performed under ultrasound guidance in order to remove pleural fluid. This fluid is analyzed and lung reexpansion is confirmed following thoracocentesis. Placement of a thoracoamniotic shunt may be indicated if rapid reaccumulation of the pleural effusion occurs. The shunt is placed as described for treatment of a CCAM with the exception that the fetal end of the shunt enters the pleural space and not the fetal lung. The same complications encountered with thoracoamniotic shunt placement for CCAM have been observed with shunt placement for IPE. Overall survival after thoracoamniotic shunt placement is significantly higher compared to that of neonates who did not have a shunt placed (6).

Cardiac Interventions

The final morphologic form of the fetal heart as well as its left and right sidedness is established by approximately 7 weeks of gestational age. Diagnostic ultrasound imaging however, only becomes possible at 12 to 14 weeks of gestation. Congenital heart defects (CHDs) can result from stenotic or atretic valves, leading to hypoplasia of the supporting ventricle that could potentially prevent the ventricle from contributing to postnatal circulation. Cardiac defects appear to result from flow abnormalities through the atrioventricular valves, increased velocities across the semi lunar valves, flow reversal in arterial/venous ducts and aortic isthmus, as well as pulmonary venous flow abnormalities (15). Therefore, the aim of in utero interventions for fetuses with abnormal cardiovascular physiology is to normalize the circulatory imbalance. There is data suggesting that restoration of normal flow promotes growth (16), and that reduction of ventricular pressures minimizes secondary damage by promoting normal development (17). An example of secondary damage is ventricular fibrosis resulting from poor coronary perfusion. Critical aortic stenosis, for example, affords little or no forward coronary artery flow from the aortic root causing coronary perfusion to be dependent on the relatively desaturated arterial duct. Resistance to coronary flow in the fetus is due in part to intraventricular pressure (75%) and myocardial contraction (25%); therefore, the increased end-diastolic ventricular pressure resulting from aortic stenosis would significantly reduce coronary perfusion and promote fibrosis (15).

Percutaneous fetal cardiac interventions that are currently performed include aortic/pulmonary valvuloplasty, balloon atrial septostomy for a restrictive or closed interatrial septum, and fetal pacing for complete heart block (18). Although sonographic guidelines have been developed to aid in selecting appropriate patients for fetal cardiac interventions, the ideal timing of the intervention remains unclear. A number of factors contribute to this uncertainty: First, the stage at which the damage becomes irreversible is unknown; and second, an immature fetus may not be able to tolerate the procedure as

the procedure-related risk of death is 10% to 20% and the risk of premature labor is 5% (19).

For most cardiac interventions, once the fetus has received intramuscular analgesia, sedation and muscle relaxation, a long needle with a flexible stylet is percutaneously introduced through the maternal abdomen, uterine wall, and into the fetal chest. Correct alignment of the needle along the axis of the outflow tract is essential, making optimal fetal lie a critical component for success. An over-the-wire coronary balloon is inflated 2 or 3 times across the valve or across the interatrial septum, as tolerated by the fetus (19).

Some fetal complications may arise from a mineralized myocardium that fails to seal at the puncture site leading to hemorrhage. This can potentially lead to cerebral ischemia, cardiac tamponade, or death (20). Of note, the success rate as defined by being able to pass a balloon through the valve has improved to greater than 80% (20); although evidence of improved neonatal outcome is more challenging.

▪ FETOSCOPY

Direct endoscopic visualization of the fetus (fetoscopy) was introduced in the 1970s. It was originally used most commonly as a diagnostic tool in order to obtain blood from fetuses with suspected hemoglobinopathies, obtain tissue biopsies, or visualize pathognomonic malformations. The initial real therapeutic application at that time was for intravascular transfusions under direct visualization.

Fetoscopy was not initially widely utilized in the United States due to the invasiveness of the procedure, limited obstetrician involvement, maternal safety concerns, uncertain procedure efficacies, and regulatory difficulties (21). As a result, it eventually became almost obsolete with the widespread introduction of ultrasound in the 1980s.

The real advance in fetoscopy began following funding of the "Eurofoetus" project in 1988, by the European Commission (22). The focus of the project was to evaluate accuracy of routine antenatal ultrasound examination in detecting malformations. The secondary consequence of the project was better collaboration between fetal medicine units and endoscopic equipment manufacturers, resulting in smaller higher quality endoscopes (23). By the 1990s fetoscopic surgery and obstetric endoscopy in combination with ultrasound, began to flourish.

An early clinical application of fetoscopy was for umbilical cord embolization under ultrasound guidance. The first endoscopic cord ligation was for an acardiac–acephalus twin, and was reported in 1993 (24). Unfortunately, a review of experiences with this procedure demonstrated a high rate of preterm premature rupture of membranes (PPROM) (25), and a high occurrence of postoperative amniotic bands (26). This procedure has since been modified to include the use of bipolar forceps, monopolar needles, and transmission of radiofrequency energy using small gauge needles. Other indications for fetoscopy are discussed in subsequent sections.

▪ PLACENTAL SHARING

The incidence of twin pregnancies is 1 in 90, of which 30% are monozygotic or identical and 70% are dizygotic or fraternal (27). Seventy-five percent of monozygotic twins are monochorionic or share a placenta. The majority of monochorionic placentas (approximately 96%) have vascular anastomoses that allow blood to flow between both fetuses (27–29). This "normal vascular connection" between the twins introduces the possibility of a blood volume imbalance with one twin becoming a donor and "losing blood volume" to the recipient twin who gains blood volume. When a circulatory imbalance occurs, this placenta sharing becomes pathologic and detrimental to one or both twins in a condition called twin–twin transfusion syndrome (TTTS).

Twin–Twin Transfusion Syndrome (TTTS)

This condition occurs in approximately 5% to 15% of monochorionic, diamniotic twin gestations with a chronic imbalance in the net flow of blood across the vascular anastomoses. The pathophysiology is usually explained on an angioarchitectural basis. Existing placental anastomoses between twins can be arterio-arterial, veno-venous, or arterio-venous. The first two anastomoses are located superficially on the placental surface and are bidirectional in nature allowing blood flow between the two fetal circulations depending on the relative interfetal vascular gradients. In contrast, arterio-venous communications occur at the capillary level, deep within a shared cotyledon, and are referred to as "deep" anastomoses (Fig. 49-1). This shared cotyledon receives its arterial supply from one twin and its venous drainage (oxygenated blood) drains to the other twin. The arterio-venous anastomoses allow blood flow in one direction only and are identified on the placental surface as unpaired arteries and veins that pierce the chorionic plate at close proximity of each other to supply the underlying shared cotyledon. This unidirectional flow can create an imbalance in interfetal blood flow resulting in twin–twin transfusion. The donor, or pump twin, from whom blood is transfused to the other twin subsequently becomes anemic, hypovolemic, hypotensive, hypoproteinemic, and develops oligohydramnios. Severe intrauterine growth restriction of the donor twin may occur; this together with accompanying oligohydramnios is responsible for this twin also being referred to as the "stuck" twin. The recipient twin however becomes polycythemic, hypervolemic, and is at risk for cardiac failure, hyperbilirubinemia, intravascular thrombosis from blood hyperviscosity, and polyhydramnios from polyuria (30). If this condition is left uncorrected, both twins are at risk for demise.

Twin–twin transfusion (TTTS) is usually diagnosed around 20 to 21 weeks' gestation although features may be observed at any time during gestation. Diagnosis is either by acute maternal symptoms of polyhydramnios such as abdominal distension, orthopnea, dyspnea, uterine contractions, or by signs observed on recommended serial follow-up ultrasound for monochorionic pregnancies. Ultrasound diagnosis of TTTS includes the presence of polyuria, polyhydramnios, and a distended bladder in the recipient twin with the deepest amniotic vertical pocket measuring at least 8 cm in a pregnancy ≤20 weeks' gestation or an amniotic pocket of 10 cm after 20 weeks' gestation. The donor twin is diagnosed by the detection of oliguric oligohydramnios and a maximum deepest vertical pocket of 2 cm (31).

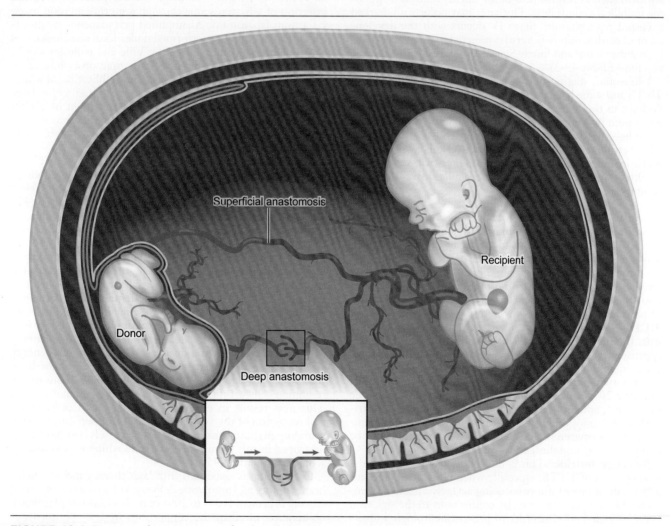

FIGURE 49-1 Diagram depicting superficial and deep anastomoses in twin–twin transfusion syndrome with the larger recipient twin on the right and the smaller donor "stuck" twin on the left, wrapped in its amniotic membrane due to oligohydramnios. Courtesy of Kenneth J. Moise, Jr., M.D.

TABLE 49-2 Quintero Staging of TTTS

Stage	Poly/ Oligohydramnios	Absent Donor Bladder	Flow Abnormalities	Hydrops	Demise
I	+	−	−	−	−
II	+	+	−	−	−
III	+	+	+	−	−
IV	+	+	+	+	−
V	+	+	+	+	+

Adapted from: Quintero RA, Morales WJ, Allen MH, et al. Staging of twin-twin transfusion syndrome. *J Perinatol* 1999;19(8 Pt 1):550–555.

A staging system for TTTS based on ultrasound and Doppler findings was developed by Quintero et al. in 1999 (32). Stage I TTTS is diagnosed by the presence of recipient twin polyhydramnios and donor twin oligohydramnios with a visible bladder in the donor twin. Stage II is also characterized by oligo–polyhydramnios but without a visible donor bladder. Stage III occurs when Doppler blood flow abnormalities exist; these flow abnormalities may include arterial abnormalities in the donor twin (absent end-diastolic velocity in the umbilical artery) or venous abnormalities in the recipient twin such as reverse flow in the ductus venosus or pulsatile umbilical venous flow. The latter may occur with marked tricuspid regurgitation. Stage IV occurs with the development of cardiac failure otherwise referred to as hydrops fetalis in either fetus; and finally Stage V is defined by the demise of a fetus (Table 49-2).

Ultrasound staging does not determine the prognosis of TTTS and some have proposed the use of echocardiographic findings in the recipient twin in conjunction with the staging system by Quintero as prognostic indicators (33–36) but these have not been found to be of prognostic value either. The treatment of TTTS has evolved over the years and currently includes serial amnioreduction, inter-twin septostomy, selective feticide, and laser photocoagulation of abnormal communicating vessels.

Treatment Options for TTTS

Amnioreduction: Under ultrasound guidance, an 18 G needle is inserted into the amniotic sac of the recipient twin and amniotic fluid is drained until the deepest vertical pocket measures approximately <5 cm. This procedure is repeated serially in order to maintain normal amniotic fluid volume until the fetus is viable, in order to reduce the likelihood of preterm labor from polyhydramnios. Large registries of TTTS pregnancies report a survival rate of 60% to 65% with this technique (37). Management of TTTS with this approach has a risk of serious neurologic sequelae which may occur in up to 20% of babies following delivery.

Inter-twin amniotic septostomy: This involves the insertion of a 20 G spinal needle through the dividing amniotic membrane, under ultrasound guidance, allowing for redistribution of amniotic fluid between the twins. Increased communication between both amniotic fluid sacs may however be complicated by umbilical cord entanglement.

Selective feticide: This is offered as a last resort in the management of TTTS, especially when both fetuses are sick as a result of one of the twins being severely affected. Complete obliteration of all vascular connections to the sick twin becomes mandatory in order to prevent neurologic impairment or demise of the less-affected twin (38).

Medical management: This has included administration of maternal digoxin in order to support cardiac function in the recipient twin. Maternal non-steroidal anti-inflammatory agents have also been used but these have not been reported to improve fetal outcome (30).

Laser photocoagulation of abnormal communicating vessels: This has become a popular indication for fetoscopy. Despite a suggestion for a potential surgical intervention for TTTS by Benirschke and Kim in 1973 (39) and a proposal to use laser energy to coagulate placental anastomoses by DeVore et al. 10 years later (40), it was not until 1990 that De Lia (41) described the technique of laser occlusion of placental vessels in TTTS. This original description involved the insertion of a hysteroscope through a uterine incision made via a mini laparotomy. A simplified percutaneous modification to this technique, performed under local anesthesia, was subsequently reported in 1995 by Ville and colleagues (42). Widespread acceptance for this fetoscopic procedure came from the "Eurotwin2twin" project and publication of a successful clinical randomized trial comparing fetoscopic laser coagulation to amnioreduction for the treatment of TTTS (31). This trial demonstrated a 25% increase in survival and a later delivery time (33.3 weeks vs. 29.0 weeks) with fetoscopic laser coagulation over amnioreduction.

Laser therapy is beneficial for Stage I and II cases of TTTS as less than 10% of cases advance beyond this stage following therapy (43), but it has also proven to be of some benefit in the therapeutic management of Stages III and IV (44). The goal of laser therapy is to selectively photocoagulate all the inter-twin placental vascular anastomoses (arterio-arterial, arterio-venous and veno-venous communications) on the chorionic plate. Under ultrasound guidance, a trocar is inserted into the uterus. A fetoscope is then passed through the trocar and a laser fiber is inserted through the operative channel of the fetoscope. Both neodymium–yttrium aluminum garnet (Nd:YAG) and diode (semiconductor) lasers are used. These lasers convert electrical or chemical energy into light energy leading to the delivery of large amount of energy to a small target area at a distance. There is optimal energy absorbance in the spectrum of hemoglobin; the light from the laser is also absorbed by the hemoglobin content of the red blood cells within the vessels producing volumetric heat. This heat results in coagulation of red blood cells, injury and retraction of the vessel wall, and is diffused into the surrounding placental tissue (Fig. 49-2). Vessels that have been destroyed in this manner demonstrate whitening on macroscopic examination (45).

Complications associated with laser therapy include membrane rupture and premature delivery. When uneven placental sharing is present (10% to 20% of monochorionic placentas), obliteration of all of the connections by laser photocoagulation may remove anastomoses that are compensating for a smaller portion of the placenta and could possibly lead to inadequate placental perfusion of the respective twin (38).

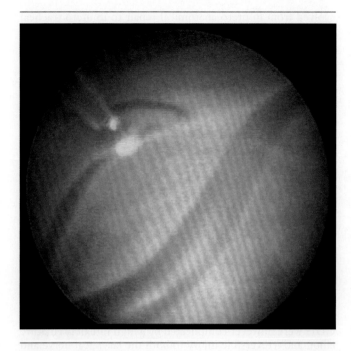

FIGURE 49-2 Arterio-venous anastomoses in twin–twin transfusion during laser therapy. Courtesy of Anthony Johnson DO.

Twin Reverse Arterial Perfusion Sequence (TRAP)

Twin reversed arterial perfusion (TRAP) sequence or "acardiac twinning" is a rare condition (incidence of approximately 1%), which is unique to monochorionic twin gestations (46). In this condition there is an acardiac twin who is kept alive by a structurally normal co-twin referred to as the "pump" twin. Superficial arterial–arterial and venous–venous anastomoses on the placenta permit the pump twin to perfuse the acardiac or recipient twin. The flow is reversed since the recipient twin receives blood via the umbilical artery instead of the umbilical vein. This reversed flow of oxygen-depleted blood from the donor to the recipient twin travels via the uterine artery/ arteries to the iliac artery/arteries and the abdominal aorta of the recipient twin. The lower limbs and abdominal organs of the recipient twin are therefore preferentially perfused and become more developed than the upper body which is commonly characterized by absent development of the heart (acardiac) and upper part of the body (anencephalic) in the recipient (47). A hemodynamic disadvantage is placed on the pump twin since this "donor" is providing cardiac output to both itself and the nonviable twin. The pump twin is therefore at increased risk of congestive heart failure from cardiac overload. The rate of perinatal mortality in the pump twin is estimated to be 50% to 75%. Mortality results mainly from polyhydramnios, congestive heart failure, and preterm labor (48). The natural course of monochorionic twin pregnancies with TRAP sequence is uncertain, making optimal management of this condition challenging to determine. The difficulty begins with identifying which pregnancies will benefit from any treatment beyond conservative or expectant management as there is a >50% perinatal mortality risk for the pump twin. Treatment should be mandatory in those cases which show the mildest deterioration in the pump twin on close surveillance scans or in cases of excessive growth of the acardiac twin (49).

Wong and Sepulveda proposed a relatively objective classification system that is based on the abdominal circumference

TABLE 49-3 Proposed Management of TRAP Sequence by Classification of Acardiac Anomaly

Type	Acardiac:pump AC Ratio (%)	Pump-twin Compromise	Management
Ia	<50	Absent	Reassess
Ib	<50	Present	Reassess
IIa	≥50	Absent	Prompt intervention
IIb	≥50	Present	Emergency intervention

Adapted from: Wong AE, Sepulveda W. Acardiac anomaly: current issues in prenatal assessment and treatment. *Prenat Diagn* 2005;25(9): 796–806.

ratio of the acardiac twin to the pump twin, and on signs of compromise in the pump twin who include polyhydramnios, cardiomegaly, and heart failure (Table 49-3). This system is intended to help direct management from expectant follow-up to emergency intervention (50). The classification uses a 50% abdominal circumference (AC) ratio to separate cases into those that may need an intervention following a 2-week follow-up reassessment and those which need prompt or emergent intervention.

Treatment options for the TRAP sequence include expectant management (observation), medical therapies (digoxin, indomethacin), selective delivery, and cord occlusion techniques (embolization, cord ligation, laser coagulation, bipolar and monopolar diathermy). In 2003, Tan and Sepulveda (49) reported on TRAP cases treated with various fetal ablation techniques. They found that following fetal cord ablation, the pump twin overall survival rate was 76%, the gestational age at delivery and median treatment to delivery interval was higher, the technical failure rate was lower, and the rate of premature delivery or rupture of membranes prior to 32 weeks' gestational age (WGA) was also lower.

Unfortunately incidental demise of the co-twin continues to be a risk in all selective termination procedures. This may occur at the time of the procedure or in the following weeks after the procedure. Other procedure-related complications include preterm labor, preterm delivery, PPROM, and placental or myometrial bleeding (51). Iatrogenic PPROM continues to be the most common complication, occurring in 10% to 30% of cases (26).

■ CONGENITAL DIAPHRAGMATIC HERNIA (CDH)

CDH is characterized by a defect in the diaphragm that permits herniation of abdominal contents into the thoracic cavity. It typically occurs on the left side (84%) although right side and bilateral defects also occur with an incidence of 13% and 2%, respectively (52). The incidence of CDH is estimated at between 1 in 3,000 and 1 in 5,000 live births (53). It is a rare anomaly that occurs in isolation in majority of cases but it may also be associated with other defects. Although CDH is described as a defect in the diaphragm, it is not clear if the primary pathology is pulmonary or diaphragmatic in origin. The clinical consequence of this lesion stems from compression of the developing lung by herniated abdominal contents leading to abnormal lung development. The ipsilateral or affected lung has fewer alveoli, thick alveolar walls, increased interstitial tissue, significantly decreased alveolar air spaces, and decreased gas exchange surface area. The pulmonary vasculature also develops abnormally with a reduced number of vessels, adventitial thickening, medial hyperplasia, and extension of the muscle layer into the smaller intra-acinar arterioles (54). Survivors of CDH often develop ventilatory insufficiency and persistent pulmonary hypertension, a result of the underlying pulmonary hypoplasia. A dangerous spiral ensues as the abnormal pulmonary vasculature demonstrates increased sensitivity to vasoconstriction, an exaggerated response to hypoxia and hypercarbia and worsening pulmonary hypertension develops and increases the right-to-left shunt. The shunted blood becomes increasingly hypoxic and acidotic which reinitiates the cycle (52).

Treatment strategies for CDH have evolved over the years (52). Previously, management consisted of aggressive hyperventilation and hyperoxygenation with emergent surgical repair. This transitioned into more gentle ventilation, or even spontaneous ventilation, with permissive hypercapnea to reduce baro- and volu-trauma until a delayed surgical repair was performed. Later, high frequency oscillatory ventilation (HFOV) emerged as a primary therapeutic option either primarily or as a bridge to extra corporeal membrane oxygenation (ECMO). The associated pulmonary hypertension in CDH has been increasingly treated early with inhaled nitric oxide as well as surfactant. These different treatment modalities have impacted the treatment of CDH but have not improved survival in very severe cases resulting in varying survival rates.

A number of features of this condition such as disproportion in ventricular size, degree of mediastinal shift, and stomach position have been considered as possible surrogate markers for indicating the severity of CDH; however, they are poorly validated prognostic indicators (52). As all the problems observed in the neonatal period of a child with CDH seemed to stem from pulmonary hypoplasia, the search began for a way to determine prognosis based on the extent of pulmonary hypoplasia. Metkus and colleagues (55) reported the use of the right lung-to-head circumference ratio (LHR) as a sonographic predictor of survival in fetal diaphragmatic hernia. The LHR is the two-dimensional area of the right lung taken at the level of the four-chamber view of the heart, divided by the head circumference. In a retrospective review of 55 fetuses with left-sided CDH, the LHR was predictive of survival at its extremes: Fetuses with low LHR values of <0.6 did not survive with postnatal therapy. In contrast, those with a value >1.35 had 100% postnatal survival with conventional postnatal therapies including ECMO (56,57). While the accuracy of LHR as described by Metkus and his group has been validated in two prospective studies (58), the LHR has not been widely adopted due to difficulty in accuracy and reproducibility of the measurement (59). It has been observed that there is a rapid growth of normal fetal lung area compared to head circumference particularly between the 12th and 32nd weeks of gestation, therefore Jani et al. (60) proposed referencing the LHR to gestational age by expressing the observed LHR as a ratio to the expected mean LHR for that gestational age. This observed-to-expected LHR ratio (O/E LHR) tends to be more accurate when measured between 32 and 33 weeks. While LHR or O/E LHR is often used to determine the prognosis of CDH, some criticize use of the measurement as it can be operator dependent.

The liver position in CDH (in the chest or in the abdomen) also correlates with survival. However, consideration of the liver as an independent variable that predicts prognosis remains controversial. In general, severely affected fetuses with CDH have an O/E LHR of 25% or less and an intrathoracic liver. Predicted survival in such affected fetuses with a left-sided CDH is approximately 15% (60).

Surgical treatments to reverse the nearly lethal condition of CDH and accompanying severe pulmonary hypoplasia have evolved from in utero anatomical repair to in utero tracheal occlusion. Initial animal studies demonstrated that intrauterine repair of the diaphragmatic defect with reversibility of pulmonary hypoplasia and hypertension was possible but the application to human fetuses was not as promising (61). The observed high maternal morbidity and poor fetal survival caused this method of intrauterine repair to be abandoned. In addition, for fetuses considered to be prime candidates for intrauterine repair due to poor prognosis (those with liver herniation into the thorax), intrauterine attempts to reposition the liver into the abdominal cavity was associated with compression or kinking of the umbilical vein.

Further animal studies demonstrated that obstruction of the trachea during pregnancy allowed for accumulation of tracheal fluid and lung-tissue stretch which in turn stimulated lung growth; thereby decreasing the morbidity and mortality associated with CDH (62). Tracheal occlusion for CDH in humans was subsequently initiated and a number of approaches were utilized including a laparotomy approach with hysterotomy, fetal neck dissection, and tracheal clipping; fetoscopic tracheal dissection and clipping, and more recently, fetoscopic balloon occlusion (52). Initial tracheal balloon occlusion techniques utilized in human fetuses with CDH were however complicated by a high rate of premature labor, and irreversible injury to both the laryngeal nerve and the trachea (58,63). A randomized trial in humans was conducted in 2003 to document the benefit of tracheal occlusion in the management of CDH (64). This study had two arms of CDH patients: Those who underwent in utero fetal tracheal occlusion and those who had postnatal surgical repair. The primary outcome of interest was survival up to 90 days of life and the secondary outcomes were measures of maternal and neonatal morbidity. The study was stopped prematurely because babies in the standard of care arm (postnatal surgery) had an unexpectedly high survival rate of 77% and those in the tracheal occlusion group had a survival rate of 73% at 90 days. It was projected that no statistically significant difference would exist between both arms of the study and it was therefore concluded that in utero tracheal occlusion did not improve postnatal survival or morbidity in neonates. In addition, infants that had in utero tracheal occlusion were noted to have premature delivery at approximately 30 weeks' gestation, while those allowed to deliver spontaneously, were carried close to term. A criticism of this study was the probability that the prematurity observed in the babies who received intrauterine therapy was due to the fact that a three-port technique was used for the fetoscopic placement of the tracheal clip. Since this early study, extensive research continued in Europe, examining different methods and types of fetoscopic procedures for CDH repair in animals (26,65,66).

Fetoscopic endoluminal tracheal occlusion (FETO) is now an established treatment offered between 26 and 28 weeks' gestation for human fetuses diagnosed with CDH in Europe (67). It is performed under ultrasound visualization for fetuses with isolated CDH and an LHR <1. The fetus's position is optimized by external manipulation and following sedation of the fetus, a trocar is inserted through the maternal abdomen and uterine wall. This trocar is exchanged for fetoscopic instruments that include a sheath loaded with an endoscope and the balloon occlusion system. The endoscope is introduced into the fetal trachea and advanced to deliver the inflatable endoluminal balloon to obstruct the trachea (see Fig. 49-3). The balloon is then inflated with fluid.

Following balloon placement, the pregnancy is allowed to continue to near term. Removal of the endoluminal balloon was initially via the EXIT procedure (see EXIT procedure later) under general anesthesia, or by fetal tracheoscopy immediately following vaginal delivery (68). However, it is

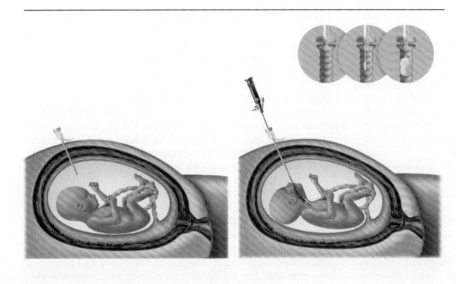

FIGURE 49-3 Cannula inserted in direction of fetal mouth. The endoscope is then advanced into the fetal pharynx and trachea. Insert: Balloon deposition (images on right). With permission from Deprest J, et al 2006 (70).

now more commonly removed prenatally via ultrasound-guided puncture of the balloon under local anesthesia at approximately 34 weeks prior to delivery (69). Women whose fetuses have undergone the FETO procedure are advised to stay close to the center in which the occlusion was performed in order to facilitate treatment by physicians adept in management of fetal airways should premature labor occur (69).

A retrospective study by Deprest and colleagues (57) documented an increase in LHR from 0.7 to 1.7 within 2 weeks of the FETO procedure and a mean gestational age at delivery of 33.5 weeks. The rate of prematurity associated with this procedure has decreased dramatically. In addition, there are few demonstrable clinical side effects of the balloon on the developing trachea except when the balloon is placed early or when complications arise at the time of balloon removal (70). While postnatal tracheomegaly has been observed in some fetuses that have undergone FETO (71), no obvious clinical impact has been documented except for a "barking cough on effort" (72). Fortunately, this widening of the trachea has been observed to become less significant overtime (73).

While FETO serves to stem progress of the lung pathophysiology in utero, definitive surgical repair of the diaphragmatic defect is still necessary following delivery of the baby.

It is estimated that FETO is successful, as measured by placement of the balloon on the first attempt, in 97% of cases. In one study, 97% of cases treated by FETO had subsequent live deliveries although only about half of these survived the subsequent surgery for repair of the diaphragmatic defect and were discharged from the hospital (74). Jani et al. (74) reported PPROM as a significant complication of FETO. It occurs in about 47% of cases, and within 3 weeks of the intervention in about 16%. The risk of PPROM can be predicted by the duration of the procedure as well as the use of general versus regional/local anesthesia; but not by operator experience, gestational age at FETO, side of diaphragmatic defect, placental location, number of FETOs performed, or O/E LHR value (74). Other maternal complications include intraamniotic hemorrhage and chorioamnionitis. Fetal complications include tracheal laceration and demise although rare.

■ FETAL PAIN AND ANESTHETIC CONSIDERATIONS IN THE FETUS

Fetal interventions have forced anesthesiologists to shift their paradigm. It was originally believed that only maternal medication was necessary for these procedures. However, the fetus is now accepted as a surgical patient in addition to the pregnant woman. Before discussing anesthesia for the fetus, we must address the issue of the presence or absence of fetal pain and the existing supporting evidence.

Fetal Pain and Analgesia

The concept of fetal analgesia warrants special discussion. Fetal perception of pain and the management thereof, remain an unresolved issue for in utero interventions. Determination of whether or not the fetus feels pain is confounded by a number of issues. First, pain is a subjective experience involving both sensory and emotional components, and it requires a sufficient level of consciousness in order for it to be recognized as "unpleasant" (75). Secondly, the experience of pain is usually associated with a nociceptive stimulus. Phantom-limb pain however, demonstrates that a nociceptive stimulus is not required in order to experience pain; and conversely, reflex withdrawal from noxious stimuli below the level of a spinal cord lesion demonstrates that the feeling of pain does not necessarily have to occur in response to a noxious stimulus (75). Finally, the emotional component of pain implies a psychological construct where conscious perception results from the presence of functional thalamocortical circuitry (76,77).

Establishment of the sensory pathway for the experience of pain begins anatomically at 7 WGA with the formation of peripheral nociceptors that connect to the spinal cord at 8 WGA, and grow C-fibers into the spinal cord by 10 WGA (78). An intact spinal reflex arc responds to non-noxious stimuli at 8 WGA and nociceptive neurons are present in the dorsal horn of the spinal cord by 19 WGA (79). A cerebral cortex, initially isolated from other brain structures, begins to form at 10 WGA (80). A cortical *sub* plate, which is specific to the fetus, and underlies the cortex from 15 WGA (81), is connected to thalamic afferent fibers around 20 to 22 WGA and subsequently regresses (82). The cerebral cortical plate undergoes a differentiation and maturation process to become the definitive cerebral cortex beginning at 17 WGA and continuing well into postnatal life (83). Penetration of the cerebral cortex by thalamic afferent fibers beginning from 23 to 24 WGA constitutes an intact anatomical pathway for pain (79).

Establishing the sensation of a stimulus and a sufficient level of consciousness, both of which are required in order to recognize the stimulus as "unpleasant," is more problematic. The very presence of anatomic nociceptive pathways does not establish that the cortex can "perceive" a stimulus and/or "recognize" it as unpleasant. In order for the cortex to "perceive" a noxious stimulus, both the cortex and the nociceptive pathways must be functional, in addition to being anatomically present. The electroencephalogram (EEG) provides a general assessment of cortical function as it measures summated synaptic potentials from the cortical neurons. A primitive EEG is discernable at 20 WGA, becomes sustained after 22 WGA, and is well characterized from 28 WGA onward (78). Unfortunately, EEG activity alone does not prove that the cortex is functional; since EEG activity may still be present even when functional neural tissue above the brainstem is missing (anencephaly) (84).

Somatosensory evoked potentials (SSEPs) demonstrate a cortical response to visceral noxious stimuli, which is transmitted from the nociceptor via the dorsal column tract of the spinal cord through the thalamus to the cortex (85). SSEPs should therefore provide evidence for both cortical and nociceptive pathway function. SSEPs may be elicited beyond 24 WGA and become well developed by 27 WGA (86), suggesting that a functional nociceptive system is present from 24 to 26 WGA.

Determination of a sufficient level of consciousness, required in order to recognize a stimulus as "unpleasant" continues to be unresolved. It has been surmised that consciousness should not be regarded as an all or nothing type of phenomenon, but rather as a continuum, where the level of consciousness may change in a manner similar to a dimmer switch (78). It is believed that consciousness is only possible after an EEG pattern indicates "wakefulness"; an arousal state mediated by the brainstem and thalamus in communication with the cerebral cortex (75). Again, unfortunately, a wakefulness EEG pattern alone does not prove consciousness as this EEG pattern may occur even during a persistent vegetative state (i.e., unconsciousness) (75).

Biophysical markers (e.g., a stress response), which would provide an objective indication of pain, are being investigated. Following a painful stimulus, a stress response (as measured by neuroendocrine or hemodynamic changes) should result and could theoretically be used to infer the perception of pain (87). For example, the plasma concentrations of neuroendocrine stress markers, that is, hormones and neurotransmitters such as cortisol, β-endorphin, and norepinephrine increase in response to a stimulus. It has been shown that following a stimulus the fetus can mount a stress response as measured by increases in both cortisol, β-endorphin (88), and noradrenaline from 18 WGA onward (89). Unfortunately, a neuroendocrine stress response does not prove the presence (or absence) of a painful stimulus as it is mediated by the autonomic nervous system and hypothalamic–pituitary–adrenal axis without conscious processing by the cortex (90). Furthermore, increased fetal plasma concentrations of these markers, for example, noradrenaline, occur following what is considered by some to be non-painful procedures such as umbilical cord transfusions (89–91).

Even though an increase in stress response hormones is not absolute proof of a painful experience, it is reasonable to interpret blunting of the stress response as a strong indication that pain was not experienced. It has been demonstrated that opioid analgesia (92) and volatile anesthesia (93) blunt the stress response to surgery in neonates with an improved outcome.

Hemodynamic changes indicating a stress response have been measured using Doppler ultrasound (94) where increased cerebral blood flow (as measured by the pulsatility index in the middle cerebral artery) occurred following venipuncture for fetal blood transfusion via the innervated abdominal wall but not via the non-innervated umbilical cord (95). This redistribution of blood flow toward the brain, at the expense of blood flow to less essential organs (intestine, kidney), referred to as "brain sparing" does not prove the presence of pain as it is also associated with fetal hypoxia (96) and intrauterine growth restriction (97).

Fetal movement in response to touch can be observed from approximately 8 WGA (98) and the experience of pain has been inappropriately attributed to these "withdrawal" movements. A flexion withdrawal response, elicited by cutaneous stimuli, is a spinal reflex that does not involve the cortex; as such, it is a reflex that occurs even in cases of anencephaly (99) and persistent vegetative states (100).

In summary, although the nociceptive pathways are both present and functioning by 24 to 26 WGA, absolute proof that the fetus experiences pain is still lacking. Nevertheless, Lee and colleagues (79) eloquently argue that "... fetal anesthesia and analgesia are still warranted for surgical procedures undertaken to promote fetal health.... evidence of fetal pain is unnecessary to justify fetal anesthesia and analgesia because they serve other purposes unrelated to pain reduction, including (1) inhibition of fetal movement during a procedure, (2)... improve surgical access to the fetus, (3) prevent hormonal stress responses associated with poor surgical outcomes in neonates, ..." Despite the ongoing and persistent debate on whether the fetus feels pain or not, most anesthesiologists will provide analgesia to the fetus during any fetal intervention in which a noxious stimulus is applied directly to the fetus.

Predominant issues for the fetal surgical patient revolve around analgesia, immobility, and hemodynamic stability. Fetal hemodynamic stability will be addressed under maternal considerations.

Anesthetic Considerations for Percutaneous Fetal Intervention in the Fetus

Medications can be administered to the fetus via three general routes: Direct administration, uptake from the amniotic fluid and lastly, via maternal transfer through the placenta. Direct administration can be via the intravenous (umbilical or hepatic vein), intramuscular, or intracardiac routes. The risks of accessing the umbilical vessels include possible compromise of the fetal circulation as a result of vessel dissection, hematoma formation, or thrombus formation. Presumed pain on accessing the hepatic vein can be alleviated with administration of fentanyl (101). The intramuscular route appears to be the preferred route for administration of medication to the fetus unless the umbilical or hepatic vessels are to be accessed for procedural purposes. Intracardiac injection has also been described (102) and may be the preferred route when fetal hemodynamic instability occurs.

Fetal immobility and analgesia is required for intrauterine fetal blood transfusion, cordocentesis, and cardiac interventions since fetal movement may increase the risk of an iatrogenic injury such as inadvertent punctures or needle cuts causing hemorrhage. In addition, access to the target anatomic site, such as is required during deployment of a shunt or balloon, or cardiac interventions may be very challenging in the presence of fetal movement. Fetal immobility and analgesia is therefore achieved with the direct intramuscular administration of nondepolarizing neuromuscular blocking agents and opioids under ultrasound guidance. Pancuronium, the preferred neuromuscular blocking agent due to its vagolytic properties and longer duration of action, can be administered via the intramuscular route (0.2 to 0.3 mg/kg). It may also be administered via the umbilical vein at a dose of 0.1 to 0.25 mg/kg. However, for majority of procedures, which typically last 1 hour, vecuronium may be administered at similar doses via the intramuscular and intraumbilical vein respectively. Opioids, commonly fentanyl (5 to 20 μg/kg) and anticholinergic agents such as atropine and glycopyrrolate can also be administered in combination with nondepolarizing neuromuscular blocking agents. The combination of these medications in a syringe is handed to the maternal–fetal intervention specialist for administration to the fetus (103).

Uptake of medications by the fetus through amniotic fluid is appealing given the low risk of complications. However, absorption of most drugs through the fetal membranes or skin has not been characterized for humans.

Placental transport of drugs administered to the mother with the intention for the shared effect on the fetus is the predominant method of administration of medication to the fetus especially during laser therapy for TTTS. Fetal/maternal ratios of select drugs are shown in Table 49-4.

TABLE 49-4 Documented Fetal/Maternal Ratios of Selected Drugs

Drug	Fetal/Maternal Ratio	Drug	Fetal/Maternal Ratio
Nitrous oxide	0.85[a]	Dexmedetomidine	0.84[r]
Isoflurane	0.71[b]	Alfentanil	0.3[s]
Etomidate	0.04–0.5[c,d]	Fentanyl (epidural)	0.37–0.94[t,u]
Ketamine	1.2[e]	Meperidine	1.0[v]
Propofol (bolus)	0.22–0.7[f–i]	Morphine	0.61[w]
Propofol (infusion)	0.5–0.76[j,i]	Remifentanil	0.73–0.88[x,y]
Thiopental	0.37–1.08[k,c,l,m]	Sufentanil	0.81[u]
Diazepam[n]	0.57–2.0[o]	Ephedrine	0.7–1.13[z,aa]
Lorazepam	1.0[p]	Phenylephrine	0.7[aa]
Midazolam	0.62[q]		

[a]Marx GF, Joshi CW, Orkin LR. Placental transmission of nitrous oxide. *Anesthesiology* 1970;32(5):429–432.

[b]Dwyer R, Fee JP, Moore J. Uptake of halothane and isoflurane by mother and baby during caesarean section. *Br J Anaesth* 1995;74(4):379–383.

[c]Esener Z, Sarihasan B, Guven H, et al. Thiopentone and etomidate concentrations in maternal and umbilical plasma, and in colostrum. *Br J Anaesth* 1992;69(6):586–588.

[d]Gregory MA, Davidson DG. Plasma etomidate levels in mother and fetus. *Anaesthesia* 1991;46(9):716–718.

[e]Ellingson A, Haram K, Sagen N, et al. Transplacental passage of ketamine after intravenous administration. *Acta Anaesthesiol Scand* 1977;21(1):41–44.

[f]Sanchez-Alcaraz A, Quintana MB, Laguarda M. Placental transfer and neonatal effects of propofol in caesarean section. *J Clin Pharm Ther* 1998;23(1):19–23.

[g]Gin T, Gregory MA, Chan K, et al. Maternal and fetal levels of propofol at caesarean section. *Anaesth Intensive Care* 1990;18(2):180–184.

[h]Valtonen M, Kanto J, Rosenberg P. Comparison of propofol and thiopentone for induction of anaesthesia for elective caesarean section. *Anaesthesia* 1989;44(9):758–762.

[i]Dailland P, Cockshott ID, Lirzin JD, et al. Intravenous propofol during cesarean section: placental transfer, concentrations in breast milk, and neonatal effects. A preliminary study. *Anesthesiology* 1989;71(6):827–834.

[j]Gin T, Yau G, Chan K, et al. Disposition of propofol infusions for caesarean section. *Can J Anaesth* 1991;38(1):31–36.

[k]Levy CJ, Owen G. Thiopentone transmission through the placenta. *Anaesthesia* 1964;19:511–513.

[l]Morgan DJ, Blackman GL, Paull JD, et al. Pharmacokinetics and plasma binding of thiopental. II: Studies at cesarean section. *Anesthesiology* 1981;54(6):474–480.

[m]Bach V, Carl P, Ravlo O, et al. A randomized comparison between midazolam and thiopental for elective cesarean section anesthesia: III. Placental transfer and elimination in neonates. *Anesth Analg* 1989;68(3):238–242.

[n]Bakke OM, Haram K, Lygre T, et al. Comparison of the placental transfer of thiopental and diazepam in caesarean section. *Eur J Clin Pharmacol* 1981;21(3):221–227.

[o]Erkkola R, Kangas L, Pekkarinen A. The transfer of diazepam across the placenta during labour. *Acta Obstet Gynecol Scand* 1973;52(2):167–170.

[p]McBride RJ, Dundee JW, Moore J, et al. A study of the plasma concentrations of lorazepam in mother and neonate. *Br J Anaesth* 1979;51(10):971–978.

[q]Wilson CM, Dundee JW, Moore J, et al. A comparison of the early pharmacokinetics of midazolam in pregnant and nonpregnant women. *Anaesthesia* 1987;42(10):1057–62.

[r]Ala-Kokko TI, Pienimaki P, Lampela E, et al. Transfer of clonidine and dexmedetomidine across the isolated perfused human placenta. *Acta Anaesthesiol Scand* 1997;41(2):313–319.

[s]Gepts E, Heytens L, Camu F. Pharmacokinetics and placental transfer of intravenous and epidural alfentanil in parturient women. *Anesth Analg* 1986;65(11):1155–1160.

[t]Bader AM, Fragneto R, Terui K, et al. Maternal and neonatal fentanyl and bupivacaine concentrations after epidural infusion during labor. *Anesth Analg* 1995;81(4):829–832.

[u]Loftus JR, Hill H, Cohen SE. Placental transfer and neonatal effects of epidural sufentanil and fentanyl administered with bupivacaine during labor. *Anesthesiology* 1995;83(2):300–308.

[v]Shnider S, Way EL, Lord MJ. Rate of appearance and disappearance of meperidine in fetal blood after administration of narcotics to the mother. *Anesthesiology* 1966;27(2):227–228.

[w]Kopecky EA, Ryan ML, Barrett JF, et al. Fetal response to maternally administered morphine. *Am J Obstet Gynecol* 2000;183(2):424–430.

[x]Kan RE, Hughes SC, Rosen MA, et al. Intravenous remifentanil: placental transfer, maternal and neonatal effects. *Anesthesiology* 1998;88(6):1467–1474.

[y]Ngan Kee WD, Khaw KS, Ma KC, et al. Maternal and neonatal effects of remifentanil at induction of general anesthesia for cesarean delivery: a randomized, double-blind, controlled trial. *Anesthesiology* 2006;104(1):14–20.

[z]Hughes SC, Ward MG, Levinson G, et al. Placental transfer of ephedrine does not affect neonatal outcome. *Anesthesiology* 1985;63(2):217–219.

[aa]Ngan Kee WD, Khaw KS, Tan PE, et al. Placental transfer and fetal metabolic effects of phenylephrine and ephedrine during spinal anesthesia for cesarean delivery. *Anesthesiology* 2009;111(3):506–512.

■ MATERNAL ANESTHESIA CONSIDERATIONS FOR PERCUTANEOUS FETAL INTERVENTION

While the fetus is considered to be the surgical patient for fetoscopic interventions, special anesthetic consideration must also be given to the mother. The anesthesiologist must first and foremost ensure maternal safety, comfort, and cooperation. The latter is paramount for fetal intervention procedures in which the mother receives only local anesthesia or conscious sedation instead of general anesthesia.

In Europe, anesthesia for fetal intervention procedures (percutaneous shunt placements, intrauterine transfusions, cordocentesis, or minimally invasive procedures such as laser photocoagulation of vessels for TTTS) occasionally involves only local anesthesia. In the United States, however, a variety of anesthetic approaches are utilized. These include conscious sedation, neuraxial anesthesia or general anesthesia; the choice depends upon preferences of the woman, maternal–fetal specialist and anesthesiologist (104).

Despite majority of these procedures being performed under conscious sedation, the possibility of conversion to a general anesthetic must be entertained and adequately prepared for. Appropriate preparation in case of need to provide general anesthesia should be completed. Conscious sedation is accomplished with local anesthesia infiltration of the mother's abdominal skin supplemented with intravenous sedatives, intermittent bolus administration of opioids such as fentanyl alone, or a combination of drugs including bolus administration of opioids, benzodiazepines, and a low-dose propofol infusion (50 to 100 mcg/kg/min). Administration of remifentanil via an infusion has also been utilized as a sedative for these minimally invasive procedures and it has been found to provide appropriate fetal immobilization at a dose of 0.1 μg/kg/min (5). A randomized double-blind trial comparing remifentanil to diazepam revealed that fetuses whose mothers received remifentanil at this dose, had significantly less intraoperative fetal movement and better operating conditions were also reported by the surgeons (5). Intravenous dexmedetomidine is used for some of these procedures outside the United States however it is currently classified as a Class C drug in the United States and its effects on the fetus have not been fully established. Conscious sedation requires a fine balance between protection of the mother's airway, prevention of an oversedated breathing pattern, and provision of adequate immobilization of the fetus and the mother in order to avoid inadvertent misdirection of the laser.

In order to perform fetoscopic procedures under local anesthesia or conscious sedation, the placenta should be located on the posterior uterine wall otherwise there is a risk of traversing the placenta upon insertion of the trocar. Occasionally when the placenta is located anteriorly, there is a small insertion "window" present that allows for safe insertion of the trocar(s) through the uterine wall without disrupting the uteroplacental unit. In the absence of a minimal insertion "window," special curved scopes (105) or trocars with side ports for laser firing (106) may be used. Alternatively, general anesthesia may be required in order to facilitate a laparoscopic approach to the uterus. With the laparoscopic approach, abdominal insufflation allows for adequate uterine manipulation in order to access a surface away from the placenta where the fetoscopic trocar(s) can be safely inserted.

Some mothers with TTTS may present with severe polyhydramnios and accompanying orthopnea. In this situation, amniocentesis may be performed prior to the fetal intervention in order to relieve the polyhydramnios. However, if the orthopnea persists, general anesthesia may be indicated, as the mother would not be able to tolerate lying supine for the procedure. General anesthesia may also be required if a fetus needs to be delivered urgently via an emergency cesarean section following an intraoperative complication in order to prevent fetal demise. Routine precautions for general anesthesia in the pregnant mother should be observed.

Neuraxial anesthesia, commonly epidural anesthesia with low concentrations of local anesthetic, can also be utilized for percutaneous fetal intervention, particularly fetoscopic laser therapy procedures that tend to last between 1 and 2 hours in duration. However, this technique may not guarantee fetal immobilization unless accompanied with small amounts of sedation such as remifentanil which easily passes to the fetus via the placenta. Neuraxial techniques may provide added benefit if a cerclage is necessary after the laser photocoagulation of the abnormal placenta vessels, in mothers who are determined to have a short cervix. Postoperative pain requirements following percutaneous fetal intervention procedures are very minimal. Therefore, postoperative pain management via an indwelling epidural catheter is not necessary.

Maternal hemodynamic stability must be maintained intraoperatively, both for the mother's safety and also for support of fetal hemodynamics. Appropriate measures to achieve hemodynamic stability in the mother and fetus include left lateral displacement of the uterus, as well as maintenance of both adequate mean arterial pressure and oxygen carrying capacity. Maternal mean arterial pressure may need to be supported by the administration of crystalloid or colloid solutions to maintain intravascular volume, and/or the administration of vasoactive agents. Finally, supplemental oxygen should be administered to the mother in order to maintain the hemoglobin oxygen saturation above 97%, and promote oxygen delivery to the fetus.

While different options abound to provide maternal anesthesia for fetal intervention procedures, maternal hypotension and intra-amniotic bleeding have been found to occur with a higher frequency in mothers who received general anesthesia for these procedures compared to those who received total intravenous anesthesia (107). This should be considered when contemplating different anesthetic options. Each specific procedure requires communication between the anesthesiologist and the surgeons in order to provide adequate operating conditions and an appropriate anesthetic for both mother and fetus.

■ OPEN FETAL SURGERY

The first open fetal surgical procedure was a lifesaving ureterostomy performed in 1981 at the University of California, San Francisco, in order to relieve LUTO in a child with congenital hydronephrosis (108). Open fetal surgery is currently reserved for a select group of fetuses who have conditions associated with very poor prognosis. This section will focus on the presentation, natural history of conditions for which open fetal surgery is performed (lung masses, sacrococcygeal teratoma [SCT], and myelomeningocele [MMC]) as well as the perioperative maternal and fetal anesthetic considerations for open fetal surgery.

Open fetal surgery has been performed for the past 20 years in the United States. Over time, performing surgery on the unborn child has steadily gained acceptance in the medical and surgical communities with an increasing number of institutions offering in utero surgery in Europe and the United States. Advances in ultrasound techniques and the capability to perform ultrafast imaging studies such as computerized tomography and magnetic resonance scans allow for quick evaluation of fetuses and detection of conditions amenable to open fetal surgery or intervention. These include nonlethal conditions such as MMC and life-threatening indications such as large lung masses and large SCTs presenting with impending cardiac failure (hydrops fetalis), a combination that can result in intrauterine death.

For fetuses with life-threatening anomalies, the risk of open fetal surgery is small in the face of possible survival. The risks to the mother are harder to quantify. While open fetal surgery may subject the mother to significant discomfort and morbidity, no maternal mortality has been reported to date. Maternal health and safety remains the priority.

Lung Masses

Lung masses, typically diagnosed by ultrasound between the 18th and 20th weeks of gestation, vary in nature and can include bronchopulmonary sequestrations, CCAMs, or rarely, pleuropulmonary blastomas which have malignant potential. Some lesions are classified as "hybrid" lesions (109); these have components of both pulmonary sequestration and cystic adenomatoid malformation.

The definitive diagnosis of a lung mass is usually made by pathology studies. Bronchogenic cysts, congenital lobar emphysema, mediastinal teratoma, and bronchial atresia are less frequently seen lung masses that may also occur (110). Expectant observation is the mode of management for majority of these lesions. Surgery is typically performed after delivery or in some cases, at delivery, via the EXIT-to-resection procedure (see section on EXIT procedure later).

Bronchopulmonary Sequestration

Bronchopulmonary sequestration (BPS) is immature, non-functional lung tissue that does not communicate with the tracheobronchial tree and has an anomalous blood supply, from the aorta (111). It can be classified into intralobar and extralobar types, based on whether the lesion is contained within the visceral pleura of the normal lung or has its own pleural involvement. Color flow Doppler ultrasonographic detection of a systemic artery from the aorta to the fetal lung lesion is a diagnostic feature of bronchopulmonary sequestration (112). Fortunately, approximately two-thirds of bronchopulmonary sequestration lesions regress and may become nearly undetectable at birth (113). Both CCAM and BPS can coexist in a hybrid lesion and result in the same pathologic effect on the fetus as a CCAM (114). The final diagnosis of the lesion is made on pathologic assessment.

Congenital Cystic Adenomatoid Malformation

This is a rare, congenital, cystic, and intraparenchymal lesion with an incidence of approximately 1 in 10,000 to 35,000 lives births. It is more common in males (115) and is characterized on histology by an abnormal proliferation of bronchiolar-like airspaces and a lack of normal alveoli. These lesions have a minute, tortuous communication with the tracheobronchial tree. This communication differentiates a CCAM from bronchopulmonary sequestration (116). Nevertheless, the lesion does not participate in gas exchange (117,118). Despite the CCAM lesion not participating in gas exchange, the connections with the tracheobronchial tree can result in air trapping which may develop during postnatal resuscitative efforts (119). Arterial supply and venous drainage arise from the normal pulmonary circulation. However, anomalous arterial and venous drainage of CCAMs have been reported (120) as well as "hybrid" CCAMs which have systemic supply (109).

CCAMs are thought to represent focal pulmonary dysplasia, failure of maturation of bronchial structures (117,118),

or bronchial obstruction (121,122). Stocker and colleagues classified CCAMs morphologically into three lesions (117): A Type I lesion is large (>2 cm diameter) and lined with ciliated pseudostratified columnar epithelium with mucus producing cells present; Type II lesions are small (<1 cm diameter) and lined with ciliated cuboidal–columnar epithelial cells without mucous producing cells; and a Type III lesion is large, bulky, non-cystic, and lined with ciliated cuboidal epithelial cells. An alternative classification of CCAMs by ultrasound evaluation is based largely on the size of the lung mass in which case CCAMs are commonly classified as macrocystic (large) or microcystic (small) (123).

As described earlier in the chapter, CCAMs may be treated with thoracentesis, stent placement for permanent thoracic drainage, or cyst aspiration to decompress the cyst and allow for growth of the surrounding pulmonary tissue (124). Approximately 15% to 20% of CCAM lesions may decrease in size during pregnancy (14,113); however, in about 10% of cases, the mass will continue to grow in the prenatal period. This expansion may result in mediastinal shift and disruption of venous return to the heart thereby precipitating nonimmune hydrops and fetal cardiac failure (Fig. 49-4) (14,125). Mortality in the fetus with CCAM and hydrops is near 100%. When CCAM occurs in the absence of hydrops, the survival rate is greater than 95% (126). With regard to the prognosis of CCAM, Crombleholme et al. (127) have suggested that a CCAM volume ratio (tumor volume normalized to head circumference), of >1.6 at presentation significantly increases the risk of hydrops.

The development of fetal hydrops is the only absolute indication for open fetal surgery for CCAM as it is nearly always a predictor of intrauterine fetal demise (119,128). The decision for open fetal surgery for CCAM is based on the presence of hydrops, gestational age of less than 32 weeks, normal karyotype, no associated congenital anomaly and no dominant cyst amenable to aspiration or drainage. The treatment algorithm for fetuses prenatally diagnosed with CCAM is shown in Figure 49-5.

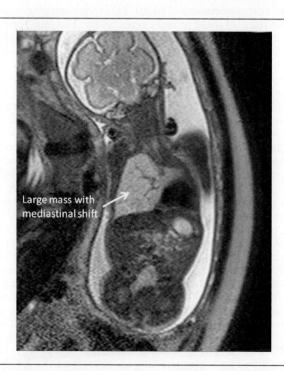

Large mass with mediastinal shift

FIGURE 49-4 Magnetic resonance image (MRI) of fetus with large lung mass causing mediastinal shift. Courtesy of Oluyinka Olutoye M.D., Ph.D.

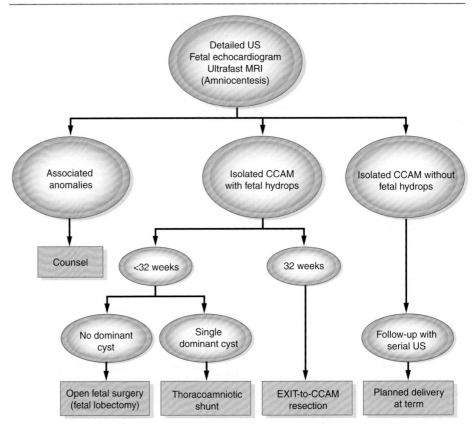

FIGURE 49-5 Treatment algorithm for fetuses prenatally diagnosed with congenital cystic adenomatoid malformation. With permission from: Adzick NS. Open fetal surgery for life-threatening fetal anomalies. *Semin Fetal Neonatal Med* 2010 (120).

Sacrococcygeal Teratoma (SCT)

SCT, the most common newborn tumor, originates from the pluripotent cells of Henson's node located inside the tail of the embryo and grows anterior to the coccyx. It occurs in approximately 1 in 40,000 live births with a 75% to 80% female preponderance (129,130). This tumor usually contains tissue from all three primary germ layers. The fetal form of this tumor is classified by the American Academy of Pediatrics Section on Surgery as Type I through Type IV depending on the anatomic location and extension of the tumor (see Fig. 49-6) (131). Type I tumors are primarily external to the pelvis with a very minimal presacral component; Type II are predominantly external but have a significant presacral portion. Type III tumors are mainly intrapelvic with intraabdominal extension but have an external component and Type IV are exclusively intrapelvic or intraabdominal without an external portion. Type IV tumors may be difficult to diagnose prenatally and may be malignant in nature when detected probably due to a delay in diagnosis of the intrapelvic tumor; they are also not amenable to fetal surgical resection. Ultrafast fetal MRI is superior in delineating the intrapelvic extension of the tumor if present (132). Fortunately, greater than 80% of SCTs are either Type I or Type II, are usually benign in nature, and are diagnosed at birth or shortly thereafter. However, these tumors may be associated with perinatal morbidity and mortality due to dystocia, fetal hydrops, polyhydramnios, and hemorrhage (133–135). In the absence of extensive secondary pathophysiologic changes, these fetuses survive; are delivered via cesarean section at or near term (Fig. 49-7) and then undergo postnatal resection. However, a prenatal diagnosis of an SCT (Fig. 49-8) is associated with an increased mortality of approximately 30% to 50% (136,137). A tumor volume to fetal weight ratio of 0.12 or greater as measured by ultrasound or MRI at 24 weeks' gestation is believed to be predictive of a poor outcome (138).

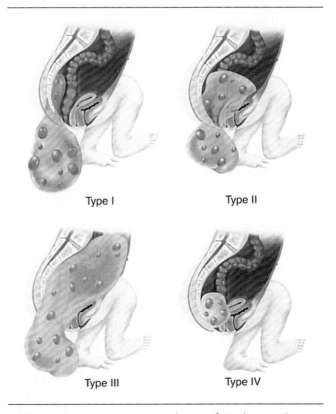

FIGURE 49-6 American Academy of Pediatrics Section of Surgery classification for sacrococcygeal teratomas. With permission from: Holzgreve, et al. The fetus with sacrococcygeal teratoma. In: Harrison MR, Golbus MS, Filly RA, eds. *The Unborn Patient*. Philadelphia, PA: WB Saunders;1991:461 (136).

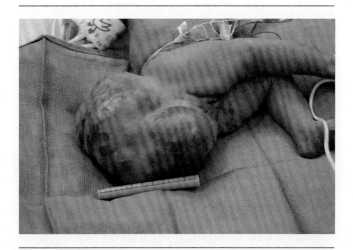

FIGURE 49-7 Sacrococcygeal teratoma following delivery prior to resection. Courtesy of Oluyinka Olutoye M.D., Ph.D.

The high mortality rate associated with fetal SCT is due to a variety of factors. Large or rapidly expanding tumors can result in a mass effect resulting in urinary tract obstruction with resultant hydronephrosis or bowel obstruction, premature delivery or dystocia. Dystocia in previously undiagnosed tumors occurs as a result of traumatic tumor rupture and hemorrhage during delivery. Large tumors may be highly vascular, with arterio-venous shunting within the tumor. Echocardiographic and Doppler assessments of these tumors have demonstrated a vascular steal phenomenon from the placenta and fetus. An actual reversal of flows in the umbilical arteries has been observed as the lower resistance present in the tumor "steals" blood from the placenta. Fetal cardiac hypertrophy results as the heart tries to keep up with the increased demands. Heart failure eventually occurs with resultant pleural and pericardial effusion, placentomegaly, and generalized body swelling or anasarca. The presence of

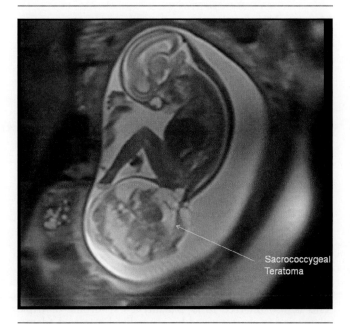

FIGURE 49-8 Prenatal MRI of fetus with sacrococcygeal teratoma. Courtesy of Oluyinka Olutoye M.D., Ph.D.

ascites in one or more fetal body cavities is defined as hydrops fetalis and this is the preterminal manifestation of high-output cardiac failure. Hydrops fetalis heralds impending fetal demise and is usually preceded by a rapid growth in tumor size. This rapid tumor growth is associated with hemorrhage into the mass. This, together with ensuing anemia, contributes to the development of high-output cardiac failure. The development of placentomegaly and hydrops may lead to the Mirror syndrome in the mother (see section on Mirror syndrome later). Intrauterine surgical resection is therefore desirable before both the fetus and mother reach this stage of decompensation.

Indications for open fetal surgery for treatment of fetal SCT include evidence of high-output cardiac failure, placentomegaly or hydrops, gestational age less than 30 weeks and favorable anatomy (Type I or II). Contraindications to surgery are fetal dilated cardiomyopathy, Type III or IV and evidence of tumor hemorrhage (139).

Myelomeningocele (MMC)

MMC is the first non-threatening fetal condition with chronic debilitating effects that has been repaired by in utero fetal surgery. It is a neural tube defect in which the spinal cord develops without a covering, thereby exposing the meninges and neural tissue to the intrauterine environment. It occurs in about 1/2,000 live births annually (140,141) and the resulting demands on the healthcare system for care of the associated morbidities is significant (142,143).

Maternal or fetal deficiency of folate is a well-known predisposing factor in the development of MMC (144). However, fetal exposure to a variety of toxins such as valproic acid, calcium channel blockers, carbamazepine, cytochalasins, and hyperthermia are also implicated in the development of MMC (145–148).

Historically, diagnosis of MMC has been based on detection of maternal serum levels of α-fetoprotein (AFP). Positive levels mandate subsequent amniocentesis and measurement of AFP in amniotic fluid (149). With the recent development of high-resolution ultrasonography, MMC can be detected as early as the first trimester of pregnancy (150). Fetal MRI techniques have also allowed for improvements in the definitive diagnosis of MMC (151). The combination of ultrasound, MRI, and maternal serum AFP levels are now used to definitively diagnose MMC (152,153).

Embryology of Myelomeningocele
Failure of closure of the neural tube during development in the third week of gestation results in the formation of MMC. This defect is considered the first insult in the two-hit phenomenon described in the pathogenesis of MMC. The second insult is subsequent injury to the exposed spinal cord as a result of exposure to the intrauterine environment (143,154,155). The lumbosacral region is a common location for this defect (153,156).

Pathophysiologic Sequelae of Myelomeningocele
Regardless of the etiology of the MMC, the defect of dorsal spinal elements and overlying tissue coverage result in the development of an overlying cerebrospinal-fluid–containing central sac, dysmorphic spinal cord, and associated nerve roots. The lack of interconnection between the dysmorphic spinal cord and the descending sensory and motor tracts which regulate sensation and voluntary movements result in some degree of lower extremity, bladder or sphincteric weakness and sensory deficits (143,152). These may lead to chronic lower extremity neurologic deficits, as well as urinary and fecal incontinence (152–154). In addition, approximately

90% and 85% of children with MMC also develop Arnold–Chiari malformation (ANC) Type II or hydrocephalus, respectively (155,157,158).

It has been postulated that fetal intervention may improve the neurologic defects associated with MMC including impaired ambulation, hydrocephalus, ANC, and can also decrease the need for ventriculoperitoneal shunting (159). A number of early animal studies supported this theory, indicating that in utero fetal intervention may prevent postnatal neurologic deficits (160–164). However, it was not until large animal studies showed similar findings (146,165) that this concept was extrapolated to management of human MMC. Human fetal interventions for MMC began in 1997 (166). Since this first attempt, there were a number of reports of in utero repair of MMC performed at different stages of gestation (167), some with no documentation on improved postnatal neurologic function (167), and some with documented reversal of pre-intervention MRI findings of hindbrain herniation and improved neurologic outcome (168,169). It appeared surgical intervention at an earlier stage of gestation may result in improved neurologic outcomes as two separate studies performed at different stages of gestation yielded different results. Adzick and colleagues (168) reported their findings on in utero closure of MMC on fetuses between 22 and 25 weeks of gestation. Of the nine patients that survived, following an average duration of 10 weeks following intervention, all had lower extremity function that was at least two or more spinal segments better than expected based on prenatal MRI. In addition, postnatal ultrafast MRI revealed ascent of the hindbrain and increased cerebrospinal fluid volume around the posterior fossa which is consistent with reversal of hindbrain herniation in utero. To date, seven (78%) of the patients who survived have required ventricular shunting (168). Another study by Bruner and colleagues (170) reported a decrease in hindbrain herniation following in utero fetal surgery performed on 29 fetuses between 24 and 30 weeks' gestation; 17 of the 29 patients (59%) required subsequent ventriculoperitoneal shunting. Also of note was that the ventriculoperitoneal shunting required was at a later age than in the control group in which a 91% shunt placement rate was observed. In this latter cohort, improved lower extremity function was not observed; this may have been due to the fact that the interventions occurred at later gestational ages and in utero biochemical or traumatic damage had already occurred. A case series of 58 patients treated over a 6-year period at the Children's Hospital of Philadelphia (171) also demonstrated resolution of hindbrain herniation in almost all patients with serial MRI evidence of ascent of hindbrain structures within 3 weeks of fetal closure. 1-, 2-, 3-, and 5-year follow-up of these patients revealed a 46% incidence of ventriculoperitoneal shunt placement, which is much less than the rate of 84% based on historical controls at that hospital between 1983 and 2000 (172).

These initial surgical interventions were criticized, for selection bias and differences in management approach that can potentially affect outcome (173). Therefore, a prospective multicenter randomized trial, the management of myelomeningocele study (MOMS) trial, was initiated in 2003 in order to validate these findings (174). The primary objective of the trial was to determine if intrauterine repair of fetal MMC at 19 to 25 weeks of gestation improved outcome, as measured by death or the need for shunting by 1 year of life, compared to postnatal MMC repair. Secondary objectives of the study were to determine whether fetal MMC repair improved the degree of Arnold–Chiari II malformation and neurologic outcome as tested by neuroimaging, neuromotor function analysis, cognitive testing, and neurodevelopment status at 12 and 30 months of age. Finally, the long-term psychological

and reproductive consequences in mothers who underwent intrauterine repair of MMC were compared to those in the postnatal repair group. The study design involved recruitment of 100 patients into each arm (in utero surgery—100 and postnatal surgery—100) with potential patients referred to one of the participating centers based on geographic criteria. This study was however stopped prematurely due to significant difference in outcomes as the prenatal surgery arm of the study showed a 40% rate of shunt placement while the postnatal surgery arm had a shunt placement rate of 82%. In addition, there was an improvement in motor function and ambulation in the prenatal surgery group at 30 months compared to the postnatal surgery group. An increased incidence of preterm delivery and uterine dehiscence was however observed in the prenatal group (174).

Preoperative Evaluation for Open Fetal Surgery
Fetal Evaluation
Once mothers carrying fetuses with problems potentially amenable to open fetal surgery are referred to a fetal treatment center, they are evaluated for possible surgery via a multidisciplinary approach. This includes (1) detailed ultrasonography to confirm diagnosis and rule out the presence of any other associated congenital anomaly, (2) ultrafast fetal magnetic resonance imaging (MRI) for additional anatomic information, (3) a fetal echocardiogram to assess fetal cardiac function and rule out congenital heart defects (the most common fetal anomaly), and (4) amniocentesis or umbilical blood sampling for fetal karyotyping (119). The presence of chromosomal abnormality, multiple gestations, and other significant anatomic abnormalities is a contraindication to open fetal surgery.

If the fetus is deemed to be a suitable candidate for open fetal surgery, preoperative imaging is performed closer to the date of surgery in order to identify any alterations in fetal physiology that may impact fetal well-being intraoperatively. This includes fetal ventricular dysfunction which can alert the anesthesiologist caring for the baby to the possibility of intraoperative fetal cardiac arrest. Ultrasonography, obtained immediately before surgery also provides an estimated fetal weight upon which intraoperative unit doses of fetal medications are based.

Maternal Evaluation
Maternal safety during open fetal surgery cannot be over emphasized regardless of the indication of the procedure. A routine medical history and physical should be obtained. Ultrasonographic documentation of the placenta size is valuable information as placentomegaly and increased placental blood flow may alter the pharmacokinetics of administered drugs and increased drug doses may be required. In addition, there are reports of the edges of a large placenta getting caught in the hysterotomy incision, resulting in massive maternal hemorrhage (175,176). While special surgical staples are used to create the hysterotomy during surgery, massive maternal hemorrhage may still occur (177). Therefore adequate preparations for maternal blood transfusion—four units of blood—should be available on the day of surgery. Maternal contraindications to open fetal surgery include medical risk factors, a history of heavy cigarette smoking, due to concern for impaired placental function, and the presence of fetal hydrops reflecting in the mother as maternal mirror syndrome.

Mirror Syndrome
This is also referred to as Ballantyne's syndrome or triple edema and is characterized by generalized maternal edema, proteinuria, and hypertension in association with fetal hydrops (178). When this condition develops, the mother

demonstrates a hyperdynamic state with associated hypertension and generalized edema. The mother clinically mirrors the features observed in the fetus hence the term "Mirror syndrome." This condition is generally associated with increased perinatal morbidity and mortality and is therefore a contraindication to open fetal surgery (119); it usually resolves with delivery of the fetus (178).

Once careful evaluation of the mother and the fetus has been completed and the decision is made to proceed, a multidisciplinary meeting including fetal/pediatric surgeons, anesthesiologists, obstetricians, a nurse coordinator, operating room nurses, and a social worker is held to discuss the nature of the anomaly with the family as well as the prognosis and alternatives to fetal intervention. The steps of the proposed surgery and postnatal care, as well as the risks, benefits, and alternatives to fetal intervention are also discussed. Potential risks associated with open fetal surgery, including (but not limited to) operative complications such as preterm labor, chorioamnionitis, rupture of uterine membranes, uterine rupture, side effects of tocolytics, risk of fetal demise, and the need for cesarean section for all subsequent pregnancies, are also clearly outlined and discussed before obtaining consent for treatment. This meeting gives the family an opportunity to ask questions and make informed decisions about management of the fetus. It is also emphasized at these meetings that the treatment option being offered is not mandatory and the ultimate decision to proceed lies with the mother. An additional factor to be considered in the decision-making process for the mother is the fact that she will be on mandatory postoperative bed rest for the remainder of the pregnancy in order to prevent preterm labor. Therefore, she will require a very strong social support system.

Intraoperative Management

Fetal Monitoring

The goal of fetal monitoring during fetal surgery is to prevent asphyxia which can be induced by cord compression as well as prevention of hypoxia and hypothermia. Recommended equipment and medications for the fetus are shown in Table 49-5. For MMC repair where the primary defect has no major impact on circulatory function and only the fetal defect is delivered into the operative field (i.e., no extremities), pulse oximetry monitoring is not routinely performed and not all the items listed in Table 49-5 will apply. However,

continuous echocardiography may be performed in order to obtain information on ventricular rate, function, and volume. For open fetal surgery procedures that involve resection of large masses, impact the circulatory function of the fetus, or involve a moderate degree of fetal exposure, for example, large lung or sacrococcygeal mass resection, continuous fetal monitoring is invaluable as it provides information on fetal oxygenation, heart rate, and intracardiac volume status. Depending on the hospital setting, an anesthesiologist dedicated to the care of the fetus during surgery is scrubbed in as part of the team on the operative field.

Fetal oxygenation depends on maternal oxygenation and placental perfusion. As changes in placental perfusion may occur in the absence of maternal hypotension, a separate pulse oximeter monitor specifically dedicated to assessment of fetal oxygen saturation should be available in the operating room. Fetal oxygen saturations are obtained by placing a regular (sterile) pulse oximeter probe on a fetal extremity (see Fig. 49.9A). It is initially challenging to get the probe to adhere firmly to the fetal skin which is wet from amniotic fluid and covered with vernix caseosa. Repeated wipe-downs with operating room sponges help dry the fetal skin. Once the probe is placed, it is covered with a piece of aluminum foil in order to prevent interference from ambient light (see Fig. 49.9B). Normal fetal oxygen saturation ranges between 50% and 70%; a value less than 50% could signal impaired placental perfusion and warrants optimization of maternal blood pressure. Umbilical cord compression could also result

TABLE 49-5 Equipment for Surgery on the Fetus

Pulse oximeter monitor and probe for monitoring of fetal oxygenation

24 G intravenous catheters

Saline flush with extension for connection to intravenous catheter

Penrose drain for use as tourniquet for intravenous catheter placement

Resuscitation medications:

  Three 1 mL syringes of epinephrine 1 μg/kg (for intravenous or umbilical cord administration)

  Two 1 mL syringes of calcium gluconate 30 mg/kg (for intravenous administration)

Fetal medication syringes with 27 G subcutaneous needles attached for intramuscular administration:

  Three syringes of unit doses of atropine, fentanyl, and pancuronium all combined in one syringe

    Array of different size endotracheal tubes with stylettes

  Two 10 mL syringes of saline

  Two 10 mL syringes of albumin

  Sixty milliliters of packed erythrocytes (Type O)

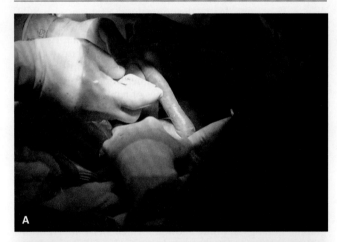

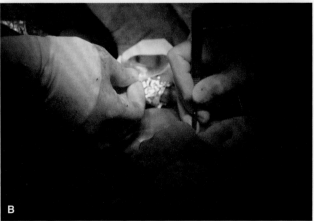

FIGURE 49-9 **A:** Pulse oximeter being applied to fetus' hand. **B:** Pulse oximeter covered with foil and tegaderm to prevent ambient light interference.

in decreased fetal oxygen saturations (<50%). A value less than 30% heralds impending cardiovascular collapse (179).

Maternal hyperoxia has been found to improve fetal oxygenation even in the face of decreased umbilical and uterine blood flow (180). However, maternal arterial oxygen concentrations of 600 mm Hg do not increase fetal arterial oxygen concentration beyond 45 to 60 mm Hg. Increased maternal oxygen concentration is therefore not associated with the development of retrolental fibroplasia or premature closure of the ductus arteriosus (181).

Continuous intraoperative fetal echocardiography by a cardiologist provides immense information about fetal well-being, namely myocardial contractility, function, as well as heart rate, and intravascular volume status. It is typically performed at the beginning of fetal exposure and is continued until uterine closure. The probe, covered by a sterile sleeve is placed on the exposed uterine wall or directly over the fetal chest and is continuously maneuvered for optimal image quality (182). This method of monitoring can be labor intensive as it requires the constant presence of a skilled cardiologist for the duration of the procedure. A study by Rychik and colleagues (182) documented cardiac changes by fetal echocardiogram in 83 fetuses undergoing fetal surgery for different indications: MMC repair, 15; resection of intrathoracic masses (ITM), 51; SCT, 4; and CDH repair, 13. They examined parameters such as heart rate, cardiac output, ductal patency, ventricular function, and valvular dysfunction, before, during, and shortly after fetal surgery. All fetuses with MMC had normal baseline cardiovascular functions. However, fetuses with ITM, CDH, and SCT had secondary cardiac malfunctions due to the anomaly; the fetuses with SCT had a high combined cardiac output while those with ITM and CDH had decreased combined cardiac output. All cases were characterized by a decrease in the combined cardiac output at the time of incision despite an increase in heart rate suggesting diminishing stroke volume. Intraoperative bradycardia was also observed in all types of fetal surgery reviewed, probably due to mechanical compression of the umbilical cord (183,184). While there was no baseline ductal constriction noted in any of the fetal surgery groups, it was observed in 27% of cases spread across the different groups. Nevertheless, there was early resolution of the constriction following surgery. This effect may be secondary to the use of the perioperative tocolytic, indomethacin, as well as the stress of surgery.

A retrospective study of open fetal surgery procedures by Keswani and colleagues (185) determined that echocardiographic findings not only allowed for beneficial interventions such as treatment for decreased ventricular filling, bradycardia, and decreased ventricular contractility but also allowed for assessment of the effectiveness of resuscitative interventions.

Prevention of fetal hypothermia is also an important consideration. The temperature of the operating room should be kept between 80 and 85°F. In addition, warm fluid continuously infused into the uterine cavity via a rapid infusion system replaces amniotic fluid losses and keeps the fetus warm. The infusion system should be primed with isotonic crystalloid (Ringer's lactate solution is commonly used). The fluid is infused into the uterus via a sterile tubing system with a dedicated person in the operating room responsible for regulating the fluid flow. In addition to keeping the fetus warm, this continuous fluid infusion serves to maintain uterine volume, prevent expulsion of the fetus or placental separation; and also serves as a cushion to prevent compression of the umbilical cord.

Fetal Anesthesia

Intraoperative management of the fetus during open fetal surgery for mass resection is more involved than that for fetuses with MMC. Items required for fetal surgery involving resection of a mass are listed in Table 49-5. Once the fetus is exposed for surgery, intramuscular medications are administered to prevent fetal stress responses, vagal responses, and to provide fetal analgesia and immobility. Specifically, a combination of fentanyl (5 to 20 mcg/kg), atropine (20 mcg/kg), and vecuronium or pancuronium (0.1 to 0.2 mg/kg) all combined in one syringe, is injected into the deltoid muscle, gluteal region, or thigh of the fetus. Adequate provision of fetal analgesia is necessary as fetal pain is believed to increase the fetal stress response, which plays a significant role in the development of preterm labor. Administration of analgesics and muscle relaxants to the fetus augment the effect of volatile anesthetics that the fetus receives via placental transfer from the mother.

While all inhaled anesthetics are lipid soluble, have low molecular weight, are nonionized and therefore easily cross the placental barrier, fetal uptake is slightly longer than that of the mother (186,187). Nevertheless, the fetus requires a lower minimum alveolar concentration (MAC) than the mother; much less than that required for uterine relaxation, so an adequate depth of maternal anesthesia should provide adequate fetal uptake and anesthesia (186,188). Once medications have been administered to the fetus, a pulse oximeter probe is placed on an extremity of the fetus as described above followed by attempts to secure peripheral intravenous access for administration of fluid and blood if necessary. Peripheral intravenous catheter placement can be challenging due to the fluid environment and presence of premature, thin-walled veins. Alternatively, intermittent administration of fluids through the umbilical cord and intraosseous administration of fluid have been used (189). Securing intravenous access for surgery involving resection of a fetal mass is important for a variety of reasons: The vascular supply to the different lesions is variable and preoperative imaging may not fully delineate every detail, hence fetal hemorrhage during thoracotomy and lung mass resection as well as during resection of a large SCT with a large arterio-venous malformation, is a real concern. During resection of large ITM, sudden relief of the compressive effect of the mass is believed to result in alteration of the preload of the heart and affect ventricular mechanics in a manner similar to what occurs following pericardiotomy for constrictive pericarditis (190). In a study of fetuses undergoing open fetal surgery for resection of ITM, 20% of them had preoperative ventricular dysfunction (182). This number increased to 80% during surgery with both ventricular and valvular dysfunction being present in almost all cases. Two-thirds of the fetuses with ITM also demonstrated bradycardia following mass resection that required vigorous resuscitation including fluid administration and cardiopulmonary resuscitation. It is therefore beneficial to increase the preload in these fetuses prior to removal of the thoracic mass. As a result of the observed hemodynamic changes during these procedures, slow removal of the tumor as well as vigilant monitoring of ventricular volumes during resection is recommended in order to decrease hemodynamic instability. Type O negative, irradiated packed red blood cells in 50 to 60 mL aliquots should be available in the operating room in the event that fetal transfusion becomes necessary.

Maternal Monitoring and Management of Anesthesia

In addition to placement of routine American Society of Anesthesiologists (ASA) monitoring for these procedures, invasive monitoring via an arterial line is utilized for close monitoring and regulation of maternal blood pressure. Placement of pneumatic compression devices should also be considered, as the mother will be on prolonged bed rest following surgery.

An epidural catheter is placed preoperatively and tested for location. The epidural is not used intraoperatively as local anesthetic-induced hypotension will augment maternal hypotension, which inevitably occurs as a result of the high volatile anesthetic concentration required for open fetal surgery.

After epidural catheter placement, the mother is positioned supine with left uterine tilt, preoxygenated and a rapid sequence induction and intubation is performed. Anesthesia is initially maintained at 1 MAC of the volatile anesthetic of choice while ultrasound is performed to ascertain fetal well-being and also to map out placenta location in relationship to the fetus before the beginning of surgery. During this time, an additional large-bore intravenous catheter, a radial arterial catheter, orogastric and urinary catheters are placed. In the absence of cardiac anomalies in the fetus, rectal indomethacin (50 mg) is administered at this time for tocolysis if it had not been administered preoperatively.

The goal of maternal anesthesia for open fetal surgery is a relaxed myometrium and maintenance of maternal blood pressure within mean awake values. The volatile agent concentration is maintained at 1 MAC until just before the surgeons are ready to make the hysterotomy incision and uterine relaxation is required. Then the concentration of volatile anesthetic is increased to approximately 2 to 3 times MAC. Volatile anesthetics at this high concentration are powerful relaxants of the myometrium and are the agents of choice for open fetal surgery. Sevoflurane, isoflurane, and desflurane have been used for open fetal surgery. The use of desflurane is attractive as its low blood-gas solubility will allow for quick emergence once surgery is completed. However, the utilization of high MAC of desflurane, for long periods of time while the patient is surgically prepped prior to the hysterotomy incision, is discouraged as a recent report by Boat et al. (191) found that fetuses who received high concentrations of desflurane during this period have a high incidence of fetal bradycardia and an increased requirement of fetal resuscitative measures. In this retrospective study, 18 mothers received high concentration of desflurane as the sole anesthetic immediately following induction of anesthesia and another 18 received intravenous infusions of propofol (150 to 200 mcg/kg/min) and remifentanil (0.2 to 0.5 mcg/kg/min) with desflurane (1 to 1.5 MAC) following induction, and immediately prior to hysterotomy they received increased concentrations of desflurane (2 to 2.5 MAC) with lower doses of supplemental propofol (50 to 75 mcg/kg/min). The amount of uterine relaxation achieved in the mothers who received an initial lower concentration of desflurane was similar to that achieved in the mothers who received high concentrations of desflurane immediately following induction of anesthesia. Fetuses of mothers who received supplemental intravenous anesthesia and a slow increase in the volatile anesthetic concentration were noted to have fewer incidences of bradycardia requiring resuscitative intervention measures compared to mothers who received high concentrations of desflurane immediately following induction of anesthesia. Fetal resuscitative measures were defined as administration of fluid boluses, epinephrine or atropine based on fetal echocardiographic findings.

The use of supplemental intravenous anesthesia with low to normal levels of volatile anesthetic agents at the beginning of the surgery is beneficial as high concentrations of volatile anesthetics decrease maternal blood pressure, uteroplacental perfusion, and subsequently fetal oxygenation.

Following resolution of the succinylcholine-induced neuromuscular blockade from induction of anesthesia, only small doses of intermediate acting muscle relaxants should be administered subsequently. This will reduce the likelihood of prolonged neuromuscular blockade from the potentiating effects of intravenous magnesium, which is given for tocolysis during uterine closure (192,193). Small amounts of intravenous opioids may also be administered for intraoperative analgesia.

It is vital to maintain maternal hemodynamics in the normal range to ensure good uteroplacental perfusion. Ephedrine had been the vasoactive agent of choice in pregnant women for many years due to its ability to increase both maternal blood pressure and uterine blood flow as it preferentially constricts the systemic vasculature and shunts blood to the uterus. However, either ephedrine or phenylephrine are acceptable choices as recent evidence does not support the supposition that phenylephrine decreases uteroplacental blood flow (194–196). Depending on the patients' hemodynamic response, an infusion of phenylephrine at a dose of 0.1 mcg/kg/min may be necessary to maintain adequate maternal blood pressure.

Once the uterus is completely exposed, adequate uterine relaxation is confirmed by the surgeon via palpation. Two sutures parallel to the intended incision site are inserted through the full thickness of the uterine wall and a hemostatic uterine stapling device (US Surgical Corporation, Norwalk, CT) is inserted through the points of suture fixation and into the amniotic cavity (14). The staples fix the amniotic membranes to the uterine wall and prevent separation which can precipitate hemorrhage. Clipping of the edge of the placenta or a loose staple may result in severe maternal hemorrhage as the uterus is completely relaxed at this stage. The specific body part of the fetus requiring surgery is positioned within the hysterotomy incision and supplemental fetal anesthesia is provided with intramuscular medications. For mass resections (thoracic mass or SCT), fetal monitoring and intravenous access is secured as described above.

Judicious administration of intravenous fluid to the mother, limited to 500 mL crystalloid, is recommended during open fetal surgery as pulmonary edema may develop from a variety of causes. Some of the warm fluid as it is continuously irrigated into the uterine cavity may be absorbed into the maternal system. Therefore this fluid needs to be closely regulated as large volumes, up to 10 L, may be used. Once the fetal surgical procedure is completed, and closure of uterine incision has begun, magnesium sulfate ($MgSO_4$) tocolysis is initiated with a loading dose of 4 to 6 g followed by a continuous infusion of 2 to 4 g/h. High serum levels of magnesium may predispose the mother to pulmonary edema in addition to fluid that may have been absorbed into the mother's system during the intraoperative continuous infusion of fluid into the uterus.

During closure of the uterine incision, analgesia is initiated with local anesthetics and opioids via the epidural catheter and the volatile anesthetic concentration is decreased. Alternatively, volatile anesthetics may actually be completely discontinued at this time and the mother can be maintained on nitrous oxide and oxygen with or without a low-dose propofol infusion until surgery is completed in order to facilitate a quick and smooth emergence at the end of surgery.

Postanesthesia Management

The woman should be closely monitored following surgery in a step down unit or intensive care unit. Capability to rapidly address any complications that may occur should be readily available. Uterine activity and irritability are continuously measured with tocodynamometers and this dictates adjustment of tocolytic therapy. Fetal well-being is periodically assessed via ultrasound in the postoperative period. The main focus in the postoperative phase is the prevention of preterm labor, which is the Achilles' heel of fetal surgery. It may occur immediately after surgery, which almost always results in fetal demise or it may occur after successful continuation of pregnancy for a few weeks following surgery. Satisfactory postoperative analgesia is paramount to preventing preterm labor. Inadequate maternal and fetal analgesia stimulate adrenocorticotrophic hormone production and subsequent cortisol release. This causes changes in the placenta resulting in fetal estrogen and prostaglandin production, both of which increase uterine activity (197). The use of epidural infusions with low concentration of local anesthetic and high-opioid concentration, such as bupivacaine 0.05% with fentanyl 10 mcg/mL, have been described (197). The high concentration of fentanyl allows for adequate fetal systemic absorption.

Prevention of uterine contractions starts about 1 hour preoperatively (preferred) or intraoperatively with the administration of 50 to 100 mg rectal indomethacin. It may also be administered every 4 to 6 hours in the postoperative period. Serial postoperative assessments of the patency of the ductus arteriosus are documented by fetal ultrasound to determine if this therapy should be continued. Intravenous $MgSO_4$ started during surgery is continued for 48 to 72 hours postoperatively. Careful monitoring of maternal serum magnesium levels is necessary as a number of side effects may result from its use including pulmonary edema, blurred vision, malaise, nausea or vomiting, muscle weakness, and respiratory impairment. Deep tendon reflexes, are depressed at $MgSO_4$ levels ≥10 mEq/L and cardiovascular collapse may occur with high levels of $MgSO_4$ (≥25 mEq/L). Intravenous calcium gluconate is administered to reverse the effects of magnesium overdose.

Additional tocolytic agents may be administered to the mother postoperatively including oral calcium channel blockers and terbutaline via oral, IV, or subcutaneous routes. The presence of maternal hypotension may however preclude the continuous use of calcium channel blockers.

■ EX UTERO INTRAPARTUM THERAPY (EXIT)

The EXIT procedure involves partial delivery of the near term or term fetus in order for intrapartum assessment and performance of lifesaving procedures on the fetus while it is still on uteroplacental support. It was originally developed as a means of removing tracheal clips in fetuses that had undergone in utero tracheal occlusion for management of pulmonary hypoplasia associated with CDH (198). However, the EXIT procedure, also referred to as the operation on placental support (OOPS) procedure (199), is currently utilized for any fetal anomaly in which resuscitation of the newborn may be compromised. This includes conditions characterized by airway obstruction, large ITM in which the EXIT-to-airway and EXIT-to-resection may be performed respectively, or other life-threatening conditions such as severe CDH and some cases of congenital cardiac disease in which immediate placement on extracorporeal membrane oxygenation will be beneficial (EXIT-to-ECMO procedure). Maneuvers critical to the infant's survival such as laryngoscopy or bronchoscopy with intubation, tracheostomy, tumor decompression and resection, or ECMO cannulation are performed while the fetus receives adequate oxygenation via uteroplacental circulation, prior to division of the umbilical cord and delivery. In contrast to previous scenarios discussed earlier in the chapter, the goal following fetal intervention in the EXIT procedure is immediate delivery of the infant. The different fetal conditions that may require delivery via the EXIT procedure are listed in Table 49-6.

Fetal Airway Obstruction

Details of each individual cause of fetal airway obstruction are beyond the scope of this section but the relatively more common lesions will be discussed briefly. Obstruction of the fetal airway can be described as extrinsic or intrinsic in nature. Extrinsic causes of fetal airway obstruction include large head

TABLE 49-6 Indications for the EXIT Procedure

Fetal cervical masses
Lymphangioma
Teratoma
Hemangioma
Neuroblastoma
Goiter
Fetal lung masses
Congenital cystic adenomatoid malformation
Bronchopulmonary sequestration
Fetal mediastinal masses
Teratoma
Lymphangioma
Congenital high airway obstruction syndrome
Tracheal atresia
Laryngeal atresia
EXIT to extracorporeal membrane oxygenation
Severe congenital diaphragmatic hernia with liver herniation into chest cavity
Congenital heart disease
Hypoplastic left heart syndrome with intact/restrictive atrial septum
Aortic stenosis with intact/restrictive atrial septum
Reversal of tracheal occlusion after tracheal clip or endoluminal balloon procedures

EXIT, ex utero intrapartum therapy.

and neck masses such as cervical teratomas, cervical lymphangiomas and less commonly, oropharyngeal tumors and congenital goiter. Intrinsic causes of airway obstruction include laryngeal atresia or congenital high airway obstruction and laryngeal web or tracheal atresia.

Cervical Teratoma

Teratomas are rare tumors that are derived from all three germ layers and occur in approximately 1 in 20,000 to 40,000 live births. Congenital cervical teratomas occur with a lesser frequency. These tumors can reach significant size at term (Fig. 49-10), and are diagnosed prenatally as a result of maternal polyhydramnios due to compression of the esophagus and impaired fetal swallowing (200). While majority of these tumors are benign, they are associated with a high morbidity and mortality mostly due to airway compression and

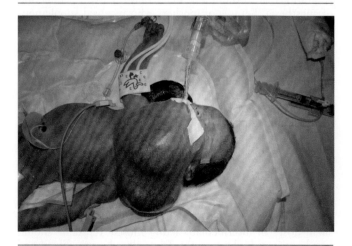

FIGURE 49-10 Cervical teratoma in newborn infant delivered via EXIT. Courtesy of Oluyinka Olutoye M.D., Ph.D.

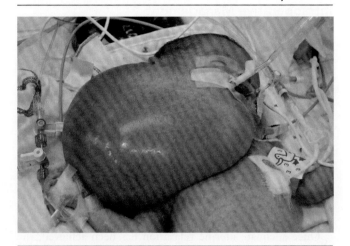

FIGURE 49-11 Cervical lymphangioma in newborn infant delivered via EXIT procedure. Courtesy of Oluyinka Olutoye M.D., Ph.D.

difficulty in securing an airway following routine delivery as the grossly distorted anatomy makes location of the trachea difficult (201–203). The EXIT procedure buys time and allows for determination of the best method of securing an airway in these infants while they are continuously oxygenated via uteroplacental perfusion.

Cervical Lymphangiomas

These are otherwise referred to as cystic hygromas and they may be located in the neck, axilla, or thorax. Large lymphangiomas located in the head and neck region will require delivery via the EXIT procedure. This mass occurs as a result of failure of the jugular sacs to join the lymphatic system early in development resulting in independent sacs that secrete lymph-like fluid and eventually compress surrounding structures (Fig. 49-11) (204). Cervical lymphangiomas may develop late in pregnancy, that is, in the third trimester. Fetuses affected in isolation have a good chance of survival following delivery provided the airway is not severely compromised. Only fetuses with isolated cervical lymphangiomas are considered to be candidates for delivery via the EXIT procedure (204). Sixty percent of fetuses diagnosed early in the prenatal period may have associated chromosomal anomalies, cardiac defects, cleft lip and palate, skeletal anomalies, and hydrops fetalis. Hydrops may develop due to compression of surrounding anatomic structures and is associated with poor prognosis.

Congenital High Airway Obstruction

This condition, commonly referred to as CHAOS, is a prenatally diagnosed clinical syndrome that occurs as a result of complete or near complete airway obstruction from laryngeal atresia, laryngeal cyst, or tracheal atresia. CHAOS is characterized by very large echogenic lungs, a dilated tracheobronchial tree, flattened or everted diaphragm, ascites, and nonimmune hydrops (Fig. 49-12) (205). The fetus diagnosed with complete airway obstruction and associated hydrops prenatally is believed to have almost 100% mortality without intervention (206). The EXIT procedure is indicated for delivery of all cases of CHAOS due to critical airway obstruction.

Intrathoracic Masses

Prenatal imaging has allowed for detailed evaluation and documentation of ITM. A wide spectrum of clinical severity

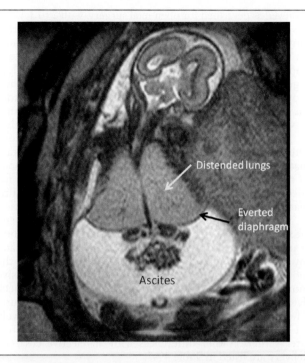

FIGURE 49-12 Prenatal MRI of fetus with congenital high airway obstruction showing large echogenic lungs and everted diaphragm. Courtesy of Oluyinka Olutoye M.D., Ph.D.

in infants with large lung masses has been observed (123). Specific types of fetal intrathoracic lung masses have been described in the section on open fetal surgery. Fetuses with slow growing intrathoracic lesions or lesions that develop late in pregnancy may be candidates for delivery via the EXIT procedure (207). Delivery via the EXIT procedure avoids acute respiratory decompensation due to mediastinal shift, air trapping, or compression of the normal lung especially if positive pressure ventilation is required following delivery and prior to resection.

Congenital Diaphragmatic Hernia (CDH) and Congenital Cardiac Disease

Severe CDH, defined as that in which the liver herniates into the chest cavity together with abdominal contents, and an ultrasonographic measurement of a lung-to-head ratio (LHR) of less than 1.0, is associated with very poor prognosis. This subset of patients as well as fetuses who have severe congenital cardiac disease may benefit from emergent ECMO after delivery. For these conditions, the EXIT-to-ECMO procedure is performed following partial delivery of the head and upper torso while the fetus is still on uteroplacental bypass.

The EXIT Procedure versus Cesarean Section

The ultimate goal of both of these procedures is the delivery of a live infant. However, the urgency with which the delivery occurs is different with each procedure. The EXIT procedure is indicated when a fetus has a specific life-threatening congenital anomaly amenable to fetal surgical intervention under controlled conditions with the assurance of adequate fetal oxygenation via continued uteroplacental infusion. Similar to open fetal surgery, fetal manipulation during the EXIT procedure is facilitated, and risk of uterine rupture is minimized with maternal uterine relaxation. Uterine relaxation is achieved as described for open fetal surgery, with 2 to 3 MAC of volatile anesthetic prior to the uterine incision or hysterotomy; hence general anesthesia is required. The hysterotomy for the EXIT procedure is performed with the use of special staples that seal the amniotic membrane and uterine edges together, thereby decreasing the risk for maternal bleeding. However, there is still an increased risk of hemorrhage from the relaxed myometrium. In addition, the high concentration of volatile anesthetics required also predisposes the mother to intraoperative hypotension requiring frequent or continuous administration of vasoactive medications to maintain maternal blood pressure within awake values. Maintenance of maternal hemodynamics within normal values allows for adequate uteroplacental perfusion, fetal perfusion, and ultimately fetal oxygenation. Unlike a routine cesarean section in which the mother usually sees her newborn baby shortly after delivery, a neonate delivered via the EXIT procedure is usually sedated, intubated, and admitted to the neonatal intensive care unit following delivery. Depending on the indication for surgery, the baby may be placed on invasive monitoring, on ECMO or may still have the head and neck deformity that necessitated delivery via the EXIT procedure. The mothers are therefore usually prepared preoperatively for the fact that they may not see their child immediately after surgery. Other differences with an elective cesarean delivery are listed in Table 49-7.

Preoperative Evaluation for EXIT Procedures

Fetal Evaluation

Preoperative evaluation of the fetus including imaging with delineation of the anomaly under consideration for intrapartum repair, exclusion of other anatomical defects, and karyotyping to rule out chromosomal anomalies, is performed before offering the EXIT procedure as a treatment option. Fetal echocardiography is also performed to rule out the presence of severe nonimmune hydrops which is associated with a poor prognosis. Immediately prior to surgery, an ultrasound assessment of the fetal weight is obtained and is used to prepare unit doses of medication to be administered to the fetus intraoperatively (see Table 49-5 for suggested equipment requirements for surgery on the fetus).

Maternal Evaluation

Obtaining a detailed history and physical examination cannot be overemphasized. Significant cardiac disease should be ruled out, as such patients may not tolerate the high concentration of volatile anesthetics required for surgery and may be unsuitable candidates for fetal intervention.

Intraoperative Management

Maternal Anesthesia and Uterine Relaxation

Monitoring as well as induction and maintenance of anesthesia is similar to that for open fetal surgery. Differences are as follows: (1) Intrathecal morphine administered preinduction is an option to placing an epidural catheter as the postoperative analgesia requirements are similar to that of a cesarean section; (2) massive polyhydramnios may require preoperative amniocentesis to improve visualization of placental edges for correct location of the hysterotomy incision (208); (3) in situations where the use of volatile anesthetics is contraindicated, the EXIT procedure may be performed under neuraxial anesthesia with the use of intravenous nitroglycerin (boluses or infusion 0.5 to 1.5 mcg/kg/min) to provide uterine relaxation. Nitroglycerin should be used cautiously as it may predispose the woman to pulmonary edema (209–211).

Once adequate uterine relaxation has been achieved, the hysterotomy incision is made with the special stapling device described previously, which uses absorbable staples to seal the amniotic membranes to the myometrium. Loss of amniotic fluid occurs once hysterotomy is performed, thereforewarm crystalloid fluids are infused continuously into the uterus to keep the uterus full and prevent expulsion of the fetus prior to completion of the procedure due to uterine contractions which can be triggered by decreased intrauterine pressure. This fluid also serves to keep the baby warm and prevents umbilical cord compression during manipulation of the fetus.

Once the indication for the EXIT procedure has been addressed (fetal airway established, thoracotomy and lung mass exteriorized/resected or baby successfully placed on ECMO), the surgeons inform the anesthesiologists for a careful coordination of clamping of the umbilical cord and administration of uterotonic agents just prior to division of the cord. The mother's concentration of volatile anesthetic is also markedly reduced at this time. Some practitioners opt to discontinue the volatile agents completely and continue the rest of the anesthetic with total intravenous anesthesia or with nitrous oxide and oxygen while simultaneously administering doses of local anesthetics and opioids through the epidural catheter previously placed for postoperative pain control.

Significant maternal hemorrhage due to uterine atony is a risk; therefore, continued communication between the surgeons and anesthesiologists during the procedure cannot be overemphasized. Oxytocin 20 units in 500 cc or 40 units in a liter of crystalloid usually suffices to restore adequate uterine tone following delivery. However, additional agents including methylergonovine, carboprost tromethamine or misoprostol should be readily available for management of postpartum

---

TABLE 49-7 Differences Between EXIT and Cesarean Delivery

	EXIT	Cesarean Delivery
Uterine tone	Goal: Maximum hypotonia for partial delivery of baby and fetal surgical intervention	Goal: Minimal hypotonia with rapid return of hypertonic uterus following delivery of baby
Preferred anesthetic	General	Regional
Anesthetic plane	Deep	Minimal to avoid neonatal depression
Infusion of warm fluid into uterus	Required	Not required
Number of anesthesiologists	2: 1 for mother, 1 for fetus	1 for mother

EXIT, ex utero intrapartum therapy.
With permission from: Garcia PJ, Olutoye OO, Ivey RT, et al. Case scenario: anesthesia for maternal-fetal surgery: the Ex Utero Intrapartum Therapy (EXIT) procedure. *Anesthesiology* 2011.

hemorrhage if this occurs. Management during the recovery period is routine, similar to that following cesarean section.

■ FETAL ANESTHESIA

Depending on the nature of the fetal anomaly, a separate room is prepared for management of the fetus following the EXIT procedure. This may be necessary in situations where the fetus has a mass and partial resection of the mass begins on mother's sterile field during the EXIT procedure. If it is anticipated that the baby's surgery will take a while to complete, the baby is transferred to a room adjacent to the mother's operating room following delivery, while the mother's abdominal incision is closed. This adjacent room dedicated to the baby's care should be predesignated for this purpose before the beginning of the EXIT procedure. The baby's operating room should include all the necessities for routine anesthetic management of a neonate. These include a warm operating room environment, crystalloid solutions infused through a fluid warming unit, an intraoperative warming device such as the Bair Hugger™, multiple dry warm towels or blankets to wipe off the vernix from the newborn baby in order to facilitate application of monitors (electrocardiogram pads) on the baby, an appropriately sized blood pressure cuff and unit doses of medications such as muscle relaxants and opioids.

Items required for the fetus during the EXIT procedure, which must be present in the mother's operating room are the same as those required during open fetal surgery (see Table 49-5). In addition to items listed in this table, a sterile self-inflating bag valve mask connected to an oxygen source and an end tidal carbon dioxide (CO_2) indicator is also required to confirm endotracheal intubation of the infant especially when the indication for the procedure is distortion of the airway by a head and neck mass.

Prior to partial delivery of the fetus, the mother's operating room is warmed to approximately 80 to 85°F. This together with the warm fluid infusing into the uterine cavity keeps the fetus warm. Depending on the hospital set-up, a pediatric anesthesiologist dedicated to baby's care scrubs and participates in the management of the fetus on the operative field. As occurs in open fetal surgery, once the surgeons have access to an upper extremity of the fetus, a pulse oximeter probe is placed on the fetus with the same considerations as previously stated. Attempts should be made at this time to also secure intravenous access in the same hand. If this cannot be easily achieved, an intramuscular injection of a combination of an opioid (fentanyl 5 to 20 mcg/kg), muscle relaxant (vecuronium or pancuronium 0.1 to 0.2 mg/kg) and an anticholinergic agent (atropine 0.02 mg/kg) is administered to supplement the anesthetic the fetus is receiving from the mother via the placenta. If necessary, during the procedure, the umbilical cord can also be accessed for direct administration of medication to the fetus. It is important for the surgeons to confirm that the umbilical cord is of sufficient length to allow for manipulation and umbilical vessel drug administration otherwise fetal bradycardia may result from excessive traction on the umbilical cord.

Fetal positioning for the required fetal intervention involves delivery of the affected body part (usually the head and neck), a small portion of the upper torso and the upper extremity in order to provide an opportunity for direct transthoracic echocardiographic monitoring. Echocardiography, performed by a cardiologist during the procedure, provides continuous assessment of fetal ventricular filling and myocardial contractility. In order to secure the fetal airway, an algorithm of direct visual laryngoscopy, bronchoscopy, and endotracheal intubation or tracheostomy is followed. Occasionally, when the indication for the EXIT procedure is a

large neck mass, partial resection may be required in order to gain access to the trachea for tracheostomy placement. If partial resection of the mass occurs while the fetus is still on uteroplacental bypass, once the cord is divided, the baby is taken to the previously prepared adjacent room as described above, in order to complete resection of the mass. At the time it is decided by the surgeons that partial resection of the mass will be necessary in order to gain access to the airway, definitive peripheral intravenous access must be secured in preparation for administration of additional medication, fluid, or blood to the fetus.

When the EXIT is performed for thoracotomy and resection of a lung mass (EXIT-to-resection), the fetus receives intramuscular opioid, muscle relaxant and anticholinergic, endotracheal intubation is performed, and intravenous access is secured for administration of additional opioids, muscle relaxants, or fluid. A fluid bolus is recommended prior to the thoracotomy incision and exteriorization of the fetal lung mass as relief of the mass compression effect can alter the preload mechanics of the heart. The fluid administered may comprise of crystalloid, colloid, or blood. If intravenous access is difficult or cannot be placed in a timely manner, intermittent needling of the umbilical cord or direct administration of fluid into the fetal heart under direct vision could be performed.

In general, once an endotracheal tube or tracheostomy has been inserted, adequate placement is confirmed with the use of an end tidal CO_2 detector as well as auscultation of equal bilateral breath sounds with a sterile stethoscope. The endotracheal tube is firmly secured by suturing it to the gums. An exception to immediate confirmation of endotracheal tube placement by manual ventilation and the use of an end tidal CO_2 detector and lung auscultation is when the indication for the EXIT is a large lung mass. In these situations, it is recommended that manual ventilation be initiated after thoracotomy incision and exteriorization of the lung mass. Ventilation of the lungs after exteriorization of the mass allows for unrestricted expansion of the lung through the incision and avoidance of further mediastinal compression.

Following clamping of the umbilical cord and delivery of the baby, the surgeons either place umbilical lines or the neonate is handed over to the neonatologists for placement of umbilical lines and subsequent transfer to the neonatal intensive care unit. Babies in whom the airway is secured via the EXIT-to-airway procedure or who have successfully undergone placement on ECMO, are transferred to the intensive care unit. Neonates requiring immediate further surgery, (completion of lung or neck mass resection) are transported in warm towels and manually ventilated with 100% oxygen en route to the adjacent operating room for completion of necessary surgery as indicated.

■ MATERNAL OUTCOMES

Future maternal fertility is not affected by the EXIT procedure (212). The low-transverse uterine hysterotomy made with special surgical staples does not preclude subsequent successful vaginal deliveries (175). Exceptions may include women who had an anterior placenta at the time of the EXIT procedure in which case the uterine incision is made at another suitable location apart from the low-transverse region. This subset of mothers may benefit from an elective cesarean section for future deliveries in order to avoid the possibility of uterine rupture.

Due to the specific challenges of the EXIT procedure and the differences between the EXIT procedure and the standard cesarean section, a coordinated multidisciplinary team effort is mandatory to ensure its success.

KEY POINTS

■ The majority of fetoscopic procedures are performed under conscious sedation. A detailed preprocedure discussion about intraoperative expectations including mild sensation of abdominal pressure, possibility of hearing ongoing conversations during the procedure etc., help allay maternal anxiety. The mother should be instructed to inform the anesthesiologist of any discomfort during the procedure so additional analgesia can be provided. While majority of procedures are performed under conscious sedation, on rare occasions, an emergent conversion to a general anesthetic might be indicated.

■ Mothers with an anterior placenta or significant polyhydramnios may require general anesthesia for fetoscopic procedures.

■ Suggested medication cocktail for fetoscopic procedures: IV Midazolam 2 to 3 mg preoperatively; Remifentanil 0.08 to 0.1 mcg/kg/min started as soon as the patient arrives in the procedure room; +/− IV Fentanyl 25 mcg bolus if the patient reacts to infiltration of local anesthetic before the beginning of the procedure. IV Benadryl may be occasionally required for persistent opioid-induced itching.

■ While the existence of fetal pain may be debated by some, the majority of practitioners administer supplemental fetal medications when instrumentation is performed on the fetus directly.

■ Uterine relaxation, provided by high concentrations of volatile anesthetics, is imperative for open fetal surgery and the EXIT procedure. While intravenous nitroglycerin may also be used to induce uterine relaxation, its effect on the uterus is not easily titratable and the side effect of pulmonary edema restricts its use to absolute conditions where the mother cannot receive volatile anesthetics.

■ Administration of local anesthetics via the epidural catheter is withheld during open fetal surgery as this will accentuate intraoperative maternal hypotension during the surgery (induced by high concentration of volatile anesthetics required for intraoperative uterine relaxation).

■ Premature labor is the "Achilles heel" of open fetal surgery therefore postoperative administration of epidural analgesia consisting of high opioid and low local anesthetic concentration such as 0.1% bupivacaine and 10 mcg/mL fentanyl is paramount. This decreases both the maternal and fetal cortisol levels which are believed to play a role in the development of preterm labor.

■ Mothers undergoing fetal surgery receive a significant amount of $MgSO_4$ for tocolysis as well as continuous intraoperative uterine crystalloid infusion. They are therefore predisposed to develop pulmonary edema. As a result, intravenous crystalloid should be administered judiciously in the intraoperative period.

■ Life-threatening fetal conditions such as large lung masses and sacrococcygeal tumors require intraoperative fetal monitoring with pulse oximetry and continuous echocardiography as well as crystalloid or blood resuscitation intraoperatively. MMC, a nonlethal condition, is not associated with significant pathophysiologic changes in the fetus hence only intraoperative echocardiography monitoring is performed and resuscitation with crystalloid or blood is hardly required.

■ The EXIT procedure differs from the cesarean section in that the baby is not urgently delivered and it involves iatrogenic uterine relaxation. The purpose of the EXIT procedure is to allow for intrapartum treatment of the fetus while it remains on uteroplacental bypass prior to delivery.

REFERENCES

1. Harrison MR, Filly RA, Golbus MS, et al. Fetal treatment 1982. *N Engl J Med* 1982;307(26):1651–1652.
2. Oepkes D, Adama van Scheltema P. Intrauterine fetal transfusions in the management of fetal anemia and fetal thrombocytopenia. *Semin Fetal Neonatal Med* 2007;12(6):432–438.
3. Moise KJ Jr. Management of rhesus alloimmunization in pregnancy. *Obstet Gynecol* 2008;112(1):164–176.
4. Van Kamp IL, Klumper FJ, Oepkes D, et al. Complications of intrauterine intravascular transfusion for fetal anemia due to maternal red-cell alloimmunization. *Am J Obstet Gynecol* 2005;192(1):171–177.
5. Van de Velde M, Van Schoubroeck D, Lewi LE, et al. Remifentanil for fetal immobilization and maternal sedation during fetoscopic surgery: a randomized, double-blind comparison with diazepam. *Anesth Analg* 2005;101(1):251–258.
6. Mann S, Johnson MP, Wilson RD. Fetal thoracic and bladder shunts. *Semin Fetal Neonatal Med* 2010;15(1):28–33.
7. Bhaya M, Schachern P, Morizono T, et al. Potters syndrome; a temporal bone histopathological study. *J Otolaryngol* 1993;22(3):195–199.
8. Housley HT, Harrison MR. Fetal urinary tract abnormalities. Natural history, pathophysiology, and treatment. *Urol Clin North Am* 1998;25(1):63–73.
9. Glick PL, Harrison MR, Golbus MS, et al. Management of the fetus with congenital hydronephrosis II: Prognostic criteria and selection for treatment. *J Pediatr Surg* 1985;20(4):376–387.
10. Wu S, Johnson MP. Fetal lower urinary tract obstruction. *Clin Perinatol* 2009;36(2):377–390, x.
11. Biard JM, Johnson MP, Carr MC, et al. Long-term outcomes in children treated by prenatal vesicoamniotic shunting for lower urinary tract obstruction. *Obstet Gynecol* 2005;106(3):503–508.
12. Wilson RD, Hedrick HL, Liechty KW, et al. Cystic adenomatoid malformation of the lung: review of genetics, prenatal diagnosis, and in utero treatment. *Am J Med Genet A* 2006;140(2):151–155.
13. Grethel EJ, Wagner AJ, Clifton MS, et al. Fetal intervention for mass lesions and hydrops improves outcome: a 15-year experience. *J Pediatr Surg* 2007;42(1):117–123.
14. Adzick NS, Harrison MR, Crombleholme TM, et al. Fetal lung lesions: management and outcome. *Am J Obstet Gynecol* 1998;179(4):884–889.
15. Gardiner HM. Progression of fetal heart disease and rationale for fetal intracardiac interventions. *Semin Fetal Neonatal Med* 2005;10(6):578–585.
16. McElhinney DB, Lock JE, Keane JF, et al. Left heart growth, function, and reintervention after balloon aortic valvuloplasty for neonatal aortic stenosis. *Circulation* 2005;111(4):451–458.
17. Hanseus K, Bjorkhem G, Lundstrom NR, et al. Cross-sectional echocardiographic measurements of right ventricular size and growth in patients with pulmonary atresia and intact ventricular septum. *Pediatr Cardiol* 1991;12(3):135–142.
18. Matsui H, Gardiner H. Fetal intervention for cardiac disease: the cutting edge of perinatal care. *Semin Fetal Neonatal Med* 2007;12(6):482–489.
19. Gardiner HM. The case for fetal cardiac intervention. *Heart* 2009;95(20):1648–1652.
20. Gardiner HM. In-utero intervention for severe congenital heart disease. *Best Pract Res Clin Obstet Gynaecol* 2008;22(1):49–61.
21. Deprest JA, Flake AW, Gratacos E, et al. The making of fetal surgery. *Prenat Diagn* 2010;30(7):653–667.
22. Grandjean H, Larroque D, Levi S. The performance of routine ultrasonographic screening of pregnancies in the Eurofetus Study. *Am J Obstet Gynecol* 1999;181(2):446–454.
23. Deprest JA, Gratacos E. Obstetrical endoscopy. *Curr Opin Obstet Gynecol* 1999;11(2):195–203.
24. McCurdy CM Jr, Childers JM, Seeds JW. Ligation of the umbilical cord of an acardiac-acephalus twin with an endoscopic intrauterine technique. *Obstet Gynecol* 1993;82(4 Pt 2 Suppl):708–711.
25. Deprest JA, Evrard VA, Van Schoubroeck D, et al. Endoscopic cord ligation in selective feticide. *Lancet* 1996;348(9031):890–891.
26. Deprest JA, Van Ballaer PP, Evrard VA, et al. Experience with fetoscopic cord ligation. *Eur J Obstet Gynecol Reprod Biol* 1998;81(2):157–164.
27. Lewi L, Van Schoubroeck D, Gratacos E, et al. Monochorionic diamniotic twins: complications and management options. *Curr Opin Obstet Gynecol* 2003;15(2):177–194.
28. Denbow ML, Cox P, Taylor M, et al. Placental angioarchitecture in monochorionic twin pregnancies: relationship to fetal growth, fetofetal transfusion syndrome, and pregnancy outcome. *Am J Obstet Gynecol* 2000;182(2):417–426.
29. Lewi L. Monochorionic diamniotic twin pregnancies pregnancy outcome, risk stratification and lessons learnt from placental examination. *Verh K Acad Geneeskd Belg* 2010;72(1–2):5–15.
30. Seng YC, Rajadurai VS. Twin-twin transfusion syndrome: a five year review. *Arch Dis Child Fetal Neonatal Ed* 2000;83(3):F168–F170.

31. Senat MV, Deprest J, Boulvain M, et al. Endoscopic laser surgery versus serial amnioreduction for severe twin-to-twin transfusion syndrome. *N Engl J Med* 2004;351(2):136–144.

32. Quintero RA, Morales WJ, Allen MH, et al. Staging of twin-twin transfusion syndrome. *J Perinatol* 1999;19(8 Pt 1):550–555.

33. Barrea C, Hornberger LK, Alkazaleh F, et al. Impact of selective laser ablation of placental anastomoses on the cardiovascular pathology of the recipient twin in severe twin-twin transfusion syndrome. *Am J Obstet Gynecol* 2006;195(5):1388–1395.

34. Michelfelder E, Gottliebson W, Border W, et al. Early manifestations and spectrum of recipient twin cardiomyopathy in twin-twin transfusion syndrome: relation to Quintero stage. *Ultrasound Obstet Gynecol* 2007;30(7):965–971.

35. Rychik J, Tian Z, Bebbington M, et al. The twin-twin transfusion syndrome: spectrum of cardiovascular abnormality and development of a cardiovascular score to assess severity of disease. *Am J Obstet Gynecol* 2007;197(4):392.e1–392.e8.

36. Stirnemann JJ, Mougeot M, Proulx F, et al. Profiling fetal cardiac function in twin-twin transfusion syndrome. *Ultrasound Obstet Gynecol* 2010;35(1):19–27.

37. Mari G, Roberts A, Detti L, et al. Perinatal morbidity and mortality rates in severe twin-twin transfusion syndrome: results of the International Amnioreduction Registry. *Am J Obstet Gynecol* 2001;185(3):708–715.

38. van Gemert MJ, Umur A, Tijssen JG, et al. Twin-twin transfusion syndrome: etiology, severity and rational management. *Curr Opin Obstet Gynecol* 2001;13(2):193–206.

39. Benirschke K, Kim CK. Multiple pregnancy. 1. *N Engl J Med* 1973;288(24):1276–1284.

40. DeVore GR, Dixon JA, Hobbins JC. Fetoscope-directed neodymium-YAG laser: a potential tool for fetal surgery. *Am J Obstet Gynecol* 1983;145(3):379–380.

41. De Lia JE, Cruikshank DP, Keye WR Jr. Fetoscopic neodymium:YAG laser occlusion of placental vessels in severe twin-twin transfusion syndrome. *Obstet Gynecol* 1990;75(6):1046–1053.

42. Ville Y, Hyett J, Hecher K, et al. Preliminary experience with endoscopic laser surgery for severe twin-twin transfusion syndrome. *N Engl J Med* 1995;332(4):224–227.

43. Bebbington MW, Tiblad E, Huesler-Charles M, et al. Outcomes in a cohort of patients with Stage I twin-to-twin transfusion syndrome. *Ultrasound Obstet Gynecol* 2010;36(1):48–51.

44. Quintero RA, Dickinson JE, Morales WJ, et al. Stage-based treatment of twin-twin transfusion syndrome. *Am J Obstet Gynecol* 2003;188(5):1333–1340.

45. Chalouhi GE, Essaoui M, Stirnemann J, et al. Laser therapy for twin-to-twin transfusion syndrome (TTTS). *Prenat Diagn* 2011;31(7):637–646.

46. James WH. A note on the epidemiology of acardiac monsters. *Teratology* 1977;16(2):211–216.

47. Van Allen MI, Smith DW, Shepard TH. Twin reversed arterial perfusion (TRAP) sequence: a study of 14 twin pregnancies with acardius. *Semin Perinatol* 1983;7(4):285–293.

48. Sogaard K, Skibsted L, Brocks V. Acardiac twins: pathophysiology, diagnosis, outcome and treatment. Six cases and review of the literature. *Fetal Diagn Ther* 1999;14(1):53–59.

49. Tan TY, Sepulveda W. Acardiac twin: a systematic review of minimally invasive treatment modalities. *Ultrasound Obstet Gynecol* 2003;22(4):409–419.

50. Wong AE, Sepulveda W. Acardiac anomaly: current issues in prenatal assessment and treatment. *Prenat Diagn* 2005;25(9):796–806.

51. Lewi L, Jani J, Deprest J. Invasive antenatal interventions in complicated multiple pregnancies. *Obstet Gynecol Clin North Am* 2005;32(1):105–126, x.

52. Done E, Gucciardo L, Van Mieghem T, et al. Prenatal diagnosis, prediction of outcome and in utero therapy of isolated congenital diaphragmatic hernia. *Prenat Diagn* 2008;28(7):581–591.

53. Puri P, Gorman F. Lethal nonpulmonary anomalies associated with congenital diaphragmatic hernia: implications for early intrauterine surgery. *J Pediatr Surg* 1984;19(1):29–32.

54. Deprest J, Jani J, Cannie M, et al. Prenatal intervention for isolated congenital diaphragmatic hernia. *Curr Opin Obstet Gynecol* 2006;18(3):355–367.

55. Metkus AP, Filly RA, Stringer MD, et al. Sonographic predictors of survival in fetal diaphragmatic hernia. *J Pediatr Surg* 1996;31(1):148–151; discussion 151–152.

56. Cannie M, Jani JC, De Keyzer F, et al. Fetal body volume: use at MR imaging to quantify relative lung volume in fetuses suspected of having pulmonary hypoplasia. *Radiology* 2006;241(3):847–853.

57. Deprest J, Jani J, Van Schoubroeck D, et al. Current consequences of prenatal diagnosis of congenital diaphragmatic hernia. *J Pediatr Surg* 2006;41(2):423–430.

58. Flake AW, Crombleholme TM, Johnson MP, et al. Treatment of severe congenital diaphragmatic hernia by fetal tracheal occlusion: clinical experience with fifteen cases. *Am J Obstet Gynecol* 2000;183(5):1059–1066.

59. Bianchi DW, Crombleholme TM, D'Alton ME, et al. Congenital diaphragmatic hernia. In: Bianchi DW, Crombleholme TM, D'Alton ME, Malone FD, eds. *Fetology*. 2nd ed. China: McGraw-Hill; 2010:278–290.

60. Jani J, Nicolaides KH, Keller RL, et al. Observed to expected lung area to head circumference ratio in the prediction of survival in fetuses with isolated diaphragmatic hernia. *Ultrasound Obstet Gynecol* 2007;30(1):67–71.

61. Harrison MR, Adzick NS, Bullard KM, et al. Correction of congenital diaphragmatic hernia in utero VII: a prospective trial. *J Pediatr Surg* 1997;32(11):1637–1642.

62. DiFiore JW, Fauza DO, Slavin R, et al. Experimental fetal tracheal ligation reverses the structural and physiological effects of pulmonary hypoplasia in congenital diaphragmatic hernia. *J Pediatr Surg* 1994;29(2):248–256; discussion 256–257.

63. Harrison MR, Sydorak RM, Farrell JA, et al. Fetoscopic temporary tracheal occlusion for congenital diaphragmatic hernia: prelude to a randomized, controlled trial. *J Pediatr Surg* 2003;38(7):1012–1020.

64. Harrison MR, Keller RL, Hawgood SB, et al. A randomized trial of fetal endoscopic tracheal occlusion for severe fetal congenital diaphragmatic hernia. *N Engl J Med* 2003;349(20):1916–1924.

65. Flageole H, Evrard VA, Vandenberghe K, et al. Tracheoscopic endotracheal occlusion in the ovine model: technique and pulmonary effects. *J Pediatr Surg* 1997;32(9):1328–1331.

66. Deprest J, Evrard VA, Verbeken EK, et al. Tracheal side effects of endoscopic balloon tracheal occlusion in the fetal lamb model. *Eur J Obstet Gynecol Reprod Biol* 2000;92(1):119–126.

67. Deprest J, Jani J, Gratacos E, et al. Fetal intervention for congenital diaphragmatic hernia: the European experience. *Semin Perinatol* 2005;29(2):94–103.

68. Deprest J, Gratacos E, Nicolaides KH, et al. Fetoscopic tracheal occlusion (FETO) for severe congenital diaphragmatic hernia: evolution of a technique and preliminary results. *Ultrasound Obstet Gynecol* 2004;24(2):121–126.

69. Deprest JA, Nicolaides K, Gratacos E. Fetal surgery for congenital diaphragmatic hernia is back from never gone. *Fetal Diagn Ther* 2011;29(1):6–17.

70. Deprest J, Breysem L, Gratacos E, et al. Tracheal side effects following fetal endoscopic tracheal occlusion for severe congenital diaphragmatic hernia. *Pediatr Radiol* 2010;40(5):670–673.

71. McHugh K, Afaq A, Broderick N, et al. Tracheomegaly: a complication of fetal endoscopic tracheal occlusion in the treatment of congenital diaphragmatic hernia. *Pediatr Radiol* 2010;40(5):674–680.

72. Fayoux P, Hosana G, Devisme L, et al. Neonatal tracheal changes following in utero fetoscopic balloon tracheal occlusion in severe congenital diaphragmatic hernia. *J Pediatr Surg* 2010;45(4):687–692.

73. Breysem L, Debeer A, Claus F, et al. Cross-sectional study of tracheomegaly in children after fetal tracheal occlusion for severe congenital diaphragmatic hernia. *Radiology* 2010;257(1):226–232.

74. Jani JC, Nicolaides KH, Gratacos E, et al. Severe diaphragmatic hernia treated by fetal endoscopic tracheal occlusion. *Ultrasound Obstet Gynecol* 2009;34(3):304–310.

75. Benatar D, Benatar M. A pain in the fetus: toward ending confusion about fetal pain. *Bioethics* 2001;15(1):57–76.

76. Derbyshire SW. Locating the beginnings of pain. *Bioethics* 1999;13(1):1–31.

77. Derbyshire SW. Fetal pain: an infantile debate. *Bioethics* 2001;15(1):77–84.

78. Glover V, Fisk NM. Fetal pain: implications for research and practice. *Br J Obstet Gynaecol* 1999;106(9):881–886.

79. Lee SJ, Ralston HJ, Drey EA, et al. Fetal pain: a systematic multidisciplinary review of the evidence. *JAMA* 2005;294(8):947–954.

80. Marin-Padilla M. Structural organization of the human cerebral cortex prior to the appearance of the cortical plate. *Anat Embryol (Berl)* 1983;168(1):21–40.

81. Kostovic I, Rakic P. Developmental history of the transient subplate zone in the visual and somatosensory cortex of the macaque monkey and human brain. *J Comp Neurol* 1990 15;297(3):441–470.

82. Hevner RF. Development of connections in the human visual system during fetal mid-gestation: a DiI-tracing study. *J Neuropathol Exp Neurol* 2000;59(5):385–392.

83. Mrzljak L, Uylings HB, Kostovic I, et al. Prenatal development of neurons in the human prefrontal cortex: I. A qualitative Golgi study. *J Comp Neurol* 1988 15;271(3):355–386.

84. Schenk VW, De Vlieger M, Hamersma K, et al. Two rhombencephalic anencephalics. A clinico-pathological and electroencephalographic study. *Brain* 1968;91(3):497–506.

85. Strigo IA, Duncan GH, Boivin M, et al. Differentiation of visceral and cutaneous pain in the human brain. *J Neurophysiol* 2003;89(6):3294–3303.

86. Klimach VJ, Cooke RW. Maturation of the neonatal somatosensory evoked response in preterm infants. *Dev Med Child Neurol* 1988;30(2):208–214.

87. Franck LS, Miaskowski C. Measurement of neonatal responses to painful stimuli: a research review. *J Pain Symptom Manage* 1997;14(6):343–378.

88. Giannakoulopoulos X, Sepulveda W, Kourtis P, et al. Fetal plasma cortisol and beta-endorphin response to intrauterine needling. *Lancet* 1994;344(8915):77–81.

89. Giannakoulopoulos X, Teixeira J, Fisk N, et al. Human fetal and maternal noradrenaline responses to invasive procedures. *Pediatr Res* 1999;45(4 Pt 1):494–499.

90. Carrasco GA, Van de Kar LD. Neuroendocrine pharmacology of stress. *Eur J Pharmacol* 2003;463(1–3):235–272.

91. Radunovic N, Lockwood CJ, Ghidini A, et al. Is fetal blood sampling associated with increased beta-endorphin release into the fetal circulation? *Am J Perinatol* 1993;10(2):112–114.

92. Anand KJ, Sippell WG, Aynsley-Green A. Randomised trial of fentanyl anaesthesia in preterm babies undergoing surgery: effects on the stress response. *Lancet* 1987;1(8527):243–248.

93. Anand KJ, Sippell WG, Schofield NM, et al. Does halothane anaesthesia decrease the metabolic and endocrine stress responses of newborn infants undergoing operation? *Br Med J (Clin Res Ed)* 1988;296(6623):668–672.

94. Teixeira J, Fogliani R, Giannakoulopoulos X, et al. Fetal haemodynamic stress response to invasive procedures. *Lancet* 1996;347(9001):624.

95. Teixeira JM, Glover V, Fisk NM. Acute cerebral redistribution in response to invasive procedures in the human fetus. *Am J Obstet Gynecol* 1999;181(4):1018–1025.

96. Woo JS, Liang ST, Lo RL, et al. Middle cerebral artery Doppler flow velocity waveforms. *Obstet Gynecol* 1987;70(4):613–616.

97. Wladimiroff JW, vd Wijngaard JA, Degani S, et al. Cerebral and umbilical arterial blood flow velocity waveforms in normal and growth-retarded pregnancies. *Obstet Gynecol* 1987;69(5):705–709.

98. Prechtl HF. Ultrasound studies of human fetal behaviour. *Early Hum Dev* 1985;12(2):91–98.

99. Ashwal S, Peabody JL, Schneider S, et al. Anencephaly: clinical determination of brain death and neuropathologic studies. *Pediatr Neurol* 1990;6(4):233–239.

100. Pilon M, Sullivan SJ. Motor profile of patients in minimally responsive and persistent vegetative states. *Brain Inj* 1996;10(6):421–437.

101. Fisk NM, Gitau R, Teixeira JM, et al. Effect of direct fetal opioid analgesia on fetal hormonal and hemodynamic stress response to intrauterine needling. *Anesthesiology* 2001;95(4):828–835.

102. Mizrahi-Arnaud A, Tworetzky W, Bulich LA, et al. Pathophysiology, management, and outcomes of fetal hemodynamic instability during prenatal cardiac intervention. *Pediatr Res* 2007;62(3):325–330.

103. Bulich LA, et al. Anesthesia for fetal cardiac intervention. In: Myers LA, Bulich LA, eds. *Anesthesia for Fetal Intervention and Surgery.* McGraw-Hill; 2005,115.

104. Myers LB, Watcha MF. Epidural versus general anesthesia for twin-twin transfusion syndrome requiring fetal surgery. *Fetal Diagn Ther* 2004;19(3):286–291.

105. Deprest JA, Van Schoubroeck D, Van Ballaer PP, et al. Alternative technique for Nd: YAG laser coagulation in twin-to-twin transfusion syndrome with anterior placenta. *Ultrasound Obstet Gynecol* 1998;11(5):347–352.

106. Quintero RA, Bornick PW, Allen MH, et al. Selective laser photocoagulation of communicating vessels in severe twin-twin transfusion syndrome in women with an anterior placenta. *Obstet Gynecol* 2001;97(3):477–481.

107. Rossi AC, Kaufman MA, Bornick PW, et al. General vs local anesthesia for the percutaneous laser treatment of twin-twin transfusion syndrome. *Am J Obstet Gynecol* 2008;199(2):137.e1–137.e7.

108. Holmes N, Harrison MR, Baskin LS. Fetal surgery for posterior urethral valves: long-term postnatal outcomes. *Pediatrics* 2001;108(1):E7.

109. Cass DL, Crombleholme TM, Howell LJ, et al. Cystic lung lesions with systemic arterial blood supply: a hybrid of congenital cystic adenomatoid malformation and bronchopulmonary sequestration. *J Pediatr Surg* 1997;32(7):986–990.

110. Stanton M, Davenport M. Management of congenital lung lesions. *Early Hum Dev* 2006;82(5):289–295.

111. Stocker JT. Sequestrations of the lung. *Semin Diagn Pathol* 1986;3(2):106–121.

112. Hernanz-Schulman M, Stein SM, Neblett WW, et al. Pulmonary sequestration: diagnosis with color Doppler sonography and a new theory of associated hydrothorax. *Radiology* 1991;180(3):817–821.

113. MacGillivray TE, Harrison MR, Goldstein RB, et al. Disappearing fetal lung lesions. *J Pediatr Surg* 1993;28(10):1321–1324; discussion 1324–1325.

114. Roggin KK, Breuer CK, Carr SR, et al. The unpredictable character of congenital cystic lung lesions. *J Pediatr Surg* 2000;35(5):801–805.

115. Laberge JM, Flageole H, Pugash D, et al. Outcome of the prenatally diagnosed congenital cystic adenomatoid lung malformation: a Canadian experience. *Fetal Diagn Ther* 2001;16(3):178–186.

116. Bianchi DW, Crombleholme T, D'Alton M, et al. Cystic adenomatoid malformation. In: Bianchi DW, Crombleholme T, D'Alton M, Malone FD, eds. *Fetology.* 2nd ed. China: McGraw-Hill; 2010;263–270.

117. Stocker JT, Madewell JE, Drake RM. Congenital cystic adenomatoid malformation of the lung. Classification and morphologic spectrum. *Hum Pathol* 1977;8(2):155–171.

118. Miller RK, Sieber WK, Yunis EJ. Congenital adenomatoid malformation of the lung. A report of 17 cases and review of the literature. *Pathol Annu* 1980;15(Pt 1):387–402.

119. Adzick NS. Open fetal surgery for life-threatening fetal anomalies. *Semin Fetal Neonatal Med* 2010;15(1):1–8.

120. Rashad F, Grisoni E, Gaglione S. Aberrant arterial supply in congenital cystic adenomatoid malformation of the lung. *J Pediatr Surg* 1988;23(11):1007–1008.

121. Demos NJ, Teresi A. Congenital lung malformations: a unified concept and a case report. *J Thorac Cardiovasc Surg* 1975;70(2):260–264.

122. Langston C. New concepts in the pathology of congenital lung malformations. *Semin Pediatr Surg* 2003;12(1):17–37.

123. Adzick NS. Management of fetal lung lesions. *Clin Perinatol* 2003;30(3):481–492.

124. Pinson CW, Harrison MW, Thornburg KL, et al. Importance of fetal fluid imbalance in congenital cystic adenomatoid malformation of the lung. *Am J Surg* 1992;163(5):510–514.

125. Adzick NS, Harrison MR, Glick PL, et al. Fetal cystic adenomatoid malformation: prenatal diagnosis and natural history. *J Pediatr Surg* 1985;20(5):483–488.

126. Vu L, Tsao K, Lee H, et al. Characteristics of congenital cystic adenomatoid malformations associated with nonimmune hydrops and outcome. *J Pediatr Surg* 2007;42(8):1351–1356.

127. Crombleholme TM, Coleman B, Hedrick H, et al. Cystic adenomatoid malformation volume ratio predicts outcome in prenatally diagnosed cystic adenomatoid malformation of the lung. *J Pediatr Surg* 2002;37(3):331–338.

128. Miller JA, Corteville JE, Langer JC. Congenital cystic adenomatoid malformation in the fetus: natural history and predictors of outcome. *J Pediatr Surg* 1996;31(6):805–808.

129. Geenberg E, Schiffer MA. Sacrococcygeal teratoma in labor and the newborn. *Am J Obstet Gynecol* 1956;72(5):1054–1062.

130. Altman RP, Randolph JG, Lilly JR. Sacrococcygeal teratoma: American Academy of Pediatrics Surgical Section Survey-1973. *J Pediatr Surg* 1974;9(3):389–398.

131. Holzgreve W, Flake AW, Langer JC. The unborn patient, prenatal diagnosis and treatment. In: Harrison MR, Golbus MS, Filly RA, eds. *The Unborn Patient.* 2nd ed. Philadelphia, PA: W.B. Saunders Company; 1991:460–469.

132. Quinn TM, Hubbard AM, Adzick NS. Prenatal magnetic resonance imaging enhances fetal diagnosis. *J Pediatr Surg* 1998;33(4):553–558.

133. Heys RF, Murray CP, Kohler HG. Obstructed labour due to foetal tumours: cervical and coccygeal teratoma. Two case reports. *Gynaecologia* 1967;164(1):43–54.

134. Bond SJ, Harrison MR, Schmidt KG, et al. Death due to high-output cardiac failure in fetal sacrococcygeal teratoma. *J Pediatr Surg* 1990;25(12):1287–1291.

135. Flake AW. Fetal sacrococcygeal teratoma. *Semin Pediatr Surg* 1993;2(2):113–120.

136. Flake AW, Harrison MR, Adzick NS, et al. Fetal sacrococcygeal teratoma. *J Pediatr Surg* 1986;21(7):563–566.

137. Holterman AX, Filiatrault D, Lallier M, et al. The natural history of sacrococcygeal teratomas diagnosed through routine obstetric sonogram: a single institution experience. *J Pediatr Surg* 1998;33(6):899–903.

138. Rodriguez MA, Cass DL, Lazar DA, et al. Tumor volume to fetal weight ratio as an early prognostic classification for fetal sacrococcygeal teratoma. *J Pediatr Surg* 2011;46(6):1182–1185.

139. Flake AW. The fetus with sacrococcygeal teratoma. In: Harrison MR, Evans MI, Adzick NA, Holzgreve W, eds. *The Unborn Patient. The Art and Science of Fetal Therapy.* 3rd ed. Orlando, FL: W.B. Saunders; 2001;591–604.

140. Lary JM, Edmonds LD. Prevalence of spina bifida at birth–United States, 1983–1990: a comparison of two surveillance systems. *MMWR CDC Surveill Summ* 1996;45(2):15–26.

141. Centers for Disease Control (CDC). Economic burden of spina bifida–United States, 1980–1990. *MMWR Morb Mortal Wkly Rep* 1989;38(15):264–267.

142. Waitzman NJ, Romano PS, Scheffler RM. Estimates of the economic costs of birth defects. *Inquiry* 1994;31(2):188–205.

143. Tulipan N, Sutton LN, Bruner JP, et al. The effect of intrauterine myelomeningocele repair on the incidence of shunt-dependent hydrocephalus. *Pediatr Neurosurg* 2003;38(1):27–33.

144. Kadir RA, Sabin C, Whitlow B, et al. Neural tube defects and periconceptional folic acid in England and Wales: retrospective study. *BMJ* 1999 10;319(7202):92–93.

145. Manning SM, Jennings R, Madsen JR. Pathophysiology, prevention, and potential treatment of neural tube defects. *Ment Retard Dev Disabil Res Rev* 2000;6(1):6–14.

146. Meuli M, Meuli-Simmen C, Yingling CD, et al. Creation of myelomeningocele in utero: a model of functional damage from spinal cord exposure in fetal sheep. *J Pediatr Surg* 1995;30(7):1028–1032; discussion 1032–1033.

147. Correia-Pinto J, Reis JL, Hutchins GM, et al. In utero meconium exposure increases spinal cord necrosis in a rat model of myelomeningocele. *J Pediatr Surg* 2002;37(3):488–492.

148. Tanyel FC. In utero meconium exposure increases spinal cord necrosis in arat model of myelomeningocele. *J Pediatr Surg* 2002;37(9):1383; author reply 1383.

149. Hogge WA, Dungan JS, Brooks MP, et al. Diagnosis and management of prenatally detected myelomeningocele: a preliminary report. *Am J Obstet Gynecol* 1990;163(3):1061–1064; discussion 1064–1065.

150. Kollias SS, Goldstein RB, Cogen PH, et al. Prenatally detected myelomeningoceles: sonographic accuracy in estimation of the spinal level. *Radiology* 1992;185(1):109–112.

151. Ertl-Wagner B, Lienemann A, Strauss A, et al. Fetal magnetic resonance imaging: indications, technique, anatomical considerations and a review of fetal abnormalities. *Eur Radiol* 2002;12(8):1931–1940.

152. Olutoye OO, Adzick NS. Fetal surgery for myelomeningocele. *Semin Perinatol* 1999;23(6):462–473.

153. Hirose S, Meuli-Simmen C, Meuli M. Fetal surgery for myelomeningocele: panacea or peril? *World J Surg* 2003;27(1):87–94.

154. Hirose S, Farmer DL, Albanese CT. Fetal surgery for myelomeningocele. *Curr Opin Obstet Gynecol* 2001;13(2):215–222.

155. Farmer DL, von Koch CS, Peacock WJ, et al. In utero repair of myelomeningocele: experimental pathophysiology, initial clinical experience, and outcomes. *Arch Surg* 2003;138(8):872–878.

156. Jobe AH. Fetal surgery for myelomeningocele. *N Engl J Med* 2002;347(4):230–231.

157. Bell JE, Gordon A, Maloney AF. The association of hydrocephalus and Arnold–Chiari malformation with spina bifida in the fetus. *Neuropathol Appl Neurobiol* 1980;6(1):29–39.

158. Dias MS, McLone DG. Hydrocephalus in the child with dysraphism. *Neurosurg Clin N Am* 1993;4(4):715–726.

159. Hirose S, Farmer DL. Fetal surgery for myelomeningocele. *Clin Perinatol* 2009;36(2):431–438, xi.

160. Michejda M. Intrauterine treatment of spina bifida: primate model. *Z Kinderchir* 1984;39(4):259–261.

161. Heffez DS, Aryanpur J, Hutchins GM, et al. The paralysis associated with myelomeningocele: clinical and experimental data implicating a preventable spinal cord injury. *Neurosurgery* 1990;26(6):987–992.

162. Heffez DS, Aryanpur J, Rotellini NA, et al. Intrauterine repair of experimental surgically created dysraphism. *Neurosurgery* 1993;32(6):1005–1010.

163. Stiefel D, Copp AJ, Meuli M. Fetal spina bifida in a mouse model: loss of neural function in utero. *J Neurosurg* 2007;106(3 Suppl):213–221.

164. Stiefel D, Meuli M. Scanning electron microscopy of fetal murine myelomeningocele reveals growth and development of the spinal cord in early gestation and neural tissue destruction around birth. *J Pediatr Surg* 2007;42(9):1561–1565.

165. Meuli M, Meuli-Simmen C, Hutchins GM, et al. In utero surgery rescues neurological function at birth in sheep with spina bifida. *Nat Med* 1995;1(4):342–347.

166. Bruner JP, Tulipan NE, Richards WO. Endoscopic coverage of fetal open myelomeningocele in utero. *Am J Obstet Gynecol* 1997;176(1 Pt 1):256–257.

167. Tulipan N, Hernanz-Schulman M, Bruner JP. Reduced hindbrain herniation after intrauterine myelomeningocele repair: A report of four cases. *Pediatr Neurosurg* 1998;29(5):274–278.

168. Adzick NS, Sutton LN, Crombleholme TM, et al. Successful fetal surgery for spina bifida. *Lancet* 1998;352(9141):1675–1676.

169. Sutton LN, Adzick NS, Bilaniuk LT, et al. Improvement in hindbrain herniation demonstrated by serial fetal magnetic resonance imaging following fetal surgery for myelomeningocele. *JAMA* 1999;282(19):1826–1831.

170. Bruner JP, Tulipan N, Paschall RL, et al. Fetal surgery for myelomeningocele and the incidence of shunt-dependent hydrocephalus. *JAMA* 1999;282(19):1819–1825.

171. Johnson MP, Sutton LN, Rintoul N, et al. Fetal myelomeningocele repair: short-term clinical outcomes. *Am J Obstet Gynecol* 2003;189(2):482–487.

172. Rintoul NE, Sutton LN, Hubbard AM, et al. A new look at myelomeningoceles: functional level, vertebral level, shunting, and the implications for fetal intervention. *Pediatrics* 2002;109(3):409–413.

173. Adzick NS. Fetal myelomeningocele: natural history, pathophysiology, and in-utero intervention. *Semin Fetal Neonatal Med* 2010;15(1):9–14.

174. Adzick NS, Thom EA, Spong CY, et al. A randomized trial of prenatal versus postnatal repair of myelomeningocele. *N Engl J Med* 2011;364(11):993–1004.

175. Bouchard S, Johnson MP, Flake AW, et al. The EXIT procedure: experience and outcome in 31 cases. *J Pediatr Surg* 2002;37(3):418–426.

176. Stevens GH, Schoot BC, Smets MJ, et al. The ex utero intrapartum treatment (EXIT) procedure in fetal neck masses: a case report and review of the literature. *Eur J Obstet Gynecol Reprod Biol* 2002;100(2):246–250.

177. Butwick A, Aleshi P, Yamout I. Obstetric hemorrhage during an EXIT procedure for severe fetal airway obstruction. *Can J Anaesth* 2009;56(6):437–442.

178. Goeden AM, Worthington D. Spontaneous resolution of mirror syndrome. *Obstet Gynecol* 2005;106(5 Pt 2):1183–1186.

179. Luks FI, Johnson BD, Papadakis K, et al. Predictive value of monitoring parameters in fetal surgery. *J Pediatr Surg* 1998;33(8):1297–1301.

180. Paulick RP, Meyers RL, Rudolph AM. Effect of maternal oxygen administration on graded reduction of umbilical or uterine blood flow in fetal sheep. *Am J Obstet Gynecol* 1992;167(1):233–239.

181. Khazin AF, Hon EH, Hehre FW. Effects of maternal hyperoxia on the fetus. I. Oxygen tension. *Am J Obstet Gynecol* 1971;109(4):628–637.

182. Rychik J, Tian Z, Cohen MS, et al. Acute cardiovascular effects of fetal surgery in the human. *Circulation* 2004;110(12):1549–1556.

183. Hon EH. The fetal heart rate patterns preceding death in utero. *Am J Obstet Gynecol* 1959;78(1):47–56.

184. Tchirikov M, Hecher K, Deprest J, et al. Doppler ultrasound measurements in the central circulation of anesthetized fetal sheep during obstruction of umbilical-placental blood flow. *Ultrasound Obstet Gynecol* 2001;18(6):656–661.

185. Keswani SG, Crombleholme TM, Rychik J, et al. Impact of continuous intraoperative monitoring on outcomes in open fetal surgery. *Fetal Diagn Ther* 2005;20(4):316–320.

186. Biehl DR, Yarnell R, Wade JG, et al. The uptake of isoflurane by the foetal lamb in utero: effect on regional blood flow. *Can Anaesth Soc J* 1983;30(6):581–586.

187. Rosen MA. Management of anesthesia for the pregnant surgical patient. *Anesthesiology* 1999;91(4):1159–1163.

188. Myers LB, Cohen D, Galinkin J, et al. Anaesthesia for fetal surgery. *Paediatr Anaesth* 2002;12(7):569–578.

189. Jennings RW, Adzick NS, Longaker MT, et al. New techniques in fetal surgery. *J Pediatr Surg* 1992;27(10):1329–1333.

190. Sunday R, Robinson LA, Bosek V. Low cardiac output complicating pericardiectomy for pericardial tamponade. *Ann Thorac Surg* 1999;67(1):228–231.

191. Boat A, Mahmoud M, Michelfelder EC, et al. Supplementing desflurane with intravenous anesthesia reduces fetal cardiac dysfunction during open fetal surgery. *Paediatr Anaesth* 2010;20(8):748–756.

192. Sinatra RS, Philip BK, Naulty JS, et al. Prolonged neuromuscular blockade with vecuronium in a patient treated with magnesium sulfate. *Anesth Analg* 1985;64(12):1220–1222.

193. Fuchs-Buder T, Tassonyi E. Magnesium sulphate enhances residual neuromuscular block induced by vecuronium. *Br J Anaesth* 1996;76(4):565–566.

194. James FM 3rd, Greiss FC Jr, Kemp RA. An evaluation of vasopressor therapy for maternal hypotension during spinal anesthesia. *Anesthesiology* 1970;33(1):25–34.

195. Lee A, Ngan Kee WD, Gin T. A quantitative, systematic review of randomized controlled trials of ephedrine versus phenylephrine for the management of hypotension during spinal anesthesia for cesarean delivery. *Anesth Analg* 2002;94(4):920–926, table of contents.

196. Reidy J, Douglas J. Vasopressors in obstetrics. *Anesthesiol Clin* 2008;26(1):75–88, vi-vii.

197. Gaiser RR, Kurth CD. Anesthetic considerations for fetal surgery. *Semin Perinatol* 1999;23(6):507–514.

198. Norris MC, Joseph J, Leighton BL. Anesthesia for perinatal surgery. *Am J Perinatol* 1989;6(1):39–40.

199. Skarsgard ED, Chitkara U, Krane EJ, et al. The OOPS procedure (operation on placental support): in utero airway management of the fetus with prenatally diagnosed tracheal obstruction. *J Pediatr Surg* 1996;31(6):826–828.

200. Bianchi DW, Crombleholme T, D'Alton M, et al. Cervical teratoma. In: Bianchi DW, Crombleholme T, D'Alton M, Malone FD, eds. *Fetology*. 2nd ed. China: McGraw-Hill; 2010:751–758.

201. Zerella JT, Finberg FJ. Obstruction of the neonatal airway from teratomas. *Surg Gynecol Obstet* 1990;170(2):126–131.

202. Myers LB, Bulich LA, Mizrahi A, et al. Ultrasonographic guidance for location of the trachea during the EXIT procedure for cervical teratoma. *J Pediatr Surg* 2003;38(4):E12.

203. Hullett BJ, Shine NP, Chambers NA. Airway management of three cases of congenital cervical teratoma. *Paediatr Anaesth* 2006;16(7):794–798.

204. Bianchi DW, Crombleholme T, D'Alton M, et al. Cystic hygroma in late pregnancy. In: Bianchi DW, Crombleholme T, D'Alton M, Malone FD, eds. *Fetology*. 2nd ed. China: McGraw-Hill; 2010:241–248.

205. Hedrick HL, Flake AW, Crombleholme TM, et al. The ex utero intrapartum therapy procedure for high-risk fetal lung lesions. *J Pediatr Surg* 2005;40(6):1038–1043; discussion 1044.

206. Hedrick MH, Ferro MM, Filly RA, et al. Congenital high airway obstruction syndrome (CHAOS): a potential for perinatal intervention. *J Pediatr Surg* 1994;29(2):271–274.

207. Bianchi DW, Crombleholme T, D'Alton M, et al. Congenital high airway obstruction syndrome. In: Bianchi DW, Crombleholme T, D'Alton M, Malone FD, eds. *Fetology*. 2nd ed. China: McGraw-Hill; 2010:231–236.

208. MacKenzie TC, Crombleholme TM, Flake AW. The ex-utero intrapartum treatment. *Curr Opin Pediatr* 2002;14(4):453–458.

209. Jorens PG, Vermeire PA, Herman AG. L-arginine-dependent nitric oxide synthase: a new metabolic pathway in the lung and airways. *Eur Respir J* 1993;6(2):258–266.

210. DiFederico EM, Harrison M, Matthay MA. Pulmonary edema in a woman following fetal surgery. *Chest* 1996;109(4):1114–1117.

211. Mulligan MS, Hevel JM, Marletta MA, et al. Tissue injury caused by deposition of immune complexes is L-arginine dependent. *Proc Natl Acad Sci USA* 1991;88(14):6338–6342.

212. Farrell JA, Albanese CT, Jennings RW, et al. Maternal fertility is not affected by fetal surgery. *Fetal Diagn Ther* 1999;14(3):190–192.

Non-obstetric Surgery during Pregnancy

Yaakov Beilin

■ INTRODUCTION

The incidence of surgery for nonobstetric procedures during pregnancy is between 0.3% and 2% (1,2). As there are approximately 4,000,000 deliveries per year in the United States this translates to 80,000 anesthetics to pregnant women per year, and most likely more due to surgery performed prior to clinical recognition of the pregnancy. Studies have demonstrated that many women presenting for surgery are unaware that they are pregnant. Unknown pregnancies in women presenting for surgery occurs in roughly 0.3% to 1.3% (3,4) of adults and 2.4% of adolescents between the age of 15 and 20 (5). For this reason a urinary pregnancy test should be considered in women of child-bearing age prior to surgery, unless an emergency clinical situation precludes this.

Surgery may be required at any time during pregnancy, though a large Swedish study of 720,000 found it was most common (2) during the first trimester (42%), followed by the second (35%), and third (24%). Appendectomy is the most frequently performed nonobstetric operation during pregnancy (6). However, almost every type of surgical procedure has been successfully performed on the pregnant patient, including open heart procedures with cardiopulmonary bypass (7), neurosurgical procedures requiring hypotension and hypothermia (8), and liver transplantation (9).

Anesthesia for the pregnant woman is one of the rare situations where the anesthesiologists must be concerned about two patients, the mother and the unborn fetus. Provision of a safe anesthetic requires an innate understanding of the physiologic changes of pregnancy and the impact of anesthesia and surgery on the developing fetus. Maternal considerations result from the physiology that affects almost every organ system (Table 50-1). Fetal concerns include the possible teratogenic effects of anesthetic agents, avoidance of intrauterine fetal asphyxia, and prevention of premature labor (Fig. 50-1).

■ PHYSIOLOGIC CHANGES OF PREGNANCY

The pregnant woman undergoes significant physiologic changes to allow adaptation for the developing fetus. The changes most pertinent to the anesthesiologist are those involving the cardiovascular, respiratory, and gastrointestinal system.

Respiratory System

Due to increased progesterone levels during the first trimester, minute ventilation is increased by almost 50% and remains so for the remainder of the pregnancy. Since anatomic dead space does not change significantly during pregnancy, at term, alveolar ventilation is increased by 70%. From 20 weeks' gestation, the functional residual capacity (FRC), expiratory reserve volume and residual volume begin to decrease as a result of upward displacement of the diaphragm by the gravid uterus; this reaches its maximum reduction of 20% by term. Vital capacity is not appreciably changed from prepregnancy levels. The increase in minute ventilation leads to a decrease in $PaCO_2$ to approximately 30 mm Hg. Arterial pH remains unchanged because of a compensatory increase in renal excretion of bicarbonate ions.

The increased alveolar ventilation and reduced FRC lead to a more rapid uptake and excretion of inhaled anesthetics. The decrease in FRC in conjunction with increases in cardiac output, metabolic rate, and oxygen consumption lead to a much greater risk of arterial hypoxemia during periods of apnea or airway obstruction. This places even greater emphasis on the value of preoxygenation prior to general anesthesia. Some have suggested that FRC is increased if the patient is positioned with the head elevated 30 degree versus supine. Whether this prolongs the time to oxygen desaturation is unknown (10).

Anatomic changes to the airway include laryngeal and pharyngeal edema that can make ventilation and tracheal intubation more difficult. In addition, mucosal capillary engorgement can cause bleeding during airway manipulation. Mallampati scores have been found to increase during pregnancy. Pilkington et al. (11) found the incidence of grade 4 airways increased by 38% from the 12th to the 38th week of pregnancy. Together with inherent weight gain and enlargement of breasts, these changes render tracheal intubation more difficult, as evidenced by failed intubation as a well-recognized cause of maternal mortality (12).

Cardiovascular System

Cardiac output is increased by 30% to 40% during the first trimester and 50% at term. This is primarily due to an increase in stroke volume (30% to 40%), and secondarily to an increase in heart rate (15%) (13). Further rises in cardiac output occur during labor and immediately postpartum, but these are beyond the scope of this chapter. Blood pressure normally decreases during pregnancy because of a fall in systemic vascular resistance due to the vasodilatory effects of estrogen and progesterone. Diastolic pressure is decreased to a greater extent (10% to 20%) than the systolic (0% to 15%). Near term, 10% to 15% of patients have a dramatic reduction in blood pressure in the supine position, often associated with diaphoresis, nausea, vomiting, pallor, and changes in cerebration. This is known as the supine hypotensive syndrome and is caused by compression of the inferior vena cava and aorta by the gravid uterus (14). This can begin as early as the second trimester and may lead to a reduction in renal and uteroplacental blood flow. Symptoms can be alleviated by tilting the patient on her left side to displace the uterus.

TABLE 50-1 Physiologic Changes of Pregnancy

Respiratory	
Minute ventilation	Increases by 50%
Tidal volume	Increases by 40%
Respiratory rate	Increases by 10%
Oxygen consumption	Increases by 20%
PaO_2	Increases by 10 mm Hg
Dead space	No change
Alveolar ventilation	Increases by 70%
$PaCO_2$	Decreases by 10 mm Hg
Arterial pH	No change
Serum HCO_3^-	Decreases by 4 mEq/L
Functional residual capacity	Decreases by 20%
Expiratory reserve volume	Decreases by 20%
Residual volume	Decreases by 20%
Vital capacity	No change
Cardiovascular	
Cardiac output	Increases by 30–40%
Heart rate	Increases by 15%
Stroke volume	Increases by 30%
Total peripheral resistance	Decreases by 15%
Femoral venous pressure	Increases by 15%
Central venous pressure	No change
Systolic blood pressure	Decreases by 0–15%
Diastolic blood pressure	Decreases by 10–20%
Intravascular volume	Increases by 45%
Plasma volume	Increases by 55%
Red blood cell volume	Increases by 30%
Gastrointestinal	
Motility	Decreases
Stomach position	More cephalad and horizontal
Transaminases	Increases
Alkaline phosphatase	Increases
Pseudocholinesterase	Decreases by 20%
Hematologic	
Hemoglobin	Decreases
Coagulation factors	Increases
Platelet count	Decreases by 20%
Lymphocyte function	Decreases
Renal	
Renal blood flow	Increases
Glomerular filtration rate	Increases
Serum creatinine and BUN	Decreases
Creatinine clearance	Increases
Glucosuria	1–10 g/day
Proteinuria	300 mg/day
Nervous System	
Minimum alveolar concentration	Decreases by 40%
Endorphin levels	Increases

Increases in cardiac output will hasten the speed of intravenous anesthesia induction. Compression of the inferior vena cava by the gravid uterus leads to dilatation of the azygos system and the epidural veins. Epidural venous engorgement decreases the volume of the epidural and intrathecal spaces, which is why the dose of drugs used in neuraxial blockade should be decreased. In addition, it is postulated that progesterone may increase the sensitivity of nerve cells to local anesthetics since neuraxial drug requirements decrease prior to uterine enlargement (15).

Gastrointestinal System

Traditionally, gastric emptying was considered prolonged in the pregnant woman by the end of the first trimester (16,17). This was thought to be related to progesterone and mechanical changes as the stomach is displaced upward by the enlarging uterus. However, recent studies using acetaminophen absorption have not found a difference in gastric emptying in pregnant women. Wong et al. found no difference in gastric emptying between term women who ingested 50 mL versus 300 mL of water in both nonobese (18) and obese women (19). This is in contrast to active labor when gastric emptying is delayed (20). Although gastric emptying per se may not be delayed until the onset of labor, when the gravid uterus enters the abdominal cavity at 20 weeks' gestation bariatric pressure is increased. In addition there is an increase in the acidity of gastric secretions (20) and a reduction in lower esophageal sphincter tone due to the influence of hormones (21). Although it is unclear when these changes are clinically relevant some consider all women at risk for aspiration of gastric content at 18 to 20 weeks (22), but certainly any woman with symptoms of acid reflux such as heartburn, a common finding in pregnancy (23), should be considered at risk.

Hematologic System

Intravascular volume is increased by 45% during pregnancy due to an increase in plasma volume. Since this increases by a greater proportion than the red blood cell volume (55% and 30%, respectively) there is a relative anemia during pregnancy. Nevertheless a hemoglobin concentration of less than 11 g/dL is considered abnormal. Most of the coagulation factors are elevated during pregnancy and consequently pregnancy is considered a hypercoagulable state, with an increased risk of thromboembolic events (24). Platelet counts generally decrease by approximately 20% during a normal pregnancy; approximately 7% of all parturients will present with a platelet count <150,000·mm^{-3}, and 0.5% to 1% will present with a platelet count <100,000·mm^{-3} (25).

Hepatic Changes

Tests of liver function (serum glutamic-oxaloacetic transaminase, lactic acid dehydrogenase, alkaline phosphatase, and cholesterol) are commonly increased during pregnancy, though this does not necessarily indicate abnormal liver function. Pseudocholinesterase activity declines by as much as 20% during the first trimester and remains at this level for the remainder of the pregnancy. However, prolonged apnea is rarely a problem following a standard dose of succinylcholine and the duration of ester-linked local anesthetics are not prolonged.

Nervous System

The minimum alveolar concentration (MAC) for inhaled anesthetics is decreased by up to 40% during pregnancy (26)

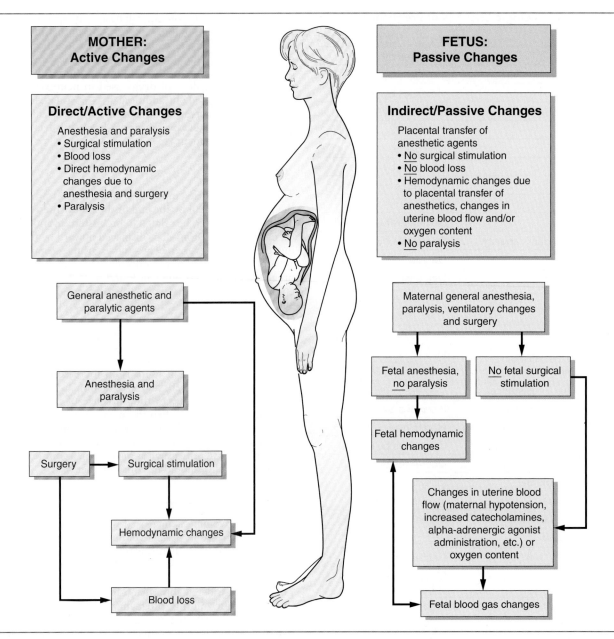

FIGURE 50-1 The effects of anesthesia and paralytic agents and surgery on the mother and fetus. Reprinted with permission from: Rosen MA. Management of anesthesia for the pregnant surgical patient. *Anesthesiology* 1999;91:1159–1163.

due to the effect of progesterone and endorphins. Accordingly, the doses of inhalational agents should be reduced. Also, as mentioned earlier, smaller doses of local anesthetics are required to produce the same dermatomal level of neuraxial anesthesia in pregnant women as compared to non-pregnant women (14). This is related to progesterone and to mechanical effects from the gravid uterus pressing on the spinal and epidural space enhancing spread of local anesthetic. This observed decrease in both MAC and neuraxial requirements begins in the first trimester.

■ FETAL CONSIDERATIONS

Drug Teratogenicity

A teratogen is a substance that produces an increase in the incidence of a particular defect that cannot be attributed to chance. In order to produce a defect, the teratogen must be

administered in a sufficient dose at a critical point in development. In humans this critical point is during organogenesis, which extends from 15 days to approximately 60 days gestational age. Each organ system has its own unique period of susceptibility. For example, the period of vulnerability for the heart is between days 18 and 40 and for the limbs is between days 24 and 34. However, the central nervous system does not fully develop until after birth, hence the critical time for this may extend beyond gestation.

Well-controlled randomized human studies are essentially impossible to perform in this domain due to the obvious ethical limitations and the large number of patients required to study these rare defects (27). Four approaches have been utilized to study the effects of anesthesia in the pregnant patient: (1) Animal studies, (2) limited retrospective human studies, (3) studies of chronic exposure of operating room personnel to trace concentrations of inhaled anesthetics, and (4) outcome studies of women who underwent surgery while pregnant.

TABLE 50-2 Teratogenic Effects of Anesthetic Agents in Animals

Anesthetic Agents	Teratogenic Effect
Thiopental	Cleft lip and cardiomyopathies
Opioids	Inguinal hernia and CNS
Local anesthetics	Cytotoxic in tissue culture only
Cocaine	GI, genitourinary, and CNS
Muscle relaxants	Musculoskeletal deformities
Potent inhaled anesthetic agents	Cleft palate and skeletal abnormalities
Nitrous oxide	Skeletal abnormalities
Benzodiazepines	Cardiac defects, spina bifida, and cleft lip
Ketamine	Neural tube defect

GI, gastrointestinal; CNS, central nervous system.

TABLE 50-4 United States Food and Drug Administration Category Ratings of Specific Anesthetic Agents

Anesthetic Agent	Classification
Induction Agents	
Etomidate	C
Ketamine	C
Methohexital	B
Propofol	B
Thiopental	C
Inhaled Agents	
Desflurane	B
Enflurane	B
Halothane	C
Isoflurane	C
Sevoflurane	B
Local Anesthetics	
2-chloroprocaine	C
Bupivacaine	C
Lidocaine	B
Ropivacaine	B
Tetracaine	C
Dexmedetomdine	C
Opioids	
Alfentanil	C
Fentanyl	C
Sufentanil	C
Meperidine	B
Morphine	C
Neuromuscular Blocking Drugs	
Atracurium	C
Cisatracurium	B
Curare	C
Mivacurium	C
Pancuronium	C
Rocuronium	B
Succinylcholine	C
Vecuronium	C
Benzodiazepines	
Diazepam	D
Midazolam	D

Almost all anesthetic agents have been found to be teratogenic in some animal models (Table 50-2). However, the results of animal studies are of limited value because of species variation, as well as the use of agents in animal studies in far greater concentrations than those used clinically. In addition, other known teratogenic factors such as hypercarbia, hypothermia, and hypoxemia were either not measured or not controlled. Species variation is particularly important. Thalidomide has no known teratogenic effects on rats and was approved by the United States Food and Drug Administration (FDA) for use in humans. However, it later became apparent that thalidomide is teratogenic in humans (28).

The United States FDA has established a risk classification system to assist physicians weigh the risks and benefits when choosing therapeutic agents for the pregnant woman (29). To date there are only five drugs known to be teratogens, and none of them are anesthetic agents. These drugs include thalidomide, isotretinoin, coumarin (warfarin), valproic acid, and folate antagonists (30). Most anesthetic agents, including the intravenous induction agents, local anesthetics, opioids, and neuromuscular blocking drugs have been assigned a Category B or C classification (Tables 50-3 and 50-4). Indeed only the benzodiazepines have been assigned as Category D (positive evidence of risk. Investigational or post-marketing data show risk to the fetus. Nevertheless, potential benefits may outweigh the potential risk). Cocaine is in Category X, or contraindicated.

■ INHALED ANESTHETICS

Nitrous oxide is a known teratogen in mammals and rapidly crosses the human placenta (31,32). It had been presumed

TABLE 50-3 United States Food and Drug Administration Category Ratings of Drugs during Pregnancy (29)

Category A: Controlled studies demonstrate no risk. Well-controlled studies in humans have not demonstrated risk to the fetus
Category B: No evidence of risks in humans. Either animal studies have found a risk but human studies have not; or animal studies are negative but adequate human studies have not been done.
Category C: Risk cannot be ruled out. Human studies have not been adequately performed and animal studies are positive or have not been conducted. Potential benefits may justify the risk.
Category D: Potential evidence of risk. Confirmed evidence of human risk. However, benefits may be acceptable despite the known risk, i.e., no other medication is available to treat a life-threatening situation.
Category X: Contraindicated in pregnancy. Human or animal studies have shown fetal risk which clearly outweighs any possible benefit to the patient.

From; Physicians' C, 64th ed. Montvale: PDR Network, LLC, 2009:215.

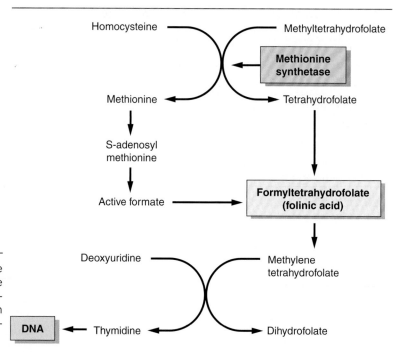

FIGURE 50-2 Nitrous oxide directly blocks the transmethylation reaction by which methionine is synthesized from homocystine and methyltetrahydrofolate. It does so by oxidizing vitamin B_{12}, the cofactor for the enzyme methionine synthetase.

that the teratogenicity of nitrous oxide in animals is related to its oxidation of vitamin B_{12}, which then cannot function as a cofactor for the enzyme methionine synthetase (Fig. 50-2)—essential for the formation of thymidine, a subunit of DNA. There is some evidence that the effects in animals of nitrous oxide are not related to these proposed effects on DNA synthesis. Pretreatment of rats exposed to nitrous oxide with folinic acid, which bypasses the methionine synthetase step in DNA synthesis, does not prevent congenital abnormalities (33), and suppression of methionine synthetase occurs at low concentrations of nitrous oxide (34)—concentrations found safe in animal studies (35). Despite these theoretical concerns, nitrous oxide has not been found to be associated with congenital abnormalities in humans (1,2,36,37). The FDA has not given nitrous oxide a category classification because it is a medical gas and not directly regulated by the FDA.

Potent inhaled anesthetic agents are commonly used during surgery. Halothane is the most studied of all the agents and the results have been mixed, some finding an association with congenital defects, cleft palate and paw defects (38), and others not (35). The same is the case with the other potent agents such as isoflurane (35,39). The clinical relevance of these findings is uncertain. Sevoflurane and desflurane are classified as Class B drugs by the FDA and there is no need to avoid using them. There may even be a theoretical benefit to using inhaled agents since they are tocolytic agents and may prevent preterm labor. In addition, in a comparative outcome study of women who underwent surgery while pregnant versus those who did not there was no difference in congenital defects between the groups and most had general anesthesia with nitrous oxide and an inhaled agent (1,2).

■ INTRAVENOUS ANESTHETIC AGENTS AND ADJUNCTS

Thiopental

Thiopental has a long track record of safety in over approximately 70 years clinical use. Although found to be teratogenic in the chick embryo it has not been specifically studied in humans and as a result of its long track record of safety is considered safe to use during pregnancy (40).

Propofol

Propofol readily crosses the placenta in almost a 1:1 fetal/maternal plasma concentration ratio (41). However, no animal or human studies have demonstrated a teratogenic effect (Category B). Interestingly, there is some controversy about its use for in vitro fertilization because of high levels of propofol in follicular fluid (42) but the same is true when thiopental is used (43) and pregnancy rates are not different between the two agents (44).

Etomidate

Etomidate crosses the placenta in a ratio of approximately 0.5 fetal to maternal concentrations (45). In rats, when given in doses 1 to 4 times the human dose, etomidate has been found to have an embryocidal effect, but not a teratogenic effect. Due to the embryocidal effect it has been given a Category C classification.

Ketamine

Ketamine crosses the placenta in a slightly higher ratio than other intravenous anesthetics (46). It has been associated with neural tube defects in the chick embryo (47) but had no effect in mice (48). There are no reports of teratogenic issues in humans. There is some controversy regarding the effects of ketamine on the developing fetal brain in rats (49), but this has not been demonstrated in humans (50) (see section regarding apoptosis).

Dexmedetomidine

Dexmedetomidine was introduced into clinical practice in 1999 primarily as a sedative agent in the intensive care unit. It has also been safely used for labor analgesia in select patients (51). Both dexmedetomidine and the related clonidine cross the placenta in small amounts (52). Tariq et al. (53) found no teratogenic or developmental effects in rats exposed to dexmedetomidine in utero. There is no controlled data in humans and the drug is given a Category C classification.

Sedative/Hypnotics

The use of sedatives, in particular benzodiazepines, in the first trimester of pregnancy is controversial. Benzodiazepines exert their action through the inhibition of gamma-aminobutyric acid (GABA) receptors in the central nervous system. GABA has been shown to inhibit palate shelf reorientation leading to cleft palate formation. Since diazepam mimics GABA it also may predispose to cleft palate formation (54). Some investigators in human retrospective studies noted an association between diazepam ingestion in the first 6 weeks of pregnancy and cleft palate (55,56). These findings have been questioned by the results of two prospective studies that did not demonstrate an association (57,58).

The concern is still apparent based on the many human studies that have ensued in this area. Laegreid et al. (59) in a case control study found an association between benzodiazepine use and cleft palate, and Dolovich et al. (60) in a meta-analysis found an association in case controlled studies but not cohort studies. Furthermore, Wikner et al. (61) used the Swedish registry and did not find an association between benzodiazepines and cleft palate but did find a weak association with pylorostenosis and alimentary tract atresia. It is important to remember that in all these studies the assessment was in women chronically exposed to benzodiazepines and not in women with a one-time low dose exposure as typically occurs during surgery. The FDA has assigned benzodiazepines a Class D designation and although controversial, and other experts do not avoid its use during pregnancy (62), this author prefers not to use benzodiazepines during nonobstetric surgery unless there is a compelling reason to do so.

Opioids

All the opioids readily cross the placenta because they are highly lipophilic (63). Opioids are teratogenic in the hamster model (64). Of interest, the maternal administration of narcotic antagonists in the rat model prevents the congenital defect suggesting that opioid-induced respiratory depression and hypercarbia caused the problem and not the narcotic itself (65). It is therefore important, when administering narcotics during pregnancy to avoid these potential side effects. Opioids, both synthetic and natural, have little to no teratogenicity in vivo and are classified as a Class C medication. They are commonly and safely used for nonobstetric surgery.

Neuromuscular Blocking Agents

Succinylcholine and all the nondepolarizing agents do not cross the placenta to any appreciable degree because of their molecular size and ionic charge and therefore have little effect on the developing fetus. Studying the effect of muscle relaxants is particularly difficult since the animal must be anesthetized and ventilated. In one study there was a suggestion of a dose dependent effect of muscle relaxants (d-tubocurarine, atracurium, vecuronium, and pancuronium) on the developing fetus, but the serum concentration was 30 times greater than those seen clinically (66). Muscle relaxants do not need to be avoided during pregnancy and most have a Category B or C classification.

Local Anesthetics

Local anesthetics act by stabilizing cell membranes and therefore might affect cell mitosis and meiosis. In vitro studies in mice and chicks suggested that prilocaine, lidocaine, and tetracaine may cause premature neural tube closure (48). However, a carefully controlled study by Fujinaga in 1998 with lidocaine in rat embryos cultured in vitro failed to demonstrate a problem until very high concentrations were used (67). In vivo studies of local anesthetics have not demonstrated any teratogenic effect (68).

■ HUMAN STUDIES

There have been two approaches to assess the effects of anesthetic agents on pregnancy outcome: large retrospective epidemiologic surveys of women chronically exposed to anesthetic gasses, and retrospective database studies comparing women who underwent surgery while pregnant to those who were not.

Epidemiologic Studies

A number of epidemiologic studies were performed in the 1970s to determine the health hazards, of chronic exposure to anesthetic gasses, including birth defects and spontaneous abortions (69,70). All the studies found similar results and the most consistent finding was that the rate of miscarriage among exposed women is approximately 25% to 30% greater than nonexposed women. Concerned by these findings, the American Society of Anesthesiologists, sponsored a large study and found similar results (71). The authors surveyed 73,496 individuals who may have been exposed to anesthetic gasses. The study population included the entire membership of the American Society of Anesthesiologists, the American Association of Nurse Anesthetists, the Association of Operating Room Nurses, and the Association of Operating Room Technicians. These personnel received questionnaires in the mail designed to gather information about the extent of their exposure and reproductive outcome. They found that operating room personnel had an increased risk of spontaneous abortions and congenital abnormalities. They recommended that a means to scavenge trace anesthetic gasses should be mandatory in all operating rooms, which is now adopted as standard. However, all these studies were later criticized for their lack of a control group, low response rate to questionnaires, recall bias, and statistical inaccuracies (72,73). An additional study with a different study design was unable to confirm these findings. Ericson and Kallen (74) used a Swedish birth registry and compared delivery outcome among nurses who worked in the operating room with those who worked on internal medicine wards. Since it is a registry study and not survey study it is not subject to the same issues as survey studies especially the problem with recall bias. They were not able to find a difference in miscarriage, perinatal deaths, or malformations among the groups.

Outcome Studies of Women who had Surgery while Pregnant

There have also been a number of retrospective studies of pregnant women who had undergone surgery to seek an association between anesthesia and surgery and congenital defects, spontaneous abortions or fetal demise. The results were remarkably similar. In 1963, Smith (75) reviewed the medical records of 67 women who had surgery while pregnant, 11 in the first trimester, and found that fetal loss was greater in the group that had surgery, and none had a congenital defect. Shnider and Webster (76) reviewed the records of 147 women who had surgery while pregnant, 47 during the first trimester, 58 during the second, and 42 during the third, and compared them with 8,926 women who did not. They found an increased rate of preterm labor, but no increase in congenital defects. They concluded that the surgical disease, not the anesthetic, was the most important determinant of preterm labor.

Brodsky et al. (1) sent questionnaires by mail to 30,272 female dental assistants and 29,514 wives of male dentists to assess the effect of occupational and surgical anesthesia exposure on the fetus. They found 287 women had surgery while pregnant, 187 during the first trimester, and 100 during the second. They found an increase in the rate of spontaneous abortion but no difference in the rate of congenital defects amongst those with either occupational exposure or surgery. The incidence of miscarriage was 8% versus 5.1% during the first trimester and 6.9% versus 1.4% in the second trimester (surgery vs. controls).

Duncan et al. (36) used health insurance data to study the entire population of Manitoba, Canada between 1971 and 1978. They matched 2,565 women who had surgery while pregnant with a similar number who did not. They did not find a difference in congenital anomalies but found a significant increase in spontaneous abortion in women having general anesthesia during the first or second trimester. The risk ratio was 1.58 with nongynecologic procedures and 2 for gynecologic procedures. They were not able to conclude whether the increased risk of spontaneous abortion was related to the anesthetic or the surgery.

The largest study to date was performed by Mazze and Kallen (2). They linked the data from three Swedish health registries—the Medical Birth Registry, the Registry of Congenital malformations, and the Hospital Discharge registry for the 9-year period 1973 to 1981. They examined the data for four adverse outcomes; congenital defects, stillborn infants, infants born alive but who died within 7 days, and infants with a birth weight <1,500 g and <2,500 g. They found 5,405 women had undergone surgery during their pregnancy from a total of 720,000 pregnancies. In their data set, most procedures were performed during the first trimester (41.6%), and the incidence decreased during the second (34.8%) and third (23.5%) trimesters. Most of the cases (54%) were done with general anesthesia, almost all of them (>98%) with nitrous oxide. They were not able to find an increase in congenital abnormalities or stillborn births among those who underwent surgery while pregnant during any trimester. However, the number of babies born with a birth weight <1,500 and 2,500 g, and the number of babies who died within 7 days of the operation was greater in those who underwent surgery while pregnant (Fig. 50-3). This was true during all three trimesters. These risks could not be linked to either the specific anesthetic agents or the anesthetic technique. The increased risk to the fetus may be due to the condition that necessitated

surgery in the first place, with the highest rate in gynecologic procedures. These same authors published the outcome from a subset of these women who underwent an appendectomy (37). They found an increase in the risk of delivery within the first week of surgery and a decrease in mean birth weight by 78 g. The increased risk of delivery did not persist beyond the first week of surgery. There was no increase in congenital anomalies or stillborn infants.

More recently, in 1993 and 2001, there were two additional studies comparing pregnant women who had surgery while pregnant to those who did not (77,78), and the results were similar to the earlier studies. Kort et al. (77) reviewed all 78 cases, between 1980 and 1989, of women who had extensive surgery while pregnant at North Carolina Memorial Hospital and Wake Medical Center and compared them to 49,489 pregnant women who did not. The most common indications for surgery were appendicitis, adnexal mass, and cholecystitis. They found an increased rate of preterm labor and preterm delivery, but not in perinatal mortality rate or congenital defects. Visser et al. (78) reviewed 77 consecutive pregnant women who had surgery between 1989 and 1996 and compared them to 40,520 women who did not. They did not find an increase in the incidence of congenital defects or perinatal mortality, but the incidence of preterm labor in the third trimester was increased.

In contrast to the results of the above studies, two separate investigators found an association between surgery and anesthesia during the first trimester and central nervous system defects (79,80). In the first study (79), using the same Swedish registry as described above (2), an increase in neural tube defects was identified in children whose mothers had surgery during weeks 4 and 5 of gestation. Sylvester et al. (80) attempted to corroborate these findings in a case control study but was not able to. They identified 694 babies who had central nervous system defects and compared them to 2,984 controls. They found an increase in the first trimester surgery and anesthesia in those with a combination of hydrocephalus and eye deficits, but not neural tube deficits. Neither of these findings were corroborated in a third study. Czeizel et al. (81) reviewed a population based data set between 1980 and 1994 in Hungary to assess the teratogenic potential of surgery under anesthesia during pregnancy. Babies with

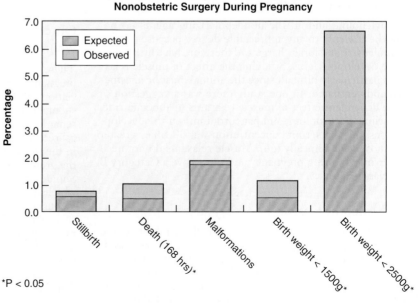

Observed vs. Expected Outcomes in Nonobstetric Surgery During Pregnancy

FIGURE 50-3 Total number of observed and expected outcomes among women having nonobstetric surgery during pregnancy. The incidence of infants with low or very low birth weight and babies who die within 168 hours were significantly increased. From: Mazze RI, Källén B. Reproductive outcome after anesthesia and operation during pregnancy: A registry study of 5405 cases. *Am J Obstet Gynecol* 1989;161:1178.

*P < 0.05

congenital defects were matched with healthy controls. Of 35,727 women whose babies did not have congenital defects, 73 (0.2%) had surgery while pregnant. Whereas, of the 20,830 women who had babies with congenital defects, 31 (0.15%) had surgery while pregnant. They found a greater incidence of low birth rate babies in those who had surgery but this was explained by those who had surgery for cervical incompetence. They did not find any difference in congenital defects between groups. They concluded that surgery under anesthesia does not present a teratogenic risk to the patient.

In summary, the data overwhelmingly indicate that surgery and anesthesia during pregnancy is not associated with an increased rate of congenital defects in the unborn child. However, it is associated with preterm labor and an increased rate of miscarriage, particularly during the first week after the surgery. Although unproven this association is most likely related to the surgery or the underlying condition rather than the anesthetic since the miscarriage rates are greatest in those having pelvic surgery.

■ BEHAVIORAL TERATOLOGY AND APOPTOSIS IN THE NEWBORN BRAIN

In 1963, Werboff and Kesner (82) used the term behavioral teratology to describe the adverse action of a drug on the behavior of the offspring to its environment. It is well known that the halogenated agents particularly halothane and enflurane cause learning deficits in rodents (83,84). Most anesthetic agents act by either blocking N-methyl-d-aspartate (NMDA) receptors or by enhancing GABA. Studies have demonstrated that when agents that act by either of these mechanisms (e.g., ketamine, nitrous oxide, midazolam, barbiturates, and volatile agents) are administered to the rodent during the period of synaptogenesis, they induce widespread neuronal apoptosis in the developing brain (50,85). Learning deficits have been described in the offspring of female rats exposed to commonly used anesthetic agents and widespread neurodegeneration was seen on histologic examination (86).

Although an association between anesthetic agents and neuronal apoptosis has been demonstrated in the animal model, extrapolation from animal studies to humans is problematic at best (51). While most organ systems have completed development by the end of the first trimester or earlier, the brain continues to develop until after delivery. The time of greatest concern is during synaptogenesis or rapid growth spurt which is from the third trimester until 3 years of age. Randomized trials to confirm apoptosis in the human brain obviously cannot be done and evaluating effect of anesthesia on the brain is complicated. Recently two separate authors assessed the effect of anesthesia and surgery on behavior later in life. One looked at learning disabilities (87) and the other deviant behavior (88). Both found an association between surgery and anesthesia and their outcome measures. The studies are far from conclusive as they were not randomized, and one was only a survey (51), but they certainly highlight the need for well-controlled studies. At this point it is premature to make any changes in anesthesia practice based on the data to date (85) and the FDA at an advisory committee meeting came to the same conclusion (89).

■ AVOIDANCE OF INTRAUTERINE FETAL ASPHYXIA

The most important consideration for the fetus during non-obstetric surgery is the maintenance of a normal intrauterine physiologic milieu and avoidance of intrauterine fetal asphyxia. Fetal oxygenation is directly dependent on maternal arterial oxygen tension, oxygen carrying capacity, oxygen affinity, and uteroplacental perfusion. It is therefore critical to maintain a normal maternal PaO_2, $PaCO_2$, and uterine blood flow.

Maternal and Fetal Oxygenation

Mild to moderate maternal hypoxemia is generally well tolerated by the fetus because fetal hemoglobin has a high affinity for oxygen. However, severe hypoxia will lead to fetal death. General anesthesia is a particular risk to the pregnant woman because management of the airway can be difficult, and the rate of hemoglobin oxygen desaturation is increased due to the decreased FRC and increased oxygen consumption. Care must also be taken during a neuraxial anesthetic because a high dermatomal level of anesthesia, a toxic local anesthetic reaction, or oversedation can also lead to a hypoxic event.

Elevated maternal oxygen tension commonly occurs during general anesthesia. Studies in isolated human placenta demonstrated vasoconstriction at increased oxygen levels suggesting that fetal oxygen levels could decrease if the mother receives high concentrations of oxygen (90). Conversely, studies of fetal scalp capillary PO_2 demonstrated that fetal levels of oxygen increase as maternal oxygen levels increase and not the opposite (91). Some have feared that increasing the inspired oxygen level to the mother could be detrimental to the fetus by causing premature closure of the ductus arteriosus or retrolental fibroplasias. However, due to placental shunting of blood, fetal PaO_2 never rises above 60 mm Hg even if maternal PaO_2 is 600 mm Hg. Therefore, maternal inspired oxygen concentration should not be limited.

Maternal Carbon Dioxide

Both maternal hypercapnia and hypocapnia can be detrimental to the fetus. Severe hypocapnia produced by excessive positive pressure ventilation may increase mean intrathoracic pressure, decrease venous return, and lead to a decrease in uterine blood flow (92). In addition, maternal alkalosis, as produced by hyperventilation, will decrease uterine blood flow by direct vasoconstriction (93), and it will decrease oxygen delivery by shifting the maternal oxyhemoglobin dissociation curve to the left (94). Severe hypercapnia is detrimental because carbon dioxide readily crosses the placenta and is associated with fetal acidosis and myocardial depression.

Uteroplacental Perfusion

Uterine blood flow is affected by both drugs and anesthetic procedures. Placental blood flow is directly proportional to the net perfusion pressure across the intervillous space and inversely proportional to the resistance. Perfusion pressure will be decreased by hypotension which may be due to the sympathectomy from local anesthetics administered as part of an epidural or spinal anesthetic, from aortocaval compression in the supine position, or from hemorrhage. Nonetheless a moderate degree of hypotension, as is occasionally needed for neurosurgical procedures, has been safely employed (8). Medications that cause vasoconstriction, e.g., α-adrenergic drugs or ketamine at doses >2 mg/kg (95), hypocapnia as may occur with hyperventilation during general anesthesia, or increased catecholamines such as occurs during pain, apprehension, or light anesthesia will increase vascular resistance and decrease uteroplacental blood flow, and should therefore be avoided. Phenylephrine used to be considered problematic because it is a vasoconstrictor and could lead to uterine vasoconstriction. However, recent data from women undergoing cesarean delivery suggest

TABLE 50-5 Guidelines for Laparoscopic Surgery during Pregnancy (100)

1. Indications for treatment of acute abdominal processes are the same in pregnant and nonpregnant patients.
2. Laparoscopy can be safely performed during any trimester of pregnancy.
3. Obstetric consultation can be obtained pre- and/or postoperatively based on the acuteness of the patient's disease and availability.
4. Pregnant patients should be placed with left uterine displacement to minimize compression of the vena cava and the aorta.
5. Fetal heart monitoring should occur pre- and postoperatively.
6. Initial access can be safely accomplished with an open or Hassan, Veress needle, or optical trocar.
7. Insufflation of 10–15 mm Hg can be safely used in the pregnant patient.
8. Intraoperative CO_2 monitoring by capnography should be used.
9. Intraoperative and postoperative pneumatic compression devices and early postoperative ambulation are recommended prophylaxis for deep venous thrombosis.
10. Tocolytic agents should not be used prophylactically, but should be considered perioperatively when signs of preterm labor are present.

From: Yumi H. Guidelines for diagnosis, treatment, and use of laparoscopy for surgical problems during pregnancy: this statement was reviewed and approved by the Board of Governors of the Society of American Gastrointestinal and Endoscopic Surgeons (SAGES), September 2007. It was prepared by the SAGES Guidelines Committee. *Surg Endosc* 2008;22:849–861.

that it may be the preferred vasopressor (96). Whether this data can be extrapolated to situations where the fetus is not being delivered, as occurs during maternal nonobstetric surgery, is unclear, but this author uses phenylephrine in this scenario.

Prevention of Premature Labor

Spontaneous abortions, premature labor, and preterm delivery are the most significant risks to the fetus during maternal surgery (1,2,36,37), and may be as great as 22% following appendectomy (37). It is unclear if this is due to the surgery, anesthetic, or underlying medical condition, but the greatest risk is during gynecologic or pelvic procedures when there is uterine manipulation (36) and the lowest risk occurs during the second trimester. The potent inhaled anesthetic agents decrease uterine tone and inhibit uterine contractions so from this perspective they may be beneficial. Also, medications that increase uterine tone such as ketamine at doses >2 mg/kg should theoretically be avoided. No study, however, has ever documented that any particular anesthetic agent or technique is associated with a greater or smaller incidence of abortion or preterm labor.

Laparoscopic Surgery

Once considered an absolute contraindication during pregnancy, laparoscopic surgery is now routinely performed (97,98). Commonly performed laparoscopic procedures include appendectomy, cholecystectomy, and surgery for adnexal masses. Reedy et al. (99) in a survey study, compared five fetal outcome variables among pregnant women who had a laparotomy (*n* = 2,181) versus those who had laparoscopy (*n* = 1,522) between the fourth and twentieth weeks of gestation, and the general pregnant population who did not undergo surgery. The outcome variables studied were birth weight, gestational duration, intrauterine growth restriction, congenital malformation, and infant survival. They found that there was an increased risk of preterm delivery and low birth weight (<2,500 g) in both surgical groups as compared to the general population. But there was no difference in any of the other outcome variables between the two surgical groups.

Specific anesthetic considerations during laparoscopy include maintaining normocarbia because carbon dioxide is commonly used to maintain a pneumoperitoneum. Adjusting maternal ventilation to maintain end-tidal carbon dioxide between 30 and 35 mm Hg should avoid hypercarbia and fetal acidosis. The Society of American Gastrointestinal and

Endoscopic Surgeons proposed guidelines for laparoscopic surgery during pregnancy. Surgical concerns include caution during placement of the trocars which can be accomplished as an open technique and maintaining low pneumoperitoneum pressures (<15 mm Hg) to maintain uterine perfusion (100) (Table 50-5).

■ FETAL HEART RATE MONITORING

Fetal heart rate (FHR) monitoring becomes feasible around 16 to 18 weeks with an external tocodynamometer, but the indication for its use intraoperatively is less well defined, and it obviously cannot be used in every case such as abdominal procedures. One issue is how to act on the information. If the fetus is not viable and the FHR tracing is concerning, all that can be done is normalize the physiologic milieu. Is this sufficient reason to use the monitor when this should be done anyway? Some believe that it is sufficient reason (101), and Katz et al. (102) reported a case in which they were able to correct an abnormal FHR in a woman who was undergoing eye surgery, by increasing the percentage of inspired oxygen given to the mother.

Another issue is who should interpret the tracing. Anesthetic agents will change the FHR baseline and decrease variability and these changes need to be distinguished from fetal compromise (101). Furthermore, if a change is noted and the fetus is viable will the obstetrician intervene with immediate delivery.

The American College of Obstetricians and Gynecologists issued a joint statement with the American Society of Anesthesiologists on this issue (103). General guidelines from the statement include:

1. A qualified individual should be readily available to interpret the FHR.
2. If the fetus is below a viable gestation, it is generally sufficient to ascertain the FHR before and after the procedure, but that in "select circumstances intraoperative monitoring may be considered to facilitate positioning or oxygenation interventions."
3. If the fetus is viable then simultaneous FHR and contraction monitoring should be performed before and after the procedure and an obstetric provider should be available and willing to intervene for fetal indications.

The statement concludes by stating, "the decision to use fetal monitoring should be individualized and ultimately, each case warrants a team approach for optimal safety of the woman and fetus."

■ GENERAL RECOMMENDATIONS FOR ANESTHETIC MANAGEMENT (FIG. 50-4)

Preoperative Management and Timing of Surgery

Whenever possible, anesthesia and surgery should be avoided during the first trimester. Although no anesthetic drug has been proven teratogenic in humans it is prudent to minimize or eliminate fetal exposure during this period of organogenesis if at all possible.

Before initiating any anesthetic an obstetrician should be consulted and FHR tones should be documented. Precautions against aspiration should be taken from as early as the 12th week and a clear nonparticulate oral antacid, H_2 receptor blocker, and metoclopramide should be considered. Ranitidine, (50 mg i.v., given approximately 60 minutes prior to general anesthesia) reduced the gastric pH in women undergoing cesarean delivery (104), and metoclopramide (10 mg i.v., given 15 to 30 minutes prior to general anesthesia) was effective in reducing gastric volume in early pregnancy (105).

Apprehension should be allayed by reassurance from the anesthesiologist rather than with premedication, if possible. The patient should be informed that there is no known risk to the baby regarding congenital malformations but that there is an increased risk of abortion or premature labor. This is a good opportunity to educate the patient as to the signs of premature labor, e.g., back pain in someone prior to term, which can occur up to 1 week after the procedure. The patient should be transported to the operating room with left uterine displacement to avoid aortocaval compression after 16 to 18 weeks' gestation.

Monitoring

In addition to the standard ASA intraoperative monitors, the FHR and uterine tone should be monitored, if at all possible.

It is the best way to assure maintenance of a normal physiologic milieu for the baby. Monitoring and interpretation should be performed by an obstetrician or someone other than the anesthesiologist with expertise in FHR interpretation. Regardless of the decision to perform intraoperative FHR monitoring, the FHR and uterine contractions should be monitored before and after the surgery.

Anesthetic Technique

The type of anesthesia should be based on maternal indications, the site and nature of the surgery, and the anesthesiologist's experience. Since MAC is decreased, the dose of all anesthetic agents for regional or general anesthesia should be reduced. Although no study has found any difference in neonatal outcome in terms of congenital defects or preterm delivery, regional anesthesia may be preferable to general anesthesia to avoid the risk of pulmonary aspiration and decrease fetal drug exposure. Also, local anesthetics have not been found teratogenic even in animal studies.

The largest risk of neuraxial anesthesia is hypotension, which reduces uteroplacental perfusion. Prevention of hypotension is difficult since prehydration does not reliably reduce the incidence of hypotension (106). If hypotension occurs ephedrine or phenylephrine can be used and there may be a benefit to phenylephrine (96). The key is not which drug is chosen but that hypotension should be treated quickly.

General anesthesia should be preceded by careful evaluation of the airway, denitrogenation, and a rapid sequence induction with the application of cricoid pressure. Edema, weight gain, and increase in breast size may make tracheal intubation technically difficult. An array of laryngoscope blades and handles, and other emergency airway management equipment should be available. Capillary engorgement of the mucosal lining of the upper airway accompanies pregnancy. This mandates extreme care during manipulation

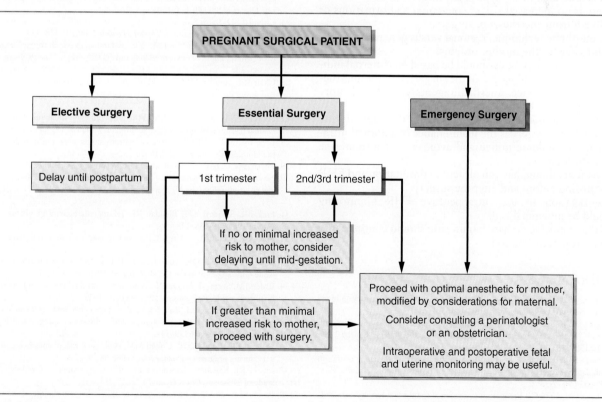

FIGURE 50-4 Summary recommendations for management of the pregnant surgical patient. Reprinted with permission from: Rosen MA. Management of anesthesia for the pregnant surgical patient. *Anesthesiology* 1999;91:1159–1163.

of the airway and the use of a smaller-than-normal tracheal tube. The use of a nasal airway and nasotracheal intubation should be avoided. A high inspired concentration of oxygen should be used (at least 50%) and $PaCO_2$ should be maintained at normal pregnancy levels (30 to 35 mm Hg). End-tidal CO_2 is an excellent approximation of $PaCO_2$ in the pregnant patient because the arterial-to-end-tidal CO_2 gradient decreases during pregnancy (107).

Postoperative Care

FHR and uterine activity monitoring should continue postoperatively. Epidural or subarachnoid opioids are an excellent choice for pain management because they cause minimal sedation and smaller doses can be utilized compared to the intramuscular or intravenous routes. Nonsteroidal anti-inflammatory drugs should be avoided because they may cause premature closure of the ductus arteriosus (108).

Regardless of the technique, attention to detail and maintenance of a normal intrauterine physiologic milieu throughout the perioperative period, including the avoidance of hypotension, hypoxemia, hypercarbia, hypocarbia, hypothermia, and acidosis is the key to a successful outcome.

KEY POINTS

- Many women will undergo surgery while pregnant.
- The risk to the mother is related to the physiologic changes of pregnancy.
- Maternal airway and cardiovascular issues are the leading cause of maternal morbidity and mortality.
- The greatest risk to the fetus is preterm labor and preterm delivery. It is unclear if the increased risk is related to the surgery, anesthesia, or underlying disease. The increased risk is unrelated to the type of anesthesia utilized.
- There is no increased risk of congenital malformations or stillbirth from anesthesia or surgery.
- No anesthetic technique, regional versus general, has been found safer for the mother or fetus.
- The choice of anesthesia should be based on maternal indications, the site and nature of the surgery, and the anesthesiologist's experience. Anesthetic agents with a long history of safety should be used.
- The most important consideration for the fetus during nonobstetric surgery is the maintenance of a normal intrauterine physiologic milieu and avoidance of intrauterine fetal asphyxia.
- All patients should have an obstetric consultation and FHR monitoring before and after the surgery.
- The decision to use intraoperative FHR monitoring should be individualized.
- FHR and uterine activity monitoring should continue into the postoperative period.

REFERENCES

1. Brodsky JB, Cohen EN, Brown BW, et al. Surgery during pregnancy and fetal outcome. *Am J Obstet Gynecol* 1980;138:1165–1167.
2. Mazze RI, Källén B. Reproductive outcome after anesthesia and operation during pregnancy: a registry study of 5405 cases. *Am J Obstet Gynecol* 1989; 161:1178–1185.
3. Manley S, de Kelaita G, Joseph NJ, et al. Preoperative pregnancy testing in ambulatory surgery. Incidence and impact of positive results. *Anesthesiology.* 1995;83:690–693.
4. Wheeler M, Coté CJ. Preoperative pregnancy testing in a tertiary care children's hospital: a medico-legal conundrum. *J Clin Anesth* 1999;11:56–63.
5. Azzam FJ, Padda GS, DeBoard JW, et al. Preoperative pregnancy testing in adolescents. *Anesth Analg* 1996;82:4–7.
6. Kort B, Katz VL, Watson WJ. The effect of nonobstetric operation during pregnancy. *Surg Gynecol Obstet* 1993;177:371–376.
7. Strickland RA, Oliver WC, Chantigian RC, et al. Subject review, anesthesia, cardiopulmonary bypass, and the pregnant patient. *Mayo Clin Proc* 1991; 66:411–429.
8. Newman B, Lam AM. Induced hypotension for clipping of a cerebral aneurysm during pregnancy. *Anesth Analg* 1986; 65:675–678.
9. Merritt WT, Dickstein R, Beattie C, et al. Liver transplantation during pregnancy: anesthesia for two procedures in the same patient with successful outcome of pregnancy. *Transplant Proc* 1991;23:1996–1997.
10. Hignett R, Fernando R, McGlennan A, et al. A randomized crossover study to determine the effect of a 30° head-up versus a supine position on the functional residual capacity of term parturients. *Anesth Analg* 2011;113:1098–1102.
11. Pilkington S, Carli F, Dakin MJ, et al. Increase in Mallampati score during pregnancy. *Br J Anaesth* 1995;74:638–642.
12. Mhyre JM, Riesner MN, Polley LS, et al. A series of anesthesia-related maternal deaths in Michigan, 1985–2003. *Anesthesiology* 2007;106:1096–1104.
13. Ueland K, Novy MJ, Peterson EW, et al. Maternal cardiovascular dynamics IV. The influence of gestational age on the maternal cardiovascular response to posture and exercise. *Am J Obstet Gynecol* 1969;104:856–864.
14. Hirabayashi Y, Shimizu R, Fukuda H, et al. Effects of the pregnant uterus on the extradural venous plexus in the supine and lateral positions, as determined by magnetic resonance imaging. *Br J Anaesth* 1997;78:317–319.
15. Fagraeus L, Urban BJ, Bromage PR. Spread of epidural analgesia in early pregnancy. *Anesthesiology* 1983;58:184–187.
16. Levy DM, Williams OA, Magides AD, et al. Gastric emptying is delayed at 8–12 weeks' gestation. *Br J Anaesth* 1994;73:237–238.
17. Simpson KH, Stakes AF, Miller M. Pregnancy delays paracetamol absorption and gastric emptying in patients undergoing surgery. *Br J Anaesth* 1988;60: 24–27.
18. Wong CA, Loffredi M, Ganchiff JN, et al. Gastric emptying of water in term pregnancy. *Anesthesiology* 2002;96:1395–1400.
19. Wong CA, McCarthy RJ, Fitzgerald PC, et al. Gastric emptying of water in obese pregnant women at term. *Anesth Analg* 2007;105:751–755.
20. Carp H, Jayaram A, Stoll M. Ultrasound examination of the stomach contents of parturients. *Anesth Analg* 1992;74:683–687.
21. Brock-Utne JG, Dow TG, Dimopoulos GE, et al. Gastric and lower oesophageal sphincter (LOS) pressures in early pregnancy. *Br J Anaesth* 1981;53:381–384.
22. Cheek TG, Baird E. Anesthesia for nonobstetric surgery: maternal and fetal considerations. *Clin Obstet Gynecol* 2009;52:535–545.
23. Fill Malfertheiner S, Malfertheiner MV, Mönkemüller K, et al. Gastroesophageal reflux disease and management in advanced pregnancy: a prospective survey. *Digestion* 2009;79:115–120.
24. Chunilal SD, Bates SM. Venous thromboembolism in pregnancy: diagnosis, management and prevention. *Thromb Haemost* 2009;101:428–438.
25. Beilin Y, Zahn J, Comerford M. Safe epidural analgesia in thirty parturients with platelet counts between 69,000 and 98,000 mm-3. *Anesth Analg* 1997; 85:385–388.
26. Chan MT, Mainland P, Gin T. Minimum alveolar concentration of halothane and enflurane are decreased in early pregnancy. *Anesthesiology* 1996;85:782–786.
27. Sullivan FM. The susceptibility of the fetus and child to chemical pollutants. Animal tests to screen for human teratogens. *Pediatrics* 1974;53:822–823.
28. Leck IM, Millar EL. Incidence of malformations since the introduction of thalidomide. *Br Med J* 1962;2:16–20.
29. Physicians' C, 64th ed. Montvale: PDR Network, LLC, 2009:215.
30. Nava-Ocampo AA, Koren G. Human teratogens and evidence-based teratogen risk counseling: the Motherisk approach. *Clin Obstet Gynecol* 2007;50:123–131.
31. Fink BR, Shepard TH, Blandau RJ. Teratogenic activity of nitrous oxide. *Nature* 1967;214:146–148.
32. Marx GF, Joshi CW, Orkin LR. Placental transmission of nitrous oxide. *Anesthesiology* 1970;32:429–432.
33. Keeling PA, Rocke DA, Nunn JF, et al. Folinic acid protection against nitrous oxide teratogenicity in the rat. *Br J Anaesth* 1986;58:528–534.
34. Baden JM, Serra M, Mazze RI. Inhibition of rat fetal methionine synthetase by nitrous oxide. *Br J Anaesth* 1987;59:1040–1043.
35. Mazze RI, Fujinaga M, Rice SA, et al. Reproductive and teratogenic effects of nitrous oxide, halothane, isoflurane and enflurane in Sprague-Dawley rats. *Anesthesiology* 1986;64:339–344.
36. Duncan PG, Pope WDB, Cohen MM, et al. Fetal risk of anesthesia and surgery during pregnancy. *Anesthesiology* 1986;64:790–794.
37. Mazze RI, Kallen B. Appendectomy during pregnancy: a Swedish registry study of 778 cases. *Obstet Gynecol* 1991;77:835–840.
38. Bashford A, Fink B. The teratogenicity of halothane in the rat. *Anesthesiology* 1968;29:1167–1173.
39. Mazze RI, Wilson AI, Rice SA, et al. Fetal development in mice exposed to isoflurane. *Teratology* 1985;32:339–345.

40. Novitt AD, Gilani SH. Abnormal embryogenesis induced by thiopental. *J Clin Pharmacol* 1979;19:697–700.

41. He YL, Seno H, Sasaki K, et al. The influences of maternal albumin concentrations on the placental transfer of propofol in human dually perfused cotyledon in vitro. *Anesth Analg* 2002;94:1312–1314.

42. Coetsier T, Dhont M, De Sutter P, et al. Propofol anaesthesia for ultrasound guided oocyte retrieval: accumulation of the anaesthetic agent in follicular fluid. *Hum Reprod* 1992;7:1422–1424.

43. Endler GC, Stout M, Magyar DM, et al. Follicular fluid concentrations of thiopental and thiamylal during laparoscopy for oocyte retrieval. *Fertil Steril* 1987;48:828–833.

44. Pierce ET, Smalky M, Alper MM, et al. Comparison of pregnancy rates following gamete intrafallopian transfer (GIFT) under general anesthesia with thiopental sodium or propofol. *J Clin Anesth* 1992;4:394–398.

45. Fresno L, Andaluz A, Moll X, et al. Placental transfer of etomidate in pregnant ewes after an intravenous bolus dose and continuous infusion. *Vet J* 2008; 175:395–402.

46. Ellingson A, Haram K, Sagen N, et al. Transplacental passage of ketamine after intravenous administration. *Acta Anaesthesiol Scand* 1977;21:41–44.

47. Lee H, Nagele RG. Neural tube defects caused by local anesthetics in early chick embryos. *Teratology* 1985;31:119–127.

48. Abdel-Rahman MS, Ismail EE. Teratogenic effect of ketamine and cocaine in CF-1 mice. *Teratology* 2000;61:291–296.

49. Young C, Jevtovic-Todorovic V, Qin YQ, et al. Potential of ketamine and midazolam individually or in combination, to induce apoptotic neurodegeneration in the infant mouse brain. *Br J Pharmacol* 2005;146:189–197.

50. Anand KJ. Anesthetic neurotoxicity in newborns: Should we change clinical practice? *Anesthesiology* 2007;107:2–4.

51. Abu-Halaweh SA, Al Oweidi AK, Abu-Malooh H, et al. Intravenous dexmedetomidine infusion for labour analgesia in patient with preeclampsia. *Eur J Anaesthesiol* 2009;26:86–87.

52. Ala-Kokko TI, Pienimäki P, Lampela E, et al. Transfer of clonidine and dexmedetomidine across the isolated perfused human placenta. *Acta Anaesthesiol Scand* 1997;41:313–319.

53. Tariq M, Cerny V, Elfaki I, et al. Effects of subchronic versus acute in utero exposure to dexmedetomidine on foetal developments in rats. *Basic Clin Pharmacol Toxicol* 2008;103:180–185.

54. Wee EL, Zimmerman EF. Involvement of GABA in palate morphogenesis and its relation to diazepam teratogenesis in two mouse strains. *Teratology* 1983;28:15–22.

55. Safra MJ, Oakley GP Jr. Association between cleft lip with or without cleft palate and prenatal exposure to diazepam. *Lancet* 1975;2:478–480.

56. Saxen I, Saxen L. Association between maternal intake of diazepam and oral cleft lip. *Lancet* 1975;2:498.

57. Shiono PH, Mills JL. Oral clefts and diazepam use during pregnancy. *NEJM* 1984; 311:919–920.

58. Rosenberg L, Mitchell AA, Parsells JL, et al. Lack of relation of oral clefts to diazepam use during pregnancy. *N Engl J Med* 1983;309:1282–1285.

59. Laegreid L, Olegård R, Conradi N, et al. Congenital malformations and maternal consumption of benzodiazepines: a case-control study. *Dev Med Child Neurol* 1990;32:432–441.

60. Dolovich LR, Addis A, Vaillancourt JM, et al. Benzodiazepine use in pregnancy and major malformations or oral cleft: meta-analysis of cohort and case-control studies. *BMJ* 1998;317:839–843.

61. Wikner BN, Stiller CO, Bergman U, et al. Use of benzodiazepines and benzodiazepine receptor agonists during pregnancy: neonatal outcome and congenital malformations. *Pharmacoepidemiol Drug Saf* 2007;16:1203–1210.

62. Rosen MA. Management of anesthesia for the pregnant surgical patient. *Anesthesiology* 1999;91:1159–1163.

63. Craft JB Jr, Coaldrake LA, Bolan JC, et al. Placental passage and uterine effects of fentanyl. *Anesth Analg* 1983; 62:894–898.

64. Geber W, Schramm L. Congenital malformations of the central nervous system produced by narcotic analgesics in the hamster. *Am J Obstet Gynecol* 1975; 123:705–713.

65. Fuginawa M, Stevenson J, Mazze R. Reproductive and teratogenic effects of fentanyl in Sprague-Dawley rats. *Teratology* 1986;34:51–57.

66. Fujinaga M, Baden JM, Mazze RI. Developmental toxicity of nondepolarizing muscle relaxants in cultured rat embryos. *Anesthesiology* 1992;76:999–1003.

67. Fujinaga M. Assessment of teratogenic effects of lidocaine in rat embryos cultured in vitro. *Anesthesiology* 1998;89:1553–1558.

68. Fujinaga M, Mazze RI. Reproductive and teratogenic effects of lidocaine in Sprague-Dawley rats. *Anesthesiology* 1986;65:626–632.

69. Cohen EN, Bellville JW, Brown BW Jr. Anesthesia, pregnancy, and miscarriage: a study of operating room nurses and anesthetists. *Anesthesiology* 1971; 35:343–347.

70. Cohen EN, Brown BW, Wu ML, et al. Occupational disease in dentistry and chronic exposure to trace anesthetic gases. *JADA* 1980;101:21–31.

71. American Society of Anesthesiologists. Ad Hoc Committee: Occupational disease among operating room personnel: A national study. *Anesthesiology* 1974;41:321–340.

72. Fink BR, Cullen BF. Anesthetic pollution: What is happening to us? *Anesthesiology* 1976;45:79–83.

73. Walts LF, Forsythe AB, Moore G. Critique: Occupational disease among operating room personnel. *Anesthesiology* 1975;42:608–611.

74. Ericson HA, Källén AJ. Hospitalization for miscarriage and delivery outcome among Swedish nurses working in operating rooms 1973–1978. *Anesth Analg* 1985;64:981–988.

75. Smith BE. Fetal prognosis after anesthesia during gestation. *Anesth Analg* 1963;42:521–526.

76. Shnider SM, Webster GM. Maternal and fetal hazards of surgery during pregnancy. *Am J Obstet Gynecol* 1965;92:891–900.

77. Kort B, Katz VL, Watson WJ. *Surg Gynecol Obstet* 1993;177:371–376.

78. Visser BC, Glasgow RE, Mulvihill KK, et al. Safety and timing of nonobstetric abdominal surgery in pregnancy. *Dig Surg* 2001;18:409–417.

79. Kallen B, Mazze RI. Neural tube defects and first trimester operations. *Teratology* 1990;41;L717–L720.

80. Sylvester GC, Khoury MJ, Lu X, et al. First-trimester anesthesia exposure and the risk of central nervous system defects: A population-based case-control studies. *Am J Public Health* 1994;84:1757–1760.

81. Czeizel AE, Pataki T, Rockenbauer M. Reproductive outcome after exposure to surgery under anesthesia during pregnancy. *Arch Gynecol Obstet* 1998; 261:193–199.

82. Werboff J, Kesner R. Learning deficits of offspring after administration of tranquilizing drugs to the mothers. *Nature* 1963;197:106–107.

83. Smith RF, Bowman RE, Katz J. Behavioral effects of exposure to halothane during early development in the rat: sensitive period during pregnancy. *Anesthesiology* 1978;49:319–323.

84. Chalon J, Tang CK, Ramanathan S, et al. Exposure to halothane and enflurane affects learning function of murine progeny. *Anesth Analg* 1981;60:794–797.

85. Jevtovic-Todorovic V, Carter LB. The anesthetics nitrous oxide and ketamine are more neurotoxic to old than to young rat brain. *Neurobiol Aging* 2005; 26:947–956.

86. Jevtovic-Todorovic V, Hartman RE, Izumi Y, et al. Early exposure to common anesthetic agents causes widespread neurodegeneration in the developing rat brain and persistent learning deficits. *J Neurosci* 2003;23:876–882.

87. Wilder RT, Flick RP, Sprung J, et al. Early exposure to anesthesia and learning disabilities in a population-based birth cohort. *Anesthesiology* 2009;110:796–804.

88. Kalkman CJ, Peelen L, Moons KG, et al. Behavior and development in children and age at the time of first anesthetic exposure. *Anesthesiology* 2009;110:805–812.

89. www.fda.gov/ohrms/dockets/ac/07/transcripts/2007-4285t1.pdf

90. Panigel M. Placental perfusion experiments. *Am J Obstet Gynecol* 1962; 84:1664–1683.

91. Khazin AF, Hon EH, Hehre FW. Effects of maternal hyperoxia on the fetus. I. Oxygen tension. *Am J Obstet Gynecol* 1971;109:628–637.

92. Levinson G, Shnider SM, de Lorimier AA, et al. Effects of maternal hyperventilation on uterine blood flow and fetal oxygenation and acid-base status. *Anesthesiology* 1974;40:340–347.

93. Motoyama EK, Rivard G, Acheson F, et al. The effect of changes in maternal pH and P-CO2 on the P-O2 of fetal lambs. *Anesthesiology* 1967;28:891–903.

94. Kamban JR, Handte RE, Brown WU, et al. The effect of normal and preeclamptic pregnancies on the oxyhemoglobin dissociation curve. *Anesthesiology* 1986;65:426–427.

95. Oats JN, Vasey DP, Waldron BA. Effects of ketamine on the pregnant uterus. *Br J Anaesth* 1979;51:1163–1166.

96. Ngan Kee WD, Khaw KS, Ng FF. Prevention of hypotension during spinal anesthesia for cesarean delivery: an effective technique using combination phenylephrine infusion and crystalloid cohydration. *Anesthesiology* 2005; 103:744–750.

97. Elerding SC. Laparoscopic cholecystectomy in pregnancy. *Am J Surg* 1993; 165:625–627.

98. Nezhat FR, Tazuke S, Nezhat CH, et al. Laparoscopy during pregnancy: a literature review. *J Soc Laparoendosc Surg* 1997;1:17–27.

99. Reedy MB, Kallen B, Kuehl TJ. Laparoscopy during pregnancy: a study of five fetal outcome parameters with use of the Swedish Health Registry. *Am J Obstet Gynecol* 1997;177:673–679.

100. Yumi H. Guidelines for diagnosis, treatment, and use of laparoscopy for surgical problems during pregnancy: this statement was reviewed and approved by the Board of Governors of the Society of American Gastrointestinal and Endoscopic Surgeons (SAGES), September 2007. It was prepared by the SAGES Guidelines Committee. *Surg Endosc* 2008;22:849–861.

101. Liu PL, Warren TM, Ostheimer GW, et al. Foetal monitoring in parturients undergoing surgery unrelated to pregnancy. *Can Anaesth Soc J* 1985;32:525–532.

102. Katz JD, Hook R, Barash PG. Fetal heart rate monitoring in pregnant patients undergoing surgery. *Am J Obstet Gynecol* 1976;125:267–269.

103. American College of Obstetricians and Gynecologists Committee on Obstetric Practice. Nonobstetric Surgery in Pregnancy. ACOG Committee Opinion No. 284, 2003. *Obstet Gynecol* 2003;102:431.

104. Rout CC, Rocke A, Gouws E. Intravenous ranitidine reduces the risk of acid aspiration of gastric contents at emergency cesarean section. *Anesth Analg* 1993;76:156–161.

105. Wyner J, Cohen SE. Gastric volume in early pregnancy. Effect of metoclopramide. *Anesthesiology* 1982;57:209–212.

106. Park GE, Hauch MA, Curlin F, et al. The effects of varying volumes of crystalloid administration before cesarean delivery on maternal hemodynamics and colloid osmotic pressure. *Anesth Analg* 1996;83:299–303.

107. Shankar KB, Moseley H, Kumar Y, et al. Arterial to end tidal carbon dioxide tension difference during caesarean section anaesthesia. *Anaesthesia* 1986;41:698–702.

108. Heymann MA, Rudolph AM. Effects of acetylsalicylic acid on the ductus arteriosus and circulation in fetal lambs in utero. *Circ Res* 1976;38:418–422.

Guidelines for Neuraxial Anesthesia in Obstetrics

These guidelines apply to the use of neuraxial anesthesia and labor anesthesia or analgesia in which local anesthetics are administered to the parturient during labor and delivery. They are intended to encourage quality patient care but cannot guarantee any specific patient outcome. Since the availability of anesthesia resources may vary, members are responsible for interpreting and establishing the guidelines for their own institutions and practices. These guidelines are subject to revision from time to time as warranted by the evolution of technology and practice.

Guideline I

Neuraxial anesthesia should be initiated and maintained only in locations in which appropriate resuscitation equipment and drugs are immediately available to manage procedurally related problems.

Resuscitation equipment should include, but is not limited to sources of oxygen and suction, equipment to maintain an airway and perform endotracheal intubation, a means to provide positive pressure ventilation, and drugs and equipment for cardiopulmonary resuscitation.

Guideline II

Neuraxial anesthesia should be initiated by a physician with appropriate privileges and maintained by or under the medical direction (1) of such an individual.

Physicians should be approved through the institutional credentialing process to initiate and direct the maintenance of obstetric anesthesia and to manage procedurally related complications.

Guideline III

Neuraxial anesthesia should not be administered until: [1] the patient has been examined by a qualified individual (2); and [2] a physician with obstetrical privileges to perform operative vaginal or cesarean delivery, who has knowledge of the maternal and fetal status and the progress of labor, and who approves the initiation of labor anesthesia, is readily available

to supervise the labor and manage any obstetric complications that may arise.

Under circumstances defined by department protocol, qualified personnel may perform the initial pelvic examination. The physician responsible for the patient's obstetrical care should be informed of her status so that a decision can be made regarding present risk and further management (2).

Guideline IV

An intravenous infusion should be established before initiation of neuraxial anesthesia and maintained throughout the duration of the neuraxial anesthetic.

Guideline V

Neuraxial anesthesia for labor and/or vaginal delivery requires that the parturient's vital signs and the fetal heart rate be monitored and documented by a qualified individual. Additional monitoring appropriate to the clinical condition of the parturient and the fetus should be employed when indicated. When extensive neuraxial blockade is administered for complicated vaginal delivery, the standards for basic anesthetic monitoring (3) should be applied.

Guideline VI

Neuraxial anesthesia for cesarean delivery requires that the standards for basic anesthetic monitoring (3) be applied and that a physician with privileges in obstetrics be immediately available.

Guideline VII

Qualified personnel, other than the anesthesiologist attending the mother, should be immediately available to assume responsibility for resuscitation of the newborn (3).

The primary responsibility of the anesthesiologist is to provide care to the mother. If the anesthesiologist is also requested to provide brief assistance in the care of the newborn, the benefit to the child must be compared to the risk to the mother.

Guideline VIII

A physician with appropriate privileges should remain readily available during the neuraxial anesthetic to manage

Committee of Origin: Obstetrical Anesthesia

Approved by the ASA House of Delegates on October 12, 1988, and last amended on October 20, 2010. Reprinted with permission of the American Society of Anesthesiologists, 520 N. Northwest Highway, Park Ridge, Illinois 60068-2573.

anesthetic complications until the patient's postanesthesia condition is satisfactory and stable.

Guideline IX

All patients recovering from neuraxial anesthesia should receive appropriate postanesthesia care. Following cesarean delivery and/or extensive neuraxial blockade, the standards for postanesthesia care (4) should be applied.

Guideline X

There should be a policy to assure availability in the facility of a physician to manage complications and to provide cardiopulmonary resuscitation for patients receiving post-anesthesia care.

REFERENCES

1. The Anesthesia Care Team (Approved by ASA House of Delegates 10/26/82 and last amended on 10/18/2006).
2. American Academy of Pediatrics and American College of Obstetricians and Gynecologists. Guidelines for Perinatal Care, 5th ed. Elk Grove Village, IL: AAP; Washington, DC: ACOG, 2002.
3. Standards for Basic Anesthetic Monitoring (Approved by ASA House of Delegates 10/21/86 and last amended on 10/25/2005).
4. Standards for Postanesthesia Care (Approved by ASA House of Delegates 10/12/88 and last amended on 10/27/04).

Practice Guidelines for Obstetric Anesthesia

An Updated Report by the American Society of Anesthesiologists Task Force on Obstetric Anesthesia*

PRACTICE guidelines are systematically developed recommendations that assist the practitioner and patient in making decisions about healthcare. These recommendations may be adopted, modified, or rejected according to clinical needs and constraints and are not intended to replace local institutional policies. In addition, practice guidelines are not intended as standards or absolute requirements, and their use cannot guarantee any specific outcome. Practice guidelines are subject to revision as warranted by the evolution of medical knowledge, technology, and practice. They provide basic recommendations that are supported by a synthesis and analysis of the current literature, expert opinion, open forum commentary, and clinical feasibility data.

This update includes data published since the "Practice Guidelines for Obstetrical Anesthesia" were adopted by the American Society of Anesthesiologists (ASA) in 1998; it also includes data and recommendations for a wider range of techniques than was previously addressed.

■ METHODOLOGY

A. Definition of Perioperative Obstetric Anesthesia

For the purposes of these guidelines, *obstetric anesthesia* refers to peripartum anesthetic and analgesic activities performed during labor and vaginal delivery, cesarean delivery, removal of retained placenta, and postpartum tubal ligation.

*Developed by the American Society of Anesthesiologists Task Force on Obstetric Anesthesia: Joy L. Hawkins, M.D. (Chair), Denver, Colorado; James F. Arens, M.D., Houston, Texas; Brenda A Bucklin, M.D., Denver, Colorado; Richard T. Connis, Ph.D., Woodinville, Washington; Patricia A. Dailey, M.D., Hillsborough, California; David R. Gambling, M.B.B.S., San Diego, California; David G. Nickinovich, Ph.D., Bellevue, Washington; Linda S. Polley, M.D., Ann Arbor, Michigan; Lawrence C. Tsen, M.D., Boston, Massachusetts; David J. Wlody, M.D., Brooklyn, New York; and Kathryn J. Zuspan, M.D., Stillwater, Minnesota.

Submitted for publication October 31, 2006. Accepted for publication October 31, 2006. Supported by the American Society of Anesthesiologists under the direction of James F. Arens, M.D., Chair, Committee on Standards and Practice Parameters. Approved by the House of Delegates on October 18, 2006. A list of the references used to develop these Guidelines is available by writing to the American Society of Anesthesiologists.

Address reprint requests to the American Society of Anesthesiologists: 520 North Northwest Highway, Park Ridge, Illinois 60068-2573. This Practice Guideline, as well as all published ASA Practice Parameters, may be obtained at no cost through the Journal Web site, www.anesthesiology.org.

B. Purposes of the Guidelines

The purposes of these guidelines are to enhance the quality of anesthetic care for obstetric patients, improve patient safety by reducing the incidence and severity of anesthesia-related complications, and increase patient satisfaction.

C. Focus

These guidelines focus on the anesthetic management of pregnant patients during labor, nonoperative delivery, operative delivery, and selected aspects of postpartum care and analgesia (i.e., neuraxial opioids for postpartum analgesia after neuraxial anesthesia for cesarean delivery). The intended patient population includes, but is not limited to, intrapartum and postpartum patients with uncomplicated pregnancies or with common obstetric problems. The guidelines do not apply to patients undergoing surgery during pregnancy, gynecologic patients, or parturients with chronic medical disease (e.g., severe cardiac, renal, or neurologic disease). In addition, these guidelines do not address (1) postpartum analgesia for vaginal delivery, (2) analgesia after tubal ligation, or (3) postoperative analgesia after general anesthesia (GA) for cesarean delivery.

D. Application

These guidelines are intended for use by anesthesiologists. They also may serve as a resource for other anesthesia providers and healthcare professionals who advise or care for patients who will receive anesthetic care during labor, delivery, and the immediate postpartum period.

E. Task Force Members and Consultants

The ASA appointed a Task Force of 11 members to (1) review the published evidence, (2) obtain the opinion of a panel of consultants including anesthesiologists and nonanesthesiologist physicians concerned with obstetric anesthesia and analgesia, and (3) obtain opinions from practitioners likely to be affected by the guidelines. The Task Force included anesthesiologists in both private and academic practices from various geographic areas of the United States and two consulting methodologists from the ASA Committee on Standards and Practice Parameters.

The Task Force developed the guidelines by means of a seven-step process. First, they reached consensus on the criteria for evidence. Second, original published research studies from peer-reviewed journals relevant to obstetric anesthesia were reviewed. Third, the panel of expert consultants was asked to (1) participate in opinion surveys on the effectiveness of various peripartum management strategies and (2) review and comment on a draft of the guidelines developed by the Task Force. Fourth, opinions about the guideline recommendations were solicited from active members of the ASA who provide obstetric anesthesia. Fifth, the Task Force held open forums at two major national meetings[†] to solicit input on its draft recommendations. Sixth, the consultants were surveyed to assess their opinions on the feasibility of implementing the guidelines. Seventh, all available information was used to build consensus within the Task Force to finalize the guidelines (Appendix 1).

F. Availability and Strength of Evidence

Preparation of these guidelines followed a rigorous methodologic process (Appendix 2). To convey the findings in a concise and easy-to-understand fashion, these guidelines use several descriptive terms. When sufficient number of studies are available for evaluation, the following terms describe the strength of the findings.

Support: Meta-analysis of a sufficient number of randomized controlled trials[‡] indicates a statistically significant relationship ($P < 0.01$) between a clinical intervention and a clinical outcome.

Suggest: Information from case reports and observational studies permits inference of a relationship between an intervention and an outcome. A meta-analytic assessment of this type of qualitative or descriptive information is not conducted.

Equivocal: Either a meta-analysis has not found significant differences among groups or conditions, or there is insufficient quantitative information to conduct a meta-analysis and information collected from case reports and observational studies does *not* permit inference of a relationship between an intervention and an outcome.

The *lack* of scientific evidence in the literature is described by the following terms.

Silent: No identified studies address the specified relationship between an intervention and outcome.

Insufficient: There are too few published studies to investigate a relationship between an intervention and outcome.

Inadequate: The available studies cannot be used to assess the relationship between an intervention and an outcome. These studies either do not meet the criteria for content as defined in the focus section of these guidelines, or do not permit a clear causal interpretation of findings due to methodologic concerns.

Formal survey information is collected from consultants and members of the ASA. The following terms describe survey responses for any specified issue. Responses are solicited on a five-point scale ranging from 1 (strongly disagree) to 5 (strongly agree), with a score of 3 being equivocal. Survey responses are summarized based on median values as follows:

Strongly Agree: Median score of 5 (at least 50% of the responses are 5)

Agree: Median score of 4 (at least 50% of the responses are 4 or 4 and 5)

Equivocal: Median score of 3 (at least 50% of the responses are 3, or no other response category or combination of similar categories contain at least 50% of the responses)

Disagree: Median score of 2 (at least 50% of the responses are 2 or 1 and 2)

Strongly Disagree: Median score of 1 (at least 50% of the responses are 1)

▪ GUIDELINES

I. Preanesthetic Evaluation

History and Physical Examination. Although comparative studies are insufficient to evaluate the peripartum impact of conducting a focused history (e.g., reviewing medical records) or a physical examination, the literature reports certain patient or clinical characteristics that may be associated with obstetric complications. These characteristics include, but are not limited to, preeclampsia, pregnancy-related hypertensive disorders, HELLP syndrome, obesity, and diabetes.

The consultants and ASA members both strongly agree that a directed history and physical examination, as well as communication between anesthetic and obstetric providers, reduces maternal, fetal, and neonatal complications.

Recommendations. The anesthesiologist should conduct a focused history and physical examination before providing anesthesia care. This should include, but is not limited to, a maternal health and anesthetic history, a relevant obstetric history, a baseline blood pressure measurement, and an airway, heart, and lung examination, consistent with the ASA "Practice Advisory for Preanesthesia Evaluation."[§] When a neuraxial anesthetic is planned or placed, the patient's back should be examined.

Recognition of significant anesthetic or obstetric risk factors should encourage consultation between the obstetrician and the anesthesiologist. A communication system should be in place to encourage early and ongoing contact between obstetric providers, anesthesiologists, and other members of the multidisciplinary team.

Intrapartum Platelet Count. The literature is insufficient to assess whether a routine platelet count can predict anesthesia-related complications in uncomplicated parturients. The literature suggests that a platelet count is clinically useful for parturients with suspected pregnancy-related hypertensive disorders, such as preeclampsia or HELLP syndrome, and for other disorders associated with coagulopathy.

The ASA members are equivocal, but the consultants agree that obtaining a routine intrapartum platelet count does *not* reduce maternal anesthetic complications. Both the consultants and ASA members agree that, for patients with suspected preeclampsia, a platelet count reduces maternal anesthetic complications. The consultants strongly agree and the ASA members agree that a platelet count reduces maternal anesthetic complications for patients with suspected coagulopathy.

Recommendations. A specific platelet count predictive of neuraxial anesthetic complications has not been determined. The anesthesiologist's decision to order or require a platelet count should be individualized and based on a patient's history, physical examination, and clinical signs. A routine platelet count is not necessary in the healthy parturient.

Blood Type and Screen. The literature is insufficient to determine whether obtaining a blood type and screen is associated with fewer maternal anesthetic complications. In addition, the literature is insufficient to determine whether a blood cross-match is necessary for healthy and uncomplicated parturients. The consultants and ASA members agree

---

[†]International Anesthesia Research Society, 80th Clinical and Scientific Congress, San Francisco, California, March 25, 2006; and Society of Obstetric Anesthesia and Perinatology 38th Annual Meeting, Hollywood, Florida, April 29, 2006.

[‡]A prospective nonrandomized controlled trial may be included in a meta-analysis under certain circumstances if specific statistical criteria are met.

[§]American Society of Anesthesiologists Task Force on Preanesthesia Evaluation: Practice advisory for preanesthesia evaluation. *Anesthesiology* 2002;96:485–496.

that an intrapartum blood sample should be sent to the blood bank for all parturients.

Recommendations. A routine blood cross-match is not necessary for healthy and uncomplicated parturients for vaginal or operative delivery. The decision whether to order or require a blood type and screen, or cross-match, should be based on maternal history, anticipated hemorrhagic complications (e.g., placenta accreta in a patient with placenta previa and previous uterine surgery), and local institutional policies.

Preanesthetic Recording of the Fetal Heart Rate. The literature suggests that anesthetic and analgesic agents may influence the fetal heart rate pattern. There is insufficient literature to demonstrate that preanesthetic recording of the fetal heart rate prevents fetal or neonatal complications. Both the consultants and ASA members agree, however, that preanesthetic recording of the fetal heart rate reduces fetal and neonatal complications.

Recommendations. The fetal heart rate should be monitored by a qualified individual before and after administration of neuraxial analgesia for labor. The Task Force recognizes that *continuous* electronic recording of the fetal heart rate may not be necessary in every clinical setting and may not be possible during initiation of neuraxial anesthesia.

II. Aspiration Prevention

Clear Liquids. There is insufficient published evidence to draw conclusions about the relationship between fasting times for clear liquids and the risk of emesis/reflux or pulmonary aspiration during labor. The consultants and ASA members both agree that oral intake of clear liquids during labor improves maternal comfort and satisfaction. Although the ASA members are equivocal, the consultants agree that oral intake of clear liquids during labor *does not* increase maternal complications.

Recommendations. The oral intake of modest amounts of clear liquids may be allowed for uncomplicated laboring patients. The uncomplicated patient undergoing elective cesarean delivery may have modest amounts of clear liquids up to 2 hours before induction of anesthesia. Examples of clear liquids include, but are not limited to, water, fruit juices without pulp, carbonated beverages, clear tea, black coffee, and sports drinks.|| The volume of liquid ingested is less important than the presence of particulate matter in the liquid ingested. However, patients with additional risk factors for aspiration (e.g., morbid obesity, diabetes, difficult airway) or patients at increased risk for operative delivery (e.g., non-reassuring fetal heart rate pattern) may have further restrictions of oral intake, determined on a case-by-case basis.

Solids. A specific fasting time for solids that is predictive of maternal anesthetic complications has not been determined. There is insufficient published evidence to address the safety of *any* particular fasting period for solids in obstetric patients. The consultants and ASA members both agree that the oral intake of solids during labor increases maternal complications. They both strongly agree that patients undergoing either elective cesarean delivery or postpartum tubal ligation should undergo a fasting period of 6 to 8 hours depending on the type of food ingested (e.g., fat content).|| The Task Force recognizes that in laboring patients the timing of delivery is uncertain; therefore, compliance with a predetermined fasting period beforwe nonelective surgical procedures is not always possible.

|| American Society of Anesthesiologists Task Force on Preoperative Fasting: Practice guidelines for preoperative fasting and the use of pharmacologic agents to reduce the risk of pulmonary aspiration. *Anesthesiology* 1999;90:896–905.

Recommendations. Solid foods should be avoided in laboring patients. The patient undergoing elective surgery (e.g., scheduled cesarean delivery or postpartum tubal ligation) should undergo a fasting period for solids of 6 to 8 hours depending on the type of food ingested (e.g., fat content).||

Antacids, H₂ Receptor Antagonists, and Metoclopramide. The literature does not sufficiently examine the relationship between reduced gastric acidity and the frequency of emesis, pulmonary aspiration, morbidity, or mortality in obstetric patients who have aspirated gastric contents. Published evidence supports the efficacy of preoperative nonparticulate antacids (e.g., sodium citrate, sodium bicarbonate) in decreasing gastric acidity during the peripartum period. However, the literature is insufficient to examine the impact of nonparticulate antacids on gastric volume. The literature suggests that H_2 receptor antagonists are effective in decreasing gastric acidity in obstetric patients and supports the efficacy of metoclopramide in reducing peripartum nausea and vomiting. The consultants and ASA members agree that the administration of a nonparticulate antacid before operative procedures reduces maternal complications.

Recommendations. Before surgical procedures (i.e., cesarean delivery, postpartum tubal ligation), practitioners should consider the timely administration of nonparticulate antacids, H_2 receptor antagonists, and/or metoclopramide for aspiration prophylaxis.

III. Anesthetic Care for Labor and Vaginal Delivery

Overview. Not all women require anesthetic care during labor or delivery. For women who request pain relief for labor and/or delivery, there are many effective analgesic techniques available. Maternal request represents sufficient justification for pain relief. In addition, maternal medical and obstetric conditions may warrant the provision of neuraxial techniques to improve maternal and neonatal outcome.

The choice of analgesic technique depends on the medical status of the patient, progress of labor, and resources at the facility. When sufficient resources (e.g., anesthesia and nursing staff) are available, neuraxial catheter techniques should be one of the analgesic options offered. The choice of a specific neuraxial block should be individualized and based on anesthetic risk factors, obstetric risk factors, patient preferences, progress of labor, and resources at the facility.

When neuraxial catheter techniques are used for analgesia during labor or vaginal delivery, the primary goal is to provide adequate maternal analgesia with minimal motor block (e.g., achieved with the administration of local anesthetics at low concentrations with or without opioids).

When a neuraxial technique is chosen, appropriate resources for the treatment of complications (e.g., hypotension, systemic toxicity, high spinal anesthesia) should be available. If an opioid is added, treatments for related complications (e.g., pruritus, nausea, respiratory depression) should be available. An intravenous infusion should be established before the initiation of neuraxial analgesia or anesthesia and maintained throughout the duration of the neuraxial analgesic or anesthetic. However, administration of a fixed volume of intravenous fluid is not required before neuraxial analgesia is initiated.

Timing of Neuraxial Analgesia and Outcome of Labor. Meta-analysis of the literature determined that the timing of neuraxial analgesia does not affect the frequency of cesarean delivery. The literature also suggests that other delivery outcomes (i.e., spontaneous or instrumented) are also unaffected. The consultants strongly agree and the ASA members agree that early initiation of epidural analgesia (i.e., at cervical dilations of less than 5 cm vs. equal to or greater than 5 cm) improves analgesia. They both *disagree* that motor block or maternal, fetal, or neonatal side effects are increased by early administration.

Recommendations. Patients in early labor (i.e., <5 cm dilation) should be given the option of neuraxial analgesia when this service is available. Neuraxial analgesia should not be withheld on the basis of achieving an arbitrary cervical dilation, and should be offered on an individualized basis. Patients may be reassured that the use of neuraxial analgesia does not increase the incidence of cesarean delivery.

Neuraxial Analgesia and Trial of Labor after Previous Cesarean Delivery. Nonrandomized comparative studies suggest that epidural analgesia may be used in a trial of labor for previous cesarean delivery patients without adversely affecting the incidence of vaginal delivery. Randomized comparisons of epidural versus other anesthetic techniques were not found. The consultants and ASA members agree that neuraxial techniques improve the likelihood of vaginal delivery for patients attempting vaginal birth after cesarean delivery.

Recommendations. Neuraxial techniques should be offered to patients attempting vaginal birth after previous cesarean delivery. For these patients, it is also appropriate to consider early placement of a neuraxial catheter that can be used later for labor analgesia, or for anesthesia in the event of operative delivery.

Early Insertion of a Spinal or Epidural Catheter for Complicated Parturients. The literature is insufficient to assess whether, when caring for the complicated parturient, the early insertion of a spinal or epidural catheter, with later administration of analgesia, improves maternal or neonatal outcomes. The consultants and ASA members agree that early insertion of a spinal or epidural catheter for complicated parturients reduces maternal complications.

Recommendations. Early insertion of a spinal or epidural catheter for obstetric (e.g., twin gestation or preeclampsia) or anesthetic indications (e.g., anticipated difficult airway or obesity) should be considered to reduce the need for GA if an emergent procedure becomes necessary. In these cases, the insertion of a spinal or epidural catheter may precede the onset of labor or a patient's request for labor analgesia.

Continuous Infusion Epidural Analgesia

CIE Compared with Parenteral Opioids. The literature suggests that the use of continuous infusion epidural (CIE) local anesthetics with or without opioids provides greater quality of analgesia compared with parenteral (i.e., intravenous or intramuscular) opioids. The consultants and ASA members strongly agree that CIE local anesthetics with or without opioids provide improved analgesia compared with parenteral opioids.

Meta-analysis of the literature indicates that there is a longer duration of labor, with an average duration of 24 minutes for the second stage, and a lower frequency of spontaneous vaginal delivery when continuous epidural local anesthetics are administered compared with *intravenous* opioids. Meta-analysis of the literature determined that there are no differences in the frequency of cesarean delivery. Neither the consultants nor ASA members agree that CIE local anesthetics compared with parenteral opioids significantly (1) increase the duration of labor, (2) decrease the chance of spontaneous delivery, (3) increase maternal side effects, or (4) increase fetal and neonatal side effects.

CIE Compared with Single-injection Spinal. There is insufficient literature to assess the analgesic efficacy of CIE local anesthetics with or without opioids compared to *single-injection spinal opioids* with or without local anesthetics. The consultants are equivocal, but the ASA members agree that CIE local anesthetics improve analgesia compared with single-injection spinal opioids; both the consultants and ASA members are equivocal regarding the frequency of motor block. The consultants are equivocal, but the ASA members disagree that the use of CIE compared with single-injection spinal opioids increases the duration of labor. They both *disagree* that CIE local anesthetics with or without opioids compared to single-injection spinal opioids with or without local anesthetics decreases the likelihood of spontaneous delivery or increases maternal, fetal, or neonatal side effects.

CIE with and without Opioids. The literature supports the *induction* of analgesia using epidural local anesthetics combined *with opioids* compared with equal concentrations of epidural local anesthetics *without opioids* for improved quality and longer duration of analgesia. The consultants strongly agree and the ASA members agree that the addition of opioids to epidural local anesthetics improves analgesia; they both disagree that fetal or neonatal side effects are increased. The consultants disagree, but the ASA members are equivocal regarding whether the addition of opioids increases maternal side effects.

The literature is insufficient to determine whether induction of analgesia using local anesthetics with opioids compared with *higher concentrations* of epidural local anesthetics without opioids provides improved quality or duration of analgesia. The consultants and ASA members are equivocal regarding improved analgesia, and they both disagree that maternal, fetal, or neonatal side effects are increased using lower concentrations of epidural local anesthetics with opioids.

For *maintenance of analgesia*, the literature suggests that there are no differences in the analgesic efficacy of *low concentrations* of epidural local anesthetics with opioids compared with *higher concentrations* of epidural local anesthetics without opioids. The Task Force notes that the addition of an opioid to a local anesthetic infusion allows an even lower concentration of local anesthetic for providing equally effective analgesia. However, the literature is insufficient to examine whether a bupivacaine infusion concentration of *less than or equal to 0.125%* with an opioid provides comparable or improved analgesia compared with a bupivacaine concentration *greater than* 0.125% without an opioid.[#] Meta-analysis of the literature determined that low concentrations of epidural local anesthetics with opioids compared with higher concentrations of epidural local anesthetics without opioids are associated with reduced motor block. No differences in the duration of labor, mode of delivery, or neonatal outcomes are found when epidural local anesthetics with opioids are compared with epidural local anesthetics without opioids. The literature is insufficient to determine the effects of epidural local anesthetics with opioids on other maternal outcomes (e.g., hypotension, nausea, pruritus, respiratory depression, urinary retention).

The consultants and ASA members both agree that maintenance of epidural analgesia using *low* concentrations of local anesthetics with opioids provides improved analgesia compared with *higher* concentrations of local anesthetics without opioids. The consultants agree, but the ASA members are equivocal regarding the improved likelihood of spontaneous delivery when lower concentrations of local anesthetics with opioids are used. The consultants strongly agree and the ASA members agree that motor block is reduced. They agree that maternal side effects are reduced with this drug combination. They are both equivocal regarding a reduction in fetal and neonatal side effects.

Recommendations. The selected analgesic/anesthetic technique should reflect patient needs and preferences, practitioner preferences or skills, and available resources. The continuous epidural infusion technique may be used for effective analgesia for labor and delivery. When a continuous

---

[#]References to bupivacaine are included for illustrative purposes only, and because bupivacaine is the most extensively studied local anesthetic for continuous infusion epidural analgesia. The Task Force recognizes that other local anesthetics are appropriate for continuous infusion epidural analgesia.

epidural infusion of local anesthetic is selected, an opioid may be added to reduce the concentration of local anesthetic, improve the quality of analgesia, and minimize motor block.

Adequate analgesia for uncomplicated labor and delivery should be administered with the secondary goal of producing as little motor block as possible by using dilute concentrations of local anesthetics with opioids. The lowest concentration of local anesthetic infusion that provides adequate maternal analgesia and satisfaction should be administered. For example, an infusion concentration greater than 0.125% bupivacaine is unnecessary for labor analgesia in most patients.

Single-injection Spinal Opioids with or without Local Anesthetics. The literature suggests that spinal opioids with or without local anesthetics provide effective analgesia during labor without altering the incidence of neonatal complications. There is insufficient literature to compare spinal opioids with parenteral opioids. There is also insufficient literature to compare single-injection spinal opioids *with* local anesthetics versus single-injection spinal opioids *without* local anesthetics.

The consultants strongly agree and the ASA members agree that spinal opioids provide improved analgesia compared with parenteral opioids. They both disagree that, compared with parenteral opioids, spinal opioids increase the duration of labor, decrease the chance of spontaneous delivery, or increase fetal and neonatal side effects. The consultants are equivocal, but the ASA members disagree that maternal side effects are increased with spinal opioids.

Compared with spinal opioids *without* local anesthetics, the consultants and ASA members both agree that spinal opioids *with* local anesthetics provide improved analgesia. They both disagree that the chance of spontaneous delivery is decreased and that fetal and neonatal side effects are increased. They are both equivocal regarding an increase in maternal side effects. However, they both agree that motor block is increased when local anesthetics are added to spinal opioids. Finally, the consultants disagree, but the ASA members are equivocal regarding an increase in the duration of labor.

Recommendations. Single-injection spinal opioids with or without local anesthetics may be used to provide effective, although time-limited, analgesia for labor when spontaneous vaginal delivery is anticipated. If labor is expected to last longer than the analgesic effects of the spinal drugs chosen or if there is a good possibility of operative delivery, a catheter technique instead of a single-injection technique should be considered. A local anesthetic may be added to a spinal opioid to increase duration and improve quality of analgesia. The Task Force notes that the rapid onset of analgesia provided by single-injection spinal techniques may be advantageous for selected patients (e.g., those in advanced labor).

Pencil-point Spinal Needles. The literature supports the use of pencil-point spinal needles compared with cutting-bevel spinal needles to reduce the frequency of post-dural puncture headache. The consultants and ASA members both strongly agree that the use of pencil-point spinal needles reduces maternal complications.

Recommendations. Pencil-point spinal needles should be used instead of cutting-bevel spinal needles to minimize the risk of post-dural puncture headache.

Combined Spinal–Epidural Analgesia. The literature supports a faster onset time and equivalent analgesia with combined spinal–epidural (CSE) local anesthetics with opioids versus epidural local anesthetics with opioids. The literature is equivocal regarding the impact of CSE versus epidural local anesthetics with opioids on maternal satisfaction with analgesia, mode of delivery, hypotension, motor block, nausea, fetal heart rate changes, and Apgar scores. Meta-analysis of the literature indicates that the frequency of pruritus is increased with CSE.

The consultants and ASA members both agree that CSE local anesthetics with opioids provide improved early analgesia compared with epidural local anesthetics with opioids. They are equivocal regarding the impact of CSE with opioids on overall analgesic efficacy, duration of labor, and motor block. The consultants and ASA members both disagree that CSE increases the risk of fetal or neonatal side effects. The consultants disagree, but the ASA members are equivocal regarding whether CSE increases the incidence of maternal side effects.

Recommendations. CSE techniques may be used to provide effective and rapid onset of analgesia for labor.

Patient-controlled Epidural Analgesia. The literature supports the efficacy of patient-controlled epidural analgesia (PCEA) versus CIE in providing equivalent analgesia with reduced drug consumption. Meta-analysis of the literature indicates that the duration of labor is longer with PCEA compared with CIE for the first stage (e.g., an average of 36 minutes) but not the second stage of labor. Meta-analysis of the literature also determined that mode of delivery, frequency of motor block, and Apgar scores are equivalent when PCEA administration is compared with CIE. The literature supports greater analgesic efficacy for PCEA with a background infusion compared with PCEA without a background infusion; meta-analysis of the literature also indicates no differences in the mode of delivery or frequency of motor block. The consultants and ASA members agree that PCEA compared with CIE improves analgesia and reduces the need for anesthetic interventions; they also agree that PCEA improves maternal satisfaction. The consultants and ASA members are equivocal regarding a reduction in motor block, an increased likelihood of spontaneous delivery, or a decrease in maternal side effects with PCEA compared with CIE. They both agree that PCEA with a background infusion improves analgesia, improves maternal satisfaction, and reduces the need for anesthetic intervention. The ASA members are equivocal, but the consultants disagree that a background infusion decreases the chance of spontaneous delivery or increases maternal side effects. The consultants and ASA members are equivocal regarding the effect of a background infusion on the incidence of motor block.

Recommendations. PCEA may be used to provide an effective and flexible approach for the maintenance of labor analgesia. The Task Force notes that the use of PCEA may be preferable to fixed-rate CIE for providing fewer anesthetic interventions and reduced dosages of local anesthetics. PCEA may be used with or without a background infusion.

IV. Removal of Retained Placenta

Anesthetic Techniques. The literature is insufficient to assess whether a particular type of anesthetic is more effective than another for removal of retained placenta. The consultants strongly agree and the ASA members agree that, if a functioning epidural catheter is in place and the patient is hemodynamically stable, epidural anesthesia is the preferred technique for the removal of retained placenta. The consultants and ASA members both agree that, in cases involving major maternal hemorrhage, GA is preferred over neuraxial anesthesia.

Recommendations. The Task Force notes that, in general, there is no preferred anesthetic technique for removal of retained placenta. However, if an epidural catheter is in place and the patient is hemodynamically stable, epidural anesthesia is preferable. Hemodynamic status should be assessed before administering neuraxial anesthesia. Aspiration prophylaxis should be considered. Sedation/analgesia should be titrated carefully due to the potential risks of respiratory depression and pulmonary aspiration during the immediate postpartum period. In cases involving major maternal hemorrhage, GA with an endotracheal tube may be preferable to neuraxial anesthesia.

Uterine Relaxation. The literature suggests that nitroglycerin is effective for uterine relaxation during the removal of retained placenta. The consultants and ASA members both agree that the administration of nitroglycerin for uterine relaxation improves success in removing a retained placenta.

Recommendations. Nitroglycerin may be used as an alternative to terbutaline sulfate or general endotracheal anesthesia with halogenated agents for uterine relaxation during removal of retained placental tissue. Initiating treatment with incremental doses of intravenous or sublingual (i.e., metered dose spray) nitroglycerin may relax the uterus sufficiently while minimizing potential complications (e.g., hypotension).

V. Anesthetic Choices for Cesarean Delivery

Equipment, Facilities, and Support Personnel
The literature is insufficient to evaluate the benefit of providing equipment, facilities and support personnel in the labor and delivery operating suite comparable to that available in the main operating suite. The consultants and ASA members strongly agree that the available equipment, facilities, and support personnel should be comparable.

Recommendations. Equipment, facilities, and support personnel available in the labor and delivery operating suite should be comparable to those available in the main operating suite. Resources for the treatment of potential complications (e.g., failed intubation, inadequate analgesia, hypotension, respiratory depression, pruritus, vomiting) should also be available in the labor and delivery operating suite. Appropriate equipment and personnel should be available to care for obstetric patients recovering from major neuraxial anesthesia or GA.

General, Epidural, Spinal, or Combined Spinal–Epidural Anesthesia
The literature suggests that induction-to-delivery times for GA are lower compared with epidural or spinal anesthesia and that a higher frequency of maternal hypotension may be associated with epidural or spinal techniques. Meta-analysis of the literature found that Apgar scores at 1 and 5 minutes are lower for GA compared with epidural anesthesia and suggests that Apgar scores are lower for GA versus spinal anesthesia. The literature is equivocal regarding differences in umbilical artery pH values when GA is compared with epidural or spinal anesthesia.

The consultants and ASA members agree that GA reduces the time to skin incision when compared with either epidural or spinal anesthesia; they also agree that GA increases maternal complications. The consultants are equivocal and the ASA members agree that GA increases fetal and neonatal complications. The consultants and ASA members both agree that epidural anesthesia increases the time to skin incision and decreases the quality of anesthesia compared with spinal anesthesia. They both disagree that epidural anesthesia increases maternal complications.

When spinal anesthesia is compared with epidural anesthesia, meta-analysis of the literature found that induction-to-delivery times are shorter for spinal anesthesia. The literature is equivocal regarding hypotension, umbilical pH values, and Apgar scores. The consultants and ASA members agree that epidural anesthesia increases time to skin incision and reduces the quality of anesthesia when compared with spinal anesthesia. They both disagree that epidural anesthesia increases maternal complications.

When CSE is compared with epidural anesthesia, meta-analysis of the literature found no differences in the frequency of hypotension or in 1 minute Apgar scores; the literature is insufficient to evaluate outcomes associated with the use of CSE compared with spinal anesthesia. The consultants and ASA members agree that CSE anesthesia improves anesthe-

sia and reduces time to skin incision when compared with *epidural* anesthesia. The ASA members are equivocal, but the consultants disagree that maternal side effects are reduced. The consultants and ASA members both disagree that CSE improves anesthesia compared with *spinal* anesthesia. The ASA members are equivocal, but the consultants disagree that maternal side effects are reduced. The consultants strongly agree and the ASA members agree that CSE compared with spinal anesthesia increases flexibility of prolonged procedures, and they both agree that the time to skin incision is increased.

Recommendations. The decision to use a particular anesthetic technique for cesarean delivery should be individualized, based on several factors. These include anesthetic, obstetric, or fetal risk factors (e.g., elective vs. emergency), the preferences of the patient, and the judgment of the anesthesiologist. Neuraxial techniques are preferred to GA for most cesarean deliveries. An indwelling epidural catheter may provide equivalent onset of anesthesia compared with initiation of spinal anesthesia for urgent cesarean delivery. If spinal anesthesia is chosen, pencil-point spinal needles should be used instead of cutting-bevel spinal needles. However, GA may be the most appropriate choice in some circumstances (e.g., profound fetal bradycardia, ruptured uterus, severe hemorrhage, severe placental abruption). Uterine displacement (usually left displacement) should be maintained until delivery regardless of the anesthetic technique used.

Intravenous Fluid Preloading
The literature supports and the consultants and ASA members agree that intravenous fluid preloading for spinal anesthesia reduces the frequency of maternal hypotension when compared with no fluid preloading.

Recommendations. Intravenous fluid preloading may be used to reduce the frequency of maternal hypotension after spinal anesthesia for cesarean delivery. Although fluid preloading reduces the frequency of maternal hypotension, initiation of spinal anesthesia should not be delayed to administer a fixed volume of intravenous fluid.

Ephedrine or Phenylephrine
The literature supports the administration of ephedrine and suggests that phenylephrine is effective in reducing maternal hypotension during neuraxial anesthesia for cesarean delivery. The literature is equivocal regarding the relative frequency of patients with breakthrough hypotension when infusions of ephedrine are compared with phenylephrine; however, lower umbilical cord pH values are reported after ephedrine administration. The consultants agree and the ASA members strongly agree that ephedrine is acceptable for treating hypotension during neuraxial anesthesia. The consultants strongly agree and the ASA members agree that phenylephrine is an acceptable agent for the treatment of hypotension.

Recommendations. Intravenous ephedrine and phenylephrine are both acceptable drugs for treating hypotension during neuraxial anesthesia. In the absence of maternal bradycardia, phenylephrine may be preferable because of improved fetal acid–base status in uncomplicated pregnancies.

Neuraxial Opioids for Postoperative Analgesia
For improved postoperative analgesia after cesarean delivery during epidural anesthesia, the literature supports the use of epidural opioids compared with intermittent injections of intravenous or intramuscular opioids. However, a higher frequency of pruritus was found with epidural opioids. The literature is insufficient to evaluate the impact of epidural opioids compared with intravenous PCA. In addition, the literature is insufficient to evaluate spinal opioids compared with parenteral opioids. The consultants strongly agree and

the ASA members agree that neuraxial opioids for postoperative analgesia improve analgesia and maternal satisfaction.

Recommendations. For postoperative analgesia after neuraxial anesthesia for cesarean delivery, neuraxial opioids are preferred over intermittent injections of parenteral opioids.

VI. Postpartum Tubal Ligation

There is insufficient literature to evaluate the benefits of neuraxial anesthesia compared with GA for postpartum tubal ligation. In addition, the literature is insufficient to evaluate the impact of the timing of a postpartum tubal ligation on maternal outcome. The consultants and ASA members both agree that neuraxial anesthesia for postpartum tubal ligation reduces complications compared with GA. The ASA members are equivocal but the consultants agree that a postpartum tubal ligation within 8 hours of delivery *does not* increase maternal complications.

Recommendations. For postpartum tubal ligation, the patient should have no oral intake of solid foods within 6 to 8 hours of the surgery, depending on the type of food ingested (e.g., fat content).‖ Aspiration prophylaxis should be considered. Both the timing of the procedure and the decision to use a particular anesthetic technique (i.e., neuraxial vs. general) should be individualized, based on anesthetic risk factors, obstetric risk factors (i.e., blood loss), and patient preferences. However, neuraxial techniques are preferred to GA for most postpartum tubal ligations. The anesthesiologist should be aware that gastric emptying will be delayed in patients who have received opioids during labor, and that an epidural catheter placed for labor may be more likely to fail with longer postdelivery time intervals. If a postpartum tubal ligation is to be performed before the patient is discharged from the hospital, the procedure should not be attempted at a time when it might compromise other aspects of patient care on the labor and delivery unit.

VII. Management of Obstetric and Anesthetic Emergencies

Resources for Management of Hemorrhagic Emergencies

Observational studies and case reports suggest that the availability of resources for hemorrhagic emergencies may be associated with reduced maternal complications. The consultants and ASA members both strongly agree that the availability of resources for managing hemorrhagic emergencies reduces maternal complications.

Recommendations. Institutions providing obstetric care should have resources available to manage hemorrhagic emergencies (Table B-1). In an emergency, the use of type-

TABLE B-1 Suggested Resources for Obstetric Hemorrhagic Emergencies

- Large-bore intravenous catheters
- Fluid warmer
- Forced-air body warmer
- Availability of blood bank resources
- Equipment for infusing intravenous fluids and blood products rapidly. Examples include, but are not limited to, hand-squeezed fluid chambers, hand-inflated pressure bags, and automatic infusion devices

The items listed represent suggestions. The items should be customized to meet the specific needs, preferences, and skills of the practitioner and healthcare facility.

TABLE B-2 Suggested Resources for Airway Management during Initial Provision of Neuraxial Anesthesia

- Laryngoscope and assorted blades
- Endotracheal tubes, with stylets
- Oxygen source
- Suction source with tubing and catheters
- Self-inflating bag and mask for positive-pressure ventilation
- Medications for blood pressure support, muscle relaxation, and hypnosis
- Qualitative carbon dioxide detector
- Pulse oximeter

The items listed represent suggestions. The items should be customized to meet the specific needs, preferences, and skills of the practitioner and healthcare facility.

specific or O negative blood is acceptable. In cases of intractable hemorrhage when banked blood is not available or the patient refuses banked blood, intraoperative cell-salvage should be considered if available.

Central Invasive Hemodynamic Monitoring

There is insufficient literature to examine whether pulmonary artery catheterization is associated with improved maternal, fetal, or neonatal outcomes in patients with pregnancy-related hypertensive disorders. The literature is silent regarding the management of obstetric patients with central venous catheterization alone. The consultants and ASA members agree that the routine use of central venous or pulmonary artery catheterization does not reduce maternal complications in severely preeclamptic patients.

Recommendations. The decision to perform invasive hemodynamic monitoring should be individualized and based on clinical indications that include the patient's medical history and cardiovascular risk factors. The Task Force recognizes that not all practitioners have access to resources for use of central venous or pulmonary artery catheters in obstetric units.

Equipment for Management of Airway Emergencies

Case reports suggest that the availability of equipment for the management of airway emergencies may be associated with reduced maternal, fetal, and neonatal complications. The consultants and ASA members both strongly agree that the immediate availability of equipment for the management of airway emergencies reduces maternal, fetal, and neonatal complications.

Recommendations. Labor and delivery units should have personnel and equipment readily available to manage airway emergencies, to include a pulse oximeter and qualitative carbon dioxide detector, consistent with the ASA Practice Guidelines for Management of the Difficult Airway.** Basic airway management equipment should be immediately available during the provision of neuraxial analgesia (Table B-2). In addition, portable equipment for difficult airway management should be readily available in the operative area of labor and delivery units (Table B-3). The anesthesiologist should have a preformulated strategy for intubation of the difficult airway. When tracheal intubation has failed, ventilation with mask and cricoid pressure, or with a laryngeal mask airway or supraglottic airway device (e.g., Combitube®, Intubating LMA [*Fastrach*™])

**American Society of Anesthesiologists Task Force on Management of the Difficult Airway: Practice guidelines for management of the difficult airway: An updated report. Anesthesiology 2003;98:1269–1277.

TABLE B-3 Suggested Contents of a Portable Storage Unit for Difficult Airway Management for Cesarean Delivery Rooms

- Rigid laryngoscope blades of alternate design and size from those routinely used
- Laryngeal mask airway
- Endotracheal tubes of assorted size
- Endotracheal tube guides. Examples include, but are not limited to, semirigid stylets with or without a hollow core for jet ventilation, light wands, and forceps designed to manipulate the distal portion of the endotracheal tube
- Retrograde intubation equipment
- At least one device suitable for emergency nonsurgical airway ventilation. Examples include, but are not limited to, a hollow jet ventilation stylet with a transtracheal jet ventilator, and a supraglottic airway device (e.g., Combitube®, Intubating LMA [*Fastrach*™])
- Fiberoptic intubation equipment
- Equipment suitable for emergency surgical airway access (e.g., cricothyrotomy)
- An exhaled carbon dioxide detector
- Topical anesthetics and vasoconstrictors

The items listed represent suggestions. The items should be customized to meet the specific needs, preferences, and skills of the practitioner and healthcare facility.

Adapted from Practice guidelines for management of the difficult airway: An updated report by the American Society of Anesthesiologists Task Force on Management of the Difficult Airway. *Anesthesiology* 2003; 98:1269–1277.

should be considered for maintaining an airway and ventilating the lungs. If it is not possible to ventilate or awaken the patient, an airway should be created surgically.

Cardiopulmonary Resuscitation. The literature is insufficient to evaluate the efficacy of cardiopulmonary resuscitation in the obstetric patient during labor and delivery. In cases of cardiac arrest, the American Heart Association has stated that 4 to 5 minutes is the maximum time rescuers will have to determine whether the arrest can be reversed by Basic Life Support and Advanced Cardiac Life Support interventions.[††] Delivery of the fetus may improve cardiopulmonary resuscitation of the mother by relieving aortocaval compression. The American Heart Association further notes that "the best survival rate for infants >24 to 25 weeks in gestation occurs when the delivery of the infant occurs no more than 5 minutes after the mother's heart stops beating. This typically requires that the provider begin the hysterotomy about 4 minutes after cardiac arrest."[††] The consultants and ASA members both strongly agree that the immediate availability of basic and advanced life-support equipment in the labor and delivery suite reduces maternal, fetal, and neonatal complications.

Recommendations. Basic and advanced life-support equipment should be immediately available in the operative area of labor and delivery units. If cardiac arrest occurs during labor and delivery, standard resuscitative measures should be initiated. In addition, uterine displacement (usually left displacement) should be maintained. If maternal circulation is not restored within 4 minutes, cesarean delivery should be performed by the obstetrics team.

[††]2005 American Heart Association guidelines for cardiopulmonary resuscitation and emergency cardiovascular care. *Circulation* 2005;112(suppl):IV1–203.

APPENDIX 1: SUMMARY OF RECOMMENDATIONS

I. Preanesthetic Evaluation

- Conduct a focused history and physical examination before providing anesthesia care
  - Maternal health and anesthetic history
  - Relevant obstetric history
  - Airway and heart and lung examination
  - Baseline blood pressure measurement
  - Back examination when neuraxial anesthesia is planned or placed
- A communication system should be in place to encourage early and ongoing contact between obstetric providers, anesthesiologists, and other members of the multidisciplinary team
- Order or require a platelet count based on a patient's history, physical examination, and clinical signs; a routine intrapartum platelet count is not necessary in the healthy parturient
- Order or require an intrapartum blood type and screen or cross-match based on maternal history, anticipated hemorrhagic complications (e.g., placenta accreta in a patient with placenta previa and previous uterine surgery), and local institutional policies; a routine blood cross-match is not necessary for *healthy and uncomplicated* parturients
- The fetal heart rate should be monitored by a qualified individual before and after administration of neuraxial analgesia for labor; *continuous* electronic recording of the fetal heart rate may not be necessary in every clinical setting and may not be possible during initiation of neuraxial anesthesia

II. Aspiration Prophylaxis

- Oral intake of modest amounts of clear liquids may be allowed for uncomplicated laboring patients
- The uncomplicated patient undergoing elective cesarean delivery may have modest amounts of clear liquids up to 2 hours before induction of anesthesia
- The volume of liquid ingested is less important than the presence of particulate matter in the liquid ingested
- Patients with additional risk factors for aspiration (e.g., morbid obesity, diabetes, difficult airway) or patients at increased risk for operative delivery (e.g., nonreassuring fetal heart rate pattern) may have further restrictions of oral intake, determined on a case-by-case basis
- Solid foods should be avoided in laboring patients
- Patients undergoing elective surgery (e.g., scheduled cesarean delivery or postpartum tubal ligation) should undergo a fasting period for solids of 6 to 8 hours depending on the type of food ingested (e.g., fat content)
- Before surgical procedures (i.e., cesarean delivery, postpartum tubal ligation), practitioners should consider timely administration of nonparticulate antacids, H_2 receptor antagonists, and/or metoclopramide for aspiration prophylaxis

III. Anesthetic Care for Labor and Delivery

Neuraxial Techniques: Availability of Resources

- When neuraxial techniques that include local anesthetics are chosen, appropriate resources for the treatment of complications (e.g., hypotension, systemic toxicity, high spinal anesthesia) should be available
- If an opioid is added, treatments for related complications (e.g., pruritus, nausea, respiratory depression) should be available
- An intravenous infusion should be established before the initiation of neuraxial analgesia or anesthesia and maintained throughout the duration of the neuraxial analgesic or anesthetic

- Administration of a fixed volume of intravenous fluid is not required before neuraxial analgesia is initiated

Timing of Neuraxial Analgesia and Outcome of Labor

- Neuraxial analgesia should not be withheld on the basis of achieving an arbitrary cervical dilation, and should be offered on an individualized basis when this service is available
- Patients may be reassured that the use of neuraxial analgesia does not increase the incidence of cesarean delivery

Neuraxial Analgesia and Trial of Labor after Previous Cesarean Delivery

- Neuraxial techniques should be offered to patients attempting vaginal birth after previous cesarean delivery
- For these patients, it is also appropriate to consider early placement of a neuraxial catheter that can be used later for labor analgesia or for anesthesia in the event of operative delivery

Early Insertion of Spinal or Epidural Catheter for Complicated Parturients

- Early insertion of a spinal or epidural catheter for obstetric (e.g., twin gestation or preeclampsia) or anesthetic indications (e.g., anticipated difficult airway or obesity) should be considered to reduce the need for general anesthesia if an emergent procedure becomes necessary
  - In these cases, the insertion of a spinal or epidural catheter may precede the onset of labor or a patient's request for labor analgesia

Continuous Infusion Epidural Analgesia

- The selected analgesic/anesthetic technique should reflect patient needs and preferences, practitioner preferences or skills, and available resources
- CIE may be used for effective analgesia for labor and delivery
- When a continuous epidural infusion of local anesthetic is selected, an opioid may be added to reduce the concentration of local anesthetic, improve the quality of analgesia, and minimize motor block
- Adequate analgesia for uncomplicated labor and delivery should be administered with the secondary goal of producing as little motor block as possible by using dilute concentrations of local anesthetics with opioids
- The lowest concentration of local anesthetic infusion that provides adequate maternal analgesia and satisfaction should be administered

Single-injection Spinal Opioids with or without Local Anesthetics

- Single-injection spinal opioids with or without local anesthetics may be used to provide effective, although time-limited, analgesia for labor when spontaneous vaginal delivery is anticipated
- If labor is expected to last longer than the analgesic effects of the spinal drugs chosen or if there is a good possibility of operative delivery, a catheter technique instead of a single-injection technique should be considered
- A local anesthetic may be added to a spinal opioid to increase duration and improve quality of analgesia

Pencil-point Spinal Needles

- Pencil-point spinal needles should be used instead of cutting-bevel spinal needles to minimize the risk of post-dural puncture headache

Combined Spinal–Epidural Anesthetics

- CSE techniques may be used to provide effective and rapid analgesia for labor

Patient-controlled Epidural Analgesia

- PCEA may be used to provide an effective and flexible approach for the maintenance of labor analgesia
- PCEA may be preferable to CIE for providing fewer anesthetic interventions, reduced dosages of local anesthetics, and less motor blockade than fixed-rate continuous epidural infusions
- PCEA may be used with or without a background infusion

IV. Removal of Retained Placenta

- In general, there is no preferred anesthetic technique for removal of retained placenta
  - If an epidural catheter is in place and the patient is hemodynamically stable, epidural anesthesia is preferable
- Hemodynamic status should be assessed before administering neuraxial anesthesia
- Aspiration prophylaxis should be considered
- Sedation/analgesia should be titrated carefully due to the potential risks of respiratory depression and pulmonary aspiration during the immediate postpartum period
- In cases involving major maternal hemorrhage, general anesthesia with an endotracheal tube may be preferable to neuraxial anesthesia
- Nitroglycerin may be used as an alternative to terbutaline sulfate or general endotracheal anesthesia with halogenated agents for uterine relaxation during removal of retained placental tissue
  - Initiating treatment with incremental doses of intravenous or sublingual (i.e., metered dose spray) nitroglycerin may relax the uterus sufficiently while minimizing potential complications (e.g., hypotension)

V. Anesthetic Choices for Cesarean Delivery

- Equipment, facilities, and support personnel available in the labor and delivery operating suite should be comparable to those available in the main operating suite
  - Resources for the treatment of potential complications (e.g., failed intubation, inadequate analgesia, hypotension, respiratory depression, pruritus, vomiting) should be available in the labor and delivery operating suite
  - Appropriate equipment and personnel should be available to care for obstetric patients recovering from major neuraxial or general anesthesia
- The decision to use a particular anesthetic technique should be individualized based on anesthetic, obstetric, or fetal risk factors (e.g., elective vs. emergency), the preferences of the patient, and the judgment of the anesthesiologist
  - Neuraxial techniques are preferred to general anesthesia for most cesarean deliveries
- An indwelling epidural catheter may provide equivalent onset of anesthesia compared with initiation of spinal anesthesia for urgent cesarean delivery
- If spinal anesthesia is chosen, pencil-point spinal needles should be used instead of cutting-bevel spinal needles
- General anesthesia may be the most appropriate choice in some circumstances (e.g., profound fetal bradycardia, ruptured uterus, severe hemorrhage, severe placental abruption)
- Uterine displacement (usually left displacement) should be maintained until delivery regardless of the anesthetic technique used

- Intravenous fluid preloading may be used to reduce the frequency of maternal hypotension after spinal anesthesia for cesarean delivery. Initiation of spinal anesthesia should not be delayed to administer a fixed volume of intravenous fluid
- Intravenous ephedrine and phenylephrine are both acceptable drugs for treating hypotension during neuraxial anesthesia
  - In the absence of maternal bradycardia, phenylephrine may be preferable because of improved fetal acid–base status in uncomplicated pregnancies
- For postoperative analgesia after neuraxial anesthesia for cesarean delivery, neuraxial opioids are preferred over intermittent injections of parenteral opioids

VI. Postpartum Tubal Ligation

- For postpartum tubal ligation, the patient should have no oral intake of solid foods within 6 to 8 hours of the surgery, depending on the type of food ingested (e.g., fat content)
- Aspiration prophylaxis should be considered
- Both the timing of the procedure and the decision to use a particular anesthetic technique (i.e., neuraxial vs. general) should be individualized, based on anesthetic risk factors, obstetric risk factors (e.g., blood loss), and patient preferences
- Neuraxial techniques are preferred to general anesthesia for most postpartum tubal ligations
  - Be aware that gastric emptying will be delayed in patients who have received opioids during labor and that an epidural catheter placed for labor may be more likely to fail with longer postdelivery time intervals
- If a postpartum tubal ligation is to be performed before the patient is discharged from the hospital, the procedure should not be attempted at a time when it might compromise other aspects of patient care on the labor and delivery unit

VII. Management of Obstetric and Anesthetic Emergencies

- Institutions providing obstetric care should have resources available to manage hemorrhagic emergencies
  - In an emergency, the use of type-specific or O negative blood is acceptable
  - In cases of intractable hemorrhage when banked blood is not available or the patient refuses banked blood, intraoperative cell-salvage should be considered if available
  - The decision to perform invasive hemodynamic monitoring should be individualized and based on clinical indications that include the patient's medical history and cardiovascular risk factors
- Labor and delivery units should have personnel and equipment readily available to manage airway emergencies, to include a pulse oximeter and qualitative carbon dioxide detector, consistent with the ASA Practice Guidelines for Management of the Difficult Airway
  - Basic airway management equipment should be immediately available during the provision of neuraxial analgesia
  - Portable equipment for difficult airway management should be readily available in the operative area of labor and delivery units
  - The anesthesiologist should have a preformulated strategy for intubation of the difficult airway
  - When tracheal intubation has failed, ventilation with mask and cricoid pressure, or with a laryngeal mask airway or supraglottic airway device (e.g., Combitube®, Intubating LMA [*Fastrach*™]) should be considered for maintaining an airway and ventilating the lungs
  - If it is not possible to ventilate or awaken the patient, an airway should be created surgically

- Basic and advanced life-support equipment should be immediately available in the operative area of labor and delivery units
- If cardiac arrest occurs during labor and delivery, standard resuscitative measures should be initiated
  - Uterine displacement (usually left displacement) should be maintained
  - If maternal circulation is not restored within 4 minutes, cesarean delivery should be performed by the obstetrics team

■ APPENDIX 2: METHODS AND ANALYSES

The scientific assessment of these guidelines was based on evidence linkages or statements regarding potential relationships between clinical interventions and outcomes. The interventions listed below were examined to assess their impact on a variety of outcomes related to obstetric anesthesia.[‡‡]

1. Preanesthetic Evaluation

  i. A directed history and physical examination
 ii. Communication between anesthetic and obstetric providers
iii. A routine intrapartum platelet count does not reduce maternal anesthetic complications
 iv. For suspected preeclampsia or coagulopathy, an intrapartum platelet count
  v. An intrapartum blood type and screen for all parturients reduces maternal complications
 vi. For healthy and uncomplicated parturients, a blood cross-match is unnecessary
vii. Preanesthetic recording of the fetal heart rate reduces fetal and neonatal complications

2. Aspiration Prophylaxis in the Obstetric Patient

  i. Oral intake of clear liquids during labor improves patient comfort and satisfaction but does not increase maternal complications
 ii. Oral intake of solids during labor increases maternal complications
iii. A fasting period for solids of 6 to 8 hours before an elective cesarean reduces maternal complications
 iv. Nonparticulate antacids versus no antacids before operative procedures (excluding operative vaginal delivery) reduces maternal complications

3. Anesthetic Care for Labor and Delivery[§§]

  i. Neuraxial techniques
    a. Prophylactic spinal or epidural catheter insertion for complicated parturients reduces maternal complications
    b. Continuous epidural infusion of local anesthetics with or without opioids versus parenteral opioids
    c. Continuous epidural infusion of local anesthetics with or without opioids versus spinal opioids with or without local anesthetics
    d. Induction of epidural analgesia using local anesthetics with opioids versus equal concentrations of epidural local anesthetics without opioids

---

[‡‡]Unless otherwise specified, outcomes for the listed interventions refer to the reduction of maternal, fetal, and neonatal complications.

[§§]Additional outcomes include improved analgesia, analgesic use, maternal comfort, and satisfaction.

e. Induction of epidural analgesia using local anesthetics with opioids versus higher concentrations of epidural local anesthetics without opioids

f. Maintenance of epidural infusion of lower concentrations of local anesthetics with opioids versus higher concentrations of local anesthetics without opioids (e.g., bupivacaine concentrations <0.125% with opioids vs. concentrations >0.125% without opioids)

g. Single-injection spinal opioids with or without local anesthetics versus parenteral opioids

h. Single-injection spinal opioids with local anesthetics versus spinal opioids without local anesthetics

ii. CSE techniques

a. CSE local anesthetics with opioids versus epidural local anesthetics with opioids

iii. PCEA

a. PCEA versus CIEs

b. PCEA with a background infusion versus PCEA without a background infusion

iv. Neuraxial analgesia, timing of initiation, and progress of labor

a. Administering epidural analgesia at cervical dilations of <5 cm (vs. >5 cm)

b. Neuraxial techniques for patients attempting vaginal birth after previous cesarean delivery

4. Removal of Retained Placenta

i. If an epidural catheter is in situ and the patient is hemodynamically stable, epidural anesthesia is preferred over general or spinal anesthesia to improve the success at removing retained placenta

ii. In cases involving major maternal hemorrhage, general anesthesia is preferred over neuraxial anesthesia to reduce maternal complications

iii. Administration of nitroglycerin for uterine relaxation improves success at removing retained placenta

5. Anesthetic Choices for Cesarean Delivery

i. Equipment, facilities, and support personnel available in the labor and delivery suite should be comparable to that available in the main operating suite

ii. General anesthesia versus epidural anesthesia

iii. General anesthesia versus spinal anesthesia

iv. Epidural anesthesia versus spinal anesthesia

v. CSE anesthesia versus epidural anesthesia

vi. CSE anesthesia versus spinal anesthesia

vii. Use of pencil-point spinal needles versus cutting-bevel spinal needles reduces maternal complications

viii. Intravenous fluid preloading versus no intravenous fluid preloading for spinal anesthesia reduces maternal hypotension

ix. Ephedrine or phenylephrine reduces maternal hypotension during neuraxial anesthesia

x. Neuraxial opioids versus parenteral opioids for postoperative analgesia after neuraxial anesthesia for cesarean delivery

6. Postpartum Tubal Ligation

i. Neuraxial anesthesia versus general anesthesia

ii. A postpartum tubal ligation within 8 hours of delivery does not increase maternal complications

7. Management of Complications

i. Availability of resources for management of hemorrhagic emergencies

ii. Immediate availability of equipment for management of airway emergencies

iii. Immediate availability of basic and advanced life-support equipment in the labor and delivery suite

iv. Invasive hemodynamic monitoring for severely pre-eclamptic patients

Scientific evidence was derived from aggregated research literature, and opinion-based evidence was obtained from surveys, open presentations, and other activities (e.g., Internet posting). For purposes of literature aggregation, potentially relevant clinical studies were identified via electronic and manual searches of the literature. The electronic and manual searches covered a 67-year period from 1940 to 2006. More than 4,000 citations were initially identified, yielding a total of 2,986 nonoverlapping articles that addressed topics related to the evidence linkages. After review of the articles, 2,549 studies did not provide direct evidence and were subsequently eliminated. A total of 437 articles contained direct linkage-related evidence.

Initially, each pertinent outcome reported in a study was classified as supporting an evidence linkage, refuting a linkage, or equivocal. The results were then summarized to obtain a directional assessment for each evidence linkage before conducting a formal meta-analysis. Literature pertaining to 11 evidence linkages contained enough studies with well-defined experimental designs and statistical information sufficient for meta-analyses. These linkages were (1) nonparticulate antacids versus no antacids, (2) continuous epidural infusion of local anesthetics with or without opioids versus parenteral opioids, (3) induction of epidural analgesia using local anesthetics with opioids versus equal concentrations of epidural local anesthetics without opioids, (4) maintenance of epidural infusion of lower concentrations of local anesthetics with opioids versus higher concentrations of local anesthetics without opioids, (5) CSE local anesthetics with opioids versus epidural local anesthetics with opioids, (6) PCEA versus CIEs, (7) general anesthesia versus epidural anesthesia for cesarean delivery, (8) CSE anesthesia versus epidural anesthesia for cesarean delivery, (9) use of pencil-point spinal needles versus cutting-bevel spinal needles, (10) ephedrine or phenylephrine reduces maternal hypotension during neuraxial anesthesia, and (11) neuraxial opioids versus parenteral opioids for postoperative analgesia after neuraxial anesthesia for cesarean delivery.

General variance-based effect-size estimates or combined probability tests were obtained for continuous outcome measures, and Mantel–Haenszel odds ratios were obtained for dichotomous outcome measures. Two combined probability tests were used as follows: (1) The Fisher combined test, producing chi-square values based on logarithmic transformations of the reported P values from the independent studies, and (2) the Stouffer combined test, providing weighted representation of the studies by weighting each of the standard normal deviates by the size of the sample. An odds ratio procedure based on the Mantel–Haenszel method for combining study results using 2×2 tables was used with outcome frequency information. An acceptable significance level was set at $P < 0.01$ (one tailed). Tests for heterogeneity of the independent studies were conducted to assure consistency among the study results. DerSimonian–Laird random-effects odds ratios were obtained when significant heterogeneity was found ($P < 0.01$). To control for potential publishing bias, a "fail-safe n" value was calculated. No search for unpublished studies was conducted, and no reliability tests for locating research results were done.

Meta-analytic results are reported in Table B-4. To be accepted as significant findings, Mantel–Haenszel odds ratios must agree with combined test results whenever both types of data are assessed. In the absence of Mantel–Haenszel

TABLE B-4 Meta-analysis Summary

Linkages	n	Fisher Chi-square	P	Weighted Stouffer Zc	P	Effect Size	Mantel–Haenszel OR	CI	Heterogeneity Significance	Heterogeneity Effect Size
Aspiration Prophylaxis										
Nonparticulate antacids vs. no antacids										
Gastric pH[a]	5	66.80	0.001	9.78	0.001	0.88	—	—	0.001	0.001
Metoclopramide vs. no metoclopramide										
Nausea	6	—	—	—	—	—	0.25	0.14–0.46	—	NS
Vomiting	6	—	—	—	—	—	0.36	0.19–0.68	—	NS
Anesthetic Care for Labor and Vaginal Delivery										
CIE local anesthetics ± opioids vs. IV opioids										
Duration of labor first stage	5	50.19	0.001	5.42	0.001	0.15	—	—	NS	NS
Duration of labor second stage	7	67.53	0.001	4.84	0.001	0.21	—	—	NS	0.001
Spontaneous delivery	8	—	—	—	—	—	0.53	0.42–0.68	—	NS
Cesarean delivery[b]	8	—	—	—	—	—	0.88	0.50–1.47	—	0.01
Fetal acidosis	5	—	—	—	—	—	0.71	0.51–0.98	—	NS
1 min Apgar	5	—	—	—	—	—	1.62	1.03–2.54	—	NS
5 min Apgar	5	—	—	—	—	—	1.17	0.41–3.32	—	NS
Epidural induction LA + O vs. equal LA doses										
Analgesia (mean, SD)	6	91.21	0.001	17.70	0.001	0.99	—	—	0.001	0.001
Analgesia (pain relief)	5	—	—	—	—	—	4.03	2.14–7.56	—	NS
Duration of labor	5	38.62	0.001	0.04	0.480	0.01	—	—	0.001	0.001
Spontaneous delivery	8	—	—	—	—	—	0.97	0.69–1.35	—	NS
Hypotension	8	—	—	—	—	—	0.79	0.44–1.44	—	NS
Motor blocka	5	—	—	—	—	—	0.44	0.24–0.81	—	NS
Pruritus	7	—	—	—	—	—	6.15	3.22–11.74	—	NS
1 min Apgar	6	—	—	—	—	—	0.82	0.45–1.51	—	NS
Epidural maintenance LA + O vs. higher LA doses										
Duration of labor	5	19.82	0.030	1.99	0.020	0.05	—	—	NS	NS
Spontaneous delivery	8	—	—	—	—	—	1.08	0.82–1.42	—	NS
Motor block	6	—	—	—	—	—	0.29	0.21–0.40	—	NS
1 min Apgar	6	—	—	—	—	—	0.94	0.60–1.47	—	NS
Pencil-point vs. cutting-bevel spinal needles										
Post-dural puncture headache	5	—	—	—	—	—	0.34	0.18–0.63	—	NS
CSE LA + O vs. epidural LA + O										
Analgesia (pain relief)[b]	7	—	—	—	—	—	1.16	0.62–1.85	—	0.010
Satisfaction with analgesia	5	—	—	—	—	—	1.45	0.89–2.34	—	NS
Analgesia (time to onset)	5	57.80	0.001	−13.33	0.001	0.90	—	—	0.001	0.001
Spontaneous delivery	13	—	—	—	—	—	0.99	0.85–1.15	—	NS
Hypotension	6	—	—	—	—	—	1.76	0.73–4.26	—	NS
Motor block	7	—	—	—	—	—	1.20	0.90–1.60	—	NS
Nausea	5	—	—	—	—	—	1.22	0.63–2.36	—	NS
Pruritus[b]	9	—	—	—	—	—	4.86	1.63–14.65	—	0.001
Motor block	7	—	—	—	—	—	1.20	0.90–1.60		NS
Fetal heart rate changes	6	—	—	—	—	—	1.25	0.92–1.70	—	NS
1 min Apgar	6	—	—	—	—	—	1.16	0.76–1.78	—	NS
5 min Apgar	6	—	—	—	—	—	1.36	0.52–3.56	—	NS
PCEA vs. CIE										
Pain relief/score	5	21.78	0.020	0.17	0.433	0.04	—	—	NS	NS
Analgesic use	7	84.98	0.001	10.74	0.001	0.85	—	—	0.001	0.001
Duration of labor first stage	5	42.42	0.001	5.24	0.001	0.44	—	—	0.008	0.001
Duration of labor second stage	6	43.08	0.001	2.01	0.022	0.18	—	—	0.001	0.001
Spontaneous delivery	13	—	—	—	—	—	1.22	0.83–1.79	—	NS
Motor block[b]	7	—	—	—	—	—	0.52	0.15–3.44	—	0.010
1 min Apgar	6	—	—	—	—	—	0.63	0.27–1.50	—	NS

(continued)

TABLE B-4 Meta-analysis Summary (*Continued*)

Linkages	n	Fisher Chi-square	P	Weighted Stouffer Zc	P	Effect Size	Mantel–Haenszel OR	CI	Heterogeneity Significance	Heterogeneity Effect Size
PCEA with background infusion vs. PCEA										
Analgesia (pain relief)	5	—	—	—	—	—	3.33	1.87–5.92	—	NS
Spontaneous delivery	5	—	—	—	—	—	0.83	0.41–1.69	—	NS
Motor block	5	—	—	—	—	—	1.18	0.47–2.97	—	NS
Early vs. late epidural										
Cesarean delivery	5	—	—	—	—	—	0.95	0.67–1.35	—	NS
Anesthetic Choices for Cesarean Delivery										
GA vs. epidural										
Umbilical pH	5	49.04	0.001	0.52	0.300	0.37	—	—	0.001	0.001
1 min Apgar	5	49.04	0.001	−2.72	0.003	0.01	—	—	0.010	0.010
5 min Apgar	5	28.40	0.005	−2.95	0.002	0.08	—	—	NS	NS
CSE vs. epidural										
Hypotension	5	—	—	—	—	—	0.92	0.44–1.94	—	NS
Umbilical pH	5	55.91	0.001	1.80	0.036	0.11	—	—	0.001	0.001
1 min Apgar	5	—	—	—	—	—	0.55	0.22–1.52	—	NS
Fluid preloading vs. no preloading										
Hypotension[a]	6	—	—	—	—	—	0.46	0.29–0.73	—	NS
Ephedrine vs. placebo										
Hypotension	7	—	—	—	—	—	0.26	0.14–0.48	—	NS
Ephedrine vs. phenylephrine										
Hypotension	6	—	—	—	—	—	1.74	0.97–3.12	—	NS
Umbilical pH	6	59.68	0.001	−7.55	0.001	0.71	—	—	0.001	0.001
Neuraxial vs. parenteral O for postoperative analgesia										
Analgesia	7	75.12	0.001	5.82	0.001	0.61	—	—	0.001	0.001
Nausea	9	—	—	—	—	—	1.13	0.57–2.22	—	NS
Vomiting	5	—	—	—	—	—	1.02	0.36–2.87	—	NS
Pruritus	9	—	—	—	—	—	6.23	3.32–11.68	—	NS

[a]Nonrandomized comparative studies included in analysis.
[b]DerSimonian–Laird random-effects odds ratio (OR).

CI, confidence interval; CIE, continuous infusion epidural; CSE, combined spinal–epidural; GA, general anesthesia; IV, intravenous; LA, local anesthetics; LA + O, local anesthetics *with opioids*; NS, not significant; O, opioids; PCEA, patient controlled epidural analgesia.

odds ratios, findings from both the Fisher and weighted Stouffer combined tests must agree with each other to be acceptable as significant.

Interobserver agreement among Task Force members and two methodologists was established by inter-rater reliability testing. Agreement levels using a k statistic for two-rater agreement pairs were as follows: (1) Type of study design, $\kappa = 0.83$–0.94; (2) type of analysis, $\kappa = 0.71$–0.93; (3) evidence linkage assignment, $\kappa = 0.87$–1.00; and (4) literature inclusion for database, $\kappa = 0.74$–1.00. Three-rater chance-corrected agreement values were (1) study design, Sav = 0.884, Var (Sav) = 0.004; (2) type of analysis, Sav = 0.805, Var (Sav) = 0.009; (3) linkage assignment, Sav = 0.911, Var (Sav) = 0.002; and (4) literature database inclusion, Sav = 0.660, Var (Sav) = 0.024. These values represent moderate to high levels of agreement.

Consensus was obtained from multiple sources, including (1) survey opinion from consultants who were selected based on their knowledge or expertise in obstetric anesthesia or maternal and fetal medicine, (2) survey opinions solicited from active members of the ASA, (3) testimony from attendees of publicly held open forums at two national anesthesia meetings, (4) Internet commentary, and (5) Task Force opinion and interpretation. The survey rate of return was 75% (n = 76 of 102) for the consultants, and 2,326 surveys were received from active ASA members. Results of the surveys are reported in Tables B-5 and B-6 and in the text of the guidelines.

The consultants were asked to indicate which, if any, of the evidence linkages would change their clinical practices if the guidelines were instituted. The rate of return was 35% (n = 36). The percent of responding consultants expecting *no change* associated with each linkage were as follows: Preanesthetic evaluation—97%; aspiration prophylaxis—83%; anesthetic care for labor and delivery—89%; removal of retained placenta—97%; anesthetic choices for cesarean delivery—97%; postpartum tubal ligation—97%; and management of complications—94%. Ninety-seven percent of the respondents indicated that the guidelines would have *no effect* on the amount of time spent on a typical case. One respondent indicated that there would be an increase of 5 minutes in the amount of time spent on a typical case with the implementation of these guidelines.

TABLE B-5 Consultant Survey Responses

		Percent Responding to Each Item				
	n	Strongly Agree	Agree	Uncertain	Disagree	Strongly Disagree
Preanesthetic Evaluation						
1. Directed history and physical examination reduces maternal, fetal, and neonatal complications	76	72.4[a]	26.3	1.3	0.0	0.0
2. Communication between anesthetic and obstetric providers reduces maternal, fetal, and neonatal complications	76	89.5[a]	10.5	0.0	0.0	0.0
3. A routine intrapartum platelet count **does not reduce** maternal anesthetic complications	75	36.0	44.0[a]	8.0	10.7	1.3
4. An intrapartum platelet count reduces maternal anesthetic complications:						
For suspected preeclampsia	76	46.1	36.8[a]	9.2	7.9	0.0
For suspected coagulopathy	76	59.2[a]	32.9	5.3	2.6	0.0
5. All parturients should have an intrapartum blood sample sent to the blood bank to reduce maternal complications	76	21.1	32.9[a]	17.1	26.3	2.6
6. Preanesthetic recording of the fetal heart rate reduces fetal and neonatal complications	76	18.4	59.2[a]	13.2	9.2	0.0
Aspiration Prophylaxis						
7a. Oral intake of clear liquids *during* labor improves patient comfort and satisfaction	76	32.9	60.5[a]	1.3	3.9	1.3
7b. Oral intake of clear liquids *during labor* **does not** increase maternal complications	75	16.0	45.3[a]	22.7	12.0	4.0
8a. Oral intake of solids *during labor* increases maternal complications	76	47.4	32.9[a]	10.5	5.3	3.9
8b. The patient undergoing elective cesarean delivery should undergo a fasting period for solids of 6–8 h depending on the type of food ingested (e.g., fat content)	76	65.8[a]	30.3	3.9	0.0	0.0
8c. The patient undergoing elective postpartum tubal ligation should undergo a fasting period for solids of 6–8 h depending on the type of food ingested (e.g., fat content)	76	56.6[a]	27.6	9.2	5.3	1.3
9. Administration of a nonparticulate antacid before operative procedures reduces maternal complications	75	29.3	45.3[a]	18.7	5.3	1.3
Anesthetic Care for Labor and Delivery						
Neuraxial techniques:						
10. Prophylactic spinal or epidural catheter insertion for complicated parturients reduces maternal complications	75	42.7	40.0[a]	16.0	1.3	0.0
11. **Continuous epidural infusion** using local anesthetics with or *without opioids* vs. **parenteral opioids:**						
Improves analgesia	75	84.0[a]	16.0	0.0	0.0	0.0
Increases the duration of labor	75	4.0	24.0	21.3	36.0[a]	14.7
Decreases the chance of spontaneous delivery	74	4.1	16.2	12.2	41.9[a]	25.7
Increases maternal side effects	75	1.3	8.0	14.7	42.7[a]	33.3
Increases fetal and neonatal side effects	75	0.0	4.0	6.7	46.7[a]	42.7
12. **Continuous epidural infusion** using local anesthetics with or *without opioids* vs. **spinal** opioids with or without local anesthetics:						
Improves analgesia	74	12.2	25.7	20.3[a]	35.1	6.8
Increases the duration of labor	75	0.0	16.0	37.3[a]	34.7	12.0
Decreases the chance of spontaneous delivery	73	0.0	9.6	26.0	45.2[a]	19.2
Increases maternal motor block	74	5.4	41.9	17.6[a]	28.4	6.8
Increases maternal side effects	74	0.0	6.8	27.0	52.7[a]	13.5
Increases fetal and neonatal side effects	75	0.0	1.3	21.3	52.0[a]	25.3
13a. **Induction** of epidural analgesia using local anesthetics *with opioids* vs. epidural analgesia with **equal concentrations** of local anesthetics *without opioids:*						
Improves analgesia	74	54.1[a]	39.2	1.4	4.1	1.4
Increases maternal side effects	74	6.8	28.4	10.8	45.9[a]	8.1
Increases fetal and neonatal side effects	74	0.0	2.7	12.2	59.5[a]	25.7
13b. Induction of epidural analgesia using low-dose local anesthetics *with opioids* vs. higher concentrations of epidural local anesthetics *without opioids:*						
Improves analgesia	74	23.0	21.6	21.6[a]	32.4	1.4
Increases maternal side effects	74	0.0	10.8	12.2	50.0[a]	27.0
Increases fetal and neonatal side effects	74	0.0	2.7	17.6	52.7[a]	27.0
14a. **Maintenance** of epidural infusion of lower concentrations of local anesthetics *with* opioids vs. higher concentrations of local anesthetics *without* opioids:						
Improves analgesia	74	21.6	28.4[a]	27.0	23.0	0.0
Reduces the duration of labor	74	4.1	35.1	40.5[a]	17.6	2.7
Improves the chance of spontaneous delivery	74	12.2	60.8[a]	14.9	10.8	1.4
Reduces maternal motor block	74	51.4[a]	43.2	5.4	0.0	0.0
Reduces maternal side effects	74	16.2	44.6[a]	23.0	16.2	0.0
Reduces fetal and neonatal side effects	74	8.1	24.3	32.4[a]	32.4	2.7

(continued)

TABLE B-5 Consultant Survey Responses (*Continued*)

		Percent Responding to Each Item				
	n	Strongly Agree	Agree	Uncertain	Disagree	Strongly Disagree
14b. **Maintenance** of epidural analgesia using bupivacaine ≤**0.125%** *with opioids* vs. bupivacaine concentrations >**0.125%** *without opioids:*						
Improves analgesia	74	21.6	33.8[a]	21.6	23.0	0.0
Reduces the duration of labor	74	6.8	33.8	45.9[a]	12.2	1.4
Improves the chance of spontaneous delivery	74	14.9	52.7[a]	24.3	8.1	0.0
Reduces maternal motor block	74	40.5	51.4[a]	5.4	2.7	0.0
Reduces maternal side effects	74	14.9	41.9[a]	25.7	17.6	0.0
Reduces fetal and neonatal side effects	74	4.1	31.1	35.1[a]	28.4	1.4
15. Single-injection **spinal** opioids with or without local anesthetics vs. **parenteral** opioids:						
Improve analgesia	74	68.9[a]	28.4	2.7	0.0	0.0
Increase the duration of labor	74	1.4	5.4	20.3	51.4[a]	21.6
Decrease the chance of spontaneous delivery	74	1.4	8.1	10.8	54.1[a]	25.7
Increase maternal side effects	74	0.0	25.7	25.7[a]	36.5	12.2
Increase fetal and neonatal side effects	74	0.0	9.5	16.2	51.4[a]	23.0
16. Single-injection spinal opioids **with** local anesthetics vs. spinal opioids **without** local anesthetics:						
Improve analgesia	74	44.6	44.6[a]	4.1	5.4	1.4
Increase the duration of labor	74	2.7	6.8	25.7	51.4[a]	13.5
Decrease the chance of spontaneous delivery	74	2.7	5.4	23.0	58.1[a]	10.8
Increase maternal motor block	74	13.5	54.1[a]	9.5	21.6	1.4
Increase maternal side effects	74	1.4	27.0	23.0[a]	40.5	8.1
Increase fetal and neonatal side effects	74	0.0	4.1	23.0	58.1[a]	14.9
Combined spinal–epidural (CSE) techniques:						
17. **CSE** local anesthetics *with opioids* vs. **epidural** local anesthetics *with opioids:*						
Improve **early** analgesia	74	48.6	35.1[a]	5.4	10.8	0.0
Improve **overall** analgesia	74	18.9	31.1	23.0[a]	25.7	1.4
Decrease the duration of labor	74	4.1	18.9	47.3[a]	29.7	0.0
Decrease the chance of spontaneous delivery	73	0.0	2.7	19.2	61.6[a]	16.4
Reduce maternal motor block	74	5.4	37.8	24.3[a]	32.4	0.0
Increase maternal side effects	74	0.0	18.9	24.3	54.1[a]	2.7
Increase fetal and neonatal side effects	74	0.0	5.4	27.0	55.4[a]	12.2
Patient-controlled epidural analgesia (PCEA):						
18. PCEA vs. continuous infusion epidurals:						
Improves analgesia	75	16.0	41.3[a]	26.7	12.0	4.0
Improves maternal satisfaction	75	41.3	46.7[a]	8.0	2.7	1.3
Reduces the need for anesthetic interventions	75	42.7	36.0[a]	10.7	9.3	1.3
Increases the chance of spontaneous delivery	74	4.1	13.5	45.9[a]	33.8	2.7
Reduces maternal motor block	75	9.3	38.7	24.0[a]	26.7	1.3
Decreases maternal side effects	75	5.3	28.0	30.7[a]	34.7	1.3
19. PCEA **with** a background infusion vs. PCEA **without** a background infusion:						
Improves analgesia	74	23.0	54.1[a]	16.2	6.8	0.0
Improves maternal satisfaction	74	24.3	43.2[a]	23.0	9.5	0.0
Reduces the need for anesthetic interventions	74	21.6	56.8[a]	12.2	9.5	0.0
Decreases the chance of spontaneous delivery	74	0.0	4.1	41.9	51.4[a]	2.7
Increases maternal motor block	74	1.4	39.2	25.7[a]	32.4	1.4
Increases maternal side effects	74	1.4	13.5	29.7	52.7[a]	2.7
Neuraxial Analgesia, Timing of Initiation, and Progress of Labor						
20. Administering epidural analgesia at cervical dilations of <5 centimeters (vs. ≥5 cm):						
Improves analgesia	75	50.7[a]	32.0	9.3	6.7	1.3
Reduces the duration of labor	75	0.0	6.7	45.3[a]	41.3	6.7
Improves the chance of spontaneous delivery	74	0.0	10.8	48.6[a]	32.4	8.1
Increases maternal motor block	75	1.3	28.0	17.3	42.7[a]	10.7
Increases maternal side effects	75	1.3	5.3	20.0	61.3[a]	12.0
Increases fetal and neonatal side effects	75	0.0	4.0	17.3	58.7[a]	20.0
21. Neuraxial techniques improve the likelihood of vaginal delivery for patients attempting vaginal birth after previous cesarean delivery	75	21.3	36.0[a]	33.3	8.0	1.3

(continued)

TABLE B-5 Consultant Survey Responses (*Continued*)

	n	Percent Responding to Each Item				
		Strongly Agree	Agree	Uncertain	Disagree	Strongly Disagree
Removal of Retained Placenta						
22. If an epidural catheter is in situ and the patient is hemodynamically stable, epidural anesthesia is the preferred technique	75	66.7[a]	30.7	2.7	0.0	0.0
23. In cases involving major maternal hemorrhage, a general endotracheal anesthetic is preferred over neuraxial anesthesia	75	30.7	48.0[a]	12.0	6.7	2.9
24. Administration of nitroglycerin for uterine relaxation improves success at removing retained placenta	75	34.7	48.0[a]	9.3	6.7	1.3
Anesthetic Choices for Cesarean Delivery						
25. Equipment, facilities, and support personnel available in the labor and delivery operating suite should be comparable to that available in the main operating suite	74	82.4[a]	16.2	1.4	0.0	0.0
26. General anesthesia vs. epidural anesthesia:						
Reduces time to skin incision	74	40.5	37.8[a]	8.1	9.5	4.1
Increases maternal complications	74	37.8	47.3[a]	9.5	5.4	0.0
Increases fetal and neonatal complications	74	14.9	28.4	24.3[a]	29.7	2.7
27. General anesthesia vs. spinal anesthesia:						
Reduces time to skin incision	74	20.3	35.1[a]	12.2	28.4	4.1
Increases maternal complications	74	33.8	50.0[a]	6.8	8.1	1.4
Increases fetal and neonatal complications	74	12.2	28.4	23.0[a]	33.8	2.7
28. Epidural anesthesia vs. spinal anesthesia:						
Increases time to skin incision	74	43.2	43.2[a]	8.1	5.4	0.0
Reduces quality of anesthesia	74	12.2	56.8[a]	9.5	17.6	4.1
Increases maternal complications	74	1.4	13.5	28.4	48.6[a]	8.1
29. CSE anesthesia vs. epidural anesthesia:						
Improves anesthesia	73	20.5	47.9[a]	20.5	11.0	0.0
Reduces time to skin incision	73	17.8	53.4[a]	12.3	16.4	0.0
Reduces maternal side effects	73	2.7	12.3	30.1	52.1[a]	2.7
30. CSE anesthesia vs. spinal anesthesia:						
Improves anesthesia	72	1.4	15.3	25.0	52.8[a]	5.6
Increases flexibility for prolonged procedures	73	61.6[a]	32.9	4.1	1.4	0.0
Increases time to skin incision	73	6.8	49.3[a]	17.8	21.9	4.1
Reduces maternal side effects	73	1.4	11.0	37.0	47.9[a]	2.9
31. Use of pencil-point spinal needles vs. cutting-bevel spinal needles reduces maternal complications	73	75.3[a]	23.3	1.4	0.0	0.0
32. Intravenous fluid preloading vs. no intravenous fluid preloading for spinal anesthesia reduces maternal hypotension	73	30.1	46.6[a]	12.3	9.6	1.4
33a. Intravenous ephedrine is an acceptable agent to treat hypotension during neuraxial anesthesia	75	48.0	49.3[a]	1.3	1.3	0.0
33b. Intravenous phenylephrine is an acceptable agent to treat hypotension during neuraxial anesthesia	75	50.7[a]	40.0	6.7	2.7	0.0
34. Neuraxial opioids vs. parenteral opioids for postoperative analgesia after regional anesthesia for cesarean delivery:						
Improves analgesia	69	60.9[a]	33.3	5.8	0.0	0.0
Improves maternal satisfaction	69	52.2[a]	33.3	8.7	5.8	0.0
Postpartum Tubal Ligation						
35. Neuraxial vs. general anesthesia **reduces** maternal complications	70	24.3	58.6[a]	12.9	2.9	1.4
36. An immediate (≤8 h) postpartum tubal ligation **does not** increase maternal complications	70	14.3	50.0[a]	22.9	11.4	1.4
Management of Complications						
37. Availability of resources for management of hemorrhagic emergencies **reduces** maternal complications	70	74.3[a]	25.7	0.0	0.0	0.0
38. Immediate availability of equipment for management of airway emergencies **reduces** maternal, fetal, and neonatal complications	70	80.0[a]	20.0	0.0	0.0	0.0
39. Immediate availability of basic and advanced life-support equipment in the labor and delivery suite **reduces** maternal, fetal, and neonatal complications	70	78.6[a]	21.4	0.0	0.0	0.0
40. Routine use of central venous or pulmonary artery catheterization **reduces** maternal complications in severely preeclamptic patients	70	0.0	10.0	12.9	55.7[a]	21.4

[a]Median.

n, number of consultants who responded to each item.

TABLE B-6 ASA Membership Survey Responses

	n	Percent Responding to Each Item				
		Strongly Agree	Agree	Uncertain	Disagree	Strongly Disagree
Preanesthetic Evaluation						
1. Directed history and physical examination reduces maternal, fetal, and neonatal complications	2,324	57.5[a]	38.3	3.0	1.0	0.1
2. Communication between anesthetic and obstetric providers reduces maternal, fetal, and neonatal complications	2,321	77.9[a]	21.3	0.6	0.2	0.1
3. A routine intrapartum platelet count **does not reduce** maternal anesthetic complications	2,320	11.9	36.2	22.3[a]	23.6	6.0
4. An intrapartum platelet count reduces maternal anesthetic complications:						
For suspected preeclampsia	2,326	35.8	47.9[a]	11.4	4.3	0.6
For suspected coagulopathy	2,323	46.8	43.5[a]	6.2	2.8	0.6
5. All parturients should have an intrapartum blood sample sent to the blood bank to reduce maternal complications	2,317	22.1	34.3[a]	19.0	21.9	2.7
6. Preanesthetic recording of the fetal heart rate reduces fetal and neonatal complications	2,319	25.0	38.5[a]	25.2	9.9	1.6
Aspiration Prophylaxis						
7a. Oral intake of clear liquids *during labor* improves patient comfort and satisfaction	2,283	15.4	65.5[a]	12.1	6.2	0.8
7b. Oral intake of clear liquids *during labor* **does not** increase maternal complications	2,285	6.7	40.2	23.6[a]	23.5	6.0
8a. Oral intake of solids *during labor* increases maternal complications	2,284	48.2	38.0[a]	9.9	2.8	1.1
8b. The patient undergoing elective cesarean delivery should undergo a fasting period for solids of 6–8 h depending on the type of food ingested (e.g., fat content)	2,283	66.8[a]	30.3	1.1	1.3	0.5
8c. The patient undergoing elective postpartum tubal ligation should undergo a fasting period for solids of 6–8 h depending on the type of food ingested (e.g., fat content)	2,281	66.9[a]	30.2	1.1	1.4	0.4
9. Administration of a nonparticulate antacid before operative procedures reduces maternal complications	2,281	24.5	43.3[a]	24.0	7.2	1.1
Anesthetic Care for Labor and Delivery						
Neuraxial techniques:						
10. Prophylactic spinal or epidural catheter insertion for complicated parturients reduces maternal complications	2,071	17.6	42.4[a]	26.9	11.8	1.2
11. **Continuous epidural infusion** using local anesthetics with or *without opioids* vs. **parenteral opioids:**						
Improves analgesia	2,170	73.6[a]	25.1	0.8	0.4	0.1
Increases the duration of labor	2,174	1.2	14.4	19.0	51.7[a]	13.8
Decreases the chance of spontaneous delivery	2,171	0.8	7.4	16.9	53.3[a]	21.6
Increases maternal side effects	2,169	0.6	12.0	9.8	58.9[a]	18.7
Increases fetal and neonatal side effects	2,168	0.3	3.0	7.5	61.3[a]	27.9
12. **Continuous epidural infusion** using local anesthetics with or *without opioids* vs. **spinal** opioids with or without local anesthetics:						
Improves analgesia	2,160	17.4	36.5[a]	24.8	20.2	1.2
Increases the duration of labor	2,161	0.8	8.9	31.8	49.7[a]	8.8
Decreases the chance of spontaneous delivery	2,158	0.6	5.8	27.7	53.7[a]	12.3
Increases maternal motor block	2,149	3.7	36.0	16.1[a]	38.7	5.4
Increases maternal side effects	2,152	0.7	10.2	21.9	58.4[a]	8.8
Increases fetal and neonatal side effects	2,153	0.4	4.2	20.9	61.2[a]	13.3
13a. **Induction** of epidural analgesia using local anesthetics *with opioids* vs. epidural analgesia with **equal concentrations** of local anesthetics *without opioids:*						
Improves analgesia	2,153	34.6	46.1[a]	6.2	10.8	2.3
Increases maternal side effects	2,150	2.6	38.0	12.8[a]	40.4	6.2
Increases fetal and neonatal side effects	2,142	0.7	7.5	17.5	63.1[a]	11.3
13b. Induction of epidural analgesia using low-dose local anesthetics *with opioids* vs. higher concentrations of epidural local anesthetics *without opioids:*						
Improves analgesia	2,155	13.1	31.7	26.9[a]	26.6	1.7
Increases maternal side effects	2,154	1.1	13.8	15.8	55.7[a]	13.6
Increases fetal and neonatal side effects	2,147	0.6	4.5	19.3	60.8[a]	14.8

(*continued*)

TABLE B-6 ASA Membership Survey Responses (*Continued*)

	n	Percent Responding to Each Item				
		Strongly Agree	Agree	Uncertain	Disagree	Strongly Disagree
14a. Maintenance of epidural infusion of lower concentrations of local anesthetics *with* opioids vs. higher concentrations of local anesthetics *without* opioids:						
Improves analgesia	1,977	17.2	38.5[a]	24.0	19.2	1.0
Reduces the duration of labor	1,980	3.9	28.0	44.9[a]	21.6	1.6
Improves the chance of spontaneous delivery	1,977	6.9	41.1	35.9[a]	15.1	1.0
Reduces maternal motor block	1,977	31.3	63.0[a]	2.9	2.4	0.4
Reduces maternal side effects	1,971	11.4	47.1[a]	26.8	14.0	0.9
Reduces fetal and neonatal side effects	1,972	7.4	34.4	38.1[a]	18.6	1.5
14b. Maintenance of epidural analgesia using bupivacaine ≤**0.125%** *with* opioids vs. bupivacaine concentrations >**0.125%** *without* opioids:						
Improves analgesia	1,973	16.5	38.6[a]	23.9	19.7	1.4
Reduces the duration of labor	1,975	4.4	25.6	46.9[a]	21.5	1.7
Improves the chance of spontaneous delivery	1,973	6.1	36.9	38.9[a]	16.7	1.4
Reduces maternal motor block	1,967	23.4	63.7[a]	5.3	6.5	1.1
Reduces maternal side effects	1,960	9.2	44.7[a]	27.0	18.1	1.0
Reduces fetal and neonatal side effects	1,957	6.3	31.3	39.0[a]	21.6	1.8
15. Single-injection **spinal** opioids with or without local anesthetics vs. **parenteral** opioids:						
Improve analgesia	1,966	36.9	50.2[a]	8.9	3.6	0.5
Increase the duration of labor	1,963	0.4	2.7	31.5	55.8[a]	9.6
Decrease the chance of spontaneous delivery	1,967	0.4	2.8	27.9	58.3[a]	10.7
Increase maternal side effects	1,958	2.1	23.7	23.1	45.1[a]	5.8
Increase fetal and neonatal side effects	1,960	0.7	7.7	25.6	55.9[a]	10.2
16. Single-injection spinal opioids **with** local anesthetics vs. spinal opioids **without** local anesthetics:						
Improve analgesia	1,961	29.2	55.6[a]	9.4	5.5	0.4
Increase the duration of labor	1,960	1.1	10.2	43.0[a]	41.2	4.6
Decrease the chance of spontaneous delivery	1,959	0.8	8.1	38.4	47.1[a]	5.7
Increase maternal motor block	1,955	12.5	59.0[a]	11.6	15.4	1.4
Increase maternal side effects	1,951	2.5	33.1	28.9[a]	33.1	2.4
Increase fetal and neonatal side effects	1,954	1.0	11.3	36.2	46.8[a]	4.7

Combined spinal–epidural (CSE) techniques:

	n					
17. CSE local anesthetics *with opioids* vs. **epidural** local anesthetics *with opioids*:						
Improve **early** analgesia	1,887	31.1	44.6[a]	11.7	11.2	1.5
Improve **overall** analgesia	1,884	14.0	26.8	27.1[a]	28.7	3.5
Decrease the duration of labor	1,884	1.5	8.8	48.2[a]	38.2	3.4
Decrease the chance of spontaneous delivery	1,882	0.3	3.1	38.5	52.1[a]	6.0
Reduce maternal motor block	1,880	4.0	23.8	27.6[a]	41.0	3.5
Increase maternal side effects	1,877	2.0	28.2	33.0[a]	34.2	2.6
Increase fetal and neonatal side effects	1,872	0.9	11.4	37.1	45.3[a]	5.2

Patient-controlled epidural analgesia (PCEA):

	n					
18. PCEA vs. continuous infusion epidurals:						
Improves analgesia	1,852	15.3	40.1[a]	29.2	14.6	0.8
Improves maternal satisfaction	1,848	27.8	46.5[a]	19.6	5.6	0.5
Reduces the need for anesthetic interventions	1,849	22.4	42.9[a]	21.4	12.1	1.1
Increases the chance of spontaneous delivery	1,845	2.6	12.1	56.9[a]	26.4	2.1
Reduces maternal motor block	1,846	4.3	34.1	40.4[a]	20.5	0.8
Decreases maternal side effects	1,838	3.8	27.0	46.5[a]	21.9	0.9
19. PCEA **with** a background infusion vs. PCEA **without** a background infusion:						
Improves analgesia	1,840	26.0	48.4[a]	20.8	4.7	0.3
Improves maternal satisfaction	1,840	25.4	46.0[a]	24.1	4.2	0.3
Reduces the need for anesthetic interventions	1,829	22.4	46.0[a]	24.7	6.6	0.3
Decreases the chance of spontaneous delivery	1,831	0.8	4.3	48.6[a]	41.6	4.8
Increases maternal motor block	1,837	1.0	27.3	40.8[a]	28.6	2.2
Increases maternal side effects	1,828	0.8	12.8	43.5[a]	39.6	3.3

(continued)

TABLE B-6 ASA Membership Survey Responses (*Continued*)

		Percent Responding to Each Item				
	n	Strongly Agree	Agree	Uncertain	Disagree	Strongly Disagree
Neuraxial Analgesia, Timing of Initiation, and Progress of Labor						
20. Administering epidural analgesia at cervical dilations of <5 cm (vs. >5 cm):						
Improves analgesia	1,831	25.9	52.7[a]	10.4	10.1	0.9
Reduces the duration of labor	1,825	1.9	13.5	40.1[a]	41.2	3.4
Improves the chance of spontaneous delivery	1,823	1.8	14.9	49.4[a]	30.9	3.0
Increases maternal motor block	1,819	0.9	20.5	21.2	53.4[a]	4.0
Increases maternal side effects	1,821	0.7	11.0	22.3	61.1[a]	5.0
Increases fetal and neonatal side effects	1,820	0.3	4.3	23.0	64.6[a]	7.7
21. Neuraxial techniques improve the likelihood of vaginal delivery for patients attempting vaginal birth after previous cesarean delivery	1,816	8.7	41.6[a]	37.9	10.1	1.7
Removal of Retained Placenta						
22. If an epidural catheter is in situ and the patient is hemodynamically stable, epidural anesthesia is the preferred technique	1,821	30.8	59.5[a]	4.3	4.4	1.0
23. In cases involving major maternal hemorrhage, a general endotracheal anesthetic is preferred over neuraxial anesthesia	1,823	36.0	48.8[a]	6.9	7.5	0.9
24. Administration of nitroglycerin for uterine relaxation improves success at removing retained placenta	1,812	15.6	54.1[a]	26.4	3.5	0.4
Anesthetic Choices for Cesarean Delivery						
25. Equipment, facilities, and support personnel available in the labor and delivery operating suite should be comparable to that available in the main operating suite	1,815	78.3[a]	20.3	0.5	0.9	0.1
26. General anesthesia vs. epidural anesthesia:						
Reduces time to skin incision	1,826	30.9	46.3[a]	6.8	14.3	1.6
Increases maternal complications	1,824	27.3	50.1[a]	10.9	9.6	2.0
Increases fetal and neonatal complications	1,825	13.9	37.5[a]	23.2	22.8	2.6
27. General anesthesia vs. spinal anesthesia:						
Reduces time to skin incision	1,823	13.1	37.2[a]	13.7	30.1	6.0
Increases maternal complications	1,815	23.8	49.6[a]	10.7	13.8	2.0
Increases fetal and neonatal complications	1,803	13.6	37.2[a]	21.9	24.6	2.8
28. Epidural anesthesia vs. spinal anesthesia:						
Increases time to skin incision	1,823	32.1	54.3[a]	3.8	8.7	1.0
Reduces quality of anesthesia	1,821	15.0	51.0[a]	8.8	21.5	3.6
Increases maternal complications	1,816	1.2	8.8	24.5	59.1[a]	6.4
29. CSE anesthesia vs. epidural anesthesia:						
Improves anesthesia	1,794	18.7	45.4[a]	22.6	12.5	0.9
Reduces time to skin incision	1,795	14.7	38.2[a]	21.7	23.2	2.3
Reduces maternal side effects	1,791	2.6	9.4	42.4[a]	43.3	2.4
30. CSE anesthesia vs. spinal anesthesia:						
Improves anesthesia	1,800	4.4	14.3	28.5	48.2[a]	4.6
Increases flexibility for prolonged procedures	1,808	32.1	54.8[a]	10.2	2.5	0.4
Increases time to skin incision	1,804	9.9	48.7[a]	17.7	22.1	1.7
Reduces maternal side effects	1,802	0.9	7.7	41.6[a]	46.1	3.7
31. Use of pencil-point spinal needles vs. cutting-bevel spinal needles reduces maternal complications	1,819	51.7[a]	39.4	5.7	2.9	0.4
32. Intravenous fluid preloading vs. no intravenous fluid preloading for spinal anesthesia reduces maternal hypotension	1,817	40.0	43.0[a]	9.0	6.5	1.4
33a. Intravenous ephedrine is an acceptable agent to treat hypotension during neuraxial anesthesia	1,819	50.7[a]	47.3	0.9	1.0	0.1
33b. Intravenous phenylephrine is an acceptable agent to treat hypotension during neuraxial anesthesia	1,820	31.9	52.8[a]	6.0	8.0	1.3
34. Neuraxial opioids vs. parenteral opioids for postoperative analgesia after regional anesthesia for cesarean delivery:						
Improves analgesia	1,822	40.1	49.7[a]	6.9	3.0	0.3
Improves maternal satisfaction	1,816	35.0	47.4[a]	13.0	4.1	0.6

(continued)

TABLE B-6 ASA Membership Survey Responses (*Continued*)

	n	Percent Responding to Each Item				
		Strongly Agree	Agree	Uncertain	Disagree	Strongly Disagree
Postpartum Tubal Ligation						
35. Neuraxial vs. general anesthesia **reduces** maternal complications	1,812	28.8	45.0[a]	15.2	9.4	1.6
36. An immediate (≤8 h) postpartum tubal ligation **does not** increase maternal complications	1,814	6.4	34.1	32.3[a]	23.0	4.2
Management of Complications						
37. Availability of resources for management of hemorrhagic emergencies **reduces** maternal complications	1,823	67.9[a]	30.8	1.0	0.3	0.0
38. Immediate availability of equipment for management of airway emergencies **reduces** maternal, fetal, and neonatal complications	1,817	77.2[a]	22.1	0.6	0.2	0.0
39. Immediate availability of basic and advanced life-support equipment in the labor and delivery suite **reduces** maternal, fetal, and neonatal complications	1,812	73.4[a]	24.8	1.6	0.2	0.0
40. Routine use of central venous or pulmonary artery catheterization **reduces** maternal complications in severely preeclamptic patients	1,822	3.2	13.3	33.0	40.8[a]	9.6

[a]Median.
ASA, American Society of Anesthesiologists; n, number of members who responded to each item.

Optimal Goals for Anesthesia Care in Obstetrics

This joint statement from the American Society of Anesthesiologists (ASA) and the American College of Obstetricians and Gynecologists (ACOG) has been designed to address issues of concern to both specialties. Good obstetric care requires the availability of qualified personnel and equipment to administer general or neuraxial anesthesia both electively and emergently. The extent and degree to which anesthesia services are available varies widely among hospitals. However, for any hospital providing obstetric care, certain optimal anesthesia goals should be sought. These include:

1. Availability of a licensed practitioner who is credentialed to administer an appropriate anesthetic whenever necessary. For many women, neuraxial anesthesia (epidural, spinal, or combined spinal epidural) will be the most appropriate anesthetic.
2. Availability of a licensed practitioner who is credentialed to maintain support of vital functions in any obstetric emergency.
3. Availability of anesthesia and surgical personnel to permit the start of a cesarean delivery within 30 minutes of the decision to perform the procedure.
4. Since the risks associated with trial of labor after cesarean delivery (TOLAC) and uterine rupture may be unpredictable, the immediate availability of appropriate facilities and personnel (including obstetric anesthesia, nursing personnel, and a physician capable of monitoring labor and performing cesarean delivery, including an emergency cesarean delivery) is optimal. When resources for immediate cesarean delivery are not available, patients considering TOLAC should discuss the hospital's resources and availability of obstetric, anesthetic, pediatric and nursing staff with their obstetric provider (1); patients should be clearly informed of the potential increase in risk and the management alternatives. The definition of immediately available personnel and facilities remains a local decision based on each institution's available resources and geographic location.
5. Appointment of a qualified anesthesiologist to be responsible for all anesthetics administered. There are many obstetric units where obstetricians or obstetrician-supervised nurse anesthetists administer labor anesthetics. The administration of general or neuraxial anesthesia requires both medical judgment and technical skills. Thus, a physician with privileges in anesthesiology should be readily available.

Persons administering or supervising obstetric anesthesia should be qualified to manage the infrequent but occasionally life-threatening complications of neuraxial anesthesia such as respiratory and cardiovascular failure, toxic local anesthetic convulsions, or vomiting and aspiration. Mastering and retaining the skills and knowledge necessary to manage these complications require adequate training and frequent application.

To ensure the safest and most effective anesthesia for obstetric patients, the Director of Anesthesia Services, with the approval of the medical staff, should develop and enforce written policies regarding provision of obstetric anesthesia. These include:

1. A qualified physician with obstetric privileges to perform operative vaginal or cesarean delivery should be readily available during administration of anesthesia. Readily available should be defined by each institution within the context of its resources and geographic location. Neuraxial and/or general anesthesia should not be administered until the patient has been examined and the fetal status and progress of labor evaluated by a qualified individual. A physician with obstetric privileges who concurs with the patient's management and has knowledge of the maternal and fetal status and the progress of labor should be readily available to deal with any obstetric complications that may arise. A physician with obstetric privileges should be responsible for midwifery back up in hospital settings that utilize certified nurse midwives/certified midwives as obstetric providers.
2. Availability of equipment, facilities, and support personnel equal to that provided in the surgical suite. This should include the availability of a properly equipped and staffed recovery room capable of receiving and caring for all patients recovering from neuraxial or general anesthesia. Birthing facilities, when used for labor anesthesia services or surgical anesthesia, must be appropriately equipped to provide safe anesthetic care during labor and delivery or postanesthesia recovery care.
3. Personnel, other than the surgical team, should be immediately available to assume responsibility for resuscitation of the depressed newborn. The surgeon and anesthesiologist are responsible for the mother and may not be able to leave her to care for the newborn, even when a neuraxial anesthetic is functioning adequately. Individuals qualified to perform neonatal resuscitation should demonstrate:
   3.1 Proficiency in rapid and accurate evaluation of the newborn condition, including Apgar scoring.
   3.2 Knowledge of the pathogenesis of a depressed newborn (acidosis, drugs, hypovolemia, trauma, anomalies, and infection), as well as specific indications for resuscitation.

Committee of Origin: Obstetrical Anesthesia

Approved by the ASA House of Delegates on October 17, 2007 and last amended on October 20, 2010. Reprinted with permission of the American Society of Anesthesiologists, 520 N. Northwest Highway, Park Ridge, Illinois 60068-2573.

3.3 Proficiency in newborn airway management, laryngoscopy, endotracheal intubations, suctioning of airways, artificial ventilation, cardiac massage, and maintenance of thermal stability.

In larger maternity units and those functioning as high-risk centers, 24-hour in-house anesthesia, obstetric and neonatal specialists are usually necessary. Preferably, the obstetric anesthesia services should be directed by an anesthesiologist with special training or experience in obstetric anesthesia. These units will also frequently require the availability of more sophisticated monitoring equipment and specially trained nursing personnel.

A survey jointly sponsored by ASA and ACOG found that many hospitals in the United States have not yet achieved the goals mentioned previously. Deficiencies were most evident in smaller delivery units. Some small delivery units are necessary because of geographic considerations. Currently, approximately 34% of hospitals providing obstetric care have fewer than 500 deliveries per year (2). Providing comprehensive care for obstetric patients in these small units is extremely inefficient, not cost-effective and frequently impossible. Thus, the following recommendations are made:

1. Whenever possible, small units should consolidate.
2. When geographic factors require the existence of smaller units, these units should be part of a well-established regional perinatal system.

The availability of appropriate personnel to assist in the management of a variety of obstetric problems is a necessary feature of good obstetric care. The presence of a pediatrician or other trained physician at a high-risk cesarean delivery to care for the newborn or the availability of an anesthesiologist during active labor and delivery when TOLAC is attempted and at a breech or multifetal delivery are examples. Frequently, these physicians spend a considerable amount of time standing by for the possibility that their services may be needed emergently, but may ultimately not be required to perform the tasks for which they are present. Reasonable compensation for these standby services is justifiable and necessary.

A variety of other mechanisms have been suggested to increase the availability and quality of anesthesia services in obstetrics. Improved hospital design, to place labor and delivery suites closer to the operating rooms, would allow for safer and more efficient anesthesia care, including supervision of nurse anesthetists. Anesthesia equipment in the labor and delivery area must be comparable to that in the operating room.

Finally, good interpersonal relations between obstetricians and anesthesiologists are important. Joint meetings between the two departments should be encouraged. Anesthesiologists should recognize the special needs and concerns of the obstetrician and obstetricians should recognize the anesthesiologist as a consultant in the management of pain and life-support measures. Both should recognize the need to provide high-quality care for all patients.

REFERENCES

1. Vaginal birth after previous cesarean delivery. ACOG Practice Bulletin No. 115. American College of Obstetricians and Gynecologists. *Obstet Gynecol* 2010;116:450–463.
2. Bucklin BA, Hawkins JL, Anderson JR, et al. Obstetric anesthesia workforce survey: twenty-year update. *Anesthesiology* 2005;103:645–653.

Intrapartum Fetal Heart Rate Monitoring: Nomenclature, Interpretation, and General Management Principles

Clinical Management Guidelines for Obstetrician–Gynecologists

The American College of Obstetricians and Gynecologists

In the most recent year for which data are available, approximately 3.4 million fetuses (85% of approximately 4 million live births) in the United States were assessed with electronic fetal monitoring (EFM), making it the most common obstetric procedure (1). Despite its widespread use, there is controversy about the efficacy of EFM, interobserver and intraobserver variability, nomenclature, systems for interpretation, and management algorithms. Moreover, there is evidence that the use of EFM increases the rate of cesarean deliveries and operative vaginal deliveries. The purpose of this document is to review nomenclature for fetal heart rate (FHR) assessment, review the data on the efficacy of EFM, delineate the strengths and shortcomings of EFM, and describe a system for EFM classification.

■ BACKGROUND

A complex interplay of antepartum complications, suboptimal uterine perfusion, placental dysfunction, and intrapartum events can result in adverse neonatal outcome. Known obstetric conditions, such as hypertensive disease, fetal growth restriction, and preterm birth, predispose fetuses to poor outcomes, but they account for a small proportion of asphyxial injury. In a study of term pregnancies with fetal asphyxia, 63% had no known risk factors (2).

The fetal brain modulates the FHR through an interplay of sympathetic and parasympathetic forces. Thus, FHR monitoring can be used to determine if a fetus is well oxygenated. It was used among 45% of laboring women in 1980, 62% in 1988, 74% in 1992, and 85% in 2002 (1).

This Practice Bulletin was developed by the ACOG Committee on Practice Bulletins with the assistance of George A. Macones, M.D. The information is designed to aid practitioners in making decisions about appropriate obstetric and gynecologic care. These guidelines should not be construed as dictating an exclusive course of treatment or procedure. Variations in practice may be warranted based on the needs of the individual patient, resources, and limitations unique to the institution or type of practice.

ACOG Practice Bulletin No. 106: Intrapartum Fetal Heart Rate Monitoring: Nomenclature, Interpretation, and General Management, Vol. 114, No. 1, July 2009. Copyright © 2009 Wolters Kluwer Health.

Despite the frequency of its use, limitations of EFM include poor interobserver and intraobserver reliability, uncertain efficacy, and a high false-positive rate.

FHR monitoring may be performed externally or internally. Most external monitors use a Doppler device with computerized logic to interpret and count the Doppler signals. Internal FHR monitoring is accomplished with a fetal electrode, which is a spiral wire placed directly on the fetal scalp or other presenting part.

Guidelines for Nomenclature and Interpretation of Electronic Fetal Heart Rate Monitoring

In 2008, the *Eunice Kennedy Shriver* National Institute of Child Health and Human Development partnered with the American College of Obstetricians and Gynecologists and the Society for Maternal–Fetal Medicine to sponsor a workshop focused on electronic FHR monitoring (3). This 2008 workshop gathered a diverse group of investigators with expertise and interest in the field to accomplish three goals: (1) To review and update the definitions for FHR pattern categorization from the prior workshop; (2) to assess existing classification systems for interpreting specific FHR patterns and make recommendations about a system for use in the United States; and, (3) to make recommendations for research priorities for EFM. A complete clinical understanding of EFM necessitates discussion of uterine contractions, baseline FHR rate and variability, presence of accelerations, periodic or episodic decelerations, and the changes in these characteristics over time. A number of assumptions and factors common to FHR interpretation in the United States are central to the proposed system of nomenclature and interpretation (3). Two such assumptions are of particular importance. First, the definitions are primarily developed for visual interpretation of FHR patterns, but should be adaptable to computerized systems of interpretation. Second, the definitions should be applied to intrapartum patterns, but also are applicable to antepartum observations.

Uterine contractions are quantified as the number of contractions present in a 10-minute window, averaged over a 30-minute period. Contraction frequency alone is a partial assessment of uterine activity. Other factors such as duration, intensity, and relaxation time between contractions are equally important in clinical practice.

Listed as follows is terminology used to describe uterine activity:

Normal: Five contractions or less in 10 minutes, averaged over a 30-minute window

Tachysystole: More than five contractions in 10 minutes, averaged over a 30-minute window

Characteristics of uterine contractions:

■ The terms hyperstimulation and hypercontractility are not defined and should be abandoned.

■ Tachysystole should always be qualified as to the presence or absence of associated FHR decelerations.

■ The term tachysystole applies to both spontaneous and stimulated labor. The clinical response to tachysystole may differ depending on whether contractions are spontaneous or stimulated.

Table D-1 provides EFM definitions and descriptions based on the 2008 National Institute of Child Health and Human Development Working Group findings. Decelerations are defined as recurrent if they occur with at least one-half of the contractions.

Classification of Fetal Heart Rate Tracings

A variety of systems for EFM interpretation have been used in the United States and worldwide (4–6). On the basis of careful review of the available options, a three-tiered system for the categorization of FHR patterns is recommended (see box). It is important to recognize that FHR tracing patterns provide information only on the current acid–base status of the fetus. Categorization of the FHR tracing evaluates the fetus at that point in time; tracing patterns can and will change. An FHR tracing may move back and forth between the categories depending on the clinical situation and management strategies used.

Category I FHR Tracings are Normal. Category I FHR tracings are strongly predictive of normal fetal acid–base status at the time of observation. Category I FHR tracings may be monitored in a routine manner, and no specific action is required.

Category II FHR Tracings are Indeterminate. Category II FHR tracings are not predictive of abnormal fetal acid–base status, yet presently there is no adequate evidence to classify these as Category I or Category III. Category II FHR tracings require evaluation and continued surveillance and reevaluation, taking into account the entire associated clinical circumstances. In some circumstances, either ancillary tests to ensure fetal well-being or intrauterine resuscitative measures may be used with Category II tracings.

Category III FHR Tracings are Abnormal. Category III tracings are associated with abnormal fetal acid–base status at the time of observation. Category III FHR tracings require prompt evaluation. Depending on the clinical situation, efforts to expeditiously resolve the abnormal FHR pattern may include but are not limited to provision of maternal oxygen, change in maternal position, discontinuation of labor stimulation, treatment of maternal hypotension, and treatment of tachysystole with FHR changes. If a Category III tracing does not resolve with these measures, delivery should be undertaken.

Three-tiered Fetal Heart Rate Interpretation System

Category I
- Category I FHR tracings include all of the following:
- Baseline rate: 110–160 beats/min
- Baseline FHR variability: Moderate
- Late or variable decelerations: Absent
- Early decelerations: Present or absent
- Accelerations: Present or absent

Category II
Category II FHR tracings include all FHR tracings not categorized as Category I or Category III. Category II tracings may represent an appreciable fraction of those encountered in clinical care. Examples of Category II FHR tracings include any of the following:

Baseline rate
- Bradycardia not accompanied by absent baseline variability
- Tachycardia

Baseline FHR variability
- Minimal baseline variability
- Absent baseline variability with no recurrent decelerations
- Marked baseline variability

Accelerations
- Absence of induced accelerations after fetal stimulation

Periodic or episodic decelerations
- Recurrent variable decelerations accompanied by minimal or moderate baseline variability
- Prolonged deceleration more than 2 minutes but less than 10 minutes
- Recurrent late decelerations with moderate baseline variability
- Variable decelerations with other characteristics such as slow return to baseline, overshoots, or "shoulders"

Category III
Category III FHR tracings include either
- Absent baseline FHR variability and any of the following:
  - Recurrent late decelerations
  - Recurrent variable decelerations
  - Bradycardia
- Sinusoidal pattern

FHR, fetal heart rate.

Macones GA, Hankins GD, Spong CY, Hauth J, Moore T. The 2008 National Institute of Child Health and Human Development workshop report on electronic fetal monitoring: update on definitions, interpretation, and research guidelines. *Obstet Gynecol* 2008;112:661–666.

Guidelines for Review of Electronic Fetal Heart Rate Monitoring

When EFM is used during labor, the nurses or physicians should review it frequently. In a patient without complications, the FHR tracing should be reviewed approximately every 30 minutes in the first stage of labor and every 15 minutes during the second stage. The corresponding frequency for patients with complications (e.g., fetal growth restriction, preeclampsia) is approximately every 15 minutes in the first stage of labor and every 5 minutes during the second stage. Healthcare providers

TABLE D-1 **Electronic Fetal Monitoring Definitions**

Pattern	Definition

Baseline	• The mean FHR rounded to increments of 5 beats/min during a 10-min segment, excluding:
	  • Periodic or episodic changes
	  • Periods of marked FHR variability
	  • Segments of baseline that differ by more than 25 beats/min
	• The baseline must be for a minimum of 2 min in any 10-min segment, or the baseline for that time period is indeterminate. In this case, one may refer to the prior 10-min window for determination of baseline
	• Normal FHR baseline: 110–160 beats/min
	• Tachycardia: FHR baseline is greater than 160 beats/min
	• Bradycardia: FHR baseline is less than 110 beats/min

Baseline variability	• Fluctuations in the baseline FHR that are irregular in amplitude and frequency
	• Variability is visually quantitated as the amplitude of peak-to-trough in beats per minute.
	  • Absent—amplitude range undetectable
	  • Minimal—amplitude range detectable but 5 beats/min or fewer
	  • Moderate (normal)—amplitude range 6–25 beats/min
	  • Marked—amplitude range greater than 25 beats/min

Acceleration	• A visually apparent abrupt increase (onset to peak in less than 30 s) in the FHR • At 32 wks of gestation and beyond, an acceleration has a peak of 15 beats/min or more above baseline, with a duration of 15 s or more but less than 2 min from onset to return • Before 32 wks of gestation, an acceleration has a peak of 10 beats/min or more above baseline, with a duration of 10 s or more but less than 2 min from onset to return • Prolonged acceleration lasts 2 min or more but less than 10 min in duration • If an acceleration lasts 10 min or longer, it is a baseline change
Early deceleration	• Visually apparent usually symmetrical gradual decrease and return of the FHR associated with a uterine contraction • A gradual FHR decrease is defined as from the onset to the FHR nadir of 30 s or more • The decrease in FHR is calculated from the onset to the nadir of the deceleration • The nadir of the deceleration occurs at the same time as the peak of the contraction • In most cases the onset, nadir, and recovery of the deceleration are coincident with the beginning, peak, and ending of the contraction, respectively
Late deceleration	• Visually apparent usually symmetrical gradual decrease and return of the FHR associated with a uterine contraction • A gradual FHR decrease is defined as from the onset to the FHR nadir of 30 s or more • The decrease in FHR is calculated from the onset to the nadir of the deceleration • The deceleration is delayed in timing, with the nadir of the deceleration occurring after the peak of the contraction • In most cases, the onset, nadir, and recovery of the deceleration occur after the beginning, peak, and ending of the contraction, respectively
Variable deceleration	• Visually apparent abrupt decrease in FHR • An abrupt FHR decrease is defined as from the onset of the deceleration to the beginning of the FHR nadir of less than 30 s • The decrease in FHR is calculated from the onset to the nadir of the deceleration • The decrease in FHR is 15 beats/min or greater, lasting 15 s or greater, and less than 2 min in duration • When variable decelerations are associated with uterine contractions, their onset, depth, and duration commonly vary with successive uterine contractions
Prolonged deceleration	• Visually apparent decrease in the FHR below the baseline • Decrease in FHR from the baseline that is 15 beats/min or more, lasting 2 min or more but less than 10 min in duration • If a deceleration lasts 10 min or longer, it is a baseline change
Sinusoidal pattern	• Visually apparent, smooth, sine wave–like undulating pattern in FHR baseline with a cycle frequency of 3–5/min which persists for 20 min or more

FHR, fetal heart rate.

Macones GA, Hankins GD, Spong CY, Hauth J, Moore T. The 2008 National Institute of Child Health and Human Development workshop report on electronic fetal monitoring: update on definitions, interpretation, and research guidelines. *Obstet Gynecol* 2008;112:661–666.

should periodically document that they have reviewed the tracing. The FHR tracing, as part of the medical record, should be labeled and available for review if the need arises. Computer storage of the FHR tracing that does not permit overwriting or revisions is reasonable, as is microfilm recording.

■ CLINICAL CONSIDERATIONS AND RECOMMENDATIONS

How efficacious is intrapartum electronic fetal heart rate monitoring?

The efficacy of EFM during labor is judged by its ability to decrease complications, such as neonatal seizures, cerebral palsy, or intrapartum fetal death, while minimizing the need for unnecessary obstetric interventions, such as operative vaginal delivery or cesarean delivery. There are no randomized clinical trials to compare the benefits of EFM with any form of monitoring during labor (7). Thus, the benefits of EFM are gauged from reports comparing it with intermittent auscultation.

A meta-analysis synthesizing the results of the randomized clinical trials comparing the modalities had the following conclusions (8):

■ The use of EFM compared with intermittent auscultation increased the overall cesarean delivery rate (relative risk [RR], 1.66; 95% confidence interval [CI], 1.30–2.13) and the cesarean delivery rate for abnormal FHR or acidosis or both (RR, 2.37; 95% CI, 1.88–3.00).
■ The use of EFM increased the risk of both vacuum and forceps operative vaginal delivery (RR, 1.16; 95% CI, 1.01–1.32).
■ The use of EFM did not reduce perinatal mortality (RR, 0.85; 95% CI, 0.59–1.23).
■ The use of EFM reduced the risk of neonatal seizures (RR, 0.50; 95% CI, 0.31–0.80).
■ The use of EFM did not reduce the risk of cerebral palsy (RR, 1.74; 95% CI, 0.97–3.11).

There is an unrealistic expectation that a nonreassuring FHR tracing is predictive of cerebral palsy. The positive predictive value of a nonreassuring pattern to predict cerebral palsy among singleton newborns with birth weights of 2,500 g or more is 0.14%, meaning that out of 1,000 fetuses with a nonreassuring FHR pattern, only one or two will develop cerebral palsy (9). The false-positive rate of EFM for predicting cerebral palsy is extremely high, at greater than 99%.

Available data, although limited in quantity, suggest that the use of EFM does not result in a reduction in cerebral palsy (8). This is consistent with data that suggest that the occurrence of cerebral palsy has been stable over time, despite the widespread introduction of EFM (10). The principal explanation for why the prevalence of cerebral palsy has not diminished despite the use of EFM is that 70% of cases occur before the onset of labor; only 4% of cases of encephalopathy can be attributed solely to intrapartum events (11,12).

Given that the available data do not show a clear benefit for the use of EFM over intermittent auscultation, either option is acceptable in a patient without complications. Logistically, it may not be feasible to adhere to guidelines for how frequently the heart rate should be auscultated. One prospective study noted that the protocol for intermittent auscultation was successfully completed in only 3% of the cases (13). The most common reasons for unsuccessful intermittent auscultation included the frequency of recording and the requirements for recording.

Intermittent auscultation may not be appropriate for all pregnancies. Most of the clinical trials that compare EFM with intermittent auscultation have excluded participants at high risk of adverse outcomes, and the relative safety of intermittent auscultation in such cases is uncertain. The labor of women with high-risk conditions (e.g., suspected fetal growth restriction, preeclampsia, and type 1 diabetes) should be monitored with continuous FHR monitoring.

There are no comparative data indicating the optimal frequency at which intermittent auscultation should be performed in the absence of risk factors. One method is to evaluate and record the FHR at least every 15 minutes in the active phase of the first stage of labor and at least every 5 minutes in the second stage (14).

What is the interobserver and intraobserver variability of intrapartum electronic fetal heart rate monitoring assessment?

There is high interobserver and intraobserver variability in the interpretation of FHR tracings. For example, when 4 obstetricians examined 50 cardiotocograms, they agreed in only 22% of the cases (15). Two months later, during the second review of the same 50 tracings, the clinicians interpreted 21% of the tracings differently than they did during the first evaluation. In another study, 5 obstetricians independently interpreted 150 cardiotocograms (16). The obstetricians interpreted the tracings similarly in 29% of the cases, suggesting poor interobserver reliability.

The interpretation of cardiotocograms is more consistent when the tracing is normal (17). With retrospective reviews, the foreknowledge of neonatal outcome may alter the reviewer's impressions of the tracing. Given the same intrapartum tracing, a reviewer is more likely to find evidence of fetal hypoxia and criticize the obstetrician's management if the outcome was poor versus good (18). Therefore, reinterpretation of the FHR tracing, especially if neonatal outcome is known, may not be reliable.

When should the very preterm fetus be monitored?

The decision to monitor the very preterm fetus requires a discussion between the obstetrician, pediatrician, and patient concerning the likelihood of survival or severe morbidity of the preterm child (based on gestational age, estimated fetal weight, and other factors) and issues related to mode of delivery. If a patient undergoes a cesarean delivery for indications related to a preterm fetus, continuous monitoring should be used rather than intermittent auscultation. The earliest gestational age that this will occur may vary.

Nonreassuring FHR patterns may occur with up to 60% of women with preterm labor, with the most common abnormality being deceleration and bradycardia, followed by tachycardia and minimal or absent baseline variability (19). Variable decelerations are more common among preterm (55% to 70%) deliveries than term (20% to 30%) deliveries (20). If FHR abnormalities are persistent, intrauterine resuscitation, ancillary tests to ensure fetal well-being, and possibly delivery should be undertaken (21).

What medications can affect the fetal heart rate?

FHR patterns can be influenced by the medications administered in the intrapartum period. Most often, these changes are transient, although they sometimes lead to obstetric interventions.

Epidural analgesia with local anesthetic agents (i.e., lidocaine, bupivacaine) can lead to sympathetic blockade, maternal hypotension, transient uteroplacental insufficiency, and alterations in the FHR. Parenteral narcotics also may affect the FHR. A randomized trial comparing epidural anesthesia with 0.25% of bupivacaine and intravenous meperidine reported that the variability was decreased, and FHR accelerations were significantly less common with parenteral analgesia compared with regional analgesia (22). The rates of decelerations and cesarean delivery for "nonreassuring" FHR tracings were similar for the two groups. A systematic review of five randomized trials and seven observational studies also noted that the rate of cesarean delivery for nonreassuring FHR was similar between those who did and those who did not receive epidural analgesia during labor (23).

Concern has been raised about combined spinal–epidural anesthesia during labor. An intent-to-treat analysis of 1,223 laboring women randomized to combined spinal–epidural anesthesia (10 mcg of intrathecal sufentanil, followed by epidural bupivacaine and fentanyl at the next request for analgesia) or intravenous meperidine (50 mg on demand, maximum 200 mg in 4 hours) noted a significantly higher rate of bradycardia and emergent cesarean delivery for abnormal FHR in the group randomized to combined spinal–epidural anesthesia (24). Neonatal outcome, however, was not significantly different between the two groups. There are some methodologic concerns with this study. Another randomized controlled trial compared the occurrence of FHR tracing abnormalities in laboring women who received combined spinal–epidural anesthesia (n = 41) to epidural anesthesia (n = 46). In this study, FHR abnormalities were more common in women receiving combined spinal–epidural anesthesia (25). Additional trials are necessary to determine the potential safety and efficacy of the combined spinal–epidural technique.

Other medications that influence FHR tracing have been studied (see Table D-2). Of note, multiple regression analysis indicated that decreased variability attributed to the use of magnesium sulfate was related to early gestational age but not the serum magnesium level (41). Studies report different findings with regard to the effect of magnesium on FHR patterns. Some show no independent effect; others show small changes in baseline or variability. In general, however, caution should be used in ascribing unfavorable findings on EFM to the use of magnesium alone.

Transient sinusoidal FHR patterns occurred in 75% of patients who received butorphanol during labor, but this was not associated with adverse outcomes (32). Fetuses exposed to cocaine did not exhibit any characteristic changes in the heart rate pattern, although they did have frequent contractions even when labor was unstimulated (34). As determined by computer analysis of cardiotocograms, a randomized trial reported that compared with meperidine, nalbuphine used for intrapartum analgesia decreased the likelihood of two 15-second accelerations over 20 minutes (45). In antepartum patients, administration of morphine decreased not only the fetal breathing movement but also the number of accelerations (28).

The effect of corticosteroids, which are used to enhance pulmonary maturity of fetuses during preterm labor, on FHR has been studied (Table D-2). Among twins (46) and singletons (36,47), the use of betamethasone transiently decreased the FHR variability, which returned to pretreatment status by the fourth to seventh day. There also may be a decrease in the rate of accelerations with the use of betamethasone. These changes, however, were not associated with increased obstetric interventions or with adverse outcomes (46). The biologic mechanism of this is unknown. Computerized analysis of the cardiotocograms indicates that use of dexamethasone is not associated with a decrease in the FHR variability (36).

What findings on EFM are consistent with normal fetal acid–base status?

The presence of FHR accelerations generally ensures that the fetus is not acidemic. The data relating FHR variability to clinical outcomes, however, are sparse. Results of an observational study suggest that moderate FHR variability is strongly associated with an arterial umbilical cord pH higher than 7.15 (48). One study reported that in the presence of late or variable decelerations, the umbilical arterial pH was higher than 7.00 in 97% of the cases if the FHR tracing had normal variability (49). In another retrospective study, most cases of adverse neonatal outcome demonstrated normal FHR variability (50). This study is limited because it did not consider other characteristics of the FHR tracing, such as the presence of accelerations or decelerations. However, in most cases, normal FHR variability provides reassurance about fetal status and the absence of metabolic acidemia.

Are there ancillary tests that can aid in the management of Category II or Category III fetal heart rate tracings?

There are some ancillary tests available that help to ensure fetal well-being in the face of a Category II or Category III

TABLE D-2 Effects of Commonly Used Medications on Fetal Heart Rate Patterns

Medications	Comments	References
Narcotics	At equivalent doses, all narcotics (with or without added antiemetics) have similar effects: A decrease in variability and a decrease in the frequency of accelerations 75 mg meperidine = 10 mg morphine = 0.1 mg fentanyl = 10 mg nalbuphine	22,26–31
Butorphanol	Transient sinusoidal FHR pattern, slight increased mean heart rate compared with meperidine	32,33
Cocaine	Decreased long-term variability	34,35
Corticosteroids	Decrease in FHR variability with betamethasone but not dexamethasone, abolishment of diurnal fetal rhythms, increased effect at greater than 29 wks of gestation	36–39
Magnesium sulfate	A significant decrease in short-term variability, clinically insignificant decrease in FHR, inhibits the increase in accelerations with advancing gestational age	40,41
Terbutaline	Increase in baseline FHR and incidence of fetal tachycardia	42,43
Zidovudine	No difference in the FHR baseline, variability, number of accelerations, or decelerations	44

FHR, fetal heart rate.

FHR tracing, thereby reducing the high false-positive rate of EFM.

In the case of an EFM tracing with minimal or absent variability and without spontaneous acceleration, an effort should be made to elicit one. A meta-analysis of 11 studies of intrapartum fetal stimulation noted that four techniques are available to stimulate the fetus: (1) Fetal scalp sampling, (2) Allis clamp scalp stimulation, (3) vibroacoustic stimulation, and (4) digital scalp stimulation (51). Since vibroacoustic stimulation and digital scalp stimulation are less invasive than the other two methods, they are the preferred methods. When there is an acceleration following stimulation, acidemia is unlikely and labor can continue.

When a Category III FHR tracing is persistent, a scalp blood sample for the determination of pH or lactate may be considered. However, the use of scalp pH assessment has decreased (52), and this test may not even be available at some tertiary hospitals (53). There are likely many reasons for this decrease, including physician experience, difficulty in obtaining and processing an adequate sample in a short amount of time, and the need for routine maintenance and calibration of laboratory equipment that may be used infrequently. More importantly, scalp stimulation, which is less invasive, provides similar information about the likelihood of fetal acidemia as does scalp pH.

In one study, the sensitivity and positive predictive value of a low scalp pH (defined in the study as less than 7.21 because it is the 75th percentile) to predict umbilical arterial pH less than 7.00 was 36% and 9%, respectively (54). More importantly, the sensitivity and positive predictive value of a low scalp pH to identify a newborn with hypoxic–ischemic encephalopathy was 50% and 3%, respectively. However, the greater utility of scalp pH is in its high negative predictive value (97% to 99%). There are some data to suggest that fetal scalp lactate levels have higher sensitivity and specificity than scalp pH (54). However, a recent large randomized clinical trial that compared the use of scalp pH assessment to scalp lactate level assessment in cases of intrapartum fetal distress did not demonstrate a difference in the rate of acidemia at birth, Apgar scores, or neonatal intensive care unit admissions (55). Although scalp stimulation has largely replaced scalp pH and scalp lactate assessment in the United States, if available, these tests may provide additional information in the setting of a Category III tracing.

Pulse oximetry has not been demonstrated to be a clinically useful test in evaluating fetal status (56–58).

Are there methods of intrauterine resuscitation that can be used for Category II or Category III tracings?

A Category II or Category III FHR tracing requires evaluation of the possible causes. Initial evaluation and treatment may include the following:

- Discontinuation of any labor stimulating agent
- Cervical examination to determine umbilical cord prolapse, rapid cervical dilation, or descent of the fetal head
- Changing maternal position to left or right lateral recumbent position, reducing compression of the vena cava and improving uteroplacental blood flow
- Monitoring maternal blood pressure level for evidence of hypotension, especially in those with regional anesthesia (if present, treatment with volume expansion or with ephedrine or both, or phenylephrine may be warranted)
- Assessment of patient for uterine tachysystole by evaluating uterine contraction frequency and duration

Supplemental maternal oxygen is commonly used in cases of an indeterminate or abnormal pattern. There are no data on the efficacy or safety of this therapy. Often, the FHR patterns persist and do not respond to change in position or oxygenation. In such cases, the use of tocolytic agents has been suggested to stop uterine contractions and perhaps avoid umbilical cord compression. A meta-analysis reported the pooled results of three randomized clinical trials that compared tocolytic therapy (terbutaline, hexoprenaline, or magnesium sulfate) with untreated controls in the management of a suspected nonreassuring FHR tracing (59). Compared with no treatment, tocolytic therapy more commonly improved the FHR tracing. However, there were no differences in rates of perinatal mortality, low 5-minute Apgar score, or admission to the neonatal intensive care unit between the groups (possibly because of the small sample size). Thus, although tocolytic therapy appears to reduce the number of FHR abnormalities, there is insufficient evidence to recommend it.

Tachysystole with associated FHR changes can be successfully treated with P_2-adrenergic drugs (hexoprenaline or terbutaline). A retrospective study suggested that 98% of such cases respond to treatment with a β-agonist (60).

When the FHR tracing includes recurrent variable decelerations, amnioinfusion to relieve umbilical cord compression may be considered (61). A meta-analysis of 12 randomized trials that allocated patients to no treatment or transcervical amnioinfusion noted that placement of fluid in the uterine cavity significantly reduced the rate of decelerations (RR, 0.54; 95% CI, 0.43–0.68) and cesarean delivery for suspected fetal distress (RR, 0.35; 95% CI, 0.24–0.52) (62). Because of the lower rate of cesarean delivery, amnioinfusion also decreased the likelihood that either the patient or the newborn will stay in the hospital more than 3 days (62). Amnioinfusion can be done by bolus or continuous infusion technique. A randomized trial compared the two techniques of amnioinfusion and concluded that both have a similar ability to relieve recurrent variable decelerations (63).

Another common cause of a Category II or Category III FHR pattern is maternal hypotension secondary to regional anesthesia. If maternal hypotension is identified and suspected to be secondary to regional anesthesia, treatment with volume expansion or intravenous ephedrine or both is warranted.

■ SUMMARY OF RECOMMENDATIONS AND CONCLUSIONS

The following recommendations and conclusions are based on good and consistent scientific evidence (Level A):

- The false-positive rate of EFM for predicting cerebral palsy is high, at greater than 99%.
- The use of EFM is associated with an increased rate of both vacuum and forceps operative vaginal delivery, and cesarean delivery for abnormal FHR patterns or acidosis or both.
- When the FHR tracing includes recurrent variable decelerations, amnioinfusion to relieve umbilical cord compression should be considered.
- Pulse oximetry has not been demonstrated to be a clinically useful test in evaluating fetal status.

The following conclusions are based on limited or inconsistent scientific evidence (Level B):

- There is high interobserver and intraobserver variability in interpretation of FHR tracing.
- Reinterpretation of the FHR tracing, especially if the neonatal outcome is known, may not be reliable.

- The use of EFM does not result in a reduction of cerebral palsy.

The following recommendations are based on expert opinion (Level C):

- A three-tiered system for the categorization of FHR patterns is recommended.
- The labor of women with high-risk conditions should be monitored with continuous FHR monitoring.
- The terms hyperstimulation and hypercontractility should be abandoned.

The MEDLINE database, the Cochrane Library, and ACOG's own internal resources and documents were used to conduct a literature search to locate relevant articles published between January 1985 and January 2009. The search was restricted to articles published in the English language. Priority was given to articles reporting results of original research, although review articles and commentaries also were consulted. Abstracts of research presented at symposia and scientific conferences were not considered adequate for inclusion in this document. Guidelines published by organizations or institutions such as the National Institutes of Health and the American College of Obstetricians and Gynecologists were reviewed, and additional studies were located by reviewing bibliographies of identified articles. When reliable research was not available, expert opinions from obstetrician–gynecologists were used.

Studies were reviewed and evaluated for quality according to the method outlined by the U.S. Preventive Services Task Force:

I   Evidence obtained from at least one properly designed randomized controlled trial.

II-1   Evidence obtained from well-designed controlled trials without randomization.

II-2   Evidence obtained from well-designed cohort or case–control analytic studies, preferably from more than one center or research group.

II-3   Evidence obtained from multiple time series with or without the intervention. Dramatic results in uncontrolled experiments also could be regarded as this type of evidence.

III   Opinions of respected authorities, based on clinical experience, descriptive studies, or reports of expert committees.

On the basis of the highest level of evidence found in the data, recommendations are provided and graded according to the following categories:

Level A—recommendations are based on good and consistent scientific evidence.

Level B—recommendations are based on limited or inconsistent scientific evidence.

Level C—recommendations are based primarily on consensus and expert opinion.

REFERENCES

1. Martin JA, Hamilton BE, Sutton PD, et al. Births: final data for 2002. *Natl Vital Stat Rep* 2003;52:1–113.

2. Low JA, Pickersgill H, Killen H, et al. The prediction and prevention of intrapartum fetal asphyxia in term pregnancies. *Am J Obstet Gynecol* 2001;184:724–730.

3. Macones GA, Hankins GD, Spong CY, et al. The 2008 National Institute of Child Health and Human Development workshop report on electronic fetal monitoring: update on definitions, interpretation, and research guidelines. *Obstet Gynecol* 2008;112:661–666.

4. Royal College of Obstetricians and Gynaecologists. The use of electronic fetal monitoring: the use and interpretation of cardiotocography in intrapartum fetal surveillance. Evidence-based Clinical Guideline No. 8. London (UK): RCOG; 2001. http://www.rcog.org.uk/files/rcog-corp/uploaded-files/NEBE FMGuidelineFinal2may2001.pdf

5. Liston R, Sawchuck D, Young D. Fetal health surveillance: antepartum and intrapartum consensus guideline. Society of Obstetrics and Gynaecologists of Canada; British Columbia Perinatal Health Program [published erratum appears in *J Obstet Gynaecol Can* 2007;29:909]. *J Obstet Gynaecol Can* 2007;29(suppl 4):S3–S56.

6. Parer JT, Ikeda T. A framework for standardized management of intrapartum fetal heart rate patterns. *Am J Obstet Gynecol* 2007;197:26.e1–26.e6.

7. Freeman RK. Problems with intrapartum fetal heart rate monitoring interpretation and patient management. *Obstet Gynecol* 2002;100:813–826.

8. Alfirevic Z, Devane D, Gyte GML. Continuous cardiotocography (CTG) as a form of electronic fetal monitoring (EFM) for fetal assessment during labour. *Cochrane Database Syst Rev.* 2006;3:CD006066. DOI: 10.1002/14651858.CD006066.

9. Nelson KB, Dambrosia JM, Ting TY, et al. Uncertain value of electronic fetal monitoring in predicting cerebral palsy. *N Engl J Med* 1996;334:613–618.

10. Clark SL, Hankins GD. Temporal and demographic trends in cerebral palsy—fact and fiction. *Am J Obstet Gynecol* 2003;188:628–633.

11. Hankins GD, Speer M. Defining the pathogenesis and pathophysiology of neonatal encephalopathy and cerebral palsy. *Obstet Gynecol* 2003;102:628–636.

12. Badawi N, Kurinczuk JJ, Keogh JM, et al. Antepartum risk factors for newborn encephalopathy: the Western Australian case-control study. *BMJ* 1998;317:1549–1553.

13. Morrison JC, Chez BF, Davis ID, et al. Intrapartum fetal heart rate assessment: monitoring by auscultation or electronic means. *Am J Obstet Gynecol* 1993;168:63–66.

14. Vintzileos AM, Nochimson DJ, Antsaklis A, et al. Comparison of intrapartum electronic fetal heart rate monitoring versus intermittent auscultation in detecting fetal acidemia at birth. *Am J Obstet Gynecol* 1995;173:1021–1024.

15. Nielsen PV, Stigsby B, Nickelsen C, et al. Intra- and inter-observer variability in the assessment of intrapartum cardiotocograms. *Acta Obstet Gynecol Scand* 1987;66:421–424.

16. Beaulieu MD, Fabia J, Leduc B, et al. The reproducibility of intrapartum cardiotocogram assessments. *Can Med Assoc J* 1982;127:214–216.

17. Blix E, Sviggum O, Koss KS, et al. Inter-observer variation in assessment of 845 labour admission tests: comparison between midwives and obstetricians in the clinical setting and two experts. *BJOG* 2003;110:1–5.

18. Zain HA, Wright JW, Parrish GE, et al. Interpreting the fetal heart rate tracing. Effect of knowledge of neonatal outcome. *J Reprod Med* 1998;43:367–370.

19. Ayoubi JM, Audibert F, Vial M, et al. Fetal heart rate and survival of the very premature newborn. *Am J Obstet Gynecol* 2002;187:1026–1030.

20. Westgren M, Holmquist P, Svenningsen NW, et al. Intrapartum fetal monitoring in preterm deliveries: prospective study. *Obstet Gynecol* 1982;60:99–106.

21. Westgren M, Hormquist P, Ingemarsson I, et al. Intrapartum fetal acidosis in preterm infants: fetal monitoring and long-term morbidity. *Obstet Gynecol* 1984;63:355–359.

22. Hill JB, Alexander JM, Sharma SK, et al. A comparison of the effects of epidural and meperidine analgesia during labor on fetal heart rate. *Obstet Gynecol* 2003;102:333–337.

23. Lieberman E, O'Donoghue C. Unintended effects of epidural analgesia during labor: a systematic review. *Am J Obstet Gynecol* 2002;186(suppl 1):S31–S68.

24. Gambling DR, Sharma SK, Ramin SM, et al. A randomized study of combined spinal-epidural analgesia versus intravenous meperidine during labor: impact on cesarean delivery rate. *Anesthesiology* 1998;89:1336–1344.

25. Abrao KC, Francisco RP, Miyadahira S, et al. Elevation of uterine basal tone and fetal heart rate abnormalities after labor analgesia: a randomized controlled trial. *Obstet Gynecol* 2009;113:41–47.

26. Panayotopoulos N, Salamalekis E, Kassanos D, et al. Intrapartum vibratory acoustic stimulation after maternal meperidine administration. *Clin Exp Obstet Gynecol* 1998;25:139–140.

27. Zimmer EZ, Divon MY, Vadasz A. Influence of meperidine on fetal movements and heart rate beat-to-beat variability in the active phase of labor. *Am J Perinatol* 1988;5:197–200.

28. Kopecky EA, Ryan ML, Barrett JF, et al. Fetal response to maternally administered morphine. *Am J Obstet Gynecol* 2000;183:424–430.

29. Rayburn W, Rathke A, Leuschen MP, et al. Fentanyl citrate analgesia during labor. *Am J Obstet Gynecol* 1989;161:202–206.

30. Nicolle E, Devillier P, Delanoy B, et al. Therapeutic monitoring of nalbuphine: transplacental transfer and estimated pharmacokinetics in the neonate. *Eur J Clin Pharmacol* 1996;49:485–489.

31. Poehlmann S, Pinette M, Stubblefield P. Effect of labor analgesia with nalbuphine hydrochloride on fetal response to vibroacoustic stimulation. *J Reprod Med* 1995;40:707–710.

32. Hatjis CG, Meis PJ. Sinusoidal fetal heart rate pattern associated with butorphanol administration. *Obstet Gynecol* 1986;67:377–380.

33. Quilligan EJ, Keegan KA, Donahue MJ. Double-blind comparison of intravenously injected butorphanol and meperidine in parturients. *Int J Gynaecol Obstet* 1980;18:363–367.

34. Chazotte C, Forman L, Gandhi J. Heart rate patterns in fetuses exposed to cocaine. *Obstet Gynecol* 1991;78:323–325.

35. Tabor BL, Soffici AR, Smith-Wallace T, et al. The effect of maternal cocaine use on the fetus: changes in antepartum fetal heart rate tracings. *Am J Obstet Gynecol* 1991;165:1278–1281.

36. Senat MV, Minoui S, Multon O, et al. Effect of dexamethasone and betamethasone on fetal heart rate variability in preterm labour: a randomised study. *Br J Obstet Gynaecol* 1998;105:749–755.

37. Rotmensch S, Liberati M, Vishne TH, et al. The effect of betamethasone and dexamethasone on fetal heart rate patterns and biophysical activities. A prospective randomized trial. *Acta Obstet Gynecol Scand* 1999;78:493–500.

38. Koenen SV, Mulder EJ, Wijnberger LD, et al. Transient loss of the diurnal rhythms of fetal movements, heart rate, and its variation after maternal betamethasone administration. *Pediatr Res* 2005;57:662–666.

39. Mulder EJ, Koenen SV, Blom I, et al. The effects of antenatal betamethasone administration on fetal heart rate and behaviour depend on gestational age. *Early Hum Dev* 2004;76:65–77.

40. Hallak M, Martinez-Poyer J, Kruger ML, et al. The effect of magnesium sulfate on fetal heart rate parameters: a randomized, placebo-controlled trial. *Am J Obstet Gynecol* 1999;181:1122–1127.

41. Wright JW, Ridgway LE, Wright BD, et al. Effect of MgSO4 on heart rate monitoring in the preterm fetus. *J Reprod Med* 1996;41:605–608.

42. Mawaldi L, Duminy P, Tamim H. Terbutaline versus nifedipine for prolongation of pregnancy in patients with preterm labor. *Int J Gynaecol Obstet* 2008;100:65–68.

43. Roth AC, Milsom I, Forssman L, et al. Effects of intravenous terbutaline on maternal circulation and fetal heart activity. *Acta Obstet Gynecol Scand* 1990;69:223–228.

44. Blackwell SC, Sahai A, Hassan SS, et al. Effects of intrapartum zidovudine therapy on fetal heart rate parameters in women with human immunodeficiency virus infection. *Fetal Diagn Ther* 2001;16:413–416.

45. Giannina G, Guzman ER, Lai YL, et al. Comparison of the effects of meperidine and nalbuphine on intrapartum fetal heart rate tracings. *Obstet Gynecol* 1995;86:441–445.

46. Ville Y, Vincent Y, Tordjman N, et al. Effect of betamethasone on the fetal heart rate pattern assessed by computerized cardiotocography in normal twin pregnancies. *Fetal Diagn Ther* 1995;10:301–306.

47. Subtil D, Tiberghien P, Devos P, et al. Immediate and delayed effects of antenatal corticosteroids on fetal heart rate: a randomized trial that compares betamethasone acetate and phosphate, betamethasone phosphate, and dexamethasone. *Am J Obstet Gynecol* 2003;188:524–531.

48. Parer JT, King T, Flanders S, et al. Fetal acidemia and electronic fetal heart rate patterns: is there evidence of an association? *J Matern Fetal Neonatal Med* 2006;19:289–294.

49. Williams KP, Galerneau F. Intrapartum fetal heart rate patterns in the prediction of neonatal acidemia. *Am J Obstet Gynecol* 2003;188:820–823.

50. Samueloff A, Langer O, Berkus M, et al. Is fetal heart rate variability a good predictor of fetal outcome? *Acta Obstet Gynecol Scand* 1994;73:39–44.

51. Skupski DW, Rosenberg CR, Eglinton GS. Intrapartum fetal stimulation tests: a meta-analysis. *Obstet Gynecol* 2002;99:129–134.

52. Goodwin TM, Milner-Masterson L, Paul RH. Elimination of fetal scalp blood sampling on a large clinical service. *Obstet Gynecol* 1994;83:971–974.

53. Hendrix NW, Chauhan SP, Scardo JA, et al. Managing nonreassuring fetal heart rate patterns before cesarean delivery. Compliance with ACOG recommendations. *J Reprod Med* 2000;45:995–999.

54. Kruger K, Hallberg B, Blennow M, et al. Predictive value of fetal scalp blood lactate concentration and pH as markers of neurologic disability. *Am J Obstet Gynecol* 1999;181:1072–1078.

55. Wiberg-Itzel E, Lipponer C, Norman M, et al. Determination of pH or lactate in fetal scalp blood in management of intrapartum fetal distress: randomised controlled multicentre trial. *BMJ* 2008;336:1284–1287.

56. Garite TJ, Dildy GA, McNamara H, et al. A multicenter controlled trial of fetal pulse oximetry in the intrapartum management of nonreassuring fetal heart rate patterns. *Am J Obstet Gynecol* 2000;183:1049–1058.

57. Bloom SL, Spong CY, Thom E, et al. Fetal pulse oximetry and cesarean delivery. National Institute of Child Health and Human Development Maternal-Fetal Medicine Units Network. *N Engl J Med* 2006;355:2195–2202.

58. East CE, Chan FY, Colditz PB, et al. Fetal pulse oximetry for fetal assessment in labour. *Cochrane Database Syst Rev* 2007;2:CD004075. DOI: 10.1002/14651858.CD004075.pub3.

59. Kulier R, Hofmeyr GJ. Tocolytics for suspected intrapartum fetal distress. *Cochrane Database Syst Rev.* 1998;2: CD000035. DOI: 10.1002/14651858.CD000035.

60. Egarter CH, Husslein PW, Rayburn WF. Uterine hyperstimulation after low-dose prostaglandin E2 therapy: tocolytic treatment in 181 cases. *Am J Obstet Gynecol* 1990;163:794–796.

61. Miyazaki FS, Taylor NA. Saline amnioinfusion for relief of variable or prolonged decelerations. A preliminary report. *Am J Obstet Gynecol* 1983;146:670–678.

62. Hofmeyr GJ. Amnioinfusion for potential or suspected umbilical cord compression in labour. *Cochrane Database Syst Rev* 1998;Issue 1:CD000013. DOI: 10.1002/14651858.CD000013.

63. Rinehart BK, Terrone DA, Barrow JH, et al. Randomized trial of intermittent or continuous amnioinfusion for variable decelerations. *Obstet Gynecol* 2000;96:571–574.

Note: Page numbers followed by f and t indicate figure and table, respectively.